Diseases of the Breast

Second Edition

Diseases of the Breast

Second Edition

Edited by

Jay R. Harris, M.D.
Professor of Radiation Oncology
Harvard Medical School
Chief, Department of Radiation Oncology
Brigham and Women's Hospital
Dana-Farber Cancer Institute
Boston, Massachusetts

Marc E. Lippman, M.D.
Professor of Pharmacology and Medicine
Director, Lombardi Cancer Center
Georgetown University Medical Center
Washington, D.C.

Monica Morrow, M.D.
Professor of Surgery
Northwestern University Medical School
Director, Lynn Sage Comprehensive Breast Program
Northwestern Memorial Hospital
Chicago, Illinois

C. Kent Osborne, M.D.
Professor of Medicine
Director, Breast Center
Baylor College of Medicine
Houston, Texas

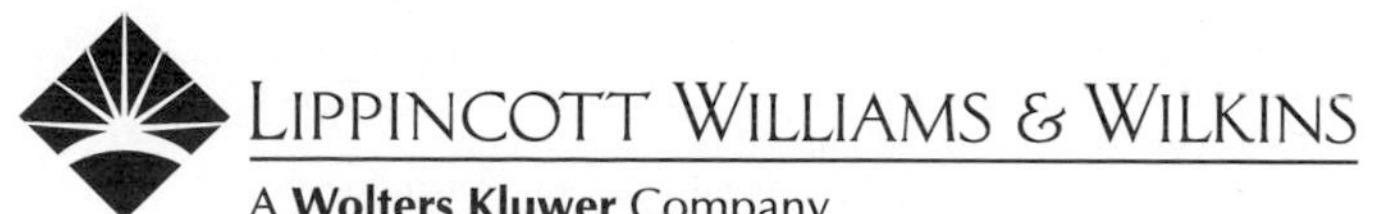

LIPPINCOTT WILLIAMS & WILKINS
A **Wolters Kluwer** Company
Philadelphia • Baltimore • New York • London
Buenos Aires • Hong Kong • Sydney • Tokyo

Acquisitions Editor: Stuart Freeman
Developmental Editor: Ellen DiFrancesco
Manufacturing Manager: Kevin Watt
Supervising Editor: Mary Ann McLaughlin
Production Editor: Allison Spearman, Silverchair Science + Communications
Cover Designer: Christine Jenny
Indexer: Linda Herr Hallinger
Compositor: Silverchair Science + Communications
Printer: Courier-Westford

Second Edition

227 East Washington Square
Philadelphia, PA 19106-3780 USA
LWW.com

Printed in the USA

Library of Congress Cataloging-in-Publication Data
Diseases of the breast / [edited by] Jay R. Harris ... [et al.]. --
2nd ed.
p. cm.
Includes bibliographical references and index.
ISBN 0-7817-1839-2
1. Breast--Diseases. I. Harris, Jay R.
[DNLM: 1. Breast Neoplasms--diagnosis. 2. Breast--pathology.
3. Breast Neoplasms--therapy. WP 870 D611 1999]
RG491.D57 1999
618.1'9--dc21
DNLM/DLC
for Library of Congress 99-29234
CIP

---

10 9 8 7 6 5 4 3 2 1

To Dr. Samuel Hellman, for his inspirational leadership in breast cancer research, his mentorship, and his friendship

Contents

SECTION XI. EVALUATION AFTER PRIMARY THERAPY

SECTION XII. MANAGEMENT OF RECURRENT BREAST CANCER

SECTION XIII. NEW BREAST CANCER THERAPEUTIC APPROACHES

SECTION XIV. SITE-SPECIFIC THERAPY OF METASTATIC BREAST CANCER

SECTION XV. BREAST CANCER IN SPECIAL POPULATIONS

SECTION XVI. ISSUES IN BREAST CANCER SURVIVORSHIP

SECTION XVII. MEDICOLEGAL CONSIDERATIONS

SECTION XVIII. BASIC TOOLS FOR ADVANCING KNOWLEDGE IN BREAST CANCER

Contributing Authors

Alan D. Aaron, M.D.
Clinical Associate Professor of Orthopaedic Surgery
Department of Orthopaedic Surgery
Georgetown University Hospital
5530 Wisconsin Avenue, Suite 604
Washington, D.C. 20815

David H. Abramson, M.D.
Clinical Professor of Ophthalmology
Department of Ophthalmology
Joan and Sanford I. Weill Medical College
New York Presbyterian Hospital - Cornell University
70 East 66th Street
New York, New York 10021

D. Craig Allred, M.D.
Professor of Pathology
Breast Center, Baylor College of Medicine
One Baylor Plaza, MS 600
Houston, Texas 77030

Deborah K. Armstrong, M.D.
Assistant Professor
Department of Oncology
Johns Hopkins University School of Medicine
600 N. Wolfe Street, Room I-121
Baltimore, Maryland 21287

Elizabeth M. Augustine, M.S., P.T.
Oncology Coordinator, Physical Therapy Section
Warren G. Magnuson Clinical Center
National Institutes of Health
10 Building, Room 6S235
Bethesda, Maryland 20892

Christine D. Berg, M.D.
Acting Chief, Lung and Upper Aerodigestive Cancer Research Group
Division of Cancer Prevention
National Cancer Institute
6130 Executive Boulevard, Suite 330G
Bethesda, Maryland 20892

Glenn D. Braunstein, M.D.
Professor of Medicine
University of California, Los Angeles, UCLA School of Medicine
Chairman, Department of Medicine
Cedars-Sinai Medical Center
Room B118
8700 Beverly Boulevard
Los Angeles, California 90048

R. James Brenner, M.D., J.D., F.A.C.R., F.C.L.M.
Clinical Professor of Radiology
University of California, Los Angeles, UCLA School of Medicine
Director, Breast Imaging
Eisenbery Keefer Breast Center
John Wayne Cancer Institute
St. John's Health Center
1328 22nd Street
Santa Monica, California 90404

W. Nils Brünner, M.D., D.M.Sc.
Associate Professor
Finsen Laboratory
Rigshospitalet
Copenhagen, DK-2100, Denmark

Nigel J. Bundred, M.D.
Reader in Surgical Oncology
Academic Department of Surgery
South Manchester University Hospital
Nell Lane
Manchester M20 8LR, United Kingdom

Harold J. Burstein, M.D., Ph.D.
Instructor in Medicine
Dana-Farber Cancer Institute
Harvard Medical School
44 Binney Street
Boston, Massachusetts 02115

François Campana, M.D.
Radiation Oncologist
Institut Curie
26 Rue D'Ulm
75231, Cedex 05
Paris, France

Martin A. Cheever, M.D.
Clinical Professor of Medicine
University of Washington School of Medicine
Vice President, Director of Medical Affairs
Corixa Corporation
1124 Columbia Street, Suite 200
Seattle, Washington 98104

Nathan I. Cherny, M.D.
Department of Medical Oncology
Shaare-Zedek Medical Center
Jerusalem, 91031, Israel

Susan E. Clare, M.D.
Assistant Professor of Surgery
Department of Surgery
Northwestern University Medical School
Lynn Sage Comprehensive Breast Program
Northwestern Memorial Hospital
Chicago, Illinois 60611

Gary M. Clark, Ph.D.
Associate Director, Breast Care Center
Baylor College of Medicine
Alkek N550, MS 600
One Baylor Plaza
Houston, Texas 77030

Robert Clarke, Ph.D.
Professor of Oncology and Physiology and Biophysics
Director, Lombardi Cancer Center Animal Research Resource
Lombardi Cancer Center
Georgetown University Medical Center
Research Building, Room W405
3970 Reservoir Road NW
Washington, D.C. 20007

Melody A. Cobleigh, M.D.
Professor of Medicine
Section of Medical Oncology
Rush Presbyterian St. Luke's Medical Center
1725 W. Harrison, Suite 821
Chicago, Illinois 60612

Graham A. Colditz, M.D., Ph.D., DADPHM
Professor of Medicine
Department of Medicine
Harvard Medical School
Channing Laboratory
181 Longwood Avenue
Boston, Massachusetts 02115

Steven E. Come, M.D.
Associate Professor of Medicine
Harvard Medical School
Director, Hematology-Oncology Units
Beth Israel Deaconess Medical Center - East Campus
330 Brookline Avenue
Boston, Massachusetts 02215

James L. Connolly, M.D.
Associate Professor of Medicine
Harvard Medical School
Director of Anatomic Pathology
Beth Israel Deaconess Medical Center - East Campus
330 Brookline Avenue
Boston, Massachusetts 02215

Alberto F. Costa, M.D.
Consultant, Breast Cancer Division
European Institute of Oncology
Via Ripamonti 435
20141 Milan, Italy

Keld Danø, M.D.
Finsen Laboratory
49 Strandboulevarden
Copenhagen, DK-2100, Denmark

Nancy E. Davidson, M.D.
Professor of Oncology
Johns Hopkins Oncology Center
Johns Hopkins University School of Medicine
600 North Wolfe Street
Baltimore, Maryland 21287

Anne de la Rochefordière, M.D.
Institut Curie
26 Rue D'Ulm
75231, Cedex 05
Paris, France

Lisa M. DeAngelis, M.D.
Chair, Department of Neurology
Memorial Sloan-Kettering Cancer Center
1275 York Avenue
New York, New York 10021

Angela DeMichele, M.D.
Assistant Professor of Medicine and Epidemiology
The University of Pennsylvania Cancer Center
16 Penn Tower
3400 Spruce Street
Philadelphia, Pennsylvania 19104

Robert B. Dickson, Ph.D.
Professor of Cell Biology and Pharmacology
Associate Director for Basic Science, Lombardi Cancer Center
Georgetown University Medical Center
Research Building
3970 Reservoir Road NW
Washington, D.C. 20007

Mary L. Disis, M.D.
Associate Professor of Medicine
Department of Medicine
Division of Oncology
University of Washington School of Medicine
Seattle, Washington 98195

J. Michael Dixon, M.D., M.B.Ch.B., F.R.C.S.
Senior Lecturer in Surgery
Edinburgh Breast Unit
Western General Hospital
Crewe Road South
Edinburgh EH4 2XU, Scotland, United Kingdom

Carl J. D'Orsi, M.D., F.A.C.R.
Professor and Vice Chairman
Director, Diagnostic Radiology
University of Massachusetts Memorial Medical Center
55 Lake Avenue North
Worcester, Massachusetts 01655

Karen Hassey Dow, Ph.D., R.N., F.A.A.N.
Associate Professor and Research Coordinator
School of Nursing, College of Health and Public Affairs
University of Central Florida
4000 Central Florida Boulevard
Orlando, Florida 32816

Richard M. Elledge, M.D.
Associate Professor of Medicine
Director, Breast Care Center
Departments of Medicine and Oncology
Baylor College of Medicine
Scurlock Tower
6560 Fannin Street, Suite 1558
Houston, Texas 77030

Matthew J. Ellis, M.B., Ph.D., M.R.C.P.
Assistant Professor of Medicine
Lombardi Cancer Center
Georgetown University Medical Center
3970 Reservoir Road NW
Washington, D.C. 20007

Geoffery Fenner, M.D.
Assistant Professor
Northwestern University Medical School
Evanston Northwestern Healthcare
1000 Central Street
Evanston, Illinois 60201

Ian S. Fentiman, M.D., F.R.C.S.
Professor of Surgical Oncology
Hedley Atkins Breast Unit
Guy's Hospital
St. Thomas's Street
London SE1 9RT, England, United Kingdom

Neil A. Fine, M.D.
Assistant Professor of Surgery
Division of Plastic Surgery
Northwestern University Medical School
707 N. Fairbanks, Suite 811
Chicago, Illinois 60611

Kathleen M. Foley, M.D.
Professor of Neurology, Neuroscience, and Clinical Pharmacology
Joan and Sanford I. Weill Medical College
New York Presbyterian Hospital - Cornell University
Chief, Pain Service
Department of Neurology
Memorial Sloan-Kettering Cancer Center
1275 York Avenue
New York, New York 10021

Roger S. Foster, Jr., M.D.
Professor of Surgery
Chief of Surgical Services
The Robert H. Woodruff Health Sciences Center
Emory University School of Medicine
Chandler Bldg. A
478 Peachtree St. NE
Atlanta, Georgia 30308

Alain Fourquet, M.D.
Department of Radiation Oncology
Institut Curie
26 Rue D'Ulm
75005 Paris, France

Stephen B. Fox, M.D.
Department of Anatomical Pathology
Christchurch Hospital
Private Bag 4710
Christchurch, New Zealand

Ronnie J. Freilich, M.B., B.S., M.D., F.R.A.C.P.
Neurologist
Department of Neurosciences
Monash Medical Centre
246 Clayton Road
Clayton, Victoria, 3168, Australia

Carl Freter, M.D., Ph.D.
Associate Professor of Medicine
Lombardi Cancer Center
Georgetown University Medical Center
3970 Reservoir Road NW
Washington, D.C.

Suzanne A. W. Fuqua, Ph.D.
Professor
Department of Medicine
Baylor College of Medicine
One Baylor Plaza
Houston, Texas 77030

Patricia A. Ganz, M.D.
Professor
University of California, Los Angeles, UCLA Schools of Medicine and Public Health
Director, Division of Cancer Prevention and Control Research
Jonsson Comprehensive Cancer Center
Box 956900, Room A2-125 CHS
Los Angeles, California 90095

Rebecca S. Gelman, Ph.D.
Associate Professor
Departments of Biostatistics and Radiation Oncology
Harvard School of Public Health
Harvard Medical School
44 Binney Street
Boston, Massachusetts 02115

Lynn H. Gerber, M.D.
Chief, Rehabilitation Medicine Department
Clinical Professor of Medicine
Georgetown University Medical Center
Reservoir Road NW
Washington, D.C. 20007

William J. Gradishar, M.D.
Associate Professor of Medicine
Director, Breast Medical Oncology
Robert H. Lurie Comprehensive Cancer Center
Northwestern University Medical School
233 E. Erie Street, Suite 700
Chicago, Illinois 60611

Anthony J. Guidi, M.D.
Director of Anatomic Pathology
Department of Pathology
North Shore Medical Center
Salem, Massachusetts 01970

Theresa A. Guise, M.D.
Associate Professor
Departments of Medicine and Endocrinology
University of Texas Health Science Center at San Antonio
7703 Floyd Curl Drive
San Antonio, Texas 78284

Susan E. Hankinson, M.P.H., Sc.D.
Assistant Professor of Medicine and Epidemiology
Harvard Medical School
Harvard School of Public Health
Channing Laboratory
181 Longwood Avenue
Boston, Massachusetts 02115

Adrian L. Harris, B.Sc., M.A., D.Phil., F.R.C.P.
Professor of Clinical Oncology
Imperial Cancer Research Fund, Medical Oncology Unit
Churchill Hospital
Headington
Oxford OX3 7LJ, England, United Kingdom

Jay R. Harris, M.D.
Professor of Radiation Oncology
Harvard Medical School
Chief, Department of Radiation Oncology
Brigham and Women's Hospital
Dana-Farber Cancer Institute
44 Binney Street, Suite 1622
Boston, Massachusetts 02115

Daniel F. Hayes, M.D.
Associate Professor of Medicine
Clinical Director, Breast Cancer Program
Lombardi Cancer Center
Georgetown University Medical Center
Research Building, Room E501
3970 Reservoir Road NW
Washington, D.C. 20007

James A. Hayman, M.D.
Department of Radiation Oncology
University of Michigan Hospital
UH-B2C490, Box 0010
1500 East Medical Center Drive
Ann Arbor, Michigan 48109

Samuel Hellman, M.D.
A. N. Pritzker Distinguished Service Professor
Department of Radiation and Cellular Oncology
Center for Advanced Medicine
University of Chicago Medical Center
5758 South Maryland Avenue, MC 9001
DCAM Room 1339
Chicago, Illinois 60637

Gabriel N. Hortobagyi, M.D.
Professor of Medicine
Department of Breast Medical Oncology
University of Texas M. D. Anderson Cancer Center
1515 Holcombe Boulevard
Houston, Texas 77030

David J. Hunter, Sc.D.
Professor of Epidemiology and Nutrition
Harvard School of Public Health
Channing Laboratory
181 Longwood Avenue
Boston, Massachusetts 02115

J. Dirk Iglehart, M.D.
Professor of Surgery
Harvard Medical School
Brigham and Women's Hospital
Dana-Farber Cancer Institute
75 Francis Street
Boston, Massachusetts 02115

Jane M. Ingham, M.B., B.S., F.R.A.C.P.
Assistant Professor of Medicine
Director of Palliative Care
Lombardi Cancer Center
Georgetown University Medical Center
3800 Reservoir Road NW
Washington, D.C. 20007

Claudine J. D. Isaacs, M.D.C.M., F.R.C.P.C.
Associate Professor of Medicine
Lombardi Cancer Center
Georgetown University Medical Center
3800 Reservoir Road NW
Washington, D.C. 20007

Michael D. Johnson, Ph.D.
Assistant Professor
Department of Oncology
Director, Transgenic Shared Resource
Lombardi Cancer Center
Georgetown University Medical Center
3970 Reservoir Road NW
Washington, D.C. 20007

V. Craig Jordan, Ph.D., D.Sc.
Professor of Cancer Pharmacology
Robert Lurie Cancer Center
Northwestern University Medical School
303 East Chicago Avenue
Chicago, Illinois 60611

Carolyn M. Kaelin, M.D.
Instructor in Surgery
Harvard Medical School
Director, Comprehensive Breast Health Center
Brigham and Women's Hospital
Dana-Farber Cancer Institute
75 Francis Street
Boston, Massachusetts 02115

Barbara Hansen Kalinowski, R.N.
Brigham and Women's Hospital
Dana-Farber Cancer Institute
75 Francis Street
Boston, Massachusetts 02146

Bella Kaufman, M.D.
Department of Oncology
Shaare-Zedek Medical Center
Jerusalem, 91031, Israel

M. John Kennedy, M.B., F.R.C.P.I.
Consultant Medical Oncologist
Department of Hematology/Oncology
St. James Hospital Dublin
HIGF, St. James Hospital, James Street
Dublin 8, Ireland

Jon F. Kerner, Ph.D.
Associate Professor
Department of Oncology
Associate Director, Lombardi Cancer Center
Georgetown University Medical Center
2233 Wisconsin Avenue NW, Suite 400
Washington, D.C. 20007

Gretchen G. Kimmick, M.D.
Assistant Professor of Medicine
Department of Internal Medicine—Hematology/Oncology
Wake Forest University School of Medicine
Medical Center Boulevard
Winston-Salem, North Carolina 27157

Daniel B. Kopans, M.D.
Department of Radiology
Massachusetts General Hospital
Zero Emerson Place
Boston, Massachusetts 02114

Fabio Leonessa, M.D.
Research Instructor
Department of Physiology and Biophysics
Georgetown University Medical Center
3970 Reservoir Road NW
Washington, D.C. 20007

Caryn Lerman, Ph.D.
Professor of Medicine
Lombardi Cancer Center
Georgetown University Medical Center
2233 Wisconsin Avenue NW, Suite 317
Washington, D.C. 20007

Robert Lerner, M.D.
Director, Lerner Lymphedema Services
360 East 57th Street
New York, New York 10022

Allen S. Lichter, M.D.
Dean, Medical School
Professor of Radiation Oncology
Department of Radiation Oncology
University of Michigan Medical School
Medical Science Building I, M7330/Box 0624
Ann Arbor, Michigan 48109

Marc E. Lippman, M.D.
Professor of Pharmacology and Medicine
Director, Lombardi Cancer Center
Georgetown University Medical Center
3970 Reservoir Road NW
Washington, D.C. 20007

David Malkin, M.D.
Associate Professor of Pediatrics
University of Toronto Faculty of Medicine
Staff Oncologist
Division of Hematology-Oncology
Scientist
Research Institute
The Hospital for Sick Children
555 University Avenue
Toronto, M5G 1X8
Ontario, Canada

Jeanne S. Mandelblatt, M.D., M.P.H.
Associate Professor of Medicine
Lombardi Cancer Center
Georgetown University Medical Center
2233 Wisconsin Avenue NW, Suite 430
Washington, D.C.

Mary Jane Massie, M.D.
Attending Psychiatrist
Director, Barbara White Fishman Center for Psychological Counseling
Department of Psychiatry and Behavioral Sciences
Memorial Sloan-Kettering Cancer Center
1275 York Avenue, Box 421
New York, New York 10021

Craig D. McColl, M.B.B.S.
Neurology Registrar
Department of Neurosciences
Monash Medical Centre
266 Clayton Road
Clayton, Victoria 3168, Australia

Beryl A. McCormick, M.D.
Senior Attending Physician
Department of Radiation Oncology
Memorial Sloan-Kettering Cancer Center
1275 York Avenue
New York, New York 10021

Steven J. Mentzer, M.D.
Associate Professor of Surgery
Department of Surgery
Division of Thoracic Surgery
Harvard Medical School
Brigham and Women's Hospital
75 Francis Street
Boston, Massachusetts 02115

Syed K. Mohsin, M.D.
Assistant Professor
Breast Center
Baylor College of Medicine
One Baylor Plaza, MS-600
Houston, Texas 77030

Anne Moore, M.D.
Professor of Clinical Medicine
Department of Hematology and Oncology
Joan and Sanford I. Weill Medical College
New York Presbyterian Hospital - Cornell University
428 East 72nd Street, Suite 300
New York, New York 10021

Monica Morrow, M.D.
Professor of Surgery
Northwestern University Medical School
Director, Lynn Sage Comprehensive Breast Program
Northwestern Memorial Hospital
675 North St. Clair Street
Galter Pavilion, 13th Floor
Chicago, Illinois 60611

Gregory R. Mundy, M.D.
Department of Medicine
University of Texas Health Science Center at San Antonio
7703 Floyd Curl Drive
San Antonio, Texas 78284

Hyman B. Muss, M.D.
Professor
Department of Medicine
University of Vermont School of Medicine
Director of Hematology/Oncology, Fletcher Allen Health Care
Associate Director, Vermont Cancer Center
MCHV Campus, Patrick 534
111 Colchester Avenue
Burlington, Vermont 05403

Thomas A. Mustoe, M.D.
Professor of Surgery
Chief, Division of Plastic Surgery
Northwestern University Medical School
707 N. Fairbanks, Suite 811
Chicago, Illinois 60611

C. Kent Osborne, M.D.
Professor of Medicine
Director, Breast Center
Baylor College of Medicine
Alkek N 550 Mail Station BCM 600
One Baylor Plaza
Houston, Texas 77030

Michael P. Osborne, M.D., F.R.C.S., F.A.C.S.
Professor of Surgery
Department of Surgery
Joan and Sanford I. Weill Medical College
New York Presbyterian Hospital - Cornell University
428 East 72nd Street
New York, New York 10021

Hilmi Ozcelik, Ph.D.
Assistant Professor
Department of Laboratory Medicine and Pathobiology
University of Toronto
Staff Scientist
Department of Pathology and Laboratory Medicine
Mount Sinai Hospital
600 University Avenue
Toronto M5G 1X5
Ontario, Canada

Beth N. Peshkin, M.S.
Assistant Professor
Department of Obstetrics and Gynecology
Certified Genetic Counselor
Lombardi Cancer Center
Georgetown University Medical Center
2233 Wisconsin Avenue NW
Washington, D.C. 20007

Jeanne A. Petrek, M.D.
Associate Professor of Surgery
Evelyn Lauder Breast Center
Memorial Sloan-Kettering Cancer Center
1275 York Avenue
New York, New York 10021

Lori J. Pierce, M.D.
Associate Professor
Director, Clinical Division
Department of Radiation Oncology
University of Michigan Medical School
1500 East Medical Center Drive
Ann Arbor, Michigan 48109

Peter M. Ravdin, M.D., Ph.D.
Associate Professor
Department of Medical Oncology
University of Texas Health Science Center at San Antonio
7703 Floyd Curl Drive
San Antonio, Texas 78284

Abram Recht, M.D.
Associate Professor
Harvard Medical School
Department of Radiation Oncology
Beth Israel Deaconess Medical Center
330 Brookline Avenue, Finard Building B25
Boston, Massachusetts 02215

Beverly Rockhill, Ph.D.
Instructor of Medicine
Harvard Medical School
Brigham and Women's Hospital
Channing Laboratory
181 Longwood Avenue
Boston, Massachusetts 02115

Lisa R. Rogers, D.O.
Associate Professor of Neurology
Wayne State University School of Medicine
Detroit, Michigan

Neal Rosen, M.D., Ph.D.
Department of Medicine, Cell Biology and Genetics
Memorial Sloan-Kettering Cancer Center
1275 York Avenue, Box 271
New York, New York 10021

Julia H. Rowland, Ph.D.
Director, Office of Cancer Survivorship
Division of Cancer Control and Population Sciences
National Cancer Institute
Bethesda, Maryland 20892

Jose Russo, M.D.
Breast Cancer Research Laboratory
Fox Chase Cancer Center
7701 Burholme Avenue
Philadelphia, Pennsylvania 19111

Norman L. Sadowsky, M.D.
Clinical Professor of Radiology
Tufts University School of Medicine
Faulkner-Sagoff Breast Imaging and Diagnostic Centre
Faulkner Hospital
1153 Centre Street
Boston, Massachusetts 02130

Stuart J. Schnitt, M.D.
Associate Professor of Pathology
Harvard Medical School
Consultant in Pathology
Brigham and Women's Hospital
Dana-Farber Cancer Institute
Director of Surgical Pathology
Beth Israel Deaconess Medical Center
330 Brookline Avenue
Boston, Massachusetts 02215

Laura Sepp-Lorenzino
Laboratory Member
Memorial Sloan-Kettering Cancer Center
1275 York Avenue
New York, NY 10021

Timothy D. Shafman, M.D.
Assistant Professor of Radiation Oncology
Harvard Medical School
Department of Radiation Oncology
Brigham and Women's Hospital
75 Francis Street
Boston, Massachusetts 02115

Lawrence N. Shulman, M.D.
Associate Professor of Medicine
Harvard Medical School
Department of Adult Oncology
Dana-Farber Cancer Institute
44 Binney Street
Boston, Massachusetts 02115

S. Eva Singletary, M.D.
Professor of Surgery
Department of Surgical Oncology
Chief, Surgical Breast Service
University of Texas M. D. Anderson Cancer Center
1515 Holcombe, Box 106
Houston, Texas 77030

Barbara L. Smith, M.D., Ph.D.
Assistant Professor of Surgery
Harvard Medical School
Gillette Center for Women's Cancers
Massachusetts General Hospital
100 Blossom Street, Cox 120
Boston, Massachusetts 02114

Robert A. Smith, Ph.D.
Director of Cancer Screening
Department of Cancer Control
American Cancer Society
1599 Clifton Road NE
Atlanta, Georgia 30329

Ross W. Stephens
Senior Research Scientist
Finsen Labratory
Copenhagen University Hospital
Copenhagen, DK-2100, Denmark

Eric A. Strom, M.D.
Associate Professor of Radiation Oncology
Department of Radiation Oncology
University of Texas M. D. Anderson Cancer Center
1515 Holcombe Boulevard
Houston, Texas 77030

David J. Sugarbaker, M.D.
Professor of Surgery
Harvard Medical School
Department of Surgery/Thoracic Surgery
Brigham and Women's Hospital
75 Francis Street
Boston, Massachusetts 02115

Mark S. Talamonti, M.D., F.A.C.S.
Associate Professor of Surgery
Director, Gastrointestinal Oncology Program
Northwestern University Medical School
300 East Superior Street, Tarry 11-703
Chicago, Illinois 60611

May Lin Tao, M.D., M.S.
Assistant Clinical Professor of Radiation Oncology
University of California, Los Angeles, UCLA Medical Center
Department of Radiation Oncology
200 UCLA Medical Plaza
Los Angeles, California 90095

Richard L. Theriault, D.O., M.B.A.
Associate Professor of Medicine
Department of Breast Medical Oncology
University of Texas M. D. Anderson Cancer Center
1515 Holcombe Boulevard, Box 56
Houston, Texas 77030

Erik W. Thompson, Ph.D.
Associate Professor of Surgery
University of Melbourne
Melbourne, Australia
Head, VBCRC Invasion and Metastasis Unit
St. Vincent's Institute of Medical Research
9 Princes Street, Fitzroy
Victoria 3065, Australia

Bruce J. Trock, Ph.D.
Associate Professor
Departments of Human Oncology and Biostatistics and Epidemiology
Lombardi Cancer Center
Georgetown University Medical Center
2233 Wisconsin Avenue NW, Suite 317
Washington, D.C. 20007

Susan L. Troyan, M.D.
Surgical Director, Breast Care Center
Instructor
Department of Surgery
Harvard Medical School
Beth Israel Deaconess Medical Center
330 Brookline Avenue
Boston, Massachusetts 02215

Luz A. Venta, M.D.
Associate Professor of Radiology
Lynn Sage Comprehensive Breast Center
Northwestern University Medical School
Medical Director, Section of Breast Imaging
Department of Radiology
Northwestern Memorial Hospital
215 E. Huron Street, Galter Pavilion 13th Floor
Chicago, Illinois 60611

Barbara L. Weber, M.D.
Professor of Medicine and Genetics
Director, Breast Cancer Program
Associate Director, Population Science and Cancer Control
The University of Pennsylvania Cancer Center
BRB II/III, Room 316-A
421 Curie Boulevard
Philadelphia, Pennsylvania 19104

Jane C. Weeks, M.D.
Associate Professor of Medicine
Harvard Medical School
Department of Adult Oncology
Dana-Farber Cancer Institute
44 Binney Street
Boston, Massachusetts 02115

Patrick Y. Wen, M.D.
Associate Professor of Neurology
Harvard Medical School
Department of Neurology
Division of Neuro-oncology
Brigham and Women's Hospital
75 Francis Street
Boston, Massachusetts 02115

Walter C. Willett, M.D., M.P.H., P.H.
Professor of Medicine
Harvard Medical School
Professor of Epidemiology and Nutrition
Chair, Department of Nutrition
Harvard School of Public Health
651 Huntington Avenue
Boston, Massachusetts 02115

Eric P. Winer, M.D.
Associate Professor of Medicine
Harvard Medical School
Department of Breast Oncology
Dana-Farber Cancer Institute
44 Binney Street
Boston, Massachusetts 02115

Toshiyuki Yoneda, Ph.D., D.D.S.
Professor of Medicine
Department of Medicine
Division of Endocrinology and Metabolism
University of Texas Health Science Center at San Antonio
7703 Floyd Curl Drive
San Antonio, Texas, 78284

Preface

The first edition of *Diseases of the Breast* was intended as an up-to-date, single-source compilation of important knowledge on breast diseases presented in a form accessible to practicing clinicians. We were gratified by the success of this effort and, for the second edition, we again invited a diverse and distinguished group of experts to summarize the current knowledge of breast diseases, including their clinical features, management, and underlying biologies and epidemiologies. We believe that by providing clinical information that can help focus their energies and talents, this book is also of value to basic and translational scientists concerned about breast cancer.

The high incidence of breast cancer in westernized countries and its common occurrence in women in their early and middle years have made it a topic of great interest, prompting intensive efforts in clinical, translational, and basic research. Clinical investigators have also helped to define various benign diseases of the breast and have described their management and relation to subsequent breast cancer development. Clinical trials performed throughout the world have contributed considerable information about the early detection and management of breast cancer using surgery, radiation therapy, and systemic therapies, including chemotherapy and hormonal interventions. Finally, rapid advances in the understanding of the molecular biology and genetics of normal tissues and cancers have raised optimism that new, more specific methods can be developed to identify a woman's risk for breast cancer, to prevent or at least detect the disease at an earlier stage, and, failing this, to cure it with minimal toxicity. The availability of testing for mutations in *BRCA1* and *BRCA2* and anti-HER2/neu therapy is a prominent example of how advances in basic science can rapidly enter the clinical arena. We believe that other advances in basic science will quickly be reflected in clinical practice. Hence, clinicians caring for patients with breast diseases should be knowledgeable about such advances.

We hope that the second edition of *Diseases of the Breast* becomes a useful resource for clinicians and scientists and fosters the understanding and communication necessary to provide optimal patient care and to achieve rapid advances in managing diseases of the breast, especially breast cancer.

Jay R. Harris, M.D.
Marc E. Lippman, M.D.
Monica Morrow, M.D.
C. Kent Osborne, M.D.

Diseases of the Breast

Second Edition

I

Diseases of the Breast, 2nd ed.,
edited by Jay R. Harris.
Lippincott Williams & Wilkins, Philadelphia © 2000.

Breast Anatomy and Development

CHAPTER 1

Breast Anatomy and Development

Michael P. Osborne

The breasts, or mammary glands, of mammals are important for the survival of the newborn and thus of the species. Nursing of the young in the animal kingdom has many physiologic advantages for the mother, such as aiding postpartum uterine involution, and for the neonate, in terms of the transfer of immunity and bonding. In humans, social influences have reduced the prevalence of breast-feeding of neonates and may have interfered with its physiologic role. It has become increasingly apparent that the advantages of nursing are substantial for both mother and child.

An understanding of the morphology and physiology of the breast and the many endocrine interrelationships of both is essential to the study of the pathophysiology of the breast and the management of benign, preneoplastic, and neoplastic disorders.

M. P. Osborne: Department of Surgery, Joan and Sanford I. Weill Medical College, Cornell University - New York Presbyterian Hospital, New York, New York

EMBRYOLOGY

During the fifth week of human fetal development, the ectodermal primitive milk streak, or "galactic band," develops from axilla to groin on the embryonic trunk.[1] In the region of the thorax, the band develops to form a mammary ridge, whereas the remaining galactic band regresses. Incomplete regression or dispersion of the primitive galactic band leads to accessory mammary tissues, found in 2% to 6% of women.

At 7 to 8 weeks' gestation, a thickening occurs in the mammary anlage (milk hill stage), followed by invagination into the chest wall mesenchyme (disc stage) and tridimensional growth (globular stage). Further invasion of the chest wall mesenchyme results in a flattening of the ridge (cone stage) at 10 to 14 weeks' gestation. Between 12 and 16 weeks' gestation, mesenchymal cells differentiate into the smooth muscle of the nipple and areola. Epithelial buds develop (budding stage) and then branch to form 15 to 25 strips of epithelium (branching stage) at 16 weeks' gestation; these strips represent the future secretory alveoli.[2] The secondary mammary anlage then develops, with differentiation of the hair follicle, sebaceous gland, and sweat gland elements, but only the sweat glands develop fully at this time. Phylogenetically, the breast parenchyma is believed to develop from sweat gland tissue. In addition, special apocrine glands develop to form the Montgomery glands around the nipple. The developments described thus far are independent of hormonal influences.

During the third trimester of pregnancy, placental sex hormones enter the fetal circulation and induce canalization of the branched epithelial tissues (canalization stage).[3,4] This process continues from the twentieth to the thirty-second week of gestation. At approximately term, 15 to 25 mammary ducts are formed, with coalescence of duct and sebaceous glands near the epidermis. Parenchymal differentiation occurs at 32 to 40 weeks with the development of lobuloalveolar structures that contain colostrum (end-vesicle stage). A fourfold increase in mammary gland mass occurs at this time, and the nipple-areolar complex develops and becomes pigmented. In the neonate, the stimulated mammary tissue secretes colostral milk (sometimes called witch's milk), which can be expressed from the nipple for 4 to 7 days postpartum in most neonates of either sex. In the newborn, colostral secretion declines over a 3- to 4-week period, owing to involution of the breast after withdrawal of placental hormones. During early childhood, the end vesicles become further canalized and develop into ductal structures by additional growth and branching.

MOLECULAR BIOLOGY OF MAMMARY GLAND DEVELOPMENT

Normal development of the mammalian breast depends on a combination of systemic mammotrophic hormones and local cell–cell interactions.[5,6] The local cellular interactions appear to be mediated by a variety of growth factors, some of which belong to the epidermal growth factor, transforming growth factor beta (TGF-β), fibroblast growth factor (FGF), and *Wnt* gene families.[7–11] Some of these growth regulators have been shown to affect mammary cell growth and differentiation in experimental systems,[10–16] whereas their differential expression in the developing breast suggests that they may act in concert with systemic hormones during normal glandular development.[7–11] Systemic hormonal alterations also combine with local cellular effects to promote involution of the mammary gland after lactation.[17]

TGF-α, a member of the epidermal growth factor family, may play a role in both ductal growth and alveolar development of the mammary gland. Ectopic expression of TGF-α causes significant alterations in mammary epithelial growth and differentiation in transgenic mice and other systems,[12–14] and the *in vivo* localization of TGF-α to actively growing end buds of the mouse mammary gland is consistent with a role in normal ductal development.[7,8] In addition, the changing temporal and spatial expression pattern of TGF-α in the breast during pregnancy suggests that it may function in mediating lobuloalveolar development.[8] TGF-α is up-regulated in both mammary ductal epithelium and stromal fibroblasts during rat and human pregnancy.[8] It is therefore possible that TGF-α functions as an autocrine or paracrine intermediate in directing hormonally induced mammary morphogenesis.[7,8,12]

Studies of the growth factors FGF-1 and FGF-2 in the mouse have suggested that they function in promoting mammary ductal development during sexual maturity.[9] At the onset of ovarian function, FGF-1 expression is up-regulated in ductal epithelium and may provide an autocrine growth stimulus for the proliferating breast. In contrast, FGF-2 is expressed in the mammary stroma, in which it may act indirectly as a ductal morphogen through its influence on extracellular matrix composition. FGF-1 and FGF-2 are well-known angiogenic factors and may also contribute to early breast development by stimulating neovascularization during ductal growth.[9]

The principal members of the TGF-β family—TGF-β1, -β2, and -β3—appear to be involved in ductal morphogenesis of the virgin mouse mammary gland and in regulating the onset of lactation.[10] TGF-β may govern early ductal development by maintaining an open ductal branching pattern that is required for subsequent alveolar development.[10] Maintenance of this ductal architecture requires suppression of lateral bud growth, and TGF-β inhibits ductal growth both *in vitro* and in transgenic mice, possibly through its effects on extracellular matrix deposition.[10,15] In addition, the TGF-β family may play a role in inhibition of lactation. TGF-β expression levels are down-regulated during lactation, and milk production is impaired in TGF-β transgenic mice.[10,16]

Several members of the *Wnt* gene family of secreted glycoproteins are expressed in the developing mouse mammary gland and may play a role in its normal development.[18,19] The first characterized member of this family, *Wnt-1*, was initially identified as an oncogene in mouse mammary tumor virus–induced mammary tumors and induces mammary hyperplasia when expressed in the mammary glands of transgenic mice.[11] Although *Wnt-1* is not expressed during normal mammary development, at least six other members of the *Wnt* family are differentially expressed in the mouse mammary gland during early development, pregnancy, and lactation.[18,19] Because some of these genes can mimic the effects of *Wnt-1* in mammary cell lines, it seems likely that they influence growth or differentiation *in vivo*.[11,20] The spatial expression patterns of these *Wnt* genes have not yet been reported, with the exception of *Wnt-2*. That expression of this gene during early mammary development has been localized to the growing epithelial end buds suggests that it may be involved in early ductal morphogenesis.[19]

The postlactational breast requires a combination of lactogenic hormone deprivation and local signals to undergo glandular involution.[17] The process of involution is characterized by apoptotic cell death and tissue remodeling.[21] Certain gene products associated with apoptosis are up-regulated during mammary involution; however, the factors that trigger the cell death pathway have not been clearly defined.[17] Local extracellular proteases involved in tissue remodeling are up-regulated during breast regression, and this may result in part from the action of TGF-α1 in the postlactational gland.[17]

The regulated expression of locally acting growth factors in the developing breast acts in combination with circulating hormones to control mammary growth, differentiation, and regression. Further investigation of the function of ligands *in vivo* will undoubtedly have importance for the understanding of both breast development and mammary tumorigenesis.

ABNORMAL BREAST DEVELOPMENT

Congenital Abnormalities

The most frequently observed abnormality seen in both sexes is an accessory nipple (polythelia). Ectopic nipple tissue may be mistaken for a pigmented nevus, and it may occur at any point along the milk streak from the axilla to the groin. Rarely, accessory true mammary glands develop. These are most often located in the axilla (polymastia). During pregnancy and lactation, an accessory breast may swell; occasionally, if it has an associated nipple, the accessory breast may function.

Hypoplasia is the underdevelopment of the breast; congenital absence of a breast is termed *amastia*. When breast tissue is lacking but a nipple is present, the condition is termed *amazia*. A wide range of breast abnormalities have been described and can be classified as follows[22,23]:

Unilateral hypoplasia, contralateral normal
Bilateral hypoplasia with asymmetry
Unilateral hyperplasia, contralateral normal
Bilateral hyperplasia with asymmetry
Unilateral hypoplasia, contralateral hyperplasia
Unilateral hypoplasia of breast, thorax, and pectoral muscles (Poland's syndrome)

Most of these abnormalities are not severe. The most severe deformity, amastia or marked breast hypoplasia, is associated with hypoplasia of the pectoral muscle in 90% of cases,[24] but the reverse does not apply. Of women with pectoral muscle abnormalities, 92% have a normal breast.[25] Congenital abnormalities of the pectoral muscle are usually manifested by the lack of the lower third of the muscle and an associated deformity of the ipsilateral rib cage. The association among absence of the pectoral muscle, chest wall deformity, and breast abnormalities was first recognized by Poland in 1841. The original description, however, did not note the concomitant abnormalities of the hand (synbrachydactyly, with hypoplasia of the middle phalanges and central skin webbing),[26] and considerable controversy has evolved concerning the validity of the eponym for this congenital syndrome.[27,28]

Acquired Abnormalities

The most common—and avoidable—cause of amazia is iatrogenic. Injudicious biopsy of a precociously developing breast results in excision of most of the breast bud and subsequent marked deformity during puberty. The use of radiation therapy in prepubertal girls to treat either hemangioma of the breast or intrathoracic disease can also result in amazia. Traumatic injury of the developing breast, such as that caused by a severe cutaneous burn, with subsequent contracture, can also result in deformity.

NORMAL BREAST DEVELOPMENT DURING PUBERTY

Puberty in girls begins at the age of 10 to 12 years as a result of the influence of hypothalamic gonadotropin-releasing hormones secreted into the hypothalamic–pituitary portal venous system. The basophilic cells of the anterior pituitary release follicle-stimulating hormone and luteinizing hormone. Follicle-stimulating hormone causes the primordial ovarian follicles to mature into graafian follicles, which secrete estrogens, primarily in the form of 17β-estradiol. These hormones induce the growth and maturation of the breasts and genital organs.[29] During the first 1 to 2 years after menarche, hypothalamic-adenohypophyseal function is unbalanced, because the maturation of the primordial ovarian follicles does not result in ovulation or a luteal phase. Therefore, ovarian estrogen synthesis predominates over luteal progesterone synthesis. The physiologic effect of estrogens on the maturing breast is to stimulate longitudinal ductal growth of ductal epithelium. Terminal ductules also form buds that precede further breast lobules. Simultaneously, periductal connective tissues increase in volume and elasticity, with enhanced vascularity and fat deposition. These initial changes are induced by estrogens synthesized in immature ovarian follicles, which are anovulatory; subsequently, mature follicles ovulate, and the corpus luteum releases progesterone. The relative role of these hormones is not clear. In experimental studies, estrogens alone induce a pronounced ductular increase, whereas progesterone alone does not. The two hormones together produce full ductular-lobular-alveolar development of mammary tissues.[29] The marked individual variation in development of the breast makes it impossible to categorize histologic changes on the basis of age.[3,4] Breast development by age has been described by external morphologic changes. The evolution of the breast from childhood to maturity has been divided into five phases by Tanner,[30] as shown in Table 1.

MORPHOLOGY

Adult Breast

The adult breast lies between the second and sixth ribs in the vertical axis and between the sternal edge and the midaxillary line in the horizontal axis (Fig. 1). The average breast measures 10 to 12 cm in diameter, and its average thickness centrally is 5 to 7 cm. Breast tissue also projects into the axilla as the axillary tail of Spence. The contour of the breast varies but is usually domelike, with a conical configuration

TABLE 1. *Phases of breast development*

Phase I Age: puberty	Preadolescent elevation of the nipple with no palpable glandular tissue or areolar pigmentation.
Phase II Age: 11.1 ± 1.1 yr	Presence of glandular tissue in the subareolar region. The nipple and breast project as a single mound from the chest wall.
Phase III Age: 12.2 ± 1.09 yr	Increase in the amount of readily palpable glandular tissue with enlargement of the breast and increased diameter and pigmentation of the areola. The contour of the breast and nipple remains in a single plane.
Phase IV Age: 13.1 ± 1.15 yr	Enlargement of the areola and increased areolar pigmentation. The nipple and areola form a secondary mound above the level of the breast.
Phase V Age: 15.3 ± 1.7 yr	Final adolescent development of a smooth contour with no projection of the areola and nipple.

From ref. 30., with permission.

in the nulliparous woman and a pendulous contour in the parous woman. The breast comprises three major structures: skin, subcutaneous tissue, and breast tissue, with the last comprising both parenchyma and stroma. The parenchyma is divided into 15 to 20 segments that converge at the nipple in a radial arrangement. The collecting ducts that drain each segment are 2 mm in diameter, with subareolar lactiferous sinuses of 5 to 8 mm in diameter. Between five and ten major collecting milk ducts open at the nipple.

The nomenclature of the duct system is varied. The branching system can be named in a logical fashion, starting with the collecting ducts in the nipple and extending to the ducts that drain each alveolus, as shown in Table 2.

Each duct drains a lobe made up of 20 to 40 lobules. Each lobule consists of ten to 100 alveoli or tubulosaccular secretory units. The microanatomy has been described in detail by Parks.[31] The stroma and subcutaneous tissues of the breast contain fat, connective tissue, blood vessels, nerves, and lymphatics.

The skin of the breast is thin and contains hair follicles, sebaceous glands, and eccrine sweat glands. The nipple, which is located over the fourth intercostal space in the nonpendulous breast, contains abundant sensory nerve endings, including Ruffini-like bodies and end bulbs of Krause. Moreover, sebaceous and apocrine sweat glands are present, but not hair follicles. The areola is circular and pigmented, measuring 15 to 60 mm in diameter. The Morgagni tubercles, located near the periphery of the areola, are elevations formed by openings of the ducts of the Montgomery glands. The Montgomery glands are large sebaceous glands capable of secreting milk; they represent an intermediate stage between sweat and mammary glands. Fascial tissues envelop the breast. The superficial pectoral fascia envelops the breast and is continuous with the superficial abdominal fascia of Camper. The undersurface of the breast lies on the deep pectoral fascia, covering the pectoralis major and anterior serratus muscles. Connecting these two fascial layers are fibrous bands (Cooper suspensory ligaments) that represent the "natural" means of support of the breast.

Blood Supply of the Breast

The principal blood supply to the breast is derived from the internal mammary and lateral thoracic arteries. Approximately 60% of the breast, mainly the medial and central parts, is supplied by the anterior perforating branches of the internal mammary artery. Approximately 30% of the breast, mainly the upper, outer quadrant, is supplied by the lateral thoracic artery. The pectoral branch of the thoracoacromial artery; the lateral branches of the third, fourth, and fifth intercostal arteries; and the subscapular and thoracodorsal arteries all make minor contributions to the blood supply.

Lymphatic Drainage of the Breast

Lymph Vessels

The subepithelial or papillary plexus of the lymphatics of the breast is confluent with the subepithelial lymphatics over the surface of the body. These valveless lymphatic vessels communicate with subdermal lymphatic vessels and merge with the Sappey subareolar plexus. The subareolar plexus receives lymphatic vessels from the nipple and areola and communicates by way of vertical lymphatic vessels equivalent to those that connect the subepithelial and subdermal plexus elsewhere.[32] Lymph flows unidirectionally from the superficial to deep plexus and from the subareolar plexus through the lymphatic vessels of the lactiferous duct to the perilobular and deep subcutaneous plexus. The periductal lymphatic vessels lie just outside the myoepithelial layer of the duct wall.[33] Flow from the deep subcutaneous and intramammary lymphatic vessels moves centrifugally toward the axillary and internal mammary lymph nodes. Injection studies with radiolabeled colloid[34] have demonstrated the physiology of lymph flow and have countered the old hypothesis of centripetal flow toward the Sappey subareolar plexus. Approximately 3% of the lymph from the breast is estimated to flow to the internal mammary chain, whereas 97% flows to the axillary nodes.[35] Drainage of lymph to the internal

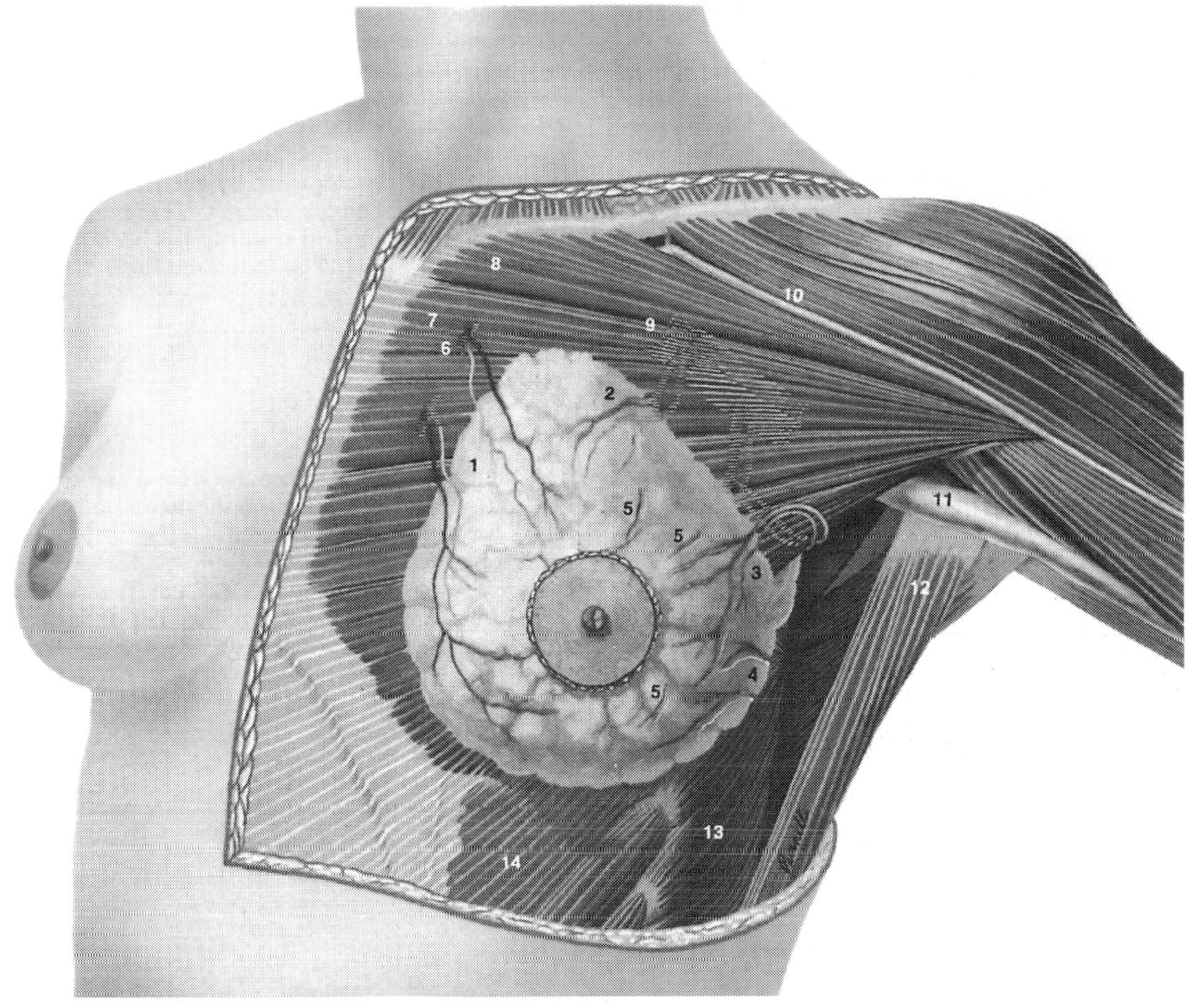

FIG. 1. Normal anatomy of the breast and pectoralis major muscle.

1. Perforating branches from internal mammary artery and vein
2. Pectoral branches from thoracoacromial artery and vein
3. External mammary branch from lateral thoracic artery and vein
4. Branches from subscapular and thoracodorsal arteries and veins
5. Lateral branches of third, fourth, and fifth intercostal arteries and veins
6. Internal mammary artery and veins
7. Sternocostal head of pectoralis major muscle
8. Clavicular head of pectoralis major muscle
9. Axillary artery and vein
10. Cephalic vein
11. Axillary sheath
12. Latissimus dorsi muscle
13. Serratus anterior muscle
14. External abdominal oblique muscle

mammary chain may be observed after injection of any quadrant of the breast.

Axillary Lymph Nodes

The topographic anatomy of the axillary lymph nodes has been studied as the major route of regional spread in primary mammary carcinoma. The anatomic arrangement of the axillary lymph nodes has been subject to many different classifications. The most detailed studies are those of Pickren,[36] which show the pathologic anatomy of tumor spread. Axillary lymph nodes can be grouped as the apical or subclavicular nodes, lying medial to the pectoralis minor muscle, and the axillary vein lymph nodes, grouped along the axillary vein from the pectoralis minor muscle to the lateral limit of the axilla; the interpectoral (Rotter) nodes, lying between the pectoralis major and minor muscles along the lateral pectoral nerve; the scapular group, comprising the nodes lying along the subscapular vessels; and the central

TABLE 2. *Nomenclature of the breast epithelial system*

Major ducts
Collecting ducts
Lactiferous sinuses
Segmental ducts
Subsegmental ducts
Terminal duct–lobular unit
Terminal ducts
Extralobular
Intralobular
Lobules
Alveoli

nodes, lying beneath the lateral border of the pectoralis major muscle and below the pectoralis minor muscle (Fig. 2). Other groups can be identified, such as the external mammary nodes lying over the axillary tail and the paramammary nodes located in the subcutaneous fat over the upper, outer quadrant of the breast.

An alternative method of delineating metastatic spread, for the purposes of determining pathologic anatomy and metastatic progression, is to divide the axillary lymph nodes into arbitrary levels.[37] Level I lymph nodes lie lateral to the lateral border of the pectoralis minor muscle, level II nodes lie behind the pectoralis minor muscle, and level III nodes are located medial to the medial border of the pectoralis minor muscle (Fig. 3). These levels can be determined accurately only by marking them with tags at the time of surgery.

Internal Mammary Lymph Nodes

The internal mammary nodes lie in the intercostal spaces in the parasternal region. The nodes lie close to the internal mammary vessels in extrapleural fat and are distributed in the intercostal spaces, as shown in Fig. 3. From the second intercostal space downward, the internal mammary nodes are separated from the pleura by a thin layer of fascia in the same plane as the transverse thoracic muscle. The number of lymph nodes described in the internal mammary chain varies. The nodes lie medial to the internal mammary vessels in the first and second intercostal spaces in 88% and 76% of cases, respectively, whereas they lie lateral to the vessels in the third intercostal space in 79% of cases. The prevalence of nodes in each intercostal space is as follows: first space, 97%; second space, 98%; third space, 82%; fourth space, 9%; fifth space, 12%; and sixth space, 62%.[38] The pathologic anatomy of this route of lymphatic drainage in the spread of breast disease has been described by Handley and Thackray[39] and Urban and Marjani.[40]

In the presence of nodal metastases, obstruction of the physiologic routes of lymphatic flow may occur, and alternative pathways may then become important. The alternative routes that have been described are deep, substernal, cross drainage to the contralateral internal mammary chain[41,42]; superficial presternal crossover, lateral intercostal, and mediastinal drainage[43]; and spread through the rectus abdominis muscle sheath to the subdiaphragmatic and subperitoneal plexus (the Gerota pathway). This last route allows the direct spread of tumor to the liver and retroperitoneal lymph nodes. Substernal crossover is demonstrable by isotope imaging of the lymph nodes[44] and may be of significance in early breast cancer.[44]

Muscular and Neural Anatomy

The important muscles in the region of the breast are the pectoralis major and minor, serratus anterior, and latissimus dorsi muscles, as well as the aponeurosis of the external oblique and rectus abdominis muscles (see Fig. 2).

The pectoralis minor muscle arises from the outer aspect of the third, fourth, and fifth ribs and is inserted into the medial border of the upper surface of the coracoid process of the scapula. The muscle is usually prefixed, rather than postfixed, and is innervated by the medial pectoral nerve, which arises mainly from the medial cord of the brachial plexus (G-8, T-1 segmental origin) and descends posteriorly to the muscle crossing the axillary vein anteriorly. The nerve enters the interpectoral space, passing through the muscle itself in 62% of cases and around the lateral border as a single branch in 38% of cases.[45] Varying numbers of branches passing through the muscle provide motor supply to the lateral part of the pectoralis major muscle. The terms *medial* and *lateral pectoral nerves* are confusing: The standard terminology refers to their brachial plexus origin rather than their anatomic positions. Changes in terminology have been proposed but have not yet been generally accepted. The arrangement of these nerves is of particular importance in performing the modified radical (Patey) mastectomy.

The serratus anterior muscle stabilizes the scapula on the chest wall. The muscle arises by a series of digitations from the upper eight ribs laterally; its origin from the first rib is in the posterior triangle of the neck. At its origin from the fifth, sixth, seventh, and eighth ribs, it interdigitates with the origin of the external oblique muscle. The muscle inserts into the vertebral border of the scapula on its costal surface and is supplied by the long thoracic nerve of Bell (the nerve to the serratus anterior muscle). The origin of this important nerve is the posterior aspect of the C-5, C-6, and C-7 roots of the brachial plexus. It passes posteriorly to the axillary vessels, emerging on the chest wall high in the medial part of the subscapular fossa. The nerve lies superficial to the deep fascia overlying the anterior serratus muscle and marks the posterior limit of dissection of the deep fascia. Preservation of the nerve to the serratus anterior muscle as it passes downward is essential to avoid "winging" of the scapula and loss of shoulder power.

The latissimus dorsi muscle, the largest muscle in the body, is characterized by a wide origin from the spinous processes and supraspinous ligaments of the seventh thoracic vertebra downward, including all the lumbar and sacral vertebrae. The muscle inserts, by a narrow tendon forming the posterior axil-

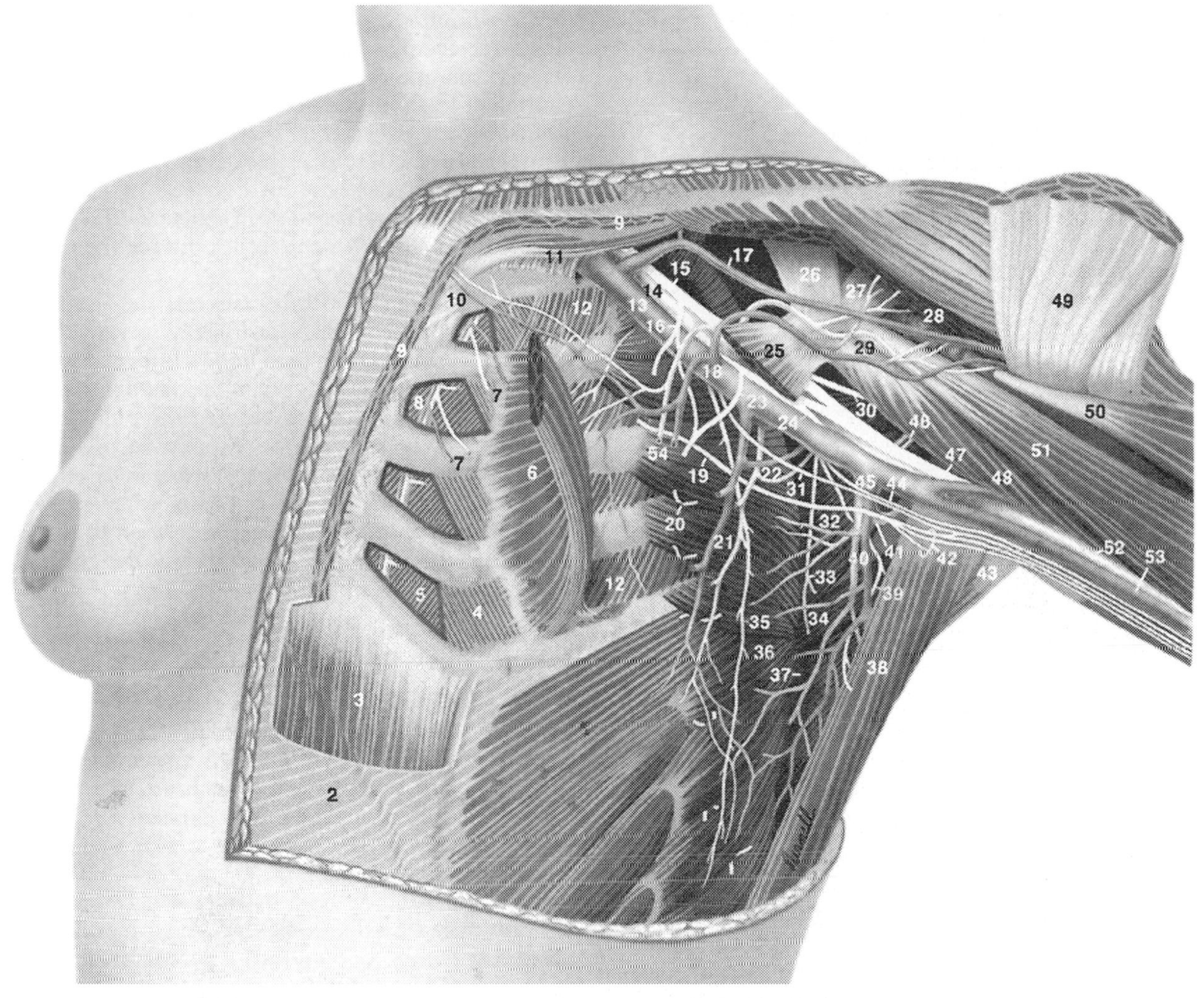

FIG. 2. Chest wall muscles and vascular anatomy.

1. External abdominal oblique muscle
2. Rectus sheath
3. Rectus abdominis muscle
4. Internal intercostal muscle
5. Transverse thoracic muscle
6. Pectoralis minor muscle
7. Perforating branches from internal mammary artery and vein
8. Internal mammary artery and vein
9. Cut edge of pectoralis major muscle
10. Sternoclavicular branch of thoracoacromial artery and vein
11. Subclavius muscle and Halsted ligament
12. External intercostal muscle
13. Axillary vein
14. Axillary artery
15. Lateral cord of brachial plexus
16. Lateral pectoral nerve (from the lateral cord)
17. Cephalic vein
18. Thoracoacromial vein
19. Intercostobrachial nerve
20. Lateral cutaneous nerves
21. Lateral thoracic artery and vein
22. Scapular branches of lateral thoracic artery and vein
23. Medial pectoral nerve (from medial cord)
24. Ulnar nerve
25. Pectoralis minor muscle
26. Coracoclavicular ligament
27. Coracoacromial ligament
28. Cut edge of deltoid muscle
29. Acromial and humeral branches of thoracoacromial artery and vein
30. Musculocutaneous nerve
31. Medial cutaneous nerve of arm
32. Subscapularis muscle
33. Lower subscapular nerve
34. Teres major muscle
35. Long thoracic nerve
36. Serratus anterior muscle
37. Latissimus dorsi muscle
38. Latissimus dorsi muscle
39. Thoracodorsal nerve
40. Thoracodorsal artery and vein
41. Scapular circumflex artery and vein
42. Branching of intercostobrachial nerve
43. Teres major muscle
44. Medial cutaneous nerve of forearm
45. Subscapular artery and vein
46. Posterior humeral circumflex artery and vein
47. Median nerve
48. Coracobrachialis muscle
49. Pectoralis major muscle
50. Biceps brachii muscle, long head
51. Biceps brachii muscle, short head
52. Brachial artery
53. Basilic vein
54. Pectoral branch of thoracoacromial artery and vein

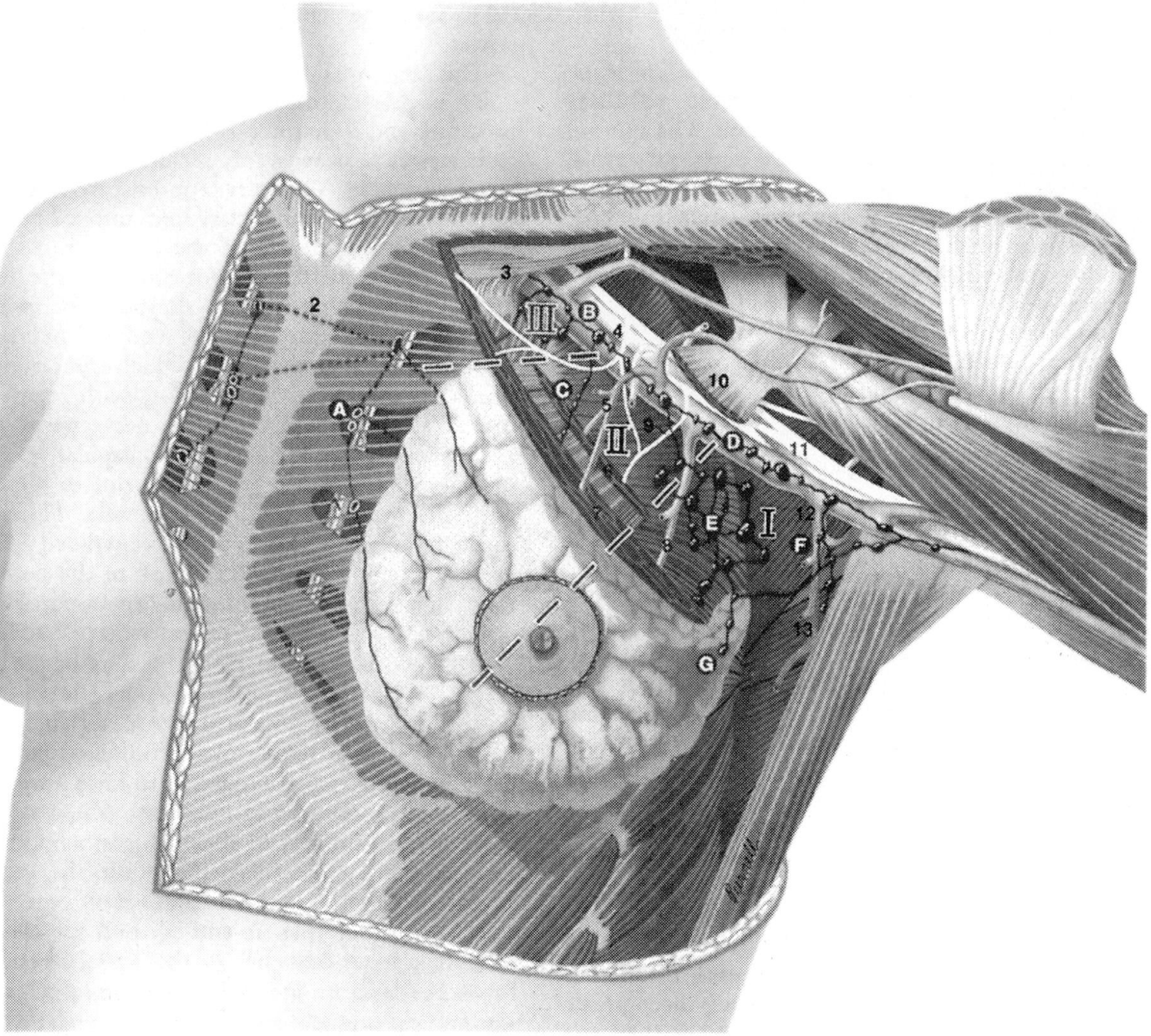

FIG. 3. Lymphatic drainage of the breast showing lymph node groups and levels.

1. Internal mammary artery and vein
2. Substernal cross drainage to contralateral internal mammary lymphatic chain
3. Subclavius muscle and Halsted ligament
4. Lateral pectoral nerve (from the lateral cord)
5. Pectoral branch from thoracoacromial vein
6. Pectoralis minor muscle
7. Pectoralis major muscle
8. Lateral thoracic vein
9. Medial pectoral nerve (from the medial cord)
10. Pectoralis minor muscle
11. Median nerve
12. Subscapular vein
13. Thoracodorsal vein

A. Internal mammary lymph nodes
B. Apical lymph nodes
C. Interpectoral (Rotter) lymph nodes
D. Axillary vein lymph nodes
E. Central lymph nodes
F. Scapular lymph nodes
G. External mammary lymph nodes

Level I lymph nodes: lateral to lateral border of pectoralis minor muscle
Level II lymph nodes: behind pectoralis minor muscle
Level III lymph nodes: medial to medial border of pectoralis minor muscle

lary fold, into a 2.5-cm insertion in the bicipital groove of the humerus. As the muscle spirals around the teres major muscle, the surfaces of the muscle become reversed to the point of insertion. The muscle is supplied by the thoracodorsal nerve (the nerve to the latissimus dorsi muscle), which arises from the posterior cord of the brachial plexus, with segmental origin from C-6, C-7, and C-8. The nerve passes behind the axillary vessels, approaches the subscapular vessels from the medial side, and then crosses anterior to these vessels to enter the medial surface of the muscle. The nerve passes through the axilla and is intimately involved in the scapular group of lymph nodes. Resection of the nerve does not result in any important cosmetic or functional defect; nevertheless, it should be preserved when possible.

An important landmark in the apex of the axilla is the origin of the subclavius muscle, which arises from the costo-

TABLE 3. *Characteristics of human breast lobules*

Lobule type	Lobule area (mm^2)	Component structures	Component area (×10^{-2}/mm^2)	No. of components/lobule	No. of components/mm^2	No. of cells/ area section
I	0.048 ± 0.0444	Alveolar bud	0.232 ± 0.090	11.20 ± 6.34	253.8 ± 50.17	32.43 ± 14.07
II	0.060 ± 0.026	Ductule	0.167 ± 0.035	47.0 ± 11.70	682.4 ± 169.0	13.14 ± 4.79
III	0.129 ± 0.049	Ductule	0.125 ± 0.029	81.0 ±16.6	560.4 ± 25.0	11.0 ± 2.0
IV	0.250 ± 0.060	Acini	0.120 ± 0.050	180.0 ± 20.8	720.0 ± 150.0	10.0 ± 2.3

From ref. 47.

chondral junction of the first rib. At the tendinous part of the lower border of this muscle, two layers of the clavipectoral fascia fuse together to form a well-developed band, the costocoracoid ligament, which stretches from the coracoid process to the first costochondral junction (the Halsted ligament). At this point, the axillary vessels (the vein being anterior to the artery) enter the thorax, passing over the first rib and beneath the clavicle. Many unnamed small branches of the axillary vein pass to its lower border from the axilla. Near the apex, a small artery, the highest thoracic artery, arises from the axillary artery and lies on the first and second ribs.

MUSCULAR ABNORMALITIES

Congenital absence of the sternocostal head of the pectoralis major muscle and its associated abnormalities has been described earlier in this chapter. In 5% of cadavers, a sternalis muscle can be found lying longitudinally between the sternal insertion of the sternocleidomastoid muscle and the rectus abdominis muscle. The pectoralis minor muscle is inserted into the head of the humerus and the coracoid process of the scapula in 15% of cases. Part of the tendon then passes between the two parts of the coracoacromial ligament to insert into the coracohumeral ligament. Rarely, the axillopectoral muscle arises as a separate part of the latissimus dorsi muscle and crosses the base of the axilla superficially, then passes deep to the pectoralis major muscle to join its insertion or to continue to the coracoid process (the Langer axillary arch). This anatomic arrangement can cause compression of the axillary vessels[46] and difficulty in orientation during axillary dissection.

Microanatomy of Breast Development

The developing breast at puberty has been described in detail by Russo and Russo[47] as growing and dividing ducts that form club-shaped terminal end buds. Growing terminal end buds form new branches, twigs, and small ductules termed *alveolar buds*. Alveolar buds subsequently differentiate into the terminal structure of the resting breast, named the *acines* by German pathologists or the *ductule* by Dawson.[3] The term *alveolus* is best applied to the resting secretory unit and *acines* to the fully developed secretory unit of pregnancy and lactation.[47]

Lobules develop during the first few years after menarche. The alveolar buds cluster around a terminal duct and form type I (virginal) lobules, comprising approximately 11 alveolar buds lined by two layers of epithelium. Full differentiation of the mammary gland proceeds through puberty, takes many years, and may not be fully completed if interrupted by pregnancies.

Detailed microanatomic studies of the breast have shown the presence of three distinct types of lobules.[47] Type I lobules, previously described, are the first generation of lobules that develop just after the menarche. The transition to type II and type III gradually results from continued sprouting of new alveolar buds. The characteristics of the four lobular types are described in Tables 3 and 4.

Microscopic Anatomy of the Adult Breast

In the immature breast, the ducts and alveoli are lined by a two-layer epithelium that consists of a basal cuboidal layer and a flattened surface layer. In the presence of estrogens at puberty and subsequently, this epithelium proliferates, becoming multilayered (Fig. 4A). Three alveolar cell types have been observed: superficial (luminal) A cells, basal B cells (chief cells), and myoepithelial cells.

Superficial, or luminal, A cells are dark, basophilic-staining cells that are rich in ribosomes. Superficial cells undergo intercellular dehiscence, with swelling of the mitochondria, and become grouped, forming buds within the lumen. Basal B cells, or chief cells, are the major cell type in mammary epithelium. They are clear, with an ovoid nucleus without

TABLE 4. *Proliferative activity of human breast terminal duct–lobular unit components as measured by DNA-labeling index*

Structure	Index
Terminal end bud	15.8 ± 5.2
Type I lobule	5.5 ± 0.5
Type II lobule	0.9 ± 1.2
Type III lobule	0.25 ± 0.3
Terminal duct	1.2 ± 0.5

From ref. 47.

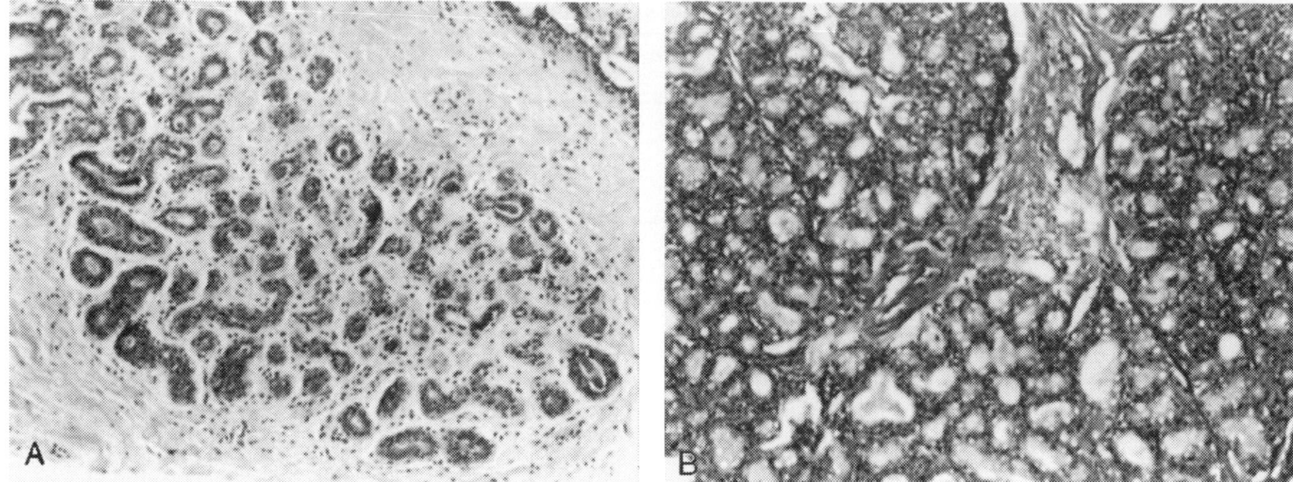

FIG. 4. A: One normal, inactive lobule from the breast of a 35-year-old woman. Alveolar cells are small and the lumina are inconspicuous. Much of the lobular space is occupied by capillaries and stroma. (Hematoxylin-eosin stain; ×40.) **B:** Portions of three adjacent, lactating lobules from the breast of a 25-year-old woman who was 3 weeks postpartum. There is cytoplasmic vacuolization of the alveolar cells, which have proliferated, leading to marked enlargement of the lobule. (Hematoxylin-eosin stain; ×40.)

nucleoli. Where the basal cells are in contact with the lumen, microvilli occur on the cell membrane. Intracytoplasmic filaments are similar to those in myoepithelial cells, suggesting their differentiation toward that cell type. Myoepithelial cells are located around alveoli and small excretory milk ducts between the inner aspect of the basement membrane and the tunica propria. Myoepithelial cells are arranged in a branching, starlike fashion. The sarcoplasm contains filaments that are 50 to 80 nm in diameter; these myofilaments are inserted by hemidesmosomes into the basal membrane. These cells are not innervated but are stimulated by the steroid hormones prolactin and oxytocin.

PHYSIOLOGY

Microscopy, Morphology, and the Menstrual Cycle

Histologic changes in the normal breast have been identified in relation to the endocrine variations of the menstrual cycle.[48] Normal menstrual cycle–dependent histologic changes in both stroma and epithelium have been observed.

Cyclic changes in the sex steroid hormone levels during the menstrual cycle profoundly influence breast morphology. Under the influence of follicle-stimulating hormone and luteinizing hormone during the follicular phase of the menstrual cycle, increasing levels of estrogen secreted by the ovarian graafian follicles stimulate breast epithelial proliferation. During this proliferative phase, the epithelium exhibits sprouting, with increased cellular mitoses, RNA synthesis, increased nuclear density, enlargement of the nucleolus, and changes in other intercellular organelles. In particular, the Golgi apparatus, ribosomes, and mitochondria increase in size or number. During the follicular phase, at the time of maximal estrogen synthesis and secretion in midcycle, ovulation occurs. A second peak occurs in the midluteal phase, when luteal progesterone synthesis is maximal. Similarly, progestogens induce changes in the mammary epithelium during the luteal phase of the ovulatory cycles. Mammary ducts dilate, and the alveolar epithelial cells differentiate into secretory cells, with a partly monolayer arrangement. The combination of these sex steroid hormones and other hormones results in the formation of lipid droplets in the alveolar cells and some intraluminal secretion.

The changes in breast epithelium in response to hormones are mediated through either intracellular steroid receptors or membrane-bound peptide receptors. The presence of steroid receptors for estrogen and progestogens in the cytosol of normal mammary epithelium has been demonstrated.[49] Through the binding of these hormones to specific receptors, the molecular changes, with their observed morphologic effects, are induced as physiologic changes. Similarly, membrane receptors are present to mediate the actions of prolactin. Increases in endogenous estrogen can also exert a histamine-like effect on the mammary microcirculation,[50] resulting in an increased, maximal blood flow 3 to 4 days before menstruation, with an average increase in breast volume of 15 to 30 cm^3.[4] Premenstrual breast fullness is attributable to increasing interlobular edema and enhanced ductular-acinar proliferation under the influence of estrogens and progestogens. With the onset of menstruation, after a rapid decline in the circulating levels of sex steroid hormones, secretory activity of the epithelium regresses.

Postmenstrually, tissue edema is reduced, and regression of the epithelium ceases as a new cycle begins, with concomitant rises in estrogen levels. Minimum breast volume is observed 5 to 7 days after menstruation. The cyclic changes in breast cellular growth rates are related to hormonal variations in the follicular and luteal phases of the menstrual cycle. Measurement of these changes can be made by observation and measurement of a variety of cellular and nuclear parameters:

- Histologic pattern
- Cellular morphology
- Nuclear morphology
- Mitoses
- Tritiated thymidine uptake
- Image cytometry
    - Nuclear area
    - Circumference
    - Boundary fluctuation
    - Chromatin granularity
    - Stain intensity
- Proliferation markers
    - Ki-67
    - PCNA
    - MIB-1

Most observations have been made from surgical specimens, which are usually from women with breast abnormalities, or from autopsy specimens, which may have resulted in inconsistent and contradictory results.

Most studies have shown that breast epithelial cell proliferation increases in the second half (luteal phase) of the menstrual cycle.[51–57]

A study of nuclear tritiated thymidine uptake in surgically excised breast tissue showed that peak uptake was during the luteal phase on days 22–24, coinciding with an increase in circulatory progesterone levels and a second peak of estrogen. The role of estrogen was considered unimportant, because the preovulatory peak of estrogen was not associated with an increase in tritiated thymidine uptake.[53] The possibility of a synergistic action between estrogen and progesterone would therefore be unlikely.

The role of estrogen and progesterone was subsequently studied in explants of human breast tissue implanted subcutaneously in nude mice.[58] An increase in epithelial cell growth was observed seven days after exposure to estrogen; progesterone had no effect, and a combination of estrogen and progesterone neither enhanced nor diminished the proliferative effect of estrogen. These observations may explain why proliferation increases during the luteal phase subsequent to the preovulatory estrogen peak.

Breast Changes during Pregnancy

During pregnancy, marked ductular, lobular, and alveolar growth occurs as a result of the influence of luteal and placental sex steroids, placental lactogen, prolactin, and chorionic gonadotropin (Fig. 4B). In experimental studies, these effects are observed when estrogen and progesterone cause a release of prolactin by reducing the hypothalamic release of prolactin-inhibiting factor (PIF).[55] Prolactin in humans is also released progressively during pregnancy and probably stimulates epithelial growth and secretion.[56,57] Prolactin increases slowly during the first half of pregnancy; during the second and third trimesters, blood levels of prolactin are three to five times higher than normal, and mammary epithelium initiates protein synthesis.

In the first 3 to 4 weeks of pregnancy, marked ductular sprouting occurs with some branching, and lobular formation occurs under estrogenic influence. At 5 to 8 weeks, breast enlargement is significant, with dilatation of the superficial veins, heaviness, and increasing pigmentation of the nipple–areolar complex. In the second trimester, lobular formation exceeds ductular sprouting under progestogenic influence. The alveoli contain colostrum but no fat, which is secreted under the influence of prolactin. From the second half of pregnancy onward, increasing breast size results not from mammary epithelial proliferation but from increasing dilatation of the alveoli with colostrum, as well as from hypertrophy of myoepithelial cells, connective tissue, and fat. If these processes are interrupted by early delivery, lactation may be adequate from 16 weeks of pregnancy onward.

At the beginning of the second trimester, the mammary alveoli, but not the milk ducts, lose the superficial layer of A cells. Before this, as in the nonpregnant woman, the two-layer structure is maintained. In the second and third trimesters, this monolayer differentiates into a colostrum–cell layer and accumulates eosinophilic cells, plasma cells, and leukocytes around the alveoli. As pregnancy continues, colostrum, composed of desquamated epithelial cells, accumulates. Aggregations of lymphocytes, round cells, and desquamated phagocytic alveolar cells (foam cells) may be found in colostrum; these are termed the *Donné corpuscles*.

Lactation

After parturition, an immediate withdrawal of placental lactogen and sex steroid hormones occurs. During pregnancy, these hormones antagonize the effect of prolactin on mammary epithelium. Concomitant to the abrupt removal of the placental hormones, luteal production of the sex steroid hormones also ceases. A nadir is reached on the fourth to fifth day postpartum; at this time, the secretion of PIF from the hypothalamus into the hypothalamoadenohypophyseal portal system decreases. This reduction in PIF secretion allows the transmembrane secretion of prolactin by pituitary lactotrophs. Sex steroid hormones are not necessary for successful lactation, and physiologic increases, such as may occur with postpartum ovulatory cycles, do not inhibit it.

Prolactin, in the presence of growth hormone, insulin, and cortisol, converts the mammary epithelial cells from a presecretory to a secretory state. During the first 4 or 5 days after birth, the breasts enlarge as a result of the accumulation of secretions in the alveoli and ducts. The initial secretion is of colostrum, a thin, serous fluid that is, at first, sticky and yellow. Colostrum contains lactoglobulin, which is identical to blood immunoglobulins. The importance of these immunoglobulins is unknown; many maternal antibodies cross the placenta, transferring passive immunity to the fetus in utero. Fatty acids, such as decadienoic acid, phospholipids, fat-soluble vitamins, and lactalbumin, in colostrum have considerable nutritional value. After colostrum secretion, transitional milk and then mature milk are elaborated.

Mechanisms of Milk Synthesis and Secretion

The effects of prolactin are mediated through membrane receptors in the mammary epithelial cells. The release of prolactin is maintained and stimulated by suckling, as is the release of corticotropin (adrenocorticotropic hormone). The mammary cells are cuboidal, depending on the degree of intracellular accumulation of secretions. The DNA and RNA of the nuclei increase, and abundant mitochondria, ribosomes, and rough endoplasmic reticulum, with a prominent Golgi apparatus, are apparent in the epithelial cells. Complex protein, mild fat, and lactose synthetic pathways are activated, as are water-ion transport mechanisms. These processes are initiated by the activation of hormone-specific membrane receptors. Changes in cyclic adenosine monophosphate stimulate milk synthesis through the induction of messenger and transfer RNA. Prolactin stimulates cyclic adenosine monophosphate–induced protein kinase activity, resulting in the phosphorylation of milk proteins. Polymerase activity and cellular transcription are enhanced.[29]

Large fat vacuoles develop and move toward the apex of the cell. At the same time, the nucleus also moves toward the apex. As the water intake of the cell increases, longitudinal cellular striations may be observed. Ultimately, the vacuoles pass from the cell along with part of the cell membrane and cytoplasm; the apical cell membrane reconstitutes as secretion takes place.

Enhanced activity occurs during suckling. Fat is secreted chiefly through an apocrine mechanism, lactose is secreted through a merocrine mechanism, and the secretion of proteins occurs as a result of a combination of mechanisms. Ions enter the milk by diffusion and active transport. Relatively little holocrine secretion is thought to take place. The end result of secretion and subsequent intraductal dilution of extracellular fluid is milk, comprising a suspension of proteins—casein, β-lactalbumin, and β-lactoglobulin—and fat in a lactose-mineral solution. The white appearance of milk is due to emulsified lipids and calcium caseinate, whereas the yellow color of butterfat is due to the presence of carotenoids.

Mechanisms of Milk Ejection

The removal of milk by suckling is aided by active ejection. Sensory nerve endings in the nipple-areolar complex are activated by tactile stimuli. Impulses pass by way of sensory nerves through the dorsal roots to the spinal cord. In the spinal cord, impulses are relayed through the dorsal, lateral, and ventral spinothalamic tracts to the mesencephalon and lateral hypothalamus. Inhibition of PIF secretion permits the unimpeded secretion of prolactin from the anterior pituitary. Simultaneously, through a different pathway in the paraventricular nucleus, the synthesis of oxytocin occurs. Oxytocin is released from the posterior pituitary neurovesicles by impulses traveling along the neurosecretory fibers of the hypothalamoneurohypophyseal tract. Oxytocin released into the systemic circulation acts on the myoepithelial cells, which contract and eject milk from the alveoli into the lactiferous ducts and sinuses. This phenomenon is specific to oxytocin, and changes in intramammary ductal pressures of 20 to 25 mm Hg may be observed in relation to peak blood levels. Oxytocin also acts on the uterus and cervix to promote involution. This effect may be stimulated by cervical dilatation and by vaginal stretching through the ascending afferent neural pathways (Ferguson reflex).

Complex neuroendocrine interactions determine normal lactation. An appreciation of these mechanisms is essential to the understanding of abnormalities and to the treatment of problems of lactation.[29]

Menopause

Declining ovarian function in late premenopause through the menopause leads to regression of epithelial structures and stroma. The duct system remains, but the lobules shrink and collapse. The last structures to appear with sexual maturity are the first ones to regress.[29]

REFERENCES

1. Hamilton NJ, Boyd JD, Mossman HW. *Human embryology*. Cambridge, UK: Heffer, 1968:428.
2. Hughes ESR. Development of mammary gland. *Ann R Coll Surg Engl* 1950;6:99.
3. Dawson EK. A histological study of the normal mamma in relation to tumour growth. I. Early development to maturity. *Edinb Med J* 1934;41:653.
4. Dabelow A. Milchdruse. In: Bargman W, ed. *Handbuch der Mikroskopishen Anatomie des Menschen*, vol 3, part 3. Berlin: Springer-Verlag, 1957.
5. Sutherland RL, Thrall OWJ, Watts CKW, Musgrave E. Estrogen and progestin regulation of cell cycle progression. *J Mamm Gland Biol Neoplasia* 1998;3:63.
6. Medina D. The mammary gland: a unique organ for the study of development and tumorigenesis. *J Mamm Gland Biol Neoplasia* 1996;1:5.
7. Snedeker SM, Brown CF, DiAugustine RP. Expression and functional properties of transforming growth factor alpha and epidermal growth factor during mouse mammary gland ductal morphogenesis. *Proc Natl Acad Sci U S A* 1991;88:2760.
8. Liscia DS, Merlo G, Ciardiello F, et al. Transforming growth factor-alpha messenger RNA localization in the developing adult rat and human mammary gland by in situ hybridization. *Dev Biol* 1990;140:123.

9. Jackson D, Bresnick J, Dickson C. A role for fibroblast growth factor signaling in the lobulo-alveolar development of the mammary gland. *J Mamm Gland Biol Neoplasia* 1997;2:385.
10. Daniel CW, Robinson S, Silberstein GB. The role of TGF-beta in patterning and growth of the mammary ductal tree. *J Mamm Gland Biol Neoplasia* 1996;1:331.
11. Nusse R, Varmus HE. Wnt genes. *Cell* 1992;69:1073.
12. Coleman S, Silberstein GB, Daniel CW. Ductal morphogenesis in the mouse mammary gland: evidence supporting a role for epidermal growth factor. *Dev Biol* 1988;127:304.
13. Vonderhaar BK. Local effects of EGF, alpha-TGF, and EGF-like growth factors on lobuloalveolar development of the mouse mammary gland in vivo. *J Cell Physiol* 1987;132:581.
14. Matsui Y, Halter SA, Holt JT, Hogan BL, Cofey RJ. Development of mammary hyperplasia and neoplasia in MMTV-TGF alpha transgenic mice. *Cell* 1990;61:1147.
15. Pierce DF Jr, Johnson MD, Matsui Y, et al. Inhibition of mammary duct development but not alveolar outgrowth during pregnancy in transgenic mice expressing active TGF-beta 1. *Genes Dev* 1993;7:2308.
16. Smith GM. TGF-β and functional differentiation. *J Mamm Gland Biol Neoplasia* 1998;1:343.
17. Strange R, Feng L, Saurer S, et al. Apoptotic cell death and tissue remodelling during mouse mammary gland involution. *Development* 1992;115:49.
18. Gavin BJ, McMahon AP. Differential regulation of the Wnt gene family during pregnancy and lactation suggests a role in postnatal development of the mammary gland. *Mol Cell Biol* 1992;12:2418.
19. Buhler TA, Dale TC, Kieback C, et al. Localization and quantification of Wnt-2 gene expression in mouse mammary development. *Dev Biol* 1993;155:87.
20. Blasband A, Schryver B, Papkoff J. The biochemical properties and transforming potential of human Wnt-2 are similar to Wnt-1. *Oncogene* 1992;7:153.
21. Pitelka DR. The mammary gland. In: Weiss L, ed. *Cell and tissue biology*. Baltimore: Urban & Schwarzenberg, 1988:877.
22. Maliniac JW. *Breast deformities and their origin*. New York: Grune & Stratton, 1950:163.
23. Simon BE, Hoffman S, Kahn S. Treatment of asymmetry of the breasts. *Clin Plast Surg* 1975;2:375.
24. Trier WC. Complete breast absence. *Plast Reconstr Surg* 1965;36:430.
25. Pers M. Aplasias of the anterior thoracic wall, the pectoral muscle, and the breast. *Scand J Plast Reconstr Surg* 1968;2:125.
26. Beals RK, Crawford S. Congenital absence of the pectoral muscles. *Clin Orthop* 1976;119:166.
27. McDowell F. On the propagation, perpetuation and parroting of erroneous eponyms such as "Poland's syndrome." *Plast Reconstr Surg* 1977;59:561.
28. Ravitch MM. Poland's syndrome: a study of an eponym. *Plast Reconstr Surg* 1977;59:508.
29. Vorherr H. *The breast: morphology, physiology and lactation*. New York: Academic Press, 1974.
30. Tanner JM. *Wachstun und Reifung des Menschen*. Stuttgart, Germany: Georg Thicme Verlag, 1962.
31. Parks AG. The micro-anatomy of the breast. *Ann R Coll Surg Engl* 1959;25:235.
32. Spratt JS, Shieber W, Dillard B. *Anatomy and surgical technique of groin dissection*. St. Louis: CV Mosby, 1965.
33. Bonsor GM, Dossett JA, Jull JW. *Human and experimental breast cancer*. Springfield, IL: Charles C. Thomas, 1961.
34. Turner-Warwick RT. The lymphatics of the breast. *Br J Surg* 1959; 46:574.
35. Hultborn KA, Larsen LG, Raghnult I. The lymph drainage from the breast to the axillary and parasternal lymph nodes: studied with the aid of colloidal Au198. *Acta Radiol* 1955;43:52.
36. Pickren JW. Lymph node metastases in carcinoma of the female mammary gland. *Bull Roswell Park Mem Inst* 1956;1:79.
37. Berg JW. The significance of axillary node levels in the study of breast carcinoma. *Cancer* 1955;8:776.
38. Stibbe EP. The internal mammary lymphatic glands. *J Anat* 1918;52:257.
39. Handley RS, Thackray AC. Invasion of internal mammary lymph nodes in carcinoma of the breast. *BMJ* 1954;1:161.
40. Urban JA, Marjani MA. Significance of internal mammary lymph node metastases in breast cancer. *Am J Roentgenol* 1971;111:130.
41. Rouviere H. *Anatomie des lymphatiques de l'homme*. Paris: Masson, 1932.
42. Ege GN. Internal mammary lymphoscintigraphy. *Radiology* 1975; 118:101.
43. Thomas JM, Redding WH, Sloane JP. The spread of breast cancer: importance of the intrathoracic lymphatic route and its relevance to treatment. *Br J Cancer* 1979;40:540.
44. Osborne MP, Jeyasingh K, Jewkes RF, et al. The preoperative detection of internal mammary lymph node metastases in breast cancer. *Br J Surg* 1979;66:813.
45. Moosman DA. Anatomy of the pectoral nerves and their preservation in modified mastectomy. *Am J Surg* 1980;139:883.
46. Boontje AH. Axillary vein entrapment. *Br J Surg* 1979;66:331.
47. Russo J, Russo IH. Development of human mammary gland. In: Neville MC, Daniel CW, eds. *The mammary gland*. New York: Plenum, 1987:67.
48. Vogel PM, Georgiade NG, Fetter BF, et al. The correlation of histologic changes in the human breast with the menstrual cycle. *Am J Pathol* 1981;104:23.
49. Wittliff JL, Lewko WM, Park DC, et al. Hormones, receptors and breast cancer. In: McGuire WL, ed. *Steroid binding proteins of mammary tissues and their clinical significance in breast cancer*, vol 10. New York: Raven, 1978:327.
50. Zeppa R. Vascular response of the breast to estrogen. *J Clin Endocrinol Metab* 1969;29:695.
51. Masters JRW, Drife JO, Scanisbrook JJ. Cyclic variation of DNA synthesis in human breast epithelium. *J Natl Cancer Inst* 1977;58: 1263.
52. Meyer JS. Cell proliferation in normal breast ducts, fibroadenomas and other ductal hyperplasias measured by nuclear labeling with tritiated thymidine. *Hum Pathol* 1977;8:67.
53. Ferguson DJP, Anderson TJ. Morphologic evaluation of cell hormone in relation to the menstrual cycle in the "resting" human breast. *Br J Cancer* 1981;44:177.
54. Longacre TA, Bartow SA. A correlative morphologic study of human breast and endometrium in the menstrual cycle. *Am J Surg Pathol* 1986;10:382.
55. Potter CS, Watson RJ, Williams GT, et al. The effect of age and menstrual cycle upon proliferative activity of the normal human breast. *Br J Cancer* 1988;58:163.
56. Going JJ, Anderson TJ, Battersby S, et al. Proliferative and secretory activity in human breast during natural and artificial menstrual cycles. *Am J Path* 1988;130:193.
57. Söderqvist G, Isaksson E, Schowltz BV, et al. Proliferation of breast epithelial cells in healthy women during the menstrual cycle. *Am J Obstet Gynecol* 1997;176:123.
58. Laidlaw IJ, Clarke RB, Howell A, et al. The proliferation of normal human breast tissue implanted into athymic nude mice is stimulated by estrogen but not progesterone. *Endocrinology* 1995;136:164.

Diseases of the Breast, 2nd ed.,
edited by Jay R. Harris.
Lippincott Williams & Wilkins, Philadelphia © 2000.

CHAPTER 2

Biochemical Control of Breast Development

Robert B. Dickson and Jose Russo

BREAST DEVELOPMENT: FROM ADOLESCENCE TO MATURITY

The development of the breast in women and of the mammary gland in all other mammalian species is controlled by a multiplicity of genetically determined hormonal and biochemical influences.[1] The inheritance of two X chromosomes is the earliest determinant of gonadal influences that become evident during embryogenesis and fetal life. During the first few months of postnatal life, the hypothalamic-pituitary-gonadal axis is transiently activated.[2] The newborn is, in addition, exposed to a variety of endogenous and exogenous maternal hormones secreted in the milk.[3]

Although breast development is under the influence of a myriad of hormones and growth factors secreted by the pituitary, adrenal, and thyroid glands, the ovary remains the leading organ in orchestrating breast development.[3] Ovarian function, in turn, is under hypothalamic control, with an early phase of central inhibition of gonadotropin-releasing hormone neuronal activity during infancy and a gradual activation of hypothalamic gonadotropin-releasing hormone pulsatile release in conjunction with the initiation of puberty.[3,4] The frequency and amplitude of secretory episodes control the synthesis and release of the pituitary gonadotropins luteinizing hormone and follicle-stimulating hormone (FSH). These hormones bind ovarian receptors, stimulating the secretion of androgens during the infantile period. In addition, the secretion of estrogens, progesterone, and the nonsteroidal glycoprotein hormones inhibin and activin are triggered from early puberty to adulthood.[2–5] In turn, the synthesis and release of pituitary FSH are regulated by inhibin and activin in feedback loops to the pituitary.[3,5] FSH and luteinizing hormone interact with pituitary growth hormone and prolactin in modulation of ovarian steroidogenesis, a function that is also influenced by epinephrine, which is secreted by the adrenal medulla.[2–5] Ductal elongation and branching, occurring during puberty, are positively regulated by pituitary growth hormone, which might act as well through its local mediator, insulinlike growth factor I (IGF-I). Normal ductal development, however, requires the additional presence of an estrogen and progesterone.[3,6,7] Estradiol and progesterone act locally in the mammary gland to stimulate DNA synthesis. This effect is likely to occur through both receptor-mediated and paracrine effects (see section Hormone Action).[3,7,8]

The most dramatic changes in breast size and shape are observed at puberty, which, in girls, occurs between the ages of 10 and 12 years.[9] The development of the breast, as evaluated by various parameters, such as its external appearance, parenchymal area, volume, degree of branching, or level of differentiation, varies greatly from woman to woman.[1,9,10] The adolescent period begins with the first signs of sexual change at puberty and terminates with sexual maturity. With the approach of puberty, the rudimentary mammae begin to show growth activity, both in the glandular tissue and in the surrounding stroma. Glandular enhancement is due to the growth and division of small bundles of primary and secondary ducts that, in turn, undergo further growth and division, ending in club-shaped terminal end buds. Cleavage of terminal end buds originates new branches and small ductules, or *alveolar buds*. Clustering of approximately 11 alveolar buds around a terminal duct constitutes the lobule type 1 (Lob 1) or virginal lobule (Fig. 1). The normal breast tissue of adult women contains two additional types of lobules, designated lobules type 2 (Lob 2) and type 3 (Lob 3) (Figs. 2 and 3). The transition from one type of lobule to the next occurs as a consequence of a gradual process of sprouting of new alveolar buds under the cyclic influence of ovarian hormones. These alveolar buds become progressively smaller and more numerous, averaging approximately 47 in Lob 2 and 80 in Lob 3, stages in which they are called *ductules* or *alveoli* (Fig. 3). The greater number of ductules results in a concomitant increase in size of the lobules, even though each individual structure is smaller.[1]

The architecture of the breast varies greatly in sexually mature women, depending on their parity history, age, and menopausal status. The breast of nulliparous women contains more undifferentiated structures, such as terminal ducts and

R. B. Dickson: Lombardi Cancer Center, Georgetown University Medical Center, Washington, D.C.
J. Russo: Breast Cancer Research Laboratory, Fox Chase Cancer Center, Philadelphia, Pennsylvania

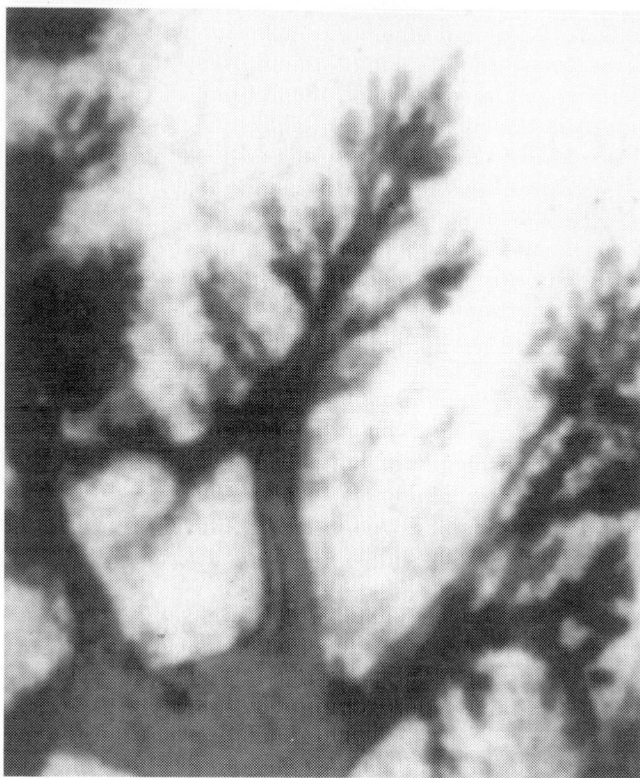

FIG. 1. Lobules type 1 (Lob 1) in the breast tissue of an 18-year-old nulliparous woman. (Whole mount preparation; toluidine blue; ×25.)

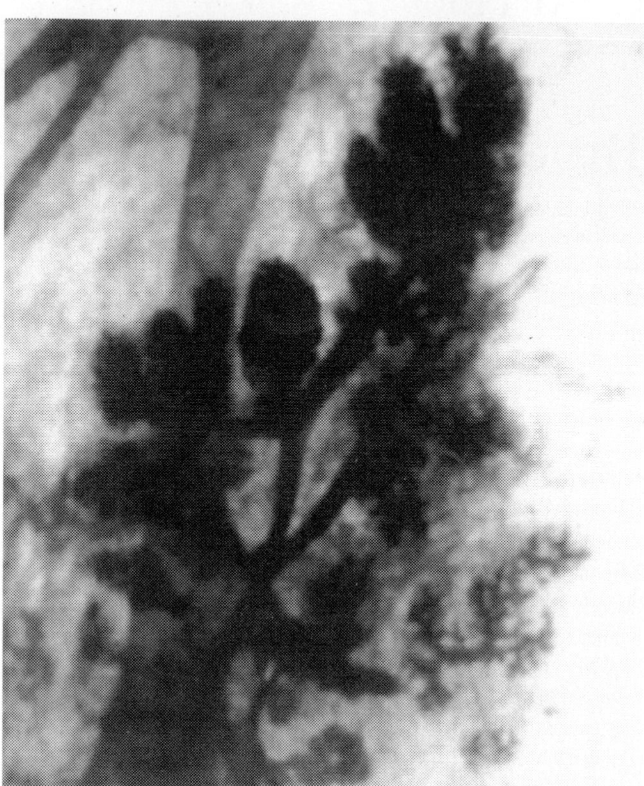

FIG. 2. Lobules type 2 (Lob 2) in the breast tissue of a 24-year-old nulliparous woman. (Whole mount preparation; toluidine blue; ×25.)

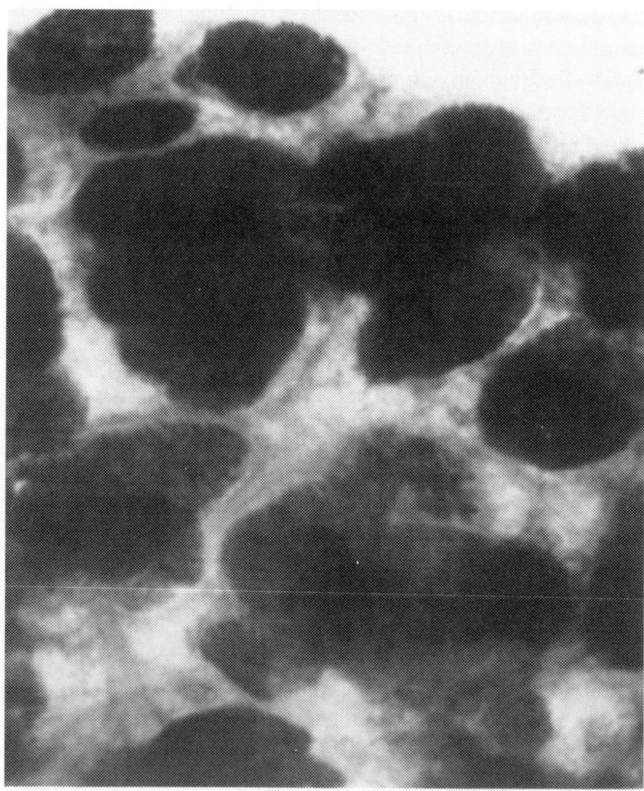

FIG. 3. Lobules type 3 (Lob 3) in the breast tissue of a 35-year-old parous woman. (Whole mount preparation; toluidine blue; ×25.)

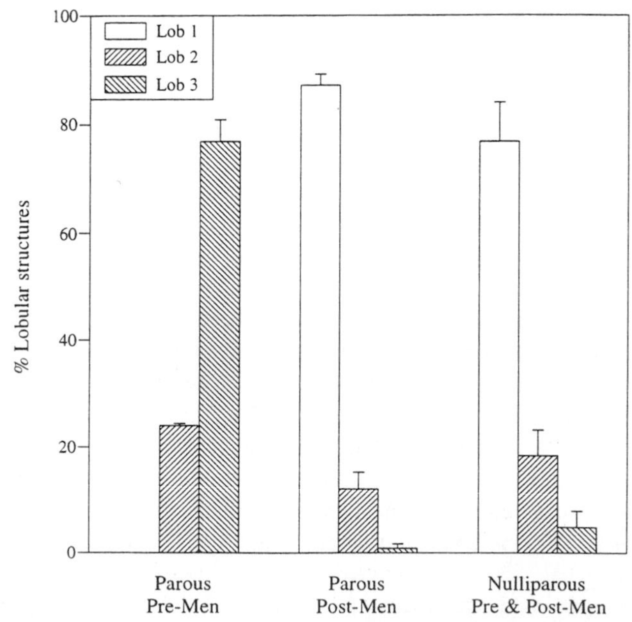

FIG. 4. Percentage of lobular structures (ordinate) in the breast of premenopausal (Pre-Men) and postmenopausal (Post-Men) parous women and pre- and postmenopausal (Pre & Post-Men) nulliparous women. Lob 1, lobules type 1; Lob 2, lobules type 2; Lob 3, lobules type 3 (abscissa).

TABLE 1. *Distribution of Ki67-, ERα-, and PgR-positive epithelial cells in the lobular structures of the human breast*

Lobule type	No. cells	Ki67	ERα	PgR	Ki67 + ERα	Ki67 + PgR
Lob 1	19,339[a]	4.72 ± 1.00[d,e]	7.46 ± 2.88[h]	5.70 ± 1.36[k]	0.48 ± 0.28[n]	0.09 ± 0.01[o]
Lob 2	8,490[b]	1.58 ± 0.45[f]	3.83 ± 2.44[i]	0.73 ± 0.57[l]	0.31 ± 0.21	0.28 ± 0.27
Lob 3	17,750[c]	0.40 ± 0.18[g]	0.76 ± 0.04[j]	0.09 ± 0.04[m]	0.01 ± 0.01	0.01 ± 0.01

[a]Total number of cells counted in lobules type 1 (Lob 1) in breast tissue samples of 12 donors; [b]Total number of cells counted in lobules type 2 (Lob 2) in breast tissue samples of 5 donors; [c]Total number of cells counted in lobules type 3 (Lob 3) in breast tissue samples of 3 donors. [d]Proliferative activity determined by the percentage of Ki67 positive cells, expressed as the mean ± standard deviation. Differences were significant in [e]Lob 1 versus [f]Lob 2 (t = 1.98, p <.05), [f]Lob 2 versus [g]Lob 3 (t = 2.27, p <.04), and [e]Lob 1 versus [g]Lob 3 (t = 2.56, p <.01). ERα positive cells were significantly different in [h]Lob 1 versus [j]Lob 3 (t = 2.04, p <.05). PgR-positive cells were significantly different in [k]Lob 1 versus [l]Lob 2 (t = 2.27, p <.05), and [k]Lob 1 versus [m]Lob 3 (t = 2.60, p <.03). [n]Percentage of cells positive for both, Ki67 and ERα, expressed as the mean ± standard deviation. [o]Percentage of cells positive for both Ki67 and PgR, expressed as the mean ± standard deviation.

Lob 1, with only occasional Lob 2 and Lob 3; all structures are found in an almost constant proportion throughout the woman's life span. In parous women, on the other hand, the predominant structure is the most differentiated structure, Lob 3, the frequency of which peaks during the early reproductive years, progressively decreasing in number after the fourth decade of life.[11] It is interesting to note that a full-term pregnancy that occurs between the ages of 14 and 20 years increases significantly the number of Lob 3, which remain present as the predominant structure until a woman reaches the age of 40 years. Thereafter, and more markedly after menopause, their number decreases, probably as a result of their involution and conversion, predominantly to Lob 1 (Fig. 4).[11]

PATTERN OF DISTRIBUTION OF PROLIFERATING AND ESTROGEN AND PROGESTERONE RECEPTOR–POSITIVE CELLS IN LOBULAR STRUCTURES

Cell proliferation is indispensable for the normal growth and development of the breast. Cell division in the mammary epithelium of both rodents and humans varies with the degree of differentiation of the mammary parenchyma.[3,12–14] The highest proliferative activity is observed in the undifferentiated Lob 1, present in the breast of young nulliparous females. The progressive differentiation of Lob 1 into Lob 2 and Lob 3, occurring under the hormonal influences of the menstrual cycle, and the full differentiation into Lob 4 during pregnancy result in a concomitant reduction in the proliferative activity of the mammary epithelium.

It is broadly accepted that the breast is a hormonally responsive organ. This postulate is supported by the presence of both estrogen and progesterone receptors (ER and PgR) in the normal mammary epithelium. This finding is an indication that epithelial cells respond to ovarian steroid hormones through a receptor-mediated mechanism. However, the relationships among cell proliferation, hormone responsiveness, and glandular differentiation are just beginning to be unraveled. Recent work has demonstrated that there are at least two types of ER. The classically studied type that is detected with most commonly available antibodies is now called *estrogen receptor alpha (ERα)*. The newly discovered receptor is termed *ERβ*.[15] The immunocytochemical detection of ERα and of PgR in the lobular structures of the breast has revealed that the content of these two types of receptors is directly proportional to the rate of cell proliferation. Maximal values for each of these three parameters are found in epithelial cells that line the undifferentiated Lob 1; they progressively decrease in Lob 2, Lob 3, and Lob 4 (Table 1).[11,13] Cell proliferation is reduced by threefold in Lob 2 and by more than tenfold in Lob 3 (see Table 1). Similar trends in the relative percentages of positive cells are observed in tissue sections incubated with antibodies directed against the proliferation marker Ki67, ERα, and PgR. Steroid hormone receptor–positive cells are found only in the epithelial component of the breast, whereas the myoepithelial and stromal components are totally devoid of such cells (see Table 1).

The use of a double immunocytochemical staining procedure for detection of proliferating cells that are positive for the nuclear antigen Ki67 and positive for ERα or PgR has allowed us to quantitate and determine in the same tissue sections the spatial relationships among those cells that were proliferating and those that expressed the steroid hormone receptors (Fig. 5). The number of cells that expressed ERα or PgR, or both, was similar to that of cells positive for Ki67 for every given lobular structure (see Table 1). The highest percentage of cells positive for the three markers was found in Lob 1. The percentages of ERα- and PgR-positive cells in Lob 1 did not differ significantly: 7.5% versus 5.7%, respectively (see Table 1). In Lob 2, the percentages of ERα- and PgR-positive cells were reduced to 3.8% and 0.7%, respectively, and in Lob 3 their numbers became negligible (see Table 1). Of interest was the observation that even though there were similarities in the relative percentages of Ki67-, ERα-, and PgR-positive cells and in the progressive reduction in the percentage of positive cells as the lobular differentiation progressed, those cells positive for Ki67 were distinct from those that reacted positively for ERα or PgR (Fig. 5; see Table 1). Very few cells, fewer than 0.5% in Lob 1 and even fewer in Lob 2 and Lob 3, appeared positive for both Ki67 and ERα (Ki67 + ERα; see Table 1). This double reactivity was identified by the staining charac-

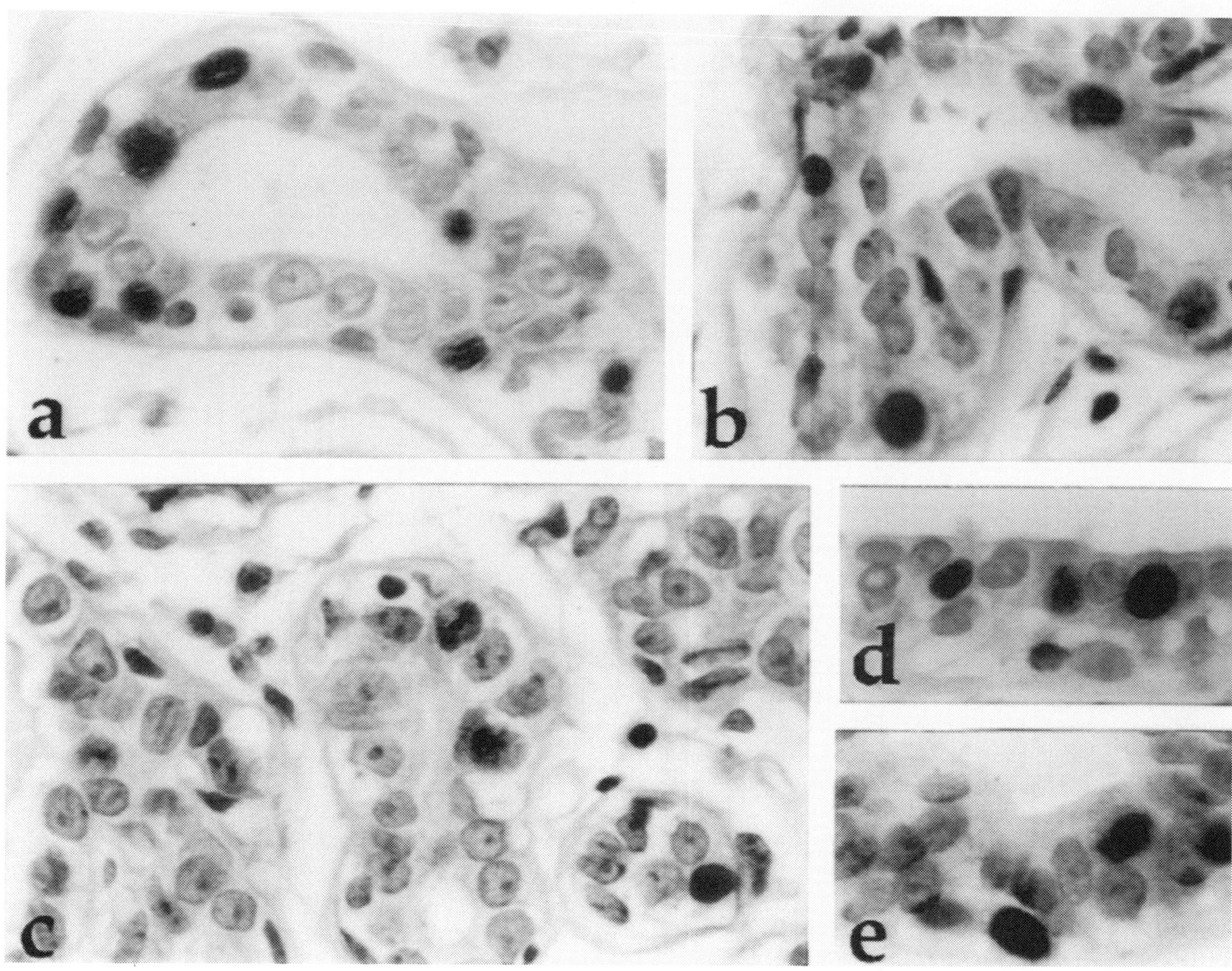

FIG. 5. Ductules of lobules type 1 of the normal breast. **A:** Single-layered epithelium containing Ki67-positive cells (brown nuclei) and ERα-positive cells (red-purple nuclei) (×40). **B:** Brown nuclei, Ki67-positive cells; red-purple nuclei, PgR-positive cells. The specificity of the reaction was verified by inverting the order of the stains. **C** and **D:** Brown, ERα-positive cells; purple-red, Ki67-positive cells. **E:** Brown nuclei, PgR-positive cells. A cell in mitosis stained purple red with Ki67.

teristics of the nuclei, which appeared dark purple-brown. The percentage of cells that exhibited double labeling with Ki67 and PgR antibodies (Ki67 + PgR; see Table 1) in Lob 1 was lower than the percentage of double-labeled ERα-positive cells. It was concluded from these studies that the expression of the receptors occurs in cells that are distinct from those that are proliferating.[3,8]

MENOPAUSAL BREAST

Menopause supervenes as the consequence of the atresia of more than 99% of the 400,000 ovarian follicles that are present at a gestational age of 5 months.[16] After menopause, the breast undergoes regression, which is manifested as an increase in the number of Lob 1 and a concomitant decline in the number of Lob 2 and Lob 3. Although this regressive phenomenon is more marked in parous women, it also occurs in nulliparous women, and by the end of the fifth decade of life, the breast tissue in these two groups of women is predominantly composed of Lob 1 (see Fig. 4).[11] These observations indicate that the understanding of breast development requires a horizontal study in which all the phases of age- and parity-related events are considered. In the breasts of nulliparous women, the predominant structure is the Lob 1, which comprises 65% to 80% of the total lobular component; its relative frequency is independent of age. Lob 2 is second in relative frequency, representing 10% to 35% of the total. The least frequently seen structure is the Lob 3, which represents only 0 to 5% of the total lobular population. In the breast of premenopausal parous women, on the other hand, the predominant lobular structure is the Lob 3, which comprises 70% to

TABLE 2. *Lobular architecture of the breast: comparison of percentages of structures found in reduction mammoplasties and breast biopsies*

Group	No. cases	Age	Lob 1(%)	Lob 2(%)	Lob 3(%)
Reduction mammoplasties (all)	33	29.4 ± 8.2	22.45 ± 23.7[1]	37.25 ± 28.61[3]	38.41 ± 34.22[5]
Reduction mammoplasties (nulliparous)	9	22.9 ± 6.7	45.87 ± 27.40	47.17 ± 22.01	6.94 ± 7.01
Reduction mammoplasties (parous)	24	31.9 ± 2.3	16.92 ± 8.26[7]	35.45 ± 3.14[9]	47.86 ± 33.4[11]
Breast biopsies (all)	45	46.6 ± 1.5	65.66 ± 34.15[2]	24.64 ± 20.64[4]	9.68 ± 6.31[6]
Breast biopsies (nulliparous)	10	42.5 ± 10.3	70.99 ± 33.3	25.26 ± 24.74	3.75 ± 1.6
Breast biopsies (parous)	35	48.9 ± 11.8	65.25 ± 37.3[8]	21.10 ± 8.07[10]	13.62 ± 3.10[12]

The percentages of lobular structures, lobules type 1 (Lob 1), lobules type 2 (Lob 2), and lobules type 3 (Lob 3) present in reduction mammoplasty specimens were compared with those present in breast biopsies. [1–12] indicates the groups in which differences are statistically significant; 1 versus 2 p <.0000005; 3 versus 4 p <.04; 5 versus 6 p <.00009; 7 versus 8 $p < 1 \times 10^{-7}$; 9 versus 10 p <.07; and 11 versus 12 p <.0003.

90% of the total lobular components. Only after menopause does their number decline; in this phase, the relative proportion of the three lobular types approaches that observed in nulliparous women. Thus, the analysis of the architecture of the breast at a single given point, without knowledge of previous reproductive history, would lead one to conclude that the breasts of nulliparous and parous women are identical. However, such a view would not take into consideration the possibility that phenomena occurring in prior years might have imprinted permanent changes in the biology of the breast that might affect the potential of the organ to develop malignancies, although they are no longer morphologically observable.[11] The difference in the pattern of development between nulliparous and parous women not only explains the protective effect induced by pregnancy but also provides a new paradigm for addressing essential questions on the differences between Lob 1 of nulliparous and parous women, such as in their abilities to metabolize estrogens or to repair any genotoxic damage. Such differences have been shown to exist and to modulate the response of the rodent mammary gland to chemically induced carcinogenesis.[17,18]

ARCHITECTURAL PATTERN OF THE ABNORMAL BREAST

The fact that the mature breast exhibits variations in the degree of differentiation, proliferative activity, and content of ER and PgR raises the question of whether benign, premalignant, and malignant lesions are a reflection of variations in the development of this organ. This question was addressed by comparing the pattern of lobular development in breast tissues obtained by reduction mammoplasties, performed in both nulliparous and parous women (Table 2) with that of breast biopsies performed because of the presence of mammographic abnormalities or clinically suspicious breast masses (breast biopsy group). The biopsies were taken from the breasts of 35 parous and ten nulliparous women (see Table 2).[19] Based on their histopathologic diagnoses, the breast biopsies (breast biopsy group) were divided into the following subgroups: normal breast or control, which consisted of biopsies with no pathology present, and abnormal breast, which comprised those biopsies that contained either ductal hyperplasia (DH), blunt duct adenosis (BDA), or sclerosing adenosis (SAD) (Figs. 6 and 7). The breast tissues of the groups classified as normal breast or control, DH, and BDA had a higher percentage of Lob 1 than Lob 2 and Lob 3. In the breast tissues of the SAD group, the highest percentage was that of Lob 2. Comparing all of the groups, the percentage of Lob 3 was significantly lower than that of Lob 1 and Lob 2; the significance of the differences was greater comparing the control group to DH biopsies than comparing control to those with the diagnosis of BDA or SAD (see Fig. 6).

In the normal breast or in the control group, the number of Ki67-positive cells was maximal in Lob 1 and significantly decreased in Lob 2 and Lob 3 (see Fig. 7). In breast biopsies containing DH, the proliferative activity in Lob 1 was higher than in Lob 1 of the control group. In breast biopsies containing BDA, on the other hand, cell proliferation was higher in Lob 2 than in Lob 1. In breast biopsies containing BDA and SAD, Lob 3 had a significantly higher proliferative activity than in the normal breast and DH groups (see Fig. 7). From these data,[19] it was concluded that those breast tissues obtained from biopsies performed because of mammographic abnormalities or clinically suspicious masses, even in cases in which no pathology or only benign lesions were diagnosed, exhibit an architectural pattern that is different from that of normal breast tissues obtained from reduction mammoplasties (see Table 2). In

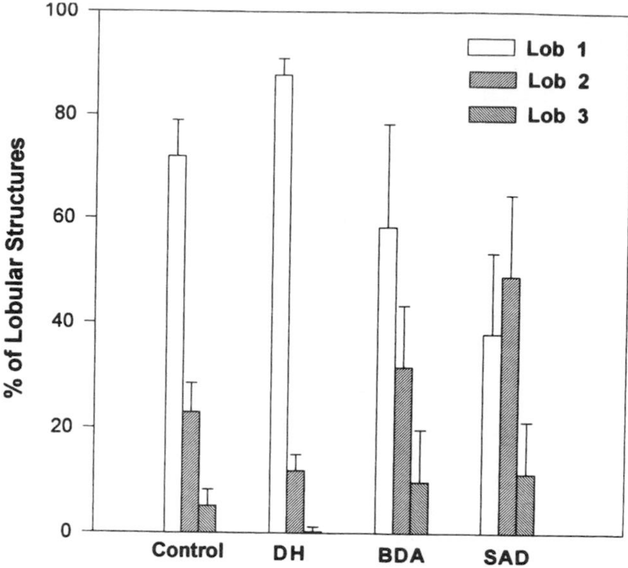

FIG. 6. Histogram showing the percentages of lobular structures found in breast biopsies. In the normal breast or control group, lobules type 1 (Lob 1) were significantly different than lobules type 2 and 3 (Lob 2 and Lob 3; $p < .0008$). The percentage of Lob 2 was significantly different from that of Lob 3 ($p < .07$). In the ductal hyperplasia (DH) group, the percentage of Lob 1 was significantly higher than the percentages of Lob 2 and Lob 3 ($p < .000001$). The percentage of Lob 2 was also significantly higher than the percentage of Lob 3 ($p < .02$). In both the blunt duct adenosis (BDA) and sclerosing adenosis (SAD) groups, the percentage of Lob 2 was significantly higher than in the normal breast or control group ($p < .07$) and the DH group ($p < .001$). The percentage of Lob 3 was significantly higher in the SAD group ($p < .05$) and in the BDA group ($p < .05$) than in those breast tissues that contained DH or in normal breast. (From ref. 19, with permission.)

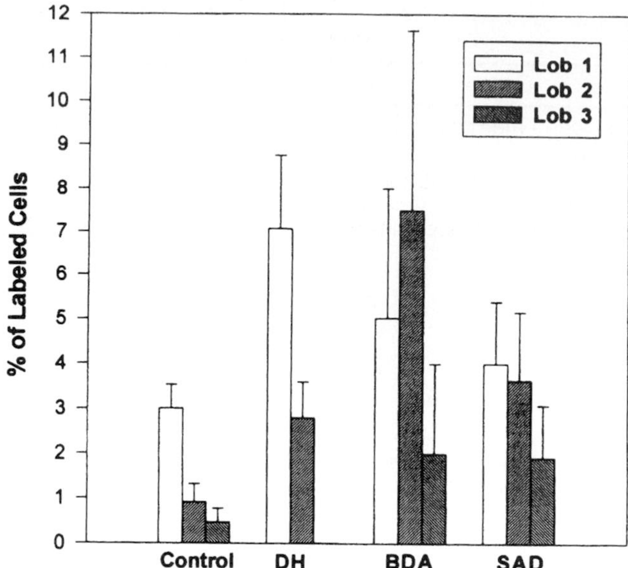

FIG. 7. Histogram showing the proliferative activity in the lobular structures of the breast biopsies of women with proliferative lesions. (From ref. 19, with permission.)

breast biopsies containing DH, the higher proliferative activity observed in Lob 1 supports previous observations, which indicate that this type of lesion originates from the Lob 1 structure. This type of lesion has also been demonstrated to be the site of origin of *in situ* ductal carcinoma.[20] The observations that Lob 2 and Lob 3 are present in higher percentages and exhibit greater rates of cell proliferation in biopsies containing BDA and SAD supports the postulate that each specific compartment of the breast gives rise to a specific type of lesion. Furthermore, the analysis of breast tissues removed by lumpectomy or mastectomy for the purpose of cancer excision revealed that the breast has an architecture similar to that of nulliparous women who are free of mammary pathology, because in both populations Lob 1 predominate.[21] Although Lob 3 predominate in reduction mammoplasty specimens of parous premenopausal women, the breasts of parous women that have developed breast cancer contain Lob 1 as their predominant structure.[21] Of interest is the fact that these women had either a late first full-term pregnancy or a family history of breast cancer. These results support the hypothesis that the degree of breast development is of importance in the susceptibility to carcinogenesis,[19–21] and that those parous women in whom breast cancer develops might exhibit a defective response to the differentiating influence of the hormones of pregnancy.

HORMONE ACTION

As mentioned in the first section of this chapter, it is well established that development and lactation of the normal breast, mammary carcinogenesis, and progression of breast cancer are regulated by hormonal factors. The endocrine steroids, peptides, and other molecules produced by the glandular tissue of the ovaries, pituitary, endocrine, pancreas, thyroid, and adrenal cortex are the best defined of these factors. After their initial interactions with their cognate nuclear or cell surface receptors, these hormones govern multiple aspects of cellular function. On a more local level of control, normal and malignant mammary tissues synthesize additional hormone-like substances. One class of these local factors is known as the *paracrine hormones*; these are factors synthesized and released by one cell type to modulate the function of neighboring mammary cells of the same or a different type. A recent variation on this theme has been described as the class of *juxtacrine factors*. Juxtacrine growth factors are growth regulatory molecules that remain exposed on the surface of a cell after their synthesis and modulate adjacent cells by contacting their receptors. A third class of local factors is known as the *autocrine* (or *intracrine*) *hormones*. These are soluble molecules, synthesized by one cell type, that act back on the same cell type through surface or intracellular receptors, respectively.

After their synthesis, polypeptide factors can be routed to multiple destinations, depending in part on features of their primary sequence. An initial point of regulation of growth factor function occurs during translation of its messenger RNA (mRNA) to protein. If there is a signal sequence encoded by

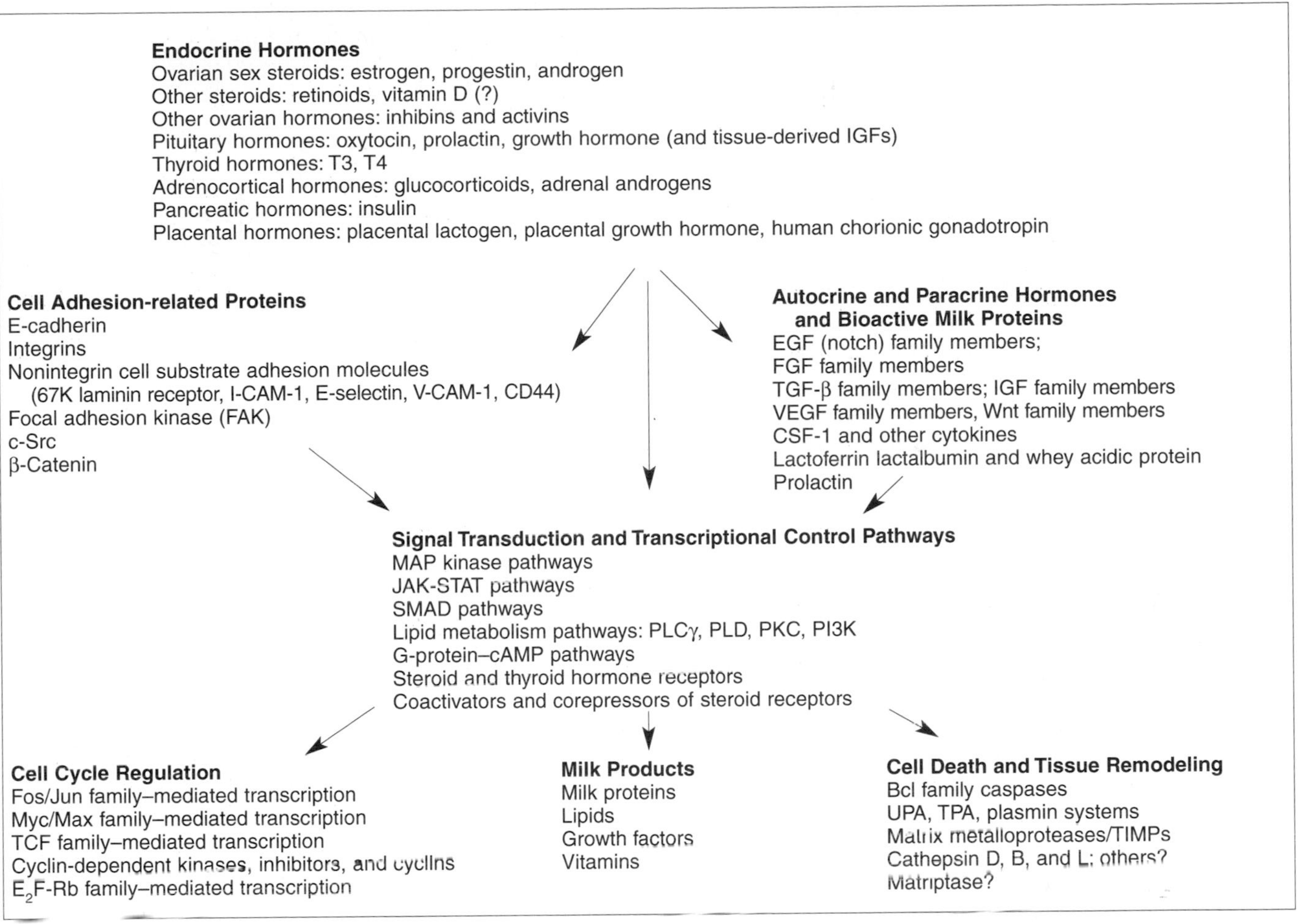

FIG. 8. Hierarchy of modulators of breast development. cAMP, cyclic adenosine monophosphate; CSF, colony-stimulating factor; EGF, epidermal growth factor; FGF, fibroblast growth factor; GF, growth factor; IGF, insulinlike growth factor; JAK-STAT, Janus kinase–signal transducers and activators of transcription; MAP, mitogen-activated protein; PI3K, phosphatidylinositol 3'-kinase; PKC, protein kinase C; PLC-γ, phospholipase Cγ; PLD, phospholipase D; TGF-β, transforming growth factor β; TIMP, tissue inhibitor metalloprotease; TPA, tissue plasminogen activator; UPA, urinary-type plasminogen activator; VEGF, vascular endothelial growth factor; Wnt, wingless.

the gene for a growth factor, then the factor is routed in the endoplasmic reticulum to a secretory pathway. There may be additional mechanisms for secretory routing of factors, such as adherence of the factor to other proteins undergoing contemporary synthesis. Some growth factors may also undergo disulfide-linked homo- or heterodimeric formation during their synthesis. During passage of a growth factor to the cell surface, carbohydrate additions (*O*- and *N*-glycosylation, glycosaminoglycan addition), proteolytic cleavages, sulfation, phosphorylation, and esterification with lipids may also occur. Some growth factors are immediately secreted after synthesis, whereas others remain on the cell surface as transmembrane molecules after their synthesis. After secretion, growth factors may adhere to extracellular matrix molecules, interact with receptors on nearby cells, enter the general circulation and exert distant effects, or perform a combination of these activities. If a growth factor is not routed for secretion or to the cell surface, it is initially synthesized and released into the cell cytoplasm. From the cytoplasm, it can accumulate in the nucleus if it has a nuclear transfer signal and a nuclear cognate binding protein. Alternatively, the factor may remain in the cytoplasm awaiting cell death for its release into the local environment.[22]

A central organizing principle of endocrine hormone action in the breast has emerged from studies indicating that systemic hormones regulate local production of growth factors in the gland. The actions of hormone-induced growth factors and the complex interactions of multiple cell surface signaling pathways with other hormone-induced gene products regulate both normal glandular function and certain dysfunctional aspects of cancer.[22,23] A corresponding hierarchy of endocrine-growth factor regulation also appears to exist for other endocrine-regulated tissues (e.g., endometrium and prostate gland) and their associated cancers (Fig. 8).[24,25]

Although polypeptide growth factors are currently among the most widely studied of the local hormonal modulators, phospholipid degradation products, such as lysophospholipids, prostaglandins, fatty acids, and other molecular classes, may serve such functions as well. Polypeptide growth factors act primarily through cell surface receptors, most of which function as homo- or heterodimeric tyrosine or serine-threonine protein kinases to add phosphate groups to protein substrates and trigger cascades of intracellular kinases and phosphatases. Other routes of peptide hormone action include additional signal transduction mechanisms, such as cyclic adenosine monophosphate, Ca^{2+} influx, lipid turnover (phospholipase C or D, phosphatidyl-3-inositol kinase), or protein kinase C. Signal transduction ultimately results in altered transcription of genes, altered stability of mRNA, regulation of protein synthesis, and modification of protein stability, function, and localization. Cellular properties under control by growth factors include cell division, differentiation, motility, glandular compartmentalization, and death. The three principal differentiated cell types of the mammary gland (stromal fibroblasts, myoepithelial cells, and epithelial cells) communicate by paracrine factors. It is clear that autocrine mechanisms may also exist, particularly for epithelial cells. Endothelial and immune inflammatory cells also play important local regulatory roles.[26]

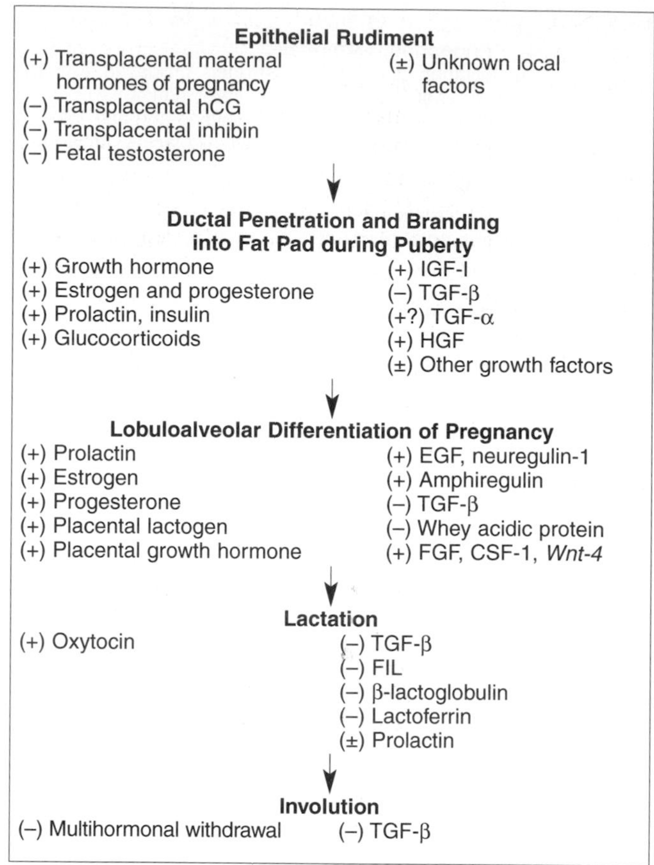

FIG. 9. Stage-by-stage action of regulatory factors on mammary epithelium. CSF, colony-stimulating factor; EGF, epidermal growth factor; FGF, fibroblast growth factor; FIL, feedback inhibitor of lactation; hCG, human chorionic gonadotropin; HGF, hepatocyte growth factor; IGF, insulinlike growth factor; TGF, transforming growth factor.

HORMONAL CONTROL OF MAMMARY DEVELOPMENT, GROWTH, AND DIFFERENTIATION

The initial development of the mammary gland involves both a prepubertal interaction between an epithelial rudiment at the nipple and the underlying fatty stroma and a response to multiple maternal hormones of pregnancy and lactation. In the female, estrogens interact with the primordial epithelial-stromal unit to promote ductal development and penetration into the fat (Fig. 9). This stromal inductive effect may be partially mimicked in a rodent model by mammary epithelial transplantation into the stroma of the embryologically related salivary gland. In the developing male, androgens interact with the epithelial-stromal unit to induce destruction of the epithelial rudiment. The exact nature of the local stromal-epithelial inductive factors for both sexes is not known.

During pubertal development, ductal elongation and branching occur. Based on studies with rodents, these processes appear to be under positive regulation by ovarian estrogen and progesterone and pituitary growth hormone. Growth hormone may mediate its effects through local production of IGF-I.[27–29] (The agricultural use of growth hormone to enhance bovine lactational productivity is an area of current public controversy due to the possibility of slightly increased levels of hormones in milk.) It has also been shown that hepatocyte growth factor is critical to branching morphogenesis at this step in development.[25,26] The most important local regulators of estrogen and progesterone in the mammary gland are not yet fully established, but likely candidates include members of the epidermal growth factor (EGF) family (e.g., EGF, TGF-α, and amphiregulin) and the transforming growth factor beta family (TGF-β1, TGF-β2, TGF-β3).[26]

The next stage of development, known as *lobuloalveolar differentiation* (see the first section of this chapter), occurs primarily during pregnancy. Lobuloalveolar development is regulated by many endocrine hormones (some of which are of placental origin): prolactin (which can be produced both systemically and locally), growth hormone (and its local mediator IGF-I), insulin, glucocorticoids, estrogen, and progesterone.[29,30] An additional, important endocrine hormone is oxytocin, which induces myoepithelial proliferation and differentiation. During completion of lobuloalveolar growth, the gland becomes competent to carry out lactation. Among the hormones of lactation, growth hormone may again play a central role, because in transgenic mouse models, the growth hormone gene can influence the gland to attain its full lactational competence in the absence of pregnancy itself.

The final, irreversible terminal differentiation of the epithelium produces secretory cells characterized by their ability to synthesize and secrete milk proteins (e.g., casein) and lipids.[29,30] As synthesis of milk products is induced, there may be direct regulatory effects of lactogenic hormones (e.g., prolactin)[31] and milk proteins, such as lactoferrin[32] and lactoglobulin, on local growth factor pathways and on epithelial proliferation. Secretion of milk is regulated by pituitary oxytocin, released in response to neural pathways, and activated by suckling. The initial mammary secretory product, colostrum, as well as milk itself are known to be very rich sources of polypeptide growth factors and growth factor–binding proteins. These regulatory molecules, in turn, may be important both in mammary growth and differentiation and in control of neonatal development, metabolism, and endocrine function.[22,33]

A significant amount of research has characterized the tissue location of various polypeptide growth factor classes during the stages of mammary development (see also Chapter 21). For example, EGF and TGF-α (a structural and functional homologue of EGF), can produce very similar biologic effects in mouse mammary explants and cultured human and mouse mammary epithelial cell lines. Their production and roles in normal and malignant mammary proliferation and differentiation have been emerging in the past few years.[33–36] It is of interest that TGF-α mRNA has been detected in mammary epithelium by *in situ* hybridization during the proliferative, lobuloalveolar development stage of rodent and human pregnancy.[36,37] A detailed study in the mouse observed TGF-α mRNA transcripts to the growing epithelial cell cap layer of the growing terminal end buds in virgin and pregnant states. High levels of TGF-α expression were not detected in lactation. In contrast, EGF mRNA transcripts were localized to inner cell layers of the end buds and to ductal luminal cells of virgin, pregnant, and lactating glands.[36,38] The mRNA for the EGF-related growth factor, amphiregulin, was expressed in stromal cells, luminal epithelial cells, myoepithelial cells of branching ducts, and epithelial cap cells in virgin and pregnant mice.[39] These EGF family growth factors are thus likely to function as regulators of all stages of mammary growth and as potentially critical components of milk. Other stimulatory factors, such as the fibroblast growth factor members FGF-1 and FGF-4, have been localized to ductal luminal cells. In contrast, FGF-2 and FGF-7 were expressed in stromal cells of the virgin mouse gland.[40] In the human gland, the FGFs also appear to have such a dual origin.[41] Some growth factors may also exert an endocrine function. Although this has been recognized for many years for the IGF factors, it may also be true of others. In this regard, it has been observed that circulating mouse salivary gland–derived EGF may promote the appearance of spontaneous mammary tumor formation in the mouse model and promote growth of the mammary tumors, if they are formed.[42,43]

Finally, growth inhibitory, differentiation-inducing TGF-β (three distinct isoforms) are all produced in mammary epithelial cells. This growth factor family, like certain FGF and EGF family members, binds heparin and is deposited into the extracellular matrix after secretion. Production of TGF-β increases during midpregnancy and lactation; it is thought that it eventually suppresses lactation and ductal budding.[44,45] Growth factor regulation of the mammary gland is almost certainly dependent on a finely controlled balance among the actions of stimulatory and inhibitory factors at the local level. In mouse and human mammary epithelial cells in culture, EGF, IGF, and FGF family members are clearly stimulatory, whereas TGF-β family members inhibit proliferation. Growth factor pellet implantation studies in the mouse mammary gland have largely confirmed these *in vitro* results *in vivo*.[46–48]

A final consideration of regulatory factors in mammary development involves the vascular endothelium and infiltrating immune cells. The growing vascular endothelial cells and immune cells may provide additional growth factors to the developing gland, although to date this area has not been adequately studied. For example, in a very interesting study, it was observed that in mice genetically deficient in the growth factor colony-stimulating factor 1, the development of the mammary gland was incomplete; lobuloalveolar development was premature, and there was a failure, not in milk protein synthesis, but in its secretion. The natural source of colony-stimulating factor 1 in the breast is unknown, but a strong candidate would be macrophages, which also secrete EGF.[49,50]

As has been shown, primarily in rodent models, an additional series of genes, termed the *Wnt family*, clearly play a vital role in gland development and tumorigenesis. Some of these genes appear to have growth factor–like function; they are differentially expressed in pregnancy and lactation, and they are transcriptionally activated as oncogenes in mouse mammary tumor virus–induced cancer.[43,50]

After the process of weaning, withdrawal of the terminally differentiated luminal epithelial cells of the lactating gland from the steroid hormones and growth factors of pregnancy results in their programmed death (a process termed *apoptosis*).[51,52] This process is characterized by triggering of a series of proteases termed *caspases*; by an influx of Ca^{2+}; and by nuclear condensation, activation of an internucleosomal nuclease, and activation of tissue transglutaminase. Cells degrade their DNA in an adenosine triphosphate–dependent fashion, the tissue undergoes autoproteolytic destruction and shrinkage, and differentiated function is lost. Whereas estrogens, progestins, and many growth factors (EGF, FGF, and IGF families) promote survival, other growth factors and cytokines [such as TGF-β and tumor necrosis factor (TNF)] are proapoptotic.[51] During this glandular involution, myoepithelial cells may play an assisting role with their increased synthesis of collagenolytic enzymes (see section Basement Membrane).

A similar, but less marked cyclicity also occurs in the proliferation and development of the mammary gland in women under regulation of the menstrual cycle. Proliferation of mammary epithelial cells is maximal in the luteal phase of the cycle, as progesterone (in the presence of estrogen) rises to a peak. This is followed by a synchronous wave of epithelial apoptosis on cessation of proliferation. This type of pattern may also exist in the shorter estrus cycles of rodents. It should be noted that the cyclic processes of proliferation and apoptosis in the mammary gland are 180 degrees out of phase with corresponding events in the endometrium (where mitoses are primarily in the follicular phase). Thus, although progesterone is a hormone that opposes the actions of estrogen on proliferation in the endometrium, the opposite is true in the breast.[52,53]

It should be clear from the discussion up to this point that, depending on the various developmental stages, different types of ovarian-controlled, hormonally dependent proliferative processes occur in the mammary gland.[50] During puberty, estrogen-dependent growth may occur by expansion of a stem cell population within the invading ductal network. These cells may give rise both to epithelial and myoepithelial cells of the gland.[54–56] As noted previously, two of the most important local growth factors during this developmental stage appear to be hepatocyte growth factor and TGF-β.[57] During the subsequent, normal reproductive cycles of pregnancy and lactation, an estrogen- and progesterone-dependent growth process may depend on expansion of a more differentiated multipotent population within the ducts and their terminal alveoli.[54] Each of these distinct, hormone-dependent proliferative processes depends on a proper epithelial-mesenchymal interaction allowing most local influences (including paracrine growth factors) to act. The central role of epithelial mesenchymal interactions in mammary development has been further emphasized using gene knockout technology in mice. Deletion of the LEF-1 transcription factor gene (in the TCF transcription factor family) impairs the development of multiple tissues, including the mammary glands, which depend on such tissue-inductive effects in their genesis.[58] Although most of the cellular and molecular studies on breast development, proliferation, differentiation, and carcinogenesis have focused on epithelial cells, recent research has included characterization of different mammary stromal cell types and their roles in hormonally regulated growth, development, and tumorigenesis.[59,60]

BASEMENT MEMBRANE

A critically important feature of mammary differentiation is the organizational influence exerted by the basement membrane. Contact with this structure through integrins polarizes epithelial cells, organizes their secretory function, and contributes to regulation of genes that are important for mammary differentiation.[61,62] This structure is a complex, lattice-like scaffolding that is synthesized and assembled at the interface of epithelium and its underlying stroma. Its principal constituents include collagen IV, laminin, fibronectin, and heparin sulfate proteoglycans. The basement membrane is undoubtedly a plastic structure, undergoing cyclic assembly and destruction (remodeling). Proteolytic enzymes of multiple classes that are capable of degrading the basement membrane have been identified in stromal fibroblasts, blood vessels, and myoepithelial cells. A good example is the matrix metalloprotease enzyme termed MMP-2. The basally located, myoepithelial cells appear to present high levels of this enzyme on their surfaces.[63] In contrast, MMP-7 has an epithelial localization.[64] The MMPs are thought to play central roles in mammary development, particularly in the apoptotic process of tissue involution, where they contribute to dissolution of unwanted milk secretory cells.[64,65] As is discussed later in the text (see section Defective Regulation of Tissue Compartmentalization in Cancer), breast cancer is characterized by progressive loss of controls of basement membrane and of hormones on proliferation and epithelial differentiation (a process termed an *epithelial-mesenchymal transition*), by genomic instability (mutations, deletions, amplifications, and chromosomal rearrangements), by alteration in nuclear matrix structure and function (to regulate gene transcription), and by loss of normal tissue organization and compartmentalization (metastasis).[63,65,66]

STEROID ACTION

As mentioned earlier (see section Patterns of Distribution of Proliferating and Estrogen and Progesterone Receptor–Positive Cells in Lobular Structures), estrogen and progesterone are well-established steroid endocrine regulators of mammary growth and differentiation. These two hormones appear to work together to promote mammary epithelial growth, differentiation, and survival.[1,52–54] Although both steroids are commonly thought to be of primary importance between the years of puberty and menopause, local aromatization of adrenal androgens provides additional estrogens in the postmenopausal years.[12] Both estrogen and progesterone act through their nuclear receptors to modulate transcription of target genes.[67–69] Genes that encode the receptors for each are members of a large superfamily of transcription-modulating factors. Although ERs may be either of two homodimeric species (alpha and beta receptors), the PgR is a heterodimeric protein. Work with each system has defined additional, alternately spliced receptor forms.[70] The biological roles of these additional variant receptor subunits are under investigation. Each steroid receptor dimer is also associated with other proteins, including heat shock proteins, to allow association with its cognate polindromic DNA elements upon ligand binding. Studies have defined coactivational and corepressive proteins, which also interact with steroid receptors and function to modulate histone acetylation and deacetylation, critical processes that are thought to allow full access of the DNA to steroid receptors. DNA interaction of steroid receptors occurs through zinc finger structures of the receptors and promotes formation of a stable initiation complex to allow promotion of transcription of responsive genes.[71–73]

Other recent studies suggest that the signal transduction pathways induced by growth factors and hormones may directly or indirectly regulate steroid receptor function. Cyclic adenosine monophosphate, EGF, and IGF-I appear to be able to modulate the activity of the ER, presumably through phosphorylation; transcription of steroid-responsive genes is induced, and steroid specificity of receptors is modulated.[68,74–76] The steroids are also well known for their abilities to modulate directly the expression of nuclear protooncogenes downstream of growth factor pathways.[23,25,26,33] These findings provide multiple mechanisms to support a role for growth factors in the progressive expression of a more malignant phenotype and escape from normal hormonal control.[48]

PEPTIDE HORMONE ACTION

At least four major types of pathways for polypeptide hormone and growth factor action have been defined for mammary epithelial cells. Most of these hormones and growth factors act through a homo- or heterodimeric cell surface receptor; for example, the EGF receptor family binds its array of receptors to trigger receptor tyrosine autophosphorylation and transphosphorylation of a variety of substrate proteins in the cytoplasm.[77,78] Several proteins, such as GRB-2, SOS, and IRS-1, bind to the tyrosine phosphorylated residues on the receptor via domains termed *SH-2* and *SH-3*. Another protein of the *ras* family then binds to help anchor the developing complex in the membrane. A cascade of subsequent serine-threonine phosphorylations of Raf-1 kinase, [a mitogen-activated protein (MAP) kinase kinase], other MAP kinase kinases and a family of downstream MAP kinases result in activation of transcription factors and in regulation of cell cycle kinases, differentiation, or cell death.[79] It is now known that at least four different MAP kinase cascades exist. These include Erkl and Erk2 (which may partially mediate cell survival), JNK and p38 (which may mediate cell death), and Bmkl/Erk5 (which may mediate proliferative effects of growth factors, such as EGF).[80,81]

A second series of pathways is triggered by TGF-β family members when they bind to their heterodimeric receptors and trigger serine-threonine kinase activities. These pathways, known as *SMADs*, also modulate proliferation, differentiation, and apoptosis.[82–89] Third, the prolactin receptor (as well as the receptors for growth hormone and some cytokines) acts by interaction with a member of the cytoplasmic JAK (Janus kinase) tyrosine kinase family. This kinase triggers transcription of genes regulating milk protein synthesis through the action of transcription factors of the STAT (signal transducers and activators of transcription) family.[50,85,86] Finally, growth factors and inflammatory cytokines (e.g., TNF) stimulate phospholipase C, phosphatidylinositol 3'-kinase, and protein kinase C in cells, leading to serine-threonine phosphorylations of multiple metabolic determinants of growth, differentiation, and apoptosis.[81,87,88]

It should be stressed that this brief summary of signal transduction is highly simplified. In particular, the potential for a broad array of diverse heterodimerization partners within many of the receptor families presents a vast potential for signal modulation.

REGULATION OF GENES ENCODING MILK PROTEINS

The principal function of the terminal differentiation state of the mammary gland is the apocrine secretion of milk. Milk consists of lipids, nutrient proteins, growth factors, and many other biologically active molecules.[89–92] Among the best-studied milk proteins are casein, lactalbumin, and the whey acidic protein. An important characteristic of the genes encoding these proteins is a consensus sequence in their promoters originally termed the *milk box*. Use of cell lines and transgenic animals has facilitated study of the detailed regulation of these genes and the nature of their mammary-specific expression.[50,93–95]

Recent work has established the nature of the transcription factor that activates milk protein synthesis in response to prolactin. This factor, originally termed *Mgf*, is a member of the STAT family of transcription factors. The regulation of expression of the casein gene depends on a balance between its activation by Mgf and its repression by other factors, such as YY1. In addition, a novel mechanism of gene regulation has been observed for beta-casein. The mRNA of beta-casein binds and sequesters a single-stranded nucleic acid–binding protein whose role is to inhibit gene expression.[50,96,97]

The ability of the mammary epithelial cells to fully differentiate and secrete milk depends not only on the proper hormonal environment but also on the proper adhesion to the basement membrane through integrins[62,98] and to each other through occludin-cytoskeletal organized tight junctions.[99]

MAMMARY EPITHELIAL CELL CYCLE AND CELL DEATH

The collection of endocrine, autocrine, and paracrine regulators of mammary epithelial proliferation is funneled to regulation of a common process, the cell cycle. This ultimate regulatory pathway consists of a series of proteins known as the *cyclin-dependent kinases* (*CDKs*); their activating subunits, the cyclins; and their inhibitory subunits, the CDK inhibitors (CDKIs). As noted earlier (see section Pattern of Distribution of Proliferating and Estrogen and Progesterone Receptor–Positive Cells in Lobular Structures), the principal proliferative cell type in the gland is the epithelial cell; indeed, most of the cancers of the breast are of epithelial origin. The early G_1 phase of the cell cycle is regulated by the cyclin D family, CDK2, CDK4, and CDK5. G_1-S is regulated by cyclin E–CDK2. S is driven by cyclin A–CDK2 and G_1M by cyclin B/A–CDC2 (also termed *CDK1*). Most of the growth factor and sex steroid pathways seem to act by modulation of the CDK4 and CDK2 complexes. Oncogenes and suppressor genes, described later in this book (see Chapter 20), also modulate the activation of these same CDK complexes, but in addition, they serve to inactivate apoptotic controls and fail-safe mechanisms (known as *checkpoints*) in the cell cycle.[100–102]

The tyrosine kinase receptor-acting growth factors (e.g., EGF) and sex steroids facilitate transit through G_1 by induction of cyclin D_1. The cyclin D_1–CDK4 complex is inhibited by a CDKI termed *p15* (INK4), by a tumor suppressor CDKI termed *p16* (MTSI), and by two recently described family members, p18 and p19. Under certain circumstances (described below), CDK4 also may be inhibited by other

CDK1s termed *p21* (Waf-1/CIPI), *p27* (Kip-1), and *p57*. To promote the G_1-S transition, cyclin E is induced and p27 is degraded. Cyclin E, p27, and an activating phosphatase termed *CDC25A* are induced by the c-Myc protein, either as a normal consequence of mitogenic growth factor or steroid action or as a pathologic consequence of amplification of overexpression of the *c-myc* gene.[103] It is of additional note that estrogen promotes the redistribution of p21 from CDK2 back to CDK4.[104] Cyclin E–CDK2 is also inhibited by p57 but not by p15, p16, p18, or p19. Synthesis of CDK4 is suppressed by the inhibitory growth factor TGF-β, and p27 and p15 are each induced by this negative factor in epithelial cells. As a part of the cellular DNA damage response (checkpoint) system, p21 is induced by the p53 protein to inhibit cellular proliferation. Correspondingly, cellular senescence is accompanied by induction of one or more CIP/Kip family members. After DNA damage and during senescence, multiple CDKs are thus simultaneously inhibited.[102–105]

Many of these CDK influences, both pathologic and physiologic, are integrated to control the activity of the principal G_1 phase checkpoint protein, pRb. pRb is phosphorylated and ultimately inactivated by the joint action of cyclin D–CDK4 and the cyclin E–CDK2 kinases; its complete phosphorylation allows release of the E_2F-1 transcription factor from its complex with pRb and results in activation of transcription of E_2F-1–responsive, S-regulatory genes, such as cyclin A.[105] It is of note that progesterone, in contrast to estrogen, seems to trigger only one cycle of mammary epithelial cell division *in vitro*; the subsequent cycle is then blocked by an induction of p21 and p27, presumably in concert with its effects to promote differentiation.[106,107] Interestingly, recent work has shown that deletion of the cyclin D_1 gene in a mouse mode results in suppression of lobuloalveolar development of the mammary gland, suggesting its selective importance in that developmental phase.[108] Another interesting aspect of cyclin D_1 is that it appears to act as a coactivator of the ER, independent of its effects on CDK4.[109]

Cell death (apoptosis) is a naturally occurring process that is triggered in the mammary epithelium after each reproductive cycle and after gestational and lactational cycles, in which it is known as *involution*.[51] Apoptosis also is induced in most normal cells after DNA damage. Apoptotic death is quite distinct from necrotic death; it requires adenosine triphosphate, the cell condenses the chromatic of its nucleus, the nucleus undergoes fragmentation, and the cell maintains an intact plasma membrane until the final stage, in which terminal cells are consumed by macrophages.[110] Estrogen acts, at least in some breast tumor cell lines and model rodent systems, to suppress apoptosis by inducing transcription of a protein termed *Bcl-2*; this characteristic may function, along with its proliferative effects, to promote mammary tumorigenesis.[101] Bcl-2 is an apoptosis-preventing protein, the prototype of an ever-growing family,[111] which forms pores in mitochondria and which interacts with multiple proteins in other cell compartments.[112] It functions, along with a homologue termed *Bcl-x_L* and other family members to suppress the function of Bax, a death-inducing protein that also forms mitochondrial pores. Other death-inducing family members exist, such as Bak, Bad, and Bcl-x_s.[113] The mitochondrial pores formed by this system somehow serve to regulate mitochondrial cytochrome C release, which modulates apoptosis through regulating activation of a cascade of cysteine proteases (caspases) within the cell.[112] These proteases cleave many important substrates, including nuclear lamins and poly(ADP)ribose polymerase, and have been recently shown to activate nuclease cleavage of DNA.[114] The apoptotic system may be triggered through cell surface receptors for cytokines (related to TNF or Fas), through DNA damage, through aberrant expression of cell cycle regulatory genes,[115–117] through external application of certain proteases (e.g., by cytotoxic T cells), through shifting the cell to a more reducing metabolic state by hypoxia, and through altered nucleotide pools. While in postlactational involution, the apoptotic process appears not to depend on the p53 tumor suppressor protein,[101] DNA damage-induced apoptosis results from induction, stabilization, and accumulation of p53.[118,119] In the latter case, p53 induces the Bax protein and suppresses expression of Bcl-2.[113]

Although the details are quite complex, the balance of life and apoptosis is critically regulated throughout glandular growth and regression. Estrogen, progesterone, TGF-α and EGF (acting through the EGF receptor family members), insulin and IGFs (acting through their receptors), and FGFs (through their respective receptors) all appear to suppress apoptosis and promote epithelial survival. In contrast, antiestrogens, antiprogestins, and TGF-β can all induce apoptosis, unless countered with a survival-promoting environmental influence. Current research is focused on how these factors suppress the apoptotic pathway(s), apparently through regulation of MAP kinase and phosphatidylinositol 3'-kinase pathways and the Bcl family of proteins.[81,101,120]

DEFECTIVE REGULATION OF BREAST EPITHELIAL GROWTH IN CANCER

The basis for our understanding of defective ovarian endocrine influences on the malignant mammary gland can be traced back to the late 1800s.[121] More recent studies have specifically identified ovarian estrogens and progesterone as the principal ovarian effectors. Studies with rodent models of carcinogen-induced and spontaneous mammary cancer have demonstrated that prolonged exposure to both progestins and estrogens is able to support initial tumor formation and early tumor growth.[122] More recent studies have also implicated growth factors. Experiments with transgenic mice have demonstrated that overexpression of several growth factors and their receptors, including those of the EGF class, is a strong risk factor for mammary cancer.[123] In rodent models, it has also been shown that early stages in spontaneous mammary neoplasia are quite sensitive to growth factor stimulation,[124] whereas the most malignant metastatic stages are characterized by overproduction of growth factors and insensitivity to their exogenous supplementation.[48]

The concept that estrogens and progestins may positively interact in proliferation of the normal rodent and human breast is based on the requirement of estrogen, acting through its receptor to induce expression of PgR. Thus, both hormones working together may regulate other genes, such as growth factors and cell cycle–associated genes.[101,125,126] Estrogenic and progestational components of the oral contraceptives are considered potential risk factors in the development of breast cancer,[52,53] although it now appears clear that the majority of women who take these drugs probably do not have a significantly increased risk of breast cancer.[127] Other established risk factors for breast cancer are known to include family history, prior patient history, a prolonged reproductively competent phase of life, late pregnancy, and excessive consumption of alcohol. Certain additional controversial, putative risk factors include a high-fat diet and cigarette smoking.[128,129] The mechanism(s) of these risk factors is not known but most likely include prolonged hormonal stimulation of proliferation, DNA damage, secretion and action of disregulated growth factors, and disregulated cell cycle–associated genes. A long-standing observation has been that an early pregnancy is protective, perhaps through induction of glandular differentiation.[13]

As noted earlier (see section Pattern of Distribution of Proliferating and Estrogen Receptor–Positive Cells in Lobular Structures),[8] ERs and PgRs have been localized by immunohistochemistry to a luminal subpopulation of ductal and lobular epithelial cells in women and rodents. These receptors are absent from epithelial cells of the terminal end buds, the most proliferative regions of the gland. It is not yet fully established that epithelial cells that contain steroid receptors serve a precursor role in breast cancer, although sex steroids are considered to be requirements for the vast majority of breast cancers in women.[130,131] Indeed, approximately one-third of breast cancers are hormonally responsive at the time they become metastatic. Although a large fraction of breast tumors may be able to respond directly to sex steroids, a body of literature strongly supports an indirect role of stromal fibroblasts (and possibly other cell types) to modulate positively steroidal growth regulation. Mechanisms of this effect are thought to involve stromal cytochrome P450–mediated metabolism systems that aromatize adrenal androgens (e.g., androstenedione) to estrogens, particularly in postmenopausal women. It is also thought that growth factors produced by the cancer (including those under hormonal control) may induce the P450 enzymes responsible for local estrogen production.[132] In analogy with normal gland growth noted earlier, growth of breast tumor cells *in vitro* in response to estrogen is also markedly enhanced *in vitro* by coculture with fibroblasts, suggesting paracrine cooperation in the hormonal response.[59,60] The biochemical nature of this paracrine control remains uncertain, although IGF-I appears to be a strong candidate.[133] Hormone responsivity of breast cancer is quite important for its treatment.[134]

ER- and PgR-negative breast cancers differ in multiple respects from their steroid receptor–positive counterparts. These differences appear to include higher proliferative and invasive rates *in vivo* and *in vitro*, altered expression of certain growth factor receptors (high levels of EGF and Erb-B2 receptors but low IGF-I receptors), elevated expression of phases I and II enzymes of drug metabolism, more aberrant nuclear morphology, increased invasiveness, and loss of certain indicators of epithelial differentiation. These differences may indicate at least two distinct stages of differentiation or two different biologic types of breast cancer.[26] Perhaps also relevant to this question is the observation that essentially all breast adenocarcinomas are characterized by expression of ductal luminal keratins.[135] These observations may support an argument that breast cancers may be derived from a luminal or luminal-committed, ER- and PgR-positive stage of differentiation and that later malignant progression could encompass phenotypic dedifferentiation from this luminal lineage.[136] Onset and progression of cancer involve multiple genetic and phenotypic changes.

BIOCHEMICAL REGULATION OF TISSUE COMPARTMENTALIZATION

As described earlier (see section Basement Membrane), the mammary epithelium has a homotypic affinity for itself and is capable of inducing production of a basement membrane in which it forms an interface with an adjacent stromal compartment. The basement membrane exerts a further influence to promote epithelial differentiation and sequestration. Proper compartmentalization of the breast thus requires cell-cell interactions and cell-substrate interactions. Both serve to regulate proper structure and differentiated function. Both types of adhesion may send intracellular signals in addition to their direct contribution to maintenance of tissue architecture.[99,137] Both homotypic adhesion of epithelial cells and heterotypic adhesion of epithelial to myoepithelial cells may be critical. In addition, the epithelial-mesenchymal interface is strongly inductive of basement membrane formation. Finally, the vascular endothelium and immune cells must be able to penetrate the tissue space and maintain sufficient plasticity to respond to the highly variable metabolic states of tissue growth, milk production, and tissue death.[138]

The principal cell-cell adhesion molecule in the mammary epithelium is the calcium-dependent E-cadherin (also termed *uvomorulin* or *L-CAM*). This molecule is proposed as a tumor-suppressor gene in the breast.[139] Cell-cell adhesion restricts motility[140] and promotes differentiation.[141] A second important interaction is that of cell-substratum. This type of interaction is mediated by the heterodimeric RGD (arginine, glycine, aspartic acid) consensus-binding transmembrane integrin class of surface molecules, as well as several nonintegrin molecules. Most integrins bind more than one ligand (collagen, fibronectin, laminin, fibrinogen, thrombospondin, and vitronectin), and a few ($\alpha_2\beta_1$, $\alpha_5\beta_1$, and $\alpha_3\beta_1$) may participate in cell-cell adhesion and cell-substrate adhesion.[142, 143]

DEFECTIVE REGULATION OF TISSUE COMPARTMENTALIZATION IN CANCER

In addition to disregulated proliferation, at least two other cellular processes seem to occur during malignant progression of breast cancer: loss of differentiated properties and loss of proper tissue compartmentalization (metastasis). It appears that loss of cell-cell attachment, altered cell substructum attachment, and altered cytoskeletal organization play a role in loss of differentiation. The same three influences, plus cell locomotion, proteolysis, survival, and proliferation at distant sites,[144] contribute to metastasis (see Chapter 21).

As noted in the previous section, the major cell-cell adhesion molecule that is thought to be involved in mammary epithelial differentiation is E-cadherin. Loss of expression of E-cadherin is associated with a more motile, fibroblastic morphology in breast cancer, with increased invasiveness and metastasis.[145] This may reflect reversion to the default pathway of tissue development.[146] A subset of breast cancer cells exists that is negative for expression of E-cadherin, expresses the mesenchymal intermediate filament vimentin (along with epithelial keratins), and expresses an even more strongly motile and invasive phenotype.[145,147] These characteristics are indicative of an epithelial mesenchymal transition (EMT) and are associated with poor histologic grade in clinical breast cancer.[148] The EMT process is known to occur frequently in other contexts during embryogenesis.[146] Loss of expression of $\alpha_2\beta_1$, $\alpha_3\beta_1$, $\alpha_5\beta_1$, and $\alpha_6\beta_1$ (also a proposed tumor suppressor) and increased expression of a 67-kd nonintegrin laminin receptor are also associated with loss of differentiation in breast cancer (reviewed in references 142 and 143). Studies have suggested that loss of expression of the ERs and PgRs may be associated with an EMT process in breast cancer.[147] The overall mechanism for induction of the EMT remains unknown, but it seems to be associated with primary defects in arrangement of desmosomal and cytoskeletal proteins.[62,145]

Attachment of cells to a matrix substratum is thus critical both for differentiation and for metastasis.[142,143] Cell substratum adhesion through the heterodimeric integrins may signal the cell through a tyrosine kinase termed *FAK* (focal adhesion kinase). This kinase is upregulated in invasive breast cancer.[149] Additional adhesion events may come into play in metastasis: expression of the vascular angiogenesis-associated integrin $\alpha_V\beta_3$, function of nonintegrin I-CAM-1, and function of the platelet–tumor cell adhesion integrin $\alpha_{IIb}\beta_3$ in embolus formation. Also, additional adhesion molecules are involved in the final metastatic stages of tumor extravasation after vascular embolus trapping: E-selectin, V-CAM-1, and CD44 (see references 142 and 143 for review).

Metastases are initially marked by local invasion of the cancer across the basement membrane to the stromal area. This transition is thought to depend on abnormal tissue remodeling (local proteolysis) and tumor cell motility. The matrix metalloprotease class of enzymes is under intense scrutiny in this respect.[64,65] Plasmin production (due to the tumor cell–secreted plasminogen activator urokinase, UPA), cathepsin D, a novel 80-kd broad substrate matrix-degrading serine protease termed *matriptase*, cathepsin B, and cathepsin L are also potentially important.[150–154] UPA and MMPs (including a specialized MMP termed *MT-MMP* that activates others) are the most widely studied enzymes for development of potential antimetastatic therapy. UPA and its inhibitor PAI-1 are now considered to be strong indicators of poor prognosis in breast cancer; they are primarily secreted by stromal cells adjacent to invasive breast cancer.[154] MMPs may also be synthesized by stromal cells in the area of the tumor and may be of prognostic use as well.[64,65] Finally, disregulation of the vasculature of the gland (angiogenesis) is of great interest in studies of the transition of the mammary gland to malignacy (see Chapter 21).[155]

SUMMARY AND FUTURE PROSPECTS

In summary, this chapter has attempted to review the multifactorial nature of breast development and its defects in cancer. Endocrine hormones are positioned at the top of a complex regulatory hierarchy. They deliver critical modulatory signals to the local tissue. Adhesion molecules and growth factors then serve as additional extremely important influences on local tissue function. Signal transduction from growth factors and adhesion molecules is now recognized to be quite diverse and complex. Finally, the combined endocrine and local influences exert their ultimate effects on cell growth, apoptosis, tissue remodeling, and milk production. Consideration of each of these topics is essential to the understanding of disregulated tissue function in breast cancer. Indeed, the cancer genes known as *oncogenes* and *suppressor genes* encode defective proteins that would otherwise serve in the normal regulation of these pathways.

REFERENCES

1. Russo J, Russo IH. Development of human mammary gland. In: Neville MC, Daniel CW, eds. *Mammary gland development regulation and function*. New York: Plenum Press, 1987:67.
2. Andersson A-M, Toppari J, Haavisto A-M, et al. Longitudinal reproductive hormone profiles in infants: peak of inhibin B levels in infant boys exceeds levels in adult men. *J Clin Endocrinol Metab* 1998;83:675.
3. Russo IH, Russo J. Role of hormones in cancer initiation and progression. *J Mammary Gland Biol Neoplasia* 1998;3:49.
4. Yen SSC. Clinical endocrinology of reproduction. In: Baulieu E-E, Kelly PA, eds. *Hormones: from molecules to disease*. New York: Chapman and Hall, 1990:445.
5. Mather JP, Moore A, Li R-H. Activins, inhibins, and follistatins: further thoughts on a growing family of regulators. *Proc Soc Exp Biol Med* 1997;215:209.
6. Brisken C, Park S, Vass T, Lydon JP, O'Malley BW, Weinberg RA. A paracrine role for the epithelial progesterone receptor in mammary gland development. *Proc Natl Acad Sci U S A* 1998;95:5076.
7. Zeps N, Bentel JM, Papadimitriou JM, D'Antuono MF, Dawkins HJ. Estrogen receptor-negative epithelial cells in mouse mammary gland development and growth. *Differentiation* 1998;62:221.
8. Russo J, Ao X, Grill C, Russo IH. Pattern of distribution of cells positive for estrogen receptor and progesterone receptor in relation to proliferating cells in the mammary gland. *Breast Cancer Res Treat* 1999;53:217.

9. Tanner JM, ed. The development of the reproductive system. In: *Growth at adolescence*. Oxford, UK: Blackwell Scientific, 1962:28.
10. Russo J, Russo IH. Development of the human breast. In: *Encyclopedia of reproduction*. New York: Academic, 1998;3:71.
11. Russo J, Rivera R, Russo IH. Influence of age and parity on the development of the human breast. *Breast Cancer Res Treat* 1992;23:211.
12. Russo J, Russo IH. Role of hormones in human breast development: the menopausal breast. In: *Progress in the management of menopause*. London: Parthenon, 1997:184.
13. Russo J, Russo IH. Role of differentiation in the pathogenesis and prevention of breast cancer. *Endocrine Rel Cancer* 1997;4:7.
14. Calaf G, Alvarado ME, Bonney GE, Amfoh KK, Russo J. Influence of lobular development on breast epithelial cell proliferation and steroid hormone receptor content. *Int J Oncol* 1995;7:1285.
15. Couse JF, Lindzey J, Grandien K, Gustafsson JA, Korach KS. Tissue distribution and quantitative analysis of estrogen receptor-alpha (ERalpha) and estrogen receptor-beta (ERbeta) messenger ribonucleic acid in the wild-type and ERalpha-knockout mouse. *Endocrinology* 1997;138:4613.
16. Edwards RG, Howles CM, Macnamee C. Clinical endocrinology of reproduction. In: Baulieu EE, Kelly PA, eds. *Hormones: from molecules to disease*. New York: Chapman and Hall, 1990:457.
17. Tay LK, Russo J. Formation and removal of 712-dimethylbenz(a)-anthracene-nucleic-acid adducts in rat mammary epithelial cells with different susceptibility to carcinogenesis. *Carcinogenesis* 1981;2:1327.
18. Tay LK, Russo J. Metabolism of 712-dimethylbenz(a)anthracene by rat mammary epithelial cells in culture. *Carcinogenesis* 1983;4:733.
19. Russo J, Russo IH. Differentiation and breast cancer development. In: Heppner G, ed. *Advances in oncobiology*, vol 2. London: Jai Press, 1998:1.
20. Russo J, Gusterson BA, Rogers A, Russo IH, Wellings SR, van Zwieten MJ. Biology of the disease. Comparative study of human and rat mammary tumorigenesis. *Lab Invest* 1990;62:244.
21. Russo J, Romero AL, Russo IH. Architectural pattern of the normal and cancerous breast under the influence of parity. *Cancer Epidemiol Biomarkers Prev* 1994;3:219.
22. Dickson RB, Lippman ME. Estrogenic regulation of growth and polypeptide growth factor secretion in human breast carcinoma. *Endocrine Rev* 1987;8:29.
23. Suchard M, Landers JP, Sandhu NP, Spelsberg TC. Steroid hormone regulation of nuclear proto-oncogenes. *Endocrine Rev* 1993;14:659.
24. Waxman J, ed. *Molecular endocrinology of cancer*. Cambridge, UK: Cambridge University Press, 1996:1.
25. Dickson RB, Salomon DS, eds. *Hormones and growth factors in development and neoplasia*. New York: Wiley-Liss, 1998:1.
26. Dickson RB, Lippman ME. Growth regulation of normal and malignant breast epithelium. In: Bland KI, Copeland EM, eds. *The breast*. Philadelphia: WB Saunders, 1998:518.
27. Daniel CW, Silberstein GB. Development of the mammary gland. In: Neville MC, Daniel CW, eds. *The mammary gland*. New York: Plenum, 1987:3.
28. Sakakura T. Mammary embryogenesis. In: Neville MC, Daniel CW, eds. *The mammary gland*. New York: Plenum, 1987:37.
29. Baserga R. The IGF-1 receptor in normal and abnormal growth. In: Dickson RB, Salomon DS, eds. *Hormones and growth factors in development and neoplasia*. New York: Wiley-Liss, 1998:269.
30. Rosen J. Milk protein gene structure. In: Neville MC, Daniel CW, eds. *The mammary gland*. New York: Plenum, 1989:301.
31. Fenton SE, Sheffield LG. Prolactin inhibits epidermal growth factor (EGF)-stimulated signaling events in mouse mammary epithelial cells by altering EGF receptor function. *Mol Biol Cell* 1993;4:773.
32. Bezault J, Bhimani R, Wiprovnick J, Furmanski P. Human lactoferrin inhibits growth of solid tumors and development of experimental metastases in mice. *Cancer Res* 1994;54:2310.
33. Dickson RB, Lippman ME. Growth factors in breast cancer. *Endocrine Rev* 1995;16:559.
34. Vonderhaar BK. Regulation of development of the normal mammary gland by hormones and growth factors. In: Lippman ME, Dickson RB, eds. *Breast cancer: cellular and molecular biology*. Boston: Kluwer, 1988:251.
35. Stampfer MR. Isolation and growth of human mammary epithelial cells. *J Tissue Cult Meth* 1985;9:107.
36. Schroeder JA, Lee DC. Dynamic expression and activation of ERBB receptors in the developing mouse mammary gland. *Cell Growth Differ* 1998;9:451.
37. Liscia DS, Merlo G, Ciardiello F, Kim N, Smith GH, Callahan RH, et al. Transforming growth factor-α messenger RNA localization in the developing adult rat and human mammary gland by in situ hybridization. *Dev Biol* 1990;140:123.
38. Snedeker SM, Brown CF, DiAugustine RP. Expression and functional properties of transforming growth factor α and epidermal growth factor during mouse mammary gland ductal morphogenesis. *Proc Natl Acad Sci U S A* 1991;88:276.
39. Kenney NJ, Dickson RB. Growth factor and sex steroid interactions in breast cancer. *J Mammary Gland Biol Neoplasia* 1996;1:189.
40. Coleman-Krnacik S, Rosen JM. Differential temporal and spatial gene expression of fibroblast growth factor family members during mouse mammary gland development. *Mol Endocrinol* 1994;8:218.
41. Johnson M, Smith K, Harris AL. WNT and fibroblast growth factor gene expression during development of the mammary gland and role of WNTs in human cancer. In: Dickson RB, Salomon DS, eds. *Hormones and growth factors in development and neoplasia*. New York: Wiley-Liss, 1998:361.
42. Oka T, Tsutsumi O, Kurachi H, Okamoto S. The role of epidermal growth factor in normal and neoplastic growth of mouse mammary epithelial cells. In: Lippman ME, Dickson RB, eds. *Breast cancer: cellular and molecular biology*. Boston: Kluwer, 1988:343.
43. Kurachi H, Okamoto S, Oka T. Evidence for the involvement of the submandibular gland epidermal growth factor in mouse mammary tumorigenesis. *Proc Natl Acad Sci U S A* 1985;81:5940.
44. Jhappan C, Geiser AG, Kordon EC, et al. Targeting expression of a transforming growth factor β1 transgene to the pregnant mammary gland inhibits alveolar development and lactation. *EMBO J* 1993;12:1835.
45. Daniel C, Silberstein GB. Local effects of growth factors. In: Lippman ME, Dickson RB, eds. *Regulatory mechanisms in breast cancer*. Boston: Kluwer, 1990:79.
46. Koli KM, Arteaga CL. Complex role of tumor cell transforming growth factor (TGF)-β on breast carcinoma progression. *J Mammary Gland Biol Neoplasia* 1996;1:373.
47. Reiss M, Barcellos-Hoff M. Transforming growth factor-β in breast cancer: a working hypothesis. *Breast Cancer Res Treat* 1997;45:81.
48. Dickson RB, Lippman ME. Molecular biology of breast cancer. In DeVita VT, Hellman S, Rosenberg SA, eds. *Principles and practice of oncology*, 5th ed. Philadelphia: JB Lippincott, 1997:1541.
49. Pollard JW, Hennighausen L. Colony stimulating factor-1 is required for mammary gland development during pregnancy. *Proc Natl Acad Sci U S A* 1994;27:9312.
50. Hennighausen L. Signal networks in the mammary gland: lessons from animal models. In: Dickson RB, Salomon DS, eds. *Hormones and growth factors in development and neoplasia*. New York: Wiley-Liss, 1998:239.
51. Strange R, Li F, Suarer S, Burkhardt A, Friis RR. Apoptotic cell death and tissue remodeling during mouse mammary gland involution. *Development* 1992;115:49.
52. Anderson TJ, Battersby S, Macintyre CCA. Proliferative and secretory activity in human breast during natural and artificial menstrual cycles. *Am J Pathol* 1988;130:193.
53. McCarty KS. Proliferative stimuli in the normal breast: estrogens or progestins. *Hum Pathol* 1989;20:1137.
54. Daniel CW, Silberstein GB. Developmental biology of the mammary gland. In: Neville MC, Daniel CW, eds. *The mammary gland*. New York: Plenum, 1987:3.
55. Chepko G, Smith GH. Three division-competent, structurally-distinct cell populations contribute to murine mammary epithelial renewal. *Tissue Cell* 1997;29:239.
56. Chepko G, Smith GH. Mammary epithelial stem cells: our current view. *J Mammary Gland Biol Neoplasia*, 1999;4:35.
57. Soriano JV, Pepper MS, Orci L, Montesano R. Roles of hepatocyte growth factor/scatter factor and transforming growth factor-beta1 in mammary gland ductal morphogenesis. *J Mammary Gland Biol Neoplasia* 1998;3:133.
58. Van Genderen C, Okamura RM, Farinas I, et al. Development of several organs that require inductive epithelial-mesenchymal interactions is impaired in LEF-1–deficient mice. *Genes Dev* 1994;8:2691.
59. Woodward TL, Xie JX, Haslam SZ. The role of mammary stroma in modulating the proliferative response to ovarian hormones in the normal mammary gland. *J Mammary Gland Biol Neoplasia* 1998;3:117.
60. Cunha GR, Hayward SW, Hom YK, et al. Growth factors as mediators of stromal-epithelial interactions in steroid hormone target

organs. In: Dickson RB, Salomon DS, eds. *Hormones and growth factors in development and neoplasia*. New York: Wiley-Liss, 1998:207.
61. Streuli CH, Bailey N, Bissell MJ. Control of mammary epithelial differentiation: basement membrane induces tissue-specific gene expression in the absence of cell-cell interaction and morphological polarity. *J Cell Biol* 1991;115:1383.
62. Streuli CH, Edwards GM. Control of normal mammary epithelial phenotype by integrins. *J Mammary Gland Biol Neoplasia* 1998;3:151.
63. Monteagudo C, Merino MJ, San-Juan J, Liotta LA, Stetler-Stevenson WG. Immunohistochemical distribution of type IV collagenase in normal, benign, and malignant breast tissue. *Am J Pathol* 1990;136:585.
64. Rudolph-Owen LA, Matrisian LM. Matrix metalloproteinases in remodeling of the normal and neoplastic mammary gland. *J Mammary Gland Biol Neoplasia* 1998;3:177.
65. Benaud C, Dickson RB, Thompson EW. Roles of matrix metalloproteases in mammary gland development and cancer. *Breast Cancer Res Treat* 1998;50:97.
66. Khanuja PS, Lehr JE, Soule HD, et al. Nuclear matrix proteins in normal and breast cancer cells. *Cancer Res* 1993;53:3394.
67. Parker MG. Transcriptional activation by oestrogen receptors. *Biochem Soc Symp* 1996;63:45.
68. Curtis SW, Korach KS. The estrogen receptor in mammalian development. In: Dickson RB, Salomon DS, eds. *Hormones and growth factors in development and neoplasia.* New York: Wiley-Liss, 1998:169.
69. Leighton JK, Wei LL. Progesterone and development. In: Dickson RB, Salomon DS, eds. *Hormones and growth factors in development and neoplasia*. New York: Wiley-Liss, 1998:177.
70. Paech K, Webb P, Kuiper GG, et al. Differential ligand activation of estrogen receptors eralpha and erbeta at ap1 sites. *Science* 1997;277:1508.
71. Green S, Chambon P. The estrogen receptor: from perception to mechanism. In: Parker MG, ed. *Nuclear hormone receptors*. London: Academic, 1991:15.
72. Read LD, Katzenellenbogen BS. Characterization and regulation of estrogen and progesterone receptors in breast cancer. In: Dickson RB, Lippman ME, eds. *Genes, oncogenes, and hormones*. Boston: Kluwer, 1992:277.
73. Spencer TE, Jenster G, Burcin MM, et al. Steroid receptor coactivator-1 is a histone acetyltransferase. *Nature* 1997;389:194.
74. Fujimoto N, Katzenellenbogen BS. Alteration in the agonist/antagonist balance of antiestrogens by activation of protein kinase A signaling pathways in breast cancer cells: antiestrogen selectivity and promoter dependence. *Mol Endocrinol* 1994;8:296.
75. Nordeen SK, Bona BJ, Moyer ML. Latent agonist activity of the steroid antagonist, RU486, is unmasked in cells treated with activators of protein kinase A. *Mol Endocrinol* 1993;7:731.
76. Gray K, Eitzman B, Washburn KR, et al. Estrogen, growth factors, and carcinogenesis in the reproductive tract. In: Dickson RB, Salomon DS, eds. *Hormones and growth factors in development and neoplasia*. New York: Wiley-Liss, 1998:311.
77. Riese II DJ, Stern DF. Specificity within the EGF family/ErbB receptor family signaling network. *Bioessays* 1998;20:41.
78. Sebastian J, Richards RG, Walker MP, et al. Activation and function of the epidermal growth factor receptor and erbB-2 during mammary gland morphogenesis. *Cell Growth Differ* 1998;9:777.
79. Hall A. A biochemical function for ras—at last. *Science* 1994;244:1413.
80. Kato Y, Tapping RI, Huang S, et al. Bmk1/Erk5 is required for cell proliferation induced by epidermal growth factor. *Nature* 1998;395:713.
81. Rosfjord EC, Dickson RB. Growth factors, apoptosis, and survival of mammary epithelial cells. *J Mammary Gland Biol Neoplasia* 1999; 4:229.
82. Alevizopouolos A, Mermod N. Transforming growth factor-β: the breaking open of a black box. *Bioessays* 1997;19:581.
83. Koli KM, Arteaga CL. Complex role of tumor cell transforming growth factor (TGF)-β on breast carcinoma progression. *J Mammary Gland Biol Neoplasia* 1996;1:373.
84. Padgett RW, Das P, Krishna S. TGF-beta signaling, smads, and tumor suppressors. *Bioessays* 1998;20:382.
85. Darnell JE, Kerr IM, Storb GR. Jak-STAT pathways and transcriptional activation in response to INFs and other extracellular signaling pathways. *Science* 1994;264:1415.
86. Clevenger CV, Chang WP, Ngo W, Pasha TL, Montone KT, Tomaszewski JE. Expression of prolactin and prolactin receptor in human breast carcinoma. Evidence for an autocrine/paracrine loop. *Am J Pathol* 1995;146:695.
87. Mangelsdorf-Soderquist A, Todderud G, Carpenter G. Elevated membrane association of phospholipase c-γ 1 in MDA-468 mammary tumor cells. *Cancer Res* 1992;52:4526.
88. Soltoff SP, Carraway KL, Priget SA, et al. $ErbB_3$ is involved in activating phosphatidylinositol 3-kinase by epidermal growth factor. *Mol Cell Biol* 1994;14:3550.
89. Mather IH, Keenan TW. The cell biology of milk secretion: historical notes. *J Mammary Gland Biol Neoplasia* 1998;3:227.
90. Grosvenor CE, Picciano MF, Baumrucker CR. Hormones and growth factors in milk. *Endocrine Rev* 1992;14:720.
91. Mather IH, Keenan TW. Origin and secretion of milk lipids. *J Mammary Gland Biol Neoplasia* 1998;3:259.
92. Burgoyne RD, Duncan JS. Secretion of milk proteins. *J Mammary Gland Biol Neoplasia* 1998;3:275.
93. Greenberg NM, Wolfe J, Rosen JM. Casein gene expression: from transfection to transgenics. In: Dickson RB, Lippman ME, eds. *Genes, oncogenes, and hormones*. Boston: Kluwer, 1991:379.
94. McKnight RA, Burdon T, Pursel VG, Shamay A, Wall RJ, Hennighausen L. The whey acidic protein. In: Dickson RB, Lippman ME, eds. *Genes, oncogenes, and hormones*. Boston: Kluwer, 1991:399.
95. Wakao H, Gouilleux F, Groner B. Mammary gland factor (Mgf) is a novel member of the cytokine regulated transcription factor gene family and confers the prolactin response. *EMBO J* 1994;13:2182.
96. Happ B, Groner B. The activated mammary gland specific nuclear factor (Mgf) enhances *in vitro* transcription of the beta-casein gene promoter. *J Steroid Biochem* 1993;47:21.
97. Altiok S, Groner B. β-casein mRNA sequesters a single-stranded nucleic acid-binding protein which negatively regulates the β-casein gene promoter. *Mol Cell Biol* 1994;14:6004.
98. Alford D, Taylor-Papadimitriou J. Cell adhesion molecules in the normal and cancerous mammary gland. *J Mammary Gland Biol Neoplasia* 1996;1:207.
99. Nguyen DD, Neville MC. Tight junction regulation in the mammary gland. *J Mammary Gland Biol Neoplasia* 1998;3:233.
100. Sutherland RL, Watts CKW, Musgrove EA. Cyclin gene expression and growth control in normal and neoplastic breast epithelium. *J Steroid Biochem Mol Biol* 1993;47:99.
101. Nass SJ, Rosfjord EC, Dickson RB. Regulation of cell cycle and cell death in breast cancer. *Breast* 1997;3:15.
102. Jacks T, Weinberg RA. The expanding role of cell cycle regulators. *Science* 1998;280:1035.
103. Prall OWJ, Rogan EM, Watts EA, Sutherland CKW, Musgrove RL. c-Myc or cyclin D1 mimics estrogen effects on cyclin E-Cdk2 activation and cell cycle reentry. *Mol Cell Biol* 1998;18:4499.
104. Plansa-Silva MD, Weinberg RA. Estrogen-dependent cyclin E-cdk2 activation through p21 redistribution. *Mol Cell Biol* 1997;17:4059.
105. Nevins JR. Toward an understanding of the functional complexity of the E2F and retinoblastoma families. *Cell Growth Differ* 1998;9:585.
106. Musgrove EA, Lee CS, Cornish AL, Swarbrick A, Sutherland RL. Antiprogestin inhibition of cell cycle progression in T47D breast cancer cells is accompanied by induction of the cyclin-dependent kinase inhibitor p21. *Mol Endocrinol* 1997;11:54.
107. Groshong SD, Owen GI, Grimison B, et al. Biphasic regulation of breast cancer cell growth by progesterone: role of the cyclin-dependent kinase inhibitors, p21 and p27 KIP1. *Mol Endocrinol* 1997;11:1593.
108. Sicinski P, Weinberg R. A specific role for cyclin D_1 in mammary gland development. *J Mammary Gland Biol Neoplasia* 1997;2:335.
109. Neuman E, Ladha MH, Lin N, et al. Cyclin D1 stimulation of estrogen receptor transcriptional activity independent of cdk4. *Mol Cell Biol* 1997;17:5338.
110. Russel P. Checkpoints on the road to mitosis. *Trends Biochem Sci* 1998;23:399.
111. Adams JM, Cory S. The Bcl-2 protein family: arbiters of cell survival. *Science* 1998;281:1322.
112. Green DR, Reed JC. Mitochondria and apoptosis. *Science* 1998; 281:1309.
113. Reed JC. Balancing cell life and death: bax, apoptosis and breast cancer. *J Clin Invest* 1996;97:2403.
114. Salvesen GS, Dixit VM. Caspases: intracellular signaling by proteolysis. *Cell* 1997;91:443.
115. Evan G, Littlewood T. A matter of life and cell death. *Science* 1998;281:1317.
116. Bates S, Phillips AC, Clark PA, et al. p14ARF links the tumour suppressors RB and p53. *Nature* 1998;395:124.

117. Palmero I, Pantoja C, Serrano M. p19ARF links the tumour suppressor p53 to Ras. *Nature* 1998;395:125.
118. Woo RA, McLure KG, Lees-Miller SP, Rancourt DE, Lee PWK. DNA-dependent protein kinase acts upstream of p53 in response to DNA damage. *Nature* 1998;394:700.
119. Elledge RM, Lee W. Life and death of p53. *Bioessays* 1995;17:923.
120. Collins MKL, Perkins GR, Gemma R-T, Nieto MA, Lopez-Rivas A. Growth factors as survival factors: regulation of apoptosis. *Bioessays* 1994;16:133.
121. Beatson GT. On the treatment of inoperable cases of carcinoma of the mamma: suggestion for a new method of treatment, with illustrative cases. *Lancet* 1986;2:104.
122. Welsch CW. Host factors affecting the growth of carcinogen-induced rat mammary carcinomas: a review and tribute to Charles Brenton Huggins. *Cancer Res* 1985;45:3415.
123. Amundadottir LT, Merlino GT, Dickson RB. Transgenic models of breast cancer. *Breast Cancer Res Treat* 1996;39:119.
124. Medina D, Kittrell FS, Oborn CJ, Schwartz M. Growth factor dependency and gene expression in preneoplastic mouse mammary epithelial cells. *Cancer Res* 1993;53:668.
125. Clarke CL, Sutherland RL. Progestin regulation of cellular proliferation. *Endocrine Rev* 1990;11:266.
126. Sutherland RL, Prall OWJ, Watts CKW, Musgrove E. Estrogen and progesterone regulation of cell cycle progression. *J Mammary Gland Biol Neoplasia* 1998;3:63.
127. Roy JA, Sawka CA, Pritchard KI. Hormone replacement therapy in women with breast cancer. Do the risks outweigh the benefits? *J Clin Oncol* 1996;14:997.
128. Willett WC, Hunter DJ, Stampfer MJ, et al. Dietary fat and fiber in relation to risk of breast cancer. *JAMA* 1992;268:2037.
129. Calle E, Miracle-McMahill HL, Thun MJ, Heath CW. Cigarette smoking and risk of fatal breast cancer. *Am J Epidemiol* 1994;139:1001.
130. Daniel CW, Silberstein GA, Strickland P. Direct action of 17β estradiol in mouse mammary ducts analyzed by sustained release implants and steroid autoradiography. *Cancer Res* 1987;47:6052.
131. Dulbecco R. Experimental studies in mammary development and cancer: relevance to human cancer. *Adv Oncol* 1990;5:3,
132. Simpson ER, Merrill JC, Hollub AJ, Graham-Lovence S, Mendelson CR. Regulation of estrogen biosynthesis by human adipose cells. *Endocrine Rev* 1984;10:136.
133. Cullen KJ, Lippman ME. Stromal-epithelial interactions in breast cancer. In: Lippman ME, Dickson RB, eds. *Genes, oncogenes, and hormones*. Boston: Kluwer, 1992:413.
134. Early Breast Cancer Trialists' Collaborative Group. Systemic treatment of early breast cancer by hormonal, cytotoxic, and immune therapy. *Lancet* 1992;339:1.
135. Taylor-Papadimitriou J, Lane EB. Keratin expression in the mammary gland. In: Neville MC, Daniel CW, eds. *The mammary gland*. New York: Plenum, 1987:181.
136. Kang KS, Morita I, Cruz A, Jeon YJ, Trosko JE, Chang CC. Expression of estrogen receptors in a normal human breast epithelial cell type with luminal and stem cell characteristics and its neoplastically transformed cell lines. *Carcinogenesis* 1997;18:251.
137. Schrocichel KL, Weaver Vas, Bissell MJ. Structural clues from the tissue microenvironment are essential determinants of the human mammary epithelial cell phenotype. *J Mammary Gland Biol Neoplasia* 1998;2:201.
138. Luscinskas FW, Lawler J. Integrins as dynamic regulators of vascular function. *FASEB J* 1994;8:929.
139. Vleminckx K, Vakaet L Jr, Mareel M, Fiers W, Roy FV. Genetic manipulation of E-cadherin expression of epithelial tumor cells reveals an invasion suppressor role. *Cell* 1991;66:107.
140. Glukhova M, Koteliansky V, Sastre X, Thiery JP. Adhesion systems in normal breast and in invasive breast carcinoma. *Am J Pathol* 1995;146:706.
141. Strange R, Li F, Friis RR, Reichmann E, Haenni B, Burri PH. Mammary epithelial differentiation *in vitro*: minimum requirements for a functional response to hormonal stimulation. *Cell Growth Differ* 1991; 2:549.
142. Rosfjord E, Dickson RB. Role of integrins in the development and malignancy of the breast. In: Bowcock A, ed. *Breast cancer*. Totowana, NJ: Humana Press, 1999:285.
143. Zutter MM, Sun H, Santoro SA. Altered integrin expression and malignant phenotype: the contribution of multiple integrated integrin receptors. *J Mammary Gland Biol Neoplasia* 1998;3:191.
144. Liotta LA, Steeg PS, Stetler-Stevenson WG. Cancer metastasis and angiogenesis: an imbalance of positive and negative regulation. *Cell* 1991;64:327.
145. Sommers CL. The role of cadherin-mediated adhesion in breast cancer. *J Mammary Gland Biol Neoplasia* 1996;1:219.
146. Frisch SM. The epithelial cell default-phenotype hypothesis and its implications for cancer. *Bioessays* 1997;19:705.
147. Thompson EW, Paik S, Brunner N, et al. Association of increased basement membrane-invasiveness with absence of estrogen receptor and expression of vimentin in human breast cancer cell lines. *J Cell Physiol* 1992;150:534.
148. Gamallo C, Palacios J, Suarez A, et al. Correlation of E-cadherin expression with differentiation grade and histological type in breast carcinoma. *Am J Pathol* 1993;142:987.
149. Weiner TM, Liu ET, Craven RJ, Cance WG. Expression of focal adhesion kinase gene and invasion cancer. *Lancet* 1993;342:1024.
150. Rochefort H, Augereau P, Capony F, et al. The 52k cathepsin D of breast cancer: structure, regulation, function, and clinical value. In: Lippman ME, Dickson RB, eds. *Breast cancer: cellular and molecular biology*. Boston: Kluwer, 1988:207.
151. Sloan BF. Cathepsin B and cystatins: evidence for a role in cancer progression. *Semin Cancer Biol* 1990;1:137.
152. Kane SE, Gottesman MM. The role of cathepsin L in malignant transformation. *Semin Cancer Biol* 1990;1:127.
153. Lin CY, Anders J, Johnson MD, Sang QA, Dickson RB. Molecular cloning of cDNA for matriptase, a matrix-degrading serine protease with trypsin-like activity. *J Biol Chem* 1999;274:18231.
154. Foekens JA, Buessecker F, Peters HA, et al. Plasminogen activator inhibitor-2: prognostic relevance in 1012 patients with primary breast cancer. *Cancer Res* 1995;55:1423.
155. Folkman J. Angiogenesis in breast cancer. In: Bland KI, Copeland EM, eds. *The breast*, 2nd ed. Philadelphia: WB Saunders, 1998:586.

II

Diseases of the Breast, 2nd ed.,
edited by Jay R. Harris.
Lippincott Williams & Wilkins, Philadelphia © 2000.

Diagnosis and Management of Benign Breast Diseases

CHAPTER 3

Physical Examination of the Breast

Monica Morrow

Obtaining a careful history is the initial step in a breast examination. Regardless of the presenting complaint, baseline information regarding menstrual status and breast cancer risk factors should be obtained. The basic elements of a breast history are listed in Table 1. In premenopausal women, knowing the date of the last menstrual period and the regularity of the cycle is useful in evaluating breast nodularity, pain, and cysts. Postmenopausal women should be questioned about use of hormone replacement therapy, given that many benign breast problems are uncommon after menopause in the absence of exogenous hormones. Specific information about the patient's presenting complaint is then elicited. A breast lump is most often the clinical breast problem that causes women to seek treatment and remains the most common presentation of breast carcinoma. Haagensen[1] observed that 65% of 2,198 breast cancer cases identified before the use of screening mammography presented as breast masses. Breast pain, a change in the size and shape of the breast, nipple discharge, and changes in the appearance of the skin are infrequent symptoms of carcinoma. The evaluation and management of these conditions are described in Chapters 4, 5, and 6. In general, the duration of symptoms, their persistence over time, and their fluctuation with the menstrual cycle should be assessed.

M. Morrow: Department of Surgery, Northwestern University Medical School, Chicago, Illinois; Lynn Sage Comprehensive Breast Program, Northwestern Memorial Hospital, Chicago, Illinois

TECHNIQUE OF BREAST EXAMINATION

A woman must be disrobed from the waist up for a complete breast examination. Although attention to modesty is appropriate and a gown or drape should be provided, inspection is an important part of the examination, and subtle abnormalities are best appreciated by comparing the appearance of both breasts. Breast examination should be done with the patient in both the sitting and supine positions, and care should be taken at all times to be gentle. The steps of a breast examination are illustrated in Fig. 1.

The breasts should initially be inspected while the patient is in the sitting position with the arms relaxed (see Fig. 1A). A comparison of breast size and shape should be made. If a size discrepancy is noted, its chronicity should be deter-

TABLE 1. *Components of the medical history of a breast problem*

All women
Age at menarche
Number of pregnancies
Number of live births
Age at first birth
Family history of breast cancer, including affected relative, age of onset, and presence of bilateral disease
History of breast biopsies (and histologic diagnosis, if available)
Premenopausal women
Date of last menstrual period
Length and regularity of cycles
Use of oral contraceptives
Postmenopausal women
Date of menopause
Use of hormone replacement therapy

mined. Many women's breasts are not identical in size, and the finding of small size discrepancies is rarely a sign of malignancy. Differences in breast size that are of recent onset or progressive in nature, however, may be due to both benign and malignant tumors and require further evaluation (Fig. 2). Alterations in breast shape, in the absence of previous surgery, are of more concern. Superficially located tumors can cause bulges in the breast contour or retraction of the overlying skin. The skin retraction seen with superficial tumors may be due to direct extension of tumor or fibrosis. Tumors deep within the substance of the breast that involve the fibrous septae (Cooper's ligaments) can also cause retraction. Retraction is not itself a prognostic factor except when due to the direct extension of tumor into the skin, and for this reason it is not a part of the clinical staging of breast cancer.[2] Although retraction is often a sign of malignancy, benign lesions of the breast, such as granular cell tumors[3] and fat necrosis,[4] also cause retraction. Other benign causes of retraction include surgical biopsy and thrombophlebitis of the thoracoepigastric vein (Mondor's disease) (Fig. 3).[5]

The skin of the breasts and the nipples should also be carefully inspected. Edema of the skin of the breast (*peau d'orange*), when present, is usually extensive and readily apparent. Localized edema is frequently most prominent in the lower half of the breast and periareolar region and is most noticeable when the patient's arms are raised. Although breast edema usually occurs as a result of obstruction of the dermal lymphatics with tumor cells, it can also be caused by extensive axillary lymph node involvement related to metastatic tumor, primary diseases of the axillary nodes, or axillary dissection. Some degree of breast edema is very common after irradiation of the breast and should not be considered abnormal in this circumstance. Erythema is another sign of pathology that is evident on inspection. It may be due to cellulitis or abscess in the breast, but a diagnosis of inflammatory carcinoma should always be considered. The erythema of inflammatory carcinoma usually involves the entire breast and is distinguished from the inflammation due to infection by the absence of breast tenderness and fever. A small percentage of large-breasted women have mild, dependent erythema of the most pendulous portion of the breast, a condition that resolves when they lie down and that is of no concern.

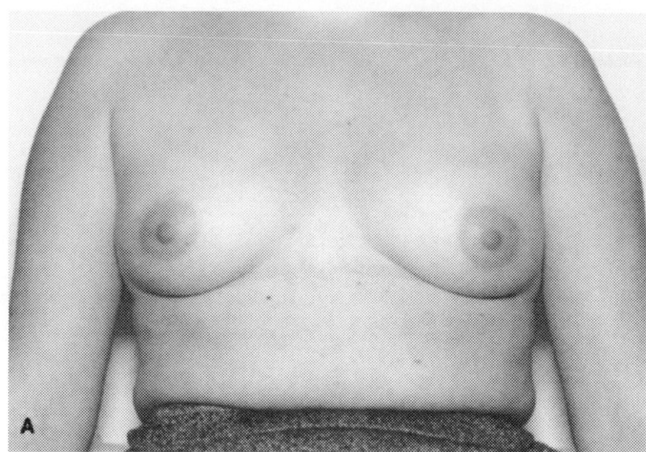

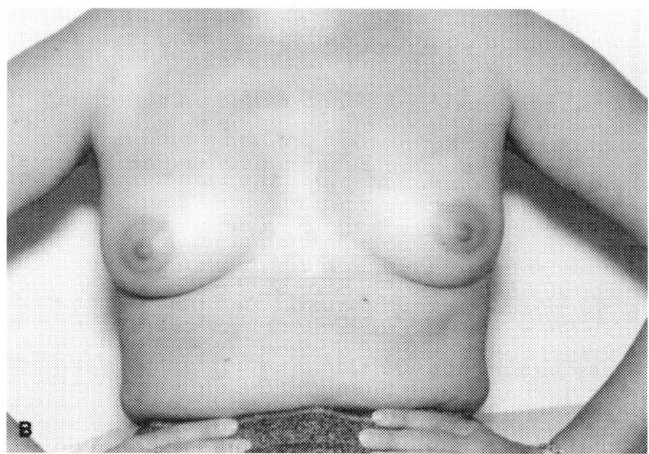

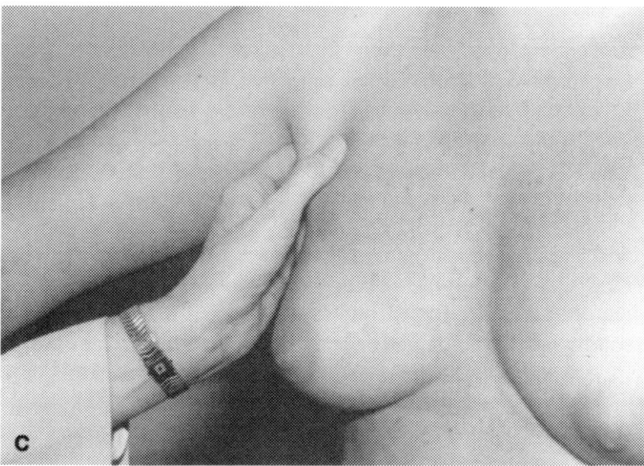

FIG. 1. Inspection of the patient in the upright position with arms relaxed **(A)** and pectoral muscles contracted **(B)**. **C:** Palpation of the axillary nodes. The patient's ipsilateral arm is supported to relax the pectoral muscle.

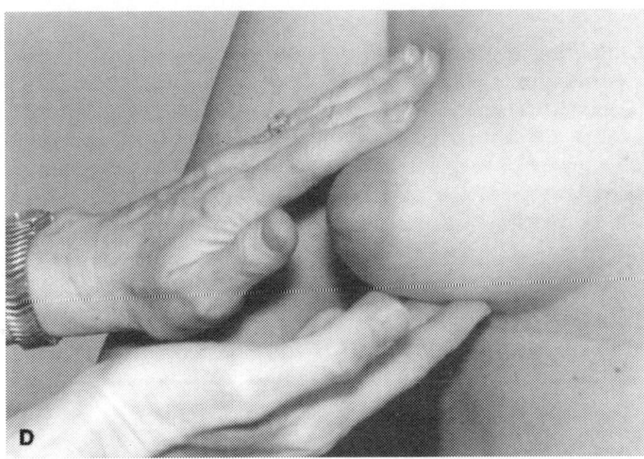

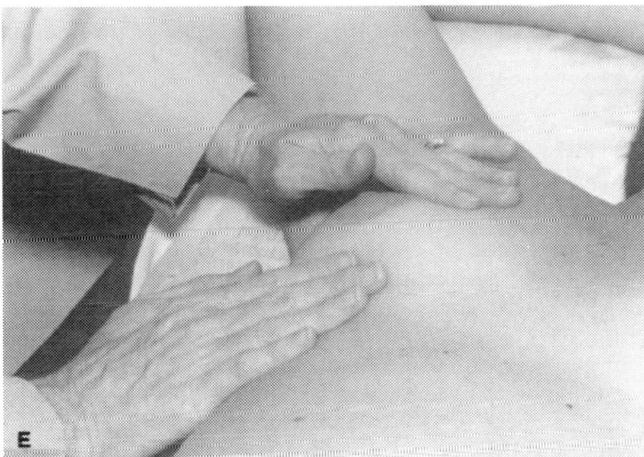

FIG. 1. *Continued.* **D:** Palpation of the breast in the upright position. **E:** Palpation of the breast in the supine position. The breast is stabilized with one hand.

Examination of the nipples should include inspection for symmetry, retraction, and changes in the character of the skin. The new onset of nipple retraction should be regarded with a high index of suspicion, except when it occurs immediately after cessation of breast-feeding. Ulceration and eczematous changes of the nipple may be the first signs of Paget's disease. The initial nipple abnormality may be limited in extent, but, if untreated, it progresses to involve the entire nipple.

After inspection with the arms relaxed, the patient should be asked to raise her arms to allow a more complete inspection of the lower half of the breasts (Fig. 4). Inspection is completed with the patient contracting the pectoral muscles by pressing her hands against her hips (see Fig. 1B). This maneuver often highlights subtle areas of retraction that are not readily apparent with the arms relaxed.

The next step in the examination is palpation of the regional nodes. Examination of the axillary and supraclavicular nodes is done optimally with the patient upright. The right axilla is examined with the physician's left hand while the patient's flexed right arm is supported (see Fig. 1C). This position allows relaxation of the pectoral muscle and access to the axillary space and is reversed to examine the left axilla. If lymph nodes are palpable, their size and character (soft, firm, tender) should be noted, as well as whether they are single, multiple, or matted together. An assessment of whether the nodes are mobile or fixed should also be made. Based on this information, the physician can assess whether the nodes are clinically suspicious. Many women have palpable axillary nodes secondary to hangnails, minor abrasions of the arm, or folliculitis of the axilla, and nodes that are small (1 cm or less), soft, and mobile (especially if bilateral) should not be regarded with a high level of suspicion. In contrast, palpable supraclavicular adenopathy is uncommon and is an indication for further evaluation.

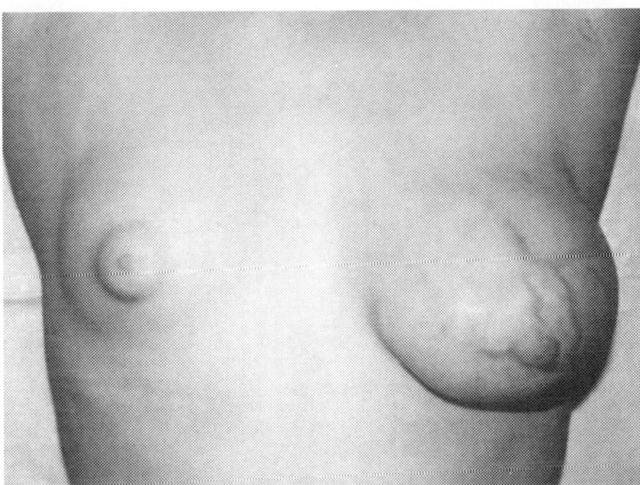

FIG. 2. Marked breast asymmetry due to a benign breast tumor.

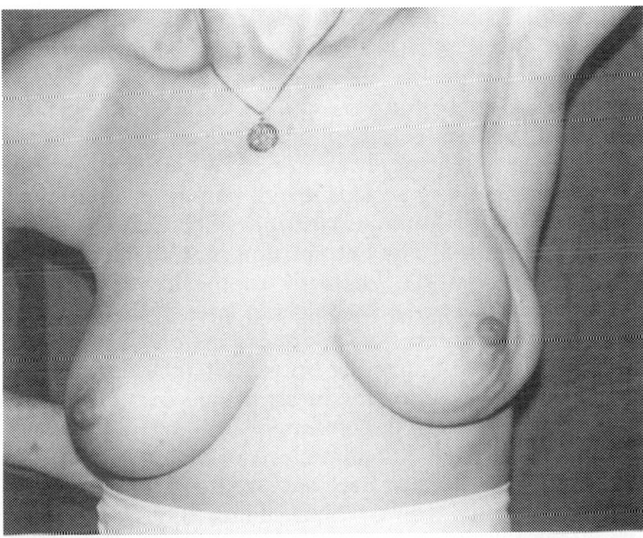

FIG. 3. Breast retraction due to thrombophlebitis of the thoracoepigastric vein (Mondor's disease). The characteristic pattern of lateral retraction superior to the nipple and crossing to the midline below the nipple is seen.

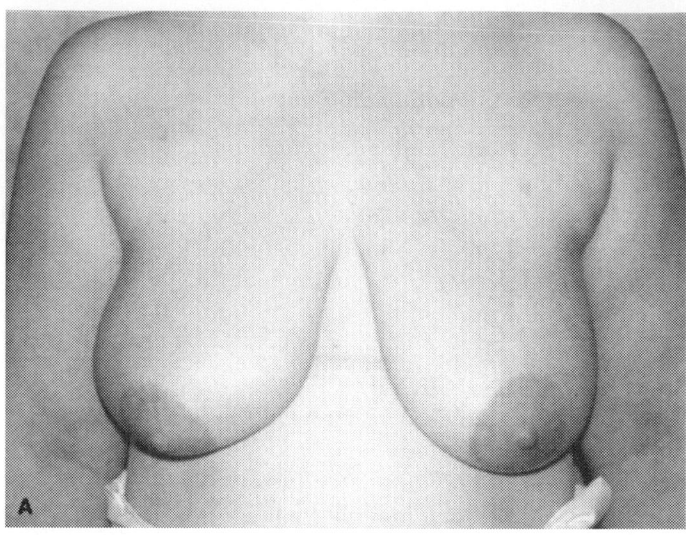

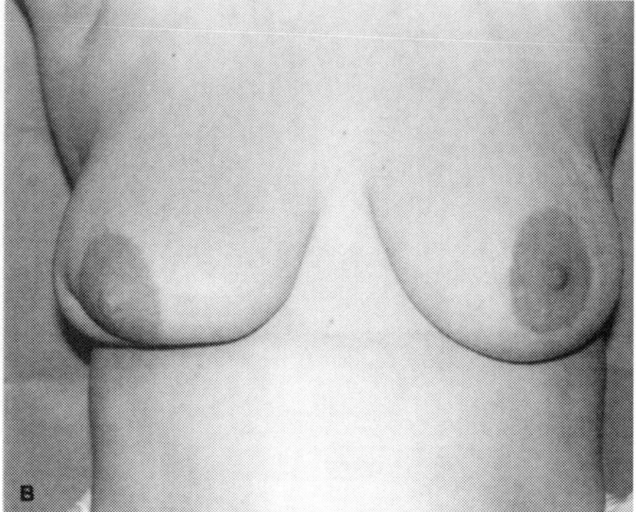

FIG. 4. A: Patient with arms at her sides. Breasts appear normal. **B:** With her arms raised, retraction in right inferior breast is readily apparent.

After the nodal evaluation is completed, palpation of the breasts should be done with the patient erect. Examination of the breast tissue in this position allows detection of lesions that might be obscured with the patient supine, such as those in the tail of the breast. The breast should be gently supported with one hand while examination is done with the flat portions of the fingers (see Fig. 1D). Pinching breast tissue between two fingers always results in the perception of a mass and is a common error of inexperienced examiners and women attempting self-examination.

The breast examination is completed with the patient in the supine position and the ipsilateral arm raised above the head (see Fig. 1E). In patients with extremely large breasts, it may be necessary to place a folded towel or a small pillow beneath the ipsilateral shoulder to elevate the breast, but this is not routinely necessary. The breast tissue is then systematically examined. Whether the examination is done using a radial search pattern or concentric circular pattern is unimportant, provided that the entire breast is examined. The examination should extend superiorly to the clavicle, inferiorly to the lower rib cage, medially to the sternal border, and laterally to the midaxillary line. Examination is done with one hand while the other hand stabilizes the breast. The amount of pressure needed to examine the breast tissue varies but should not cause the patient discomfort.

One of the most difficult aspects of breast examination results from the nodular, irregular texture of normal breasts in premenopausal women. Normal breasts tend to be most nodular in the upper outer quadrants where the glandular tissue is concentrated, in the inframammary ridge area, and in the subareolar region. The characteristics that distinguish a dominant breast mass include the absence of other abnormalities of a similar character, density that differs from the surrounding breast tissue, and three dimensions. Generalized lumpiness is not a pathologic finding. Comparing the breasts is often helpful in determining whether a questionable area requires further evaluation. If the patient notices a mass that is not evident to the examiner, she should be asked to indicate the area of concern. The location of the perceived abnormality and the character of the breast tissue in the region should be described in the medical record. If uncertainty remains regarding the significance of an area of nodular breast tissue in a premenopausal woman, a repeat examination at a different time during the menstrual cycle may clarify the issue. If a dominant mass is identified, it should be measured, and its location, mobility, and character should be described in the medical record. The identification of a dominant mass is an indication for further evaluation. The steps in the evaluation of a palpable mass are described in Chapter 4.

REFERENCES

1. Haagensen CD. *Diseases of the breast*. Philadelphia: WB Saunders, 1986:502.
2. American Joint Committee on Cancer. *Manual for staging of cancer*, 3rd ed. Philadelphia: JB Lippincott, 1988:145.
3. Gold DA, Hermann G, Schwartz IS, et al. Granular cell tumor of the breast. *Breast Dis* 1989;2:211.
4. Adair F, Munzer J. Fat necrosis of the female breast. *Am J Surg* 1947;74:117.
5. Tabar L, Dean P. Mondor's disease: clinical, mammographic and pathologic features. *Breast* 1981;7:17.

CHAPTER 4

Diseases of the Breast, 2nd ed.,
edited by Jay R. Harris.
Lippincott Williams & Wilkins, Philadelphia © 2000.

Management of the Palpable Breast Mass

Susan E. Clare and Monica Morrow

The discovery of a breast lump is one of the most anxiety-provoking occurrences in a woman's life. To assuage this anxiety, the diagnostic evaluation must be carried out as expeditiously as possible, while ensuring that accuracy and reliability are not sacrificed for speed. In addition, the diagnostic evaluation must incur minimal morbidity, and it must preserve the maximum number of options for treatment.

The initial purpose of a surgical consultation is to determine whether a true mass exists. The majority of breast masses are self-discovered or are identified by a primary care provider. A study conducted at Northwestern University Medical School[1] on the evaluation of breast masses in 605 women younger than age 40 sought to determine how often the report of a breast mass by a patient or primary care provider was confirmed by surgical evaluation. In 484 (80%), the mass was self-detected, either as part of a routine monthly breast examination or as an incidental finding. In the remaining 121 patients, the mass was identified on an office visit to a primary care provider and was unknown to the patient before the time of the examination. Using surgeon confirmation of the presence of a dominant mass as the standard of evaluation, the positive predictive value (PPV) of a mass identified by the patient was 36%, as compared to 29% for masses identified by the primary care providers, a difference that was not statistically significant. Using pathologic confirmation of a dominant breast mass as the standard of evaluation, the PPV of a mass identified by the patient was 29%, significantly higher than the PPV of 19% of masses identified by a primary care provider.

HISTORY AND PHYSICAL EXAMINATION

A thorough history and physical examination are the initial indispensable parts of the diagnostic evaluation. The following questions should be included in the history: When was the mass discovered? What brought the mass to the patient's or physician's attention? Is pain associated with the lesion? Does the pain change as a function of phase of the menstrual cycle? Has the lesion changed in size since its discovery, or does it fluctuate with the menstrual cycle? Has the patient had previous biopsies or cyst aspirations, or both? In premenopausal women, the date of the last menstrual period and any history of menstrual irregularity should also be determined. Breast masses are three-dimensional, distinct from surrounding tissues, and generally asymmetric when compared to the other breast.[2] Certain characteristics are more often associated with malignant lesions; these include hardness, indistinct borders, and attachment to the skin or pectoral fascia. Benign lesions generally are mobile and have borders that are well demarcated. These characteristics, however, are not mutually exclusive and should not be used without other studies to make a diagnosis when physical examination confirms the presence of a dominant mass.

S. E. Clare: Department of Surgery, Northwestern University Medical School, Chicago, Illinois; Lynn Sage Comprehensive Breast Program, Northwestern Memorial Hospital, Chicago, Illinois

M. Morrow: Department of Surgery, Northwestern University Medical School, Chicago, Illinois; Lynn Sage Comprehensive Breast Program, Northwestern Memorial Hospital, Chicago, Illinois

CYSTS

If the presence of a mass is confirmed by a clinical breast examination (CBE), the first question to be addressed is whether the mass is solid or cystic. Cysts are thought to be the result of cystic lobular involution. Acini within a lobule distend to become microcysts, which may in turn provide the basis for the development of macrocysts. Cystic change in the breast is a common finding at autopsy. Davies and associates[3] reported necropsy results of 725 women: 58% had microcysts and 21% had cysts greater than 1 cm in diameter. Dupont and Page[4] reviewed 10,542 breast biopsies performed on 3,303 women and found that 32% had microcysts and 23% had cysts larger than 1 cm in diameter. Clinically apparent cysts, however, occur much less frequently. Haagensen's[5] estimate was that breast cysts develop in 7% of women in the Western world, the same percentage as reported in a study by Sterns.[6] Cysts often fluctuate with the menstrual cycle. They are usually well demarcated from the surrounding tissue, mobile, and firm, characteristics that can make them difficult to distinguish from solid, benign lesions on physical examination. They occur at any age, but are most common in women in their 40s and those who are perimenopausal. Cysts are uncommon in postmenopausal women who are not receiving

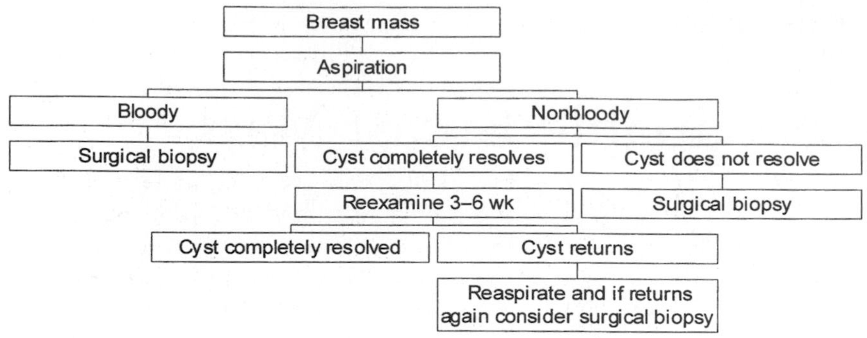

FIG. 1. Management of a cystic breast lesion.

hormone replacement therapy and, therefore, should be regarded with suspicion, as they may be secondary to ductal obstruction by a malignant lesion.

The question of solid versus cystic can be resolved using fine-needle aspiration (FNA) or ultrasound. Aspiration is a straightforward and inexpensive means of immediately distinguishing a cyst from a solid mass. In a premenopausal woman, if fluid is obtained, if it is nonbloody, and if the mass disappears completely, no further evaluation is required. The routine submission of cyst fluid for cytologic evaluation is not recommended. The yield of a malignant result has been shown to be less than 1%.[7–11] If the cyst fluid is bloody, if the palpable abnormality does not resolve completely, or if the same cyst recurs multiple times within a short interval, a biopsy to exclude intracystic carcinoma is indicated (Fig. 1). In postmenopausal women, aspiration is also the first step in the diagnostic evaluation, and the qualifications enumerated for premenopausal women (i.e., nonbloody fluid and complete resolution of the palpable mass) still apply. However, a repeat examination 4 to 6 weeks after the aspiration is essential to rule out a recurrence of the cyst. If ultrasound is elected and a simple cyst is identified, no further intervention is usually necessary. Painful cysts are often aspirated for relief of symptoms. Cystic lesions, which do not have the classic appearance of simple cysts on ultrasound, should be aspirated. Complex masses that clearly have a solid component within a cyst require biopsy and should not be aspirated, as collapsing the cyst could render the remaining lesion nonpalpable.

SOLID MASSES

Failure to aspirate cyst fluid suggests a solid mass; in addition, there are masses that are obviously solid on the basis of physical examination. A tissue or imaging study, or both, is required to make the diagnosis of these lesions.

Fibroadenoma

Fibroadenomas have long been considered to be benign tumors of the breast; however, investigators have advanced the concept that they are the result of a minor aberration of the normal process of lobular development.[12] Autopsy studies have shown fibroadenomas to be present in 9% to 10% of women.[13,14] They are found in 7% to 13% of patients examined in breast clinics.[15] They comprise approximately 50% of breast biopsies, and this rate rises to 75% for biopsies in women younger than age 20.[16,17] On clinical examination, fibroadenomas are rubbery, round, or lobulated masses that are nontender and mobile. They share these characteristics with several other breast lesions, and a clinical diagnosis of fibroadenoma is accurate in only one-half to two-thirds of cases.[18,19] They are usually solitary, but may present as multiple lesions in 10% to 15% of patients.[20] Of these multiple lesions, equal proportions are detected synchronously and metachronously in the same and opposite breast.[21] Foster and associates[22] found that 30% of metachronous fibroadenomas developed in the same quadrant as the first fibroadenoma after a mean interval of approximately 4 years. The left breast is affected slightly more often than the right, and the most frequent location is the upper, outer quadrant.[21]

Sonographic criteria that are used to diagnose a fibroadenoma are a round or oval, circumscribed, homogeneous solid mass with low-level internal echoes in a uniform distribution and intermediate acoustic attenuation.[23] However, fibroadenomas may evidence ultrasound characteristics of carcinoma: Approximately one-fourth of fibroadenomas display irregular margins,[23,24] and 6% to 10% show acoustic shadowing.[24–26] Other benign processes can also mimic the sonographic features of "classic" fibroadenoma. To redress these problems, rather than relying on a single or a few sonographic criteria, a number of investigators have developed combinations of multiple sonographic characteristics or descriptors.[26,27] Principal in the design of these studies is the requirement that malignant lesions not be classified as benign by sonography; therefore, these studies accept high false-positive rates. Both of the referenced studies used high-frequency (7.5–10.0 MHz) probes. The six descriptors that were combined in the Skaane and Engedal study[26] were shape, contour, echo texture, echogenicity, sound transmission, and surrounding tissue. The negative predictive value using all six descriptors was 100% in palpable and 96% in nonpalpable tumors. It is estimated that by using combinations such as these, the number of biopsies done for fibroadenoma could be reduced by as much as 60%.[27] These studies are promising; however, whether they can be reproduced within the majority of clinical practice remains to be seen. To be reproduced, the descriptors must be unambiguous and reliably determined; additionally, the incidence of breast carcinoma in the population being studied must be similar to that in these studies.

Assuming the predicate that, in general, fibroadenomas are oval in shape and infiltrating ductal carcinomas round in shape, attempts have been made to quantify the shape of lesions using sonographic measurements. Fornage et al.[24] advanced the possibility that the ratio of the length (L) to the anteroposterior diameter (AP) could be used as a measure of elongation and to differentiate fibroadenomas from infiltrating ductal carcinomas. A subsequent study by Adler et al.[28] failed to find a significant difference between carcinomas and fibroadenomas when comparing the L to AP ratio. Although ultrasonography is a useful technique in the evaluation of masses suspected of being fibroadenomas, biopsy-proven fibroadenomas have been demonstrated to be sonographically "invisible" in 18% to 20% of cases.[23]

The ability to follow the natural history of fibroadenomas became a realistic possibility only with the advent of FNA. Cytologic characteristics that are considered to be diagnostic of fibroadenoma are abundant bipolar stromal cells, usually seen as bare nuclei; irregular flat sheets of epithelium composed of uniform, evenly spaced polygonal cells; so-called antler-horn clusters; and fenestrated or "honeycomb" sheets composed of similar cells.[29]

FNA permits a relatively reliable diagnosis to be made without removal of the lesion. Haagensen[30] believed that most fibroadenomas grew to 2 to 3 cm in size and then remained static. However, more recent studies have revealed that between 16% and 59% of fibroadenomas resolve spontaneously.[15,31–33] One study reported that 12% of those that do not resolve became smaller over 13 to 24 months, 25% had no alteration in size, and 32% grew in size.[20]

Knowledge of the relationship between fibroadenomas and breast carcinoma is useful in developing a management strategy for these lesions. Two questions must be addressed: (a) whether fibroadenoma is a marker of increased risk of breast cancer and (b) whether breast carcinoma can evolve from the epithelial component of fibroadenomas. The answer to the first question appears to be that there is a small but definite increased risk for breast cancer development. This is predicated on three population-based, retrospective cohort studies[34–36] and two prospective cohort studies.[37,38] The relative risk reported in these studies ranged between 1.2 and 3.0, and unlike other lesions, such as atypical hyperplasia, for which the risk decreases over time,[39] the risk associated with fibroadenoma appears to persist over time.[19] Odds ratios such as these should prompt continued interest in the relationship of fibroadenomas to invasive ductal carcinoma, but they should have little impact on clinical management.

A 1994 study by Dupont and colleagues[40] attempted to identify subgroups of patients with fibroadenoma who were at particularly high risk of developing breast cancer. They identified a number of histologic variants of fibroadenoma, which were associated with roughly comparable increased risks of invasive breast cancer, and they grouped these lesions together under the rubric "complex fibroadenoma." Included in this group were fibroadenomas that contained cysts larger than 3 mm, sclerosing adenosis, epithelial calcifications, and papillary apocrine changes. The relative risk of invasive breast cancer for patients whose fibroadenomas displayed these histologic variations was 2.6; in those with a family history of breast cancer, it was 3.72. This risk persists for more than three decades. It is interesting to note that, if these histologic features were discovered within the breast parenchyma and not within a fibroadenoma, they would confer little or no increased risk of breast carcinoma.[4] This single study is insufficient to recommend any major changes in follow-up or treatment of women with these lesions at this time. It should be recommended that women with significant family histories of breast carcinoma (i.e., breast cancer in a first-degree relative) have increased surveillance regardless of whether they have had a biopsy with the diagnosis of a fibroadenoma. A distinct second group of patients who were identified to be at increased risk were those whose biopsies displayed proliferative disease in the parenchyma adjacent to the fibroadenoma. Proliferative disease in the breast epithelium is an established risk factor for breast cancer.[4,34–36] The relative risk for patients with proliferative disease in the parenchyma adjacent to the fibroadenoma was similar to the risk reported for patients with proliferative disease but no fibroadenoma; therefore, discussion of the risk with the patient should be based on the presence of atypia within the proliferative disease and on the patient's family history.

In contrast, the transformation of the epithelial component of a fibroadenoma to a carcinoma is a rare event. The incidence of a carcinoma arising within a fibroadenoma is reported to be 0.002% to 0.125%.[41,42] Approximately 50% of these tumors were lobular carcinoma *in situ*, 20% were infiltrating lobular carcinoma, 20% were ductal carcinoma *in situ*, and the remaining 10% were infiltrating ductal carcinoma.[43] The clinical, mammographic, and sonographic characteristics of fibroadenomas containing carcinoma are usually similar to those of benign fibroadenomas.[44,45] Carcinoma is most often an incidental finding when a fibroadenoma is removed from a woman in her mid-40s, although these lesions have been discovered in women ranging in age from the late teens to the 70s.

Juvenile Fibroadenoma

Juvenile fibroadenomas account for approximately 4% of all fibroadenomas.[46] These patients tend to be younger than the average age for adult fibroadenoma, with the majority younger than 20 years of age.[46,47] In the study of Pike and Oberman,[47] the most common time for presentation of the

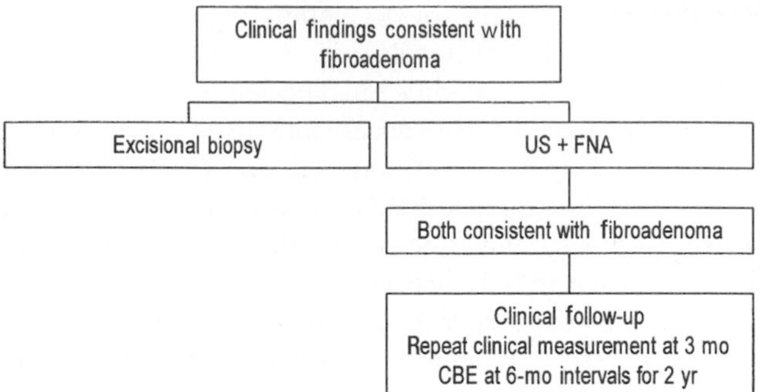

FIG. 2. Management of solid breast masses that are clinically consistent with fibroadenoma. CBE, clinical breast examination; FNA, fine-needle aspiration; US, ultrasound.

tumors was within 1 to 3 years after menarche. Most patients present with a single, painless, discrete, and mobile mass that may enlarge rapidly and sometimes becomes large enough to stretch the skin and cause marked breast asymmetry. Juvenile fibroadenomas have prominent stromal cellularity[46] and epithelial hyperplasia[48] and usually have a pericanalicular or mixed periintracanalicular pattern of growth.[46] Solitary juvenile fibroadenomas are treated by enucleation. Care should be taken to preserve the central breast bud. In Pike and Oberman's series of 13 patients,[47] there were no recurrences. In those cases in which subsequent breast development was described, it was reported to be normal with contour similar to that of the unaffected breast. This was true even in those patients who had large tumors occupying most of the breast. Six of the patients in this study presented with multiple tumors in both breasts, and all subsequently manifested recurrent fibroadenomas. Multiple excisions result in multiple scars and the potential for breast deformity and asymmetry. Patients who present with multiple fibroadenomas can be managed in one of two ways. One is to excise the largest and most worrisome of the fibroadenomas and follow the remainder of the masses with clinical examinations and ultrasound. The second option is to perform a core-needle biopsy on all palpable lesions and to confirm that any nonpalpable lesions have ultrasound characteristics consistent with a fibroadenoma. Excisional biopsy is mandatory for any lesion for which the diagnosis is in question.

Management

When a lesion is identified on physical examination that is consistent with a fibroadenoma, the surgeon has two options (Fig. 2). One option is to excise the lesion. This method has the advantage of producing a definitive diagnosis and relieving any patient anxiety associated with the presence of a clinical breast abnormality. It also avoids the need for frequent follow-up visits and problems of patient compliance. It has the disadvantages of removing a benign lesion that was unlikely to have had an impact on the patient's health and mortality, producing unbecoming cosmesis, and, given the relative frequency of this lesion in the population, adopting a policy of surgical removal of every suspected fibroadenoma, which would unnecessarily drive up health care costs. A second option is to use the combination of physical examination, ultrasonography, and FNA to select patients who require biopsy and use clinical follow-up for the remainder. Before selecting this option, the surgeon needs to be knowledgeable of the accuracy of this method and particularly its reliability in distinguishing a carcinoma from a fibroadenoma. Physical examination provides an accurate diagnosis of fibroadenoma in only one-half to two-thirds of cases studied.[18,19] FNA combined with the clinical diagnosis of a fibroadenoma can improve the sensitivity of the diagnosis to 86% and the specificity to 76%.[24] However, it is insufficient to know only the accuracy of this method to correctly identify a fibroadenoma. The clinician must be aware of the sensitivity of FNA to correctly diagnose a malignant neoplasm at his or her institution, because the critical differentiation to be made is the one between benign and malignant. A significant false-negative rate in the diagnosis of breast carcinoma should prompt the surgeon to proceed to excisional biopsy. For comparison, the sensitivity of FNA to detect a malignant neoplasm is reported to be 97.5% at the M. D. Anderson Hospital[49] in Houston and 96% at the Department of Pathology at the University of Cape Town.[50] Therefore, given these sensitivities and specificities, although aspiration cytology may misdiagnose a fibroadenoma as another of the benign breast lesions, failure to diagnose a malignancy is a rare event.

The accuracy of all three modalities combined—clinical examination, FNA, and ultrasonography—is 70% to 80%, but they provide a 95% accurate differentiation between a benign and malignant lesion.[43] This combined accuracy might lead to the conclusion that ultrasound adds little to the accuracy of the diagnosis; however, the improvement in the accuracy of ultrasound to diagnose fibroadenoma, as evidenced in the studies of Skaane and Engedal and of Stavros et al.,[27] will ultimately be reflected in an improved accuracy of all three modalities combined. Which patients with a breast mass that is clinically consistent with a fibroadenoma can be managed by the triple modalities of physical examination, sonography, and FNA? Knowledge of the frequency of occurrence of these lesions as a function of age can be helpful in making this clinical decision. Fibroadenomas are the most common cause of breast masses in women younger than 25 years of age.[24] A review of all surgical pathology reports of breast biopsies conducted at the Los Angeles County/University of Southern California Medical Center from 1986 to 1989 revealed 486 cases of fibroadenoma. The peak incidence occurred in the 5 years between ages 21 and 25.[51] The peak age incidence for black patients with fibroadenoma was between ages 16 and 20.[52] In contrast, Surveillance, Epidemiology, and End Results Program (SEER) data[53] show that the age-specific incidence of invasive breast cancer in the United States begins to increase steeply after age 40 and peaks in the 5-year period from ages

70 to 74. Carcinoma is a rare occurrence in women younger than age 30.

A study by Cant and colleagues[50] examined the risk of missing a carcinoma using FNA as a function of the patient's age. Comparing annual frequency of carcinoma to that of fibroadenoma and assuming a 4% false-negative rate of aspiration cytology for carcinoma, they calculated the risk for women aged 20 to 24 to be 1 to 3,313 and for women 25 to 29 to be 1 to 229. Based on these results, they recommended triple-modality diagnostic workup of women 25 years old or younger. Other authors have recommended 35 years of age for the cutoff.[54] A report by Greenberg et al.[43] recommends that if all three modalities are consistent with the diagnosis, the patient should be followed with clinical examination every 6 months to age 35. Morrow and associates[1] recommend a similar algorithm but would offer triple-modality workup to patients younger than 40 who have clinically benign masses. If an observational approach is to be used, the results of the FNA and the ultrasound must demonstrate findings consistent with fibroadenoma. A cytologic aspirate that reveals only fat or blood does not contribute to the diagnostic evaluation. Patients must be educated regarding the small but real risk of a delay in diagnosis of carcinoma and the need for clinical follow-up. We generally have patients return 3 to 4 months after their initial evaluation for a repeat measurement of the lesion and then see them at 6-month intervals for 2 years. The need for repeat ultrasound of clinical lesions that are stable has not been established.

Hamartomas

Hamartomas are lesions that are composed of an abnormal mixture of tissue elements or an abnormal proportion of a single element that is usually present at that site.[55] Hamartomas of the breast are composed of variable amounts of glandular tissue, fat, and fibrous connective tissue. The two common variants of mammary hamartoma are adenolipoma and chondrolipoma. Hamartoma is a relatively uncommon lesion, diagnosed only 16 times in 10,000 consecutive mammograms performed from 1967 to 1976 at the University of Lausanne.[56] These lesions most often occur in postmenopausal women,[57] and the peak incidence is approximately two decades after that of fibroadenomas.[56] On clinical examination, they may be well defined or indistinct but are usually soft and do not differ in texture from the surrounding breast parenchyma. Hamartomas can have a classic mammographic appearance that is virtually diagnostic. The lesion is circumscribed and contains both fat and soft-tissue density surrounded by a thin radiopaque capsule that is visible when fat is present on both sides.[56,58–60] When the classic mammographic appearance is present, no further intervention is necessary. In those cases in which the lesion is not visualized or in which the appearance is not classic, an excisional biopsy is warranted. These lesions have not been reported to recur.

Hematomas

Hematoma of the breast can result from blunt or penetrating trauma and from iatrogenic causes, including image-guided needle biopsy and excisional biopsy. Patients usually present with ecchymosis and a painful breast mass. The trauma may have been relatively minor and considered inconsequential by the patient, and a detailed history may be necessary to elicit a probable cause. When a patient with a breast mass and a history of trauma to the breast is evaluated, the differential diagnosis must always include infiltrating ductal carcinoma, as 9% to 11% of women with breast cancer attribute their lesions to antecedent trauma.[61]

Automobile accidents are responsible for 60% of all traumatic injuries in the United States and are believed to cause most cases of breast trauma as well. For the occupant restrained with a lap belt and shoulder harness, the force of impact determines a range of injury. For moderate-impact accidents, contusion/hematoma may result, and ecchymosis may be present in a bandlike distribution across the chest. For the driver, the upper central to inner half of the left or the lower inner quadrant, or both, of the right breast are most frequently involved; for a front-seat passenger, it is the upper inner quadrant of the right breast or the lower inner quadrant, or both, of the left breast.[62] These injuries can produce characteristic linear appearances on mammogram.[62] In high-speed accidents that result in considerable force, subcutaneous rupture of the breast has been reported.[63,64] The mechanism of injury is believed to be compression of the breast tissue between the seat belt and the bony thorax by the force of deceleration. Ecchymosis along the course of the seat belt and a visible furrow in the breast at the site of rupture are present. Fat necrosis is often a sequela of seat belt injury and can result in significant deformity that necessitates cosmetic surgery. In the case of the unrestrained driver, injury can result from impact with the steering wheel or dashboard, or both, and, therefore, the hematoma may be present in any quadrant of the breast.

A trauma that results in force that is great enough to cause significant injury to the breast is very likely to have caused significant intrathoracic injury. Significant breast injury should reflexively alert the examiner to the possible coexistence of pulmonary contusions, pneumothorax, hemothorax, flail chest, and blunt cardiac injuries.

With regard to the iatrogenic causes of hematoma, a 1997 study that looked at stereotactic, 14-gauge vacuum biopsy revealed mammographic evidence of a hematoma in 60% of these biopsies[65]; using sonography to monitor the formation of hematoma after image-guided core biopsy, 19% of biopsy cavities were shown to have evidence of hematoma.[66] However, the majority of these hematomas were not clinically evident. The incidence of postoperative hematoma after excisional breast biopsy ranges from 0.5% to 4.0%.[67–70] Breast carcinoma may present with spontaneous hemorrhage and hematoma in the absence of a history of breast trauma, although this is extremely uncommon.

Acutely, hematomas appear as ill-defined soft-tissue masses on mammography that may raise the concern of a carcinoma. They may increase in size in the immediate post-trauma period; however, they decrease over time and usually resolve completely.[71]

The management of a breast hematoma varies with the clinical presentation. The majority of iatrogenically caused hematomas are clinically insignificant. For small hematomas or diffuse contusion in the breast, support with a brassiere, analgesics, and observation represent the therapy of choice. Imaging studies are not routinely indicated in the patient with a history of trauma and an examination consistent with a hematoma and, in fact, should be avoided because they often raise unwarranted concerns about malignancy. In clinically suspicious cases, aspiration cytology may be helpful in establishing a diagnosis of malignancy. Even if the results of the aspiration cytology are negative, careful follow-up is indicated to ensure that an underlying breast mass is not present. Repeated spontaneous hemorrhage in the same area of the breast is an indication for an excisional biopsy. A patient who presents with an enlarging hematoma within hours of an excisional biopsy should be returned to the operating room for evacuation of the hematoma and ligation or cauterization of the bleeding vessel.

Fat Necrosis

Fat necrosis in the breast may be the sequela of trauma to the breast, including motor vehicle accident, assault, crush injury, a fall, kicking, or pinching; breast biopsy or needle aspiration; lumpectomy; reduction mammoplasty; breast reconstruction; infection; duct ectasia; or radiation therapy. It is the result of aseptic saponification of the fat by means of blood and tissue lipase.[72] Fat necrosis was first described in 1920 by Lee and Adair.[73] In a subsequent report, Adair and Munzer[74] observed that 44% of these patients with fat necrosis had experienced antecedent trauma to the breast. In a later study, Haagensen[75] reported trauma in 32% of the patients, and in 1998 Soo and associates[72] determined that antecedent trauma to the breast had occurred in 65% of their patients with fat necrosis. In the update by Adair and Munzer,[74] fat necrosis accounted for 0.6% of all breast problems seen between 1924 and 1946 at New York's Memorial Hospital and for 2.75% of benign tumors.

Fat necrosis occurs most frequently in overweight women and in women with pendulous breasts.[76] The mean age of presentation in the Adair and Munzer series[74] was in the 40s, and in Haagensen's[75] study the mean was 52 years with a range of 27 to 80 years. Patients typically present with a firm, painless, ill-defined, and immobile lesion. The tumors tend to be small, averaging 2 cm.[75] Fat necrosis is located in the superficial breast tissue and may be accompanied by retraction or dimpling of the overlying skin. The skin is frequently thickened clinically and radiographically. Fat necrosis most frequently occurs in the subareolar and periareolar areas but is not limited to these regions. Clinically, fat necrosis cannot be reliably distinguished from carcinoma.

Many of the mammographic findings of fat necrosis also mimic those of infiltrating ductal carcinoma, including spiculated masses, microcalcifications, architectural distortion and skin thickening, retraction, or a combination of these.[77] A common and characteristic finding of fat necrosis is a circumscribed mass with a calcified or noncalcified rim of radiolucent or mixed fat and soft-tissue density, known as a *lipid* or *oil cyst*.[76,78,79] Lipid or oil cysts are the only mammographic finding that reliably indicates fat necrosis.

A spectrum of ultrasound findings is associated with fat necrosis. The only finding that may be a specific sonographic sign of fat necrosis is a fluid-filled mass, which contains an echogenic band that shifts in orientation with changes in the patient's position. The band may correspond to a mixture of liquefied fat and serosanguineous fluid that is echogenic owing to multiple interfaces between the two types of droplets.[72]

In those cases in which there is unequivocal evidence of trauma to the breast or the characteristic mammographic features of a lipid cyst are present, or both, observation of the mass is appropriate. However, in the majority of cases, because the clinical and radiologic characteristics of fat necrosis resemble those of carcinoma, a needle localization or excisional biopsy is required.

TRIPLE DIAGNOSIS

Only approximately 20% of all excisional biopsies reveal a malignancy.[80] For the purposes of avoiding patient morbidity and decreasing health care costs, attempts have been made to accurately identify a subset of patients with palpable breast lesions whose lesions are very probably benign and who, therefore, can be followed clinically and without excisional biopsy (Fig. 3). *Triple diagnosis* refers to a combination of three diagnostic modalities for the evaluation of a palpable lesion: CBE, mammography, and FNA. The false-negative rate of each of these modalities is too high to justify its use as a sole criterion to make a diagnosis. However, if all three are indicative of a benign lesion, the probability of a diagnostic error has been shown to be less than 1%.[81–84]

CBE uses the palpable characteristics of the lesion enumerated previously to dichotomize lesions into clinically benign and clinically suspicious. If a lesion is clinically benign, mammography is the second stage in the diagnostic evaluation. Mammography should occur before FNA to avoid interpretation difficulties that arise when a hematoma results from an FNA. It is an absolute requirement that the clinician who palpated the lesion personally review the mammograms to correlate the palpable abnormality with any mammographic abnormality. It must be verified, based on location, that the two findings are the same. A mammogram that fails to show the palpable abnormality renders the

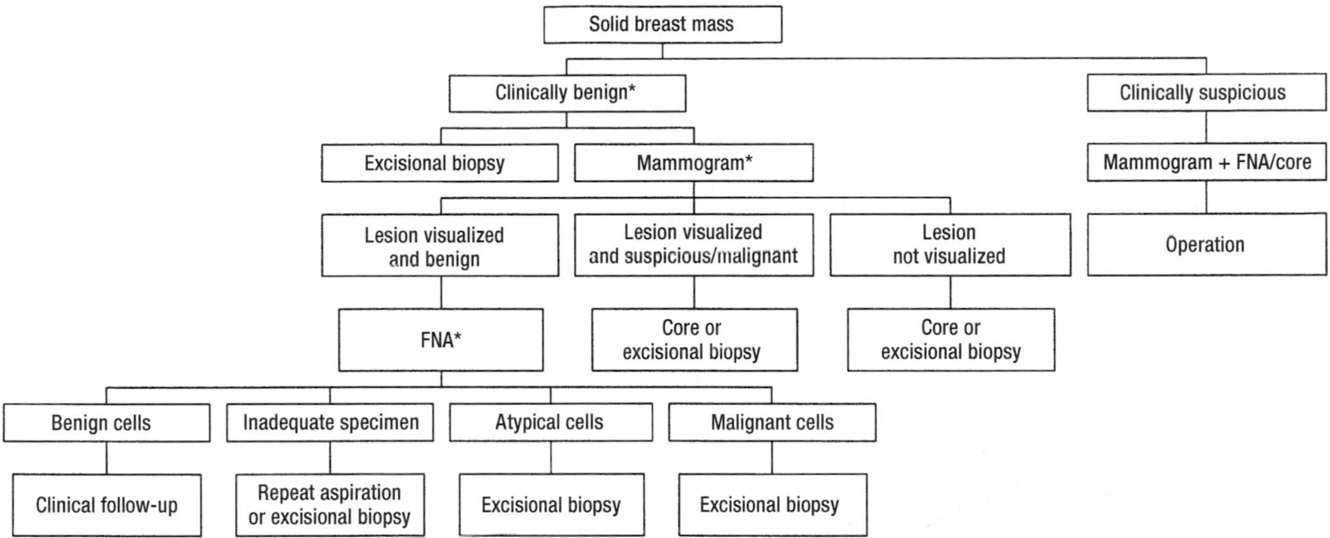

FIG. 3. Management of solid breast masses. Decisions regarding biopsy of clinical follow-up should consider the patient's risk factors for breast carcinoma, including but not limited to age, family history, and any previous biopsy results. The patient and clinician should be cognizant of the fact that follow-up has a small but not zero risk of missing cancer. FNA, fine-needle aspiration. *The three modalities of triple diagnosis.

patient ineligible for triple diagnosis, because accuracy depends on mammographic visualization of the lesion and its demonstration of certain benign characteristics.

The third stage of triple diagnosis is FNA biopsy. Two requirements must be met for FNA to be successful. First, the clinician should be experienced in the technique of FNA, as there is a learning curve, and initial attempts at FNA frequently produce acellular specimens. The second requirement is that the cytopathologist be experienced. It is the responsibility of the clinician to determine the sensitivity of FNA to diagnose breast carcinoma at his or her institution. Sensitivities range between 90%[80] and 97.9%[81] at the institutions that report false-negative rates of less than 1% for triple diagnosis of benign lesions. For the diagnostic accuracy of triple diagnosis to be greater than 99%, all three of the modalities (i.e., CBE, mammography, and FNA) must be benign. If discordance exists between any of the three diagnostic modalities, excisional biopsy should be done.

Patients who choose triple diagnosis are usually seen for at least one follow-up visit at 3 months, and return visits can then be spaced at 3- to 6-month intervals if CBE determines that the lesion is stable. The mass should be monitored by the same examiner at intervals for at least 1 year. The natural history of many of these lesions is resolution over time. Any change in the mass as determined by CBE or mammography, or both, necessitates excisional biopsy.

MANAGEMENT SUMMARY

The initial purpose of a surgical consultation is to determine whether a breast mass exists.

Once a breast mass has been identified, the first determination to be made is whether it is cystic or solid; neither CBE nor mammography can make this determination.

The diagnosis of a fibroadenoma can be made using excisional biopsy or the combined modalities of CBE, ultrasound, and FNA. Excisional biopsy remains the "gold standard."

Any cytologic specimen that is inadequate must be repeated or an excisional biopsy performed.

Hamartomas can produce a classic mammographic image that is virtually diagnostic.

Because the clinical and radiologic characteristics of fat necrosis resemble those of carcinoma in the majority of cases, a needle localization or excisional biopsy is required.

Triple diagnosis requires that the palpable abnormality be visualized by mammography, and the surgeon must know the sensitivity of FNA to diagnose breast carcinoma at his or her institution.

When biopsy is deferred after triple diagnosis, careful follow-up is mandatory.

REFERENCES

1. Morrow M, Wong S, Venta L. The evaluation of breast masses in women younger than forty years of age. *Surgery* 1998;124:634.
2. Donegan WL. Evaluation of a palpable mass. *N Engl J Med* 1992; 327:937.
3. Davies HH, Simons M, Davis JB. Cystic disease of the breast. Relationship to carcinoma. *Cancer* 1964;17:957.
4. Dupont WD, Page DL. Risk factors for breast cancer in women with proliferative breast disease. *N Engl J Med* 1985;312:146.
5. Haagensen CD. *Diseases of the breast.* Philadelphia: WB Saunders, 1986:251.
6. Sterns EE. The natural history of macroscopic cysts in the breast. *Surg Gynecol Obstet* 1992;174:36.

7. Kinnaird DW. Results of cytological study of aspirated fluid from breast cysts. *Am Surg* 1975;41:505.
8. McSwain GR, Valicenti JF Jr, O'Brien PH. Cytologic evaluation of breast cysts. *Surg Gynecol Obstet* 1978;146:921.
9. Cowen PN, Benson EA. Cytological study of fluid from breast cysts. *Br J Surg* 1979;66:209.
10. Solla JA, Walters MJ, Rosenthal D. Breast cyst aspiration cytology. *Mil Med* 1986;151:653.
11. Smith DN, Kaelin CM, Korbin CD, Ko W, Meyer JE, Carter GR. Impalpable breast cysts: utility of cytologic examination of fluid obtained with radiologically guided aspiration. *Radiology* 1997;204:149.
12. Hughes LE. The ANDI concept and classification of benign breast disorders: an update. *Br J Clin Pract Suppl* 1989;68:1.
13. Franyz VK, Pickern JW, Melcher GW, Auchincoloss JR. Incidence of chronic cystic disease in so-called normal breast: a study based on 225 post mortem examinations. *Cancer* 1951;4:762.
14. Gadd MA, Souba WW. Evaluation and treatment of benign breast disorders. In: Bland KI, Copeland EM III, eds. *The breast. Comprehensive management of benign and malignant diseases*, 2nd ed. Philadelphia: WB Saunders, 1998:236.
15. Dent DM, Hacking EA, Wilkie W. Benign breast disease clinical classification and disease distribution. *Br J Clin Pract* 1988;42[Suppl 56]:69.
16. Schuerch C III, Rosen PP, Hirota T, et al. A pathologic study of benign breast diseases in Tokyo and New York. *Cancer* 1982;50:1899.
17. Onuigbo WI. Adolescent breast masses in Nigerian Igbos. *Am J Surg* 1979;137:367.
18. Wilkinson S, Anderson TJ, Rifkind E, Chetty U, Forrest AP. Fibroadenoma of the breast: a follow-up of conservative management. *Br J Surg* 1989;76:390.
19. Cant PJ, Learmouth GM, Dent DM. When can fibroadenoma be managed conservatively? *Br J Clin Pract* 1988;42[Suppl 56]:62.
20. Dent DM, Cant PJ. Fibroadenoma. *World J Surg* 1989;13:706.
21. Rosen PP. Fibroepithelial neoplasms. In: *Breast pathology.* Philadelphia: Lippincott–Raven,1997;144.
22. Foster ME, Garrahan N, Williams S. Fibroadenoma of the breast: a clinical and pathological study. *J R Coll Surg Edinb* 1988;33:16.
23. Cole-Beugler C, Soriano RZ, Kurtz AB, Goldberg BB. Fibroadenoma of the breast: sonomammography correlated with pathology in 122 patients. *AJR Am J Roentgenol* 1983;140:369.
24. Fornage BD, Lorigan JG, Andry E. Fibroadenoma of the breast: sonographic appearance. *Radiology* 1989;172:671.
25. Guyer PB, Dewbury KC, Warwick D, Smallwood J, Taylor I. Direct contact B-scan ultrasound in the diagnosis of solid breast masses. *Clin Radiol* 1986;37:451.
26. Skaane P, Engedal K. Analysis of sonographic features in the differentiation of fibroadenoma and invasive ductal carcinoma. *AJR Am J Roentgenol* 1998;170:109.
27. Stavros AT, Thickman D, Rapp CL, Dennis MA, Parker SH, Sisney GA. Solid breast nodules: use of sonography to distinguish between benign and malignant lesions. *Radiology* 1995;196:123.
28. Adler DD, Hyde DL, Ikeda DM. Quantitative sonographic parameters as a means of distinguishing breast cancers from benign solid breast masses. *J Ultrasound Med* 1991;10:505.
29. Rosen PP. Fibroepithelial neoplasms. In: *Breast pathology.* Philadelphia: Lippincott–Raven, 1997;154.
30. Haagensen CD. *Diseases of the breast*, 2nd ed. Philadelphia: WB Saunders, 1971:213.
31. Smallwood JA, Roberts A, Guyer DP, Taylor I. The natural history of fibroadenomas. *Br J Clin Pract* 1988;56[Suppl]:86.
32. Wilkinson S, Forrest APM, Rifkind E, Chetty U, Anderson TJ. Natural history of fibroadenomas of the breast. *Br J Clin Pract* 1988;56[Suppl]:67.
33. Sainsbury JRC, Nicholson S, Needham GK, Wadehra A, Farndon JR. Natural history of the benign breast lump. *Br J Surg* 1988;75:1080.
34. Dupont WD, Parl FF, Hartmann WH, et al. Breast cancer risk associated with proliferative breast disease and atypical hyperplasia. *Cancer* 1993;71:1258.
35. London SJ, Connolly JL, Schnitt SJ, Colditz GA. A prospective study of benign breast disease and the risk of breast cancer. *JAMA* 1992;267:941.
36. McDivitt RW, Stevens JA, Lee NC, Wingo PA, Rubin GL, Gersell D. Histologic types of benign breast disease and the risk for breast cancer. The Cancer and Steroid Hormone Study Group. *Cancer* 1992;69:1408.
37. Carter CL, Corle DK, Micozzi MS, Schatzkin A, Taylor PR. A prospective study of the development of breast cancer in 16,692 women with benign breast disease. *Am J Epidemiol* 1988;128:467.
38. Krieger N, Hiatt RA. Risk of breast cancer after benign breast diseases. Variation by histologic type, degree of atypia, age at biopsy, and length of follow-up. *Am J Epidemiol* 1992;135:619.
39. Dupont WD, Page DL. Relative risk of breast cancer varies with time since diagnosis of atypical hyperplasia. *Hum Pathol* 1989;20:723.
40. Dupont WD, Page DL, Parl FF, et al. Long-term risk of breast cancer in women with fibroadenoma. *N Engl J Med* 1994;331:10.
41. Deschenes L, Jacob S, Fabia J, Christen A. Beware of breast fibroadenomas in middle-aged women. *Can J Surg* 1985;28:372.
42. Buzanowski-Konakry K, Harrison EG Jr, Payne WS. Lobular carcinoma arising in fibroadenoma of the breast. *Cancer* 1975;35:450.
43. Greenberg R, Skornick Y, Kaplan O. Management of breast fibroadenomas. *J Gen Intern Med* 1998;13:640.
44. Pick PW, Iossifides IA. Occurrence of breast carcinoma within a fibroadenoma. A review. *Arch Pathol Lab Med* 1984;108:590.
45. Ozzello L, Gump FE. The management of patients with carcinomas in fibroadenomatous tumors of the breast. *Surg Gynecol Obstet* 1985;160:99.
46. Fekete P, Petrek J, Majmudar B, Someren A, Sandberg W. Fibroadenomas with stromal cellularity. A clinicopathologic study of 21 patients. *Arch Pathol Lab Med* 1987;111:427.
47. Pike AM, Oberman HA. Juvenile (cellular) adenofibromas. A clinicopathologic study. *Am J Surg Pathol* 1985;9:730.
48. Rosen PP. *Breast pathology.* Philadelphia: Lippincott–Raven, 1997:152.
49. Ballo MS, Sneige N. Can core needle biopsy replace fine-needle aspiration cytology in the diagnosis of palpable breast carcinoma? A comparative study of 124 women. *Cancer* 1996;78:773.
50. Cant PJ, Madden MV, Close PM, Learmonth GM, Hacking EA, Dent DM. Case for conservative management of selected fibro-adenomas of the breast. *Br J Surg* 1987;74(9):857.
51. Hindle WH, Alonzo LJ. Conservative management of breast fibroadenomas. *Am J Obstet Gynecol* 1991;164:1647.
52. Oluwole SF, Freeman HP. Analysis of benign breast lesions in blacks. *Am J Surg* 1979;137:786.
53. Miller BA, Gloeckler Ries LA, Hankey BF, et al., eds. *SEER Cancer Statistics Review, 1973–1990.* Section IV: Breast. US Department of Health and Human Services, Public Health Service, National Institutes of Health, National Cancer Institute. Bethesda, MD: National Institutes of Health, 1991:6. Publication No. 93-2789.
54. Wilkinson S, Anderson TJ, Rifkind E, Chetty U, Forrest AP. Fibroadenoma of the breast: a follow-up of conservative management. *Br J Surg* 1989;76:390.
55. Spraycar M, ed. *Stedman's medical dictionary*, 26th ed. Baltimore: Williams & Wilkins, 1995:760.
56. Hessler C, Schnyder P, Ozzello L. Hamartoma of the breast: diagnostic observation of 16 cases. *Radiology* 1978;126:95.
57. Rosen PP. *Breast pathology.* Philadelphia: Lippincott–Raven, 1997:676.
58. Andersson I, Hildell J, Linell F, Ljungqvist U. Mammary hamartomas. *Acta Radiol* 1979;20:712.
59. Crothers JG, Butler NF, Fortt RW, Gravelle IH. Fibroadenolipoma of the breast. *Br J Radiol* 1985;58:191.
60. Helvie MA, Adler DD, Rebner M, Oberman HA. Breast hamartomas: variable mammographic appearance. *Radiology* 1989;170:417.
61. Wynder EL, Bross IJ, Hirayama T. A study of the epidemiology of cancer of the breast. *Cancer* 1960;13:573.
62. DiPiro PJ, Meyer JE, Frenna TH, Denison CM. Seat belt injuries of the breast: findings on mammography and sonography. *AJR Am J Roentgenol* 1995;164:317.
63. Eastwood DS. Subcutaneous rupture of the breast: a seat-belt injury. *Br J Surg* 1972;59:491.
64. Dawes RF, Smallwood JA, Taylor I. Seat belt injury to the female breast. *Br J Surg* 1986;73:106.
65. Liberman L, Hann LE, Dershaw DD, Morris EA, Abramson AF, Rosen PP. Mammographic findings after stereotactic 14-gauge vacuum biopsy. *Radiology* 1997;203:343.
66. Harlow CL, Schackmuth EM, Bregman PS, Zeligman BE, Coffin CT. Sonographic detection of hematomas and fluid after imaging guided core breast biopsy. *J Ultrasound Med* 1994;13:877.
67. Landercasper J, Gundersen SB Jr, Gundersen AL, Cogbill TH, Travelli R, Strutt P. Needle localization and biopsy of nonpalpable lesions of the breast. *Surg Gynecol Obstet* 1987;164:399.

68. Ostrow LB, DuBois JJ, Hoefer RA Jr, Brant WE. Needle-localized biopsy of occult breast lesions. *South Med J* 1987;80:29.
69. Homer MJ, Smith TJ, Marchant DJ. Outpatient needle localization and biopsy for nonpalpable breast lesions. *JAMA* 1984;252:2452.
70. Kaelin CM, Smith TJ, Homer MJ, et al. Safety, accuracy, and diagnostic yield of needle localization biopsy of the breast performed using local anesthesia. *J Am Coll Surg* 1994;179:267.
71. Jackson VP, Jahan R, Fu YS. Benign breast lesions. In: Bassett LW, Jackson VP, Jahan R, Fu YS, Gold RH. *Diagnosis of diseases of the breast*. Philadelphia: WB Saunders,1997:372.
72. Soo MS, Kornguth PJ, Hertzberg BS. Fat necrosis in the breast: sonographic features. *Radiology* 1998;206:261.
73. Lee B, Adair F. Traumatic fat necrosis of the female breast and its differentiation from carcinoma. *Ann Surg* 1920;72:188.
74. Adair F, Munzer J. Fat necrosis of the female breast. *Am J Surg* 1947;74:117.
75. Haagensen CD. *Diseases of the breast*, 2nd ed. Philadelphia: WB Saunders, 1971:202.
76. Rosen PP. *Breast pathology*. Philadelphia: Lippincott–Raven, 1997:23.
77. Bassett LW, Gold RH, Cove HC. Mammographic spectrum of traumatic fat necrosis: the fallibility of "pathognomonic" signs of carcinoma. *AJR Am J Roentgenol* 1978;130:119.
78. Bassett LW, Gold RH, Mirra JM. Nonneoplastic breast calcifications in lipid cysts: development after excision and primary irradiation. *AJR Am J Roentgenol* 1982;138:335.
79. Evers K, Troupin RH. Lipid cyst: classic and atypical appearances. *AJR Am J Roentgenol* 1991;157:271.
80. Butler JA, Vargas HI, Worthen N, Wilson SE. Accuracy of combined clinical-mammographic-cytologic diagnosis of dominant breast masses. A prospective study. *Arch Surg* 1990;125:893.
81. Kreuzer G, Boquoi E. Aspiration biopsy cytology, mammography and clinical exploration: a modern set up in diagnosis of tumors of the breast. *Acta Cytol* 1976;20:319.
82. Hermansen C, Skovgaard Poulsen H, Jensen J, et al. Diagnostic reliability of combined physical examination, mammography, and fine-needle puncture ("triple-test") in breast tumors. A prospective study. *Cancer* 1987;60:1866.
83. Kaufman Z, Shpitz B, Shapiro M, Rona R, Lew S, Dinbar A. Triple approach in the diagnosis of dominant breast masses: combined physical examination, mammography, and fine-needle aspiration. *J Surg Oncol* 1994;56:254.
84. van Wyk WF, Dent DM, Hacking EA, et al. Combined assessment (aspiration cytology and mammography) of clinically suspicious breast masses. *S Afr Med J* 1995;85:81.

Diseases of the Breast, 2nd ed.,
edited by Jay R. Harris.
Lippincott Williams & Wilkins, Philadelphia © 2000.

CHAPTER 5

Management of Disorders of the Ductal System and Infections

J. Michael Dixon and Nigel J. Bundred

Disorders of the ductal system can present as nipple discharge, nipple inversion, breast mass, or periareolar infection.

NIPPLE DISCHARGE

Nipple discharge accounts for approximately 5% of referrals to breast clinics.[1] It is a frightening symptom because of the fear of breast cancer. Approximately 95% of women presenting to the hospital with nipple discharge have a benign cause for the discharge.[2] Discharge associated with significant underlying pathology is spontaneous, arises from a single duct, is persistent or troublesome, and is bloodstained or contains blood on testing. For this reason, the physician must establish whether the discharge is spontaneous or induced, whether it arises from a single or multiple ducts, and whether it is from one or both breasts. The characteristics of the discharge also need to be defined: whether it is viscous or watery and whether it is serous, serosanguinous, bloody, clear, milky, green, or blue-black. The frequency of discharge and the amount of fluid also need to be assessed; this assessment is important for milky discharge, which should be considered to be galactorrhea only if it is copious in amount and arises from multiple ducts of both breasts.[3]

Investigations

Assessment includes performance of a complete physical examination to identify the presence or absence of a breast mass. During the examination, firm pressure should be applied around the areola to identify the site of any dilated duct (pressure over the dilated duct will produce the discharge); this is helpful in defining where an incision should be made for any subsequent surgery. The nipple is squeezed with firm digital pressure, and if fluid is expressed, the site and character of the discharge are recorded. Testing of the discharge for hemoglobin determines whether blood is present. Fewer than 10% of patients who have a bloodstained discharge or who have a discharge containing moderate or large amounts of blood have an underlying malignancy. Age is an important predictor of malignancy; in one series, 3% of patients younger than 40, 10% of patients between ages 40 and 60, and 32% of patients older than 60 who presented with nipple discharge as their only symptom were found to have cancers.[4] Cytology of nipple discharge is of little value in determining whether duct excision should be performed. In two studies of 1,009 and 338 patients with nipple discharge, cytology had a sensitivity for malignancy of 34.6%[2] and 46.5%,[5] respectively. Ductography or galactography can identify lesions within the ductal tree. Although this investigation has only a 60% sensitivity for malignancy, a filling defect or duct cutoff has a high positive predictive value for the presence of either a papilloma or a carcinoma.[2,6] Because patients who have significant pathology have persistent or troublesome discharge, neither cytology nor ductography has a role in the routine management of patients with nipple discharge (Fig. 1). Ductography is indicated only for patients with minimal symptoms when avoidance of surgery is desired or for a young patient in cases in which localization of any abnormality allows limited surgery to preserve the ability to breast-feed.

If clinical examination demonstrates a mass lesion or mammography raises suspicion of malignancy, then cytology or core biopsy of the lesion should be performed. Otherwise, when no abnormality is found on clinical or mammographic examination, patients are managed according to whether the discharge is from a single duct or multiple ducts (see Fig. 1). Surgery is indicated in cases of spontaneous discharge from a single duct that is confirmed on clinical examination and has one of the following characteristics:

- Is bloodstained or contains moderate or large amounts of blood on testing
- Is persistent (occurs on at least two occasions per week)

J. M. Dixon: Edinburgh Breast Unit, Western General Hospital, Edinburgh, Scotland, United Kingdom

N. J. Bundred: Academic Department of Surgery, South Manchester University Hospital, Manchester, England, United Kingdom

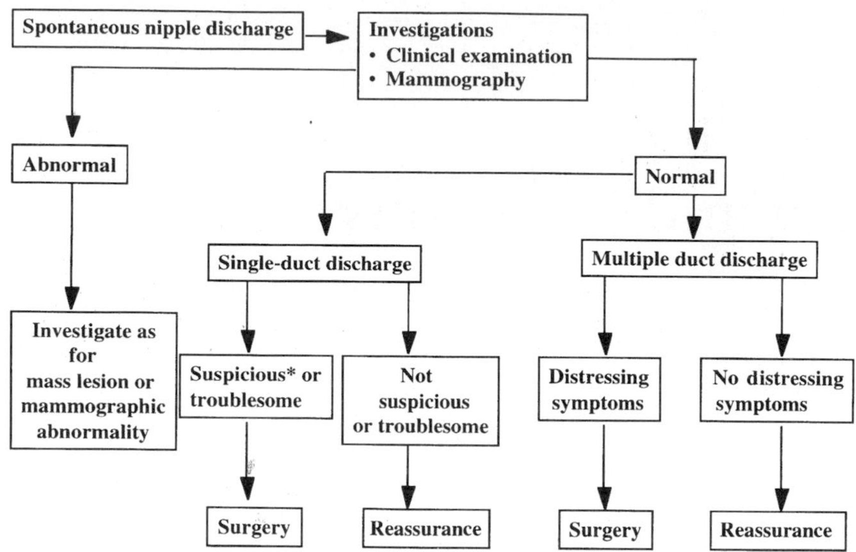

FIG. 1. Investigation of nipple discharge. Suspicious (*) means discharge that is bloodstained or contains moderate or large amounts of blood on testing, is associated with a mass, or is a new development in women older than age 50 and is not thick or cheesy.

- Is associated with a mass
- Is a new development in a woman older than 40 years of age but is not thick or cheesy

Discharge from multiple ducts normally requires surgery only when it causes distressing symptoms, such as persistent staining of the clothes.[1,7] Some breast units adopt an age-related policy: Patients younger than age 30 who have serous, serosanguinous, or watery discharge are observed, with microdochectomy reserved for cases in which discharge persists at review some months later[8]; patients older than age 45 are treated by a formal excision of the major duct system on the affected side; patients between ages 30 and 45 are deemed suitable for either approach.[8] Other units adopt an expectant policy for patients with single-duct discharge and normal mammograms; this practice is based on a review of 98 consecutive patients undergoing microdochectomy, of whom 8 patients had ductal carcinoma *in situ* and 6 had abnormal mammography.[9]

Causes of Nipple Discharge

Physiologic Causes

In two-thirds of nonlactating women, a small quantity of fluid can be expressed from the ducts of the nipple if the nipple is cleaned and gentle bimanual pressure is applied.[10,11] This fluid is physiologic secretion and varies in color from white to yellow to green to brown to blue-black[1]; it is thought to represent apocrine secretion, the breast being a modified apocrine gland. Physiologic secretion usually emanates from multiple ducts, and the discharge from each duct can vary in color. Women often first notice discharge after a warm bath or after nipple manipulation, and the discharge is not usually spontaneous or bloodstained. Once this condition is diagnosed, no specific treatment is required, and reassurance should be given.

Intraductal Papilloma

A true intraductal papilloma develops in one of the major subareolar ducts and is the most common lesion causing a serous or serosanguinous discharge. In approximately one-half of women with papillomas, the discharge is bloody; in the other one-half of cases, it is serous.[8] Papillomas should be differentiated from papillary hyperplasia, which affects the terminal duct lobular unit and can also cause nipple discharge. Central papillomas consist of epithelium covering arborescent fronds of fibrovascular stroma attached to the wall of the duct by a stalk. The covering epithelium has a two-cell population, with lining cuboidal or columnar cells covering an underlying layer of myoepithelial cells. A mass may be felt on examination in as many as one-third of cases.[9] Occasionally, the papilloma is so close to the nipple that it can be seen in the orifice of the duct at the nipple. The treatment of choice is microdochectomy. A solitary papilloma is not thought to be a premalignant lesion[12] and is considered by some to be an aberration rather than a true disease process.[1]

Multiple Intraductal Papillomas

In approximately 10% of cases of intraductal papilloma, the lesions are found to be multiple; usually, two or three occur, often in the same duct. The term *multiple intraductal papilloma syndrome* is reserved for a rare and distinctive group of patients in whom one duct system is involved by large and often palpable papillomas with a peripheral distribution.[10] Nipple discharge is less common in this group than in patients with a solitary intraductal papilloma. In one study, multiple papillomas were found to be associated with an increased risk of breast cancer,[12] but any increased risk is almost certainly associated with areas of atypical epithelial hyperplasia rather than with the papillomas themselves.[13]

Juvenile Papillomatosis

Juvenile papillomatosis is a rare condition that affects women between the ages of 10 and 44.[14] The patient usually presents with a discrete mass lesion. In one series of 13 patients, 11 had a peripheral and two a central lesion.[15] Three of the 13 presented with nipple discharge; in two, the discharge was associated with a peripheral mass lesion, and the third had nipple discharge alone. Treatment is by complete excision. Patients with this condition may be at some increased risk of subsequent breast cancer, and close clinical surveillance of any woman with this condition is indicated.[16]

Carcinoma

An invasive or noninvasive cancer can cause nipple discharge. Only rarely does an invasive cancer cause nipple discharge in the absence of a clinical mass. In most series, ductal carcinoma *in situ* (DCIS) is responsible for up to 10% of unilateral nipple discharges.[2] Nipple discharge alone or in association with a mass or Paget's disease is the presenting feature in approximately one-third of symptomatic *in situ* cancers.[17] With the advent of mammography, increasing numbers of noninvasive cancers are being detected, and overall nipple discharge is the presenting symptom in 7% to 8% of all cases of DCIS. Scanty data exist on the frequency with which these *in situ* cancers are visible on mammography. Although one study visualized on mammography 6 of 8 cases of DCIS presenting as nipple discharge,[9] other more recent studies have found that the majority are not visible on mammography and that mammography is unreliable in this situation.[18–20] A diagnosis of invasive or noninvasive cancer is often established only by microdochectomy, which is rarely, if ever, therapeutic.

Bloody Nipple Discharge in Pregnancy

Nipple discharge with blood present either visibly or cytologically during pregnancy or lactation is common. In 20% of women with nipple discharge during pregnancy, blood can be confirmed by analysis of nipple secretion.[21] The likely cause is hypervascularity of developing breast tissue. The condition is benign and requires no specific treatment.[22]

Galactorrhea

A woman should be considered to have galactorrhea if she has copious bilateral milky discharge not associated with pregnancy or breast feeding. A careful drug history should be taken from such women, because a number of drugs, particularly psychotropic agents, cause hyperprolactinemia. Blood should be taken to test for prolactin, and if prolactin levels are significantly elevated (greater than 1,000 mU/L) in the absence of any drug cause, then a search for a pituitary tumor should be instituted.[7] The diagnosis of hyperprolactinemia is suggested by a history of galactorrhea, amenorrhea, and relative infertility. The galactorrhea disappears after appropriate drug therapy or surgical removal of the adenoma. Appropriate drug therapy includes administration of bromocriptine mesylate, which produces significant side effects in up to one-third of patients, or the newer agent cabergoline. For patients with troublesome galactorrhea who are intolerant of medication, bilateral total duct ligation appears successful.[27]

Periductal Mastitis and Duct Ectasia

A variety of terms have been applied to the conditions now known as *periductal mastitis* and *duct ectasia*. Haagensen first introduced the term *duct ectasia* and considered the condition to be an age-related phenomenon; he believed that breast ducts dilated with age and that stagnant secretions in these dilated ducts leaked into surrounding tissues to cause periductal mastitis.[23] This description of events ignores the findings of all other authors that periductal inflammation predominates in young women, whereas duct dilatation increases in frequency with advancing age, so the sequence of events described by Haagensen must be incorrect.[24,25] If periductal mastitis and duct ectasia are related, then one would expect patients with duct ectasia to have a past history of episodes of periductal mastitis. In one study of 186 patients with the clinical syndrome of duct ectasia, only one (0.5%) had a history of previous periductal mastitis; in contrast, 97 (70%) of 139 patients with the clinical syndrome of periductal mastitis reported a previous clinical episode of periductal mastitis.[26]

Clinical Syndromes

Periductal mastitis is characterized clinically by episodes of periareolar inflammation with or without an associated mass, a periareolar abscess, and a mammary duct fistula. Nipple retraction can be seen early at the site of the affected duct and is often subtle.[28] Nipple discharge can also occur and is often purulent.

The clinical features of duct ectasia include nipple retraction at the site of the shortened duct or ducts and cheesy, viscous, toothpastelike nipple discharge. Patients with multiple duct green discharge are often said to have duct ectasia, but the majority of these have leaking physiologic breast secretion. These clinical syndromes affect different age groups; in one large series, periductal mastitis affected women between the ages of 18 and 48, whereas patients presented with duct ectasia between the ages of 42 and 85.[26]

Etiology

Although parity and breast-feeding were thought at one time to be important factors in the etiology of duct dilatation,[24] subsequent studies have not demonstrated any association between these factors and periductal mastitis or duct ectasia.[29] Age is an important factor in the etiology of duct ectasia; the frequency of the condition increases with age, and in one postmortem study, 48% of women age 60 or older had pathologic evidence of duct ectasia.[30] Although early studies suggested that the lesions of both periductal mastitis and duct ectasia are sterile,[23] when appropriate transport media are used, bacteria can be isolated from 83% of periareolar inflammatory masses and 100% of nonlactational abscesses and mammary duct fistulae.[31] The organisms isolated are frequently anaerobic. In contrast, a study of duct ectasia lesions identified bacteria in only one of 11 patients, a finding indicating that these lesions are usually sterile.[32]

An association between smoking and recurrent periareolar abscesses was first reported in 1988.[33] A subsequent study showed that heavy smokers are more likely to develop abscess recurrence or a subsequent mammary duct fistula than light smokers or nonsmokers.[34] Studies with carefully matched case controls have shown a significant excess of smokers among patients with the clinical syndrome of periductal mastitis but no excess of smokers among women with clinically diagnosed duct ectasia.[26,35] Women with periductal mastitis are also more likely to be heavy smokers.[35] How cigarette smoking causes periductal mastitis is unclear. Substances in cigarette smoke may either directly or indirectly damage the wall of subareolar ducts. Accumulation of toxic metabolites, such as lipid peroxidase, epoxides, nicotine, and cotinine in breast ducts, has been demonstrated to occur within 15 minutes of a woman's starting to breast-feed.[36,37] Smoking has also been shown to inhibit growth of gram-positive bacteria *in vivo* and *in vitro*, leading to an overgrowth of gram-negative bacteria.[38] This may affect the normal bacterial flora and allow overgrowth of pathogenic aerobic and anaerobic gram-negative bacteria and would explain the presence of these organisms in the lesions of periductal mastitis. Microvascular changes have also been recorded and may cause local ischemia.[39] The combination of damage due to toxins with leakage into the surrounding tissues, microvascular damage by lipid peroxidases, and altered bacterial flora may be responsible for the clinical manifestations of periductal mastitis.

Etiologic data suggest that periductal mastitis and duct ectasia are separate conditions with different causes. Duct ectasia appears to be an involutionary phenomenon, whereas periductal mastitis is a disease in which smoking and bacteria are important causal factors.

Other Causes of "Nipple" Discharge

Other diseases of the nipple-areolar complex can present with "nipple" discharge, including nipple adenoma, eczema, Paget's disease, ulcerating carcinoma, and long-standing nipple inversion with maceration.[9] Nipple adenoma is rare but easy to diagnose. It usually presents with a bloodstained discharge or change in contour or color of the nipple. Occasionally, an ulcer develops. Clinically, it is an indiscrete mass in the substance of the superficial layer of the nipple. Definitive treatment is complete excision.[7] Eczema or dermatitis can affect the nipple and is usually caused by irritation from chemicals on clothes or cosmetics. Eczema can be differentiated from Paget's disease in that eczema affects primarily the areola and only rarely spreads onto the nipple.[40] In contrast, Paget's disease affects the nipple first and only secondarily affects the areola. Treatment for eczema is removal of any aggravating factor, such as perfumed soap or detergents, by the use of hypoallergenic washing materials for clothes and skin and prescription of a short course of topical corticosteroids.

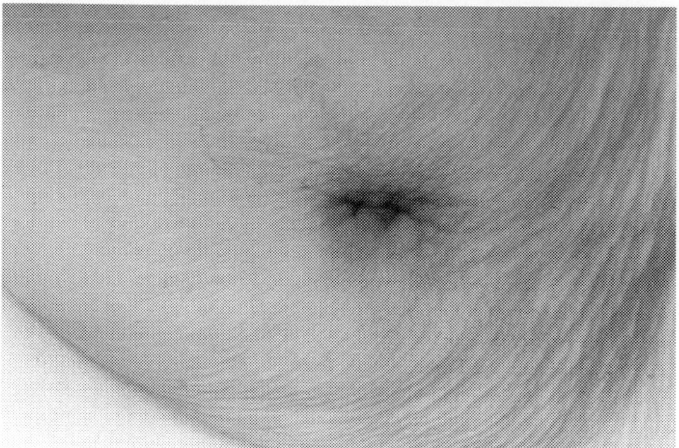

FIG. 2. Nipple inversion from breast cancer.

Long-standing nipple inversion with maceration is rare but is seen in elderly people.[9] The injured skin produces a discharge, which can be purulent. Treatment is by careful cleaning of the affected area.

NIPPLE INVERSION OR RETRACTION

The terms *inversion* and *retraction* are often used interchangeably, although some call the condition *inversion* only when the whole nipple is pulled in (Fig. 2) and use the term *retraction* when part of the nipple is drawn in at the site of a

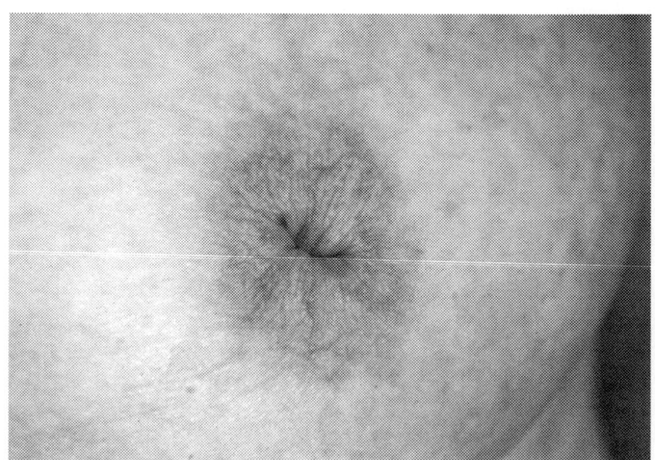

FIG. 3. Slitlike nipple retraction from duct ectasia.

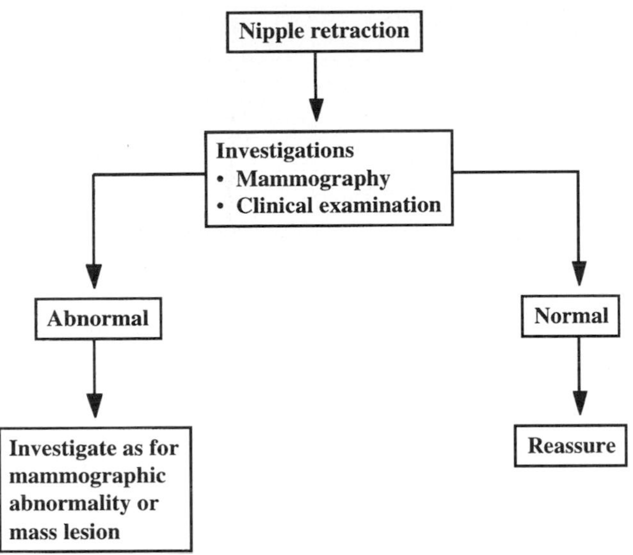

FIG. 4. Management of nipple retraction.

single duct to produce a slitlike appearance (Fig. 3).[1] These changes can be congenital or acquired. The acquired causes, in order of frequency, are duct ectasia, periductal mastitis, carcinoma, and tuberculosis.

All patients with acquired nipple inversion or retraction should have a full clinical examination and, if the patient is older than 35 years, a mammogram.[41] Management depends on the presence or absence of a clinical or mammographic abnormality (Fig. 4). Central symmetric transverse slitlike retraction is characteristic of benign disease; nipple inversion occurring in association with either breast cancer or inflammatory breast disease is more likely to involve the whole of the nipple and, in a breast cancer, to be associated with distortion of the areola when the breast is examined in different positions (see Figs. 2 and 3). Benign nipple retraction requires no specific treatment but can be corrected surgically if the patient requests it and the surgeon considers the operation appropriate. Usually, division or excision of the underlying breast ducts (total duct division or excision) is required, and patients should be warned that they cannot breast-feed after this procedure.

OPERATIONS FOR NIPPLE DISCHARGE OR RETRACTION

Microdochectomy

Microdochectomy can be performed either through a radial incision across the areola or through a circumareolar incision centered over the discharging duct. A circumareolar incision leaves a better cosmetic scar. After the discharging duct is cannulated with a probe, the abnormal duct containing the probe is identified on the undersurface of the nipple. The duct is dissected distally into the breast; a portion of the duct over a distance of at least 2 to 3 cm is removed, as almost all significant pathology affects the proximal 5 cm.[8] If the remaining duct appears abnormal and dilated after the proximal portion of the duct is removed, then the distal duct can be opened and any pathologic lesion in the remaining duct can be visualized and excised. Drains are not necessary after this procedure, and the skin is closed in layers with an absorbable suture.

Total Duct Excision or Division

Because the lesions of periductal mastitis usually contain organisms, patients having operations for this condition should receive appropriate antibiotic treatment during the operation and continuing for 5 days after surgery. Options for antibiotic therapy include co-amoxyclav or a combination of erythromycin and metronidazole hydrochloride. A circumareolar incision based at the 6-o'clock position is used unless a previous scar exists, in which case it can be reopened. Dissection is performed under the areola down either side of the major ducts. Curved tissue forceps are then passed around the ducts, and these are delivered into the wound. The ducts are divided from the undersurface of the nipple, and if a total duct excision is being performed, a 2-cm portion of ducts is excised.[42] If the operation is being performed for periductal mastitis, the back of the nipple must be cleared of all ducts up to the nipple skin, because recurrence of this condition is well described and occurs when residual diseased ductal tissue is left.[42] No sutures need to be placed in the breast. If the nipple was inverted before the operation, it is manually everted; only rarely must sutures be placed under the nipple to maintain nipple eversion. No drains are placed, and the wound is closed in layers with an absorbable suture. Patients should be warned that this operation results in significantly reduced nipple sensitivity in almost 40% of women.[43]

BREAST INFECTION

Breast infection is much less common than it used to be. It is occasionally seen in neonates but most commonly affects women between the ages of 18 and 50. In the adult, breast infection can be considered lactational or nonlactational. Infection can also affect the skin overlying the breast, and occurs either as a primary event or secondary to a lesion within the skin, such as a sebaceous cyst, or a more generalized condition, such as hidradenitis suppurativa. The organisms responsible for different types of breast infection and the most appropriate antibiotics with activity against these organisms are summarized in Table 1.[44] The guiding principle in treating breast infection is to give antibiotics as early as possible to stop abscess formation; if the infection fails to resolve after one course of antibiotics, then abscess formation or an underlying cancer should be suspected.[45]

TABLE 1. *Organisms responsible for different types of breast infection and appropriate antibiotics*

Type of infection	Organism	No penicillin allergy	Penicillin allergy
Neonatal Lactational Skin associated	*Staphylococcus aureus*	Co-amoxyclav	Erythromycin
Nonlactational infection Hidradenitis suppurativa	*S. aureus* *Enterococcus* species Anaerobic organisms *Streptococcus* species *Bacteroides* species	Co-amoxyclav	Combination of cephradine or erythromycin and metronidazole hydrochloride

Mastitis Neonatorum

Continued enlargement of the breast bud in the first week or two of life occurs in approximately 60% of newborn babies, and the gland may reach several centimeters in size before regressing. The enlarged breast bud can become infected, usually by *Staphylococcus aureus*, although *Escherichia coli* can sometimes cause this infection. In the early stage, antibiotics (flucloxacillin) can control infection; however, if fluctuation is evident, incision and drainage performed as peripherally as possible so as not to affect the breast bud are usually effective at producing resolution.

Lactational Infection

Lactational infection is less common in developed countries than it used to be, but it is still a frequent problem in many parts of the world. The infection is usually caused by *S. aureus*, but it can also be due to *Staphylococcus epidermidis* and *Streptococcus* species. Usually, the patient has a history of a cracked nipple or a skin abrasion, which results in a break in the body's defense mechanisms and an increase in the number of bacteria over the skin of the breast. These increased numbers of bacteria can enter the breast through the nipple and infect poorly draining segments. Infection most commonly occurs in the first 6 weeks of breast-feeding or during weaning. Patients present with pain, erythema, swelling, tenderness, or systemic signs of infection. Clinically, the breast is swollen, tender, and erythematous; if an abscess is present, a fluctuant mass with overlying shiny red skin may be noted.[43] Axillary lymphadenopathy is not usually a feature. Patients can be toxic with pyrexia, tachycardia, and leucocytosis.

Antibiotics given at an early stage usually control the infection and stop abscess formation. Because more than 80% of staphylococci are resistant to penicillin, flucloxacillin, co-amoxyclav or, in patients with a penicillin sensitivity, erythromycin or clarithromycin should be given. Tetracycline, ciprofloxacin, and chloramphenicol should not be used to treat infection in breast-feeding women, as they enter breast milk and may harm the child.[43] Patients whose condition does not improve rapidly on antibiotic therapy require further investigation and assessment with either ultrasonography or fine-needle aspiration to determine whether pus is present and to exclude an underlying neoplasm. Inflammatory cancers can be difficult to differentiate from abscesses. If an abscess is suspected clinically or on ultrasonography, aspiration to dryness should be performed. If no pus is aspirated, cells are removed for cytology. Provided the skin overlying the abscess is not thinned or shiny, repeated aspiration combined with oral antibiotics is the treatment of choice.[46] Aspiration should be repeated every 2 to 3 days until no further pus is obtained. Characteristically, the aspirate changes from pus to blood and then to milk. If the skin overlying the abscess is thinned and pus is present on aspiration or visible on ultrasonography, then local anesthetic cream is applied to the thinned skin and a small incision (mini-incision) is made over the point of maximum fluctuation, and the pus is drained.[44] The cavity is then irrigated with local anesthetic solution, which produces instant pain relief. Thereafter, the cavity is lavaged with saline to wash out all the pus. Irrigation is continued daily, until the site of incision closes. If the skin overlying the abscess is necrotic, then the necrotic skin is excised, which allows the pus to drain. Few lactational abscesses require drainage under general anesthesia, and neither the placement of drains nor wound packing after incision is necessary. Breast-feeding should be continued if possible, as this promotes drainage of the engorged segment and helps resolve infection. The infant is not harmed by bacteria in the milk, nor by the flucloxacillin, co-amoxyclav, or erythromycin. Patients who have incision and drainage of their breast abscesses performed under general anesthesia usually must stop breast-feeding, but those who are treated by mini-incision or aspiration and antibiotic therapy can usually continue to breast-feed if they wish. Only rarely is it necessary to suppress lactation in patients with breast infection.

Nonlactational Infection

Nonlactational infections can be divided into those occurring centrally in the breast in the periareolar region and those affecting peripheral breast tissue.

Periareolar Infection

Periareolar infection is most commonly seen in young women; the mean age of occurrence is 32, and the majority of these patients are smokers. The underlying pathology is usually periductal mastitis.[44,47] It can present as periareolar inflammation with or without a mass, a periareolar abscess, or a mammary duct fistula. Associated nipple retraction, which can be quite subtle, may also be seen at the site of the diseased duct,[38] and nipple discharge, which can be purulent, may be present. A patient presenting with periareolar inflammation without a mass should be treated by co-amoxyclav or, if the patient has a penicillin allergy, by a combination of erythromycin and metronidazole hydrochloride.[48] These antibiotics are active against both the aerobic and anaerobic bacteria seen in these lesions (see Table 1). If the infection does not resolve after one course of antibiotics, investigations should be undertaken to exclude an underlying abscess or neoplasm. A patient who presents with or develops an abscess is treated as for a lactational abscess by recurrent aspiration and continuation of oral antibiotics or incision and drainage under local anesthesia. After resolution of the infective episode, patients older than age 35 years should have mammography performed, as very rarely infection can develop in association with comedo necrosis in an area of ductal carcinoma *in situ*. Up to one-half of patients with periareolar sepsis develop recurrent episodes of infection; the only effective long-term treatment for these women is removal of all the affected ducts (total duct excision). If this operation is performed carefully, it is usually curative.[42]

Mammary Duct Fistula

A mammary duct fistula is a communication between the skin, usually in the periareolar region, and a major subareolar breast duct (Fig. 5).[44] It is most commonly seen after incision and drainage of a nonlactational breast abscess, although it can occur after spontaneous discharge of a periareolar inflammatory mass or after biopsy of an area of periductal mastitis.[49] Patients usually have preceding episodes of recurrent abscess formation and pussy discharge, both through the nipple and through the fistula opening. Occasionally, one or more external openings are noted at the areolar margin, either from a single duct or from multiple affected ducts.

Treatment is surgical and consists of either opening up the fistula tract and leaving it to granulate[50] or excising the fistula and affected duct or ducts (a total duct excision is usually required) and closing the wound primarily under antibiotic cover.[51] The latter is the preferred management method, as it produces a much more satisfactory cosmetic outcome.[51]

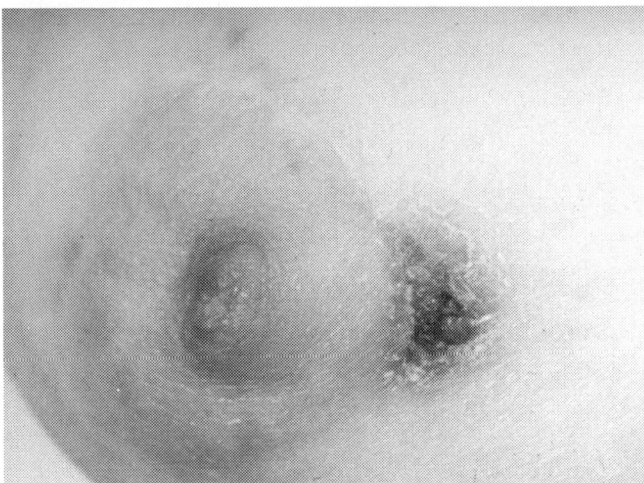

FIG. 5. Mammary duct fistula. The fistula is discharging in the periareolar region at one end of a circumareolar scar, which is at the site of a previous abscess drainage. The affected duct is pulled toward the fistula site scar.

Peripheral Nonlactational Breast Abscess

Peripheral nonlactational breast abscesses are less common than periareolar abscesses and are often associated with an underlying disease state, such as diabetes, rheumatoid arthritis, steroid treatment, or trauma.[52] *S. aureus* is the organism usually responsible, but some abscesses contain anaerobic organisms. Peripheral nonlactational breast abscesses are three times more common in premenopausal women than in menopausal or postmenopausal women. Systemic evidence of malaise and fever is usually absent. Management is the same as for lactational abscesses, with aspiration or incision and drainage.

Skin Associated Infection

Cellulitis of the breast with or without abscess formation is common, particularly in patients who are overweight, have large breasts, or have had previous surgery or radiotherapy.[44] It is most common in the lower one-half of the breast, where sweat accumulates and intertrigo develops. *S. aureus* is the organism most commonly responsible for skin infection. Skin-associated infection can also occur in association with sebaceous cysts in the skin over the breast or can be seen in association with hidradenitis suppurativa.[53] Women with hidradenitis become infected with the same organisms seen in periductal sepsis (see Table 1). Excision of the affected skin and grafting is effective in up to 50% of cases.[44] For some women with large breasts and recurrent skin infection, reduction mammoplasty can be effective at preventing further episodes of infection.

Acute episodes of infection should be treated with appropriate antibiotics, and when an abscess is present, aspiration or incision and drainage should be performed. In patients with recurrent infections affecting the lower one-half of the breast, the area should be kept as clean and dry as possible; the area should be washed twice a day, creams and talcum powders should be avoided, and cotton bras or a cotton T-shirt or vest worn inside the bra should be used.[44]

Other Rare Infections

Tuberculosis

Tuberculosis is rare in Western countries. The breast can be the primary site, but tuberculosis more commonly reaches the breast through lymphatic spread from axillary, mediastinal, or cervical nodes or directly from underlying structures, such as the ribs. Tuberculosis predominantly affects women in the latter part of their childbearing years. An axillary or breast sinus is present in up to 50% of patients. The most common presentation is that of an acute abscess resulting from infection of an area of tuberculosis by pyogenic organisms.[44] Treatment is with local surgery and antitubercular drug therapy.

Granulomatous Lobular Mastitis

Granulomatous lobular mastitis is characterized by non-caseating granulomata and microabscesses confined to the breast lobule.[54,55] The condition presents as a firm mass, which is often indistinguishable from breast cancer, or as multiple or recurrent abscesses. Young, parous women are most frequently affected. Although organisms can be found in these lesions, they do not appear to have a primary causative role.[55] In patients presenting with a breast mass, once a diagnosis is established by cytologic examination of fine-needle aspirate or core biopsy, excision of the mass should be avoided, as it is often followed by persistent wound discharge and failure of the wound to heal. Any abscesses that develop require aspiration or mini-incision and drainage. Some patients with granulomatous lobular mastitis report that their breasts are tender. A strong tendency is seen for this condition to recur, but eventually it does spontaneously resolve without treatment.[44] The cause is unknown. Steroids have been tried without consistent success.[55]

Factitial Disease

Cases of factitious abscess are occasionally seen. These patients generally have psychiatric problems, but some cases can appear quite plausible. Factitial disease should be suspected when peripheral abscesses persist or recur despite appropriate treatment.[53] The condition can be difficult to treat, as patients are often resistant to help and may be very manipulative.

REFERENCES

1. Dixon JM, Mansel RE. Symptoms, assessment and guidelines for referral. ABC of breast diseases. *BMJ* 1994;309:722.
2. Ambrogetti D, Berni D, Catarzi S, Ciatto S. The role of ductal galactography in the differential diagnosis of breast carcinoma. *Radiologia Medica* 1996;91:198.
3. Kleinberg D, Noel G, Frantz A. Galactorrhoea: a study of 235 cases including 48 with pituitary tumors. *N Engl J Med* 1977;296:589.
4. Selzer MH, Perloff LJ, Kelley RI, Fitts WT. Significance of age in patients with nipple discharge. *Surg Gynecol Obstet* 1970;131:519.
5. Groves AM, Carr M, Wadhera V, Lennard TWJ. An audit of cytology in the evaluation of nipple discharge: a retrospective study of 10 years' experience. *Breast* 1996;5:96.
6. Van Zee KJ, Ortega Perez G, Minnard E, Cohen MA. Preoperative galactography increases the diagnostic yield of major duct excision for nipple discharge. *Cancer* 1998;82:1874.
7. Chetty U. Nipple discharge. In: Smallwood JA, Taylor I, eds. *Benign breast disease*. London: Edward Arnold, 1990:85.
8. Hughes LE, Mansel RE, Webster DJT. Nipple discharge. In: *Benign disorders and diseases of the breast: concepts and clinical management*. London: Bailliere Tindall, 1989:142.
9. Locker AP, Galea MH, Ellis IO, et al. Microdochectomy for single-duct discharge from the nipple. *Br J Surg* 1988;75:700.
10. Sartorius OW, Smith HS, Morris P, Benedict D, Friesen L. Cytologic evaluation of breast fluid in the detection of breast disease. *J Natl Cancer Inst* 1977;59:1073.
11. Wynder EL, Hill P, Laakso K, Lettner R, Kettrinen K. Breast secretion in Finnish women. *Cancer* 1981;47:1444.
12. Haagensen CD, Bodian C, Haagensen DE. *Breast carcinoma risk and detection*. Philadelphia: WB Saunders, 1981:146.
13. Page DL, Anderson TJ. *Diagnostic histopathology of the breast*. Edinburgh, UK: Churchill Livingstone, 1987.
14. Rosen PP, Holmes G, Lesser ML, Kinne DW, Beattie EJ. Juvenile papillomatosis and breast carcinoma. *Cancer* 1985;55:1345.
15. Bazzocchi F, Santini D, Martinelli G, et al. Juvenile papillomatosis (epitheliosis) of the breast: a clinical and pathologic study of 13 cases. *Am J Clin Pathol* 1986;86:745.
16. Rosen PP, Cantrell B, Mullen DL, DePalo A. Juvenile papillomatosis (Swiss cheese disease) of the breast. *Am J Surg Pathol* 1980;4:3.
17. Bonser GM, Dossett JA, Jull JW. *Human and experimental breast cancer*. London: Pitman Medical, 1961.
18. Ito Y, Tamaki Y, Nakano Y, et al. Nonpalpable breast cancer with nipple discharge: how should it be treated? *Anticancer Res* 1997;17:791.
19. Fung A, Rayter Z, Fisher C, et al. Preoperative cytology and mammography in patients with single-duct nipple discharge treated by surgery. *Br J Surg* 1990;77:1211.
20. Welsh M, Durrant D, Gonzales J, et al. Microdochectomy for discharge from single lactiferous duct. *Br J Surg* 1990;77:1213.
21. Kline TS, Lash SR. The bleeding nipple of pregnancy and postpartum: a cytologic and histologic study. *Am J Pathol* 1964;8:336.
22. Lafreniere R. Bloody nipple discharge during pregnancy: a rationale for conservative treatment. *J Surg Oncol* 1990;43:228.
23. Haagensen CD. Mammary-duct ectasia: a disease which may simulate carcinoma. *Cancer* 1951;4:749.
24. Bonser GM, Dossett JA, Jull JW. *Human and experimental breast cancer*. London: Pitman Medical 1961:237.
25. Dixon JM. Periductal mastitis/duct ectasia. *World J Surg* 1989; 13:715.
26. Dixon JM, Ravi Sekar O, Chetty U, Anderson TJ. Periductal mastitis and duct ectasia: different conditions with different aetiologies. *Br J Surg* 1996;83:820.
27. Dixon JM. Duct surgery: microdochectomy and total duct excision. In: Dixon JM, Veronesi U, Kinne D, eds. *Operative breast surgery*. Edinburgh, UK: Churchill Livingstone, 1999 (*in press*).
28. Rees BI, Gravelle IH, Hughes LE. Nipple retraction in duct ectasia. *Br J Surg* 1977;64:577.
29. Dixon JM, Anderson TJ, Lumsden AB, Elton RA, Roberts MM, Forrest APM. Mammary duct ectasia. *Br J Surg* 1983;70:60.
30. Frantz VK, Pickren JW, Melcher GW, Auchincloss H. Incidence of chronic cystic disease in so-called normal breast. *Cancer* 1950;4:762.
31. Bundred NJ, Dixon JM, Lumsden AB, et al. Are the lesions of duct ectasia sterile? *Br J Surg* 1985;72:844.
32. Aitken RJ, Hood J, Going JJ, Miles RS, Forrest APM. Bacteriology of mammary duct ectasia. *Br J Surg* 1988;75:1040.
33. Schafer P, Furrer G, Mermillod B. An association of cigarette smoking with recurrent subareolar breast abscesses. *Int J Epidemiol* 1988;17:810.

34. Bundred NJ, Dover MS, Coley S, Morrison JM. Breast abscesses and cigarette smoking. *Br J Surg* 1992;79:58.
35. Bundred NJ, Dover MS, Aluwihare N, Faragher EB, Morrison JM. Smoking and periductal mastitis. *BMJ* 1993;307:772.
36. Wynder EL, Hill P. Nicotine and cotinine in breast fluid. *Cancer Lett* 1979;6:251.
37. Petrakis NL, Maack CA, Lee RE, Lyer M. Mutagenic activity of nipple aspirates of breast fluid. *Cancer Res* 1980;40:188.
38. Ertel A, Eng R, Smith SM. The differential effect of cigarette smoke on the growth of bacteria found in humans. *Chest* 1991;100:628.
39. Bundred NJ. Surgical management of periductal mastitis. *Breast* 1988;7:79.
40. Dixon JM, Sainsbury JRC, Rodger A. Breast cancer: treatment of elderly patients and uncommon conditions. ABC of breast diseases. *BMJ* 1994;309:1292.
41. Kalbhen CL, Kezdi-Rogus PC, Dowling MP, Flisak ME. Mammography in the evaluation of nipple inversion. *AJR Am J Roentgenol* 1998;170:117.
42. Dixon JM, Kohlhardt SR, Dillon P. Total duct excision. *Breast* 1998; 7:216.
43. Dixon JM. Breast surgery. In: Taylor EW, ed. *Infection in surgical practice*. Oxford, UK: Oxford Medical Publications, 1992:187.
44. Dixon JM. Breast infection. ABC of breast diseases. *BMJ* 1994;309:946.
45. Hughes LE, Mansel RE, Webster DJT. Infection of the breast. In: *Benign disorders and diseases of the breast: current concepts and clinical management*. London: Bailliere Tindall, 1989:143.
46. Dixon JM. Repeated aspiration of breast abscesses in lactating women. *BMJ* 1988;297:1517.
47. Dixon JM. Periductal mastitis and duct ectasia: an update. *Breast* 1998;7:128.
48. Dixon JM, Lee ECG, Greenall MJ. Treatment of periareolar inflammation associated with periductal mastitis using metronidazole and flucloxacillin: a preliminary report. *Br J Clin Pract* 1988;42:78.
49. Bundred NJ, Dixon JM, Chetty U, Forrest APM. Mammillary fistula. *Br J Surg* 1987;74:466.
50. Atkins HJB. Mammillary fistula. *BMJ* 1955;2:1473.
51. Dixon JM, Thompson AM. Effective surgical treatment for mammillary fistula. *Br J Surg* 1991;78:1185.
52. Rogers K. Breast abscess and problems with lactation. In: Smallwood JA, Taylor I, eds. *Benign breast disease*. London: Edward Arnold, 1990:96.
53. Hughes LE, Mansel RE, Webster DJT. Miscellaneous conditions. In: *Benign disorders and disease of the breast: current concepts and clinical management*. London: Bailliere Tindall, 1989:175.
54. Going JJ, Anderson TJ, Wilkinson S, Chetty U. Granulomatous lobular mastitis. *J Clin Pathol* 1987;40:535.
55. Howell JD, Barker F, Gazet J-C. Granulomatous lobular mastitis: report of a further two cases and a comprehensive literature review. *Breast* 1994;3:119.

Diseases of the Breast, 2nd ed.,
edited by Jay R. Harris.
Lippincott Williams & Wilkins, Philadelphia © 2000.

CHAPTER 6

Management of Breast Pain

Ian S. Fentiman

Breast pain is a common problem in the setting of both primary care and breast clinics. For the majority of women, it is a self-limiting condition that requires no treatment other than reassurance. Nevertheless, in a few cases, severe, prolonged cyclical or noncyclical breast pain may cause major disturbance to social, sexual, and working aspects of life. A survey of women interviewed at a mammographic screening indicates that 69% experienced severe breast pain, but only 3% sought treatment.[1] Confronted with patients complaining of breast pain, clinicians have to determine whether it arises from a mammary or an extramammary source. If the problem originates from the breast, further management depends on its nature, severity, and duration. Only rarely are specific endocrine interventions required, but, after appropriate patient selection, some may derive great benefit from treatment. Devil's advocates suggest that, because no consistent histologic, endocrine, or behavioral factors have been identified in women with severe breast pain, and because no good measures of assessment are available, cyclical mastalgia, such as fibroadenosis, is not a clinical condition.[2] The Atlantic has been the main divide, with many American surgeons being skeptical, so that almost all the randomized trials of treatment have been carried out in Europe.

ETIOLOGY

In premenopausal women, breast fullness is an almost invariable event in the late luteal phase of the cycle, sometimes associated with discomfort or pain. Cyclical mastalgia is a more extreme form of this change; hence, many studies have sought endocrine abnormalities in those with severe breast pain, particularly examining estradiol, progesterone, and prolactin. Sitruk-Ware et al.[3] suggest that inadequate corpus luteal function is an etiologic factor in women with benign breast disease. The term *benign breast disease* has been used as a *portmanteau* into which all nonmalignant breast conditions have been cast, thereby blurring the distinction between a variety of benign breast conditions.[4] The Cardiff group has proposed a classification of benign conditions, aberrations of normal development and involution, in which mastalgia is a benign disorder that arises from hormonal activity.[5]

When Walsh and associates[6] measured serum progesterone levels in women with and without breast pain, they found no evidence of deficiency during the luteal phase in those with mastalgia. No consistent abnormality of estradiol has been reported in women with cyclical mastalgia, with some finding normal levels[7] and others reporting elevation of estradiol during the luteal phase.[8] In terms of prolactin, baseline levels have been reported as either normal or marginally elevated,[7,8] but when prolactin storage was measured after domperidone stimulation, significantly elevated levels were found in those with severe cyclical mastalgia.[9] This may be a preexisting abnormality, but it could represent a stress response to prolonged pain.

CLASSIFICATION

Based on a series of patients treated at a breast pain clinic, Preece et al.[10] proposed a classification with six subgroups: cyclical mastalgia, duct ectasia, Tietze's syndrome, trauma, sclerosing adenosis, and cancer. Subsequently, this was simplified by dividing patients with noncyclical pain into two groups: those with true noncyclical breast pain and those with other causes of chest wall pain.[11] Although an accurate diagnosis should be achieved on the basis of history and examination, patients with breast pain can simply be assigned to one of three groups: cyclical breast pain, noncyclical breast pain, or extramammary pain.[12]

EVALUATION

Important aspects of history-taking from women with breast pain include the type of pain, relationship to menses, duration, location, and nature of any other medical problems. It is important to establish whether the patient's main concern is that her symptoms are due to sinister underlying breast pathology or, alternatively, that she is

I. S. Fentiman: Department of Surgical Oncology, Hedley Atkins Breast Unit, Guy's Hospital, London, England, United Kingdom

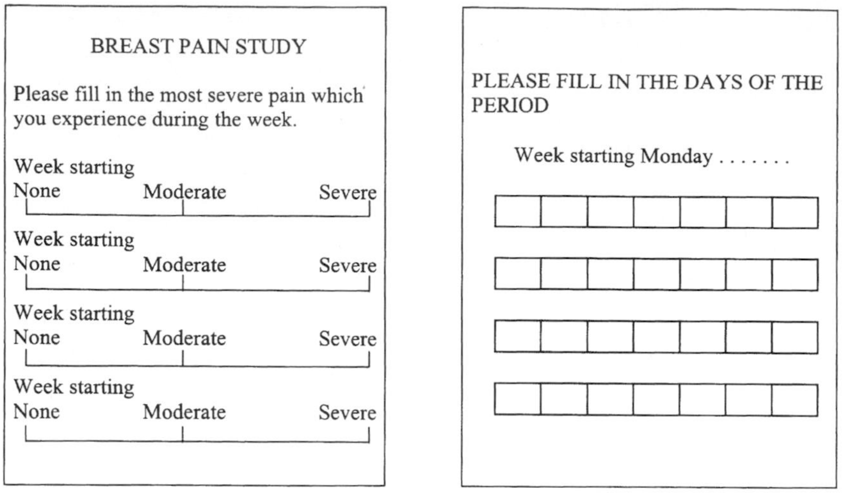

BREAST PAIN STUDY

Please fill in the most severe pain which you experience during the week.

Week starting
None Moderate Severe

Week starting
None Moderate Severe

Week starting
None Moderate Severe

Week starting
None Moderate Severe

PLEASE FILL IN THE DAYS OF THE PERIOD

Week starting Monday . . . .

FIG. 1. Guy's Hospital breast pain chart (obverse and reverse).

sufficiently affected by the pain that she wants some specific treatment. In almost all cases, the former consideration predominates.

The first aspect of the breast examination after inspection should be a very gentle palpation of the breasts once the patient has indicated the site(s) of the pain. After this first check, to exclude discrete masses, a more probing evaluation should be performed, focusing on the site(s) of pain. After turning the patient half on her side, so that the breast tissue falls away from the chest wall, it is often possible to identify, particularly in postmenopausal women, that the pain is arising from the underlying rib and indeed to reproduce the pain (once) with a fingertip on the affected rib. This can demonstrate to the patient that the pain is extramammary in origin.

In women with severe mastalgia, nodularity may be associated with the pain, but the extent of nodularity bears no relation to the extent of the pain, and some women who are severely distressed with pain may have minimal signs other than exquisite tenderness. If it is apparent that the pain, whether cyclical or noncyclical, is mammary in origin, the decision to treat is based on the subjective assessment of pain together with the duration of symptoms. Unless the pain has been present for a minimum of 6 months, treatment should be by reassurance alone. If the patient still wishes to have treatment, she should be given a pain analogue card to complete, keeping a daily or weekly record of pain and also the menstrual history. The card used at Guy's Hospital is shown in Fig. 1. For simplicity, the patient is asked to give a weekly analogue score on a 10-cm scale of her most severe pain and to indicate the days of menstruation, when appropriate. It is important to note that a disproportionate number of women with breast pain have had a previous hysterectomy, so the menstrual relationship of the pain may not be apparent.[13]

ROLE OF RADIOLOGY

The average age of women entered into trials of treatment for severe mastalgia is 32 years. Under these circumstances, mammography would not be used as a standard adjunct to clinical evaluation. Additionally, in the absence of a discrete lump or localized nodularity, ultrasound is unlikely to yield information of clinical value. Breast pain associated with a lump needs evaluation on its own merits. Women older than age 35 usually have mammography as part of their workup, although there is no evidence to show that this is of value in either detection of breast cancer or reduction in mortality from the disease in premenopausal women. No specific radiologic signs are associated with mastalgia, although very rarely a subclinical carcinoma is found to be the underlying cause of the pain.[14]

MONDOR'S DISEASE

Mondor's disease is a rare cause of breast pain, with clinical features of local pain associated with a tender, palpable subcutaneous cord or linear skin dimpling[15] (see Fig. 3-3). The cause is superficial thrombophlebitis of the lateral thoracic vein or a tributary thereof. Almost invariably, the condition resolves spontaneously, but nonsteroidal antiinflammatory drugs may help to relieve symptoms. Mondor's disease may cause serious alarm for some patients who assume that the skin tethering is secondary to an underlying carcinoma, and they are greatly relieved when informed of the benign nature of the condition.

In a series of 63 cases of Mondor's disease, no underlying pathology was found in 31 cases.[16] Of the remaining 32, local trauma or surgical intervention was responsible in 15 (47%), an inflammatory process in six (19%), and carcinoma in eight (25%). In view of this, mammography should be carried out in women with Mondor's disease who are age 35 or older to exclude an impalpable breast cancer.

PSYCHOSOCIAL ASPECTS

Surgeons, such as Sir Hedley Atkins and David Patey, who originally studied women with breast pain, believed that most of these patients had a psychological basis for their symptoms.[17,18] Preece and associates[19] used the Middlesex Hospital questionnaire to compare patients with mastalgia, psychiatric patients, and women undergoing varicose vein surgery. This instrument measured personality type rather than mood and did not show any significant difference between those undergoing varicose vein surgery and those with mastalgia, although a subgroup with treatment-resistant pain had morbidity similar to that of psychiatric patients. In a subsequent study of 25 women with severe mastalgia, using the Composite International Diagnostic Interview, a total of 45 diagnoses were made in 21 patients (84%): anxiety (17), panic disorder (5), somatization disorder (7), and major depression (16).[20]

Using the Hospital Anxiety and Depression scale (HAD), Downey and associates[21] found high levels of both anxiety and depression in 20 women with severe mastalgia compared with 12 symptom-free control subjects. The HAD scale was also used in a series of 54 women with mastalgia seen at Guy's Hospital.[22] Of these, 33 had severe mastalgia, with levels of anxiety and depression similar to those seen in women with breast cancer on the morning of their surgery. Fox and colleagues[23] conducted a randomized trial of 45 women with mastalgia that warranted treatment; all of these patients kept a pain diary for 12 weeks, with half the women randomized to listen daily to a relaxation tape during weeks 5 to 8. Abnormal or borderline HAD scores were found at entry in 54%. Complete or substantial reduction in analogue pain score was measured in 25% of the control group and 61% of those randomized to relaxation therapy (p <.005).

TREATMENT TRIALS

A variety of agents have been used in women with "benign breast disease," some of whom had nothing more than nodularity with or without some tenderness. In terms of assessment of quality of studies, women with well-defined cases who had breast pain should have been entered and measured with visual analogue scales (VAS), using each patient as her own control. Because of relatively high spontaneous remission rates, pain should have been present for a minimum of 6 months. Trials should be of double-blind, placebo-controlled randomized design and include a minimum of 20 patients. Many trials have met these criteria and have shown those drugs or interventions that can significantly reduce cyclical mastalgia.

Danazol, an antigonadotropin that acts as an impeded androgen, may relieve pain in up to 93% of cases.[24,25] Unfortunately, this is achieved in the face of side effects, including nausea, depression, menstrual irregularity, and headaches, which occur in up to two-thirds of patients and sometimes lead to discontinuation of treatment. Bromocriptine, a prolactin inhibitor, can also significantly reduce mastalgia.[26–28] In a multicenter European study of 272 women that compared bromocriptine, 2.5 mg twice a day, with placebo, significant symptom relief occurred in those who received active treatment, but 29% dropped out because of side effects, particularly nausea and dizziness.[29] Hinton and associates[30] conducted a double-blind study in 47 women with severe breast pain who were treated with either danazol, bromocriptine, or placebo. Those who received bromocriptine and danazol had significantly better pain relief than those given placebo, but the danazol-treated group demonstrated the best response as measured by VAS.

Because progesterone deficiency has been reported as being responsible for mastalgia, the efficacy of progesterone vaginal cream has been investigated in two randomized trials.[31,32] In a trial comprised of 32 women, McFadyen and associates[31] reported a small but nonsignificant benefit for those women given the placebo cream. In a larger trial with 80 participants, a greater than 50% reduction in pain on VAS was recorded in 22% of the placebo group and in 65% of those who received progesterone-containing cream.[32] Maddox and colleagues[33] compared medroxyprogesterone acetate tablets, 20 mg per day, in the luteal phase of the cycle with placebo and found no difference in response rate or side effects in 26 women. In a multicenter, double-blind randomized trial, Peters[34] administered the synthetic 19-norsteroid gestrinone to 73 women and placebo to 72 others, all of whom had cyclical mastalgia. As assessed by VAS, a significantly greater reduction in breast pain was seen in the gestrinone group. Side effects were reported by 44% of the treated patients and 14% of the control group.

The agent tamoxifen, a partial antiestrogen and partial estrogen agonist, has been shown to be effective in treating breast pain. An outline of the randomized trials and results is given in Table 1.[35–40] In the first double-blind, crossover randomized trial that was conducted at Guy's Hospital, pain relief occurred in 71% of those given tamoxifen and 38% of patients who received placebo.[35] After 3 months, nonresponders switched to the alternate treatment arm, and mastalgia pain control was achieved in 75% of those who received tamoxifen and 33% of those given placebo. The most common side effect of tamoxifen was hot flashes, which occurred in 27%.

A similar placebo response was seen in the trial run by Messinis and Lolis,[36] but among the group that received tamoxifen, 10 mg, breast pain was controlled in 89%. In two trials that compared tamoxifen, 10 mg, with 20 mg, similar response rates were seen, but side effects in those given the lower dose were substantially reduced (21% versus 64%).[13,37] When tamoxifen was compared with danazol, similar response rates were seen, but Powles and associates[38] reported significantly more side effects in those given danazol (90% versus 50%). Kontostolis and colleagues[39] reported

TABLE 1. *Randomized trials of tamoxifen in women with mastalgia*

Design	Response rate	Response rate	Response rate	Reference
Tamoxifen, 20 mg vs placebo	Tamoxifen 22/31 (71%)	Placebo 11/29 (38%)	—	35
Tamoxifen, 10 mg vs placebo	Tamoxifen 16/18 (89%)	Placebo 6/16 (38%)	—	36
Tamoxifen, 10 mg vs 20 mg	10 mg 26/29 (90%)	20 mg 24/28 (86%)	—	13
Tamoxifen, 10 mg vs 20 mg	10 mg 127/155 (82%)	20 mg 107/142 (75%)	—	37
Tamoxifen, 20 mg, vs danazol, 100 mg	20 mg 24/25(96%)	100 mg 23/25 (92%)	—	38
Tamoxifen, 10 mg, vs danazol vs placebo	10 mg 23/32 (72%)	Danazol 21/32 (66%)	Placebo 11/29 (38%)	39
Tamoxifen, 10 mg, vs bromocriptine, 7.5 mg	10 mg 18/20 (90%)	7.5 mg 17/20(85%)	—	40

hot flashes in 25% of those given tamoxifen, 10 mg, and weight gain in 31% of the danazol-treated group.

Several agents have been tested in controlled trials and found to be no better than placebo. These include vitamin E,[41] lynestrenol,[42] mefenamic acid,[43] and caffeine reduction.[44] As an alternative, more complex approach, reduction in dietary fat can significantly reduce cyclical breast pain.[45] Boyd and associates[45] entered 21 women with a minimum of 5 years of breast pain into a trial in which 11 were shown how to reduce their dietary fat content to 15% of total calories and 10 received general dietary advice. Those who were in the fat-reduction group had a significant reduction in breast pain, as measured by their daily diary. Although a nondrug intervention may appeal to some patients, long-term dietary change may be unacceptable to many others. The long chain fatty acid gamma-linolenic acid, present in evening primrose oil (EPO) and starflower oil, may provide a nonendocrine approach but with an efficacy that is still in dispute. Preece and colleagues[46] entered 103 women with mastalgia into a double-blind crossover study comparing EPO with placebo for 3 months, after which both groups received EPO capsules for a further 3 months. Only 72 patients were assessable, of whom 41 had cyclical and 31 had noncyclical mastalgia. Cyclical pain was significantly diminished in those given EPO, but no effect was seen in those with noncyclical mastalgia.

MANAGEMENT

The essentials of management of women with breast pain are to exclude the presence of serious underlying pathology, make a diagnosis, and communicate this to the patient in simple terms so that reassurance is achieved for the majority (Fig. 2). Only a small proportion, fewer than 10% of women with mastalgia, have problems of such severity and duration that specific treatment is necessary. For patients with moderate or severe pain that has been present for less than 6 months, there is still a high probability of spontaneous remission after reassurance, and specific treatment other than gamma-linolenic acid should not be given. The small group with severe prolonged pain should be encouraged to keep a pain chart and return after 6 weeks. If the pain persists, treatment should be started with either tamoxifen or danazol. The former has fewer side effects and can be very effective but is not licensed specifically for treatment of mastalgia. Nevertheless, tamoxifen can be prescribed for women with no abnormality other than a family history of breast cancer; therefore, using this drug for severe breast pain is a very reasonable approach. Treatment should be given at a dosage of 10 mg per day for 3 months. If this achieves pain relief, the dose can be further reduced to 10 mg on alternate days for a further 3 months. For the few who do not respond, a higher dosage of 20 mg per day should be given. The very few who do not respond to this treatment should be switched to danazol or bromocriptine, but there is little likelihood of response. Severely distressed women who have not responded to any treatment may ask for mastectomy. This course of action should not be undertaken before a full psychiatric assessment has been sought. Without careful selection, surgical intervention can damage body image without achieving relief of the pain.

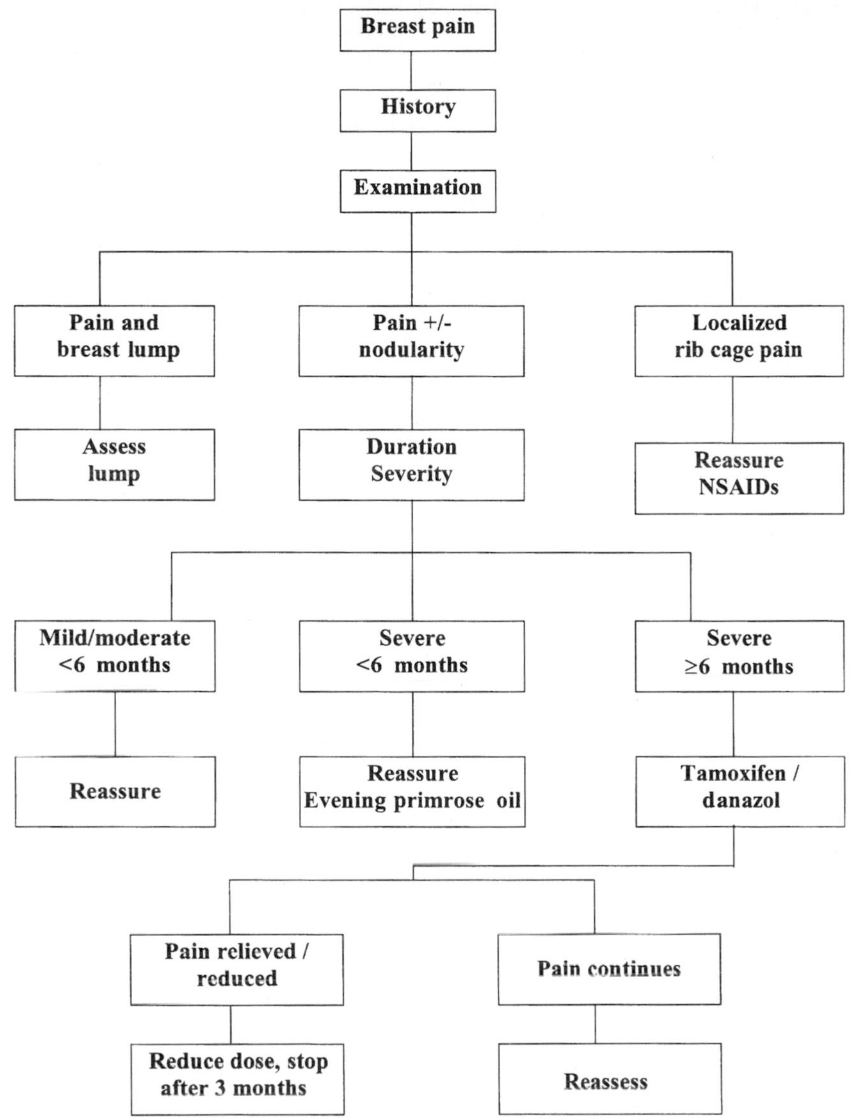

FIG. 2. Management of women with breast pain. NSAIDs, nonsteroidal antiinflammatory drugs.

REFERENCES

1. Leinster SJ, Whitehouse GH, Walsh PV. Cyclical mastalgia; clinical and mammographic observations in a screened population. *Br J Surg* 1987;74:220.
2. Love SM, Gelman RS, Silen W. Fibrocystic "disease" of the breast—a nondisease. *N Engl J Med* 1982;307:1010.
3. Sitruk-Ware LR, Sterkers N, Mowszowics I, Mauvais-Jarvis P. Inadequate corpus luteal function in women with benign breast disease. *J Clin Endocrinol Metab* 1977;44:771.
4. Wang DY, Fentiman IS. Epidemiology and endocrinology of benign breast disease. *Breast Cancer Res Treat* 1985;6:5.
5. Hughes LE, Mansel RE, Webster DJT. Aberrations of normal development and involution (ANDI): a new perspective on pathogenesis and nomenclature of benign breast disorders. *Lancet* 1987;2:1316.
6. Walsh PV, Bulbrook RD, Stell PM, Wang DY, McDicken IW, George WD. Serum progesterone concentration during the luteal phase in women with benign breast disease. *Eur J Cancer Clin Oncol* 1984;20:1339.
7. Watt-Boolsen S, Andersen AN, Blichert-Toft M. Serum prolactin and oestradiol levels in women with cyclical mastalgia. *Horm Metab Res* 1981;13:700.
8. Walsh PV, McDicken IW, Bulbrook RD, Moore JW, Taylor WH, George WD. Serum oestradiol-17β and prolactin concentrations during the luteal phase in women with benign breast disease. *Eur J Cancer Clin Oncol* 1984;20:1345.
9. Kumar S, Mansel RE, Hughes LE, et al. Prolactin response to thyrotropin-releasing hormone stimulation and dopaminergic inhibition in benign breast disease. *Cancer* 1984;53:1311.
10. Preece PE, Hughes LE, Mansel RE, Baum M, Bolton PM, Gravelle IH. Clinical syndromes of mastalgia. *Lancet* 1976;2:670.

11. Maddox PR, Harrison BJ, Mansel RE, Hughes LE. Non-cyclical mastalgia: an improved classification and treatment. *Br J Surg* 1989;76:901.
12. Fentiman IS. Tamoxifen and mastalgia: an emerging indication. *Drugs* 1986;32:477.
13. Fentiman IS, Caleffi M, Hamed H, Chaudary MA. Dosage and duration of tamoxifen treatment for mastalgia: a controlled trial. *Br J Surg* 1988:75:845.
14. Preece PE, Baum M, Mansel RE, et al. Importance of mastalgia in operable breast cancer. *BMJ* 1982;284:1299.
15. Mondor H. Tronculite sous-cutane subaigue de la paroi thoracique antéro-latérale. *Mem Acad Chir Paris* 1939;65:1271.
16. Catania S, Zurrida S, Veronesi P, Galimberti V, Bono A, Pluchinotta A. Mondor's disease and breast cancer. *Cancer* 1992;69:2267.
17. Atkins HJB. Chronic mastitis. *Lancet* 1938;1:707.
18. Patey DH. Two common non-malignant conditions of the breast. The clinical features of cystic disease and the pain syndrome. *BMJ* 1949; 1:96.
19. Preece PE, Mansel RE, Hughes LE. Mastalgia: psychoneurosis or organic disease? *BMJ* 1978;1:29.
20. Jenkins PL, Jamil N, Gateley C, Mansel RE. Psychiatric illness in patients with severe treatment-resistant mastalgia. *Gen Hosp Psych* 1993;15:55.
21. Downey HM, Deadman JM, Davis C, Leinster SJ. Psychological characteristics of women with cyclicai mastalgia. *Breast Dis* 1993; 6:99.
22. Ramirez AJ, Jarrett SR, Hamed H, Smith P, Fentiman IS. Psychological adjustment of women with mastalgia. *Breast* 1995;4:48.
23. Fox H, Walker LG, Heys SD, Ah-See AK, Eremin O. Are patients with mastalgia anxious, and does relaxation help? *Breast* 1997;6:138.
24. Mansel RE, Wisbey JR, Hughes LE. Controlled trial of the antigonadotrophin danazol in painful nodular benign breast disease. *Lancet* 1982;1:928.
25. Doberl A, Tobiassen T, Rasmussen T. Treatment of recurrent cyclical mastodynia in patients with fibrocystic breast disease. *Acta Obstet Gynecol Scand Suppl* 1984;123:177.
26. Mansel RE, Preece PE, Hughes LE. A double-blind trial of the prolactin inhibitor bromocriptine in painful benign breast disease. *Br J Surg* 1978;65:724.
27. Blichert-Toft M, Nyobe Andersen AN, Hendriksen OB, Mygind T. Treatment of mastalgia with bromocriptine: a double-blind cross-over study. *BMJ* 1979;1:237.
28. Durning P, Sellwood RA. Bromocriptine in severe cyclical breast pain. *Br J Surg* 1982;69:248.
29. Mansel RE, Dogliotti L. European multicentre trial of bromocriptine in cyclical mastalgia. *Lancet* 1990;335:190.
30. Hinton CP, Bishop HM, Holliday HW, Doyle PJ, Blamey RW. A double-blind controlled trial of danazol and bromocriptine in the management of severe cyclical breast pain. *Br J Clin Prac* 1986;40:326.
31. McFadyen IJ, Raab GM, Macintyre CCA, Forrest APM. Progesterone cream for cyclic breast pain. *BMJ* 1989;298:931.
32. Nappi C, Affinito P, Di Carlo C, Esposito G, Montemagno U. Double-blind controlled trial of progesterone vaginal cream treatment for cyclical mastodynia in women with benign breast disease. *J Endocrinol Invest* 1992;15:801.
33. Maddox PR, Harrison BJ, Horobin JM, et al. A randomised controlled trial of medroxyprogesterone acetate in mastalgia. *Ann R Coll Surg Engl* 1990;72:71.
34. Peters F. Multicentre study of gestrinone in cyclical breast pain. *Lancet* 1992;339:205.
35. Fentiman IS, Caleffi M, Brame K, Chaudary MA, Hayward JL. Double-blind controlled trial of tamoxifen therapy for mastalgia. *Lancet* 1986;1:287.
36. Messinis IE, Lolis D. Treatment of premenstrual mastalgia with tamoxifen. *Acta Obstet Gynecol Scand* 1988;67:307.
37. GEMB (Grupo de Estudio de Mastopatias Benignas). Tamoxifen therapy for cyclical mastalgia: dose randomized trial. *Breast* 1997;5:212.
38. Powles TJ, Ford HT, Gazet J-C. A randomised trial to compare tamoxifen with danazol for treatment of benign mammary dysplasia. *Breast Dis* 1987;2:1.
39. Kontostolis E, Stefanidis K, Navrozoglou I, Lolis D. Comparison of tamoxifen with danazol for treatment of cyclical mastalgia. *Gynecol Endocrinol* 1997;11:393.
40. Sandrucci S, Mussa A, Festa V, Borrè A, Grosso M, Dogliotti L. Comparison of tamoxifen and bromocriptine in management of fibrocystic breast disease: a randomized blind study. *Ann N Y Acad Sci* 1990;586:626.
41. Ernster VL, Goodson WH, Hunt TK, Petrakis NL, Sickles EA, Miike R. Vitamin E and benign breast "disease": a double-blind randomized trial. *Surgery* 1984;97:490.
42. Colin C, Gaspard U, Lambotte R. Relationship of mastodynia with its endocrine environment and treatment in a double-blind trial with lynestrenol. *Arch Gynakol* 1978;225:7.
43. Gunston KD. Premenstrual syndrome in Capetown. Part II. A double-blind placebo-controlled study of the efficacy of mefenamic acid. *S Afr Med J* 1986;70:159.
44. Ernster VL, Mason L, Goodson WH, et al. Effects of caffeine-free diet on benign breast disease: a randomized trial. *Surgery* 1982;91:263.
45. Boyd NF, Shannon P, Kriukov V, et al. Effect of a low-fat high-carbohydrate diet on symptoms of cyclical mastopathy. *Lancet* 1988;2:128.
46. Preece PE, Hanslip JI, Gilbert L, et al. Evening primrose oil (Efamol) for mastalgia. In: Horrobin D, ed. *Clinical uses of essential fatty acids.* Montreal: Eden Press, 1982.

Diseases of the Breast, 2nd ed.,
edited by Jay R. Harris.
Lippincott Williams & Wilkins, Philadelphia © 2000.

CHAPTER 7

Abnormalities of the Breast in Pregnancy and Lactation

Jeanne A. Petrek

CLINICAL BREAST EXAMINATION

The finding of a thickness or possible mass on physical examination during pregnancy brings different considerations than in the nonpregnant young woman. In the menstruating woman, one often reexamines the patient just after her next menstrual period(s). In the pregnant woman, however, no cycle exists, and the hormonal milieu intensifies steadily, causing greater breast volume and firmness. A follow-up physical examination in a pregnant woman in 2 to 4 weeks for a questionable or suspicious area is advisable (Fig. 1).

If the opportunity presents itself before pregnancy, a careful physical examination and a baseline (or interval screening) mammography, as indicated by a patient's age and risk factors, are helpful and reassuring during the subsequent pregnancy. The more common circumstance is the chance to perform a thorough breast examination at the first obstetric visit when the breasts have undergone the least physiologic changes. With progression of pregnancy, the breasts increase greatly in volume, firmness, and nodularity, which is the reason for a short-interval follow-up on physical examination of any questionable area. As the pregnancy continues, the mass may feel similar to the normal hypertrophic thickness, or the mass may be deeper in the breast due to the generalized greater volume, causing it to be nonpalpable.

BREAST IMAGING

It has been conventional wisdom that mammograms are not routinely performed, since little information can be gained. It is intuitive that the increased vascularity, cellularity, and water content of the pregnant breast and the additional presence of milk in the lactating breast would all contribute to a generalized radiographic parenchymal density with loss of the contrasting fatty tissue. However, a small 1998 series compared the mammograms of 18 women who were pregnant, currently lactating, or recently lactating with mammograms obtained before pregnancy in the same women.[1] Using the four categories of breast density from the Breast Imaging Reporting and Data System, surprisingly few women had an increased density category compared to their baseline.

There are several small series of breast imaging in pregnancy-associated breast cancer. At Memorial Sloan-Kettering Hospital, 78% of mammograms in 23 women with clinically evident pregnancy-associated breast cancer demonstrated radiologic signs of the cancer.[2] All of six ultrasonographic examinations performed in these patients with a palpable abnormality revealed a solid mass. In 1998, at the Princess Margaret Hospital, breast cancer found on physical examination was demonstrated in five of eight women with pregnancy-associated breast cancer who underwent mammography.[3] Ultrasonography was suspicious for cancer in two of four of these women who underwent this examination. In an older series, negative mammograms were found in six of eight pregnant patients with breast mass and subsequent biopsy-proven cancer.[4] If mammography is necessary in the lactating woman, it should be performed immediately after the breast is emptied by nursing or pumping and a serviceable radiographic image can be produced.

Ionizing radiation absorbed by the fetus is minimal with a standard two-view study if the abdomen is shielded, and should expose the embryo to less than 50 mrads (500 mGy).[5] Nevertheless, fetal radiation dose must be considered as well as the unknown but theoretical carcinogenic potential for future increased risk of breast cancer from mammography during the hyperstimulated state of pregnancy or lactation.

Breast ultrasonography is accurate and safe—as it is in nonpregnant women—in differentiating whether a palpable mass is fluid-filled or solid. Aspiration, obtaining fluid, and noting the disappearance of the mass readily serve to differentiate a fluid-filled cyst or galactocele from a solid tumor. It is not pos-

J. A. Petrek: Evelyn Lauder Breast Center, Memorial Sloan-Kettering Cancer Center, New York, New York

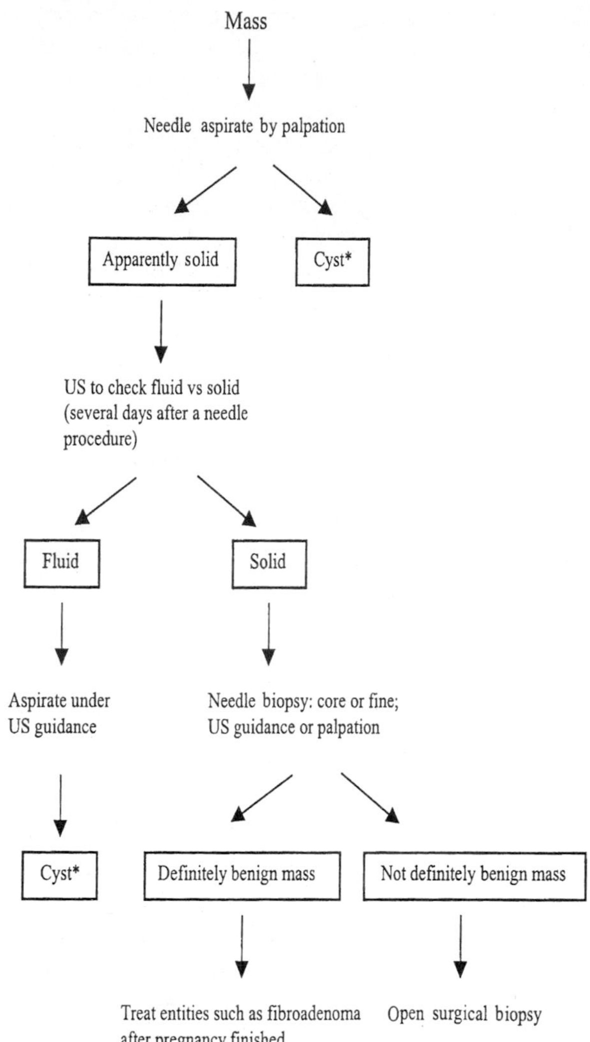

FIG. 1. Suggestions for diagnostic workup of a palpable mass during pregnancy. *Send for cytology of fluid using guidelines in Chapter 4. US, ultrasound.

sible to distinguish benign solid masses from malignant. Furthermore, there is no published literature on the normal gestational breast appearance that would aid the ultrasonographic diagnosis of a questionable mass on physical examination.

Magnetic resonance imaging (MRI) may be deemed useful in the future, but there are no data on the normal image of the pregnant or lactating breast thus far. As stated by the Safety Committee of the Society for the Magnetic Resonance Imaging, "the safety of MR imaging during pregnancy has not been proven."[6] It is plausible to think that the changes of pregnancy and lactation, especially the vascularity, may cause physiologic enhancement and decrease the accuracy of MRI.

FINE-NEEDLE ASPIRATION AND CORE-NEEDLE BIOPSY

With the ever-increasing popularity of fine-needle aspiration cytology in routine breast masses, several small reports concerning pregnancy and lactation address inherent problems.[7–9] The largest report concerns 331 women from New Zealand and finds the technique successful.[10] The women ranged from 8 weeks of gestation to 30 weeks postpartum while lactating. Cancer did not develop in any of the patients with benign fine-needle biopsy diagnosis in a follow-up period of 1.5 to 2.0 years. Ten women in this large group with the cytodiagnosis of cancer had surgical confirmation. Nevertheless, false-positive aspiration cytodiagnosis for benign breast tissue has been documented during gestation and may be relatively common due to frequent mitosis, increased cellularity, anisonucleosis, prominent nucleoli, and variable granular chromatin within a proteinaceous background. An experienced aspiration cytopathologist with specific knowledge of the pregnancy is required. With these caveats, aspiration cytology has a place in the workup of abnormalities in pregnant and lactating breasts. Furthermore, as can occur in any patient, the needle tip can miss and aspirate cells adjacent to the mass, thereby causing false reassurance. Core biopsy may be more accurate, but there has now been a report of milk fistula, a complication known well in open surgical biopsy in the lactating breast.[11]

DELAY IN DIAGNOSTIC BIOPSY

Many authors have attributed to delay of diagnosis the advanced disease and thereby the poor prognosis that are often characteristic of gestational breast cancer. Delays longer than those in the case of nonpregnant women seem to be common.[12–14] After a thickness or possible mass is found, the postponement of a surgical biopsy may be due to the greater complication rate expected in the pregnant or lactating woman.

A study of 63 patients diagnosed while pregnant or within 1 year postpartum at Memorial Sloan-Kettering Hospital suggests the reluctance to biopsy during pregnancy.[14] Fewer than 20% of such patients were diagnosed during pregnancy, and almost half were diagnosed within 12 weeks after delivery for a mass noted during pregnancy. Even in those with previously undocumented masses, the large size of the cancers at the time of postpartum diagnosis (median of 3.5 cm) makes it likely that a smaller mass was palpable during pregnancy.

SPECIAL CONSIDERATIONS OF BIOPSY IN THE PREGNANT OR LACTATING BREAST

In the pregnant woman, local anesthesia is theoretically always safer.[15] Monitored sedation or even general anesthesia (with an anesthesiologist experienced in obstetrics) may be rarely required and is acceptable, especially in the later phases of pregnancy when teratogenesis is not of great concern. Further discussion of anesthesia effects are to be found in Chapter 44.

Although excisional biopsies under local anesthesia during pregnancy are occasionally difficult, depending on the individual breast, an incisional biopsy is also an alternative.

Excellent hemostasis is necessary because of the increased vascularity and likelihood of postoperative hematoma.

The patient should cease breast-feeding before biopsy is performed because of the significant risk of milk fistula or infection, or both (because milk is a good culture medium). Binding the breast and using ice packs may help. Lowering prolactin by use of bromocriptine has not been associated with breast cancer and has been advocated.[16]

If a woman will not stop nursing but will accept the risk of fistula or infection (best recorded in writing), the physician can proceed with biopsy, depending on the individual factors. Although there appear to be no published data, it is surmisable that the risk of milk fistula increases from low in peripheral biopsies to high in central biopsies. Because the large ducts intercommunicate, an operative infection can involve the whole breast.

As concerns infection, if the woman stops nursing briefly, preoperative antibiotics can be given. The milk, containing the mother's antibiotics, can be expressed by breast pump and discarded. After a brief period of bottle-feeding, the infant can resume breast-feeding, assuming a benign diagnosis. However, the milk may be bloody, and the risk of milk fistula probably remains.

PATHOLOGIC DIAGNOSIS OF BREAST LUMPS DURING PREGNANCY AND LACTATION

In the largest series with 105 benign biopsies during pregnancy, 71% of patients had conditions also found in nonpregnant women, and only a small proportion had changes peculiar to pregnancy, including lobular hyperplasia, galactocele, and lactational mastitis.[17] Benign lesions during pregnancy, in decreasing order of frequency, include fibroadenomas, lipomas, papillomas, fibrocystic disease, galactoceles, and inflammatory lesions. Moreover, localized breast infarcts can cause mass lesions during pregnancy, either from overgrowth of a preexisting fibroadenoma or spontaneously.[18–21] The likelihood of diagnosing cancer is similar to that in a nonpregnant population: Byrd and associates[17] report that 22% of breast biopsies in pregnancy showed malignancy, compared with 19% in overall patients.

A 1993 report also notes that the majority of breast lumps excised during the pregnancy were preexisting (although growth rate may be stimulated during pregnancy).[22] Morphologically, a preexisting underlying lesion was readily identified in 18 cases (7 fibroadenomas, 5 tubular adenomas, and 6 hamartomas). The other 12 cases were lobular hyperplasia and inflammation with no evidence of a prepartum lesion.

BLOOD IN NIPPLE DISCHARGE

Nipple discharge with blood present either visibly or cytologically during pregnancy or lactation is rather common. In 20% of women with nipple discharge during pregnancy, and in 15% of asymptomatic lactating women, blood was confirmed by cytologic analysis of the nipple secretion.[23,24]

Two authors present long-term follow-up of 12 women[12] and of 5 women[25] with bloody nipple discharge while pregnant in whom neither cancer nor a benign lesion, such as intraductal papilloma, developed on postpartum follow-up. The possible etiology as related to rapid ductal proliferation and hypervascularity is discussed.[12,23–25]

The clinical follow-up to bloody nipple discharge with a nonsuspicious physical examination includes nipple secretion cytology. As is noted previously, it is important that the cytologist be aware of the clinical setting. If repeated cytologic analyses reveal no malignant cells, close follow-up is suggested. Women should be advised not to squeeze the nipple, since they often "check to see what's there" and may be reinjuring the duct structure. If cytologic analyses demonstrate malignant cells, then mammography, ultrasonography, and possibly a galactogram are indicated to localize the source.

INFECTION

Infection is uncommon during pregnancy but occurs relatively often during breast-feeding. The symptoms of suppurative mastitis seldom appear before the first week after birth, and infection does not become common until the third or fourth week. With infection, the patient becomes febrile, and the whole breast becomes hard, reddened, and painful. In a small group of women, infection is subacute or almost chronic, and the first clinical indication is a fluctuant mass.

The organism that most commonly causes infection is *Staphylococcus aureus*, and streptococcal groups are second. Toxic shock has been reported.[26] The source is nearly always the nursing infant's nose and throat. The bacterial colonization of the infant may be totally asymptomatic or, in the neonate, may involve the umbilicus or the skin. The organism is thought to enter through the nipple at a fissure or a minute abrasion. The possibility of entrance through the lactiferous ducts with intact integument has also been considered.[27] The organism can nearly always be cultured from breast milk.

Antibiotic therapy should be started as soon as possible after breast milk is obtained for culture. The initial choice of antibiotic will undoubtedly be influenced by the current experiences with staphylococcal and streptococcal infections in the hospital and neighborhood area.[15,27] Nursing should be discontinued, because it is painful and the infant harbors the organism and can cause reinfection. Once established, resistant staphylococcal infections tend to recur in the family.

Repeated aspiration of an abscess coupled with antibiotics often suffices as treatment for the infection. Formal incision and drainage may also be necessary when a trial of repeated aspirations fails.[15] An incision, usually radial, should be placed over the most dependent area of the fluctuance overlying the infected ducts. The operation should ideally be performed under general anesthesia, allowing the manual breakdown of the loculations. The resulting cavity is loosely packed with gauze.

INFLAMMATORY CANCER VERSUS INFECTION

Inflammatory cancer probably arises no more frequently in pregnant patients than in others,[28,29] despite earlier opinions to the contrary. Notwithstanding referral patterns that might attract more severe cases, only 3% of pregnant patients with breast cancer at Memorial Sloan-Kettering Hospital had inflammatory breast cancer.[14] Nevertheless, the surgeon must not make the dire error of mistaking inflammatory cancer for the quite common lactational mastitis or abscess, and it is useful to biopsy the skin and the indurated breast tissue at the time of incision and drainage.[30]

MANAGEMENT SUMMARY

Before pregnancy, a careful physical examination and mammography, as indicated by the patient risk factors, are useful. The great majority of benign masses excised during pregnancy are present before pregnancy. Most often, however, the opportunity for an exacting physical examination exists only on the first obstetric visit.

During pregnancy, the workup of a palpable abnormality can include the same techniques that are used in the non-pregnant woman, although the mammary changes of pregnancy bring special considerations.

1. *Mammography*. Radiographic images in the presence of gestational changes may or may not be useful.
2. *Ultrasonography*. No reports define the range of normal gestational appearance, although the differentiation of simple cysts from solid masses is successful.
3. *MRI*. No reports related to the pregnant or lactating breast exist.
4. *Fine-needle aspiration*. The gestational cellular changes are hyperproliferative and may be misdiagnosed if the cytologist is unaware of the pregnancy.
5. *Open surgical biopsy*. The hypervascularity and increased volume of the breast in the setting of local anesthesia make these procedures difficult, although open surgical biopsy is usually necessary for palpable abnormalities.

REFERENCES

1. Swinford AE, Adler DD, Garver KA. Mammographic appearance of the breasts during pregnancy and lactation: false assumptions. *Acad Radiol* 1998;5:467.
2. Liberman L, Giess CS, Dershaw DD, Deutch BM, Petrek JA. Imaging of pregnancy-associated breast cancer. *Radiology* 1994;191:245.
3. Samuels TH, Liu F, Yaffe M, Haider M. Gestational breast cancer. *Can Assoc Radiol J* 1998;49:172.
4. Max MH, Klamer TW. Pregnancy and breast cancer. *South Med J* 1983;76:1008.
5. Wagner LK, Lester RG, Saldana L, eds. The amount of radiation absorbed by the conceptus. In: *Exposure of the pregnant patient to diagnostic radiation: a guide to medical management*. Philadelphia: JB Lippincott, 1985:40.
6. Kanal E. Pregnancy and the safety of magnetic resonance imaging. *Magn Reson Imaging Clin N Am* 1994;2:309.
7. Bottles K, Taylor RN. Diagnosis of breast masses in pregnant and lactating women by aspiration cytology. *Obstet Gynecol* 1985;66:76S.
8. Gupta RK, McHutchinson AGR, Dowle CS, Simpson JS. Fine-needle aspiration cytodiagnosis of breast masses in pregnant and lactating women and its impact on management. *Diagn Cytopathol* 1993;9:156.
9. Novotny DB, Maygarden SJ, Shermer RW, Frable WJ. Fine needle aspiration of benign and malignant breast masses associated with pregnancy. *Acta Cytol* 1991;35(6):676.
10. Gupta RK. The diagnostic impact of aspiration cytodiagnosis of breast masses in association with pregnancy and lactation with an emphasis on clinical decision making. *Breast J* 1997;3(3):131.
11. Schackmuth EM, Harlow CL, Norton LW. Milk fistula: a complication after core biopsy. *Am J Roentgenol* 1993;161:961.
12. Haagenson CD. Carcinoma of the breast in pregnancy. In: Haagensen CD, ed. *Diseases of the breast*, 2nd ed. Philadelphia: WB Saunders, 1971.
13. Zemlickis D, Lishner M, Degendorfer P, et al. Maternal and fetal outcome after breast cancer in pregnancy. *Am J Obstet Gynecol* 1992;166:781.
14. Petrek JA, Dukoff R, Rogatko A. Pregnancy-associated breast cancer. *Cancer* 1991;67:869.
15. Canter JW, Oliver GC, Zaloudek CJ. Surgical diseases of the breast during pregnancy. *Clin Obstet Gynecol* 1983;26:853.
16. Anderson JM. Mammary cancers and pregnancy. *BMJ* 1979;1:1124.
17. Byrd BF, Bayer DS, Robertson JC, et al. Treatment of breast tumors associated with pregnancy and lactation. *Ann Surg* 1962;155:940.
18. Rickert RR, Rajan S. Localized breast infarcts associated with pregnancy. *Arch Pathol* 1974;97:159.
19. Jiminez JF, Rickey RO, Cohen C. Spontaneous breast infarction associated with pregnancy presenting as a palpable mass. *J Surg Oncol* 1986;32:174.
20. Majmudar B, Rosales-Quintana S. Infarction of breast fibroadenomas during pregnancy. *JAMA* 1975;231:963.
21. O'Hara MF, Page DL. Adenomas of the breast and ectopic breast under lactational influences. *Hum Pathol* 1985;16:707.
22. Slavin JL, Billson R, Ostor AG. Nodular breast lesions during pregnancy and lactation. *Histopathology* 1993;22:481.
23. Kline TS, Lash SR. The bleeding nipple of pregnancy and postpartum. A cytologic and histologic study. *Am J Pathol* 1964;8:336.
24. Kline TS, Lash S. Nipple secretion in pregnancy. A cytologic and histologic study. *Am J Clin Pathol* 1962;37:626.
25. Lafreniere R. Bloody nipple discharge during pregnancy: a rationale for conservative treatment. *J Surg Oncol* 1990;43:228.
26. Dixey JJ, Swanson DC, Williams TD, et al. Toxic-shock syndrome: four cases in a London hospital. *BMJ* 1982;285:342.
27. Cunningham I, Gary F, Williams JW. *Williams' obstetrics*, 19th ed. Norwalk, CT: Appleton & Lange, 1993.
28. Wallack MK, Wolf JA Jr, Bedwinek J, et al. Gestational carcinoma of the female breast. *Curr Probl Cancer* 1983;7:1.
29. Donegan WL. Pregnancy and breast cancer. *Obstet Gynecol* 1977;50:244.
30. White TT. Carcinoma of the breast in the pregnant and the nursing patient. *Am J Obstet Gynecol* 1955;69:1277.

CHAPTER 8

Diseases of the Breast, 2nd ed.,
edited by Jay R. Harris.
Lippincott Williams & Wilkins, Philadelphia © 2000.

Management of Gynecomastia

Glenn D. Braunstein

Benign proliferation of the glandular tissue of the male breast constitutes the histologic hallmark of gynecomastia, which, if great enough, appears clinically as palpable or visual enlargement of the breast. This condition, which is exceedingly common, may be a sign of a serious underlying pathologic condition, may cause physical or emotional discomfort, or may be confused with other breast problems, most significantly carcinoma.

PREVALENCE

Breast glandular proliferation commonly occurs in infancy, during puberty, and in older age. It has been estimated that between 60% and 90% of infants exhibit the transient development of palpable breast tissue due to estrogenic stimulation from the maternal-placental-fetal unit. This stimulus for breast growth ceases as the estrogens are cleared from the neonatal circulation, and the breast tissue gradually regresses over a 2- to 3-week period. Although population studies have shown that the prevalence of pubertal gynecomastia varies widely, most have indicated that 30% to 60% of pubertal boys exhibit gynecomastia, which generally begins between 10 and 12 years of age, with the highest prevalence between 13 and 14 years of age (corresponding to Tanner stage III or IV of pubertal development), followed by involution that is generally complete by age 16 to 17 years.[1–10] The percentage of men who exhibit gynecomastia increases with advancing age, with the highest prevalence found in the 50- to 80-year age range (Fig. 1). The prevalence of the condition in men ranges between 24% and 65%, with the differences between series being accounted for by the defining criteria and by the population studied.[10–17]

PATHOGENESIS

No inherent differences appear to exist in the hormonal responsiveness of the male or female breast glandular tissue.[9,18] The hormonal milieu, the duration and intensity of stimulation, and the individual's breast tissue sensitivity determine the type and degree of glandular proliferation. Under the influence of estrogens, the ducts elongate and branch, the ductal epithelium becomes hyperplastic, the periductal fibroblasts proliferate, and the vascularity increases. This histologic picture is found early in the course of gynecomastia and is often referred to as the *florid stage.* Acinar development is not seen in males, because it requires the presence of progesterone in concentrations found during the luteal phase of the menstrual cycle.[19] Androgens exert an antiestrogen effect on rodent breast cancer models and the human MCF-7 breast cancer cell line and are thought to antagonize at least some of the effects of estrogens in normal breast tissue.[20] Accordingly, gynecomastia is generally considered to represent an imbalance between the breast stimulatory effects of estrogen and the inhibitory effects of androgens. In fact, alterations in the estrogen-androgen ratio have been found in many of the conditions associated with gynecomastia. Such alterations can occur through a variety of mechanisms (Table 1).

In men, the testes secrete 95% of the testosterone, 15% of the estradiol, and less than 5% of the estrone produced daily. Most of the circulating estrogens are derived from the extraglandular conversion of estrogen precursors by extragonadal tissues, including the liver, skin, fat, muscle, bone, and kidney (Fig. 2). These tissues contain the aromatase enzyme that converts testosterone to estradiol and androstenedione, an androgen primarily secreted by the adrenal glands, to estrone. Estradiol and estrone are interconverted in extragonadal tissues through the activity of the 17-ketosteroid reductase enzyme. This enzyme is also responsible for the interconversion of testosterone and androstenedione. When androgens and estrogens enter the circulation, either through direct secretion from gonadal tissues or from the sites of extragonadal metabolism, most are bound to sex hormone–binding globulin (SHBG), a protein derived primarily from the liver and one that has a greater affinity for androgens than for estrogens. The non-SHBG sex hormones circulate either in the free or

G. D. Braunstein: Department of Medicine, University of California, Los Angeles, UCLA School of Medicine, Los Angeles, California; Cedars-Sinai Medical Center, Los Angeles, California

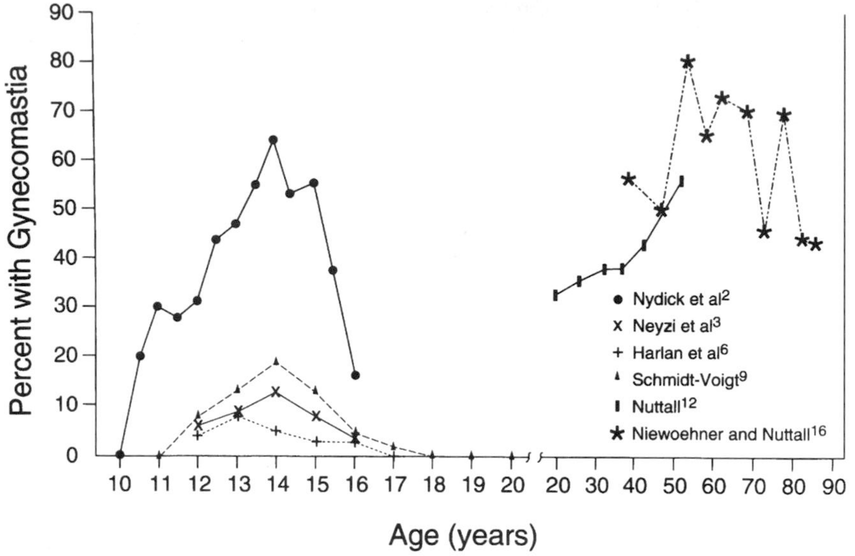

FIG. 1. Prevalence of gynecomastia at various chronologic ages. Data were derived from multiple population studies.[2,3,6,9,12,16] (Adapted from ref. 25.)

unbound state or are weakly bound to albumin. These fractions are able to cross the plasma membrane of target cells and are bound to cytoplasmic steroid receptors. In some target tissues, testosterone is converted to dihydrotestosterone through the action of the 5α-reductase enzyme. Testosterone and dihydrotestosterone bind to the same androgen receptor and are translocated into the nucleus. Each also binds to the hormone-responsive element of the appropriate genes, resulting in the initiation of transcription and hormone action. A similar sequence of events occurs after the binding of estradiol or estrone to the cytoplasmic estrogen receptor.[19]

From a pathophysiologic standpoint, an imbalance between estrogen and androgen concentrations or effects can occur as a result of abnormalities at several levels (see Table 1). Overproduction of estrogens from testicular or adrenal neoplasms or enhanced extraglandular conversion of estrogen precursors to estrogens can elevate the total estrogen concentration. Such extraglandular conversion may occur directly in the breast tissue. Indeed, increased aromatization of androgens to estrogens has been noted in pubic skin fibroblasts from some patients with idiopathic gynecomastia.[21] Elevations of the absolute quantity of circulating free estrogens can occur if estrogen metabolism is slowed or if SHBG-bound estrogens are displaced from the protein. Conversely, decreased secretion of androgens from the testes—due to primary defects in the testes or secondary to loss of tonic stimulation by pituitary gonadotropins, enhanced metabolic degradation of androgens, or increased binding of androgens to SHBG—results in decreases in free androgens that could antagonize the effect of estrogens on the breast glandular tissue. As was noted previously, androgen and estrogen balance depend not only on the amount and availability of free androgens and estrogens but also on their ability to act at the target tissue level. Thus, defects in the androgen receptor or displacement of androgens from their receptors by drugs with antiandrogenic effects (e.g., spironolactone) result in decreased androgen action and, hence, decreased estrogen antagonism at the breast glandular cell level. Finally, the inherent sensitivity of an individual's breast tissue to estrogen or androgen action may predispose some persons to development of gynecomastia even in the presence of apparently normal concentrations of estrogens and androgens.

ASSOCIATED CONDITIONS

Tables 1 and 2 list the various conditions and drugs that have been associated with gynecomastia. Although the list is relatively long, almost two-thirds of the patients have either pubertal gynecomastia (approximately 25%), drug-induced gynecomastia (10% to 20%), or no underlying abnormality detected (idiopathic gynecomastia, approximately 25%). Most of the remainder have cirrhosis or malnutrition (8%), primary hypogonadism (8%), testicular tumors (3%), secondary hypogonadism (2%), hyperthyroidism (1.5%), or renal disease (1%).[22] For most pathologic conditions, alterations in the balance between estrogen and androgen levels or action occur through several of the pathophysiologic mechanisms outlined in Table 1. One of the best examples is the gynecomastia associated with spironolactone. This aldosterone antagonist inhibits the testicular biosynthesis of testosterone, enhances the conversion of testosterone to the less potent androgen androstenedione, increases the aromatization of testosterone to estradiol, displaces testosterone from SHBG (leading to an increase in its metabolic clearance rate), and binds to the androgen receptors in target tissues, thereby

TABLE 1. *Conditions associated with gynecomastia and their primary pathophysiologic mechanisms*

- Physiologic
  - Neonatal
  - Pubertal
  - Aging
- Pathologic
  - Idiopathic
  - Drug induced (see Table 2)
  - Increased serum estrogen
    - Increased aromatization (peripheral and glandular)
      - Sertoli cell (sex cord) tumors
      - Testicular germ cell tumors
      - Leydig cell tumors
      - Adrenocortical carcinoma
      - Hermaphroditism
      - Obesity
      - Hyperthyroidism
      - Liver disease
      - Testicular feminization
      - Refeeding after starvation
      - Primary aromatase excess
    - Displacement of estrogen from sex hormone–binding globulin
      - Spironolactone
      - Ketoconazole
    - Decreased estrogen metabolism
      - Cirrhosis (?)
    - Exogenous sources
      - Topical estrogen creams and lotions
      - Ingestion of estrogen
    - Eutopic human chorionic gonadotropin (hCG) production
      - Choriocarcinoma
    - Ectopic hCG production
      - Lung carcinoma
      - Liver carcinoma
      - Gastric carcinoma
      - Kidney carcinoma
  - Decreased testosterone synthesis
    - Primary gonadal failure, congenital
      - Anorchia
      - Klinefelter's syndrome
      - Hermaphroditism
      - Hereditary defects in testosterone synthesis
    - Primary gonadal failure, acquired
      - Viral orchitis
      - Castration
      - Granulomatous diseases (including leprosy)
    - Testicular failure due to hypothalamic and/or pituitary disease
  - Androgen resistance due to androgen receptor defects
  - Other
    - Chronic renal failure
    - Chronic illness
    - Spinal cord injury
    - Human immunodeficiency virus
    - Enhanced breast tissue sensitivity

Adapted from ref. 26.

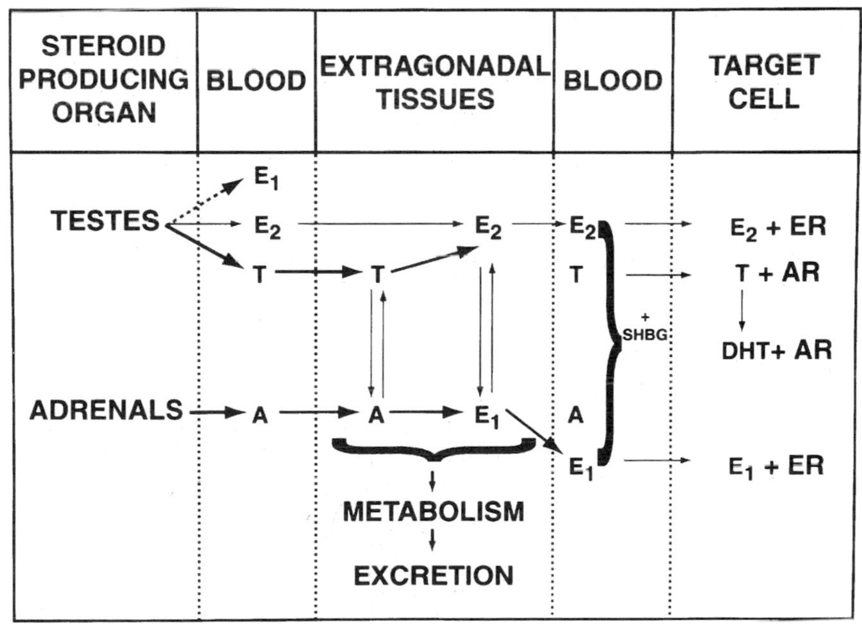

FIG. 2. Pathways of estrogen and androgen production, action, and metabolism. A, androstenedione; AR, androgen receptor; DHT, dihydrotestosterone; E_1, estrone; E_2, estradiol; ER, estrogen receptor; SHBG, sex hormone–binding globulin; T, testosterone. (Adapted from ref. 26.)

TABLE 2. *Drugs associated with gynecomastia*

Hormones	Psychoactive agents
Androgens and anabolic steroids*	Diazepam
Chorionic gonadotropin*	Haloperidol
Estrogens and estrogen agonists*	Phenothiazine
Growth hormone	Tricyclic antidepressants
Antiandrogens or inhibitors of androgen synthesis	Drugs of abuse
Bicalutamide*	Alcohol
Cyproterone*	Amphetamines
Flutamide*	Heroin
Gonadotropin-releasing hormone agonists*	Marijuana
Antibiotics	Methadone
Ethionamide	Other
Isoniazid	Auranofin
Ketoconazole*	Diethylpropion
Metronidazole	Domperidone
Minocycline	Etretinate
Antiulcer medications	Metoclopramide
Cimetidine*	Penicillamine
Omeprazole	Phenytoin
Ranitidine	Sulindac
Cancer chemotherapeutic agents	Theophylline
Alkylating agents*	
Methotrexate	
Vinca alkaloids	
Combination chemotherapy	
Cardiovascular drugs	
Amiodarone	
Captopril	
Digitoxin*	
Digoxin	
Diltiazem	
Enalapril	
Methyldopa	
Nifedipine	
Reserpine	
Spironolactone*	
Verapamil	

*A strong relation has been established. Other relations have been proposed on the basis of epidemiologic studies or challenge-rechallenge studies of individual patients or small groups of patients.

acting as an antiandrogen.[23] For an in-depth discussion of the pathophysiology of gynecomastia associated with each of the conditions listed in Tables 1 and 2, the reader is referred to several reviews.[14,18,19,22,24–27]

EVALUATION

Most patients with gynecomastia are asymptomatic, with the condition detected during a physical examination. Patients with recent onset of gynecomastia due to drugs or one of the pathologic conditions noted in Tables 1 and 2, however, may present with breast or nipple pain and tenderness. Approximately 10% to 15% of patients recall a history of breast trauma just before or at the time of discovery of the breast enlargement.[18,27] It is unclear whether breast trauma itself causes gynecomastia. It is likely that, in many patients with an antecedent history of trauma, the breast irritation from the trauma actually led to the discovery of preexisting gynecomastia. Although one-half of patients have clinically apparent bilateral gynecomastia, histologic studies have shown that virtually all patients have bilateral involvement.[15] This discrepancy may be explained by asynchronous growth of the two breasts and differences in the amount of breast glandular and stromal proliferation.

Gynecomastia must be differentiated from other conditions that cause breast enlargement. Although neurofibromas, dermoid cysts, lipomas, hematomas, and lymphangiomas may enlarge portions of the breast, these abnormalities are usually easily distinguished from gynecomastia on historical or clinical grounds. The two conditions that are most important to differentiate are pseudogynecomastia and breast carcinoma. *Pseudogynecomastia* refers to enlargement of the breasts due to fat deposition rather than to glandular proliferation. Patients with this condition often have generalized obesity and do not complain of breast pain or tenderness. Additionally, the breast examination should allow the correct diagnosis. The breasts are best examined while the patient is lying on the back with hands behind the head. The examiner places a thumb on one side of the breast and the second finger on the other side. The fingers are then gradually brought together without more than superficial pressure being applied to the skin. Patients with gynecomastia have a rubbery or firm disc of tissue that extends concentrically out from the nipple and that either is easily palpated or offers some resistance to the apposition of the fingers, whereas those with pseudogynecomastia exhibit no such mound of tissue, and no resistance is felt as the fingers are brought together.

Differentiation of gynecomastia from breast carcinoma usually can be accomplished through careful physical examination. Carcinoma of the breast in men is usually eccentric in location and unilateral (rather than subareolar and bilateral) and is hard or firm, whereas gynecomastia tends to be rubbery to firm in texture. Patients with carcinoma may also exhibit skin dimpling and nipple retraction, are more likely to have a nipple discharge (60%) than are patients with gynecomastia (2%), and may present with axillary lymphadenopathy.[27] If the two conditions cannot be differentiated on clinical grounds, then mammography, fine-needle aspiration for cytologic examination, or open biopsy should be done. With the exception of Klinefelter's syndrome (XXY genotype), no well-established data indicate that gynecomastia predisposes to the development of carcinoma. Patients with Klinefelter's syndrome do have a 16-fold higher risk of developing breast carcinoma than do men without the syndrome.[28]

After a clinical diagnosis of gynecomastia has been made, several etiologies should be investigated through a thorough history and physical examination. A careful history of medication use is essential, specifically regarding ingestion of the drugs listed in Table 2. A history of liver or renal disease, especially if the patient has been receiving hemodialysis for the latter, may point to the underlying etiology. A history of weight loss, tachycardia, tremulousness, diaphoresis, heat intolerance, and hyperdefecation, with or without the presence of a goiter, raises the possibility of hyperthyroidism. The patient should be evaluated for the signs and symptoms of hypogonadism, including loss of libido, impotence, decreased strength, and testicular atrophy. A careful examination for abdominal masses, which may be present in nearly one-half the patients with adrenocortical carcinoma, and a meticulous examination for testicular masses are essential parts of the evaluation.

The next step depends on the results of the clinical evaluation. If any of the drugs listed in Table 2 have been ingested, they should be discontinued and the patient reexamined in 1 month. If the drug was the inciting agent, then a decrease in breast pain and tenderness should occur during that time. If the patient is of pubertal age and has an otherwise normal general physical and testicular examination, he probably has transient or persistent pubertal gynecomastia. Reexamination at 6-month intervals should determine whether the condition is transient or persistent. At this time, medical or surgical therapy should be considered. If, during routine clinical examination, an adult is found to have asymptomatic gynecomastia without the presence of underlying disease, biochemical assessments of liver, kidney, and thyroid function should be performed. In a patient with normal results, no further tests are necessary, but he should be reevaluated in 6 months. Conversely, if the gynecomastia is of recent onset or if the patient complains of pain or tenderness, additional studies—including measurements of serum concentrations of human chorionic gonadotropin, estradiol, testosterone, and luteinizing hormone—should be done.

The algorithm outlined in Fig. 3 can be used to discern the underlying abnormality, if any, that is responsible for the breast enlargement.[22] An elevated level of human chorionic gonadotropin in the serum indicates the presence of a testicular or nongonadal germ cell tumor or, rarely, a nontrophoblastic neoplasm that secretes the hormone ectopically. A testicular ultrasound should be done, and, if no testicular mass is found, a chest radiograph and abdominal computed tomographic scan or magnetic resonance imaging study should be performed in an effort to localize an extragonadal human chorionic gonadotropin–producing tumor. Most nontro-

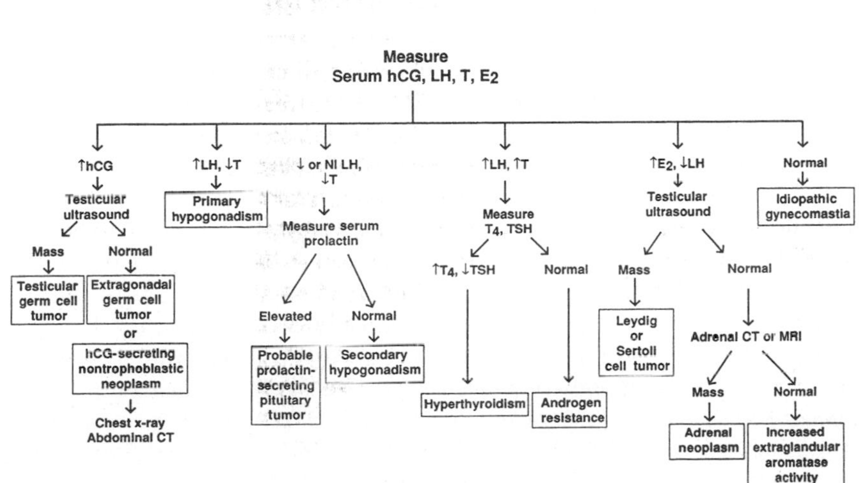

FIG. 3. Algorithm providing interpretation of serum hormone levels and recommendations for further evaluation of patients with gynecomastia. CT, computed tomography; E_2, estradiol; hCG, human chorionic gonadotropin; LH, luteinizing hormone; MRI, magnetic resonance imaging; Nl, normal; T, testosterone; T_4, thyroxine; TSH, thyroid-stimulating hormone. (From ref. 22.)

phoblastic tumors that secrete the hormone are bronchogenic, gastric, renal cell, or hepatic carcinomas. An elevated serum concentration of luteinizing hormone associated with a low testosterone level is indicative of primary hypogonadism, whereas a low testosterone level and a low or normal luteinizing hormone level suggest secondary hypogonadism due to a hypothalamic or pituitary abnormality. Serum prolactin concentration should be determined in this situation to rule out a prolactin-secreting pituitary adenoma, which can cause hypogonadotropic hypogonadism. Elevated serum concentrations of luteinizing hormone and testosterone are found with hyperthyroidism and in patients with various forms of androgen resistance due to androgen receptor disorders. Thyroid function tests can distinguish between these conditions.

If an elevated serum estradiol level is found along with a normal or suppressed concentration of luteinizing hormone, a testicular ultrasound is indicated to rule out a Leydig cell, Sertoli cell, or sex cord testicular tumor. If the ultrasound is normal, a computed tomographic scan or magnetic resonance imaging scan of the adrenal glands should be done to detect an estrogen-secreting adrenal neoplasm. If both the testes and adrenal glands appear normal, the increased estradiol level is probably due to enhanced extraglandular aromatization of estrogen precursors to estrogens. In this situation, estrone levels are often relatively higher than estradiol concentrations. Finally, if all of these endocrine measurements are normal, the patient is considered to have idiopathic gynecomastia.

PREVENTION

Two situations exist in which gynecomastia can be prevented. The first is in patients who require a medication. Avoidance of the drugs listed in Table 2 decreases the risk for drug-induced breast stimulation. Also, not all the therapeutic agents within the drug groups listed in the table cause gynecomastia to the same extent. For example, when considering the use of a calcium channel blocker in an older man, the clinician should remember that nifedipine has been associated with the highest frequency of gynecomastia, followed by verapamil, with diltiazem having the lowest association.[24,29] Similarly, the incidence of gynecomastia in patients receiving histamine receptor or parietal cell proton-pump blockers is highest with cimetidine, then ranitidine, and least with omeprazole.[24,30] The second area of prevention occurs among patients with prostate cancer who are about to receive estrogens. Numerous studies have shown that prophylactic administration of low-dose radiation (900 rad) greatly reduces the appearance of gynecomastia.[31]

TREATMENT

Discontinuation of the offending drug or correction of the underlying condition that altered the estrogen-androgen balance results in regression of gynecomastia in recent-onset breast growth. As was noted previously, histologic studies of the breast tissue from men with gynecomastia have shown a marked duct epithelial cell proliferation, inflammatory cell infiltration, increase in stromal fibroblasts, and enhanced vascularity early in the course of the disorder. It is during this proliferative, or florid, stage that patients may complain of breast pain and tenderness. This stage persists for a variable period but usually lasts less than a year and is followed by spontaneous resolution or enters an inactive stage. There is a reduction in the epithelial proliferation, dilatation of the ducts, and hyalinization and fibrosis of the stroma.[11,15,32] The inactive stage is usually asymptomatic. This histologic picture predominates in men whose gynecomastia is detected during a routine physical examination. When considering therapeutic approaches, it is important to appreciate that, after the inactive stage is reached, the gynecomastia is unlikely to spontaneously regress and is also unlikely to respond to medical therapies. Another important factor to consider is that most gynecomastia regresses spontaneously. Indeed, pubertal gynecomastia develops in a large proportion of boys, but very few exhibit persistent breast glandular enlargement. Similarly, in a group of patients with gynecomastia from various causes, 85% of untreated patients had spontaneous improvement.[27] This finding emphasizes the difficulties in assessing the response to any medical intervention.

The indications for therapy are severe pain, tenderness, or embarrassment sufficient to interfere with the patient's normal daily activities. Surgical removal of the breast glandular and stromal tissue has been the mainstay of interventional therapy. Subcutaneous mastectomy through a periareolar incision with contouring of the breast by suction-assisted lipectomy to remove the subglandular adipose tissue is currently the surgical procedure that is usually performed.[33] Alternatively, the glandular tissue can be removed by pulling it through two incisions located on one side of the inframammary fold and one in the anterior axillary region, thus avoiding an areolar scar.[34] These techniques should be used as primary therapy in patients with long-standing gynecomastia and as definitive therapy in patients who fail to respond to a series of medical therapies.

Three types of medical therapy—androgens, antiestrogens, and aromatase inhibitors—have been tested in patients with gynecomastia. Because this condition has a high frequency of spontaneous regression, the decision of when to treat is often difficult. It is also difficult to assess the use of most medications that have been tried, given the small sample sizes and nonblinded uncontrolled designs of most studies. Nevertheless, with the exception of early pubertal gynecomastia that has been present for less than 3 months, a trial of medical therapy for patients with moderate to severe symptoms is recommended.

Testosterone administration has not been shown to be more effective than placebo in patients with pubertal or idiopathic gynecomastia and carries the risk of exacerbating the condition by being aromatized to estradiol.[27] However, micronized testosterone has been shown in a double-blind, placebo-controlled trial to reduce the prevalence of gynecomastia in men with liver cirrhosis after 6 months of therapy.[35] Dihydrotestosterone, a nonaromatizable androgen, given either by injection or percutaneously, has been followed by a reduction in breast volume in 75% of patients, with complete resolution in approximately one-fourth.[36] Responders had a decrease in breast tenderness within 1 to 2 weeks without side effects. The androgenic progestogen danazol has also been tried in uncontrolled trials and a single placebo-controlled study, with the latter showing a complete resolution in 23% of patients who received danazol and only a 12% response in those given placebo.[37] Although the investigators believed that this drug was safe and well tolerated, other studies using danazol to treat other conditions have noted side effects, including edema, weight gain, acne, nausea, and muscle cramps.

The two antiestrogens that have been tested are clomiphene citrate and tamoxifen. Response rates of 36% to 95% have been reported for clomiphene citrate, but two of the three systematic studies indicate that fewer than one-half of patients had a decrease in breast volume of 20% or more or were satisfied with the results.[38–40] No side effects were noted by the investigators when the drug was used in dosages of 50 to 100 mg per day orally. In other settings, the drug has been associated with gastrointestinal distress and visual problems. Tamoxifen, given in dosages of 10 mg orally twice a day, has been studied in two randomized double-blind studies in a combined total of 16 patients.[41,42] This therapy was associated with a statistically significant reduction in pain and breast size, although neither study reported complete remissions. A complete response was reported in 80% of patients studied in an uncontrolled trial.[43] None of the studies has reported any side effects from tamoxifen given in these doses, and, in view of its safety, the author usually recommends a 3-month trial of the drug for patients with painful gynecomastia.

The aromatase inhibitor testolactone has been given to a small number of patients with pubertal gynecomastia for up to 6 months at a dose of 450 mg per day orally without side effects.[44] The authors of this uncontrolled study report a decrease in breast size after 2 months of therapy, but insufficient data currently exist to recommend this drug as a first-line agent. On theoretical grounds, however, a more potent member of this class of medications, such as anastrozole or letrozole, would appear to be beneficial in patients whose gynecomastia is primarily the result of enhanced extraglandular aromatization of estrogen precursors.

A Chinese herbal product, Gegen-Teng (Tsumura & Co., Ltd., Tokyo, Japan), was given to four patients with gynecomastia, who had a decrease in pain and induration but no decrease in the size of the glandular tissue.[45] Obviously, more experience is needed to assess this type of therapy.

REFERENCES

1. Jung FT, Shafton AL. Mastitis, mazoplasia, mastalgia, and gynecomastia in normal adolescent males. *Ill Med J* 1938;73:115.
2. Nydick M, Bustos J, Dale JH Jr, et al. Gynecomastia in adolescent boys. *JAMA* 1961;178:449.
3. Neyzi O, Alp H, Yalcindag A, et al. Sexual maturation in Turkish boys. *Ann Hum Biol* 1975;2:251.
4. Lee PA. The relationship of concentrations of serum hormones to pubertal gynecomastia. *J Pediatr* 1975;86:212.
5. Fara GM, DelCorvo G, Bernuzzi S, et al. Epidemic of breast enlargement in an Italian school. *Lancet* 1979;2:295.
6. Harlan WR, Grillo GP, Cornoni-Huntley J, et al. Secondary sex characteristics of boys 12 to 17 years of age: the U.S. Health Examination Survey. *J Pediatr* 1979;95:293.
7. Moore DC, Schlaepfer LV, Paunier L, et al. Hormonal changes during puberty. V. Transient pubertal gynecomastia: abnormal androgen-estrogen ratios. *J Clin Endocrinol Metab* 1984;58:492.
8. Biro FM, Lucky AW, Huster GA, et al. Hormonal studies and physical maturation in adolescent gynecomastia. *J Pediatr* 1990;116:450.
9. Schmidt-Voigt J. Brustdruenschwellungen bei mannlichen Jugendlichen des Pubertatsalters (Pubertatsmakromastie). *Z Kinderheilkd* 1941;62:590.
10. Georgiadis E, Papandreou L, Evangelopoulou C, et al. Incidence of gynaecomastia in 954 young males and its relationship to somatometric parameters. *Ann Hum Biol* 1994;21:579.
11. Williams MJ. Gynecomastia: its incidence, recognition and host characterization in 447 autopsy cases. *Am J Med* 1963;34:103.
12. Nuttall FQ. Gynecomastia as a physical finding in normal men. *J Clin Endocrinol Metab* 1979;48:338.
13. Ley SB, Mozaffarian GA, Leonard JM, et al. Palpable breast tissue versus gynecomastia as a normal physical finding. *Clin Res* 1980;28:24A.
14. Carlson HE. Gynecomastia. *N Engl J Med* 1980;303:795.
15. Andersen JA, Gram JB. Male breast at autopsy. *APMIS* 1982;90:191.
16. Niewoehner CB, Nuttall FQ. Gynecomastia in a hospitalized male population. *Am J Med* 1984;77:633.
17. Murray NP, Daly MJ. Gynaecomastia and heart failure: adverse drug reaction or disease process? *J Clin Pharm Ther* 1991;16:275.
18. Hall PF. *Gynaecomastia*. Glebe, Australia: Australasian Medical Publishing Company, 1959.
19. Wilson JD, Aiman J, MacDonald PC. The pathogenesis of gynecomastia. *Adv Intern Med* 1980;29:1.
20. Rochefort H, Garcia M. The estrogenic and antiestrogenic activities of androgens in female target tissues. *Pharmacol Ther* 1984;23:193.
21. Bulard J, Mowszowicz I, Schaison G. Increased aromatase activity in pubic skin fibroblasts from patients with isolated gynecomastia. *J Clin Endocrinol Metab* 1987;64:618.
22. Braunstein GD. Gynecomastia. *N Engl J Med* 1993;328:490.
23. Rose LI, Underwood RH, Newmark SR, et al. Pathophysiology of spironolactone-induced gynecomastia. *Ann Intern Med* 1977;87:398.
24. Thompson DF, Carter JR. Drug-induced gynecomastia. *Pharmacotherapy* 1993;13:37.
25. Braunstein GD. Pubertal gynecomastia. In: Lifshitz F, ed. *Pediatric endocrinology*. New York: Marcel Dekker, 1996:197.
26. Mathur R, Braunstein GD. Gynecomastia: pathomechanisms and treatment strategies. *Horm Res* 1997;48:95.
27. Treves N. Gynecomastia. The origins of mammary swelling in the male: an analysis of 406 patients with breast hypertrophy, 525 with testicular tumors, and 13 with adrenal neoplasms. *Cancer* 1958;11:1083.
28. Fentiman IS. Male breast cancer. In: *Detection and treatment of early breast cancer*. Philadelphia: JB Lippincott, 1990:207.
29. Tanner LA, Bosco LA. Gynecomastia associated with calcium channel blocker therapy. *Arch Intern Med* 1988;148:379.
30. Lindquist M, Edwards IR. Endocrine adverse effects of omeprazole. *BMJ* 1992;305:451.
31. Waterfall NB, Glaser MG. A study of the effects of radiation on prevention of gynaecomastia due to oestrogen therapy. *Clin Oncol (R Coll Radiol)* 1979;5:257.
32. Nicolis GL, Modlinger RS, Gabrilove JL. A study of the histopathology of human gynecomastia. *J Clin Endocrinol Metab* 1971;32:173.

33. Braunstein GD, Glassman HA. Gynecomastia. In: Bardin CW, ed. *Current therapy in endocrinology and metabolism*. Philadelphia: CV Mosby, 1997;401.
34. Morselli PG. "Pull-through": a new technique for breast reduction in gynecomastia. *Plast Reconstr Surg* 1996;97:450.
35. The Copenhagen Study Group for Liver Diseases. Testosterone treatment of men with alcoholic cirrhosis: a double-blind study. *Hepatology* 1986;6:807.
36. Kuhn JM, Roca R, Laudat MH, et al. Studies on the treatment of idiopathic gynaecomastia with percutaneous dihydrotestosterone. *Clin Endocrinol (Oxf)* 1983;19:513.
37. Jones DJ, Davison DJ, Holt SD, et al. A comparison of danazol and placebo in the treatment of adult idiopathic gynaecomastia: results of a prospective study in 55 patients. *Ann R Coll Surg Engl* 1990;72:296.
38. Stepanas AV, Burnet RB, Harding PE. Clomiphene in the treatment of pubertal-adolescent gynecomastia: a preliminary report. *J Pediatr* 1977;90:651.
39. Plourde PV, Kulin HE, Santner SJ. Clomiphene in the treatment of adolescent gynecomastia: clinical and endocrine studies. *Am J Dis Child* 1983;137:1080.
40. LeRoith D, Sobel R, Glick SM. The effect of clomiphene citrate on pubertal gynaecomastia. *Acta Endocrinol (Copenh)* 1980;95:177.
41. Parker LN, Gray DR, Lai MK, et al. Treatment of gynecomastia with tamoxifen: a double-blind crossover study. *Metabolism* 1986;35:705.
42. McDermott MT, Hofeldt FD, Kidd GS. Tamoxifen therapy for painful idiopathic gynecomastia. *South Med J* 1990;83:1283.
43. Alagaratnam TT. Idiopathic gynecomastia treated with tamoxifen: a preliminary report. *Clin Ther* 1987;9:483.
44. Zachmann M, Eiholzer U, Muritano M, et al. Treatment of pubertal gynaecomastia with testolactone. *Acta Endocrinol (Copenh)* 1986;279(Suppl):218.
45. Motoo Y, Taga H, Su S-B, Sawabu N. Effect of Gegen-Tang on painful gynecomastia in patients with liver cirrhosis: a brief report. *Am J Chinese Med* 1997;25:317.

Diseases of the Breast, 2nd ed.,
edited by Jay R. Harris.
Lippincott Williams & Wilkins, Philadelphia © 2000.

CHAPTER 9

Pathology of Benign Breast Disorders

Stuart J. Schnitt and James L. Connolly

Benign breast disorders are a heterogeneous group of lesions that clinically and radiographically span the entire spectrum of breast abnormalities. Some benign lesions present on physical examination or imaging studies with findings that are similar to those of breast cancer, and a biopsy or an excision is required to make the distinction.

Once a breast lesion has been shown to be benign on pathologic examination, the most important clinical consideration is the risk of subsequent breast cancer associated with that lesion. Physicians have known for many years that some benign breast lesions are more highly associated with breast cancer than are others. Two types of studies have evaluated this relationship. In the first type, the prevalence of benign alterations in breasts with cancer was compared with their prevalence in breasts without cancer.[1,2] Although these studies demonstrated that some benign lesions are more common in cancer-containing breasts, the histologic coexistence of certain benign breast lesions with breast cancer is not sufficient to establish that those benign lesions impart an increased cancer risk.

Studies from the late 1970s to the late 1990s have evaluated the subsequent risk of developing breast cancer in patients who have had a benign breast biopsy and for whom long-term follow-up is available.[3–13] In these studies, the benign biopsies were reviewed, and the type of benign lesion present was recorded and related to the risk of breast cancer. In some of these studies, the interaction of the histologic findings with other factors, such as family history of breast cancer, time since biopsy, and menopausal status, could also be examined in determining cancer risk. The results of these studies have provided important information regarding the risk of breast cancer associated with benign breast lesions, and this information is useful in patient management, counseling, and follow-up. These studies have further indicated that terms such as *fibrocystic disease*, *chronic cystic mastitis*, and *mammary dysplasia* are not clinically meaningful, because they encompass a heterogeneous group of processes, some physiologic and some pathologic, with widely varying cancer risks.[2,14,15]

The seminal study evaluating benign breast disease and cancer risk is the retrospective cohort study reported by Dupont and Page[4] and Page et al.[16] In this study, the slides of benign breast biopsies from more than 3,000 women in Nashville were reviewed, and the histologic lesions present were categorized using strictly defined criteria[4,16,17] into one of three categories: nonproliferative lesions, proliferative lesions without atypia, and atypical hyperplasias (Table 1). The risk of developing breast cancer was then determined for each of these groups. This system provides a pragmatic, clinically relevant approach to benign breast lesions and has been supported by a consensus conference of the College of American Pathologists.[18,18a] Studies from other groups have largely confirmed the initial observations of the Nashville group and have extended these findings by providing important new information regarding benign breast disease and breast cancer risk.[7,8,11,13]

NONPROLIFERATIVE LESIONS

Nonproliferative lesions, as defined by Dupont and Page,[4] include cysts, papillary apocrine change, epithelial-related calcifications, and mild hyperplasia of the usual type. *Cysts* are fluid-filled round to ovoid structures that vary in size from microscopic to grossly evident (Fig. 1). *Gross cysts*, as defined by Haagensen, are those that are large enough to produce palpable masses.[19] Cysts are derived from the terminal duct lobular unit. The epithelium usually consists of two layers: an inner (luminal) epithelial layer and an outer myoepithelial layer. In some cysts, the epithelium is markedly attenuated or absent; in others, the lining epithelium shows apocrine metaplasia, characterized by granular eosinophilic cytoplasm and apical cytoplasmic protrusions ("snouts"). *Papillary apocrine change* is characterized by a proliferation of ductal epithelial cells, in which all of the cells show apocrine features. *Epithelial-related calcifications* are frequently observed in breast tissue and may be seen in normal ducts and lobules or in virtually any pathologic condition in the breast. Calcifications may also be seen in the breast stroma and blood vessel walls. *Mild hyperplasia of the usual type* is defined as an increase in the number of epithelial cells within

S. J. Schnitt: Department of Pathology, Harvard Medical School, Brigham and Women's Hospital, Dana-Farber Cancer Institute, Boston, Massachusetts; Department of Surgical Pathology, Beth Israel Deaconess Medical Center, Boston, Massachusetts

J. L. Connolly: Department of Medicine, Harvard Medical School, Beth Israel Deaconess Medical Center, Boston, Massachusetts

TABLE 1. *Categorization of benign breast lesions according to the criteria of Dupont, Page, and Rogers*[4,16,17]

Nonproliferative
Cysts
Papillary apocrine change
Epithelial-related calcifications
Mild hyperplasia of the usual type
Proliferative lesions without atypia
Moderate or florid ductal hyperplasia of the usual type
Intraductal papilloma
Sclerosing adenosis
Fibroadenoma
Atypical hyperplasia
Atypical ductal hyperplasia
Atypical lobular hyperplasia

a duct that is less than four epithelial cells in depth. In this type of hyperplasia, the epithelial cells do not cross the lumen of the involved space.

In the study of Dupont and Page,[4] 70% of the biopsies showed nonproliferative lesions. The risk of subsequent breast cancer among these patients was no greater than that of women who had had no breast biopsy (relative risk, 0.89), even in patients with a family history of breast cancer (in a mother, sister, or daughter). The patients with lesions in the nonproliferative category who had an increased risk of developing breast cancer were those who had gross cysts plus a family history of breast cancer. The relative risk with gross cysts alone was 1.5, but the relative risk in patients with gross cysts and a family history of breast cancer was 3.0. Although Dupont and Page initially included fibroadenomas among the nonproliferative lesions, the results of a 1994 study by these investigators indicated a higher relative risk of breast cancer among patients with fibroadenoma than among patients with nonproliferative lesions.[20] As a result, fibroadenomas are now included among the proliferative lesions without atypia (see the section Fibroadenomas).

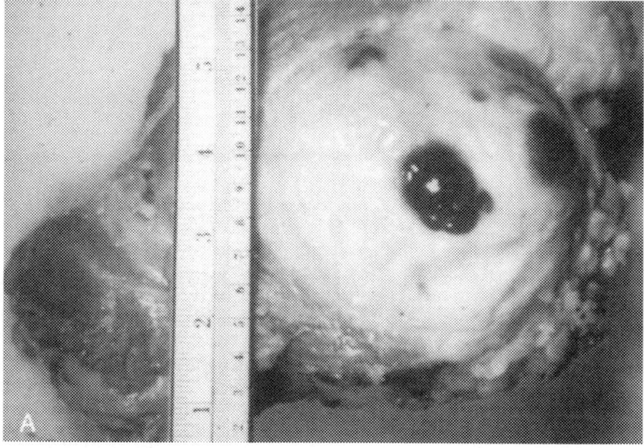

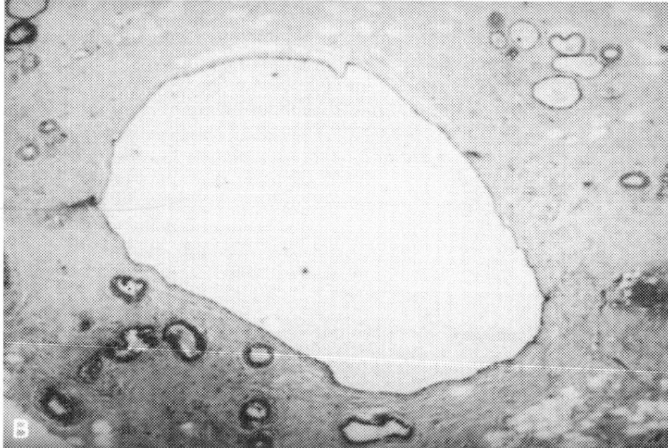

FIG. 1. A: This fibrotic breast tissue contains grossly apparent cysts. The cysts are often blue in the fresh state; hence, their designation as *blue dome cysts.* **B:** Photomicrograph shows breast tissue containing a cyst that is surrounded by fibrous stroma and is lined by a flattened layer of epithelial cells.

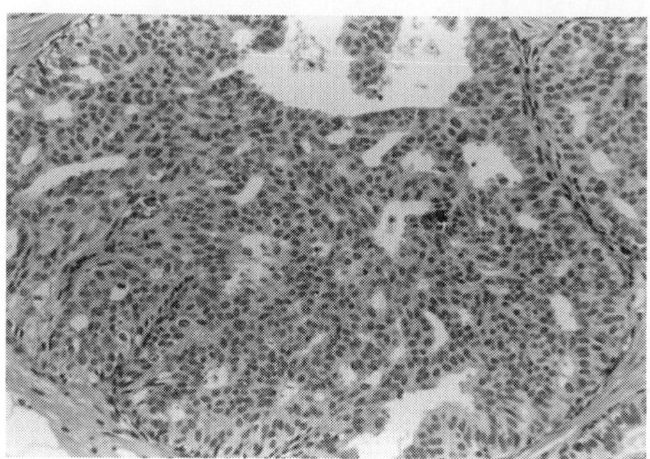

FIG. 2. Florid intraductal hyperplasia is characterized by a proliferation of cytologically benign epithelial cells that fill and distend the duct. The nuclei vary in size, shape, and orientation. The spaces within the duct are also variable in size and contour.

PROLIFERATIVE LESIONS WITHOUT ATYPIA

Included within the group of proliferative lesions without atypia are moderate or florid hyperplasias of the usual type, intraductal papillomas, and sclerosing adenosis.[4,21] As noted in the previous paragraph, fibroadenomas are now included in this category. *Moderate* or *florid hyperplasias of the usual type* are intraductal epithelial proliferations more than four epithelial cells in depth. They are characterized by a tendency to bridge and often distend the involved space. The proliferation may have a solid, fenestrated, or papillary architecture. If spaces remain within the duct lumen, they are irregular and variable in shape. The cells comprising this type of proliferation are cytologically benign and variable in size, shape, and orientation (Fig. 2). Two distinct cell populations can often be discerned: epithelial cells and myoepithelial cells. A fibrovascular stroma is sometimes present. *Intraductal papillomas* are discussed in the section Intra-

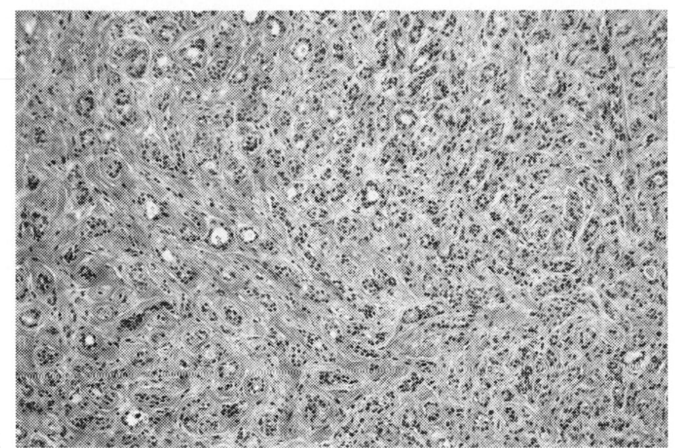

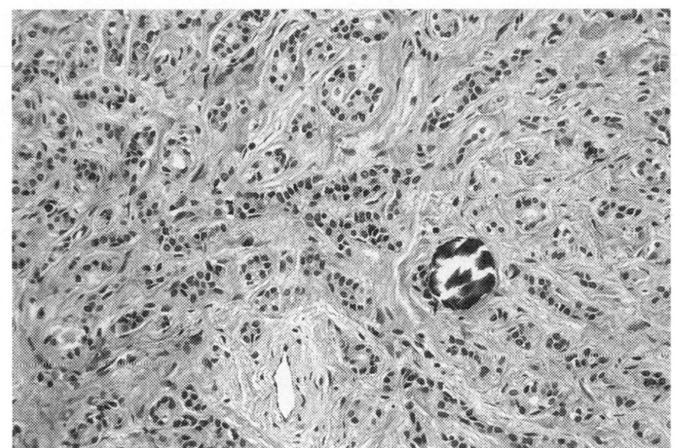

FIG. 3. Sclerosing adenosis. **A:** Low-power photomicrograph demonstrates a lobulocentric proliferation of stromal and epithelial elements. **B:** High-power examination reveals epithelial cells entrapped in a fibrotic stroma. The cells are cytologically benign, but the pattern simulates that of invasive carcinoma.

ductal Papillomas. *Sclerosing adenosis* is most often an incidental microscopic finding, but it may present as a palpable mass (the "adenosis tumor"). Microscopically, these lesions consist of a proliferation of glandular (acinar) structures and stroma in a lobulocentric configuration. Particularly in the center of such lesions, the stroma may compress and distort the glandular elements, producing a pattern that may mimic infiltrating carcinoma (Fig. 3). In some cases, the epithelial cells in sclerosing adenosis show prominent apocrine features (apocrine adenosis).[22] Many examples of sclerosing adenosis are associated with calcifications, which may, in turn, be seen on mammograms.

Women who have had a benign breast biopsy showing proliferative lesions without atypia, as defined earlier, have a mildly elevated breast cancer risk, 1.5 to 2.0 times that of the reference population (Table 2).

ATYPICAL HYPERPLASIAS

Atypical hyperplasias are proliferative lesions of the breast that possess some, but not all, of the features of carcinoma *in situ*.[4,16,17] Thus, an understanding of the histologic features of atypical hyperplasia requires familiarity with the histologic features of carcinoma *in situ* (Table 3). Atypical hyperplasias are categorized as either ductal or lobular. *Atypical ductal hyperplasias* are lesions that have some of the architectural and cytologic features of ductal carcinoma *in situ* (DCIS), such as nuclear monomorphism, regular cell placement, and round regular spaces, in at least part of the involved space (Fig. 4). *Atypical lobular hyperplasias* are characterized by changes similar to those of lobular carcinoma *in situ* but lack the complete criteria for that diagnosis (Fig. 5). In addition to involving lobular units, the cells of atypical lobular hyperplasia may involve ducts.[23]

With the increasing use of mammographic screening, atypical hyperplasias are being diagnosed more frequently than in the past. For example, when a biopsy is performed because of a palpable mass, atypical hyperplasia is seen in only 2% to 4% of cases.[4,24] In contrast, atypical hyperplasia is identified in 12% to 17% of biopsies performed because of the presence of microcalcifications on mammography.[25,26]

TABLE 2. *Relative risk of breast cancer according to histologic category of benign breast disease in studies using the criteria of Dupont, Page, and Rogers*[4,16,17]

Study	Study design	Histologic category: Nonproliferative	Proliferative without atypia	Atypical hyperplasia
Nashville[4]	Retrospective cohort	1	1.9 (1.0–2.3)	5.3 (3.1–8.8)
Nurses' Health Study[13]	Case control	1	1.6 (1.2–2.2)	3.9 (2.6–5.9)
Breast Cancer Detection Demonstration Project[11]	Case control	1	1.3 (0.77–2.20)	4.3 (1.7–11.0)
Florence, Italy[7]	Case control	1	1.3 (0.5–3.5)	13.0 (4.1–41.7)

Numbers in parentheses represent 95% confidence intervals.

TABLE 3. *Histologic criteria for diagnosis of carcinoma* in situ

	Nuclei	Cells	Pattern
Ductal[a]	Round or oval Monotonous Hyperchromatic	Round-cuboidal or polygonal Distinct cell borders (usually) Evenly spaced At least two spaces completely involved with same cell population	No swirls or streaming Round, regular, and smooth spaces or micropapillae with narrow base Rigid, geometric configuration, bridges lacking attenuation
Lobular	Round Monotonous Hyperchromatic (usually)	Round-cuboidal or polygonal Evenly spaced	One-half of acini in lobular unit completely filled, distorted, and distended with characteristic cells

[a]Low-grade types.
Adapted from ref. 16 with permission.

Women who have had a benign breast biopsy that demonstrates atypical hyperplasia are at a substantially increased risk for developing breast cancer—3.5 to 5.0 times that of the reference population (see Table 2). However, in both the Nashville study[16] and the Nurses' Health Study,[13] the risk associated with atypical lobular hyperplasia was greater than that associated with atypical ductal hyperplasia (Table 4). Furthermore, patients whose biopsies showed atypical lobular hyperplasia involving both lobules and ducts had a higher relative risk of developing cancer (6.8) than those with either atypical lobular hyperplasia alone (relative risk, 4.3) or those with only ductal involvement by atypical lobular hyperplasia cells (relative risk, 2.1).[23]

These studies of benign breast disease and breast cancer risk have also demonstrated that the risk of breast cancer in patients with atypical hyperplasia (of both ductal and lobular types) is approximately equal in both breasts.[7,27] This finding suggests that atypical hyperplasia is best considered a marker of generalized increased risk.

FACTORS MODIFYING BREAST CANCER RISK IN WOMEN WITH BIOPSY-PROVEN BENIGN BREAST DISEASE

A number of factors appear to modify the breast cancer risk associated with biopsy-proven benign breast disease,

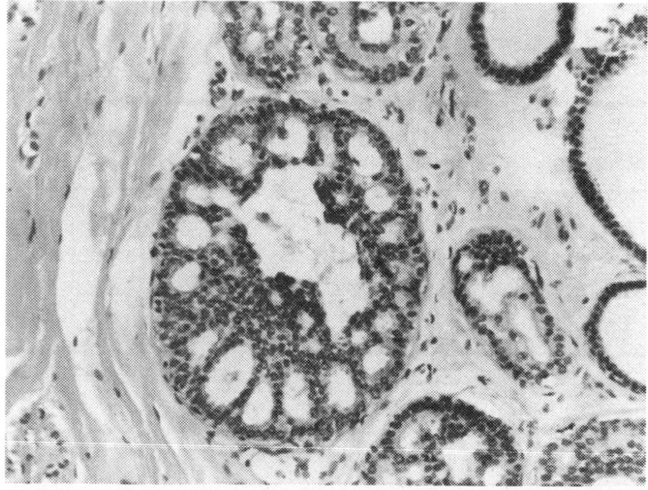

FIG. 4. Atypical ductal hyperplasia. Near the center of this space is a proliferation of relatively uniform epithelial cells with monomorphic, round nuclei. However, this proliferation involves only a portion of the space. In other areas, the proliferating epithelial cells maintain their orientation to one another. Thus, this lesion has some of the features of low-grade ductal carcinoma *in situ* and is best categorized as atypical ductal hyperplasia.

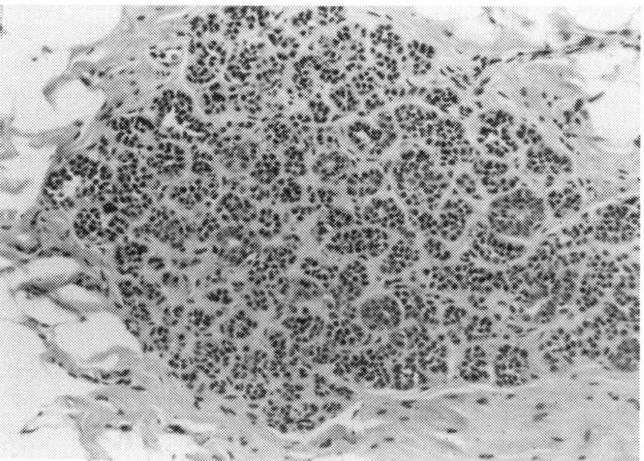

FIG. 5. Atypical lobular hyperplasia. The acini contain a proliferation of small, uniform cells, which are discohesive in some areas; however, the involved acinar structures are not distended by this proliferation. Because this lesion has some features of lobular carcinoma *in situ*, it is most appropriately categorized as atypical lobular hyperplasia.

TABLE 4. *Relative risk of breast cancer according to type of atypical hyperplasia*

Study	All atypical hyperplasia	Atypical ductal hyperplasia	Atypical lobular hyperplasia
Nashville[16]	5.3 (3.1–8.8)	4.7 (2.5–8.9)	5.8 (3.0–11.0)
Nurses' Health Study[13]	3.4 (2.0–5.9)	2.4 (1.3–4.5)	5.3 (2.7–10.4)

Numbers in parentheses represent 95% confidence intervals.

including a family history of breast cancer, time since biopsy, and menopausal status.

Family History

General agreement exists that the presence of a family history of breast cancer in a first degree relative (mother, sister, or daughter) is associated with a slight increase in the breast cancer risk in women with proliferative lesions without atypia (Table 5).[4,11,16] However, the influence of family history on breast cancer risk in women with atypical hyperplasia is somewhat less clear. Dupont and Page[4] and Page et al.[16] reported that the risk among patients with both atypical hyperplasia and a family history of breast cancer was twice that of women with atypical hyperplasia without a family history. Similarly, in the Breast Cancer Detection Demonstration Project (BCDDP) study, the presence of a positive family history substantially increased the breast cancer risk among women with atypical hyperplasia.[11] However, these studies included few women who had both atypical hyperplasia and a positive family history, and the 95% confidence intervals for these risk estimates are broad (see Table 5). In an update of the Nurses' Health Study, the presence of a positive family history was not associated with the dramatic increase in breast cancer risk among women with atypical hyperplasia seen in the Nashville and BCDDP studies (see Table 5). The reason for this discrepancy is not clear but may be related at least in part to differences in the age or menopausal status of the patients in the various studies. For example, it is plausible that a positive family history primarily increases breast cancer risk in younger or premenopausal women with atypical hyperplasia, at least some of whom may have a genetic predisposition to breast cancer. Therefore, studies with greater numbers of younger, premenopausal women may be more apt to show an influence of family history on breast cancer risk in women with atypical hyperplasia than studies with fewer such women. Additional studies are needed to clarify this important issue.

Time Since Biopsy

The risk of developing breast cancer does not appear to be constant over time. For example, in the Nashville study, women with proliferative lesions without atypia who remained free of breast cancer for 10 years after their benign breast biopsy were at no greater breast cancer risk than women of similar age without such a history. In addition, the breast cancer risk among women with atypical hyperplasia was greatest (9.8) in the first 10 years after the benign breast biopsy and fell to 3.6 after 10 years.[28] A similar decrease in breast cancer risk beyond 10 years was also observed in the Nurses' Health Study cohort among women with atypical lobular hyperplasia, but not among those with atypical ductal hyperplasia. More data are needed to clarify the relationship between time since biopsy and breast cancer risk for women with atypical hyperplasia.

Menopausal Status

The risk of breast cancer among women with atypical hyperplasia appears to be influenced by the patient's menopausal status. In the BCDDP study, premenopausal women with a biopsy showing atypical hyperplasia were at a substantially higher breast cancer risk (relative risk, 12; 95% confidence interval, 1.0–68.0) than postmenopausal women with that diagnosis (relative risk, 3.3; 95% confidence interval, 1.1–10.0).[11] In the Nurses' Health Study, women with atypical hyperplasia had a higher relative risk of premenopausal breast cancer (relative risk, 5.3; 95% confidence interval, 2.6–10.7) than postmenopausal breast cancer (rela-

TABLE 5. *Effect of family history of breast cancer in a first-degree relative on relative risk of breast cancer*

Study	Proliferative without atypia		Atypical hyperplasia	
	No family history	Family history	No family history	Family history
Nashville[4]	1.9 (1.2–3.0)	2.7 (1.4–5.3)	4.3 (2.4–7.8)	8.4 (2.6–27.0)
Nurses' Health Study[a]	1.6 (1.1–2.2)	2.4 (1.4–4.2)	4.1 (2.6–6.4)	4.7 (2.1–10.4)
Breast Cancer Detection Demonstration Project[11]	1.7 (0.9–3.2)	2.6 (1.0–6.4)	4.2 (1.4–12.0)	22.0 (2.4–20.3)

Numbers in parentheses represent 95% confidence intervals.
[a]Unpublished data, May 1998.

tive risk, 3.7; 95% confidence interval, 2.1–6.6). Of note, in the BCDDP study and the Nurses' Health Study, the breast cancer risk among women with proliferative lesions without atypia did not vary with menopausal status.

Another issue of clinical importance is the influence of postmenopausal hormone replacement therapy on the risk of breast cancer in women with biopsy-proven benign breast disease. Clinical follow-up studies have shown that women who take hormone replacement therapy are at increased risk for developing breast cancer.[29] However, the use of hormone replacement does not appear to further increase the risk in women with proliferative breast disease without atypia or in those with atypical hyperplasia.[30,30a] In an analysis from the Nurses' Health Study, the relative risks of breast cancer among women with proliferative lesions without atypia were 1.3, 1.3, and 1.5 for women who never used postmenopausal hormones, past users, and current users, respectively. Among women with atypical hyperplasia, the relative breast cancer risks were 3.4 for those who had not used hormone replacement, 3.0 for past users, and 2.5 for current users. Thus, the available data suggest that the use of hormone replacement therapy is not contraindicated in women with a history of biopsy-proven benign breast disease.[30]

The foregoing data provide compelling evidence that breast cancer risk varies with the histologic category of benign breast disease. They further indicate that the risk among women with biopsy-proven benign breast disease is influenced by other factors. However, for proper counseling of individual patients, the difference between relative risk and absolute risk must be understood.[31] The *relative risk* for breast cancer represents the incidence of breast cancer among women within a certain subpopulation divided by the incidence of breast cancer in the reference population. The magnitude of the relative risk is highly dependent on the breast cancer incidence in both the study group and the reference population. In contrast, a woman's *absolute risk* of breast cancer is her probability of developing breast cancer during some specified time period. For example, whereas the relative risk for patients with atypical hyperplasia and a family history of breast cancer in the study of Dupont and Page was 8.9, only 20% of patients in this group had developed breast cancer 15 years after their benign biopsy. Eight percent of patients with atypical hyperplasia but no family history, 4% of patients with proliferative lesions without atypia, and 2% of women with nonproliferative lesions developed breast cancer in 15 years.[4]

CONSISTENCY OF HISTOLOGIC CLASSIFICATION

Given the apparent clinical importance of distinguishing among the various types of benign breast disease, the ability of pathologists to accurately and reproducibly categorize such lesions and to distinguish them from carcinoma *in situ* is a matter of legitimate concern. This problem has been addressed in several studies.[32–34] In one of these studies, conducted by Rosai, five highly respected breast pathologists were asked to apply the criteria they used in their daily practice to categorize a series of proliferative breast lesions. Under these conditions, there was not a single case in which all five pathologists arrived at the same diagnosis, and in only 18% of the cases did four of the five pathologists agree.[32] The results of another study suggest that, with standardization of histologic criteria among pathologists, interobserver variability in the diagnosis of proliferative breast lesions can be reduced. In that study, six experienced breast pathologists were instructed to use the same diagnostic criteria (i.e., those of Page et al.[4,16,17]) for categorizing a series of proliferative breast lesions. Complete agreement among all six pathologists was observed in 58% of the cases, and all but one pathologist arrived at the same diagnosis in 71%.[33] The results of these studies indicate that, although the use of standardized histologic criteria improves interobserver concordance in the diagnosis of these lesions, even under these circumstances, some proliferative lesions defy reproducible categorization. Some authors have suggested that quantitative criteria should also be used to aid in distinguishing between atypical ductal hyperplasia and DCIS. For example, Page et al. require that all of the features of DCIS be uniformly present throughout at least two separate spaces before DCIS is diagnosed.[16] Lesions that have the qualitative features of low-grade DCIS that do not fulfill this quantitative criterion are categorized as atypical hyperplasias. Tavassoli and Norris have suggested that the risk of breast cancer associated with very small foci of low-grade DCIS (i.e., less than 2 mm) is similar to that associated with atypical ductal hyperplasia; therefore, they classify lesions that fulfill the qualitative criteria for low-grade DCIS but that are less than 2 mm in size as atypical ductal hyperplasias.[6] Whereas these quantitative criteria are of some value in the categorization of very small lesions that have been widely excised, they should not be used when such lesions are identified at or near the margin of an excision specimen or in a core-needle biopsy specimen.

To overcome some of the limitations of morphology, studies have attempted to identify biological or genetic markers that may be useful adjuncts to histopathology in distinguishing among these various proliferative lesions. In particular, a marker to aid in the distinction between atypical ductal hyperplasia and low-grade DCIS would be particularly valuable. Unfortunately, atypical ductal hyperplasia and low-grade DCIS share similar immunophenotypes for most markers evaluated. For example, both lesions are typically estrogen receptor–positive,[35] lack overexpression of the HER-2/neu oncogene,[35,36] lack accumulation of the p53 protein,[35,37–41] and show Bcl-2 protein expression.[41] The only marker reported to date that has been claimed to be useful for distinguishing between these two lesions is cyclin D_1 messenger RNA (mRNA) overexpression. In a study using *in situ* hybridization for mRNA using formalin-fixed, paraffin-embedded material, cyclin D_1 overexpression was observed in 18% of cases of atypical ductal hyperplasia. In contrast, overexpression was seen in 76% of cases of low-grade DCIS, a frequency similar to that seen in high-grade DCIS and invasive cancer.[42] However, in a later study, a similar proportion of cases of atypical ductal hyperplasia and low-grade DCIS showed overexpression of the cyclin D_1 protein by immunohistochemistry (39% and 45%, respectively).[43] Therefore, cyclin D_1 overexpression, at least at the protein level, does not appear to be useful as a diagnostic aid to distinguish between atypical ductal hyperplasia and low-grade DCIS.

Active effort is also being made to determine if biological markers in benign breast biopsies might be useful in predicting breast cancer risk, either alone or in combination with histopathology. To date, a number of markers have been studied in this regard, including estrogen receptor, angiogenesis, p53 expression, and HER-2/neu expression. In a study of estrogen receptor expression in benign breast tissue, Khan et al. found that the odds ratio for breast cancer in women with estrogen receptor–positive benign epithelium was 3.2 in comparison with women with estrogen receptor–negative benign breast tissue.[44] In a small pilot study, Guinebretiere et al. found that increased angiogenesis in benign breast biopsies was associated with a significantly increased breast cancer risk, independent of the presence of atypical hyperplasia.[45] One study suggested that p53 protein accumulation in benign breast tissue was associated with an increased breast cancer risk (relative risk, 2.55), even after adjustment for other breast cancer risk factors. In that study, no significant association was seen between HER-2/neu protein expression in benign breast tissue and increased breast cancer risk.[46] However, in another study, *HER-2/neu* gene amplification in benign breast tissue, as determined by polymerase chain reaction, was associated with an increase in breast cancer risk.[47] A number of studies have also evaluated loss of heterozygosity and microsatellite instability at various chromosomal loci in benign breast lesions. These studies have shown that at least some examples of florid ductal hyperplasia and atypical hyperplasia exhibit loss of heterozygosity, microsatellite instability, or both at a number of different genetic loci.[48–52] The clinical significance of these observations is not yet clear.[51] Nonetheless, studies such as these may ultimately provide important new information regarding the molecular and genetic alterations involved in both neoplastic progression and breast cancer risk in women with benign breast lesions. This subject is discussed in greater detail in Chapter 24.

A number of follow-up studies evaluating benign breast disease and breast cancer risk have used diagnostic criteria other than those of the Nashville group for categorizing benign breast lesions.[3,5,9,10,12] In general, the breast cancer risk in the highest risk groups in these studies is not as great as the risk found in the studies that have used the combined histologic-cytologic criteria outlined by Dupont, Page, and Rogers.[4,16,17]

In summary, the results of clinical follow-up studies indicate that the majority of women who have a benign breast biopsy are not at increased risk for developing breast cancer. A substantially increased breast cancer risk is seen only in the small percentage of patients whose benign breast biopsies show atypical hyperplasia using strictly defined histologic and cytologic criteria. The role of biological and molecular markers to help in distinguishing among the various proliferative breast lesions and to assess breast cancer risk is not yet well defined but remains an area of active investigation.

BENIGN NEOPLASMS AND PROLIFERATIVE LESIONS

Fibroadenomas

The clinical and epidemiologic features of fibroadenomas and their management are discussed in Chapter 4.

On gross examination, fibroadenomas are pseudoencapsulated and sharply delimited from the surrounding breast tissue. They are usually spheric or ovoid but may be multilobulated. When cut, the tumor bulges above the level of the surrounding breast tissue. The cut surface is most typically grey-white, and small, punctate, yellow-to-pink soft areas and slitlike spaces are commonly observed. Occasionally, the tumor has a gelatinous, mucoid consistency.

Microscopically, fibroadenomas have both an epithelial and stromal component. The histologic pattern depends on which of these components predominates. In general, the epithelial component consists of well-defined glandlike and ductlike spaces lined by cuboidal or columnar cells with uniform nuclei. Varying degrees of epithelial hyperplasia are frequently observed. The stromal component consists of connective tissue that has a variable content of acid mucopolysaccharides and collagen (Fig. 6). In older lesions and in postmenopausal patients, the stroma may become

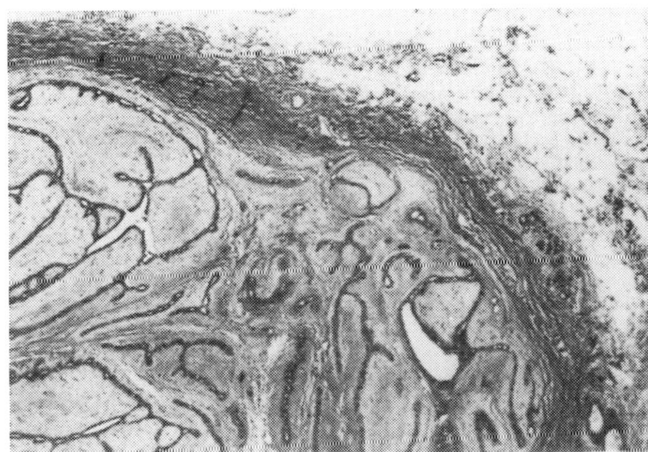

FIG. 6. In this fibroadenoma, the tumor is well circumscribed and is separated from the adjacent breast tissue by a rim of dense collagen. Both glandular and stomal elements are apparent.

hyalinized, calcified, or even ossified (ancient fibroadenoma). On rare occasions, mature adipose tissue or smooth muscle may comprise a portion of the stroma.[53,54] The term *intracanalicular* has been used to describe tumors in which the stromal component compresses the glands into slitlike spaces, whereas *pericanalicular* tumors are those in which the rounded configuration of the glandular structures is maintained. In fact, these two patterns often coexist in the same lesion, and this distinction has no clinical significance.

Complex Fibroadenomas

Fibroadenomas that contain cysts larger than 3 mm in diameter, sclerosing adenosis, epithelial calcifications, or papillary apocrine change have been designated *complex fibroadenomas*. In a review of almost 2,500 fibroadenomas, such changes were seen in 23% of cases. In one clinical follow-up study, complex fibroadenomas were reported to be associated with a greater subsequent breast cancer risk than fibroadenomas that lack such changes.[55]

Juvenile Fibroadenomas

Most fibroadenomas in adolescents and younger women are the same type usually seen in older patients. A minority present a different clinical and pathologic picture and are termed *juvenile fibroadenomas*.[56–59] Unfortunately, this term has been used by different authors to describe different lesions. Some authors use the term to refer to fibroadenomatous lesions that grow rapidly and may show venous dilatation in the overlying skin. Such lesions may clinically resemble virginal hypertrophy, and only surgical exploration reveals a circumscribed tumor.[56–59] On microscopic examination, these lesions are more floridly glandular and have greater stromal cellularity than the more common adult-type fibroadenoma. Mies and Rosen use the term *juvenile fibroadenomas* to refer to fibroadenomatous lesions demonstrating severe epithelial hyperplasia that may border on carcinoma *in situ*.[59] Nevertheless, these lesions behave in a clinically benign fashion.

Giant Fibroadenomas

Some tumors that histologically are typical fibroadenomas may attain great size. Unfortunately, several authors have used the terms *giant fibroadenoma* and *benign cystosarcoma phyllodes* synonymously and have created considerable confusion regarding these entities. A lesion that has the microscopic appearance of a conventional fibroadenoma but that is large should still be classified as a fibroadenoma and may be treated adequately by enucleation. The major feature distinguishing a cystosarcoma phyllodes (preferably called a *phyllodes tumor*) from a giant fibroadenoma is the cellularity of the stromal component in the former.[53] However, making the distinction between these two entities may be extremely difficult in some cases, as discussed in Chapter 41. Because juvenile fibroadenomas may attain great size, some authors consider them to be variants of giant fibroadenomas.[58]

Infarction

Fibroadenomas may undergo partial, subtotal, or total infarction. Pregnancy and lactation are the most common predisposing factors. A relative vascular insufficiency in the face of increased metabolic activity in the breast has been postulated to underlie this phenomenon.[53]

Involvement of Fibroadenomas by Carcinoma

The involvement of fibroadenomas by carcinoma has been reviewed by Azzopardi[53] and by Pick and Iossifides.[60] Infrequently, carcinoma may occur in association with a fibroadenoma. The most frequent type of carcinoma involving fibroadenomas is lobular carcinoma *in situ*, but DCIS, infiltrating ductal carcinomas, and infiltrating lobular carcinomas have also been observed. In almost one-half of the reported cases, the malignant tumor also involves the surrounding breast tissue. The prognosis of carcinoma limited to a fibroadenoma is excellent.

Adenomas

Adenomas of the breast are well-circumscribed tumors composed of benign epithelial elements with sparse, inconspicuous stroma.[61] The last feature differentiates these lesions from fibroadenomas, in which the stroma is an integral part of the tumor. For practical purposes, adenomas may be divided into two major groups: tubular adenomas and lactating adenomas.

Tubular Adenomas

Tubular adenomas present in young women as well-defined, freely movable nodules that clinically resemble fibroadenomas.[61] Gross examination reveals a well-circumscribed, tan-yellow, firm tumor. On microscopic examination, tubular adenomas are seen to be separated from the adjacent breast tissue by a pseudocapsule and are composed of a proliferation of uniform, small tubular structures with a scant amount of intervening stroma. The tubules consist of an inner epithelial layer and an outer myoepithelial layer, and resemble normal breast acini on light-microscope and ultrastructural examination. In some cases, this pattern is mixed with that of a fibroadenoma, suggesting a relationship between the two tumors.

Lactating Adenomas (Nodular Lactational Hyperplasia)

Lactating adenomas present as one or more freely movable masses during pregnancy or the postpartum period.[61] On a gross level, they are well circumscribed and lobulated, and on cut section they appear tan and softer than tubular adenomas. On microscopic examination, these lesions show lobulated borders and are composed of glands lined by cuboidal cells with secretory activity, identical to the lactational changes normally observed in breast tissue during pregnancy and the puerperium. Although some authors believe that these lesions are the result of lactational changes superimposed on a preexisting tubular adenoma, others have suggested that they represent *de novo* lesions and are merely nodular foci of hyperplasia in the lactating breast.

O'Hara and Page reviewed 42 cases of breast adenomas that demonstrated lactational changes.[62] They observed an overlapping spectrum of morphologic features in fibroadenomas with lactational changes and in lactating and tubular adenomas. These authors suggested that all these lesions may have a common pathogenesis.

Rarely, adenomatous tumors resembling dermal sweat-gland neoplasms are observed as primary lesions in the breast parenchyma (e.g., clear cell hidradenoma and eccrine spiradenoma)[52,60] or nipple (e.g., syringomatous adenoma).[63,64] Pleomorphic adenomas, histologically identical to those seen in the salivary glands and skin, have also been described in the breast.[65–68] Although some of these lesions appear to arise from the breast tissue *de novo*, others appear to represent variants of intraductal papillomas.[68]

Adenoma of the Nipple

Adenoma of the nipple has been described under a variety of names, including *florid papillomatosis of the nipple ducts*,[69] *subareolar duct papillomatosis*,[53] *papillary adenoma of the nipple*,[70] and *erosive adenomatosis of the nipple*.[71] It is not, strictly speaking, a true adenoma of the breast, as defined by Hertel et al.,[61] because of its prominent stromal component. The clinical features of this lesion are discussed in Chapter 5.

On macroscopic examination, some adenomas of the nipple appear as solid, grey-tan, poorly demarcated tumors in the nipple and subareolar region; in other cases, no gross lesion is evident. Microscopically, the dominant feature is a proliferation of small glandlike structures. Solid and papillary proliferation of ductal epithelium is usually evident as well; however, the papillary pattern may be inconspicuous or totally absent. In advanced lesions, glandular epithelium extends out onto the surface of the nipple. This phenomenon results in the clinically apparent, reddish, granular appearance. Squamous epithelium frequently extends into the superficial regions of the involved ducts, sometimes with the formation of keratinaceous cysts. The lesions usually show considerable stromal fibrosis. This connective tissue may distort and entrap the epithelial elements, resulting in a pattern mimicking invasive carcinoma. The lesion is distinguishable from carcinoma by the preservation of a double layer of epithelium in the proliferating glands (an inner epithelial and outer myoepithelial layer), minimal nuclear atypicality, absence of necrosis, and the overall configuration on low-power microscopy. In problematic cases, immunohistochemical stains for actin may be of value in distinguishing a nipple adenoma (the glands of which are surrounded by actin-positive myoepithelial cells) from invasive carcinoma (which lacks an actin-positive myoepithelial cell component).[72]

A few cases of carcinoma associated with adenomas of the nipple have been reported.[73–75] In the majority of cases, however, the lesion is entirely benign. Reports of recurrence probably represent cases in which the initial resection failed to remove the lesion completely.

Intraductal Papillomas

A variety of lesions in the breast are characterized by a papillary configuration on gross or microscopic examination (or both). These include solitary intraductal papillomas, multiple (peripheral) papillomas, and papillomatosis. *Solitary intraductal papilloma* represents a distinct clinicopathologic entity, as described below and in Chapter 5. *Papillomatosis* is a term used to describe microscopic foci of intraductal hyperplasia that have a papillary architecture and are, therefore, included by Dupont and Page in the category of proliferative lesions without atypia.[4] *Multiple (peripheral) papillomas* are lesions that are less uniformly recognized. Although some authors include these in the category of papillomatosis, others recognize a separate clinicopathologic entity characterized clinically by an indistinct mass with or without nipple discharge and pathologically by multiple small, but grossly evident, papillary lesions.[19]

Solitary Intraductal Papillomas

Solitary intraductal papillomas are tumors of the major lactiferous ducts, most frequently observed in women 30 to 50 years of age. The clinical findings are presented in Chapter 5. These lesions are generally smaller than 1 cm in diameter and usually measure 3 mm to 4 mm. Occasionally, they may be as large as 4 or 5 cm. On gross examination, intraductal papillomas are tan-pink, friable tumors within a dilatated duct or cyst. A frankly papillary configuration may or may not be apparent. The tumor is usually attached to the wall of the involved duct by a delicate stalk, but it may be sessile. To identify the papilloma, the involved duct should be opened carefully, using a fine pair of scissors, until the tumor is exposed. Identification of the lesion may be facilitated by the placement of a suture at the end of the involved duct nearest the nipple. Randomly slicing through

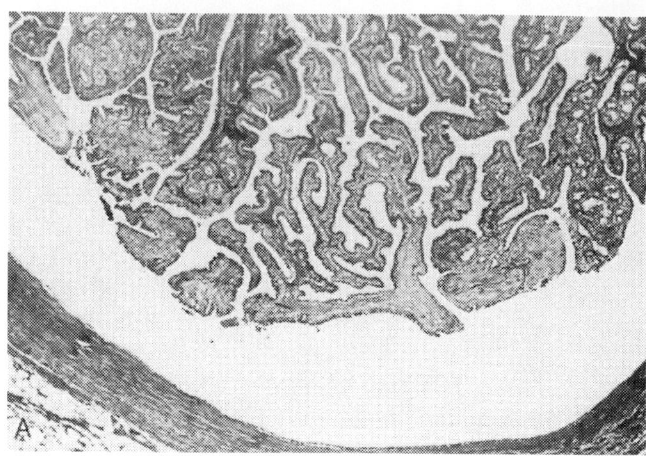

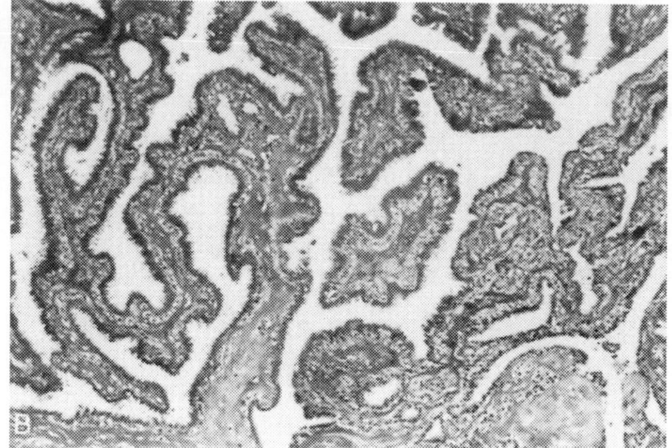

FIG. 7. Intraductal papilloma. **A:** Low-power photomicrograph demonstrates the papillary lesion within a dilatated duct. **B:** Higher-power view demonstrates that the papillae are composed of central fibrovascular cores covered by two layers of cells, a myoepithelial layer (lying closer to the cores) and an epithelial layer (lying closer to the duct lumen).

the excised tissue is not recommended, as a small lesion may be missed.

Microscopically, these tumors are composed of multiple, branching, and interanastomosing papillae, each with a central fibrovascular core and a covering layer of cuboidal to columnar epithelial cells. A myoepithelial cell layer is often discernible between the epithelial cells and the connective tissue stalk (Fig. 7). In some areas, the complex growth pattern of the papillae results in the formation of glandlike spaces. Variable amounts of fibrosis may result in the entrapment of epithelial elements, producing a pseudoinfiltrative pattern. Many lesions, designated by some authors as "ductal adenomas," appear to represent extensively sclerotic intraductal papillomas.[76,77] In addition, florid epithelial proliferation is sometimes observed in intraductal papillomas. At times, the epithelial cell hyperplasia or fibrosis (or both) and the architectural distortion make it extremely difficult to distinguish between benign papilloma and papillary carcinoma. Features helpful in making this distinction have been elucidated by Kraus and Neubecker[78] and by Azzopardi.[53] In general, benign lesions are characterized by a proliferation composed of two cell types (epithelial and myoepithelial); lack of nuclear hyperchromasia or monomorphism; scant mitotic activity; prominent connective tissue stroma; apocrine metaplasia; lack of necrosis; and the presence of benign proliferative lesions, such as intraductal hyperplasia and sclerosing adenosis, in the adjacent breast tissue. Immunohistochemical staining for a variety of antigens has been used as an aid in distinguishing benign from malignant papillary lesions. Although differences in the distribution of actin-positive myoepithelial cells, carcinoembryonic antigen, and some keratin proteins have been noted,[79,80] such studies still must be considered as adjuncts to routine evaluation by light microscope. One study has also suggested that the epithelial cells of benign intraductal papillomas are monoclonal in origin,[81] which indicates that even clonal analysis is unlikely to be helpful in distinguishing benign from malignant papillary lesions. The foregoing description should make it apparent that careful evaluation of intraductal papillomas can be accomplished only with paraffin-embedded sections. Therefore, frozen-section evaluation of papillary lesions of the breast is strongly discouraged.

Several additional features of intraductal papillomas deserve emphasis. Papillomas may undergo partial or total infarction, often accompanied by distortion of the adjacent, viable epithelium and production of a pattern that may simulate invasive carcinoma. Squamous metaplasia has been observed in intraductal papillomas. In some cases, it accompanies infarction, but it has also been observed in the absence of infarction. This phenomenon may also result in a disturbing growth pattern that may be confused with carcinoma.[82] Finally, some intraductal papillomas exhibit areas of atypia that range from foci resembling atypical ductal hyperplasia to areas qualitatively similar to low-grade ductal carcinoma *in situ*. In one study, the subsequent breast cancer risk associated with the presence of atypical ductal hyperplasia or limited (less than 3-mm) low-grade ductal carcinoma *in situ* within a papilloma was similar to that of patients with atypical hyperplasia in the breast parenchyma (fourfold to fivefold relative risk). The breast cancer risk in these patients was largely confined to the ipsilateral breast, in the area of the original papilloma.[83]

Multiple (Peripheral) Intraductal Papillomas

Compared to solitary intraductal papillomas, multiple intraductal papillomas tend to occur in younger patients, are less often associated with nipple discharge, are more frequently peripheral, and are more often bilateral. Most important, these lesions appear to be susceptible to the development of carcinoma. In Haagensen's series of 68 patients with multiple papillomas, simultaneous or subsequent carcinoma of the apocrine papillary and cribriform types was observed in 22 patients (32%).[19] A study from another group, in which surgically excised specimens from patients with intraductal papillomas were subjected to three-dimensional reconstruction, confirms these observations.[84] All 16 cases of multiple papillomas in the series were found to originate in the most peripheral portion of the duct system, the terminal duct lobular unit. Furthermore, carcinoma was associated with these multiple peripheral papillomas in six cases (37.5%). In contrast, no cases of carcinoma were found to be associated with solitary papillomas involving the large ducts. These findings suggest that peripheral papillomas, in contrast to solitary central papillomas, may be highly susceptible to malignant transformation.

Papillomatosis

Foci of moderate or florid hyperplasia may grow in a papillary configuration. Such lesions have the same significance as other types of moderate and florid hyperplasia (see section Proliferative Lesions without Atypia).

Juvenile Papillomatosis (Swiss Cheese Disease)

Juvenile papillomatosis was first recognized as a clinicopathologic entity by Rosen et al. in 1980.[85] This lesion occurs most commonly in adolescents and young women (mean age of 23 years), but it has been seen in women up to 48 years of age. Patients typically present with a painless mass that, on physical examination, is circumscribed, easily movable, and most often considered to be a fibroadenoma.

On gross pathologic examination, the lesions range in size from 1 to 8 cm. Multiple cysts of up to 1 cm in diameter are generally apparent. The microscopic features of juvenile papillomatosis are not unique to this entity and are all components described as part of "fibrocystic disease." The constellation of histologic features, however, forms a characteristic complex. These lesions appear to be well circumscribed but not encapsulated and are characterized by the following elements: duct papillomatosis, presence of apocrine and nonapocrine cysts, papillary apocrine hyperplasia, sclerosing adenosis, and duct stasis. The epithelial proliferation in these lesions may be quite marked, and the cytologic and architectural features may approach those of DCIS.

Follow-up studies have suggested that juvenile papillomatosis is associated with an increased risk of breast cancer in the patient's female relatives, and that the patient herself may be at increased risk for developing carcinoma, particularly if the lesion is bilateral and the patient has a family history of breast cancer.[86–89] The clinical significance of juvenile papillomatosis is discussed in more detail in Chapter 5.

Microglandular Adenosis

Microglandular adenosis (MGA) is an uncommon lesion that may be identified as an incidental finding in breast tissue excised for a variety of other lesions, or it may present as a palpable mass. Most women in whom this lesion has been reported are older than 40 years, but patients as young as 28 years and as old as 82 years have been reported to have MGA. The pathologic features of MGA have been reviewed by Millis and Eusebi.[90] MGA has generally been described to appear on gross examination as an ill-defined area of firm, rubbery tissue that is usually 3 to 4 cm in diameter. The importance of this lesion is that it may be mistaken for a well-differentiated (tubular) carcinoma on histologic examination. Microscopically, the lesion of MGA is characterized by a poorly circumscribed, haphazard proliferation of small, round glands in the breast stroma and adipose tissue. Unlike sclerosing adenosis, MGA does not have a lobulocentric, organoid configuration. The glands are composed of a single layer of cuboidal epithelial cells with clear to slightly eosinophilic cytoplasm and small, regular nuclei. The cells stain strongly for S100 protein, and the glands are surrounded by basement membrane material.[91,92] Eosinophilic secretions are frequently present within the glandular lumina. The stroma is typically composed of dense, relatively acellular collagen, which usually demarcates the lesion from the adjacent parenchyma. In some areas, the stroma is minimal and the proliferating glands lie exposed in adipose tissue (Fig. 8).

The relationship between MGA and cancer has been addressed in several studies. Simultaneous or subsequent carcinoma was reported in 4 of the 13 patients originally described by Rosen,[93] 1 of the 11 patients described by Tavassoli and Norris,[94] and none of the six patients reported by Clement and Azzopardi.[95] Rosenblum et al. described seven cases of MGA associated with carcinoma.[96] Most recently, James et al. noted carcinoma arising in or in conjunction with MGA in 14 of 60 cases (23%).[97] Thus, in some cases, MGA may be associated with carcinoma. At the present time, the recommended approach to the management of patients with MGA is complete, local excision of the lesion and careful follow-up.

Radial Scars

Radial scars have been described in the literature by a variety of names, including *sclerosing papillary proliferation*, *nonencapsulated sclerosing lesion*, *indurative mastopathy*, and *radial sclerosing lesion*.[68,98–101] The importance of these lesions is twofold. First, they may, on mam-

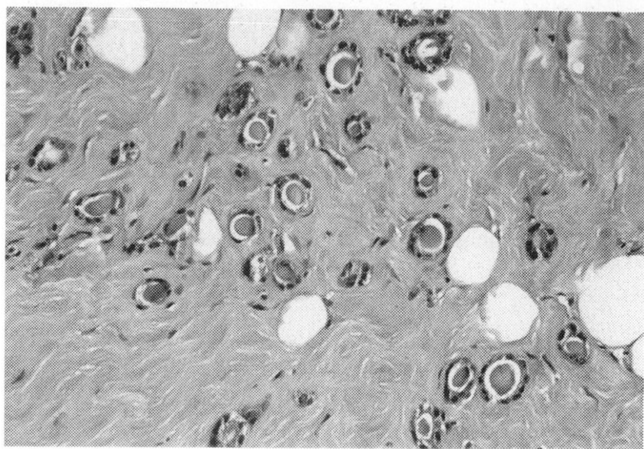

FIG. 8. Microglandular adenosis is characterized by a proliferation of small, glandular structures composed of a single layer of epithelial cells. The cells have clear to eosinophilic cytoplasm. The glands are round, and many contain eosinophilic secretions within their lumina.

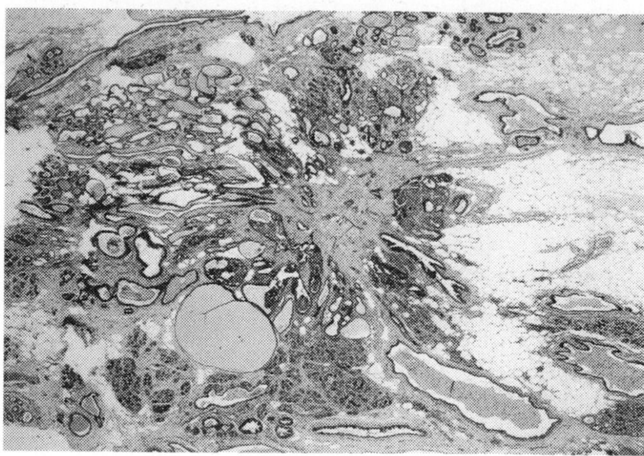

FIG. 9. Radial scar. This lesion is characterized by a central fibroelastotic core containing entrapped glandular elements. Radiating from this core are ducts and lobules that show a variety of changes, including cysts and hyperplasia.

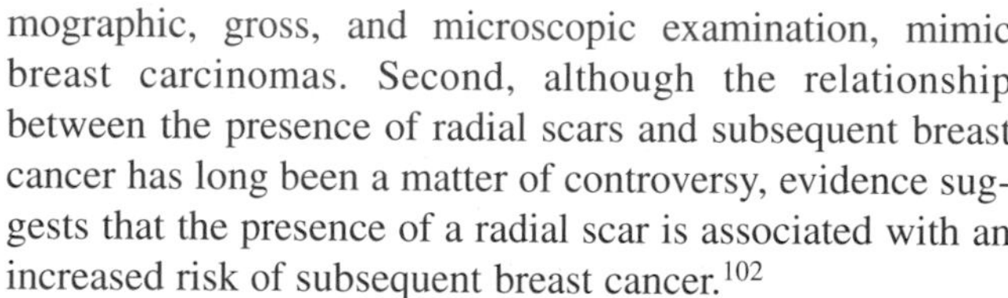

mographic, gross, and microscopic examination, mimic breast carcinomas. Second, although the relationship between the presence of radial scars and subsequent breast cancer has long been a matter of controversy, evidence suggests that the presence of a radial scar is associated with an increased risk of subsequent breast cancer.[102]

Radial scars are most frequently incidental findings in breast tissue excised because of another abnormality. They are often multiple, with as many as 31 lesions having been observed in a single breast.[103] Occasionally, they are large enough to be detected by mammography, on which they appear as spiculated masses that cannot be reliably distinguished from carcinomas. These lesions are typically less than 1 cm in diameter and, on gross examination, are irregular, grey-white, and indurated with central retraction—an appearance identical to that of scirrhous carcinoma. Similar lesions of greater size (i.e., larger than 1 cm) have been termed *complex sclerosing lesions*.[104]

Microscopically, the lesion has a stellate configuration and consists of a central, fibroelastotic core containing entrapped glandular elements. Radiating from this core are ducts with varying degrees of epithelial hyperplasia and papillomatosis. Ducts at the periphery may be dilatated cystically (Fig. 9). Sclerosing adenosis and apocrine metaplasia frequently accompany the lesion. The surrounding breast tissue typically shows varying degrees of intraductal hyperplasia and adenosis. The entrapped glands in the center of the lesion may be confused with the glands of tubular carcinoma. The configuration of the lesion on low-power microscopy permits the correct diagnosis.

The significance of radial scars with regard to the subsequent development of breast carcinoma is controversial. Some authors have argued that these lesions may represent incipient tubular carcinomas[99] or a stage in the development of many invasive breast cancers.[105] An autopsy study has demonstrated that these lesions are significantly more common in breasts of cancer patients than in noncancerous breasts[103]; however, this result is clearly not sufficient evidence to prove that these lesions are precancerous. To define further the relationship between radial scars and breast cancer, Sloane and Mayers reviewed 126 cases of radial scars and complex sclerosing lesions.[106] They found that carcinoma and atypical hyperplasia were more common in radial scars larger than 6 to 7 mm than in smaller radial scars and were more common in radial scars in women older than 50 years than in younger women.

Although several follow-up studies have failed to show an increased incidence of breast cancer in patients who have had a radial scar excised, these studies have been limited by small numbers of patients and lack of a suitable control group.[98,101,107] The results of a case-control study suggest that women with a biopsy-proven radial scar are at increased risk for subsequent breast cancer. In that study, the presence of a radial scar was associated with a twofold increase in breast cancer risk, independent of the histologic category of benign breast disease.[102] Moreover, the presence of a radial scar further increased the breast cancer risk in women with other types of proliferative breast disease, particularly those with proliferative lesions without atypia. In particular, among women with proliferative lesions without atypia, those with a radial scar had a relative risk of breast cancer of 3.0, whereas the relative risk of breast cancer in those without a radial scar was 1.5.

Granular Cell Tumors

Granular cell tumors are uncommonly found in the breast but, when present, simulate carcinoma on clinical, mammographic, and pathologic examination.[108,109] These tumors occur more commonly in African-Americans than in whites; they also typically appear between puberty and menopause, so that some hormonal factor appears implicated in their development. Granular cell tumors of the breast most commonly occur in the upper, inner quadrant in contrast to carcinomas, which occur most frequently in the upper, outer quadrant. Patients present with a palpable mass that may be associated with skin retraction or fixation to skeletal muscles of the chest wall. The similarity of granular cell tumors to carcinoma is also evident on mammographic examination, on which they resemble scirrhous carcinoma. Gross examination of the lesion reveals a grey-white to tan, firm tumor that may be gritty when cut with a knife; these features further support the impression of carcinoma. Microscopically, these lesions are identical to granular cell tumors in other sites and consist of a poorly circumscribed proliferation of clusters of cells in which the most characteristic feature is prominent granularity of the cytoplasm. On electron microscopic examination, these granules correspond to secondary lysosomes. The nuclei are small and uniform and lack the features of malignant disease.

Granular cell tumors are almost invariably benign and are adequately treated by wide local excision. Rare cases of malignant granular cell tumors have been reported in both the breast and extramammary sites.

Granular cell tumors were initially considered to be myogenic in origin (hence, their earlier designation as granular cell myoblastomas), but ultrastructural and immunohistochemical evidence support a neurogenic origin for these tumors.[109,110]

Fibromatosis

Fibromatosis of the breast is analogous to fibromatosis at other sites (e.g., desmoid tumors of the abdominal wall) and is characterized by a locally invasive, nonencapsulated proliferation of well-differentiated spindle cells.[111–116] These tumors can recur locally if inadequately excised, but they do not metastasize. Patients typically present with a palpable mass that is sometimes associated with skin retraction or fixation to the underlying pectoral muscle. On mammography, these lesions are indistinguishable from carcinomas. Gross pathologic examination reveals an ill-defined, firm, grey-white lesion. Microscopically, fibromatoses consist of interlacing bundles of spindle-shaped cells surrounded by collagen. The cells show minimal to no cytologic atypism, and mitoses are only infrequently encountered. The proliferation tends to surround and entrap preexisting ducts and lobules without destroying them. The edges of the lesion infiltrate irregularly into the adjacent parenchyma. On electron microscopic and immunohistochemical examination, many of the tumor cells have the features of myofibroblasts.

The proper treatment for these lesions is wide local excision. Although metastases have not been reported, lesions may recur locally. Zayid and Dehmis described a case in which a patient was treated with mastectomy and subsequently developed multiple tumor recurrences in the chest wall, which ultimately resulted in her death.[117]

Interestingly, a few of the reported cases of fibromatosis of the breast have been associated with Gardner's syndrome.[113] Another case occurred in a patient with familial multicentric fibromatosis.[117]

Miscellaneous Benign Lesions

Lipomas consist of encapsulated nodules of mature adipose tissue. Although true lipomas occur in the breast, many lesions designated "lipoma" probably represent foci of fatty breast tissue without a true capsule. *Adenolipoma* is a term applied to a benign fatty tumor of the breast containing entrapped lobular epithelial elements[53]; however, the distinction between this lesion and breast tissue with prominent stromal adipose tissue is often unclear.

Benign vascular lesions of the breast parenchyma are relatively uncommon and most often represent incidental microscopic findings. In a series of 550 mastectomy specimens from patients with breast carcinoma, the incidence of benign hemangiomas was 1.2%.[118] Benign vascular lesions of the breast may be divided into four major categories: *perilobular hemangiomas*, *angiomatoses*, *venous hemangiomas*, and *hemangiomas involving the mammary subcutaneous tissue*.[119–122] The major significance of these lesions is that they must be distinguished from angiosarcomas.[123] Benign angiomatous lesions are almost always microscopic in size and lack interanastomosing channels, endothelial proliferation, and atypia. Complete excision is recommended for all vascular lesions of the breast. Atypical vascular lesions have been described in the skin of the breast and the mammary parenchyma in women who have been treated with conservative surgery and radiation therapy for breast cancer.[124] *Pseudoangiomatous hyperplasia of the mammary stroma* is a benign stromal proliferation that simulates a vascular lesion.[125–127] The lesion is often seen as an incidental microscopic finding but may present as a palpable mass. Microscopic examination reveals complex interanastomosing spaces, some of which have spindle-shaped stromal cells at their margins simulating endothelial cells. However, ultrastructural examinations have demonstrated that the spaces appear to be caused by separation and disruption of collagen fibers and that the associated spindle cells are fibroblasts. The significance of this lesion is that it must be distinguished from angiosarcoma.

Chondromatous lesions of the breast are uncommon. Although chondromatous changes are most often seen in breast carcinomas and sarcomas, chondroid metaplasia may rarely be observed in fibroadenomas and intraductal papillomas. A few cases of *chondrolipoma* have also been reported,[128,129] as has a single case of *choristoma* containing cartilage.[130]

Leiomyomas of the breast are most often seen in the areolar region and rarely occur in the breast parenchyma.[53] The histologic characteristics are the same as those of leiomyomas in other tissue.

Neurofibromas and *neurilemomas* (*Schwannomas*) are benign nerve sheath tumors. These lesions are most frequently seen in the breast in patients with neurofibromatosis and are most common in the areolar area.[131]

Adenomyoepitheliomas are uncommon lesions composed of a combination of epithelial and myoepithelial elements. These lesions present as palpable masses and are adequately treated by complete local excision.[132–135] Lesions composed exclusively of myoepithelial cells (*myoepitheliomas*) have also been described.[134,135]

Hamartomas of the breast present as well-defined masses on physical examination and on mammography. Microscopically, these lesions are composed of an admixture of ducts, lobules, fibrous stroma, and adipose tissue in varying proportions.[136,137] Occasional lesions also contain smooth muscle (*myoid hamartomas*).[138] These lesions frequently go unrecognized by the pathologist, because they histologically resemble other benign or physiologic changes in the breast.

Mucocele-like lesions are characterized by accumulations of extravasated mucus within the breast stroma, often accompanied by mucin-filled cysts.[139–141] The mucoid character of these lesions is usually evident on gross examination. Microscopically, the epithelium lining these cysts may assume a variety of histologic appearances, including that of flat, cuboidal epithelium, papillary hyperplasia, atypical ductal hyperplasia, and DCIS. These lesions must be completely excised and carefully examined histologically to rule out the possibility of an invasive mucinous carcinoma.[139–143]

Myofibroblastomas are uncommon benign mesenchymal tumors occurring more often in males than in females. These lesions are typically well circumscribed and are composed of a proliferation of relatively uniform-appearing spindle cells in a densely collagenized stroma. The cells comprising the tumor show features of myofibroblasts on ultrastructural and immunohistochemical examination.[144,145]

Collagenous spherulosis is a lesion detected incidentally during microscopic examination of breast tissue removed because of another abnormality. It is characterized by a fenestrated proliferation of epithelial and myoepithelial cells and intraluminal spherules composed of variable amounts of basement membrane–like material and collagen. This lesion is important to recognize because it must be distinguished from adenoid cystic carcinoma and DCIS.[146]

REACTIVE AND INFLAMMATORY LESIONS

Mammary Duct Ectasia (Periductal Mastitis)

Mammary duct ectasia occurs primarily in perimenopausal and postmenopausal women and is characterized by dilatation of the subareolar ducts.[19] Considerable controversy exists regarding the most appropriate name for this condition. This controversy has arisen from the fact that some authors consider ductal dilatation to be the primary event, whereas others consider the ectatic ducts to be the consequence of prior periductal inflammation.

Duct ectasia is a frequent pathologic finding in breast tissue obtained at autopsy and in surgically excised material. It has been observed on microscopic examination in 30% to 40% of women older than 50 years. Clinically evident disease occurs much less frequently, however.[147] Details regarding the clinical presentation of patients with duct ectasia are presented in Chapter 5.

A wide spectrum of pathologic changes is observed in this condition. Cut section of the gross specimen often reveals dilatated, thick-walled ducts that contain pasty, yellow-brown secretions. The intervening stroma may be fibrotic. On microscopic examination, some cases show prominent inspissation of lipid-rich material within ducts, accompanied by periductal inflammation. Rupture or leakage of the ducts results in release of this material into the adjacent stroma, with subsequent inflammation and fat necrosis. Plasma cells may be a prominent component of the periductal and stromal inflammatory infiltrate. Many cases previously designated as plasma cell mastitis probably represent a stage in the evolution of duct ectasia. In other cases, the histologic picture is dominated by periductal fibrosis and ductal dilatation with minimal inflammation.

As alluded to earlier in this section, the pathogenesis of this condition has not been fully established. Dixon et al. previously suggested that the primary event is periductal inflammation and that duct ectasia is the ultimate outcome of this disorder. In support of this premise, they observed that inflammation around nondilatated ducts predominates in younger patients with this condition, whereas duct dilatation and nipple retraction are more common in older patients.[147] Thus, their postulated sequence of events in the evolution of this disease was that periductal inflammation leads to periductal fibrosis, which subsequently results in ductal dilatation. However, in a 1996 study, this group of investigators has suggested that periductal mastitis and duct ectasia should be considered as two separate entities, based on differences among women with these two disorders with regard to age, clinical history, and smoking history.[148]

Fat Necrosis

Fat necrosis is important because it may closely mimic carcinoma, both clinically and on mammographic examination.[19,149] The clinical features are presented in Chapter 4.

The macroscopic appearance of fat necrosis depends on its age. In early lesions, hemorrhage and indurated fat are seen. With time, a rounded, firm tumor is formed. The cut surface of the lesion at this stage has a variegated, yellow-grey appearance with focal hemorrhage. Cavitation may

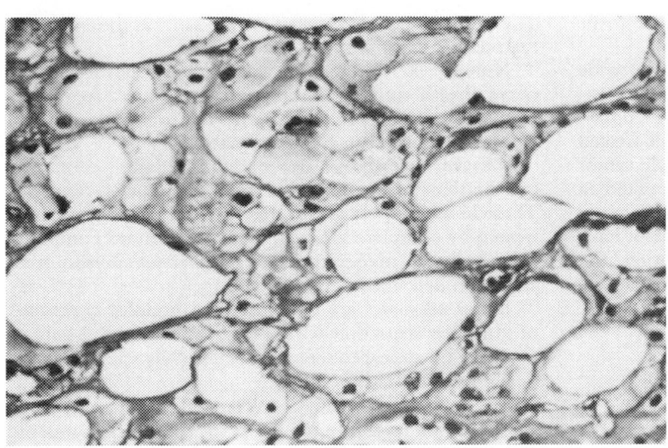

FIG. 10. Fat necrosis. The fatty breast tissue is infiltrated by histiocytes containing foamy cytoplasm.

subsequently occur, owing to liquefactive necrosis. The lesion may eventually be converted to a dense, fibrous scar or may remain a cystic cavity with calcification of its walls.

On microscopic examination, early lesions show cystic spaces surrounded by lipid-laden macrophages and foreign body–type giant cells with foamy cytoplasm (Fig. 10). A variable, acute inflammatory cell infiltrate may be present, and focal hemorrhage may be noted. With time, fibroblastic proliferation with deposition of collagen occurs. Scattered, chronic inflammatory cells are usually present, and focal hemosiderin deposition may be observed. Even in older lesions, scattered, foamy histiocytes and foreign-body giant cells are usually discernible.

A similar pathologic appearance may be noted after surgical trauma to the breast and after radiation therapy for carcinoma (see the following section, Pathologic Changes Associated with Radiation Therapy for Carcinoma).

Reactions to Foreign Material

Foreign body–type granulomatous inflammation has been described after injection within the breast of a variety of substances, including paraffin and silicone. Clinically, these lesions generally appear as firm nodules that may be tender.[149]

A variety of tissue reactions have been reported in association with mammary implants.[150–154] One of these is the formation of a fibrous capsule in the surrounding tissue. In 10% to 40% of patients, contracture of this capsule occurs; this contracture results in breast tightness or firmness and deformation of the implant, necessitating either capsulotomy or removal of the implant and the surrounding capsule. Histologic examination of the capsular tissue shows varying degrees of fibrosis, chronic inflammation, fat necrosis, presence of granulation tissue, fibrin deposition, and presence of histiocytes and foreign-body giant cells, often with demonstrable silicone (and, in some cases in which it has been used as part of the implant shell, polyurethane). In some cases, the capsule surrounding breast implants develops a cellular lining that histologically, immunohistochemically, and ultrastructurally resembles either normal synovium or synovium with papillary hyperplasia (proliferative synovitis) and that has physiologic properties similar to synovium.[155–158] This change has been variously described as "pseudoepithelialization," "synovial metaplasia," and "capsular synovial hyperplasia." The factors associated with development of synovial-type metaplasia in this setting are not known. Some have suggested that this is a consequence of mechanical forces (e.g., micromotion and friction) between the implant and the surrounding tissue.

Mondor's Disease (Phlebitis of the Thoracoepigastric Vein)

Mondor's disease, or phlebitis of the thoracoepigastric vein, has been considered rare; however, it is increasingly being recognized.[159–161] The clinical features are discussed in Chapter 6. On pathologic examination, phlebitis and periphlebitis are noted. The obliterative endophlebitis is associated with varying degrees of thrombosis, and the adventitia and media may be completely destroyed in advanced cases.

Pathologic Changes Associated with Radiation Therapy for Carcinoma

Breast-conserving surgery followed by radiation therapy is now a common treatment for patients with early-stage breast cancer. The effects of therapeutic doses of ionizing radiation on the skin of the breast have been well described and are identical to the radiation-induced alterations occurring in skin at any irradiated site.[162]

Fat necrosis may occur in the breast after local excision and radiation therapy for carcinoma. These lesions may be indistinguishable from carcinoma by clinical and radiographic examination, so that a complete histologic examination is required for accurate diagnosis.[163] The most characteristic pathologic finding in breast tissue excised after breast-conserving surgery and radiation therapy for carcinoma is epithelial cell atypicality in the terminal duct lobular unit, usually associated with varying degrees of lobular sclerosis and atrophy (Fig. 11).[164] These changes may be distinguished from carcinoma involving the terminal duct lobular unit by the preservation of polarity and cohesion and by the absence of cellular proliferation and distention of the involved terminal duct lobular unit in areas of radiation-induced change. Similar epithelial changes have been described in patients treated with chemotherapy before tumor excision.[165] Less frequently, epithelial atypia in large (extralobular) ducts, atypical fibroblasts in the stroma, and radiation-related vascular changes may be observed. Interestingly, stromal fibrosis, a characteristic feature of radiation effect in other organs, is so variable among both

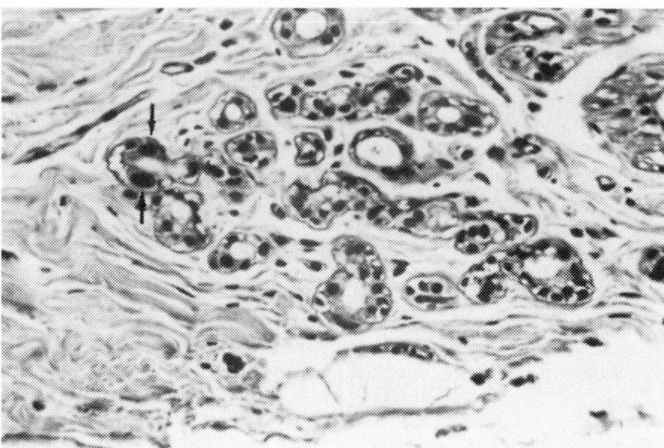

FIG. 11. Radiation effects. This terminal duct lobular unit contains scattered, enlarged epithelial cells with large, diffusely hyperchromatic nuclei (*arrows*). Cellular polarity is maintained, and no evidence of epithelial cell proliferation is present.

irradiated patients and nonirradiated control subjects that it is not, by itself, a reliable marker for radiation-induced injury in the breast.

Sarcoidosis

Involvement of the breast by sarcoidosis is rare but, when present, may clinically simulate a neoplasm.[166–168] Histologically, the lesions consist of typical, noncaseating granulomas with varying numbers of giant cells, which are present in the interlobular and intralobular connective tissue. A diagnosis of sarcoidosis should be made only after the exclusion of other causes of granulomatous inflammation, such as mycobacterial, fungal, and parasitic infections or reactions to foreign materials. Sarcoidosis should also be distinguished from granulomatous mastitis, a lesion in which the granulomas are associated with microabscesses and which may respond to corticosteroid therapy.[169–172]

Diabetic Mastopathy

Insulin-dependent diabetic patients occasionally develop breast masses that on histologic examination show a characteristic constellation of features.[173–175] These include dense, keloidlike fibrosis, lymphocytic infiltrates in association with ducts and lobules (lymphocytic ductitis and lobulitis), lymphocytic vasculitis, and epithelioid fibroblasts in the stroma. The pathogenesis of this lesion is unknown; it may represent an autoimmune reaction.

REFERENCES

1. Page DL, Dupont WD. Anatomic indicators (histologic and cytologic) of increased breast cancer risk. *Breast Cancer Res Treat* 1993;28:157.
2. Love SM, Gelman RS, Silen W. Fibrocystic "disease" of the breast—a nondisease? *N Engl J Med* 1982;307:1010.
3. Kodlin D, Winger EE, Morganstern NL, Chen U. Chronic mastopathy and breast cancer: a follow-up study. *Cancer* 1977;39:2603.
4. Dupont WD, Page DL. Risk factors for breast cancer in women with proliferative breast disease. *N Engl J Med* 1985;312:146.
5. Carter CL, Cook DK, Micozzi MS, Schatzkin A, Taylor PR. A prospective study of the development of breast cancer in 16,692 women with benign breast disease. *Am J Epidemiol* 1988;128:467.
6. Tavassoli FA, Norris HF. A comparison of long-term follow-up for atypical intraductal hyperplasia and intraductal hyperplasia of the breast. *Cancer* 1990;65:518.
7. Palli D, Del Turco MR, Simoncini R, Bianchi S. Benign breast disease and breast cancer: a case-control study in a cohort in Italy. *Int J Cancer* 1991;47:703.
8. London SJ, Connolly JL, Schnitt SJ, Colditz GA. A prospective study of benign breast disease and the risk of breast cancer. *JAMA* 1992; 267:941.
9. Krieger N, Hiatt RA. Risk of breast cancer after benign breast diseases: variation by histologic type, degree of atypia, age at biopsy and length of follow-up. *Am J Epidemiol* 1992;135:619.
10. McDivitt RW, Stevens JA, Lee NC, et al. Histologic types of benign breast disease and the risk of breast cancer. *Cancer* 1992;69:1408.
11. Dupont WD, Parl FF, Hartmann WH, et al. Breast cancer risk associated with proliferative breast disease and atypical hyperplasia. *Cancer* 1993;71:1258.
12. Bodian CA, Perzin KH, Lattes R, Hoffman P, Abernathy TG. Prognostic significance of benign proliferative breast disease. *Cancer* 1993;71:3896.
13. Marshall LM, Hunter DJ, Connolly JL, et al. Risk of breast cancer associated with atypical hyperplasia of lobular and ductal types. *Cancer Epidemiol Biomarkers Prev* 1997;6:297.
14. Hutter RVP. Goodbye to "fibrocystic disease." *N Engl J Med* 1985; 312:179.
15. Hughes LE, Mansel RE, Webster DJT. Aberrations of normal development and involution (ANDI): a new perspective on pathogenesis and nomenclature of benign breast disorders. *Lancet* 1987;2:1316.
16. Page DL, Dupont WD, Rogers LW, et al. Atypical hyperplastic lesions of the female breast: a long-term follow-up study. *Cancer* 1985;55:2698.
17. Page DL, Rogers LW. Combined histologic and cytologic criteria for the diagnosis of mammary atypical ductal hyperplasia. *Hum Pathol* 1992;23:1095.
18. Consensus Meeting: Is "fibrocystic disease" of the breast precancerous? *Arch Pathol Lab Med* 1986;110:171.

18a. Fitzgibbons PL, Henson DE, Hutter RVP. Benign breast changes and the risk for subsequent breast cancer. An update of the 1985 consensus statement. *Arch Pathol Lab Med* 1998;122:1053.

19. Haagensen CD. *Diseases of the breast*, 3rd ed. Philadelphia: WB Saunders, 1986.
20. Dupont WD, Page DL, Parl FF, et al. Long-term risk of breast cancer in women with fibroadenoma. *N Engl J Med* 1994;331:10.
21. Jensen RA, Page DL, Dupont WD, Rogers LW. Invasive breast cancer risk in women with sclerosing adenosis. *Cancer* 1989;64:1977.
22. Eusebi V, Damiani S, Losi L, Millis RR. Apocrine differentiation in breast epithelium. *Adv Anat Pathol* 1997;4:139.
23. Page DL, Dupont WD, Rogers LW. Ductal involvement by cells of atypical lobular hyperplasia: a long-term follow-up study of cancer risk. *Hum Pathol* 1988;19:201.
24. Schnitt SJ, Wang HH. Histologic sampling of grossly benign breast biopsies. How much is enough? *Am J Surg Pathol* 1989;13:505.
25. Owings DV, Hann L, Schnitt SJ. How thoroughly should needle localization breast biopsies be sampled for microscopic examination? A prospective mammographic-pathologic correlative study. *Am J Surg Pathol* 1990;14:578.
26. Rubin E, Visscher DW, Alexander RW, Urist MM, Maddox WA. Proliferative disease and atypia in biopsies performed for nonpalpable lesions detected mammographically. *Cancer* 1988;61:2077.
27. Connolly JL, Schnitt SJ, London S, Dupont W, Colditz G, Page D. Both atypical lobular hyperplasia (ALH) and atypical ductal hyperplasia (ADH) predict for bilateral breast cancer risk. *Lab Invest* 1992;66:13A.
28. Dupont WD, Page DL. Relative risk of breast cancer varies with time since diagnosis of atypical hyperplasia. *Hum Pathol* 1989;20:723.
29. Collaborative Group on Hormonal Factors in Breast Cancer. Breast cancer and hormone replacement therapy: collaborative reanalysis of data from 51 epidemiological studies of 52,705 women with breast cancer and 10,8411 women without breast cancer. *Lancet* 1997;350:1047.
30. Dupont WD, Page DL, Rogers LW, Parl FF. Influence of exogenous estrogens, proliferative breast disease, and other variables on breast cancer risk. *Cancer* 1989;63:948.

30a. Dupont WD, Page DL, Parl FF, et al. Estrogen replacement therapy in women with a history of proliferative breast disease. *Cancer* 1999; 85:1277.
31. Dupont WD, Plummer WD. Understanding the relationship between relative and absolute risk. *Cancer* 1996;77:193.
32. Rosai J. Borderline epithelial lesions of the breast. *Am J Surg Pathol* 1991;15:209.
33. Schnitt SJ, Connolly JL, Tavassoli FA, et al. Interobserver reproducibility in the diagnosis of ductal proliferative breast lesions using standardized criteria. *Am J Surg Pathol* 1992;16:1133.
34. Bodian CA, Perzin KH, Lattes R, Hoffman P. Reproducibility and validity of pathologic classifications of benign breast disease and implications for clinical applications. *Cancer* 1993;71:3908.
35. Gillett CE, Lee AH, Millis RR, Barnes DM. Cyclin D1 and associated proteins in mammary ductal carcinoma in situ and atypical ductal hyperplasia. *J Pathol* 1998;184:396.
36. Lodato RF, Maguire HC, Greene MI, et al. Immunohistochemical evaluation of c-erbB-2 oncogene expression in ductal carcinoma in situ and atypical ductal hyperplasia of the breast. *Mod Pathol* 1990;3:449.
37. Millikan R, Hulka B, Thor A, et al. P53 mutations in benign breast tissue. *J Clin Oncol* 1995;13:2293.
38. Humphrey PA, Franquemont DW, Geary WA, et al. Immunodetection of p53 protein in noninvasive epithelial proliferative breast disease. *Appl Immunohistochem* 1994;2:22.
39. Eriksson ET, Schimmelpenning H, Aspenblad U, et al. Immunohistochemical expression of the mutant p53 protein and nuclear DNA content during the transition from benign to malignant breast disease. *Hum Pathol* 1994;25:1228.
40. Younes M, Lebovitz RM, Bommer KE, et al. P53 accumulation in benign breast biopsy specimens. *Hum Pathol* 1995;26:155.
41. Siziopikou KP, Prioleau JE, Harris JR, Schnitt SJ. Bcl-2 expression in the spectrum of preinvasive breast lesions. *Cancer* 1996;77:499.
42. Weinstat-Saslow D, Merino MJ, Manrow RE, et al. Overexpression of cyclin D1 mRNA distinguishes invasive and in situ breast carcinomas from non-malignant lesions. *Nature Med* 1995;1:1257.
43. Alle KM, Henshall SM, Field AS, Sutherland RL. Cyclin D1 protein is overexpressed in hyperplasia and intraductal carcinoma of the breast. *Clin Cancer Res* 1998;4:847.
44. Khan SA, Rogers MAM, Khurana KK, et al. Estrogen receptor expression in benign breast epithelium and breast cancer risk. *J Natl Cancer Inst* 1998;90:37.
45. Guinebretiere J-M, Monique GL, Bahi J, Contesso G. Angiogenesis and risk of breast cancer in women with fibrocystic disease (letter). *J Natl Cancer Inst* 1994;86:635.
46. Rohan TE, Hartwick W, Miller AB, Kandel RA. Immunohistochemical detection of c-erbB-2 and p53 in benign breast disease and breast cancer risk. *J Natl Cancer Inst* 1998;90:1262.
47. Stark A, Hulka B, Joens S, et al. Her-2 amplification in benign breast tissue increases the risk for subsequent breast cancer. *Proc Annu Meet Am Assoc Cancer Res* 1997;38:A4156.
48. Steeg PS, Clare SE, Lawrence JA, Zhou Q. Molecular analysis of premalignant and carcinoma in situ lesions of the human breast. *Am J Pathol* 1996;149:733.
49. Lakhani SR, Stack DN, Hamoudi RA, et al. Detection of allelic imbalance indicates that a proportion of mammary hyperplasia of the usual type are clonal, neoplastic proliferations. *Lab Invest* 1996;74:129.
50. Chuaqui RF, Zhuang Z, Emmert-Buck MR, et al. Analysis of loss of heterozygosity on chromosome 11q13 in atypical ductal hyperplasia and in situ carcinoma of the breast. *Am J Pathol* 1997;150:297.
51. Kasami M, Vnencak-Jones CL, Manning S, et al. Loss of heterozygosity and microsatellite instability in breast hyperplasia. No obligate correlation of these genetic alterations with subsequent malignancy. *Am J Pathol* 1997;10:1925.
52. O'Connell P, Pekkel V, Fuqua SAW, et al. Analysis of loss of heterozygosity in 399 premalignant breast lesions at 15 genetic loci. *J Natl Cancer Inst* 1998;90:696.
53. Azzopardi JG. *Problems in breast pathology*. Philadelphia: WB Saunders, 1979.
54. Goodman ZD, Taxy JB. Fibroadenomas of the breast with prominent smooth muscle. *Am J Surg Pathol* 1981;5:99.
55. Dupont WD, Page DL, Parl FF, et al. Long-term risk of breast cancer in women with fibroadenoma. *N Engl J Med* 1994;331:10.
56. Oberman HA. Breast lesions in the adolescent female. In: Sommers SC, Rosen PP, eds. *Pathology annual, part 1*. Norwalk, CT: Appleton-Century-Crofts, 1979.
57. Nambiar R, Kutty K. Giant fibroadenoma (cytosarcoma phyllodes) in adolescent females—a clinicopathologic study. *Br J Surg* 1974;61:113.
58. Ashikari R, Farrow JH, O'Hara J. Fibroadenomas in the breast of juveniles. *Surg Gynecol Obstet* 1971;132:259.
59. Mies C, Rosen PP. Juvenile fibroadenoma with atypical epithelial hyperplasia. *Am J Surg Pathol* 1987;11:184.
60. Pick PW, Iossifides IA. Occurrence of breast carcinoma within a fibroadenoma: a review. *Arch Pathol Lab Med* 1984;108:590.
61. Hertel BF, Zaloudek C, Kempson RL. Breast adenomas. *Cancer* 1976;37:2891.
62. O'Hara MF, Page DL. Adenomas of the breast and ectopic breast under lactational influences. *Hum Pathol* 1985;16:707.
63. Rosen PP. Syringomatous adenoma of the nipple. *Am J Surg Pathol* 1983;7:739.
64. Jones MW, Norris HJ, Snyder RC. Infiltrating syringomatous adenoma of the nipple. A clinical and pathological study of 11 cases. *Am J Surg Pathol* 1989;13:197.
65. Chen KTK. Pleomorphic adenoma of the breast. *Am J Clin Pathol* 1990;93:792.
66. Moran CA, Suster S, Carter D. Benign mixed tumors (pleomorphic adenomas) of the breast. *Am J Surg Pathol* 1990;14:913.
67. Ballance WA, Ro JY, El-Naggar AK, et al. Pleomorphic adenoma (benign mixed tumor) of the breast. An immunohistochemical, flow cytometric, and ultrastructural study and review of the literature. *Am J Clin Pathol* 1990;93:795.
68. Rosen PP, Oberman HA. *Tumors of the mammary gland*, Third Series Fascicle 7. Washington: Armed Forces Institute of Pathology, 1993.
69. Jones DB. Florid papillomatosis of the nipple ducts. *Cancer* 1955;8:315.
70. Perzin KH, Lattes R. Papillary adenoma of the nipple (florid papillomatosis, adenoma, adenomatosis). A clinicopathologic study. *Cancer* 1972;29:996.
71. Smith EJ, Kron SD, Gross PR. Erosive adenomatosis of the nipple. *Arch Dermatol* 1970;102:330.
72. Diaz NM, Palmer JO, Wick MR. Erosive adenomatosis of the nipple: histology, immunohistology, and differential diagnosis. *Mod Pathol* 1992;5:179.
73. Gudjonsdottir A, Hagerstrand I, Ostberg G. Adenoma of the nipple with carcinomatous development. *Acta Pathol Microbiol Scand [A]* 1971;79:676.
74. Bhagavan BS, Patchevsky AS, Koss LG. Florid subareolar duct papillomatosis (nipple adenoma) and mammary carcinoma: report of three cases. *Hum Pathol* 1973;4:289.
75. Rosen PP, Caicco JA. Florid papillomatosis of the nipple. A study of 51 patients, including nine with mammary carcinoma. *Am J Surg Pathol* 1986;102:87.
76. Azzopardi JG, Salm P. Ductal adenoma of the breast: a lesion which can mimic carcinoma. *J Pathol* 1984;144:15.
77. Lammie GA, Millis RR. Ductal adenoma of the breast—a review of 15 cases. *Hum Pathol* 1989;20:903.
78. Kraus FT, Neubecker RD. The differential diagnosis of papillary lesions of the breast. *Cancer* 1962;25:444.
79. Papotti M, Eusebi V, Gugliotta P, Bussolati G. Immunohistochemical analysis of benign and malignant papillary lesions of the breast. *Am J Surg Pathol* 1983;7:451.
80. Jarasch E-D, Nagle RB, Kaufmann M, et al. Differential diagnosis of benign epithelial proliferations and carcinomas of the breast using antibodies to cytokeratins. *Hum Pathol* 1988;19:276.
81. Noguchi S, Motomura K, Inaji H, et al. Clonal analysis of solitary intraductal papilloma of the breast by means of polymerase chain reaction. *Am J Pathol* 1994;144:1320.
82. Flint A, Oberman HA. Infarction and squamous metaplasia of intraductal papilloma. A benign breast lesion that may simulate carcinoma. *Hum Pathol* 1984;15:764.
83. Page DL, Salhany KE, Jensen RA, Dupont WD. Subsequent breast carcinoma risk after biopsy with atypia in a breast papilloma. *Cancer* 1996;78:258.
84. Ohuchi N, Abe R, Kasai M. Possible cancerous change of intraductal papillomas of the breast. A 3-D reconstruction study of 25 cases. *Cancer* 1984;54:605.
85. Rosen PP, Cantrell B, Mullen DL, et al. Juvenile papillomatosis (Swiss cheese disease) of the breast. *Am J Surg Pathol* 1980;4:3.
86. Rosen PP, Lyngholm B, Kinne DW, et al. Juvenile papillomatosis and family history of breast carcinoma. *Cancer* 1982;49:2591.
87. Rosen PP, Holmes G, Lesser ML, et al. Juvenile papillomatosis and breast carcinoma. *Cancer* 1985;55:1345.

88. Bazzochi F, Santini D, Martinelli G, et al. Juvenile papillomatosis (epitheliosis) of the breast. A clinical pathological study of 13 cases. *Am J Clin Pathol* 1986;86:745.
89. Rosen PP, Kimmel M. Juvenile papillomatosis of the breast. A follow-up study of 41 patients having biopsies before 1979. *Am J Clin Pathol* 1990;93:599.
90. Millis RR, Eusebi V. Microglandular adenosis of the breast. *Adv Anat Pathol* 1995;2:10.
91. Diaz NM, McDivitt RW, Wick MR. Microglandular adenosis of the breast. An immunohistochemical comparison with tubular carcinoma. *Arch Pathol Lab Med* 1991;115:578.
92. Tavassoli FA, Bratthauer GL. Immunohistochemical profile and differential diagnosis of microglandular adenosis. *Mod Pathol* 1993;6:318.
93. Rosen PP. Microglandular adenosis. A benign lesion simulating invasive mammary carcinoma. *Am J Surg Pathol* 1983;7:137.
94. Tavassoli FA, Norris HJ. Microglandular adenosis of the breast. A clinicopathologic study of 11 cases with ultrastructural observations. *Am J Surg Pathol* 1983;7:731.
95. Clement PB, Azzopardi JG. Microglandular adenosis of the breast—a lesion simulating tubular carcinoma. *Histopathol* 1983;7:169.
96. Rosenblum MK, Purrazzella R, Rosen PP. Is microglandular adenosis a precancerous disease? A study of carcinoma arising in microglandular adenosis. *Lab Invest* 1985;52:57A.
97. James BA, Cranor ML, Rosen PP. Carcinoma of the breast arising in microglandular adenosis. *Am J Clin Pathol* 1993;100:507.
98. Fenoglio C, Lattes R. Sclerosing papillary proliferations in the female breast. A benign lesion often mistaken for carcinoma. *Cancer* 1974;33:691.
99. Fisher ER, Palekar AS, Kotwal N, et al. A nonencapsulated sclerosing lesion of the breast. *Am J Clin Pathol* 1979;71:240.
100. Rickert RR, Kalisher L, Hutter RVP. Indurative mastopathy: a benign sclerosing lesion of breast with elastosis which may simulate carcinoma. *Cancer* 1981;47:561.
101. Andersen JA, Gram JB. Radial scar in the female breast. A long-term follow-up study of 32 cases. *Cancer* 1984;53:2557.
102. Jacobs TW, Byrne C, Colditz G, et al. Radial scars and breast cancer risk: a case-control study. *N Engl J Med* 1999;340:430.
103. Wellings SR, Alpers CE. Subgross pathologic features and incidence of radial scars in the breast. *Hum Pathol* 1984;15:475.
104. Page DL, Anderson TJ. *Diagnostic histopathology of the breast*. Edinburgh, UK: Churchill Livingstone, 1987.
105. Linell F, Ljungberg O, Andersson I. Breast carcinoma: aspects of early stages, progression and related problems. *Acta Pathol Microbiol Scand* 1980;272(Suppl):14.
106. Sloane JP, Mayers MM. Carcinoma and atypical hyperplasia in radial scars and complex sclerosing lesions: importance of lesion size and patient age. *Histopathology* 1993;23:225.
107. Nielsen M, Christensen L, Andersen J. Radial scars in women with breast cancer. *Cancer* 1987;59:1019.
108. DeMay RM, Kay S. Granular cell tumors of the breast. In: Sommers SC, Rosen PP, eds. *Pathology annual, part 1*. Norwalk, CT: Appleton-Century-Crofts, 1984.
109. Damiani S, Koerner FC, Dickersin GR, Cook MG, Eusebi V. Granular cell tumor of the breast. *Virchows Arch [A] Pathol Anat Histopathol* 1992;420:219.
110. Ingram DL, Mossler JA, Snowhite J, et al. Granular cell tumors of the breast. Steroid receptor analysis and localization of carcinoembryonic antigen, myoglobin and S100 protein. *Arch Pathol Lab Med* 1984;108:897.
111. Gump FE, Sternschein MJ, Wolff M. Fibromatosis of the breast. *Surg Gynecol Obstet* 1981;153:57.
112. Ali M, Fayemi AO, Braun EV, et al. Fibromatosis of the breast. *Am J Surg Pathol* 1979;3:501.
113. Rosen Y, Sozos CP, Gardner B. Fibromatosis of the breast. *Cancer* 1978;41:1409.
114. Hanna WM, Jambrosic J, Fish E. Aggressive fibromatosis of the breast. *Arch Pathol Lab Med* 1985;109:260.
115. Wargotz ES, Norris HJ, Austin RM, Enzinger FM. Fibromatosis of the breast. A clinical and pathological study of 28 cases. *Am J Surg Pathol* 1987;11:38.
116. Rosen PP, Ernsberger D. Mammary fibromatosis. A benign spindle-cell tumor with significant risk for local recurrence. *Cancer* 1989;63:1363.
117. Zayid I, Dehmis C. Familial multicentric fibromatosis-desmoids. *Cancer* 1969;24:786.
118. Rosen PP, Ridolfi RL. The perilobular hemangioma. A benign microscopic vascular lesion of the breast. *Am J Clin Pathol* 1977;68:21.
119. Jozefczyk MA, Rosen PP. Vascular tumors of the breast II. Perilobular hemangiomas and hemangiomas. *Am J Surg Pathol* 1985;9:491.
120. Rosen PP. Vascular tumors of the breast III. Angiomatosis. *Am J Surg Pathol* 1985;9:652.
121. Rosen PP. Vascular tumors of the breast IV. The venous hemangioma. *Am J Surg Pathol* 1985;9:659.
122. Rosen PP. Vascular tumors of the breast V. Nonparenchymal hemangiomas of mammary subcutaneous tissues. *Am J Surg Pathol* 1985;9:723.
123. Donnell RM, Rosen PP, Lieberman PH, et al. Angiosarcoma and other vascular tumors of the breast: pathologic analysis as a guide to prognosis. *Am J Surg Pathol* 1981;5:629.
124. Fineberg S, Rosen PP. Cutaneous angiosarcoma and atypical vascular lesions of the skin and breast after radiation therapy for breast carcinoma. *Am J Clin Pathol* 1994;102:757.
125. Vuitch MF, Rosen PP, Erlandson RA. Pseudoangiomatous hyperplasia of mammary stroma. *Hum Pathol* 1986;17:185.
126. Ibrahim RE, Sciotto CG, Weidner N. Pseudoangiomatous hyperplasia of mammary stroma. Some observations regarding its clinicopathologic spectrum. *Cancer* 1989;63:1154.
127. Powell CM, Cranor ML, Rosen PP. Pseudo angiomatous stromal hyperplasia (PASH). A mammary stromal tumor with myofibroblastic differentiation. *Am J Surg Pathol* 1995;19:270.
128. Kaplan L, Walts A. Benign chondrolipomatous tumor of the human female breast. *Arch Pathol Lab Med* 1977;101:149.
129. Marsh WL, Lucas JG, Olsen J. Chondrolipomas of the breast. *Arch Pathol Lab Med* 1989;113:369.
130. Metcalf JS, Ellis B. Choristoma of the breast. *Hum Pathol* 1985;16:739.
131. Cohen MB, Fisher PE. Schwann cell tumors of the breast and mammary region. *Surg Pathol* 1991;4:47.
132. Rosen PP. Adenomyoepithelioma of the breast. *Hum Pathol* 1987;18:1232.
133. Young RH, Clement PB. Adenomyoepithelioma of the breast. A report of three cases and review of the literature. *Am J Clin Pathol* 1988;89:308.
134. Tavassoli FA. Myoepithelial lesions of the breast. Myoepitheliosis, adenomyoepithelioma, and myoepithelial carcinoma. *Am J Surg Pathol* 1991;15:554.
135. Erlandson RA, Rosen PP. Infiltrating myoepithelioma of the breast. *Am J Surg Pathol* 1982;6:795.
136. Oberman HA. Hamartoma and hamartoma variants of the breast. *Semin Diagn Pathol* 1989;6:135.
137. Daya D, Trus T, D'Souza TJ, et al. Hamartoma of the breast, an underrecognized breast lesion. A clinicopathologic and radiographic study of 25 cases. *Am J Clin Pathol* 1995;103:685.
138. Daroca PJ, Reed RJ, Love GJ. Myoid hamartomas of the breast. *Hum Pathol* 1985;16:212.
139. Rosen PP. Mucocele-like tumors of the breast. *Am J Surg Pathol* 1986;10:464.
140. Ro J, Sahin A, Sneige N, Silva A, Ayala A. Mucocele-like tumor (MLT) of the breast. A clinicopathological study. *Lab Invest* 1990;62:83A.
141. Hamele-Bena D, Cranor ML, Rosen PP. Mammary mucocele-like lesions. Benign and malignant. *Am J Surg Pathol* 1996;20:1081.
142. Weaver MG, Abdul-Karim FK, Al-Kaisi N. Mucinous lesions of the breast. A pathological continuum. *Path Res Pract* 1993;189:873.
143. Fisher ER, Palekar AS, Stoner F, Costantino J. Mucocele-like lesions and mucinous carcinoma of the breast. *Int J Surg Pathol* 1994;1:213.
144. Wargotz ES, Weiss SW, Norris HJ. Myofibroblastoma of the breast. Sixteen cases of a distinctive benign mesenchymal tumor. *Am J Surg Pathol* 1987;11:493.
145. Hamele-Bena D, Cranor ML, Sciotto C, et al. Uncommon presentation of mammary myofibroblastoma. *Mod Pathol* 1996;9:786.
146. Clement PB, Young RH, Azzopardi JG. Collagenous spherulosis of the breast. *Am J Surg Pathol* 1987;11:411.
147. Dixon JM, Anderson TJ, Lumsden AB, et al. Mammary duct ectasia. *Br J Surg* 1983;70:601.
148. Dixon JM, Ravisekar O, Chetty U, Anderson TJ. Periductal mastitis and duct ectasia: different conditions with different aetiologies. *Br J Surg* 1996;83:820.
149. Symmers W. The breasts. In: Symmers W. *Systematic pathology*. Edinburgh, UK: Churchill Livingstone, 1978.
150. Sanchez-Guerrero J, Schur PH, Sergent JS, Liang HM. Silicone breast implants and rheumatic disease. Clinical, immunologic, and epidemiologic studies. *Arthr Rheum* 1994;37:158.

151. Bridges AJ, Vasey FB. Silicone breast implants. History, safety and potential complications. *Arch Intern Med* 1993;153:2638.
152. Carter D. Tissue reactions to breast implants. *Am J Clin Pathol* 1994;102:565.
153. Schnitt SJ. Tissue reactions to mammary implants: a capsule summary. *Adv Anat Pathol* 1995;2:24.
154. Noone RB. A review of the possible health implications of silicone breast implants. *Cancer* 1997;79:1747.
155. Chase DR, Oberg KC, Chase RL, Malott RL, Weeks DA. Pseudoepithelialization of breast implant capsules. *Int J Surg Pathol* 1994;1:151.
156. Raso DS, Crymes LW, Metcalf JS. Histological assessment of fifty breast capsules from smooth and textured augmentation and reconstruction mammoplasty prostheses with emphasis on the role of synovial metaplasia. *Mod Pathol* 1994;7:310.
157. Emery JA, Spanier SS, Kasnic G, Hardt NS. The synovial structure of breast implant-associated bursae. *Mod Pathol* 1994;7:728.
158. Hameed MR, Erlandson R, Rosen PP. Capsular synovial-like hyperplasia around mammary implants similar to detritic synovitis. A morphologic and immunohistochemical study of 15 cases. *Am J Surg Pathol* 1995;19:433.
159. Honig C, Rado R. Mondor's disease—superficial phlebitis of the chest wall: a review of seven cases. *Ann Surg* 1961;153:589.
160. Fischl RA, Kahn S, Simon BE. Mondor's disease. *Plastic Reconstr Surg* 1975;56:319.
161. Tabar L, Dean PB. Mondor's diesease: clinical, mammographic, and pathologic features. *Breast* 1981;7:18.
162. Fajardo LJ. *Pathology of radiation injury*. New York: Masson Publishing, 1982.
163. Clarke D, Curtin JL, Martínez A, et al. Fat necrosis of the breast simulating recurrent carcinoma after primary radiotherapy in the management of early stage breast carcinoma. *Cancer* 1983;52:442.
164. Schnitt SJ, Connolly JL, Harris JR, et al. Radiation-induced changes in the breast. *Hum Pathol* 1984;15:545.
165. Kennedy SM, Merino MJ. Histological evaluation of the effects of chemotherapy and hormonal therapy in residual and tumoral breast tissues: their significance in diagnoses. *Lab Invest* 1988;58:47A.
166. Gansler TS, Wheeler JE. Mammary sarcoidosis. Two cases and literature review. *Arch Pathol Lab Med* 1984;108:673.
167. Ross MJ, Merino MJ. Sarcoidosis of the breast. *Hum Pathol* 1985;16:185.
168. Fitzgibbons PL, Smiley DF, Kern WH. Sarcoidosis presenting initially as breast mass: report of two cases. *Hum Pathol* 1985;16:851.
169. Kessler E, Wolloch Y. Granulomatous mastitis: a lesion clinically simulating carcinoma. *Am J Clin Pathol* 1972;58:642.
170. Dettertogh DA, Rossof AH, Harris AA, Economou SG. Prednisone management of granulomatous mastitis. *N Engl J Med* 1980;303:799.
171. Fletcher A, Magrath IM, Riddell RH, Talbot IC. Granulomatous mastitis: a report of seven cases. *J Clin Pathol* 1982;35:941.
172. Kessler EI, Katzav JA. Lobular granulomatous mastitis. *Surg Pathol* 1990;3:115.
173. Tomaszewski JE, Brooks JSJ, Hicks D, LiVolsi VA. Diabetic mastopathy: a distinctive clinicopathologic entity. *Hum Pathol* 1992;23:780.
174. Seidman JD, Schnapper LA, Phillips LE. Mastopathy in insulin-requiring diabetes mellitus. *Hum Pathol* 1994;25:819.
175. Morgan MC, Weaver MG, Crowe JP, Abdul-Karim FW. Diabetic mastopathy: a clinicopathologic study in palpable and nonpalpable breast lesions. *Mod Pathol* 1995;8:349.

CHAPTER 10

Diseases of the Breast, 2nd ed.,
edited by Jay R. Harris.
Lippincott Williams & Wilkins, Philadelphia © 2000.

Techniques of Diagnosis of Palpable Breast Masses

Roger S. Foster, Jr.

When physical examination of the breast shows a suspicious abnormality, either a definite mass or a thickening that is not unequivocally within the normal range, a biopsy for pathologic diagnosis should be performed. Four techniques are used to obtain pathologic material from a palpable lesion: fine-needle aspiration biopsy (FNAB), core-cutting needle biopsy, excisional biopsy, and incisional biopsy. Each of these procedures has advantages that may make it the most suitable for a particular patient. FNABs are usually done without anesthesia or with local anesthesia in the skin. Core-cutting needle biopsies and incisional biopsies require a local anesthetic. With appropriate technique, excisional biopsies may almost always be done comfortably while the patient is under local anesthesia. Some surgeons prefer to use a general anesthetic for most excisional breast biopsies.

Most patients are treated using a two-step procedure. The first step is the biopsy, which can be followed by a more extensive workup and an informed discussion with the patient; the second step is the definitive surgical treatment. Costs are less when the two-step procedure is accomplished using FNAB than when an excisional biopsy is used, particularly if the excisional biopsy is done using general anesthesia.[1–3]

Prior to the 1970s, one of the rationales for the one-step procedure was an emergency theory of the behavior of breast cancer; any delay in treatment was thought to adversely affect the patient's prognosis. Concern also existed that the biopsy procedure might disturb the cancer and lead to a lower survival rate if definitive surgery was not performed. Retrospective studies and data from large prospective clinical trials show no difference in the survival rates for one-step and two-step procedures.[4–7] Moreover, no evidence from these studies has shown that delays of a month or even more between biopsy and definitive surgery lead to a poorer outcome. Making the breast cancer diagnosis by needle biopsy and leaving the primary breast cancer in place may be advantageous if the patient is to have a sentinel node procedure for regional node staging. Several studies have reported higher success rates for sentinel node identification in patients when the cancer has been diagnosed by needle biopsy rather than excisional biopsy.[8]

R. S. Foster, Jr.: Department of Surgery, The Robert H. Woodruff Health Sciences Center, Emory University School of Medicine, Atlanta, Georgia

FINE-NEEDLE ASPIRATION AND FINE-NEEDLE ASPIRATION BIOPSY

Fine-needle aspiration and FNAB of the breast are complementary procedures. Fine-needle aspiration of gross breast cysts is both diagnostic and therapeutic. If the suspected cyst proves to be a solid lesion, material for FNAB may be obtained instead. Even if excision of a probably benign mass is planned and FNAB is believed to be redundant—as, for example, in a young woman with a dominant mass that is presumed to be a fibroadenoma—performing an aspiration before the excision is appropriate to exclude a tense cyst that may mimic a fibroadenoma on physical examination. An alternative to attempted aspiration to exclude the presence of a cyst would be an ultrasonographic examination to show whether the lesion is solid.

FNAB has been used for more than six decades for the diagnosis of breast lesions and has been an established procedure in Europe for many years.[9–12] Only since the 1970s and 1980s, however, has it become more widely accepted and used in the United States. When a skilled cytopathologist is available for interpretation of the specimen, FNAB has many advantages. For palpable breast masses, the advantages of FNAB include simplicity, good accuracy, low morbidity, minimal patient discomfort, low cost, and immediate availability as an office procedure that can be performed at the time the patient is first seen in the surgeon's office.[13]

If skilled cytopathologists are provided with adequate material, the diagnostic accuracy of FNAB should be high.[14] The apparent simplicity of FNAB, however, can lead to its application in unskilled hands.[15] A review of 31,340 FNABs in the medical literature indicates that the sensitivity and specificity of FNAB vary widely among reporting groups.[16] In that review, the reported sensitivity ranged from 65% to 98%, and the specificity ranged from 34% to 100%. No cytopathologist can make a reading unless adequate cellular material is aspirated from the lesion.

Before an FNAB diagnosis of breast malignancy is used as the basis for definitive patient management, the track record of the cytopathologist should be known. A false-positive FNAB diagnosis by a skilled cytopathologist should be very rare. Among experienced cytopathologists, the rate of false-positive results ranges from 0.0% to 0.4%, with an overall average of approximately 0.17%.[13,15,17,18] Rare false-positive readings also occur with open breast biopsies.

FNAB cannot usually distinguish between an invasive carcinoma and noninvasive ductal carcinoma *in situ*. Pathologists should be encouraged to stratify their malignant diagnoses into "definite malignancy" and "probable malignancy," with only a definite diagnosis of malignancy supporting definitive therapy.[19] Histologic confirmation is required for the "probable malignancy" group. This approach not only avoids false-positive results but also tends to place *in situ* carcinomas and low-grade carcinomas requiring special clinical management into the "probable" group, ensuring that they are recognized before definitive treatment is begun.

False-negative rates in various series have ranged from 0% to 4%.[13,14,20] A greater possibility of a false-negative interpretation exists for well-differentiated tumors, such as tubular carcinomas and papillary carcinomas, and for cases in which the tumor is paucicellular.[21] Most false-negative results are due to sampling errors, which tend to be associated with small tumor size, rather than to misinterpretation by the cytopathologist.[13] The FNAB report needs to be interpreted in relation to the clinical examination and mammographic findings. If the clinical examination or mammogram is suggestive of possible malignancy, an incisional or excisional biopsy should be performed.

Triple-Negative Diagnostic Test

The FNAB has been recommended as part of a triad of diagnostic procedures in women who present with asymmetric, thickened areas of the breast that clinically are thought to be probably benign yet raise a small element of suspicion.[22–24]

If mammographic results are not suggestive of cancer, a negative FNAB that shows normal breast epithelial cells can provide additional reassurance. An FNAB that is acellular does not provide satisfactory reassurance that the sampling was adequate and usually should be repeated. The cytopathologist may indicate that the aspirate was nondiagnostic. A fatty area may well be acellular, and a judgment not to repeat the fine-needle aspiration may be appropriate. If a question exists as to whether sufficient cellular material was obtained for an adequate cytologic interpretation, then a repeat fine-needle aspiration may be appropriate.

The triple test has also been used in younger women to document that a palpable mass can be followed with observation rather than surgically removed. For example, in women under the age of 40 years, a mass is probably benign if the clinical examination shows the characteristics of a benign mass, the imaging examination (either ultrasonography or mammogram) shows a benign appearance, and the FNA demonstrates benign cytology.[25]

Fine-Needle Aspiration Biopsy of Surgical Scar Lesions

Properly performed FNAB can be useful in evaluating lesions detected in the scars after breast-conserving surgery or total mastectomy. The sensitivity, specificity, and positive and negative predictive values are similar to those for FNAB in patients with primary breast cancer.[26] Open biopsies of lesions in a breast that has been irradiated are associated with a relatively high rate of wound-healing complications.[27]

Technique of Fine-Needle Aspiration of Cysts

For fine-needle aspiration of cysts, the skin of the breast is first treated with alcohol or an iodophor. A local anesthetic is not generally used, because it requires a needle puncture, and the typical cyst can be aspirated in a single pass. Brief application of ethyl chloride spray, insufficient to freeze the skin but sufficient to distract the patient, can be used if available. A 1-inch no. 21 needle is satisfactory for aspiration of most cysts. The size of the syringe chosen depends on the suspected volume of the cyst. Usual syringe sizes are 3 to 10 mL. Using universal precautions, the operator stabilizes the cyst between two fingers of the nondominant hand so the cyst may be punctured and aspirated with the dominant hand. The needle should be rotated as it is slowly withdrawn toward the completion of the aspiration to be certain that any cyst wall impinging on the bevel of the needle does not prevent complete aspiration. Palpation with the fingers of the nondominant hand can be used to determine whether the cyst has been completely emptied and whether an adjacent mass exists. Typical cyst fluid is thin and slightly opalescent, and varies from light tan to very dark green. The fluid in a long-standing cyst may occasionally become thick and require a larger needle for complete evacuation. After aspiration, the patient is instructed to maintain pressure on the site for at least 5 minutes to prevent bleeding into the cyst cavity. Typical cyst fluid is discarded, because large studies have shown that cytologic examination of typical cyst fluid is of little use.[10,28,29] When malignant lesions are cystic, additional clinical factors usually indicate that the abnormality is not a typical gross cyst. In such cases, the fluid is bloody, or a residual mass is present after aspiration of the fluid. On rare occasions, an unsuspected nonpalpable ductal or lobular carcinoma *in situ* has been detected on examination of apparently normal cyst fluid, just as such lesions sometimes are serendipitously identified adjacent to benign lesions that have been excised. If a bloody cyst is encountered, the fluid should be sent for cytologic examination to rule out cystic carcinoma.[30]

A benign cystic mass should disappear completely after aspiration. A persistent residual mass, multiple recurrences after aspiration of the same cyst, and a bloody aspirate are all indications for obtaining adequate material for pathologic examination.

Technique of Fine-Needle Aspiration Breast Biopsy

Adequate FNAB depends on skillful technique by both the operator and the cytopathologist. The operator must have the expertise to ascertain that the needle is within the lesion and that sufficient material for an adequate cytologic examination is obtained. Depending on the needs of the cytopathologist, the aspirated material must immediately be smeared on microscope slides or placed into a fixative for cell-block or cytospin preparations. The cytopathologist may request that the slides be immediately wet-fixed in 95% ethyl alcohol with no air drying, that they be air-dried, or that both types of preparations be done.

FNAB is performed after the skin has been cleaned with an antiseptic. The needle used for FNAB may vary in size from no. 21 to no. 27. If a cyst has been anticipated but the lesion proves to be solid, the no. 21 needle may be used to obtain the cytologic material. If the lesion is believed to be solid, use of a no. 25 needle may lead to less admixture of blood with the cells from the lesion. Some operators use a 20-mL syringe in a special holder designed to stabilize the syringe barrel to aid one-handed withdrawal of the plunger, which creates the vacuum for aspirations. Others find it simpler to use a one-handed technique to withdraw the plunger of a standard 3-, 5-, or 10-mL hypodermic syringe. The needle is passed in and out of the lesion 3 to 10 times in various directions. A slight rotary motion allows the bevel of the needle to cut additional cells from the mass. The appearance of the aspirated material in the hub of the needle usually signals that an adequate amount of material has been aspirated. The suction on the plunger is released, and, after equilibration, the needle and syringe are withdrawn. The needle is disconnected from the syringe, and the syringe is filled with air. The needle is replaced, and a drop of the material is carefully expressed onto a glass microscopic slide and immediately spread with another slide. Slides are either immediately wet-fixed or air-dried, as discussed in the paragraph above.

CORE-CUTTING NEEDLE BIOPSY

Core-cutting needle biopsies provide histologic material that is usually suitable for interpretation by any pathologist[18,31] and does not require the special skills of a cytopathologist. Core-cutting needle biopsies may be processed for permanent or frozen sections.

False-positive diagnoses obtained using core-cutting needle biopsies are rare but could occur with sclerosing ductal proliferations such as radial scars, which show a pseudoinvasive mingling of proliferating epithelium and stroma that is easier to diagnose using open biopsies, which include the entire lesion. False-negative diagnoses with core-cutting needle biopsies are related to the same sampling problems encountered with FNAB. Sampling problems may even be slightly greater because of increased resistance to penetration of the larger needle into the tumor. In such cases, the needle may be deflected and may thus sample tissue adjacent to, rather than within, the tumor.[32] Occasionally, the core biopsy sample may not provide sufficient material for diagnosis because of extreme desmoplasia or necrosis.

Although the likelihood of seeding the needle track with tumor cells during FNAB appears very low, some reports have described needle-track seeding from core-needle breast biopsies.[33] Prudence dictates that, when possible, the biopsy track should be placed so the definitive treatment includes it. The depth of the biopsy should be adjusted to eliminate any chance of carrying malignant tissue into the chest wall or into other areas of the breast that would not be removed in the planned surgical procedure.

Core-needle biopsies may be obtained using disposable needles, such as the Tru-Cut (Baxter Healthcare, Deerfield, IL) (Fig. 1), or spring-loaded core-cutting needle devices. The advantages of Tru-Cut needles are their ready availability and relatively low cost. The advantages of the spring-loaded devices are decreased pain, a slightly higher sampling success rate, a greater diagnostic sensitivity, and a somewhat better specimen quality than for the Tru-Cut.[34] The spring-loaded devices are relatively expensive, however, and therefore are less likely to be available in the outpatient office. The two general types of spring-loaded core-biopsy devices are disposable devices and reusable devices. The reusable guns have permanent firing devices into which disposable needles are fitted.

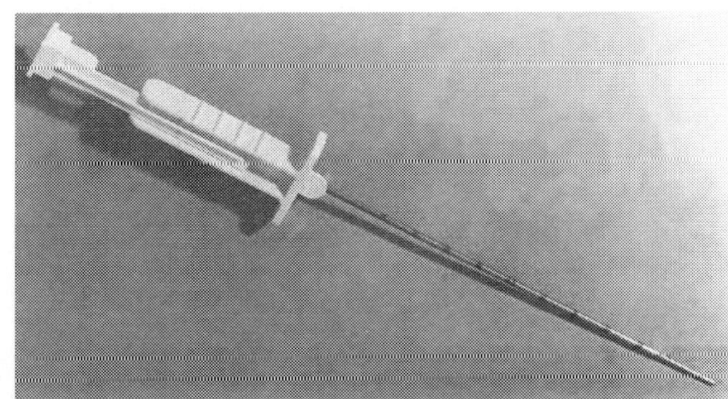

FIG. 1. The Tru-Cut (Baxter Healthcare, Deerfield, IL) disposable core-cutting needle may be used for obtaining core biopsies of solid breast masses.

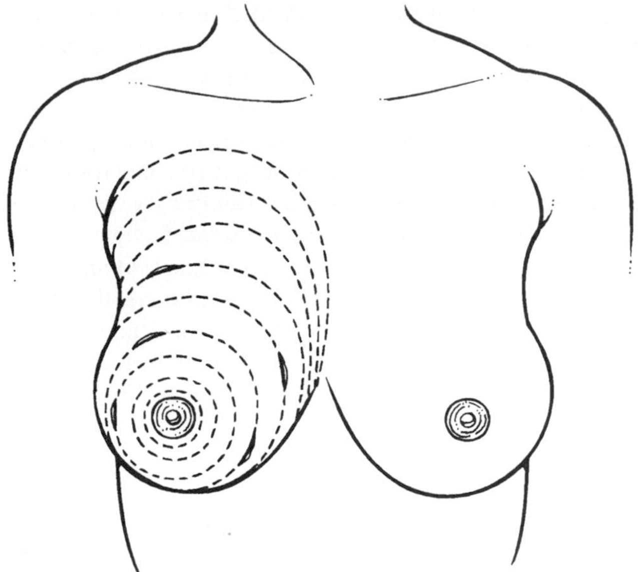

FIG. 2. Langer's lines are the natural lines of skin tension and skin creasing. Incisions placed along Langer's lines usually produce the optimum cosmetic result. For larger lesions in the lower half of the breast, radial incisions may produce better cosmesis (see Fig. 3).

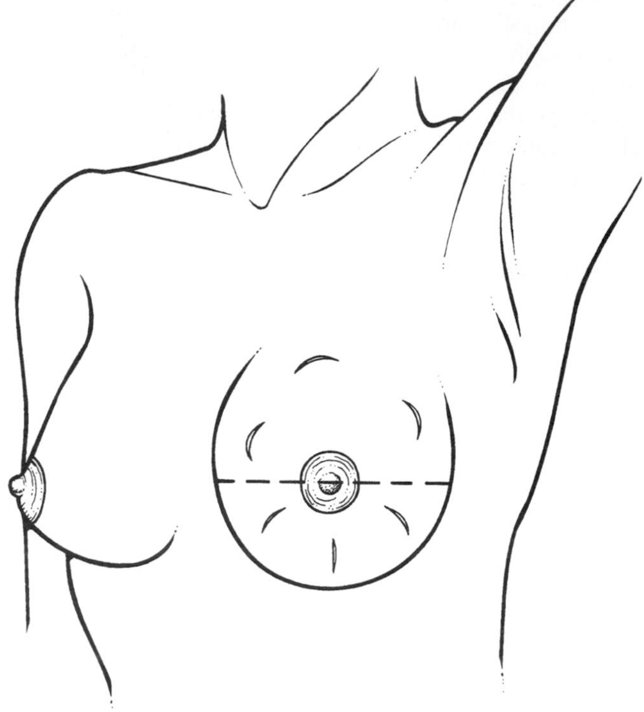

FIG. 3. For larger excisions or when skin must be excised, radial incisions in the lower half of the breast and curvilinear incisions along Langer's lines in the upper half of the breast tend to provide the best cosmesis.

EXCISIONAL BIOPSY

Excisional breast biopsy is the complete removal of a lesion, with or without a rim of surrounding normal parenchyma. Excisional biopsy is usually the definitive treatment for benign lesions. For malignant lesions, if a margin of normal tissue has been removed and if the pathologic examination confirms that the margins are not involved by cancer, no further breast surgery may be necessary. A lumpectomy will have been performed.

Local anesthesia, with or without supplemental sedation, can be used for excisional breast biopsies. The use of general anesthesia entails greater cost, a slightly longer period of disability for the patient, and a small but finite risk of fatalities. Use of local anesthesia requires that the surgeon be skilled in infiltrating the anesthetic in a manner that causes minimal discomfort, that the surgeon be willing to communicate with the patient during the procedure, and that the surgery be done with minimal traction.

Adding 1 mL of 8.5% sodium bicarbonate to each 10 mL of 1% lidocaine without epinephrine creates a more neutral pH that causes less discomfort during infiltration. Discomfort can also be minimized by slowing the rate of infiltration, particularly during infiltration of the skin.

Although placing the breast biopsy incision so as to obtain the best cosmetic result is desirable, consideration should also be given to further surgical management of the patient if the lesion is suspected to be malignant. Liberal use of fine-needle aspirations before excisional biopsy minimizes the number of unexpected malignancies. Incisions along Langer's lines usually produce the best cosmesis, particularly in the upper half of the breast (Fig. 2). In young women, in whom the lesion is most likely a benign fibroadenoma, use of a periareolar incision may be appropriate, even when the incision is a considerable distance from the areola. Incisions overlying the sternal area are particularly prone to the development of a hypertrophic scar. Most malignant lesions in the central and upper portions of the breast are best excised with transverse curvilinear incisions that are placed over the lesion. A radial incision is frequently preferred for malignant lesions in the lower half of the breast (Fig. 3). For larger lesions, the potential problem with incisions along Langer's lines in the lower half of the breast is that a greater cosmetic deformity is created if the removal of skin or tissue causes a shortening of the distance between the nipple-areolar complex and the inframammary crease than if the same volume of tissue removal causes a slight narrowing of the breast.

The biopsy should be performed using a cold knife rather than electrocautery. Thermal injury may confound histologic interpretation of the biopsy results, particularly assessment of the margins of excision. The heat from electrocautery can also cause degradation of the estrogen-receptor protein, leading to a falsely low or negative result. Specific bleeding encountered during the dissection may be managed by electrocoagulation if necessary. After the lesion has been removed, hemostasis may be obtained with electrocoagulation.

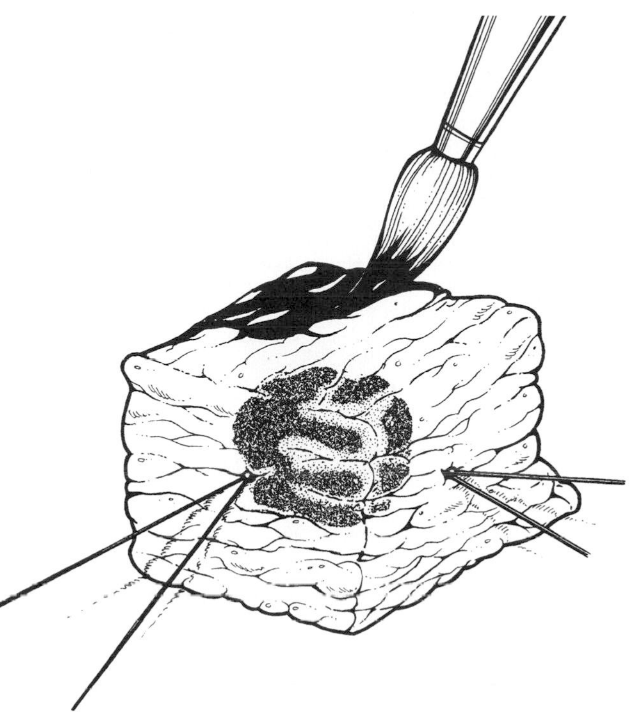

FIG. 4. Specimen should remain intact and should be marked so that the dorsal, ventral, cephalad, caudad, medial, and lateral surfaces can be identified by the pathologist. Rectangular margins are easier to orient than are ellipsoid margins. One convention for marking the specimen is to place a long suture on the lateral margin and a short suture on the superior (cephalad) margin.

Fibroadenomas may be excised with a small rim of normal breast tissue, or they may be enucleated, provided care is taken so that the lesion is not morcellated.

Lesions that are shown or suspected to be malignant should be excised with a margin of apparently normal tissue. If malignancy is clearly established and if tumor-free margins exist, the patient will probably have had an adequate resection, should breast conservation be done. The author prefers to remove a rectangular portion of apparently normal breast parenchyma around the lesion rather than a spheroid rim. The rectangular resection makes orientation of the margins easier and simplifies location of any area that requires reexcision because the margin is not tumor free.

If the excisional biopsy includes a rim of apparently normal tissue around the lesion, orientation of the specimen margins relative to their location in the residual breast should be maintained. The specimen must be marked so that the cephalad (superior), caudad (inferior), dorsal, ventral, medial, and lateral margins can be identified by the pathologist. One method is to use two sutures, one long lateral suture and one short superior suture (Fig. 4).

The intact specimen should be examined by the surgeon to confirm that the biopsy contains the lesion. By moving the normal surrounding tissue over a suspected malignancy, the surgeon can usually determine whether an adequate margin has been removed. The surgeon should also manually examine the biopsy cavity to make sure no additional lesions are present.

After hemostasis is established, the incision is closed without a drain. The best approach is almost always not to try to approximate the breast parenchyma, as this creates distortion of the breast and poorer cosmesis. If the initial incision has been carried down through the subcutaneous fat and the superficial layer of the superficial fascia, closure of the superficial fascia provides good restoration of breast form. The skin is closed with a subcuticular suture.

INCISIONAL BIOPSY

Incisional biopsy is a diagnostic biopsy that removes a portion of a mass for pathologic examination in cases in which complete removal of the mass is unnecessary or might compromise future mastectomy. Unless larger amounts of tissue are required for pathologic examination, adequate material for diagnosis may be obtained more simply through FNAB or core-needle biopsy.

SKIN BIOPSY

Skin biopsy for histologic examination may be appropriate when lesions either are primary in the skin of the breast or originate within the breast but involve the skin. An incisional biopsy of the skin may sometimes be included when an incisional biopsy of an underlying breast mass is being performed.

An excellent technique for obtaining a full-thickness skin specimen is to use a disposable punch biopsy tool. Biopsy specimens obtained with this tool range in size from 2 to 6 mm, and the procedure is simple to perform with the patient under local anesthesia (Fig. 5). The circular biopsy hole assumes an elliptic shape in the direction of Langer's lines.

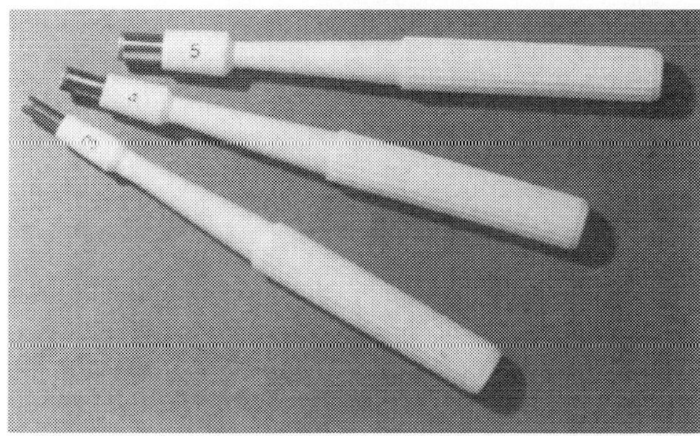

FIG. 5. Disposable punch biopsies can be used for full-thickness biopsy of skin lesions.

The small biopsy incision can be closed with one or two fine sutures or with sterile tape.

BIOPSY OF REGIONAL ADENOPATHY OR CHEST WALL RECURRENCE

All of the techniques described here can be used to obtain pathologic material for the evaluation of regional adenopathy that develops either in the absence of a breast mass or after previous treatment of the primary mass. The judgments regarding the selection of the optimum biopsy procedure are similar. Frequently, FNAB is used as the initial diagnostic procedure for regional adenopathy or subcutaneous recurrence. Punch biopsies are useful for obtaining histologic confirmation of a suspected cutaneous recurrence.

REFERENCES

1. Walker GM, Foster RS Jr, McKegney CP, McKegney FP. Breast biopsy. A comparison of outpatient and inpatient experience. *Arch Surg* 1978;113:942.
2. Layfield LJ, Chrischilles EA, Cohen MB, Bottles K. The palpable breast nodule. A cost-effectiveness analysis of alternate diagnostic approaches. *Cancer* 1993;72:1642.
3. Koss LG. The palpable breast nodule. A cost-effectiveness analysis of alternate diagnostic approaches. The role of the needle aspiration biopsy. *Cancer* 1993;72:1499.
4. Jackson PP, Pitts HH. Biopsy with delayed radical mastectomy for carcinoma of the breast. *Am J Surg* 1959;98:184.
5. Abramson DJ. Delayed mastectomy after outpatient biopsy. *Am J Surg* 1976;132:596.
6. Fisher ER, Sass R, Fisher B. Biologic considerations regarding the one and two step procedures in the management of patients with invasive carcinoma of the breast. *Surg Gynecol Obstet* 1985;161:245.
7. Bertario L, Reduzzi D, Piromalli D, et al. Outpatient biopsy of breast cancer. Influence on survival. *Ann Surg* 1985;201:64.
8. Krag D, Weaver D, Ashikaga T, et al. The sentinel node in breast cancer—a multi-center validation study. *N Engl J Med* 1998;339:941.
9. Martin HE, Ellis EB. Biopsy by needle puncture and aspiration. *Ann Surg* 1930;92:169.
10. Franzen S, Zajicek J. Aspiration biopsy in diagnosis of palpable lesions of the breast. Critical review of 3479 consecutive biopsies. *Acta Radial Ther Phys Biol* 1968;7:241.
11. Zajdela A, Ghossein NA, Pilleron JP, Ennuyer A. The value of aspiration cytology in the diagnosis of breast cancer: experience at the Foundation Curie. *Cancer* 1975;35:499.
12. Zajicek J, Caspersson T, Jakobsson, et al. Cytologic diagnosis of mammary tumors from aspiration biopsy smears. Comparison of cytologic and histologic findings in 2111 lesions and diagnostic use of cytophotometry. *Acta Cytol* 1970;14:370.
13. Abati A, Abele J, Bacus S, et al. National Cancer Institute Conference, Bethesda, MD, October, 1997. The uniform approach to breast fine-needle aspiration biopsy. *Am J Surg* 1997;174:371.
14. Wollenberg NJ, Caya JB, Clowry LJ. Fine needle aspiration cytology of the breast. A review of 321 cases with statistical evaluation. *Acta Cytol* 1985;29:425.
15. Lee KR, Foster RS Jr, Papillo JL. Fine needle aspirate of the breast. Importance of the aspirator. *Acta Cytol* 1987;31:281.
16. Hermans J. The value of aspiration cytologic examination of the breast. A statistical review of the medical literature. *Cancer* 1992;69:2104.
17. Feldman PS, Covell JL. *Fine needle aspiration cytology and its clinical application: breast and lung*. Chicago: American Society of Clinical Pathologists Press, 1985:27.
18. Innes DJ Jr, Feldman PS. Comparison of diagnostic results obtained by fine needle aspiration cytology and Tru-Cut or open biopsies. *Acta Cytol* 1983;27:350.
19. Casey TT, Rodgers WH, Baxter JW, et al. Stratified diagnostic approach to fine needle aspiration of the breast. *Am J Surg* 1992;163:305.
20. Lannin DR, Silverman JF, Walker C, Pories WJ. Cost-effectiveness of fine needle biopsy of the breast. *Ann Surg* 1986;203:474.
21. O'Malley F, Casey TT, Winfield AC, et al. Clinical correlates of false-negative fine needle aspirations of the breast in a consecutive series of 1005 patients. *Surg Gynecol Obstet* 1993;176:360.
22. Wanebo HJ, Feldman PS, Wilhelm MC, et al. Fine-needle aspiration cytology in lieu of open biopsy in management of breast cancer. *Ann Surg* 1984;199:569.
23. Ulanow RM, Galblum L, Canter JW. Fine needle aspiration in the diagnosis and management of solid breast lesions. *Am J Surg* 1984; 148:653.
24. Painter RW, Clark WE II, Deckers PJ. Negative findings on fine-needle aspiration biopsy of solid breast masses: patient management. *Am J Surg* 1988;155:387.
25. Morrow M, Wong S, Venta L. The evaluation of breast masses in women younger than forty years of age. *Surgery* 1998;124:634.
26. Malberger E, Edoute Y, Toledano O, Sapir D. Fine-needle aspiration and cytologic findings of surgical scar lesions in women with breast cancer. *Cancer* 1992;69:148.
27. Pezner RD, Lorant JA, Terz J, et al. Wound-healing complications following biopsy of the irradiated breast. *Arch Surg* 1992;127:321.
28. Kline TS, Joshi LP, Neal MS. Fine-needle aspiration of the breast: diagnosis and pitfalls. A review of 3545 cases. *Cancer* 1979;44:1458.
29. Cowen PN, Benson GA. Cytologic study of fluid from benign breast cysts. *Br J Surg* 1979;66:209.
30. Devitt JE, Barr JR. The clinical recognition of cystic carcinoma of the breast. *Surg Gynecol Obstet* 1984;159:130.
31. Foster RS Jr. Core cutting needle biopsy for the diagnosis of breast cancer. *Am J Surg* 1982;143:622.
32. Shabot MM, Goldberg IM, Schick P, et al. Aspiration cytology is superior to "Tru-Cut" needle biopsy in establishing the diagnosis of clinically suspicious breast masses. *Ann Surg* 1982;196:122.
33. Harter LP, Curtis JS, Ponto G, Craig PH. Malignant seeding of the needle track during stereotaxic core needle breast biopsy. *Radiology* 1992;185:713.
34. McMahon AJ, Lutfy AM, Matthew A, et al. Needle core biopsy of the breast with a spring-loaded device. *Br J Surg* 1992;79:1042.

III

Diseases of the Breast, 2nd ed.,
edited by Jay R. Harris.
Lippincott Williams & Wilkins, Philadelphia © 2000.

Breast Imaging and Image-Guided Biopsy Techniques

CHAPTER 11

Screening for Breast Cancer

Robert A. Smith and Carl J. D'Orsi

The importance of detecting localized breast cancer was recognized in the mid-eighteenth century by Henri François LeDran, who proposed that breast cancer originated as a localized disease that subsequently spread via the lymphatics to the general circulation. According to Donegan,[1] this pivotal concept established the idea that surgery, if performed early, offered the potential to cure breast cancer. However, it was not until the early twentieth century that experimental work with x-rays by Salomon and others demonstrated the detection of occult breast disease, thereby establishing the potential for diagnosis before the earliest detection of a palpable mass.[1,2] These important discoveries ushered in the technology and the public health impetus to screen for breast cancer.

Once the efficacy of breast cancer screening was confirmed by early results from the Health Insurance Plan of Greater New York randomized trial (HIP), more fundamental questions about organized screening began to be asked.[3] Could mammography and clinical breast examination (CBE) achieve the same results at the community level as had been demonstrated in the HIP trial? Would women and their doctors participate in regular screening for breast cancer? To answer these questions, the American Cancer Society (ACS) and the National Cancer Institute (NCI) cosponsored the Breast Cancer Detection Demonstration Project (BCDDP), which screened more than 280,000 women at 29 centers between 1973 and 1980.[4] Participation rates were high over the course of the study, and nearly one-half of all breast cancers were found by mammography alone. Furthermore, the distribution of stage at diagnosis was much more favorable among study participants compared with incident cases in the NCI's Surveillance Epidemiology and End Results program during the same time period; overall long-term survival likewise has been better.[5] These results, in combination with the findings from the HIP study, were sufficiently persuasive to justify promotion of routine breast cancer screening, a public health initiative that continues to be a high priority. In addition to the HIP and BCDDP studies, seven additional randomized trials have contributed evidence related to screening for breast cancer with mammography.[6–10]

R. A. Smith: Cancer Screening, Department of Cancer Control, American Cancer Society, Atlanta, Georgia

C. J. D'Orsi: Diagnostic Radiology, University of Massachusetts Memorial Medical Center, Worchester, Massachusetts

There is widespread acceptance of the value of regular breast cancer screening as the single most important public health strategy to reduce mortality from breast cancer. In 1981, Illinois passed the first legislation that required insurance companies to address health insurance coverage for mammography as part of their health plans, and now nearly all states have legislation requiring that routine mammography be offered as part of a basic benefits package.[11] The Health Insurance Financing Administration (HCFA) now provides for annual mammography for all Medicare beneficiaries aged 40 and older and waives the Part B deductible.[12] Surveys of physicians reveal support for the value of mammography for their patients, and the most recent survey results show that a majority of women aged 40 and older report having had a mammogram in the previous 2 years.[13–16]

The control of breast cancer has historically relied entirely on successful treatment, which has been measurably improved by favorable shifts in stage at diagnosis brought about by screening as well as gains in treatment regimens.[17] However, continued progress in our understanding of the epidemiology of breast cancer, and the recent results of the Breast Cancer Prevention trial showing a 49% reduction in breast cancer incidence among a higher-risk cohort of women who took tamoxifen, suggest that over time, primary prevention strategies will begin to provide a greater and more direct contribution to breast cancer control.[18–20] Yet, however encouraging, the overall potential for breast cancer prevention in average- and higher-risk women through either lifestyle modification or chemoprevention is uncertain at this time. For this reason, early detection and appropriate treatment will remain the cornerstones of the disease control strategy for the foreseeable future.

In this chapter, we discuss breast cancer screening in the context of basic screening principles, methodologic issues related to the evaluation of screening, the current evidence of screening efficacy, and practical and clinical aspects of modern breast cancer screening.

PRINCIPLES OF CANCER SCREENING

The decision to screen an asymptomatic population for preclinical disease is based on well-established, although not specific, criteria that relate to the disease in question and the characteristics of applicable screening test(s).[21] The first goal of screening for breast cancer on an individual or population basis is to distinguish among those who are likely and not likely to have the disease.[22] The emphasis on *likelihood* underscores the limits of what can be expected of screening (i.e., screening is not a diagnostic process). It is inherent to the concept of screening that a person identified with an abnormality is then referred for further diagnostic testing to determine whether the disease truly is present. Further, the emphasis on likelihood also is important because screening programs have inherent limitations that are a function of the specific disease, differences between individuals, available technology, and finally, the basic criteria for the acceptability of a screening test—in other words, its ability to efficiently test a large asymptomatic population at an acceptable cost. In the case of breast cancer screening, the majority of screening interpretations are accurate, but it is inevitable that some women will be identified as possibly having breast cancer when they do not, and screening tests will fail to identify some women who do have the disease.[23]

Before large numbers of asymptomatic individuals undergo routine testing for the presence of a chronic disease, certain conventional criteria should be met.[24] First, the disease should be an important health problem. Second, there should be a period when the disease is detectable in an asymptomatic individual (i.e., a detectable preclinical phase). Treatment at this early stage should offer better outcomes than if the disease were treated at a later stage. Third, the screening test must be effective, reasonably accurate, and affordable or at least not prohibitively expensive. With respect to accuracy, ideally the test should achieve acceptable levels of sensitivity and specificity. The importance of accuracy is unquestionable, but the comparative consequence of a false-positive or false-negative test result may also be a consideration when determining thresholds of acceptability. Moreover, the complements of sensitivity and specificity (i.e., false-negatives and false-positives) provide insights not only into what is being achieved in a screening program but also how accuracy can be improved and, thus, what potentially is *achievable* in a screening program. Finally, the test must be acceptable to targeted individuals and referring physicians.

Screening for breast cancer meets each of these criteria well enough, although current data indicate that screening may not be equally effective among all age groups, an observation that has been a source of ongoing health policy debate. The controversy over the value of screening women between the ages of 40 to 49 is well known, but there are also differences of opinion about the benefit of screening women older than age 70 and different ideas about recommended screening intervals for women of different ages.[25–29] There are also concerns about various costs associated with screening. These costs, both financial and psychosocial, include the proportion of women who receive false-positive results, the anxiety experienced by women whose mammograms are interpreted as abnormal and those who undergo avoidable biopsy, and the rate of diagnosis of ductal carcinomas *in situ* (DCIS), some of which would not eventually progress to invasive disease.[26,30–33] These costs are regarded by some as too high, by others as acceptable or at least unavoidable, and by others as evidence of a need to strive for better performance.[32,34–37] We address each of the previously mentioned criteria as a basis for summarizing what we know about the effectiveness of screening, as well as key issues related to the status of breast cancer screening in clinical practice today.

DISEASE BURDEN

By a sizable margin, breast cancer is the most common malignancy diagnosed in American women and the second leading cause of death from cancer.[38,39] According to current incidence and mortality estimates, in a hypothetical cohort of women, approximately 1 in 8 will be diagnosed with breast cancer in her lifetime, and 1 in 29 will die from this disease.[39] Breast cancer is the second most common cause of person-years of life lost to cancer among men and women, accounting for an estimated 841,000 years of premature mortality.[39] On average, a woman who dies of breast cancer has lost 19.3 years of life that she might have had if she had not died of this disease.[39] This count does not include the years of diminished quality of life and lower productivity from the time of diagnosis, which are difficult to factor into disease burden measures but nonetheless are important to acknowledge. As noted here, and in greater detail in Chapter 15, breast cancer is among the more serious threats to health that a woman experiences in her lifetime.

SOJOURN TIME AND THE INFLUENCE OF EARLY INTERVENTION

The detectable preclinical phase, also known as the *sojourn time*, is the estimated duration of time that an occult tumor can be detected before the onset of symptoms.[40] The *lead time* is the amount of time actually gained by screening before the onset of symptoms. The breast cancer sojourn time, and therefore the lead time, varies in individuals, and analysis of trial data has shown that the mean sojourn time and mean lead time also vary by age and, in postmenopausal women, also by histology.[41] Tabar and colleagues[8] have estimated that the mean sojourn time is 1.7 years in women aged 40 to 49, 3.3 years in women aged 50 to 59, and 3.8 years in women aged 60 to 69.

In a perfect world, the lead time would always nearly equal the sojourn time, meaning that there would be a coincidence between the occasion of a screening test and the onset of the detectable preclinical period. This is rarely the case, but knowledge of sojourn time is important for determining screening intervals in a breast cancer screening program, because the sojourn time defines the upper limit of the lead time that might be gained.[40] When a screening interval exceeds the mean sojourn time, there is increased potential for a higher rate of interval cancers and thus poorer prognosis in that subset of incident cases. Early evidence of the influence of mean sojourn time on the interval cancer rate was seen in the Swedish Two-County study, which reported nearly twice the interval cancer rate in women aged 40 to 49 compared with women aged 50 and older when both groups were screened at intervals of 24 or more months.[42]

Stage at diagnosis is an important factor in prognosis. When breast cancer is detected while still localized to the breast, 5-year survival is markedly improved compared with a diagnosis of regional disease or the presence of distant metastases. For cases diagnosed during the period 1986 to 1993, 5-year survival among women in the United States for localized diseased was 97.4%, compared with 77.4% for regional disease and 21.2% for women diagnosed with distant metastases.[39] Smart and colleagues[5] recently reported adjusted survival rates after 20 years of follow-up cases diagnosed in the BCDDP; survival for women diagnosed with stage I disease was 86.8%, compared with 40.3% for women diagnosed with stage III disease. Data on long-term survival are remarkably consistent between surveillance programs, trials, and demonstration projects, with each showing an inverse association between tumor size and long-term survival.[5,8,10,43] When grouped by stage at diagnosis, long-term survival is similar in all age groups of women.[43]

EVALUATION OF BREAST CANCER SCREENING

The efficacy of a screening test is best evaluated with a population-based, randomized clinical trial with a mortality end point. Randomized trials eliminate the potential biases in observational studies that may influence comparative survival among screen-detected and nonscreen-detected cases, most notably lead-time bias, length-bias sampling, and selection bias. As Miller[44] notes, in most instances screen-detected cases have better survival than cases diagnosed after the onset of clinical symptoms. It is therefore important to distinguish the actual improvements in survival from apparent improvements. As noted previously, the goal of screening is to gain lead time. If treatment before the onset of symptoms offers greater benefits, then improvements in survival should be associated with lead time gained, and mortality should be lower in cases diagnosed by screening. On the other hand, if lead time only advances the time of diagnosis and life is not extended because death occurs at the same point in the natural history of the disease among screen-detected and nonscreen-detected cases, then there is only the appearance of a greater survival duration. *Lead-time bias* occurs when increased survival is a function only of the time gained *before* the point at which diagnosis would have occurred in the absence of screening. *Length-bias sampling* refers to the tendency for screening to detect more slow-growing, less aggressive disease and to be less successful at detecting more aggressive, faster-growing disease. If screening selectively identifies cases at a lower risk of death, length-bias sampling may influence end results. *Selection bias* refers to the tendency for individuals who are healthier, or more health conscious, and with a different probability of developing and/or dying from cancer, to participate in screening.

In a population-based randomized trial, these biases are eliminated, because randomization should result in equal distributions of these confounding factors in the groups invited and not invited to several rounds of screening. Lead-time bias is eliminated, because disease-specific mortality in the group invited to screening is compared with mortality in the group not invited to screening at some future date after the starting point of the study, which is the same for both groups. Length-bias sampling and selection bias are eliminated, because randomization should ensure the same distribution of individuals with underlying probabilities of developing cancer, with faster- and slower-growing tumors, and with similar overall health status into each group in the study. Because the analysis is based on mortality differences in the two groups and not on the basis of the sub-

TABLE 1. *Summary of randomized controlled trials of breast cancer screening*

Study (duration)	Screening protocol CBE (yes/no)	Frequency (no. rounds)	Study population				Years of follow-up	Relative risk (95% CI)
			Age (yr)	Subgroup	Invited	Control		
HIP study (1963–1969)	2 V MM CBE	12 mo 4 rounds	40–64	40–49	14,432	14,701	18	0.77 (0.53–1.11)
				50–64	16,568	16,299	18	0.80 (0.59–1.08)
Edinburgh (1979–1988)	1 or 2 V MM CBE (initial)	24 mo 4 rounds	45–64	45–49	11,755[a]	10,641[a]	12.6	0.81[a] (0.54–1.20)
				50–64	11,245	12,359	10	0.85 (0.62–1.15)
Kopparberg (1977–1985)	1 V MM	24 mo 4 rounds	40–74	40–49	9,650	5,009	15.2	0.67 (0.37–1.22)
				50–74	28,939	13,551	11	0.58 (0.43–0.78)
Ostergotland (1977–1985)	1 V MM	24 mo 4 rounds	40–74	40–49	10,240	10,411	14.2	1.02 (0.59–1.77)
				50–74	28,229	26,830	11	0.73 (0.56–0.97)
Malmö (1976–1990)	1 or 2 V MM	18–24 mo 5 rounds	45–69	45–49[b]	13,528	12,242	12.7	0.64[b] (0.45–0.89)
				50–69	17,134	17,165	9	0.86 (0.64–1.16)
Stockholm (1981–1985)	1 V MM	28 mo 2 rounds	40–64	40–49	14,185	7,985	11.4	1.01 (0.51–2.02)
				50–64	25,815	12,015	7	0.65 (0.4–1.08)
Gothenburg (1982–1988)	2 V MM	18 mo 5 rounds	39–59	39–49	11,724	14,217	12	0.56 (0.32–0.98)
				50–59	9,276	16,394	5	0.91 (0.62–1.52)
CNBSS-1 (1980–1987)	2 V MM CBE	12 mo 4–5 rounds	40–49	40–49	25,214	25,216	10.5	1.14 (0.83–1.56)
CNBSS-2 (1980–1987)	2 V MM CBE	12 mo 4–5 rounds	50–59	50–59	19,711	19,694	7.0	0.97 (0.62–1.52)

CBE, clinical breast examination; CI, confidence interval; CNBSS, Canadian National Breast Screening Study; HIP, Health Insurance Plan of Greater New York; 1 V MM, one-view mammography of each breast; 2 V MM, two-view mammography of each breast

[a]The Edinburgh trial included three separate groups of women aged 45 to 49 at entry: The first had 5,949 women in the invited group and 5,818 in the control group (with 14 years' follow-up); the next had 2,545 in the invited group and 2,482 in the control group (12 years' follow-up); the third had 3,261 in the invited group and 2,341 in the control group (10 years' follow-up). Only the first group's results had been reported previously.

[b]The Malmö trial included two groups of women aged 45 to 49 at entry: One group (Malmö Mammographic Screening Trial I, or MMST-I) received first-round screening in 1977 to 1978 and had 3,954 women in the invited group and 4,030 women in the control group; the second group (MMST-II) received first-round screening from 1978 to 1990 and had 9,574 women in the invited group and 8,212 women the control group. Only the first group's results had been reported previously.

groups that were and were not screened, most known and unknown biases can be minimized.

MAMMOGRAPHY TRIALS AND META-ANALYSES

Following are brief summaries of the major randomized trials of breast cancer screening (Table 1). They represent study designs in which a large group of women was randomly assigned to a group that either would or would not receive an invitation to be screened for breast cancer. As can be seen, the first of these studies was initiated in the early 1960s, and for some, follow-up still continues. Each followed a somewhat different protocol, and the outcome in each has been influenced by a number of factors that have important implications for the interpretation of study results. These factors include the study methodology, the clinical protocol, participation rates in the study group (compliance), screening rates in the control group (contamination), and the number of screening rounds before an invitation was extended to the control group. Other factors that likely influenced end results include the quality of the screening process, thresholds for diagnosis, and follow-up mechanisms for women with an abnormality. For these factors, we have few insights into individual trials.[6,45,46] It is also the case that, with the exception of the randomized trials conducted in Canada (NBSS-I and -II), which, as noted in the description of the Canadian trials below, have been controversial, none was specifically designed to evaluate the efficacy of breast cancer screening in age-specific subgroups (e.g., women aged 40 to 49). The availability of data in each of the trials has provided the opportunity for retrospective analysis of screening efficacy by age; however, limitations in statistical power and questions regarding the appropriateness of applying the same screening protocol to pre- and postmenopausal women have been the focus of debate over whether health policy could reliably be informed by the existing data.

Health Insurance Plan of New York Randomized Clinical Trial

The HIP study was initiated in December 1963.[3] It was the first randomized, controlled trial to evaluate the efficacy of breast cancer screening with CBE and mammography. Approximately 62,000 women aged 40 to 64 were randomly assigned to two groups: The study group would be offered annual CBE and two-view mammography (craniocaudal and mediolateral views) for 4 years, and the control group would receive usual care. After 10 years from entry into the study, approximately 30% fewer breast cancer deaths occurred in the study group compared with the control group.[47] At 18 years of follow-up, there were 23% fewer deaths. Mammography and CBE contributed independently to breast cancer detection, with 33% of cases detected by mammography alone, 45% with CBE alone, and 22% with combined modalities.[48]

Swedish Two-County Study

The largest randomized trial of breast cancer screening is the Swedish Two-County study, so-called because women were randomized into study and control groups within two counties in Sweden, Kopparberg and Ostergötland.[7] The trial consisted of approximately 133,000 women aged 40 to 74 years, with approximately 77,000 women invited to the screening. The screening intervals differed by age, with women aged 40 to 49 invited every 24 months and women aged 50 and older invited every 33 months. The screening examination included only single-view mammography (mediolateral oblique view) and did not include CBE. After 8, 11, and 14 years of follow-up, approximately 30% fewer breast cancer deaths occurred in the study group invited to the screening compared with the control group.[7,8,49]

Malmö

In Malmö, Sweden, a randomized trial to evaluate the efficacy of breast cancer screening was initiated in 1976, designated the *Malmö Mammographic Screening Trial I*.[50] Approximately 42,000 women aged 45 to 69 were randomized on the basis of birth cohort (women born between 1927 and 1932) into study and control groups. The study group was invited to receive two-view mammography (craniocaudal and oblique views) at 18- to 24-month intervals for five rounds. CBE was not part of the screening regimen. No overall reduction in deaths was observed in the study group compared with the control group at 8 and 11 years of follow-up, although a nonsignificant 20% lower breast cancer death rate was observed for women aged 55 and older. Among the explanations that have been offered for these results is the finding that approximately 25% of the control group was screened with mammography during the study period, and a similar percentage were nonattenders in the study group, thus diluting the differences between the original allocation. A second cohort of women born between 1933 and 1945, designated *Malmö Mammographic Screening Trial II*, were invited to be screened between 1978 and 1990. The most recent update reports only results of the combined cohorts for women younger than age 50 at the time of randomization. The investigators observed a statistically significant 36% reduction in breast cancer mortality among the group invited to the screening.[51]

Stockholm

The Stockholm randomized trial of breast cancer screening was initiated in 1981. Sixty thousand women aged 40 to 64 were randomized on the basis of birth date into a study group of approximately 40,000 women who would receive invitations to screening and a control group of 20,000 women.[52] The study consisted of only two rounds of screening with single-view mammography (oblique view) without CBE at a 28-month interval and observed a nonsignificant 29% reduction in breast cancer mortality in the group invited to the screening.

Gothenburg

The Gothenburg randomized trial of breast cancer screening was initiated in 1982.[53] Approximately 52,000 women aged 39 to 59 years were randomized into groups to be invited and not to be invited to five screening rounds. The screening interval was 18 months, and usually women were screened with two-view mammography (craniocaudal and mediolateral oblique views), unless prior screening examinations indicated such low breast density that single-view mammography was justified (approximately 30% of mammograms). CBE was not part of the screening regimen. The investigators observed a 44% statistically significant reduction in breast cancer mortality among women aged 39 to 49 after 11 years of follow-up.

Edinburgh

The Edinburgh trial was initiated in 1979 and was an evaluation of the efficacy of CBE and, initially, two-view mammography (depending on initial findings, single-view mammography was often performed in subsequent screening rounds).[54] CBE was done annually and mammography every 2 years. Eighty-seven general practices representing approximately 45,000 women were randomized into study and control groups, which led to unanticipated confounding by socioeconomic status. Women aged 45 to 64 in the study group received invitations to four rounds of screening with mammography. At 7 years of follow-up, 17% fewer breast cancer deaths had occurred in the study group compared with the control group, a difference that was not statistically significant.[55]

Canada–National Breast Screening Study 1

The Canadian randomized trial of the efficacy of breast cancer screening in women aged 40 to 49 was initiated in 1980.[56] It was designed to specifically test the efficacy of breast cancer screening in women in their 40s and consisted of four to five rounds of annual CBE and mammography, depending on time of entry into the study. After a physical examination that included CBE, women were invited to participate in the study, and volunteers were then randomized into a study group or control group. Approximately 50,000 women participated in the study, with virtually equal numbers randomized to study and control groups. At 7 years of follow-up, approximately 36% more breast cancer deaths had occurred in the study group than in the control group. At 10.5 years of follow-up, the rate of excess mortality had declined to 14%.[57] This study and its conclusions have been controversial for a number of reasons, including study design (all study participants received a high-quality CBE before randomization), questions about the randomization process, the quality of mammography, and the observation that there was a significant excess of patients with advanced tumors in the group invited to screening compared with the usual care group.[45,58–60] More specifically, Tarone[61] has shown that the excess of patients in the National Breast Screening Study 1 (NBSS-1) who had four or more positive nodes in the screening arm is statistically significant and inconsistent with the stage distribution of disease in other trials, both in the first round and at the conclusion of the study. There is no known explanation for the excess of advanced tumors in the group invited to the screening, and a review of the randomization process did not uncover any irregularities.[62] However, it is apparent that this yet unexplained excess of advanced cancers accounts for the higher breast cancer death rate in the screening arm.

Canada–National Breast Screening Study 2

The National Breast Screening Study 2 (NBSS-2) was also initiated in 1980 and was a trial of the efficacy of breast cancer screening in women aged 50 to 59.[63] It was designed to test specifically the efficacy of breast cancer screening in this age group with mammography and CBE versus CBE alone and consisted of four rounds of annual examinations in the study and control groups. As with the NBSS-1, after a physical examination that included CBE, women were invited to participate in the study. Volunteers were then randomized into a study group or control group. Approximately 39,000 women participated in the study, with virtually equal numbers randomized to study and control groups. At 7 years of follow-up, only 3% fewer deaths had occurred from breast cancer in the study group than in the control group. This particular study has received less attention than the study of women aged 40 to 49, but many of the same critiques apply.

Metaanalyses

Before 1997 both the HIP study and the Swedish Two-County study provided clear and early evidence that mammography could reduce breast cancer mortality in women aged 50 and older, providing a sound basis for the promotion of screening for this age group. Evidence supporting the value of screening for women in their 40s was less clear. Although there was indirect evidence of a benefit both from the trials and observational studies, until recently no single trial had shown a statistically significant reduction in breast cancer deaths among women randomized to an invitation to screening in their 40s. Whereas the absence of definitive evidence of a benefit was troubling to some, especially in light of early findings of an excess of breast cancer deaths in the NBSS-1, others were persuaded that the absence of a benefit was an artifact of methodologic shortcomings, in particular low statistical power in the trials for subgroup analysis.[45,64,65]

To overcome the limits of small sample sizes, investigators began to conduct meta-analyses of trial data, combining age-specific results from the various studies to overcome the limits of small sample sizes.[66–72] There are two important observations about these meta-analyses. First, as was the case with individual trials, benefits for women aged 50 and older appear early in the follow-up period, whereas they occur later for women aged 40 to 49. Second, with accumulating years of follow-up in the 40 to 49 group, the relative risk of mortality steadily improved. As shown in Fig. 1, with an average follow-up of 12.7 years, the meta-analysis using the most current data shows a relative risk of 0.82 (18% fewer breast cancer deaths) when all trials are combined, a relative risk of 0.74 (26% fewer deaths) when only population-based trials are combined (not shown), and a relative risk of 0.71 (29% fewer deaths) for all five Swedish randomized controlled trials. Each point estimate is statistically significant at the 95% confidence level, although the all-trial meta-analysis has the lowest relative risk of breast cancer mortality because of the excess rate of breast cancer deaths in the NBSS-1 in the group invited to screening. The meta-analysis of Swedish trials is

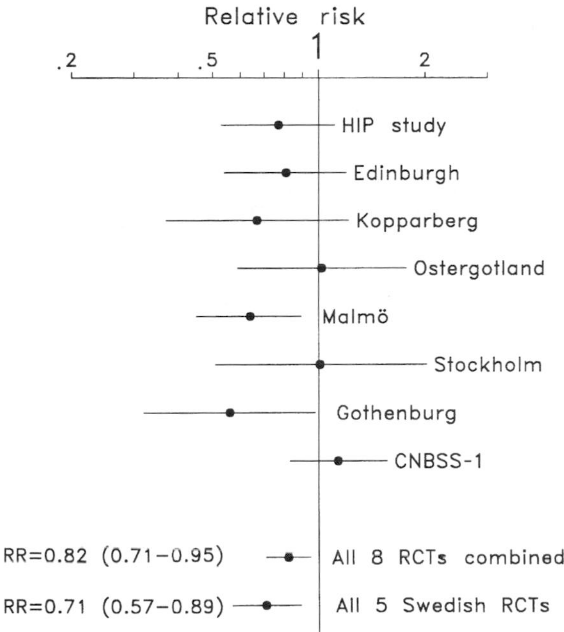

FIG. 1. All randomized controlled trials (RCTs) of women aged 40 to 49. CNBSS, Canadian National Breast Screening Study; HIP, Health Insurance Plan of Greater New York; RR, relative risk. (From ref. 72, with permission.)

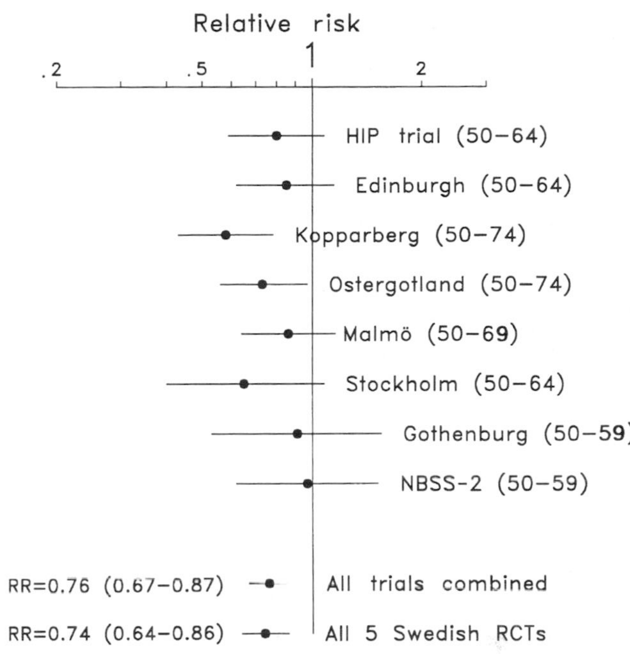

FIG. 2. All randomized controlled trials (RCTs) of women aged 50 to 74. HIP, Health Insurance Plan of Greater New York; NBSS, National Breast Screening Study; RR, relative risk.

included in this comparison because they represent a more homogeneous group and because they include the two second-generation trials (i.e., Gothenburg and Malmö), which applied more advanced screening protocols and observed 44% and 36% fewer breast cancer deaths in the invited groups compared with the control groups.

As shown in Fig. 2, when the same meta-analyses are conducted for women aged 50 and older, the point estimates are 0.76 (24% fewer deaths) for all trials combined, 0.73 (27% fewer deaths) when only population-based trials are combined (not shown), and 0.74 (26% fewer deaths) when combining only the five Swedish trials. What is evident in these meta-analyses is that they show very similar mortality reductions among women younger and older than age 50 who were invited to the screening.

The one analysis that stands apart from the others is the all-trial meta-analysis of women in their 40s, in which the size of the NBSS-1 and the excess rate of deaths in the group invited to screening measurably reduce the estimated benefit. Because irregularities in the NBSS-1 have yet to be explained, the consistency of results in the other meta-analyses and the recent results from Gothenburg and Malmö suggest that it is reasonable to regard the potential benefit of screening in younger versus older women as more similar than different, especially if recommended screening intervals are tailored to the age-specific estimated sojourn time.

As mentioned at the beginning of this section, there are notable differences in the cumulative trial mortality trends for women younger and older than age 50, and reasons for this difference have been an ongoing source of debate—long on conjecture but short of a clear explanation. Some have argued that the observed delay in benefit was simply a function of small sample sizes and overall better survival in younger compared with older women.[73] By this argument, it doesn't matter when a mortality reduction appears, because screening is beneficial if it averts deaths from breast cancer in the near or long term. However, others have argued that the delayed benefit was a methodologic artifact of trial design, in which mortality reductions attributed to women in their 40s actually were due to diagnoses after age 50 among women randomized in their 40s.[74] Because the analysis of age-specific mortality differences in trials is based on age at randomization (not age at diagnosis), at the time of analysis the group randomized in their 40s includes patients diagnosed *after* they have had a fiftieth birthday. According to this hypothesis, if a benefit from screening truly begins at age 50, then the observation of benefit for women in their 40s is more apparent than real, because it must be due to the benefit of diagnosing breast cancer after age 50 among women randomized in their 40s. Thus, a benefit later in the follow-up period would be due to the time required to accumulate the age migration cases. Likewise, for women randomized in their 50s, the benefit from screening was seen earlier in the follow-up period because they were already at an age when mammography is beneficial. In effect, this argument was a call for analysis of trial data by age at diagnosis.

Although it seems logical, analysis of trial data by age at diagnosis has a built-in bias, because the purpose of screening is to diagnosis breast cancer earlier in its natural history, which means, for any individual who develops breast cancer at a

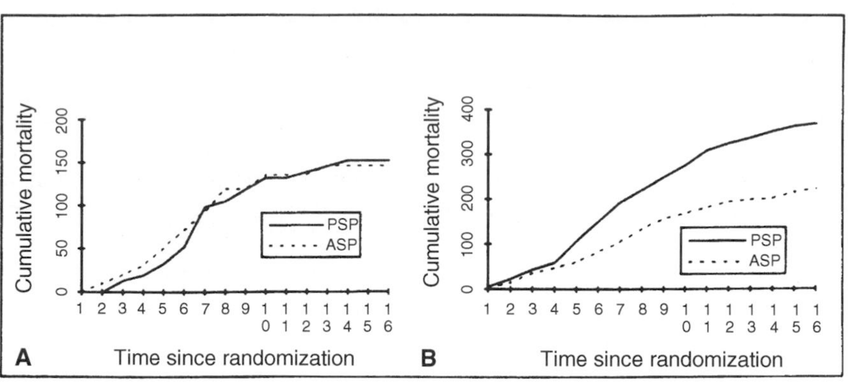

FIG. 3. Cumulative mortality from breast cancer for ductal grade 3 carcinoma by age, Swedish Two-County trial. **A:** Age, 40–49 years; relative risk = 0.95 (0.55–1.64). **B:** Age, 50–74 years; relative risk = 0.61 (0.47–0.78). ASP, active study population; PSP, passive study population. (From ref. 77, with permission.)

younger age than when symptoms would be expected to appear. Because age at diagnosis is influenced by the study intervention (i.e., mammography), it is regarded as a pseudovariable.[75] By introducing lead-time bias, it complicates comparisons between the invited and not-invited group and is therefore methodologically inappropriate. The question of age-specific benefits is important, but to be properly addressed a trial would need to randomize a narrow age range of women (i.e., women aged 40 to 41) to an invited and not-invited group and follow them for the duration of interest (i.e., until age 50), thus avoiding "age-creep." Still, this question has been pursued.

In 1995, de Koning and colleagues[76] published data from the Swedish Two-County trial arguing that age migration in the group randomized in their 40s could account for 70% of the observed benefit and thus explain the late onset of benefit in this age group. In an accompanying editorial, it was argued that this kind of analysis actually violates the underlying logic of trial data analysis as noted in the previous paragraph, but if it were to be pursued, analysis of actual trial data rather than modeling would be the logical approach. Tabar and colleagues[9] subsequently evaluated Swedish Two-County data by age at randomization and age at diagnosis and observed no support for this hypothesis. In fact, the relative mortality reduction among women randomized in their 40s was greater among women diagnosed before their fiftieth birthday than in women diagnosed after age 50. No support for this hypothesis was observed in a similar analysis of Gothenburg trial data.[53]

Recent analysis of Swedish Two-County data provides a clearer and more clinically intuitive explanation for the delay in benefit observed in the individual trials and meta-analyses based on an assessment of the effect of the trial screening protocols on mortality trends by tumor histology.[10,29] As described in the section Sojourn Time and the Influence of Early Intervention, the mean breast cancer sojourn time (i.e., potential lead time) is shorter in women younger than age 50 than in women older than age 50.[10,27] Because the majority of the world's trials screened women aged 40 to 49 at randomization at an interval of 24 months, faster tumor progression in women in this age group meant that they were less likely to benefit from mammography than would women aged 50 and older. The consequence of screening all women at the same 24-month interval becomes further evident when cumulative mortality trends are examined by age and tumor histology. When cumulative mortality trends are compared for ductal grade 3 tumors, a benefit begins to appear after 5 years among women aged 50 to 74 but is not evident in the follow-up period among women aged 40 to 49 (Fig. 3). These higher malignancy grade tumors are more aggressive, have a worse prognosis, and, compared with ductal grade 2, medullary, and invasive lobular cancers, account for a higher proportion of breast cancer deaths that occur sooner after diagnosis. When comparing trends in the invited versus control group in the trial for ductal, grade 2, lobular, and medullary carcinoma, women aged 40 to 49 and 50 to 74 showed similar trends in cumulative mortality (Fig. 4). Fur-

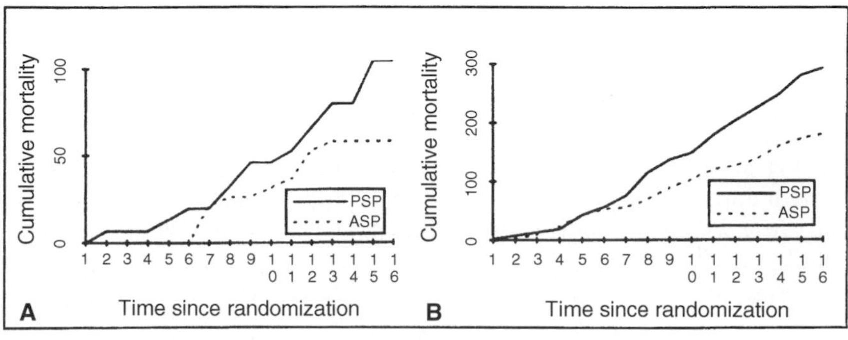

FIG. 4. Cumulative mortality from breast cancer for ductal grade 2, lobular, and medullary carcinoma by age, Swedish Two-County trial. **A:** Age, 40–49 years; relative risk = 0.64 (0.30–1.41). **B:** Age, 50–74 years; relative risk = 0.64 (0.48–0.86). ASP, active study population; PSP, passive study population. (From ref. 77, with permission.)

thermore, for both women younger and older than age 50 who were diagnosed with these less aggressive cancers, the mortality benefit does not appear until after 7 to 8 years of follow-up, consistent with the observation that survival is better for these tumor types and that associated mortality occurs later. When examining the overall trend in cumulative mortality by age, these same trends are evident; in other words, for the groups invited to screening, a mortality benefit begins to emerge after approximately 5 years for women aged 50 to 74 and after 8 years for women aged 40 to 49.

The organizers of the Falun meeting concluded that the screening interval of 24 or more months was differentially effective in reducing mortality among women aged 40 to 49 versus women aged 50 and older.[53] Whereas this interval was equally effective in both age groups for grade 2, medullary, and invasive lobular tumors, and effective in reducing deaths among grade 3 tumors diagnosed in women aged 50 and older, it was entirely ineffective for grade 3 tumors diagnosed in women aged 40 to 49. New results from Gothenburg, which screened women aged 39 to 49 at 18-month intervals, show that the timing of the benefit, which appears at 6 to 8 years, is similar to that observed for women aged 50 and older. Additional insights into these observations come from earlier analysis of Swedish Two-County data comparing long-term survival by tumor size, extent of disease, and histologic grade. When tumors are grouped by size, grade, and nodal involvement, there is little difference in observed survival by age.[78] However, Tabar and colleagues[41] have also observed that the likelihood that a tumor will have progressed to grade 3 at the time of diagnosis is higher in women younger than age 50 than in women aged 50 and older, indicating that one important difference between breast cancer in premenopausal women compared with postmenopausal women is the greater likelihood of tumor dedifferentiation to less favorable histology. As shown in earlier work, the influence of tumor grade on survival becomes increasingly pronounced once tumors are greater than 10 mm in size.[78,79] As a general rule, it is important to diagnose tumors at the earliest opportunity, but these data suggest that this goal is especially important in premenopausal women.

The fundamental conclusion that can be drawn from these data is that the common screening interval of 2 or more years in the trials contributed to sufficiently favorable lead times for most tumor types in women aged 50 and older and failed to provide that same benefit to the more aggressive tumors in women younger than age 50.[29,41] More than any other explanation, a mismatch between the estimated mean sojourn time and the screening interval contributed to poorer performance in the trials among women aged 40 to 49 and also to the longer period of observation required to see a benefit. The observation that some eventual benefit accrued to women aged 40 to 49 who were invited to the screening is a function of the heterogeneity of breast cancer. Although the wide screening interval provided little benefit to women in their 40s in whom aggressive tumors developed, the detection of less aggressive tumors was still beneficial and appeared later in the follow-up period.

If the screening interval is greater than the mean sojourn time, the potential for the program to reduce the rate of advanced disease is compromised, because a higher proportion of cancers will progress undetected to the point at which they become clinically evident and appear as interval cancers. In Gothenburg, which screened women aged 40 to 49 every 18 months and showed a 44% reduction in breast cancer mortality, the proportional interval cancer incidence was only 18% in the first 12 months after a negative screen but increased to more than 50% in the period from 12 to 18 months.[53] In the University of California at San Francisco screening program, sensitivity declined at twice the rate in the interval between 1 and 2 years for women in their 40s compared with women aged 50 and older, reflecting faster growth rates for women in their 40s.[36] According to Sickles,[36] interval cancer rates for women aged 40 to 49 with annual screening are approximately equivalent to interval cancer rates in women aged 50 years and older who are screened every 2 years.

SENSITIVITY, SPECIFICITY, AND POSITIVE PREDICTIVE VALUE

The interpretation of a screening examination ultimately falls into one of two categories: normal or abnormal. These judgments, in turn, ultimately are divided among four categories based on either the determination or estimation of the underlying reality of having or not having breast cancer at the time of screening. A normal interpretation may be a *true-negative* or a *false-negative*. A positive interpretation may be a *true-positive* or a *false-positive*. As noted in the introduction, screening tests for breast cancer divide women into those who are likely to have the disease and those who are unlikely to have the disease. By convention, each of these initial findings is given a summary determination on the basis of the patient's status at 1 year after the screening examination and are defined as follows[80]: *true-positive* (*TP*)—cancer diagnosed within 1 year after biopsy recommendation based on an abnormal mammogram; *true-negative* (*TN*)—no known cancer diagnosed within 1 year of a normal mammogram; *false-negative* (*FN*)—cancer diagnosed within 1 year of a normal mammogram; *false-positive* (*FP*)—no known cancer diagnosed within 1 year of an abnormal mammogram. There are three definitions of false-positives: FP_1 refers to a case recalled for additional imaging evaluation of an abnormal finding on a screening mammogram in which no cancer was found within 1 year or a recalled case was not shown to be malignant within 1 year. The additional imaging may take place at the same time as the screening examination or at a later date.[81–83] FP_2 refers to a case in which no known cancer was diagnosed within 1 year after an abnormal mammogram and recommendation for biopsy or surgical consultation. This definition is based on the recommendation for biopsy alone—a biopsy may or may not be done.[81,84] FP_3 refers to a case in which benign disease is found at biopsy within 1 year after an abnormal mammogram and biopsy.[82,84–86] This last definition of *FP* is similar to the definition proposed by the American College of Radiology (ACR) breast imaging reporting and data system, described later in the section on Quality Assurance.[87]

These summary categories are the basis elements for measuring the performance of screening programs. Because the large majority of women who undergo mammography examinations do not have breast cancer, nearly all normal interpretations (true-negatives) are accurate. True-positives are obviously measured in the near term by biopsy results. False-negatives or false-positives are based on the assumption that cancer would have been detected, or was not present, on the basis of the presence or absence of histologic confirmation of disease within 1 year.

Sensitivity is a measure of the probability of detecting breast cancer when it is truly present. It is the proportion of patients found to have breast cancer within 1 year of screening who were identified as having an abnormality at the time of screening [sensitivity = TP/(TP + FN)]. Another method of measuring sensitivity has been outlined by Day and Walter[88] and is based on the ratio of observed (invited group) to expected (control group) rates after omitting results from the first screening round as a basis for estimating the proportion of cases that would be expected to appear as clinical cancers. *Specificity* is the probability of correctly identifying a patient as normal when no cancer exists and is the proportion of all patients not found to have breast cancer within 1 year of screening who had a normal interpretation at the time of screening [specificity = TN/(TN + FP)]. *Positive predictive value* (*PPV*) of a screening test is the proportion of all screening cases that result in a diagnosis of cancer and varies according to the criteria for a false-positive interpretation ($PPV_{1-3} = TP/TP + FP_{1-3}$). PPV_1 is the rate of cancer diagnosis among all women with an abnormal mammogram (FP_1).[82,85,86,89–91] PPV_2 is the rate of cancer based on the subset of women with abnormal mammograms who receive a recommendation for biopsy or surgical consultation (FP_2).[84] PPV_3 is the proportion of all screening examinations that result in a diagnosis of cancer based on biopsies performed (FP_3).[82,84–86,92] According to the Agency for Health Care Policy and Research (AHCPR), approximate targets for PPV_1 are 5% to 10%, whereas for PPV_2 or PPV_3 the target is 25% to 40%.[80]

Sensitivity estimates derived from the trials have shown that the sensitivity of mammography was higher in women aged 50 and older than in women aged 40 to 49. For women in their 40s, sensitivity ranged from 53% to 81%, whereas for women who were 50 and older it ranged from 73% to 88%.[64] These sensitivity estimates are based on a variety of screening protocols and screening intervals, of which the latter is likely to be the major factor in observed age group differences. If the screening interval is wider than the estimated mean sojourn time, the false-negative rate (the complement of sensitivity) is adversely influenced due to the comparatively higher rate of interval cancers that arise within the screening interval. When Swedish Two-County data are adjusted for the screening interval and estimated age-specific mean sojourn time, the magnitude of these differences diminishes, with sensitivity estimated to be 86% for women aged 40 to 49 and approximately 93% for women aged 50 to 59.[8] Furthermore, service screening programs offer a glimpse into current estimates of sensitivity when screening intervals are actually tailored to the estimated sojourn time. When women are screened for breast cancer at appropriate intervals, the estimated differences in sensitivity between younger and older women diminish considerably.[36,77,93,94] In a screening program in Albuquerque, New Mexico, representing more than 100,000 women, sensitivity was 85.3% for women aged 40 to 49 and 87.7% for women aged 50 and older.[93] In the University of California at San Francisco screening program, the sensitivity was 86.7% for women aged 40 to 49 and 93.6% for women aged 50 to 59.[36] In each of these instances, a difference in the sensitivity of mammography in younger versus older women is still seen, but the data show that the sensitivity of the test in the two age groups is more similar than different when screening intervals reflect the underlying mean sojourn time. In each case, the large majority of cancers are detected at the time of screening.

Specificity is also an important measure of the efficacy of a screening program, and even small differences in program specificity can mean a large difference in program efficacy and costs. Data from the Centers for Disease Control and Prevention's (CDC) National Breast and Cervical Cancer Early Detection Program, representing more than 200,000 women in hundreds of facilities across the United States, provides a good picture of comparative program specificity by age. The rate of abnormal mammograms among women aged 40 to 49 was 5.8%, and among women aged 50 to 59 it was 5.6%.[95] In the series from San Francisco mentioned previously, the abnormal rate among women aged 40 to 49 was 6.4%, and among women aged 50 to 59 it was 6.8%.[36] Other data series show similar patterns. These series also show a similar pattern in specificity for false-positives based on biopsy results and thus higher PPV with increasing age. Because the prevalence of disease is lower in women in their 40s, the yield of cancers from these procedures is naturally lower. Thus, although the rate of false-positive results based on additional mammographic views and referral for biopsy is very similar in younger and older women, the cost-effectiveness of screening improves with increasing age.[36,96]

GUIDELINES AND RISK-BASED SCREENING

By convention, in the United States, most guidelines for breast cancer screening recommend that women begin

TABLE 2. *Breast cancer screening guidelines*

Age group (update)	ACS (1997)	ACR (1997)	NCI (1997)	USPSTF (1996)
18–39	Monthly BSE; CBE every 3 yr	Monthly BSE; CBE every 3 yr	No recommendation	No recommendation
40–49	Begin annual mammography and yearly CBE at age 40 Women at higher risk should consult with their physician about beginning screening before age 40 and to determine their mammography schedule in their 40s	Begin annual mammography and yearly CBE at age 40 Women at higher risk should consult with their physician about beginning screening before age 40 and to determine their mammography schedule in their 40s	Mammography every 1–2 yr for women in their 40s at average risk of breast cancer Women at higher risk should consult with their physician about beginning screening before age 40 and to determine their mammography schedule in their 40s	Insufficient evidence to recommend for or against mammography
50+	Annual mammography and CBE and monthly BSE No upper age limit as long as a woman is in good health	Annual mammography and CBE and monthly BSE No upper age limit as long as a woman is in good health	Mammography every 1–2 yr Upper age limit not addressed	Mammography every 1–2 yr with or without annual CBE for women aged 50–69 Insufficient evidence to recommend for or against screening after age 70

ACR, American College of Radiology; ACS, American Cancer Society; BSE, breast self-examination; CBE, clinical breast examination; NCI, National Cancer Institute; USPSTF, United States Preventive Services Task Force.

screening at age 40 or at some time in their 40s. Guidelines that recommend screening beginning at age 50 are based more on previous debates over efficacy of screening before age 50 than on disease burden. The age of 40 is admittedly arbitrary and based on the legacy of methodologic decisions related to choosing study populations for the trials. Shapiro and colleagues[48] included women age 40 and older after they observed that more than one-third of the premature mortality from breast cancer occurred in women diagnosed between the ages of 40 and 49. Since 1997, the ACS, NCI, and ACR have released updated guidelines for breast cancer screening, in large part informed by new data published in 1997.[97,98] Each organization recommends that women begin regular screening mammography in their 40s (Table 2). The United States Preventive Services Task Force currently recommends mammography every 1 to 2 years for women beginning at age 50, having concluded that there is insufficient evidence to recommend for or against breast cancer screening before the age of 50. However, their last guidelines update was published in 1996, before the availability of more recent individual trial and meta-analysis findings.[99] NCI recommendations differ from those of the ACS and ACR by not specifying a specific age to begin screening. The NCI guidelines also recommend screening at intervals of 1 to 2 years versus annual screening and encourage women at higher risk to consult with their physicians about establishing an interval for periodic screening that is appropriate in their individual case. Current differences in breast cancer screening guidelines are a function of the timing of evidence-based literature reviews and different approaches to evidence-based medicine.

Some have questioned the value of screening women older than age 70, based on both lack of evidence from randomized trials (only one trial included women over the age of 70) and lower cost-effectiveness.[27,28] On the issue of a lack of data, the U.S. Preventive Services Task Force found little evidence to conclude that breast cancer screening would be any less beneficial in women older than age 70.[99] Further, although comorbidity increases with increasing age, a significant percentage (71%) of the population older than age 65 rate their health as excellent, very good, or good.[100] Given the high breast cancer incidence and mortality among women older than age 65, it is a mistake to presume that screening is not beneficial to this group. The ACS has asserted that there is no upper age limit for screening mammography, and as a general rule as long as a woman is in reasonably good health and does not have such significant comorbidity that she would not be a candidate for surgery, screening is recommended.[97]

Whereas some organizations recommend breast self-examination (BSE) and CBE in their guidelines, others do not, mostly because of the lack of clear evidence of their efficacy as a stand-alone examination or in combination with mammography. Randomized trials of screening have shown mortality reductions among women invited to screening that included either mammography or mammography in combination with CBE.[7,101] In the HIP study and the BCDDP, CBE was responsible for finding some cancers not detected by mammography.[48,102] However, it is unclear what CBE contributes to breast cancer detection apart from mammography, although few would question the value of CBE as a complementary modality. Some breast cancers cannot be seen on a mammogram, or the mammographic examination may be enhanced if there is awareness of a palpable mass detected by CBE. For this reason, the ACS has recommended that CBE should occur close to and before the occasion of a screening mammogram.[97] Furthermore, recommendations from the AHCPR's *Quality Determinants of Mammography*[80] strongly assert that a negative mammogram in the presence of a palpable mass does not rule out breast cancer. It should be stressed, however, that the value of CBE is determined by the quality of the examination, which is addressed in Chapter 3.

The value of BSE is similar to that of CBE—that is, it is a form of low-cost surveillance for breast changes that should be brought to the attention of a physician. For women younger than age 40 who are at average risk, routine BSE can heighten awareness of the normal composition of the breasts. This benefit continues after a woman begins undergoing routine mammography, although the greater advantage is the potential to be alert to a palpable mass that may have been missed by recent mammography or a lesion that is fast growing. One methodologic problem associated with the evaluation of BSE relates to whether self-detected tumors are found during BSE or at some other time. However, the more important issue is awareness of an abnormality rather than the occasion of detection (i.e., self-discovery versus BSE).

It is doubtful that new studies will provide additional insights into the value of these examinations; for this reason, the most pragmatic approach is to view these physical examinations in the context of their age-specific relevance. For women younger than age 40, when breast cancer incidence is comparatively lower, regular BSE and periodic CBE provide an opportunity to identify the emergence of a palpable mass earlier rather than later. After a woman begins having regular mammograms, CBE and BSE provide a safeguard against the limitations of mammography.

Mammography participation rates rose rapidly in the late 1980s and have continued to increase during the last decade. Among states (n = 50, plus the District of Columbia) participating in the CDC's Behavioral Risk Factor Surveillance System, the median percentage of women age 40 and older who reported ever having had a mammogram is 84% (range, 71.8 to 91.4).[103] The median percentage of women reporting a recent mammogram is lower and declines with increasing age. Among women aged 40 to 49, the median percentage reporting a mammogram in the past 2 years is 65.4% (range, 50.2 to 74.4). Although not directly comparable, the median proportion of women aged 50 and older who reported having had a mammogram in the past year is 57% (range, 41.8 to 70.1), and for women 65 and older, the median proportion is 54.1% (range, 38.3 to 67.7).

As noted previously in the section Principles of Cancer Screening, an important factor in planning a screening program is identifying a population with sufficient prevalence of occult disease. It would seem logical, then, that breast cancer risk factors other than age might prove useful in improving the efficiency of screening programs. This potential could extend to determining when to begin screening, which women should be screened at shorter or wider screening intervals, and, ideally, organizing screening programs on the basis of risk so that a truly low-risk population could be excluded from routine testing. What, then, is the potential for making individual decisions about screening based on risk apart from the recommendations or guidelines issued by medical organizations? When answering these questions, it is important to distinguish between program considerations relating to cost-effectiveness and the decision reached by an individual woman based on her unique circumstances.

For women at very high risk, due to a significant family history in first-degree relatives diagnosed premenopausally, a family history suggestive of an inherited predisposition to breast cancer, or confirmation of an inherited mutation of known significance on a breast cancer susceptibility gene, more aggressive surveillance has been recommended based on expert opinion (Table 3).[104] Women with a prior diagnosis of breast cancer, DCIS, lobular neoplasia, or atypical hyperplasia might also reach a decision with their physician to establish a program of more aggressive surveillance. For women who do not fall into these higher-risk categories, it also has been proposed that informed decisions about screening should be made weighing comparative risks (e.g., cost, inconvenience, anxiety associated with false-positive results, harm associated with avoidable biopsy) and benefits.[26,105,106] The underlying message in this recommendation is that women should understand their risk of breast cancer, the benefit of screening, and the comparative risk of harm associated with screening. Because the majority of women are not diagnosed with breast cancer in their lifetimes, they could choose to not be screened, be screened less often, or delay screening in order to reduce their higher risk of a false-positive examination compared with a lower likelihood of being diagnosed with breast cancer. It is not an entirely unreasonable recommendation, provided that

TABLE 3. *Options for breast cancer surveillance for carriers of BRCA1 and BRCA2 mutations*

Intervention	Provisional recommendation	Quality of evidence	Cautions
BSE	Education regarding monthly BSE, beginning at age 18	Expert opinion	Benefit not proven
CBE	Annually or semiannually beginning at age 25–35	Expert opinion	Benefit not proven
Mammography	Annually, beginning at age 25–35	Expert opinion	Benefit not proven

BSE, breast self-examination; CBE, clinical breast examination;

TABLE 4. *Risk to age 90 years for a white U.S. woman aged 40 years based on various combinations of known risk factors**

Age at menarche	Age at first live birth	No. of first-degree relatives with breast cancer	No. of biopsies/atypical hyperplasia (y/n)	Risk to age 90 (%)
15	16	0	0	6.7
13	22	0	0	9.0
12	20	0	0	9.0
12	25	0	0	11.1
12	25	1	0	18.8
12	25	0	1/y	13.5
12	30	0	0	13.6
12	30	2	0	26.8
12	30	2	1/y	52.0

*Including age at menarche, age at first live birth, family history of breast cancer, and history of breast biopsy.
From ref. 107, with permission.

women fully understand the issues and implications of their choices and the fact that third-party payers do not make these choices for them. Further, individuals vary in the degree to which they wish to make individual decisions about screening and in the degree to which various methods of information delivery and kinds of information fully communicate the issues in a manner that ensures complete understanding. In other words, we face an immense challenge in assisting those women who wish to make informed decisions about screening to do so.

Because breast cancer risk increases with increasing age, concerns about comparative risks and benefits associated with breast cancer screening have been raised. At an age when breast cancer risk is comparatively low, Gail and Rimer[105] have proposed that a woman's risk factor profile could be used to make decisions about whether to begin screening before age 50. Their model, which is derived from BCDDP data, is based on the assumption that regular mammographic screening is justified for a 50-year-old woman with none of the important risk factors. Regular screening would be justified for women in their 40s if they have a prior history of breast cancer; atypical hyperplasia on a previous breast biopsy; two or more breast biopsies even with benign results; a known mutation on a breast cancer susceptibility gene; a mother, sister, or daughter previously diagnosed with breast cancer; or if they are age 45 to 49 with at least 75% breast density. For women in their 40s who do not fall into any of these categories, age at menarche, number of previous breast biopsies, and age at first live birth would be the basis for an informed decision about screening. For example, according to the authors, in a woman in her early 40s with no history of breast biopsies and age at first live birth younger than 30 years, delay would be an option. Based on their estimates, only approximately 10% of 40-year-old women would make a decision to be screened if this model were followed, compared with 68% by age 45 and 95% by age 49. Because breast cancer risk increases with increasing age, their model may prove useful for women who wish to make an informed, risk-based decision about when to begin screening. No data are included with this model to estimate the proportion of incident cases within specific ages that would be identified if all women followed this approach. Although this kind of information is more immediately relevant for program planning, it is unknown whether it would be useful for making an informed decision at the individual level.

Another tool available to help women understand their individual risk is an interactive computer program for breast cancer risk assessment that has come to be known as the *risk disk*. This risk assessment tool is available from NCI and was developed to determine eligibility for participation in the Breast Cancer Prevention Trial.[107] This program cannot estimate risk for women with a prior history of breast cancer, a history of DCIS or lobular neoplasia, or an inherited mutation on a known breast cancer susceptibility gene. However, for women who do not fall into these higher-risk categories, absolute risk can be estimated for the next 5 years or to age 90, compared with a woman with no risk factors, based on current age, age at menarche, age at first live birth, and number of offspring; family history of breast cancer in first-degree relatives; and history of breast biopsy, including the presence of atypical hyperplasia (Table 4). It is important to keep in mind that the comparison group with no risk factors does not represent an average woman. This woman's risk to age 90 is 6.7%, whereas an average woman's risk is closer to 9%.[39]

These tools may have their greatest value in helping women understand individual risk against the backdrop of health education messages and articles in the popular press that emphasize risk as a basis for raising awareness about breast cancer prevention and early detection. Although well intentioned, there is concern that these messages have heightened anxiety far past the point at which they become sufficiently motivational at the individual level.

Are risk factors other than age useful for establishing screening intervals? No study has shown an association between a breast cancer risk factor and the length of the detectable preclinical phase. Thus, any attempt to decide on the basis of risk factors whether to be screened more or less frequently than recommended guidelines would be a decision based on the underlying probability of disease, not the underlying probability of having a longer or shorter sojourn time. It may also be a decision based on one's concern about the risk of an abnormal mammogram and potential interventions that ultimately may be false-positives. In this case, less frequent screening may reduce the risk of an avoidable intervention based on a false-positive result simply based on exposure to screening. However, that might not prove true, because specificity tends to be lower at the prevalent screen, and therefore it is by no means certain that less frequent screening reduces the odds of false-positive results. Here again, a woman would need to reconcile the greater odds of a false-positive examination compared with the lower odds of developing breast cancer and consider the relative benefits and potential costs associated with her decision.

On a population basis, risk-based screening for breast cancer has never been shown to have much potential to identify the majority of new cases by screening a subgroup of women at higher risk. In 1984, Solin et al.[108] reported on the screening experience of 17,543 women, for whom data on eight risk factors were collected (including any family history, prior breast biopsy, menstrual history, pregnancy history, lactation, and hormone use). They concluded that more than one-half of the 246 cases diagnosed would not have been detected if the program had only screened women with either prior breast biopsy or family history and that more than 40% would have been missed if the program had been limited to any one of the listed risk factors.

In 1987, Alexander and colleagues[109] reported similar findings from the analysis of Edinburgh trial data; by screening the 20% of the population at higher risk due to having had a prior biopsy or a family history in a mother or sister, only 30% of the first-round cancers would have been detected. When menopausal status or nulliparity/first birth after age 30 were included, the proportion of new cases that would have been detected in the first round increased to 29.6%. Again, concentrating on the more important risk factors would fail to identify the majority of prevalent cancers in an asymptomatic population.

Madigan et al.[110] recently reported population-attributable risk estimates for breast cancer using data from the National Health and Nutrition Examination Survey Epidemiologic Follow-Up Study. Using well-established risk factors, such as later age at first live birth, nulliparity, higher family income, and family history of breast cancer in first-degree relatives, these risk factors were associated with approximately 41% of breast cancer cases in the United States[110] In each of these instances, it is estimated that fewer than one-half of breast cancer cases would be identified by a risk-based screening strategy applying well-established risk factors.

QUALITY ASSURANCE

The usefulness of mammography is dependent on the proper use of dedicated mammography equipment, the diagnostic skills of the interpreter, and assessing and diminishing barriers to its regular use. These issues have been and are currently being addressed in an effort to promote safe and effective mass screening for early-stage breast cancer.

As knowledge and use of mammography slowly increased after the beginning of early promotion efforts, the Nationwide Evaluation of X-Ray Trends demonstrated a great variation in dose and image quality among mammography sites.[111] This report emerged at the time that the ACS was initiating its National Breast Cancer Awareness Screening Program. Troubled by the Nationwide Evaluation of X-Ray Trends report and hoping to alleviate the problems it identified, the ACS approached the ACR to stimulate the development of quality standards for mammography facilities. With funding from the ACS, the voluntary ACR Mammography Accreditation Program was established and began to accredit mammography facilities in August 1987.[112] The application process included a questionnaire to obtain information about personnel, volume, and type of examinations performed; the imaging system through evaluation of phantom images and dose delivery; and, most important, assessment of clinical images to evaluate positioning, contrast, compression, and image-label identifiers. The process of clinical image evaluation was performed by a group of radiologists with extensive experience in mammography who were trained to identify problems in clinical images that would hinder or prevent identification of early breast cancer. Evaluation of the image processing was later added when it was learned that many problems identified by clinical image review could be traced to faulty processor performance. Over time, greater understanding of the link between high-quality mammography and the goals of breast cancer screening led to new regulatory initiatives.

Maryland was the first state to pass legislation pertaining to quality assurance in mammography. In 1986, legislation was passed that required mammography examinations to be performed with machinery designed and built only for mammography. These dedicated units were vastly superior to mammography performed on general purpose machines in terms of dose and image quality. By 1993, 41 states and the District of Columbia had either passed legislation or established regulations addressing quality mammography.[113]

Toward the end of 1990, Congress added mammography to the benefit package for Medicare-eligible women and included quality standards for sites approved to provide services to Medicare beneficiaries.[114] These standards were heavily influenced by the ACR Mammography Accreditation Program standards. Also in that year, Congress passed the Breast and Cervical Cancer Mortality Prevention Act of 1990 (PL 101-354), appropriating funds to the CDC for state programs to provide breast and cervical cancer screening to low-income women. Recognizing the importance of high-quality mammography, the CDC required facilities that provided services under this program to be certified by the Health Insurance Financing Administration and to have ACR accreditation. By this time, a mammography facility could have been operating under a state standard, a federal standard, and a voluntary standard, each of which could vary on important criteria related to quality. On the other hand, a facility might have operated with little or no oversight, because ACR accreditation was voluntary, and the facility might choose not to offer screening to Medicare beneficiaries or to participate in the CDC program. Although a majority of states had regulations governing mammography quality assurance, state oversight was inconsistent at best. Thus, even with the emergence of new quality-oriented programs, the majority of facilities still had uneven adherence to quality standards. In order to ensure that women could depend on a uniform set of quality standards in all mammography facilities, in 1992 Congress passed the Mammography Quality Standards Act (MQSA), which was signed by President George Bush in October of that year. Under MQSA, all facilities offering mammography services would be required to be accredited by a private accrediting body, undergo an annual on-site inspection, and be certified by an agency designated by the Secretary of Health and Human Services. The following year, the Food and Drug Administration was assigned the task of enforcing MQSA by establishing standards, regulations, inspection processes, compliant mechanisms, and penalties for failure to comply with the regulations.

At approximately the same time as MQSA was being enacted, the AHCPR convened a panel to produce clinical practice guidelines on the quality determinants of mammography for interpreting physicians, clinicians, and consumers.[80] The panel considered the entire process involved in providing quality mammography to consumers, including (a) actions before the examination related to scheduling, including triaging patients into screening or diagnostic examinations; (b) appropriate data to collect for the patient's history; (c) the role of the imaging team, including qualifications; (d) machinery standards, dose limitations, quality control procedures, and the importance of routine evaluation of clinical images and the imaging system; and (c) the communication of results to patients. The development of these clinical practice guidelines underscores the importance of factors beyond image quality that contribute to a high-quality examination. Among the most important of these factors is communication with patients and referring physicians.

Many studies have demonstrated that clinicians often fail to communicate mammography results to patients.[115,116] In part, this pattern has been influenced by a tradition of "no news is good news," but there also is evidence of a failure to communicate abnormal findings. The panel strongly recommended that all women, regardless of whether their mammograms were negative, be informed by the imaging facility of their results. The preferred route suggested was use of a series of standardized letters that stressed subsequent steps, if any, to be taken by the woman, but the panel strongly urged that the method of communication should be tailored to the results of the examination. For example, the panel firmly discouraged notification of abnormal results initially by mail. Because the advocacy community regarded direct reporting as an important factor in the overall quality assurance of an examination, the requirement for direct reporting was included in the 1998 reauthorization of the MQSA.

In addition to determinants of a high-quality examination, the AHCPR panel addressed the critical issue of assessing outcome data from mammography facilities by use of medical audits. Data (both collected and derived) required for the basic medical audit include (a) the number and type of mammography examinations performed; (b) the recall rate from screening mammography for further evaluation; (c) the PPV of screening mammography, as well as the PPV of patients sent to biopsy for a mammographic abnormality; and (d) the stage of disease at diagnosis and the breast cancer detection rate per 1,000 women screened. A more advanced audit requires linkage to a breast cancer registry, which is not possible in most areas in the United States.[117] Here, one would also evaluate the sensitivity and specificity of screening mammography. The document also established goals for many of these outcome parameters as a guideline for facilities, noting, however, that outcome data vary based on the size of the practice or number of audits in the database and by the underlying characteristics of the population being screened. Although a more complete review of the document is not within the scope of this chapter, the interested reader is urged to review this set of guidelines.[80]

The final and arguably most critical step toward quality mammography is interpretation. A major barrier toward this educational goal had been the absence of any standardized language for mammographic features. Through the efforts of the ACR, with support from various clinical colleges, including the American College of Surgeons (ACS) and the American College of Obstetrics and Gynecology, a multidisciplinary committee was established in the early 1990s to address the suboptimal and often confusing terminology used in mammography reports. The document produced by this committee is the Breast Imaging Reporting and Data System (BI-RADS).[87] BI-RADS is designed to standardize mammographic reporting, reduce confusion in breast imaging interpretations, and facilitate outcome monitoring. The system is divided into four sections:

1. *Breast imaging lexicon.* An illustrated review of all the findings seen on a mammogram with suggested terminology as well as guidance regarding whether the findings are worrisome for malignancy, are probably benign, or are definitely benign.
2. *Reporting system.* Provides an organized approach to image interpretation and reporting. Several sample reports are included to illustrate the suggested format for different mammographic scenarios.
3. *Follow-up outcome monitoring.* Describes minimum data to be collected and used to calculate important audit measures, allowing each radiologist to assess his or her overall performance in mammography interpretation.
4. *ACR National Mammography Database.* A preliminary effort for collection of national data that will ultimately allow groups to adjust their thresholds by comparison with pooled national data.[87]

There are six categories in BI-RADS that cover all possible initial and summary interpretations. Category 0 is "assessment is incomplete." This category should be used on reports of screening mammograms that require further evaluation. After this evaluation is complete or in the case of screening examinations that do not require assessment, there are five final categories. Category 1 is a "negative" examination. It does not require comment, and the patient is encouraged to return for routine screening in 1 year. Category 2 is a "benign finding." This is also a negative examination, but the interpreting physician may wish to describe a benign feature for subsequent reviewers. The patient is encouraged to return for routine screening in 1 year. Category 3 is for a "probably benign finding." This category is reserved for findings that have an extremely low probability of malignancy (i.e., 2% or less).[118] It is not intended as an intermediate category between benign and malignant, but rather to denote a finding that has such a low probability of malignancy that a short-term follow-up, usually 6 months, is more appropriate than further diagnostic interventions. The interpreting physician, referring physician, and patient all have an interest in assuring compliance with this recommendation, because neglecting the short-term follow-up results in adverse consequences in a small percentage of cases. The next two categories are those that warrant a biopsy. Category 4, "suspicious abnormality—biopsy should be considered," is for a lesion that has a definite probability of being malignant; category 5, "highly suggestive of malignancy—appropriate action should be taken," is for a lesion that is very characteristic for malignancy.

At a time after significant progress has been made in lowering dose and improving image quality, a greater understanding of factors associated with higher mammographic accuracy should be a priority for greater data collection and research. With the advent of a standardized lexicon and a more complete understanding of the benefits of a medical audit, obtaining data on the status of interpretation in the United States is a necessary first step.[117] Successful methods of education focused on interpretation skills must be developed and tested both in initial small groups and subsequently in actual practice. Finally, we must develop outcome measures of interpretive performance and identify where weaknesses exist. Elmore et al.[119] describe the variability of mammographic interpretation between radiologists and the variability in specificity by age 35. If one examines the variability that they describe, one sees from the receiver operating curves presented that it is along the curve rather than above or below it. This suggests that improvement in interpretive skills to better define features and criteria for biopsy will have a significant beneficial impact on this variability.[120]

Inasmuch as breast cancer is among women's greatest health concerns, test results suggesting that a woman may have breast cancer are likely to cause anxiety, and the anxiety may be greater and more lasting the further along the diagnostic chain her evaluation proceeds. However, in terms of the consequences and resulting anxiety, from a measurement standpoint there is no justification for treating all false-positive results (i.e., FP_{1-3} or PPV_{1-3}), as equivalent. Elmore reviewed mammographic recall and biopsy data over a 10-year period and observed that 23.8% of women had at least one false-positive mammogram and 31.7% had either a false-positive mammogram or CBE. Although relatively high over time (2,227 women had 9,762 examinations over the study period), the rate of false-positive findings by examination was much lower. In other words, the likelihood of a false-positive result is considerably lower per screening event than over the duration of screening events. This is to be expected, and Elmore's study highlights not only that a higher rate of false-positives can be expected with sporadic, opportunistic screening but also the need to identify best practices in order to reduce the rate of avoidable false-positives. Because women are worried about breast cancer, providers must handle any need for extra procedures with great sensitivity. Although avoiding mammography because of the risk of false-positive results has been proposed, a more valuable strategy would assure that women who undergo screening know what to expect.[23,24] New programs are needed to improve the overall quality of screening and follow-up services, including greater attention to the psychosocial needs of women who have abnormal findings.

An encouraging report and actually the first glimpse of mammography as performed on a national level was presented by May et al.[95] As noted in the discussion of specificity, the report summarizes findings for 230,143 women who underwent mammography during the first 4 years of the National Breast and Cervical Cancer Early Detection Program. When biopsy was recommended from mammography, the PPV was 26%. The suggested goal from the AHCPR panel is 25% to 40%. The rate of prevalent cancers found was 5.1 in 1,000, and the rate of incident cancers was 2.0 per 1,000, a little lower than the AHCPR suggested goals for these parameters of 6 to 10 per 1,000 and 2 to 4 per 1,000, respectively, but overall the CDC screening population was skewed in early years toward a younger population of women. The recall rate was 5%, and the suggested goal is no greater than 10%. Finally, minimal cancers (invasive tumors less than 1.0 cm and DCIS) comprised 45% of the cancers, with a suggested goal of more than 30%. Thus, what we see from this report is a first view of screening results in the United States that is not limited to academic centers but is probably representative of a broad cross section of our screening efforts. The fact that overall performance by facilities participating in the CDC program falls within the target ranges that were established by the AHCPR panel is encouraging.

OTHER SCREENING TESTS

The search for alternative methods of screening for breast cancer is stimulated by a desire to increase accuracy and to overcome some of the technical barriers associated with film screen mammography. We do not address adjunctive modalities but discuss only those with a possible use as a breast cancer screening tool. Many screening methods have and are being suggested, including electrical impedance, light scanning, and infrared imaging of the breast. There has been no substantiation of a benefit accruing from these technologies for detection of early breast cancer in a screening situation. However, digital full-field mammography and magnetic resonance (MR) mammography seem to hold promise in this regard.

All current routine screening of the breast is performed with dedicated equipment, due to the requirement of high spatial resolution and contrast for mammography. Digital techniques promise to fulfill these requirements. There are two general techniques of performing digital mammography. The first and less desirable method is digitizing a film screen mammogram. Although this allows for some of the desirable features of digital mammography, it also preserves some undesirable attributes of the film screen technique. The second method replaces the film screen cassette combination with a specialized detector capable of transforming the latent x-ray image into an electronic digital image. There are major benefits and significant barriers to digital mammography use for routine screening. Because there is no film processing involved, image acquisition is much faster, producing a mammogram in approximately 6 seconds as compared to the 90 to120 seconds required for film development. In a situation in which 40 or more screening examinations are done per day, this higher performance could increase throughput. Once a digital image is acquired, it can be manipulated to adjust contrast and brightness to the individual patient. Regions of interest may also be magnified. This can all be accomplished with the single x-ray exposure used to produce the original image and may be particularly useful in the dense breast, in which a masking effect for early cancer detection can exist.[121]

Issues of concern associated with screening mammography are the variability of interpretation and the false-positive rate involved with screening.[35,119] With the evolution of digital screening mammography, computer video diagnosis and computer-aided detection (CAD) is becoming a reality.[122,123] Using detection algorithms for specific mammographic features associated with malignancy, this software is able to indicate these findings on the digital image. However, this benefit is balanced by the indication of densities that may be fictitious or due to overlapping structures within the breast. Thus, if there were too many false-positives, CAD would lose its use. However, if these false-positives could be kept to a minimum, perhaps one to two per image, and detect a high degree of true findings, perhaps 85% to 90%, then real benefit could be realized. Recent presentations indicate that these factors are real. CAD could then function as a second reader and possibly have a positive impact on variability and false-positive diagnoses while not diminishing the high sensitivity of screening mammography. Underserved areas, especially rural settings and remote facilities that provide mammographic services, could benefit from the ability to transport digital images almost anywhere. This can be done without loss of image fidelity and rapidly enough to be of clinical use. Preliminary results from a screening trial comparing routine film screen images with digital images on the same patient suggest at least equivalence in detection of breast cancer and a significantly lower recall and false-positive rate for digital screening mammography.[124]

Significant barriers to use of a digital technique for screening mammograms exist and must be addressed before its full potential can be realized. In order to attain the benefit of image processing, the digital images must be viewed on specialized monitors. These must have the ability to present the entire image at full resolution with a small pixel size. At present, these are prohibitively expensive, and one would require at least two monitors in routine practice. Additionally, the brightness of these monitors does not approach that of a mammographic view box. This could affect detection, especially microcalcifications, which can be an important finding of DCIS. Additionally, although the ability to portray many more levels of grey increases soft-tissue display, the monitor only allows for small segments of this enhanced grey-scale display per monitor image. Thus, image manipulation is required, which could increase the time required for interpretation. These problems are currently being addressed by novel new methods of displaying digital images and improving workstation software. Finally, at present, full-field digital screening mammography units are very costly. Because these units are prototypes, costs can range as high as $400,000 to $500,000 per unit. In this age of cost-containment coupled with the extremely small reimbursement for screening mammography, there is little consumer (i.e., mammography providers) interest in purchasing these units. It is hoped that as more data concerning digital screening mammography emerge and the cost of wet processing, film, cassettes, and x-ray film storage are eliminated, consumer demand will increase and price will decline.

The mammogram is a sensitive method for detection of early breast cancer in a screening population. However, it frequently lacks the specificity to separate benign from malignant lesions. These limitations have fueled the interest for magnetic resonance mammography (MRM). Initial examinations were performed without contrast enhancement, and separation of benign from malignant lesions was marginal. However, with the use of contrast agents specifically tailored for MR imaging, improvement in sensitivity and specificity over nonenhanced MRM has been realized.[125]

The basis for contrast-enhanced MR imaging of the breast centers on the vascularity and vessel permeability difference of benign and malignant tumors. Benign lesions frequently are sparsely vascularized, whereas malignant breast tumors require additional blood supply, as they grow much over 1 cm in size.[126,127] The contrast agents used for MR imaging are paramagnetic agents and tend to concentrate in tissue with more abundant vasculature.[128] Because these agents alter the MR signatures, the conspicuity of areas with greater blood supply than normal is enhanced. This neovascularity associated with malignant tumors is only a partial explanation for their concentration of paramagnetic agents.

In addition, increased capillary permeability and local changes in osmolar pressure also contribute to the enhancement characteristics of breast cancer.[129]

General screening for breast cancer with MRM deserves special mention. Screening implies the testing of a large population to identify the small subset that may have preclinical disease. As noted in the section Principles of Cancer Screening, just as the decision to screen an asymptomatic population for disease must meet well-defined benchmarks, so too does the introduction of a new screening technology if it is to replace the existing standard-bearer. MRM as a screening test does not meet these conventional criteria as well as conventional mammography. We do not have sufficient data regarding sensitivity and specificity, and MRM is also much more costly at present than mammography and is an invasive technique that requires injection of paramagnetic contrast agents. Thus, MR imaging should not be used in a pure screening setting until more data concerning test accuracy and reproducibility are available. Furthermore, MRM would need to undergo the same degree of quality assurance scrutiny and standard setting related to quality control procedures and personnel standards as has screen-film mammography under MQSA. For the interested reader, the article by Weinreb and Newstead[130] is an excellent overview of MR imaging of the breast.

We do not specifically address ultrasound in this chapter, because its use is strictly adjunctive and not meant to be used for screening purposes. However, a recent article by Kolb et al.[131] reports on 11,220 consecutive patients prospectively examined with screening ultrasound, in which all 3,626 women with dense breasts and negative clinical and mammographic exams were included. In this group, 11 cancers (0.30%) were found by ultrasound only, and the cancer detection rate in this group was increased 17%. Although this is an intriguing report, ultrasound requires further evaluation and validation by multiple centers before it can be recommended as a screening tool, even in a subset of extremely dense breasts.

CONCLUSION

The decision to screen women for breast cancer is based on the importance of the disease as a public health problem and the demonstrated ability of screening tests to meet acceptable levels of performance and reduce morbidity and mortality. However, although great progress has been made over the last decade, the full potential of breast cancer screening as a disease control strategy remains unfulfilled. Although a majority of women aged 40 and older have had a mammogram, most women are not screened at recommended intervals. Data also suggest that improvements are needed to ensure timely screening according to recommended intervals. In the United States, screening is commonly opportunistic rather than organized, and access is still a significant problem for medically underserved women. Once the decision to screen has been reached, screening programs should be carefully monitored, and attention should be devoted to using results to improve performance. In general, a breast cancer screening program must have high levels of participation and must achieve acceptable levels of performance in terms of sensitivity and specificity. More fundamentally, for screening to be effective, the program must reduce the incidence rate of advanced breast cancer in a population so that more successful treatment is assured. In the coming years, there must be renewed efforts to make the most of the technology at hand as we anticipate newer screening modalities and emerging preventive strategies.

REFERENCES

1. Donegan WL. Introduction to the history of breast cancer. In: Donegan WL, Spratt JS, eds. *Cancer of the breast*. Philadelphia: WB Saunders, 1995:1.
2. Bassett LW, Gold RH, Kimme-Smith C. History of the technical development of mammography. In: Haus AG, Yaffe MJ, eds. *Syllabus: a categorical course in physics: technical aspects of breast imaging*. Chicago: Radiological Society of North America, 1993:9.
3. Shapiro S, Strax P, Venet L. Periodic breast cancer screening in reducing mortality from breast cancer. *JAMA* 1971;215:1777.
4. Baker L. Breast Cancer Detection Demonstration Project: five year summary report. *CA Cancer J Clin* 1982;32:196.
5. Smart CR, Byrne C, Smith RA, et al. Twenty-year follow-up of the breast cancers diagnosed during the Breast Cancer Detection Demonstration Project [See comments]. *CA Cancer J Clin* 1997;47:134.
6. Hurley SF, Kaldor JM. The benefits and risks of mammographic screening for breast cancer. *Epidemiol Rev* 1992;14:101.
7. Tabar L, Fagerberg CJ, Gad A, et al. Reduction in mortality from breast cancer after mass screening with mammography. Randomised trial from the Breast Cancer Screening Working Group of the Swedish National Board of Health and Welfare. *Lancet* 1985;1:829.
8. Tabar L, Fagerberg G, Chen HH, et al. Efficacy of breast cancer screening by age. New results from the Swedish Two-County Trial. *Cancer* 1995;75:2507.
9. Tabar L, Duffy SW, Chen FM. Re: Quantitative interpretation of age-specific mortality reductions from the Swedish Breast Cancer-Screening Trials [Letter; comment]. *J Natl Cancer Inst* 1996;88:52.
10. Tabar L, Chen HH, Fagerberg G, Duffy SW, Smith TC. Recent results from the Swedish Two-County Trial: the effects of age, histologic type, and mode of detection on the efficacy of breast cancer screening. *J Natl Cancer Inst Monogr* 1997;22:43.
11. Calder K. Access to screening mammography: patient concerns about insurance. *Women's Health Issues* 1992;2:189.
12. Health Care Financing Administration. Medicare covers mammograms, 1997. Available at: http://www.hcfa.gov/news/pr1997/ncireq.htm.
13. American Cancer Society. Survey of physicians' attitudes and practices in early cancer detection. *CA Cancer J Clin* 1990;40:77.
14. American Cancer Society. *Cancer risk report: prevention and control, 1997*. Atlanta: American Cancer Society, 1998.
15. Czaja R, McFall SL, Warnecke RB, Ford L, Kaluzny AD. Preferences of community physicians for cancer screening guidelines. *Ann Intern Med* 1994;120:602.
16. Young J, Ward J, Sladden M. Do the beliefs of Australian general practitioners about the effectiveness of cancer screening accord with the evidence? *J Med Screen* 1998;5:67.
17. Chu KC, Tarone RE, Kessler LG, et al. Recent trends in U.S. breast cancer incidence, survival, and mortality rates [See comments]. *J Natl Cancer Inst* 1996;88:1571.
18. Brinton LA, Bernstein L, Colditz GA. Summary of the workshop: workshop on physical activity and breast cancer, November 13–14, 1997. *Cancer* 1998;83:595.
19. Huang Z, Hankinson SE, Colditz GA, et al. Dual effects of weight and weight gain on breast cancer risk [See comments]. *JAMA* 1997; 278:1407.
20. Fisher B, Costantino JP, Wickerham DL, et al. Tamoxifen for prevention of breast cancer: report of the National Surgical Adjuvant Breast and Bowel Project P-1 Study. *J Natl Cancer Inst* 1998;90:137.

21. Wilson JMG, Junger G. *Principles and practice of screening for disease*. Geneva, Switzerland: World Health Organization, 1968.
22. Morrison A. *Screening in chronic disease*. New York: Oxford University Press, 1992.
23. Smith RA. Screening fundamentals. *Monogr Natl Cancer Inst* 1997;22:15.
24. Eddy D. ACS report on the cancer-related health checkup. *CA Cancer J Clin* 1980;30:193.
25. Healy BP. Screening mammography for women in their forties: the panel of Babel. *J Women's Health* 1997;6:1.
26. National Institutes of Health Consensus Development Panel. National Institutes of Health Consensus Development conference statement: breast cancer screening for women ages 40–49, January 21–23, 1997. *J Natl Cancer Inst* 1997;89:1015.
27. Welch HG, Fisher ES. Diagnostic testing following screening mammography in the elderly. *J Natl Cancer Inst* 1998;90:1389.
28. Smith-Bindman R, Kerlikowske K. Is there a downside to elderly women undergoing screening mammography? *J Natl Cancer Inst* 1998;90:1322.
29. Organizing committee and collaborators. Breast cancer screening with mammography in women aged 40–49 years—report of the organizing committee and collaborators, Falun meeting, Falun, Sweden (March 21–22, 1996). *Cancer* 1996;68:693.
30. Rimer BK. Putting the "informed" in informed consent about mammography [Editorial; comment]. *J Natl Cancer Inst* 1995;87:703.
31. Harris RP, Fletcher SW, Gonzalez JJ, et al. Mammography and age: Are we targeting the wrong women? A community survey of women and physicians. *Cancer* 1991;67:2010.
32. Fletcher SW. Whither scientific deliberation in health policy recommendations? Alice in the Wonderland of breast-cancer screening [See comments]. *N Engl J Med* 1997;336:1180.
33. Ernster VL, Barclay J, Kerlikowske K, Grady D, Henderson C. Incidence of and treatment for ductal carcinoma in situ of the breast [See comments]. *JAMA* 1996;275:913.
34. Sox RC. Benefit and harm associated with screening for breast cancer [Editorial; comment]. *N Engl J Med* 1998;338:1145.
35. Elmore JG, Barton MB, Moceri VM, Polk S, Arena PJ, Fletcher SW. Ten-year risk of false positive screening mammograms and clinical breast examinations [See comments]. *N Engl J Med* 1998;338:1089.
36. Sickles EA. Breast cancer screening outcomes in women ages 40–49: clinical experience with service screening using modem mammography. *J Natl Cancer Inst Monogr* 1997;22:99.
37. Linver M. Meet high expectations for mammography with high-quality services. *Diagn Imaging* 1998;20:89.
38. Landis SH, Murray T, Bolden S, Wingo PA. Cancer statistics, 1998 [Published erratum appears in *CA Cancer J Clin* 1998;48:192]. *CA Cancer J Clin* 1998;48:6.
39. Ries L, Kosary C, Hankey B, et al. *SEER cancer statistics review, 1973–1995*. Bethesda, MD: National Cancer Institute, 1998.
40. Duffy SW, Chen HH, Tabar L, Day NE. Estimation of mean sojourn time in breast cancer screening using a Markov chain model of both entry to and exit from the preclinical detectable phase. *Stat Med* 1995;14:1531.
41. Tabar L, Fagerberg G, Chen HH, Duffy SW, Gad A. Tumour development, histology and grade of breast cancers: prognosis and progression. *Int J Cancer* 1996;66:413.
42. Tabar L, Fagerberg G, Day NE, Holmberg L. What is the optimum interval between mammographic screening examinations? An analysis based on the latest results of the Swedish two-county breast cancer screening trial. *Br J Cancer* 1987;55:547.
43. Ries L, Henson D, Harras A. Survival from breast cancer according to tumor size and nodal status. *Surg Oncol Clin N Am* 1994;3:35.
44. Miller AB. Fundamentals of screening. In: Miller AB, ed. *Screening for cancer*. Orlando: Academic, 1985:3.
45. Kopans DB. An overview of the breast cancer screening controversy. *J Natl Cancer Inst Monogr* 1997;22:1.
46. Sickles EA, Kopans DB. Deficiencies in the analysis of breast cancer screening data [Editorial; comment; see comments]. *J Natl Cancer Inst* 1993;85:1621.
47. Shapiro S, Venet W, Strax P, Venet L, Roeser R. Ten- to fourteen-year effect of screening on breast cancer mortality. *J Natl Cancer Inst* 1982;69:349.
48. Shapiro S, Venet W, Strax P, Venet L. *Periodic screening for breast cancer: the health insurance plan project and its sequelae*. Baltimore: Johns Hopkins Press, 1988.
49. Tabar L, Fagerberg G, Duffy SW, Day NE. The Swedish two county trial of mammographic screening for breast cancer: recent results and calculation of benefit. *J Epidemiol Community Health* 1989;43:107.
50. Andersson I, Aspegren K, Janzon L, et al. Mammographic screening and mortality from breast cancer: the Malmo mammographic screening trial. *BMJ* 1988;297:943.
51. Andersson I, Janzon L. Reduced breast cancer mortality in women under age 50: updated results from the Malmo mammographic screening program. *J Natl Cancer Inst Monogr* 1997;22:63.
52. Frisell J, Eklund G, Hellstrom L, Lidbrink E, Rutqvist LE, Somell A. Randomized study of mammography screening—preliminary report on mortality in the Stockholm trial. *Breast Cancer Res Treat* 1991;18:49.
53. Bjurstam N, Bjomeld L, Duffy SW, et al. The Gothenburg breast screening trial: first results on mortality, incidence, and mode of detection for women ages 39–49 years at randomization [See comments]. *Cancer* 1997;80:2091.
54. Roberts MM, Alexander FE, Anderson TJ, et al. The Edinburgh randomised trial of screening for breast cancer: description of method. *Br J Cancer* 1984;50:1.
55. Alexander FE, Anderson TJ, Brown HK, et al. The Edinburgh randomised trial of breast cancer screening: results after 10 years of follow-up. *Br J Cancer* 1994;70:542.
56. Miller AB, Baines CJ, To T, Wall C. Canadian national breast screening study. 1. Breast cancer detection and death rates among women aged 40 to 49 years [Published erratum appears in *Can Med Assoc J* 1993;148:718; see comments]. *Can Med Assoc J* 1992;147:1459.
57. Miller AB, To T, Baines CJ, Wall C. The Canadian National Breast Screening Study: update on breast cancer mortality. *Monogr Natl Cancer Inst* 1997;22:37.
58. Kopans DB, Feig SA. The Canadian National Breast Screening Study: a critical review. *AJR Am J Roentgenol* 1993;161:755.
59. Mettlin CJ, Smart CR. The Canadian National Breast Screening Study. An appraisal and implications for early detection policy. *Cancer* 1993;72:1461.
60. Burhenne LJ, Burhenne HJ. The Canadian National Breast Screening Study: a Canadian critique. *AJR Am J Roentgenol* 1993;161:761.
61. Tarone RE. The excess of patients with advanced breast cancer in young women screened with mammography in the Canadian National Breast Screening Study. *Cancer* 1995;75:997.
62. Bailar JC, MacMahon B. Randomization in the Canadian National Breast Cancer Screening Study. Report of a review team appointed by the National Cancer Institute of Canada. *Can Med Assoc J* 1997;156:213.
63. Miller AB, Baines CJ, To T, Wall C. Canadian National Breast Screening Study. 2. Breast cancer detection and death rates among women aged 50 to 59 years [Published erratum appears in *Can Med Assoc J* 1993;148:7181; see comments]. *Can Med Assoc J* 1992;147:1477.
64. Fletcher SW, Black W, Harris R, Rimer BK, Shapiro S. Report of the International Workshop on Screening for Breast Cancer [See comments]. *J Natl Cancer Inst* 1993;85:1644.
65. Kopans DB. Screening for breast cancer and mortality reduction among women 40–49 years of age. *Cancer* 1994;74:311.
66. Wald N, Chamberlain J, Hackshaw A. Report of the European Society of Mastology Breast Cancer Screening Committee. *Breast* 1993;2:209.
67. Eckhardt S, Badellino F, Murphy GP. UICC meeting on breast-cancer screening in pre-menopausal women in developed countries. Geneva, 29 September–1 October 1993. *Int J Cancer* 1994;56:1.
68. Elwood JM, Cox B, Richardson AK. The effectiveness of breast cancer screening by mammography in younger women [Published errata appear in *Online J Curr Clin Trials* March 5, 1993; doc 34 and March 31, 1994; doc 121; see comments]. *Online J Curr Clin Trials* 1993; doc 32. Accessed 25 February 1993.
69. Elwood K, Cox B, Richardson A. The effectiveness of breast cancer screening by mammography in younger women: correction [Letter]. *Online J Curr Clin Trials* 1994; doc 121. Accessed 25 February 1993.
70. Smart CR, Hendrick RE, Rutledge JH, Smith RA. Benefit of mammography screening in women ages 40 to 49 years. Current evidence from randomized controlled trials [Published erratum appears in *Cancer* 1995;75:11]. *Cancer* 1995;75:1619.
71. Kerlikowske K, Grady D, Rubin SM, Sandrock C, Ernster VL. Efficacy of screening mammography. A meta-analysis [See comments]. *JAMA* 1995;273:1,49.

72. Hendrick RE, Smith RA, Rutledge JH 3rd, Smart CR. Benefit of screening mammography in women aged 40–49: a new meta-analysis of randomized controlled trials. *J Natl Cancer Inst Monogr* 1997;22:87.
73. Kopans DB. Mammography screening and the controversy concerning women aged 40 to 49. *Radiol Clin North Am* 1995;33:1273.
74. Foffest AP, Alexander FE. A question that will not go away: at what age should mammographic screening begin? [Editorial; comment]. *J Natl Cancer Inst* 1995;87:1195.
75. Prorok PC, Hankey BF, Bundy BN. Concepts and problems in the evaluation of screening programs. *J Chron Dis* 1981;34:159.
76. de Koning HJ, Boer R, Warmerdam PG, Beemsterboer PM, van der Maas PJ. Quantitative interpretation of age-specific mortality reductions from the Swedish breast cancer-screening trials [See comments]. *J Natl Cancer Inst* 1995;87:1217.
77. Duffy SW, Day NE, Tabar L, Chen RH, Smith TC. Markov models of breast tumor progression: some age-specific results. *J Natl Cancer Inst Monogr* 1997;22:93.
78. Tabar L, Duffy SW, Burhenne LW. New Swedish breast cancer detection results for women aged 40–49. *Cancer* 1993;72:1437.
79. Tabar L, Fagerberg G, Duffy SW, Day NE, Gad A, Grontoft O. Update of the Swedish two-county program of mammographic screening for breast cancer. *Radiol Clin North Am* 1992;30:187.
80. Bassett LW, Hendrick RE, Bassford TI, et al. *Quality determinants of mammography*. Clinical practice guidelines, No. 13. Publication No. 95-00632. Rockville, MD: Agency for Health Care Policy and Research Public Health Service, US Department of Health and Human Services, 1994.
81. Bird RE. Analysis of cancers missed at screening mammography. *Radiology* 1989;171:87.
82. Burhenne LW, Hislop TG, Burhenne H. Xeromammographic diagnosis of carcinoma of the breast in office practice. *Surg Gynecol Obst* 1987;164:452.
83. Reinig JW, Strait CJ. Professional mammographic quality assessment program for a community hospital. *Radiology* 1991;180:393.
84. Linver MN, Paster SB, Rosenberg RD, Key CR, Stidley CA, King WV. Improvement in mammography interpretation skills in a community radiology practice after dedicated teaching courses: 2-year medical audit of 38,633 cases [Published erratum appears in *Radiology* 1992;184:878]. *Radiology* 1992;184:39.
85. Sickles EA, Oniinsky SH, Sollitto RA, Galvin BB, Monticciolo DL. Medical audit of a rapid-throughput mammography screening practice: methodology and results of 27,114 examinations. *Radiology* 1990;175:323.
86. Sickles EA. Quality assurance: how to audit your own mammography practice. *Radiol Clin North Am* 1992;30:265.
87. American College of Radiology. *Illustrated breast imaging reporting and data system (BI-RADS)*. Reston, VA: American College of Radiology, 1998.
88. Day NE, Walter SD. Simplified models of screening for chronic disease: estimation procedures from mass screening programmes. *Biometrics* 1984;40:1.
89. Baines CJ, Miller AB, Wall C, et al. Sensitivity and specificity of first screen mammography in the Canadian National Breast Screening Study: a preliminary report from five centers. *Radiology* 1986;160:295.
90. Lynde JL. A community program of low-cost screening mammography: the results of 21,141 consecutive examinations. *South Med J* 1993;86:338.
91. Robertson CL. A private breast imaging practice: medical audit of 25,788 screening and 1,077 diagnostic examinations. *Radiology* 1993;187:75.
92. Mosenson D. Audit of mammography in a community setting. *Am J Surg* 1992;163:544.
93. Linver MN, Paster SB. Mammography outcomes in a practice setting by age: prognostic factors, sensitivity, and positive biopsy rate. *J Natl Cancer Inst Monogr* 1997;22:113.
94. Duffy SW, Chen HH, Tabar L, Fagerberg G, Paci E. Sojourn time, sensitivity and positive predictive value of mammography screening for breast cancer in women aged 40–49. *Int J Epidemiol* 1996;25:1139.
95. May D, Lee N, Nadel M, et al. The National Breast and Cervical Cancer Early Detection Program: report on the first 4 years of mammography provided to medically underserved women. *Am J Radiol* 1998;170:97.
96. Rosenquist CJ, Lindfors KK. Screening mammography beginning at age 40 years: a reappraisal of cost-effectiveness. *Cancer* 1998;82:2235.
97. Leitch AM, Dodd GD, Costanza M, et al. American Cancer Society guidelines for the early detection of breast cancer: update 1997. *CA Cancer J Clin* 1997;47:150.
98. National Cancer Institute. *Statement from the National Cancer Institute on the National Cancer Advisory Board recommendations on mammography*. Bethesda, MD: National Cancer Institute, 1997.
99. U.S. Preventive Services Task Force. *Guide to clinical preventive services*. Baltimore: Williams & Wilkins, 1996.
100. U.S. Senate Special Committee on Aging. *Aging America*. Washington, DC: U.S. Department of Health and Human Services, 1991.
101. Shapiro S. Evidence on screening for breast cancer from a randomized trial. *Cancer* 1977;39:2772.
102. Smart CR. Highlights of the evidence of benefit for women aged 40–49 years from the 14-year follow-up of the Breast Cancer Detection Demonstration Project. *Cancer* 1994;74:296.
103. American Cancer Society. *Cancer risk report: prevention and control, 1999*. Atlanta: American Cancer Society, 1999.
104. Burke W, Daly M, Garber J, et al. Recommendations for follow-up care of individuals with an inherited predisposition to cancer. 11. BRCA1 and BRCA2. Cancer Genetics Studies Consortium [See comments]. *JAMA* 1997;277:997.
105. Gail M, Rimer B. Risk-based recommendations for mammographic screening for women in their forties. *J Clin Oncol* 1998;16:3105.
106. Berry DA. Benefits and risks of screening mammography for women in their forties: a statistical appraisal. *J Natl Cancer Inst* 1998;90:1431.
107. National Cancer Institute. *Breast cancer risk assessment tool 1999*. Bethesda, MD: National Cancer Institute, 1998.
108. Solin L, Schwartz G, Feig S, Shaber G, Patchefsky A. Risk factors as criteria for inclusion in breast cancer screening programs. In: Ames F, Blumenschein G, Montague E, eds. *Current controversies in breast cancer*. Austin, TX: University of Texas Press, 1984.
109. Alexander F, Roberts K, Huggins A. Risk factors for breast cancer with applications to selection for the prevalence screen. *J Epidemiol Community Health* 1987;41:101.
110. Madigan W, Ziegler RG, Benichou J, Byme C, Hoover RN. Proportion of breast cancer cases in the United States explained by well-established risk factors. *J Natl Cancer Inst* 1995;87:1681.
111. Conway BJ, McCrohan JL, Rueter FG, Suleiman OH. Mammography in the eighties. *Radiology* 1990;177:335.
112. McLelland R, Hendrick RE, Zinniger MD, Wilcox PA. The American College of Radiology mammography accreditation program [See comments]. *AJR Am J Roentgenol* 1991;157:473.
113. Fintor L, Alciati NM, Fischer R. Legislative and regulatory mandates for mammography quality assurance. *J Public Health Policy* 1995;16:81.
114. Hendrick RE, Smith RA, Wilcox PA. ACR accreditation and legislative issues in mammography. In: Haus AG, Yaffee MJ, eds. *Syllabus: a categorical course in physics: technical aspects of breast imaging*. Chicago: Radiological Society of North America, 1993:137.
115. Cardenosa G, Eklund GW. Rate of compliance with recommendations for additional mammographic views and biopsies. *Radiology* 1991;181:359.
116. Monsees B, Destouet JM, Evens RG. The self-referred mammography patient: a new responsibility for radiologists. *Radiology* 1988;166:69.
117. Smith RA, Osuch JR, Linver MN. A national breast cancer database. *Radiol Clin North Am* 1995;33:1247.
118. Sickles EA. Management of probably benign lesions of the breast. *Radiology* 1996;193:582.
119. Elmore JG, Wells CF, Carol MPH, et al. Variability in radiologists' interpretation of mammograms. *N Engl J Med* 1993;331:99.
120. D'Orsi CJ, Swets JA. Letter to the editor. *N Engl J Med* 1995; 132.1172.
121. Van Gils CH, Otten JD, Verbeek AL, Hendricks JH. Mammographic breast density and risk of breast cancer: masking bias or causability? *Eur J Epidemiol* 1998;14:315.
122. Qian W, Clarke L. Digital mammography: computer-assisted diagnosis method for mass detection with multi-orientation and multi-resolution wavelet transforms. *Acad Radiol* 1997;4:724.
123. Kalman BL, Reinus WR, Kwasny SC, Laine A, Kotner L. Prescreening entire mammograms for masses with artificial neural networks: preliminary results. *Acad Radiol* 1997;4:405.

124. Lewin JM, Hendrick RE, D'Orsi CJ, Moss LJ, Sisney GE, Karellas A. *Clinical evaluation of a full-field digital mammography prototype for cancer detection in a screening setting—work in progress*. Presented at the 84th Scientific Assembly and Annual Meeting of the Radiological Society of North America, 1998.
125. Heywang SH, Hahn D, Schmidt H, et al. MR imaging of the breast using gadolinium-DTPA. *J Comput Assist Tomogr* 1986;10:199.
126. Cosgrove DO, Kedar RP, Bamber JC, et al. Breast diseases: color Doppler US in differential diagnosis [See comments]. *Radiology* 1993;189:99.
127. Folkman J, Shing Y. Angiogenesis. *J Biol Chem* 1992;267:10931.
128. Strich G, Hagan PL, Gerber KH, Slutsky RA. Tissue distribution and magnetic resonance spin lattice relaxation effects of gadolinium-DTPA. *Radiology* 1985;154:723.
129. Brasch RC, Weinmann HJ, Wesbey GE. Contrast-enhanced NMR imaging: animal studies using gadolinium-DTPA complex. *AJR Am J Roentgenol* 1984;142:625.
130. Weinreb JC, Newstead G. MR imaging of the breast. *Radiology* 1995;196:593.
131. Kolb TM, Lichy J, Newhouse JE. Occult cancer in women with dense breasts: detection with screening ultrasound—diagnostic yield and tumor characteristics. *Radiology* 1998;207:191.

Diseases of the Breast, 2nd ed.,
edited by Jay R. Harris.
Lippincott Williams & Wilkins, Philadelphia © 2000.

CHAPTER 12

Imaging Analysis of Breast Lesions

Daniel B. Kopans

One of the most exciting aspects of health care at the end of the twentieth century was the literal explosion in body imaging technology. Over a 20-year period, ultrasound went from being a way to detect submarines to being a highly developed way to image virtually every organ system. Computed tomography made exploratory surgery obsolete. Magnetic resonance imaging (MRI) was able to reveal just about every anatomic detail (although, as the author's colleague, Peter Mueller, once said, "but where is the soul?"), and digital x-ray imaging became practical. The use of radioactive tracers led to the evolution of tomographic techniques and the beginning of metabolic studies using positron emission tomography (PET). As each of these technologies evolved, each was applied to analysis of the breast.

Breast evaluation with these multiple modalities would have little clinical value except that the 1960s through the turn of the century witnessed the validation through randomized, controlled clinical trials that early detection for breast cancer through the screening of asymptomatic "healthy" women offered the opportunity to reduce the rate of death from mammary malignancy in the same way that cervical cancer screening reduced deaths from cancer of the uterus.

The only test that has proved efficacy for screening is x-ray mammography. The ability of x-ray imaging to detect nonpalpable cancers will be enhanced when solid-state x-ray photon detectors are substituted for the conventional film/screen combinations and digital mammography replaces film-based systems. Digital mammography will open additional avenues of exploration that will enhance the ability to detect early cancers using dual energy subtraction techniques, as well as limited angle tomography and tomosynthesis and contrast subtraction techniques, to detect and evaluate neovascularity.

Ultrasound is the most useful adjunct to mammography because of its ability to differentiate cysts from solid masses and to guide needle biopsy procedures. Some data suggest that certain ultrasound characteristics can be used to differentiate a number of benign breast lesions from those that are malignant. Basic philosophy and cost-benefit analyses will determine whether any imaging test that does not approach 100% in at least being able not to dismiss cancer can be safely substituted for a breast biopsy (needle or open), because a breast biopsy is one of the safest procedures to perform.

Ultrasound has a very high false-positive rate and, in older studies, missed many cancers that were either palpable or visible by mammography. A few studies using modern equipment have raised the possibility that ultrasound may be able to find occult cancers in radiographically dense breasts, and trials are under way to see if modern ultrasound technology can have efficacy as a second-level screening test for these women.

Computed tomography has been overlooked in its usefulness for evaluating breast problems, and the first years of the twentieth century should see its increasing value using faster, high-resolution three-dimensional scanners.

Except for its cost and limited access, MRI of the breast would likely supplant ultrasound as the most useful adjunct to mammography. Not only can it be used as an expensive method of determining that a lesion is a cyst, but it is also, perhaps, the most exciting technology because it offers the ability to detect cancers that are occult to mammography and clinical examination. As MRI becomes less expensive, it will become a second-level screening test for high-risk women whose breast tissue is difficult to evaluate by mammography.

This chapter reviews these technologies, but, because x-ray mammography is the most valuable in terms of actually saving lives, x-ray imaging is stressed.

HIGH-QUALITY SCREENING AT REDUCED COST

The primary reason for evaluating the breast is to achieve earlier detection of breast cancer in an effort to prevent it from spreading to other organ systems. The screening of asymptomatic women to detect breast cancer earlier has been shown, in randomized controlled trials (RCT), to reduce the death rate by 20% to 30%.[1] This has been almost

D. B. Kopans: Department of Radiology, Massachusetts General Hospital, Boston, Massachusetts

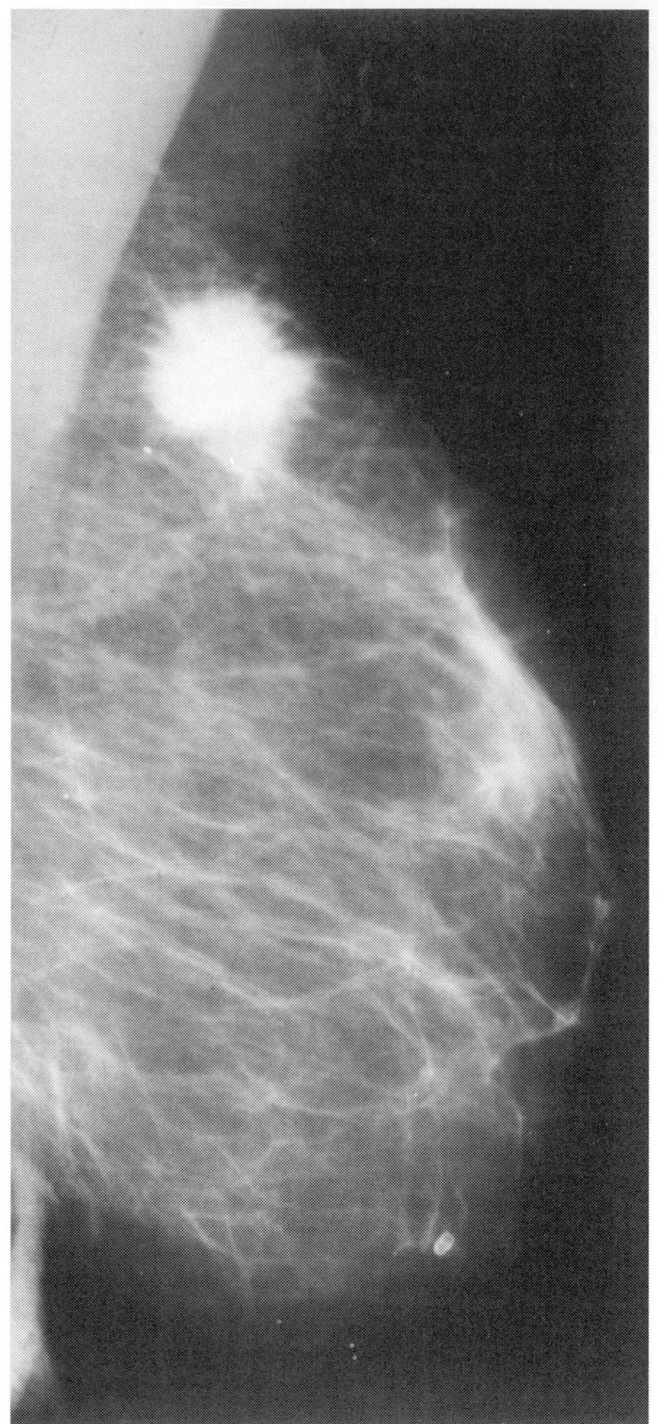

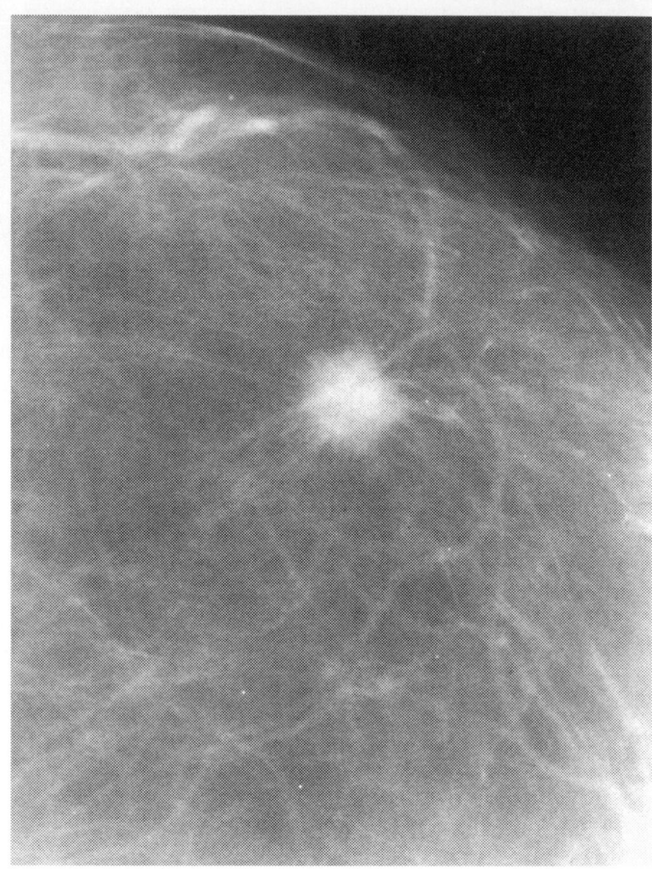

FIG. 1. A: Large palpable cancer with a typical spiculated appearance. **B:** This mammographically detected, spiculated, invasive ductal cancer is smaller than 1 cm in diameter.

universally accepted. The screening controversy as to whether women aged 40 to 49 years can benefit from earlier detection was the result of inappropriate analyses[2] and data manipulation.[3] Even though the trials were not designed to permit analysis of women aged 40 to 49 as a separate group, the data show a statistically significant mortality reduction of as high as 45% for screening women in their 40s.[4] Women should therefore be advised to begin screening on an annual basis by the age of 40.

SCREENING VERSUS DIAGNOSIS

The value of mammography for screening is well established. Although it is frequently used to evaluate women with signs or symptoms of breast cancer, the use of mammography as a "diagnostic" procedure is less efficacious. In 1979, Moskowitz was the first to emphasize the difference between *detection* (screening) and *diagnosis*.[5] Detection is the process of finding abnormalities in the breast that may

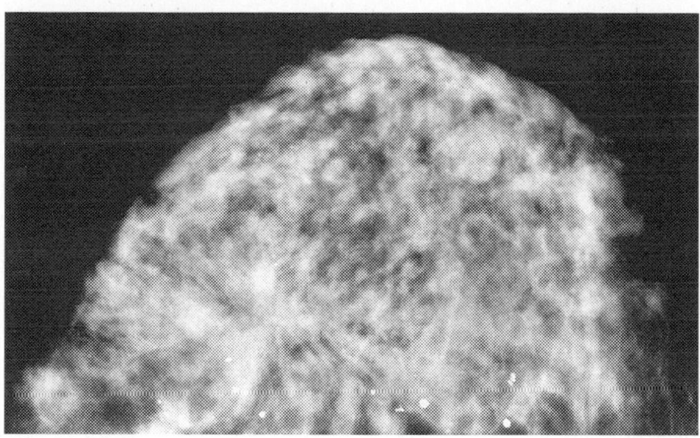

FIG. 2. Spiculated architectural distortion is present in the lateral aspect of the right breast that could be due to cancer, but in this case it is a persistent postsurgical scar.

be breast cancer. Diagnosis is the process of determining which of the abnormalities actually is cancer. Understanding this simple distinction is critical for the proper use of mammography and other breast imaging techniques.

Mammography is unsurpassed in enabling the detection of anomalies in the breast, many of which are early breast cancer, but it is much less useful as a diagnostic method of differentiating benign from malignant lesions. It is a technique that provides the radiologist only with morphologic and x-ray attenuation information. Radiologists have a fairly complete understanding of the underlying histopathologic changes that account for most mammographic findings, but the problem remains that many benign and malignant lesions share similar morphologic characteristics on mammograms. The differentiation is often insufficient to obviate the need for a tissue diagnosis.

Because tissue diagnosis (a breast biopsy) is relatively safe and the consequences of early breast cancer detection are so critical, the accuracy of a noninvasive diagnostic study that is substituted for a biopsy should be extremely high. However, with the exception of the ultrasonic differentiation of a cyst from a solid mass, no imaging technologies are sufficiently accurate to obviate the need for a biopsy when a lesion is deemed suspicious by mammography.

As with any test, the likelihood that a given finding represents malignancy is a statistical probability. Many morphologic criteria have a high probability of malignancy. A spiculated mass (Fig. 1) is virtually certain to indicate a malignant process. Spiculated architectural distortion may be a very early sign of cancer if the patient has not had previous breast surgery to account for the finding (Fig. 2). Nevertheless, benign idiopathic lesions, such as a radial scar, may have the same appearance. A tissue diagnosis is the only way to differentiate the two. Other lesions, such as the solitary round or oval circumscribed mass (Fig. 3), have such a low probability of malignancy that many would argue that a tissue diagnosis is not justified and that monitoring the lesion at short intervals to assess its stability and permit early intervention, should it change, is a more reasonable approach.[6] Still other findings are always due to benign processes and only coincidentally are ever associated with cancer.

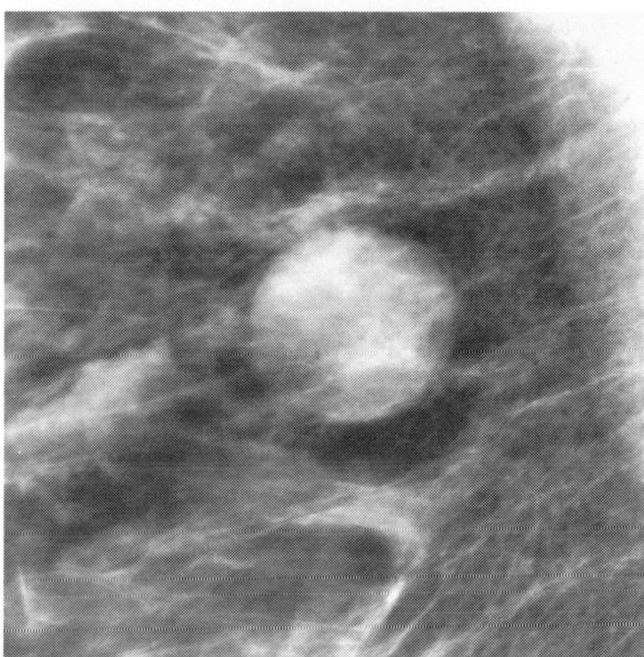

FIG. 3. Solitary circumscribed mass that proved to be a cyst.

Mammography is the only technique with proven efficacy for breast cancer screening. Only one of the RCT, the Health Insurance Plan of New York trial, has shown a benefit from routine clinical breast examination.[7] Nevertheless, a number of cancers are not detected by mammography but are evident on clinical examination, and complete breast examination is still advisable.

Screening is far from perfect. It does not detect all cancers and does not detect all cancers early enough to prevent death. If 100 women with cancer were screened today using mammography and clinical examination, 80 of the cancers would be detected. Among these, 68 (85%) would be detected by mammography, and another 12 (15%) would be detected only by clinical examination. Over the course of the next year, 20 more (20% of the original 100) would become clinically evident (detectable by the patient or her physician). Presumably, these 20 "interval cancers" (cancers found between screens) would have been present at the time of the screen but were undetectable by mammography or clinical examination.[8]

Despite the fact that mammography does not find all cancers and does not find all cancers early enough, it is the most effective method that is available, and it can reduce the death rate by at least 30%. If screening in the United States became universal, more than 12,000 lives might be saved each year.

In an era of diminishing health care resources, a major concern for the initiation of any type of screening is cost. For the benefits of screening to be available to *all* women, the cost of mammography needs to be kept as low as possible. Because the quality of the mammographic image is directly related to the ability to detect cancers earlier, cost reduction must not result in reduced image quality.

An efficient approach to screening can maintain quality and reduce cost. As has been shown in Europe and the United States, costs can be reduced by separating screening from the more costly evaluation of women who have a clinically evident problem or a problem detected by mammographic screening (*diagnosis*).[9,10] The screening mammogram is performed at a center dedicated to breast cancer screening (or in a mobile facility). The quality of the study is assured by expertly trained technologists, and then the patient leaves. Using this approach, one woman can be screened every 15 minutes.

To enhance the productivity of the radiologist, the screening studies are interpreted later, in batches. This approach is similar to that used for cervical cancer screening, and, although the psychological implications differ, mammography is the "Pap" test for the breast.

Batch interpretation has the disadvantage that the patient does not receive an immediate report. This is more than offset by the reduced expense from efficient screening and the added advantage that reading mammograms on an alternator, in batches, permits double reading.

DOUBLE READING

As has been shown in the interpretation of chest x-rays and other image interpretation, the perception of an abnormality is complicated by the psychovisual phenomenon that guarantees that significant abnormalities, visible in retrospect, are periodically overlooked by even the most experienced observer.[11] The failure to perceive an abnormality differs between observers. Errors can be reduced by having more than one "reader." Mammographic interpretation is no exception. Double reading has been shown to improve the breast cancer detection rate by 5% to 15%.[12–14]

Unless performed efficiently, however, double reading can increase the cost of screening, because both reviewers must be paid. A surprising amount of time is wasted handling films. Removing films from their envelope, organizing them on view boxes, replacing them in their folders, and dealing with paperwork can account for several minutes for each case. This can amount to an hour or more (depending on the number of films being reviewed) of time spent that is not directly involved in film interpretation. If this work is duplicated by each radiologist, then the time and cost become prohibitive.

There has been a great deal of misdirected effort in the United States to urge women to demand an immediate analysis of the mammogram. Although a psychological benefit is derived from having the radiologist on site and providing the patient with a review and summary of her mammogram, this is not the best use of resources. The value of mammography lies in detecting breast cancers earlier. It is well established that mammography cannot be used to exclude breast cancer; thus, having the radiologist reassure the patient that a study is negative has no real value. Resources would be better spent increasing the ability to detect early lesions through double reading. This is best accomplished by delaying the interpretation and mounting mammograms on an alternator (multiviewer), in batches, permitting multiple reviews with little increase in cost.

In our own experience, double reading increases our breast cancer detection rate by 7%. This is accomplished by having the first reader review films that were preloaded on a multiviewer, methodically, as well as completing all of the paperwork involved in film interpretation. A second reader can then concentrate completely on film review and accomplish a second reading, in a fraction of the time required by the first reader, by reviewing the cases in rapid succession. In our study of 5,900 screening mammograms, 39 cancers were identified. The methodical reader detected eight more cancers than the rapid reader, but the rapid reader detected an additional three cancers that were not appreciated by the methodical reader. Through efficient organization, and a slight delay (24 hours) for the patient in receiving her report, the false-negative rate can be reduced with virtually no increase in cost.

Although the psychology differs, the analogy to cervical screening is appropriate. As with the Papanicolaou test, screening mammograms should, ideally, be read in batches and double read. Women need to be educated as to the benefit of this approach rather than insisting on the false sense of security and unnecessary increased cost that come from an immediate interpretation.

COMPUTER-AIDED DETECTION AND DIAGNOSIS

When it became possible to convert images into data that could be evaluated by a computer, efforts began to develop computer-aided detection and computer-aided diagnosis (CAD). Although they have the same acronym, computer-aided detection and computer-aided diagnosis are distinctly different. *Computer-aided detection* is the use of a computer to assist the radiologist in detecting abnormalities that might represent malignancy, whereas *CAD* is the use of a computer to determine whether a detected abnormality is benign or malignant. The increased detection rates afforded by double reading stimulated efforts to develop computer assistance in the detection of breast cancer, and commercial systems have become available to assist the radiologist in detecting lesions. Although no large prospective study has been published, Schmidt, at the University of Chicago, has reported that CAD systems have been able to point out cancers that were overlooked by radiologists interpreting screening films.

Until primary digital mammographic systems become common, CAD requires that the film mammogram be digitized so it can be evaluated by the computer. This can be time consuming, because the level of resolution needed to detect microcalcifications is high, and digitizing x-rays at high resolution takes time and large amounts of computer memory. A single film mammogram digitized at 100 mm (the size of the pixel defining each point on the image) would require more than ten megabytes of memory. As memory has become less expensive, these systems have become feasible.

These systems are not useful if they are cumbersome and too distracting. If there are too many false-positive calls by the computer that end up merely distracting the radiologist, then the systems are turned off and not used. Consequently, developers have focused on maintaining a high detection rate while reducing the false-positive calls. As computer power and algorithms have improved, the ability of the programs to detect cancers without too many false-positive calls has improved. These systems make it possible for every radiologist to have a "second" reader and help reduce false-negative interpretations.

Once a lesion has been detected, the radiologist must determine its significance: Is it benign or malignant? Computers can help in this effort as well (CAD). Such approaches as neural networks, in which the computer is able to "learn" as it is exposed to more and more examples of different lesions, can provide the radiologist with probabilities of cancer that are based on images remembered by the computer that have a similar appearance. The computer may, ultimately, have an advantage, because it has a perfect memory, and other data can be integrated into the analysis, including age and family history, in ways that the radiologist cannot do.

It does not appear that the radiologist will be eliminated from the analysis of mammograms (at least in the near term), but the computer will become a greater and greater aid in image analysis. Once mammograms are acquired directly as digital images, computer-aided detection and diagnosis will become an important component of breast cancer detection and diagnosis.

DETECTION THRESHOLDS

As with many medical procedures, screening and the earlier detection of breast cancer are a combination of science and art. The vagaries of perception and the importance of double reading have already been discussed, but an additional factor enters into the success of a screening program. This element is the threshold at which the radiologist recommends intervention. Because many of the ways that breast cancer appears on a mammogram overlap with the presentation of benign lesions, many of these lesions have a low probability of malignancy (fewer than 5%). There is legitimate disagreement as to how aggressively these low-probability lesions should be pursued. The influence of detection threshold was demonstrated in a highly publicized study involving ten radiologists who were asked to review a series of 150 mammographic studies without the knowledge that they included 27 cancer cases.[15] Almost one-third of the cancers were these borderline lesions. The radiologist who had the highest true-positive rate (detected the highest percentage of cancers) also had the highest false-positive rate (was concerned about many lesions that proved not to be cancer), whereas the radiologist who had the lowest false-positive rate also had the highest false-negative rate and missed most of the cancers.[16] Unless one radiologist knows a secret way to differentiate benign from malignant lesions, most experienced radiologists operate on the same receiver operating characteristic curve. This means that the only way to reduce the false-positive call rate is to allow cancers to pass through the screen. A high threshold for intervention can reduce the call-back rate but misses cancers, whereas a low threshold increases the yield of cancer at the cost of an increased call-back rate. This has led to a major disagreement. Health planners are most concerned with high call-back rates, whereas the goal of most radiologists is to find as many early cancers as possible.

MONITORING RESULTS: BREAST IMAGING AUDIT

The best method for determining the success of a screening program is an audit that evaluates the cancer detection rate and the types of cancers detected. The Mammography Quality Standards Act, passed by Congress and administered by the U.S. Food and Drug Administration (FDA), became effective in October 1994. As part of the requirement for licensure, mammography facilities must monitor the results of their breast cancer detection programs. Sickles et al. describe an audit of a screening practice in great detail.[17] Each facility should monitor, among other parameters, the number of women screened, the number recalled for additional evaluation, the number recommended for biopsy, the positive predictive value for biopsies recommended, and the number, size, and stage of cancers detected. Because many of these factors vary with the population being screened and the prior probability of cancer in a particular population, there are no absolute figures for these data. In our own practice, in which we screen women beginning by age 40, we recall approximately 7% of women for additional evaluation after their first screen (prevalence). This drops to fewer than 4% on subsequent screens. Approximately 2% to 3% of women are recommended for a biopsy based on their first mammogram. This drops to 1% to 2% on subsequent screens. We detect approximately eight cancers per 1,000 women in the first screen and two to three per 1,000 in subsequent screens. Approximately 30% of the cancers detected are ductal carcinoma *in situ* (DCIS). Among the invasive cancers, approximately 50% are 1 cm or smaller, and fewer than 20% of the women diagnosed with breast cancer have positive axillary lymph nodes. These are not necessarily optimal figures, but by evaluating the results of a screening effort, thresholds can be adjusted to improve the success of the program.

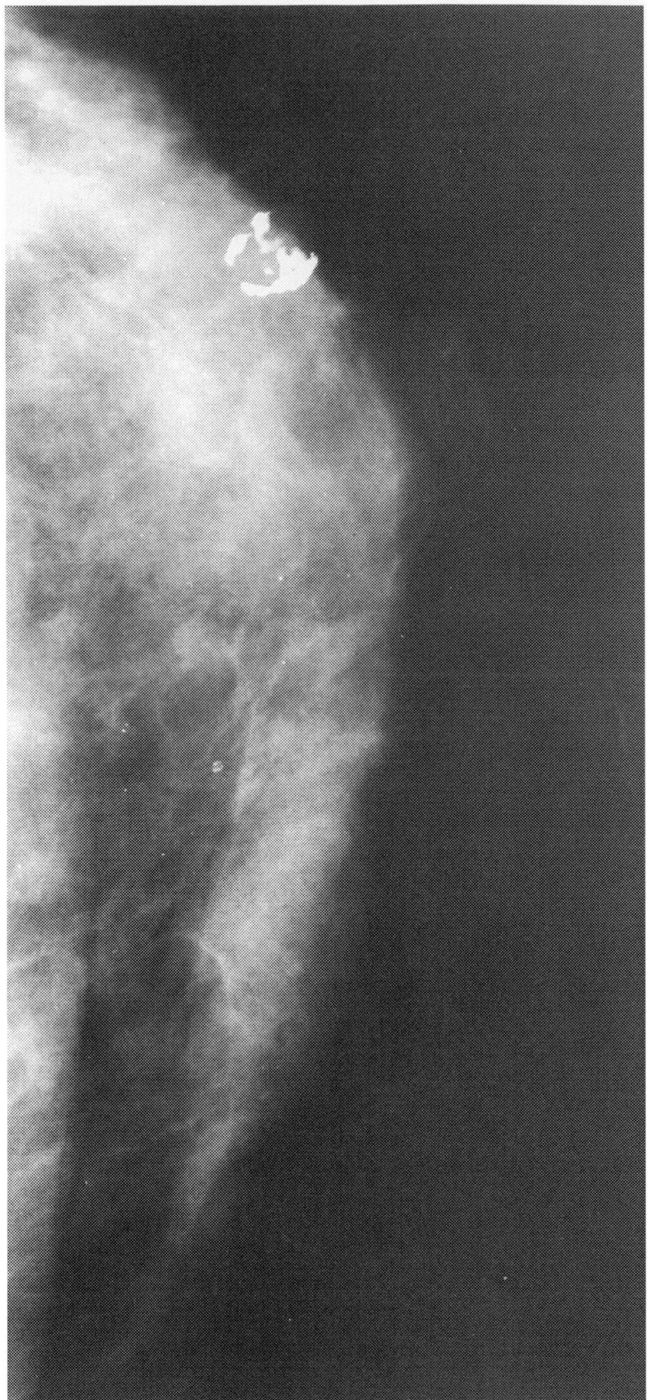

FIG. 4. Calcified fibroadenoma that is so characteristic it does not require any further evaluation.

MAMMOGRAPHY

The primary role of mammography is to screen asymptomatic women with the goal of detecting breast cancer at a smaller size and earlier stage than the woman's own surveillance or her doctor's routine examination might ordinarily achieve. Mammography is also used to evaluate women with palpable abnormalities; however, its use in this setting is limited.[18] The mammogram may reinforce the diagnosis of cancer and help avoid overlooking a malignancy.[19] On rare occasions, the mammogram demonstrates a clearly benign lesion, and a biopsy can be avoided (Fig. 4), but, because some palpable cancers are not visible by mammography, the study cannot be used to exclude cancer. If the clinical examination raises concern, *a negative mammogram should not delay further investigation.*

It is best to always think of mammography as being primarily a screening study. Management of a clinically apparent lesion must ultimately be determined by the clinical evaluation. Even among symptomatic women, mammography is primarily for screening. Because mammography cannot be used to exclude breast cancer, and the mammographic findings are frequently not specific in the symptomatic woman, its primary value for these patients is to survey the remainder of the ipsilateral breast and screen the contralateral breast to detect clinically occult cancer.[20]

ANALYZING LESIONS DETECTED BY MAMMOGRAPHY

Mammographic analysis should be systematic and should proceed according to the following simple sequence:

Find it.
Is it real?
Where is it?
What is it?
What should be done about it?

Find It

The ability to detect early cancers is related to the quality of the mammogram. Cancers cannot be detected if they are not imaged because of poor positioning or because the film is not properly exposed or properly processed. High-quality mammography is required. Double reading should be encouraged.

If previous mammograms are available, they should be compared to the present mammographic study to look for changes. New masses or new indeterminate calcifications should be evaluated carefully, because the breast is relatively stable on mammograms from year to year. Because changes may be slow to evolve and difficult to appreciate from one year to the next, we have found it best to compare the present study to one from at least 2 years previous.

The mammographic tissue pattern of the breast is important. High attenuation (dense) breast tissue is normal, but it can hide cancers, and the referring physician should be alerted to this fact, because the clinical examination becomes more important if the mammographic pattern is dense. There are a range of patterns, from those that appear to be almost entirely fat and like window glass on a mammogram, to breasts that contain some fibroglandular densities, to breasts that are heterogeneously dense, to those that are extremely dense.

Is It Real?

Because a mammogram is the projection of three-dimensional structures on a two-dimensional image, many findings that elicit concern on a screening study prove to be benign superimpositions of normal structures on follow-up imaging. Before significant concern is raised, the radiologist should determine that a perceived abnormality is, in fact, three-dimensionally real. Methods have been developed to accomplish this,[21] including repositioning the breast and magnification mammography.

Where Is It?

Once a lesion has been found and confirmed as three-dimensionally real, its location in the breast should be established if further evaluation is indicated. This can be accomplished using altered mammographic positions,[22] ultrasound,[23] or even computed tomography.[24]

What Is It?

Is It Benign?

The first major step in mammographic analysis is to try to determine whether the detected change can be categorized as a benign finding. If its morphology clearly indicates a benign structure, further evaluation is unnecessary. If it is not clearly benign, then analysis should proceed.

What Should Be Done About It?

This is the basis of imaging analysis that often ends with the need for a tissue diagnosis.

REPORTING MAMMOGRAPHIC FINDINGS

The American College of Radiology designed a Breast Imaging Reporting and Data System (BI-RADS) to create a universal language and format for radiologists to report mammographic findings. Radiologists are encouraged to use BI-RADs to reduce ambiguity and confusion. BI-RADS provides a dictionary of terminology and a report organization that ends in a decision-oriented final assessment of a mammogram.[25] Five assessment categories have been defined for grouping findings:

1. A negative mammogram. There is no abnormality to report.
2. A benign finding: negative. This indicates that there is a lesion, such as a calcifying fibroadenoma, that the radiologist wishes to document so a less experienced observer will not mistake it as a significant abnormality. The overall mammogram, however, shows no evidence of cancer.
3. There is a finding that is probably benign, but short interval follow-up is recommended. This assessment is directly comparable to the clinical situation in which the clinician palpates an abnormality and believes that it is a benign change but wishes to evaluate it over several months to confirm its regression or stability.
4. There is an abnormality that is indeterminate, but the risk of cancer is measurable, and a biopsy should be considered. This is an incompletely defined category that may contain lesions that have a 2% to 5% probability of malignancy (the solitary circumscribed mass) up to as high as perhaps 40% to 50% probability. If the radiologist has sufficient data to permit accurate figures, the use of probabilities may be helpful for the patient and her physician.
5. There is a lesion that has a morphologic appearance that makes it likely to be breast cancer. This lesion needs to be biopsied.

The first, second, and last categories are fairly straightforward. Benign changes require no further evaluation. Changes that suggest malignancy require intervention. There are no data other than anecdotal that the high-probability lesion requires additional evaluation other than a tissue diagnosis. Some suggest that, in cases in which conservation therapy (lumpectomy and radiation therapy) is to be used, additional evaluation in high-probability lesions may involve magnification views in an attempt to better define the extent of a lesion[26] or to search for multifocality.

BI-RADS identifies a category 0 that is used when the analysis is incomplete. This category is used if immediate additional evaluation, such as ultrasound, or magnification views are needed before a complete assessment can be rendered. In general, every mammographic report should ultimately be placed in categories 1 through 5 so there is no ambiguity as to the level of concern of the interpreting radiologist.

MAMMOGRAPHIC APPEARANCE OF BREAST CANCER

Breast cancer usually presents in one or a combination of the following:

1. A mass
2. Associated calcifications
3. Architectural distortion
4. Asymmetry of architecture, tissue density, or duct dilatation
5. Skin or nipple changes

Skin thickening or retraction and nipple retraction or inversion are generally changes associated with later-stage cancers and are usually evident on clinical inspection. The mammogram should be performed to emphasize the analysis of the breast tissues. High-contrast mammograms maximize the perception of breast cancer, and images should be obtained to permit assessment of the breast parenchyma, with imaging of the skin and nipples secondary in importance.

ANALYZING MASSES

Masses should be evaluated based on their size, shape, margins, location, and x-ray attenuation.

Size

The size of a cancer at the time of diagnosis is a significant prognostic indicator.[27] Although the traditional staging of breast cancer uses 2 cm as the cutoff for stage I infiltrating cancers, even within stage I lesions, there is a significant difference in prognosis that improves with the diminishing diameter of the tumor.[28] Many years ago, Gallager and Martin demonstrated the benefit of finding infiltrating cancers of 5 mm or smaller.[29] This is a desirable goal, but it is difficult to achieve, even with mammography. A number of studies have looked at 1 cm as a threshold and have shown that finding infiltrating cancers smaller than 1 cm has a survival benefit that is almost as high as a 5-mm threshold.[30–32] This is an achievable goal. In our own screen of detected cancers since 1978, 57% of the infiltrating lesions have been smaller than 1 cm. Certainly for spiculated and ill-defined masses there should be no size threshold, and a biopsy should be recommended at any size for these lesions, but for the "most likely benign" circumscribed mass, a threshold for investigation (ultrasound, aspiration, or biopsy) should be considered for solitary lesions that approach 1 cm.

Shape

Masses can be divided into round, oval, lobulated, or irregular shapes (Fig. 5). The probability of malignancy increases with these variations, depending on the appearance of a lesion's margin. An area of architectural distortion not associated with a mass in an area in which no prior surgery has been performed frequently is due to an underlying malignancy.

Margins

The interface between a lesion and the surrounding tissue is one of the most important factors in determining the significance of a mass (Fig. 6). Circumscribed masses whose margins form a sharp, abrupt transition with the surrounding tissue are almost always benign (Fig. 7). Magnification

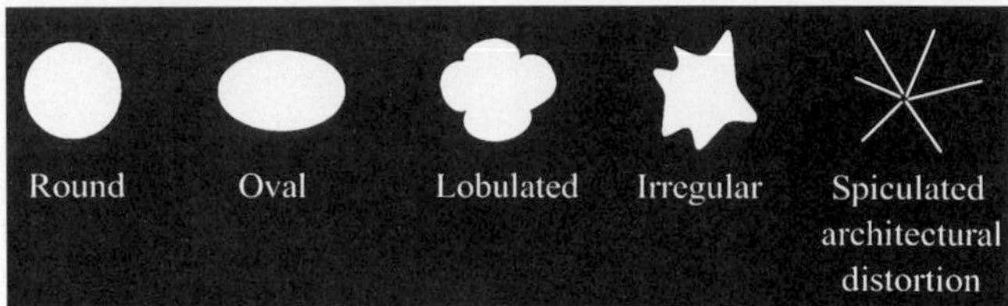

FIG. 5. The shapes of masses are important. These have been divided into round, oval, lobulated, irregular, or spiculated architectural distortion. The last two are strongly associated with malignancy.

mammography with increased resolution can increase the confidence of circumscription or reveal a less well-defined margin that should increase concern.

The microlobulated margin reflects the irregular surface that can be produced by a breast cancer. The irregular protrusions that form at a tumor's edge can form short undulations at the surface of the lesion when seen on the mammogram.

An obscured margin occurs when the normal surrounding tissue hides the true edge of the lesion. The interpreter must decide whether a lesion's margin is obscured or truly infiltrative. The latter raises the level of concern.

The vast majority of breast cancers have an irregular interface as they invade the surrounding tissue. This produces the truly ill-defined margin that should raise concern. The probability of malignancy is high in lesions with ill-defined margins, although benign masses including cysts and fibroadenomas may have ill-defined margins.

The classic breast cancer has a spiculated margin. This is due to fibrous projections extending from the main tumor mass. Careful microscopic analysis of these projections reveals associated cancer cells, although, by convention, the diameter of a cancer is measured across the tumor mass and excludes the spicules. Spiculated masses or areas of architectural distortion that appear spiculated should always be biopsied, unless the distortion can be directly attributed to previous surgery. The analysis of breast lesions is thus aided by having some historical information. Knowledge of previous surgery, the site of the inci-

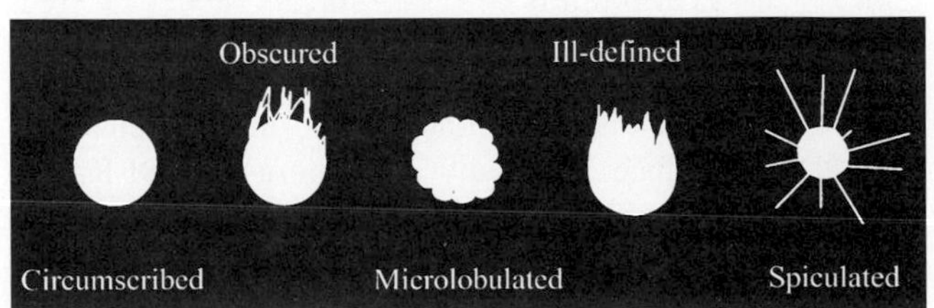

FIG. 6. The margins of lesions help to determine their significance. These have been divided into sharply circumscribed, obscured (believed to be well defined but the overlying tissue is covering them), microlobulated, ill defined, and spiculated. The last three are strongly associated with malignancy.

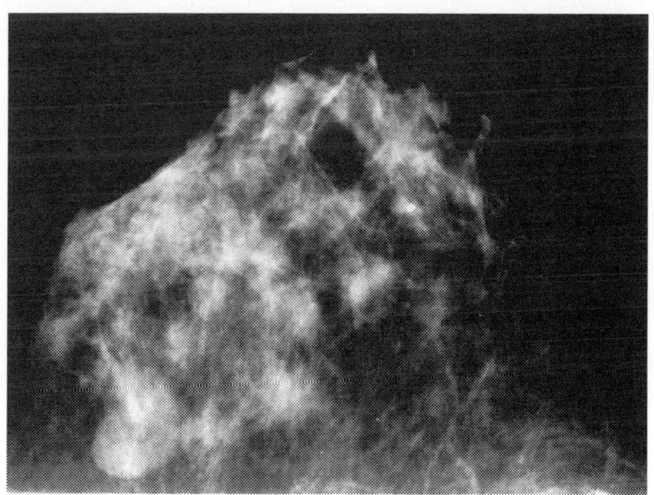

FIG. 7. The sharply defined mass deep in the right breast has a partially obscured margin. It proved to be a cyst.

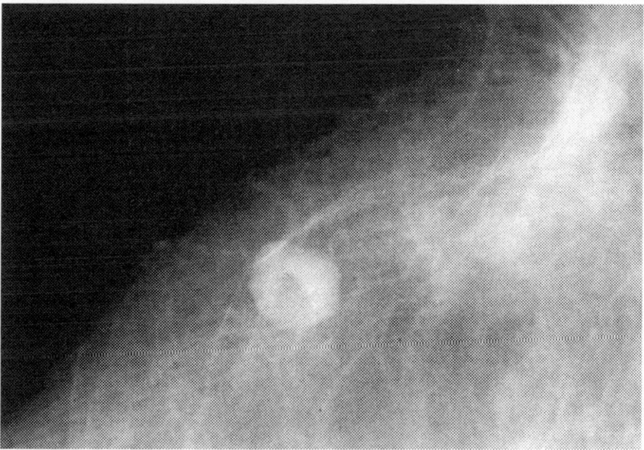

FIG. 8. Typical intramammary lymph node found in the lateral breast tissues. Note that it has a fatty hilar notch.

sion, and, in particular, the site from which tissue was removed is important for the interpretation of masses and calcifications. Architectural distortion is not uncommon during the first year after any form of breast surgery, but this should resolve in almost all cases within 12 to 18 months.[33] Complete healing may be delayed if the breast has been irradiated. Postsurgical fat necrosis can produce calcifications that can at times be confusing.[34]

Sclerosing duct hyperplasia (radial scar) may produce spicules, and its likelihood can be suggested from morphologic criteria, but a biopsy is still required to make a safe diagnosis.[35]

Location

Knowledge of the location is primarily useful when the morphology of a mass suggests an intramammary lymph node. This is an extremely common finding and is recognizably visible in approximately 5% of all mammograms. Typically, these are reniform masses, smaller than 1 cm in size and with a lucent notch (Fig. 8), that occur at the edge of the breast tissue in the outer portions of the breast. They may be found as far as two-thirds to three-fourths of the way from the chest wall to the nipple.

X-Ray Attenuation

Lesions that truly contain fat (do not just appear to have fat or trap fat) are never malignant. The "oil cyst" form of fat necrosis that contains gelatinized fat defined by a thin capsule is characteristic. Lipomas and high fat content galactoceles present no diagnostic dilemma and are always benign. Similarly, the mixed-density hamartoma is always benign.

Most breast cancers have a higher x-ray attenuation than an equal volume of fibroglandular tissue. This is likely due to the dense fibrosis associated with these lesions. Many cancers are isodense, and occasionally some, such as colloid cancers, are less attenuating, so this characteristic does not have a perfect correlation. Benign lesions can also have higher attenuation. Cysts that contain blood are frequently dense for their size.

Other Findings

Other features involved in the assessment of a mass include skin and nipple changes and associated calcifications. Skin changes are occasionally useful, although they are usually equally or more evident on clinical evaluation. Often, skin thickening or nipple changes are late findings in breast cancer, and only rarely are skin changes the predominant finding in an early breast cancer.

Pleomorphic calcifications smaller than 0.5 mm that are found in association with a mass are of concern, just as they would be if no mass were present. The presence of large (>0.5 mm) calcifications in a mass makes it more likely to be a benign lesion, such as an involuting fibroadenoma or papilloma.

ANALYZING CALCIFICATIONS

Analysis of calcifications includes an evaluation of their location, size, number, morphology, and distribution. A major determination is whether calcifications are truly intramammary or in the skin. This may seem trivial, yet numerous women have undergone truly unnecessary surgery to try to remove calcifications that were in fact benign skin deposits.[36] Tangential views of the skin that contains the calcifications can confirm the location of these particles.

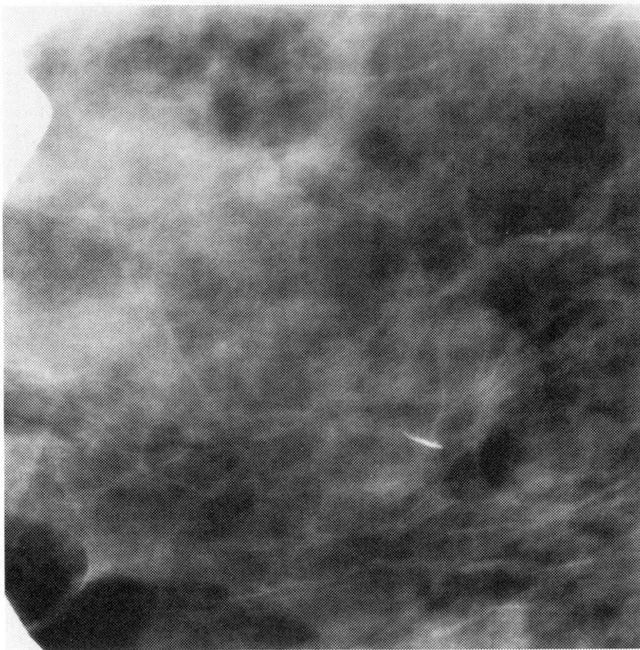

FIG. 9. Milk of calcium. This curvilinear calcification is actually a fine powder that is layered in the dependent portion of a cyst whose contour can just barely be seen in this horizontal beam lateral projection. This is a clear indication of a benign process.

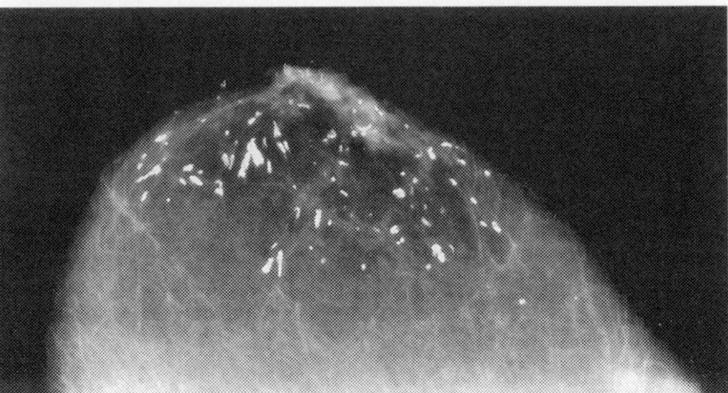

FIG. 10. These large rod-shaped calcifications are benign secretory deposits.

Size

Breast cancers rarely produce calcifications larger than 1 mm, and most calcifications associated with breast cancer are smaller than 0.5 mm in diameter.

Number

The use of a threshold number to categorize suspicious groupings of calcifications has caused much discussion. The number 5 in a cubic centimeter has been derived from general experience and from a large series published by Egan et al., in which the probability of malignancy was zero when there were fewer than five calcific particles in a volume of tissue.[37] Obviously, this is an observational phenomenon and not a fact of nature. There are undoubtedly cancers that indicate their presence by forming fewer than five calcifications, but on a statistical basis, the probability of malignancy increases with the number of calcifications. The morphology and distribution of the calcifications must be taken into account when assessing their significance.

Morphology

Morphology is the most important element in the analysis of calcifications. The shapes of the particles and heterogeneity of the shapes and sizes are frequently valuable in determining the likely cause of the deposits. A better understanding of the microscopic histologic and pathologic environment in which calcifications form can also help in understanding the morphologic changes seen on mammography.[38] Calcifications that can be categorized as due to benign processes need no further evaluation.

Calcifications that form in the acinar structures of the lobule are virtually always benign. Probably due to the mold in which they form (the dilated acini), these calcifications are often smooth and round. Solid or lucent-centered spheres are almost always due to benign processes. Sedimented calcium that settles to the bottom of cysts formed by dilated acini are also benign forms of calcium deposits. The appearance of crescent-shaped calcifications that are concave up on the horizontal beam lateral (Fig. 9) can secure a benign diagnosis on the mammogram.[39]

Other lucent-centered calcifications include those that may form around the benign debris that can accumulate in ducts. Skin calcifications may also appear as lucent-centered calcifications.

Solid rod-shaped calcifications (Fig. 10), as well as lucent-centered, tubular forms, are usually due to calcifications within or around normal or ectatic ducts.[40] These forms of benign secretory calcification are almost always larger than 0.5 mm in diameter and can rarely be confused with malignant calcifications.

Very thin deposits associated with the rim of breast cysts are another form of calcification that should not elicit concern. These "eggshell" calcifications are only serendipitously associated with breast cancer. Thicker "spherical" deposits are usually due to fat necrosis (Fig. 11).

Vascular calcifications, with their distinctive parallel track appearance, have such typical morphologic characteristics that they can be ignored.

The initial assessment of calcifications is made to determine if they conform to these well-established benign morphologies. If the characteristics of the calcifications are such that they cannot be reliably classified as being due to benign processes, then

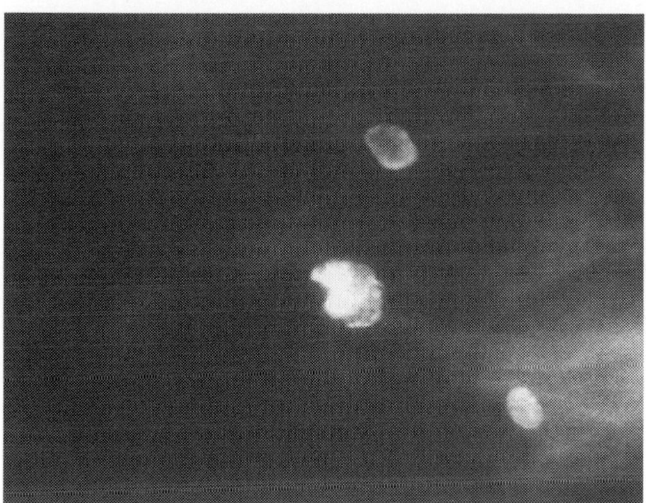

FIG. 11. These spheric, lucent-centered calcifications are due to fat necrosis.

additional evaluation is indicated. Magnification mammography is the primary technique used to further analyze calcifications. A clearer appreciation of the morphology and distribution of the calcifications is afforded by magnification, and this is used to ultimately decide, using objective criteria, whether a biopsy to establish a firm diagnosis is needed.

The shapes of calcifications are the key to their analysis (Fig. 12). Calcifications that vary in size (most smaller than 0.5 mm) and shape are a cause for concern. Calcifications due to breast cancer are either caused by cellular secretion or the calcification of necrotic cancer cells. Virtually all calcifications that form in breast cancers (including invasive lesions) form in the intraductal portion of the cancer. Although the multiplying cells can expand the duct, the necrosis usually occurs irregularly in the center of the duct. One study suggests that this happens when the tumor diameter enlarges beyond 180 mm.[41] The cells in the center become hypoxic as their distance from their blood supply increases, and eventually the center of the tumor becomes necrotic. Because this is an irregular process at the center of the intraductal cancer, the calcifications formed are very small and irregular. Although these calcifications have been termed *casting*, they are actually the result of irregular patterns of tissue necrosis within cancers in a duct. Their distribution, however, is guided by the course of the duct, giving a sometimes distinctive linear branching pattern (Fig. 13A). In many cases of DCIS, the calcifications are pleomorphic and clustered, with no other defining characteristics (Fig. 13B).

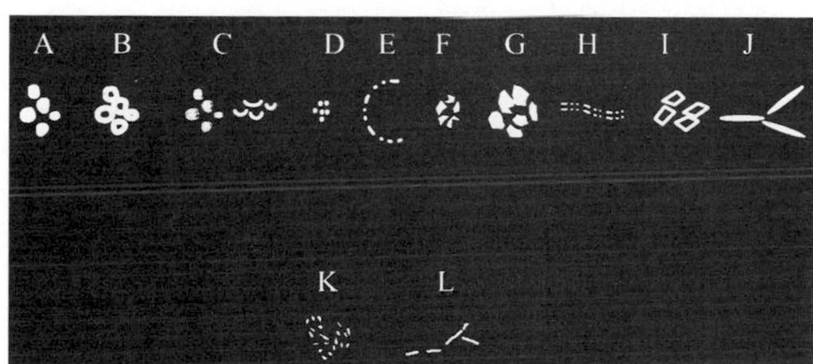

FIG. 12. Calcifications are analyzed based on their size, number, distribution, and morphology. A, round regular calcifications; B, lucent-centered, spherical calcifications; C, milk of calcium; D, punctate; E, rim deposits; F, early deposits of an involuting fibroadenoma; G, late deposits of an involuting fibroadenoma; H, vascular deposits; I, dermal deposits; J, secretory deposits; K, pleomorphic clustered calcifications; L, fine linear branching calcifications.

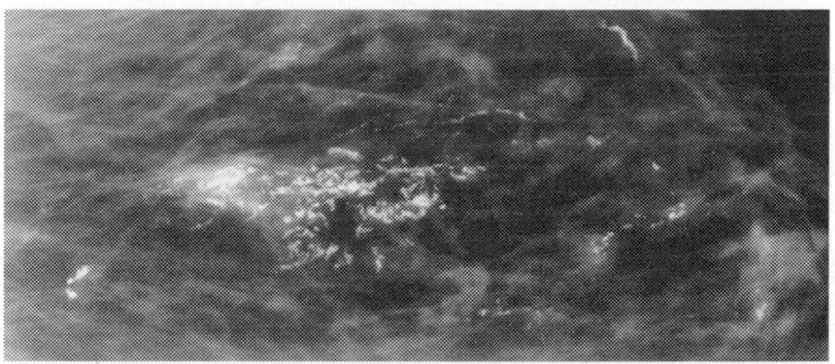

A

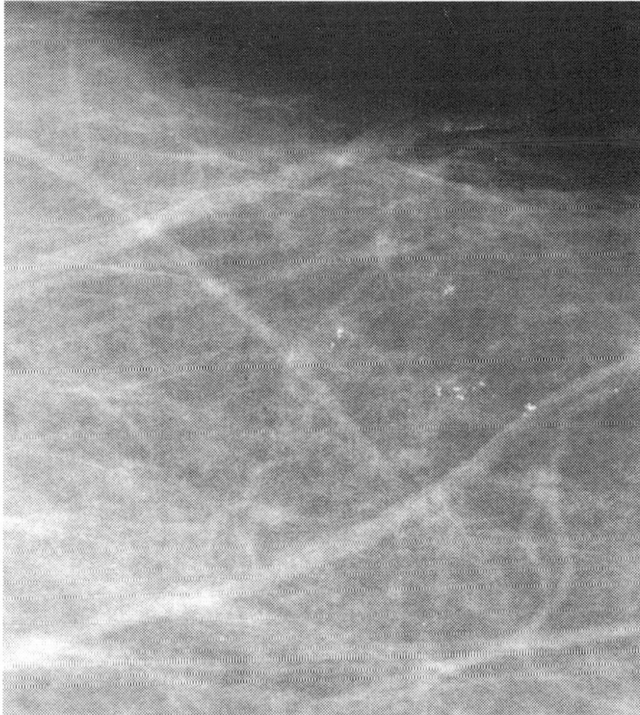

B

FIG. 13. A: Linear branching calcifications that are typical of comedonecrosis in ductal carcinoma *in situ*. **B:** Pleomorphic calcifications caused by ductal carcinoma *in situ*.

Distribution

The distribution of calcifications can assist in their assessment (Fig. 14).

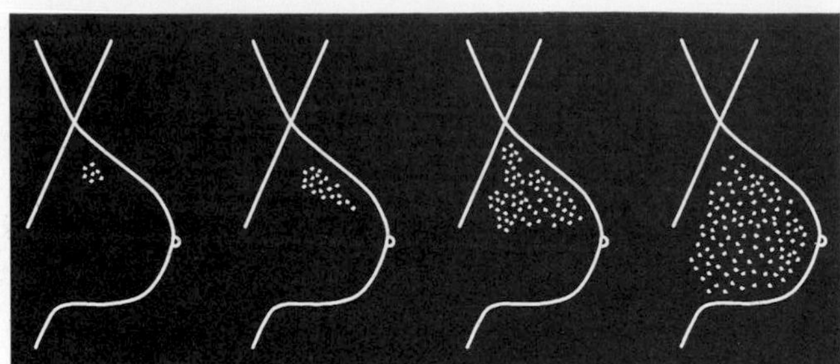

FIG. 14. The distribution of calcifications is useful in their analysis. Geographically distributed and diffusely scattered calcifications are rarely due to malignancy.

Clustered

Many cancer calcifications form in nonspecific clusters. These are the types of calcifications that are the most difficult to analyze accurately and are the cause of most benign biopsies. Many define a cluster of calcifications as a group of five or more particles in a cubic centimeter of tissue. Heterogeneous calcifications that cannot be accurately placed in benign categories may still be due to benign processes. Clusters may be caused by adenosis, peripheral duct papillomas, hyperplasia, and other benign breast conditions. Unfortunately, cancer can also produce these "clusters" of calcifications, and biopsy is needed to establish an accurate diagnosis.

Segmental

Segmental distribution is thought to represent calcifications within a single duct network. A lobe or segment of the breast is defined by the major duct opening on the nipple and its branches spreading into the breast that terminate in its lobules. Many believe that breast cancer is a process that initially is confined to a single duct network. True multicentric cancer (multiple duct networks involved) is unusual, whereas multifocality (cancer at multiple sites within one duct network) appears to be relatively common.[42] Calcifications whose distribution suggests a duct network are of concern.

Regional or Diffusely Scattered Calcifications

Calcifications that appear randomly distributed throughout large volumes or throughout the breast are almost always benign. Although breast cancer can be extensive, this is very unusual, and diffusely scattered calcifications are almost always due to benign processes.

ADJUNCTIVE ASSESSMENT

To arrive at a final assessment, additional techniques beyond the standard two-view mammogram are useful. Magnification mammography results in an absolute increase in resolving capability. The morphology and number of calcifications are better appreciated using magnification. The margins of masses are seen with greater clarity, and this may aid in the assessment of these lesions. One should use magnification carefully. The focal spot must be sufficiently small to permit the amount of magnification desired without creating geometric unsharpness. The use of the spot compression device to better spread overlapping structures can be combined with magnification, but the operator should recognize the possibility that spot compression can squeeze a true lesion out of the field of view, and if a suspicious lesion seems to disappear with spot compression this possibility should be considered. We have also noted that, for as yet unexplained reasons, true architectural distortion may not be as evident on magnification, and we prefer to use spot compression without magnification as the first step in evaluating an area of architectural distortion. Other special views can be used to better visualize questionable lesions by rolling the breast[43] or angling the tube.

DIGITAL MAMMOGRAPHY

As in all aspects of imaging, the development of the electronic acquisition and computer rendering of an image has been applied to mammography. Several vendors have developed mammographic systems that convert the x-rays passing through the breast into an electronic signal that can then be processed by a computer. These systems essentially count the number of x-ray photons passing through the breast at every point and provide a number (digits) for each point that indicates the count. By reducing the size of the area in which the photons are counted (the pixel size), the resolution of the image can be increased.

Because the film in conventional film/screen mammography is both the detector (acquires the image) and the display medium, the characteristics of the film and its development determine the exposure requirements of the process. Because a computer display of an image can be adjusted after it has been acquired, the primary digital acquisition of the image permits optimization of that acquisition. A film mammogram can be under- and overexposed, and information can be lost. A digital mammogram can be adjusted after it has been acquired so that repeat exposure to the patient is not needed.

A film mammogram is the only copy of the study. It is difficult to copy film mammograms, because information is lost on the copy. Once an image is in digital form, however, it can be duplicated as many times as needed and transmitted any where in the world, and identical copies can be saved electronically in a number of places so that it is unlikely to be lost. In addition, as noted in the section Computer-Aided Detection and Diagnoses, computers can be used to analyze the images and assist the radiologist in detection and diagnosis.

A number of technologies are being developed to permit digital mammography. Several involve the conversion of x-ray photons into visible light by a fluorescent screen and then conduction of these light photons through fiberoptic coupling devices to charged coupled devices that convert the light to an electrical signal. Because charge coupled devices are relatively small, they need to be either scanned under the breast or tiled together to form a large area detector.

Other approaches involve the conversion of the photons to light and the measurement of this light at each pixel by solid-state detectors in a matrix over a large area. Direct conversion of photons to electrical signal is also being developed to eliminate the need to convert the photons to light. Digital mammography should become available by the end of 2000 or in 2001, unless politics at the FDA continue to delay it.

ULTRASOUND

Ultrasound Should Not Be Used for Screening outside of a Clinical Trial

Ultrasound technology has evolved over many years. Original hopes that ultrasound could be effective as a screening technique did not survive scientific scrutiny. Rigorous evaluation of whole-breast ultrasound proved that not only was ultrasound incapable of detecting early-stage cancers with any reliability, but scanning the breast with ultrasound also resulted in concern being raised for suspicious areas that never proved to be malignant.[44]

Ultrasound instrumentation has improved significantly, however. Several articles have suggested that there are some cancers that can be seen by ultrasound but are not evident on clinical examination or mammography.[45,46] These preliminary results need to be confirmed in larger prospective trials, however, before there is any efficacious role for ultrasound in the evaluation of asymptomatic women. Consequently, ultrasound should not be used to survey breast tissue but to evaluate specific areas of concern raised by mammography and perhaps clinical examination.

Ultrasound Is Not as Reliable as Biopsy in the Differentiation of Benign from Malignant Solid Masses

Several studies have attempted to show that ultrasound can be used to differentiate benign from malignant lesions.[47,48] The only reason to use ultrasound in the evaluation of lesions that are spiculated on mammography is to determine whether they are amenable to ultrasound-guided needle biopsy or localization. These lesions are almost certain to be cancer, and a tissue diagnosis cannot be replaced safely by an imaging study.

The primary situation in which some use ultrasound to avoid a tissue diagnosis is in the evaluation of lesions that are circumscribed on the mammogram or those that are palpable solid masses that are well defined ovals or are smoothly lobulated on ultrasound. Because most invasive breast cancers infiltrate into normal tissue in an irregular fashion, as on mammograms, a lesion that is oval or lobulated with a sharply defined margin (a clear abrupt demarcation between its edge and the surrounding tissue) by ultrasound is likely to be benign. Because the prior probability of cancer increases with increasing age, the likelihood that an oval or lobulated mass seen on ultrasound is benign increases with decreasing age of the patient. Unfortunately, although the number of cases is small, there are exceptions to every rule, and some cancers are sharply defined, oval, or smoothly lobulated.

Other characteristics have been used to differentiate benign from malignant circumscribed masses. Fornage[49] developed a ratio of the length of a lesion to its height. The length is measured as the longest axis that parallels the skin, whereas the height is perpendicular to the skin and chest wall. He found virtually no cancers that had a ratio of 1.4 to 1 or greater (we have seen a few), and most cancers had a ratio that was less than 1.0 to 1 (they are "vertically" oriented as, however, are some benign masses).

Another sign that has been used to suggest that a lesion is benign is the appearance of a notch in the upper surface of a sharply defined lobulated mass. This *usually* suggests that the lesion represents a fibroadenoma.

A third "benign" finding is the appearance of a thin echogenic "rim" delineating the margin of an oval or smoothly lobulated mass. This has the appearance of a pseudocapsule.

The reviews that argue in support of ultrasound as a diagnostic test suffered from a lack of blinding to the mammographic findings and other methodologic biases that compromised the significance of the findings. Those who rely on the observations noted to separate benign from malignant lesions have statistics on their side. Most circumscribed masses are not cancer. It becomes a philosophic (and medicolegal) issue as to what level of certainty is appropriate. Because a biopsy is so safe and relatively simple, it may be difficult to justify substituting an imaging test that has a false-negative rate for a biopsy that has a much lower error rate.

It remains to be shown in a scientific fashion that improvements in ultrasound imaging technology have had any significant effect on the sensitivity or specificity of ultrasound.

Doppler Ultrasound

Investigators have, for many years, hoped that the ultrasound measurement of blood flow using the Doppler effect would increase the ability of ultrasound to differentiate benign from malignant lesions. Because many breast cancers appear to have a substantial neovasculature (at the microscopic level), and most benign lesions do not have increased blood flow, the rationale for "Doppler" ultrasound would appear to make sense. Unfortunately, the clinical results have not been particularly convincing. Many cancers can be shown to have increased blood flow, particularly at their periphery. High-velocity flow seems to be almost only found in breast cancers.[50] Although preliminary reports suggested a high sensitivity and specificity for Doppler,[51] other studies were not as successful, suggesting poor discrimination between normal and cancerous tissues.[52] The most optimistic report concluded, "Color Doppler signal in a lesion otherwise thought to be benign should prompt a biopsy, while the absence of signals in an indeterminate lesion is reassuring."[53] The clinical application of this is not particularly useful. Because benign lesions may exhibit increased flow and, more importantly, a significant number of cancers do not exhibit evidence of abnormal flow,[54] particularly lesions smaller than 1 cm,[55] Doppler is not yet reliable for distinguishing benign from malignant lesions. Given the safety and accuracy in a breast biopsy and the overlap of benign and malignant characteristics with Doppler, it is difficult to rely on Doppler analysis. Thus, at this time, Doppler is not a clinically useful test for evaluating breast lesions.

Although continued investigation and development of ultrasound are strongly urged, it is likely that the sonographic characteristics of normal and abnormal breast tissues are such that the modality itself will never have greater use than for solid cyst differentiation and as a guide for selected interventional procedures.[56–58]

ULTRASOUND AND PALPABLE MASSES

The routine use of ultrasound in the evaluation of palpable masses is controversial. If a palpable mass is shown to be a cyst by ultrasound, there is no reason to aspirate it. If the ultrasound demonstration of a cyst averts any further intervention, then its use to evaluate palpable lesions is efficacious. Some physicians, however, argue that a palpable cyst interferes with the clinical evaluation of the tissue under it, and they aspirate these lesions. Other palpable cysts are aspirated because they are uncomfortable or even painful for the patient, and still others are aspirated because the patient does not like to have a lump. Aspiration has the advantage that the problem is diagnosed and eliminated simultaneously. If a lesion is to be aspirated, despite the demonstration that it is a cyst by ultrasound, then the ultrasound will have been superfluous.

From a purely scientific perspective, the use of ultrasound to evaluate palpable masses should be limited to those that have resisted aspiration but are still believed to be cysts. On occasion, a cyst may have a thick wall or be sufficiently mobile to defy clinically guided aspiration. The demonstration by ultrasound that these lesions are indeed cysts can avoid an excisional biopsy. Unfortunately, because a number of medicolegal cases have been decided or settled against radiologists who did not use ultrasound for palpable masses, many now practice defensively and examine all palpable masses with ultrasound.

LESION ANALYSIS USING ULTRASOUND

High-frequency transducers (7.5 mHz or higher) should be used for breast ultrasound. These should be focusable from the skin to 3 to 4 cm beneath the skin so that most of the tissue in most breasts can be imaged. The patient is examined in the supine position with the ipsilateral arm extended behind the head to flatten the breast against the chest wall. Transverse and longitudinal scans are recommended as standard. Some advocate radial scanning extending from the nipple, but there has never been any scientific justification for this. Clearly, the transducer should be rotated and angled to provide the most complete and detailed evaluation of the tissue being evaluated.

The gain settings should be adjusted to provide a moderately wide grey scale but with the preservation of contrast. Fat is less echogenic than fibroglandular breast tissue. Ideally, the settings will permit the sometimes subtle differentiation of a hypoechoic solid mass from fat.

Cysts

The primary role for ultrasound is to differentiate cysts from solid masses and to guide needle procedures. A cyst should be round, ovoid, or smoothly lobulated. It should have no internal echoes, and the retrocystic echoes should be enhanced. What appear to be septations in cysts are of no consequence. They generally represent two cysts abutting one another or a cyst that has preserved some of its acinar origin.

Solid Masses

Solid masses can have a wide range of appearances. Most masses, whether benign or malignant, are hypoechoic. Generally, masses that are round, oval, or smoothly lobulated with a uniform internal texture, echogenic rim (pseudocapsule), and enhanced through transmission of sound are benign. Unfortunately, on occasion, cancers can have the same appearances.

Masses that are irregular in shape with heterogeneous internal echoes and retrotumoral shadowing are usually malignant, although, on occasion, a benign lesion can have the same appearance. Many breast cancers seem to be more vertically oriented (Fig. 15) with respect to the skin, whereas benign lesions are more horizontal in their orientation.[58]

Unfortunately, none of these descriptions is perfect for the characterization of a given lesion. If it is important to obtain the true histology of a lesion, then the only way to do this is through a biopsy.

Abscesses

Ultrasound can be of value in analyzing what is thought to be an infection. It can reveal an abscess and facilitate its drainage to hasten recovery.

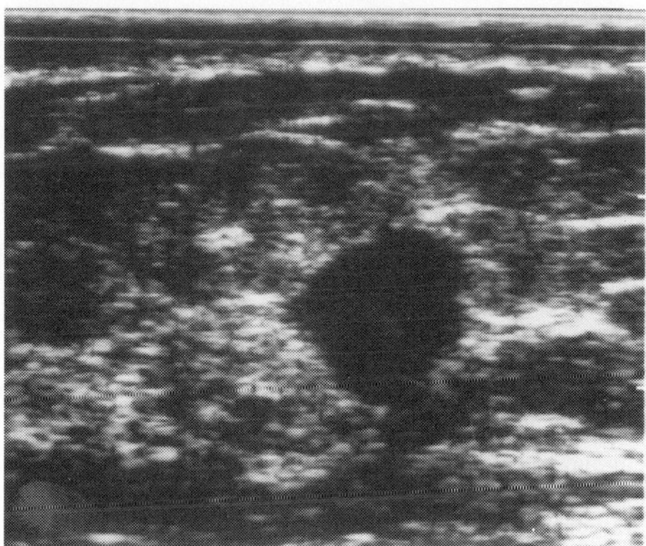

FIG. 15. This hypoechoic mass is an invasive breast cancer that is taller than it is wide. Most benign masses, on the other hand, are wider than they are tall. Unfortunately, there is an overlap, and these are not perfect correlations.

Ultrasound of Implants

Some use ultrasound to evaluate implants for rupture. The importance of discovering a ruptured implant remains controversial. Ultrasound is not as sensitive as MRI for the detection of implant rupture, but the collapse of the silicone rubber implant envelope into the gel may be visible on the mammogram as causing a "stepladder" appearance,[60] or silicone outside the implant may cause a "snowstorm" appearance.[61]

MAGNETIC RESONANCE IMAGING

MRI of the breast is gradually gaining clinical use. MRI is the best method for evaluating implants to determine whether they are ruptured. Although many still believe that MRI for lesion analysis is experimental, some now incorporate MRI into the clinical management of breast lesions using the intravenous administration of gadolinium. The pattern of enhancement, as well as the morphology of a lesion, can be used to try to determine the extent of breast cancer, to search for a primary lesion when metastatic disease has been found, and to detect intramammary recurrence after primary conservation therapy.

The vast majority of invasive ductal cancers demonstrate enhancement after the intravenous administration of gadolinium. Some use the lack of enhancement to reinforce the likelihood that a specific lesion is not an invasive breast cancer. This approach, however, has yet to be demonstrated in sufficiently large, prospective series that include, in particular, small (<1 cm) nonpalpable cancers. Potentially compounding the reliance on MRI to exclude cancer is the fact that normal tissues and a number of benign lesions enhance. A further problem is that ductal carcinoma *in situ* may not always enhance.

Basic Magnetic Resonance Imaging Pulse Sequences

MRI requires dedicated breast coils because these provide a better signal to noise resolution than a body coil. Imaging both breasts simultaneously permits comparison of both sides; however, some coils are designed such that only one breast can be imaged at a time. The imaging is improved if the patient lies in the prone position with the breasts pendent in the coil. The effect of gravity helps to separate the tissues and provides a greater understanding of anatomic relationships than if the patient were lying supine with the breast flattened on the chest wall.

A variety of techniques and pulse sequences have proved useful. One of the simplest sequences includes a T1-weighted gradient echo localizer with a flip angle of 30 degrees, a T2-weighted fast-spin echo sequence. When an implant is being analyzed, we add a T2-weighted fast-spin echo sequence with water suppression.[62] Implant imaging should be performed to enhance the signal from silicone. Because silicone and water have similar signal intensity on T2-weighted imaging, water suppression allows for differentiating cysts and other fluid collections from extruded silicone.

When the breast is being evaluated for cancer, the T1 sequences are repeated after the intravenous administration of gadolinium. The faster the postcontrast scans can be performed, the better. It is the degree and rate of enhancement after the bolus that are most useful for evaluating masses. For most lesions, the enhancement occurs within 1.0 and 1.5 minutes.

This group of sequences is fast, allowing completion of an examination within 30 minutes. Because fat and silicone both have bright signal intensity, fat suppression methods such as inversion recovery or three-point Dixon techniques can be added to decrease the fat signal relative to the silicone for better silicone imaging.[63] Silicone selective pulse sequences have been used[64,65] as well as inversion recovery techniques for fat suppression and a chemical shift selective excitation pulse for water suppression.[12]

Fat suppression is useful when evaluating breast lesions to appreciate tissue enhancement. If fat suppression is not available, then precontrast images must be subtracted from those obtained after contrast to determine what tissues have enhanced. This requires very accurate registration, which is complicated by any patient motion.

Magnetic Resonance Imaging of Breast Implants

It has been estimated that between 1 and 2 million women in the United States have had breast augmentation or reconstruction with silicone gel implants. The FDA blocked the sale of silicone implants as a result of health concerns that had been raised. Despite the fact that large cohort studies have not reported any significant association between silicone implants and connective tissue diseases,[66] concern persists among women about the health effects of these implants. Most now agree that if the detection of an implant rupture is important, MRI is the best method for evaluating silicone gel breast implants when an implant rupture is suspected.

Most implants stimulate the formation of a fibrous capsule around the implant. This capsule can contract, causing the implant to feel hard and distorted. The demonstration of implant rupture by mammography, however, may be difficult, because silicone is highly attenuating and blocks most of the low-energy x-rays used in mammography. Consequently, only the contour of the silicone gel is visible on the mammogram. If a capsule has formed around the implant, the envelope may have completely disintegrated, but the implant appears intact on the mammogram because the gel is contained by the fibrous capsule.

Because MRI is a cross-sectional technique that can differentiate the low signal intensity of the silicone rubber envelope and fibrous capsule from the high signal intensity of the silicone gel, imaging of these structures is possible. As a consequence of this capability, MRI has been shown to be able to diagnose many ruptures. Although ultrasound has been used for implant imaging,[67] the overall anatomic and structural detail provided by MRI appears to be superior to that of ultrasound for implant evaluation.[68]

Because of the ongoing concern about the safety of silicone implants, only saline-filled implants have been available for aesthetic augmentation since April 1992.[69] However, silicone implants are available for patients with a certified medical need who are enrolled in clinical trials. Silicone implants are also allowed for patients with temporary expanders who are awaiting permanent placement, those patients who are undergoing reconstructive surgery at the time of mastectomy, and those patients with ruptured implants that need replacement.

Normal implants usually have a smooth implant/tissue interface on MRI. The silicone rubber envelope and reactive fibrous capsule around the implant envelope produce a low signal intensity band surrounding the implant. Undulations of the implant contour are common due to normal, surrounding tissue pressures. Without other MR abnormalities, and without gross asymmetry between the two sides, these are not considered abnormal. Some implants (especially those with a polyurethane coating and often with saline implants) have linear and curvilinear, low signal intensity structures that protrude into the gel or saline from the surface in a radial fashion. These "radial folds" are merely creases in the implant envelope due to tissue pressure or contraction of the fibrous capsule. They appear as low signal intensity linear bands extending from the periphery of the implant into the gel or saline.

Silicone shows the lowest signal intensity on T1-weighted images because of its long T1 value and appears bright on T2-weighted images because of its long T2 value. Fat can be distinguished due to its relatively shorter T1 value (high signal intensity on T1-weighted images) and longer T2 value. Breast parenchyma is of intermediate signal intensity on both T1- and T2-weighted images, and muscle has intermediate signal intensity on T1-weighted images and low signal intensity on T2-weighted images.

The complications involving breast implants are varied (Fig. 16). An *intracapsular rupture* is defined as a disruption of the implant envelope with the implant contents contained by the surrounding fibrous capsule. As noted earlier in this section, the fibrous capsule may become discontinuous, allowing protrusion of the implant through the opening with an intact implant envelope, resulting in herniation. If both the fibrous capsule and implant envelope are disrupted, free silicone gel extrudes into the surrounding tissue, termed an *extracapsular rupture*.

Postoperative complications after implantation are fairly common. In a study of 749 women, 27.8% underwent "implant-related" surgery over a mean follow-up period of 7.8 years.[70] The most common problem, found in 15% of the women, was capsular contracture. Ruptured implants occurred in 3.9%. A number of problems occur early after implantation and include hematomas and abscess formation. In capsular contraction, myofibroblasts may be responsible for pain and capsule formation, which can produce a hard implant. However, because there are no proven correlates of capsular contracture on imaging, the diagnosis remains a clinical one.

The MR appearance of intracapsular rupture was described by Gorczyca et al.[71] The ruptured silicone envelope sinks into the gel and is seen on the MR image as a fine, serpentine, low signal intensity linear band within the silicone gel. In cross section, it has been thought to look like a piece of pasta weaving back and forth on a plate and was termed the *linguine sign*. Others call it the *fallen envelope sign*[72,73] (Fig. 17). In an intracapsular rupture, the implant gel is held in place by the fibrous capsule, which may or may not be identified on the MR images. The MRI of extracapsular rupture includes globules of silicone outside the expected location of the implant either separate or contiguous with the implant. Without an associated fallen envelope and where the protruding silicone surface is continuous with the implant, herniation may remain difficult to distinguish from extracapsular rupture. The linguine sign represents the best evidence of a ruptured implant. Several series show a high correlation of the linguine sign with rupture, reporting 76% to 94% sensitivities (predictive of rupture) and 97% to 100% specificities (no rupture when the sign is not present).[74–76]

In addition to implant analysis, other specific uses for breast MRI are emerging. These include staging of local disease by determining the extent of tumor involvement and evaluation of women who have already been treated for can-

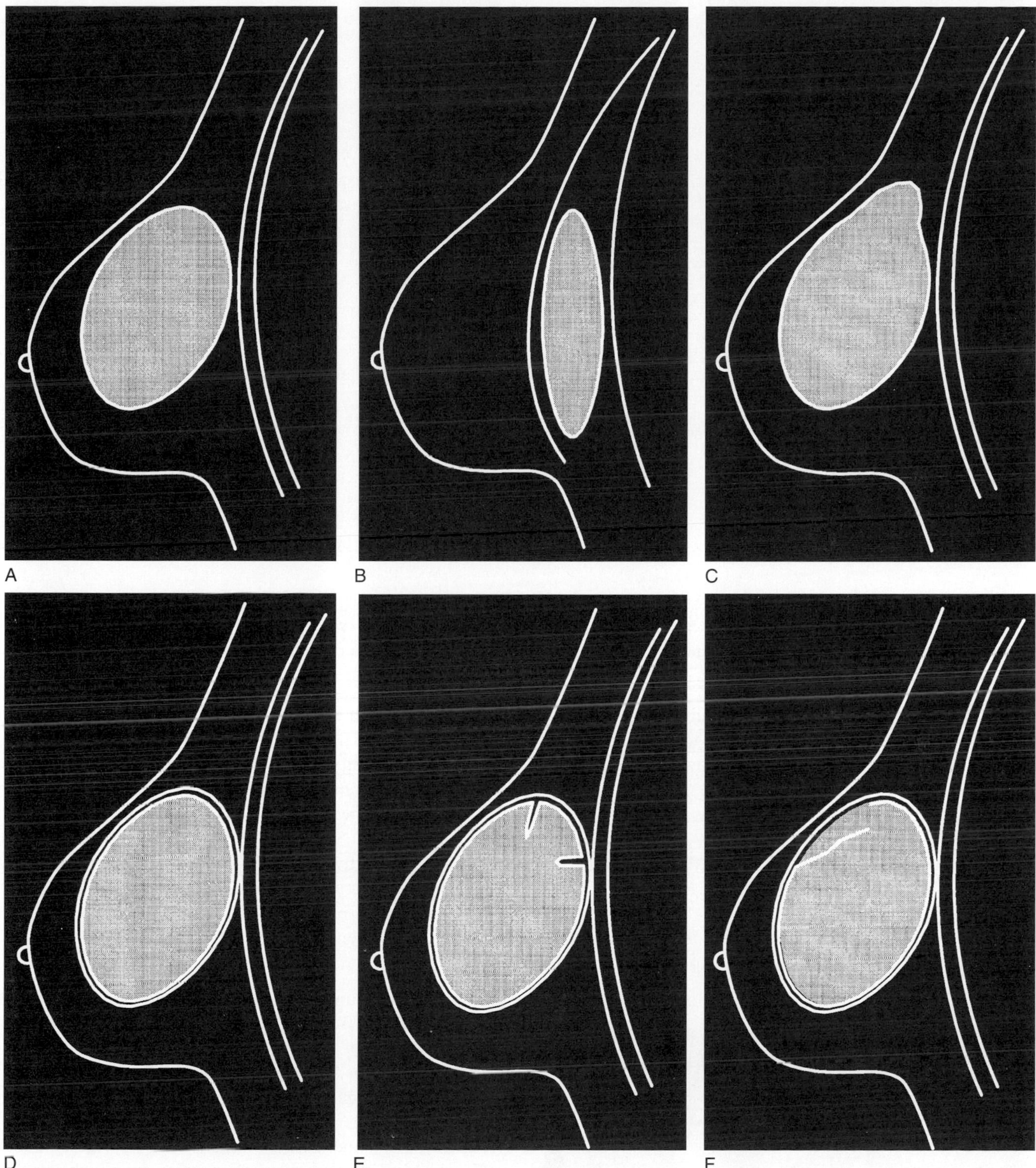

FIG. 16. Schematics representing some of the variations that can occur with silicone implants. **A:** Implant that is in front of the pectoralis major muscle. **B:** Implant that is in a retropectoral location. **C:** Implant is bulging, but its envelope is intact. **D:** Most implants develop a fibrous capsule that surrounds them. **E:** Because implants are patulous, normal tissue pressures can cause folds to form. **F:** If the fibrous capsule is intact, a ruptured implant may not be apparent by mammography, which only shows the shadow caused by the silicone gel. (*continued*)

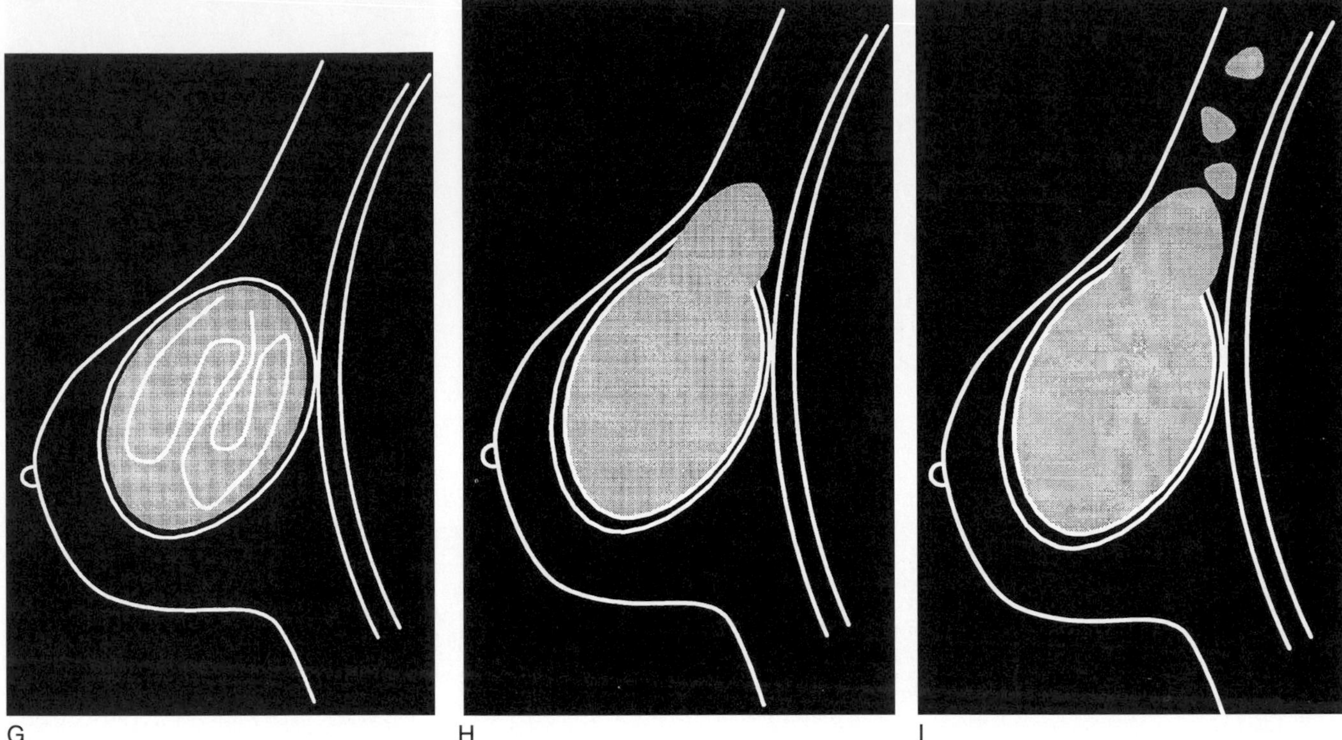

FIG. 16. *Continued* **G:** The ruptured silicone envelope may sink into the gel and look like a piece of pasta on cross-sectional imaging such as magnetic resonance imaging. This has been termed the *linguine sign.* **H:** Free silicone may preserve a smooth contour yet bulge through a torn envelope and capsule. **I:** A rupture is apparent when free silicone can be seen in the soft tissues.

cer in an effort to detect local tumor recurrence in the postsurgical scar site.[77–81] MRI also appears to be the best way to detect an occult primary breast cancer when a patient presents with metastatic disease.

USING MAGNETIC RESONANCE IMAGING TO DETERMINE THE EXTENT OF A CANCER

MRI appears to be the most effective imaging technique for demonstrating additional occult foci of breast cancer in a breast in which a cancer has been detected. Some have begun to use MRI to establish the extent of the lesion for treatment planning. This becomes somewhat more difficult in that benign lesions may also enhance, and, although sensitivity is high, specificity of MRI is moderate to low using just enhancement. Separating true positive foci of cancer from falsely positive tissue is problematic. Efforts to measure the time course of tissue enhancement have had variable results, but breast cancer appears to enhance more rapidly than do benign lesions.

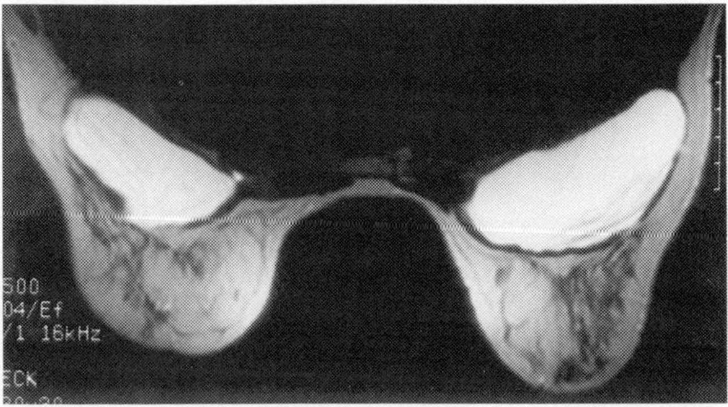

FIG. 17. The curvilinear low signal intensity structures in the bright silicone gel are the ruptured envelopes that have collapsed into the gel.

Magnetic Resonance Enhancement Behavior of Breast Lesions: Telling Benign from Malignant

There has been a great deal of interest in using MRI to differentiate benign lesions from malignant. Almost all invasive malignancies enhance with gadolinium (Gd)-DTPA (Fig. 18), and some research has shown that, with dynamic MR imaging techniques, malignancies may enhance at much more rapid initial rates than benign lesions.[82–88] This rapid initial enhancement rate of malignancies is likely due to tumor angiogenesis. Malignant lesions are known to require the recruitment of a large concentration of tumor neovessels to permit their continued growth beyond a few millimeters.[89] New vessels recruited by the tumors also have abnormal basement membranes. This results in vessel leakiness and an increase in surrounding interstitial fluid pres-

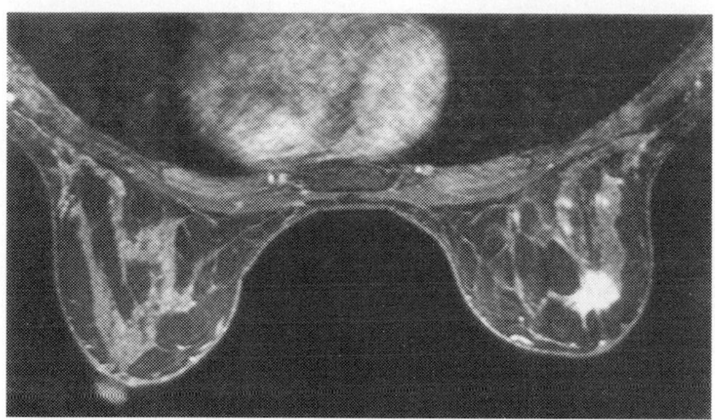

FIG. 18. Invasive ductal carcinoma in the right breast shows marked enhancement on this T1-weighted image after the infusion of gadolinium.

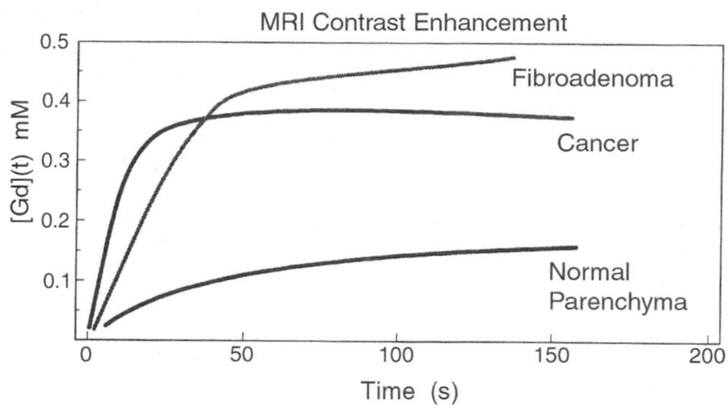

FIG. 19. As portrayed schematically, many cancers enhance rapidly after a bolus injection of gadolinium. Some benign lesions also enhance, but their pattern of enhancement usually differs from that of cancer. MRI, magnetic resonance imaging.

sure.[90] The increased concentration of vessels at the tumor site and their leakiness likely account for the rapid accumulation of Gd-DTPA in breast cancers. Some benign breast lesions also enhance with Gd-DTPA. This may also be due to higher vascularity, although whether the enhancement is due to increased concentrations of neovessels or large feeding vessels in some benign entities is not clear. The initial enhancement rate (within the first minute) is usually less rapid in benign diagnoses than in malignancies, offering the opportunity of distinguishing benign lesions from malignant by their enhancement pattern[91–97] (Fig. 19). It is important to note that if MR imaging is delayed and scanning begins even only minutes after the injection of Gd-DTPA, some benign lesions will show a higher signal intensity than malignant lesions. It is not the absolute enhancement that may permit separation of benign from malignant lesions but the dynamics of the enhancement. It should be remembered that if the goal is to use MRI to differentiate benign from malignant lesions, the analysis of the enhancement soon after injection of the contrast appears to be critical.

Some investigators have disputed the consistency of early dynamic MR in distinguishing benign from malignant lesions, as several benign lesions demonstrated a more rapid rate of enhancement than expected.[98–101] Furthermore, several invasive cancers, including several infiltrating lobular carcinomas, two malignant phylloides tumors, one tubular carcinoma, and colloid and mucinous carcinomas, have been reported as having slow enhancement profiles.[102–106] Although differences in vessel density may be the explanation for such variation, studies correlating low vessel density with slow enhancement of certain cancer cell types have not been performed. However, pathologic studies have shown a low expression of endothelial growth factor receptor messenger RNAs in infiltrating lobular carcinomas (as opposed to strong expression in invasive ductal carcinomas), which may account for decreased vascularity of this cell type.[107]

Some of these variations in enhancement may also be the result of the MR technique used to calculate enhancement. If conventional techniques are used and simple change in enhancement (or percent enhancement) from pre- and post-contrast scans are calculated, an overlap in benign and malignant values may result, as this method does not account for the varying baseline of the T1 values of benign and malignant lesions before injection (the reason that MR could not distinguish benign from malignant lesions without Gd-DTPA). For example, a lesion with a longer baseline T1 value would show greater relative enhancement than a lesion with a shorter baseline T1 value at 1 minute, even though the concentration of Gd-DTPA within the first lesion (longer T1) may be less than the concentration of Gd-DTPA in the second lesion (shorter T1). As some benign lesions have longer initial T1 values than cancers, this baseline T1 variation may explain the overlap described by some researchers. Improved techniques for estimating the actual concentration of Gd-DTPA in lesions and accounting for baseline T1 values, as well as correlation with vessel density, are under investigation.[108–110]

Some authors report that the morphology of the lesion and its pattern of enhancement may permit the separation of benign from malignant processes.[111–115] As has been shown by mammography and ultrasound, cancers demonstrate more irregularly shaped borders than do benign tumors. However, because neither mammography nor ultrasound has been able to differentiate many lesions morphologically with sufficient accuracy to avoid a tissue diagnosis, it is unlikely that MRI will be any more successful. Nevertheless, morphologic studies using MRI bear careful evaluation, because MRI provides cross-sectional morphology, which, combined with enhancement dynamics, may improve its accuracy. Numes et al. constructed a flow chart model to try to use these enhancement and architectural characteristics to differentiate benign lesions from malignant.[116] They used the results from 98 cases to produce the model and then tested it on 94 different cases. They found that a lesion was likely to be cancer, primarily, if it enhanced. A high degree of enhancement, an irregular pattern of enhancement, irregular borders, and the lack of any internal septations were associated with malignancy. Cancer was very unlikely if the lesion was not visible after gadolinium infusion, if its borders were smooth or lobulated, or if the mass was regular in shape or it had nonenhancing internal septations.

The early results from trials are frequently the most successful. More work is necessary in applying patterns of enhancement shape, rate, or combination of MR data with mammography and sonography before benign and malignant lesions can be distinguished with sufficient accuracy to avoid a safe tissue diagnosis.

Magnetic Resonance Imaging and Ductal Carcinoma *In Situ*

The MR behavior of DCIS is less clear, as enhancement varies from a rapid rate to no enhancement. This variation in enhancement behavior may be due to the variation of neovessel recruitment in DCIS. Despite the fact that these are intraductal lesions, some DCIS can stimulate neovascularity.[117,118] Soderstrom et al. suggest that virtually all DCIS can be detected.[119] Others have not been as successful, because some cases of DCIS do not appear to enhance. In a review of 13 patients with pure DCIS, Orel et al.[120] were able to identify ten of the lesions on MRI scans. In six cases, curvilinear enhancement was termed *ductal*. In three of the cases there was segmental or "regional" enhancement, and in one case the enhancement was termed *peripheral*. Three lesions were not evident on their scans, and two other lesions were not identified in six additional patients who had both invasive and intraductal cancer.[120] Giles et al.[121] evaluated 36 women with DCIS and contrast enhancement evaluation using the subtraction technique. They were able to identify 34 of the lesions but failed to demonstrate two cases of comedocarcinoma. One problem that complicates some of the studies is the fact that there is a difference between knowing where DCIS was found, histologically, and "finding" it on an imaging study versus identifying the lesion prospectively and having it confirmed by the imaging.

The ability of MRI to detect DCIS, particularly poorly differentiated DCIS, is important. Not only do these lesions tend to progress to invasion sooner, but it is also critical for assessing the extent of the cancer. If DCIS is not recognized extending away from a primary invasive tumor, then excision, or even destroying the primary tumor *in vivo* (e.g., laser, cryotherapy, high-frequency ultrasound), will be likely to fail to achieve local control because residual, undetected (and hence untreated) tumor will lead to high recurrence rates.

Specific Applications of Breast Magnetic Resonance Lesion Imaging

The roles for MR in evaluating breast lesions are being defined. The ability to distinguish benign from malignant lesions on the basis of their dynamic enhancement pattern or their morphologic characteristics, or both, using the variety of techniques discussed previously remains under investigation in the United States.

MR imaging is already being used by some in the following specific areas:

1. Tumor staging to determine the extent of disease within the breast, which is important in permitting complete excision or tumor destruction if conservation therapy is chosen.
2. The differentiation of scar from cancer recurrence. Sometimes, a patient who has undergone lumpectomy or radiation therapy, or both, for cancer may later present with a suspicious mammogram or physical examination in the region of prior surgery. Some of these patients undergo reexcision of the scar due to the concern for local recurrence, although local recurrence only occurs in 1% of such patients each year.[122] MRI may be useful in distinguishing scar tissue from local recurrence at the specified postoperative time interval. Although immediately after surgery and during the course of radiation therapy, a high density of new vessels from wound healing can result in enhancement on MR imaging, recent small series have suggested that scar tissue does not enhance with Gd-DTPA on MR. Dao et al. have suggested that MR imaging can be used to follow up women treated conservatively with excision and irradiation.[123] Areas of surgery frequently enhance if they are studied within 6 to 12 months after treatment. After that period of healing, fixed fibrosis does not enhance, but recurrent breast cancer frequently does.[124] If any enhancement is visualized in a scar older than 12 months, the possibility of recurrence increases. Although the early detection of recurrence in the breast may have useful therapeutic value, it has yet to be shown that detecting recurrences earlier alters mortality. Nevertheless, in the absence of data, early detection of recurrent breast cancer would seem to be a good idea.

Chest wall imaging, searching for a primary malignancy, and following the response of breast cancers to chemotherapy are other areas in which some find MR imaging of the breast to be useful. As noted earlier, we and others have found MR imaging to also be useful in searching for a primary breast cancer in patients with metastatic disease of unknown origin or in those with axillary adenopathy that is highly suspicious for a breast malignancy.

The evaluation of local tumor response to chemotherapy with MR breast imaging may also provide useful information to oncologists or surgeons who are employing neoadjuvant chemotherapy and wish to monitor tumor response.

Magnetic Resonance Imaging as a Possible Second-Level Screen

Another possibility, which has yet to be proved, is the use of MRI to detect breast cancer in asymptomatic, healthy-appearing women with negative mammograms. We have found a surprising number of mammographically and clinically occult synchronous breast cancers in the contralateral breasts of women with breast cancer detected only by MRI (4 of 17).

In addition, among eight women who presented with metastatic disease, six had their clinically and mammographically occult breast cancers detected by MRI. These anecdotal cases suggest the possibility of MRI as a second-level screening technology that may be able to detect early cancers that, at present, are mammographically as well as clinically occult.

Despite the fact that the experience with contrast-enhanced MRI of the breast has greatly increased, many of the data are anecdotal. The lack of large prospective studies to define scientifically the efficacy of MRI in breast evaluation has kept it largely as a research tool. The cost of the study and limited access to the magnets have greatly slowed the research. Before MRI can be applied to screening, much work is needed to validate its efficacy.

NUCLEAR MEDICINE BREAST IMAGING: TECHNETIUM 99M SESTAMIBI

Interest has been raised in the use of radionuclides for evaluating breast lesions. Tracers that were originally developed for myocardial imaging have been found to concentrate in many breast malignancies. Thallium-201 has been used to image some breast malignancies. More recently, the myocardial imaging tracer, technetium 99m sestamibi, has been found to have similar properties as thallium and to concentrate in some breast cancers.

Based on preliminary observations, a large nonblinded evaluation of sestamibi was undertaken that culminated in its approval for breast imaging by the FDA under the trade name *Miraluma*. One review of sestamibi included 387 women and 3 men[125] who were evaluated for mammographically or clinically detected abnormalities. Included in the study were 182 palpable abnormalities, 222 nonpalpable lesions, and 20 "normal" volunteers. The smallest mass was 8 mm. The patients received 20 mCi technetium 99m sestamibi intravenously by hand injection. The breasts were imaged sequentially from the lateral side while the patient lay prone with the breast imaged while pendent and as close to the camera as possible. Five minutes after the injection, the breast was imaged for 10 minutes. The investigators considered a focal area of uptake as significant. Mild diffuse uptake or none at all was negative. The authors report that the scans correctly identified 90% of the cancers with a 3% false-negative rate and a 7% false-positive rate.

Our own evaluation of sestamibi was less encouraging.[126] We evaluated a group of 31 patients with lesions detected only by mammography (nonpalpable). The lesions consisted of 14 groups of calcifications, 12 masses, and five areas of architectural distortion. There were seven malignancies and 24 benign lesions. The sensitivity of the sestamibi was only 29%, with a specificity of 83%. Three invasive cancers and two cases of DCIS were falsely negative, and there were four falsely positive scans. These results raise serious doubts concerning the efficacy of the tracer for evaluating nonpalpable early lesions.

The agent appears to delineate cancers in two ways. Circulating in the blood, it is likely more concentrated where there is a high density of blood vessels, such as the neovascularity that develops in many cancers. This is similar to the early enhancement of cancers that is seen after the intravenous administration of iodinated contrast and the enhancement by gadolinium on MRI. It also appears that there is some active uptake by the mitochondria of the cells.

Although sestamibi has FDA approval, its role in breast evaluation has yet to be defined. There are no data to support its use for screening. Use of the agent for axillary staging has not been studied in any rigorous fashion. Because it cannot be used to differentiate benign lesions from malignant, its efficacy remains to be defined.

POSITRON EMISSION TOMOGRAPHIC SCANNING

PET requires highly specialized equipment. Early results suggest that breast cancers have elevated metabolic activity. This can be detected through the use of fluorine 18–labeled glucose (FDG).[127] Preliminary information suggests that PET may be a method for staging breast cancers by assessing the axillary nodal status and possible distant metastatic spread. PET may also be valuable in assessing the possibility of recurrence after breast cancer treatment. Large trials are necessary to establish any efficacy in the screening of asymptomatic women for breast cancer. This application for PET will likely be limited by the requirement for the injection of radioactive material, which is difficult to produce because it must be made using a cyclotron. Investigators are considering the possibility of using FDG with single photon emission computed tomography scanning to take advantage of the metabolism of FDG without the need for an expensive PET scanner.

The risk from present-day tracers is greatest for the bladder due to clearance in the urine. This will likely limit the usefulness of PET to older women.

PET scanning offers the opportunity to not only determine whether a lesion is benign or malignant but also to assess some metabolic parameters that might be of prognostic value by their use or by incorporation of the labeled molecule. The isotopes that are used, however, are very short lived and must be produced by an on-site accelerator, increasing the cost of performing PET studies.

Glucose labeled with fluorine 18 to form 2-[fluorine 18]-fluoro-2-deoxy-D-glucose (FDG) is one of the more widely studied molecules. This agent has been used to demonstrate lesions that are metabolically active and have an increased use of glucose. Early results suggest that many breast cancers have elevated metabolic activity that can be detected through the use of FDG. Wahl et al. found increased uptake in ten out of ten primary breast cancers.[127] Adler et al. studied 28 women with 35 masses that were larger than 1 cm and found increased uptake in 26 of the 27 malignant lesions (sensitivity of 96%), with no false-positive scans (specificity of 100%).[128] These authors were also able to identify increased activity in the axillae in nine of the ten women who were shown to have positive axillary nodes.

The evaluation of PET for breast imaging has, thus far, been limited. This is in part due to limited access to scanners and the need for agents with short half-lives that must be generated by a nearby cyclotron. It remains to be seen whether PET will be accepted as a diagnostic technique to differentiate benign from malignant lesions to obviate the need for needle or open biopsy.

The few studies that have been published have used PET to image large cancers. Its ability to evaluate small cancers is questionable. Although our own experience is very limited, we have already seen a 7-mm invasive breast cancer that was not evident on the PET scan.

Adler et al.[128] compared the normalized activity of the lesions with the nuclear grade of the cancers, and their data indicate that higher-grade (poorly differentiated) lesions exhibit greater activity. This suggests that PET may be useful as a prognostic test.

EVALUATION OF PALPABLE AND NONPALPABLE FINDINGS

It is often overlooked that mammography is primarily a screening test. Its major value is in the detection of cancers that are not clinically evident. If a patient has a sign or symptom of breast cancer, a negative mammogram does not mean that the patient does not have breast cancer, and the clinical abnormality needs to be satisfactorily resolved.

The evaluation of a patient who has a palpable abnormality is initially determined by her age. A woman in her late teens or early 20s who has a palpable mass that is freely moveable and has definable margins on clinical examination has a benign fibroadenoma. Other histologies are possible but extremely rare. Even cysts, which become increasingly common with increasing age, are extremely rare in women younger than age 25 to 30. Only 2% of the women of this age group who are referred to us for imaging have a cyst (presumably, some others had aspirations and were not referred). Breast cancer occurs but is so uncommon in women younger than age 25 that it is not a serious consideration. As the age of the individual increases, however, the possibility of breast cancer increases. Because breast cancer begins to appear in women in their late 20s, and because many of these cancers are visible by mammography,[129] we recommend a mammogram for anyone in her late 20s or older who has a sign or symptom. The reader should be aware of the fact that the efficacy of mammography, in terms of lives saved, has not been shown for anyone younger than age 40, because younger women were not included in the randomized controlled trials of screening. However, the results of mammography may influence the management of the problem[130] and is primarily useful to search for unexpected cancer elsewhere in the same breast or in the contralateral breast.[131]

If a palpable abnormality feels like a possible cyst, the most expeditious and cost-effective management is to insert a needle and aspirate it. This has the advantage of making the diagnosis and eliminating the mass in a single step. It is usually less expensive than ultrasound. For some reason, clinically guided aspiration is being used less and less, and most women with a "lump" are now sent for ultrasound. If the individual's age is appropriate, we would first obtain a mammogram to be sure that no other area needed ultrasound evaluation. If the ultrasound demonstrates a simple cyst, then no further evaluation is needed. If the lesion is solid, many believe that a biopsy is indicated (either imaging or clinically guided needle biopsy or excisional biopsy). Some rely on the ultrasound characteristics of the mass. If the lesion is well defined, with its long axis parallel to the skin with smooth or smoothly lobulated margins, a uniform echo texture, and an echogenic pseudocapsule, and is good or enhanced through transmission of sound, the likelihood of a benign lesion (fibroadenoma) is very high. The younger the woman, the more often this is true (on a statistical basis alone). Many now merely follow these lesions. (One problem with this approach is that whenever these women change doctors, many are reevaluated.) There are no prospective studies in which the ultrasound evaluation has been blinded to provide accurate measures of the safety of this approach, but it is becoming increasingly common.

Mammography is usually only valuable if it demonstrates a finding. If a palpable lesion is not visible by mammography the clinician must decide its significance based on the clinical assessment. A negative mammogram should rarely influence the decision as to whether to intervene unless it clearly demonstrates a benign lesion, such as a fat-containing mass (lipoma, hamartoma, oil cyst) or a calcified involuting fibroadenoma.

When a lesion has been detected mammographically, the evaluation should be guided by the radiologist. A number of alternatives are dictated by the findings. Most abnormalities prove to be of no consequence. This can frequently be determined by a few additional mammographic projections. Special magnification mammograms are obtained to provide a clearer view of the findings and are especially useful for the evaluation of calcifications. If calcifications are being evaluated, at least one of the images should be a horizontal beam lateral magnification view, because this can show that the deposits are benign milk of calcium.

If the mammographic finding is a possible mass, then ultrasound is useful. If the mass is a simple cyst by ultrasound, then no further evaluation is needed. If it is solid, then biopsy should be considered. The same ultrasound characteristics of lesions that are probably benign apply, as noted previously.

If the lesion does warrant a biopsy, then the radiologist must determine the best approach. If it is visible by ultrasound, then ultrasound-guided needle biopsy may be possible. If x-ray imaging is needed, and the lesion is "targetable," then stereotactically guided biopsy can be used. Needle localization and excisional biopsy are always options. Although the latter is more expensive and traumatic, if performed properly, it is the most accurate method for diagnosing an occult breast cancer.

Some are beginning to use MRI to assist in management. If a lesion proves to be cancer, MRI can better define its extent than another imaging modality. The actual value of MRI for patient management, however, is unproven. If a lesion shows no enhancement after intravenous contrast administration, then it is very unlikely to be a breast cancer. This has never been tested in a prospective fashion, however, and most tissues show some enhancement; therefore, the value of MRI remains unproven.

In general, if a lesion does not have benign characteristics, a tissue diagnosis (needle biopsy or excision) is usually indicated. The results of the biopsy should be concordant with the expectations from the imaging and clinical evaluation. If they are not, then rebiopsy will likely be needed.

REFERENCES

1. Shapiro S. Screening: assessment of current studies. *Cancer* 1994;74: 231–238.
2. Kopans DB. The breast cancer screening controversy: lessons to be learned. *J Surg Oncol* 1998;67:143–150.
3. Kopans DB, Moore RH, McCarthy KA, Hall DA, Hulka C, Whitman GJ, Slanetz PJ, Halpern EF. Biasing the interpretation of mammography screening data by age grouping: nothing changes abruptly at age 50. *The Breast Journal* 1998;4:139–145.
4. Hendrick RE, Smith RA, Rutledge JH, Smart CR. Benefit of screening mammography in women ages 40–49: a new meta-analysis of randomized controlled trials. *J Natl Cancer Inst Monogr* 1997;22:87–92.
5. Moskowitz M. Screening is not diagnosis. *Radiology* 1979;133:265–268.
6. Sickles EA. Periodic mammographic follow-up of probably benign lesions: results of 3184 consecutive cases. *Radiology* 1991;179: 463–468.
7. Shapiro S, Venet W, Strax P, Venet L. *Periodic screening for breast cancer: the Health Insurance Plan Project and its sequelae, 1963–1986*. Baltimore: The Johns Hopkins University Press, 1988.
8. Baker LH. Breast cancer detection demonstration project. five-year summary report. *CA Cancer J Clin* 1982;32(4):194–225.
9. Sickles EA, Weber WN, Galvin HB, Ominsky SH, Sollitto RA. Mammographic screening: how to operate successfully at low cost. *Radiology* 1986;160:95–97.
10. Bird RE, McLelland R. How to initiate and operate a low–cost screening mammography center. *Radiology* 1986;161:43–47.
11. Revesz G, Kundel HL. Psychophysical studies of detection errors in chest radiology. *Radiology* 1977;123:559–562.
12. Bird RE. Professional quality assurance for mammographic screening programs. *Radiology* 1990;177:587.
13. Tabar L, Fagerberg G, Duffy S, Day N, Gad A, Grontoft O. Update of the Swedish two-county program of mammographic screening for breast cancer. *Radiol Clin N Am* 1992;30:187–210.
14. Thurfjell EL, Lernevall KA, Taube AAS. Benefit of independent double reading in a population-based mammography screening program. *Radiology* 1994;191:241–244.
15. Elmore JG, Wells CK, Lee CH, Howard DH, Feinstein AR. Variability in radiologists' interpretations of mammograms. *N Engl J Med* 1994;331:1493–1499.
16. Kopans DB. The accuracy of mammographic interpretation. *N Engl J Med* 1994;331:1521–1522.
17. Sickles EA, Ominsky SH, Sollitto RA, Galvin HB, Monticciolo DL. Medical audit of a rapid-throughput mammography screening practice: methodology and results of 27,114 examinations. *Radiology* 1990;175:323–327.
18. Kopans DB. Breast imaging and the "standard of care" for the "symptomatic" patient. *Radiology* 1993;187:608–611.
19. Meyer JE, Kopans DB. Analysis of mammographically obvious breast carcinomas with benign results on initial biopsy. *Surg Gynecol Obstet* 1981;153:570–572.
20. Kopans DB, Meyer JE, Cohen AM, Wood WC. Palpable breast masses: the importance of preoperative mammography. *JAMA* 1981;246:2819–2822.
21. Kopans DB. *Breast imaging*, 2nd ed. Philadelphia: Lippincott–Raven, 1997.
22. Swann CA, Kopans DB, McCarthy KA, White G, Hall DA. Localization of occult breast lesions: practical solutions to problems of triangulation. *Radiology* 1987;163:577–579.
23. Kopans DB, Meyer JE, Lindfors KK, Bucchianeri SS. Breast sonography to guide aspiration of cysts and preoperative localization of occult breast lesions. *AJR Am J Roentgenol* 1984;143:489–492.
24. Kopans DB, Meyer JE. Computed tomography guided localization of clinically occult breast carcinoma: the "N" skin guide. *Radiology* 1982;145:211–212
25. D'Orsi CJ, Kopans DB. Mammographic feature analysis. *Semin Roentgenol* 1993;28:204–230.
26. Sadowsky NL, Semine A, Harris JR. Breast imaging: a critical aspect of breast conserving treatment. *Cancer* 1990;65(9):2113–2118.
27. Carter CL, Allen C, Henson DE. Relation of tumor size, lymph node status, and survival in 24,740 breast cancer cases. *Cancer* 1989;63:181–187.
28. Rosen PP, Groshen PE, Kinne DW, Hellman S. A long-term follow-up study of survival in stage I (T1N0M0) and stage II (T1N1M0) breast carcinoma. *J Clin Oncol* 1989;7:355–366.
29. Gallager HS, Martin JE. Early phases in the development of breast cancer. *CA Cancer J Clin* 1969;24(6):1170 1178.
30. Fisher B, Slack NH, Bross IDJ, et al. Cancer of the breast: size of neoplasm and prognosis. *Cancer* 1969;24:1071–1080.
31. Tabar L, Duffy SW, Krusemo UB. Detection method, tumour size and node metastases in breast cancers diagnosed during a trial of breast cancer screening. *Eur J Cancer Clin Oncol* 1987;23(7):959–962.
32. Rosner D, Lane WW. Node-negative minimal invasive breast cancer patients are not candidates for routine systemic adjuvant therapy. *Cancer* 1990;66:199–205,
33. Sickles EA, Herzog KA. Mammography of the postsurgical breast. *AJR Am J Roentgenol* 1981;136:585–588.
34. Bassett LW, Gold RH, Cove HC. Mammographic spectrum of traumatic fat necrosis: the fallibility of "pathognomonic" signs of carcinoma. *AJR Am J Roentgenol* 1978;130:119–122.
35. Mitnick JS, Vazquez MF, Harris MN, Roses DF. Differentiation of radial scar from scirrhous carcinoma of the breast: mammographic-pathologic correlation. *Radiology* 1989;173:697–700.
36. Kopans DB, Meyer JE, Homer MJ, Grabbe J. Dermal deposits mistaken for breast calcifications. *Radiology* 1983;149:592–594.
37. Egan RL, McSweency MB, Sewell CW. Intrammary calcifications without an associated mass in benign and malignant diseases. *Radiology* 1980;137:1–7.
38. Kopans DB. *Breast imaging*. Philadelphia: JB Lippincott, 1989.
39. Sickles EA, Abele JS. Milk of calcium within tiny benign breast cysts. *Radiology* 1981;141:655–658.
40. Levitan LH, Witten DM, Harrison KG. Calcification in breast disease: mammographic-pathologic correlation. *Radiology* 1964;92(1):29–39.
41. Mayr NA, Staples JJ, Robinson RA, Vanmetre JE, Hussey DH. Morphometric studies in intraductal breast carcinoma using computerized image analysis. *Cancer* 1991;67:2805–2812.
42. Holland R, Hendriks JHCL, Verbeck ALM, Mravunac M, Schuurmans, Stekhoven JH. Extent, distribution, and mammographic/histological correlations of breast ductal carcinoma in situ. *Lancet* 1990;335:519–522.
43. Swann CA, Kopans DB, McCarthy KA, White G, Hall DA. Practical solutions to problems of triangulation and preoperative localization of breast lesions. *Radiology* 1987;163:577–579.

44. Kopans DB, Meyer JE, Lindfors KK. Whole breast ultrasound imaging: four year follow up. *Radiology* 1985;157:505–507.
45. Gordon PB, Goldenberg SL. Malignant breast masses detected only by ultrasound: a retrospective review. *Cancer* 1995;76:626–630.
46. Kolb TM, Lichy J, Newhouse JH. Occult cancer in women with dense breasts: detection with screening US—diagnostic yield and tumor characteristics. *Radiology* 1998;207:191–199.
47. Stavros AT, Thickman D, Rapp CL, Dennis MA, Parker SH, Sisney GA. Solid breast nodules: use of sonography to distinguish between benign and malignant lesions. *Radiology* 1995;196:123–134.
48. Skaane P, Engedal K. Analysis of sonographic features in the differentiation of fibroadenoma and invasive ductal carcinoma. *AJR Am J Roentgenol* 1998;170:109–114.
49. Fornage BD, Lorigan JG, Andry E. Fibroadenoma of the Breast: Sonographic Appearance. *Radiology* 1989;172:671–675.
50. Cosgrove DO, Bamber JC, Davey JB, McKinna JA, Sinnett HD. Color doppler signals from breast tumors. *Radiology* 1990;176: 175–180.
51. Schoenberger SG, Sutherland CM, Robinson AK. Breast neoplasms: duplex sonographic imaging as as adjunct in diagnosis. *Radiology* 1988;168:665–668.
52. Adler DD, Carson PL, Rubin JM, Quinn-Reid D. Doppler ultrasound color flow imaging in the study of breast cancer: preliminary findings. *Ultrasound Med Biol* 1990;16:553–559.
53. Cosgrove DO, Kedar RP, Bamber JC, et al. Breast diseases: color doppler US in differential diagnosis. *Radiology* 1993;189:99–104.
54. Dock W. Duplex sonography of mammary tumors: a prospective study of 75 patients. *J Ultrasound Med* 1993;2:79–82.
55. Dixon JM, Walsh J, Paterson D, Chetty U. Colour doppler ultrasonography studies of benign and malignant breast lesions. *Br J Surg* 1992;79:259–260.
56. Bassett LW, Kimme-Smith C. Breast sonography. *AJR Am J Roentgenol* 1991;449–455.
57. Jackson VP. The role of US in breast imaging. *Radiology* 1990;177:305–311.
58. Fornage BD, Faroux MJ, Simatos A. Breast masses: US-guided fineneedle aspiration biopsy. *Radiology* 1987;162:409–414.
59. Fornage BD, Lorigan JG, Andry E. Fibroadenoma of the breast: sonographic appearance. *Radiology* 1989;172:671–675.
60. DeBruhl ND, Gorczyca, Ahn CY, Shaw WW, Bassett LW. Silicone breast implants: US evaluation. *Radiology* 1993;189:95–98.
61. Ganott MA, Harris KM, Ilkhanipour ZS, Costa-Greco MA. Augmentation mammoplasty: normal and abnormal findings with mammography and US. *Radiographics* 1992;12:281–295.
62. Gorczyca DP, Sinha S, Ahn C, et al. Silicone breast implants in vivo: MR imaging. *Radiology* 1992;185:407–410.
63. Gorczyca DP, Schneider E, DeBruhl ND. Silicone breast implant rupture: comparison between three-point Dixon and fast spin-echo MR imaging. *AJR Am J Roentgenol* 1994;162:305–310.
64. Garrido L, Kwong K, Pfleiderer B. Echo-planar chemical shift imaging of silicone gel prostheses. *MRI* 1993;11:625–634.
65. Monticciolo DL, Nelson RC, Dixon WT, Bostwick J, Mukundan S, Hester RT. MR detection of leakage from silicone breast implants: value of a silicone selective pulse sequence. *AJR Am J Roentgenol* 1994;163;51–56.
66. Sanchez-Guerrero J, Colditz GA, Karlson EW, Hunter DJ, Speizer FE, Liang MH. Silicone breast implants and the risk of connective-tissue diseases and symptoms. *N Engl J Med* 1995:332:1666–1670.
67. Harris KM, Ganott MA, Shestak KC, Losken HW, Tobon H. Silicone implant rupture: detection with ultrasound. *Radiology* 1993;187: 761–768.
68. Gorczyca DP, DeBruhl ND, Ahn CY. Silicone breast implant ruptures in an animal model: comparison of mammography, MR imaging, US, and CT. *Radiology* 1994;190:227–232.
69. Kessler, DA. The basis of the FDA's decision on breast implants. *N Engl J Med* 1992:326:1713–1715.
70. Gabriel SE, Woods JE, O'Fallon M, Beard CM, Kurland LT, Melton LJ. Complications leading to surgery after breast implantation. *N Engl J Med* 1997;336:677–682.
71. Gorczyca DP, Sinha S, Ahn C, et al. Silicone breast implants in vivo: MR imaging. *Radiology* 1992;185:407–410.
72. Gylbert L, Asplund O, Jurell G. Capsular contracture after breast reconstruction with silicone and saline-filled implants: a 6-year follow-up. *Plast Reconstr Surg* 1990;85:373–377.
73. Kessler, DA. The basis of the FDA's decision on breast implants. *N Engl J Med* 1992:326:1713–5.
74. Gorczyca DP, Sinha S, Ahn C, et al. Silicone breast implants in vivo: MR imaging. *Radiology* 1992;185:407–410.
75. Gorczyca DP, Schneider E, DeBruhl ND, et al. Silicone breast implant rupture: comparison between three-point Dixon and fast spin-echo MR imaging. *AJR Am J Roentgenol* 1994;162:305–310.
76. Monticciolo DL, Nelson RC, Dixon WT, Bostwick J, Mukundan S, Hester RT. MR detection of leakage from silicone breast implants: value of a silicone selective pulse sequence. *AJR Am J Roentgenol* 1994;163;51–56.
77. Gorczyca DP, Sinha S, Ahn C, et al. Silicone breast implants in vivo: MR imaging. *Radiology* 1992;185:407–410.
78. Orel SG, Schnall MD, Powell CM, et al. Staging of suspected breast cancer: effect of MR imaging and MR-guided biopsy. *Radiology* 1995;196:115–112.
79. Dao TH, Rahmouni A Campana F, Laurent M, Asselain B, Fourquet A. Tumor recurrence versus fibrosis in the irradiated breast: differentiation with dynamic gadolinium-enhanced MR imaging. *Radiology* 1993;187:751–755.
80. Gilles R, Guinebretiere JM, Shapeero LG, et al. Assessment of breast cancer recurrence with contrast enhanced subtraction MR imaging: preliminary results in 26 patients. *Radiology* 1993;188:473–478.
81. Heywang SH, Hilbertz T, Beck R, Bauer WM, Eiermann W, Permanetter W. Gd-DTPA enhanced MR imaging of the breast in patients with postoperative scarring and silicone implants. *J Comput Assist Tomogr* 1990;14:348–356.
82. Kaiser WA, Zeitler E. MR imaging of the breast: fast imaging sequences with and without Gd-DTPA. *Radiology* 1989;170:681–686.
83. Gorczyca DP, Sinha S, Ahn C, et al. Silicone breast implants in vivo: MR imaging. *Radiology* 1992;185:407–410.
84. Dao TH, Rahmouni A, Campana F, Laurent M, Asselain B, Fourquet A. Tumor recurrence versus fibrosis in the irradiated breast: differentiation with dynamic gadolinium-enhanced MR imaging. *Radiology* 1993;187:751–755.
85. Stack JP, Redmond OM, Codd MB, Dervan PA, Ennis JT. Breast disease: tissue characterization with Gd-DTPA enhancement profiles. *Radiology* 1990;174:491–494.
86. Hachiya J, Seki T, Okada M, Nitatori T, Korenaga T, Furuya Y. MR imaging of the breast with Gd-DTPA enhancement: comparison with mammography and ultrasonography. *Radiat Med* 1991;9(6): 232–240.
87. Gilles R, Guinebretiere JM, Lucidarme O, et al. Nonpalpable breast tumors: diagnosis with contrast-enhanced subtraction dynamic MR imaging. *Radiology* 1994;191:625–631.
88. Fobben ES, Rubin CZ, Kalisher L, Dembner AG, Seltzer MH, Santoro EJ. Breast MRI techniques with commercially available techniques: radiologic-pathologic correlation. *Radiology* 1995;196:143–152.
89. Folkman, J. What is the evidence that tumors are angiogenesis dependent? *J Natl Cancer Inst* 1990;82:4–6.
90. Negendank WG, Brown TR, Evelhoch JL, Griffiths JR, Liotta LA, Margulis AR, et al. Proceedings of a national cancer institute workshop: MR spectroscopy and tumor cell biology. *Radiology* 1992;185:875–883.
91. Kaiser WA, Zeitler E. MR imaging of the breast: fast imaging sequences with and without Gd-DTPA. *Radiology* 1989;170:681–686.
92. Gilles R, Guinebretiere JM, Shapeero LG, et al. Assessment of breast cancer recurrence with contrast enhanced subtraction MR imaging: preliminary results in 26 patients. *Radiology* 1993;188:473–478.
93. Dao TH, Rahmouni A Campana F, Laurent M, Asselain B, Fourquet A. Tumor recurrence versus fibrosis in the irradiated breast: differentiation with dynamic gadolinium–enhanced MR imaging. *Radiology* 1993;187:751–755.
94. Cohen MS, Weisskoff RM. Ultra-fast imaging. *MRI* 1991;9:1–37.
95. Hulka CA, Smith BL, Sgroi DC, et al. Benign and malignant breast lesions: differentiation with echo planar imaging. *Radiology* 1995;197:33–38.
96. Kaiser WA, Zeitler E. MR imaging of the breast: fast imaging sequences with and without Gd-DTPA. *Radiology* 1989;170:681–686.
97. Gorczyca DP, Sinha S, Ahn C, et al. Silicone breast implants in vivo: MR imaging. *Radiology* 1992;185:407–410.
98. Gilles R, Guinebretiere JM, Shapeero LG, et al. Assessment of breast cancer recurrence with contrast enhanced subtraction MR imaging: preliminary results in 26 patients. *Radiology* 1993;188:473–478.

99. Kelcz F, Santyr G, Mongin S, Fairbanks E. *Reducing false positive gadolinium enhanced breast MRI results through parameter analysis of the enhancement profile*. New York: 1993:121.
100. Schnall M, Orel S, Muenz L. *Analysis of time intensity curves for enhancing lesions*. New York: 1993:120.
101. Orel SG, Schnall MD, LiVolsi VA, Troupin RH. Suspicious breast lesions: MR imaging with radiologic-pathologic correlation. *Radiology* 1994;190:485–493.
102. Gilles R, Guinebretiere JM, Shapeero LG, et al. Assessment of breast cancer recurrence with contrast enhanced subtraction MR imaging: preliminary results in 26 patients. *Radiology* 1993;188:473–478.
103. Hulka CA, Smith BL, Sgroi DC, et al. Benign and malignant breast lesions: differentiation with echo planar imaging. *Radiology* 1995;197:33–38.
104. Kaiser WA, Zeitler E. MR imaging of the breast: fast imaging sequences with and without Gd-DTPA. *Radiology* 1989;170: 681–686.
105. Boetes C, Barentsz JO, Mus RD, et al. MR characterization of suspicious breast lesions with a gadolinium-enhanced turboFLASH subtraction technique. *Radiology* 1994;193:777–781.
106. Piccoli CW, Mitchell DG, Schwartz GF, Vinitski S. Contrast-enhanced breast MR imaging with dynamic and fat-suppression techniques. In: Society for Magnetic Imaging 1993 annual meeting program. San Francisco, 1993:47–48.
107. Brown LF, Berse B, Jackman RW, et al. Expression of vascular permeability factor (vascular endothelial growth factor) and its receptors in breast cancer. *Hum Pathol* 1995;26:86–91.
108. Dao TH, Rahmouni A, Campana F, Laurent M, Asselain B, Fourquet A. Tumor recurrence versus fibrosis in the irradiated breast: differentiation with dynamic gadolinium-enhanced MR imaging. *Radiology* 1993;187:751–755.
109. Cohen MS, Weisskoff RM. Ultra-fast imaging. *MRI* 1991;9:1–37.
110. Hulka CA, Smith BL, Sgroi DC, et al. Benign and malignant breast lesions: differentiation with echo planar imaging. *Radiology* 1995; 197:33–38.
111. Orel SG, Schnall MD, Powell CM, et al. Staging of suspected breast cancer: effect of MR imaging and MR-guided biopsy. *Radiology* 1995;196:115–112.
112. Heywang-Koebrunner SH, Haustein J, Pohl C, et al. Contrast-enhanced MR imaging of the breast: comparison of two different doses of gadopentate dimeglumine. *Radiology* 1994;191:639–646.
113. Weinreb JC, Newstead G. MR imaging of the breast. *Radiology* 1995;196:593–610.
114. Kaiser WA, Zeitler E. MR imaging of the breast: fast imaging sequences with and without Gd–DTPA. *Radiology* 1989;170:681–686.
115. Kaiser WA, Zeitler E. MR imaging of the breast: fast imaging sequences with and without Gd–DTPA. *Radiology* 1989;170:681–686.
116. Numes LW, Schnall MD, Orel SG. Breast MR imaging: interpretation model. *Radiology* 1997;202:833–841.
117. Gilles R, Guinebretiere JM, Shapeero LG, et al. Assessment of breast cancer recurrence with contrast enhanced subtraction MR imaging: preliminary results in 26 patients. *Radiology* 1993;188:473–478.
118. Guidi AJ, Fischer L, Harris JR, Schnitt SJ. Microvessel density and distribution in ductal carcinoma in situ of the breast. *J Natl Cancer Inst* 1994;86:614–619.
119. Soderstrom CE, Harms SE, Copit DS, et al. Three dimensional RODEO MR imaging of lesions containing DCIS. *Radiology* 1996;201:427–432.
120. Orel SG, Mendonca MH, Reynolds C, Schnall MD, Solin LJ, Sullivan DC. MR imaging of ductal carcinoma in situ. *Radiology* 1997;202:413–420.
121. Giles R, Zanfrani B, Guinebretiere J, et al. Ductal carcinoma in situ: MR imaging-histopathologic correlation. *Radiology* 1995;196:415–419.
122. Kurtz JM, Amalric R, Brandone H, et al. Local recurrence after breast-conserving surgery and radiotherapy: frequency, time-course, and prognosis. *Cancer* 1989;63:1912–1917.
123. Dao T, Rahmouni A, Scrvios V, Nguyen–Tan T. MR imaging of the breast in the follow-up evalaution of conservatively treated breast cancer. *Magn Reson Imaging Clin N Am* 1994;2:605–622.
124. Dao TH, Rahmouni A, Campana F, Laurent M, Asselain B, Fourquet A. Tumor recurrence versus fibrosis in the irradiated breast: differentiation with dynamic gadolinium-enhanced MR imaging. *Radiology* 1993;187:751–755.
125. Diggles L, Mena I, Khalkhali I. Technical aspects of prone dependent-breast scintimammography. *J Nucl Med Tech* 1994;22:165–170.
126. Whitman GJ, Fischman AJ, Lee JM, Barrow SA, Moore RH, Kopans DB. Sestamibi breast imaging with histopathologic findings in 31 nonpalpable breast lesions. Presented to the 82nd Scientific Assembly of the Radiological Society of North America. Chicago, 1996.
127. Wahl RL, Cody RL, Hutchins GD, Mudgett EE. Primary and metastatic breast carcinoma: initial clinical evaluation with PET with the radiolabeled glucose analogue 2-[F-18]-fluoro-2-deoxy-D-glucose. *Radiology* 1991;179:765–770.
128. Adler LE, Crowe JP, Al-Kaisi NK, Sunshine JL. Evaluation of breast masses and axillary lymph nodes with [F–18] 2-deoxy-2-fluoro-D-glucose PET. *Radiology* 1993;187:743–750.
129. Meyer JE, Kopans DB, Oot R. Mammographic visualization of breast cancer in patients under 35 years of age. *Radiology* 1983;147:93–94.
130. Meyer JE, Kopans DB. Analysis of mammographically obvious breast carcinomas with benign results on initial biopsy. *Surg Gynecol Obstet* 1981;153:570–572.
131. Kopans DB, Meyer JE, Cohen AM, and Wood WC. Palpable breast masses: the importance of preoperative mammography. *JAMA* 1981;246:2819–2822.

CHAPTER 13

Diseases of the Breast, 2nd ed.,
edited by Jay R. Harris.
Lippincott Williams & Wilkins, Philadelphia © 2000.

Image-Guided Biopsy of Nonpalpable Breast Lesions

Luz A. Venta

Improved mammographic detection of small and subtle nonpalpable abnormalities has resulted in increased detection of small cancers and an approximately 30% reduction in mortality from breast cancer.[1] A criticism of the increased use of screening mammography in the United States is the relatively high cost involved in diagnosing each cancer, primarily due to the large number of benign surgical biopsies that result from detection of indeterminate mammographic lesions.[2–4] It is estimated that if all eligible women in the United States were to follow the American Cancer Society's recommendations for screening mammography, approximately 1 million breast biopsies would be recommended per year for mammographically detected abnormalities.[3,5] Positive biopsy rates of 10% to 40% have been reported for excisional biopsy, so that 600,000 to 900,000 would be expected to be benign.[5–7] Surgical excisional biopsy after preoperative needle localization can be the most expensive component of mammography screening programs.[8] Although surgical excision with prior preoperative needle localization is a proven safe procedure with low complication rates, recent studies have demonstrated that needle biopsy of nonpalpable lesions is an equally accurate technique. Most needle biopsy procedures are easy to perform, have a very low complication rate, and are well tolerated by patients. Needle biopsy, when used appropriately, can avoid surgical biopsy in a large number of patients while maintaining the goal of early breast cancer detection. Thus, it is not only an alternative in diagnosis but also an improvement in patient management.

This chapter reviews the current methods available for needle biopsy of nonpalpable lesions, emphasizing aspects of the procedure that are clinically significant and impact patient management. A discussion of the basic technical procedural aspects is included to familiarize the reader with important considerations in patient selection and to present technical limitations.

L. A. Venta: Department of Radiology, Lynn Sage Comprehensive Breast Program, Northwestern University Medical School, Chicago, Illinois; Section of Breast Imaging, Department of Radiology, Northwestern Memorial Hospital, Chicago, Illinois

FINE-NEEDLE ASPIRATION

Fine-needle aspiration (FNA) guided by physical examination has been used effectively for years to evaluate patients with palpable breast lumps. A review of 3,000 cases of nonpalpable lesions evaluated by FNA with histologic follow-up concluded that the results were comparable to FNA of palpable breast lumps. The sensitivity of FNA for palpable lesions ranged between 72% and 99% and for nonpalpable lesions between 82% and 100%.[9] Multiple other studies have compared the accuracy of FNA for evaluating nonpalpable breast lesions with results from surgical biopsy. These studies have yielded mixed and conflicting results.[10–12] The reported sensitivity has varied from 68% to 93% and the specificity from 88% to 100%. The false-negative rate for FNA of nonpalpable lesions ranges from 0 to 32%[5,13,14] and may be due to inaccurate lesion localization, small lesion size, deflection of the fine needle by firm masses, or a combination of these. Reported false-positive rates in nonpalpable lesions vary from 0 to 6%.[12,15–22] This is usually due to misinterpretation of atypical abnormalities found in areas of proliferative breast changes.

Perhaps the single most important impediment to the wide-scale implementation of FNA for nonpalpable lesions has been the relatively high rate of inadequate or nondiagnostic cytologic samples. The rate of inadequate samples in palpable abnormalities ranges between 4% and 13%, whereas FNA of nonpalpable lesions yielded an insufficient sample in 2% to 36%. This higher rate of insufficient samples on cytology of nonpalpable lesions is an important and significant difference.[9,23] There are several explanations for this different and higher rate of insufficient samples. First, nonpalpable lesions are often low in cellularity and tend to yield scant cellular material that is insufficient for diagnosis.[15,18] Hann and colleagues[18] found that 40% of inadequate cases were from fibrotic and hypocellular abnormalities from which a low cellular yield would be anticipated. Among lesions associated with a low cellular yield are commonly encountered nonpalpable benign lesions, such as sclerosing adenosis and fibroadenomas.[5] Among malignant lesions, the histologic tumor type plays a role in the cellularity of the aspirate, with medullary and mucinous types yielding a more cellular sample than infiltrating lobular carcinoma.

Other explanations for scant cellularity in the aspirate of nonpalpable lesions are the smaller lesion size or aspiration technique, or both. FNA guided by the clinical examination is performed by directing the needle in multiple directions so that different areas of the palpable lump can be sampled. This is impractical in smaller nonpalpable lesions, in which brisk needle motion easily results in needle displacement outside the lesion and into surrounding normal tissue.

FINE-NEEDLE ASPIRATION VERSUS CORE BIOPSY

Conflicting reports regarding the diagnostic accuracy of FNA compared with core biopsy are found in the older literature.[24–27] However, these studies compared multiple-pass FNA with single-pass core biopsy. The core biopsies were performed without automated devices and without imaging guidance, and most studies evaluated palpable lesions. Thus, the results of these studies are not applicable to image-guided needle biopsy of nonpalpable lesions. More recent reports have proved core biopsy to be superior to FNA for the evaluation of nonpalpable lesions in several aspects. Core biopsy offers a more definitive histologic diagnosis, avoids inadequate samples, and allows differentiation between invasive and *in situ* carcinoma.[13,28–32] The high rate of inadequate cytologic samples in aspirates of nonpalpable lesions has led many to abandon this method and adopt core biopsy with a large cutting needle preferentially.[13] The advantages and disadvantages of FNA and core biopsy are summarized in Table 1.

TABLE 1. *Comparison of fine-needle aspiration and core biopsy for nonpalpable breast lesions*

	Fine-needle aspiration	Core biopsy
Needle size (gauge)	20–22	11–14
Imaging modality used to guide procedure	Ultrasound or stereotactic	Ultrasound or stereotactic
Pathologic evaluation of the sampled material	Cytology	Histology
Rate of inadequate samples	0–37%	<1%
Can differentiate *in situ* from invasive cancer?	No	Yes
Cost[a]	$	$$

[a]The cost per procedure predominantly depends on the choice of imaging method used for guidance. Cost of the needle employed contributes to the overall cost in that 22-gauge hypodermic needles used for FNA cost are relatively inexpensive. The automated biopsy guns uses needles of variable gauge, ranging from 14 to 21, and are intermediate in price. The 11-gauge core biopsy needles used with the vacuum-assisted biopsy probe are most expensive, costing approximately $200 each.

The type of needle used for lesion sampling is different for FNA and for core biopsy and results in significantly different specimen material. Core biopsy is performed with a large cutting needle, usually 14 gauge, deployed into the breast by a rapid-fire, spring-loaded, automated biopsy instrument, commonly called a *biopsy gun*. The sampled material consists of a core of tissue suitable for standard histologic analysis, familiar to most pathologists. Insufficient sampling is infrequent with core biopsy, because more tissue is removed and the tissue cores are easily seen during the procedure so that more tissue can be obtained if the sample is visibly inadequate. In contrast, FNA is performed with a 20- to 22-gauge needle manually inserted into the breast. The fine needle yields cellular material suitable for cytologic evaluation. Accurate cytologic interpretation requires an experienced cytopathologist, which may not be available in all sites. The material extracted with FNA is smaller and prone to be insufficient for diagnosis.

IMAGING MODALITY USED TO GUIDE NEEDLE BIOPSY

Breast needle biopsies of nonpalpable lesions, be they FNA or core biopsy, require imaging to guide needle placement. Imaging guidance can be performed with stereotactic mammography or ultrasound. Both imaging modalities are widely available. The choice of imaging technique used for guidance depends on the visibility of the lesion and does not affect the accuracy of the procedure. Generally, ultrasound guidance is preferred for masses visualized with ultrasound, as it is faster and does not require breast compression, making it better tolerated by most patients. Stereotactic biopsy is used for mammographically detected lesions not identified with ultrasound.

STEREOTACTIC BIOPSY

Historical Perspective

Stereotactic mammography was introduced in Sweden in 1976.[33] Studies using combined mammographic and stereotactic FNA of 2,594 breast lesions reported 77% to be benign and not require surgical evaluation, whereas of those recommended for surgery, 76% were malignant.[29] Dr. Kambiz Dowlatshahi introduced the first dedicated prone stereotactic table in the United States at the University of Chicago in the mid-1980s. Stereotactic FNA preceding needle localization and excisional biopsy resulted in the correct diagnosis in 11 of 12 malignant cases, but the sampled aspirate was reported to be inadequate in 14 of 84 cases.[34] The high rate of inadequate cytologic aspirates and the lack of availability of expert cytopathologists prevented widespread implementation of needle biopsy of nonpalpable lesions until 1989, when Dr. Steve Parker reported on stereotactic biopsy using an automated biopsy gun and a large-gauge needle. Of 102 core biopsies performed, histologic agreement between core biopsy and surgical excision resulted in 97% of cases, with no inadequate samples.[32] By overcoming the high rate of inadequate samples and the need for expert cytopathologists, core biopsy became rapidly accepted as an alternative to surgical excision in most practices. A national survey in the United States reported in 1997 found image-guided core biopsy to be performed in 81% of sites responding to the survey.[35]

Equipment

The cost of stereotactic biopsy equipment is significant, and a high patient volume is needed to justify its use. The two main types of stereotactic biopsy units currently available are the dedicated prone tables and the "add-on" adapted upright units. The add-on stereotactic units attach to standard mammography equipment and were developed in an effort to keep cost at a minimum. The add-on units are less expensive, require less space, and, when not in use, allow the equipment to be used for standard mammography. With the add-on units, the patient is seated and able to see the biopsy procedure. As a result, patients can experience vasovagal reactions or move inadvertently. The dedicated prone tables have several advantages. These include less patient motion and very few vasovagal reactions. The patient lies prone with the breast placed through an opening in the table and is mostly unaware of the biopsy procedure going on under the table. Prone stereotactic tables are more expensive and require a dedicated room. As it became apparent that motion was a critical issue and patient comfort was necessary, dedicated prone tables began to dominate the market. Irrespective of the type of stereotactic unit used, mammographic breast compression is needed during the entire procedure, and a motionless, cooperative patient is essential to ensure accurate targeting and lesion sampling.

Technical Aspects

Stereotactic localization uses the principle of parallax to determine the lesion position in three-dimensional space. Two angled radiographic views (stereotactic pair) acquired with the x-ray beam 15 degrees on either side of the center are used to determine the location of a mammographic lesion. A computer algorithm uses simple geometric relations to calculate the position of the lesion based on the lesion "shift" between the two acquired views. Calculations are based on the targeting information provided by the physician performing the procedure (Fig. 1).

Stereotactic localizations are accurate to 1 mm.[33,34,36] Lesion location is expressed in terms of a coordinate system (x = horizontal, y = vertical, and z = depth). The biopsy needle apparatus is supported by a stage attached to the stereotactic equipment and moved to the calculated coordinates with a push of a button. Orientation of the needle parallel to the chest wall eliminates the concern of needle excursion into the chest wall or thorax. Histologic samples obtained with core biopsy needles are preserved in formalin and interpreted by a histopathologist.

Advances in stereotactic equipment during the 1990s resulted in the development of digital image acquisition. The ability to acquire and display mammographic lesions digitally has greatly increased the speed of the procedure and reduced patient discomfort by decreasing the amount of time the breast is held in mammographic compression. Depending on the type of lesion being sampled, most stereotactic procedures require 20 minutes to 1 hour to perform.

Core Biopsy Needles

Two devices are commonly used to obtain core breast biopsies: automated biopsy guns and the directional, vacuum-assisted biopsy device. Automated biopsy guns use a double-action needle that consists of an inner trocar with a sample notch and an outer cutting cannula. The needle is preloaded into the biopsy gun and placed a few millimeters proximal to the lesion and is ready to be "fired" by simply pushing a button. The spring-loaded, double-action biopsy gun rapidly advances the needle into the breast, taking a core of tissue during its excursion. As the gun is fired, a sample of tissue is cut off by the outer cannula and stored in the sample notch. The needle is then removed from the breast, and the tissue sample is retrieved from the needle. The powerful needle motion allows penetration of dense breast tissue without displacing lesions out of the needle's path. The nearly instantaneous sample withdrawal also reduces patient discomfort. The first guns used for breast biopsy used 18- to 20-gauge needles and a short throw or excursion.[37] However, specimens were not always diagnostic, and difficulties were often encountered when small lesions were targeted. Biopsy guns using 14-gauge needles and a longer needle throw produced more reliable specimens and proved to be as accurate as surgical excisional biopsy for most cases.[31,38]

Multiple core biopsy samples are necessary to ensure accurate sampling of different areas of the lesion. In most cases, accurate lesion sampling can be achieved by obtaining five core samples for masses and five to ten core samples for microcalcifications.[39] Automated biopsy gun devices require multiple needle insertions to retrieve multiple core samples. Every time the gun is deployed, a single core sample is obtained, and the needle is removed from the breast in order to retrieve the core of tissue. In contrast, the directional, vacuum-assisted biopsy instrument (Mammotome, Biopsys Medical, Irvine, CA) is inserted once and rotated while in the breast to obtain samples from different areas of the lesion. By avoiding the need for needle reinsertion, the biopsy time is markedly reduced. A vacuum

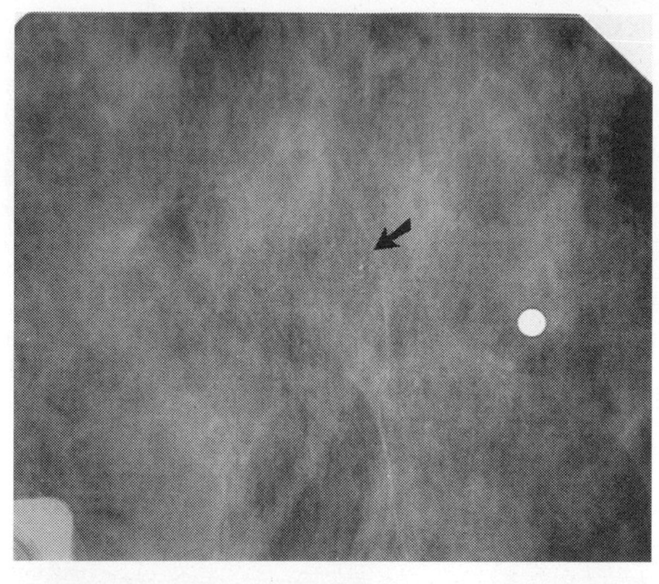
A

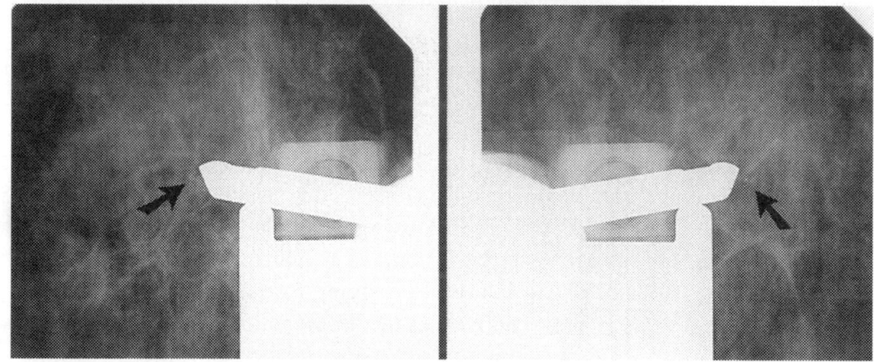
B

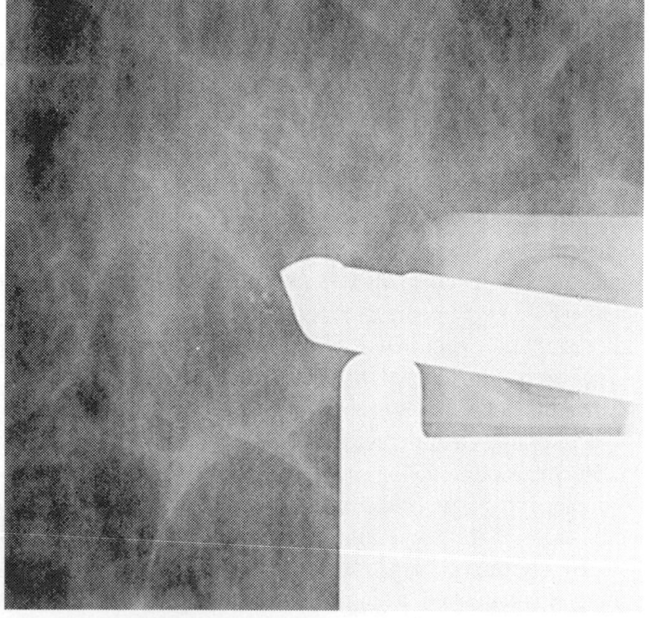
C

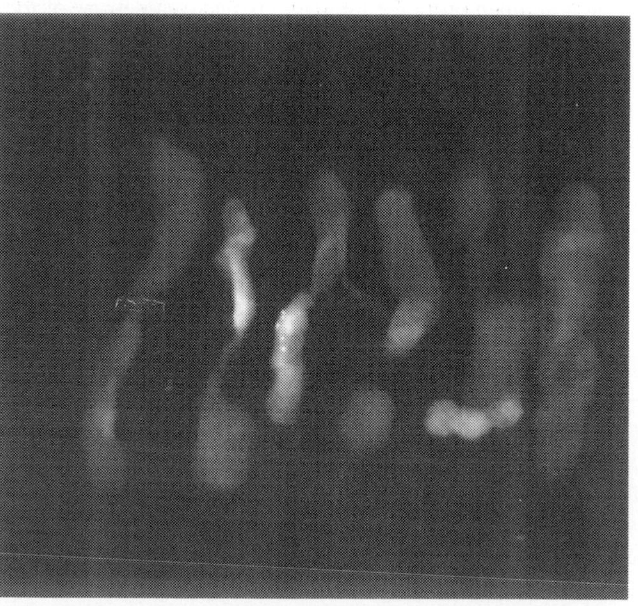
D

FIG. 1. Stereotactic needle biopsy. **A:** The lesion is a small cluster of indeterminate calcifications (Breast Imaging Reporting and Data System category 4) (*arrow*). **B:** Stereotactic pair obtained with the needle positioned in front of the targeted cluster (*arrows*). Adequate needle placement is confirmed by the symmetry of the needle tip–lesion distance in each of the two stereo pairs. The needle used is an 11-gauge vacuum-assisted probe. **C:** Close-up of the needle and the targeted calcifications from **(B)**. **D:** Core specimen radiograph demonstrates multiple calcifications to be present. *Continued.*

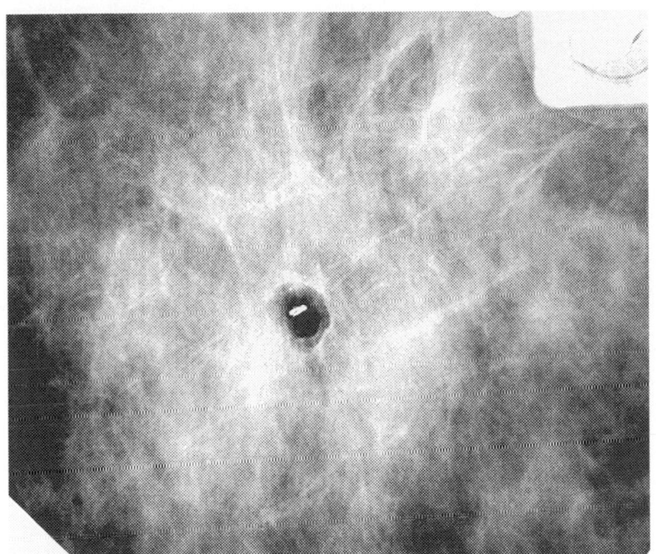

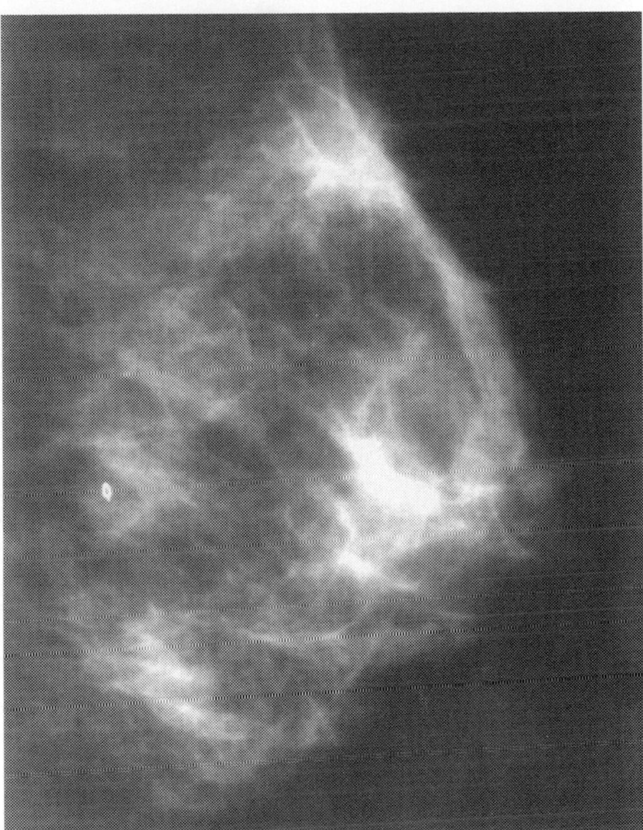

FIG. 1. *Continued.* **E:** Postprocedure stereotactic view shows biopsy cavity filled with air and the deployed metallic clip in the upper aspect of the cavity. **F:** Mediolateral mammogram shows complete removal of the cluster of calcifications. The metallic clip marks the biopsy site. Histology: ductal hyperplasia without atypia.

is used to pull tissue into the sample notch, where it is cut and transported back through the needle and out to the collection chamber. Multiple tissue samples are collected without removing the needle from the breast. The needle or "probe" consists of an outer hollow sleeve with a notch at the end, an inner hollow cutting cannula that is manually advanced to cut the tissue, and an inner vacuum stylet. The probes come in 14- and 11-gauge sizes. The samples obtained using the vacuum-assisted device are larger than those obtained using automated guns.[40,41] A study has shown improved sampling of microcalcifications with the vacuum-assisted biopsy instrument.[42] Because the vacuum-assisted biopsy instrument is larger and cumbersome to handle manually, it is most often used for sampling of stereotactically guided procedures and not for free hand procedures performed with ultrasound guidance.

ULTRASOUND GUIDANCE

The use of ultrasound to guide needles into breast lesions has been used increasingly since the 1980s.[43] Ultrasound-guided core biopsies can be performed for any masses that are sonographically evident. This approach is an alternative to stereotactic core biopsy and is preferred by patients due to the lack of breast compression, more comfortable positioning, and lack of radiation. Radiologists who have mastered this technique also find it faster and easier than stereotactic biopsy. Additionally, ultrasound allows real-time observation of needle passage within the lesion breast, thereby assuring adequate sampling.

Lesion visibility is the limiting step in using ultrasound guidance to sample all nonpalpable breast lesions. Studies comparing ultrasound guidance and stereotactic biopsy have reported that more than 50% of all lesions requiring biopsy could not be visualized with ultrasound, in particular small masses measuring less than 6 mm, calcifications, and architectural distortions.[44,45] The introduction of higher-frequency transducers during the mid- to late 1990s have improved sonographic visualization of small masses, making ultrasound guidance possible for an increasing number of lesions.

Equipment requirements for interventional ultrasound-guided procedures are the same as for diagnostic ultrasound imaging. The ultrasound transducer selected should have the maximum resolution possible that allows penetration of the beam to the desired depth. A linear array transducer with a frequency of at least 7.5 MHz is required, with many centers currently using 10-MHz transducers. The linear shape of the ultrasound beam allows better visualization of the needle and the lesion during the procedure. Simultaneous imaging of the needle and the lesion is a key factor in determining accurate needle placement and documenting adequate lesion sampling.

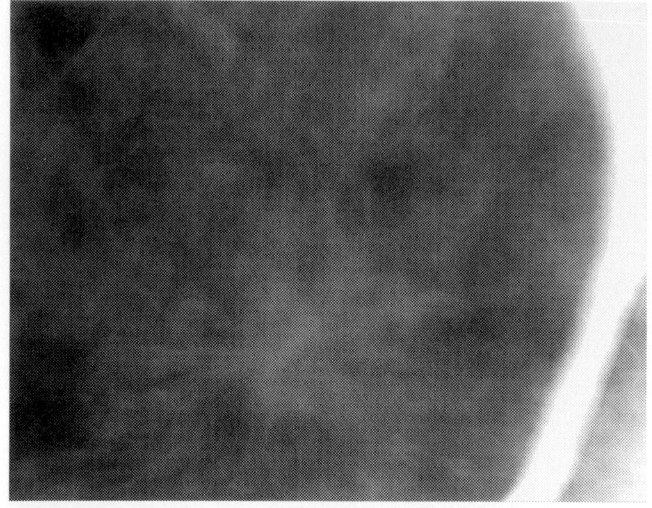

A

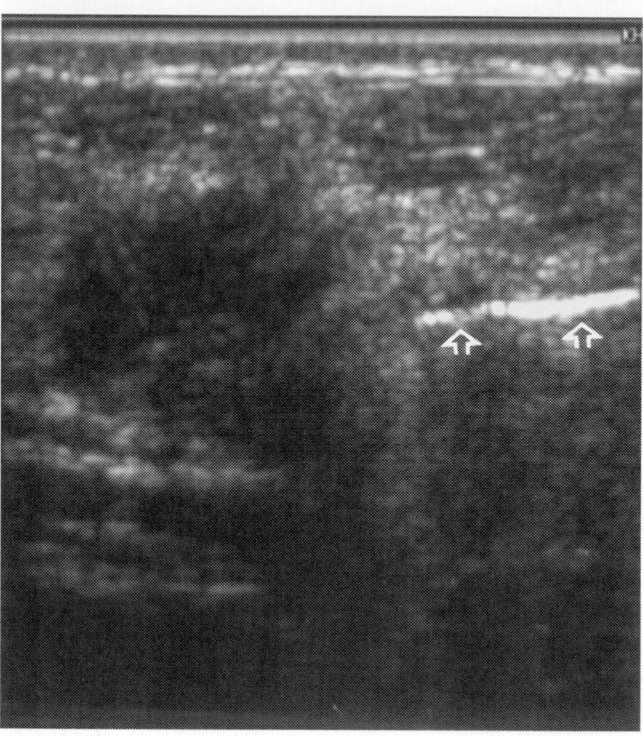

B

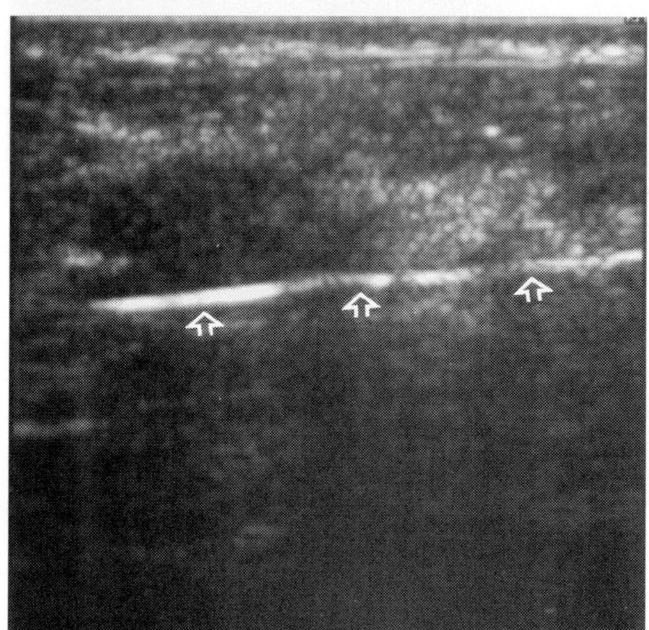

C

FIG. 2. Ultrasound-guided core biopsy. **A:** Spot magnification view in craniocaudal projection demonstrates a spiculated mass, highly suspicious for malignancy (Breast Imaging Reporting and Data System category 5). **B:** Ultrasound shows the needle (*arrows*) placed in front of the mass before deployment. **C:** Ultrasound image after automated needle deployment confirms needle placement through the mass (*arrows*). Histology: invasive ductal carcinoma.

The technical aspects involved in performing ultrasound-guided procedures with a free hand approach have been described previously.[43,46,47] The technique used consists of the following steps: imaging the lesion, finding the needle in the longitudinal plane through the lesion, maximally visualizing the needle tip, and placing the needle in the lesion. Development of good hand-eye coordination is key to a successful lesion sampling. Practicing ultrasound-guided procedures on phantoms improves needle placement and results in faster and more secure initial clinical experience.[48] A review article on different manufacturers' phantoms and homemade phantoms is summarized by Georgian-Smith and Lyon.[49] Once needle placement is mastered, even small lesions measuring 3 to 4 mm in diameter can be accurately sampled.

The needle and spring-loaded deployment casting or biopsy gun commonly selected for ultrasound-guided core biopsy has a needle excursion of approximately 2 cm. Because the tip of the needle will end up 2 cm beyond the initial placement after deployment, this tissue is scanned to ensure that important structures, such as pectoral muscle or major vessels, are not inadvertently punctured with deployment. Provided that this precaution is taken and the needle trajectory is kept parallel to the chest wall, core biopsies can be performed accurately and safely. During the sampling process, the three-dimensional location of the needle is determined before removal of the needle by turning the transducer 90 degrees to the trajectory. Visualizing the needle track within the lesion at the end of the procedure also confirms adequate sampling of the lesion (Fig. 2).

Most lesions selected for ultrasound-guided biopsy are solid masses that can be sampled with 14-gauge core needles. Complex cysts that cannot be distinguished from solid masses by sonographic criteria alone have been managed in the past with ultrasound-guided aspiration to confirm the cystic nature of the lesion.[50,51] Little has been written regarding the need for aspiration of complex cysts. In a review of 4,562 consecutive

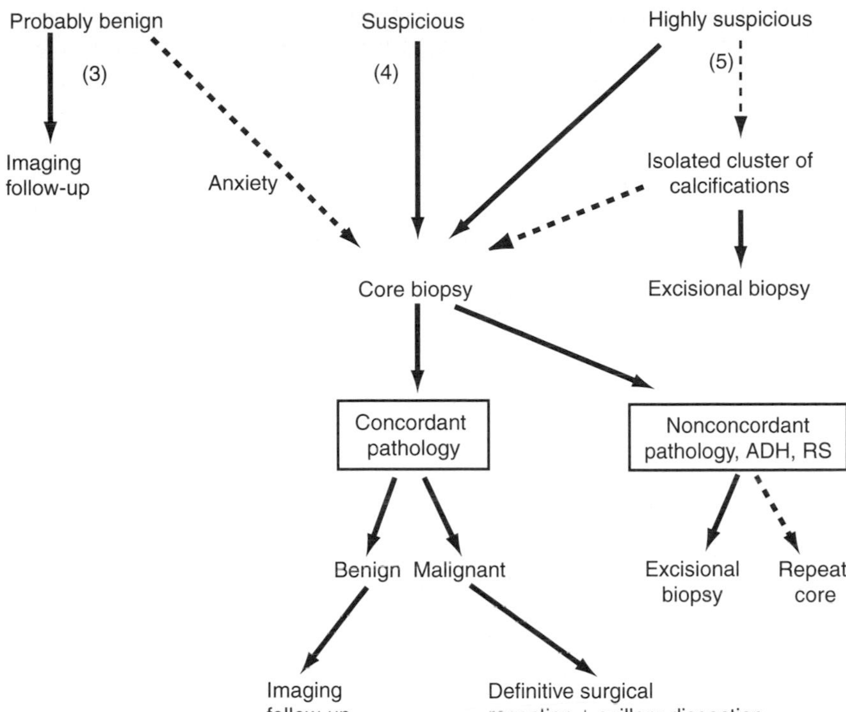

FIG. 3. Lesion selection and patient management based on the mammographic degree of suspicion. Nonpalpable lesions can be classified according to these imaging features into Breast Imaging Reporting and Data System (BI-RADS) categories based on the degree of suspicion for malignancy. - - - - - -, infrequent events; ———, commonly encountered events; ( ), BI-RADS category; ADH, atypical ductal hyperplasia; RS, radial scar.

breast ultrasounds in our center, 308 complex cysts were prospectively diagnosed. Management recommendations were varied and reflect the lack of consensus on optimal management of complex cysts. Recommendations were as follows: 1-year follow-up imaging studies in 13, 6-month follow-up in 148, ultrasound-guided aspiration in 81, aspiration with possible core biopsy in 62, and excisional biopsy in 3. The number of malignancies encountered among lesions classified as complex cysts in this series was 0.3% (1 out of 308). This malignancy rate is lower than that encountered among lesions classified as probably benign using mammographic criteria. The accepted standard practice of probably benign lesions [Breast Imaging Reporting and Data System (BI-RADS) category 3; see the following section, Lesion Selection] is follow-up imaging studies.[52] The low yield of malignancy in our series suggests that complex cysts can also be managed with periodic follow-up imaging studies instead of intervention.[53]

Ultrasound-guided procedures require close mammographic correlation to ensure that the lesion sampled corresponds to the suspicious mammographic lesion. A 10% misidentification rate between the mammographic mass and sonographic lesion has been reported.[54]

INDICATIONS

It is possible to perform image-guided FNA or core biopsy on most patients with nonpalpable suspicious or indeterminate lesions detected with mammography for which surgical biopsy would be considered. However, needle biopsy should not replace imaging workup. It is unlikely that an abnormality detected with screening mammography should undergo needle biopsy without the intervening step of diagnostic mammographic workup—that is, spot compression and magnification views of the area of concern and high-resolution ultrasound as needed. This imaging workup is essential to completely analyze the abnormality, assess the degree of suspicion, and exclude multiple lesions. Assessing the degree of suspicion is indispensable in evaluating mammographic-pathologic concordance after the procedure, when the histologic diagnosis becomes available (Fig. 3).

Lesions referred for stereotactic sampling because they are seen in only one view may end up being "pseudolesions" once further imaging has been performed. If this is unrecognized and the core biopsy is performed inappropriately, progressive invasive procedures may follow, as the histologic diagnosis of normal tissue resulting from the core biopsy is deemed nonconcordant. A review of 89 canceled stereotactic core-needle biopsies reported the reasons for cancellation to be lack of a recognizable lesion in 29%, reassessment of the lesion as benign in 19%, and benign cysts in 25%.[55] This study reports that a complete imaging workup including ultrasound would have avoided the delay in diagnosis and anxiety produced by scheduling (and canceling) a stereotactic biopsy in 48% of patients.

LESION SELECTION

Careful logic should be used to determine which patients could benefit from needle biopsy. The American College of Radiology BI-RADS has developed a lexicon for mammography in an effort to standardize mammographic reporting, reduce confusion in breast imaging interpretation, and facilitate outcome monitoring.[56] According to this standard, a final mammographic assessment should be included in each mammographic report. The five final assessment BI-RADS categories are (1) negative (N), (2) benign finding (B), (3) probably benign finding (P), (4) suspicious abnormality (S), and (5) highly suggestive of malignancy (M). Lesions categorized as P are usually managed by 6-month follow-up mammography, whereas lesions in categories 4 and 5 (i.e., suspicious or highly suggestive of malignancy) require histologic sampling.

Using mammographic degree of suspicion, a patient treatment algorithm can be developed that defines the role of needle biopsy (see Fig. 3). Patients with "probably benign" nonpalpable mammographic lesions (a less than 2% chance of malignancy) need not undergo needle biopsy. Studies have proved that lesions in category 3 can be safely followed mammographically, so that needle biopsy is unnecessary and only adds to the cost of screening.[52,57] Although some advocate needle biopsy of low-suspicion lesions to lower the anxiety of nervous women who do not wish to undergo follow-up, a study assessing patient stress reports the overall stress experience by women who underwent core biopsy to be significantly greater than that reported in the group who were followed up with mammography.[58] Percutaneous biopsy of intermediate-suspicion lesions yields the greatest cost benefit, as most of these are found to be benign, and the patients are spared the possible breast deformity associated with surgical biopsy.

Image-guided needle biopsy can also decrease the number of operations performed in women with breast cancer. Many women who undergo open surgical biopsy for cancer diagnosis require a second surgery for definitive therapy and axillary lymph node dissection. If the cancer diagnosis is made by preoperative core-needle biopsy, definitive therapy and axillary dissection can be performed in a single operation. Jackman et al.[59] report that a single surgical procedure was performed in 90% of patients whose cancers were diagnosed by percutaneous biopsy versus 24% of patients whose cancers were diagnosed by surgical biopsy. Other studies have shown similar results.[60,61] In our institution, we prospectively compared the number of surgical procedures to completion of local therapy after core biopsy and surgical biopsy on the basis of lesion type, degree of suspicion, and type of local therapy for 1,854 abnormalities in 1,550 consecutive patients. The benefit of core biopsy in reducing the number of surgical procedures was seen in patients who had mastectomy or axillary surgery. In patients who had lumpectomy alone, surgical biopsy was as likely as core-needle biopsy followed by lumpectomy to be the definitive surgical procedure.[62] A single surgery based on frozen section analysis has been used to combine separate surgeries for diagnosis and definitive therapy. However, this method is flawed by the inaccuracies of frozen section diagnosis.[63] In addition, with this method patients must agree to the possibility of extensive surgery before obtaining a tissue diagnosis. When a preoperative tissue diagnosis is obtained by a percutaneous core-needle biopsy, the patient can consider all of the therapeutic options before treatment, as receptor status and the presence of biomarkers can be determined from core biopsy samples.

The usefulness of core biopsy in obtaining clear surgical margins in subsequent lumpectomy is debatable. A retrospective review of 197 nonpalpable carcinomas diagnosed with core-needle biopsy or surgical biopsy after needle localization compared the frequency of tumor at the margins of the lumpectomy specimen.[60] Tumor was present at the lumpectomy margins in 8% of cases diagnosed preoperatively with image-guided core biopsy and in 5% of cases diagnosed with surgical biopsy. This difference was not statistically significant. In contrast, a similar report comparing 171 patients undergoing image-guided core biopsy or preoperative needle localization found the incidence of positive margins to be less in the group diagnosed with core biopsy (29% versus 65%, $p < .0001$).[64] This higher rate of negative margins in the group diagnosed with needle biopsy was likely related to the larger specimen volume in that group of patients (as volume of excision was statistically significantly greater in the group diagnosed with core biopsy: 106 cm^3 versus 52 cm^3). In patients undergoing needle biopsy of high-suspicion lesions, only a malignant result is accepted, as all benign results are considered nonconcordant with the mammographic appearance. As noted in Fig. 3 and in the section Concordance, the role of core biopsy in evaluating highly suspicious masses is to facilitate a single and definitive surgical procedure by histologically confirming invasive carcinoma. Thus, the role of core biopsy in evaluating highly suspicious small clusters of calcifications likely representing ductal carcinoma *in situ* (DCIS) is not clear, as subsequent surgical excision of the lesion is necessary and axillary dissection will not be performed. In these cases, core biopsy adds a step to the diagnostic management and results in only a modest cost savings.[65]

Core-needle biopsy is extremely useful in the evaluation of patients with multiple suspicious lesions. Tissue samples can be obtained without having to perform multiple surgical biopsies. Establishing the extent of a patient's cancer allows surgical mapping; optimal resection can help determine the most appropriate therapy (i.e., mastectomy or breast conservation). A report of stereotactic core-needle biopsy of multiple sites found malignant histology in 60% of patients, with 40% having more than one malignant site.[66] Multisite stereotactic core biopsy had a positive effect on patient care in 80% of patients by either helping confirm the need for mastectomy without intervening needle localization biopsy or by documenting benign disease and sparing preoperative needle localization of multiple lesions.

PATIENT SELECTION

There are certain limiting patient and mammographic factors that must be considered during the selection of patients

TABLE 2. *Accuracy rate: core biopsy compared with surgical excision*

Author	Year	No. of pts.	No. of cancers	Sensitivity (%)	Needle gauge	Imaging guidance	Nondiagnostic (%)
Dowlatshahi et al[37]	1991	250[a]	76	71	20	Stereo	8
Parker et al[31]	1991	102	23	96	14	Stereo	0
Dronkers[123]	1992	53	45	91	18	Stereo	6
Elvecrog et al[44]	1993	100	35	100[b]	14	Stereo	0
Parker et al[116]	1993	49	34	100	14	US	0
Gisvold et al[124]	1994	104[c]	65	92	14	Stereo	<1
Parker et al[68]	1994	1,363	910	98	14	Stereo[d] and US	0
Meyer et al[125]	1996	103	61	100	14	Stereo	1[e]
Brenner et al[110]	1996	230	140	96	14	Stereo	3[f]

Stereo, stereotactic; US, ultrasound.
[a]Fine-needle aspiration only in the first 130 cases.
[b]Core biopsy and surgical excision each missed one cancer.
[c]Cases with five or more cores obtained.
[d]77% stereotactic and 23.9% ultrasound guidance.
[e]Repeated core biopsy to reevaluate diagnosis of normal tissue resulted in a specific benign histology.
[f]Correct diagnosis not achieved within the five-core sample limit of this study.

for stereotactic needle biopsy. A report on canceled stereotactic biopsies found 8% of cancellations caused by the patients' inability to tolerate the procedure.[55] Patient cooperation is key to successful lesion sampling, as she must remain motionless for the duration of the procedure, often for 20 to 40 minutes. Patients with severe coughing or anxiety may move too much to allow accurate targeting. Patients who are unable to lie prone because of abdominal or spinal problems may not be able to undergo stereotactic biopsy. Stereotactic tables have a patient weight limit that, if exceeded, can result in damage to the motorized table-moving apparatus. The weight limit varies between manufacturers but is often approximately 300 lb (135 kg). Patients who exceed this weight cannot be sampled stereotactically.

It can be difficult to perform stereotactic biopsy of breast lesions that are very superficial or near the nipple due to the inability to place the area in proper compression. Lesions that are near the chest wall cannot be targeted, as it is difficult to image very posterior tissue using the prone biopsy tables. Patients with very thin breasts may not have enough tissue to allow for needle excursion. Lesion location and small-sized breasts accounted for 4% and 8%, respectively, of canceled core biopsies in one report.[55] The factors described here do not apply to ultrasound-guided needle biopsies, which are only limited by lesion visibility.

ACCURACY RATE

The accuracy of image-guided core-needle biopsy as compared to surgical biopsy has been reported by several authors (Table 2). Based on the data collected, it is clear that experienced operators can obtain adequate samples most of the time and achieve an accuracy rate comparable to that of surgical biopsy.[67] Most interventional mammographers performing core biopsy are using automated 14-gauge biopsy devices, for which the sensitivity is reported to be between 92% and 100%. Parker et al.[68] report a miss rate of core biopsy of 1.1% among 1,363 lesions that were evaluated with both core biopsy and excisional biopsy. The miss rate with core biopsy is similar to the 2% to 9% that has been reported with surgical biopsy.[7,69]

CONCORDANCE

Correlation of the radiographic findings with the pathologic diagnosis is essential in avoiding missed cancers. For low- and intermediate-suspicion lesions, if the radiographic finding and pathologic diagnosis are benign and concordant, the patient is spared the need for surgical biopsy, and she may return to routine mammographic surveillance. If a benign diagnosis is obtained for a highly suspicious radiographic abnormality, surgical biopsy or repeat core biopsy must be performed to avoid missing a potential cancer (see Fig. 3). For low- to intermediate-suspicion lesions in which a nonspecific but benign diagnosis is made, mammographic follow-up in 6 months, after the standard protocol for probably benign lesions, can be performed. This should only be done if accurate targeting during the biopsy can be assured.

Concordance and adequate lesion sampling are easier to assess when the targeted lesion contains microcalcifications. Tissue removed from calcified lesions is examined with specimen radiography to confirm the presence of microcalcifications, which are also specifically described in the pathology report. If the pathologist does not see microcalcifications, it may be necessary to obtain deeper cuts through the paraffin blocks, as the microcalcifications may not have been included in the sectioned slides. In a series of 100 patients reported by Elvecrog and associates,[44] three lesions were missed with stereotactic biopsy, one of which was a carcinoma presenting with mammographic calcifications. In that case, no calcifications were reported histologically. A specimen radiograph was not performed, but this experience prompted the authors to recommend routine specimen radiography of lesions containing calcifications. Specimen radiography is standard practice to ensure adequate sampling of lesions that contain calcifications.

Discordant imaging and histopathologic results are an indication for repeat biopsy. Discordance was reported as the cause for repeat biopsy in 27% of patients.[70] Rebiopsy in these patients revealed malignancy in 47%, again emphasizing the need for concordance and accurate assessment of degree of suspicion. Another report found benign discordant findings in 5% of cancers not diagnosed at stereotactic core biopsy.[71] Review of these cases revealed inaccurate lesion targeting in 71% of cases, most of which were performed during the first 9 months after introduction of stereotactic biopsy in clinical practice.[71] In a multicenter study of 6,152 core biopsies, 280 patients with negative core results but suspicious mammographic findings underwent surgical biopsy, and 5.4% were malignant.[68]

Partial concordance is encountered when the degree of carcinoma is underestimated. In cases in which DCIS is diagnosed, core-needle biopsy can confirm the presence of invasion but cannot exclude it.[68,72] As many as 20% of patients diagnosed with DCIS by 14-gauge stereotactic biopsy are found to have foci of invasion at surgery.[73] This may require that the patient undergo a second separate surgical procedure for axillary lymph node dissection. The accuracy of stereotactic core-needle biopsy in correctly diagnosing atypical ductal hyperplasia (ADH) and DCIS has increased with the use of the 14-gauge vacuum-assisted biopsy instrument.[74,75] The rate of complete concordance will most likely improve even further with the use of the 11-gauge vacuum-assisted biopsy probe, but this remains to be proved.

CONTROVERSIAL MANAGEMENT ISSUES

Partial or Complete Lesion Removal

Lesion removal may occur inadvertently during core sampling of a small lesion. This occurrence is of no concern when the pathology is benign but has important practical implications if ensuing surgical excision is necessary due to a pathology report of atypia or malignancy. Mammographic changes, such as air or hematoma from 14-gauge core-needles or 14-gauge vacuum biopsy probes, resolve completely in time, leaving no residual mark at the site of the biopsy.[76–78] If a 14-gauge needle is used for the needle biopsy, it is important not to remove the lesion entirely so that the area can be localized if surgical excision is ultimately necessary.

This problem has been addressed with the 11-gauge vacuum-assisted biopsy probe, which allows placement of a small metallic clip at the biopsy site. Clip placement identifies the biopsy site for subsequent surgical excision even if the mammographic lesion has been completely removed. Reports on the accuracy of clip placement have found the distance between the clip and the residual lesion or biopsy site to be less than 1 cm in 95% of cases.[79] Potentially clinically meaningful misplacement rates with a distance of more than 24 mm from the targeted lesion have been reported in 7% to 11% of cases.[80] Identification of clip misplacement during the needle biopsy procedure dictates rapid surgical reexcision if it is deemed necessary based on the histologic result, so that postbiopsy changes can be used to gũide preoperative wire localization. In our own practice, review of 74 stereotactic core biopsies with the 11-gauge vacuum-assisted probe and clip replacement revealed clip positioning within 10 mm of the lesion in 84% of cases. The targeted lesion was completely removed by the 11-gauge vacuum-assisted probe in 58% of cases in which a clip was deployed. In two cases, the distance between the clip and this lesion was between 10 and 20 cm, and in three cases, the distance was greater than 30 mm. These large displacements occurred along the needle tract and can be seen in association with hematomas at the biopsy site.[81] Hematomas are important to recognize at the time of the procedure, as they can obscure the targeted lesion and pose difficulties in subsequent localizations, should surgical intervention be needed. Metallic clips can also be placed under ultrasound guidance when small suspicious lesions are sampled to mark the lesion site.[82] Early experience with this technique has yielded accurate clip placement with pathologic confirmation of the clip location at the lesion site.

A potential result of partial lesion removal with core-needle biopsy is inaccuracies in the final estimate of tumor size in cases of invasive carcinoma. Tumor removal in fragments, rather than in a single intact specimen, can lead to underestimation of the tumor size and, thus, final cancer staging. This is more relevant for smaller cancers, as the volume of tissue removed from these lesions can represent a significant percentage of the total tumor burden present. Final estimates of the tumor size in excised surgical specimens in cases diagnosed with prior core-needle biopsy should incorporate the volume of tumor found in the core samples, so that the estimated size is accurate and tumor understaging is avoided. When a significant portion (or all) of the tumor has been removed by the needle biopsy, a final tumor size estimate is obtained by combining the tumor volume in the core tissue sample with the residual tumor in the excisional surgical specimen. In our institution, the pathologist routinely reports the maximum tumor length in the core samples to give a preoperative estimate of the tumor diameter. The pathologic method used in the calculation of final tumor size is similar to that used to calculate final tumor burden from combined tumor measurements in surgical excisional specimens and residual tumor in the reexcision or mastectomy specimens. Patients undergoing core-needle biopsy and final lumpectomy or mastectomy in different institutions pose a dilemma, as review of both the core samples and the surgical specimen is needed for accurate size estimation. In such cases, review of the imaging studies obtained before core biopsy can be helpful, as microscopic measurement of small breast carcinomas shows the best correlation with mammographic tumor size measurements.[83]

A device called the *Advanced Breast Biopsy Instrumentation (ABBI) system* (U.S. Surgical Corporation, Norwalk, CT) has been developed to perform automated stereotactic biopsy and was granted Food and Drug Administration approval in 1996. This device offers cannula sizes of 0.5 to 2.0 cm in diameter, which remove cylinders of tissue of the selected diameter size. It is more expensive and more invasive than core-needle biopsy and involves cautery and wound suturing. In theory, the potential advantage of this system may be the ability to remove an entire small lesion in a single specimen rather than multiple fragments and avoid the need for follow-up studies. Although not approved by the Food and Drug Administration for this function, in certain cases the ABBI biopsy could serve as an excisional biopsy and obviate the need for additional surgery. A review of 58 cases involving the use of the ABBI system reported a 43% failure rate (25 cases). The procedure could not be completed in 2 patients, 9 patients were eliminated because of technical issues, and 14 patients were converted to open surgical excision.[84] The number of lesions for which percutaneous removal by this device is desired is limited, because there are few indications for removal of benign nonpalpable lesions. Most important, the ability of this procedure to obtain clean margins during cancer biopsy has yet to be determined in a large study. If, after the ABBI procedure, patients also require surgical biopsy, the procedure has added considerable cost without significant benefit. The procedure is then, in effect, a more expensive and more invasive core biopsy method for obtaining diagnosis with little current practical application. Clearly, clinical studies are needed to determine what, if any, is the role for this device.

Atypical Hyperplasia

The distinction between cytologic atypia and the histologic diagnosis of atypical hyperplasia is an important one. Cytologic atypia result from FNA of solid breast masses in 12% to 17% of aspirations.[85,86] Some breast lesions are particularly difficult to diagnose cytologically, such as lobular and papillary lesions, and result in a higher proportion of atypical samples. Atypical hyperplasia represents a diagnostic challenge and limitation for the cytopathologist.[87] Excisional biopsy is advocated for cases diagnosed as atypical or suspicious on FNA.[88–90]

ADH is a histologic diagnosis that is made on tissue sampling, be it excisional biopsy or core biopsy. There are substantial degrees of subjectivity and disagreement in making this diagnosis histologically.[91–93] Isolated ADH is a benign histologic diagnosis on excisional biopsy. When ADH is encountered in core samples, surgical excision of the lesion is indicated, as it may coexist with adjacent DCIS or invasive ductal carcinoma.[94] A study found the most common reason for recommending rebiopsy after stereotactic biopsy to be ductal atypia.[70] A histologic diagnosis of ADH has been reported in 4.2% to 10.0% of patients undergoing core biopsy, and 18% to 50% of patients with ADH have cancer found at surgery.[70,74,95] The diagnosis of ADH occurs more often when biopsy is performed for microcalcifications rather than masses.[71] The frequent diagnosis of ADH when sampling a carcinoma is likely due to the difficulties the pathologist faces in distinguishing ADH from DCIS in small specimens. The frequency with which a cancer yields atypical hyperplasia at stereotactic biopsy is dependent on the mammographic findings and the final histologic diagnosis. A study reported the frequency of ADH to be higher for calcifications than for masses, for DCIS than for invasive carcinoma, and for noncomedo than for comedo DCIS.[71] The rate of ADH on core biopsy varies depending on the confidence and experience of the pathologist in evaluating core samples and the type of needle used. A review of 500 cores in our practice obtained with 14-gauge and 11-gauge needles revealed ADH as the histologic diagnosis in 3.4% of the cases. Subsequent excisional biopsy revealed DCIS in only 19% of the patients.

A diagnosis of lobular neoplasia at core-needle biopsy appears to be an incidental finding that is unrelated to the mammographic abnormality that initiated the biopsy. Lobular "neoplasia," which includes atypical lobular hyperplasia and lobular carcinoma *in situ*, is considered a risk factor and does not necessarily require subsequent biopsy. Women with this diagnosis on core biopsy should be managed on an individual basis after consultation with the pathologist and the surgeon to ensure that the histologic findings are clearly distinct from solid-type DCIS and that there is concordance with the mammographic lesion.

Radial Scar

A radial scar (equivalent terms: *complex sclerosing lesion, sclerosing ductal lesion*) is a complex lesion of hyperplasia that mimics the architectural features of an infiltrating ductal carcinoma.[96–99] The central area of the lesion contains dense collagen, and the more peripheral ducts are often dilated and hyperplastic, often exhibiting combinations of ductal hyperplasia (with or without atypia), adenosis, papillomas, lobular neoplasia, and, occasionally, DCIS. Radial scars appear as stellate masses with multiple, fine low-density spicules.[100] It is not possible to differentiate mammographic radial scars from an infiltrating tumor.[101]

Potential radial scars are best surgically excised rather than evaluated with core-needle biopsy. The coexistence of complex epithelial changes makes histologic evaluation of the entire lesion necessary. In addition, radial scars may be difficult to differentiate from tubular carcinoma in small core specimens, often requiring histologic evaluation of the entire lesion.[102,103]

Histologic Specimen Interpretation

Pathologists interpreting surgical biopsy specimens in which a prior core-needle biopsy was performed should be aware of the phenomenon of epithelial displacement.[104] Displacement of DCIS into the adjacent parenchyma after needle biopsy can sometimes be mistaken for invasion in the surgical specimen. This can be avoided if the pathologist notes findings suggestive of epithelial displacement, such as fragments of epithelium in artificial spaces accompanied by hemorrhage, inflammation, and granulation tissue.

Only a few cases of tumor cells seeding the needle track have been reported in the literature, one including seeding after needle biopsy of a mucinous carcinoma.[105] However, seeding of the needle track with tumor after core-needle biopsy may occur more frequently than initially expected. In our institution, a review of 352 surgically resected specimens identified the needle track from a prior core biopsy in 325 cases.[106] Histologic evaluation of the needle track revealed 114 cases of tumor displacement, in which tumor cell clusters lodged in benign fibrous or fatty stroma in or adjacent to the needle tract were identified. In 76 of 114 cases demonstrating tumor displacement, the dislodgment was limited to one to two cell clusters. Tumor displacement was encountered more frequently in cases in which the lesion was sampled using sonographic guidance with a 14-gauge biopsy gun than when the lesion was sampled stereotactically using a vacuum-assisted device. One possible explanation for the observed difference in frequency of cellular displacement is needle reinsertion used with biopsies using biopsy guns. As the needle moves in and out of the tumor multiple times and traverses the adjacent breast tissue, tumor cells are displaced into the adjacent tissue. In contrast, the vacuum-assisted biopsy needle is inserted only once and rotated in place, thereby reducing the number of times the needle traverses the tumor and the adjacent breast parenchyma. This theory is supported by the fact that tumor displacement is seen in 40% of palpable lesions sampled with core biopsy. Needle sampling of palpable lesions has been standard clinical practice for some time without apparent adverse effect on prognosis.[24–26]

Interestingly, we found tumor displacement to be more prevalent in cases in which the time interval between core biopsy and excision was short. Tumor displacement was seen in 42% of cases with an interval between biopsy and excision of fewer than 15 days, in 31% of cases with an interval of 15–28 days, and in 15% of tumors excised more than 28 days after core biopsy ($p < .005$). This observation suggests that tumor cells do not survive displacement.

Complications

Complications for needle biopsy are similar to those of needle localization procedures and may include bleeding, infection, and vasovagal reactions.[107] Using a 14-gauge needle, the estimated frequencies of hematoma and infection are each less than 2 in 1,000.[38,40] The complication rates with the 14-gauge vacuum-assisted biopsy are similar to those with 14-gauge automated biopsy guns.[78] Bruising at the biopsy site and mild tenderness are expected symptoms and are of no clinical concern. Permanent mammographic scarring or architectural distortion has not been observed as a result of core-needle biopsies.[78] Pneumothorax after ultrasound-guided core biopsy is possible but extremely rare.

Hematomas are more likely to occur in patients with bleeding disorders or those receiving anticoagulant medication, such as warfarin (Coumadin) and aspirin. For patients receiving Coumadin, close consultation with the referring physician is advised to determine if discontinuing the drug for 3 days before the needle biopsy is medically indicated. Patients receiving high-dose aspirin or antiinflammatories may also have prolonged bleeding and, if feasible, should discontinue the medication 5 to 7 days before the procedure. A large hematoma resulting from stereotactic core biopsy of a 5-mm invasive carcinoma with a 14-gauge needle was reported in a patient subsequently diagnosed with factor XI deficiency.[108] The hematoma, although of no clinical significance in and of itself, obscured the small carcinoma, posing a management dilemma. In this case, the patient underwent lumpectomy after the hematoma reabsorbed to 3 cm, 12 weeks after the stereotactic biopsy. This clinical scenario is rarely encountered in patients with normal bleeding times.

Patients with prosthetic valves who need prophylactic antibiotics before procedures in the mouth do not routinely need prebiopsy antibiotics, provided that the core biopsy is performed using sterile techniques. Patients with severe valvular disease may be an exception to this rule, so that consultation between the physician performing the needle biopsy and the referring clinician is prudent.

UNRESOLVED ISSUES

The rapid widespread use of image-guided needle biopsy of nonpalpable lesions has defrayed cost[109] and improved patient care by eliminating cosmetic deformity but has led to several issues that are currently unresolved. Among these, three are of primary clinical importance: (a) required credentials for physicians performing the procedure, (b) appropriate lesion selection, and (c) length and interval of follow-up after the procedure.

A national survey of practice patterns in the United States found that although core biopsy was widespread in use, there was considerable variability among sites regarding the credential requirements, practice patterns, and follow-up after the image-guided biopsy procedures.[35] In this report, 85% of procedures were performed by radiologists, 13% by radiologists and surgeons either jointly or separately, 1% by surgeons, 0.3% by pathologists, and 0.3% by radiologists and pathologists. The number of needle biopsies performed weekly ranged from 0.1 to 30.0. Performing a large number of needle biopsies has been reported to lead to increased procedural accuracy,[110] so that a significantly lower accuracy rate may be seen in centers that perform very few procedures. Of physicians performing core biopsy, 61% had no special credentials, whereas the remainder had variable requirements, without any consistent pattern. The survey also found wide variability with regard to practice patterns in terms of patient and lesion selection. In lesions categorized as probably benign, low suspicion, and intermediate to high suspicion, both masses and calcifications were included as indications for core biopsy. Probably benign masses have a low probability of malignancy and are usually managed with periodic imaging follow-up studies.[52] These masses were included as lesions indicated for core biopsy in 55% of respondents, despite strong evidence that they can be safely followed.[111,112]

Core biopsy is a sampling method, so that patient follow-up subsequent to the procedure is important, particularly in cases in which the histologic diagnosis is benign but nonspecific, as this histology can be encountered in sampling of normal (or adjacent) breast tissue. It is agreed that patient tracking for follow-up imaging studies is the responsibility of the physician performing the procedure, although there is lack of consensus regarding the length of follow-up required. A report found the median follow-up to be 12 months (range, 1–60 months), and 12% of physicians reported tracking patients indefinitely.[35] Protocols for imaging follow-up are described in two multiinstitutional studies. Parker and associates[68] describe follow-up mammography at 6 months for benign biopsy results concordant with the imaging findings. Brenner et al.[110] describe a follow-up program for patients with benign core results with mammograms at 6, 12, 24, and 36 months. The appropriate interval and duration of follow-up in patients with benign core results depend on the degree of specificity of the histologic diagnosis and the mammographic degree of suspicion.

Compliance with follow-up recommendations among patients undergoing breast procedures is higher for patients recommended for surgical excision than for those recommended for imaging follow-up (74% versus 54%, respectively).[113] Noncompliance with recommended follow-up after percutaneous breast biopsy is a major problem, despite rigorous tracking and a quality assurance outcome program.[113,114] Patient compliance with recommended follow-up is essential to optimize the benefits of image-guided core biopsy and to avoid delay in diagnosing missed cancers.[115,116] Despite the apparent diagnostic reliability of core biopsies (see Table 2), maintaining mammographic follow-up after benign core biopsy is critical to uncover false-negative results.[117,118]

SUMMARY

Image-guided percutaneous breast biopsy has become an acceptable alternative to open surgical biopsy in the evaluation of most nonpalpable breast lesions. It is well tolerated by patients and can be performed under stereotactic or ultrasound guidance.

Percutaneous breast biopsy has several advantages over open surgical biopsy. Percutaneous biopsy is fast and inexpensive and avoids the scarring and breast deformity that are associated with surgical biopsy. It has been estimated that as much as 32% of the total cost of screening mammography programs can be attributed to surgical biopsies for benign disease.[119] A benign concordant needle biopsy result avoids a surgical biopsy. Even though a small percentage of women who undergo percutaneous biopsy also require a surgical biopsy due to insufficient sampling, indeterminate results, or radiographic-histopathologic discordance, studies have shown a cost savings of 23% to 50% with the use of needle-core biopsy instead of surgery.[120,121]

As expected, the introduction and widespread use of core-needle biopsy to sample nonpalpable lesions have had a major impact on clinical practice. The ratio of interventional procedures in our practice has shifted from 50% core biopsy and 50% preoperative needle localization 2 years ago to 66% and 33%, respectively, presently. Core-needle biopsy is an important part of patient care, but it must be considered in terms of what is best for the patient. Anxious patients who have decided on surgical excision as the management choice for a nonpalpable lesion should not be evaluated with core biopsy, as it only adds another procedure to the diagnostic and treatment process. Image-guided needle biopsy contributes to the management of patients with breast cancer only after careful planning of surgical treatment options. For example, core biopsy of multiple lesions affects patient management only if breast conservation, not mastectomy, is preferred by the patient.

In the future, standardization of the equipment, physician credentials, and lesion selection criteria will improve clinical management of patients by providing uniform quality of care. The American College of Radiology has developed a program for personnel credentials, equipment quality control, and radiation dose measurements to facilitate standardization.[122] Ultimately, minimally invasive percutaneous biopsy techniques may involve not only cancer diagnosis but also cancer therapy. Tumor ablation methods using focused ultrasound, laser, and cryoablation through a needle placed percutaneously into the breast cancer are currently being studied.

REFERENCES

1. Tabar L, Fagerberg CJG, Gad H, et al. Reduction in mortality from breast cancer after mass screening with mammography. *Lancet* 1985;1:829.
2. Eddy DM. Screening for breast cancer. *Ann Intern Med* 1989; 111:389.
3. Hall F. Screening mammography: potential problems on the horizon. *N Engl J Med* 1986;31:53.
4. Tersegno MM. Mammography positive value and true-positive biopsy rate. *AJR Am J Roentgenol* 1993;160:660.
5. Hall FM, Storella JM, Silverstone DZ, et al. Nonpalpable breast lesions: recommendations for biopsy based on suspicion of carcinoma at mammography. *Radiology* 1988;167:353.
6. Bernstein JR. Role of stereotactic breast biopsy. *Semin Surg Oncol* 1996;12:290.

7. Yankaskas BC, Knelson MH, Abernathy ML, et al. Needle localization biopsy of occult lesion of the breast. Experience in 199 cases. *Invest Radiol* 1988;23:729.
8. Yim JH, Premsri W, Weber B, et al. Mammographically detected breast cancer: benefits of stereotactic core versus wire localization biopsy. *Ann Surg* 1996;223:688.
9. Masood S. Fine needle aspiration biopsy of nonpalpable breast lesions. In: Schmidt W, ed. *Cytopathology annual 1993*. Baltimore: Williams & Wilkins, 1994.
10. Fornage BD, Faroux MJ, Simatos A. Breast masses: US-guided fine-needle aspiration biopsy. *Radiology* 1987;162:409.
11. Evans WP, Cade SH. Needle localization and fine needle aspiration biopsy of nonpalpable breast lesions with use of standard and stereotactic equipment. *Radiology* 1989;173:53.
12. Helvie MA, Baker D, Adler DD, et al. Radiographically guided fine-needle aspiration of nonpalpable breast lesions. *Radiology* 1990;174:657.
13. Lofgren M, Andersson I, Bondenson L, et al. X-ray guided fine needle aspiration for the cytologic diagnosis of nonpalpable breast lesions. *Cancer* 1988;61:1032.
14. Svane G, Silfversward C. Stereotaxic needle biopsy of nonpalpable breast lesions: cytologic and histologic findings. *Acta Radiol (Stockh)* 1983;24:283.
15. Bibbo M, Scheiber M, Cajulis R, et al. Stereotaxic fine needle aspiration cytology of occult malignant and premalignant breast lesions. *Acta Cytol* 1988;32:193.
16. Masood S, Frykberg ER, McLellan GL, et al. Prospective evaluation of radiologically detected fine needle aspiration biopsy of nonpalpable breast lesions. *Cancer* 1990;66:1480.
17. Ciatto S, Cataliotti L, Distante V. Nonpalpable lesions detected with mammography: review of 512 consecutive cases. *Radiology* 1987; 165:99.
18. Hann L, Ducatman BS, Wang HH, et al. Nonpalpable breast lesions: evaluation by means of fine needle aspiration cytology. *Radiology* 1989;171:373.
19. Arishita GI, Cruz BK, Harding CL, et al. Mammogram-directed fine needle aspiration of nonpalpable breast lesions. *J Surg Oncol* 1991;48:153.
20. Dent DM, Kirkpatrick AE, McGoogan E, et al. Stereotaxic localization and aspiration cytology in nonpalpable breast lesions. *Clin Radiol* 1989;40:380.
21. Lofgren M, Anderson J, Lindholm K. Stereotaxic fine needle aspiration for cytologic diagnosis of nonpalpable breast lesions. *AJR Am J Roentgenol* 1990;154:1191.
22. Fajardo LL, Davis JR, Weins JL, et al. Mammography guided stereotactic fine needle aspiration cytology of nonpalpable breast lesions: perspective comparison with surgical biopsy results. *AJR Am J Roentgenol* 1990;155:977.
23. Masood S. Occult breast lesions and aspiration biopsy: a new challenge. *Diagn Cytopathol* 1993;9:611.
24. Elston CW, Cotton RE, Davies DJ, et al. A comparison of the use of the "Tru-Cut" needle and fine needle aspiration cytology in the preoperative diagnosis of carcinoma of the breast. *Histopathology* 1978;2:239.
25. Vorherr H. Breast aspiration biopsy with multihole needles for histologic and cytologic examination. *Am J Obstet Gynecol* 1985;151:70.
26. Pederson L, Guldhammer B, Kamby C, et al. Fine needle aspiration and Tru-Cut biopsy in the diagnosis of soft tissue metastases in breast cancer. *Eur J Cancer Clin Oncol* 1986;22:1045.
27. Shabot MM, Goldberg IM, Schick P, et al. Aspiration cytology is superior to Tru-Cut needle biopsy in establishing the diagnosis of clinically suspicious breast masses. *Ann Surg* 1982;196:122.
28. Gent HJ. Stereotaxic needle localization and cytological diagnosis of occult breast lesions. *Ann Surg* 1986;204:580.
29. Azavedo E, Svane G, Auer G. Stereotactic fine needle biopsy in 2594 mammographically detected nonpalpable lesions. *Lancet* 1989;1:1033.
30. Ciatto S, Del Turco, Bravetti B. Non-palpable breast lesions: stereotaxic fine needle aspiration cytology. *Radiology* 1989;173:57.
31. Parker SH, Lovin JD, Jobe WE, et al. Nonpalpable breast lesions: stereotactic automated large core biopsies. *Radiology* 1991;180:403.
32. Parker SH, Lovin JD, Jobe WE, el al. Stereotactic breast biopsy with a biopsy gun. *Radiology* 1990;176:741.
33. Bulmgren J, Jacobson B, Nordenstrom B. Stereotaxis instrument for needle biopsy of the mamma. *AJR Am J Roentgenol* 1977;129:121.
34. Dowlatshahi K, Jokich PM, Schmidt R, et al. Cytologic diagnosis of occult breast lesions using stereotaxic needle aspiration. *Arch Surg* 1987;122:1343.
35. March DE, Raslavicus A, Coughlin BF, et al. Use of breast core biopsy in the United States: results of a national survey. *AJR Am J Roentgenol* 1997;169:697.
36. Nordenstrom B, Zajicek J. Stereotaxic needle biopsy and preoperative indication of non-palpable mammary lesions. *Acta Cytologica* 1977;21:350.
37. Dowlatshahi K, Yaremko NL, Kluskens LF, et al. Nonpalpable breast lesions: findings of stereotaxic needle core biopsy and fine needle aspiration cytology. *Radiology* 1991;181:745.
38. Myer JE. Value of large core biopsy of occult breast lesions. *AJR Am J Roentgenol* 1992;158:991.
39. Liberman L, Dershaw DD, Rosen PP, et al. Stereotaxic 14-gauge breast biopsy: how many core biopsy specimens are needed? *Radiology* 1994;192:793.
40. Burbank F. Stereotactic breast biopsy: comparison of 14 and 11 gauge Mammotome probe performance and complication rates. *Am Surg* 1997;63:988.
41. Berg WA, Krebs TL, Campassi C, et al. Evaluation of 14 and 11 gauge directional, vacuum-assisted biopsy probes and 14 gauge biopsy alms in a breast parenchymal model. *Radiology* 1997;205:203.
42. Meyer JE, Smith DN, Dipiro PJ, et al. Stereotactic breast biopsy of clustered microcalcifications with a directional, vacuum-assisted device. *Radiology* 1997;204:575.
43. Kopans D, Meyer J, Lindfors K, et al. Breast sonography to guide cyst aspiration and wire localization of occult solid lesions. *AJR Am J Roentgenol* 1984;143:89.
44. Elvecrog EL, Lechner MC, Nelson MT. Nonpalpable breast lesions: correlation of stereotaxic large-core needle biopsy and surgical results. *Radiology* 1993;188:453.
45. Fornage BD, Coan JD, David CL. Ultrasound-guided needle biopsy of the breast and other interventional procedures. *Radiol Clin North Am* 1992;30:167.
46. Georgian-Smith D, Shiels W. Freehand invasive sonography in breast: basic principles and clinical application. *Radiographics* 1996;16:149.
47. Fornage B. A simple phantom for training in ultrasound-guided needle biopsy using the freehand technique. *J Ultrasound Med* 1989;8:701.
48. Georgian-Smith D. Interventional breast ultrasound: training experience on a tissue model. In: Madjar H, Teubner J, Hackeloer B, eds. *Breast ultrasound update: proceedings of the eighth annual international congress on the ultrasonic examination of the breast*. Heidelberg, Germany: Basel and Karger, 1993;276.
49. Georgian-Smith D, Lyon R. A smorgasbord of interventional phantoms. *Semin Interv Radiol* 1997;14:377.
50. Georgian-Smith D. Variable appearance of breast cysts on ultrasound and suggested management. *Mammography Matters* 1996;3:22.
51. Georgian-Smith D, Yassin R. Solidified benign breast cyst. *J Ultrasound Med* 1996;15:165.
52. Sickles EA. Periodic mammographic follow-up of probably benign lesions: results in 3,184 consecutive cases. *Radiology* 1991;179:463.
53. Venta LA, Kim JP, Pelloski CE, Morrow M. Management of complex breast cysts. *AJR Am J Roentgenol* 1999 *(in press)*.
54. Conway WF, Hayes CW, Brewer WH. Occult breast masses: use of a mammographic localizing grid for US evaluation. *Radiology* 1991;181:143.
55. Philpotts LE, Lee CH, Horvath LJ, et al. Canceled stereotactic core-needle biopsy of the breast: analysis of 89 cases. *Radiology* 1997;205:423.
56. American College of Radiology. *Breast imaging reporting and date system (BI-RADS)*, 2nd ed. Reston, VA: American College of Radiology, 1995.
57. Sickles EA. Nonpalpable, circumscribed, noncalcified solid breast masses: likelihood of malignancy based on lesion size and age of patient. *Radiology* 1994;192:439.
58. Lindfors KK, O'Connor J, Acredolo CR, et al. Short-interval follow up mammography versus immediate core biopsy of benign breast lesions: assessment of patient stress. *AJR Am J Roentgenol* 1998;171:55.
59. Jackman RJ, Marzoni FA, Finkelstein SL, et al. Benefits of diagnosing nonpalpable breast cancer with stereotactic large-core needle biopsy. Lower costs and fewer operations. *Radiology* 1996;201:311.
60. Liberman L, LaTrenta LR, Dershaw DD, et al. Impact of core biopsy on the surgical management of impalpable breast cancer. *AJR Am J Roentgenol* 1997;168:495.
61. Smith DN, Christian R, Meyer JE. Large-core needle biopsy of nonpalpable breast cancers: the impact on subsequent surgical excision. *Arch Surg* 1997;132:256.

62. Morrow M, Venta L, Stinson T, Shih L, Oquendo A, Bennett C. *Is core biopsy (Cbx) the diagnostic procedure of choice for all mammographic abnormalities*? Paper presented at the 35th Annual Meeting of the American Society of Clinical Oncology, May 1999, Atlanta.
63. Bianchi S, Palli D, Ciatto S, et al. Accuracy and reliability of frozen section diagnosis in a series of 672 nonpalpable breast lesions. *Am J Clin Pathol* 1995;103:199.
64. Whitten TM, Wallace TW, Bird RE, et al. Image-guided core biopsy has advantages over needle localization biopsy for the diagnosis of nonpalpable breast cancer. *Am Surg* 1997;63:1072.
65. Liberman L, LaTrenta LR, Van Zee KJ, et al. Stereotactic core biopsy of calcifications highly suggestive of malignancy. *Radiology* 1997;203:673.
66. Rosenblatt R, Fineberg SA, Sparano JA, et al. Stereotactic core needle biopsy of multiple sites in the breast: efficacy and effect on patient care. *Radiology* 1996;201:67.
67. Schmidt RA. Stereotactic breast biopsy. *CA Cancer J Clin* 1994;44:172.
68. Parker SH, Burbank F, Jackman RJ, et al. Percutaneous large-core breast biopsy: a multi-institutional study. *Radiology* 1994;193:359.
69. Haselgren P, Hummel RP, Georgia-Smith P, et al. Breast biopsy with needle localization accuracy of specimen x-ray and management of missed lesions. *Surgery* 1993;114:836.
70. Dershaw DD, Morris EA, Liberman L, et al. Nondiagnostic stereotaxic core breast biopsy: results of re-biopsy. *Radiology* 1996;198:323.
71. Liberman L, Dershaw DD, Glassman JR, et al. Analysis of cancers not diagnosed at stereotactic core breast biopsy. *Radiology* 1997;203:151.
72. Jackman RJ, Nowels KW, Shepard MJ, et al. Stereotaxic large-core needle biopsy of 450 non-palpable breast lesions with surgical correlation in lesions with cancer or atypical hyperplasia. *Radiology* 1994;193:91.
73. Liberman L, Dershaw DD, Rosen PP, et al. Stereotaxic core biopsy of breast carcinoma: accuracy at predicting invasion. *Radiology* 1995;194:379.
74. Jackman RJ, Burbank F, Parker SH, et al. Atypical ductal hyperplasia diagnosed at stereotactic breast biopsy: improved reliability with 14 gauge, directional, vacuum-assisted biopsy. *Radiology* 1997;204:485.
75. Burbank F. Stereotactic breast biopsy of atypical ductal hyperplasia and ductal carcinoma in situ lesions: improved accuracy with a directional, vacuum-assisted biopsy instrument. *Radiology* 1997;202:843.
76. Kaye MD, Vicinanza-Adami CA, Sullivan MI. Mammographic findings after stereotaxic biopsy of the breast performed with large-core needles. *Radiology* 1994;192:149.
77. Burbank F. Mammographic findings after 14 gauge automated needle and 14 gauge directional vacuum assisted stereotactic breast biopsies. *Radiology* 1997;204:153.
78. Liberman L, Hann LE, Dershaw DD, et al. Mammographic findings after stereotactic 14-gauge vacuum biopsy. *Radiology* 1997;203:343.
79. Liberman L, Dershaw D, Morris EA, et al. Clip placement after stereotactic vacuum-assisted breast biopsy. *Radiology* 1997;205:417.
80. Burbank F, Forcier N. Tissue marking clip for stereotactic breast biopsy: initial placement accuracy. Long-term stability, and usefulness as a guide for wire localization. *Radiology* 1997;205:407.
81. Comstock CE, Phillips SW, Venta LA. Accuracy of clip placement after 11-gauge stereotactic vacuum-assisted breast biopsy. *AJR Am J Roentgenol* 1999;172[suppl]:10.
82. Phillips SW, Gabriel H, Venta LA. Preliminary experience with sonographically guided metallic clip placement. *AJR Am J Roentgenol* 1999;172[suppl]:87.
83. Wiley EL, Arnell P, Rivera CE, Gehl JJ, DeLeon P, Venta L. Tumor staging of mammographically detected breast carcinoma: is gross tumor measurement accurate for staging? *Mod Pathol* 1999;12:33A.
84. Ferzli GS, Hurwitz JB, Puza T, et al. Advanced breast biopsy instrumentation: a critique. *J Am Coll Surg* 1997,185:145.
85. Hann L, Ducatman BS, Wang HH, et al. Non palpable breast lesions: evaluation by means of fine needle aspiration cytology. *Radiology* 1989;171:373.
86. Hayes MK, DeBruhl ND, Hirshowitz S, et al. Mammographically guided fine-needle aspiration cytology of the breast: reducing the rate of insufficient specimens. *AJR Am J Roentgenol* 1996;167:381.
87. Masood S. Pathological interpretation of fine needle aspiration cytology. In: Fajardo LL, Willison KM, Pizzutiello RJ, eds. *A comprehensive approach to stereotactic breast biopsy*. Boston: Blackwell Science, 1996:232.
88. Silverman J, Masood S, Ducatman BS, et al. Can FNA biopsy separate atypical hyperplasia, carcinoma in situ, and invasive carcinoma of the breast? Cytomorphologic criteria and limitations in diagnosis. *Diagn Cytopathol* 1993;9:713.
89. Shiels LA, Mulford D, Dawson AG. Cytomorphology of proliferative breast disease. *Acta Cytol* 1993;37:768.
90. Stanley MW, Henry-Stanley MJ, Zera R. Prospective study of high risk proliferative lesions of breast duct epithelium by fine needle aspiration. *Acta Cytol* 1991;35:611.
91. Beck JS. Observer variability in reporting breast lesions. *J Clin Pathol* 1985;38:1358.
92. Rosai J. Borderline epithelial lesions of the breast. *Am J Surg Pathol* 1991;15:209.
93. Scnitt SJ, Connolly JL, Tavassoli FA, et al. Intraobserver reproducibility in the diagnosis of ductal proliferative breast lesions using standardized criteria. *Am J Surg Pathol* 1992;16:1133.
94. Sneige N, Fornage BD, Saleh G. Ultrasound-guided fine needle aspiration of non-palpable breast lesions. Cytologic and histologic findings. *Am J Clin Pathol* 1994;102:98.
95. Liberman L, Cohen MA, Dershaw DD, et al. Atypical ductal hyperplasia diagnosed at stereotaxic core biopsy of breast lesions: an indication for surgical biopsy. *AJR Am J Roentgenol* 1995;164:1111.
96. Azzopardi JG. *Problems in breast pathology*. Philadelphia: WB Saunders, 1979:174.
97. Fenoglio C, Lattes R. Sclerosing papillary proliferations in the female breast. A benign lesion often mistaken for carcinoma. *Cancer* 1974;33:691.
98. Fisher ER, Palekar AS, Kotwal N, et al. A nonencapsulated sclerosing lesion of the breast. *Am J Clin Pathol* 1979;71:240.
99. Andersen JA, Gram JB. Radial scar in the female breast. A long term follow-up study of 32 cases. *Cancer* 1984;53:2557.
100. Nielsen M, Jensen J, Andersen JA. An autopsy study of radial scar in the female breast. *Histopathology* 1985;9:287.
101. Adler DD, Helvie AH, Oberman HA, et al. Radial sclerosing lesion of the breast. Mammographic features. *Radiology* 1990;176:737.
102. de la Torre A, Lindholm K, Lingren A. Fine needle aspiration cytology of tubular breast carcinoma and radial scar. *Acta Cytol* 1994;38:884.
103. Jackman RJ, Finkelstein SL, Marzoni FA. Stereotaxic large-core needle biopsy of histologically benign nonpalpable breast lesions: false-negative results and failed follow-up. *Radiology* 1995;197:203.
104. Youngson BJ, Liberman L, Rosen PP. Displacement of carcinomatous epithelium in surgical breast specimens following stereotaxic core biopsy. *Am J Clin Pathol* 1995;103:598.
105. Harter LP, Curtis JS, Ponto G, et al. Malignant seeding of the needle track during stereotactic core needle breast biopsy. *Radiology* 1992;185:713.
106. Diaz LK, Wiley EL. Are malignant cells displaced by large-gauge needle core biopsies of the breast? *AJR Am J Roentgenol* 1999 (*in press*).
107. Helvie MA, Ikeda DM, Adler DD. Localization and needle aspiration of breast lesions: complications in 370 cases. *AJR Am J Roentgenol* 1991;157:711.
108. Deutch BM, Schwartz MR, Tomasine F, et al. Stereotactic core breast biopsy of a minimal carcinoma complicated by a large hematoma: a management dilemma. *Radiology* 1997;202:431.
109. Lee CH, Egglin RK, Philpotts L, et al. Cost-effectiveness of stereotactic core needle biopsy: analysis by means of mammographic findings. *Radiology* 1997;202:849.
110. Brenner RJ, Fajardo L, Fisher PR, et al. Percutaneous core biopsy of the breast. Effect of operator experience and number of samples on diagnostic accuracy. *AJR Am J Roentgenol* 1996,166:341.
111. Sickles EA, Parker SH. Appropriate role of core biopsy in the management of probably benign lesions (Editorial). *Radiology* 1993;188:315.
112. Logan-Young WW, Janus JA, Destounis SV, et al. Appropriate role of core biopsy in the management of probably benign lesions. *Radiology* 1994;190:313.
113. Goodman KA, Birdwell RL, Ikeda DM. Compliance with recommended follow-up after percutaneous breast core biopsy. *AJR Am J Roentgenol* 1998;170:89.
114. Pal S, Ikeda DM, Birdwell RL. Compliance with recommended follow-up after fine-needle aspiration biopsy of nonpalpable breast lesions: a retrospective study. *Radiology* 1996;201:71.

115. Helvie MA, Pennes DR, Rebner M, et al. Mammographic follow-up of low-suspicion lesions compliance rate and diagnostic yield. *Radiology* 1991;178:155.
116. Parker SH, Jobe WE, Dennis MA, et al. US-guided automated large-core breast biopsy. *Radiology* 1993;187:507.
117. Morrow M. When can stereotactic core biopsy replace excisional biopsy? A clinical perspective. *Breast Cancer Res Treat* 1995;36:1.
118. Kopans DB. Caution on core. *Radiology* 1994;193:325.
119. Cyrlak D. Induced costs of low-cost screening mammography. *Radiology* 1988;168:661.
120. Lindfors KK, Rosenquist CJ. Needle core biopsy guided with mammography. A study of cost effectiveness. *Radiology* 1994; 190:217.
121. Liberman L, Fahs MC, Dershaw DD, et al. Impact of stereotaxic core biopsy on cost of diagnosis. *Radiology* 1995;195:633.
122. America College of Radiology. *Stereotactic breast biopsy accreditation program*. Reston, VA: American College of Radiology, 1996.
123. Dronkers DJ. Stereotaxic core biopsy of breast lesions. *Radiology* 1992;183:631.
124. Gisvold JJ, Goeliner JR, Grant CS, et al. Breast biopsy: a comparative study of stereotaxically guided core and excisional techniques. *AJR Am J Roentgenol* 1994;162:815.
125. Meyer JE, Christian RL, Lester SC. Evaluation of nonpalpable solid breast masses with stereotaxic large needle core biopsy using a dedicated unit. *AJR Am J Roentgenol* 1996;167:179.

CHAPTER 14

Diseases of the Breast, 2nd ed.,
edited by Jay R. Harris.
Lippincott Williams & Wilkins, Philadelphia © 2000.

Preoperative Imaging-Guided Needle Localization and Biopsy of Nonpalpable Breast Lesions

Daniel B. Kopans and Barbara L. Smith

Randomized, controlled trials of breast cancer screening, as well as large-scale screening projects, have demonstrated that periodic screening of women who lack any signs or symptoms of breast cancer can lead to earlier detection of breast cancer, reduction in the size and stage at which cancers are diagnosed, and reduction in the absolute mortality from breast cancer by 25% to 30%.[1–3] This benefit has been shown to apply to women who begin screening by the age of 40.[4]

Mammography is the only screening modality that has been shown in large prospective trials to detect clinically occult malignancy reliably in asymptomatic women. Cancers detected by mammography alone are more likely to be of a smaller size and earlier stage than clinically evident cancers and have a correspondingly more favorable prognosis.[5]

Although mammography is the best method of detecting early breast cancer, many of the lesions that are detected on the mammogram and raise the physician's concern prove to be benign. A number of efforts are under way to develop noninvasive methods of distinguishing benign from malignant lesions; surgical removal and histologic analysis, however, remain the most accurate way of making a diagnosis.

Fine-needle aspiration cytology and core-needle biopsy have increasingly become used in an effort to reduce the cost and trauma of differentiating benign lesions from those that are malignant. Fine-needle aspiration requires interpretation by experienced cytopathologists and is not available at all institutions. Although fine-needle aspiration has a low false-positive rate, even in experienced hands the false-negative rate is significant. Fine-needle aspiration has the additional disadvantage of being unable to distinguish *in situ* from invasive breast cancer and can only occasionally provide specific tissue diagnosis of benign lesions. As a result, imaging-guided core-needle biopsy has become the predominant needle-biopsy diagnostic technique because it is more automated, less operator dependent, and is interpreted using standard histologic criteria rather than cytologic analysis. The use of needle biopsy can reduce the number of operations needed to treat cancer successfully and, if performed accurately, permit avoidance of surgery for benign lesions.

Despite the widespread adoption of needle biopsy, the false-negative rate for the procedure has never been accurately determined in any large prospective study series, although small prospective series suggest a relatively low miss rate.[6–8] The actual degree of sampling error (cancers missed because the needle did not sample the proper volume of tissue) remains a major unresolved question. The available data suggest that the false-negative rate for breast cancer using stereotactically guided needle biopsy is 3% to 5%.

The most accurate method of arriving at a tissue diagnosis remains the surgical removal of the suspected tissue. Properly performed needle localization and surgical excision has a less than 1% error rate for breast cancer, and these misses are usually evident when the lesion is not visible on the specimen radiograph. Because these lesions are not evident to the surgeon, excision of these nonpalpable lesions using preoperative needle localization requires the coordinated efforts of the radiologist, surgeon, and pathologist.

PREOPERATIVE NEEDLE LOCALIZATION FOR SURGICAL EXCISION

Excisional biopsy after imaging-guided needle localization remains the gold standard for the diagnosis of clinically occult lesions detected by mammography. It is the most accurate method of separating benign from malignant lesions and is the only method that permits the pathologist to fully characterize malignant lesions. The combined procedure should be performed with the objectives of safety and accuracy paramount. Whether the biopsy is performed for primary diagnostic purposes, for diagnosis after a nondiagnostic needle biopsy, or as

D. B. Kopans: Department of Radiology, Massachusetts General Hospital, Boston, Massachusetts

B. L. Smith: Harvard Medical School, Gillette Center for Women's Cancers, Massachusetts General Hospital, Boston, Massachusetts

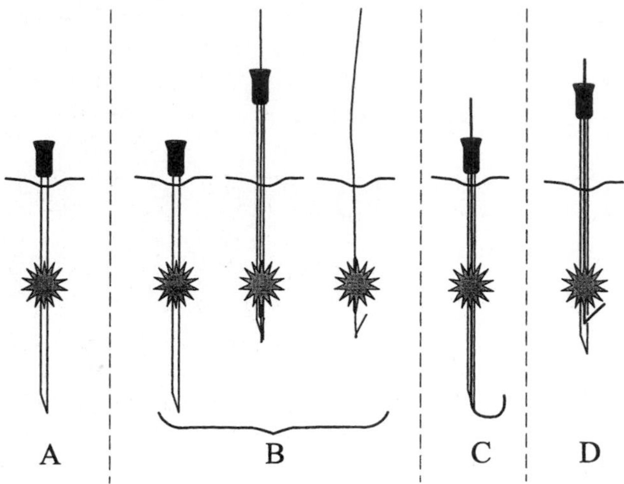

FIG. 1. Types of guides. **A:** A simple hypodermic needle can be used, transfixing or placed alongside a suspicious abnormality. **B:** Hookwires can be placed through needles that are first positioned in appropriate relationship to the lesion; the hook is then engaged, leaving a flexible wire for the surgeon to follow. **C:** Curved wires can be used to anchor needles, but their holding power is limited. **D:** Wires projecting from the side of a needle can be used to anchor a needle in position.

therapy after a needle biopsy diagnosis of malignancy, the positioning of guides for the surgeon, and the excision itself, should be planned carefully and performed with the goal of minimizing the trauma for the patient while providing accurate and complete characterization of the mammographic lesion.

Guide placement for the majority of clinically occult mammographically detected lesions can be accomplished easily using mammography. Ultrasonography[9] and computed tomography (CT)[10] can also be used to place guides for the surgeon. Quadrant resection to remove nonpalpable lesions without imaging guidance is inappropriate. It is inaccurate and results in the removal of unnecessarily large amounts of tissue.

The radiologist and surgeon should recognize the difficulty of deducing the actual position of a lesion when the patient is lying supine on the operating table using mammograms obtained with the breast vigorously compressed and pulled away from the chest wall. Skin markers are thus reliable only if the lesion is immediately beneath the skin.

To minimize the volume of tissue excised, accurate preoperative localization should position the guide through or alongside the lesion. The technique described in the section Mammographically Guided Preoperative Needle Localization allows a needle to be routinely placed within 5 mm of a lesion.[11] Placement at any greater distance from a lesion should be unacceptable, and if the guide is not within 5 mm of the abnormality, it should be repositioned or replaced.

Choice of Guide

Numerous guides with varying advantages and disadvantages have been developed to assist the surgeon in resecting a lesion that cannot be palpated even after the tissues have been entered (Fig. 1). These guides rely on the positioning of a needle under imaging observation and guidance. The actual choice of a guide depends on the preferences of the radiologist and surgeon. Many systems are available, ranging from standard hypodermic needles to specially designed localization devices.[12]

Hookwire Systems

The guides most commonly used feature a wire with a hook on the end. The hookwires can be passed through a needle; the hook re-forms when the needle is withdrawn over the wire, anchoring the wire in the tissue.[13] The needle is first positioned (or repositioned) to achieve a satisfactory relationship to the lesion; then the wire is engaged in the appropriate tissue volume. These devices can also be stiffened when a cannula is slid over them in the operating room.[14]

The length of the wire guide is important. Wires that are too short should not be used, because they may be enveloped by the breast when it changes position. Wires must be long enough that the wire is not drawn beneath the skin when the breast is in its natural position. The length of the wire should exceed by several centimeters the distance from the skin entry site to the lesion. If the length of wire is chosen properly and insertion is performed parallel to the chest wall, the protruding end of the wire need not be anchored. Firmly anchoring the wire is actually undesirable, because traction from breast movement may cause it to be pulled out of the lesion. These guides should be taped loosely to the skin so movement of the breast does not cause them to be inadvertently dislodged.

Introduction of Dyes

The injection of vital dyes[15] or the deposition of inert carbon particles at a suspicious lesion[16] and staining of the tissues to provide a track from the lesion to the skin have been found useful by some for guiding biopsies. The issue of the stability of materials in the tissue has generated some debate. Introduction of dyes fairly close to the time of surgery is probably a good idea to prevent their absorption or diffusion into a large volume of tissue. Injecting very small quantities of dye reduces the likelihood of diffusion into a large tissue volume. The surgeon may have difficulty following a thin trail of dye to the lesion, and many who use this technique also leave a needle or wire guide in position.

MAMMOGRAPHICALLY GUIDED PREOPERATIVE NEEDLE LOCALIZATION

Location of an Occult Lesion

Before recommending a biopsy, the radiologist must have an accurate idea of the three-dimensional location of a lesion and be confident of the ability to place a needle tip at the lesion. Methods have been described that assist in confirmation and triangulation when the location is not certain.[17,18] Lesions that are not clearly identified on two projections can often be localized using a parallax method.[19] If mammographic methods fail, ultrasonography[20] or CT can be used to direct the placement of guides.[21]

Because the standard screening lateral projection is the mediolateral oblique, an additional straight lateral image (orthogonal to the craniocaudal) should be obtained before needle placement to provide true perpendicular coordinates to the craniocaudal view.

Occasionally, multiple localizing wires are required to mark multiple lesions or to facilitate complete removal of a large area of calcifications. Careful planning is required for appropriate placement of wires in these cases.

Patient Preparation

The procedure should be explained to the patient in detail so the patient may be fully informed. Compassionate support should be provided for the patient, because these procedures are uncomfortable and can generate a great deal of anxiety. The patient should be attended at all times, because vasovagal reactions, although rare, should be anticipated. Premedication is not recommended if it reduces the patient's ability to be fully cooperative for the localization procedure. Local anesthesia may be used, but for the majority of patients it is not needed and may be more painful than the localization procedure itself.[22]

General Considerations

The radiologist, surgeon, and pathologist must work closely together. The radiologist should try to minimize the amount of dissection needed by choosing the shortest distance to the lesion that is feasible. Careful surgical dissection will avoid dislodging needles or cutting wires.

All methods available require the placement of a needle either through or alongside the target lesion. From a surgical perspective, excision would be easiest if the wires were placed from the front of the breast, so the wire could be followed directly to the lesion using the shortest, most direct route. This is generally difficult to do with a high degree of accuracy. It requires a freehand needle localization that is extremely dependent on operator skill, and routinely positioning guides within 0.5 cm of a lesion using the freehand method is difficult. Positioning guides from the front of the breast also runs the risk of causing a pneumothorax or entrance into the mediastinum.[23] If the lesion can be seen by ultrasonography, however, then a more direct, anterior route can be achieved with the needle under direct ultrasonic observation to avoid the inadvertent penetration of the pectoralis musculature or the thorax.

Regardless of the type of guide used, the development of dedicated mammography equipment has resulted in the ability to position needles very accurately into or alongside the smallest mammographically detected abnormalities.[24] This is accomplished most accurately and most safely by introducing the needle with the breast held in the mammographic compression system and the needle introduced parallel to the chest wall. Compression plates are used that have a series of holes or a fenestration permitting access to the breast and to a lesion while the breast is held in compression. The lesion is accessible through the fenestration. A single fenestration with calibrations along the sides is the most convenient and accurate to use. Provided the appropriate technique is used, the shaft of the needle should rarely if ever be more than 5 mm from the lesion.[25]

Wires with a 2-cm thickened segment just proximal to the hook are helpful for the surgeon. With these wires, the hook is ideally engaged 1.5 cm beyond the lesion so the lesion is on the thickened segment just proximal to the hook. By placing the thickened segment of hookwire systems through or alongside the lesion, the surgeon can use it as a marker to indicate that the level of the lesion has been reached and the hook is 2 cm beyond. Placing a radiopaque marker (BB) at the wire entry point on the skin to be included in the final picture of the wire and lesion is also helpful to assist the surgeon in anticipating the depth of the lesion (allowing for distortion from the mammographic compression).

ULTRASONOGRAPHICALLY GUIDED NEEDLE PLACEMENT

With the appropriate ultrasonic device, needles and lesions can be imaged. The course of the needle can be observed in real time as it is positioned through or alongside a breast lesion. If the lesion is visible by ultrasonography, then a needle biopsy needle or a localization guide can be placed under ultrasonographic guidance. On occasion, calcifications are visible under ultrasonography, but this is uncommon. For the most part, ultrasonographically guided needle procedures are performed to guide the biopsy or excision of masses, whereas mammography or stereotactic mammography is used to guide the biopsy of calcifications. Ultrasonographically guided localizations have the advantage of being more comfortable for the patient (breast compression is not needed) and, when localizations are performed, often provide a more direct route for the surgeon because the guide can be placed from the front of the breast.

The procedure should be carefully explained to the patient, and the patient's questions should be answered. Because ultrasonographically guided procedures are directed back toward the chest wall, discussion of the possibility of pneumothorax (extremely rare), as well as the potential need for a chest tube if a pneumothorax were to occur, is probably best. Hematomas are fairly common. The possibility of infection, although also extremely rare, should probably also be mentioned.

Patient Positioning for Ultrasonographically Guided Procedures

Most ultrasonographically guided procedures can be performed with the patient lying fairly comfortably in the supine position. The patient should be rolled into whichever oblique position causes the portion of the breast that contains the lesion to be as thin as possible against the chest wall to reduce the amount of tissue that the ultrasonic beam and the needle must traverse. Placing a bolster behind the patient can help the patient maintain the appropriate position. The breast can be further thinned on the chest wall by having the patient extend the arm, placing the palm of the hand behind the head. Tightening the tissues against the chest wall in this fashion also helps to hold the lesion and prevent it from being pushed aside by the needle.

General Considerations

Various methods of using ultrasonography to guide needle placement have been described.[26–28] With the appropriate ultrasonic equipment, the needle and its tip can be followed as it is passed through the breast tissue and into a tumor. Fine-needle aspiration or core-needle biopsy of solid masses can be performed, and wires can be placed to guide surgical excision under direct ultrasonographic observation.

Alcohol or sterile saline is preferred as the coupling medium during these procedures so the breast does not become slippery, which makes it difficult to maintain transducer position. A 7.5- or 10-mHz linear array transducer is preferred.

The authors use pressure and a small straw to mark a point over the lesion and another point at the site for needle insertion. These impressions provide constant references that are clearly evident on the skin during the procedure, even after sterile preparation. Sterile preparation of the skin is performed in the usual manner, and a fenestrated sterile drape is placed over the breast, leaving the skin over the lesion and the needle entry point exposed. This provides a sterile field.

Although very few cases of infection have been reported, placing a sterile cover over the transducer head, with coupling gel inside the cover, is prudent. Some use a sterile condom to cover the transducers, whereas others merely cleanse the transducer with an iodinated cleaner.

The lesion is located under the transducer. The skin entry can be numbed using a local anesthetic. Although the pain sensors in the breast tissues are usually sparse, some prefer also to anesthetize the deep tissues down to the lesion. The needle is introduced just off the end of the long axis of the transducer so that its tip can be monitored as it passes through the skin and is advanced into the field of view of the transducer. It is directed toward the lesion and, under ultrasonographic observation, rapidly and smoothly introduced into or alongside the targeted tissue. The operator should be able to monitor the tip of the needle at all times. If it is not visible, the orientation of the transducer or the direction of the needle should be adjusted so the location of needle tip is visible to avoid inadvertently passing the needle into the chest wall. At times, a more horizontal course for the needle, providing a more perpendicular direction for the sound reflection, may improve the visibility of the needle.

Many breast lesions are relatively superficial, and positioning the patient supine and oblique with the ipsilateral arm behind the head allows the breast tissue to be thinned so that the needle penetrates a minimum of tissue. This benefits the patient and the surgeon when a localizing wire is placed. For localization, the needle should be passed through or immediately alongside the lesion so the tip is 0.5 to 1.0 cm beyond the lesion.

Once the needle is positioned in or alongside the lesion, a spring-hookwire can be deployed and the needle removed. During removal of the needle and deployment of the hookwire, an assistant should hold the breast around the needle down against the chest wall so the lesion is not pulled off the needle before the hook is engaged.

A follow-up mammogram is sometimes useful to confirm the relation of the wire to the lesion. The wire must be long enough that it is not enveloped completely by the breast when the patient sits up. If the lesion was visible by mammography, the location of the wire relative to the lesion can be confirmed using a single mammographic view with compression perpendicular to the course of the wire (compression in the direction of the wire is not a good idea). The wire is then taped loosely, the skin entry is protected by a sterile bandage, and the patient is sent to the operating room.

COMPUTED TOMOGRAPHIC GUIDANCE FOR NEEDLE LOCALIZATION OF OCCULT BREAST LESIONS

CT is used most often when a lesion is visible on only one mammographic projection and is not visible on any other mammographic projection. This situation frequently occurs when the lesion is visible in the lateral mammographic projection and the lesion is close to the chest wall. Thus, its three-dimensional location cannot be determined. If the lesion cannot be triangulated by mammography, CT can be used to triangulate the lesion and position guides for surgical biopsy.

The patient is placed within the scanner so that the breasts are symmetrically positioned and aligned with the plane of scan. This permits the comparison of symmetric areas so asymmetric areas can be detected. The breast is scanned in 1-cm thick slices at 1-cm intervals covering the portion of the breast in which the lesion is anticipated to be found based on the mammogram. If contrast enhancement is needed, as for lesions found using magnetic resonance imaging (MRI), the patient should not move between the precontrast and postcontrast scans, so areas of enhancement can be identified.

Once the lesion is located, a needle for fine-needle aspiration or a wire guide for preoperative localization can be placed at the lesion using the scanner.[29] The patient preferably should remain within the scanner during the localization procedure to avoid shifting of the breast on the chest wall with table movement. The skin is prepared in a sterile manner, and a sterile piece of wire or thin needle is taped sagittally over the expected region of the lesion. This fiducial wire should be visible on the scanner but should not be thick enough to cause artifacts. This wire remains in place during the procedure as a constant reference.

The patient is then positioned in the gantry with the arm extended and the body rotated so that a minimum amount of breast tissue overlies the lesion. If the lesion is close to the chest wall, rotating the patient so that the needle passes parallel to the chest wall might be preferable to avoid passing the needle into the chest wall or deeper. The lesion is again located by scanning and accurately triangulated using thinner slices. Thin slices (5 mm or less) should be used when positioning needles so that the tip and hub are visible within the scan plane. This avoids angling of the needle through the plane, which gives the appearance that the tip is further from the chest wall than it actually is. Measurement of the location of the lesion relative to the reference wire on the skin, along with the depth of the lesion on the scan, allows a needle to be introduced using the laser and the skin wire to triangulate the point of entry and depth of insertion. Care should be taken to avoid entering the pectoralis or thorax. A hookwire can be engaged when the needle tip is satisfactorily positioned just deep to the lesion.

Because the needle is placed from the front of the breast and the wire is engaged with the patient supine, a long wire should be used, as the breast will reexpand when the patient sits up. The wire may be engulfed by the breast and should be long enough that it will not disappear completely into the breast. The external wire is then loosely taped to the skin, and a sterile gauze is placed over the entry site.

LOCALIZATION OF LESIONS DETECTED BY MAGNETIC RESONANCE IMAGING

The use of MRI for breast evaluation continues to increase. MRI appears to be very sensitive for the detection of breast cancer, but many benign lesions are also detected by contrast-enhanced MRI. Biopsy of these is needed to determine their benign etiology. Some techniques have been developed for guiding needle positioning while the patient is in the MR device. However, most MRI systems do not have easy methods for positioning needles or guides.

In the absence of these devices, CT scanning can be used to guide the positioning of needles. Chang et al. have shown that many breast cancers enhance after the intravenous administration of iodinated contrast material.[30] The mechanism of iodine enhancement is similar to that of gadolinium enhancement. Most lesions that enhance with gadolinium during MRI also enhance on CT scanning after the intravenous administration of an iodinated contrast agent. Once the enhanced lesion is identified, a guide wire can be placed using CT as described above[31] and surgical removal accomplished.

IMAGING OF EXCISED TISSUE AFTER LOCALIZATION AND EXCISION: SPECIMEN RADIOGRAPHY

The excised tissue from all "localized" biopsies should be sent for imaging confirmation. Instances of missed cancers have been noted in which the surgeon thought that the lesion was palpable and did not send the tissue for specimen radiography, causing a delay in diagnosis.

Imaging is easiest if the excised tissue is placed in a plastic bag. This permits imaging of the excised tissue without the need for handling exposed tissues and the attendant biohazard. When a plastic bag is used, the tissue can be placed on ice in the operating room, if desired. Use of a plastic bag makes handling of the tissue safer and easier for specimen radiography. When the lesion is in the bag, it can be placed in a mammography unit or specimen x-ray unit under mild compression, and radiographs can be obtained (Fig. 2). Magnification is helpful to improve the visualization of subtle details. In addition to confirming the lesion's removal, the radiologist should alert the surgeon if the excised lesion appears to be close to a margin. If the lesion had been visible only by ultrasonography, ultrasonographic imaging of the specimen directly through the plastic bag can be used to confirm the removal of the lesion.

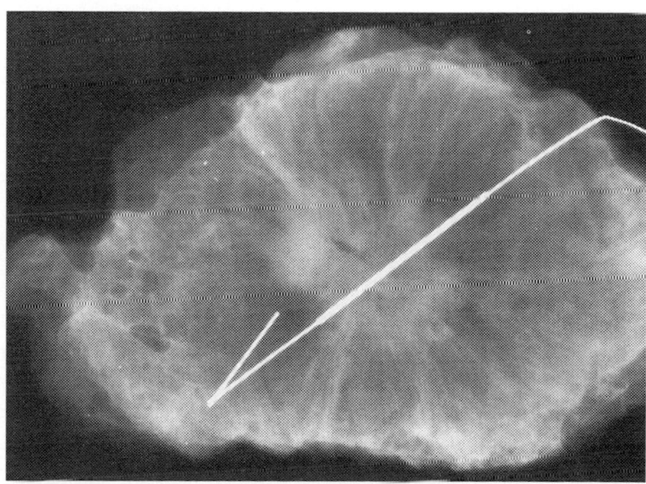

FIG. 2. This specimen radiograph shows the lesion and wire centered in the tissue sample with a rim of normal surrounding breast tissue. If the lesion is malignant, this placement helps in obtaining clear margins.

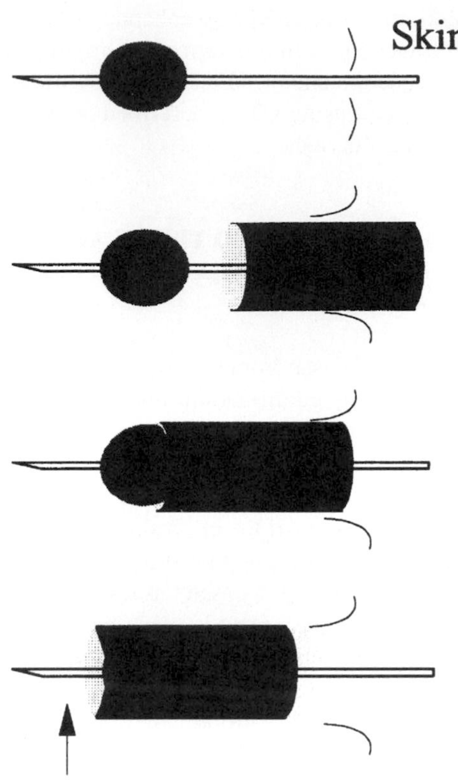

FIG. 3. In large-core imaging-guided tissue removal, a guide is placed through the target tissue to hold the tissue in place. A large-core biopsy system is introduced through a surgical incision. The tissue is cut to include the entire suspected lesion and some surrounding tissue.

LARGE-CORE EXCISIONAL BIOPSY

To reduce the sampling error that can occur using needle biopsy techniques (fine-needle aspiration and core-needle biopsy), cutting devices based on an apple coring–like mechanism have been devised to remove larger volumes of breast tissue. The first commercially available system is called the Advanced Breast Biopsy Device (ABBI, U.S. Surgical, Norwalk, Connecticut); a similar device is named the SiteSelect (Imagyn Surgical, Newport Beach, California).

Both devices operate on a similar principle. They are cylindrical cutters (Fig. 3) that, when rotated or oscillated, cut a core of tissue that is 0.5 cm to 2.0 cm in diameter (depending on the size of cutter chosen). The goal in devising these instruments was to permit the complete excision of a lesion with high accuracy when the target was under direct observation in a stereotactic mammography system. The theory was a good one, but the practice has not lived up to expectations. A lesion must be ideally located to permit such a biopsy. If insufficient tissue exists around the lesion, a biopsy cannot be performed. Because of the elasticity and resilience of breast tissue and difficulty in cutting it, complete removal of a small lesion is very hard to achieve. Lesions may be completely missed or, more often, end up at the edge of the excised tissue.

Large-core excisional biopsies are actually surgical procedures, and the sterility and support of an operating room are required. The complication rates (bleeding and infection) are higher than those occurring with imaging-guided core-needle biopsy. Electrocautery is used, as with any excisional procedure in the breast. A guide is positioned through or alongside the targeted lesion in the breast under stereotactic observation. The guide is anchored just beyond the lesion. A surgical incision is made through the skin. In the early development of the ABBI system, the coring device was then advanced and a cylinder of tissue was cored from just beneath the skin to just beyond the depth of the lesion. A spring-loaded wire garrote was then released, cutting the sample at the base of the core. Because removing tissue from the skin down is not necessary, the ABBI and SiteSelect devices can be advanced further into the tissue to remove a shorter core to preserve normal tissue.

A significant amount of bleeding generally occurs with these procedures, and cautery is used. Once the core has been removed, the patient is moved into the supine position so the surgeon can achieve hemostasis. The wound is sutured closed, as with any surgical breast lesion excision.

Preliminary tests have not demonstrated these devices to be capable of complete lesion excision with clear margins.[32] Consequently, their advantage has not been established. Although imaging-guided core-needle biopsy is somewhat less accurate than needle localization and excisional biopsy, at the present time, core-needle biopsy appears to be more accurate, less traumatic, and less expensive than these large core–biopsy procedures.[33]

SURGICAL APPROACH TO BIOPSY OF NONPALPABLE LESIONS

Anesthetic Techniques

Nearly all needle-localized breast biopsies can be performed under local anesthesia or local anesthesia plus intravenous sedation. Use of general anesthesia should be limited to patients who require biopsies of multiple sites or those who have a deep central lesion in a very large breast so that the volume of tissue to be anesthetized raises concerns of toxicity due to the amount of local anesthesia required. Only rarely does a patient require a general anesthesia because of extreme anxiety.

Accurate Localization for Accurate Excision

The accurate placement of guides by the radiologist is critical. As described in Mammographically Guided Preoperative Needle Localization, the needle or wire should either be through the lesion, or no more than 5 mm from it. This reduces the amount of tissue that must be removed and diminishes the probability that the lesion will be missed at surgery. The literature suggesting that as much as 40 mL of tissue must be removed during needle-localized biopsy comes from series in which freehand localizations were performed, and the wire was frequently 1 cm or more from the lesion. This method required larger volumes of tissue to be removed and increased the likelihood that a cancer would be missed at surgical excision.[34] In addition to permitting removal of less tissue, precise wire placement should keep failure to excise a breast cancer at less than 1%. In the authors' experience in excising 1,000 cancers, in only 5 cancers (0.5%) did the first localization result in a failure to excise that necessitated a repeat needle localization and surgical excision.

Communication between the radiologist and surgeon is critical to permit accurate biopsy. The position of the breast in the operating room with the patient supine is different from the position of the breast during the localization procedure. In the supine position, the breast often falls laterally, altering the alignment of the wire and potentially drawing additional wire length into the breast. Therefore, although precise wire localization of the lesion by the radiologist is critical, sending the mammograms to the operating room is equally important to allow the surgeon to determine the three-dimensional location of the lesion in the breast when the patient is supine, as well as the position of the lesion relative to the wire. Two images are used to orient the surgeon and should be available in the operating room: the image looking down the needle and the final, orthogonal image of the wire in place. A diagram drawn by the radiologist marking the positions of the wire and the lesion within the breast helps with this orientation. The orientation process is also greatly facilitated by marking the skin entry site and the nipple clearly on the films. Providing the surgeon with an estimate of the distance in centimeters between the lesion and the skin entry site is also helpful.

The position of the wire's hook relative to the nipple remains fairly constant, even with the movement of the breast into the supine position, and this can be used to estimate the location of the lesion within the breast. The skin incision can then be placed as directly as possible over the lesion. The lesion itself should also be marked on the films, so its distance from the wire and position relative to the wire can be determined easily. This allows the surgeon to gauge how much tissue to remove around the wire and on what side of the wire the greatest tissue volume should be excised. The use of wires with thickened segments is especially helpful in judgment of distances along the length of the wire and the distance to the hook within the breast tissue.[35]

Surgical Principles

Although the excision of a nonpalpable needle-localized breast lesion is technically more difficult than excision of a palpable lesion, the same general principles apply to the former as to the latter. Each lesion should be treated as if it is a malignancy and excised through an incision that could be contained within a mastectomy incision or converted into a cosmetically acceptable partial mastectomy (lumpectomy) incision. As most lesions requiring needle localization are small, an effort should be made to excise the lesion completely, with a rim of surrounding normal tissue. However, the majority of needle-localized breast lesions ultimately prove to be benign. The volume of tissue excised should therefore be as small as possible; wide excision should be reserved for lesions for which malignancy is strongly suspected or those already identified as malignant by needle biopsy techniques.

With these principles in mind, the rules for the placement of the incision in needle-localized biopsy of a breast lesion are similar to those for a biopsy of a palpable lesion. The incision should be placed directly over the lesion; excessive tunneling through breast tissue should be avoided, because it increases the volume of tissue that must receive a radiation boost. If the wire takes a long course through the breast tissue to reach the lesion, the incision should be moved along the expected course of the wire, away from the skin entry of the wire and closer to the expected location of the lesion (Fig. 4). The surgeon then dissects down to identify the wire within breast tissue and follows it to the thickened segment.

Circumareolar incisions should be used only when the lesion is close to the areolar border. Curvilinear incisions parallel to the areolar border are preferable for most locations; radial incisions are reserved for very medial or very lateral lesions. The incision should be sufficiently long to provide adequate exposure, as the vigorous retraction required with a very small incision may cause the wire to become dislodged. Skin should not be included in the biopsy specimen, even when the wire entry site is included in the incision.

The course of the wire is identified and followed to the thick segment. The tissue is then removed around the thick segment to encompass the lesion and a small amount of surrounding normal tissue (Fig. 5). For lesions known to be malignant by fine-needle or core biopsy, an appropriately wide margin should be obtained. If the thick portion of the wire is encountered, the surgeon knows that he or she is very close to the lesion and can adjust the dissection accordingly.

Once the appropriate portion of the wire has been identified, tissue on either side of the wire is grasped with clamps, and a cylinder of tissue is taken around the wire. Caution must be used to avoid dividing the wire with scissors or cautery during the dissection. The amount of tissue taken around the wire depends on the actual distance of the lesion from the wire as indicated on the localization films. In some cases, the lesion is palpable once its general position is identified by the wire. In such cases, complete excision of the lesion with a grossly clean margin is appropriate. If the preoperative placement of the guide has been accurate, only a small total volume of tissue need be excised.[24] Excising a

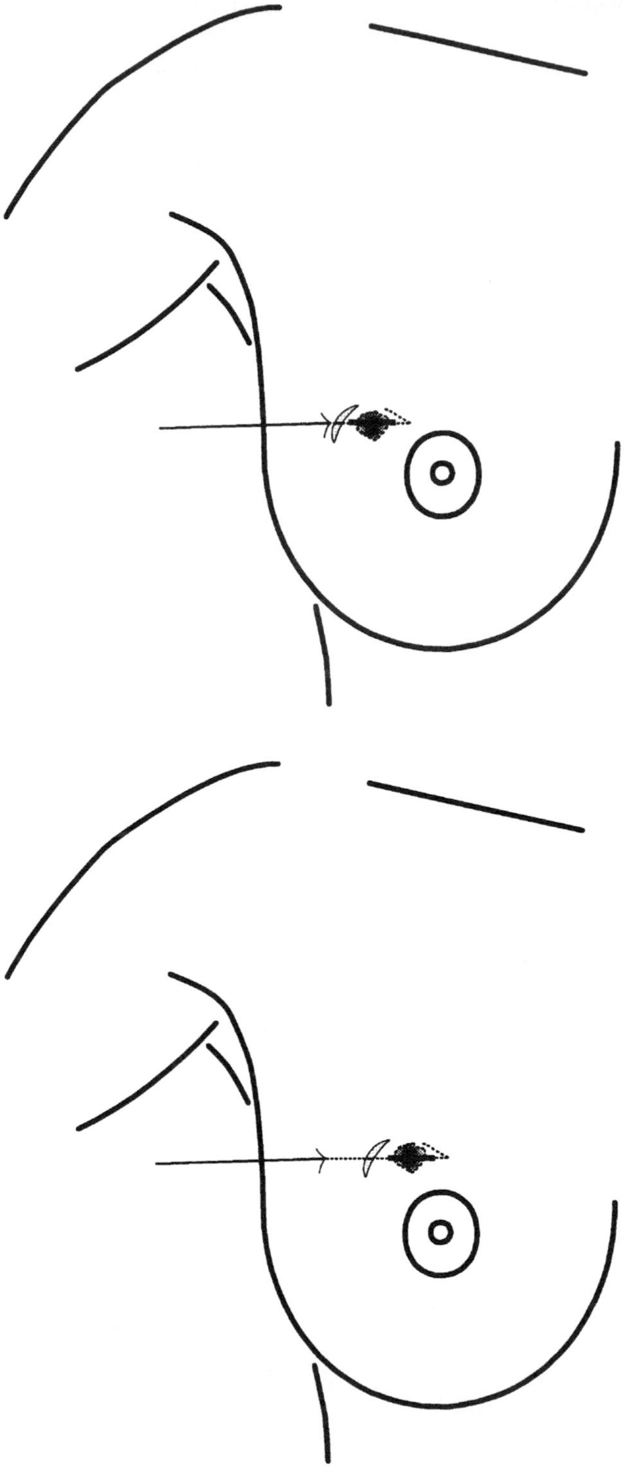

A

B

FIG. 4. Approach to localized lesions. **A:** If the lesion is close to the skin entry site, then the incision can be made to follow the wire directly to the lesion. **B:** If the distance from the entry to the lesion is considerable, the surgeon can cut down onto the wire from a point that is closer to the lesion and then dissect along the wire to the lesion to remove it and a small amount of surrounding tissue.

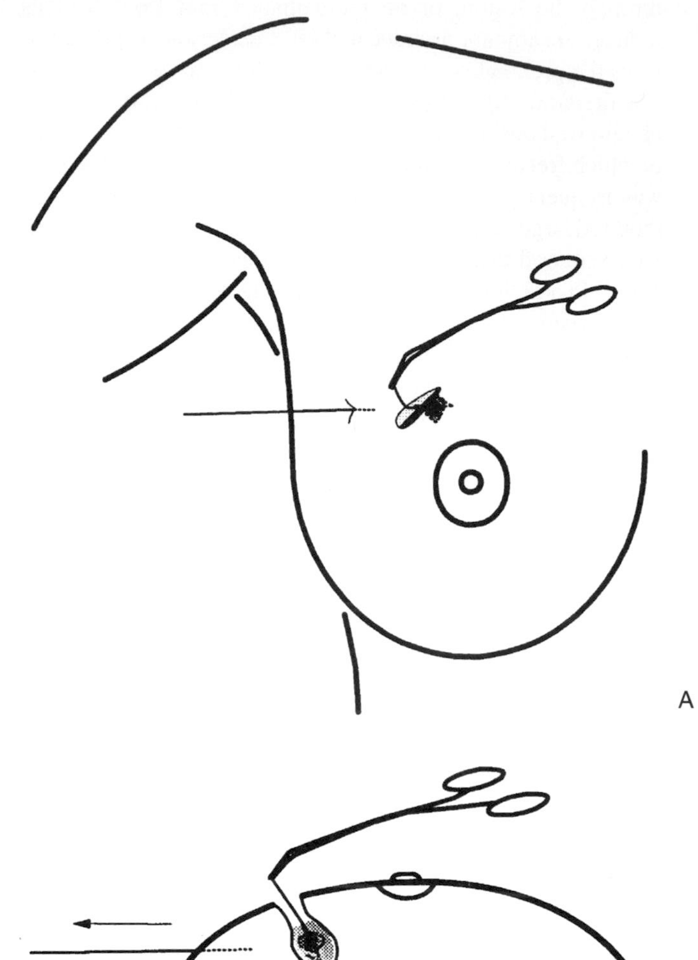

FIG. 5. In excision of a localized lesion, the wire is delivered into the incision **(A)** and dissection is carried out **(B)** to remove the lesion and wire with a rim of normal surrounding tissue.

cylinder of tissue along the entire course of the wire is not necessary. Doing so takes a larger tissue sample than required and necessitates a larger reexcision should the lesion prove to be malignant. Excision should be focused on the segment of wire nearest the lesion. Closure of the incision should strive for a good cosmetic result using a subcuticular closure rather than staples or nylon sutures.

Excised Specimen

Immediately after the surgical excision, the specimen should be radiographed with some compression and magnification to confirm that the targeted abnormality has been removed. For lesions identified by ultrasonography alone, ultrasonographic imaging of the excised specimen should be performed to confirm that the lesion is in the specimen.

If the radiologist does not see the lesion in the specimen, and the surgeon does not feel that the lesion was a cyst that ruptured during the excision, the surgeon may excise additional tissue around the track of the wire. If there has been traction on the wire, the lesion may be further along the previous course of the wire. If the lesion is not contained within the second specimen, the best course generally is to close and obtain repeat mammographic views at a later time, rather than excising an excessive amount of tissue. In most cases, the patient is able to tolerate a mammogram within 2 to 3 weeks after the initial biopsy attempt. Waiting several months before reimaging a patient when the lesion may have been missed is neither necessary nor appropriate. On occasion, these repeat views show that the lesion has, in fact, been removed. If the lesion remains, another localization and biopsy should be performed expeditiously.

Once excision of the lesion has been documented, both the biopsy specimen and the specimen radiograph should be sent to the pathologist. As is the case for any breast biopsy, the margins of the specimen should be inked. If the lesion proves to be malignant, the specimen should be analyzed for hormone receptors and other appropriate markers.

The specimen radiograph helps the pathologist ensure that the area of the specimen containing the mammographic abnormality is appropriately sampled. If the biopsy was performed for calcifications, the pathologists must be sure that the calcifications are visualized in histologic tissue sections to be sure that the area containing the lesion has been examined. If the calcifications are not found on routine examination of tissue sections, radiographic images may be obtained of the paraffin-embedded tissue blocks to identify the sections containing the calcifications. Imaging the block on its side[36] can demonstrate that suspicious calcifications are deep in the block so that appropriate sections at deeper levels may be obtained.

If an area showing calcifications is found to contain a malignancy, many believe it is important to ensure that all the calcifications are removed in the definitive wide excision. Magnification views of the biopsied breast are suggested if any concern exists that calcifications remain. Any calcifications that remain may be wire localized for subsequent wide excision.

CONCLUSION

Accurate positioning of guides for the surgical removal of clinically occult lesions is required to ensure the safety of the patient and the accurate diagnosis of breast abnormalities with minimal cosmetic deformity. The radiologist, surgeon, and pathologist should have a close working relationship to ensure that the lesion is removed and appropriately analyzed. As with any interventional technique, a thoughtful approach to the particular lesion in question and an understanding of the procedures and their possible problems minimize the likelihood of complications.

REFERENCES

1. Fletcher SW, Black W, Harris R, Rimer BK, Shapiro S. Report of the International Workshop on Screening for Breast Cancer. *J Natl Cancer Inst* 1993;85:1644.
2. Smart CR. Highlights of the evidence of benefit for women aged 40-49 years from the 14-year follow-up of the Breast Cancer Detection Demonstration Project. *Cancer* 1994;74:296.
3. Fletcher SW, Black W, Harris R, Rimer BK, Shapiro S. Report of the International Workshop on Screening for Breast Cancer. *J Natl Cancer Inst* 1993;85:1644.
4. Hendrick RE, Smith RA, Rutledge JH, Smart CR. Benefit of screening mammography in women ages 40-49: a new meta-analysis of randomized controlled trials. *Monogr Natl Cancer Inst* 1997; 22:87.
5. Bassett LW, Liu TH, Giuliano AE, Gold RH. The prevalence of carcinoma in palpable versus impalpable mammographically detected lesions. *AJR Am J Roentgenol* 1991;157:21.
6. Parker SH, Lovin JD, Jobe WE, Burke BJ, Hopper KD, Yakes WF. Nonpalpable breast lesions: stereotactic automated large-core biopsies. *Radiology* 1991;180:403.
7. Parker SH, Jobe WE, Dennis MA, et al. US-guided automated large-core breast biopsy. *Radiology* 1993;187:507.
8. Elvecrog EL, Lechner MC, Nelson MT. Nonpalpable breast lesions: correlation of stereotaxic large-core needle biopsy and surgical biopsy results. *Radiology* 1993;188:453.
9. Kopans DB, Meyer JE, Lindfors KK, Bucchianeri SS. Breast sonography to guide aspiration of cysts and preoperative localization of occult breast lesions. *AJR Am J Roentgenol* 1984;143:489.
10. Kopans DB, Meyer JE. Computed tomography guided localization of clinically occult breast carcinoma—the "N" skin guide. *Radiology* 1982;145:211.
11. Gallagher WJ, Cardenosa G, Rubens JR, McCarthy KA, Kopans DB. Minimal-volume excision of nonpalpable breast lesions. *AJR Am J Roentgenol* 1989;153:957.
12. Kopans DB, Swann CA. Preoperative imaging-guided needle placement and localization of clinically occult breast lesions. *AJR Am J Roentgenol* 1989;152:1.
13. Kopans DB, Deluca S. A modified needle-hookwire technique to simplify the preoperative localization of occult breast lesions. *Radiology* 1980;134:781.
14. Kopans DB, Meyer JE. The versatile spring-hookwire breast lesion localizer. *AJR Am J Roentgenol* 1982;138:586.
15. Horns JW, Arndt RD. Percutaneous spot localization of nonpalpable breast lesions. *AJR Am J Roentgenol* 1976;127:253.
16. Svane G. A stereotaxic technique for preoperative marking of nonpalpable breast lesions. *Acta Radiol* 1983;24:145.
17. Berkowitz JE, Gatewood OMB, Gayler BW. Equivocal mammographic findings: evaluation with spot compression. *Radiology* 1989;171:369.
18. Swann CA, Kopans DB, McCarthy KA, White G, Hall DA. Practical solutions to problems of triangulation and preoperative localization of breast lesions. *Radiology* 1987;163:577.
19. Kopans DB, Waitzkin ED, Linetsky L, et al. Localization of breast lesions identified on only one mammographic view. *AJR Am J Roentgenol* 1987;149:39.
20. Kopans DB. *Breast imaging*. Philadelphia: Lippincott–Raven, 1997: 692.
21. Kopans DB, Meyer JE. Computed tomography–guided localization of clinically occult breast carcinoma—the "N" skin guide. *Radiology* 1982;145:211.
22. Reynolds HE, Jackson VP, Musnick BS. Preoperative needle localization in the breast: utility of local anesthesia. *Radiology* 1993; 187:503.
23. Bristol JB, Jones PA. Transgression of localizing wire into the pleural cavity prior to mammography. *Br J Radiol* 1981;54:139.
24. Kopans DB, Meyer JE, Lindfors KK, McCarthy KA. Spring-hookwire breast lesion localizer: use with rigid compression mammographic systems. *Radiology* 1985;157:505.
25. Gallagher WJ, Cardenosa G, Rubens JR, McCarthy KA, Kopans DB. Minimal-volume excision of nonpalpable breast lesions. *AJR Am J Roentgenol* 1989;153:957.
26. Davros WJ, Madsen EL, Zagzebski JA. Breast mass detection by US: a phantom study. Radiology 1985;156:773.
27. Fornage BD, Fariux MJ, Simatos A. Breast masses: US-guided fine-needle aspiration biopsy. *Radiology* 1987;162:409.

28. Parker SH, Jobe WE, Dennis MA, et al. US-guided automated large-core breast biopsy. *Radiology* 1993;187:507.
29. Kopans DB. *Breast imaging*. Philadelphia: Lippincott–Raven, 1998.
30. Chang CHJ, Nesbit DE, Fisher DR, et al. Computed tomographic mammography using a conventional body scanner. *AJR Am J Roentgenol* 1982;138:553.
31. Slanetz PJ, Jain R, Kline JL, et al. CT-guided preoperative needle localization of MR imaging-detected mammographically occult lesions. *AJR Am J Roentgenol* 1999;172:160.
32. Leibman AJ, Frager D, Choi P. Experience with breast biopsies using the advanced breast biopsy instrumentation system. *AJR Am J Roentgenol* 1999;172:1409.
33. Liberman L. Advanced Breast Biopsy Instrumentation (ABBI): analysis of published experience. *AJR Am J Roentgenol* 1999;172: 1413.
34. Tinnemans JGM, Wobbes T, Hendricks JHCL, van der Sluis RF, Lubbers EJC, de Boer HHM. Localization and excision of nonpalpable breast lesions: a surgical evaluation of three methods. *Arch Surg* 1987;122:802.
35. Kopans DB, Meyer JE. The versatile spring-hookwire breast lesion localizer. *AJR Am J Roentgenol* 1982;138:586.
36. Cardenosa G, Eklund GW. Paraffin block radiography following breast biopsies: use of orthogonal views. *Radiology* 1991;180: 873.

IV

Diseases of the Breast, 2nd ed.,
edited by Jay R. Harris.
Lippincott Williams & Wilkins, Philadelphia © 2000.

Epidemiology and Assessing and Managing Risk

CHAPTER 15

Epidemiology and Nongenetic Causes of Breast Cancer

Walter C. Willett, Beverly Rockhill, Susan E. Hankinson, David J. Hunter, and Graham A. Colditz

Breast cancer has an enormous impact on the health of women.[1] Approximately 180,000 women are diagnosed with breast cancer annually in the United States, and breast cancer accounts for approximately 30% of all incident cancers among women. Each year, 44,000 women die of breast cancer, making it the second leading cause of cancer deaths among American women, after lung cancer, and the leading cause of death among women aged 40 to 55 years. Breast cancer is rare among men, with only 1,600 incident cases and 400 deaths estimated for the United States in 1998.[1] The lifetime risk through age 85 years of being diagnosed with breast cancer for an American woman is approximately 1 in 8, or 12.5%, whereas the lifetime risk of dying from breast cancer is approximately 3.4%.[1]

This chapter begins with a description of the marked variations in breast cancer rates among populations and over time. Decades of research have led to a substantial understanding of the factors involved in the development of breast cancer; known and suspected risk factors are reviewed and considered in relation to etiologic mechanisms leading to breast cancer. The contribution that known risk factors make to the existing variations in rates is considered; this contribution is central to the question of whether unidentified pollutants or dietary factors explain the present high rates in the United States. Because of the major investments in breast cancer research, the means for preventing a substantial fraction of breast cancer now exist; strategies that can be adopted by individual women, their health care providers, and societies and governments as a whole are examined.

W. C. Willett: Harvard Medical School, Boston, Massachusetts; Department of Nutrition, Harvard School of Public Health, Boston, Massachusetts

B. Rockhill: Harvard Medical School, Brigham and Women's Hospital, Boston, Massachusetts

S. E. Hankinson: Departments of Medicine and Epidemiology, Harvard Medical School and Harvard School of Public Health, Boston Massachusetts

D. J. Hunter: Departments of Epidemiology and Nutrition, Harvard School of Public Health, Boston, Massachussetts

G. A. Colditz: Department of Medicine, Harvard Medical School, Boston, Massachussetts

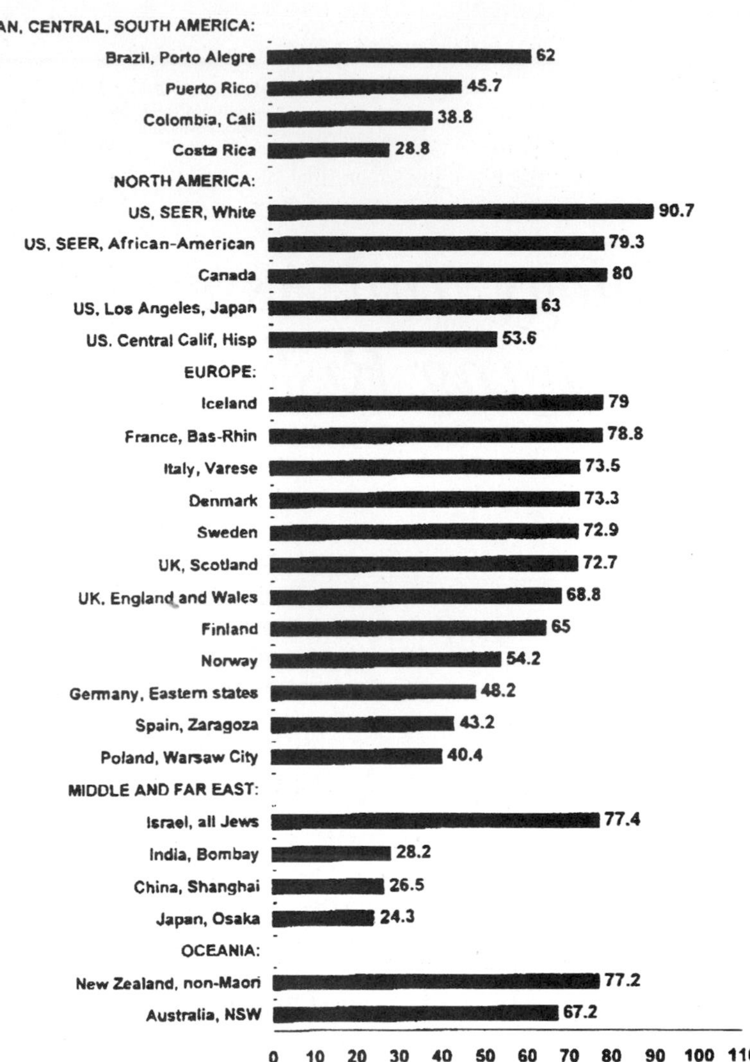

FIG. 1. International variation in breast cancer incidence among women, 1988 to 1993, per 100,000 woman-years, age-adjusted to the world standard. SEER, Surveillance, Epidemiology, and End Results Program. (Data from Parkin DM, Whelan SL, Ferlay J, et al. *Cancer incidence in five continents.* No. 143. Vol. VII. Lyons, France: International Agency for Research on Cancer Scientific Publications, 1997.)

DESCRIPTIVE EPIDEMIOLOGY OF BREAST CANCER

High-Risk and Low-Risk Populations

The incidence of female breast cancer varies markedly between countries. It is highest in the United States and Northern Europe, intermediate in Southern and Eastern Europe and South America, and lowest in Asia.[2] During 1983 to 1987, the age-adjusted incidence of breast cancer varied by approximately a factor of five among countries (Fig. 1). However, rates have been rising in traditionally low-incidence Asian countries, particularly in Japan, Singapore, and urban areas of China, as these regions make the transition toward a Western-style economy and pattern of reproductive behavior.[3,4] As a result of unfavorable trends in these countries, the international gap in breast cancer incidence has narrowed since 1970.[5]

Age-Incidence Curve of Breast Cancer Risk

Breast cancer is extremely rare among women younger than age 20 years and is uncommon among women younger than age 30 years. Incidence increases sharply with age, however, and becomes substantial before age 50. During 1991 to 1995, the incidence of breast cancer among American women aged 30 to 34 years was 25 per 100,000 and increased to 200 per 100,000 among women aged 45 to 49 years. The rate of increase in breast cancer incidence continues throughout life but slows somewhat between ages 45 and 50 years. This finding strongly suggests the involvement of reproductive hormones in breast cancer etiology, because non–hormone-dependent cancers do not exhibit this change in slope of the incidence curve around the time of menopause.[6] The incidence of breast cancer among American women aged 70 to 74 years rises to 463 per 100,000.[1] The shape of the age-incidence curve in low-risk and intermediate-risk populations

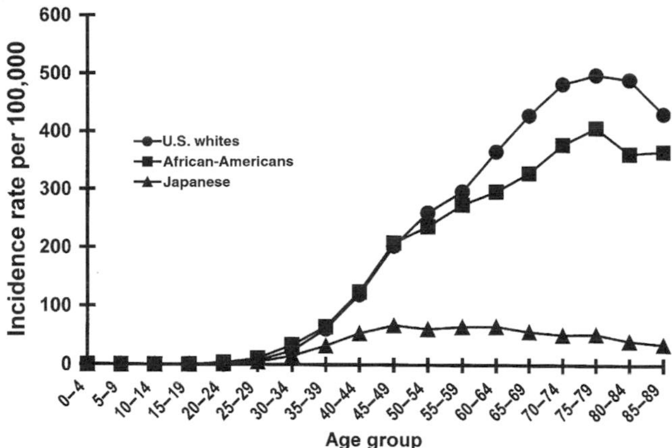

FIG. 2. Incidence of breast cancer by age group for American and Japanese women. (Data for U.S. women from ref. 1; data for Japanese women from ref. 7.)

is similar to that in the United States, although the absolute rates are lower at each age (Fig. 2).[7]

Racial and Ethnic Groups within the United States and Studies of Migrants

According to data from the Surveillance, Epidemiology, and End Results (SEER) Program registries,[1] the lifetime risk of breast cancer for white women in the United States is 13.1%, slightly higher than 1 in 8, whereas that for African-American women is 9.6%, slightly less than 1 in 10. In 1995, the overall age-adjusted incidence of breast cancer among white women in the United States was 115 per 100,000 women, whereas the corresponding rate among African-American women was 101 per 100,000 women.[1] These age-adjusted figures conceal a crossover pattern, however, in which the risk of breast cancer at a young age is modestly higher among African-American women than among white women. At older ages, breast cancer rates for white women are substantially higher than for African-American women (see Fig. 2).

Unlike most other illnesses, the lifetime risk of breast cancer is positively associated with higher socioeconomic status. This association is largely explained by the known reproductive risk factors[8]; women in lower socioeconomic strata are more likely to have more children and to have them at a younger age than women in higher socioeconomic strata. Much, if not all, of the differences in breast cancer rates between African-Americans and whites in older age groups are likely to reflect racial differences in social class distribution,[9] and thus in the distribution of established reproductive risk factors. The modestly higher incidences of breast cancer among young African-American women relative to young white women is consistent with the hypothesis of a short-term increase in breast cancer risk immediately after pregnancy,[10] whereas the overall lower lifetime risk of breast cancer among African-American women is consistent with the hypothesis of a long-term benefit of early and repeated pregnancy.[10] The effect of these reproductive factors on breast cancer risk is described in greater detail in the section Models of Reproductive Factors and Breast Cancer Incidence. Although African-American women have a lower probability of developing breast cancer over their lifetimes, their risk of dying from breast cancer is the same as, or perhaps even slightly higher than, that of white women (3.6% for African-American women, compared with 3.5% for white women). African-American women have poorer 5-year survival rates from breast cancer at all ages of diagnosis compared with white women.[1] This poorer survival can be attributed, in part, to the tendency for African-American women to be diagnosed at later stages of disease.[1]

Breast cancer rates are considerably lower among Asian, Hispanic, and American Indian women in the United States than among (non-Hispanic) white women.[1] The magnitude of the difference in incidence among various ethnic groups often depends on migrant status. For instance, breast cancer incidence for Chinese-American and Japanese-American women during 1973 to 1986 was approximately 50% lower for those born in Asia and approximately 25% lower for those born in the United States compared with U.S.-born white women.[11] Among Filipino residents of the United States, the incidence of breast cancer was nearly identical for foreign-born and U.S.-born women, and rates for both were less than one-half the rates for U.S.-born white women. Compared with Chinese women living in the mainland, Singapore, and Hong Kong, Asian-born Chinese women living in the United States had an almost twofold higher annual rate of breast cancer, and U.S.-born Chinese women had a rate that was higher still.[2,11] The pattern for Japanese women was similar.[11]

These findings are consistent with a large body of literature showing increases in breast cancer incidence after migration from a low-risk country to the United States.[12–17] Ziegler et al.[12] noted a sixfold gradient in risk of breast cancer among Asian women, depending on recency of migration. Asian-American women with three or four grandparents born in the West were at highest risk, whereas women who were born in rural areas of Asia and whose length of residence in the United States was a decade or less were at lowest risk. Whereas the studies of breast cancer risk among migrants have focused almost exclusively on migrants from low-risk to high-risk countries and have shown convergence of rates, some data also suggest that a convergence of rates similarly occurs when migrants move from high-risk to low-risk countries. For instance, Kliewer and Smith,[18] reporting on immigrants to Australia and Canada, noted that immigrant groups coming from countries in which breast cancer mortality rates were higher than those of native-born women often showed a decrease in mortality. Such findings strongly suggest that factors associated with the lifestyle or environment of the destination country influence breast cancer risk and are consistent with a positive relationship between length of time in the destination country and adoption of that country's lifestyle. For example, among immigrants, the fertility rate as well as average number of children born tend to converge to the rates of the destination country.[19,20]

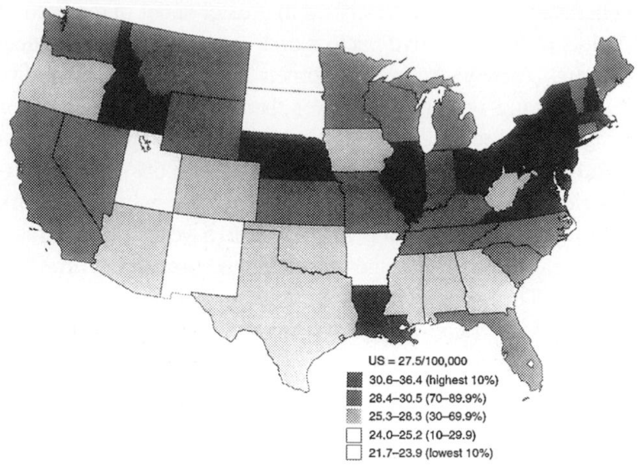

FIG. 3. Age-adjusted breast cancer mortality rates for women (of all races) by state in 1990. (From ref. 5. Reprinted with permission from Lippincott–Raven.)

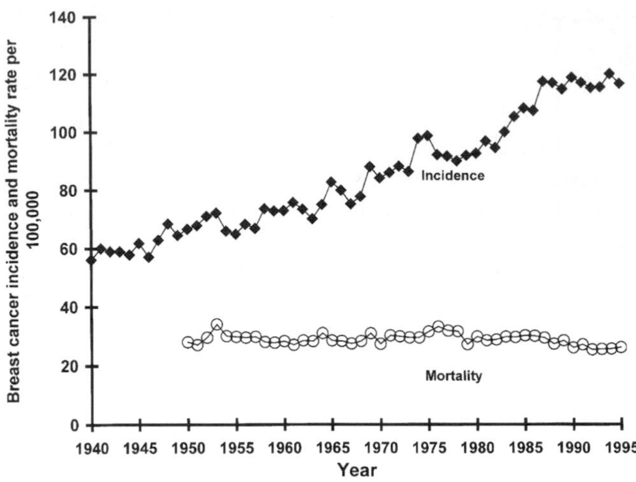

FIG. 4. Age-standardized incidence of breast cancer and mortality rates in Connecticut from 1940 to 1995. [Data are from the Surveillance, Epidemiology, and End Results Program (data for 1989–1995 provided by B. Miller, written communication, October 1998). Reprinted from ref. 76 with permission of the *New England Journal of Medicine.*]

Geographic Variation within the United States

Breast cancer incidence and mortality rates vary within the United States, although to a much smaller degree than among countries. During the 1980s, the incidence of breast cancer in the San Francisco Bay area was somewhat higher than that in the rest of the United States, and international comparisons based on data from this time period led to an often-quoted statement that white women in the San Francisco Bay area had the highest incidence of breast cancer in the world.[2,21] Based on the SEER data,[1] the age-adjusted annual incidence among white women in the San Francisco area (127 per 100,000) is now surpassed by that of white women in Hawaii, where the age-adjusted incidence is 128 per 100,000. The incidence of breast cancer is also higher than the national average among white women in the northeastern United States (age-adjusted incidence for Connecticut, 119 per 100,000).[1] Reports have concluded that the high incidence of breast cancer in the San Francisco area and in the Northeast can probably be accounted for by regional differences in the prevalence of known risk factors, including parity, age at first full-term pregnancy, age at menarche, and age at menopause.[21–23]

Among the 11 SEER registry sites, the lowest age-adjusted incidences among white women are found in Utah (98 per 100,000) and New Mexico (99 per 100,000). Again, regional differences in reproductive risk factors probably largely explain these lower rates. Seven of the 11 SEER registry sites have data on incidence among African-American women. The variation in age-adjusted rates for African-American women across the geographic sites is relatively small, ranging from 94 per 100,000 in Connecticut to 106 per 100,000 in metropolitan Atlanta.

Geographic differences in breast cancer mortality parallel those in incidence. Mortality is highest in the urban Northeast and West, and lowest in the South and Midwest.[1] Figure 3 illustrates these regional differences for 1990. These differences have remained remarkably constant over the past 50 years. In 1940, before the introduction of DDT, polychlorinated biphenyls (PCBs), and other environmental causes postulated to be linked to geographic differences in breast cancer risk, the Northeast and western areas of the United States tended to have the highest age-adjusted mortality rates, whereas the South had the lowest.[5] Again, geographic differences in the prevalence of established risk factors explain much of the geographic differences in mortality. In 1987, age-adjusted mortality ratios among women aged 50 years and older were 1.15, 1.18, and 1.30 in the West, Midwest, and Northeast, respectively, compared with the South. After adjustment for established breast cancer risk factors, these mortality ratios fell to 1.13, 1.08, and 1.13, respectively.[22]

Trends in Incidence and Mortality in the United States

Rates of breast cancer have been steadily increasing in the United States since formal record-keeping began in Connecticut in the 1930s (Fig. 4). Between 1940 and 1982, the age-adjusted incidence rose by an average of 1.2% per year in this state,[24] which has the oldest cancer registry in continuous operation. This represents a cumulative increase of approximately 65% over the 42 years. During the 1980s, incidences rose more sharply. Data from the SEER program, which began collecting data from different registries across the country in 1973, confirm the trends in incidence portrayed in the Connecticut registry since that time. Increases have occurred in all age groups since 1935, although the magnitude of increase has been greater for older women. In recent decades, rates have increased more sharply among African-American women than among white women. According to SEER data,[1] between 1973 and 1995, incidence among

African-American women younger than 50 years of age increased by 34% compared with a cumulative increase of 10% for white women under age 50 years. Among women 50 years of age and older, the cumulative increase was 51% for African-American women and 45% for white women.

Several studies have examined whether the increase in breast cancer incidence in the United States has been due to the increasing use of screening mammography.[24–29] Because screening causes at most a transient increase in incidence, and because its use was limited before the 1980s, it can explain little of the long-term increase between the 1930s and the 1980s. During the 1980s, however, the increased incidence was due almost entirely to an increase in localized disease and in tumors measuring less than 2 cm in diameter; the incidence of tumors 2 cm or larger remained stable. These findings, as well as the observed decrease in mortality for white women (discussed in the following paragraph), suggest that the increase in use of screening mammography accounts for part of the increase in breast cancer incidence in the 1980s and 1990s.[27,30]

Trends in breast cancer mortality are of major public health interest, but their interpretation is complex, because they reflect the combined effects of trends in underlying risk of breast cancer, changes in screening practices, and effectiveness of treatment. Furthermore, mortality rates lag behind changes in breast cancer risk, screening, and treatment by at least 5 to 10 years.[31] Age-adjusted mortality rates in the United States were relatively stable between the 1950s and the late 1980s, when an overall decline was first noted.[30] These overall trends obscure important variation by age and race, however. Since the 1970s, mortality rates have fallen for younger white women, and this decline has accelerated since the late 1980s. From 1973 to 1995, the cumulative decline in mortality rates for white women younger than age 60 was more than 20%, with much of this decline occurring since 1988. In contrast to these trends among younger white women, mortality rates for white women aged 60 years and older increased slowly during the 1970s and 1980s, although since the late 1980s mortality has also begun to decline in this group.[30,31] The trends in breast cancer mortality among African-American women have been unfavorable; since the 1970s, mortality rates have increased for African-American women in all age groups, and no evidence is seen of a recent decline in mortality, as has been noted for white women[31] (Fig. 5).

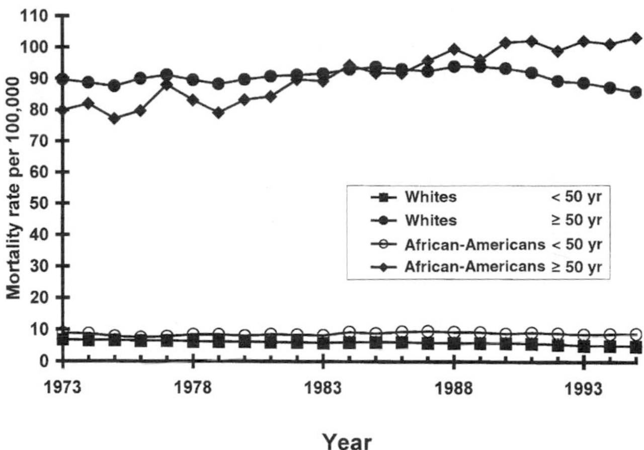

FIG. 5. Trends in breast cancer mortality for white and African-American women in the United States by age group. (Data from ref. 1, with permission.)

Trends in Incidence and Mortality around the World

Since the 1950s, breast cancer incidence has been increasing in many of the lower-risk countries and in high-risk Western countries. Some of the recent increases in incidence in high-risk populations may be due to greater use of mammography, as in the United States. This appears to be the case in Sweden,[32] as well as in England and Wales.[33] In Norway, however, a substantial increase in breast cancer incidence occurred between 1983 and 1993 despite low use of mammographic screening.[34] Breast cancer rates have nearly doubled since the 1950s in traditionally low-risk countries such as Japan[4,7] and Singapore,[3] and in the urban areas of China.[35] Dramatic changes in lifestyle in such regions brought about by growing economies, increasing affluence, and increases in the proportion of women in the industrial workforce have had an impact on the population distribution of established breast cancer risk factors, including age at menarche and fertility, and nutritional status. These changes have resulted in a convergence toward the risk factor profile of Western countries.

Trends in breast cancer mortality around the world have largely paralleled the trends in incidence. Since the 1960s, mortality has been increasing in both high-risk and lower-risk populations, although a slight decline in mortality has been observed since 1990 in the United Kingdom, The Netherlands, and Sweden, similar to the decline over the same time period in the United States.[36] As in the United States, some of the downturn in mortality in these countries may be due to more widespread use of screening mammography and adjuvant chemotherapy during the 1980s.[36,37] Countries with a recent downturn in mortality are generally those with the highest incidence and mortality rates, whereas those countries with mortality rates that are still increasing tend to be those with the lowest mortality.[36] For instance, among European countries, Poland and Spain have had the lowest mortality rates, and these rates are continuing to rise. Thus, a convergence of breast cancer mortality rates may be occurring internationally, in part reflecting an international convergence of reproductive factors.[36]

REPRODUCTIVE FACTORS

This section addresses reproductive factors during the course of a woman's life in relation to risk of breast cancer. An underlying concept is that ovarian hormones initiate breast development and that subsequent monthly menstrual cycles induce regular breast cell proliferation. This pattern of cell division terminates with a natural menopause, as indicated by cessation of ovulation and menstrual periods.

Age at Menarche

Menarche represents the development of the mature hormonal environment of a young woman, and the onset of monthly cycling of hormones that induce ovulation, menstruation, and cell proliferation within the breast and endometrium. Earlier age at menarche has been consistently associated with increased risk of breast cancer.[38] Most studies suggest that age at menarche is related to both premenopausal and postmenopausal breast cancer risk.

Although menarche is most clearly related to the onset of ovulation, some, but not all, studies suggest that hormone levels may be higher through the reproductive years among women who have early menarche.[39] In addition, early menarche may be associated with more rapid onset of regular, ovulatory menstrual cycles and hence greater lifetime exposure to endogenous hormones.[40] Whether the levels of ovarian hormones or their cyclic characteristics are the underlying influence on breast cancer risk is undetermined[6]; both likely play a role.

Menstrual Cycle Characteristics

Shorter cycle length has been quite consistently related to greater risk of breast cancer,[38] although not all studies support this relation.[41] Shorter cycle length during ages 20 to 39 years may be associated with higher risk of breast cancer, perhaps because the shorter cycle length is associated with a greater number of cycles and more time spent in the luteal phase, when both estrogen and progesterone levels are high. Long and irregular cycles may also be related to reduced risk of breast cancer.[41]

Ovulatory infertility, an indicator of infertility due to hormonal causes, has not been consistently related to risk of breast cancer, although one cohort study suggested a substantially lower risk among women with this condition (relative risk of 0.4 compared with women with no infertility history).[41] The significant inverse association seen in this study may be due to the young age of the cohort and thoroughness of investigation of the cause of infertility in this group of health professionals.

Pregnancy and Age at First Full-Term Pregnancy

Nulliparous women are at increased risk of breast cancer compared with parous women. This risk is evident after age 40 to 45 years, but not for breast cancer diagnosed at younger ages. In the majority of epidemiologic studies, a younger age at first full-term pregnancy predicts a lower lifetime risk of breast cancer.[38] The reduction in risk after pregnancy compared with nulliparity is not immediate but takes 10 to 15 years to manifest.[42] In fact, risk of breast cancer is increased for the first decade after the first pregnancy.[43–45] The proliferation of breast cells during the first pregnancy results in differentiation into mature breast cells prepared for lactation; this may also lead to growth of mutated cells and excess risk over the next decade. Epidemiologic evidence for the transient excess risk after the first pregnancy is consistent. Less clear is the presence of a transient increase in risk after subsequent pregnancies; some studies suggest an adverse effect,[46] but others do not.[44]

The first pregnancy is associated with permanent changes in the glandular epithelium and with changes in the biological properties of the mammary cells. After the differentiation of pregnancy, epithelial cells have a longer cell cycle and spend more time in G_1, the phase that allows for DNA repair.[47] The longer the interval from menarche to first pregnancy, the greater the adverse effect of the first pregnancy.[45] The later the age at first full-term pregnancy, the more likely that DNA mistakes have occurred that will be propagated with the proliferation of mammary cells during pregnancy. The susceptibility of mammary tissue to carcinogens decreases after the first pregnancy, reflecting the differentiation of the mammary gland. This is seen in the age-dependent susceptibility of the breast to radiation, reviewed in the section Ionizing Radiation.

Number and Spacing of Births

A higher number of births is consistently related to lower risk of breast cancer; each additional birth beyond the first reduces long-term risk of breast cancer. Although in some analyses this has not been independent of earlier age at first birth, the overall evidence indicates an independent effect of greater parity.[48] In addition to a protective effect of higher parity, several studies indicate that more closely spaced births are associated with lower lifetime risk of breast cancer.[44,49] This may be due to the breast's having less time to accumulate DNA damage before it attains maximal differentiation by repeated pregnancies.

Lactation

As early as 1926, the proposal was made that a breast never used for lactation is more likely to become cancerous.[50] This hypothesis is consistent with knowledge of breast physiology and breast carcinogenesis,[51] as well as with patterns of international variation in breast cancer incidence: Rates are lower in populations in which breast-feeding is both common and of long duration. The overall evidence from case control and cohort studies supports a reduction in risk with longer duration of breast-feeding, but the findings have varied substantially in the level of risk reduction. A review of 32 studies published through 1998 (R. Blum and G. Colditz, *personal communication*, 1998) showed that only 2 were prospective, and only 16 of 32 demonstrated a statistically significant lower risk with longer duration of breast-feeding.[51] The strongest results supported at least a 50% reduction in risk for women who breast-fed for 2 or more years,[52] but this was in the setting of extremely high parity. Some of the differences may relate to the pattern of breast-feeding, for example, whether feeding was exclusively from the breast or supplemented with other food; this needs to be evaluated further.

Social norms regarding parity and breast-feeding in American culture have limited the ability even to study this potential preventive behavior; the population that breast-feeds at all is small, and the group that breast-feeds over an extended period is even smaller. For example, despite the strong recommendation of the American Academy of Pediatrics that infants be breast-fed through the first 6 months of life because of unequivocal benefit to the infant,[53] in 1988 breast-feeding was practiced by only 32% of new mothers.[54] Although low, this still represents a doubling since 1970.

Spontaneous and Induced Abortion

Close to one-quarter of all clinically identified pregnancies in the United States end as induced abortions,[55] and for women whose pregnancies continue for 8 to 28 weeks, the probability of spontaneous abortion ranges from 8% to 12%.[56] It has been suggested that breast cells are the most vulnerable to mutation when breast tissue consists of rapidly growing and undifferentiated cells, such as during adolescence and pregnancy. In early pregnancy, the number of undifferentiated cells increases as rapid growth of the breast epithelium takes place. If the pregnancy continues to term, these cells differentiate by the third trimester; thus, the number of cells susceptible to malignancy decreases. The interruption of the differentiation of breast cells that takes place as a result of spontaneous and induced abortions has been hypothesized to increase a woman's risk of developing breast cancer.[57] This hypothesis appears to be supported by a meta-analysis that included data from 28 published reports on induced abortion and breast cancer incidence.[58] This analysis, however, based largely on case control studies, contains the underlying serious potential for bias in retrospective studies of the relationship between abortion and breast cancer. Induced abortion can be an extremely sensitive topic, and reporting on abortion history by women with a life-threatening condition such as breast cancer may be more complete than reporting by women without breast cancer.

Other studies provide a different picture of the association between breast cancer and abortion. In a hospital-based case control study including 1,803 women with breast cancer, the relative risk among parous women was 1.1 (95% confidence interval of 0.9 to 1.5) for women with a history of any induced abortion compared with women who had never had induced or spontaneous abortion.[59] The relative risk associated with induced abortions in nulliparous women was 1.3 (95% confidence interval, 0.9 to 1.9). Spontaneous abortions similarly were not associated with increased breast cancer risk. Although selection bias could not be ruled out, this large study provided little support for an increase in breast cancer risk in association with spontaneous or induced abortion. In another large case control study,[60] only abortions performed before they were legal in the United States were associated with risk of breast cancer, thus supporting the likelihood of bias in case control studies. Given these concerns regarding recall bias in case control studies of induced abortion and risk of breast cancer, greater weight must be placed on the results from prospective studies that are by design free from such recall bias.

By far the strongest study on the association between breast cancer and abortion was a population-based cohort study made up of 1.5 million Danish women born April 1, 1935 through March 31, 1978.[61] Of these women, 280,965 (18.4%) had had one or more induced abortions. After adjusting for potential confounders of age, parity, age at delivery of first child, and calendar period, the risk of breast cancer for women with a history of induced abortion was no different from that for women who had not had an induced abortion (relative risk, 1.0; 95% confidence interval, 0.94 to 1.06). The number of induced abortions in a woman's history also had no significant relation to risk of breast cancer. A statistically significant increase in risk was found among the very small number of women with a history of second-trimester abortion. Results from this population-based prospective cohort thus provide strong evidence against an increase in risk of breast cancer among women with a history of induced abortion during the first trimester. Taken as a whole, and accounting for the limitations of the case control study design, the available evidence does not support any important relation between induced abortion and risk of breast cancer.

Age at Menopause

Early studies of age at menopause and risk of breast cancer focused on women who had undergone bilateral oophorectomy at a young age; these women have a greatly reduced risk of breast cancer.[62,63] Women who underwent bilateral oophorectomy before age 45 years have approximately one-half the risk of breast cancer of those who had a natural menopause at age 55 years or older. On average, the risk of breast cancer increases by some 3% per year of delay in age at menopause. Although some studies suggest that the effect of age at menopause decreases with advancing age at breast cancer diagnosis,[64] this may reflect greater error in recall of age at menopause as women are further removed from the event.[65] Adjustment for error in recall removes this apparent decrease in the effect of menopause with advancing age.

The reduction in risk of breast cancer with early menopause is probably due to the cessation of breast cell division with the termination of menstrual cycles and the decline in endogenous hormone levels, which become substantially lower than during the premenopausal years.

Models of Reproductive Factors and Breast Cancer Incidence

Biomathematical models relating epidemiologic risk factors of breast cancer can provide a structure to view the process of carcinogenesis. In addition, such models summarize the impact of multiple variables and provide a means of identifying areas that require more research.[66] The classic models of carcinogenesis proposed by Armitage and Doll[67] and by Moolgavkar and Knudson[68] are the best known. Pike et al. reviewed the epidemiologic evidence in the early 1980s and proposed a model of tissue aging that accounted for the relationship between reproductive risk factors and breast cancer incidence.[43] Ultimately, models ideally will be developed that take into account all known risk factors.

The mathematical model proposed by Pike was based on the observed age-incidence curve and on the known relation of the age at menarche, first birth, and menopause to the risk of breast cancer.[43] The Pike model built on earlier work by Moolgavkar et al., who fitted mathematical parameters to breast cancer incidence data from several countries. The Pike model related breast cancer rates to the growth of the breast. The model allowed a short-term increase in risk with first pregnancy followed by a subsequent decrease in risk. Finally, at menopause, the breast begins an involutional process that is thought to reflect a decrease in cell turnover and eventual disappearance of epithelium. The original Pike model, however, did not include terms for the second or subsequent births or for the spacing of pregnancies, nor did it easily accommodate pregnancies after age 40 years. Although controversy has existed about whether the bearing of additional children beyond the first reduces the risk of breast cancer, substantial evidence (reviewed in the section Number and Spacing of Births) indicates that both the number of births and their spacing are associated with risk: The greater the number of births and the more closely they are spaced, the lower a woman's risk of breast cancer.

An extension of the Pike model of breast cancer incidence used prospective data from the Nurses' Health Study[44,45] and added a term to summarize the spacing of births. Nonlinear models produced parameters that were difficult to interpret,[44] but a subsequent modification allowed ready estimation of relative risks,[45] thus making the results more accessible to epidemiologists and clinicians familiar with the relative risk as a measure of the relation between an exposure and disease. Before menopause, the incidence of breast cancer increased 1.7% for each 1-year increase in age at first birth. Closer spacing of births was related to significantly reduced risk of breast cancer. For each additional year of delay between the first and second births, for example, the risk of breast cancer increased by 0.4%. The increase in risk with first pregnancy originally observed with this modified Pike model has since been documented in a prospective study from Sweden[46] and in an analysis from an international case control study.[69] The effects of age at first and subsequent births on breast cancer incidence were still greater after menopause (Table 1).

According to the extended Pike model, a parous woman with a single birth at age 35 years has a 34% increase in breast cancer incidence at the time of the birth relative to a nulliparous woman. The excess risk goes down very slowly over time. Even at age 70 years, such a woman has a 19% excess risk relative to a nulliparous woman. Conversely, a parous woman who had first birth at an early age and multiple births conceived at a young age has a slight excess risk immediately after the first birth relative to the nulliparous woman (relative risk, 1.10); this risk slowly diminishes over time, reaching equality with the nulliparous woman at age 32 years and continuing to decline until menopause (age 50), at which time the relative risk is 0.82. Because the relationship between breast cancer incidence and reproductive

TABLE 1. *Breast cancer incidence (per 100,000) by age, for three hypothetical groups of women*

			Age at birth(s) (yr)			
	Nulliparous		35		20, 23, 26	
Age (yr)	Incidence	RR	Incidence	RR	Incidence	RR
20	21	1.0	21	1.0	23	1.10
25	31	1.0	31	1.0	33	1.07
30	46	1.0	46	1.0	47	1.02
35	70	1.0	93	1.34	67	0.96
40	105	1.0	138	1.31	96	0.91
45	158	1.0	203	1.29	136	0.86
50	237	1.0	300	1.27	194	0.82
55	303	1.0	378	1.25	229	0.76
60	389	1.0	477	1.23	271	0.70
65	498	1.0	602	1.21	320	0.64
70	638	1.0	760	1.19	378	0.59
13–70	10,032	1.0	12,128	1.21	7,571	0.75

For all examples, age at menarche is considered to be 13 years, and age at menopause is considered to be 50 years.
RR, relative risk compared with nulliparous women.

history changes with age, cumulative incidence rather than age-specific incidence is a useful summary (see Table 1). A woman with one birth at age 35 years has a 21% excess risk over the age period of 30 to 70 years compared with a nulliparous woman, whereas a woman with births at ages 20, 23, and 26 years has a 25% decrease in risk over the same age period[45] compared with a nulliparous woman.

In the original Pike model,[43] factors associated with reduced risk of breast cancer were each considered to slow the rate of "breast tissue aging," which correlates with the accumulation of molecular damage in the pathway to breast cancer. In the Rosner and Colditz extension of the Pike model,[45] the rate of tissue aging was highest between menarche and first birth, consistent with the hypothesis that this is the period when the breast is most vulnerable to mutagenesis. The transient increase in the risk of breast cancer associated with the first pregnancy is followed by a 20% decrease in the rate of breast tissue aging.[45] This observation helps explain the crossover effect in certain subgroups of women: Around menopause, rates of one subgroup that were initially higher drop below rates of a second subgroup. For instance, using data from New York State, Janerich and Hoff showed a crossover in breast cancer incidence between single and married women at age 42 years, such that married women had a higher incidence before this age and lower mortality thereafter.[70] A similar crossover of incidence has been reported for African-American and white women in the United States,[9,71] consistent with the distribution of age at first birth by race. Over many decades, pregnancy rates have been higher and age at first birth has been younger for African-American women than for white women.[72]

The age-incidence curve from biomathematical models of reproductive events and breast cancer incidence also mirrors the observed patterns of breast cancer incidence in many countries. In China and many developing countries, the estimated number of births in the early 1960s was 6.5 births per woman[73] and is not associated with a late age at first birth. Also, the average age at menarche in China was approximately 17 years, even through the 1960s.[74] When the Rosner model is fitted with menarche at age 16 years, first birth at age 19 years, 6 births spaced a year apart, and menopause at age 50 years, the annual rate of breast cancer incidence for 65-year-old women in China is estimated to be 93.6 per 100,000. For the cohort of U.S. women born from 1921 to 1925, the average age at menarche was approximately 13.5 years, the median age at first birth was 23 years, the mean number of children was 3, and the mean interval between births was 3 years.[72] Considering these characteristics, and holding age at menopause constant at 50 years, the annual rate of breast cancer incidence predicted for 65-year-old U.S. women is 279 per 100,000—close to the observed SEER rate of 300 per 100,000 for women of this age, and approximately three times the rate for Chinese women. Applying this model to typical reproductive patterns for women from low-incidence countries suggests that that reproductive factors alone account for more than one-half of the international variation in the risk of breast cancer.[75] Further development of these models to include other risk factors will provide an increasingly comprehensive prediction of breast cancer risk.

ENDOGENOUS SEX HORMONE LEVELS

Several lines of evidence have long suggested that sex hormones play a central role in the etiology of breast cancer. As noted in the section Age-Incidence Curve of Breast Cancer Risk, rates of breast cancer increase rapidly in the premenopausal years, but the rate of increase slows sharply at the time of menopause, when endogenous hormone levels decline rapidly. In addition, several reproductive variables that alter estrogen status affect risk of breast cancer; for example, early age at menarche and late age at menopause are associated with increased risk of breast cancer. After menopause, adipose tissue is the major source of estrogen, and obese postmenopausal women have both higher levels of endogenous estrogen and a higher risk of breast cancer.[76,77] In animals, estrogens and progesterone promote mammary tumors. Also, hormonal manipulations, such as administration of antiestrogens (e.g., tamoxifen citrate), are useful in the treatment of breast cancer and reduce breast cancer incidence in high-risk women.[78] Despite this strong body of evidence suggesting a central role of endogenous estrogen, studies directly relating blood or urinary hormone levels to risk of breast cancer have largely been inconsistent. Only with the availability of large prospective studies has a clearer picture emerged.

Methodologic Issues in Studies of Endogenous Hormones and Breast Cancer Risk

In contrast to clinical determinations, in which discerning grossly abnormal from normal hormone levels is the focus, epidemiologic studies are usually aimed at detecting modest differences within the normal range of levels. Considerable laboratory error has been reported in studies of assay reproducibility, and several hormones are measured quite poorly by some laboratories.[79,80] Low reproducibility could result in failure to detect true (and important) exposure-disease associations. Varying sensitivities and specificities of different laboratory assays also have made comparison of results between studies difficult. For example, in studies of plasma estradiol levels, mean levels in control subjects have ranged from 9 pg per mL[81] to 28 pg per mL.[82] Although these differences may result in part from differences in the characteristics of study subjects (i.e., differences in adiposity), a substantial component is probably due to the use of varying laboratory methods.

Several hormones, particularly estrogens, fluctuate markedly over the menstrual cycle. In some early studies, hormone levels were measured in samples collected without regard to the menstrual cycle phase, thus adding considerable noise to the comparison of hormone levels between breast cancer cases and controls. This noise could mask true associations or, because of chance differences in the distribution of cycle phase between cases and controls, could result in associations that do not truly exist. Wih better understanding of such methodologic issues, studies have begun to collect all samples at approximately the same time in the cycle, have matched on cycle day, or have carefully controlled for cycle day in the analysis—all appropriate strategies.

For both logistic and financial reasons, in most epidemiologic studies, only a single blood sample can be collected per study subject. Whether a single sample can reflect long-term hormone levels (generally the exposure of greatest etiologic interest) is therefore an important issue. In several studies, repeated blood samples were collected over a 1- to 3-year period in postmenopausal women, and the correlation between the samples was calculated. Overall, levels of steroid hormones were reasonably stable, with intraclass correlations ranging from 0.5 to 0.9.[83–86] This level of reproducibility is similar to that found for other biological variables, such as blood pressure and serum cholesterol measurements, all parameters that are considered reasonably measured and that are consistent predictors of disease in epidemiologic studies. Data on premenopausal women are much more limited, although androgen levels have been noted to be reasonably correlated over a several-year period.[85,86]

The complexity and expense of hormone assays, coupled with the need to collect urine or blood samples from study subjects (and timed samples in premenopausal subjects) have resulted in both a limited number of epidemiologic studies of these issues and small sample sizes. These factors, in conjunction with error in the laboratory assays, have likely contributed to the lack of consistent findings. A summary, which relies when possible predominantly on the larger studies and those using a prospective design, is provided in the sections below.

Estrogens

Estradiol, considered the most biologically active endogenous estrogen, circulates in blood either unbound ("free") or bound to sex hormone–binding globulin or albumin. Free or bioavailable (free plus albumin-bound) estradiol is thought to be readily available to breast tissue and thus may be more strongly related to risk than total estradiol. Postmenopausally, estrone is the source of most circulating estradiol, and estrone sulfate is the most abundant circulating estrogen.[87] Both normal and malignant breast cells have sulfatase and aromatase activity,[88] so estrone and estrone sulfate could serve as a ready source of intracellular estradiol.

Among postmenopausal women, the most consistent finding is a positive relationship between total estradiol and risk of breast cancer (Table 2). In a meta-analysis of six prospective studies, breast cancer patients had mean estradiol levels that were 15% higher (p <.001) than those of healthy controls.[89] Similarly, among 16 case control studies, breast cancer patients were noted to have mean levels 24% higher than levels in controls, although substantial heterogeneity in results was noted among these studies.

TABLE 2. *Ratio of plasma estradiol levels in cases to controls—data from prospective studies*

Study	No. of cases/ controls	Ratio	95% Confidence interval
Garland et al.[357]	15/400	0.87	0.66–1.14
Helzlsouer et al.[91]	29/58	0.96	0.74–1.24
Toniolo et al.[82]	130/251	1.21	1.07–1.37
Berrino et al.[105]	24/88	1.09	0.92–1.30
Dorgan et al.[104]	71/133	1.17	0.93–1.46
Thomas et al.[92]	60/175	1.30	1.08–1.57
Hankinson et al.[81]	154/308	1.12[a]	1.00–1.25
	83/190	1.25[b]	1.07–1.45

[a]Ratio = 1.12 among all postmenopausal women.
[b]Ratio = 1.25 among the subset of postmenopausal women who never used postmenopausal hormones.

Results of the largest prospective study have been published since this meta-analysis.[81] Blood samples were collected from 32,826 women in the Nurses' Health Study from 1989 to 1990; among postmenopausal women not using hormone replacement therapy at blood collection, 156 women were diagnosed with breast cancer after blood collection. Two controls were selected per case, matched on age, menopausal status, and time of blood collection. A significant positive association between plasma estradiol level and risk of breast cancer was seen (top versus bottom quartile comparisons: multivariate relative risk, 1.9; 95% confidence interval, 1.2 to 3.5). Among women with no prior use of postmenopausal hormone therapy (for whom the single plasma hormone measure would best reflect past hormone levels), the association was markedly stronger (relative risk, 3.8; 95% confidence interval, 1.6 to 8.7). The comparable relative risk for women with high levels of plasma estrone sulfate was 4.3 (95% confidence interval, 1.9 to 10.1).

Other estrogens and estrogen fractions have not been as thoroughly evaluated as total estradiol. Percent free estradiol has been assessed in four prospective studies; a positive relationship was noted in three[82,90,91] but not in the fourth.[81] Percent bioavailable estradiol was positively associated with risk in one study[82] but not in a second.[81] Higher estrone levels were significantly associated with increased breast cancer risk in several studies[81,82] but not in all. Similarly, findings for estrone sulfate (evaluated in only three studies) have been somewhat inconsistent.

Overall, the epidemiologic data now provide strong evidence for an influence of plasma estrogens on breast cancer risk in postmenopausal women based largely on the substantial evidence for total estradiol.[89] However, the specific estrogens and estrogen fractions most related to risk, and the dose-response relationship, remain to be defined.

Data on premenopausal estrogen levels and breast cancer risk are more limited, in large part because of the complexities related to sampling during the menstrual cycle. Data from several case control studies, but not others, suggest that high levels of estradiol in premenopausal women increase the risk of breast cancer.[40] In the largest prospective analysis to date, involving 61 cases, estradiol levels were 12% higher in women who developed breast cancer than in controls.[92] A second prospective study, with 22 cases, reported a nonsignificant increased risk for women with higher estrone and estradiol levels in the follicular phase but not the luteal phase of the menstrual cycle,[91] whereas a third study found no association.[93] To date, few studies have evaluated free or bioavailable estradiol levels in premenopausal women.[40]

Estrogen Metabolites

A woman's pattern of estrogen metabolism has also been hypothesized to influence her breast cancer risk. Estradiol and estrone can be metabolized through one of two mutually exclusive pathways, the 16α and 2-hydroxy pathways.[94] Products of these two pathways have markedly different biological properties, and opposing hypotheses have been proposed concerning their influence on risk.[94]

The epidemiologic studies that evaluated associations between levels of estrogen metabolites and breast cancer risk have been small (the largest had 42 cases), and results are inconsistent. In the only study of premenopausal women (with 19 cases), the 2-hydroxyestrone to 16α-hydroxyestrone ratio was not associated with breast cancer risk, although in postmenopausal women an inverse relation was observed.[95] In another study of perimenopausal and postmenopausal women, percent oxidation by 16α-hydroxylation was significantly greater and oxidation by 2-hydroxylation nonsignificantly greater in cases than in controls.[96] Similar results were observed in several,[97,98] but not all,[99] other case control studies of postmenopausal women. These associations have not been evaluated in prospective studies. Overall, limited data exist to address these hypotheses, and no conclusions can yet be drawn.

Androgens

Androgens have been hypothesized to increase breast cancer risk either directly, by increasing the growth and proliferation of breast cancer cells, or indirectly, by their conversion to estrogen.[40] Administration of dehydroepiandrosterone (DHEA) to rodents can decrease the risk of spontaneous and chemically induced cancers.[100] In humans, DHEA may act like an antiestrogen premenopausally but an estrogen postmenopausally in stimulating cell growth,[101] in part because of the estrogenic effect of its metabolite, 5-androstene-3β,17β-diol,[102] which also can bind to the estrogen receptor.[102]

In postmenopausal women, higher testosterone levels have been positively associated with breast cancer in most,[92,103–105] but not all,[93] studies. The association has tended to be attenuated, however, after plasma estrogen levels are taken into account.[40,92] In the largest prospective study, the modest, nonsignificant association with testosterone level was substantially attenuated after the investigators controlled for estrogen levels.[81] Postmenopausal dehydroepiandrosulfate (DHEAS) levels were generally associated with either significant[81] or nonsignificant[103,105–107] increases in breast cancer risk in previous prospective studies. In three previous prospective assessments of DHEA, significant positive associations were observed in two,[106,107] whereas no association was observed in the third.[81] In the only previous study of 5-androstene-3β,17β-diol[107] among postmenopausal women, women in the top quartile of levels had a significant threefold higher risk of breast cancer; women in the highest quartile for both DHEA and 5-androstene-3β,17β-diol (compared with the lowest for both) had a sixfold higher risk.

Overall, higher levels of testosterone may have a modest, but probably indirect, association with postmenopausal breast cancer through its conversion to estradiol. Most studies have noted at least a modest positive association with DHEA and DHEAS; further delineation of the exact nature of these associations is required.

Among premenopausal women, no association was found between testosterone level and breast cancer risk in two prospective studies.[92,93] Strong positive associations have been noted in several case control studies, with RRs ranging from 3.4 to 10.2 for women in the top category of plasma testosterone.[40] Results from studies addressing androstenedione levels and breast cancer are inconsistent.[40] The only prospective study of DHEA and DHEAS levels and breast cancer in premenopausal women had just 15 cases.[108] Again, the data are too limited to draw any firm conclusions relating androgen levels to breast cancer risk in premenopausal women.

Progesterone

Progesterone exerts powerful influences on breast physiology and can influence tumor development in rodents.[109] Based largely on indirect evidence, progesterone has been hypothesized both to decrease breast cancer risk by opposing estrogenic stimulation of the breast[109] and to increase risk because breast mitotic rates are highest in the luteal (high-progesterone) phase of the menstrual cycle.[40] In one prospective study, serum progesterone was 95% higher in cases compared with controls in the luteal phase and 20% higher in the follicular phase[91]; however, the study was small (22 cases), and the differences were not statistically significant. A nonsignificant inverse association between progesterone and breast cancer has been reported in an addi-

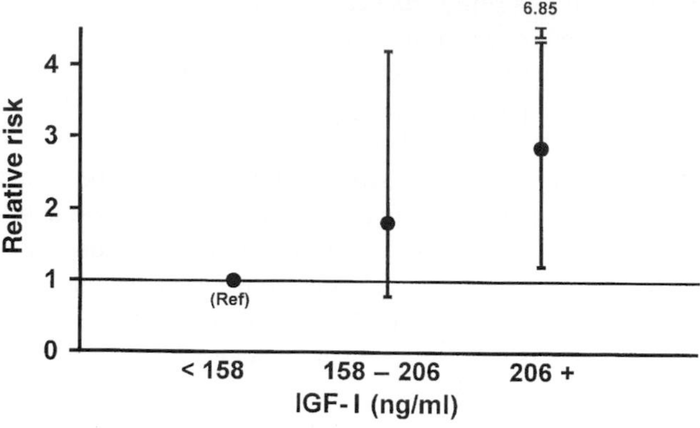

FIG. 6. Plasma levels of type I insulinlike growth factor (IGF-I) and risk of breast cancer in premenopausal women. (From ref. 129, with permission.)

tional prospective analysis.[92] Additional larger studies are needed to address this relationship in detail.

Prolactin

Indirect evidence suggests that prolactin could play a role in breast carcinogenesis. Prolactin receptors have been found in more than 50% of breast tumors,[110] and prolactin increases the growth of both normal and malignant breast cells *in vitro*,[111] although these findings have not been entirely consistent.[112] Prolactin administration is well documented to increase mammary tumor rates in mice.

A number of case control studies of prolactin levels and breast cancer risk have been conducted, although the largest of these included just 66 cases. Also, because prolactin is influenced by both physical and emotional stress,[113,114] levels in women with breast cancer may not reflect their predisease levels. Thus, evaluation of this association in prospective studies is particularly important. Only two prospective studies have been conducted. In the first, which included 40 postmenopausal breast cancer cases,[115] women in the top quintile of prolactin levels had a nonsignificant 63% higher risk of breast cancer compared with those in the bottom quintile. In a prospective analysis of prolactin and breast cancer risk from the Nurses' Health Study that included 306 postmenopausal cases and 448 postmenopausal controls, a significant positive association was seen (top versus bottom quartile comparison: relative risk, 2.0; 95% confidence interval, 1.2 to 3.3; p for trend = .01).[116]

Epidemiologic data on premenopausal prolactin levels and breast cancer risk are more sparse, and results are inconsistent. In the only prospective study, with 71 cases,[115] no relationship was observed, although confidence limits were wide (top versus bottom quintile comparison: relative risk, 1.1; 95% confidence interval, 0.5 to 2.2). Thus, no conclusion can be drawn as to the relationship between prolactin levels and breast cancer risk in premenopausal women.

Insulinlike Growth Factor

Insulinlike growth factor type I (IGF-I) is a polypeptide hormone with structural homology to insulin, and it is regulated primarily by growth hormone.[117] Evidence is increasing that the growth hormone–IGF-I axis stimulates proliferation of both breast cancer[118,119] and normal breast epithelial cells.[120] Transgenic mice that overexpress growth hormone exhibit a high frequency of breast cancer,[121] and rhesus monkeys treated with growth hormone or IGF-I show histologic evidence of mammary gland hyperplasia.[122] In addition, positive associations have been observed between breast cancer and both birth weight[123] and height,[124] which are both positively correlated with IGF-I level.[125,126]

The relationships between blood levels of IGF-I and its major binding protein, insulinlike growth factor binding protein 3 (IGFBP-3), have been evaluated in several epidemiologic studies. In two case control studies, a positive relationship was noted between plasma IGF-I levels and breast cancer risk.[127,128] In the larger of the two studies (with 109 cases),[127] the relationship was strongest among premenopausal women. In the Nurses' Health Study, plasma levels in 397 women with invasive breast cancer (diagnosed after they provided a blood sample) were compared with those of 620 age-matched controls.[129] No association was noted between IGF-I level and risk in postmenopausal women. A positive relationship was observed, however, between premenopausal IGF-I levels and risk (top versus bottom tertile, controlling for IGFBP-3: relative risk, 2.9; 95% confidence interval,1.2 to 6.9) (Fig. 6); this relationship was particularly strong among premenopausal women under age 50 years (relative risk, 7.3; 95% confidence interval, 2.4 to 22.0), although these analyses included few cases.

The difference in RRs between premenopausal and postmenopausal women, observed in two of the three studies published to date, may reflect a relatively important effect of the growth hormone–IGF-I axis earlier in life after breast development. Alternatively, IGF-I levels may be specifically relevant to risk of premenopausal breast cancer, perhaps because estradiol may enhance IGF-I activity in the breast.[130] Although these findings relating plasma levels of IGF-I (and IGFBP-3) to breast cancer are promising, they require further confirmation in larger studies, particularly in studies among premenopausal women.

Prenatal Risk Factors

In utero exposure to circulating hormones has been hypothesized to influence the fetus's breast cancer risk in adulthood, perhaps through the influence of these levels on the number and degree of differentiation of breast stem cells.[131] To address this hypothesis, factors such as birth weight and occurrence of preeclampsia, known to be associated with hormone levels during pregnancy, have been evaluated in relation to breast cancer risk. Data are relatively consistent in showing a positive association between birth weight and breast cancer.[123,132] Strong inverse associations between preeclampsia and disease risk also have been reported.[132] Findings for other measures of *in utero* hormone exposure, however (e.g., maternal smoking behavior, birth order), have been less consistent. Overall, increasing evidence suggests some influence of *in utero* exposures on subsequent risk of breast cancer.

ORAL CONTRACEPTIVES

Since oral contraceptives were first introduced in the 1960s, they have been used by many millions of women. In 1988, more than 10.7 million U.S. women were current oral contraceptive users.[133] Most combined oral contraceptives contain ethinyl estradiol (or mestranol, which is metabolized to ethinyl estradiol) and a progestin. The estrogen dose in oral contraceptives has ranged from 100 or more μg in 1960 to 20 to 30 μg, the doses most commonly used today; during this same time period, at least nine different progestins have been used.[134] Patterns of use also have changed considerably over time, with both increasing durations of use and a trend toward earlier age at first use. More than 50 epidemiologic studies have evaluated the relationship between oral contraceptive use and breast cancer risk.

Any Use of Oral Contraceptives

In several meta analyses,[135,136] reviews,[137] and a large pooled analysis[64] studying women who had "ever used" oral contraceptives, use of oral contraceptives was not found to be associated with breast cancer risk. Although this finding is reassuring, defining oral contraceptive use this way is misleading, because women in the "ever use" category are a mixture of women with long-term and short-term use, so any true relationship with one particular aspect of oral contraceptive use may be missed.

Duration of Use

Most studies have observed no significant increase in breast cancer risk with long durations of use of oral contraceptives. Individual data from 54 epidemiologic studies were collected and analyzed centrally.[64] In this large pooled analysis, data from 53,297 women with breast cancer and 100,239 women without breast cancer were evaluated, and no overall relationship was observed between duration of use and risk of breast cancer. These analyses, in which women of all ages were combined, provide considerable evidence against any material adverse effect of long-term oral contraceptive use overall. Similar results were generally observed when long-term use was evaluated among either postmenopausal women or women older than 45 years of age. Findings have not been quite as consistent or reassuring, however, in analyses of long-term use in young women. Summary relative risks for long duration of use in young women were 1.5 in one meta-analysis[136] and 1.4 in another.[135] The greatest increase tended to be observed in the youngest women, generally women younger than 35 years of age.

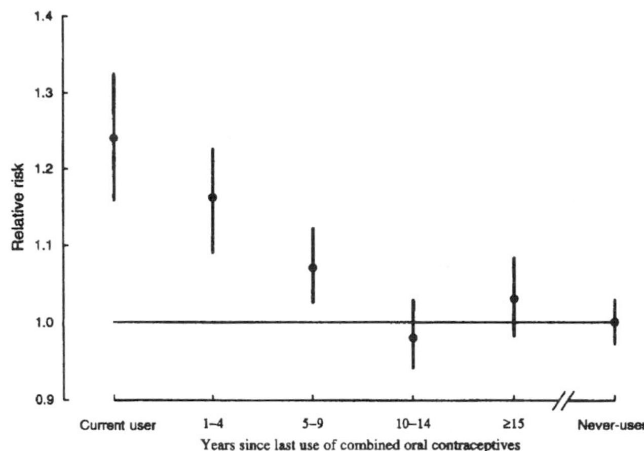

FIG. 7. Relative risk of breast cancer by time since last use of combined oral contraceptives. Relative risk (with 95% confidence interval) is shown in comparison with those who never used oral contraceptives, stratified by study, age at diagnosis, parity, age at first birth, and age at which risk of conception ceased. (Reprinted from ref. 64 with permission of *The Lancet*.)

Several cohort studies also have evaluated these relationships.[138–140] In the Oxford Family Planning Association study,[138] no association was observed with increasing duration of use among women 25 to 44 years, although only 14 cases were younger than 35 years. In the Royal College of General Practitioners cohort,[139] a substantial increased risk was observed among women aged 30 to 34 years. These results must be interpreted cautiously, however, because few cases of breast cancer occurred among women aged 30 to 34 years, the follow-up rate in this cohort was low, and the incidence among the youngest women who did not use oral contraceptives was considerably lower than the age-specific national breast cancer rates. In the Nurses' Health Study cohort, no positive association was noted among women older than 35 years of age.[140,141] Both the Oxford study and the Nurses' Health Study have provided considerable reassurance that no substantial increase in risk occurs among women older than 35 years who used oral contraceptives for extended durations. However, neither of these cohorts included a sufficient number of women younger than 35 years to evaluate the risk in this specific group, and thus further study is needed.

In the large pooled analysis,[64] current and recent users of oral contraceptives were found to have an increased risk of breast cancer (relative risk for current users versus those who never used oral contraceptives was 1.24; 95% confidence interval, 1.15 to 1.33). This increased risk subsided within 10 years of stopping oral contraceptive use (relative risk by years since stopping use versus no use: 1 to 4 years, 1.16; 5 to 9 years, 1.07; 10 to 14 years, 0.98; more than 15 years, 1.03) (Fig. 7). Importantly, the authors observed a modestly increased risk of breast cancer only among current and recent oral contraceptive users, and did not observe any independent effect of long duration of use on risk of breast cancer, even among very young women. Thus, the increased risk of breast cancer observed among young, long-term oral contraceptive users in past individual studies appears to be due primarily to recency of oral contraceptive use rather than to duration of use. These data suggest that oral contraceptives may act as late-stage promoters.

Use before a First Full-Term Pregnancy or at an Early Age

Because any influence of oral contraceptives on the breast has been hypothesized to be greatest before the cellular differentiation that occurs with a full-term pregnancy,[142] a number of investigators have evaluated the effect of oral contraceptive use before a first full-term pregnancy. In both meta-analyses, the summary relative risk indicated a modest increase in risk with long-term use. In several studies not included in these meta-analyses,[143,144] no increase in risk was observed. In the pooled analysis,[64] a significant trend of increasing risk with first use before age 20 years was observed. Among women diagnosed at ages 30 to 34 years, the relative risk associated with recent oral contraceptive use was 1.54 if use began before age 20 years and 1.13 if use began at age 20 years or older.

Type and Dosage of Oral Contraceptives

The specific oral contraceptive formulation might be important in determining cancer risk, but studies of this issue are difficult to perform, because study participants may not be able to remember specific formulations and may use a number of formulations over time, because very large studies are needed to have sufficient statistical power to examine individual brands, and because no satisfactory classification system exists for categorizing specific oral contraceptive formulations by their effect on breast tissue. Although only a few studies have evaluated this issue, overall, no consistent evidence is seen of a differential effect according to type or dosage of either estrogen or progestin.[40] Limited data exist regarding the influence of the newer oral contraceptive formulations on breast cancer risk.[64]

Interactions with Other Breast Cancer Risk Factors

Interactions of oral contraceptive use with other breast cancer risk factors have been evaluated in many studies. However, limited statistical power in these analyses has resulted in wide confidence limits and thus a limited ability to detect true differences; moreover, the categorization of oral contraceptive use was generally "ever use" versus "never use," a crude and uninformative exposure definition. Possible interactions with other breast cancer risk factors were first evaluated in detail, with oral contraceptive use defined in terms of recency and age at first use, in the collaborative pooling project.[145] Overall, the relationship between oral contraceptive use and breast cancer did not vary appreciably with family history of breast cancer, weight, alcohol intake, or other breast cancer risk factors.

Progestin-Only Contraceptives

Progestin-only contraceptives include progestin-only pills ("minipill"), depot-medroxyprogesterone (DMPA), and implantable levonorgestrel (Norplant). Although the progestin-only pill has been evaluated in few studies, no increase in breast cancer risk has been observed for women who have "ever used" this contraceptive.[146] In the studies in which duration of use was evaluated, longer-term users were observed to have either a similar or lower risk of breast cancer compared with those who had never used this contraceptive.[146] DMPA, an injectable contraceptive, also has received limited study in relation to breast cancer risk. In the most comprehensive study of this relationship,[147] no significant increase in risk was observed with increasing duration of use (relative risk for more than 3 years of use versus no use was 0.9; 95% confidence interval, 0.6 to 1.4), although both long-term users who began use before age 25 years and users younger than age 35 years overall were observed to have a modest increase in breast cancer risk. Levonorgestrel, a long-acting contraceptive that is implanted subdermally, was introduced in the United States in 1990. No epidemiologic data have been published on levonorgestrel's effect, if any, on breast cancer risk. Further epidemiologic research is needed for each of these drugs, particularly DMPA and levonorgestrel.

Summary of Oral Contraceptives and Breast Cancer Risk

Results of more than 50 studies have provided considerable reassurance that breast cancer risk increases little, if any, with oral contraceptive use in general, even among women who have used oral contraceptives for 10 or more years. A relatively consistent finding among previous case control studies, however, is an increase in risk among young women who used oral contraceptives for extended durations. This observation has not been confirmed by the larger prospective studies, although these studies included few very young women (younger than 35 years of age), the age group in which the increased relative risk was most consistently observed. In the recent pooled analysis, however, long-term use among young women was not independently associated with an increase in breast cancer risk. Rather, current users and recent users (those with fewer than 10 years since last use) were observed to have a modest elevation in risk compared with those who had never used oral contraceptives. This relationship most likely could not be discerned from the individual studies, because duration of use, rather than recency of use, was often reported. Among young women, the long-term users are more likely to be recent users, and thus large data sets (e.g., the pooled analysis) are needed to determine the independent effect of these variables.

Current and recent users, the group that appears to have a modest increase in risk, are generally young (younger than 45 years of age) and thus have a low absolute risk of breast cancer. Hence, a modest increase in their risk results in few additional cases of breast cancer. Nevertheless, this apparent increased risk among current and recent users should be considered in the overall decision of whether to use oral contraceptives.

POSTMENOPAUSAL HORMONE USE

By the mid-1970s, almost 30 million prescriptions for postmenopausal hormones were being filled annually in the United States.[148] A challenge in studying the relationship between postmenopausal hormone use and breast cancer is the substantial variation in formulations and patterns of use that has occurred over time. By the time sufficient use of one type of hormone has occurred to allow a detailed epidemiologic evaluation, new formulations are already being introduced.

The possible relation between postmenopausal estrogen use and risk of breast cancer has been investigated in more than three dozen epidemiologic studies over the past 20 years. Most of these studies have been summarized in six meta-analyses[149–154] and a large pooled analysis.[155] A summary of these findings, plus a more detailed discussion of several of the most important and most recent studies, is provided in the following subsections on postmenopausal hormones.

Any Use

All meta-analyses have concluded that, overall, women who have ever used postmenopausal estrogens have little or no increase in risk of breast cancer compared with women who have never used this therapy. Depending on the inclusion criteria for the meta-analyses, the relative risk estimates across studies range from 1.01 to 1.07. The relative risk observed in the pooled analysis[155] was 1.14. As with oral contraceptive use, however, "ever use" is a poor measure of exposure, because it fails to distinguish between short and long duration and recent and past users.

Duration of Use

In the meta-analyses, significant increases in risk of 30% to 45% with more than 5 years of use have been observed. Results of several large case control studies have become available since the publication of the meta-analyses.[156,157] A significant positive association between postmenopausal hormone use and breast cancer risk was not seen, even among long-term users, but the 95% CIs were broad enough to encompass the elevated RRs observed in the meta-analyses. One potential difficulty in interpreting the results of case control studies is the impact of nonparticipation, particularly among the controls. In the general population, estrogen users tend to have a somewhat higher socioeconomic status on average,[158] and typically, better-educated individuals are more likely to participate as controls in health-related research studies.

In updated results from the Nurses' Health Study,[159] which included 1,935 breast cancer cases, an excess risk of breast cancer was limited to women with current or very recent use of postmenopausal hormones. The risk increased with increasing duration of use and was statistically significant among current users of 5 or more years duration (e.g., compared with those who never used postmenopausal hormones, relative risk for those with 10 or more years of use was 1.47; 95% confidence interval, 1.22 to 1.76).[160]

Recency of Use

Data on recency of use have been sparse, because many studies did not distinguish current from past users. One meta-analysis calculated a relative risk for current use of 1.63 for women with natural menopause and 1.48 for women with surgical menopause. In a second, the summary relative risk was 1.40 (95% confidence interval, 1.20 to 1.63) for current users compared with those who had never taken menopausal hormones. In the report from the Nurses' Health Study cohort,[159] an excess risk of breast cancer was limited to women with current or very recent use of postmenopausal hormones. In the Breast Cancer Detection Demonstration Project cohort (BCDDP), a positive association with invasive breast cancer was noted among current users of 5 to 15 or more years' duration that varied little by duration of use (relative risks ranged from 1.0 to 1.4).[161]

These relationships were evaluated in considerable detail in the pooled analysis that combined results of 51 epidemiologic studies.[155] Importantly, women whose age at menopause was uncertain (e.g., women with simple hysterectomies) were excluded from these analyses, because inadequate accounting for age at menopause in the analysis can lead to substantial attenuation of the observed relationships between postmenopausal hormone use and breast cancer risk. The investigators observed a statistically significant association between current or recent use of postmenopausal hormones and risk of breast cancer; the positive association was strongest among those with the longest duration of use (Fig. 8). For example, among women who used postmenopausal hormones within the previous 5 years (compared with those who never used postmenopausal hormones), the relative risks for duration of use were 1.08 for 1 to 4 years of use, 1.31 for 5 to 9 years, 1.24 for 10 to 14 years, and 1.56 for 15 or more years of use. No significant increase in breast cancer risk was noted for women who had quit using postmenopausal hormones 5 or more years in the past, regardless of the duration of use.

Some investigators have suggested that the increased risk observed in many of the studies is an artifact of increased surveillance for breast cancer among women taking hormones. Consistent with such a possibility, a higher relative risk has

Duration of use and time since last use	Cases/controls	RR (FSE)	RR and 99% FCI
Never used	12,467/23,568	1.00 (0.021)	
Last use <5 years before diagnosis			
Duration <1 year	368/860	0.99 (0.085)	
Duration 1–4 years	891/2,037	1.08 (0.060)	
Duration 5–9 years	588/1,279	1.31 (0.079)	
Duration 10–14 years	304/633	1.24 (0.108)	
Duration ≥15 years	294/514	1.56 (0.128)	
Last use ≥5 years before diagnosis			
Duration <1 year	437/890	1.12 (0.079)	
Duration 1–4 years	566/1256	1.12 (0.068)	
Duration 5–9 years	151/374	0.90 (0.115)	
Duration ≥10 years	93/233	0.95 (0.145)	

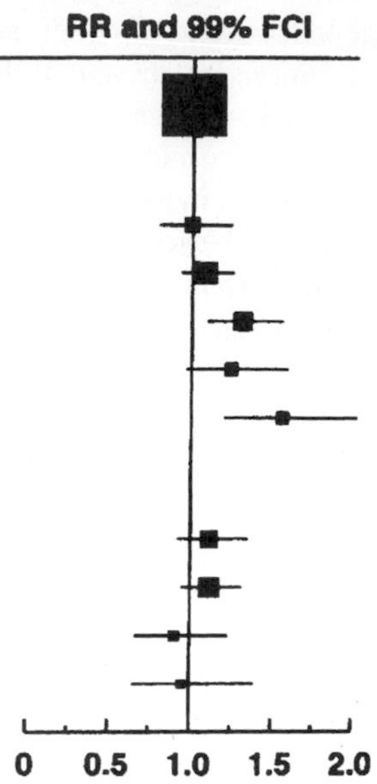

0 0.5 1.0 1.5 2.0

FIG. 8. Relative risk (RR) of breast cancer for different durations of use of hormone replacement. Relative risk is shown in comparison with those who never used hormone replacement therapy, stratified by study, age at diagnosis, time since menopause, body mass index, parity, and the age of the woman at the time her first child was born. "Last use ≥5 years before diagnosis" includes current users. Floated standard error (FSE) and floated confidence interval (FCI) were calculated from floated variance for each exposure category (see methods in ref. 64). Any comparison between groups must take variation into account. Each analysis is based on aggregate data from all studies. Black squares indicate relative risk, area of which is proportional to amount of information contributed (i.e., to inverse of variance of logarithm of relative risk). Lines indicate 99% FCI (lines are white when 99% FCIs are so narrow as to be entirely within width of square). (From ref. 155, with permission.)

been found to be associated with *in situ* disease than with invasive disease.[159,161] In the studies with this finding, however, a significant positive (although weaker) association was noted when only invasive breast cancer cases were considered. Also, in the Nurses' Health Study, mammography rates were uniformly high, exceeding 90% even among women who never used hormones. Moreover, past users and current users of short duration were not observed to have an elevated risk, despite higher mammography rates than among those who had never used postmenopausal hormones. Finally, an elevated death rate from breast cancer was observed among current users who had used hormones for 10 or more years at the time of diagnosis. This latter analysis provides further evidence that the association cannot be explained simply as an artifact of screening.

Type, Dosage, and Mode of Delivery of Estrogen

Limited data are available regarding the effects of dosage or type of estrogen on breast cancer risk. Again, the best data come from the pooled analysis.[155] No significant differences in relative risks were observed according to either the type of estrogen used (conjugated estrogen versus other) or estrogen dose (less than 0.625 mg versus 1.25 mg or more), although some modest differences in estimates suggested that further evaluation is warranted.

Although the effect of estrogen use on breast cancer risk could be reasonably hypothesized to vary by mode of estrogen delivery (e.g., patch estrogen, by avoiding the first-pass effect in the liver, does not increase sex hormone–binding globulin to the extent that oral preparations do), insufficient data are available to evaluate these potential differences.

Risk According to Breast Cancer Risk Factor Profile

The risk associated with postmenopausal hormone use was assessed in a number of specific subgroups in the pooled analysis.[155] Risk did not appear to vary according to reproductive history, alcohol or smoking history, or family history of breast cancer. However, the relative risks associated with 5 or more years of postmenopausal hormone use were highest among the leanest women (p for heterogeneity = .001); this interaction has been consistently observed.[77]

Use of Estrogen Plus Progestin

The addition of a progestin to estrogen regimens has become increasingly common, because it minimizes or eliminates the increased risk of endometrial hyperplasia and cancer associated with the use of unopposed estrogens. In the United States, by the mid-1980s, almost 30% of postmenopausal hormone prescriptions included a prescription for progestin.[162] The impact, if any, of an added progestin on the risk of breast cancer was first evaluated in 1983[163] and remains controversial.

Two of the first studies to assess this relationship suggested that the addition of a progestin could decrease breast cancer risk.[163,164] These studies were small, however, and potentially important confounders (e.g., age, parity) were not accounted for in the analyses. Since that time, several additional studies have assessed this relationship, and together these studies indicate that a protective effect of the dosages typically used in postmenopausal hormone therapy can be ruled out.[155] Only two prospective studies have reported on this relationship, and their findings were similar. Bergkvist et al. observed a relative risk of 4.4 (95% confidence interval, 0.9 to 22.4) among women who used estrogen plus progestin for 6 or more years compared with those who had never used progestin.[165] Women using hormones for shorter duration did not appear at an increased risk, but CIs again were wide and did not exclude either a modest increase or decrease in risk. In findings from the Nurses' Health Study[166] in which, among women using progestins, approximately two-thirds used 10 mg of medroxyprogesterone for 14 or fewer days per month, the relative risk associated with current use of estrogen plus progestin versus no previous use was 1.4 (95% confidence interval, 1.2 to 1.7). In the pooled analysis,[155] data on postmenopausal hormone formulation were available from only 39% of women, and only 12% of these reported using estrogen plus a progestin. The relative risk associated with 5 or more years of recent use, relative to no previous use, was 1.53. The comparable relative risk for estrogen use alone was 1.34. Data from the Nurses' Health Study[167] indicate that the addition of a progestin appears to increase risk beyond that for estrogen use alone. Because widespread use of estrogen plus progestin is so recent, few data are available to evaluate the effect of different formulations, dosages, or schedules of use on risk of breast cancer.

Summary of Postmenopausal Hormone Use and Breast Cancer Risk

Although some aspects of the relationship between postmenopausal hormone use and breast cancer risk remain unresolved, several areas of agreement have emerged. The finding of no increase in risk of users compared with those who never used postmenopausal hormones is consistent and reassuring. Much of that observation, however, reflects the experience among short-term users and hormone use in the past. Among these groups, most studies are in agreement that little if any excess risk is present.

Overall, the findings also indicate an increased risk in two important subgroups of users: users of long duration and current users. In general, users of long duration are more likely to be current users, so in many studies these two groups overlap substantially. From a biological perspective, these are the groups one would most expect to demonstrate a relation with breast cancer risk, because exogenous estrogens appear to act at a very late stage, perhaps stimulating growth of tumors that are already present but undiagnosed. Although limited data exist, the increase in breast cancer risk associated with the use of estrogen plus progestin may be greater than that for use of estrogen alone; this is an important issue that needs further evaluation.

LOW-PENETRANCE GENOTYPES AND GENE-ENVIRONMENT INTERACTIONS

Family history of breast cancer in a first-degree relative is a consistent risk factor; risk increases with earlier age at diagnosis in first-degree relatives and with the number of relatives affected. In the Nurses' Health Study, for instance, the relative risk associated with a maternal diagnosis before age 40 years was 2.1, and the relative risk associated with maternal diagnosis after age 70 years was 1.5. The relative risk was 2.5 for women with both an affected mother and at least one affected sister.[168] Most women with breast cancer do not have a family history of the disease in a first-degree relative; however, only 5% to 10% of breast cancers are estimated to be attributable to the inheritance of rare, highly penetrant, germ-line mutations in genes, although this proportion is higher at younger ages of diagnosis. Mutations in *BRCA1* and *BRCA2* are responsible for most of these inherited breast cancers; mutations in the gene for the tumor protein p53 (causing Li-Fraumeni syndrome) and in *PTEN* (causing Cowden disease) account for a small proportion of inherited breast cancers. Mutations in each of these genes occur in fewer than 1% of the population. These genes and their clinical implications are reviewed in detail in Chapter 16.

Polymorphisms are usually defined as a sequence variant in a gene that occurs in more than 1% of alleles. Polymorphisms in genes that code for enzymes, receptors, or other proteins that act in metabolic pathways of potential relevance to breast cancer may influence the function of these proteins and thus create between-person differences in metabolic activity that may alter risk of breast cancer. Candidates include genes for carcinogen-metabolizing enzymes, steroid hormone–metabolizing enzymes, and receptors such as the estrogen and progesterone receptors. If these polymorphisms cause only modest increases in risk, or confer risk only in conjunction with exposure to carcinogens, they would not cause noticeable familial aggregation. Because these polymorphisms may be very common (the homozygous deletion in the glutathione-*S*-transferase *mu* gene occurs in approximately 50% of whites), their population-attributable risks may be large even if the relative risks are modest.

Carcinogen-Metabolizing Genes

Most exogenous carcinogens are metabolized by enzymes, which may change them to more DNA-damaging forms or detoxify them, often by attaching glutathione or other groups that promote excretion of the modified compounds. Many of the genes that encode these enzymes display phenotypic variation (individuals differ in the activity of the enzymes), and for many of these enzymes, the alterations in DNA sequence that are responsible for the phenotypic variation are known. A growing number of studies have examined whether these different genotypes are associated with breast cancer risk or interact with environmental exposures (e.g., cigarette smoking).

N-Acetyltransferases

Cigarette smoking is a route of exposure to aryl aromatic amine carcinogens that can be activated by the cytochrome *P450 1A2* (*CYP1A2*) and *NAT1* and *NAT2* (*N*-acetyltransferase 1 and 2) genes. The *NAT2* gene has four major alleles in whites. Individuals homozygous for any combination of the three slow acetylator alleles are phenotypically slow at the acetylation step; those who have at least one copy of the rapid acetylator allele are rapid acetylators (approximately 45% of whites).[169] In more than 10 studies, the prevalence of slow acetylators was similar among cases of breast cancer and among controls; thus, no independent main effect of this genotype is seen. In a case control study of 185 postmenopausal cases and 213 controls,[170] among women who were slow acetylators, those in the highest quartile of number of cigarettes smoked were at increased breast cancer risk (odds ratio, 4.4; 95% confidence interval, 1.3 to 14.8), suggesting that smoking was a risk factor for breast cancer among slow acetylators. Subsequent studies that included 466 cases[171] and 498 cases[172] did not confirm this finding; indeed, in the latter study, an increased risk was observed among rapid acetylators who were recent smokers. The latter study also examined a polymorphism in *NAT1* that may code for a rapid acetylation form of this enzyme; no main effect was observed, although among postmenopausal women an increase in risk was observed among recent smokers with the putative rapid allele. *NAT2* is also important in the metabolic activation of heterocyclic amines formed during the high-temperature cooking of animal protein, and heterocyclic amines have been found to be mammary carcinogens in some rodent models. In the two published studies, however, no interaction was seen between meat intake and *NAT2* genotype.[173,174]

CYP1A1

Polycyclic aromatic hydrocarbons are animal mammary carcinogens also found in cigarette smoke. The cytochrome *P450 1A1* (*CYP1A1*) gene product is involved in metabolism of polycyclic aromatic hydrocarbons and is polymorphic, although the exact functional significance of these polymorphisms is unclear. No association was observed with a variant in exon 7 among 96 cases of breast cancer.[175] In data based on 216 cases, a significant increase in risk among postmenopausal women with the exon 7 variant was observed,[176] and the increase in risk was greater among lighter than among heavier smokers. In a study of 466 cases, no main effect of the exon 7 polymorphism was observed, and little evidence was found of an interaction with pack-years of smoking.[177] This study, however, showed a suggestion of an interaction between an *MspI* polymorphism and smoking: Both long duration and early onset of smoking were associated with increased risk among carriers of this polymorphism. No main effect of either of these polymorphisms or two additional polymorphisms was observed among 164 white and 59 African-American cases.[178] Thus, no polymorphisms in *CYP1A1* have been independently associated with breast cancer risk; larger studies are needed to assess potential interactions with cigarette smoking.

Glutathione-*S*-Transferases

The glutathione-*S*-transferases are involved in the detoxification of carcinogens. Several related genes exist; the most studied are the μ, τ, and π classes. The homozygous deletion in *GSTμ* is common, occurring in 50% of whites. No association with breast cancer was seen in studies of 212 cases,[176] 245 cases,[179] 232 cases,[178] and 361 cases.[180] In a study of 110 cases,[181] an increased risk for the *GSTμ* null genotype was observed (odds ratio, 2.1; 95% confidence interval, 1.2 to 3.6), along with nonsignificant elevations in risk for the homozygous deletion in *GSTτ* and for an isoleucine-valine substitution polymorphism in *GSTπ*. No interactions with cigarette smoking were seen for these genotypes in studies that reported data on this issue.

Hormone-Metabolizing Genes

Because steroid hormones, particularly estrogens and progesterone, are so strongly implicated in breast carcinogenesis, genes involved in the steroidogenic pathway are natural candidates in the search for polymorphic variants that influence breast cancer risk.[182] This pathway includes many enzymes, and many of them are large and have complex tissue-specific patterns of gene expression and alternate coding and splicing forms; much work needs to be done to define potential polymorphic variants with definite functional significance.

CYP17

The *CYP17* gene encodes the rate-limiting step in androgen production in the ovary and adrenal glands. A polymorphism in the 5' untranslated region designated the *A2* allele was initially associated with a nonsignificant elevation in breast cancer risk and a significant increase in risk of advanced breast cancer (odds ratio, 2.5; 95% confidence interval, 1.1 to 5.9).[183] Subsequent larger studies have not observed any increase in risk overall, or among cases of more advanced breast cancer.[184–186]

Catechol-*O*-Methyltransferase

The catechol-*O*-methyltransferase (COMT) enzyme inactivates catechol estrogens and is polymorphic, with approximately 25% of whites being homozygous for the low activity allele of the enzyme (LL). In a study including 112 cases, the LL genotype was associated with increased breast cancer risk among postmenopausal women (odds ratio, 2.2; 95% confidence interval, 0.9 to 5.1).[187] In another study, this risk was inversely associated with risk among postmenopausal women (odds ratio, 0.3; 95% confidence interval, 0.1 to 0.7) but was positively associated with risk among premenopausal women (odds ratio, 2.1; 95% confidence interval, 1.4 to 4.3).[188]

CYP19

The aromatase coded by the *CYP19* gene is responsible for the conversion of C19 steroids to estrogens and plays a major role in the production of estrogens in postmenopausal women. A polymorphic tetranucleotide (TTTA) repeat in intron 5 was studied among 182 sporadic and 185 familial breast cancer cases in Scandinavia.[189] A relatively rare allele containing the longest repeat (12 TTTA repeats) was found significantly more frequently in women with breast cancer than in controls (odds ratio, 2.4; 95% confidence interval, 1.0 to 5.8).

HRAS1

A region linked to the *HRAS1* protooncogene, consisting of 30 to 100 copies of a 28 base-pair repeat, has been studied with respect to risk of a wide variety of cancers. Several alleles (repeat lengths) are common, and a large number of rare alleles of varying length are found. Among women with at least one rare allele, risk of breast and a number of other cancers was approximately doubled.[190] In a case control study with 160 cases, a similar elevation in risk was seen, and a stronger association was observed among African-Americans than among white women.[191] The functional significance of these rare alleles is uncertain.

Ataxia-Telangiectasia Gene

Analyses of pedigrees from families in which autosomal recessive transmission of ataxia-telangiectasia had been demonstrated suggested that women who were heterozygous for the ataxia-telangiectasia gene (*ATM*) were at approximately fivefold increased risk of breast cancer.[192] The gene has been cloned, but it is very large and detection of mutations is difficult. In an analysis that detected mutations causing protein truncation, these mutations were detected in 2 of 401 women with early-onset breast cancer and 2 of 202 controls[193]; these results suggest that heterozygosity for the *ATM* gene is unlikely to be an important cause of breast cancer at young age.

Summary of Low-Penetrance Genotypes and Breast Cancer Risk

No low-penetrance genes may be confidently associated with breast cancer risk. This is perhaps not surprising, as only a limited number of candidate genes have been examined, and for most of these only one or two polymorphisms have been tested. Other relevant candidate genes remain to be studied, and undoubtedly many candidates have yet to be discovered and cloned. The difficulty of assessing the functional significance of polymorphisms remains a barrier to selection of the most promising polymorphisms to examine. To assess gene-environment interactions, large studies with high-quality data on the environmental exposures are required; few such studies exist.

DIETARY FACTORS

Nutritional factors have been prominent among the environmental determinants of breast cancer hypothesized to account for the large variation in breast cancer incidence around the world and the large increases in rates among the offspring of migrants from countries with low incidence to countries with high incidence. The dominant hypothesis has been that high fat intake increases risk. In this section, evidence for this relationship is reviewed, and alternative hypotheses are suggested.

Dietary Fat

Animal Studies

High-fat diets have long been known to increase the occurrence of mammary tumors in rodents. The interpretation of these and other animal data is controversial, however. Fat is the most energy-dense macronutrient (9 kcal/g compared with 4 kcal/g for protein and carbohydrate); thus, high-fat diets tend to be higher in energy intake unless care is taken to keep energy intake constant. Many animal experiments have not done this, so fat consumption is confounded by energy intake. In a meta-analysis of diet and mammary cancer experiments in mice, Albanes[194] observed a weak inverse association with fat composition (adjusted for energy), whereas total energy intake was positively associated with mammary tumor incidence. Freedman et al.[195]

conducted a similar meta-analysis of experiments in rats and mice and reported that higher fat intake and higher caloric intake independently increase mammary tumor incidence. In studies specifically designed to determine the independent effects of fat and energy intake, the effect of fat was either weak[196] or nonexistent[197] in relation to that of energy intake. Furthermore, the relevance to human experience of rodent models, in which animals are given high doses of specific carcinogens to which humans are rarely exposed, is questionable. Notably, in a very large study of rats and mice fed substantially different amounts of corn oil without administration of a carcinogen, no effect of fat intake was found on spontaneous mammary cancer incidence.[198] In a case control study in dogs, fat intake, which ranged from 10% to 70% of energy, was not associated with risk of breast cancer.[199] The clearest message from the animal data is the importance of total energy intake and the need to consider energy balance in epidemiologic studies.

International Correlation (Ecologic) Studies

The dietary fat hypothesis is based largely on the observation that national per capita fat consumption is highly correlated with breast cancer mortality rates.[200] A serious problem with ecologic comparisons of diet and breast cancer is the potential for confounding by known and suspected breast cancer risk factors. National fat consumption per capita is highly correlated with level of economic development; thus, any factor that characterizes affluent Western countries would also be correlated with national rates of breast cancer. Prentice et al.[201] have found that the ecologic relation between fat disappearance and breast cancer incidences was still statistically significant after adjustment for gross national product per capita and average age at menarche. Other breast cancer risk factors, however, such as low parity, late age at first birth, greater body fat, and lower levels of physical activity, are more prevalent in Western countries and would be expected to confound the association with dietary fat. Thus, good reason exists to question whether the international correlation between fat intake and breast cancer represents a causal relationship.

Secular Trends

Estimates of per capita fat consumption based on "food-disappearance" data (the food available rather than the amount actually eaten) and breast cancer incidences increased substantially in the United States during the twentieth century. Surveys based on measures of individual intake, rather than food disappearance, however, indicate that consumption of fat as a percentage of energy has actually declined in the last several decades, a time during which breast cancer incidence has increased. Higher dietary fat consumption has been implicated in the increase in breast cancer incidence in Japan since 1950. However, this increase could also be due to the increasing prevalence of reproductive and other risk factors that characterize Western populations.

The famine that occurred in Norway during World War II provided a natural experiment on the effects of nutritional deprivation on breast cancer risk.[202] Women who were adolescents during the famine have subsequently experienced a reduction in breast cancer risk (approximately 13% lower) at all ages. These data on time trends indicate the sensitivity of breast cancer rates to nutritional and lifestyle factors but do not specifically support a role of dietary fat.

Data from special populations with distinct dietary patterns are valuable, because adherence to a particular diet over many years may represent a more stable long-term exposure than that of most free-living adults, whose diet may change substantially over time. Because these populations often have unusual distributions of nondietary potential risk factors, such as alcohol consumption, smoking, and reproductive behavior, care must be taken in attributing differences in cancer rates to diet alone. Seventh-Day Adventists, who consume relatively small amounts of meat and other animal products, have substantially lower rates of colon cancer but only slightly lower breast cancer rates than other U.S. white women of similar socioeconomic status.[203] Breast cancer rates among British nuns who ate no or very little meat were similar to rates among single women from the general population,[204] findings also suggesting that no substantial association exists between animal fat and risk of breast cancer.

Case Control Studies

In a typical case control study of diet and breast cancer, the diet before diagnosis reported by women with breast cancer (cases) is compared with the diet reported by women who have not been diagnosed with breast cancer (controls). The largest such study is that of Graham et al.,[205] who used a food frequency questionnaire to compare the fat intake of 2,024 women with breast cancer to that of 1,463 female controls seen at the hospital with benign conditions. Animal fat and total fat intake were almost identical in the two groups. In a meta-analysis, Howe et al.[206] summarized the results from 12 smaller case control studies comprising a total of 4,312 cases and 5,978 controls. The overall pooled relative risk for a 100-g increase in daily total fat intake was 1.35; the risk was somewhat stronger for postmenopausal women (relative risk, 1.48). Because average total fat consumption is approximately 70 g per day for U.S. women, a reduction in fat intake as large as 100 g would be impossible for almost all women. The results of this pooled analysis suggest that, even if the reported positive association were correct, the relative risk for readily achievable changes in total fat intake would be relatively small; for example, the reduction in risk for a 20 g per day decrease among postmenopausal women (corre-

TABLE 3. *Results from large prospective studies of total and saturated fat intake and risk of breast cancer*

Study	Total no. in cohort	Years of follow-up	No. of cases	Relative risk (95% confidence interval) (high vs low category)	
				Total fat	Saturated fat
Nurses' Health Study[235]	89,494	8	1,439	0.86 (0.67–1.08)	0.86 (0.73–1.02)
Canadian study[358]	56,837	5	519	1.30 (0.90–1.88)	1.08 (0.73–1.59)
New York State cohort[244]	17,401	7	344	1.00 (0.59–1.70)	1.12 (0.78–1.61)[a]
Iowa women's study[359]	32,080	4	408	1.13 (0.84–1.51)	1.10 (0.83–1.46)
Dutch health study[360]	62,573	3	471	1.08 (0.73–1.59)	1.39 (0.94–2.06)
Adventists health study[361]	20,341	6	193		1.21 (0.81–1.81)
Swedish mammography screening cohort[362]	61,471	6	674	1.00 (0.76–1.32)	1.09 (0.83–1.42)

[a]Animal fat.

sponding to a decrease from 40% to 29% of calories for a typical middle-aged woman), would be only approximately 0.9. Furthermore, in case control studies, relative risks of this magnitude may easily be due to selection bias (the controls are drawn from a population with a different distribution of fat intake than the distribution in the population that gave rise to the cases) or recall bias (the cases, knowing their diagnosis, differentially misreport their prediagnosis diet).[207]

Cohort Studies

In a cohort (prospective) study, the diets of a large group of women are measured, and the subsequent rates of breast cancer among those with different levels of dietary factors are compared. Selection bias should not be a problem, because the population that gave rise to the cases is known (the starting members of the cohort); recall bias should not occur, because dietary information is collected before knowledge of disease. The results for postmenopausal breast cancer (for which fat intake has been hypothesized to be strongest, because the international differences are largest for this group) from prospective studies with at least 200 incident cases of breast cancer are shown in Table 3. The number of breast cancer cases in these studies is similar to the number in the pooled analysis of case control studies referred to above, and the size of the comparison series (i.e., noncases) is much larger. In not a single study was a significant association with total fat intake observed (when the highest and lowest categories of total fat intake were compared). A collaborative pooled analysis of 4,980 cases of breast cancer (among 337,819 women) has been conducted on all the prospective studies included in Table 3.[208] In addition to providing great statistical precision, the pooled analysis allowed the application of standard analytic approaches to all studies, an examination of a wider range of fat intake, and a detailed evaluation of interactions with other breast cancer risk factors. Overall, no association was observed between intake of total, saturated, monounsaturated, or polyunsaturated fat and risk of breast cancer. As noted in Fig. 9, no reduction in risk was seen even for fat intakes as low as 20% of energy. When the relatively few women with fat intake lower than 15% of energy were examined, their risk of breast cancer was actually increased twofold; this could not be accounted for by other dietary or nondietary factors.

Substudies were available for each cohort in the pooled analysis in which the measurement errors of the dietary questionnaires were quantified, and these were used to adjust the overall relative risks and confidence intervals to take into

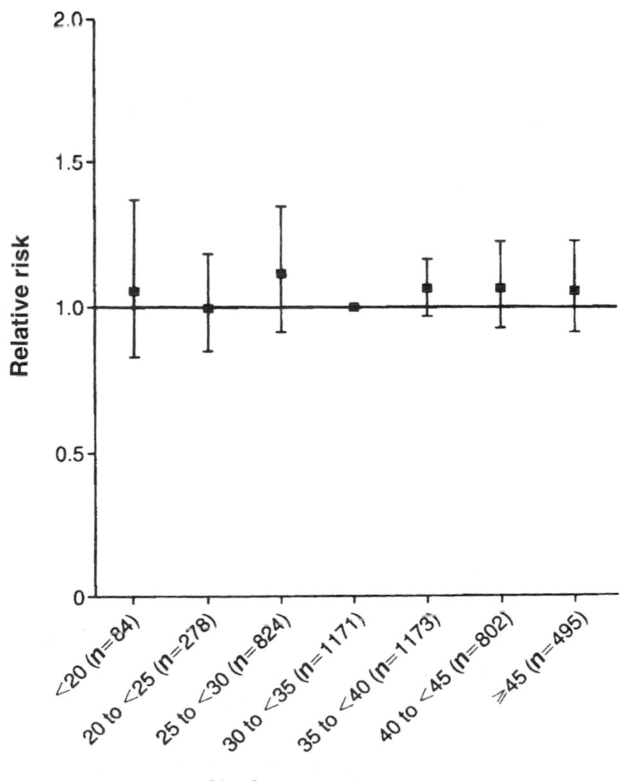

FIG. 9. Pooled relative breast cancer risk and 95% confidence intervals associated with percentage of energy derived from fat intake. (Reprinted from ref. 208 with permission from the *New England Journal of Medicine.*)

account errors in measuring diet. Without correction, the relative risk for an increment of 25 g per day in fat intake was 1.02 (95% confidence interval, 0.94 to 1.11). After accounting for measurement error, the relative risk was 1.07 (95% confidence interval, 0.86 to 1.34). The upper bound of the adjusted 95% confidence interval excludes the relative risk of 1.4 to 1.5 predicted by the international correlations. In calculations based on a series of theoretical assumptions, Prentice has claimed that the pooled analysis of breast cancer failed to find a positive association because the measurement error correction did not account for underreporting of fat intake by more obese women.[209] Actual studies do not support this assumption, however, and the other predictions based on this theoretical model are not supported by the data.[210] Thus, these theoretical concerns appear groundless. In the Nurses' Health Study, additional analyses have been conducted with 8 years (1,439 cases of breast cancer) and 14 years (2,956 cases) of follow-up.[211] In the 14-year analysis, up to four assessments of fat intake were available, which substantially improved the measurement of long-term dietary intake. The relative risk for a 5% increase in percentage of energy from total fat was 0.97 (95% confidence interval, 0.94 to 1.00); the overall weak inverse trend was actually statistically significant. No suggestion of any reduction in risk was seen for fat intakes even lower than 20% of energy.[211] Thus, the prospective studies provide strong evidence that no major relation exists between total dietary fat intake over a wide range during midlife and breast cancer incidence. Although it remains possible that dietary fat intake during childhood or early adult life may affect breast cancer risk decades later, no evidence exists for this.

Intervention Studies

Some have suggested that the relationship between dietary fat and breast cancer can be established only by randomized trials of fat reduction. The Women's Health Initiative sponsored by the U.S. National Institutes of Health has been developed with the goal of enrolling and randomizing several tens of thousands of women, one-half of whom will be instructed on how to reduce their total fat intake to 20% of calories from fat. However, the difficulty of maintaining compliance with a diet very different from prevailing food consumption habits, as well as the gradual secular decline in total fat consumption already under way, which may reduce the size of the comparison in fat intake between intervention groups and controls, may compromise the ability of any trial to address the effect of reducing percentage of energy from fat. Furthermore, as pointed out by the Women's Health Initiative investigators, "women in the dietary intervention group will be counseled to adopt a dietary pattern that is high in fruits, vegetables, and grain products and low in total fat and saturated fat."[212] Thus, the trial would be unable to distinguish between a decrease in risk due to increased intake of fruits, vegetables, and grains, and a decrease due to lower fat intake. Also, this trial will not answer whether dietary fat reduction at an early age may reduce breast cancer risk decades later.

Type of Fat

In addition to overall fat intake, intake of specific types of fat could differentially affect risk of breast cancer. In most animal studies, diets high in polyunsaturated fat (linoleic acid), but typically at levels beyond human exposure, have clearly increased the occurrence of mammary tumors. As noted, a positive association has not been found in prospective epidemiologic studies.

Some animal studies have suggested that monounsaturated fat, in the form of olive oil, may be protective relative to other sources of energy.[213] In a Spanish study specifically undertaken because of the high consumption of olive oil and low breast cancer rates in this population, no association was observed between breast cancer rates and total fat intake.[214] Higher intake of olive oil was associated with reduced risk of breast cancer, however. Similar inverse associations with consumption of olive oil or monounsaturated fat were seen in case control studies in Greece, Italy, and elsewhere in Spain[215]; in the Italian study, intake of polyunsaturated oils was also related to lower risk.

High intake of omega-3 fatty acids from marine oils has inhibited the occurrence of mammary tumors in animals. Case control and cohort studies, however, have in general found little relation between intake of omega-3 fatty acids or fish (the major source of extra-long-chain omega-3 fatty acids) and risk of breast cancer.[215]

Height and Weight

As noted under Animal Studies, energy restriction powerfully reduces mammary tumor incidence in rodents.[194,195] This relationship is difficult to evaluate directly in humans, because estimates by adults of their energy intake, especially during childhood, are unlikely to be sufficiently precise, and any analysis would also need to account for physical activity with high accuracy. However, because children who experience energy deprivation during growth do not attain their full potential height, attained height may be used as a proxy for childhood energy intake. Nevertheless, this is not a specific indicator, because protein restriction and genetic factors also affect stature. In Japan, for instance, a substantial increase in average height occurred during the twentieth century, presumably due to improved nutrition. Among countries, height is positively correlated with breast cancer rates,[216] supporting the hypothesis that childhood and adolescent energy intake may influence breast cancer rates decades later.

Most of the case control and cohort studies of attained height and risk of breast cancer suggest a modest positive association[124] (Fig. 10). In a follow-up of 7,259 postmenopausal women in the Netherlands, a more than twofold increase in risk was observed for a 15-cm difference in height. In a follow-up of the National Health and Nutrition Examination Survey I (NHANES I) population, in which women at risk for malnutrition had been over-

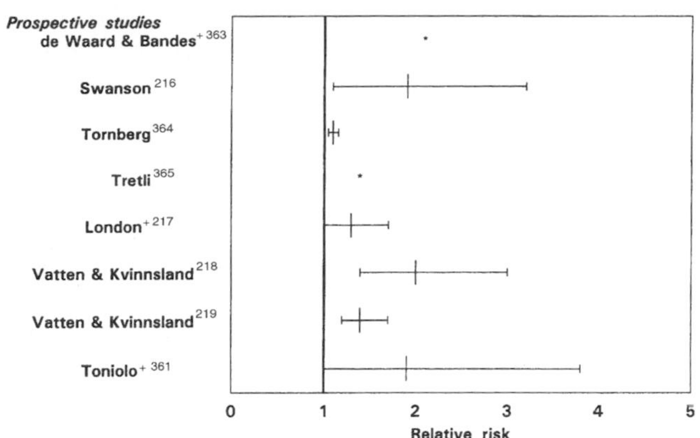

FIG. 10. Results of prospective studies of the association between height and breast cancer risk. Vertical bars and asterisks represent the relative risks for the highest category of height versus the lowest; error bars represent the 95% confidence intervals. +, results for postmenopausal women only.

sampled, a similar increase in risk was observed.[217] In the NHANES I study, height was positively associated with later age at menarche (protective against breast cancer) and late age at first birth, low parity, higher socioeconomic status, and alcohol use (risk factors for breast cancer); these findings suggest that height may be confounded by other cancer risk factors.[217] Controlling for these variables in multivariate analyses, however, had little influence on the association between height and breast cancer. Among women in the Nurses' Health Study, a significant positive association was seen between height and breast cancer among postmenopausal women but not among premenopausal women.[218] Several large cohort studies have been conducted in Scandinavia, and in all of them significant associations have been observed, ranging from 1.1 (for a 5-cm increment) to 2.0 (for an increment larger than 8 cm). In the studies of Vatten and Kvinnsland,[219,220] the positive trend between height and risk of breast cancer was most nearly linear in the birth cohort of women (1929 to 1932) who lived through their peripubertal period during World War II, a time in which food was scarce and average attained height was reduced. Collectively, these data provide convincing evidence that attained height is associated with a modest increase of breast cancer.

Age at menarche, an established risk factor for breast cancer, provides a second indirect indicator of energy balance during childhood. Nutritional factors—in particular, energy balance—appear to be the major determinants of age at menarche. In prospective studies among young girls, the major predictors of age at menarche were weight, height, and body fatness.[221–223] A marginally significant inverse association between dietary fat and age at menarche was seen in one study,[224] but no relation was observed in the others. The potential for energy balance to influence breast cancer risk through age at menarche is greater than might be appreciated by examining the distribution of this variable in modern Western countries. Although the average age at menarche in these countries is now 12 to 13 years, in rural China the typical age has been 17 to 18 years,[74] similar to that of Western countries 200 years ago. An effect of growth rate on breast cancer risk may begin even before birth, as an inverse relation between birth weight and breast cancer risk has been observed in one study of mainly premenopausal women.[123]

The mechanisms by which age at menarche and attained height are related to risk of breast cancer are probably multiple. Early onset of menstrual cycles exposes the breast to ovarian hormones at a younger age and for a longer duration over a lifetime. Also, in several studies, an early menarche has been associated with higher estrogen levels at later ages.[224] Height has been suggested to be a surrogate for mammary gland mass,[225] which may be related to higher risk. IGF-I could be a key intermediary, because this hormone is directly involved in regulation of growth during childhood, and plasma levels in premenopausal women have been associated with risk of breast cancer.[129] The temporal nature of this relationship remains unclear, because an effect of IGF-I on breast cancer risk could be mediated entirely during the years of growth and development, with the association between adult levels and breast cancer risk only reflecting the correlation of blood levels over time. Alternatively, the blood IGF-I levels may have a temporally more proximate relation to risk, so that reductions in levels during adulthood would reduce risk of breast cancer. The determinants of blood IGF-I levels in humans are not known and may be both genetic and nutritional. In animals, energy restriction reduces IGF-I levels,[226] and infusion of IGF-I appears to negate the effects of energy restriction on bowel tumors in mice.[226]

Weight and Weight Change during Adulthood

Attained weight and weight change in adults provide sensitive measures of the balance between long-term energy intake and expenditure. Although the relationship between these variables and breast cancer risk has been complex and confusing, recent findings provide a coherent picture and indicate a major contribution of weight gain to risk of postmenopausal breast cancer risk. Two reproducible findings have been particularly enigmatic: (a) In affluent Western populations with high rates of breast cancer, measures of body fatness have been *inversely* related to risk of premenopausal breast cancer, and (b) body fatness has been only weakly related to postmenopausal breast cancer risk despite strong associations between body fat and endogenous estrogen levels.

The inverse relationship between body weight [typically considered as body mass index (BMI), calculated as weight in kilograms divided by the square of height in meters, to account for variation in height] and incidence of premenopausal breast cancer has been consistently seen in prospective studies[77] and in a meta-analysis of case control and cohort studies.[227] Little relationship of BMI to breast cancer mortality has been observed in premenopausal women, probably because delayed detection and diagnosis in heavier women counterbalances the lower incidence among heavier women. Heavier premenopausal women, even at the upper limits of what are considered to be healthy weights, have more irregular menstrual cycles and increased rates of anovulatory infertility,[228] findings suggesting that their lower risk may be due to fewer ovulatory cycles and less exposure to ovarian hormones. Increased rates of menstrual irregularity and anovulatory infertility are also seen among very lean women, but such women are uncommon in Western populations. In case control studies, a consistent relationship between menstrual cycle regularity and breast cancer risk has not emerged, which could cast doubt on this explanation, but this may be due to the indirect relationship between menstrual regularity and ovulation and to difficulties in remote recall. In a prospective study among younger women, both shorter and longer or irregular cycles, compared with regular cycles of approximately 28 days, were associated with reduced risk of breast cancer[41]; this finding lends support to irregular anovulation as the explanation for the lower risk in heavier women.

In case control and prospective studies conducted in affluent Western countries, the association between BMI and risk of breast cancer among postmenopausal women has been only weakly positive or nonexistent.[124,206] The lack of a stronger association has been surprising, because obese postmenopausal women have plasma levels of endogenous estrogens nearly twice those of lean women, due to conversion of androstenedione to estrogens in adipose tissue and also to lower levels of sex hormone–binding globulin.[229] The lack of a stronger positive association now appears to be due to two factors. First, as with the protective effect of early pregnancy, the reduction in breast cancer risk associated with being overweight in early adult life appears to persist throughout later life.[77,230] Thus, an elevated BMI in a postmenopausal woman represents two opposing risks: a protective effect due to the correlation between early weight and postmenopausal weight, and an adverse effect due to elevated estrogen levels after menopause. For this reason, weight *gain* from early adult life to after menopause should be more strongly related to postmenopausal breast cancer risk than attained weight. Indeed, a positive association between weight gain and increased risk of postmenopausal breast cancer has been consistently supported by both case control[231] and prospective studies.[77,230,232] A second reason for the failure to appreciate a greater adverse effect of excessive weight or weight gain on risk of postmenopausal breast cancer is that the use of postmenopausal hormones obscures the variation in endogenous estrogens due to adiposity and elevates breast cancer risk regardless of body weight.[77] To appreciate fully the impact of weight or weight gain, an analysis should be limited to women who never used postmenopausal hormones. Thus, among women who never used postmenopausal hormones in the Nurses' Health Study, those who gained 25 kg or more after age 18 had double the risk of breast cancer compared with women who maintained their weight within 2 kg[77] (Fig. 11). In this population, the combination of using postmenopausal hormones or gaining weight after age 18 years accounted for one-third of postmenopausal breast cancer cases.

The relationship between body weight and breast cancer risk in lower-risk, mainly non-Western, countries has been

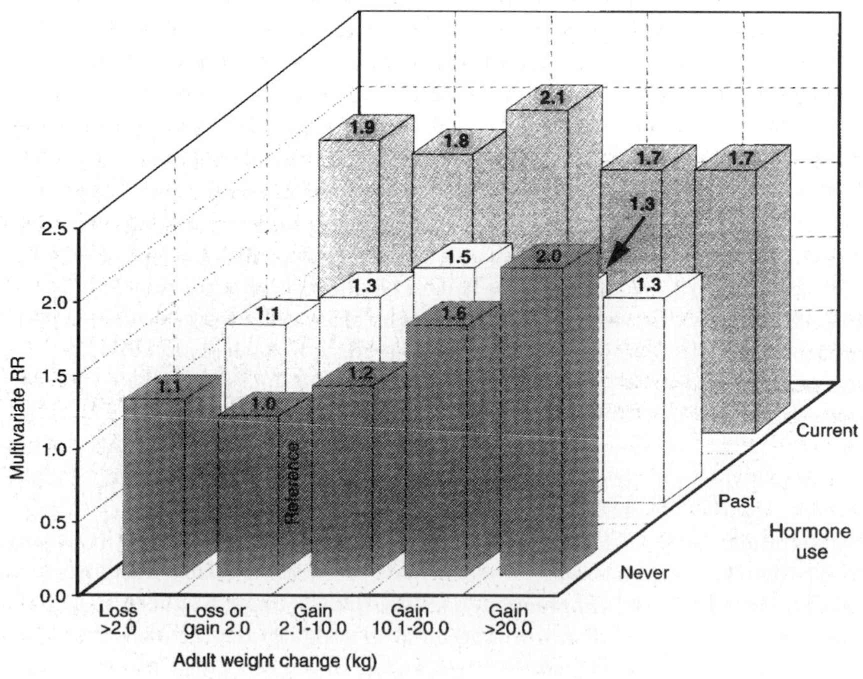

FIG. 11. Relative risk (RR) of breast cancer by adult weight change and hormone use among postmenopausal women. Relative risk was adjusted for age, height, history of benign breast disease, family history of breast cancer, age at menarche, parity, age at first birth, age at menopause, and body mass index at age 18 years. (Reprinted from ref. 77 with permission of the *Journal of the American Medical Association.*)

observed to be somewhat different than that in higher-risk countries.[233] In general, the inverse relationship between weight and premenopausal breast cancer risk has not been observed, and the association between weight and postmenopausal risk has been stronger. This difference is likely to be due to the lower prevalence of overweight among premenopausal women in these low-risk countries; few women are likely to be sufficiently overweight to cause anovulation and a reduction in premenopausal breast cancer risk. As a result, BMI after menopause would reflect only the adverse effects of high levels of endogenous estrogens, unopposed by a residual protective effect due to correlation with overweight in early adult life.

In summary, as in animal studies, energy balance appears to play an important but complex role in the causation of breast cancer in humans. During childhood, rapid growth rates accelerate the occurrence of menarche, an established risk factor, and result in greater attained stature, which has been consistently associated with increased risk. During early adult life, overweight is associated with a lower incidence of breast cancer before menopause, but no reduction in breast cancer mortality. Weight gain after age 18 years, however, is associated with a graded and substantial increase in postmenopausal breast cancer that is seen most clearly in the absence of hormone replacement therapy.

Dietary Fiber

Diets high in fiber have been hypothesized to protect against breast cancer, perhaps due to inhibition of the intestinal reabsorption of estrogens excreted via the biliary system. A high-fiber diet has been found to be associated with reduced incidence of mammary cancer in animals.[213] Dietary fiber includes crude fiber that is excreted unchanged and various soluble fiber fractions that may have different biological effects. Epidemiologic assessment of fiber intake has been difficult due to the scarcity of data on the fiber content of individual foods as well as controversy about the most appropriate methods of biochemical analysis to determine fiber content. In a meta-analysis of 10 case control studies in which dietary fiber intake was estimated, a statistically significant relative risk of 0.85 for a 20 g per day increase in dietary fiber was observed.[206] Prospective studies have been less supportive, however. In a Canadian prospective study including 519 cases,[234] a marginally significant inverse association between dietary fiber and breast cancer risk was seen; in another prospective study with a cohort of 344 cases, no suggestion of a protective effect was found.[235] In the Nurses' Health Study, the association between total dietary fiber intake and subsequent breast cancer incidence (1,439 cases) was very close to null,[236] which suggests that any protective effect of dietary fiber is unlikely to be large. The possibility remains, however, that certain subfractions of fiber intake may be relevant to breast cancer causation.

Micronutrients

Vitamin A

Vitamin A consists of preformed vitamin A (retinol, retinyl esters, and related compounds) from animal sources and certain carotenoids found primarily in fruits and vegetables that are partially converted to retinol in the intestinal epithelium (carotenoid vitamin A). Many carotenoids are potent antioxidants and thus may provide a cellular defense against reactive oxygen species that damage DNA. Vitamin A is also a regulator of cell differentiation and may prevent the emergence of cells with a malignant phenotype. Retinol inhibits the growth of human breast carcinoma cells *in vitro*,[237] and retinyl acetate reduces breast cancer incidence in some rodent models.[238]

Human studies of vitamin A intake and breast cancer risk have been mostly case control studies; thus, their interpretation is limited by uncertainty about the extent to which selection and recall bias may have altered the observed estimates of effect. In the earliest and the largest case control study of total vitamin A intake (retinol plus carotenoid vitamin A),[205] a relative risk of 0.8 was seen between women with the highest quartile of vitamin A consumption and the lowest, and a significant inverse trend in risk was noted with increased vitamin A consumption. In a meta-analysis of nine other case control studies with data on vitamin A intake,[206] a significant protective effect of total vitamin A intake on breast cancer was reported. When preformed vitamin A and carotenoids were examined separately, however, the data from these case control studies are more strongly supportive of a protective association for carotenoid vitamin A than for preformed vitamin A. In 1996, specific carotenoids were examined in a case control study that used the USDA–National Cancer Institute carotenoid database.[239] Inverse associations were observed between dietary intake of β-carotene and lutein-zeaxanthin, and risk of breast cancer in premenopausal women.

The limited available prospective data suggest a possible modest inverse association between vitamin A intake and breast cancer.[124] In two cohorts with 123 and 344 cases of breast cancer, a weak inverse association or no association was observed. In a cohort of Canadian women (519 cases),[234] a marginally significant protective association between total vitamin A intake and breast cancer was seen, with both preformed vitamin A and β-carotene contributing to the inverse association. In the 8-year analysis of the Nurses' Health Study, which included 1,439 cases, a modest (relative risk, 0.8) but significant protective association for total vitamin A was apparent. At 14 years of follow-up (2,697 cases), the inverse association with total vitamin A intake was limited to premenopausal women.[240] This inverse association was accounted for primarily by carotenoid sources of vitamin A; when specific carotenoids were examined, intake of β-carotene and lutein-zeaxanthin were found to be associated with reduced risk, but intake of lycopene was not. The inverse associations with specific carotenoids were strongest among women with a family history of breast cancer.

An alternative to the dietary assessment of vitamin A intake is the measurement of vitamin A compounds in blood. Most studies have assessed blood retinol, however, which is uninformative about vitamin A intake in well-nourished populations, because the liver maintains relatively constant blood retinol concentrations. Blood levels of β-carotene do reflect β-carotene intake, however. Unfortunately, little consistency is seen among the studies examining this compound,[124,241] probably related in part to their small size.

Thus, available data are suggestive, but not conclusive, of a modest protective association between vitamin A intake and breast cancer. The evidence is stronger for benefits of carotenoid sources of vitamin A. Also, evidence of benefit is stronger for premenopausal women. Other anticarcinogens in vegetables and fruits, including carotenoids such as lutein, may be responsible for the apparent benefits. The effect of vitamin A supplements, either in the form of preformed vitamin A or carotenoids, should be evaluated in randomized trials. A randomized trial of fenretinide, a powerful synthetic retinoid, in the prevention of contralateral breast cancer in women already diagnosed with a first breast cancer is under way in Italy. The Women's Health Study of 40,000 female health professionals is a randomized trial designed to test whether β-carotene or vitamin E supplements reduces breast cancer risk. The β-carotene arm was terminated in 1996, however, after reports from trials in Finland and the United States that β-carotene supplements appeared to increase the risk of lung cancer among smoking men. Thus, data from randomized trials on specific carotenoids and breast cancer risk, particularly among premenopausal women, may never be available.

Vitamin E

Vitamin E is also an antioxidant and has inhibited mammary tumors in rodents in some, but not all, experiments.[242] Relatively few studies are available to assess the association between dietary vitamin E intake and breast cancer, and none of the published prospective studies has reported a significant inverse association.[234,240,243] In the largest of these,[240] no evidence of a protective effect was seen with use of vitamin E supplements, even at high doses for long duration.

Vitamin C

Vitamin C (ascorbic acid) is also an antioxidant and can block the formation of carcinogenic nitrosamines. Few animal studies have assessed the effect of vitamin C on mammary cancer; in a study in rats, ascorbic acid had no effect on the growth of either transplanted or dimethylbenzanthracene-induced mammary tumors.[244]

In the largest case control study reported,[205] no effect for vitamin C was observed; however, in a subsequent study by the same group,[245] a significant protective effect was present (relative risk of 0.6 for highest versus lowest quartile). In a meta-analysis of nine other case control studies with data on vitamin C,[206] a significant inverse association (relative risk of 0.7 for each 300 mg per day increase in vitamin C) was observed. In prospective studies, however, no significant association between intake of vitamin C and breast cancer was observed.[234,235,240,243,246] In the 14-year follow-up of the Nurses' Health Study, no evidence of any reduction in risk was seen with long-term use of vitamin C supplements.[240] Thus, the existing data on intake of vitamin C and breast cancer risk are somewhat inconsistent. However, the available prospective data do not support benefits of high vitamin C intake for reducing breast cancer risk.

Selenium

Selenium is an important component of the antioxidant enzyme glutathione peroxidase, inhibits cell proliferation, and, in animal studies, has been shown to protect against a variety of cancers, although usually at high levels of intake.[247] In the United States, ecological studies have shown strong inverse associations between county-specific and national measures of selenium exposure and breast cancer rates.[248] Selenium intake cannot be measured accurately by means of dietary assessment in geographically dispersed populations, because the selenium content of individual foods varies greatly depending on the geographic area in which the foods were grown. Selenium levels in tissues such as blood and toenails do reflect selenium intake,[249] however, and thus provide an informative measure of diet.

Several studies using these biomarkers of selenium intake have been performed. In one relatively small study, a nonsignificant positive association was observed between erythrocyte selenium level and breast cancer.[250] In the largest prospective study, Hunter et al.[251] observed no association between selenium levels in toenail and risk of breast cancer during 4 years of follow-up. Of the other prospective studies, only the study of Knekt et al.[252] from Finland showed any evidence of an increased risk among women in the lowest category of selenium level. As women in Finland at that time had extremely low selenium intakes, this observation is consistent with the possibility that a threshold exists below which low selenium intake does increase breast cancer risk. In a small randomized trial, breast cancer was the only malignancy that occurred more frequently among those receiving selenium supplements.[253] Taken together, these data suggest that increases in selenium intake are unlikely to reduce risk of breast cancer for most women in countries with existing moderate or high levels of selenium intake.

Other Dietary Constituents

Alcohol

Although the association between alcohol consumption and breast cancer risk has been controversial, substantial evi-

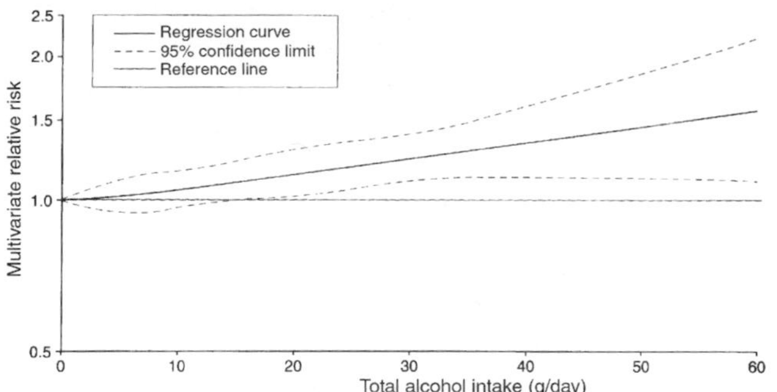

FIG. 12. Nonparametric regression for the relationship between total alcohol intake and breast cancer. One drink of beer, wine, or liquor equals 12–15 g alcohol. (Reprinted from ref. 254 with permission from the *Journal of the American Medical Association.*)

dence has accumulated to support the existence of a positive association. In a meta-analysis of 38 case control and cohort studies, Longnecker[254] estimated relative risks of 1.1 (95% confidence interval, 1.1 to 1.2) for 1 drink per day, 1.2 (1.1 to 1.3) for 2 drinks per day, and 1.4 (1.2 to 1.6) for 3 drinks per day. In the five largest prospective studies, all controlled for major breast cancer risk factors, relative risks for the highest category of alcohol consumption compared with zero consumption were 3.3 (95% confidence interval, 1.2 to 9.3) based on 303 cases, 1.6 (1.0 to 2.6) based on 2,933 cases, 1.5 (1.0 to 2.0) based on 493 cases, 1.2 (0.8 to 1.9) based on 519 cases, and 1.7 (p for trend = .05) based on 422 cases[124]

In a pooled analysis of the six cohort studies examining data on alcohol and dietary factors that included 200 or more cases,[255] the risk of breast cancer increased monotonically with increasing intake of alcohol (Fig. 12), with no statistical evidence of heterogeneity among studies. The multivariate relative risk for a 10 g per day increase in alcohol was 1.09 (95% confidence interval, 1.04 to 1.13). In this and other analyses, adjustment for known breast cancer risk factors and dietary variables hypothesized to be related to breast cancer had little impact on the association with alcohol. In the collective literature, beer, wine, and liquor all contribute to the positive association,[241,255] which strongly suggests that alcohol *per se* is responsible for the increased risk.

Whether reducing alcohol consumption in middle life decreases risk of breast cancer is an important practical issue. In a 1987 report,[256] women who drank before age 30 years and later stopped experienced a similar elevation in risk to those who continued to drink. In a large study designed to address this issue,[257] however, recent consumption of three or more drinks per day was associated with a relative risk of 2.2, whereas the relative risk was 0.9 for consumption of three or more drinks per day from ages 16 to 29 years. This suggests that recent adult drinking may be more important than drinking patterns earlier in life and that reductions in consumption in midlife should reduce risks of breast cancer.

In intervention studies, consumption of approximately two alcoholic drinks per day increased total and bioavailable estrogen levels in premenopausal women,[258] and single doses of alcohol acutely increased plasma estradiol levels in postmenopausal women.[259] These findings suggest a mechanism by which alcohol may increase breast cancer risk. In a cross-sectional study, alcohol intake was associated with elevated plasma levels of estrone sulfate, a long-term indication of estrogen status,[229] which in turn was associated with future risk of breast cancer.[81] In a large prospective analysis, high intake of folic acid appeared to mitigate completely the excess risk of breast cancer due to alcohol, although folic acid intake was not associated with breast cancer risk among nondrinkers. Because alcohol metabolites inactivate folic acid and low folate levels are associated with increased misincorporation of uracil into DNA, this finding suggests another mechanism for the adverse effects of alcohol.

Of all the associations between dietary factors and breast cancer risk, the relationship with alcohol is by far the most consistent. This association has been observed in many diverse populations and cultures, and rigorous attempts to account for this relationship by other variables have been unsuccessful. Moreover, the effect of alcohol on endogenous estrogen levels provides a plausible mechanism. Together, this body of data provides strong evidence for a causal relationship between alcohol consumption and breast cancer risk. The public health implications of this knowledge, however, are complicated by the fact that consumption of one to two alcoholic beverages per day is almost certainly protective against cardiovascular disease. Because cardiovascular disease is the leading cause of death among women, moderate drinking is associated overall with a modest reduction in total mortality.[260] Although the situation is still complex, reduction of daily alcohol consumption appears to be one of relatively few methods of actively reducing breast cancer risk, whereas many methods exist for reducing the risk of cardiovascular disease.

Caffeine

Considerable speculation that caffeine may be a risk factor for breast cancer followed a report that women with benign breast disease experienced relief from symptoms after eliminating caffeine from their diets. Most case control studies, however, have not observed evidence of a positive association with breast cancer. In prospective studies, no increase in breast cancer risk has been seen,[235,261–263] and in one[264] a weak, but significant, inverse association between caffeine consumption and breast cancer risk was observed. Similarly, no evidence for an association between tea consumption and risk of breast cancer has been seen in epidemiologic studies.[241] Thus, the epidemiologic evidence is not compatible with any substantial increase in breast cancer risk associated with drinking coffee or tea.

Phytoestrogens

A wide variety of compounds in fruits and vegetables, other than those discussed here, have potential anticarcinogenic activity *in vitro*.[265] Phytoestrogens in soy products have attracted scientific and popular attention, in part because they are highly consumed in Asian countries, such as Japan and China, that have low rates of cancer. These compounds, which include daidzen and genistein, can bind estrogen receptors but are much less potent than estradiol. In principle, these substances may thus act like tamoxifen by blocking the action of endogenous estrogens to reduce breast cancer risk. Dietary supplementation with a large amount of soy protein slightly lengthens menstrual cycle length,[266] an effect that would be predicted to decrease breast cancer risk only minimally. Also, soy protein consumption is not the primary explanation for low rates of breast cancer in Japan and China, because rates are similarly low in some parts of China, elsewhere in Asia, and in many developing countries in which soy and related foods are not consumed regularly. In a case control study in Singapore,[267] intake of soy products was associated with lower risk of breast cancer. However, in two case control studies in China that were particularly informative because they encompassed a wide range in levels of soy protein consumption, little relation was seen.[268] Conceivably, phytoestrogens could even increase overall estrogenic activity among postmenopausal women with low levels of endogenous estrogens. Another group of compounds formed from glucosinolates found in cruciferous vegetables is hypothesized to alter the balance of estrogen metabolism toward less potent forms, but relevant human data are minimal. The possibility that phytochemicals that block estrogen function or modulate estrogen metabolism may provide a nontoxic means of altering breast cancer risk deserves further study, but the available evidence is insufficient.

Specific Foods

Foods contain an extremely complex mix of essential nutrients and other compounds that could individually or collectively influence breast cancer risk in ways that may not be detected by the study of individual nutrients. Thus, an examination of foods and food groups in relation to risk of breast cancer could be informative. Because the foods examined in most studies are too numerous to be reported individually, however, published results are likely to reflect a bias toward reporting findings that are statistically significant or that fit preexisting hypotheses.

Despite the potential for biases, inverse associations between intakes of fruits and vegetables and breast cancer risk have been reported in a notably large number of case control studies.[241] These associations have been more consistent for vegetables than for fruits, and for green vegetables in particular. In two cohort studies, however, only weak and nonsignificant inverse associations were seen with consumption of fruits and vegetables.[241] In the 14-year follow-up of the Nurses' Health Study, evidence for a protective effect of vegetable intake was limited to premenopausal women (relative risk of 0.6 for highest versus lowest intakes; 95% confidence interval, 0.4 to 1.0)[240]; little relation was seen with fruit consumption.

Associations between red meat consumption and risk of breast cancer have been reported sporadically.[269] In the largest cohort study, however, no relationship was seen,[236] despite a strong association between red meat consumption and risk of colon cancer in the same population. In the few studies that have examined poultry consumption, little relationship with risk of breast cancer was observed.[241] Although a protective effect of fish consumption has been suggested in a few studies, the overall evidence from case control and cohort studies suggests little relationship.[215] Intake of nuts and legumes has received limited attention in reports on diet and breast cancer, but in general no relationship has been seen.[241]

Diet and Breast Cancer Survival

Regardless of whether diet is related to the occurrence of breast cancer, if postdiagnosis diet were related to risk of recurrence or survival, then dietary modifications might assist in breast cancer treatment. Several studies[270] have examined dietary fat intake before breast cancer diagnosis in relation to survival by following up the cases from breast cancer case control studies; results have been inconsistent. Because the original interest was the relation of diet to breast cancer incidence, the investigators were at pains to assess diet before diagnosis. This approach is unsatisfactory, however, if the question is whether diet after diagnosis has an influence on survival, because women may make major changes in their diets after receiving the diagnosis. In one study of diet after diagnosis (albeit in the 1 to 5 months immediately after the diagnosis), no association was seen between dietary fat intake and survival.[271] In a larger study, diet was assessed both before and after breast cancer diagnosis.[272] Fat intake after diagnosis was not associated with survival. However, higher protein consumption, mainly from poultry, fish, and dairy sources, was related to a better prognosis, even after controlling for protein consumption before diagnosis. In the same study, neither alcohol consumption nor vitamin A intake was associated with survival. A randomized trial of a low-fat intervention diet among breast cancer patients is under way.[273] However, other aspects of diet also merit further examination in relation to breast cancer survival.

Summary of Diet and Breast Cancer Risk

The role of specific dietary factors in breast cancer causation is not completely resolved. Enthusiasm for the hypothesis that dietary fat intake is responsible for the high breast cancer rates in Western countries was based largely on the weakest form of epidemiologic evidence—ecologic correlation studies. Results from prospective studies do not support the concept that fat intake in middle life has a major relationship to breast cancer risk during up to 14 years of follow-up. High energy intake in relation to physical activity, which accelerates growth and the onset of menstruation during childhood and leads to weight gain in middle life, contributes substantially to breast cancer risk. These effects of energy balance clearly account for an important part of international differences in breast cancer rates. Although the responsible constituents are not clear, considerable evidence suggests that low intake of vegetables modestly increases the risk of breast cancer. The possibility that vitamin A or other compounds in vitamin A–rich foods are protective deserves further consideration. Alcohol intake is the best-established specific dietary risk factor for breast cancer, and studies demonstrating that even moderate alcohol intake increases endogenous estrogen levels provide a potential mechanism, thus supporting a causal interpretation. Hypotheses relating childhood and adolescent diet to breast cancer risk decades later will be more difficult to test unless novel data sources or methods for measuring diet in the distant past are developed, or unless radiographic, histologic, or other markers of breast cancer risk are found and validated for use as intermediate markers of breast cancer. Nevertheless, available evidence is strong that breast cancer risk can be reduced by avoiding weight gain during adult years, limiting alcohol consumption, and consuming an abundant amount of vegetables and fruits. Some evidence suggests that replacing saturated fat with monounsaturated fat may reduce risk of breast cancer, and this will reduce risk of coronary heart disease.

PHYSICAL ACTIVITY

Regular physical activity has been hypothesized to prevent breast cancer, largely by reducing circulating levels of sex hormones. The mechanisms by which physical activity reduces exposure to hormones vary by period of life. Young girls participating in strenuous athletic training, such as running and ballet dancing, have delayed menarche,[274–276] which is known to reduce risk of breast cancer, and even moderate-intensity physical activity may delay menstruation.[223] This effect of activity at young ages may be reflected in lower body weight and body fat, both of which are determinants of delayed menstruation.[221,276] A later menarche is associated with a later onset of regular ovulatory cycles as well as lower serum estrogen concentrations during adolescence.[277] Once menstruation has been established, anovulatory and irregular menstrual cycles may be more frequent among moderately and strenuously active women than among inactive women,[274,278,279] although disagreement exists regarding the degree to which the intensity of physical activity influences menstrual abnormalities.[280] Furthermore, a substantial degree of ovarian dysfunction may occur, even among physically active women who appear to have normal menstrual cycles.[281] Among older women, levels of past and current physical activity influence fat stores,[275,276,281–284] which after menopause are the locus of conversion of androstenedione to estrogen.[285,286]

Despite the evidence that higher levels of physical activity are associated with lower levels of circulating ovarian hormones, epidemiologic studies relating physical activity to risk of breast cancer show inconsistent results.[287] Methodologic differences in physical activity assessment are likely to have contributed to these inconsistencies. Studies have differed in the ages at which physical activity was assessed; methods for measuring intensity, frequency, and duration of physical activity; definition and categorization of physical activity levels; and age of breast cancer diagnosis. Furthermore, ranges of physical activity typically studied are very limited in comparison with the levels of hard labor typically practiced by women in traditional agrarian societies.

Figure 13 displays relative risks and associated 95% confidence intervals from 17 published studies that have evaluated the association between recreational physical activity and breast cancer. The period of life to which the activity assessment pertains is listed after the author's name, and the menopausal status of the study population is indicated by the symbol locating the relative risk. Many studies are represented by more than one bar, because they included assessment of physical activity at more than one period in life. This figure demonstrates that not all the studies measured the same exposure; some studies measured physical activity early in life, others focused on relatively long-term adult physical activity levels, and many have been limited to measures of physical activity in the period immediately preceding study enrollment. Results have varied, however, even among studies that measured physical activity at similar periods in life.

The strongest reduction in breast cancer risk associated with increased physical activity was reported in a population-based case control study of women younger than age 40.[288] The relative risk was 0.42 (95% confidence interval, 0.27 to 0.64) for women with a lifetime average of 3.8 hours or more of physical activity per week compared those with an average of 0 hours per week. This has been the only study explicitly devoted to the relationship between physical activity and breast cancer, and it used a detailed physical activity assessment instrument to quantify the average number of hours per week of recreational physical activity over the reproductive life span, beginning at menarche. Activities such as housework, gardening, and easy walking not for the explicit purpose of physical exercise were not counted in the measure of physical activity. These researchers concluded from their various analyses that lifelong physical activity is the critical factor of interest with regard to breast cancer risk.

In contrast to the detailed measurement instrument used in the study described in the previous paragraph, a relatively simple measure of physical activity was used in a prospective

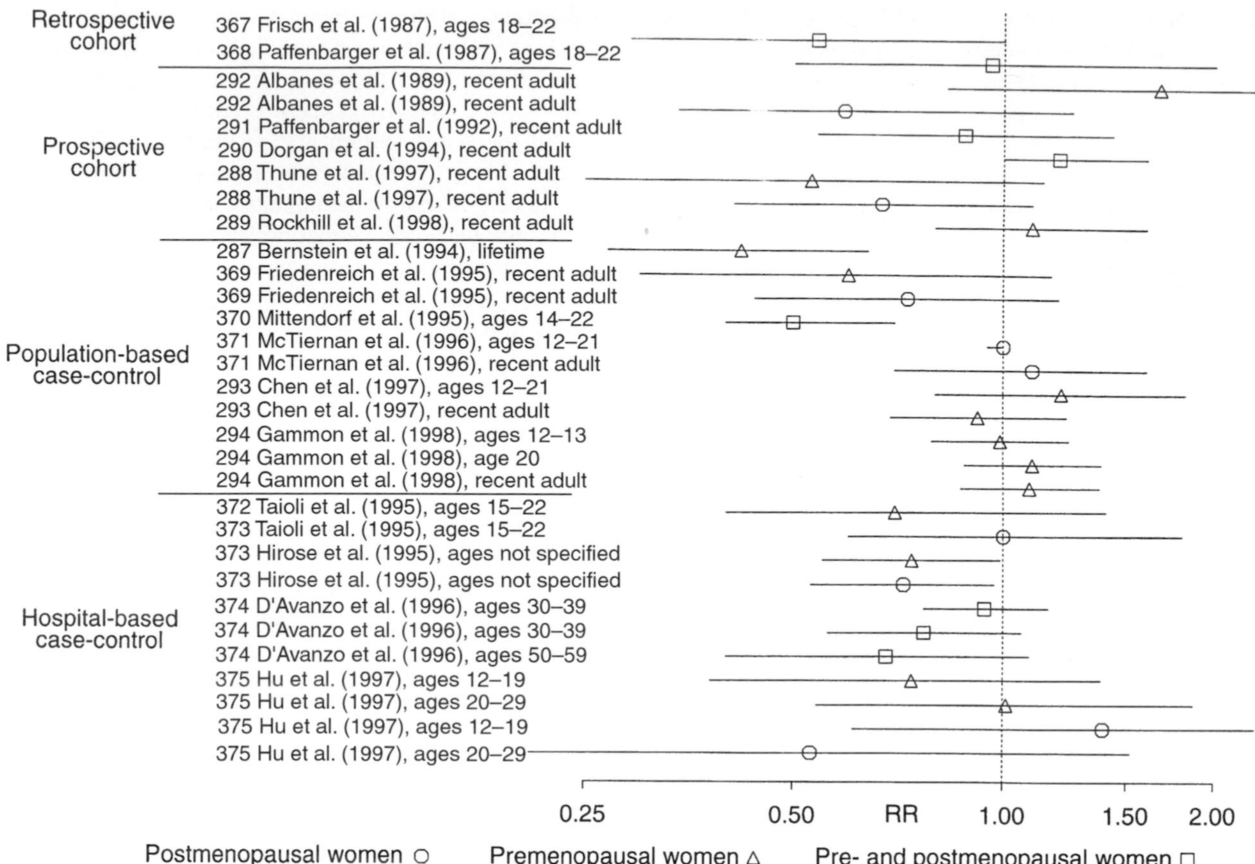

FIG. 13. Results of studies of the relative risk of breast cancer associated with various levels of physical activity for premenopausal and postmenopausal women. Bars represent 95% confidence intervals. See text for further explanation. (Reprinted from ref. 289 with permission of the *Journal of the National Cancer Institute*.)

cohort study of Norwegian women aged 20 to 54 years at baseline.[289] Over a period of 3 to 5 years, women were administered two surveys about their patterns of physical activity during leisure hours. The relative risk was 0.63 (95% confidence interval, 0.42 to 0.95) for consistently active women compared with consistently sedentary women, which is the second-strongest inverse association reported in the literature. This study is also the only prospective cohort study of those reported[289–293] to find a substantial inverse association between physical activity and breast cancer risk.

Most studies fall between these two[288,289] with regard to the detail of physical activity measurement and categorization. For instance, in two population-based case control studies[294,295] conducted among younger women, physical activity both early in life and in the period immediately before the interview was assessed. However, neither of these studies found an inverse association between physical activity (in either period) and breast cancer risk, despite defining physical activity categories in various ways.

Because of the potential public health significance of an association between a modifiable lifestyle risk factor such as physical activity and breast cancer, studies need to address important methodologic issues surrounding physical activity measurement. These issues include the resolution of whether a critical time period exists during which increased physical activity exerts its strongest effect on breast cancer risk, or whether, as hypothesized by Bernstein et al.,[288] lifetime physical activity is the critical exposure of interest. A second important issue relates to the quantification of physical activity and how information on frequency, intensity, duration, and time span of activity should be combined into a single measure. A third issue pertains to the validity of women's reports of past physical activity. In case control studies, random error in recall of past activity levels that is not dependent on disease status would be expected, on average, to dilute any inverse association that might truly exist. If errors are differential by disease status, however, findings may be biased in either direction away from their true point estimates. A fourth issue concerns the need to consider recreational and occupational physical activity together. As with the studies of recreational physical activity summarized in Fig. 13, those examining the relationship between occupational physical activity and breast cancer risk are inconsistent, although overall a modest reduction in risk is suggested.[296] In studies of occupational physical activity, the results can potentially be confounded by reproductive characteristics, because women in physically active jobs may be more likely to be of lower socioeconomic status and thus may be more likely to have a lower-risk reproductive profile. Several studies of occupational activity were unable to control for such potential confounders. Finally, although a hormonal mechanism has been postulated, few data exist relating physical activity over sustained periods of time to lower endogenous ovarian hormone levels. Available studies have been very short term, have been based on small numbers of women, and often have been limited to comparisons between young women who engage in high levels of activity and inactive young women.

Although the relationship between physical activity and risk of breast cancer remains unsettled, indirect evidence relating higher physical activity levels to decreased risk of postmenopausal breast cancer is strong because of the important role of activity in controlling weight gain, an important cause of postmenopausal breast cancer. This, in addition to many other benefits of staying lean and fit, provides sufficient justification for including regular physical activity in daily life.

IONIZING RADIATION

Ionizing radiation to the chest in moderate to high doses (e.g., 1 to 3 Gy) at a young age substantially increases breast cancer risk. Among survivors of the atomic bombing of Hiroshima and Nagasaki,[297] breast cancer risk was strongly associated with estimated breast tissue dose of radiation. Further, the relative risk of breast cancer associated with each radiation dose depended heavily on age at the time of the bombing; risk was highest for women exposed before age 10 years.

Studies of radiation therapy have revealed a similar pattern of excess risk of breast cancer associated both with higher doses and with younger ages at exposure. In a study of women who received substantial radiation to the chest as a result of repeated fluoroscopic examinations for tuberculosis,[298] the maximum excess risk was among women with first exposure between the ages of 10 and 14 years, whereas women first exposed at age 35 years or older had virtually no excess risk. In a study of women exposed to radiation therapy to the chest as treatment for Hodgkin's disease,[299] the excess risk of breast cancer was similarly dependent on dose and age at irradiation. In a study of radiation treatment of breast cancer and development of second breast cancers,[300] risk of second cases was significantly elevated (above its already high level) among women who underwent radiation at ages younger than 45 years.

In these studies, attained age and age at time of exposure were correlated. However, radiation exposure at a young age was associated with excess relative risk of early-onset breast cancer, and within categories of current age, the excess relative risks associated with early age of exposure are apparent.[297] These findings support the notion of age-dependent susceptibility to breast carcinogenesis and the hypothesis that undifferentiated breast cells are more vulnerable to cancer initiation than differentiated cells.[301]

The risk associated with low-dose radiation exposure to the chest has been difficult to quantify, because the expected excess of breast cancers is small relative to the background risk.[298] Thus, the risk of breast cancer associated with low-dose radiation as in mammography has been estimated by extrapolating the dose-response relationship from studies of women exposed to higher doses of radiation.[302] In this way, fewer than 1% of all cases of breast cancer have been estimated to result from diagnostic radiography.[302]

ENVIRONMENTAL POLLUTION

Evidence of geographic variation in incidence and mortality rates of breast cancer within the United States, the steady increase in incidence over time, and the identification of suspected breast cancer clusters have stimulated interest in the possibility that industrial chemicals or electromagnetic fields may be environmental risk factors for breast cancer. The experimental and epidemiologic evidence for associations of certain specific synthetic chemicals with breast cancer are considered in the following sections and have been comprehensively reviewed with detailed citations elsewhere.[303,304]

Organochlorines

Epidemiologic studies of breast cancer and environmental exposure to synthetic chemicals have concentrated on biologically persistent organochlorines. This class of compounds includes pesticides such as DDT, chlordane, hexachlorocyclohexane (HCH, lindane), hexachlorobenzene (HCB), kepone, and mirex; industrial chemicals such as polychlorinated biphenyls (PCBs) and polybrominated biphenyls (PBBs); and dioxins [polychlorinated dibenzofurans (PCDFs) and polychlorinated dibenzodioxins (PCDDs)], compounds produced as combustion by-products of PCBs or contaminants of pesticides. Many of these chemicals are weak estrogens and are therefore hypothesized to increase breast cancer risk by mimicking endogenous estradiol. Furthermore, they are excreted in breast milk, which suggests that ductal and other cells in the breast are directly exposed. Other compounds, specifically the dioxins and some PCB congeners, exhibit antiestrogenic activity; therefore, despite the established carcinogenicity of dioxin at other anatomic sites in animal tests, they might be protective against breast cancer.

The organochlorines are highly lipophilic and resistant to metabolism. Thus, many of these compounds bioaccumulate in the food chain and persist in the body. These chemicals can be measured in breast milk, adipose tissue, and blood.

Most of the epidemiologic literature on organochlorines focuses on DDT, DDE [1,1-dichloro-2,2,-bis(*p*-dichlorophenyl)ethylene, the main metabolite of DDT], and PCBs, because they are among the most persistent in humans. The general population was thought to be exposed to these compounds predominantly through ingestion of fish, dairy products, and meat. Almost everyone in the United States has had some measurable exposure; however, the average body burden of some of these chemicals (e.g., DDT) has been decreasing with time since the cessation of their production in this country (1972 for DDT and 1977 for PCBs).

Although a positive correlation of age-specific breast cancer mortality rates in Israel with trends in DDT and other pesticide contamination in milk has been reported,[305] estimates were based on only 2 years of data. When more extensive mortality and incidence data were analyzed, no association was observed.[306] In a study of PCB-contaminated fatty fish from the Baltic Sea, breast cancer rates among fishermen's wives from the contaminated east coast were higher than rates among fishermen's wives from the noncontaminated west coast (relative risk, 1.35; 95% confidence interval, 0.98 to 1.86).[307] However, there was no control for other known breast cancer risk factors. An accidental explosion in 1976 at a chemical plant near Seveso, Italy, provided the opportunity to evaluate exposure to high levels of dioxin. Breast cancer incidence during the decade after the accident in the areas closest to the accident was slightly but not significantly lower than expected.[308]

Studies of occupational exposure to organochlorines have not supported an association with increased breast cancer risk. Fewer cases were observed than expected in studies of women occupationally exposed to phenoxy herbicides and PCBs. A twofold increase in breast cancer mortality was found in facilities with herbicide and dioxin exposures,[309] but only 7% of the subjects worked in high-exposure areas. These studies are limited by difficulties of exposure assessment and the small numbers of women employed in the occupations with greatest exposure.

The results of small case control studies of organochlorine levels and breast cancer risk have been mixed. In a large European case control study (265 cases), a significant inverse relationship between levels of adipose DDE and risk of breast cancer was observed after controlling for known breast cancer risk factors; the authors did not evaluate PCBs.[310] In a case control study in Buffalo, New York, lipid-adjusted serum levels of DDE, HCB, Mirex, and total PCBs were evaluated among 154 incident breast cancer cases and 192 community controls. No evidence was seen of a positive association between levels of any of these compounds and breast cancer risk, with the possible exception of the less-chlorinated PCBs.[311] Lopez-Carrillo et al. analyzed serum DDE levels in a case control study in Mexico, where the pesticide DDT is still in use.[312] Serum DDE levels were not associated with risk of breast cancer. In one small study, however, contrary to expectation, the levels of octachlorinated dibenzo-*p*-dioxin (OCDD) were slightly elevated in the cancer cases,[313] although no differences were observed for six other polychlorinated dibenzo-*p*-dioxin isomers.

Three prospective studies have used stored blood samples collected before diagnosis to evaluate the relationship between DDE and total PCBs, and breast cancer.[314–316] In a cohort of 14,290 women in New York City[315] (80% of whom were white), levels in sera from 58 women diagnosed with breast cancer within 1 to 6 months of blood collection were compared with levels among 171 controls. After adjusting for known risk factors, the odds ratio for women in the tenth decile of DDE levels compared with those in the first was 4.08 (95% confidence interval, 1.49 to 11.20), and the positive trend was statistically significant. The equivalent odds ratio associated with PCB level was not statistically significant. In a prospective study of 57,040 San Francisco Bay area women who had provided blood in the late 1960s, when DDT and PCBs were still in production,[314] 50 white women, 50 African-American women, and 50 Asian-American women with breast cancer occurring after blood draw and before 1991 were selected and compared with 150 control women matched for age and ethnicity. Risk of breast cancer was not associated with either DDE or PCB level when all ethnic groups were combined, although nonsignificant elevated risks were observed for DDE for African-Americans and whites. Among 236 women with breast cancer and their matched controls in the Nurses' Health Study, no evidence was found of a positive association between breast cancer and either DDE or PCBs.[316] The multivariate relative risks for women in the highest quintile compared with women in the lowest were 0.72 (95% confidence interval, 0.4 to 1.4) for DDE and 0.66 (95% confidence interval, 0.32 to 1.37) for PCBs. For women in the highest quintiles of both DDE and PCB levels, the relative risk was 0.43 (95% confidence interval, 0.13 to 1.44) for joint exposure.

In summary, most large studies have not found evidence of increased breast cancer risk associated with blood levels of DDE or total PCBs; however, a small effect will always be difficult to exclude. All available studies address exposure to organochlorines in the decade or two before enrollment; it will be very difficult to obtain data to address the hypothesis that childhood or even *in utero* exposure is associated with breast cancer risk 50 or more years afterward. Nonetheless, organochlorines appear unlikely to be major breast cancer risk factors or the explanation for rising breast cancer rates.

Electromagnetic Fields

Electromagnetic fields (EMFs) have been proposed to alter breast cancer risk, perhaps by altering melatonin secretion by the pineal gland. Although animal evidence is suggestive, few data address the relationship of melatonin levels to human breast cancer risk. Exposure to light at night has been shown to suppress melatonin secretion, and in some studies breast cancer risk has been lower among blind women.[317,318] Gathering high-quality epidemiologic data on EMF and nocturnal light exposure is challenging, and these questions are unlikely to be resolved definitively in the near future. Evidence of an elevated risk of male breast cancer associated with presumed occupational EMF exposure based on job title has been observed in some studies, but these results are based on small numbers of cases. No evidence of an increased risk of breast cancer was observed in the studies that also included female employees. In case control studies designed specifically to study occupational exposure to EMF and breast cancer in women, small increases in risk have been inconsistently observed. However, in those studies, misclassification of exposure is a major concern. Because classifications are based on subjects' "usual" occupation, often obtained from death certificates, duration of exposure and personal work tasks could not be accounted for in most of the studies, and adjustment for known breast cancer risk factors was limited or entirely absent.

The general population is exposed to EMFs primarily from power lines, transformer substations, and electrical appliance use. In an initial 1987 study of mortality from all cancer subtypes and residential wiring configurations, a statistically significant elevation in female breast cancer incidence was associated with magnitude of exposure at the current residence.[319] Other studies in Britain, the Netherlands, and Taiwan, however, did not observe an association between female breast cancer deaths and residence in the vicinity of electricity transmission facilities. Again, these studies are limited by the indirect methods used to assess EMF exposure.

Use of electric blankets (produced before 1990) throughout the night approximately doubles an individual's average exposure to EMFs, because the blanket is placed close to the body. In one case control study, the use of electric blankets continuously throughout the night was associated with marginally significant increases for breast cancer in postmenopausal women (odds ratio, 1.46; 95% confidence interval, 0.96 to 2.20)[320] and for premenopausal women (odds ratio, 1.43; 95% confidence interval, 0.94 to 2.17).[321] In a large case control study of breast cancer in women younger than age 55 years, however, no association was seen.[322] Additional studies of electric blanket exposure and other residential exposures to EMFs and breast cancer risk are ongoing, but the biological plausibility and epidemiologic support for an important relation between EMF exposure and breast cancer risk are weak.

Active and Passive Smoking

The relationship between active cigarette smoking and risk of breast cancer has been extensively evaluated in both case control and cohort studies; collectively, the data provide strong evidence against any major overall relationship. Initiation of smoking early in adolescence, when breast tissue may be maximally sensitive to carcinogenic influences, has been associated with an increased risk in a large case control study.[323] However, in the largest case control study to date, no association with smoking at an early age was observed.[324]

Passive smoking has been suggested to be an important risk for breast cancer, in part because sidestream smoke contains more carcinogenic activity per milligram than mainstream smoke. In a cohort study of cancer mortality among Japanese women exposed to passive smoke at home, a slight and insignificant risk elevation was seen (crude relative risk, 1.3; 95% confidence interval, 0.8 to 2.0).[325,326] In several case control studies, increases in risk of breast cancer have been seen, but usually without evidence of a dose response. Despite these positive associations, the absence of an effect of heavy smoking for decades is difficult to reconcile with an effect of exposure to much lower amounts of environmental smoke. A likely explanation for the positive association seen in case control studies is methodologic bias related to the selection of controls or the retrospective recall of exposure to passive smoke. However, data from large prospective studies is required to resolve the issue.

Silicone Breast Implants

Most studies examining the relation of silicone breast implants to breast cancer risk have actually reported lower rates of breast cancer among women with implants[327–330], thus, a direct association between silicone breast implants and the occurrence of breast cancer is unlikely.

Summary of Evidence on Environmental Pollution and Breast Cancer Risk

In general, evidence does not support any substantial relationship between exposure to humanmade chemicals or electrical fields in the environment and breast cancer risk. The most recent evidence in prospective analyses does not support an association between exposure to organochlorines and breast cancer risk. Although occupational studies of EMF exposure have been inconclusive, residential studies imply that no risk is associated with overhead power lines. Measurable increases in breast cancer risk due to passive smoke seem implausible because of the lack of effect of active smoking, but prospective data are needed.

Although other environmental exposures that have not been identified may warrant evaluation, with the exception of ionizing radiation, no environmental exposure can be confidently labeled as a cause of breast cancer.

OCCUPATION

A review of 115 studies conducted between 1971 and 1994[331] found little support for an association between specific occupations and breast cancer risk. Limited evidence suggested that cosmetologists, beauticians, and pharmaceutical manufacturing workers had a modestly elevated risk of breast cancer, but conclusions were not possible due to lack of adequate exposure data. Although ionizing radiation is a recognized risk factor for breast cancer, none of the studies of radiation workers, including those of x-ray technicians and workers at uranium fuel plants and atomic energy plants, found an elevation of breast cancer risk among women in these occupations. The few studies carried out on specific occupational agents have not provided any evidence of association. In particular, although organic solvents may increase risk of various cancers in animals, women who worked in dry cleaning or shoe manufacturing, or who were exposed to trichloroethylene did not have an elevated risk of breast cancer.[331]

Despite the large literature on occupation as a risk factor, most studies have simply examined associations between occupational title and breast cancer risk; specific information on exposure to potential carcinogens was collected in only a few studies. Although some studies collected detailed information on lifetime occupational history, often broad occupational groupings representing only the most recent occupation were used in analyses. Furthermore, most studies have not controlled adequately for known breast cancer risk factors—reproductive factors, in particular—that are likely to confound any observed association with occupation.[332] Employment outside the home, and in a specific occupation, is likely to be highly correlated with educational attainment and socioeconomic status, and thus with reproductive characteristics. In the few studies that have controlled for sociodemographic and reproductive risk, breast cancer risk was not found to vary across occupational groups. In contrast, a consistent finding across studies that were unable to control for important confounding factors has been an increased breast cancer risk among more highly educated women, rather than a consistently observed association with any specific occupation. Thus, further analyses of occupational titles without consideration of known breast cancer risk factors or actual workplace exposures are unlikely to be informative.

MEDICAL HISTORY

A variety of diseases and medications are known or suspected to cause or be associated with modifications of hormones or growth factors and thus may influence breast cancer risk.[333] Type 2 diabetes mellitus has been suggested to increase risk of breast cancer. Hyperinsulinemia, as occurs in type 2 diabetes mellitus, may promote breast cancer, because insulin may be a growth factor for human breast cancer cells.[334] Furthermore, insulin levels are inversely related to levels of sex hormone–binding globulin, and thus are positively related to levels of available estrogens and androgens.[333] Many studies have lacked information about the type and severity of diabetes, which makes the interpretation of the various findings difficult.[333] In a case control investigation of subclinical diabetes, hyperinsulinemia with insulin resistance was a significant risk factor for breast cancer, independent of weight or body fat distribution.[335] Results of a case control study published in 1997 showed that a history of type 2 diabetes mellitus was associated with a 50% increase in postmenopausal breast cancer, again independent of weight.[333] Further studies of the relationship between breast cancer and insulin resistance are warranted, because insulin resistance is modifiable through increases in physical activity, dietary changes, and maintenance of a lean body weight.

A relationship between thyroid disease and breast cancer has been suggested, but again, findings are inconsistent. Reports of a moderate increase in breast cancer risk after a diagnosis of thyroid cancer may reflect the effect of increased medical surveillance of thyroid cancer patients, as well as socioeconomic and reproductive risk factors that are shared by the two cancers. Most epidemiologic studies of prior diagnosis of thyroid disease have not found an association with breast cancer risk.

Strong evidence suggests that the use of nonsteroidal anti-inflammatory drugs (NSAIDs), including aspirin, inhibits colon carcinogenesis in humans[336,337]; this provides a rationale to investigate an inhibitory role of NSAIDs in breast carcinogenesis. Some epidemiologic studies have shown modest reductions in risk of breast cancer associated with NSAID use, whereas others have found none. Because most NSAID use is sporadic, it may be difficult to capture patterns of use on a questionnaire. Unanswered questions remain regarding the effect of regular NSAID use for long durations, the effect of different dosages, and the effects of different NSAIDs (in particular, aspirin versus nonaspirin).[338]

A history of eclampsia, preeclampsia, or pregnancy-induced hypertension has been associated with a reduced risk of breast cancer in parous women in at least two case control studies.[339,340] Explanations for these findings have focused on hormone-related factors: Women who develop preeclampsia have been found to have relatively low estrogen levels during pregnancy. However, nonspecific cellular immune responses may be involved as well.[341,342]

An elevated risk of breast cancer associated with the use of antidepressants has been seen in at least one case control study,[343] but this finding was based on a small number of participants. The literature on the effect of antidepressants on cancer in humans and in experimental animal models is conflicting, however. Future epidemiologic studies of this topic must control for possibly strong confounding factors, such as alcohol use, which may be associated with use of antidepressants. Furthermore, the indication for antidepressant use may itself be associated with increased cancer risk, and depression may possibly be an early symptom of occult cancer.

Cytotoxic drugs used in the treatment of cancer may exert their own carcinogenic effects. One category of cytotoxic drugs, alkylating agents, may lead to an increased risk of solid tumors, including breast cancer, although evidence for this hypothesis is weak.[344]

TABLE 4. *Risk factors for breast cancer and approximate strength of association*

Reproductive factors		Hormonal factors		Nutritional factors		Other factors	
Age at first period (≥15 vs 11)	–	Estrogen replacement (<5 yr vs none)	+	Monounsaturated fat[a]	–	Family history (mother *and* sister)[b]	+++
Age at first birth (≥35 vs ≤20)	++	OC use (current use vs none)	+	Physical activity (≥3 hr/wk)	–	Family history (first-degree relative)[c]	++
No. of births (0 or 1 child)	+	Estrogen replacement (≥5 yr vs none)	+	Saturated fat[a]	+	Jewish heritage (yes vs no)	+
Age at menopause (5-yr increment)	+	High blood estrogens (past menopause)	+++	Height (>5'7")	+	Ionizing radiation (yes vs no)	+
Breast-feeding (>1 yr vs none)	–	High blood IGF-I (premenopausal)	+++	Vegetables[a]		Benign breast disease[d] (MD diagnosed)	++
		High blood prolactin	++	Obesity (premenopausal) (>27 BMI vs <21 BMI)	–		
				Obesity (postmenopausal) (>27 BMI vs <21 BMI)	+		
				Alcohol (>1 drink/day vs none)	+		

BMI, body mass index; IGF-I, insulinlike growth factor type I; OC, oral contraceptive; +, relative risk (RR) = 1.1–1.4; ++, RR = 1.5–2.9; +++, RR = 3.0–6.9; –, RR = 0.7–0.8.

[a]Upper quartile (top 25%) versus lower quartile (lowest 25%).

[b]Two first-degree relatives who have a history of breast cancer before age 65 years versus no relatives.

[c]First-degree relative who has a history of breast cancer before age 65 years versus no relative.

[d]Clinically recognized chronic cystic, fibrocystic, or other benign breast disease versus none.

ETIOLOGIC SUMMARY

Much is known about the behavioral factors that influence breast cancer risk, and the links between these factors and the pathophysiology of the disease are becoming clearer. Known and suspected risk factors are described in Table 4, grouped by reproductive, hormonal, nutritional, and other variables. Approximate strengths of association are also given for specific comparisons. These comparisons are somewhat arbitrary, because many of these risk factors are continuous variables, and the relative risks depend on the levels chosen for comparison. For example, for age at menarche, 15 years has been compared with 11 years, but the relative risk would be stronger if age 17 were contrasted with age 11. Although most of these risk factors are established with a high degree of certainty, some—such as high prolactin levels, low physical activity, and low consumption of monounsaturated fat—require further research for confirmation.

Mechanisms linking confirmed and suspected risk factors to the development of breast cancer are known with varying levels of certainty. Early events involve mutations of breast stem cells. These mutations can be inherited (e.g., mutations in *BRCA1*, *BRCA2*, or the p53 gene) or acquired, such as by exposure to ionizing radiation. Little evidence exists that classic chemical carcinogens play an important role in human breast cancer by causing early mutations. Oxidative damage from endogenous metabolism is hypothesized to contribute to DNA damage,[345] but the importance of this mechanism is difficult to quantify. To the extent that oxidative damage is important, antioxidants in vegetables and fruits may account in part for the apparent protective effects seen with higher intake of these foods, and higher intake of monounsaturated fat results in cell structures that are less easily oxidized. Low availability of folic acid, which is exacerbated by high alcohol intake, leads to the incorporation of uracil rather than thymine into DNA and can also be a cause of mutations. Pregnancy appears to render the breast substantially less susceptible to somatic mutations, although the exact mechanisms are unclear; thus, earlier first pregnancies minimize the period of susceptibility. Vitamin A also plays a role in maintaining cell differentiation, but it may be that only quite low intakes are related to increased risk.

High endogenous estrogen levels are now well established as an important cause of breast cancer, and many known risk factors operate through this pathway. The additional contributions of cyclical estrogen exposure (as opposed to continuously high levels) and progestins are less clear, but available evidence suggests that progestins add to breast cancer risk. Factors that increase lifetime exposure to estrogens and progestins include early age at menarche, regular ovulation, and late menopause. Lactation and overweight during young adult life result in anovulation, and this probably accounts for most of their protective effects. Extreme underweight also causes anovulation and would be expected to reduce risk, but direct evidence is lacking. Alcohol consumption increases endogenous estrogen levels, and this may, at least in part, account for the observed increase in risk among regular drinkers. The increased risk of breast cancer among current or recent users of older high-dose oral contraceptives is also presumably due to their estrogenic (and possible progestational) effects. After menopause, the major determinants of estrogen exposure are the amount of body fat and use of postmenopausal hormones; these are important risk factors for breast cancer. Increases in physical activity can delay the onset of menarche and can also reduce risk of breast cancer by helping to control weight gain and possibly by reducing ovulation and endogenous estrogen levels among premenopausal women.

Estrogens, by their mitotic effect on breast cells, appear to accelerate the development of breast cancer at many points along the progression from early mutation to metastasis and death. By increasing cell multiplication, estrogens may also increase the probability that DNA lesions become mutations. Although earlier exposure to high estrogen levels during adolescence increases risk decades later, reduction in levels late in life abruptly reduces risk, whether this be by oophorectomy, cessation of postmenopausal hormones, or the administration of antiestrogens. Other growth factors in addition to estrogens, particularly IGF-I and prolactin, also appear to contribute to risk of breast cancer, but these relationships are less firmly established.

Although this broad outline of breast carcinogenesis is unlikely to change substantially with further research, many details are incomplete, and other contributing factors will probably be documented. For example, genetic polymorphisms yet to be identified are likely to contribute to variation in endogenous levels of, or responsiveness to, estrogens, IGF-I, and prolactin. Dietary and other behavioral determinants of these factors are incompletely defined. Also, other molecular mechanisms, such as DNA repair and apoptosis, are thought to be important in carcinogenesis in general, but the extent to which exogenous factors influence these processes in the context of human breast cancer is not known.

ATTRIBUTABLE RISK: THE QUANTITATIVE CONTRIBUTION OF KNOWN RISK FACTORS

As noted in the first section of this chapter, the search for specific breast cancer risk factors has been stimulated by the large differences in rates of breast cancer among countries, and by changes in rates among migrating populations and within countries over time. The extent to which known risk factors account for these differences in rates is therefore of considerable interest. An often-quoted estimate is that only 30% of breast cancer cases are explained by known risk factors.[193,346] This estimate has been widely used to suggest that other major risk factors remain to be discovered, in part fueling the search for environmental pollutants that may be responsible. A study of population-attributable risks in a nationwide survey, however, estimated that at least 45% to 55% of breast cancer cases in the United States may be explained by later age at first birth, nulliparity, family history of breast cancer, higher socioeconomic status, earlier age at menarche, and prior benign breast disease.[347] In another analysis, parity and age at menarche, first birth, and menopause appeared to explain more than one-half of the difference between breast cancer rates in China and the United States.[75] Among postmenopausal women, just the combination of weight gain after age 18 years and use of postmenopausal hormones accounted for approximately one-third of breast cancer cases.[77] Combined with the reproductive variables, this would clearly account for a large majority of the international differences.

A precise determination of the degree to which changes in the prevalences of known breast cancer risk factors account for the increases in breast cancer rates over time is difficult. Changes in age at first birth do not appear to account for appreciable increases in overall U.S. breast cancer rates through 1990, although more delayed childbearing by women born after 1950 should ultimately contribute to an approximately 9% increase in rates.[348] Since the 1940s, however, obesity, use of postmenopausal hormones, and alcohol consumption by women have increased dramatically. Although further work is needed to quantify these contributions to the secular trends, novel risk factors are not required to account for substantial increases in breast cancer rates.

COMMUNICATION OF RISK TO PATIENTS

Women and their health care providers are increasingly exposed to information on epidemiologic risk factors for breast cancer, benefits of prevention strategies, and treatment options. The Gail model of breast cancer risk prediction[349] is increasingly used by clinicians to assess breast cancer risk of women with differing risk factor profiles. Evidence suggests that the understanding of risk is poor, however. For example, in a sample of women with a family history of breast cancer, more than two-thirds of women overestimated their lifetime risk of breast cancer, even after participating in a counseling session.[350] The overestimation of risk was substantial and perhaps could lead to inappropriate behaviors, such as overscreening, excessive breast self-examination, or inappropriate decisions regarding prophylactic mastectomy or other strategies.

Factors that appear to influence perception of risk include numeracy.[351] Women with higher numeracy scores had significantly higher accuracy in gauging the benefits of mammography. Importantly, when risk and risk reduction are discussed with an individual, research indicates that both absolute risk and relative risk must be included in the message to maximize the accuracy of risk perception. Although more effective formats for presentation of risk and benefits are required, the evidence supports discussion of the "risk in 1,000 women exactly like you," as well as the magnitude of risk reduction, perhaps given as a percentage.

PREVENTION OF BREAST CANCER

Approaches for the primary prevention of breast cancer according to period of life are discussed here briefly and are considered in more detail elsewhere.[301] Although the major reasons for the high rates of breast cancer in affluent Western populations are largely known, this knowledge does not necessarily translate easily into strategies for breast cancer prevention. Some risk factors (e.g., age at menarche) are well established but are difficult to modify; some (e.g., postmenopausal hormone use) are well established but have other important benefits; and others (e.g., replacement of saturated fat with monounsaturated fat) are unproven although suggested by available data and have other strong benefits that justify the strategy, with reduction in breast cancer being a possible additional benefit. Also, known risk factors for breast cancer are modest in magnitude; relative risks are usually in the range of 1.3 to 1.8 for attainable changes. Although these relative risks are far less dramatic than those involving smoking and lung cancer, they should still be considered important. To provide perspective, the relative risk of death from breast cancer for women who do not have mammography compared with those who receive regular mammograms is approximately 1.3. Just as great emphasis and resources are given to the provision of mammography, the avoidance of a risk factor with a similar magnitude of effect should have even higher priority, because this prevents both the occurrence and need for treatment of breast cancer as well as death. When considering primary prevention, one must remember that even small changes at the individual level can produce substantial changes in the population rates of disease.[352]

Some strategies for prevention can be implemented by individuals themselves, but the health system, as well as governments and society as a whole, can take actions that strongly influence rates of breast cancer. Table 5 lists possible prevention strategies, along with actions that can be taken at these different levels to reduce rates of breast cancer.

Early onset of menarche in the United States and other affluent countries is largely the result of rapid growth and weight gain of children related to an abundant food supply, excellent sanitation, and low levels of physical activity (including sitting in school). Much of this is desirable for many reasons, and no reasonable expectation exists that one could, or would, want to increase the average age at menarche to 17 years, as has been typical in rural China. Yet generally desirable increases in physical activity, such as greater recreational activities, have been associated with modest delays in age at menarche[223,353] and should thus contribute to reductions in breast cancer. The amount of time spent watching television is a major determinant of excessive weight gain by children[354] and is therefore an appropriate focus for reducing risk of breast cancer and future cardiovascular disease. Society, through the provision of daily physical activity in schools and safe environ-

TABLE 5. *Possible strategies and levels of action for primary prevention of breast cancer*

Strategy	Individual	Health system	Society/government
Delay menarche.	Provide parental support for recreational activity and limit television watching.	Encourage regular activity.	Provide daily physical activity in schools, safe play environment.
Breast-feed.	Breast-feed at least 6 months per pregnancy.	Encourage lactation.	Provide infant child care at work and/or long maternal leaves.
Limit alcohol.	Limit intake to several drinks per week.	Provide education.	Develop social norms for low alcohol intake by women.
Avoid long-term estrogen therapy.	Limit use to treatment of symptoms.	Educate patients on risks and benefits.	—
Avoid adult weight gain.	Engage in regular physical activity, moderately restrain total calorie intake.	Counsel patients on importance of avoiding weight gain.	Provide safe environment for pedestrians and bicycle riding. Provide worksite and community recreational facilities.
Eat five servings of fruits and vegetables per day. Replace saturated fat with olive, canola, and other oils high in monounsaturated fats.	Make healthy dietary choices.	Encourage healthy diets.	Provide healthy choices in worksite and schools, and provide best current information on diet and health.

ments for recreational activity, must play a major role in these efforts.

Early age at first birth substantially reduces breast cancer, but the societal trends are in the opposite direction because of delay of childbirth until after advanced educational programs are completed and careers are established. Furthermore, unplanned early pregnancies and an average of more than two completed pregnancies per woman have undesirable social and ecologic consequences. Nevertheless, a social norm that encouraged carefully planned first pregnancies at the beginning of advanced education and career development would reduce breast cancer rates. Major behavioral changes and social supports, such as the provision of child care, would be required for this to be practical on a widespread basis; because of the complex social changes needed for it to be a practical strategy for breast cancer prevention, it has not been included in Table 5.

At least 6 months of lactation are recommended for optimal infant health,[53] and evidence suggests that this modestly reduces risk of breast cancer, particularly among premenopausal women. Improved physician counseling[355] can encourage this practice, but changes at workplaces to allow breast-feeding and longer maternity leaves are also needed for many women to adopt this practice.

Alcohol consumption has a complex mix of desirable and adverse health effects, one being an increase in breast cancer. Individuals should make decisions considering all the risks and benefits, but for a middle-aged woman who drinks alcohol on a daily basis, reducing intake is one of relatively few behavioral changes that is likely to reduce risk of breast cancer. Taking a multiple vitamin containing folic acid greatly reduces risks of neural tube defects and may prevent coronary heart disease[356] and colon cancer, and one study suggests this may also mitigate the excess risk of breast cancer due to alcohol. Thus, taking a multiple vitamin appears sensible for women who do elect to drink regularly.

Postmenopausal hormone use, like alcohol consumption, involves a complex trade-off of benefits and risks. From the standpoint of breast cancer risk, the optimal strategy would be to use estrogens not at all, or at most for a few years to relieve menopausal symptoms. The range of options is rapidly increasing, however, with the availability of selective estrogen receptor modulators, such as tamoxifen citrate and raloxifene hydrochloride, that can prevent the progression of osteoporosis and simultaneously reduce risk of breast cancer. Physicians need to play a key role in advising women in this rapidly evolving field.

Avoiding weight gain during adult life can importantly reduce risk of postmenopausal breast cancer as well as of cardiovascular disease and many other conditions. Individual women can reduce weight gain by exercising regularly and moderately restricting caloric intake. Health care providers play an important role in counseling patients throughout adult life about the importance of weight control. The incorporation of greater physical activity into daily life will be difficult for many persons, however, unless governments provide a safer and more accessible environment for pedestrians and bicycle riders. The provision of worksite and community exercise facilities can also contribute importantly.

Specific aspects of diet that influence risk of breast cancer are not yet well established, but available evidence generally suggests that increasing intake of vegetables can modestly reduce risk and that replacing saturated and *trans* fat with monounsaturated fat may reduce risk. These are reasonable strategies to pursue, because they reduce risk of cardiovascular and other diseases, and reduced risk of breast cancer may be an added benefit. Physicians can assess dietary habits and provide guidance. Governmental policies also influence diet in many ways. Providing the best current information on diet and health is one such way.

With demonstration that tamoxifen citrate, and probably other selective estrogen receptor modulators, can be effective in the primary prevention of breast cancer,[78] chemoprevention has become an option for women at elevated risk. Many other pharmacologic agents are being evaluated and are likely to increase the number of alternatives. The availability of effective chemopreventive agents raises many questions about the optimal criteria for use of these drugs. Evaluation of an individual woman's risk of breast cancer has become much more important, because this risk can now be modified. Until the mid-1990s, risk had been based primarily on an evaluation of family and reproductive history and history of benign breast disease. New information on risk based on genotype, detailed histologic characteristics of benign breast disease,[357] and serum hormone levels[81] now allows a much more powerful prediction of risk for an individual woman. Screening for elevated estrogen levels in postmenopausal women to help identify those who would most benefit from an estrogen antagonist, as is done for serum cholesterol, may become part of medical practice. Physicians will play a key role in keeping abreast of this rapidly developing area and counseling patients appropriately.

In summary, available evidence provides a basis for a number of strategies that can reduce risk of breast cancer, although some of these represent complex decision making. Attainable changes can have an important impact on individual risk of breast cancer. However, the collective implementation of all lifestyle strategies will not reduce population rates of breast cancer to the very low levels seen in traditional poor societies, because the magnitude of the necessary changes is unrealistic or undesirable. Thus, a role will exist for hormonal and other chemopreventive interventions, which may be appropriate for women at particularly high risk and, potentially, for wide segments of the population, as few women can be considered to have very low risk. Together, the modification of nutritional and lifestyle risk factors and the judicious use of chemopreventive agents can have a major impact on incidence of this important disease.

ACKNOWLEDGMENTS

The authors thank Elizabeth Lenart and Alice Smythe for research assistance.

REFERENCES

1. National Center for Health Statistics. *SEER cancer statistics review, 1973–1995*. Bethesda, MD: US National Cancer Institute, 1998.
2. Parkin DM, Muir C, Whelan SL, et al. *Cancer incidence in five continents,* vol VI. Lyon, France: International Agency for Research on Cancer Scientific Publications, 1992.
3. Seow A, Duffy S, McGee M, et al. Breast cancer in Singapore: trends in incidence 1968–1992. *Int J Epidemiol* 1996;25:40–45.
4. Nagata C, Kawakami N, Shimizu H. Trends in the incidence rate and risk factors for breast cancer in Japan. *Breast Cancer Res Treat* 1997;44:75–82.
5. Hoover R. Breast cancer: geographic, migrant, and time-trend patterns. In: Fortner JSP, ed. *Accomplishments in cancer research.* New York: Lippincott–Raven, 1996.
6. Pike MC, Spicer DV, Dalimoush L, Press MF. Estrogens, progestogens, normal breast cell proliferation, and breast cancer risk. *Epidemiol Rev* 1991;15:48–65.
7. Tominaga S, Aoki K, Fujimoto I, Kurihara M. *Cancer mortality and morbidity statistics: Japan and the world—1994*. Tokyo: Japan Scientific Societies Press, 1994.
8. Heck KE, Pamuk ER. Explaining the relation between education and postmenopausal breast cancer. *Am J Epidemiol* 1997;145:366–372.
9. Krieger N. Social class and the black/white crossover in the age-specific incidence of breast cancer: a study linking census-derived data to population-based registry records. *Am J Epidemiol* 1990;131:804–814.
10. Rosner B, Colditz G. Nurses' health study: log-incidence mathematic model of breast cancer incidence. *J Natl Cancer Inst* 1996;88:359–364.
11. Stanford J, Herrinton L, Schwartz S, Weiss N. Breast cancer incidence in Asian migrants to the United States and their descendants. *Epidemiology* 1995;6:1819–1827.
12. Ziegler RG, Hoover RN, Pike MC, et al. Migration patterns and breast cancer risk in Asian-American women. *J Natl Cancer Inst* 1993;85: 1819–1827.
13. Kolonel L. Cancer patterns of four ethnic groups in Hawaii. *J Natl Cancer Inst* 1980;65:1127–1139.
14. Dunn J. Cancer epidemiology in populations of the United States—with emphasis on Hawaii and California—and Japan. *Cancer Res* 1975;35:3240–3245.
15. Yu H, Harris R, Gao Y, Gao R, Wynder E. Comparative epidemiology of cancers of the colon, rectum, prostate, and breast in Shanghai: China versus the United States. *Int J Epidemiol* 1991;20:76–81.
16. Shimizu H, Ross RK, Bernstein L, Yatani R. Henderson BE, Mack TM. Cancers of the prostate and breast among Japanese and white immigrants in Los Angeles County. *Br J Cancer* 1991;63:963–966.
17. Tominaga S. Cancer incidence in Japanese in Japan, Hawaii, and western United States. *Natl Cancer Inst Monogr* 1985;69:83–92.
18. Kliewer E, Smith K. Breast cancer mortality among immigrants in Australia and Canada. *J Natl Cancer Inst* 1995;97:1154–1161.
19. Young C. Changes in demographic behaviour of migrants in Australia and the transition between generations. *Population Studies* 1991;45: 67–89.
20. Bouchardy C. Cancer in Italian migrant populations: France. *IARC Sci Publ* 1993;123:149–159.
21. Robbins A, Brescianini S, Kelsey J. Regional differences in known risk factors and the higher incidence of breast cancer in San Francisico. *J Natl Cancer Inst* 1997;89:960–965.
22. Sturgeon S, Schairer C, Gail M, McAdams M, Brinton L, Hoover R. Geographic variation in mortality from breast cancer among white women in the United States. *J Natl Cancer Inst* 1995;87:1846–1853.
23. Centers for Disease Control and Prevention. Breast cancer on Long Island, New York. Washington: U.S. Department of Health and Human Services, 1992.
24. White E, Lee C, Kristal A. Evaluation of the increase in breast cancer incidence in relation to mammography use. *J Natl Cancer Inst* 1990;82:1546–1552.
25. Liff J, Sung J, Chow W, Greenberg R, Flanders W. Does increased detection account for the rising incidence of breast cancer? *Am J Public Health* 1991;81:462–465.
26. Lantz P, Remington P, Newcomb P. Mammography screening and increased incidence of breast cancer in Wisconsin. *J Natl Cancer Inst* 1991;83:1540–1546.
27. Miller BA, Feuer EJ, Hankey BF. The increasing incidence of breast cancer since 1982: relevance of early detection. *Cancer Causes Control* 1991;2:67–74.
28. Feuer E, Wun M. How much of the recent rise in breast cancer incidence can be explained by increases in mammography utilization: a dynamic population model approach. *Am J Epidemiol* 1992;136:1423–1436.
29. Miller BA, Feuer EJ, Hankey BF. Recent incidence trends for breast cancer in women and the relevance of early detection: an update. *CA Cancer J Clin* 1993;43:27–41.
30. Chu K, Tarone R, Kessler L. Recent trends in breast cancer incidence, survival, and mortality rates. *J Natl Cancer Inst* 1996;88:1571–1579.
31. Chevarley F, White E. Recent trends in breast cancer mortality among white and black US women. *Am J Public Health* 1997;87:775–781.
32. Persson L, Bergstrom R, Barlow L, Adami H-O. Recent trends in breast cancer incidence in Sweden. *Br J Cancer* 1998;77:167–169.
33. Quinn M, Allen E. Changes in incidence of and mortality from breast cancer in England and Wales since introduction of screening. *BMJ* 1995;311:1391–1395.
34. Matheson I, Tretli S. Changes in breast cancer incidence among Norwegian women under 50. *Lancet* 1996;348:900–901.
35. Jin F, Shu X-O, Devesa S, Zheng W, Blot W, Gao Y-T. Incidence trends for cancers of the breast, ovary, and corpus uteri in urban Shanghai, 1972–1989. *Cancer Causes Control* 1993;4:355–360.
36. Hermon C, Beral V. Breast cancer mortality rates are levelling off or beginning to decline in many western countries: analysis of time trends, age-cohort and age-period models of breast cancer mortality in 20 countries. *Br J Cancer* 1996;73:955–960.
37. Beral V, Hermon C, Reeves G, Peto R. Sudden fall in breast cancer death rates in England and Wales. *Lancet* 1995;345:1642–1611.
38. Kelsey JL, Gammon MD, John EM. Reproductive factors and breast cancer. *Epidemiol Rev* 1993;15:233–243.
39. MacMahon B, Trichopoulos D, Brown J. Age at menarche, urine estrogens and breast cancer risk. *Int J Cancer* 1982;30:427–431.
40. Bernstein L, Ross R. Endogenous hormones and breast cancer risk. *Epidemiol Rev* 1993;15:48–62.
41. Garland M, Hunter DJ, Colditz GA, et al. Menstrual cycle characteristics and history of ovulatory infertility in relation to breast cancer risk in a large cohort of women. *Am J Epidemiol* 1998;147: 636–643.
42. Bruzzi P, Negri E, La Vecchia C. Short term increase in risk of breast cancer after full term pregnancy. *BMJ* 1988;47:757–762.
43. Pike MC, Krailo MD, Henderson BE, Casagrande JT, Hoel DG. "Hormonal" risk factors, "breast tissue age," and the age-incidence of breast cancer. *Nature* 1983;303:767–770.
44. Rosner B, Colditz GA, Willett WC. Reproductive risk factors in a prospective study of breast cancer: the Nurses' Health Study. *Am J Epidemiol* 1994;139:819–835.
45. Rosner B, Colditz G. Extended mathematical model of breast cancer incidence in the Nurses' Health Study. *J Natl Cancer Inst* 1996;88: 359–364.
46. Lambe M, Hsieh C,Trichopoulos D, Ekbom A, Pavia A, Adami H-O. Transient increase in risk of breast cancer after giving birth. *N Engl J Med* 1994;331:5–9.
47. Russo J, Tay LK, Russo IK. Differentiation of the mammary gland and susceptibility to carcinogenesis. *Breast Cancer Res Treat* 1982;2:5–73.
48. La Vecchia C, Negri E, Boyle P. Reproductive factors and breast cancer: an overview. *Soz Praventivmed* 1989;34:101–107.
49. Trichopoulos D, Hsieh C, MacMahon B, Lin T, Lowe C, Mirra A. Age at any birth and breast cancer risk. *Int J Cancer* 1983;31: 701–704.
50. Lane-Claypon JE. A further report on cancer of the breast, with special reference to its associated antecedent conditions. London: Ministry of Health, 1926.
51. Russo J, Russo IH. The etiopathogenesis of breast cancer prevention. *Cancer Lett* 1995;90:81–89.
52. Romieu I, Hemandez-Avila M, Lazcano E, Lopez L, Romero-Jaime R. Breast cancer and lactation history in Mexican women. *Am J Epidemiol* 1996;132:17–26.

53. Committee on Nutrition, American Academy of Pediatrics. *Pediatric nutrition handbook*, 3rd ed. LA Baness, ed. Elk Grove Village, IL: American Academy of Pediatrics, 1993.
54. Gordon A, Nelson L. Characteristics and outcomes of WIC participants and non-participants: analysis of the 1988 National Maternal and Infant Health Survey. Alexandria, VA: US Department of Agriculture, 1995.
55. Ventura S, Taffel S, Mosher W, Wilson J, Hensiiax AS. Trends in pregnancies and pregnancy rates: estimates for the United States, 1980–92. Monthly vital statistics report 43[Suppl]:11. Hyattsville, MD: National Center for Health Statistics; 1995.
56. Kline J, Stein Z, Susser M. *Conception to birth: epidemiology of prenatal development*. New York: Oxford University Press, 1989.
57. Krieger N. Exposure, susceptibility, and breast cancer risk: a hypothesis regarding exogenous carcinogens, breast tissue development, and social gradients, including black/white differences in breast cancer incidence. *Breast Cancer Res Treat* 1989;13:205–223.
58. Brind J, Chinchilli V, Severs W, Summy-Long J. Induced abortion as an independent risk factor for breast cancer: a comprehensive review and meta-analysis. *J Epidemiol Community Health* 1996;50: 481–496.
59. Palmer J, Rosenberg L, Rao R. Induced and spontaneous abortion in relation to risk of breast cancer (United States). *Cancer Causes Control* 1997;8:841–849.
60. Newcomb P, Storer B, Longnecker M, Mittendorf R, Greenberg E, Willett W. Pregnancy termination in relation to risk of breast cancer. *JAMA* 1996;275:283–287.
61. Melbye M, Wohlfahrt J, Olsen J. Induced abortion and the risk of breast cancer. *N Engl J Med* 1997;336:81–85.
62. Trichopoulos D, MacMahon B, Cole P. Menopause and breast cancer risk. *J Natl Cancer Inst* 1972;48:605–6l3.
63. Lilienfeld AM. The relationship of cancer of the female breast to artificial menopause and marital status. *Cancer* 1956;9:927–934.
64. Collaborative Group on Hormonal Factors in Breast Cancer. Breast cancer and hormonal contraceptives: collaborative reanalysis of individual data on 53,297 women with breast cancer and 100,239 women without breast cancer—from 54 epidemiological studies. *Lancet* 1996;47:1713–1727.
65. Colditz GA, Stampfer MJ, Willett WC, et al. Reproducibility and validity of self-reported menopausal status in a prospective cohort study. *Am J Epidemiol* 1987;126:319–325.
66. Moolgavkar S. Cancer models. *Epidemiology* 1990;1:419–420.
67. Armitage P, Doll R. The age distribution of cancer and a multistage theory of carcinogenesis. *Br J Cancer* 1954;8:1–12.
68. Moolgavkar S, Knudson A, Jr. Mutation and cancer: a model for human carcinogenesis. *J Natl Cancer Inst* 1981;66:1037–1052.
69. Hsieh C, Pavia M, Lambe M. Dual effect of parity on breast cancer risk. *Eur J Cancer* 1994;30A:969–973.
70. Janerich DT, Hoff MB. Evidence for a crossover in breast cancer risk factors. *Am J Epidemiol* 1982;116:737–742.
71. Gray GE, Henderson BE, Pike MC. Changing ratio of breast cancer incidence rates with age of black females compared with white females in the United States. *J Natl Cancer Inst* 1980;64:461–463.
72. U.S. Department of Commerce, Bureau of the Census. Fertility of American women: June 1983. Current Population Report. Series P-20, population characteristics, no 395. Washington: U.S. Bureau of the Census; 1983.
73. Bank W. *Social indicators of development 1993*. Baltimore: The Johns Hopkins University Press; 1991.
74. Chen J, Campbell TC, Junyao L, Peto R. *Diet, life-style, and mortality in China: a study of the characteristics of 65 Chinese counties*. Oxford: Oxford University Press, 1990.
75. Colditz GA. A blomathematical model of breast cancer incidence: the contribution of reproductive factors to variation in breast cancer incidence. In: Fortner JG, Sharp PA, eds. *Accomplishments in cancer research 1996*. Philadelphia: Lippincott–Raven, 1997: 116–121.
76. Harris JR, Lippman ME, Veronesi U, Willett WC. Breast cancer. *N Engl J Med* 1992;327:319–328.
77. Huang Z, Hankinson SE, Colditz GA, et al. Dual effects of weight and weight gain on breast cancer risk. *JAMA* 1997;278:1407–141
78. Fisher B, Costantino JP, Wickerham DL, et al. Tamoxifen for prevention of breast cancer. Report of the National Surgical Adjuvant Breast and Bowel Project P-1. *J Natl Cancer Inst* 1998;90:1371–1388.
79. Hankinson SE, Manson JE, London SJ, Willett WC, Speizer FE. Laboratory reproducibility of endogenous hormone levels in postmenopausal women. *Cancer Epidemiol Biomarkers Prev* 1994;3: 51–56.
80. Potischman N, Falk RT, Liaming VA, Siiteri PK, Hoover RN. Reproducibility of laboratory assays for steroid hormones and sex-hormone binding globulin. *Cancer Res* 1994;54:5363–5367.
81. Hankinson SE, Willett WC, Manson JE, et al. Plasma sex steroid hormone levels and risk of breast cancer in postmenopausal women. *J Natl Cancer Inst* 1998;90:1292–1299.
82. Toniolo PG, Levitz M, Zeleniuch-Jacquotte A, et al. A prospective study of endogenous estrogens and breast cancer in postmenopausal women. *J Natl Cancer Inst* 1995;87:190–197.
83. Toniolo P, Koenig KL, Pasternack BS, et al. Reliability of measurements of total, protein-bound, and unbound estradiol in serum and plasma. *Cancer Epidemiol Biomarkers Prev* 1994;3:47–50.
84. Hankinson SE, Manson JE, Spiegelman D, Willett WC, Longcope C, Speizer FE. Reproducibility of plasma hormone levels in postmenopausal women over a 2–3 year period. *Cancer Epidemiol Biomarkers Prev* 1995;4:649–654.
85. Micheli A, Muti P, Pisani P, et al. Repeated serum and urinary androgen measurements in premenopausal and postmenopausal women. *J Clin Epidemiol* 1991;44:1055–1061.
86. Muti P, Trevisan M, Micheli A, et al. Reliability of serum hormones in premenopausal and postmenopausal women over a one-year period. *Cancer Epidemiol Biomarkers Prev* 1996;5:917–922.
87. Roberts KD, Rochefort JG, Bleau G, Chapdelaine A. Plasma oestrone sulphate concentrations in postmenopausal women. *Steroids* 1980;35: 179–186.
88. Pasqualini JR, Chetrite G, Blacker C, et al. Concentrations of estrone, estradiol and estrone sulfate and evaluation of sulfatase and aromatase activities in pre- and postmenopausal breast cancer patients. *J Clin Endrocrinol Metab* 1996:1460–1464.
89. Thomas HV, Reeves GK, Key TJA. Endogenous estrogen and postmenopausal breast cancer: a quantitative review. *Cancer Causes Control* 1997;8:922–928.
90. Moore JW, Clark GM, Bulbrook RD, et al. Serum concentrations of total and nonprotein-bound oestradiol in patients with breast cancer and in normal controls. *Int J Cancer* 1982;29:17–21.
91. Helzlsouer KJ, Alberg AJ, Bush TL, Longcope C, Gordon GB, Comstock GW. A prospective study of endogenous hormones and breast cancer. *Cancer Detect Prev* 1994;18:79–85.
92. Thomas HV, Key TJ, Allen DS, et al. A prospective study of endogenous serum hormone concentrations and breast cancer risk in premenopausal women on the island of Guernsey. *Br J Cancer* 1997;75:1075–1079.
93. Wysowski DK, Comstock GW, Helsing KJ, Lau HL. Sex hormone levels in serum in relation to the development of breast cancer. *Am J Epidemiol* 1987;125:791–799.
94. Yager JD, Liehr JG. Molecular mechanisms of estrogen carcinogenesis. *Annu Rev Pharmacol Toxicol* 1996;136:203–232.
95. Kabat GC, Chang CJ, Sparano JA, et al. Urinary estrogen metabolites and breast cancer: a case-control study. *Cancer Epidemiol Biomarkers Prev* 1997;6:505–509.
96. Fishman J, Schneider J, Hershcopf RJ, Bradlow HL. Increased estrogen-16 alpha-hydroxylase activity in women with breast and endometrial cancer: a case-control study. *J Steroid Biochem* 1984;20:1077–1081.
97. Schneider J, Kinne D, Fracchia A, et al. Abnormal oxidative metabolism of estradiol in women with breast cancer. *Proc Natl Acad Sci U S A* 1982;79:3047–3051.
98. Zheng W, Dunning L, Jin F, Holtzman J. Urinary estrogen metabolites and breast cancer: a case-control study. *Cancer Epidemiol Biomarkers Prev* 1998:7:85–86.
99. Adlercreutz H, Fotsis T, Hockerstedt K, et al. Diet and urinary estrogen profile in premenopausal omnivorous and vegetarian women and in premenopausal women with breast cancer. *J Steroid Biochem* 1989;34:527–530.
100. Gordon GB, Shantz LM, Talalay P. Modulation of growth differentiation and carcinogenesis by dehydroepiandrosterone. *Adv Enzyme Regul* 1987;26:355–382.
101. Ebeling P, Koivisto VA. Physiological importance of dehydroepiandrosterone. *Lancet* 1994;343:1479–1481.
102. Seymbur-Munn K, Adams J. Estrogenic effects of 5-androstene-3beta, 17beta-diol at physiological concentrations and its possible implication in the etiology of breast cancer. *Endocrinology* 1983,112: 486–491.

103. Zeleniuch-Jacquotte A, Bruning PF, Bonfrer JMG, Koenig KL, Shore RE, Kim MY. Relation of serum levels of testosterone and dehydroepiandrosterone sulfate to risk of breast cancer in postmenopausal women. *Am J Epidemiol* 1997;145:1030–1038.
104. Dorgan JF, Longcope C, Stephenson HE, et al. Relation of prediagnostic serum estrogen and androgen levels to breast cancer risk. *Cancer Epidemiol Biomarkers Prev* 1996;5:533–539.
105. Berrino F, Muti P, Micheli A, et al. Serum sex hormone levels after menopause and subsequent breast cancer. *J Natl Cancer Inst* 1996:98:291–296.
106. Gordon GB, Bush TL, Helzlsouer KJ, Miller SR, Comstock GW. Relationship of serum levels of dehydroepiandrosterone and dehydroepiandrosterone sulfate to the risk of developing postmenopausal breast cancer. *Cancer Res* 1990;50:3859–3862.
107. Dorgan JF, Stanczyk FZ, Longcope C, et al. Relationship of serum dehydroepiandrosterone (DHEA), DHEA sulfite, and 5-androstene-3-beta, 17-beta-diol to risk of breast cancer in postmenopausal women. *Cancer Epidemiol Biomarkers Prev* 1997;6:177–181.
108. Helzlsouer KJ, Gordon GB, Alberg AJ, Bush TL, Comstock GW. Relationship of prediagnostic serum levels of dehydroepiandrosterone and dehydroepiandrosterone sulfate to the risk of developing premenopausal breast cancer. *Cancer Res* 1992;52:1–4.
109. Kelsey JL. A review of the epidemiology of human breast cancer. *Epidemiol Rev* 1979;1:74–109.
110. Partridge RK, Hahnel R. Prolactin receptors in human breast carcinoma. *Cancer* 1979;43:643–646.
111. Malarkey WB, Kennedy M, Allred LE, Lo G. Physiological concentrations of prolactin can promote the growth of human breast tumor cells in culture. *J Clin Endocrinol Metab* 1983;56:673–677.
112. Beedy DI, Easty GC, Gazet JC, Grigor K, Neville AM. An assessment of the effects of hormones on short term organ cultures of human breast carcinoma. *Br J Cancer* 1975; 31:317–328.
113. Herman V, Kalk WJ, de Moor NG, Levin J. Serum prolactin after chest wall surgery: elevated levels after mastectomy. *J Clin Endocrinol Metab* 1981;52:148–151.
114. Yen SSC, Jaffe RB. *Reproductive endocrinology*. Philadelphia: WB Saunders, 1991.
115. Wang DY, De Stavola BL, Bulbrook RD, et al. Relationship of blood prolactin levels and the risk of subsequent breast cancer. *Int J Epidemiol* 1992;21:214–221.
116. Hankinson SE, Willett WC, Michaud DS, et al. Plasma prolactin levels and subsequent risk of breast cancer in postmenopausal women. *J Natl Cancer Inst* 1999;91:629–634.
117. Zapf J, Froesch ER. Insulin-like growth factors; somatomedins: structure, secretion, biological actions and physiological role. *Horm Res* 1986;24:121–130.
118. Yang XF, Beamer W, Huynh HT, Pollak M. Reduced growth of human breast cancer xenografts in hosts homozygous for the lit mutation. *Cancer Res* 1996;56:1509–1511.
119. Pollak M, Costantino J, Polychronakos C, et al. Effect of tamoxifen on serum insulinlike growth factor I levels in stage I breast cancer patients. *J Natl Cancer Inst* 1990;82:1693–1697.
120. Ruan W, Newman C, Kleinberg D. Intact and amino-terminally shortened forms of insulin-like growth factor I induce mammary gland differentiation and development. *Proc Natl Acad Sci U S A* 1992;89: 10872–10876.
121. Tomell J, Carlsson B, Pohjanen P, Wennbo H, Rymo L, Isaksson OGP. High frequency of mammary adenocarcinomas in metallothionein promoter-human growth hormone transgenic mice created from two different strains of mice. *J Steroid Biochem Mol Biol* 1992;43:237–242.
122. Ng S, Zhou J, Adesanya OO, Wang J, LeRoith D, Bondy CA. Growth hormone treatment induces mammary gland hyperplasia in aging primates. *Nature (Medicine)* 1997;3:1141–1144.
123. Michels KB, Trichopoulos D, Robins JM, et al. Birthweight as a risk factor for breast cancer. *Lancet* 1996;348:1542–1546.
124. Hunter DJ, Willett WC. Diet, body size, and breast cancer. *Epidemiol Rev* 1993;15:110–132.
125. Lassarre C, Hardouin S, Daffos F, Forestier F, Frankenne F, Binoux M. Serum insulin-like growth factors and insulin-like growth factor binding proteins in the human fetus: relationships with growth in normal subjects and in subjects with intrauterine growth retardation. *Pediatr Res* 1991;29:219–225.
126. Juul A, Bang P, Hertel NT, et al. Serum insulin-like growth factor-I in 1030 healthy children, adolescents, and adults: relation to age, sex, stage of puberty, testicular size, and body mass index. *J Clin Endocrinol Metab* 1994;78:744–752.
127. Bruning PF, Van Doom J, Bonfrer JMG. Insulin-like growth-factor-binding protein 3 is decreased in early-stage operable premenopausal breast cancer. *Int J Cancer* 1995;62:266–270.
128. Peyrat JP, Bonneterre J, Hecquet B, Hondermarck H, Adenis A. Plasma IGF-I concentrations in human breast cancer. *Eur J Cancer* 1993;29a:492–497.
129. Hankinson SE, Willett WC, Colditz GA, et al. Circulating concentrations of insulin-like growth factor-I and risk of breast cancer. *Lancet* 1998;351:1393–1396.
130. Ruan W, Catanese V, Wieczorek R, Feldman M, Kleinberg DL. Estradiol enhances the stimulatory effect of insulin-like growth factor-I (IGF-I) on mammary development and growth hormone-induced IGF-I messenger ribonucleic acid. *Endocrinology* 1995:36:1296–1302.
131. Trichopoulos D. Hypothesis: does breast cancer originate in utero? *Lancet* 1990;335:939–940.
132. Ekbom A, Hsieh CC, Lipworth L, Adami HQ. Trichopoulos D. Intrauterine environment and breast cancer risk in women: a population-based study. *J Natl Cancer Inst* 1997;89:71–76.
133. Institute of Medicine, Committee on the Relationship Between Oral Contraceptives and Breast Cancer. *Oral contraceptives and breast cancer*. Washington: National Academy Press; 1991.
134. Annegers JF. Patterns of oral contraceptive use in the United States. *Br J Rheumatol* 1989;28 [Suppl 1]:48–50.
135. Thomas DB. Oral contraceptives and breast cancer: review of the epidemiologic literature. *Contraception* 1991;43:597–642.
136. Romieu I, Berlin JA, Colditz GA. Oral contraceptives and breast cancer: review and meta-analysis. *Cancer* 1990;66:2253–2263.
137. Malone KE, Daling JR, Weiss NS. Oral contraceptives in relation to breast cancer. *Epidemiol Rev* 1993;15:80–97.
138. Vessey MP, McPherson K, Villard-Mackintosh L, Yeates D. Oral contraceptives and breast cancer: latest findings in a large cohort study. *Br J Cancer* 1989;59:613–617.
139. Kay CR, Hannaford PC. Breast cancer and the pill—a further report from the Royal College of General Practitioners' oral contraception study. *Br J Cancer* 1988;58.675–680.
140. Romieu I, Willett WC, Colditz GA, et al. A prospective study of oral contraceptive use and the risk of breast cancer in women. *J Natl Cancer Inst* 1989;81:1313–21.
141. Hankinson SE, Colditz GA, Manson JE, et al. A prospective study of oral contraceptive use and risk of breast cancer (Nurses' Health Study, United States). *Cancer Causes Control* 1997;8:65–72.
142. Russo J, Gusterson BA, Rogers AE, Russo IH, Wellings SR, van Zwieten MJ. Biology of disease: comparison study of human and rat mammary tumorigenesis. *Lab Invest* 1990;62:244–278.
143. Wingo PA, Lee NC, Orv HW, Beral V, Peterson HB, Rhodes P. Age-specific differences in the relationship between oral contraceptive use and breast cancer. *Obstet Gynecol* 1991;78:161–170.
144. White E, Malone KE, Weiss NS. Breast cancer among young U.S. women in relation to oral contraceptive use. *J Natl Cancer Inst* 1994;86:505–514.
145. Collaborative Group on Hormonal Factors in Beast Cancer. Breast cancer and hormonal contraceptives: further results. *Contraception* 1996;54[Suppl]:1S–106S.
146. Stanford JL, Thomas DB. Exogenous progestin and breast cancer. *Epidemiol Rev* 1993;15:98–107.
147. WHO Collaborative Study of Neoplasia and Steroid Contraceptives. Breast cancer and depot-medroxyprogesterone acetate: a multinational study. *Lancet* 1991;338:833–838.
148. Kennedy DL, Baum C. Noncontraceptive estrogen and progestins: use patterns over time. *Obstet Gynecol* 1985,65:441–446.
149. Dupont WD, Page DL. Menopausal estrogen replacement therapy and breast cancer. *Arch Intern Med* 1991;151:67–72.
150. Steinberg KK, Thacker SB, Smith SJ, et al. A meta-analysis of the effect of estrogen replacement therapy on the risk of breast cancer. *JAMA* 1991;265:1985–1990.
151. Sillero-Arenas M, Delgado-Rodriguez M, Rodigues-Canteras R, Bueno-Cavnillas A, Galvez-Vargas R. Menopausal hormone replacement therapy and breast cancer: a metaanalysis. *Obstet Gynecol* 1992;79:286–294.
152. Colditz GA, Egan KM, Stampfer MJ. Hormone replacement therapy and risk of breast cancer: results from epidemiologic studies. *Am J Obstet Gynecol* 1993;168:1473–1480.

153. Steinberg KK, Smith SJ, Thacker SB, Stroup DF. Breast cancer risk and duration of estrogen use: the role of study design in meta-analysis. *Epidemiology* 1994;5:415–421.
154. Grady D, Rubin SM, Petitti DB, et al. Hormone therapy to prevent disease and prolong life in postmenopausal women. *Ann Intern Med* 1992;117:1016–1036.
155. Collaborative Group on Hormonal Factors in Breast Cancer. Breast cancer and hormone replacement therapy: collaborative reanalysis of data from 51 epidemiologic studies of 52,705 women with breast cancer and 108,411 women without breast cancer. *Lancet* 1997;350:1047–1059.
156. Newcomb PA, Longnecker MP, Storer BE, et al. Long-term hormone replacement therapy and risk of breast cancer in postmenopausal women. *Am J Epidemiol* 1995;332:1589–1593.
157. Stanford JL, Weiss NS, Voigt LF, Daling JR, Habel LA, Rossing MA. Combined estrogen and progestin hormone replacement therapy in relation to risk of breast cancer in middle-aged women. *JAMA* 1995;274:137–142.
158. Egeland GM, Matthews KA, Kuller LH, Kelsey SF. Characteristics of noncontraceptive hormone users. *Prev Med* 1988;17:403–411.
159. Colditz GA, Hankinson SE, Hunter DJ, et al. The use of estrogens and progestins and the risk of breast cancer in postmenopausal women. *N Engl J Med* 1995;332:1589–1593.
160. Colditz GA, Willett WC, Speizer FE. The use of estrogens and progestins and the risk of breast cancer in postmenopausal women [Letter to the Editor, errata]. *N Engl J Med* 1995;333:1357–1358.
161. Schairer C, Byme C, Keyl PM, Brinton LA, Sturgeon SR, Hoover RN. Menopausal estrogen and estrogen-progestin replacement therapy and risk of breast cancer (United States). *Cancer Causes Control* 1994;5:491–500.
162. Hemminki E, Kennedy DL, Baum C, McKinlay SM. Prescribing of noncontraceptive estrogens and progestins in the United States, 1974–1986. *Am J Public Health* 1988;78:1479–1481.
163. Gambrell RD Jr, Maier RC, Sanders BI. Decreased incidence of breast cancer in postmenopausal estrogen-progestogen users. *Obstet Gynecol* 1983;62:435–443.
164. Nachtigall LE, Nachtigall RH, Nachtigall RD, Beckman EM. Estrogen replacement therapy, II: a prospective study in the relationship to carcinoma and cardiovascular and metabolic problems. *Obstet Gynecol* 1979;54:74–79.
165. Bergkvist L, Adami HO, Persson I, Hoover R, Schairer C. The risk of breast cancer after estrogen and estrogen-progestin replacement. *N Engl J Med* 1989;321:293–297.
166. Colditz GA, Stampfer MJ, Willett WC, Hennekens CH, Rosner B, Speizer FE. Prospective study of estrogen replacement therapy and risk of breast cancer in postmenopausal women. *JAMA* 1990;264: 2648–2653.
167. Colditz GA, Rosner B (for the Nurses' Health Study Research Group). Use of estrogen plus progestin is associated with greater increase in breast cancer risk than estrogen alone. *Am J Epidemiol* 1998;147[Suppl]:648.
168. Colditz GA, Willett WC, Hunter DJ, et al. Family history, age, and risk of breast cancer. *JAMA* 1993;270:338–343.
169. Lin HJ, Han C-Y, Lin BK, Hardy S. Slow acetylator mutations in the human polymorphic N-acetyltransferase gene in 786 Asians, blacks, Hispanics, and whites: application to metabolic epidemiology. *Am J Hum Genet* 1993;52:827–834.
170. Ambrosone CB, Freudenheim JL, Graham S, et al. Cigarette smoking, N-acetyltransferase 2, genetic polymorphisms, and breast cancer risk. *JAMA* 1996;276:1494–1501.
171. Hunter DJ, Hankinson SE, Hough H, et al. A prospective study of NAT2 acetylation genotype, cigarette smoking, and risk of breast cancer. *Carcinogenesis* 1997;18:2127–2132.
172. Millikan RC, Pittman GS, Newman B, et al. Cigarette smoking, N-acetyltransferases 1 and 2, and breast cancer risk. *Cancer Epidemiol Biomarkers Prev* 1998;7:371–378.
173. Ambrosone CB, Freudenheim JL, Sinha R, et al. Breast cancer risk, meat consumption and N-acetyltransferase (NAT2) genetic polymorphisms. *Int J Cancer* 1998;75:825–830.
174. Gertig DM, Hankinson S, Hough H, et al. N-acetyltransferase 2 genotypes, meat intake and breast cancer risk. *Int J Cancer* 1999;80:13–17.
175. Rebbeck TR, Rosvold EA, Duggan DJ, Zhang J, Buetow KH. Genetics of CYP1A1: coamplification of specific alleles by polymerase chain reaction and association with breast cancer. *Cancer Epidemiol Biomarkers Prev* 1994,3:511–514.
176. Ambrosone CB, Freudenheim JL, Graham S, et al. Cytochrome P4501A1 and glutathione S-transferase (M1) genetic polymorphisms and postmenopausal breast cancer risk. *Cancer Res* 1995;55: 3483–3485.
177. Ishibe N, Hankinson SE, Colditz GA, et al. Cigarette smoking, cytochrome P450 1A1 polymorphisms, and breast cancer risk in the Nurses' Health Study. *Cancer Res* 1998;58:667–671.
178. Bailey LR, Roodi N, Verrier CS, Yee CJ, Dupont WD, Parl FF. Breast cancer and CYP1A1, GSTM1, and GSTT1 polymorphisms: evidence of a lack of association in Caucasians and African-Americans. *Cancer Res* 1999:58:65–70.
179. Kelsey KT, Hankinson SE, Colditz GA, et al. Glutathione S-transferase class mu deletion polymorphism and breast cancer: results from prevalent versus incident cases. *Cancer Epidemiol Biomarkers Prev* 1997;6:511–51.
180. Maugard CM, Charrier J, Bignon YJ. Allelic detection at glutathione S-transferase M1 locus and its association with breast cancer susceptibility. *Chem Biol Interact* 1998;111–112:365–375.
181. Helzlsouer KJ, Selmin O, Huang HY, et al. Association between glutathione S-transferase M1, P1, and T1 genetic polymorphisms and development of breast cancer. *J Natl Cancer Inst* 1998;90:512–518.
182. Feigelson HS, Ross RK, Yu MC, Coetzee GA, Reichardt JK, Henderson BE. Genetic susceptibility to cancer from exogenous and endogenous exposures. *J Cell Biochem* 1996;25S:15–22.
183. Feigelson HS, Coetzee GA, Kolenel LN, Ross RK. Henderson BE. A polymorphism in the CYP17 gene increases the risk of breast cancer. *Cancer Res* 1997;57:1063–1065.
184. Dunning AM, Healey CS, Pharoah PD, et al. No association between a polymorphism in the steroid metabolism gene CYP17 and risk of breast cancer. *Br J Cancer* 1998;77:2045–2047.
185. Helzlsouer KJ, Huang HY, Strickland PT, et al. Association between CYP17 polymorphisms and the development of breast cancer. *Cancer Epidemiol Biomarkers Prev* 1998;7:945–949.
186. Weston A, Pan C, Bleiweiss IJ, et al. CYP17 genotype and breast cancer risk. *Cancer Epidemiol Biomarkers Prev* 1998;7:941–944.
187. Lavigne JA, Helzlsouer KJ, Huang HY, et al. An association between the allele coding for a low activity variant of catechol-O-methyltransferase and the risk for breast cancer. *Cancer Res* 1997;57:5493–5497.
188. Thompson PA, Shields PG, Freudenheim JL, et al. Genetic polymorphisms in catechol-O-methyltransferase, menopausal status, and breast cancer risk. *Cancer Res* 1998;58:2107–2110.
189. Kristensen VN, Andersen TI, Lindblom A, Erikstein B, Magnus P, Borresen-Dale AL. A rare CYP19 (aromatase) variant may increase the risk of breast cancer. *Pharmacogenetics* 1998;8:43–48.
190. Krontiris TG, Karp DD, Robert NJ, Risch N. An association between the risk of cancer and mutations in the HRAS1 minisatellite locus. *N Engl J Med* 1993;329:517–523.
191. Garrett PA, Hulka BS, Kim YL, Farber RA. HRAS protooncogene polymorphism and breast cancer. *Cancer Epidemiol Biomarkers Prev* 1993;2:131–138.
192. Swift M, Morrell D, Massey RB, Chase CL. Incidence of cancer in 161 families affected by ataxia-telangiectasia. *N Engl J Med* 1991;26:1831–1836.
193. FitzGerald MG, Bean JM, Hegde SR, et al. Heterozygous ATM mutations do not contribute to early onset of breast cancer. *Nat Genet* 1997;15:307–310.
194. Albanes D. Total calories, body weight, and tumor incidence in mice. *Cancer Res* 1987;47:1987–92.
195. Freedman LS, Clifford C, Messina M. Analysis of dietary fat, calories, body weight, and the development of mammary tumors in rats and mice: a review. *Cancer Res* 1990;50:5710–5719.
196. Ip C. Quantitative assessment of fat and calorie as risk factors in mammary carcinogenesis in an experimental model. In: Mettlin CJ, Aoki K, eds. *Recent progress in research on nutrition and cancer: proceedings of a workshop sponsored by the International Union Against Cancer, held in Nagoya, Japan, November 1–3, 1989*. New York: Wiley-Liss, 1990:107–117.
197. Beth M, Berger MR, Aksoy M, Schmahl D. Comparison between the effects of dietary fat level and of calorie intake on methylnitrosourea-induced mammary carcinogenesis in female SD-rats. *Int J Cancer* 1987;39:737–744.
198. Appleton BS, Landers RE. Oil gavage effects on tumor incidence in the National Toxicology Program's 2-year carcinogenesis bioassay. *Adv Exp Med Biol* 1986;206:99–104.

199. Sonnenschein E, Glickman L, Goldschmidt M, McKee L. Body conformation, diet, and risk of breast cancer in pet dogs: a case-control study. *Am J Epidemiol* 1991;133:694–703.
200. Armstrong B, Doll R. Environmental factors and cancer incidence and mortality in different countries, with special references to dietary practices. *Int J Cancer* 1975;15:617–631.
201. Prentice RL, Kakar F, Hursting S, Sheppard L, Klein R, Kushi LH. Aspects of the rationale for the Women's Health Trial. *J Natl Cancer Inst* 1988;80:802–814.
202. Tretli S, Gaard M. Lifestyle changes during adolescence and risk of breast cancer: an ecologic study of the effect of World War II in Norway. *Cancer Causes Control* 1996;7:507–512.
203. Phillips RL, Garfinkel L, Kuzma JW, Beeson WL, Lotz T, Brin B. Mortality among California Seventh-Day Adventists for selected cancer sites. *J Natl Cancer Inst* 1980;65:1097–1107.
204. Kinlen LJ. Meat and fat consumption and cancer mortality: a study of strict religious orders in Britain. *Lancet* 1982;1:946–949.
205. Graham S, Marshall J, Mettlin C, Rzepka T, Nemoto T, Byers T. Diet in the epidemiology of breast cancer. *Am J Epidemiol* 1982;116:68–75.
206. Howe GR, Hirohata T, Hislop TG, et al. Dietary N factors and risk of breast cancer: combined analysis of 12 case-control studies. *J Natl Cancer Inst* 1990;82:561–569.
207. Giovannucci E, Stampfer MJ, Colditz GA, et al. A comparlson of prospective and retrospective assessments of diet in the study of breast cancer. *Am J Epidemiol* 1993;137:502–511.
208. Hunter DJ, Spiegelman D, Adami HO, et al. Cohort studies of fat intake and the risk of breast cancer: a pooled analysis. *N Engl J Med* 1996;334:356–361.
209. Prentice RL. Measurement error and results from analytic epidemiology: dietary fat and breast cancer. *J Natl Cancer Inst* 1996;88: 1738–1747.
210. Holmes MD, Hunter DJ, Stampfer MJ, et al. Types of dietary fat and the risk of breast cancer. *Am J Epidemiol* 1998;147[Suppl]:S88.
211. Freedman LS, Prentice RL, Clifford C, et al. Dietary fat and breast cancer: where we are. *J Natl Cancer Inst* 1993;85:764–765.
212. Cohen LA, Kendall ME, Zang E, Meschter C, Rose DP. Modulation of N-nitrosomethylurea-induced mammary tumor promotion by dietary fiber and fat. *J Natl Cancer Inst* 1991;83:496–501.
213. Martin-Moreno JM, Willett WC, Gorgojo L, et al. Dietary fat, olive oil intake and breast cancer risk. *Int J Cancer* 1994;58:774–780.
214. Willett WC. Specific fatty acids and risks of breast and prostate cancer: dietary intake. *Am J Clin Nutr* 1997;66[Suppl]:1557s–1563s.
215. Micozzi MS. Nutrition, body size, and breast cancer. *Yearbook of Physical Anthropology* 1985;28:175–206.
216. Swanson CA, Jones DY, Schatzkin A, Brinton LA, Ziegler RG. Breast cancer risk assessed by anthropometry in the NHANES I epidemiological follow-up study. *Cancer Res* 1988;48:5363–5367.
217. London SJ, Colditz GA, Stampfer MJ, Willett WC, Rosner B, Speizer FE. Prospective study of relative weight, height and the risk of breast cancer. *JAMA* 1989;262:2853–2858.
218. Vatten LJ, Kvinnsland S. Body height and risk of breast cancer: a prospective study of 23,831 Norwegian women. *Br J Cancer* 1990; 61:881–885.
219. Vatten LJ, Kvinnsland S. Prospective study of height, body mass index and risk of breast cancer. *Acta Oncol* 1992;31:195–200.
220. Meyer F, Moisan J, Marcoux D, Bouchard C. Dietary and physical determinants of menarche. *Epidemiology* 1990;1:377–81.
221. Maclure M, Travis LB, Willett WC, MacMahon B. A prospective cohort study of nutrient intake and age at menarche. *Am J Clin Nutr* 1991;54:649–656.
222. Merzenich H, Boeing H, Wahrendorf J. Dietary fat and sports activity as determinants for age at menarche. *Am J Epidemiol* 1993;138: 217–224.
223. Kelsey JL, Horn-Ross PL. Introduction: magnitude of the problem and descriptive epidemiology. *Epidemiol Rev* 1993;15:7–16.
224. Trichopoulos D, Lipman R. Mammary gland mass and breast cancer risk. *Epidemiology* 1992;3:523–526.
225. Dunn SE, Kari FW, French J, et al. Dietary restriction reduces insulin-like growth factor I levels, which modulates apoptosis, cell proliferation, and tumor progression in p53-deficient mice. *Cancer Res* 1997; 57:4667–4672.
226. Ursin G, Longnecker MP, Halies RW, Greenland S. A meta-analysis of body mass index and risk of premenopausal breast cancer epidemiology. *Epidemiology* 1995;6:137–141.
227. Rich-Edwards JW, Goldman MB, Willett WC, et al. Adolescent body mass index and ovulatory infertility. *Am J Obstet Gynecol* 1994;171:171–177.
228. Hankinson SE, Willett WC, Manson JE, et al. Alcohol, height, and adiposity in relation to estrogen and prolactin levels in postmenopausal women. *J Natl Cancer Inst* 1995;87:1297–1302.
229. Bames-Josiah D, Potter JD, Sellers TA, Himes JH. Early body size and subsequent weight gain as predictors of breast cancer incidence (Iowa, United States). *Cancer Causes Control* 1995;6:112–118.
230. Ziegler RG, Hoover RN, Nomura AMY, et al. Relative weight, weight change, height, and breast cancer risk in Asian-American women. *J Natl Cancer Inst* 1996;88:650–660.
231. Le Marchand L, Kolonel LN, Earle ME, Mi MP. Body size at different periods of life and breast cancer risk. *Am J Epidemiol* 1988;128:137–152.
232. Pathak DR, Whittemore AS. Combined effects of body size, parity, and menstrual events on breast cancer incidence in seven countries. *Am J Epidemiol* 1992;135:153–168.
233. Rohan TE, Howe GR, Friedenreich CM, Jain M, Miller AB. Dietary fiber, vitamins A, C, and E, and risk of breast cancer: a cohort study. *Cancer Causes Control* 1993;4:29–37.
234. Graham S, Zielezny M, Marshall J, et al. Diet in the epidemiology of postmenopausal breast cancer in the New York State cohort. *Am J Epidemiol* 1992;136:1327–1337.
235. Willett WC, Hunter DJ, Stampfer MJ, et al. Dietary fat and fiber in relation to risk of breast cancer: an 8-year follow-up. *JAMA* 1992;68: 2037–2044.
236. Fraker LD, Halter SA, Forbes JT. Growth inhibition by retinol of a human breast carcinoma cell line in vitro and in athymic mice. *Cancer Res* 1984;44:5757–5763.
237. Moon RC, McCormick DL, Mehta RG. Inhibition of carcinogenesis by retinoids. *Cancer Res* 1983;43:2469.
238. Freudenheim JL, Marshall JR, Vena JE, et al. Premenopausal breast cancer risk and intake of vegetables, fruits, and related nutrients. *J Natl Cancer Inst* 1996;88:340–348.
239. Zhang S, Hunter DJ, Forman MR, et al. Dietary carotenoids and vitamins A, C, and E and risk of breast cancer. *J Natl Cancer Inst* 1999; 91:547–556.
240. American Institute for Cancer Research, World Cancer Research Fund. Food, nutrition and the prevention of cancer: a global perspective. Washington: American Institute for Cancer Research; 1997.
241. King MM, McCay PB. Modulation of tumor incidence and possible mechanism of mammary carcinogenesis by dietary antioxidants. *Cancer Res* 1981;43:2485s.
242. Verhoeven DTH, Assen N, Goldbohm RA, et al. Vitamins C and E, retinol, beta-carotene and dietary fiber in relation to breast cancer risk: a prospective cohort study. *Br J Cancer* 1997;75:149–155.
243. Abdul-Hajj YJ, Kelliher M. Failure of ascorbic acid to inhibit growth of transplantable and dimethylbenzanthracene induced rat mammary tumors. *Cancer Lett* 1982;17:67–73.
244. Graham S, Hellmann R, Marshall J, et al. Nutritional epidemiology of postmenopausal breast cancer in western New York. *Am J Epidemiol* 1991;134:552–566.
245. Kushi LH, Fee RM, Sellers TA, Zheng W, Folsom AR. Intake of vitamin A, C, and E and postmenopausal breast cancer. *Am J Epidemiol* 1996;144:165–174.
246. Ip C. The chemopreventive role of selenium in carcinogenesis. *J Am Coll Toxicol* 1986;5:7–20.
247. Clark LC. The epidemiology of selenium and cancer. *Fed Proc* 1985;44:2584–2589.
248. Hunter DJ. Biochemical indicators of dietary intake. In: Willett WC, ed. *Nutritional epidemiology*. New York: Oxford University Press, 1990:143–216.
249. Meyer F, Verreault R. Erythrocyte selenium and breast cancer risk. *Am J Epidemiol* 1987;125:917–919.
250. Hunter DJ, Morris JS, Stampfer MJ, Colditz GA, Speizer FE, Willett WC. A prospective study of selenium status and breast cancer risk. *JAMA* 1990;264:1128–1131.
251. Knekt P, Aromaa A, Maatela J, et al. Serum vitamin A and the subsequent risk of cancer: cancer incidence follow-up of the Finnish Mobile Clinic Health Examination Survey. *Am J Epidemiol* 1990;132:857–870.
252. Clark LC, Combs GF Jr, Turnbull BW, et al. Effects of selenium supplementation for cancer prevention in patients with carcinoma of the

skin. A randomized controlled trial. Nutritional Prevention of Cancer Study Group. *JAMA* 1996;276:1957–1963.
253. Longnecker MP. Alcoholic beverage consumption in relation to risk of breast cancer: meta-analysis and review. *Cancer Causes Control* 1994;5:73–82.
254. Smith-Warner SA, Spiegelman D, Yaun S-S, et al. Alcohol and breast cancer in women: a pooled analysis of cohort studies. *JAMA* 1998; 279:535–540.
255. Harvey EB, Schairer C, Brinton LA, Hoover RN, Fraumeni JF Jr. Alcohol consumption and breast cancer. *J Natl Cancer Inst* 1987;78:657–661.
256. Longnecker MP, Newcomb PA, Mittendorf R, et al. Risk of breast cancer in relation to lifetime alcohol consumption. *J Natl Cancer Inst* 1995:87:923–929.
257. Reichman ME, Judd JT, Longcope C, et al. Effects of alcohol consumption on plasma and urinary hormone concentrations in premenopausal women. *J Natl Cancer Inst* 1993;85:722–727.
258. Ginsburg ES, Walsh BW, Gao XP, Gleason RE, Feltmate C, Barbieri RL. The effect of acute ethanol ingestion on estrogen levels in postmenopausal women using transdermal estradiol. *J Soc Gynecol Invest* 1995;2:26–29.
259. Fuchs CS, Stampfer MJ, Colditz GA, et al. Alcohol consumption and mortality among women. *N Engl J Med* 1995;332:1245–1250.
260. Snowden DA, Phillips RL. Coffee consumption and the risk of fatal cancers. *Am J Public Health* 1984;74:820–823.
261. Folsom AR, McKenzie DR, Bisgard KM, Kushi LH, Sellers TA. No association between caffeine intake and postmenopausal breast cancer incidence in the Iowa Women's Health Study. *Am J Epidemiol* 1993;138:380–383.
262. Vatten LJ, Solvoll K, Loken EB. Coffee consumption and the risk of breast cancer: a prospective study of 14,593 Norwegian women. *Br J Cancer* 1990;62:267–270.
263. Hunter DJ, Manson JE, Stampfer MJ, et al. A prospective study of caffeine, coffee, tea, and breast cancer [Abstract]. *Am J Epidemiol* 1992;136:1000–1001.
264. Steinmetz KA, Potter JD. Vegetables, fruit, and cancer. II. Mechanisms. *Cancer Causes Control* 1991;2:427–442.
265. Cassidy A, Bingham S, Carlson J, Setchell KD. Biological effects of plant estrogens in premenopausal women [Abstract]. *FASEB J* 1993;7:A866.
266. Lee HP, Gourley L, Duffy SW, Esteve J, Lee J, Day NE. Dietary effects on breast cancer risk in Singapore. *Lancet* 1991;337:1197–1200.
267. Yuan J-M, Yu MC, Ross RK, et al. Risk factors for breast cancer in Chinese women in Shanghai. *Cancer Res* 1988;48:1949–1953.
268. Toniolo P, Riboll E, Shore RE, Pasternack BS. Consumption of meat, animal products, protein, and fat and risk of breast cancer—a prospective cohort study in New York. *Epidemiology* 1994;5:391–397.
269. Holmes M, Hunter DJ, Willett WC. Dietary guidelines. In: Stoll BA, ed. *Reducing breast cancer risk in women*, vol. 75. Boston: Kluwer Academic, 1995:248.
270. Newman SC, Miller AB, Howe GR. A study of the effect of weight and dietary fat on breast cancer survival time. *Am J Epidemiol* 1986;123:767–774.
271. Holmes MD, Stampfer MJ, Rosner B, Hunter DJ, Willett WC, Colditz GA. Dietary factors affecting survival of women with breast cancer [Abstract]. *Am J Epidemiol* 1997;145[Suppl]:S46.
272. Chlebowski RT, Nixon DW, Blackburn GL, et al. A breast cancer nutrition adjuvant study (NAS): protocol design and initial patient adherence. *Breast Cancer Res Treat* 1987;10:21.
273. Malina R, Spirduso E, Tate C, Baylor A. Age at menarche and selected menstrual characteristics in athletes at different competitive levels and in different sports. *Med Sci Sports Exerc* 1978,10:218–222.
274. Frisch RE, Wyshak G, Vincent L. Delayed menarche and amenorrhea in ballet dancers. *N Engl J Med* 1980;303:17–19.
275. Frisch RE, Gotz–Welbergen AV, McArthur JW, et al. Delayed menarche and amenorrhea of college athletes in relation to age of onset of training. *JAMA* 1981;246:1559–1563.
276. Apter D, Vihko R. Early menarche, a risk factor for breast cancer, indicates early onset of ovulatory cycles. *J Clin Endocrinol Metab* 1983;57:82–86.
277. Bernstein L, Ross R, Lobo R, Hanisch R, Krailo M, Henderson B. The effects of moderate physical activity on menstrual cycle patterns in adolescence: implications for breast cancer prevention. *Br J Cancer* 1987;55:681–685.
278. Harlow S, Matanoski G. The association between weight, physical activity and stress and variation in the length of the menstrual cycle. *Am J Epidemiol* 1991;133:38–49.
279. Cumming D, Wheeler G, Harber V. Physical activity, nutrition, and reproduction. *Ann N Y Acad Sci* 1994;709:55–76.
280. Broocks A, Pirke KM, Schweiger U, et al. Cyclic ovarian function in recreational athletes. *J Appl Physiol* 1990;68:2083–2086.
281. Feicht CB, Johnson TS, Martin BJ, Sparkes KE, Wagner WW Jr. Secondary amenorrhoea in athletes [Letter]. *Lancet* 1978;2:1145–1146.
282. Builen BA, Skrinar GS, Beitins IZ, von Mering G, Turnbull BA, McArthur JW. Induction of menstrual disorders by strenuous exercise in untrained women. *N Engl J Med* 1985;312:1349–1353.
283. Russell JB, Mitchell D, Musey PI, Collins DC. The relationship of exercise to anovulatory cycles in female athletes: hormonal and physical characteristics. *Obstet Gynecol* 1984;63:452–456.
284. Siiteri PK. Adipose tissue as a source of hormones. *Am J Clin Nutr* 1987;45[Suppl]:277–282.
285. Cauley JA, Gutai JP, Kuller LH, LeDonne D, Powell JG. The epidemiology of serum sex hormones in postmenopausal women. *Am J Epidemiol* 1989;129:1120–1131.
286. Brinton L, Bernstein L, Colditz G. Summary of workshop on physical activity and breast cancer, November 13–14, 1997. *Cancer* 1998;83[Suppl]:595–599.
287. Bernstein L, Henderson BE, Hanisch R, Sullivan-Hailey J, Ross RK. Physical exercise and reduced risk of breast cancer in young women. *J Natl Cancer Inst* 1994;86:1403–1408.
288. Thune I, Brenn T, Lund E, Gaard M. Physical activity and the risk of breast cancer. *N Engl J Med* 1997;336:1269–1275.
289. Rockhill B, Willett WC, Hunter DJ, et al. Physical activity and breast cancer risk in a cohort of young women. *J Natl Cancer Inst* 1998;90:1155–1160.
290. Dorgan JF, Brown C, Barrett M, et al. Physical activity and risk of breast cancer in the Framingham heart study. *Am J Epidemiol* 1994;139:662–669.
291. Paffenbarger RS Jr, Lee I-M, Wing AL. The influence of physical activity on the incidence of site-specific cancers in college alumni. In: Jacobs MM, ed. *Exercise, calories, fat and cancer*. New York: Plenum, 1992;7–15.
292. Albanes D, Blair A, Taylor PR. Physical activity and risk of cancer in the NHANES I population. *Am J Public Health* 1989;79:744–750.
293. Chen CL, White E, Malone KE, Daling JR. Leisure-time physical activity in relation to breast cancer among young women (Washington, United States). *Cancer Causes Control* 1997;8:77–84.
294. Gammon MD, Schoenberg JB, Britton JA. Recreational physical activity and breast cancer risk among women under age 45 years. *Am J Epidemiol* 1998;147:273–280.
295. Gammon MD, John EM, Britton JA. Recreational and occupational physical activities and risk of breast cancer. *J Natl Cancer Inst* 1998;90:100–117.
296. Tokunaga M, Land C, Tokuoka S, Nishimori I, Soda M, Akiba S. Incidence of female breast cancer among atomic bomb survivors 1950–1985. *Radiat Res* 1994;138:209–223.
297. Miller AB, Howe GR, Sherman GJ, et al. Mortality from breast cancer after irradiation during fluoroscopic examinations in patients being treated for tuberculosis. *N Engl J Med* 1989;321: 1285–1289.
298. Hancock S, Tucker M, Hoppe R. Breast cancer after treatment of Hodgkin's disease. *J Natl Cancer Inst* 1993;85:25–31.
299. Boice J, Harvey E, Blettner M, Stovall M, Flannery J. Cancer in the contralateral breast after radiotherapy for breast cancer. *N Engl J Med* 1992;326:781–785.
300. Colditz G, Frazier A. Models of breast cancer show that risk is set by events of early life: prevention efforts must shift focus. *Cancer Epidemiol Biomarkers Prev* 1995;4:567–571.
301. Evans J, Wennberg J, McNeil B. The influence of diagnostic radiography on the incidence of breast cancer and leukemia. *N Engl J Med* 1986;315:810–815.
302. Adami H-O, Lipworth L, Titus-Ernstoff L, et al. Organochlorine compounds and estrogen-related cancers in women. *Cancer Causes Control* 1995;6:551–566.
303. Laden F, Hunter DJ. Environmental risk factors and female breast cancer. *Annu Rev Public Health* 1998;19:101–123.
304. Westin JB, Richter E. The Israeli Breast-Cancer Anomaly. *Ann N Y Acad Sci* 1990;609:269–276.

305. Shames LS, Munekata MT, Pike MC. Re: Blood levels of organochlorine residues and risk of breast cancer [Correspondence]. *J Natl Cancer Inst* 1994;86:1642–1643.
306. Rylander L, Hagmar L. Mortality and cancer incidence among women with a high consumption of fatty fish contaminated with persistent organochloride compounds. *Scand J Work Environ Health* 1995; 21:419–426.
307. Bertazzi PA, Pesatori AC, Consonni D, Tironi A, Landi MT, Zocchetti C. Cancer incidence in a population accidentally exposed to 2,3,7,8-tetrachlorodibenzo-para-dioxin. *Epidemiology* 1993;4:398–406.
308. Manz A, Berger J, Dwyer JH, Flesch-Janys D, Nagel S, Waltsgott H. Cancer mortality among workers in a chemical plant contaminated with dioxin. *Lancet* 1991;338:959–964.
309. van't Veer P, Lobbezoo IE, Martin-Moreno JM, et al. DDT (dicophane) and postmenopausal breast cancer in Europe: case-control study. *BMJ* 1997;315:81–85.
310. Moysich KB, Ambrosone CB, Vena JE, et al. Environmental organochlorine exposure and postmenopausal breast cancer risk. *Cancer Epidemiol Biomarkers Prev* 1998;7:181–188.
311. Lopez-Carrillo L, Blair A, Lopez-Cervantes M, et al. DDT serum levels and breast cancer risk: a case-control study from Mexico [Abstract]. *Epidemiology* 1997;8:S24.
312. Hardell L, Lindstrom G, Liljegren G, Dahl P, Magnuson A. Increased concentrations of octachlorodibenzo-p-dioxin in cases with breast cancer—results from a case-control study. *Eur J Cancer Prev* 1996;5: 351–357.
313. Krieger N, Wolff MS, Hiatt RA, Rivera M, Vogelman J, Orentrelch N. Breast cancer and serum organochlorines: a prospective study among white, black, and Asian women. *J Natl Cancer Inst* 1994;86:589–599.
314. Wolff MS, Toniolo PG, Lee EW, Rivera M, Dubin N. Blood levels of organochlorine residues and risk of breast cancer. *J Natl Cancer Inst* 1993;85:648–652.
315. Hunter DJ, Hankinson SE, Laden F, et al. Plasma organochlorine levels and the risk of breast cancer. *N Engl J Med* 1997;337:1253–1258.
316. Hahn RA. Profound bilateral blindness and the incidence of breast cancer. *Epidemiology* 1991;2:208–210.
317. Feychting M, Osterlund B, Ahlbom A. Reduced cancer incidence among the blind. *Epidemiology* 1998;9:490–494.
318. Wertheimer N, Leeper E. Magnetic field exposure related to cancer subtypes. *Ann N Y Acad Sci* 1987;502:43–54.
319. Vena JE, Graham S, Hellmann R, Swanson M, Brasure J. Use of electric blankets and risk of postmenopausal breast cancer. *Am J Epidemiol* 1991;134:180–185.
320. Vena JE, Freudenheim JL, Marshall JR, Laughlin R, Swanson M, Graham S. Risk of premenopausal breast cancer and use of electric blankets. *Am J Epidemiol* 1994;140:974–979.
321. Gammon MD, Schoenberg JB, Britton JA, et al. Electric blanket use and breast cancer risk among younger women. *Am J Epidemiol* 1998;148:556–563.
322. Palmer JR, Rosenberg L, Clarke EA, et al. Breast cancer and cigarette smoking: a hypothesis. *Am J Epidemiol* 1991;134:1–13.
323. Baron JA, Newcomb PA, Longnecker MP, et al. Cigarette smoking and breast cancer. *Cancer Epidemiol Biomarkers Prev* 1996;5:399–403.
324. Hirayama T. Cancer mortality in nonsmoking women with smoking husbands based on a large-scale cohort study in Japan. *Prev Med* 1984;13:680–690.
325. Wells AJ. Breast cancer, cigarette smoking, and passive smoking. *Am J Epidemiol* 1991;133:208–210.
326. Brinton LA, Brown SL. Breast implants and cancer. *J Natl Cancer Inst* 1997;89:1341–1349.
327. Deapen DM, Bernstein L, Brody GS. Are breast implants anticarcinogenic? A 14-year follow-up of the Los Angeles Study. *Plast Reconstr Surg* 1997;99:1346–1353.
328. Brinton LA, Malone KE, Coates RJ, et al. Breast enlargement and reduction: results from a breast cancer case-control study. *Plast Reconstr Surg* 1996;97:269–275.
329. Bryant H, Brasher P. Breast implants and breast cancer—reanalysis of a linkage study. *N Engl J Med* 1995;332:1535–1539.
330. Goldberg M, Labreche F. Occupational risk factors for female breast cancer: a review. *Occup Environ Med* 1996;53:145–156.
331. Calle E, Murphy T, Rodriguez C, Thun M, Heath C. Occupation and breast cancer mortality in a prospective cohort of US women. *Am J Epidemiol* 1998;148:191–197.
332. Talamini R, Franceschi S, Favero A, Negri E, Parazzini F, La Vecchia C. Selected medical conditions and risk of breast cancer. *Br J Cancer* 1997;75:1699–1703.
333. Freiss G, Prebois C, Rochefort H, Vignon F, Anti-steroidal and anti-growth factor activities of anti-estrogens. *J Steroid Biochem* 1990;37:777–791.
334. Bruning P, Bonfrer J, van Noord P, Hart A, DeJong-Baker M, Nooijen W. Insulin resistance and breast cancer risk. *Int J Cancer* 1992;52:511–516.
335. Rosenberg L, Palmer J, Zauber A, Warshauer M, Stolley P, Shapiro S. A hypothesis: nonsteroidal anti-inflammatory drugs reduce the incidence of large-bowel cancer. *J Natl Cancer Inst* 1991;83:355–358.
336. Giovannucci E, Egan KM, Hunter DJ, et al. Aspirin and the risk of colorectal cancer in women. *N Engl J Med* 1995;333:609–614.
337. Rosenberg L. Aspirin and breast cancer: no surprises yet. *J Natl Cancer Inst* 1996;88:941–942.
338. Polednak A, Janerich D. Characteristics of first pregnancy in relation to early breast cancer: a case-control study. *J Reproduct Med* 1983;28:314–318.
339. Thompson W, Jacobson H, Negrini B, Janerich D. Hypertension, pregnancy, and risk of breast cancer. *J Natl Cancer Inst* 1989;81:1571–1574.
340. Pacheco-Sanchez M, Grunewald KK. Body fat deposition: effects of dietary fat and two exercise protocols. *J Am Coll Nutr* 1994;13:601–607.
341. Polednak A. Pre-eclampsia, autoimmune diseases and breast cancer etiology. *Med Hypotheses* 1995;44:414–418.
342. Wallace R, Sherman B, Bean J. A case-control study of breast cancer and psychotropic drug use. *Oncology* 1982;39:279–283.
343. Schottenfeld D, Fraumeni JF Jr. *Cancer epidemiology and prevention.* New York: Oxford University Press, 1996:1521.
344. Ames BN, Gold LS, Willett WC. The causes and prevention of cancer. *Proc Natl Acad Sci U S A* 1995;92:5258–5265.
345. Davis DL, Bradlow HL. Can environmental estrogens cause breast cancer? *Sci Am* 1995;273:166–172.
346. Madigan MP, Ziegler RG, Benichou J, Byrne C, Hoover RN. Proportion of breast cancer cases in the United States explained by well-established risk factors. *J Natl Cancer Inst* 1995;87:1681–1685.
347. White E. Projected changes in breast cancer incidence due to the trend toward delayed childbearing. *Am J Public Health* 1987;77:495–497.
348. Gail MH, Brinton LA, Byar DP, et al. Projecting individualized probabilities of developing breast cancer for white females who are being examined annually. *J Natl Cancer Inst* 1989;81:1879–1886.
349. Lerman C, Lustbader E, Rimer B, et al. Effects of individualized breast cancer risk counseling: a randomized trial. *J Natl Cancer Inst* 1995;87:286–292.
350. Schwartz LM, Woloshin S, Black WC, Welch HG. The role of numeracy in understanding the benefit of screening mammography. *Ann Intern Med* 1997;127:966–972.
351. Rose G. Strategy of prevention: lessons from cardiovascular disease. *BMJ* 1981;282:1847–1851.
352. Mosian J, Meyer F, Gingras S. Leisure, physical activity and age at menarche. *Med Sci Sports Exerc* 1991;23(10):1170–1175.
353. Gortmaker SL, Dietz WH, Cheung LW. Inactivity, diet, and the fattening of America. *J Am Diet Assoc* 1990:90:1247–1252.
354. Freed GL, Clark SJ, Sorensen J, Lohr JA, Celalo R, Curtis P. National assessment of physicians' breastfeeding knowledge, attitudes, training, and experience. *JAMA* 1995;273:472–476.
355. Rimm E, Willett W, Manson J, Speizer F, Hennekens C, Stampfer M. Folate and vitamin B6 intake and risk of myocardial infarction among US women [Abstract]. *Am J Epidemiol* 1996;143[Suppl].S36.
356. Jacobs TW, Byme C, Colditz G, Connolly JL, Schnitt SJ. Radial scars and breast cancer risk: a case-control study. *N Engl J Med* 1998 *(in press).*
357. Garland C, Friedlander N, Barrett-Connor E, Khaw K. Sex hormones and postmenopausal breast cancer: a prospective in an adult community. *Am J Epidemiol* 1992;135:1220–1230.
358. Howe GR, Friedenreich CM, Jain M, Miller AB. A cohort study of fat intake and risk of breast cancer. *J Natl Cancer Inst* 1991;83:336–340.
359. Kushi LH, Sellers TA, Potter JD, et al. Dietary fat and postmenopausal breast cancer. *J Natl Cancer Inst* 1992;84:1092–1099.
360. Van den Brandt PA, Van't Veer P, Goldbohm RA, et al. A prospective cohort study on dietary fat and the risk of postmenopausal breast cancer. *Cancer Res* 1993;53:75–82.
361. Mills PK, Beeson WL, Phillips RL, Fraser GE. Dietary habits and breast cancer incidence among Seventh-Day Adventists. *Cancer* 1989;64:582–590.
362. Wolk A, Bergstrom R, Hunter D, et al. A prospective study of associ-

ation of monounsaturated and other types of fat with risk of breast cancer. *Arch Intern Med* 1998;158:41–45.
363. de Waard F, Baanders-van Halewijn EA. A prospective study in general practice on breast-cancer risk in postmenopausal women. *Int J Cancer* 1974;14:153–160.
364. Tornberg SA, Holm LE, Carstensen JM. Breast cancer risk in relation to serum cholesterol, serum beta-lipoprotein, height, weight, and blood pressure. *Acta Oncologica* 1988;27:31–37.
365. Tretli S. Height and weight in relation to breast cancer morbidity and mortality. A prospective study of 570,000 women in Norway. *Int J Cancer* 1989;44:23–30.
366. Toniolo P, Riboli E, Shore RE, Pasternack BS. Consumption of meat, animal products, protein, and fat and risk of breast cancer—a prospective cohort study in New York. *Epidemiol* 1994;5:391–397.
367. Frisch RE, Wyshak G, Albright NL, et al. Lower lifetime occurrence of breast cancer and cancers of the reproductive system amang former college athletes. *Am J Clin Nutr* 1987;45[Suppl]:328–335.
368. Paffenbarger RSJ, Hyde RT, Wing AL. Physical activity and incidence of cancer in diverse populations: a preliminary report. *Am J Clin Nutr* 1987;45[Suppl]:312–317.
369. Friedenreich CM, Rohan TE. Physical activity and risk of breast cancer. *Eur J Cancer Prev* 1995;4:145–151.
370. Mittendorf R, Longnecker MP, Newcomb PA, et al. Strenuous physical activity in young adulthood and risk of breast cancer (United States). *Cancer Causes Control* 1995;6:347–353.
371. McTiernan A, Stanford JL, Weiss NS, Daling JR, Voigt LF. Occurrence of breast cancer in relation to recreational exercise in women age 50–64 years. *Epidemiology* 1996;7:598–604.
372. Taioli E, Barone J, Wynder E. A case-control study on breast cancer and body mass. *Eur J Cancer* 1995;4:145–151.
373. Hirose K, Tajima K, Hamajima N, et al. A large-scale, hospital-based case-control study of risk factors of breast cancer according to menopausal status. *Jpn J Cancer Res* 1995;86:146–154.
374. D'Avanzo B, Nanni O, La Vecchia C, et al. Physical activity and breast cancer risk. *Cancer Epidemiol Biomarkers Prev* 1996;5: 155–160.
375. Hu Y, Nagata C, Shimizu H, Kaneda N, Kashiki Y. Association of body mass index, physical activity, and reproductive histories with breast cancer: a case-control study in Gifu, Japan. *Breast Cancer Res Treat* 1997;43:65–72.

Diseases of the Breast, 2nd ed.,
edited by Jay R. Harris.
Lippincott Williams & Wilkins, Philadelphia © 2000.

CHAPTER 16

Inherited Genetic Factors

Angela DeMichele and Barbara L. Weber

Although noninherited factors certainly play a major role in familial clustering of breast cancer, breast cancer susceptibility genes appear directly responsible for 5% to 10% of all breast cancer.[1] Much remains to be understood about the heritable factors involved; however, enormous strides have been made in understanding inherited susceptibility to breast cancer with the discovery and characterization of a number of genes responsible for the clustering of breast cancer in certain families. Nevertheless, almost nothing is known about the interaction of various genes and the interaction of genes and environmental factors, both exogenous (e.g., pesticides) and endogenous (e.g., estrogen).

EPIDEMIOLOGIC STUDIES OF FAMILIAL BREAST CANCER

The first attempts to determine the influence of family history on breast cancer risk were published in the first half of the twentieth century.[2–5] Although many of these studies have methodological flaws, they consistently demonstrated a twofold to threefold increase in breast cancer risk in mothers and sisters of breast cancer patients. The largest population-based study to estimate breast cancer risk associated with a family history was a study conducted in Sweden that involved 2,660 women.[6] Within this study cohort, women with an affected relative had a relative breast cancer risk of 1.7. Relative risks of a similar magnitude were found in a Canadian population-based study[7] and in the U.S. Nurses' Health Study.[8]

Preliminary data from the population-based Carolina Breast Cancer Study have been released recently. Although information on controls has not yet been published, in this series, 20% of individuals with breast cancer reported a first-degree relative with breast cancer, and 49% reported breast cancer in at least one relative of any type.[1] Although information on controls is needed before relative risks of family history in this cohort can be calculated, the familial component to breast cancer is likely to be even greater than has been appreciated in the past. These data also suggest that increased breast cancer incidence in this population compared with that in the previously cited historical studies, as well as increases in both public awareness and the likelihood that women will discuss a diagnosis of breast cancer with family members, has contributed to higher reporting of affected family members.

Anderson[9] was among the first to suggest that breast cancer was not a homogeneous disease and that the occurrence of breast cancer was not influenced by genetic factors in a uniform manner. In such a setting, a small subset of families with a very high risk of developing breast cancer as the result of a single genetic defect might be obscured in studies in which the majority of breast cancer cases were multifactorial in origin. To emphasize the hereditary component, Anderson therefore assembled a database enriched for kindreds with a family history of breast cancer.[9,10] The primary factors that increased risk within families were premenopausal status at time of diagnosis and bilateral disease.

By 1980, a significant body of evidence had accumulated to support the presence of inherited factors responsible for familial clustering of breast cancer, and efforts shifted to determining the inheritance pattern of breast cancer within these families. In 1984, Williams and Anderson[11] examined 200 Danish pedigrees and provided the first evidence for an autosomal dominant breast cancer susceptibility gene with an age-related penetrance, as was supported in 1988 by Newman et al.[12]

FAMILIAL BREAST CANCER IN NONWHITE POPULATIONS

Even though researchers are beginning to understand the influence of genetic factors on the incidence of breast cancer in largely white, Western populations of women, very little is known about breast cancer risk attributable to inherited factors in other populations. The few studies that have examined breast cancer risk in African-American women have concluded that a family history of breast cancer confers a magnitude of increased risk similar to that seen in white population–based

A. DeMichele: Departments of Medicine and Epidemiology, The University of Pennsylvania Cancer Center, Philadelphia, Pennsylvania

B. L. Weber: Departments of Medicine and Genetics, Breast Cancer Program, Population Science and Cancer Control, The University of Pennsylvania Cancer Center, Philadelphia, Pennsylvania

studies.[13–15] Few African-American families in whom breast cancer fits an autosomal dominant pattern of inheritance have been described in the literature.[16–19] This lack could reflect a low prevalence of breast cancer–related inherited mutations in African-Americans, but it is equally likely to be due to selection or referral biases. In fact, some of these families are now known to carry *BRCA1* or *BRCA2* mutations,[18,19] but a cohort ascertained for the purpose of estimating population frequencies has not been assembled.

Only one study of familial breast cancer clustering in North American Hispanic individuals has been conducted. This study of Hispanic women living in Laredo, Texas, from 1870 to 1981 suggested that familial clustering of breast cancer also appears in this population.[20] However, the study design allowed for a significant margin of error, predominantly from underreporting of cases. No epidemiologic information from outside the United States is available on Hispanic populations; however, estimates are available from Spain on *BRCA1* and *BRCA2* mutation prevalence in a breast cancer population. These data[21–24] suggest that the incidence of *BRCA1* mutations is similar to that seen in other European populations. Thus, breast cancer susceptibility gene mutations may be equally prevalent throughout South America, as Spain provided many of the founders of the white population on that continent.

One study of family history of breast cancer in Japanese women living in Japan has been reported in the English medical literature.[25] In this study, the relative risk of developing breast cancer of women with two or more affected relatives was 2, comparable to that in studies involving primarily white women. Reports of *BRCA1* germ-line mutations in Japan[26,27] suggest that the prevalence of *BRCA1* mutations may be lower than in Western countries, but *BRCA2* mutation rates may be similar to those seen in Western populations.[28,29] Finally, a study of breast cancer in Arab women included 73 breast cancer cases identified at a single hospital in Israel and found 15 patients (20%) who reported at least one affected family member.[30] This study again suggests that breast cancer risk attributable to inherited susceptibility genes of high or moderate penetrance may be relatively uniform throughout the world; yet, once again, the work needed to genetically characterize these populations has not been done.

HOW MUCH BREAST CANCER IS INHERITED?

Two groups[31,32] have analyzed data from the Cancer and Steroid Hormone (CASH) Study, a large case-control study initiated in 1981. In this study group, 11% of breast cancer patients reported a first-degree relative with breast cancer, compared with 5% of control individuals.[31] Using these data, Claus estimated that 36% of breast cancer among women aged 20–29 years is attributable to a single dominant susceptibility gene, with this fraction decreasing to less than 1% for women aged 80 years.[33] Analysis of women diagnosed with breast cancer before age 40 years suggests that approximately 10% of such American women have a *BRCA1* mutation,[34,35] whereas the prevalence of *BRCA2* mutations may be much lower in this group.[36] Results from the only population-based case-control study of *BRCA1* mutations suggest that *BRCA1* accounted for 3.3% of breast cancer in a group of women not selected for early age of onset.[1] In summary, current estimates place the percentage of breast cancer cases directly attributable to inherited factors at 5% to 10%; further studies are needed to refine these estimates.

AUTOSOMAL DOMINANT INHERITANCE

Mendelian diseases are defined as those diseases that are the result of a single mutated gene inherited in the simple pattern described by Mendel in 1865 during his study of hybrid garden peas. In his 1901 text *Versuche uber Pflanzenhybriden*, Mendel described these principles as follows: "Those characteristics that are transmitted entire, or almost unchanged by hybridization . . . are termed dominant, and those that become latent in the process are termed recessive." To date, all studies of inherited susceptibility to breast cancer have suggested that the predominant breast cancer susceptibility genes are transmitted in an autosomal dominant manner, and the identification of at least five such genes has born out this hypothesis.

Many of the most common genetic disorders of adult life are autosomal dominant diseases; these include familial colon cancer syndromes, polycystic kidney disease, familial hypercholesterolemia, Huntington's disease, and neurofibromatosis. The pattern of autosomal dominant inheritance is illustrated in Fig. 1. In this setting, an individual could have one of three possible genotypes: carrier of two nonmutant gene copies, called *alleles* (homozygous normal), or carrier of one (heterozygous) or two (homozygous) mutant alleles and therefore affected or at risk of being affected based on the penetrance of the gene. Penetrance is the likelihood that the effect of a mutation will become clinically apparent. Individuals carrying two copies of an autosomal dominant disease-related gene are extremely rare, partly because of the mathematical probability of mating between heterozygotes and partly because of the potential for a lethal defect in a homozygous affected fetus.

During meiosis, each germ cell (sperm or egg) generated carries a single copy of each gene, resulting in a 50% chance that any one offspring will inherit a mutant copy from the heterozygous parent. Thus, on average, 50% of the related individuals in a family carry the mutant gene. If the penetrance of the gene is high, the pedigree pattern for an autosomal dominant disease is quite striking, with vertical inheritance and half the children of an affected parent being affected, whereas none of the offspring of a homozygous normal parent are affected. This pedigree pattern also presupposes a low risk in the general population, which is not the case for breast cancer. As a result, breast cancer in women from families that have a known *BRCA1* mutation but who do not themselves carry the mutation is not uncom-

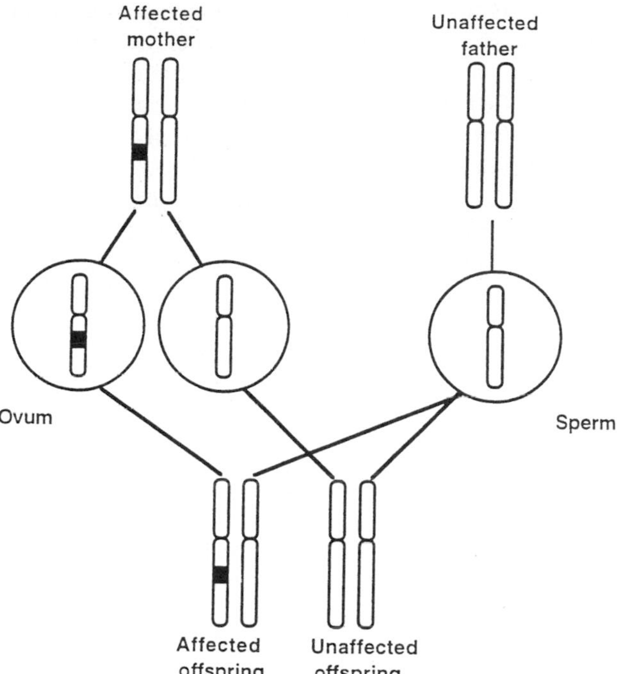

FIG. 1. Autosomal dominant inheritance. A pair of chromosomes is shown from each parent. During gametogenesis, germ cells are formed that carry only one member of a chromosomal pair. In this example, all sperm are equivalent because the father is unaffected. In the genesis of ovum, one-half of the germ cells carry a disease-related mutation and one-half do not. In the case of dominant inheritance, all offspring inheriting the disease-related mutation from the affected mother also are affected (assuming 100% penetrance). In the case of recessive inheritance, offspring must inherit two copies of a disease-related mutation, one from each carrier parent, to be affected.

mon. Such women are termed *phenocopies*—they have the phenotype associated with the gene mutation but are noncarriers. This situation is illustrated in the pedigree shown in Fig. 2, a typical pedigree of a family known to carry a mutation in the breast cancer susceptibility gene *BRCA1*.

TUMOR-SUPPRESSOR GENES

Two fundamental types of genetic damage responsible for the development of the malignant phenotype are found in cancer cells: (a) activation of proto-oncogenes producing a "gain of function" in the affected cell, and (b) inactivation of tumor-suppressor genes producing a "loss of function" in the cell. Some tumor-suppressor genes appear to be important in cell cycle regulation, normally functioning as checks on cell growth; others are critical elements in the cellular response to DNA damage, preventing the propagation of mutations in other critical genes. Mutated tumor-suppressor genes are thought to lose these regulatory functions, leading to malignant transformation. However, because all individuals are born with two copies of every gene, an explanation was needed for the development of cancer in large numbers of individuals who had only a single inherited mutation in a tumor-suppressor gene. In 1971, Knudson put forth the "two-hit hypothesis," suggesting that cancer arises as a result of two genetic events occurring in the same cell, inactivating both copies of a given tumor-suppressor gene.[37] In the case of sporadic, or noninherited, cancer, the likelihood that two events would occur in the same cell is quite low. However, individuals from "cancer families" inherit an inactivating mutation in one allele of the implicated tumor-suppressor gene in all cells (i.e., a germ-line mutation); therefore, only one somatic (noninherited) event is required to inactivate the single remaining copy, making the development of cancer a much more common event than in individuals born without the "first hit."

HEREDITARY BREAST CANCER SYNDROMES

The study of clinical syndromes that include an increased incidence of breast cancer has provided insight into the mechanisms by which genetic mutations result in the development of breast cancer. The most frequently identified pedigrees contain site-specific breast cancer (i.e., breast can-

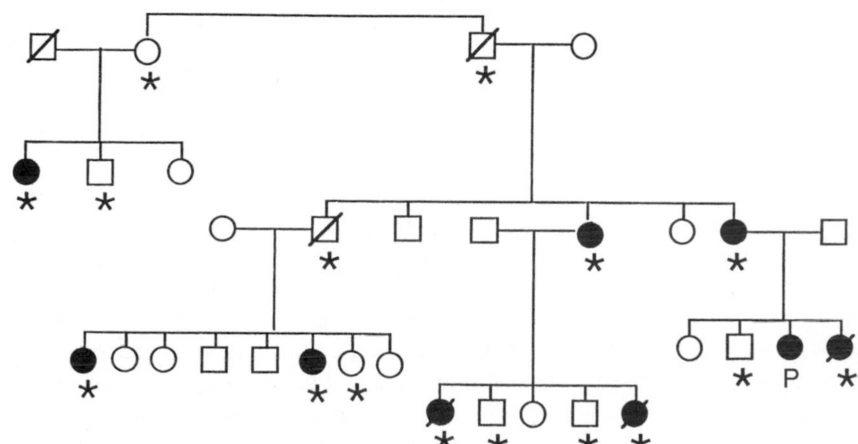

FIG. 2. Kindred with a *BRCA1* mutation. □ unaffected males; ○ unaffected females; ● females with breast or ovarian cancer; * denotes known *BRCA1* mutation carriers. Deceased individuals are indicated with a diagonal line through the symbol. A pheno copy is seen in the third generation, marked with a *P*.

cer in these families is not found in association with inherited susceptibility to other cancers, such as ovarian) and are thought to represent the effect of a single genetic abnormality. *BRCA1* and *BRCA2* are examples, and others are likely to be identified in the future. Breast cancer also has been noted to occur in association with other cancers. The occurrence of breast cancer in association with diverse childhood neoplasms in the Li-Fraumeni/SBLA (*s*oft tissue and bony sarcomas, *b*rain tumors, *l*eukemias, and *a*drenocortical carcinomas) syndrome and the association between breast and ovarian cancer represent some of the most intensively studied examples. Finally, an increased frequency of breast cancer may occur in patients with hereditary syndromes that include nonmalignant manifestations as well, such as Cowden disease and Muir-Torre syndrome.

BRCA1

In 1990, chromosome 17q21 was identified as the location of a susceptibility gene for early-onset breast cancer, now termed *BRCA1*.[38] Shortly thereafter, linkage between the genetic marker D17S74 on 17q21 and the appearance of ovarian cancer in several large kindreds was also demonstrated.[39] Initial estimates suggested that *BRCA1* mutations were responsible for more than 90% of breast cancer cases in families with apparent autosomal dominant transmission of breast cancer and at least one case of ovarian cancer, and 45% of cases in families with breast cancer only. However, the percentage of site-specific breast cancer cases attributed to *BRCA1* mutations rose to almost 70% if the median age of onset of breast cancer in the families was younger than 45 years.[40]

Using direct mutation testing, several groups have attempted to refine the estimates of mutation prevalence and breast cancer penetrance in *BRCA1* carriers found in less striking families.[1,41,42] In families identified through clinics treating high-risk breast cancer, *BRCA1* mutations appear to be responsible for 20% to 30% of breast cancer cases and 10% to 20% of ovarian cancer cases.[35,43–45] Estimates of *BRCA1* prevalence in unselected breast cancer patients are not well documented, although initial studies suggest that the proportion is in the range of 3% as defined by two different studies.[1,42]

Population Genetics of *BRCA1* and *BRCA2*

The population genetics of *BRCA1* and *BRCA2* reflect several basic human evolutionary principles. It is postulated that each gene has undergone multiple mutations, and that these mutations have migrated with the people in which they occur. Certain "founder mutations" are now known to exist in *BRCA1* and *BRCA2*. These are ancient mutations that have occurred in specific ethnic populations many generations in the past. They are thought to persist because the development of disease normally occurs after childbearing age, so that individuals carrying these mutations are able to pass them on to subsequent generations with little impact of the mutated alleles on survival of the species. Founder mutations so far have been identified in at least nine separate ethnic subpopulations, including those in Iceland,[46] Finland,[47] Hungary,[48] Russia,[49] France,[43] Holland and Belgium,[50] Israel,[51] Sweden and Denmark,[52] and Norway.[53] A comprehensive review of these studies by Szabo and King[54] reveals the similarities and differences in mutation rate, penetrance, and nature of the mutations among various population groups. The proportion of high-risk families with breast or ovarian cancer appears to vary widely by population group; mutations in *BRCA1* are most common in Russia (79% of families with breast/ovarian cancer), followed by Israel (47% of families) and Italy (29%). Moreover, the population dynamics of the groups are very different; only a small number of different mutations are seen in the Russian and Israeli populations, whereas a large number of unique mutations are found in the Italian population. Thus, the number of families affected does not accurately reflect the number of different mutations present. *BRCA2* mutations appear to be more common than *BRCA1* mutations only in Iceland, where a single mutation accounts for virtually all of the *BRCA2*-associated breast and ovarian cancer.[55,56]

The *BRCA1* and *BRCA2* mutations among the Ashkenazi Jewish population have been studied most intensively. The two most common mutations in *BRCA1* are 185delAG and 5382insC, each accounting for approximately 10% of the total. These two mutations, along with a mutation in *BRCA2*, 6174delT, have been identified with the highest frequency in the Ashkenazi Jewish population. The mutations 185delAG and 5382insC have been shown to occur in individuals of Ashkenazi descent with a combined frequency of approximately 1%[57,58]; the estimated frequency of *BRCA1* mutations in an unselected white population is less than 0.1%.[42] This observation has subsequently been expanded to include the Moroccan, Iraqi, and Yemenite Jewish populations.[59] Analysis of germ-line *BRCA1* mutations in several cohorts of Jewish women suggests that just over 20% of Jewish women developing breast cancer before age 40 carry the 185delAG mutation.[34,60] Even more strikingly, estimates suggest that 30% to 60% of all Ashkenazi Jewish women with ovarian cancer carry either a common *BRCA1* or *BRCA2* germ-line mutation.[51,61,62] Other *BRCA1* mutations have also been detected in the Jewish population but at much lower levels.[63]

Other Types of Cancers Associated with Mutations in *BRCA1*

Risk for cancers other than breast and ovarian cancer also appears to be increased in the presence of an inherited *BRCA1* mutation. The first such indication came from the study of a large Icelandic family group with breast and ovarian cancer, which suggested that prostate cancer also is a component of the *BRCA1* syndrome.[64] Subsequently, the Breast Cancer

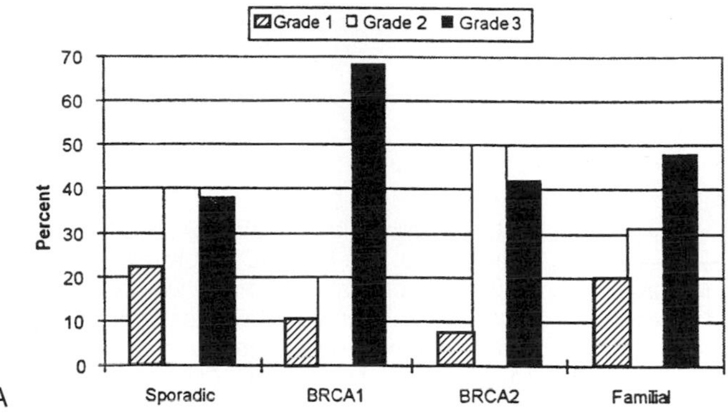

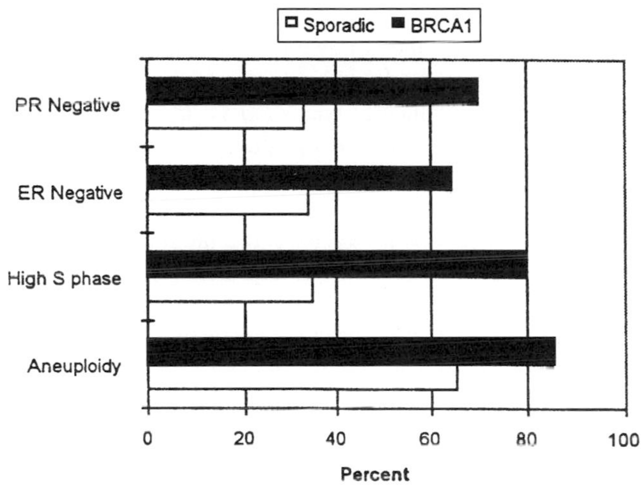

FIG. 3. Pathologic features of *BRCA1* and *BRCA2* breast cancers. **A:** Grade distribution of sporadic, *BRCA1*, *BRCA2*, and combined familial breast tumors.[67] **B:** Frequency of pathobiological characteristics of sporadic and *BRCA1*-related breast tumors.[68–72] ER, estrogen receptor; PR, progesterone receptor.

Linkage Consortium estimated a relative risk of 3.33 for prostate cancer and a relative risk of 4.11 for colon cancer in males thought to carry *BRCA1* germ-line mutations. However, the excess colon cancer risk in this study reflects the experience of only a few families, which suggests either very low penetrance with regard to colon cancer or a limited number of specific mutations that increase colon cancer risk. No significant excesses were observed for cancers originating from other anatomic sites,[65] and male breast cancer is only rarely associated with *BRCA1* germ-line mutations.

Pathobiology of *BRCA1*-Associated Breast Tumors

The relationship between *BRCA1* and tumor prognosis is one of the key clinical questions that followed the identification of *BRCA1*. In the first study to address this question, Lynch et al. analyzed 180 tumors from families with hereditary breast/ovarian or site-specific breast cancer.[66] Ninety-eight of the 180 tumors they studied were classified as the "*BRCA1* group." These tumors were thought to have the highest likelihood of arising as a result of *BRCA1* mutations but were not directly tested for mutations. The *BRCA1* group was found to include more aneuploid and more high S-phase tumors; however, surprisingly, disease-free survival was longer for patients whose tumors were of this type than for those whose tumors were thought less likely to have *BRCA1* mutations. Subsequent studies have verified that *BRCA1*-associated tumors are often high grade and tend to be estrogen-receptor and progesterone-receptor negative (Fig. 3).[67–72] Genetic studies of *BRCA1*-related breast and ovarian tumors further indicate that these tumors are both genetically unstable and highly proliferative.[73,74]

Whether the aggressive pathologic features described in association with *BRCA1*-associated breast tumors translate into reduced survival or lack of response to standard treatment strategies is not yet clear, but data are accumulating that these high-grade lesions behave as would be expected.[75,76] In addition, a study of Ashkenazi Jewish *BRCA1* mutation carriers suggested that a *BRCA1* mutation is an adverse prognostic factor in its own right.[77] Ongoing large-scale studies are currently under way to address this issue in mutation carriers, in the context of other known prognostic factors.

BRCA1 Gene Structure and Mutation Spectrum

The *BRCA1* gene is composed of 24 exons, or coding regions, and is translated into a protein consisting of 1,863 amino acids (Fig. 4). This is important from a clinical standpoint in the context of genetic testing, because this very large size makes screening the entire gene for mutations technically demanding and costly. The entire gene covers approximately 100 kb of genomic sequence, and in the case of *BRCA1*, this region contains a large number of repetitive elements called *Alu repeats*. Of clinical importance, these repetitive elements facilitate the generation of large deletions and duplications in *BRCA1*, creating disease-associated mutations that are not detectable by methods in current use in commercial testing laboratories. The prevalence of these mutations in the United States is not known yet, but three such mutations account for 36% of *BRCA1* mutations in the Netherlands.[50] These mutations clearly represent a potential source of a significant number of false-negative *BRCA1* tests.

Now that *BRCA1* has been identified, more than 500 coding region sequence variations have been detected. A listing and description of most known *BRCA1* mutations is available on the Breast Cancer Information Core (BIC) website: (http://www.nhgri.nih.gov/dir/Intramural_research/Lab_transfer/Bic/index.html). Surprisingly, almost all described mutations are found in the germ line. Somatic *BRCA1* mutations are rare in sporadic breast and ovarian tumors,[78–81] a finding which suggests that *BRCA1* coding region mutations

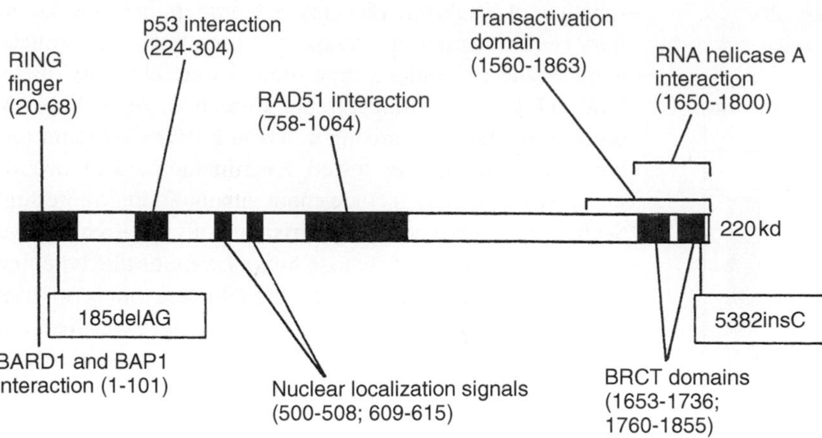

FIG. 4. Functional domains of *BRCA1*. Idiogram of the 220-kd *BRCA1* protein depicts known functional domains. Domains are shown as filled areas within the diagram. The two common mutations found in the Ashkenazi Jewish population (185delAG and 5382insC) are indicated.

play a limited role in the development of sporadic breast cancer. Whereas only one report of an individual with two *BRCA1* mutations exists in the literature,[82] a number of individuals who carry both *BRCA1* and *BRCA2* mutations have been described.[83]

Preliminary work has begun to identify possible correlations between specific *BRCA1* mutations and the types of cancers that subsequently develop. Two studies[59,84] have suggested that mutations in the 5' half of *BRCA1* predispose to both breast and ovarian cancer, whereas mutations closer to the 3' portion of the gene are predominantly associated with site-specific breast cancer. This correlation has been observed in several European studies but is rarely seen in the *BRCA1* population in the United States. It appears to be due largely to the reduced penetrance of ovarian cancer associated with these mutations rather than to an increased incidence of breast cancer arising in association with mutations in the 5' end of the gene. Finally, mutations occurring at either end of *BRCA1* may be associated with a more severe phenotype, as defined by high tumor grade,[85] suggesting that these two regions may be important for the control of mammary cell growth. Identification of these specific genotype/phenotype correlations will ultimately aid clinicians in recommending appropriate screening, prevention, and treatment strategies in women with known *BRCA1* mutations, but at present these data are too preliminary to be used in counseling women with known mutations.

Biological Function of BRCA1

To date, numerous studies have linked normal BRCA1 function to the cellular processes involved in transcription, apoptosis (programmed cell death), cell cycling, DNA repair, and developmental biology. The evidence supporting each of these functions for BRCA1 is summarized in the sections that follow.

Convincing evidence now exists that BRCA1 is a nuclear protein, and it is likely to play a role in altering the expression of other genes and in the response to DNA damage.[86–89] Some controversy arose with the report of the presence of a granin motif in BRCA1, which is characteristic of secreted molecules normally found in the cytoplasm and membrane of cells.[90] However, overwhelming evidence now suggests that BRCA1 is not secreted; and that the observations made suggesting that BRCA1 is a secreted molecule may have arisen due to a lack of specificity of the early BRCA1 antibodies.[91]

For the most part, BRCA1 protein does not display homology to any other known motif or gene. The two exceptions are the RING finger domain at the beginning of BRCA1 and the BRCT motif at the end of the gene. The 126 base pair region of homology to a RING finger motif near the amino terminus of the protein binds zinc and is thought to be involved in protein-protein interactions.[92] Two novel proteins, BAP1 (BRCA1 activator protein 1) and BARD1 (BRCA1-associated RING domain protein 1), have now been identified that bind the BRCA1 RING finger.[93,94] BAP1 is thought to enhance BRCA1-mediated cell growth suppression, whereas BARD1 may be involved in response to DNA damage. Further study of the function of both BARD1 and BAP1 should help define the function of BRCA1.

BRCA1 and Transcription

Evidence is mounting in support of a role for BRCA1 as a transcriptional coactivator—a protein that facilitates transcription of genes in the presence of direct transcriptional activators. First, BRCA1 has been shown to interact with two key components of the cell's transcription machinery—the RNA polymerase holoenzyme[95] and the transcription factor CREB binding protein.[96] In addition, two groups have characterized a transcriptional activation domain in the carboxy terminus of the BRCA1 protein.[97,98] Finally, BRCA1 has been shown to bind p53, a critical component of response to DNA damage that is itself known to be a direct transcriptional activator.[99,100] The interaction between BRCA1 and p53 has been associated with activation of p21 expression; this leads to a cell cycle pause,[101] which may be necessary for DNA damage repair to take place. Without this pause, which could perhaps not occur if BRCA1 was absent or mutated, mutations in additional genes could accumulate, facilitating malignant transformation.

BRCA1 and Development

Wild-type BRCA1 appears to play a critical role in both mouse and human development. The first studies of the role of BRCA1 in development were performed by *in situ* hybridization of mouse embryos and indicated that BRCA1 was widely expressed in many developing tissues.[102] These investigations also demonstrated that BRCA1 was highly expressed in the mouse mammary gland during development and pregnancy. Proof that BRCA1 is necessary for normal mouse development was provided by the derivation of four BRCA1 "knockout" mouse strains, each of which died in early embryonic development.[103–106] The mechanisms by which BRCA1 exerts an effect on mouse development and its role in human development remain unclear; however, this pathway provides another means of defining BRCA1 function.

BRCA1 and Cell Cycling

BRCA1 has been associated with the orderly and efficient progression of the cell through the cell cycle, as originally suggested by studies of breast cancer cell lines demonstrating that BRCA1 and cyclin A RNA levels increased in parallel in response to hormone treatment.[107] BRCA1 also has been shown to be phosphorylated in a cell cycle–dependent manner.[108] Thus, BRCA1 may play a role in G_1/S-phase checkpoint control or may be up-regulated during the cell cycle in response to cellular messages.

BRCA1 and Response to DNA Damage

Finally, BRCA1 appears to play an important role in response to DNA damage. BRCA1 complexes with Rad51[109] and BRCA2,[110] both of which have been associated with the cellular response to double-strand DNA breaks. Rad51 is the human homologue to an *Escherichia coli* recombination and repair protein, RecA.[111] Additional work in this area suggests a role for BRCA1 not just in response to damaged DNA, but also in the control of normal recombination and thus in genome integrity.[109]

In further evaluating the role of BRCA1 and Rad51 in response to DNA damage, foci containing both proteins were visualized in the cell nucleus and shown to disperse in response to the presence of hydroxyurea, ultraviolet radiation, mitomycin C, and gamma radiation—all agents that induce double-strand breaks in DNA.[112] After dispersal, BRCA1, BARD1, and Rad51 all accumulated in structures known to play a role in repairing damaged DNA. Further attempts to identify clinically relevant damaging agents and repair pathways involving BRCA1 showed that doxorubicin and ultraviolet radiation down-regulate BRCA1 expression in a mutant p53 ovarian cancer cell line,[113] suggesting that BRCA1-associated DNA repair may be dependent on p53 function. Resistance to *cis*-diamine dichloroplatinum (CDDP) also has been associated with induction of BRCA1 expression, and antisense BRCA1 expression has been associated with CDDP sensitivity.[114] Finally, BRCA1 nullizygous mouse embryonic stem cells have been shown to be hypersensitive to ionizing radiation and hydrogen peroxide and are unable to perform preferential transcription–coupled repair of oxidative DNA damage.[115] Taken together, these data suggest that BRCA1 and BRCA2 associate with Rad51 and play a role in response to DNA damage, and they suggest a role for BRCA1 as a key guardian against malignant transformation. Why breast and ovarian cancer are the primary manifestations of BRCA1 mutations, and not widespread malignancy, remains an intriguing mystery.

BRCA2

Initial progress toward the identification of a second breast cancer susceptibility gene came from a linkage analysis of 22 families with multiple cases of early-onset female breast cancer and at least one case of male breast cancer. Linkage between male breast cancer and polymorphic genetic markers on band 13q12-13 identified the *BRCA2* locus.[116] In 1995, the partial sequence of BRCA2[117] and six germ-line mutations that truncated the putative BRCA2 protein were published, and shortly thereafter, the complete DNA coding sequence and exonic structure of *BRCA2* was published by another collaborative group.[118]

Frequency of *BRCA2*-Associated Breast Cancer

No studies have been performed on *BRCA2* in the general population because of the difficulty in screening the entire coding sequence for mutations. However, one study of selected breast cancer patients identified *BRCA2* mutations in only 2.7% of women with breast cancer younger than 32 years.[36] This finding suggests that *BRCA2* mutations may contribute to fewer cases of early-onset breast cancer than do *BRCA1* mutations. This observation is supported by studies identifying *BRCA2* mutations in 10% to 20% of families at high risk for breast and ovarian cancer.[41,43,45,51,62,119–122]

In contrast to *BRCA1* mutations, in association with which almost all breast cancer appears in women, *BRCA2* mutations are associated with a 6% lifetime risk of male breast cancer.[123] Although in absolute terms this represents significantly less cancer risk to men than to women, the relative risk represents a similar 100-fold increase over the general population risk. The first study to examine this issue after *BRCA2* was identified estimated that *BRCA2* mutations account for

14% of all male breast cancer.[120] However, these estimates were generated from a cohort heavily weighted toward male breast cancer cases with a significant family history of female breast cancer; thus, 15% was thought to be an overestimate of attributable risk of male breast cancer for an unselected population. The only population-based study of the frequency of *BRCA2* mutations in men with breast cancer who were unselected for family history supports this hypothesis. This study demonstrated a 4% prevalence of *BRCA2* mutations in men identified from a cancer registry.[122] However, this was a small study, and 30% of the subjects reported a family history of female breast or ovarian cancer, potentially biasing the results of this study as well. The lack of more conclusive data reflects the fact that familial male breast cancer is very difficult to study because of the rarity of breast cancer in men and the even smaller number of cases that occur in first-degree or second-degree male relatives. In the past 100 years, only 16 families with two or more cases of male breast cancer have been reported in the literature.[124,125] Analysis of these families suggests that familial male breast cancer is likely to be as heterogeneous as familial female breast cancer. In addition, more than one-half of these families with male breast cancer include first-degree relatives with other types of cancers, such as oropharyngeal, ovarian, and female breast cancer.[124] Nine of the families for which data were available reported cases of female breast cancer.[125] In these families, average age at diagnosis of breast cancer in female relatives was 46 years; this is considerably younger than the average age at diagnosis in the general population (57 years)[126] and is consistent with the findings in studies of familial breast cancer in females. Thus, the data from families with combined male and female breast cancer argue strongly for the existence of at least one additional male breast cancer susceptibility gene. One potential candidate, a germ-line mutation in the androgen receptor gene, has been identified in two families to date,[127,128] supporting the belief that this is a very rare cause of inherited male breast cancer. More work is needed to further clarify the role of *BRCA2* and other genes in susceptibility to male breast cancer; this currently remains an area of intensive study.

Other Types of Cancer Associated with Mutations in *BRCA2*

BRCA2 mutations are associated with elevated risks for the development of a variety of other cancers. Higher than expected rates of prostate cancer, pancreatic cancer, non-Hodgkin's lymphoma, basal cell carcinoma, fallopian tube tumors, and bladder carcinoma have been reported in association with *BRCA2* mutations.[121,129,130] However, the full spectrum of cancers associated with *BRCA2* remains poorly defined.

One approach to defining the risk of other cancers associated with *BRCA1* and *BRCA2* mutations is the study of women with multiple primary cancers. In the initial report of such a study, 63 women with multiple primary cancers (of which one was breast cancer) were analyzed for *BRCA1* and *BRCA2* mutations.[131] Seven (17.9%) of the 39 women with breast cancer and a nonovarian second primary cancer had either a *BRCA1* or *BRCA2* mutation. Second cancers included two cases of unspecified skin cancers; a single case each of uterine leiomyosarcoma, brain cancer, bladder cancer, leukemia; and both thyroid and colon cancer in one proband. Overall, 29 (46%) of 63 families screened had a mutation in either the *BRCA1* or *BRCA2* gene. These data suggest that cancer susceptibility in general is increased in carriers of these mutations.

Pathobiology of *BRCA2*-Associated Breast Cancer

One study found that, unlike *BRCA1*-associated tumors, *BRCA2*-associated tumors are similar to sporadic tumors in the number of mitoses, degree of pleomorphism, and proportion classified as medullary.[67] In this study, the proportion of tubular carcinomas was significantly lower in the *BRCA2*-associated group than the sporadic group, whereas rates of invasive ductal carcinoma, invasive lobular carcinoma, and ductal carcinoma *in situ* were no different in the *BRCA2*-associated and the sporadic groups. However, other researchers who compared 85 cases presumed to be *BRCA2*-related (familial, *BRCA1* negative) with 90 *BRCA1*-confirmed cases and 187 sporadic cases found that the *BRCA2* group had a significantly greater proportion of tubular cancers.[68] Little is known yet about the natural history of breast cancer due to *BRCA2* mutations; prospective longitudinal studies are under way to attempt to address this question.

BRCA2 Gene Structure and Mutation Spectrum

The coding region of *BRCA2* is 11.2 kb in length and is comprised of 26 exons. This is approximately twice as large as *BRCA1*, itself one of the largest genes isolated to date. This size adds to the difficulties associated with mutation analysis in both the clinical and research settings. Unlike *BRCA1*, the genomic region of *BRCA2* is not rich in repetitive elements, and genomic deletions as the underlying basis of disease-associated germ-line *BRCA2* mutations have not been described. Like *BRCA1*, *BRCA2* is expressed in most tissues at very low levels, with higher expression in testis and thymus.[118] *BRCA2* cDNA has no significant homology to any previously described gene, and the protein contains no previously defined functional domains (Fig. 5). However, eight copies of a 30- to 80-amino-acid repeat (BRC repeat) are encoded by exon 11. The functional significance of the conserved repeats remains controversial, but at least some of the repeats form the binding site for the interaction between BRCA2 and Rad51.

More than 250 *BRCA2* mutations have been identified to date.[117,118,120,129,130,132–135] A tabulated list of these mutations can be found on the BIC website (http://www.nhgri.nih.gov/dir/Intramural_research/Lab_transfer/Bic/index.html). Inter-

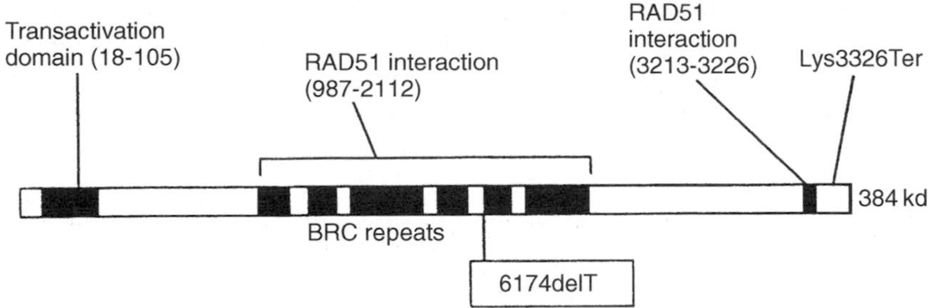

FIG. 5. Functional domains of *BRCA2.* The known functional domains of the BRCA2 protein, including the N-terminal transactivation domain, the C-terminal Rad51-binding site, and the central Rad51-binding BRC repeats are depicted as filled areas within the diagram. The common mutation (6174delT) found in the Ashkenazi Jewish population is indicated.

estingly, several similarities with *BRCA1* are apparent. First, *BRCA2* mutations span the entire coding region of the gene, adding little information on important functional regions and making mutation screening difficult in this very large gene. No mutation hot spots have been detected. Second, most mutations reported to date are truncating mutations, again adding little in the way of clues for defining functional regions. Finally, as with *BRCA1*, few mutations have been identified in the *BRCA2* gene in sporadic breast or ovarian cancers, suggesting that mutations in coding regions in *BRCA2* do not play a role in sporadic breast cancer pathogenesis.[129]

Several founder mutations have been identified in the *BRCA2* gene in specific populations. As discussed previously, the 6174delT mutation has been found in the Ashkenazi Jewish population at a prevalence of 1.2%, with more than 2.5% of the entire Ashkenazi Jewish population now thought to carry one of three specific *BRCA1* and *BRCA2* mutations.[58,132,136] No cases of patients carrying two mutated copies of *BRCA2* have been reported, which suggests that this combination may be incompatible with life. However, several groups have reported patients found to have one *BRCA1* mutation and one *BRCA2* mutation (*unpublished data*, Breast Cancer Linkage Consortium meeting, 1997).

Studies of the *BRCA2* gene in the Icelandic population have determined that a founder effect also exists in that population; the majority of high-risk breast and ovarian cancer patients share a common haplotype flanking *BRCA2*,[137] which is associated with 999del5 mutation.[55] Research also has shown that 8.5% of breast cancer patients, 7.9% of ovarian cancer patients, and 2.7% of prostate cancer patients under 65 years of age in Iceland carry the 999del5 mutation. Finally, founder mutations have been identified in Finland. These include the 9346-2A>G mutation and the 999del5 mutation, which suggests that individuals from Finland might have introduced this mutation into Iceland.[47] Analysis of haplotypes associated with nine recurrent mutations in *BRCA2* suggested that all are ancestral, as no evidence was found of multiple origins of common *BRCA2* mutations.[138]

Biological Function of *BRCA2*

The biological function of the *BRCA2* gene is not yet well understood, but like *BRCA1*, it is thought to play a role in DNA damage response, possibly within some of the same pathways. Importantly, BRCA1 and BRCA2 are now known to be associated with one another, a finding that confirms their function in the same cellular pathways.[139] The regions of the gene that appear to be very similar in human *BRCA2* and murine *Brca2* have been studied by several groups. Interestingly, both *Brca1* and *Brca2* are expressed in the mouse mammary gland concurrently, with the steady-state levels of their respective messenger RNAs both up-regulated during pregnancy.[140] Like BRCA1, BRCA2 has been localized to the cell nucleus.[110,141]

BRCA2 and Transcription

An N-terminal transactivation domain, consisting of repression and activation components, has been identified in BRCA2.[142] Unlike BRCA1, however, BRCA2 has not been shown to interact with the RNA polymerase II holoenzyme, although studies have demonstrated that BRCA2 interacts with both BRCA1 and RAD51.[110,143] BRCA2 does bind directly to RAD51,[143,144] which in turn has been shown to bind to both p53 and the RNA polymerase II holoenzyme. These observations suggest a possible role for BRCA2 in regulation of transcription, although no direct BRCA2-DNA interactions have yet been reported.

BRCA2 and Development

BRCA2 hybridization using mouse embryonic tissue showed widespread expression in many developing tissues, suggesting that *BRCA2* may play a role in tissue development.[145] Sharan et al. produced the first *Brca2* nullizygous mice. The null allele resulted in embryonic lethality at day 8.5 of embryogenesis, the same time that *Brca2* expression levels became detectable in the normal animals.[146] Heterozygous mice were healthy and fertile. Suzuki et al. also demonstrated that embryos lacking functional *Brca2* die before day 9.5 of development.[147] The death of the *Brca2* nullizygous mice during early postimplantation suggests a role for *Brca2* in cellular proliferation and development by Sharan and Suzuki.

The mouse models described carried *Brca2* mutations that truncated the protein in the region encoded by exon 10 or early exon 11, eliminating the BRC repeats. However, viable mice with two copies of truncated *Brca2* have been generated by two groups.[148,149] In these animals, truncation of *Brca2* occurred in regions more toward the 3' portion of the gene than in previous models. The allele described by Connor et al. contained seven of the eight BRC repeats.[149] The Friedman et al.[148] mice retained three of the four BRC repeats, were sickly and growth retarded, but survived to adulthood. Some developed thymic lymphomas. Interestingly, these mice also had a marked defect in chromosomal segregation; cultured fibroblasts demonstrated generation of bizarre chromosomal forms in only three to four passages. These data provide support for the hypothesis that BRCA2 is important in recombination, as suggested by high expression levels in the thymus and testes.

BRCA2 and Cell Cycling

Shortly after the identification of *BRCA2*, the gene was shown to be regulated in a cell cycle–dependent manner and to be associated with cellular proliferation.[107,143,150] Levels of BRCA2 are low in the G_1 phase of the cell cycle but increase as the cell approaches the G_1-S boundary. The highest levels of BRCA2 are detected in S phase, as with BRCA1. The cell cycle kinetics of BRCA2 appear to be very similar to the kinetics of BRCA1; this suggests that these proteins may be coordinately regulated, consistent with the finding that they interact with each other.

BRCA2 and Response to DNA Damage

Several experiments have supported the hypothesis that BRCA2 plays a role in double-strand break repair.[151] First, Morimatsu et al. successfully identified RAD51 as a binding partner of mouse Brca2.[152] Subsequently, Hasty and other researchers demonstrated that Rad51 binds to human BRCA2 (residues 3196-3232)[112,144,146] Rad51 is known to be critical for mitotic and meiotic recombination and double-strand DNA break repair.[111] These amino acids are 95% conserved between mouse and human BRCA2, suggesting that the domain is important for BRCA2 function.

Further evidence supporting a role for BRCA2 in DNA damage repair has been provided by studies of *Brca2*-mutant embryos, which display hypersensitivity to ionizing radiation.[153] After mutant embryos were exposed to gamma radiation, the inner cell mass outgrowth of these embryos was completely ablated, an effect not seen in heterozygous or normal embryos. Mouse embryo fibroblasts from viable *Brca2* homozygous mutant animals with mutations toward the 3' portion of the BRC repeats also are hypersensitive to agents that create double-strand DNA breaks.[149,152,154]

Studies in a pancreatic cancer cell line (CAPAN-1) with both copies of *BRCA2* deleted have shown that the lack of these repeats leads to hypersensitivity to methyl methanesulfonate treatment. This sensitivity persists with the introduction of *BRCA2* containing mutated BRC repeats but is reversed by the introduction of wild-type *BRCA2*. In addition, CAPAN-1 cells were demonstrated to be highly sensitive to drugs inducing double-strand DNA breaks, such as etoposide, and to ionizing radiation.[155] Tumors in mice derived from CAPAN-1 cell implantation also demonstrated hypersensitivity to radiation and mitoxantrone; this finding suggests that irradiation or treatment with DNA-damaging agents may be a useful method for elimination of *BRCA2*-null cells—a suggestion with clear potential clinical significance for women with *BRCA2*-related breast cancer.

LI-FRAUMENI SYNDROME

Li-Fraumeni syndrome was first identified in 1969 in a description of four kindreds identified through children with sarcomas whose cousins or siblings also had childhood soft-tissue sarcomas and whose other relatives had excessive cancer occurrence.[156] Subsequent epidemiologic efforts have identified the major component neoplasms, including breast cancer, soft-tissue sarcomas and osteosarcomas, brain tumors, leukemia, and adrenocortical carcinomas; several additional tumor types are likely to merit inclusion.[157,158] Segregation analysis of families identified through a family member with sarcoma confirmed the autosomal dominant pattern of transmission of cancer susceptibility, with age-specific penetrance estimated to reach 90% by age 70.[159] Nearly 30% of tumors in reported families occur before age 15 years.[158]

The pattern of breast cancer in families with Li-Fraumeni syndrome is remarkable. In one report, among 24 families with the syndrome, 44 women had breast cancer, of whom 77% were between the ages of 22 and 45 years.[160] Bilateral disease was documented in 25% of these women; 11% had additional primary tumors. Men may have later-onset tumors in Li-Fraumeni syndrome families because they do not get breast cancer, which is so dramatic among female family members with the syndrome.

In 1990, germ-line mutations were identified in the p53 tumor-suppressor gene in affected members of Li-Fraumeni syndrome families, identifying p53 mutations as the cause of the syndrome.[161,162] Approximately 50% of such carefully defined families have alterations identified in the p53 gene. Also, p53 genes ostensibly normal by sequencing but with abnormal functional assays or expression have been observed.[163–165] The prevalence of germ-line p53 mutations in women with breast cancer diagnosed before age 40 has been estimated at approximately 1%.[166,167] It is therefore not a very common explanation for breast cancer occurrence in the population; nonetheless, p53 mutations formed the basis for the first predisposition testing programs for breast cancer susceptibility.

Ataxia-Telangiectasia

Ataxia-telangiectasia is an autosomal recessive disorder characterized by oculocutaneous telangiectasias, cerebellar ataxia, immune deficiency, and a predisposition to leukemia and lymphoma. *ATM* (A-T, mutated) is the gene mutated in ataxia-telangiectasia patients.[168] It is a member of a large family of protein kinases, and it appears to function as a checkpoint in response to DNA damage. Two approaches have been used to address the question of whether female *ATM* heterozygotes may have an increased risk for breast cancer. The first type of study, which looks at family members of patients with ataxia-telangiectasia, has observed an increased number of breast cancer cases in obligate and predicted heterozygotes.[169–171] However, the controls in the two largest studies had an unusually low incidence of breast cancer. A study using linkage analysis in these families to clearly determine heterozygote status showed an increase in breast cancer risk of 3.8-fold.[172] Interestingly, no trend was noted toward an early age at diagnosis; in fact, the odds ratio was highest in women older than age 60. The second approach is to examine families with clustering of early-onset breast cancer cases and to use linkage or mutational analysis in those groups to define the role of *ATM* in familial breast cancer. The first study using mutational analysis of *ATM* in 88 families with at least two cases of breast as well as lymphoma, leukemia, or gastric cancer in the family showed an increased frequency of *ATM* heterozygotes (4.3%) compared with the observed carrier frequency in the population (0.2% to 1.0%).[173] However, a study of 100 women affected with breast cancer who had at least one additional relative affected with breast cancer did not find an increased prevalence of *ATM* mutations.[174] In addition, the tumors of patients carrying *ATM* mutations were examined and displayed no loss of *ATM*, suggesting that either *ATM* was not acting as a tumor-suppressor gene or that it was not involved in the etiology of breast cancer. Finally, in a study of 401 women diagnosed with breast cancer earlier than age 40, the prevalence of mutations in *ATM* was the same as that in 202 controls, lending further credence to the hypothesis that mutations in *ATM* do not contribute significantly to breast cancer susceptibility.[175]

One controversy that has emerged as a result of the question of breast cancer risk in *ATM* heterozygotes is the use of mammography in women younger than age 50. Concern was raised over repeated mammography, because *ATM* homozygotes have increased DNA damage from ionizing radiation. This biologic defect suggests that the use of mammography for cancer detection should be weighed against the possibility of cancer induction as a result of radiation exposure. However, the increased risk of breast cancer due to mammography in *ATM* heterozygotes is unknown and is presumably small, and the benefit of detecting a neoplasm in its early stages is large. Thus, agreement has been almost uniform that screening mammography should be initiated when clinically appropriate.

Cowden Disease

Multiple hamartoma syndrome, or Cowden disease, is a rare genetic syndrome with multiple clinical features. The most consistent and characteristic findings are mucocutaneous lesions, including multiple facial trichilemmomas, papillomatosis of the lips and oral mucosa, and acral keratoses.[176] Benign proliferations in other organ systems, including thyroid goiter and adenomata, gastrointestinal polyps, uterine leiomyomata, and lipomata, are common in patients with Cowden disease. Nonmalignant abnormalities of the breast are similarly noted in these patients and include fibroadenomas, fibrocystic lesions, areolar and nipple malformations, and ductal epithelial hyperplasia.[176,177]

A marked increase in breast cancer incidence compared with that in the general population was observed in an early series of cases of Cowden disease.[176] Breast neoplasms occurred in 10 of the 21 female patients; lesions were bilateral in 4 women. Additional cases of Cowden syndrome now have been published, bringing the total number of reported patients to 83, of whom 51 are female.[177] The total number of women with breast cancer and Cowden syndrome totals 15 (29%). Because many of the women in these families are still alive and are at risk of developing breast cancer, the number of Cowden syndrome women with breast cancer is likely to increase, raising current estimates for the lifetime risk of developing breast cancer for women with this syndrome.

The gene for Cowden disease was mapped to band 10q22-23 in 1996.[178] In 1997, *PTEN/MMAC1/TEP1* (phosphatase and tensin homologue/mutated in multiple advanced cancers 1/transforming growth factor β–regulated and epithelial cell–enriched phosphatase 1) was identified as the responsible gene.[179–181]

The wild-type PTEN protein has been shown to be a "dual-specificity" phosphatase. These proteins remove phosphate groups from other proteins, an important regulatory function that often reversibly inactivates proteins.[182] Tyrosine phosphatases have been postulated to act as tumor suppressors by offsetting the oncogenic, growth-promoting action of tyrosine kinases—proteins that put phosphate groups onto proteins, often activating them. PTEN also has homology to tensin, a cytoskeletal protein that binds actin in focal adhesions.[179] The biological significance of this finding has yet to be determined, but further study of this gene product should provide additional insight into the factors that result in malignant transformation.

Peutz-Jeghers Syndrome

Peutz-Jeghers syndrome, first described in the 1920s, is characterized by the occurrence of hamartomatous polyps in the small bowel and pigmented macules of the buccal mucosa, lips, fingers, and toes.[183,184] It is an autosomal dominant disorder that has been reported to occur in approximately 1 in 20,000 live births. More recently, it has been associated with an excess incidence of tumors involving the breast, gastrointestinal tract, ovary, testis, and uterine cervix.[185,186] Two studies have attempted to define the degree of cancer risk associated with the syndrome. Giardiello et al. described a cohort of 31 patients followed from 1973 to 1985. Forty-eight percent of the patients developed cancer in that interval: Four developed gastrointestinal cancer and ten developed nongastrointestinal cancer, representing a relative risk 18 times that of the general population.[185] Subsequently, another group of investigators reported an elevated risk of breast and gynecologic cancers in women with Peutz-Jeghers syndrome. In this cohort of 34 patients, the affected women had a relative risk of cancer of approximately 20, whereas male patients had a lower cancer risk, approximately sixfold that of the general population.[186] These findings suggest that, despite its rare occurrence, Peutz-Jeghers syndrome is associated with a markedly increased risk of breast cancer. The gene mutated in Peutz-Jeghers syndrome was recently identified on chromosome 19[187] and is now known to be *STKII/LKB1*, a putative tumor-suppressor gene that encodes a protein kinase. The association between mutations in *STKII/LKB1* and Peutz-Jeghers syndrome was subsequently confirmed in 20 additional families.[188]

Muir-Torre Syndrome

Muir-Torre syndrome, a variant of hereditary nonpolyposis colon cancer (HNPCC, also called *Lynch Type II syndrome*) is the eponym given to the association between multiple skin tumors and multiple benign and malignant tumors of the upper and lower gastrointestinal and genitourinary tracts.[189–191] Many of the manifestations of Muir-Torre syndrome are common lesions (basal cell carcinomas, keratoacanthomas, and colonic diverticula) in distributions similar to that in the general population but with earlier age of onset in affected individuals. Females with the syndrome reportedly have an increased tendency to breast cancer, particularly after menopause, although lifetime risk has not been calculated.[191] Multiple genes responsible for HNPCC have been described, including *MLH1* and *MSH2*.[192–195] Mutations in these genes are thought to lead to development of HNPCC through accumulation of DNA replication errors and associated subsequent genome instability.[194] Confirmation that Muir-Torre syndrome is a variant of HNPCC occurred with the identification of germ-line mutations in *MHS2* in individuals with the syndrome.[190,196] A truncating mutation in *MLH1* also has been detected in a Muir-Torre syndrome family.[197]

FUTURE DIRECTIONS IN BREAST CANCER GENETICS

Elucidation of the basic mechanisms involved in the pathogenesis of breast cancer and numerous potential applications await further study of *BRCA1*, *BRCA2*, and other breast cancer susceptibility genes. Patients carrying germ-line mutations in such genes might be targeted for interventions designed to reduce or eliminate risk. Questions of genetic heterogeneity can be addressed, such as whether various hereditary and nonhereditary forms of the disease involve the same or different loci. The mechanisms of the development of other cancers in the various clinical syndromes associated with familial breast cancer also may be clarified. Finally, the influence of exogenous exposures is being addressed. The next several years should bring exciting developments in genetic epidemiology and molecular biology that may revolutionize present thinking about the role of hereditary factors in breast cancer and provide new tools for the diagnosis and treatment of breast cancer in women affected with both inherited and sporadic forms of breast cancer.

REFERENCES

1. Newman B, Mu H, Butler LM, Millikan RC, Moorman PG, King MC. Frequency of breast cancer attributable to BRCA1 in a population-based series of American women [See comments]. *JAMA* 1998;279:915.
2. Lane-Clayton J. A further report on cancer of the breast, with special reference to its associated antecedent conditions. Reports of the Ministry of Health. London: His Majesty's Stationary Office, 1926–1932.
3. Wasink W. Cancer et heredite. *Genetika* 1935;17:103.
4. Penrose L, MacKenzie HJ, Karn MNA. Genetical study of human mammary cancer. *Ann Eugenics* 1948;14:234.
5. Anderson V, Goodman K, Reed S. *Variables related to human breast cancer*. Minneapolis, MN: University of Minnesota Press, 1950.
6. Adami HO, Hansen J, Jung B, Rimsten A. Characteristics of familial breast cancer in Sweden—absence of relation to age and unilateral versus bilateral disease. *Cancer* 1981;48:1688.
7. Lubin JH, Burns PE, Blot WJ, et al. Risk factors for breast cancer in women in northern Alberta, Canada, as related to age at diagnosis. *J Natl Cancer Inst* 1982;68:211.
8. Bain C, Speizer FE, Rosner B, Belanger C, Hennekens CH. Family history of breast cancer as a risk indicator for the disease. *Am J Epidemiol* 1980;111:301.
9. Anderson DE. Some characteristics of familial breast cancer. *Cancer* 1971;28:1500.
10. Anderson DE. Breast cancer in families. *Cancer* 1977;140[Suppl 4]: 1855.
11. Williams WR, Anderson DE. Genetic epidemiology of breast cancer: segregation analysis of 200 Danish pedigrees. *Genet Epidemiol* 1984;11(l):7.
12. Newman B, Austin MA, Lee M, King MC. Inheritance of human breast cancer: evidence for autosomal dominant transmission in high-risk families. *Proc Natl Acad Sci U S A* 1988;85:3044.
13. Amos Cl, Goldstein AM, Harris EL. Familiality of breast cancer and socioeconomic status in blacks. *Cancer Res* 1991;51:1793.
14. Schatzkin A, Palmer JR, Rosenberg L, et al. Risk factors for breast cancer in black women. *J Natl Cancer Inst* 1987;78:213.
15. Bondy M. Ethnic differences in familial breast cancer. *Proc Am Assoc Cancer Res* 1991;[Suppl]:Al316.
16. Siraganian PA, LeNine PR, Madigan P, Mulvihill JJ. Familial breast cancer in black Americans. *Cancer* 1987;60:1657.
17. Chamberlain JS, Boehnke M, Frank TS, et al. BRCA1 maps proximal to DI 7S579 on chromosome 17q2l by genetic analysis. *Am J Hum Genet* 1993;52:792.
18. Arena J, Smith S, Plewinska M, et al. BRCA1 mutations in African-American women. *Am J Hum Genet* 1996;59[Suppl]:A34.
19. Gao Q, Neuhausen S, Cummings S, Luce M, Olopade OI. Recurrent germ-line BRCA1 mutations in extended African American families with early-onset breast cancer [Letter]. *Am J Hum Genet* 1997;160:1233.
20. Weiss KM, Chakraborty R, Smouse PE, Buchanan AV, Strong LC. Familial aggregation of cancer in Laredo, Texas: a generally low-risk Mexican-American population. *Genet Epidemiol* 1986;3:121.
21. Osorio A, Robledo M, San Roinan JM, et al. Mutation analysis of the BRCA2 gene in breast/ovarian cancer Spanish families: identification of two new mutations. *Cancer Lett* 1997;1121:115.

22. Osorio A, Robledo M, Albertos J, et al. Molecular analysis of the six most recurrent mutations in the BRCA1 gene in 87 Spanish breast/ovarian cancer families. *Cancer Lett* 1998;123:153.
23. Garcia-Patino E, Gomendio B, Provencio M, et al. Germline BRCA1 mutations in women with sporadic breast cancer: clinical correlations. *J Clin Oncol* 1998;16(1):115.
24. Garcia-Patino E, Gomendio B, Silva JM, et al. BRCA1 mutations in patients with familial risk of breast cancer [Letter]. *Acta Oncol* 1998;37:299.
25. Kato I, Miura S, Kasurmi F, et al. A case-control study of breast cancer among Japanese women: with special reference to family history and reproductive and dietary factors. *Breast Cancer Res Treat* 1992;24(1):51.
26. Katagiri T, Emi M, Ito I, et al. Mutations in the BRCA1 gene in Japanese breast cancer patients. *Hum Mutat* 1996;7:334.
27. Takano M, Aida H, Tsuneki I, et al. Mutational analysis of BRCA1 gene in ovarian and breast-ovarian cancer families in Japan. *Jpn J Cancer Res* 1997;88:407.
28. Inoue R, Ushijima T, Fukutomi T, et al. BRCA2 germ-line mutations in Japanese breast cancer families. *Int J Cancer* 1997;74:199.
29. Inoue R, Fulcutomi T, Ushijima T, Matsumoto Y, Sugimura T, Nagao M. Germline mutation of BRCA1 in Japanese breast cancer families. *Cancer Res* 1995;55:3521.
30. Zidan J, Diab M, Robinson E. [Familial breast cancer in Arabs]. *Harefuah* 1992;122:767–769, 819.
31. Sattin RW, Rubin GL, Webster LA, et al. Family history and the risk of breast cancer. *JAMA* 1985;253:1908.
32. Claus EB, Risch N, Thompson AD. Genetic analysis of breast cancer in the Cancer and Steroid Hormone Study. *Am J Hum Genet* 1991;48:232.
33. Claus EB, Schildkraut JM, Thompson WD, Risch NJ. The genetic attributable risk of breast and ovarian cancer. *Cancer* 1996;77:18.
34. Fitzgerald MG, MacDonald DJ, Krainer M, et al. Germ-line BRCA1 mutations in Jewish and non-Jewish women with early-onset breast cancer [See comments]. *N Engl J Med* 1996;334:143.
35. Couch FJ, DeShano ML, Blackwood MA, et al. BRCA1 mutations in women attending clinics that evaluate the risk of breast cancer [See comments]. *N Engl J Med* 1997;336:1409.
36. Krainer M, Silva-Arrieta S, Fitzgerald MG, et al. Differential contributions of BRCA1 and BRCA2 to early-onset breast cancer [See comments]. *N Engl J Med* 1997;336:1416.
37. Knudson AG Jr. Mutation and cancer: statistical study of retinoblastoma. *Proc Natl Acad Sci U S A* 1971;68:820.
38. Hall JM, Lee MK, Newman B, et al. Linkage of early-onset familial breast cancer to chromosome 17q21. *Science* 1990;250(4988):1684.
39. Narod SA, Feunteun J, Lynch HT, et al. Familial breast-ovarian cancer locus on chromosome 17ql2-q23 [See comments]. *Lancet* 1991;338(8759):82.
40. Easton DF, Bishop DT, Ford D, Crockford GP. Genetic linkage analysis in familial breast and ovarian cancer results from 214 families. The Breast Cancer Linkage Consortium. *Am J Hum Genet* 1993;52:678.
41. Struewing JP, Hartge P, Wacholder S, et al. The risk of cancer associated with specific mutations of BRCA1 and BRCA2 among Ashkenazi Jews [See comments]. *N Engl J Med* 1997;336:1401.
42. Whittemore AS, Gong G, Itnyre J. Prevalence and contribution of BRCA1 mutations in breast cancer and ovarian cancer: results from three U.S. population-based case-control studies of ovarian cancer. *Am J Hum Genet* 1997;160:496.
43. Stoppa-Lyonnet D, Laurent-Puig P, Essioux L, et al. BRCA1 sequence variations in 160 individuals referred to a breast/ovarian family cancer clinic. Institut Curie Breast Cancer Group [See comments]. *Am J Hum Genet* 1997;60:1021.
44. Shattuck-Eidens D, Oliphant A, McClure M, et al. BRCA1 sequence analysis in women at high risk for susceptibility mutations. Risk factor analysis and implications for genetic testing [See comments]. *JAMA* 1997;278:1242.
45. Frank TS, Manley SA, Olopade OI, et al. Sequence analysis of BRCA1 and BRCA2: correlation of mutations with family history and ovarian cancer risk. *J Clin Oncol* 1998;16:2417.
46. Bergthorsson JT, Johannsdottir J, Jonasdottir A, et al. Chromosome imbalance at the 3pl4 region in human breast tumours: high frequency in patients with inherited predisposition due to BRCA2. *Eur J Cancer* 1998;34(1):142.
47. Huusko P, Paakkonen K, Launonen V, et al. Evidence of founder mutations in Finnish BRCA1 and BRCA2 families [Letter]. *Am J Hum Genet* 1998;62:1544.
48. Ramus SJ, Kote-Jarai Z, Friedman LS, et al. Analysis of BRCA1 and BRCA2 mutations in Hungarian families with breast or breast-ovarian cancer [Letter]. *Am J Hum Genet* 1997;60:1242.
49. Gayther SA, Mangion J, Russell P, et al. Variation of risks of breast and ovarian cancer associated with different germline mutations of the BRCA2 gene. *Nat Genet* 1997;15(1):103.
50. Petrij-Bosch A, Peelen T, van Vliet M, et al. BRCA1 genomic deletions are major founder mutations in Dutch breast cancer patients [Published erratum appears in *Nat Genet* 1997;17:503]. *Nat Genet* 1997;17:341.
51. Levy-Lahad E, Catane R, Eisenberg S, et al. Founder BRCA1 and BRCA2 mutations in Ashkenazi Jews in Israel: frequency and differential penetrance in ovarian cancer and in breast-ovarian cancer families [See comments]. *Am J Hum Genet* 1997;160:1059.
52. Johannsson O, Ostermever EA, Hakansson S, et al. Founding BRCA1 mutations in hereditary breast and ovarian cancer in southern Sweden. *Am J Hum Genet* 1996;158:441.
53. Dorum A, Moller P, Kamsteeg EJ, et al. A BRCA1 founder mutation, identified with haplotype analysis, allowing genotype/phenotype determination and predictive testing. *Eur J Cancer* 1997;33:2390.
54. Szabo CI, King MC. Population genetics of BRCA1 and BRCA2 [Editorial; comment]. *Am J Hum Genet* 1997;60:1013.
55. Thorlacius S, Olafsdottir G, Tryggvadottir L, et al. A single BRCA2 mutation in male and female breast cancer families from Iceland with varied cancer phenotypes [See comments]. *Nat Genet* 1996;13(1):117.
56. Couch FJ, Weber BL. Mutations and polymorphisms in the familial early-onset breast cancer (BRCA1) gene. *Hum Mutat* 1996;8(1):8.
57. Tonin P, Serova O, Lenoir G, et al. BRCA1 mutations in Ashkenazi Jewish women [Letter]. *Am J Hum Genet* 1995;57(1):189.
58. Struewing JP, Abehovich D, Peretz T, et al. The carrier frequency of the BRCA1 185delAG mutation is approximately 1 percent in Ashkenazi Jewish individuals [See comments; published erratum appears in *Nat Genet* 1996;12(1):110]. *Nat Genet* 1995;11:198.
59. Gayther SA, Warren W, Mazoyer S, et al. Germline mutations of the BRCA1 gene in breast and ovarian cancer families provide evidence for a genotype-phenotype correlation. *Nat Genet* 1995;11:428.
60. Offit K, Gilewski T, McGuire P, et al. Germline BRCA1 185detAG mutations in Jewish women with breast cancer [See comments]. *Lancet* 1996;347(9016):1643.
61. Muto MG, Cramer DW, Tangir J, Berkowitz R, Mok S. Frequency of the BRCA1 185delAG mutation among Jewish women with ovarian cancer and matched population controls. *Cancer Res* 1996;56:1250.
62. Abeliovich D, Kaduri L, Lerer I, et al. The founder mutations 185delAG and 5382insC in BRCA1 and 6174delT in BRCA2 appear in 60% of ovarian cancer and 30% of early-onset breast cancer patients among Ashkenazi women. *Am J Hum Genet* 1997;60:505.
63. Berman DB, Wagner-Costalas J, Schultz DC, Lynch HT, Daly M, Godwin AK. Two distinct origins of a common BRCA1 mutation in breast-ovarian cancer families: a genetic study of 15 185delAG-mutation kindreds. *Am J Hum Genet* 1996;58:1166.
64. Arason A, Barkardottir RB, Eglisson V. Linkage analysis of chromosome 17q markers and breast-ovarian cancer in Icelandic families, and possible relationship to prostatic cancer. *Am J Hum Genet* 1993; 52:711.
65. Ford D, Easton DF, Bishop DT, Narod SA, Goldgar DE. Risks of cancer in BRCA1-mutation carriers. Breast Cancer Linkage Consortium. *Lancet* 1994;343(8899):692.
66. Lynch HT, Marcus J, Watson P, Page D. Distinctive clinicopathologic features of BRCA1-linked hereditary breast cancer. *Proc Am Soc Clin Oncol* 1994;13:56.
67. Anonymous. Pathology of familial breast cancer: differences between breast cancers in carriers of BRCA1 or BRCA2 mutations and sporadic cases. Breast Cancer Linkage Consortium [See comments]. *Lancet* 1997;349(9064):1505.
68. Marcus JN, Watson P, Page DL, et al. Hereditary breast cancer: pathobiology, prognosis, and BRCA1 and BRCA2 gene linkage [See comments]. *Cancer* 1996;77:697.
69. Karp SE, Tonin PN, Begin LR, et al. Influence of BRCA1 mutations on nuclear grade and estrogen receptor status of breast carcinoma in Ashkenazi Jewish women. *Cancer* 1997;80:435.
70. Robson M, Rajan P, Rosen PP, et al. BRCA-associated breast cancer: absence of a characteristic immunophenotype. *Cancer Res* 1998; 58:1839.
71. Wagner TM, Moslinger RA, Muhr D, et al. BRCA1-related breast cancer in Austrian breast and ovarian cancer families: specific BRCA1 mutations and pathological characteristics. *Int J Cancer* 1998;77:354.

72. Eisinger F, Stoppa-Lyonnet D, Longy M, et al. Germ line mutation at BRCA1 affects the histoprognostic grade in hereditary breast cancer. *Cancer Res* 1996;56:471.
73. Tirkkonen M, Johannsson O, Agnarsson BA, et al. Distinct somatic genetic changes associated with tumor progression in carriers of BRCA1 and BRCA2 germ-line mutations. *Cancer Res* 1997;57:1222.
74. Tapper J, Sarantaus L, Vahteristo P, et al. Genetic changes in inherited and sporadic ovarian carcinomas by comparative genomic hybridization: extensive similarity except for a difference at chromosome 2q24-q32. *Cancer Res* 1998;58:2715.
75. Johannsson OT, Ranstam J, Borg A, Olsson H. Survival of BRCA1 breast and ovarian cancer patients: a population-based study from southern Sweden [See comments]. *J Clin Oncol* 1998;16:397.
76. Verhoog LC, Brekelmans CT, Seynaeve C, et al. Survival and tumour characteristics of breast-cancer patients with germline mutations of BRCA1. *Lancet* 1998;351(9099):316.
77. Foulkes WD, Wong N, Rozen F, Brunet JS, Narod SA. Survival of patients with breast cancer and BRCA1 mutations [Letter]. *Lancet* 1998;351(9112):1359.
78. Merajver SD, Pham TM, Caduff RF, et al. Somatic mutations in the BRCA1 gene in sporadic ovarian tumours. *Nat Genet* 1995;9:439.
79. Hosking L, Trowsdate J, Nicolai H, et al. A somatic BRCA1 mutation in an ovarian tumour [Letter]. *Nat Genet* 1995;9:343.
80. Takahashi H, Behbakht K, McGovern PE, et al. Mutation analysis of the BRCA1 gene in ovarian cancers. *Cancer Res* 1995;55:2998.
81. Matsushima M, Kobayashi K, Emi M, et al. Mutation analysis of the BRCA1 gene in 76 Japanese ovarian cancer patients: four germline mutations, but no evidence of somatic mutation. *Hum Mol Genet* 1995;4:1953.
82. Boyd M, Harris F, McFarlane R, Davidson HR, Black DM. A human BRCA1 gene knockout [Letter]. *Nature* 1995;375(6532):541.
83. Tsongalis GJ, Linfert DR, Johnson RC, Ackroyd R, Berman MM, Ricci A Jr. Double heterozygosity for mutations in the BRCA1 and BRCA2 genes in a breast cancer patient. *Arch Pathol Lab Med* 1998;1122:548.
84. Holt JT, Thompson ME, Szabo C, et al. Growth retardation and tumour inhibition by BRCA1 [See comments]. *Nat Genet* 1996;12:298.
85. Sobol H, Stoppa-Lyonnet D, Bressac-de-Paillerets B, et al. Truncation at conserved terminal regions of BRCA1 protein is associated with highly proliferating hereditary breast cancers. *Cancer Res* 1996;56:3216.
86. Chen Y, Chen CF, Riley DJ, et al. Aberrant subcellular localization of BRCA1 in breast cancer [See comments; published erratum appears in *Science* 1995;270(5241):1424]. *Science* 1995;270(5237):789.
87. Scully R, Ganesan S, Brown M, et al. Localization of BRCA1 in human breast and ovarian cancer cells. *Science* 1996;272:122.
88. Thakur S, Zhang HB, Peng Y, et al. Localization of BRCA1 and a splice variant identifies the nuclear localization signal. *Mol Cell Biol* 1997;17(l):444.
89. Wilson CA, Payton MN, Elliott GS, et al. Differential subcellular localization, expression and biological toxicity of BRCA1 and the splice variant BRCA1-deltal lb. *Oncogene* 1997;14:1.
90. Jensen RA, Thompson ME, Jetton TL, et al. BRCA1 secreted and exhibits properties of a granin [See comments]. *Nat Genet* 1996;12:303.
91. Wilson CA, Payton MN, Pekar SK, et al. BRCA1 protein products: antibody specificity. *Nat Genet* 1996;13:264.
92. Roehm PC, Berg JM. Sequential metal binding by the RING finger domain of BRCA1. *Biochemistry* 1997;36:10240.
93. Jensen DE, Proctor M, Marquis ST, et al. BAP1: a novel ubiquitin hydrolase which binds to the BRCA1 RING finger and enhances BRCA1-mediated cell growth suppression. *Oncogene* 1998;16:1097.
94. Wu LC, Wang ZW, Tsan JT, et al. Identification of a RING protein that can interact in vivo with the BRCA1 gene product. *Nat Genet* 1996;14:430.
95. Scully R, Anderson SF, Chao DM, et al. BRCA1 is a component of the RNA polymerase 11 holoenzyme. *Proc Natl Acad Sci U S A* 1997;94:5605.
96. Cui JQ, Shao N, Chai Y, Wang K, Reddy ES, Pao VN. BRCA1 splice variants BRCA1a and BRCA1b associate with CBP co-activator. *Oncol Rep* 1998;5:591.
97. Chapman MS, Verma IM. Transcriptional activation by BRCA1 [Letter; comment]. *Nature* 1996;382:678.
98. Monteiro AN, August A, Hanafusa H. Evidence for a transcriptional activation function of BRCA1 C-terminal region. *Proc Natl Acad Sci U S A* 1996;93:13595.
99. Zhang H, Somasundaram K, Peng Y, et al. BRCA1 physically associates with p53 and stimulates its transcriptional activity. *Oncogene* 1998;16:1713.
100. Ouchi T, Monteiro AN, August A, Aaronson SA, Hanafusa H. BRCA1 regulates p53-dependent gene expression. *Proc Natl Acad Sci U S A* 1998;95:2302.
101. Somasundaram K, Zhang K, Zeng YX, et al. Arrest of the cell cycle by the tumour-suppressor BRCA1 requires the CDK-inhibitor p21WAF1/CiP1. *Nature* 1997;389:187.
102. Marquis ST, Rajan JV, Wynshaw-Boris A, et al. The developmental pattern of Brca1 expression implies a role in differentiation of the breast and other tissues. *Nat Genet* 1995;111:17.
103. Gowen LC, Johnson BL, Latour AM, Sulik KK, Koller BH. Brca1 deficiency results in early embryonic lethality characterized by neuroepithelial abnormalities. *Nat Genet* 1996;12:191.
104. Hakem R, de la Pompa JL, Strard C, et al. The tumor suppressor gene Brca1 is required for embryonic cellular proliferation in the mouse. *Cell* 1996;85:1009.
105. Liu CY, Flesken-Nikitin A, Li S, Zeng Y, Lee WH. Inactivation of the mouse Brca1 gene leads to failure in the morphogenesis of the egg cylinder in early postimplantation development. *Genes Dev* 1996;10:1835.
106. Ludwig T, Chapman DL, Papaioannou VE, Efstratiadis A. Targeted mutations of breast cancer susceptibility gene homologs in mice: lethal phenotypes of Brca1, Brca2, Brca1/Brca2, Brca1/p53, and Brea2/p53 nullizygous embryos. *Genes Dev* 1997;11:1226.
107. Gudas JM, Nguyen H, Li T, Cowan KE. Hormone-dependent regulation of BRCA1 in human breast cancer cells. *Cancer Res* 1995;55:4561.
108. Chen Y, Farmer AA, Chen CF, Jones DC, Chen PL, Lee NVH. BRCA1 is a 220-kDa nuclear phosphoprotein that is expressed and phosphorylated in a cell cycle-dependent manner [Published erratum appears in *Cancer Res* 1996;1156:4074]. *Cancer Res* 1996;56:3168.
109. Scully R, Chen J, Plug A, et al. Association of BRCA1 with Rad51 in mitotic and meiotic cells. *Cell* 1997;88:265.
110. Chen J, Silver D, Walpita D, et al. Stable interaction between products of BRCA1 and BRCA2 tumor suppressor genes in mitotic and meiotic cells. *Molecular Cell* 1998;2:317.
111. Shinohara A, Ogawa H, Ogawa T. Rad51 protein involved in repair and recombination in *S. cermislae* is a RecA-like protein [Published erratum appears in *Cell* 1992;71]. *Cell* 1992;69:457.
112. Scully R, Chen J, Ochs RL, et al. Dynamic changes of BRCA1 subnuclear location and phosphorylation state are initiated by DNA damage. *Cell* 1997;90:425.
113. Fan S, Twu NF, Wang JA, et al. Down-regulation of BRCA1 and BRCA2 in human ovarian cancer cells exposed to adriamycin and ultraviolet radiation. *Int J Cancer* 1998;77:600.
114. Husain A, He G, Venkatraman ES, Spriggs DR. BRCA1 up-regulation is associated with repair-mediated resistance to cis-diaminedichloroplatinum (II). *Cancer Res* 1998;58:1120.
115. Gowen LC, Avrutskaya AV, Latour AM, Koller BH, Leadon SA. BRCA1 required for transcription-coupled repair of oxidative DNA damage. *Science* 1998;281:1009.
116. Wooster R, Neuhausen SL, Mangion J, et al. Location of a breast cancer susceptibility gene, BRCA2, to chromosome 13ql2-13. *Science* 1994;265:2088.
117. Wooster R, Bignell G, Lancaster J, et al. Identification of the breast cancer susceptibility gene BRCA2 [See comments; published erratum appears in *Nature* 1996;379:749]. *Nature* 1995;378:789.
118. Tavtigian SV, Simard J, Rommens J, et al. The complete BRCA2 gene and mutations in chromosome 13q-linked kindreds [See comments]. *Nat Genet* 1996;12:333.
119. Hakansson S, Johannsson O, Johansson U, et al. Moderate frequency of BRCA1 and BRCA2 germ-line mutations in Scandinavian familial breast cancer [See comments]. *Am J Hum Genet* 1997;60:1068.
120. Couch FJ, Farid LM, DeShano ML, et al. BRCA2 germline mutations in male breast cancer cases and breast cancer families. *Nat Genet* 1996;13:123.
121. Schubert EL, Lee MY, Mefford HC, et al. BRCA2 in American families with four or more cases of breast or ovarian cancer: recurrent and novel mutations, variable expression, penetrance, and the possibility of families whose cancer is not attributable to BRCA1 or BRCA2 [See comments]. *Am J Hum Genet* 1997;60:1031.
122. Friedman LS, Gayther SA, Kurosaki T, et al. Mutation analysis of BRCA1 and BRCA2 in a male breast cancer population. *Am J Hum Genet* 1997;60:313.
123. Wooster R, Bignell G, Lancaster J. Identification of the breast cancer susceptibility gene BRCA2. *Nature* 1995;378:789.

124. Kozak FK, Hall JG, Baird PA. Familial breast cancer in males. A case report and review of the literature. *Cancer* 1986;58:2736.
125. Hauser A, Lemer I, King R. Familial male breast cancer. *Am J Med Genet* 1992;44:839.
126. Nemoto TVJ, Bedwani R, Baker HW, McGregor FH, Murphy GP. Management and survival of female breast cancer: results of a national survey by the American College of Physicians. *Cancer* 1980,45:2917.
127. Wooster R, Mangion J, Eeles R, et al. A germline mutation in the androgen receptor gene in two brothers with breast cancer and Reifenstein syndrome. *Nat Genet* 1992;2:132.
128. Lobaccaro J, Lumbroso S, Belon C, et al. Male breast cancer and the androgen receptor gene [Letter]. *Nat Genet* 1993;5:109.
129. Teng DH, Bogden R, Mitchell J, et al. Low incidence of BRCA2 mutations in breast carcinoma and other cancers. *Nat Genet* 1996;113:241.
130. Phelan CM, Lancaster JM, Tonin P, et al. Mutation analysis of the BRCA2 gene in 49 site-specific breast cancer families [See comments; published erratum appears in *Nat Genet* 1996;13:374]. *Nat Genet* 1996;13:120.
131. Shih K, Antin-Ozerkis D, Nathanson K, Rebbeck T, Weber B. Multiple primary cancers are associated with BRCA1 or BRCA2 mutations. *Am J Hum Genet* 1998;63[Suppl 4]:A86.
132. Neuhausen S, Gilewski T, Norton L, et al. Recurrent BRCA2 6174delT mutations in Ashkenazi Jewish women affected by breast cancer. *Nat Genet* 1996;13:126.
133. Lancaster JM, Wooster R, Mangion J, et al. BRCA2 mutations in primary breast and ovarian cancers. *Nat Genet* 1996;13:238.
134. Miki Y, Katagiri T, Kasumi F, Yoshimoto T, Nakamura Y. Mutation analysis in the BRCA2 gene in primary breast cancers. *Nat Genet* 1996;13:245.
135. Takahashi K, Chiu HC, Bandera CA, et al. Mutations of the BRCA2 gene in ovarian carcinomas. *Cancer Res* 1996;56:2738.
136. Tonin P, Weber B, Offit K, et al. Frequency of recurrent BRCA1 and BRCA2 mutations in Ashkenazi Jewish breast cancer families [See comments]. *Nat Med* 1996;2:1179.
137. Gudmundsson J, Johannesdottir G, Arason A, et al. Frequent occurrence of BRCA2 linkage in Icelandic breast cancer families and segregation of a common BRCA2 haplotype. *Am J Hum Genet* 1996;58:749.
138. Neuhausen SL, Godwin AK, Gershoni-Baruch R, et al. Haplotype and phenotype analysis of nine recurrent BRCA2 mutations in 111 families: results of an international study. *Am J Hum Genet* 1998;62:1381.
139. Chen J, Silver D, Walpita D, et al. Stable interaction between products of BRCA1 and BRCA2 tumor suppressor genes in mitotic and meiotic cells. *Molecular Cell* 1998;2:317.
140. Rajan JV, Wang M, Marquis ST, Chodosh LA. Brca2 is coordinately regulated with Brca1 during proliferation and differentiation in mammary epithelial cells. *Proc Natl Acad Sci U S A* 1996;93:13078.
141. Bertwistle D, Swift S, Marston NJ, et al. Nuclear location and cell cycle regulation of the BRCA2 protein. *Cancer Res* 1997;57:5485.
142. Milner J, Ponder B, Hughes-Davies L, Seltmann M, Kouzarides T. Transcriptional activation functions in BRCA2 [Letter; see comments]. *Nature* 1997;386:772.
143. Wong AKC, Pero R, Ormonde PA, Tavtigian SV, Bartel PL. RAD51 interacts with the evolutionarily conserved BRC motifs in the human breast cancer susceptibility gene brca2. *J Biol Chem* 1997;272:31941.
144. Mizuta R, LaSalle JM, Cheng HL, et al. RAB22 and RAB163/mouse BRCA2: proteins that specifically interact with the RAD51 protein. *Proc Natl Acad Sci U S A* 1997;94:6927.
145. Rajan TV, Marquis ST, Gardner HP, Chodosh LA. Developmental expression of Brca2 colocalizes with Brca1 and is associated with proliferation and differentiation in multiple tissues. *Dev Biol* 1997;1184:385.
146. Sharan SK, Morimatsu M, Albrecht U, et al. Embryonic lethality and radiation hypersensitivity mediated by Rad51 in mice lacking Brca2 [See comments]. *Nature* 1997;386:804.
147. Suzuki A, de la Pompa JL, Hakem R, et al. Brca2 is required for embryonic cellular proliferation in the mouse. *Genes Dev* 1997;511:1242.
148. Friedman LS, Thistlethwaite FC, Patel KJ, et al. Thymic lymphomas in mice with a truncating mutation in Brca2. *Cancer Res* 1998;58:1338.
149. Connor F, Bertwistle D, Mee PJ, et al. Tumorigenesis and a DNA repair defect in mice with a truncating Brca2 mutation. *Nat Genet* 1997; 17:423.
150. Gudas JM, Li T, Nguyen H, Jensen D, Rauscher FJ, Cowan KH. Cell cycle regulation of BRCA1 messenger RNA in human breast epithelial cells. *Cell Growth Differ* 1996;7:717.
151. Lim DS, Hasty P. A mutation in mouse rad51 results in an early embryonic lethal that is suppressed by a mutation in p53. *Mol Cell Biol* 1996;16:7133.
152. Morimatsu M, Donoho G, Hasty P. Cells deleted for Brca2 COOH terminus exhibit hypersensitivity to gamma-radiation and premature senescence. *Cancer Res* 1998;58:3441.
153. McAllister KA, Haugen-Strano A, Hagevik S, et al. Characterization of the rat and mouse homologues of the BRCA2 breast cancer susceptibility gene. *Cancer Res* 1997;57:3121.
154. Patel KJ, Vu VP, Lee K, et al. Involvement of Brca2 in DNA repair. *J Clin Monit Comput* 1998;1:347.
155. Abbott DW, Freeman ML, Holt JT. Double-strand break repair deficiency and radiation sensitivity in BRCA2 mutant cancer cells [See comments]. *J Natl Cancer Inst* 1998;90:978.
156. Li FP, Fraumeni JF. Soft-tissue sarcomas, breast cancer, and other neoplasms: familial syndrome? *Ann Intern Med* 1969;71:747.
157. Li FP, Fraumeni JF, Mulvihill JJ. A cancer family syndrome in 24 kindreds. *Cancer Res* 1988;48:5358.
158. Strong LC, Williams WR, Tainsky MA. The Li-Fraumeni syndrome: from clinical epidemiology to molecular genetics. *Am J Epidemiol* 1992;135:190.
159. Williams W, Strong L. Genetic epidemiology of soft tissue sarcomas in children. In: Muller H, Weber W, eds. *Familial cancer: first international research conference*. Basel, Switzerland: Karger, 1985:151.
160. Garber JE, Goldstein AM, Kantor AF, Dreyfus MG, Fraumeni JF Jr, Li FP. Follow-up study of twenty-four families with Li-Fraumeni syndrome. *Cancer Res* 1991;51:6094.
161. Malkin D, Li FP, Strong LC, et al. Germ line p53 mutations in a familial syndrome of breast cancer, sarcomas, and other neoplasms [See comments]. *Science* 1990;250:1233.
162. Srivasta S, Zou ZQ, Pirollo K, Blattner W, Chang EH. Germ-line transmission of a mutated p53 gene in a cancer-prone family with Li-Fraumeni syndrome [See comments]. *Nature* 1990;348:747.
163. Frebourg T, Kassel J, Lam KT, et al. Germ-line mutations of the p53 tumor suppressor gene in patients with high risk for cancer inactivate the p53 protein. *Proc Natl Acad Sci U S A* 1992;89:6413.
164. Bames DM, Hanby AM, Gillett CE, et al. Abnormal expression of wild type p53 protein in normal cells of a cancer family patient. *Lancet* 1992;340:259.
165. Toguchida J, Yamaguchi T, Dayton SK, et al. Prevalence and spectrum of germline mutations of the p53 gene among patients with sarcoma [See comments]. *N Engl J Med* 1992;326:1301.
166. Sidransky D, Tokino T, Helzlsouer K, et al. Inherited p53 gene mutations in breast cancer. *Cancer Res* 1992;52:2984.
167. Borresen AL, Andersen TI, Garber J, et al. Screening for germ line TP53 mutations in breast cancer patients. *Cancer Res* 1992;52:3234.
168. Savitsky K, Sfez S, Tagle DA, et al. The complete sequence of the coding region of the ATM gene reveals similarity to cell cycle regulators in different species. *Hum Mol Genet* 1995;14:2025.
169. Swift M, Reltnauer PJ, Morrell D, Chase CL. Breast and other cancers in families with ataxia-telangiectasia. *N Engl J Med* 1987; 316:1289.
170. Swift M, Morrell D, Massey RB, Chase CL. Incidence of cancer in 161 families affected by ataxia-telangiectasia [See comments]. *N Engl J Med* 1991;325:1831.
171. Easton DF. Cancer risks in A-T heterozygotes. *Int J Radiat Biol* 1994;66[Suppl 6]:S177.
172. Athma P, Rappaport R, Swift M. Molecular genotyping shows that ataxia-telangiectasia heterozygotes are predisposed to breast cancer. *Cancer Genet Cytogenet* 1996;92:1304.
173. Vorechovsky I, Rasio D, Luo L, et al. The ATM gene and susceptibility to breast cancer: analysis of 38 breast tumors reveals no evidence for mutation. *Cancer Res* 1996;56:2726.
174. Chen J, Birkholtz GG, Lindblom P, Rubio C, Lindblom A. The role of ataxia-telangiectasia heterozygotes in familial breast cancer. *Cancer Res* 1998;58:1376.
175. Fitzgerald MG, Bean JM, Hegde SR, et al. Heterozygous ATM mutations do not contribute to early onset of breast cancer [See comments]. *Nat Genet* 1997;15:307.
176. Brownstein MH, Wolf M, Bikowski JB. Cowden's disease: a cutaneous marker of breast cancer. *Cancer* 1978;41:2393.
177. Starink TM. Cowden's disease: analysis of fourteen new cases. *J Am Acad Dermatol* 1984;11:1127.
178. Nelen MR, Padberg GW, Peeters EA, et al. Localization of the gene for Cowden disease to chromosome 10q22-23. *Nat Genet* 1996;13:114.

179. Liaw D, Marsh DJ, Li J, et al. Germline mutations of the PTEN gene in Cowden disease, an inherited breast and thyroid cancer syndrome. *Nat Genet* 1997;16:64.
180. Nelen MR, van Staveren WC, Peeters EA, et al. Germline mutations in the PTEN/MMAC1 gene in patients with Cowden disease. *Hum Mol Genet* 1997;6:1383.
181. Tsou HC, Teng DH, Ping XL, et al. The role of MMAC1 mutations in early-onset breast cancer: causative in association with Cowden syndrome and excluded in BRCA1-negative cases. *Am J Hum Genet* 1997;61:1036.
182. Li DM, Sun H. TEP1, encoded by a candidate tumor suppressor locus, is a novel protein tyrosine phosphatase regulated by transforming growth factor beta. *Cancer Res* 1997;57:2124.
183. Jeghers K, McKusick V, Katz K. Generalized intestinal polyposis and melanin spots of the oral mucosa, lips and digits: a syndrome of diagnostic significance. *N Engl J Med* 1949;241:992.
184. Peutz J. On a very remarkable case of familial polyposis of the mucous membrane of the intestinal tract and nasopharynx accompanied by peculiar pigmentation of the skin and mucous membrane. *Ned Tijdschr Geneeskd* 1921;110:134.
185. Giardiello FM, Welsh SB, Hamilton SR, et al. Increased risk of cancer in the Peutz-Jeghers syndrome. *N Engl J Med* 1987;316:1511.
186. Boardman LA, Thibodeau SN, Schaid DJ, et al. Increased risk for cancer in patients with the Peutz-Jeghers syndrome. *Ann Intern Med* 1998;128:896.
187. Hemminki A, Tomlinson I, Markie D. Localization of a susceptibility locus for PJS to 19p using comparative genomic hybridization and targeted linkage analysis. *Nat Genet* 1997;115:87.
188. Olschwang S, Markle D. Peutz-Jeghers disease: most, but not all, families are compatible with linkage to 19p13.3. *J Med Genet* 1998;35:42.
189. Muir EG, Bell AJ, Barlow KA. Multiple primary carcinomata of the colon, duodenum, and larynx associated with kerato-acanthomata of the face. *Br J Surg* 1967;54:191.
190. Hall NR, Williams MA, Murday VA, Newton JA, Bishop DT. Muir-Torre syndrome: a variant of the cancer family syndrome. *J Med Genet* 1994;31:627.
191. Anderson DE. An inherited form of large bowel cancer: Muir's syndrome. *Cancer* 1980;45[Suppl 5]:1103.
192. Fishel R, Lescoe MK, Rao MR, et al. The human mutator gene homolog MSH2 and its association with hereditary nonpolyposis colon cancer [Published erratum appears in *Cell* 1994;77:167]. *Cell* 1993;75:1027.
193. Leach FS, Nicolaides NC, Papadopoulos N, et al. Mutations of a mutS homolog in hereditary nonpolyposis colorectal cancer. *Cell* 1993;75:1215.
194. Papadopoulos N, Nicolaides NC, Wei YF, et al. Mutation of a mutL homolog in hereditary colon cancer [See comments]. *Science* 1994;263:1625.
195. Bronner CE, Baker SM, Morrison PT, et al. Mutation in the DNA mismatch repair gene homologue hMLH1 is associated with hereditary non-polyposis colon cancer. *Nature* 1994;368:258.
196. Kolodner PD, Hall NR, Lipford J, et al. Structure of the human MSH2 locus and analysis of two Muir-Torre kindreds for msh2 mutations [Published erratum appears in *Genomics* 1995;28:613]. *Genomics* 1994;24:516.
197. Bapat B, Xia L, Madlensky L, et al. The genetic basis of Muir-Torre syndrome includes the hMH1 locus [Letter]. *Am J Hum Genet* 1996;59:736.

Diseases of the Breast, 2nd ed.,
edited by Jay R. Harris.
Lippincott Williams & Wilkins, Philadelphia © 2000.

CHAPTER 17

Evaluation and Management of Women with a Strong Family History of Breast Cancer

Claudine J. D. Isaacs, Beth N. Peshkin, and Caryn Lerman

As breast cancer risk factors, including the impact of a positive family history, become better understood, genetic counseling and testing are being increasingly integrated into the management of women at high risk for this disease. When family histories suggest transmission of genetic risk, high-risk women and their family members may benefit from participation in counseling and testing programs. High-risk women potentially can reduce their risk of cancer morbidity and mortality through increased surveillance and adoption of risk-reducing strategies. Noncarriers of risk-conferring mutations may be relieved of persistent worry. Despite these possible benefits, testing carries a number of psychological and social risks that patients and providers must consider. These include adverse psychological effects in individuals and families and the chance of insurance discrimination.

Although genetic counseling and testing for breast cancer are diffusing into mainstream oncologic care, critical questions regarding cancer risks, the benefits of genetic testing, and the efficacy of management options remain unanswered. These limitations in knowledge create challenges for the providers who must counsel patients about these issues and for the patients who face these decisions. This chapter provides an overview of the medical and psychosocial issues relevant to this process. The chapter focuses on high-risk patients who have family histories consistent with inherited susceptibility to breast cancer and who have been deemed appropriate candidates for genetic testing by major medical organizations.[1] The evaluation and management of women with less suggestive family histories are also addressed. The assessment of the likelihood that a family harbors a breast cancer–predisposing mutation is first examined, followed by a discussion of cancer risks in mutation carriers. The genetic counseling process and laboratory testing issues are then reviewed. Finally, the medical and psychosocial management issues for high-risk individuals and families are discussed.

C. J. D. Isaacs: Lombardi Cancer Center, Georgetown University Medical Center, Washington, D.C.

B. N. Peshkin: Department of Obstetrics and Gynecology, Lombardi Cancer Center, Georgetown University Medical Center, Washington, D.C.

C. Lerman: Lombardi Cancer Center, Georgetown University Medical Center, Washington, D.C.

ASSESSMENT OF THE PROBABILITY OF INHERITED SUSCEPTIBILITY

Of the many factors known to influence a woman's risk of breast cancer, family history and increasing age are among the most significant. Estimates are that 20% to 30% of women with breast cancer have at least one relative with this disease,[2,3] and 5% to 10% have a true hereditary predisposition to breast cancer.[4] Thus, the majority of women with a family history of the disease do not have hereditary breast cancer but rather have a familial basis to their disease. Most hereditary breast cancers arise from mutations in *BRCA1* and *BRCA2*. Registry-identified families with deleterious mutations in these genes often have cancer histories extending over many generations and thus provide unmistakable clues about the hallmarks of hereditary breast cancer. As illustrated in Fig. 1, these features include the presence of multiple relatives affected with breast or ovarian cancer, usually with a predominance of early-onset cases; the presence of women with more than one primary cancer, such as bilateral breast cancer or breast and ovarian cancer; and vertical transmission, including transmission in two or more generations as well as through male relatives (consistent with autosomal dominant inheritance). In addition, the occurrence of rare malignancies or certain hallmark features may be suggestive of a specific syndrome or gene mutation. For example, early-onset sarcomas and breast cancers are suggestive of Li-Fraumeni syndrome, whereas the presence of hamartomas is suggestive of Cowden disease.

When performing risk assessments for hereditary breast cancer, in addition to obtaining family medical history, the clinician should also inquire about the patient's ethnic background, as specific mutations in *BRCA1* and *BRCA2* have been found to occur with increased frequency in certain populations. For example, two *BRCA1* mutations, 185delAG and 5382insC, and one *BRCA2* mutation, 6174delT, have been found with increased frequency in individuals of

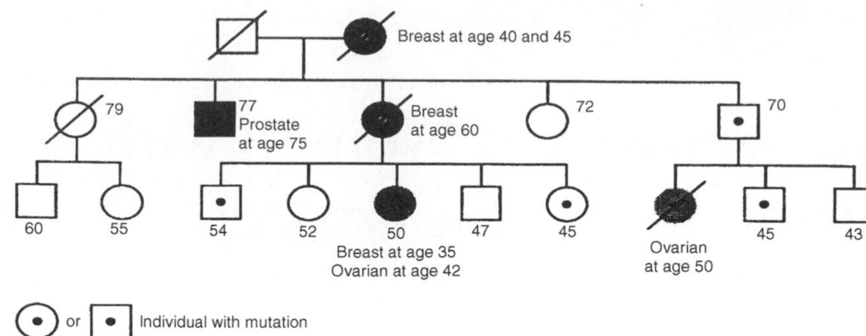

FIG. 1. This pedigree illustrates classic features of hereditary breast cancer. An autosomal dominant pattern of inheritance is clearly demonstrated; three generations are affected, and approximately 50% of offspring at risk carry the mutation. Other characteristic features of hereditary breast cancer include early onset of breast and ovarian cancer, bilateral breast cancer, and multiple primary cancers in the same individual. Note that transmission through men is also possible.

Ashkenazi Jewish descent.[5] The impact of founder mutations on the likelihood of detecting a mutation in *BRCA1* or *BRCA2* is discussed in greater detail below.

In practice, the ability to discern a pattern of hereditary breast cancer may be hampered by a variety of factors. These include the genes' variable expressivity and incomplete penetrance. In addition, many individuals have limited knowledge about their family histories. Kindreds may also be small in size or may not be highly informative. For example, families may contain many men relative to women at risk, women who died young, or individuals not yet old enough to exhibit the phenotype.

Given all of these considerations, when a patient's family history is deemed to be suggestive of hereditary breast cancer, risk assessment is based on probabilistic estimates of finding a gene mutation, the chance that the individual is a gene carrier based on Mendelian analysis, and the risk of cancer based on estimates of gene penetrance. In cases in which a patient's history is not highly suggestive of hereditary breast cancer, however, empiric models are available to estimate risk of breast cancer.

Empiric Models of Risk Assessment

The Cancer and Steroid Hormone (CASH) Study, a population-based, case-control study, fit genetic models to derive age-specific breast cancer risk estimates for women with at least one relative with breast cancer.[6] Risk tables from this model are available that allow the clinician to assess risk based on the relatives' age at diagnosis and the degree of relationship of these relatives. For example, a woman with one first-degree relative with breast cancer diagnosed in her thirties is estimated to have a 16% lifetime risk of developing breast cancer. This model also predicted breast cancer risk of women with a very strong family history of the disease. Thus, a woman with two first-degree relatives with breast cancer, one diagnosed at age 45 and the other at age 52, is predicted to have a lifetime risk of breast cancer of approximately 30%. However, if both these relatives were diagnosed in their twenties, the woman's risk is estimated to be approximately 48%. One must remember that this model predated the identification of *BRCA1* and *BRCA2* and is based on the possibility that a rare autosomal dominant allele is segregating in the family. Now that *BRCA1* and *BRCA2* have been cloned, the probabilistic models described below may also be useful for assessing the likelihood that an individual with a strong family history of breast cancer harbors a mutation in one of these genes. This information, in turn, can be used to estimate her risk of cancer.

Another model, known as the Gail model, is based on data from the Breast Cancer Detection Demonstration Project. This model uses the following risk factor information to derive age-specific breast cancer risk estimates: age at menarche, age at first live birth, number of previous biopsies, presence of atypical hyperplasia or lobular carcinoma *in situ*, and number of first-degree relatives with breast cancer.[7] Data for an individual patient can be analyzed using a computer program developed by the National Cancer Institute or extrapolated from graphs.[8] For example, a 45-year-old woman with menarche at age 11, a first full-term pregnancy at age 26, one first-degree relative with breast cancer, and no prior breast biopsies is estimated to have a 1.8% 5-year risk and a 19% lifetime risk (to age 90) of breast cancer. If this woman had two first-degree relatives with breast cancer rather than just one, her 5-year risk of breast cancer would increase to 3.1% and her lifetime risk to 32%. If, on the other hand, this woman had no relatives with breast cancer, her 5-year risk of cancer is estimated at 1%, and her lifetime risk is estimated at 12%. Limitations of this model are the inclusion of a nonbiological variable (i.e., the number of breast biopsies may be influenced by patient or physician concern due to family history) and the exclusion of more extensive family history information, including information from all paternal relatives and the ages at diagnosis of cancer. Whereas the inclusion of any biopsy history may falsely elevate risk, omission of family history data may lead to a sizable underestimation of risk. Validation studies of this model revealed that, in certain circumstances, it overestimated cancer risk. Data from the Nurses' Health Study found that the Gail model overpredicted the absolute risk of breast cancer by 33% for women between 25 and 61 years of age who did not undergo annual mammography screening.[9] A second study found that the Gail model provided a good estimation of cancer risk for women who participated in regular cancer screening; however, it overpredicted the risk for women not adhering to screening recommendations as well as for those under the age of 60, and underpredicted the risk for those over age 60.[10]

Risk estimates for the same woman based on CASH and Gail models have been compared and were found to be discordant in several circumstances, in part because of the different parameters of the models.[11] Thus, no model is appropriate for every patient. However, the information may be interpreted qualitatively to get a sense of whether the patient is at a somewhat higher risk of developing breast cancer or at a very high risk for the disease. Screening and prevention programs may then be tailored to the risk level of the patient.

Probabilistic Estimates and Models of Risk Assessment for Individuals with Family Histories Suggestive of Hereditary Breast Cancer

Founder Mutations

An important aspect of accurate assessment of hereditary risk is documentation of the pedigree and the patient's ethnic background. For example, the carrier frequency for *BRCA1* mutations in the general population is between 1 in 500 and 1 in 800[12] and is lower for *BRCA2*; however, in individuals of Ashkenazi Jewish descent, two *BRCA1* mutations (185delAG and 5382insC) and one *BRCA2* mutation (6174delT) occur with a background frequency of 2.3%,[13] In light of this high background frequency, it is not surprising that 50% to 90% of Jewish families with strong histories of breast and ovarian cancer harbor one of these founder mutations.[5,14] In addition, studies have been performed in breast and ovarian cancer patients of Ashkenazi Jewish descent who were unselected for family history. Those with breast cancer diagnosed at age 40 or younger were found to have a 21% chance of carrying the 185delAG mutation,[15] and 38% of ovarian cancer patients diagnosed before age 50 carried the 185delAG mutation.[16] Another study conducted in Israel examined the frequency of the three common founder mutations in 199 Ashkenazi Jewish women with breast or ovarian cancer (or both).[17] Of these women, 99 had no family history of breast or ovarian cancer. Thirty percent of the breast cancer patients younger than age 40 and 62% of the ovarian cancer patients tested positive for one of the three mutations. Thus, for Jewish individuals, one case alone of early-onset breast or ovarian cancer is sufficient history to warrant consideration of *BRCA1* and *BRCA2* testing.

As reviewed by Szabo and King, founder mutations have been identified in other ethnic subpopulations, including those in Iceland, Finland, France, Holland/Belgium, Russia, Sweden, and Denmark.[18] The attributable risk of *BRCA* mutations in these populations varied considerably. For example, in Russia, 79% of families with breast and ovarian cancer had one of two common *BRCA1* mutations; one of these, 5382insC, occurs quite frequently in Europeans in general, including Ashkenazi Jews. The other mutation, 4153delA, appears to occur only in Russians. Similarly, in Israel, the three Jewish founder mutations accounted for a high proportion (47%) of hereditary breast and ovarian cancer, as would be expected. However, in Italy, only 29% of high-risk families had a *BRCA1* mutation, and almost all of them were unique mutations. As additional studies are undertaken, a pattern of recurrent mutations may emerge in additional populations, as suggested by some preliminary data from African-American families.[19] In addition, a study showed that six *BRCA1* and *BRCA2* mutations were found in 40% of high-risk French Canadian families.[20] Overall, *BRCA2* mutations occur less frequently than *BRCA1* mutations. However, in Iceland, a single *BRCA2* mutation, 999del5, accounted for a substantial proportion of breast and ovarian cancer cases in that country.[21,22] Thus, information about the genetic epidemiology of *BRCA1* and *BRCA2* in different populations may assist the clinician in determining the likelihood of a hereditary susceptibility to breast cancer as well as the type, extent, or sequence of testing to be performed in particular subsets of patients.

Probabilistic Models

In addition to assessments related to ethnic ancestry, probabilistic models have been developed to assist the clinician in determining the likelihood that an individual harbors a *BRCA1* or *BRCA2* mutation. One study used a logistic regression analysis to predict the probability of detecting a *BRCA1* mutation given various factors in a woman's medical and family history.[23] Twenty institutions in North America and Europe pooled *BRCA1* data on 798 high-risk women from distinct families. In 102 women, a deleterious mutation was identified. The age of the proband, personal cancer history, Ashkenazi Jewish ancestry, and family history were all found to significantly influence the likelihood that these mutations would be detected. The odds of detecting a *BRCA1* mutation decreased by 8% with each year added to the proband's age at diagnosis. The odds were increased by personal cancer history, strong family history, and Ashkenazi Jewish ancestry. When women with unilateral breast cancer were used as the comparison group, the odds were found to increase 3.7-fold for those with bilateral breast cancer, 5.4-fold for those with ovarian cancer, and 8-fold for those with unilateral breast cancer and ovarian cancer. Odds also increased 2.9-fold for each relative with ovarian cancer, 5.3-fold for each relative with both breast and ovarian cancer, and 1.4-fold for each relative with breast cancer alone. In addition, an Ashkenazi Jewish woman's chance of carrying a deleterious mutation was 4.1 times that of a non-Ashkenazi woman. For example, in Jewish families with at least two cases of breast cancer and one case of ovarian cancer, the chance of finding a *BRCA1* mutation is 75%. In non-Ashkenazi families with the same history, the probability drops to 33%. A smaller study of 169 women referred to a

TABLE 1. *Modeled probabilities of detecting a* BRCA1 *or* BRCA2 *mutation*

Family history parameter	Likelihood of *BRCA1* mutation	Likelihood of *BRCA2* mutation
Single affected individuals (no other family history)		
Breast cancer at <30 yr	12%	n/a
Breast cancer at <40 yr	6%	n/a
Jewish woman with breast cancer at <40 yr	33%	n/a
Two or more cases of breast/ovarian cancer in FDR or SDR		
≥2 breast cancers at ≥50 yr	2%	n/a
1 breast cancer at 40–50 yr and 1 breast cancer at <50 yr	10%	14.5%
1 breast cancer at 40–50 yr and FDR or SDR with ovarian cancer	23%	12.5%
1 breast cancer case at 40–50 yr with bilateral breast cancer or ovarian cancer and FDR or SDR with breast cancer at <50 yr	42%	10%
1 breast case cancer at 40–50 yr with bilateral breast cancer or ovarian cancer and FDR or SDR with ovarian cancer	65%	6%

FDR, first-degree relative; n/a, not available; SDR, second-degree relative.
Adapted from refs. 23 and 25.

high-risk clinic also found that breast cancer diagnosis at an early age, the presence of ovarian cancer, the occurrence of breast and ovarian cancer in the same individual, and Ashkenazi Jewish ancestry were all associated with an increased risk of detecting a *BRCA1* mutation.[24]

Newer models have been developed since the cloning of *BRCA2*. The most extensive model is based on a study of 238 women with breast cancer diagnosed before age 50 or ovarian cancer diagnosed at any age and a positive family history.[25] This model demonstrated that the presence of ovarian cancer within families significantly increases the chance of finding a *BRCA1* or *BRCA2* mutation. For example, the model predicts that if two women with breast cancer diagnosed before age 50 are first- or second-degree relatives of one another, the probability of finding a *BRCA1* mutation is approximately 10%, and the chance of finding a *BRCA2* mutation is approximately 15%; thus, the combined probability of finding a mutation in one or the other gene is 25%. However, if one of these relatives also had ovarian cancer, the chance of finding a mutation doubles to approximately 50% (a 42% chance of finding a *BRCA1* mutation and a 10% chance of finding a *BRCA2* mutation). An early age of onset for breast cancer (younger than 40 years) and a diagnosis of ovarian cancer in the same woman, in combination with a family history of breast and ovarian cancer, increases the likelihood of finding a *BRCA1* or *BRCA2* mutation to almost 90%. Additional examples are highlighted in Table 1. Although the issue was not addressed quantitatively in the aforementioned study, in a family presenting with rare cancers, such as those of the pancreas or male breast, the clinician may suspect the likelihood of finding a *BRCA2* mutation to be higher.[26,27] In general, however, *BRCA2* mutations account for a lower proportion of hereditary breast cancer cases than *BRCA1* mutations.

Despite the fact that other studies have found Ashkenazi ancestry to be associated with a significantly increased chance of finding a *BRCA1* or *BRCA2* mutation, the model by Frank et al. did not confirm this finding.[25] The authors hypothesized that this may be due to the fact that only families with strong histories of breast and ovarian cancer were included; thus, probability estimates may not be significantly impacted by ethnicity in the setting of a strong family history.

A substantial proportion of individuals with a very strong family history of breast and ovarian cancer are not found to have mutations in either *BRCA1* or *BRCA2*.[24,25] The most probable explanation for this finding is that other as yet undefined genes account for the cancers seen in these families. In addition, methods of testing are unable to detect all disease-conferring mutations in *BRCA1* and *BRCA2*.

In summary, the models outlined provide patients with an estimate of their risk status and the likelihood that *BRCA1* and *BRCA2* gene testing will be informative. In accordance with guidelines set forth by the American Society of Clinical Oncology, individuals with family histories consistent with at least a 10% chance of finding a mutation in a breast cancer susceptibility gene[1] are considered at high risk for breast cancer on the basis of family history and are appropriate candidates for genetic testing. Individuals who have at least one first-degree relative with breast cancer but who do not have a family history strong enough to be consistent with at least a 10% chance of harboring a mutation in *BRCA1* or *BRCA2* or those with at least a 1.66% 5-year risk of breast cancer as determined by the Gail model are considered at moderate risk of breast cancer. Importantly, factors related to family history are only one aspect to be considered by patients in deciding whether to undergo genetic testing. As outlined in the section on Genetic Counseling Process, individuals with a strong family history of breast or ovarian cancer must seriously weigh the benefits, limitations, and risks of testing before deciding whether to pursue testing.

CLINICAL CHARACTERISTICS OF HEREDITARY BREAST CANCER

The majority of cases of hereditary breast cancer is due to mutations in *BRCA1* and *BRCA2*. Rare syndromes that

TABLE 2. *Estimated cancer risks associated with* BRCA1 *and* BRCA2 *mutations*

Type of cancer	Estimated lifetime risk in *BRCA1* mutation carriers[13,28–30,33]	Estimated lifetime risk in *BRCA2* mutation carriers[5,25–27,31,32]	Lifetime risk in general population
Breast cancer	55%–85%	37%–85%	12.5%
Contralateral breast cancer	Up to 65%	Possibly similar to *BRCA1* risks	0.5%–1.0% per year
Ovarian cancer	15%–60%	15%–27%	1.4%
Ovarian cancer after breast cancer	Up to 30%–55%	Significantly elevated	2%–3% (approximately twice the average risk)
Colon cancer	Possible relative risk of 4	Possible increased risk	Approximately 6%
Prostate cancer	Increased risk, possibly up to a relative risk of 3	Probable increased risk	At least 10%, but risk is difficult to quantify partially owing to the presence of clinically undetectable cancers
Male breast cancer	A few reported cases	Approximately 6%	Extremely rare
Pancreatic cancer	Not increased	Associations noted	Rare

These risks are cumulative and are not mutation specific. In general, early ages of onset have been associated primarily with female breast cancer and ovarian cancer. However, some cases of early-onset pancreatic cancer associated with *BRCA2* alterations have been reported. Relative risks, such as those associated with prostate and colon cancer in *BRCA1* carriers, are not directly translatable to absolute risks. Figures for general population risks include some patients with hereditary cancer. All risks must be evaluated in the context of the patient's medical and family history.
Modified from ref. 61.

account for substantially less than 1% of all cases of breast cancer include the Li-Fraumeni syndrome, Cowden disease, Peutz-Jeghers syndrome, Muir-Torre syndrome, and possibly ataxia-telangiectasia heterozygosity. The cancer risks of individuals with hereditary breast cancer are summarized below.

BRCA1 and *BRCA2*

Cancer Risks

BRCA1 and *BRCA2* carriers have been found to have a wide range of cancer risks (Table 2). The initial studies assessing cancer risks were performed in very highly selected families with multiple cases of breast and ovarian cancer. In these studies, the risk of breast cancer in *BRCA1* and *BRCA2* carriers was estimated to be up to 85%.[27,28–31] *BRCA1* and *BRCA2* carriers have been found to have an early age of onset of breast cancer in comparison with the general population. Approximately 20% of *BRCA1* carriers develop breast cancer before the age of 40; one-half of carriers develop it by the age of 50.[28] *BRCA2* carriers may have a slightly older age of onset of breast cancer than do *BRCA1* carriers. A study found that 32% of *BRCA2* carriers had developed breast cancer by age 50 and 53% by age 60.[31] In these individuals, the average age of onset of breast cancer was found to be 41 years.[26] The risk of ovarian cancer by age 70 was estimated at close to 60% for *BRCA1* carriers[28,29] and at up to 27% for *BRCA2* carriers.[29] Subsequently, population-based studies were performed and demonstrated lower cancer risks. The family history information obtained from population-based studies is often incomplete. Thus, these studies may underestimate cancer risks. A study of 5,000 individuals of Ashkenazi Jewish descent not selected for a family history of breast or ovarian cancer estimated that the risk of breast cancer was 56% by age 70 for carriers of two *BRCA1* mutations, 185delAG and 5382insC, and one *BRCA2* mutation, 6174delT.[13] The risk of ovarian cancer in this population was found to be 15%. Another population-based study performed in Iceland, which obtained family history only on first-degree relatives, found that carriers of the 999del5 *BRCA2* mutation had a 37% risk of breast cancer by age 70.[32] Therefore, for *BRCA1* carriers, the breast cancer risk varies between 55% and 85%, and for *BRCA2* carriers, the risk may be as low as 37% or as high as 85%. The risk of ovarian cancer is estimated to be 15% to 60% for *BRCA1* carriers and between 15% and 27% for *BRCA2* carriers.

Mutation carriers also face an increased risk of second malignancy. *BRCA1* carriers who are affected with breast cancer have been estimated to have a 38% 10-year risk and up to a 65% cumulative risk of contralateral breast cancer.[28,33] In comparison, individuals with sporadic breast cancer have a 0.5% to 1.0% annual risk of contralateral breast cancer. No conclusive information exists on the risk of ipsilateral recurrence in mutation carriers with breast cancer after breast-conserving surgery and radiation therapy. This subject is discussed in greater detail in Chapter 33. In addition to the increased risk of a second primary breast cancer, the risk for ovarian cancer in *BRCA1* carriers affected with breast cancer has been estimated to be as high as 44% by age 70.[28] This compares to a risk of approximately 3% in patients with sporadic breast cancer. *BRCA2* carriers' risk of ovarian cancer after a diagnosis of breast cancer has been estimated to be ten times greater than that of women with sporadic breast cancer.[25]

Results from a population-based study indicated that men with *BRCA1* and *BRCA2* mutations have a 16% risk of prostate cancer by age 70.[13] Noncarriers were found to have a risk of 4%. Typically, the age of onset of prostate cancer is the same in *BRCA1* and *BRCA2* carriers as in the general population. In addition, men with a *BRCA2* mutation have been estimated to have up to a 6% chance of developing breast cancer.[27] Some studies have also suggested that colon cancer is associated with *BRCA1* mutations[30] and pancreatic cancer with *BRCA2* mutations.[5,26]

In summary, the precise cancer risks for any one mutation carrier are difficult to define. These risks should be interpreted within the context of the individual's own family history. In addition, specific *BRCA1* or *BRCA2* mutations may be associated with different cancer risks.

Cancer Risk Modifiers

Individuals within the same family carrying the same mutation may show significant differences in the age of onset and type of cancer developed. For instance, one woman may develop breast cancer in her thirties; her sister may develop both early-onset breast cancer and ovarian cancer; and a third mutation-positive relative may be healthy in her seventies. This variable penetrance and expressivity of *BRCA1* and *BRCA2* has led investigators to examine the role of environmental risk factors and other genes in modifying the cancer risks of carriers.

A study of the reproductive history of 333 women with *BRCA1* mutations was conducted to shed some light on possible environmental risk modifiers.[34] The risk of breast cancer was found to be increased in those who experienced menarche before age 12 (relative risk, 1.57) and in those with parity of less than three (relative risk, 2). Age at first full-term pregnancy was not found to influence the risk of breast cancer. In distinction to what is seen in the general population, the risk of ovarian cancer was found to be higher in those with increased parity, with each additional birth resulting in an increased relative risk of 1.4. However, a protective effect was found for a later age at last birth. Women whose last birth was at age 30 or older had a 48% reduction in risk of ovarian cancer compared with those who were 29 years or younger at last birth.

A case-control study examined the effects of oral contraceptive use on the risk of ovarian cancer in mutation carriers.[35] Known mutation carriers with a history of ovarian cancer were compared with their sister controls. The results suggested that oral contraceptive use may reduce the risk of ovarian cancer by as much as one-half in *BRCA1* and *BRCA2* carriers. However, the sister-control group included mutation carriers, noncarriers, and individuals whose mutation status was unknown. In addition, 42% of the control group had undergone prophylactic oophorectomy. The heterogeneity of the control group and the presence of confounding factors, such as prophylactic surgery, make it difficult to ascertain the true impact of oral contraceptive use in mutation carriers. Nonetheless, this study does suggest that oral contraceptive use offers protection against ovarian cancer in this patient population. A study of 50 young Ashkenazi Jewish breast cancer patients, however, indicated that long-term oral contraceptive use (more than 48 months), particularly before a first full-term pregnancy, was associated with a higher chance of being classified as a *BRCA1* or *BRCA2* carrier; this finding suggests that oral contraceptive use may increase breast cancer risk more in *BRCA1* and *BRCA2* mutation carriers than in noncarriers.[36] Thus, in mutation carriers, oral contraceptives may possibly provide protection against ovarian cancer but may also increase the risk of breast cancer. Further studies are needed to address this issue.

Modifier genes may also affect gene penetrance. For example, one group found that the risk of ovarian cancer in *BRCA1* carriers with one or two rare *HRAS1* alleles was approximately two times greater than in carriers with only common *HRAS1* alleles.[37] Another study examined allelic variants of *CYP1A1*, a gene involved in the metabolism of polyaromatic hydrocarbons and in the hydroxylation of estradiol, in *BRCA1* and *BRCA2* mutation carriers with and without breast cancer.[38] In this study, a particular allelic variant was found in 14% of carriers with cancer and in 22% of unaffected carriers and reduced the risk of breast cancer by approximately 40%. Studies addressing the role of other gene-gene interactions are under way.

Ideally, to best address the impact of gene-gene or gene-environment interactions on the risk of cancer in mutation carriers, studies should be performed only in individuals with a defined *BRCA1* or *BRCA2* mutation. Study designs of this type would allow a clearer evaluation of the effect of a possible risk modifier on cancer incidence in mutation carriers. To date, identification of enough affected and unaffected carriers to carry out studies in this fashion has not been possible. Therefore, further studies are needed to validate the observations from the studies discussed in this chapter. If these findings are substantiated, it may be possible to more specifically determine an individual carrier's cancer risks and to devise tailored risk-reduction strategies.

Li-Fraumeni Syndrome

Li-Fraumeni syndrome is an autosomal dominant condition characterized by soft-tissue sarcomas, osteosarcomas, leukemias, brain tumors, adrenocortical malignancies, and early-onset breast cancer. Estimates are that 50% of carriers develop some form of cancer by age 30 years and 90% by age 70 years.[39] In particular, the occurrence of breast cancer in these families is remarkable. In a study of 24 Li-Fraumeni syndrome families including 200 individuals, 45 women were found to have developed breast cancer, of whom 73% were diagnosed before age 45.[40] Multiple breast cancers were diagnosed in approximately 25% of these women, and more than 25% had had other additional primary tumors. Mutations in the tumor-suppressor gene p53 have been documented in up to 70% of families with Li-Fraumeni syndrome; however, estimates vary depending on the ascertainment criteria used and the extent of gene testing performed.[41] When a mutation is identified, predictive testing may be available to family members at risk. Screening for most of the component cancers of this syndrome is not available, but informing women at risk for Li-Fraumeni syndrome about options for early detection and prevention of breast cancer is critical.

Ataxia-Telangiectasia

Ataxia-telangiectasia is an autosomal recessive condition characterized by immunodeficiency, cerebellar degeneration, oculocutaneous telangiectasias, and a markedly elevated risk of solid tumors and hematologic malignancies, such as leukemia and lymphoma. The causative gene, *ATM*, is located on chromosome arm 11q, and the carrier frequency of mutations is estimated at 1%.[42] A study of female relatives of known *ATM* heterozygotes found that carriers had a fourfold greater risk of breast cancer than did noncarriers.[43] A previous study had also indicated that the risk of breast cancer in female heterozygotes may be further increased by exposure to ionizing radiation.[44] This issue remains controversial, however, as other studies have not demonstrated a link between *ATM* heterozygosity and an elevated breast cancer risk.[45] Further research is needed to clarify the clinical implications associated with *ATM* mutations.

Cowden Syndrome

Cowden syndrome is a rare autosomal dominant condition characterized by multiple hamartomatous lesions and an increased risk of early-onset breast cancer and thyroid cancer.[46] The hamartomas seen in association with this condition are present in skin, oral mucosa, breast, and intestine. The mucocutaneous hamartomas include papillomas of the lips and mucous membranes, acral keratoses of the skin, and rough-surfaced facial papules called *trichilemmomas*. The majority of individuals affected with Cowden syndrome develop skin lesions by age 20. Breast cancer may affect 25% to 50% of females with Cowden syndrome. Many of these women will be diagnosed premenopausally, and the majority do not appear to have a family history of breast cancer.[47] Schrager et al. noted that the malignant tumors are usually ductal in origin and are often surrounded by densely collagenized hamartomatous lesions.[47] Also, an increased incidence of bilateral disease has been observed for benign and malignant conditions.[47] For example, the benign conditions associated with Cowden syndrome, which may occur in up to 75% of affected women, include ductal hyperplasia, intraductal papillomatosis, adenosis, lobular atrophy, fibroadenomas, and fibrocystic changes.[46,47] Management of breast cancer risk includes monthly breast self-examination, annual breast examinations by a physician, and mammography at age 30 or 5 years earlier than the youngest age of breast cancer onset in the family.[46] Another common feature of Cowden syndrome is nonmedullary thyroid cancer, which may be observed in up to 10% of individuals with this disorder.[46] In addition, more than one-half of those affected with Cowden syndrome have follicular adenomas or multinodular goiter of the thyroid.[46] Germ-line mutations in the *PTEN* (phosphatase and tensin homologue) gene have been identified in patients with Cowden syndrome, and predictive testing may be available for some individuals if a mutation is identified.[46,48] Because of the complex presentation of this disorder, patients are usually managed by a multidisciplinary team including surgeons, gynecologists, and dermatologists.[46]

Peutz-Jeghers Syndrome

Peutz-Jeghers syndrome is an autosomal dominant condition characterized by hamartomatous polyps in the gastrointestinal tract and by mucocutaneous melanin deposits in the buccal mucosa, lips, fingers, and toes. Studies have described an increased risk of both gastrointestinal and extraintestinal cancer associated with this syndrome, including some rare genital tumors.[49] Although only a limited number of cases have been reported, Boardman et al. observed an excess number of women with Peutz-Jeghers syndrome who were affected with breast cancer, with an average age at diagnosis of 39.[49] These data were derived from 34 patients in 31 kindreds. A study of 31 patients from 13 families studied at Johns Hopkins University revealed that 15 (48%) of the affected patients developed cancer, of whom 2 developed ductal cancer of the breast at ages 41 and 56.[50] Thus, in addition to the special surveillance for colon disorders and other associated findings, women with this syndrome need, at a minimum, routine surveillance for breast cancer. Genetic studies have shown that many, but not all, Peutz-Jeghers syndrome families are characterized by mutations at the chromosome locus 19p13.3[51]; germ-line mutations in STK11, a serine/threonine kinase gene, have been identified in several affected individuals.[52]

Muir-Torre Syndrome

Muir-Torre syndrome is another rare autosomal dominant condition that is considered to be a variant of hereditary nonpolyposis colorectal cancer (HNPCC). The hallmark of this condition is multiple sebaceous gland and skin tumors, including keratoacanthomas and basal cell carcinomas. These cutaneous manifestations are typically seen in association with tumors of the small and large bowel. In addition, tumors of the larynx, stomach, endometrium, kidney, bladder, ovaries, and breast are observed. One review noted that the world literature contains 162 cases of Muir-Torre syndrome, with 316 internal malignancies documented.[53] Ninety percent of these were gastrointestinal, urogenital, or breast cancers. Overall, the average age of diagnosis of Muir-Torre syndrome is 55 years, and the diagnosis is usually based on dermatologic findings.[54] Little specific information is available to characterize further the nature of the breast cancers in affected individuals. Mutations in the DNA mismatch-repair genes *MSH2* and *MLH1*, the major genes implicated in HNPCC, are associated with this condition; thus, predictive testing may be possible for some families.[55,56] As with other complex cancer predisposition syndromes, specific management plans have been developed, and affected or at-risk individuals are often followed by a multidisciplinary team.[54,57]

GENETIC COUNSELING PROCESS

Genetic counseling for high-risk individuals is critical, especially when genetic testing is an option. In the latter case, both pretest and posttest counseling are important because of the complexities in test result interpretation and medical management options and the potential emotional ramifications of test results.[58] The process of genetic counseling, as outlined in Fig. 2, may help individuals to make informed decisions about whether they would like to pursue testing based on the potential benefits, risks, and limitations. In addition, they are also afforded an opportunity to contemplate how the information may impact them and their families.

Initial, or pretest, genetic counseling sessions involve a detailed review of the patient's family and medical history. The family history may be conveniently recorded in the form of a pedigree and updated as needed. Pedigrees recorded for the purpose of cancer risk assessment should include information about maternal and paternal relatives, preferably covering three generations. With respect to cancer history, the practitioner should record and document, where possible, all cancer or precancer diagnoses, ages of the individuals at diagnosis, laterality, treatment, and history of prophylactic surgery. Relevant environmental and exposure history is also important to note, as is ethnic ancestry. In addition, current ages of living family members, ages and causes of death of deceased individuals, and other chronic medical conditions of unaffected and affected individuals should be indicated on the pedigree. Analysis of the pedigree for hallmark features of hereditary cancer provides the basis for an accurate risk assessment.

Many patients overestimate the contribution of single gene mutations to breast and ovarian cancer, and many unaffected women in particular overestimate their risk of developing these cancers.[59,60] Thus, it is valuable to tell patients whether the features of the family history are suggestive of hereditary

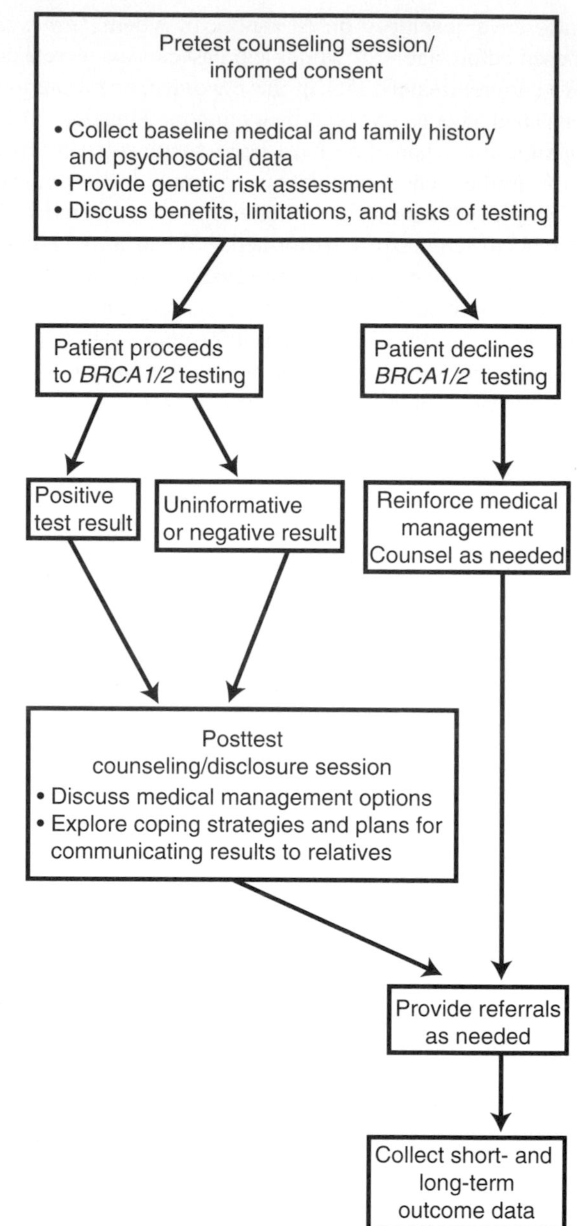

FIG. 2. Flow diagram depicting the process of genetic counseling.

breast cancer, and, if so, what the likelihood is that testing will provide a clinically meaningful result. For some families, a sizable difference may exist between the likelihood that the cancers in the family are hereditary and the probability that a mutation will be detected.[61] Although various models and methods are available for evaluating the chance that testing for the two major breast cancer genes, *BRCA1* and *BRCA2*, will yield a positive result, these data need to be interpreted in the context of a specific pedigree. Patients also must weigh the financial cost of testing if this service is not offered as part of a research protocol. A discussion of inheritance patterns (usually autosomal dominance) is also very important. This risk should be contrasted with the cancer risks associated with mutations in predisposing genes, and an individualized explanation of available medical management options should be given.

Another important aspect of pretest counseling is the review of the possible benefits, risks, and limitations of genetic testing. Although no individual can imagine fully how he or she might react on learning a test result, engaging in this discussion beforehand can at least begin to prepare individuals for different responses and enable them to mobilize coping, support, and informational resources ahead of time.

Potential benefits of testing include the reduction of uncertainty due to increased knowledge. In addition, results may help facilitate more informed decision making about medical options, including prophylactic surgery. Although such surgery may be undertaken by women who have never had a diagnosis of cancer, data regarding the risk of ipsilateral and contralateral breast cancers in *BRCA1* and *BRCA2* carriers could potentially impact the surgical decision making of high-risk patients newly diagnosed with breast cancer who choose to learn their genetic status preoperatively.[62] Frequently, the choice to be tested may also be motivated by a desire to obtain information for other family members. In some instances, the medical implications for cancer patients who are the first in their families to pursue testing may not be highly significant, but the knowledge obtained for relatives could be substantial.

Limitations of testing include the possibility that results may not be informative. Even when test results are positive, broad or uncertain ranges of cancer risks combined with the lack of long-term outcome data regarding management strategies may complicate medical decision making. Although no substantial physical risks are associated with genetic testing, the psychosocial risks may be considerable. A common reason for declining genetic testing is the fear of genetic discrimination in the areas of health and life insurance, and employment.[63] The existing federal legislation does not apply to all individuals, and the provisions that are available usually apply to health insurance but not life insurance. Therefore, even those who do choose to obtain test results often exercise caution about how and with whom the information is shared.

Although studies have not demonstrated significant adverse emotional effects of testing, as described in the section Psychosocial Issues, carriers normally experience some level of distress, anxiety, or sadness.[64] Although many individuals pursue testing for the sake of obtaining information for family members,[63] the decision to disseminate one's test results and the ensuing ramifications can cause strain among relatives. It is not uncommon for those with true negative results to feel a combination of relief and "survivor guilt" for being spared a burden that other relatives may experience. In addition, the role of information gatekeeper may be overwhelming for some individuals as they try to attend also to their own needs for support. Registry-based and clinic-based studies of large families have demonstrated that most individuals, carriers and noncarriers, do opt to share their results with relatives at risk[65]; however, a provider cannot understand or know the multitude of dynamics within families that may result in either open or impeded communication regarding risk.[66] Nevertheless, the genetic counselor should tell patients what the implications to family members may be, identify individuals at risk based on the pedigree structure, and encourage patients to share this information with their relatives.[67]

Thus, because of the possible significance of these issues to patients, an integral part of the informed-consent process is discussion of these issues before genetic testing. Posttest genetic counseling provides an opportunity to review pertinent information and may also serve to help individuals begin to assimilate their results. Specially trained genetic counselors and nurses are now available in most areas of the country who can provide these services to interested patients, often in combination with a multidisciplinary team of professionals, such as oncologists, surgeons, geneticists, and psychologists.

ISSUES IN TEST RESULT INTERPRETATION

Regardless of which hereditary breast cancer syndrome is suspected within a family, the degree to which testing will be informative is always maximized by first testing the individual in the family who is most likely to carry a mutation (i.e., usually a woman with breast or ovarian cancer diagnosed at a young age). The most complete and most expensive method of gene testing is direct sequencing of exons and adjacent noncoding introns. This method is thought to have the highest degree of sensitivity and specificity. For example, a commercial laboratory has estimated that the sensitivity of *BRCA1* and *BRCA2* sequencing is greater than 98%.[68] However, because sequencing cannot detect deletions of complete exons or genes or some errors in RNA processing, up to 15% of mutations in *BRCA1* and *BRCA2* may be missed. This estimate is based in part on findings from families showing evidence for linkage to *BRCA1* and *BRCA2* in which no deleterious mutation could be identified.[69,70] Other assays for full gene analysis are available that vary in sensitivity (e.g., conformation-sensitive gel electrophoresis).[71] To date, no systematic, blinded studies have been conducted to directly compare these alternative methods of testing for sensitivity and specificity.

Techniques designed to identify specific mutations are very accurate. These include allele-specific oligonucleotide (ASO) and allele-specific polymerase chain reaction (PCR) assays and fluorogenic PCR allelic discrimination assays.[13,72] These methods may be used to test for familial mutations or to test for panels of common mutations. However, when a first attempt is made to identify a mutation in a family, negative test results from partial testing methods such as these must be considered inconclusive. For example, although three *BRCA1* and *BRCA2* mutations account for the majority of alterations found in individuals of Ashkenazi Jewish descent, novel mutations have been reported that would require further analysis to detect.[25]

Testing can have many possible outcomes. The most unambiguous results are either "true positives" or "true negatives." "True positive" results refer to nonsense or frameshift mutations (due to deletions or insertions) that lead to protein truncation. In addition, some alterations, including some missense mutations, are known to be deleterious based on functional assays or RNA studies.[73–75] A catalogue of reported mutations is also available on-line, which, together with published reports, reveals that some mutations have been identified in numerous high-risk families.[23,25,76] In the future, it may be possible to correlate cancer risks with specific mutations; at present, however, such data are too preliminary to be useful in clinical counseling. "True negative" results refer to the case in which an individual tests negative for the mutation identified in his or her family, usually in a close relative. The standard practice is to test these relatives only for the presence or absence of the familial mutation; the exception is individuals of Ashkenazi Jewish descent, for whom all three founder mutations should be analyzed, given the high background frequency of these mutations.[5] The finding of a "true negative" result has significant implications, as these individuals usually can be reassured that their cancer risks are approximately the same as those of other individuals in the general population, and therefore only routine screening is warranted.

The most difficult results to interpret are those in which no deleterious mutations are identified after full testing, or those in which an alteration of uncertain clinical significance is found. If an affected high-risk individual is the first to be tested in the family, a negative result could arise for a number of reasons; for example, (a) a mutation could be present (e.g., in a regulatory region) but is not detectable by available methods; (b) another gene that is rare or not yet isolated could be implicated; or (c) the individual tested could have developed sporadic cancer. In many cases, distinguishing which of these possibilities accounts for the negative finding is difficult. Also, genetic variants, termed *mutations of uncertain clinical significance*, may be found that do not overtly affect the gene's protein product. Such alterations are usually missense mutations (single base pair changes). Missense mutations may be presumed to be of little clinical consequence if they occur in noncritical domains of the gene, result in a single amino acid's being substituted with a similar amino acid, or occur in conjunction with known deleterious mutations. However, in the absence of functional tests or multiple segregation analyses, these determinations remain only speculative. Proper interpretation of test results is critical, because individuals may use this information, interpreted in the context of their medical and family histories, to make significant decisions regarding medical management.

PSYCHOSOCIAL ISSUES

Patient Decision Making about Genetic Testing

To make an informed decision about genetic testing, patients must be educated about the benefits, limitations, and risks of testing as described previously. Given the complexities and challenges inherent in this decision, the fact that preliminary data suggest that many high-risk individuals choose not to learn their genetic status is not surprising. In a prospective cohort study of *BRCA1* testing in 279 members of families with hereditary breast and ovarian cancer,[63] only 43% decided to receive their test results. Individuals with health insurance, those who had a greater number of affected relatives, and those who were more knowledgeable about breast cancer genetics were more likely to participate. Reasons cited for wanting the testing included the desire to learn about their children's risks, the wish to be reassured, and the need to make decisions about screening and surgery. Reasons for not wanting testing included possible insurance discrimination, potential emotional effects on self and family, and concerns about test accuracy. In addition to these factors, evidence exists that psychological distress motivates desire for genetic testing for breast cancer susceptibility.[77] This finding is worrisome, because it suggests that the individuals most likely to request testing may be more psychologically vulnerable. These data underscore the importance of discussing these psychosocial aspects of the testing decision with patients, in addition to addressing genetic and medical issues.

Disclosure of Genetic Test Results

With the identification of the major breast cancer susceptibility genes, early reports warned of the potential for adverse psychosocial consequences of disclosure of genetic information.[58,78] Several controlled investigations of the psychosocial impact of *BRCA1* testing have now been initiated, and data are available to address this question.

The first of these studies focused on the psychosocial effects of testing in a large hereditary breast cancer kindred in Utah. The study protocol and measures were described previously.[79] An analysis of the first 60 women who received *BRCA1* mutation test results found no evidence of significant adverse psychological effects.[80] No significant change was seen in the level of general anxiety reported by carriers. Among noncarriers, a small but significant decline in anxiety was noted. However, on a measure of stress responses specific to genetic testing, one group showed significantly higher levels of stress compared with the other participants. Specifically, women with no history of cancer or prophylactic surgery reported higher levels of stress after genetic testing. In contrast, mutation carriers who had already experienced cancer or prophylactic surgery showed no more stress than noncarriers. Overall, however, levels of stress responses were not substantially elevated above the norm.

A second prospective cohort study focused on several extended families in a hereditary breast cancer registry.[63] The study sample included 46 carriers of *BRCA1* mutations, 50 noncarriers, and 44 individuals who declined *BRCA1* testing. At baseline and 1-month follow-up, all three groups scored in the normal ranges on measures of depression and functional health status. Noncarriers of *BRCA1* mutations exhibited significant decreases in depressive symptoms and role impairment and marginally significant decreases in sexual impairment, compared with carriers and those who declined testing. Carriers and those who declined testing did not exhibit changes in any of these distress outcomes. Six-month follow-up data from this cohort suggest that this pattern of responses is maintained over time.[81]

Although these two initial reports do not provide evidence for significant or pervasive adverse psychological effects of *BRCA1* testing, caution is warranted in generalizing these findings to other populations and settings. Participants in these studies were members of high-risk families in hereditary cancer registries, many of whom were involved in prior cancer genetics studies. These families had been included in the registries because of their unusually high cancer rates. Because study participants had witnessed cancer in many close family members, their emotional responses may have been blunted. In addition, most unaffected individuals in these high-risk families reported before testing that they expected to be mutation carriers. Thus, receiving a positive test result may have confirmed what they believed to be true all along. In some cases, worrying about the possibility of being a mutation carrier may be no less distressing than having that belief confirmed. Individuals who have less significant family histories, and who do not expect to receive positive results, may be more vulnerable to adverse psychological sequelae of *BRCA1* testing. All individuals in these studies were white (all of the Utah subjects were Mormon), and most had a high school education. In addition, all testing was provided free of charge as part of research protocols with extensive education and counseling.

Although these initial studies have not found evidence for significant psychological morbidity, emotional responses to testing may vary widely. One study examined the use of a brief precounseling assessment to identify individuals at risk for adverse psychological effects of genetic testing for breast cancer susceptibility.[82] The results showed that the presence of cancer-related stress symptoms was highly predictive of subsequent depression in a subgroup of hereditary breast cancer family members. However, contrary to predictions, these adverse effects were seen primarily in individuals who were offered but declined genetic counseling and testing. These results suggest that members of families in which a mutation is identified who decline genetic testing should also be monitored for adverse effects, especially if they manifest cancer-related stress symptoms. The development of depression in these individuals may be minimized by their participation in genetics education and counseling programs, even if they ultimately decline to be tested.

Medical Decision Making

For *BRCA1* and *BRCA2* testing to lead to the anticipated reductions in breast and ovarian cancer mortality, mutation carriers must adopt recommendations for intensive and frequent surveillance. However, relatively less attention has been focused on understanding psychological issues in medical decision making in these high-risk patients. Data from the cohort study of hereditary breast cancer family members suggest that adherence to screening regimens is suboptimal.[81] Only 60% of eligible carriers had the recommended mammograms during the 6 months after testing, and fewer than 10% had transvaginal ultrasound or the serum tumor marker CA-125.

In lieu of participating in frequent and intensive surveillance, many high-risk women seek counseling about whether to obtain prophylactic surgery. In the cohort study described above, among unaffected female *BRCA1* carriers, 18% intended to obtain prophylactic mastectomies and 33% intended to obtain prophylactic oophorectomies.[63] Among carriers of cancer-predisposing genes, prophylactic surgery may have psychological benefits, such as the reduction of chronic worry.[83] However, such procedures also carry psychological risks.[84] One study suggested that breast cancer–related distress may also influence prophylactic mastectomy decisions.[85] In this study, women were presented with vignettes that described a woman at high risk for breast cancer who was deciding whether to obtain a prophylactic mastectomy or to have close breast cancer follow-up. Women were asked to indicate what their choice would be in that situation. Women who had higher levels of perceived personal risk and higher levels of breast cancer worries were significantly more likely to select prophylactic mastectomy over close follow-up. Younger women and women selecting prophylactic mastectomy reported less confidence in their choices.

For women at high risk for breast cancer, another important decision concerns whether to participate in chemoprevention trials. As yet, however, the factors that influence the decisions of high-risk women regarding participation in such trials are poorly understood. One study of recruitment of high-risk women to a breast cancer health promotion trial suggested that the timing of the recommendation may be an important determinant. In this study, women with a higher level of formal education were more likely to participate if they were approached within the first 2 months after the breast cancer diagnosis of a close relative.[86] Familial polyposis patients also were more likely to participate in a colon cancer chemoprevention program if they had been diagnosed more recently.[87] During the initial period after a personal cancer diagnosis or diagnosis in a close relative, heightened perceived risk or distress may motivate risk-reduction behaviors, such as participation in a chemoprevention or health promotion trial.

Preliminary data suggest that reproductive plans and choices may also be altered by genetic testing for breast cancer susceptibility. In a survey of 56 women aged 40 years and younger who had a family history of breast cancer, 22%

reported that they would be less likely to have children if they tested positive for a *BRCA1* mutation, and 17% reported being uncertain as to whether they would complete a pregnancy under these circumstances.[88]

The findings reviewed in this section suggest that psychological support may be important for high-risk women faced with difficult medical management decisions. Psychosocial interventions for women at high risk of breast cancer have been reviewed elsewhere.[89,90] Research conducted with breast cancer patients suggests that training in structured decision-making strategies can enhance medical decision making and psychological adjustment.[91] These strategies, developed and evaluated in the nursing literature, could be adapted easily to assist high-risk women in deciding whether to undergo prophylactic surgery or to participate in chemoprevention trials. Although such educational approaches may be sufficient for some patients, others may require referral to more formal psychological counseling services. Thus, health care providers who may lack the time or the training to deliver psychosocial counseling should establish mechanisms for referral of their patients to psychiatrists, psychologists, or other mental health professionals.

MEDICAL MANAGEMENT OF HIGH-RISK INDIVIDUALS

At present, few proven methods exist for cancer screening or prevention for high-risk women or those with an inherited susceptibility to cancer. Studies are currently under way that address the impact of some of these strategies on the cancer risk of mutation carriers. High-risk women must fully understand their various cancer screening and prevention options so that they can make informed decisions about their medical care. These options are outlined in the following paragraphs.

Breast Cancer

Screening Options

Little data exist to document the benefit of screening interventions in mutation carriers or other high-risk individuals. The current breast cancer screening guidelines for women with a known inherited susceptibility to cancer who do not elect to have prophylactic surgery include monthly breast self-examinations, semiannual or annual clinician-performed breast examinations beginning at age 25 to 35, and annual mammograms beginning at age 25 to 35.[92] Controversy exists about the age at which mammographic screening should commence and the intervals at which it should be repeated; most of this controversy relates to the use of mammography in women younger than 40. Although the risk exists of false-positive results or false reassurance from negative results, particularly in this age group, some series have demonstrated the value of screening mammography in women younger than 40.[93,94] In addition, preliminary evidence suggests that the mammographic appearance of *BRCA1*-associated breast cancers is similar to that of sporadic cancers.[95] Because of concerns that *BRCA* tumors may have a faster growth rate than sporadic tumors, and to allay patient anxiety, some clinicians recommend mammography every 6 months to carriers beginning at age 25 to 35.[96] However, because of theoretical concerns about the role of mammography in breast carcinogenesis in carriers[97–98] and the lack of data, the use of mammography more than once per year is generally discouraged in the absence of a specific indication. Most experts, however, believe that the benefit of early detection with annual mammograms beginning at age 25 to 35 outweighs the potential for adverse effects.[92,99] Clinical trials of other imaging techniques, such as magnetic resonance imaging, may lead to the development of more sensitive methods of early detection without the associated radiation exposure.

For women at moderate risk of breast cancer, monthly breast self-examination and semiannual or annual clinician-performed breast examinations are recommended. Despite the controversy about the benefit of screening mammography for women between the ages of 40 and 49, annual mammograms beginning at age 40 in this moderate-risk group are recommended.

Prevention Options

Prophylactic Mastectomy

A study by Hartmann et al. evaluated the efficacy of prophylactic mastectomy in women with a family history of breast cancer.[100] This study included more than 600 women who were either at moderate or high risk of breast cancer on the basis of their family histories. Women with any family history of breast cancer were considered at moderate risk. Approximately two-thirds of the women included in this moderate-risk group had at least one first-degree relative with breast cancer. The definition of high risk in this study was quite broad, and other data[24] suggest that, at most, 10% of these women would be carriers of *BRCA1* mutations.

For the 425 moderate-risk women, the investigators used the Gail model to predict the expected numbers of cases of breast cancer. With a median follow-up of 14 years, the Gail model predicted 37 cases of breast cancer, and four were seen. This highly statistically significant difference translated into a 90% reduction in the incidence of breast cancer. To evaluate the efficacy of prophylactic mastectomy in high-risk women, their untreated sisters served as controls. This approach demonstrated that prophylactic mastectomy reduced the risk of breast cancer in high-risk women by at least 90%. In addition, breast cancer–related mortality was reduced by at least 81% in the high-risk group and by 100%

in the moderate-risk group. This study demonstrated that prophylactic mastectomy significantly reduced breast cancer incidence in women at increased risk for this disease. Women entered in this study received both prophylactic subcutaneous and total mastectomy. Subcutaneous mastectomy is no longer considered the procedure of choice due to the fact that a significant amount of breast tissue is found in the nipple-areolar complex. With the availability of improved surgical techniques, including skin-sparing mastectomies and newer methods of reconstruction, most surgeons now recommend prophylactic total mastectomy (see Chapter 18).

Schrag et al. used decision-analysis tools to predict the benefits of prophylactic surgery in mutation carriers.[101] They modeled an 85% reduction in risk of breast cancer for carriers undergoing prophylactic mastectomy and found that a 30-year-old female mutation carrier would gain 2.9 to 5.3 years of life expectancy from this surgery. Although there is reason to be optimistic about the benefits of prophylactic mastectomy in *BRCA1* and *BRCA2* mutation carriers, currently published studies have not specifically addressed this issue. Thus, caution should be used when extrapolating results of these studies to mutation carriers. Studies focusing on mutation carriers are under way and should provide clearer answers on the efficacy of this approach in this patient population.

Prophylactic Oophorectomy

In individuals with hereditary breast cancer, one study demonstrated that healthy *BRCA1* carriers who had undergone prophylactic bilateral oophorectomy had a significant reduction in their risk of breast cancer.[102] Overall, the risk of breast cancer was reduced by more than 70% in those undergoing prophylactic oophorectomy. Thus, in *BRCA1* and *BRCA2* carriers, prophylactic oophorectomy likely reduces the risk not only of ovarian cancer but also of breast cancer. No data exist on the impact of this procedure in other moderate-risk or high-risk women.

Chemoprevention

The Breast Cancer Prevention Trial randomized more than 13,000 healthy high-risk women into groups receiving 5 years of tamoxifen (tamoxifen citrate) therapy or placebo.[103] Eligible women included any woman age 60 or older, those between the ages of 35 and 59 with a predicted 5-year risk of breast cancer of 1.66% or higher, and anyone older than age 35 with lobular carcinoma *in situ*. Of the study participants, 56% had one first-degree relative with breast cancer, 16% had two affected first-degree relatives, and 3% had three affected first-degree relatives. With a median follow-up of 4.5 years, tamoxifen was found to halve the risk of invasive estrogen receptor–positive tumors and noninvasive breast cancer. No reduction in risk of estrogen receptor–negative tumors was seen. The reduction in breast cancer risk was seen for all family history constellations and all age groups of women, as well as those with lobular carcinoma *in situ* and atypical ductal hyperplasia. Based on the results of this study, the Food and Drug Administration approved the use of tamoxifen for reducing the incidence of breast cancer in women at high risk for developing the disease. In contrast to the Breast Cancer Prevention Trial, the Royal Marsden Hospital tamoxifen randomized chemoprevention trial failed to demonstrate a decreased incidence of breast cancer in the tamoxifen group.[104] In this study, a total of 2,471 women with at least one first-degree relative younger than age 50 with breast cancer were randomized into treatment and nontreatment groups. Of note, a significant proportion of women took hormone replacement therapy at some point during this trial. The disparity of results seen in these two studies has not yet been fully explained. It has been postulated that some of the differences may be due to the fact that tamoxifen is not effective as a chemoprevention agent in patients with familial or hereditary breast cancer. The Breast Cancer Prevention Trial is currently performing a subgroup analysis and is genotyping a subset of participants to determine the effectiveness of tamoxifen in preventing breast cancer in *BRCA1* and *BRCA2* mutation carriers. Thus, at present, a reasonable approach is to consider the use of tamoxifen for breast cancer prevention in women who fit the eligibility criteria of the study and to exercise greater caution when considering this therapy for those with an inherited susceptibility to breast cancer. The benefits in the latter group will become clearer when the results of the subgroup analysis are available. In general, health care providers are advised to carefully evaluate the benefits and risks for any individual patient before prescribing this drug.

Other chemoprevention trials are under way. These include the Study of Tamoxifen and Raloxifene (STAR) trial, in which postmenopausal moderate-risk and high-risk women will be randomized to treatment with tamoxifen or raloxifene (raloxifene hydrochloride), a selective estrogen-receptor modulator. In addition, trials in known mutation carriers are also planned. Chemoprevention is discussed in detail in Chapter 19.

Hormone Replacement Therapy and Other Options

Postmenopausal women generally consider taking hormone replacement therapy (HRT) to reduce their risk of cardiovascular disease and osteoporosis and to treat postmenopausal symptoms. However, long-term use of HRT in women in the general population increases the risk of breast cancer (relative risk, 1.2–1.5).[105,106] Concern exists that this risk would be magnified in women with a family history of breast cancer and in those with *BRCA1* or *BRCA2* mutations. Several studies have addressed whether family history influences the risk of breast cancer in users of HRT. These studies have varied from showing no effect to finding a 3.4-fold excess risk of breast cancer in those with a positive family history.[107] Little information exists on the effect of HRT in women who are *BRCA1* or *BRCA2* carriers. Thus, the decision to take HRT for protection against heart and bone disease and for relief from menopausal symptoms is often a difficult one both for women with a positive family history of breast cancer and for those with *BRCA1* or *BRCA2* mutations. This issue may be of particular concern to *BRCA1* or *BRCA2* carriers who are considering or have undergone prophylactic oophorectomy and thus are faced with the consequences of premature menopause. At present, little information is available to guide patients and their physicians who are considering this option. In general, the recommendation is that *BRCA1* or *BRCA2* carriers avoid this therapy and that women with a low to moderate risk of breast cancer based on family history carefully consider the risk to benefit ratio of such treatment.

Several other treatment options are now available to reduce a woman's risk of cardiac disease and osteoporotic fracture. These include the selective estrogen-receptor modulators tamoxifen and raloxifene. Tamoxifen and raloxifene lower both total cholesterol and low-density-lipoprotein cholesterol,[108,109] and tamoxifen may reduce the risk of coronary heart disease.[110,111] Tamoxifen has been demonstrated to increase bone mineral density in the lumbar spine both in healthy women[112] and in breast cancer patients[113] and to decrease hip and Colles' fractures in healthy women.[103] Randomized trials have demonstrated that raloxifene is effective at preventing bone loss, although neither raloxifene nor tamoxifen is as potent as HRT.[109,114] Like tamoxifen, raloxifene appears to have antiestrogenic activity at the level of the breast. A combined analysis of placebo-controlled trials in healthy postmenopausal women indicated that women receiving raloxifene had a 55% reduction in risk of developing invasive breast cancer.[115] Thus, tamoxifen and raloxifene may be useful alternatives to HRT in this patient population. Not only do they reduce the risk of osteoporosis and possibly heart disease, but they also appear to protect against breast cancer. Unfortunately, both of these agents tend to worsen hot flashes and provide little if any relief from other postmenopausal symptoms, such as vaginal dryness. In addition to the selective estrogen-receptor modulators, bisphosphonates and calcitonin can be used safely in this patient population to prevent or treat osteoporosis.

Individuals with documented *BRCA1* or *BRCA2* mutations also face increased risks of other cancers, including ovarian cancer, prostate cancer, and possibly colon cancer. The screening and prevention options for these malignancies are outlined in the following paragraphs.

Ovarian Cancer

Screening Options

For mutation carriers who have not had prophylactic oophorectomy, semiannual or annual transvaginal ultrasonography with color Doppler and CA-125 is recommended beginning at age 25 to 35.[92] The benefits of these screening options for mutation carriers are unknown. In the general population, these measures have not been proven very effective. However, these measures may possibly have a higher predictive value in mutation carriers, given the high incidence of ovarian cancer in this patient group.

Prevention Options

Prophylactic Oophorectomy

Prophylactic oophorectomy should be considered in mutation carriers; however, the efficacy of such an approach in high-risk women and mutation carriers is unknown. Clearly, a residual risk of primary peritoneal carcinomatosis exists. Two studies shed some light on this risk. Of the 324 women from the Gilda Radner Familial Ovarian Cancer Registry who had undergone prophylactic bilateral oophorectomy, 6 (2%) developed primary peritoneal carcinomatosis 1 to 27 years after this procedure.[116] A second study found that members of high-risk families who had undergone prophylactic oophorectomy had a 13-fold excess risk of "ovarian" cancer as compared with a 24-fold excess risk of ovarian cancer in those family members who had not had prophylactic surgery.[117] Thus, these studies suggest that prophylactic surgery reduces the risk of ovarian cancer in members of high-risk families, but that residual risks remain. Further research is under way addressing the impact of this surgery in known mutation carriers.

Chemoprevention

Oral contraceptive use is known to decrease the risk of ovarian cancer in the general population.[118] As discussed in the section on Cancer Risk Modifiers, one case-control study suggested that oral contraceptive use also significantly reduced the risk of ovarian cancer in *BRCA1* and *BRCA2* carriers.[35] However, some concern exists that oral contraceptive use may increase the risk of breast cancer in mutation carriers.[36] Given the limited knowledge, mutation carriers face a difficult decision as they balance the potential risks and benefits of the pill.

Prostate Cancer

Typically, the age of onset of prostate cancer in mutation carriers is similar to that in individuals with sporadic disease. Thus, the screening recommendations are the same as those for the general population and include annual rectal examination and prostate-specific antigen testing beginning at age 50.

Colon Cancer

Individuals with a *BRCA1* or *BRCA2* mutation should follow the screening guidelines for the general population.

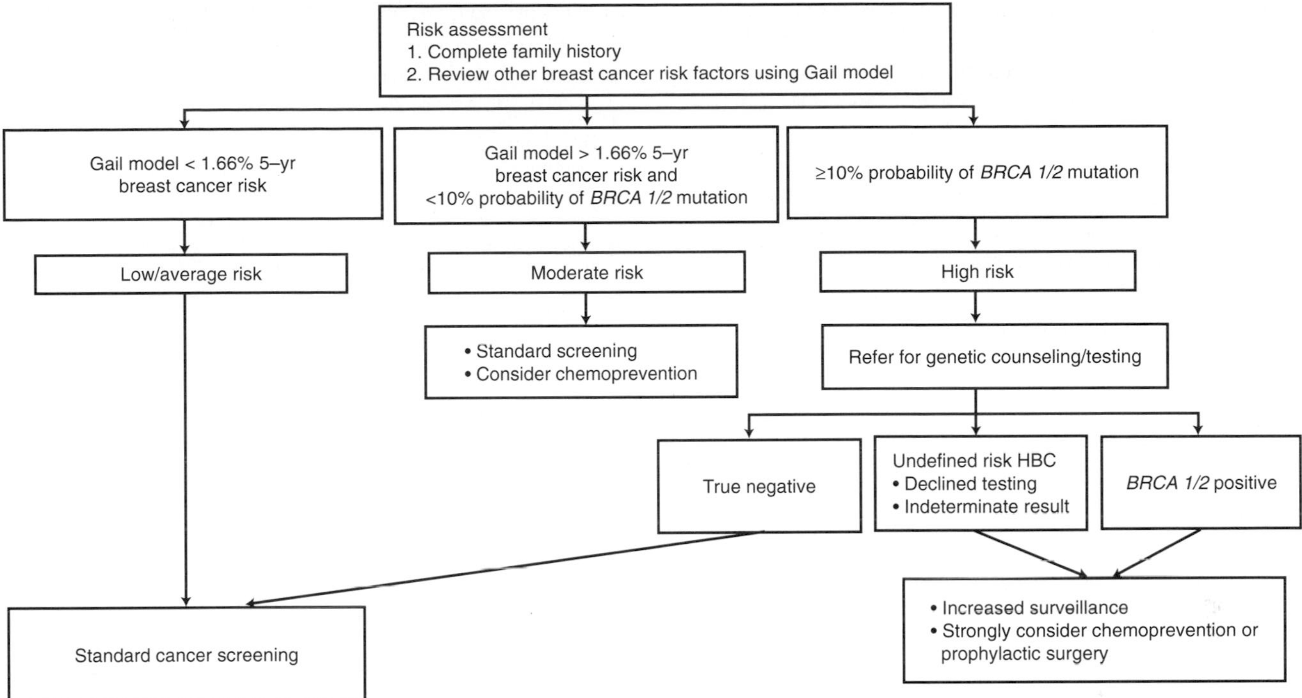

FIG. 3. Flow diagram depicting the process of risk evaluation and management of women with a family history of breast cancer. HBC, hereditary breast cancer.

These include fecal occult blood test annually and flexible sigmoidoscopy or colonoscopy every 3 to 5 years beginning at age 50.

Individualizing Screening and Prevention Programs

High-risk women, particularly those found to be mutation carriers, must understand that no proven means of cancer prevention or screening exist. Thus, each woman should be encouraged to take the time to weigh fully the implications of different management approaches before deciding on a particular plan. Not infrequently, an individual's approach changes over time. For example, a young woman with a *BRCA1* mutation may choose surveillance for ovarian cancer if she has not yet completed childbearing. Once her family is complete, she may then wish to consider prophylactic surgery. High-risk women should be strongly encouraged to participate in clinical trials addressing the efficacy of cancer screening and prevention strategies.

SUMMARY

Most individuals with a family history of breast cancer have a familial rather than hereditary basis to their disease. Among women with hereditary breast cancer, *BRCA1* and *BRCA2* mutations account for the majority of cases. Mutations in these genes are associated with a significantly elevated risk of early-onset breast and ovarian cancer. In addition, other cancers may be seen with an increased frequency in mutation carriers. Models based on cancer history, family history, and ethnic background are available to guide clinicians in estimating the likelihood that an individual harbors a risk-conferring mutation. Due to the complexities involved in decision making about genetic testing and medical management, genetic counseling is critical before testing is carried out. The process of risk evaluation and management for women with a family history of breast cancer is outlined in Fig. 3. Studies on genetic and environmental cancer risk modifiers, genotype-phenotype correlations, and the impact of cancer screening and prevention options are under way and will continue to provide further insight into the features and management of high-risk individuals.

REFERENCES

1. Statement of the American Society of Clinical Oncology. Genetic testing for cancer susceptibility. *J Clin Oncol* 1996;14:1730.
2. Slattery ML, Kerber RA. A comprehensive evaluation of family history and breast cancer risk. *JAMA* 1993;270:1563.
3. Claus EB, Risch N, Thompson WD. Age at onset as an indicator of familial risk of breast cancer. *Am J Epidemiol* 1990;131:961.
4. Claus EB, Schildkraut JM, Thompson WD, Risch NJ. The genetic attributable risk of breast and ovarian cancer. *Cancer* 1996;77:2318.
5. Tonin P, Weber B, Offit K, et al. Frequency of recurrent BRCA1 and BRCA2 mutations in Ashkenazi Jewish breast cancer families. *Nat Med* 1996;2:1179.

6. Claus EG, Risch N, Thompson WD. Autosomal dominant inheritance of early-onset breast cancer: implications for risk prediction. *Cancer* 1994;73:643.
7. Gail MH, Brinton LA, Byar DP, et al. Projecting individualized probabilities of developing breast cancer for white females who are being examined annually. *J Natl Cancer Inst* 1989;81:1879.
8. Benichou J, Gail MH, Mulvihill JJ. Graphs to estimate an individualized risk of breast cancer. *J Clin Oncol* 1996;14:103.
9. Spiegelman D, Colditz GA, Hunter D, Hertzmark E. Validation of the Gail et al model for predicting individual breast cancer risk. *J Natl Cancer Inst* 1994;86:600.
10. Bondy M, Lustbader ED, Halabi S, Ross E, Vogel VG. Validation of a breast cancer risk assessment model in women with a positive family history. *J Natl Cancer Inst* 1994;86:620.
11. McGuigan KA, Ganz PA, Breant C. Agreement between breast cancer risk estimation methods. *J Natl Cancer Inst* 1996;88:1315.
12. Ford D, Easton DF, Peto J. Estimates of the gene frequency of BRCA1 and its contribution to breast and ovarian cancer incidence. *Am J Hum Genet* 1995;57:1457.
13. Struewing JP, Hartge P, Wacholder S, et al. The risk of cancer associated with specific mutations of BRCA1 and BRCA2 among Ashkenazi Jews. *N Engl J Med* 1997;336:1401.
14. Schubert EL, Mefford HC, Dann JL, Argonza RH, Hull J, King M-C. BRCA1 and BRCA2 mutations in Ashkenazi Jewish families with breast and ovarian cancer. *Genetic Testing* 1997;1:41.
15. FitzGerald MG, MacDonald DJ, Krainer M, et al. Germ-line BRCA1 mutations in Jewish and non-Jewish women with early onset breast cancer. *N Engl J Med* 1996;334:143.
16. Muto MG, Cramer DW, Tangir J, Berkowitz R, Mok S. Frequency of the BRCA1 185delAG mutation among Jewish women with ovarian cancer and matched population controls. *Cancer Res* 1996;56:1250.
17. Abeliovich D, Kaduri L, Lerer I, et al. The founder mutations 185delAG and 5382insC in BRCA1 and 6174delT in BRCA2 appear in 60% of ovarian cancer and 30% of early-onset breast cancer patients among Ashkenazi Jewish women. *Am J Hum Genet* 1997;60:505.
18. Szabo CI, King M-C. Invited editorial: population genetics of BRCA1 and BRCA2. *Am J Hum Genet* 1997;60:1013.
19. Gao Q, Neuhausen S, Cummings S, et al. Recurrent germ-line BRCA1 mutations in extended African American families with early-onset breast cancer. *Am J Hum Genet* 1997;60:1233.
20. Tonin PN, Mes-Masson A-M, Futreal PA, et al. Founder BRCA1 and BRCA2 mutations in French Canadian breast and ovarian cancer families. *Am J Hum Genet* 1998;63:1341.
21. Thorlacius S, Olafsdottir G, Tryggvadottir L, et al. A single BRCA2 mutation in male and female breast cancer families from Iceland with varied cancer phenotypes. *Nat Genet* 1996;13:117.
22. Johannesdottir G, Gudmundsson J, Bergthorsson JT, et al. High prevalence of the 999del5 mutation in Icelandic breast and ovarian cancer patients. *Cancer Res* 1996;56:3663.
23. Shattuck-Eidens D, Oliphant A, McClure M, et al. BRCA1 sequence analysis in women at high risk for susceptibility mutations: risk factor analysis and implications for genetic testing. *JAMA* 1997;278:1242.
24. Couch FJ, DeShano ML, Blackwood A, et al. BRCA1 mutations in women attending clinics that evaluate the risk of breast cancer. *N Engl J Med* 1997;336:1409.
25. Frank TS, Manley SA, Olopade OI, et al. Sequence analysis of BRCA1 and BRCA2: correlation of mutations with family history and ovarian cancer risk. *J Clin Oncol* 1998;16:2417.
26. Phelan CM, Lancaster JM, Tonin P, et al. Mutation analysis of the BRCA2 gene in 49 site-specific breast cancer families. *Nat Genet* 1996; 13:120.
27. Easton DF, Steele L, Fields P, et al. Cancer risks in two large breast cancer families linked to BRCA2 on chromosome 13q 12-13. *Am J Hum Genet* 1997;61:120.
28. Easton DF, Ford D, Bishop T, and the Breast Cancer Linkage Consortium. Breast and ovarian cancer incidence in BRCA1-mutation carriers. *Am J Hum Genet* 1995;56:265.
29. Ford D, Easton DF, Stratton M, et al. Genetic heterogeneity and penetrance analysis of the BRCA1 and BRCA2 genes in breast cancer families. *Am J Hum Genet* 1998;62:676.
30. Ford D, Easton DF, Bishop DT, Narod SA, Goldgar DE, and the Breast Cancer Linkage Consortium. Risks of cancer in BRCA1-mutation carriers. *Lancet* 1994;343:692.
31. Schubert EL, Lee MK, Mefford HC, et al. BRCA2 in American families with four or more cases of breast or ovarian cancer; recurrent and novel mutations, variable expression, penetrance, and the possibility of families whose cancer is not attributable to BRCA1 or BRCA2. *Am J Hum Genet* 1997;60:1031.
32. Thorlacius S, Struewing JP, Hartge P, et al. Population-based study of risk of breast cancer in carriers of BRCA2 mutation. *Lancet* 1998;352:1337.
33. Marcus JN, Watson P, Page DL, et al. Hereditary breast cancer: pathobiology, prognosis, and BRCA1 and BRCA2 gene linkage. *Cancer* 1996;77:697.
34. Narod SA, Goldgar D, Cannon-Albright L, et al. Risk modifiers in carriers of BRCA1 mutations. *Int J Cancer* 1995;64:394.
35. Narod SA, Risch H, Moslehi R, et al. Oral contraceptives and the risk of hereditary ovarian cancer. *N Engl J Med* 1998;339:424.
36. Ursin G, Henderson BE, Haile RW, et al. Does oral contraceptive use increase the risk of breast cancer in women with BRCA1/2 mutations more than other women? *Cancer Res* 1997;57:3678.
37. Phelan CM, Rebbeck TR, Weber BL, et al. Ovarian cancer risk in BRCA1 carriers is modified by the *HRAS1* variable number of tandem repeat (VNTR) locus. *Nat Genet* 1996;12:309.
38. Brunet JS, Vesprini D, Abrahamson J, Neuhausen S, Narod S. Breast cancer risk in BRCA1/BRCA2 carriers is modified by the CYP1A1 gene. *Am J Hum Genet* 1998;63:A247.
39. Malkin D. The Li-Fraumeni syndrome. *Principles and Practice of Oncology Updates* 1993;7:1.
40. Hisada M, Garber JE, Fung CY, Fraumeni JF, Li FP. Multiple primary cancers in families with Li-Fraumeni syndrome. *J Natl Cancer Inst* 1998;90:606.
41. Varley JM, McGown G, Throncroft M, et al. Germ-line mutations of p53 in Li-Fraumeni families: an extended study of 39 families. *Cancer Res* 1997;57:3245.
42. Savitsky K, Bar-Shira A, Gilad S, et al. A single ataxia telangiectasia gene with a product similar to PI-3 kinase. *Science* 1995;268:1749.
43. Athma P, Rappaport R, Swift M. Molecular genotyping shows ataxia telangiectasia heterozygotes are predisposed to breast cancer. *Cancer Genet Cytogenet* 1996;92:130.
44. Swift M, Morrell D, Massey RB, Chase CL. Incidence of cancer in 161 families affected by ataxia-telangiectasia. *N Engl J Med* 1991; 325:1831.
45. FitzGerald MG, Bean JM, Hegde SR, et al. Heterozygous ATM mutations do not contribute to early onset breast cancer. *Nat Genet* 1997;15:307.
46. Eng C. Genetics of Cowden syndrome: through the looking glass of oncology (review). *Int J Oncol* 1998;12:701.
47. Schrager CA, Schneider D, Gruener A, Tsou H, Peacocke M. Clinical and pathological features of breast disease in Cowden's syndrome: an underrecognized syndrome with an increased risk of breast cancer. *Hum Pathol* 1998;29:47.
48. Nelen MR, van Staveren WC, Peeters EA, et al. Germline mutations in the PTEN/MMAC1 gene in patients with Cowden disease. *Hum Mol Genet* 1997;6:1383.
49. Boardman LA, Thibodeau SN, Schaid DJ, et al. Increased risk for cancer in patients with the Peutz-Jeghers syndrome. *Ann Intern Med* 1998;128:896.
50. Giardello FM, Welsh SB, Hamilton SR, et al. Increased risk of cancer in the Peutz-Jeghers syndrome. *N Engl J Med* 1987;316:1511.
51. Olschwang S, Markie D, Seal S, et al. Peutz-Jeghers disease: most, but not all, families are compatible with linkage to 19p13.3. *J Med Genet* 1998;35:42.
52. Jenne DE, Reimann H, Nezu J, et al. Peutz-Jeghers syndrome is caused by mutations in a novel serine threonine kinase. *Nat Genet* 1998;18:38.
53. Serleth HJ, Kisken WA. A Muir-Torre syndrome family. *Am Surg* 1998;64:365.
54. Schwartz RA, Torre DP. The Muir-Torre syndrome: a 25-year retrospect. *J Am Acad Dermatol* 1995;33:90.
55. Kruse R, Rütten A, Lamberti C, et al. Muir-Torre phenotype has a frequency of DNA mismatch-repair-gene mutations similar to that in hereditary nonpolyposis colorectal cancer families defined by the Amsterdam criteria. *Am J Hum Genet* 1998;63:63.
56. Bapat B, Xia L, Madlensky L, et al. The genetic basis of Muir-Torre syndrome includes the hMLH1 locus. *Am J Hum Genet* 1996;59:736.
57. Cohen PR, Kohn SR, Davis DA, Kurzrock R. Muir-Torre syndrome. *Dermatol Clin* 1995;13:79.
58. Biesecker BB, Boehnke M, Calzone K, et al. Genetic counseling for families with inherited susceptibility to breast and ovarian cancer. *JAMA* 1993;269:1970.

59. Iglehart JD, Miron A, Rimer BK, Winer E, Berry D, Schildkraut JM. Overestimation of hereditary breast cancer risk. *Ann Surg* 1998;228:375.
60. Sagi M, Kaduri L, Zlotogora J, Peretz T. The effect of genetic counseling on knowledge and perceptions regarding risks for breast cancer. *J Genet Couns* 1998;7:417.
61. Matloff ET, Peshkin BN. Complexities in cancer genetic counseling: breast and ovarian cancer. *Principles and Practice of Oncology Updates* 1998;12(1):1.
62. Matloff ET, Peshkin BN, Ward BA. The impact of genetic screening on surgical decision-making in breast cancer. In: Szabó Z, Lewis JE, Fantini GA, Savalgi RS, eds. *Surgical technology international VII: international developments in surgery and surgical research.* San Francisco: Universal Medical Press, 1998:333.
63. Lerman C, Narod S, Schulman K, et al. BRCA1 testing in families with hereditary breast-ovarian cancer: a prospective study of patient decision-making and outcomes. *JAMA* 1996;275:1885.
64. Lynch HT, Lemon SJ, Durham C, et al. A descriptive study of BRCA1 testing and reactions to disclosure of test results. *Cancer* 1997;79:2219.
65. Lerman C, Peshkin BN, Hughes C, Isaacs C. Family disclosure in genetic testing for cancer susceptibility: determinants and consequences. *J Health Care Law and Policy* 1998;1:353.
66. Green J, Richards M, Murton F, Statham H, Hallowell N. Family communication and genetic counseling: the case of hereditary breast and ovarian cancer. *J Genet Couns* 1997;6:45.
67. American Society of Human Genetics Social Issues Subcommittee on Familial Disclosure. ASHG statement: professional disclosure of familial genetic information. *Am J Hum Genet* 1998; 62:474.
68. Myriad Genetic Laboratories. BRACAnalysis Technical Specifications. Updated May 5, 1999.
69. Easton DF, Bishop DT, Ford D, et al. Genetic linkage analysis in familial breast and ovarian cancer: results from 214 families. *Am J Hum Genet* 1992;52:678.
70. Wooster R, Bignell G, Lancaster J, et al. Identification of the breast cancer susceptibility gene BRCA2. *Nature* 1995;378:789.
71. Ganguly T, Dhulipala R, Godmilow L, Ganguly A. High throughput fluorescence-based conformation sensitive gel electrophoresis (F-CSGE) identifies six unique BRCA2 mutations and an overall low incidence of BRCA2 mutations in high-risk BRCA1-negative breast cancer families. *Hum Genet U S A* 1998;102:549.
72. Abbaszadegan MR, Struewing JP, Brown KM, et al. Automated detection of prevalent mutations in BRCA1 and BRCA2 genes, using a fluorogenic PCR allelic discrimination assay. *Genetic Testing* 1997/1998;1:171.
73. Wu LC, Want ZW, Tsan J, et al. Identification of a RING protein that can interact *in vivo* with the BRCA1 gene product. *Nat Genet* 1996;14:430.
74. Humphrey JS, Salim A, Erdos M, Collins FS, Brody LC, Klausner RD. Human *BRCA1* inhibits growth in yeast: potential use in diagnostic testing. *Proc Natl Acad Sci* 1997;94:5820.
75. Maquat LE. Invited editorial: defects in RNA splicing and the consequence of shortened translational reading frames. *Am J Hum Genet* 1996;59:279.
76. The National Human Genome Research Institute. 1999 Breast cancer information core. Available at: http://www.nhgri.nih.gov/intramural_research/ Lab_transfer/Bic. Accessed March 24, 1999.
77. Lerman C, Schwartz MD, Lin TH, et al. The influence of psychological distress on use of genetic testing for cancer risk. *J Consult Clin Psychol* 1997;65:414.
78. Lynch HT, Watson P, Conway TA. DNA screening for breast/ovarian cancer susceptibility on linked markers: a family study. *Arch Intern Med* 1993;153:1979.
79. Botkin JR, Croyle RT, Smith KR, et al. A model protocol for evaluating the behavioral and psychological effects of BRCA1 testing. *J Natl Cancer Inst* 1996;88:872.
80. Croyle RT, Smith KR, Botkin JR, et al. Psychological responses to BRCA1 mutation testing: preliminary findings. *Health Psychol* 1997;16:63.
81. Lerman C, Hughes C, Lemon S, et al. Outcomes study of BRCA1/2 testing in members of hereditary breast ovarian cancer (HBOC) families. *Breast Cancer Res Treat* 1997;46:10a.
82. Lerman C, Hughes C, Lemon SJ, et al. What you don't know can hurt you: adverse psychologic effects in members of BRCA1-linked and BRCA2-linked families who decline genetic testing. *J Clin Oncol* 1998;16:1650.
83. Lerman C, Croyle R. Psychological issues in genetic testing for breast cancer susceptibility. *Arch Intern Med* 1994;154:609.
84. Stefanek ME. Bilateral prophylactic mastectomy: issues and concerns. *J Natl Cancer Inst Monographs* 1995;17:37.
85. Stefanek M, Lerman C. Prophylactic mastectomy decision making. Presented to the Society of Behavioral Medicine; March 1996; Washington, DC.
86. Rimer BK, Schildkraut JM, Lerman C, et al. Participation in a women's breast cancer risk counseling trial. Who participates? Who declines? *Cancer* 1996;77:2348.
87. Miller HH, Bauman LJ, Friedman DR, DeCosse JJ. Psychosocial adjustment of familial polyposis patients and participation in a chemoprevention trial. *Int J Psychiatry Med* 1986–1987;16:211.
88. Lerman C, Audrain J, Croyle RT. DNA-testing for heritable breast cancer risk: lessons from traditional genetic counseling. *Ann Behav Med* 1994;16:327.
89. Kash KM, Lerman C. Psychological, social, and ethical issues in gene testing. In: Holland J, Massey MJ, eds. *Psycho-Oncology*. New York: Oxford University Press, 1998:196.
90. Lerman C, Croyle RT. Emotional and behavioral responses to genetic testing for susceptibility to cancer. *Oncology* 1996;10:191.
91. Owens RG, Ashcroft JJ, Leinster SF. Informal decision analysis with breast cancer patients: an aid to psychological preparation for surgery. *J Psychosocial Oncology* 1987;5:23.
92. Burke W, Daly M, Garber J, et al. Recommendations for follow-up care of individuals with an inherited predisposition to cancer: II. BRCA1 and BRCA2. *JAMA* 1997;277:997.
93. Meyer JE, Kopans DB, Oot R. Breast cancer visualized by mammography in patients under 35. *Radiology* 1983;147:93.
94. Cohen MI, Mintzer RA, Matthies HJ, Bernstein JR. Mammography in women less than 40 years of age. *Surg Gynecol Obstet* 1985;160:220.
95. Helvie MA, Bouridoux MA, Weber BL, Merajver SD. Mammography of breast carcinoma in women who have mutations of the breast cancer gene BRCA1: initial experience. *Am J Radiol* 1997;168:1599.
96. Hoskins KF, Stopfer JE, Calzone K, et al. Assessment and counseling for women with a family history of breast cancer: a guide for clinicians. *JAMA* 1995;273:577.
97. den Otter W, Merchant TE, Beijerinck D, Koten JW. Breast cancer induction due to mammographic screening in hereditarily affected women. *Anticancer Res* 1996;16:3173.
98. Law J. Cancers detected and induced in mammographic screening: new screening schedules and younger women with family history. *Br J Radiol* 1997;70:62.
99. Lynch HT, Conway T, Watson P, et al. Extremely early onset hereditary breast cancer (HBC): surveillance/management implications. *Neb Med J* 1988;73:97.
100. Hartmann LC, Schaid DJ, Woods JE, et al. Efficacy of bilateral prophylactic mastectomy in women with a family history of breast cancer. *N Engl J Med* 1999;340:77.
101. Schrag D, Kuntz KM, Garber JE, Weeks JC. Decision analysis—effects of prophylactic mastectomy and oophorectomy on life expectancy among women with BRCA1 or BRCA2 mutations. *N Engl J Med* 1997;336:1465.
102. Rebbeck TR, Levin A, Daly M, et al. Cancer risk reduction by prophylactic surgery in BRCA1 and BRCA2 mutation carriers. *Am J Hum Genet* 1998;63:A249.
103. Fisher B, Costantino JP, Wickerham DL, et al. Tamoxifen for prevention of breast cancer: report of the National Surgical Adjuvant Breast and Bowel Project P-1 study. *J Natl Cancer Inst* 1998;90:1371.
104. Powles T, Eeles R, Ashley S, et al. Interim analysis of the incidence of breast cancer in the Royal Marsden Hospital tamoxifen randomized chemoprevention trial. *Lancet* 1998;352:98.
105. Grady D, Rubin SM, Petitti DB, et al. Hormone therapy to prevent disease and prolong life in postmenopausal women. *Ann Int Med* 1992;117:1016.
106. Colditz GA, Hankinson SE, Hunter DJ, et al. The use of estrogens and progestins and the risk of breast cancer in postmenopausal women. *N Engl J Med* 1995;332:1589.
107. Roy JA, Sawka CA, Pritchard KI. Hormone replacement therapy in women with breast cancer: do the risks outweigh the benefits? *J Clin Oncol* 1996;14:997.
108. Love RR, Wiebe DA, Newcomb PA, et al. Effects of tamoxifen on cardiovascular risk factors in postmenopausal women. *Ann Int Med* 1991;115:860.
109. Delmas P, Bjarnason N, Mitlak B, et al. Effects of raloxifene on bone mineral density, serum cholesterol concentrations, and uterine endometrium in postmenopausal women. *N Engl J Med* 1997; 337:1641.
110. McDonald CC, Stewart HJ. Fatal myocardial infarction in the Scottish adjuvant tamoxifen trial. The Scottish Breast Cancer Committee. *BMJ* 1991;303:435.

111. Constantino JP, Kuller LH, Ives DG, Fisher B, Dignam J. Coronary heart disease mortality and adjuvant tamoxifen. *J Natl Cancer Inst* 1997;89:776.
112. Grey AB, Stapleton JP, Evans MC, Tatnell MA, Ames RW, Reid IR. The effect of the antiestrogen tamoxifen on bone mineral density in normal late postmenopausal women. *Am J Med* 1995;99:636.
113. Love RR, Mazess RB, Barden HS, et al. Effects of tamoxifen on bone mineral density in postmenopausal women with breast cancer. *N Engl J Med* 1992;326:852.
114. Lufkin EG, Whitaker MD, Nickelsen T, et al. Treatment of established postmenopausal osteoporosis with raloxifene: a randomized trial. *J Bone Miner Res* 1998;13:1747.
115. Jordan VC, Glusman JE, Eckert S, et al. Raloxifene reduces incident primary breast cancers: integrated data from multicenter double-blind placebo-controlled randomized trials in postmenopausal women. *Breast Cancer Res Treat* 1998;50:2a.
116. Piver MS, Jishi MF, Tsukada Y, Nava G. Primary peritoneal carcinoma after prophylactic oophorectomy in women with a family history of ovarian cancer. *Cancer* 1993;71:2751.
117. Struewing JP, Watson P, Easton DF, Ponder BA, Lynch HT, Tucker MA. Prophylactic oophorectomy in inherited breast/ovarian cancer families. *J Natl Cancer Inst Monogr* 1995;17:33.
118. Rosenberg L, Palmer JR, Zauber AG, et al. A case-control study of oral contraceptive use and invasive epithelial ovarian cancer. *Am J Epidemiol* 1994;139:654.

Diseases of the Breast, 2nd ed.,
edited by Jay R. Harris.
Lippincott Williams & Wilkins, Philadelphia © 2000.

CHAPTER 18

Prophylactic Mastectomy

J. Dirk Iglehart

Prophylactic mastectomy is the removal of a normal breast to prevent the future occurrence of malignancy. This surgical procedure is reserved for women with an increased risk of breast cancer in one of two clinical scenarios. In the first situation, a woman who has never had breast cancer contemplates bilateral mastectomy to avoid cancer. In the second, a woman considers a prophylactic contralateral mastectomy after having a breast cancer in one breast. Prior to 1990, contralateral mastectomy was a more common procedure. The procedure was frequently performed at the time of a therapeutic mastectomy on the affected side, usually because of a perceived increased risk of cancer in the healthy breast. With the popularity of breast-conserving procedures, and with better risk assessment, contralateral mastectomy is performed much less frequently.

Prophylactic mastectomy includes two basic procedures: total mastectomy and subcutaneous mastectomy. *Total mastectomy*, or *simple mastectomy*, usually refers to complete removal of the glandular breast and the nipple and areola, with or without an ellipse of surrounding skin. In *subcutaneous mastectomy*, the glandular breast is removed, but the overlying skin and the nipple-areolar complex are preserved. These preventive procedures are usually combined with breast reconstruction using one of several surgical approaches. Common procedures for mastectomy and reconstruction and are covered in more detail in Chapters 34 and 35.

Risk assessment is at the heart of the clinical decision for or against prophylactic mastectomy in the asymptomatic patient. In modern practice, highest risks are conferred by dominant breast cancer susceptibility genes, a mutated allele of either *BRCA1* or *BRCA2*. Women who have a strong family history of breast cancer but do not carry a mutation in either of the two known susceptibility genes also have an increased risk of breast cancer. These women may harbor undiscovered genetic factors. Finally, susceptibility may be the result of a combination of genetic and nongenetic factors, which in aggregate cross a threshold of risk in the judgment of the patient or her physicians. This chapter presents the range of surgical procedures briefly, describes risk factors in detail, and discusses the effectiveness of prophylactic procedures in preventing breast cancer.

J. D. Iglehart: Department of Surgery, Brigham and Women's Hospital, Dana-Farber Cancer Institute, Harvard Medical School, Boston, Massachusetts

PROPHYLACTIC PROCEDURES

Total Mastectomy (Simple Mastectomy)

Prophylactic total mastectomy is similar to therapeutic total mastectomy, which is used to treat certain types of breast cancers. The postoperative result is similar in appearance to that of a therapeutic operation for breast cancer. Lymph nodes in the ipsilateral axilla are not included in a prophylactic procedure; however, the subcutaneous dissection extends into the low axilla to complete the removal of the breast. Figure 1 displays the initial skin incisions commonly used for simple mastectomy. As shown in Fig. 1A, the nipple-areolar complex is removed with an ellipse of surrounding central skin. This procedure is most familiar to general surgeons who perform therapeutic mastectomy. Without reconstruction, the result is a flat chest wall with a single transverse incision. Many surgeons consider this procedure the best for providing access to the entire glandular breast and completely removing subareolar ductal tissue.

A variation of the standard total mastectomy procedure is shown in Fig. 1B. In this procedure, termed a *skin-sparing mastectomy*, the nipple and areola are removed, exposing the breast tissue through the incision around the areola.[1] A lateral extension of the incision, as shown in the figure, is used to assist the subcutaneous dissection. The standard simple mastectomy or the skin-sparing mastectomy can be combined with breast reconstruction, as described in Chapter 34.

Subcutaneous Mastectomy

In subcutaneous mastectomy, the glandular breast is removed through a single surgical incision, usually placed in

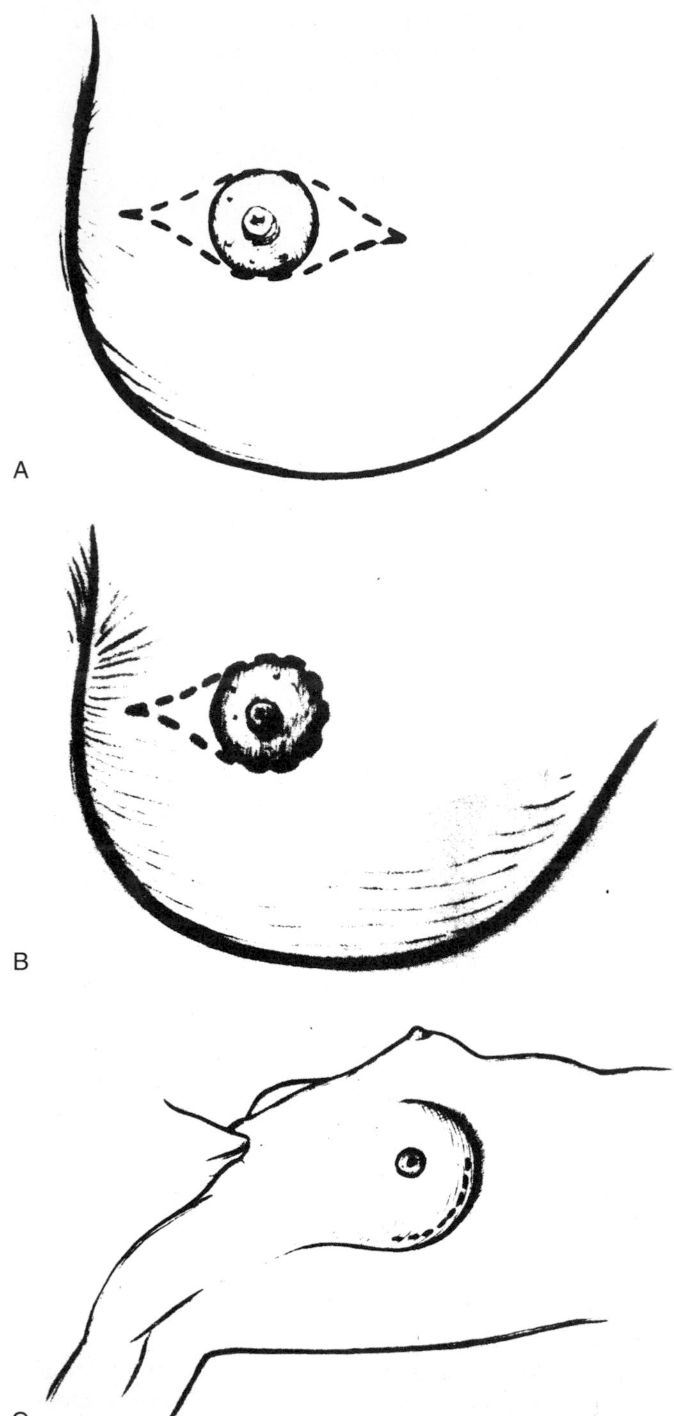

FIG. 1. Procedures commonly performed for prophylactic mastectomy. **A:** Total mastectomy (simple mastectomy), performed through an elliptical incision around the entire nipple-areolar complex, including the central skin of the breast. **B:** Skin-sparing mastectomy, performed through a keyhole incision around the areola. The incision is tapered laterally. Frequently, the lateral extension is a single surgical opening directed outward from an incision completely encircling the areola. **C:** Subcutaneous mastectomy, commonly performed through a single incision in the inframammary crease, leaving the nipple-areolar complex and the complete skin envelope of the breast.

the inframammary crease (see Fig. 1C). This procedure conserves the entire skin envelope of the breast and preserves the nipple and areola.[2] The breast form may be reconstructed with a prosthetic implant. Pedicle or free muscle flaps are also used to provide a breast mound under the skin envelope of the breast. Complete removal of the glandular breast tissue is not as easily performed by this procedure. After a subcutaneous mastectomy, residual breast tissue may be left under the nipple and at the periphery of the dissection.[3] Certain patients with a favorable chest wall configuration may be candidates for this procedure, however. The central plateau of the nipple can be removed with the larger ducts immediately under the nipple (*nipple coring*), and the areolar skin can be preserved. This procedure has been advocated to increase the completeness of subcutaneous mastectomy. Breast ducts may be found within the dermis of the areolar skin, however, a fact that underscores the difficulty of removing all at-risk tissue by subcutaneous mastectomy.[4] For the patient who wishes to reduce her risk by the greatest degree, total mastectomy, as depicted in Figs. 1A and 1B, is recommended.

RISK FACTORS

Genetic Risk Factors for Breast Cancer

The accurate assessment of breast cancer risk, both in the asymptomatic woman and in the patient with unilateral breast cancer, is critical to successful detection and prevention, and to prophylactic strategies. In general, the higher the risk of cancer, the greater the motivation for prophylactic intervention. As discussed later, however, in Evidence for Effectiveness of Prophylactic Mastectomy, prophylactic surgery is neither 100% effective nor free of complications.

In asymptomatic women, risk factors include family history and genetic predisposition, the presence of benign proliferative breast disease, and hormonal and reproductive history. Exposure to radiation is an important risk factor for breast cancer. Therapeutic radiation, commonly for the treatment of Hodgkin's disease, increases the risk of breast cancer and is a more potent hazard when used in younger women.[5,6] A more complete discussion of nongenetic risk factors is found in Chapter 15.

The highest risk estimates are for those women who carry mutations in either of the two known predisposition genes, *BRCA1* and *BRCA2*. For these women, the lifetime probability of developing breast cancer is very high, although estimates vary and our knowledge is incomplete. Very high estimates were derived from study of the families used to map and identify these genes, which usually contained many cases of breast or ovarian cancer. For members of these families, the lifelong risk of breast cancer for gene carriers varied between 75% and 87%.[7–10] In these kindreds, chosen because of the high number of cancer cases, other genetic or environmental factors might be operating to increase the observed penetrance. Unbiased population samples, not

TABLE 1. *Cumulative risk of breast cancer by attained age for* BRCA1 *or* BRCA2 *carriers*

	Cumulative risk (%)		
Attained age	Highest estimates[a]	Population-based estimates[b]	U.S. population from SEER data[c]
30	3.2	<2	0.16
40	19.1	15	1.0
50	50.8	33	3.0
60	54.2	50	5.7
70 (lifetime)	85.0	56–68	8.9

[a]From refs. 7, 8, 9, and 10.
[b]From refs. 11 and 12.
[c]General population estimates from Surveillance, Epidemiology, and End Results (SEER) Program. Feuer EJ, et al. The lifetime risk of developing breast cancer. *J Natl Cancer Inst* 1993;85:892–897.

selected solely because of striking family histories, yield more moderate estimates of cancer risks for gene carriers.[11–13] In the study of Struewing et al., 5,318 Jewish men and women were tested for two common mutations in *BRCA1* and one mutation in *BRCA2*. In this group, the risk of breast cancer among carriers was 56%, with a 95% confidence interval of 40% to 73%.[11]

Risk estimates in these studies are projected over a lifetime until a theoretical age has been attained, usually age 70. For the purpose of advising women about prophylactic surgery, presenting information in intervals of time that are meaningful to individual women is useful. Table 1 presents the cumulative risk of breast cancer for women carrying mutations in *BRCA1* and *BRCA2* according to attained age. Both the highest risk estimates from the initial linkage families and the moderate estimates from population-based studies are tabulated. When physicians counsel women who carry *BRCA1* or *BRCA2* mutations and who are considering prophylactic surgery, the inclusion of lower risk estimates from population-based studies has been advised.[13] Furthermore, the timing of surgery is an important consideration, from the standpoint both of breast cancer risk and the effect of breast removal in women of different ages. Table 1 shows that, even at the highest estimates of penetrance, the risk of breast cancer in women younger than age 30 is small, and the risk is moderate for women who are younger than age 40. Based on comparable risks—for instance, recurrence rates after breast-conserving treatments—delay of preventive mastectomy well past age 30 seems reasonable.

BRCA1 and *BRCA2* carriers are a special case and represent a particularly high-risk group of women. However, unaffected women with a strong family history of breast or ovarian cancer are at increased risk for breast cancer even if they do not carry a detectable mutation in *BRCA1* or *BRCA2*. Although the majority of families segregating both breast and ovarian cancer carry mutations in the two known predisposing genes, a significant number test negatively for disease-associated mutations. One study reported on 238 women with early-onset breast cancer or ovarian cancer who were tested for *BRCA1* or *BRCA2* mutations by complete sequencing.[14] Of 117 affected women who belonged to families with both breast and ovarian cancer, 58 (50%) had no detectable deleterious mutations in either gene. In families with breast cancer, but without ovarian cancer, an even higher number of breast cancer cases cannot be explained by *BRCA1* or *BRCA2* mutations. These two genes were completely sequenced in 21 affected women with more than 3 relatives with breast cancer; 13 (62%) carried no detectable mutation in either gene. These data are corroborated by surveys in the United States,[15] among French Canadians,[16] and in Finland.[17] In studies carried out at Duke University in Durham, NC, 100 women with a personal history of breast cancer were offered genetic testing. The probability that these women carried a dominant gene with the characteristics of *BRCA1* and *BRCA2* was computed using a statistical model.[18,19] Fifteen women in this high-risk population were identified who had a carrier probability of greater than 75% and yet tested negatively.[20] These studies and other similar experiences indicate that a negative test for *BRCA1* or *BRCA2* does not exclude a powerful genetic component to the disease.

Two models of breast cancer risk are available to estimate the probability that unaffected women will develop cancer. The Gail model, drawing on data from the Breast Cancer Detection Demonstration Project (BCDDP), is based on factors including age, reproductive history, and a history of breast cancer in first-degree relatives.[21] The model does not take into account the breast cancer history of second-degree relatives and therefore ignores paternal transmission. Claus et al. developed a second model to account for the autosomal dominant inheritance of breast cancer. This model considers both the number of breast cancers and the age of onset of cancer in relatives on both sides of the family.[22] Neither model provides an entirely comprehensive estimate of risk using genetic and nongenetic risk factors together in one counseling tool. The Gail model has been used to determine eligibility for preventive treatment with tamoxifen citrate in the National Surgical Adjuvant Breast and Bowel Project (NSABP) P-1 trial.[23] The Claus-Risch model is useful for women who have a family history of breast cancer and whose *BRCA1* and *BRCA2* status is not determined. Table 2 provides examples of risk computations for an unaffected 30-year-old woman under several different family cancer situations, based on the Claus-Risch model.

Composite Risk Factors in the Asymptomatic Patient

BRCA1 or *BRCA2* mutation is an example of a single risk factor that provides a quantitative estimate of breast cancer risk. The magnitude of this risk is large and dominates other individual risk factors. A combination of predisposing factors, however, when added together, may achieve a risk that rivals in magnitude the risk from mutation in *BRCA* genes.

TABLE 2. *Risk of breast cancer for a 30-year-old woman according to family history*

	Relatives with breast cancer aged 40–49 yr			
Interval of life (from age 30 yr)	1 first-degree[a]	2 first-degree	1 second-degree[b]	1 first-degree, 1 second-degree
Next 10 yr	0.9	3.4	0.5	3.3
Next 20 yr	2.9	10.4	1.9	9.8
Lifetime (to age 79 yr)	13.0	34.0	10.2	33.0

Table shows chance of getting breast cancer over specified interval, expressed as percent.
[a]Primary relatives are mothers, sisters, and daughters.
[b]Secondary relatives are aunts, cousins, and grandparents on either paternal or maternal side. When multiple relatives are specified, they are assumed to be on the same side of the family.
From ref. 22, with permission.

The Gail model is an attempt to account for multiple risk factors and provide age-specific hazard rates for breast cancer for individual women.[21]

The Gail model was derived from the BCDDP population of predominately white American women who participated in sponsored breast cancer screening on an annual basis.[21,24] The major predictors of breast cancer risk eventually included in the composite model were a family history of breast cancer in first-degree relatives, age at first childbirth, age at the time of menarche, and a history of multiple previous breast biopsies (for benign disease). The model can compute risk for an individual woman who has attained a specific age over a subsequent interval of life. A multiplier is added for a diagnosis of atypical ductal or lobular hyperplasia (see below).

The Gail model provides probabilities that are being used to counsel women, particularly in screening and the development of preventive strategies. However, the range of calculated risks in the Gail model overlaps those estimated for carriers of *BRCA1* and *BRCA2* mutations. For instance, a 40-year-old woman with several risk factors might accumulate a probability of breast cancer in the 30% to 40% range, close to the lower limits of risk for *BRCA1* or *BRCA2* carriers. Future improvements in risk assessment models may incorporate history of lobular carcinoma *in situ*, history of contralateral breast cancers, and augmented family history information. Certain women may ask for information about prophylactic surgery based on the constellation of risk factors in their individual situations. Although risk assessment models are useful, they should be applied in clinical practice with caution.

Histologic Risk Factors

In the Gail model, atypical epithelial hyperplasia occurring in ducts or lobules is recognized as a risk factor for eventual breast cancer. In the BCDDP population studied by Gail et al., the relative risk of atypical hyperplasia was 1.96, with a 95% confidence interval of 1.51 to 2.54.[21] In an earlier study of atypical hyperplasia using the same nested cohort of women undergoing breast biopsy for benign lesions in the BCDDP, the same team of investigators observed a relative risk of atypical hyperplasia of 3.0 compared with normal subjects.[25] Young women with atypical hyperplasia were at a particularly increased risk of breast cancer (relative risk of 5.7 compared with normal subjects). Somewhat higher estimates were reported by Dupont and Page, who found the risk of contracting breast cancer in women with atypical hyperplasia to be 5.3 times that of women who underwent breast biopsy for benign lesions that revealed only nonproliferative changes.[26] Later work by these investigators compared risks for women with different states of proliferative disease with risks for women in the Connecticut tumor registry. In this later analysis, atypical hyperplasia was found to increase risk by a factor of 4.0.[27] Interaction of atypical hyperplasia with other factors, such as parity and family history, was noted by Dupont and Page. Combining atypical hyperplasia with a family history of breast cancer in first-degree relatives produced a projected risk of breast cancer of 20% at 15 years of follow-up. Age of onset of breast cancer in relatives, paternal transmission, ovarian cancer in relatives, and the number of relatives with cancer were not factored into these studies. Refined models capable of combining a number of risk factors may give individual projections high enough to make prophylactic mastectomy a realistic consideration for some women. Risk projections for women with atypical hyperplasia, however, range from 1.96 to 5.30. Because of this variability, the integration of atypical hyperplasia into composite estimates of breast cancer risk that are used to counsel patients about irreversible surgery is hard to recommend.

Lobular carcinoma *in situ* (LCIS) is a histologic lesion found in the breasts of younger women. Although this lesion was once treated by unilateral mastectomy, accumulating data suggest that LCIS is either a precursor lesion or a histologic risk factor. Early data from a study at Memorial Hospital, with an average follow-up of 24 years, projected a ninefold increase in risk of breast cancer after a diagnosis of LCIS. Significantly, subsequent cancers were distributed nearly evenly in the ipsilateral and contralateral breast.[28] Other data sets have produced lower estimates or have not noted an increased number of contralateral cancers.[29,30] NSABP Protocol B-17 followed 182 women with LCIS treated by biopsy only for a mean of 5 years.[31] Four cases of ipsilateral invasive cancer (2.2%) and two cases of con-

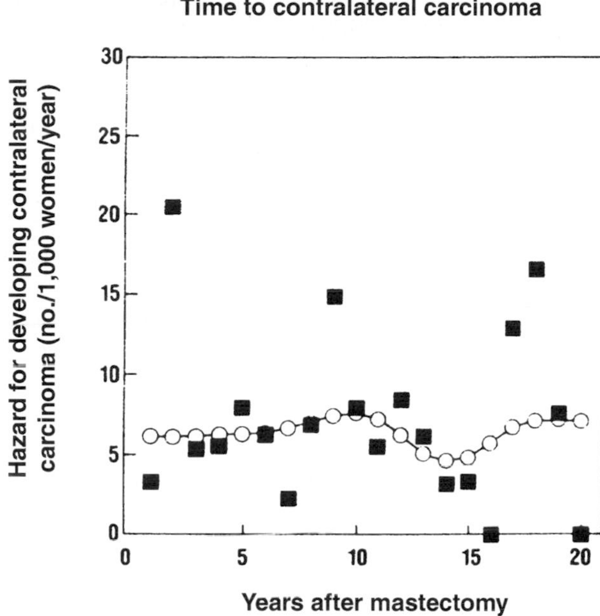

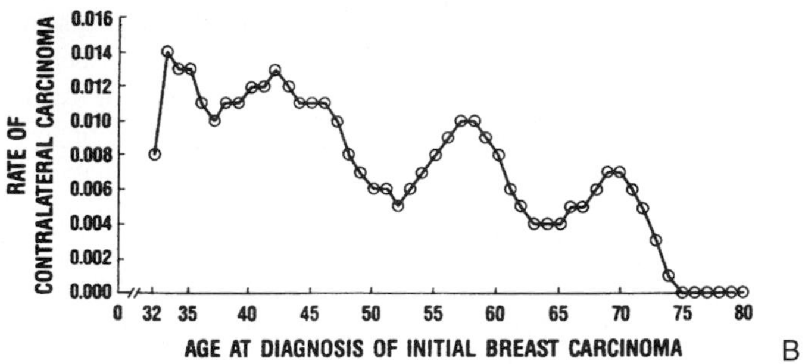

FIG. 2. Contralateral breast cancer risk. **A:** Yearly hazard rate for development of contralateral breast cancer after a cancer in the first breast. (*Squares*, raw data for each year; *circles*, smoothed data for each year.) **B:** Rate of contralateral carcinoma as a function of age at the time of diagnosis of the initial breast carcinoma. The data have been smoothed to show the downward trend in contralateral cancer with increasing age at the time of the first breast cancer. (From ref. 36, with permission.)

tralateral breast cancer (1.1%) were recorded. The ipsilateral recurrences were in the same quadrant as the initial LCIS, suggesting that the LCIS lesions served as precursor or premalignant lesions rather than as true risk factors. Longer follow-up in the NSABP study may reveal more breast cancers and alter the conclusions made up to this point. Two European studies conducted in the same time frame and with approximately the same follow-up time found a higher ipsilateral occurrence of breast cancer but tended to confirm the low incidence of contralateral breast cancer.[30,32] Therefore, based on current data, bilateral prophylactic mastectomy for a diagnosis of LCIS seems hard to justify in the absence of other risk factors. In fact, in some cases, LCIS may be a precursor lesion with a low biological potential.

Cancer in the Contralateral Breast

A history of previous cancer in one breast is a strong risk factor for cancer in the opposite breast. The magnitude of this risk, frequently quoted in clinical practice, is between 0.5% and 1.0% during each year of follow-up.[33–35] Six hundred and forty-four patients with T1 N0 M0 and T1 N1 M0 cancers who were treated at Memorial Sloan-Kettering Cancer Center were followed for a median of 18.2 years. The average annual incidence of contralateral breast cancer was 8 per 1,000 patients per year of follow-up (0.8% per year).[36] Significantly, the hazard rate was relatively constant throughout two decades of follow-up, as shown in Fig. 2A. Age was an important determiner of risk; the annual hazard rate generally declined as the age at the time of first breast cancer diagnosis increased. As shown in Fig. 2B, women younger than age 45 at diagnosis of first breast cancer have an average annual rate of contralateral breast cancer of approximately 1% (0.8–1.4%). In women older than age 50 at first diagnosis, the annualized risk falls to approximately 0.5% (≤1%). A 35-year-old woman assumed to be cured of her first breast cancer may face a lifetime risk of cancer in the opposite breast of 30% to 40%. This risk is similar in magnitude to the risk imparted by mutations in dominant susceptibility genes.

Although the risk of cancer is high, several factors mitigate the need for a prophylactic removal of the opposite breast. A risk of eventual cancer in the range of 0.5% to 1.0% per year is similar to the risk of ipsilateral local recurrence after breast-conserving procedures.[37,38] Risks of this magnitude are routinely accepted by patients choosing breast-conserving treatment, with the encouragement of surgeons and radiotherapists. As with ipsilateral recurrence, overall mortality is determined by distant disease and not by local failure. Contralateral breast cancer accounts for only a small fraction of overall failures after a first breast cancer, and overall mortality is determined largely by the first cancer. For instance, in the work from Memorial Sloan-Kettering Cancer Center, contralateral cancers were found to be responsible for only 5.1% of all recurrences and 2.6% of cancer deaths.[36] Finally, breast cancer mortality is relatively low in a population of women undergoing vigilant screening. In the BCDDP population, the overall breast cancer–adjusted survival rate (counting only deaths due to breast cancer) was 80.5% after 20 years of follow-up.[24] For a woman with invasive breast cancer in the first breast, who is at risk for distant disease and death, the occurrence of a second breast cancer (in the opposite breast) accounts for 5% of all recurrences. Assuming vigilant screening of the opposite breast, cure is expected for 80% of new primary cancers during 20 years of follow-up. Therefore, such a woman can reasonably expect to face a 1% chance of dying of a second breast cancer that occurs in the opposite breast, assuming that the first cancer was cured. For most patients with invasive breast cancer in one breast, a preventive operation on the unaffected side is hard to justify.

The example above assumes an invasive breast cancer of unspecified histology. Certain histologic types, however, have been associated with a higher risk of contralateral breast cancer. Invasive lobular carcinoma, with or without concomitant LCIS, has been advanced as increasing the risk of subsequent contralateral cancer.[39,40] Other studies have failed to find a higher rate of cancers in the opposite breast in patients with lobular carcinoma.[41–43] The risk of bilateral cancer after the diagnosis of ductal carcinoma *in situ* (DCIS) is usually presumed to be the same as after invasive ductal cancers. Some surgeons have worried that diffuse and multifocal DCIS may be different and may portend a higher risk for the opposite breast. At least one study failed to show an increased incidence of cancer in the opposite breast after a primary diagnosis of DCIS.[44] Whether a multifocal or diffuse intraductal cancer is associated with increased risk is open to question. Identifying a particular histologic type of breast cancer in the first breast that justifies preventive surgery on the opposite breast is not possible.

PROPHYLACTIC MASTECTOMY IN CLINICAL PRACTICE

Interest in prophylactic mastectomy as a means of reducing breast cancer risk remains high among patients and their doctors. This is particularly true when concern is voiced about the contralateral, unaffected breast after treatment of the first cancer. Interest in bilateral prophylactic mastectomy to prevent breast cancer is also high among health care providers and their patients. Before the identification of *BRCA1* and *BRCA2*, 250 oncologists and nurses were surveyed about their attitudes toward a hypothetical woman who has two primary relatives with early-onset breast cancer, both of whom died from the disease.[45] Nearly one-third of the physicians selected bilateral mastectomy as the optimal treatment for this patient, whose risk of developing breast cancer is in the range of 30% to 40% (see Table 2). In addition, when female respondents were asked to consider themselves as the patient in this example, an even higher proportion selected bilateral mastectomy as the optimal course of prevention that they would pursue. These attitudes were confirmed by Houn et al., who surveyed Maryland surgeons for their opinions about and recommendations for bilateral mastectomy for their high-risk patients.[46] Although more plastic surgeons agreed that prophylactic surgery played a role in breast cancer risk reduction (84.6%), a substantial number of general surgeons and gynecologists also agreed (47.0% and 38.3%, respectively). A large proportion of plastic surgeons recommended the surgery to their patients (81%), whereas 38.8% of general surgeons and 17.7% of gynecologists recommended the surgery. These studies, directed at women and their health care providers, confirm an interest in this procedure. The evidence for effectiveness of prophylactic mastectomy needs to be critically reviewed, however.

Evidence for Effectiveness of Prophylactic Mastectomy

Evidence for the effectiveness of prophylactic mastectomy in asymptomatic patients must address three issues: (a) Is the procedure likely to reduce the incidence of breast cancer? (b) How does the procedure compare with vigilant screening as a mode of reducing breast cancer mortality? (c) Is the procedure acceptable to women who choose to undergo removal of both breasts?

Does prophylactic mastectomy reduce the incidence of breast cancer? This question has been addressed by several strategies. Early investigations modeled prophylactic mastectomy in experimental animals, using the model of rodent mammary cancer induced by chemical carcinogens first described by Huggins and Yang in 1962.[47] In the first series of experiments, the breast tissue–bearing ventral surface of the experimental animals was divided into quadrants, and the mammary tissue was cleared surgically in two or three quadrants. These animals were then compared with sham, non–surgically treated control animals.[48] The overall risk of an animal's developing breast cancer after carcinogen administration was not affected by the volume of mammary tissue removed surgically. The incidence of tumors in the nonsurgical quadrants was increased in proportion to the amount of mammary tissue removed; the risk of cancer increased in the remaining tissue. A second series of experiments compared partial to total mastectomy in all four breast tissue–bearing quadrants.[49] In these experiments, the onset of cancer was delayed but not prevented in the operated animals. The total number of cancers per animal was not significantly different in the experimental groups than in control, nonoperated animals. The investigators concluded that residual breast tissue left after mastectomy harbored an increased risk of cancer that defeated the overall effectiveness of the surgery.

These animal experiments, although not directly germane to human breast cancer, point out the danger of incomplete mastectomy. This danger has been illustrated in anecdotal reports of the occurrence of breast cancer after subcutaneous mastectomy, which admittedly does not remove all glandular tissue at risk.[50,51] In distinction to the animal experiments, however, subcutaneous mastectomy did appear to reduce the incidence of breast cancer in at least one long-term study. Pennisi and Capozzi reported results from a registry of patients on whom subcutaneous mastectomy was performed between 1975 and 1986 by 165 plastic surgeons. Seventy percent of the women were followed for an average of 9 years.[52] Six cancers developed during follow-up, an incidence of 0.57% among the 1,050 women for whom data

TABLE 3. *Incidence of and death from breast cancer in women undergoing prophylactic mastectomy*

Events in sisters[a] (control group)	Breast cancer events (occurrence or death) Number expected (from sisters)	Number observed (in mastectomy group)	Reduction in events (%)
All breast cancers (before and after patient's prophylactic mastectomy) from age 18 to end of follow-up[b]	30.0	3	90.0 (70.8–97.9)
Breast cancers after patient's prophylactic mastectomy	37.4	3	92.0 (76.6–98.3)
Deaths from breast cancer after patient's prophylactic mastectomy	10.5	2	80.9 (31.4–97.7)

Numbers in parentheses are 95% confidence intervals.
[a]Control group consisted of sisters of women undergoing prophylactic surgery. Expected incidence of breast cancer was determined by analysis of cancer occurring in sisters before or after the mastectomy in patients, as indicated.
[b]Incidence was adjusted for ascertainment bias.
Adapted from ref. 53.

were complete. Twenty percent of these women had a history of breast cancer in a first-degree relative (mother, sister, or daughter), but age of onset was not specified. Although risk reduction was not calculated, 1,000 moderate-risk women would have a 10-year breast cancer incidence of approximately 50 cases based on Gail model estimates.[21] Therefore, a risk reduction of more than 80% can be estimated for women who had subcutaneous bilateral mastectomy compared with a moderate-risk untreated population.

These estimates agree with the results of a review of 639 asymptomatic women, all with a family history of breast cancer, who underwent prophylactic bilateral mastectomy at the Mayo Clinic between 1960 and 1993.[53] Seven breast cancers were detected during a median follow-up of 14 years. All seven were in 575 women who underwent subcutaneous mastectomy; no cancers occurred in 64 women who had bilateral total mastectomy. Although these data imply a lower rate for women with total mastectomy, statistical power was too weak to differentiate between these two procedures ($p = .38$). In this study of familial breast cancer, nonoperated sisters of study subjects were used as a control group, and the data were adjusted in two different ways. Because the occurrence of cancer in a first-degree relative may influence the decision to undergo prophylactic mastectomy, this would lead to a selection bias in favor of cancer in the sisters of women who seek mastectomy. In the first correction, only breast cancers occurring in the nonoperated sisters after the prophylactic surgery in the study subjects were included in the study. Second, because women with multiple breast cancers in their families are more likely to seek prophylactic mastectomy, an adjustment was made for this ascertainment bias. The observed and expected numbers of breast cancers and the deaths due to breast cancer are shown in Table 3, which is taken directly from the work of Hartmann et al.[53]

These two retrospective reviews—Pennisi and Capozzi,[52] and Hartmann et al.[53]—measured significant reductions in breast cancer incidence after bilateral prophylactic mastectomy, in the range of 80% to 90%. These two investigations involved populations of women who had a moderate risk of breast cancer. Both cohorts were treated before the discovery of susceptibility genes or the widespread recognition of histologic risk factors. Assuming a constant reduction in breast cancer incidence after bilateral prophylactic surgery (of 80% to 90%), two separate groups of investigators constructed statistical models to estimate the gain in survival for women who carry disease-producing mutations in *BRCA1* or *BRCA2*.[54,55] These models produced similar age-specific estimates for the improvement in survival afforded to carriers of *BRCA* gene mutations. A study by Schrag et al. modeled oophorectomy, mastectomy, or a combination of these procedures.[54] Immediate or delayed surgery was also modeled in the work of Schrag et al. A study by Grann et al. added gains or losses in quality of life and quality-adjusted life-years.[55] In both models, improvements in survival were dependent on the estimates of cancer risk and declined with advancing age at the time of prophylactic surgery. For 30-year-old women in the study of Schrag et al., gains in life expectancy from 2.9 to 5.3 years were calculated for women undergoing prophylactic mastectomy, depending on the level of initial breast cancer risk. To aid clinicians advising young women about the irrevocable decision of preventive mastectomy, this study examined the effect of delaying the procedure on survival of breast cancer. For women at age 30, delays of up to 10 years (until age 40) are tolerated without appreciable effect on survival. Preventive total mastectomy at age 50, however, produced gains of only 1.0 to 2.3 years, calculated according to the cumulative estimates of risk for carriers of *BRCA1* or *BRCA2*.[54]

Balancing of Risks and Benefits

Although bilateral mastectomy is effective in reducing the incidence and mortality of breast cancer, the choice for individual high-risk women is not based simply on medical effectiveness. The use of prophylactic mastectomy is determined by balancing the negative effects of breast removal against the reduction of breast cancer incidence. Furthermore, preventive surgery may be weighed against the chances that a diagnosis of breast cancer will lead to premature death. In the decision models described previously, the risk of dying of breast cancer was determined from the National Cancer Institute's Surveillance, Epidemiology, and End Results (SEER) Program for the years 1973 to 1992. This 20-year interval spans the introduction of film-screen mammography and its widespread application in the U.S. population. A modern cohort of women, screened annually by modern techniques, may display better overall survival after the diagnosis of breast cancer, thus diminishing the beneficial effect of preventive surgery on overall survival.[56] As noted, breast cancer mortality in a screened population from the BCDDP was less than 20%. Patients whose cancers were detected by mammography had an overall 20-year adjusted survival of 85.1%.[24] Therefore, the additional benefits of preventive mastectomy are likely to diminish if the figures are compared with those for a screened population of women.

Although women report satisfaction with prophylactic mastectomy, definite disadvantages exist. Surgical reconstruction is complex and carries a significant complication rate. Prosthetic implantation is probably the simplest means of reconstructing the chest wall after mastectomy. However, an overall complication rate of 23.8% was reported among 749 women undergoing prosthetic implantation at the Mayo Clinic.[57] For reconstruction after prophylactic mastectomy, complication rates were higher (17.3% at 1 year and 34% at 5 years). The most common complication was capsular contraction; rupture, hematoma, and infection followed in order of frequency. Quoted complication rates for muscle transfer procedures generally exceed those for implantation, primarily because of the complexity of the surgery involved. Finally, the reconstructed breast is insensitive and devoid of nipple and areolar reflexes, no matter how normal the breast may appear after reconstruction.

In decision analysis of prophylactic mastectomy performed by Grann et al., the benefits of mastectomy, measured in additional quality-adjusted life-years, were apparent only in the highest-risk scenario (85% lifelong risk of breast cancer for *BRCA1* and *BRCA2* carriers).[55] These quality-of-life estimates were determined by the time trade-off technique and based on interviews with women and on published data. For *BRCA1* or *BRCA2* carriers whose estimated risk of breast cancer was moderate or low, gains in quality-adjusted life-years resulting from prophylactic mastectomy were nullified or even reversed. The reasons for this are undoubtedly complex and personal for each patient. For individual women, fear of breast cancer is weighed against the effects of losing the breasts. These effects are both psychological and cosmetic; in addition, mastectomy involves loss of the normal physiologic functions performed by the human mammary glands. Although risk estimates will improve with the availability of better data and statistical models, the effect of preventive mastectomy on quality of life must be determined by probing discussions with each patient.

One group of investigators is using the time trade-off method of comparing two medical outcomes—in this case, living with risk and undergoing breast cancer screening versus living with a prophylactic mastectomy.[58] The time trade-off method of assessing quality of life allows patients to compare the time spent in one health state (e.g., with bilateral mastectomies) with the time spent in other states of health (e.g., at risk for breast cancer). This technique of determining preferences may be useful for women who are considering prophylactic surgery.[58] However, the psychological effects of bilateral mastectomy have not been determined for large groups of asymptomatic women undergoing this procedure to prevent breast cancer. The extensive literature regarding psychological adjustment to mastectomy pertains to patients with breast cancer. For the most part, declarations of psychological impairment or benefit represent estimates given by women before mastectomy or by health care providers who draw on observations of their patients with breast cancer. Few studies have been undertaken among asymptomatic women who have undergone bilateral mastectomy to prevent breast cancer.

Two studies have addressed the issue of preventive mastectomy. Among 370 women who underwent a bilateral prophylactic mastectomy and volunteered to be included in a registry, only 5% expressed regrets about having the procedure.[59] The authors of this study qualify their results by recognizing that this registry was voluntary and retrospective. A smaller prospective study of the first-degree relatives of women with breast cancer examined the satisfaction of these unaffected women with their treatment decisions.[60] Only 14 of 164 women decided to undergo bilateral prophylactic surgery. Fifty-eight women reported no interest in prophylactic mastectomy; 92 were interested but decided against surgery. In general, the women choosing surgery were at a higher risk than those who were not interested in surgery and were satisfied with their decisions. Eleven of 14 women who chose surgery were either "quite a bit" or "very much" satisfied with their decision. In this study, the factors that influenced decisions about preemptive surgery were fear of breast cancer, a history of having had investigative biopsies, and the perception of risk level. Although our knowledge after the fact of bilateral mastectomy is incomplete, probing patients who are deciding whether to have surgery about a range of possible scenarios is wise. These include living with physical alterations, possible barriers to sexual activity, altered chest wall sensation, and postmastectomy pain. Many research questions remain unanswered.[61] If prophylactic mastectomy becomes more common, research in the field of health education and psychology will make valuable contributions to clinical care.

MANAGEMENT SUMMARY

The following statements are suggested guidelines for counseling high-risk women who are candidates for preventive surgery. These assertions represent the author's opinions; reasonable clinicians may take a different approach to high-risk patients.

- There are no clinical situations in which prophylactic mastectomy is required; preventive mastectomy is only a choice.
- The possibility of preemptive surgery should be presented to women seeking information about lowering their risks in the context of other options. These options include vigilance, chemoprevention, genetic testing, and modification of diet and lifestyle.
- Vigilance is considered the optimal strategy at the current time. Women who practice breast self-examination, obtain annual mammograms, and see a competent and concerned physician on a regular basis should be told that their chances of dying from breast cancer are very low.
- At present, chemoprevention must be considered unproven.
- Genetic testing is reserved for women who have a very strong family history of breast cancer. Testing within a family should be offered to women affected by breast cancer before it is used in asymptomatic women.
- Under most circumstances, women who choose mastectomy should be referred to a plastic and reconstructive surgeon for a discussion of the restorative procedures available. In many circumstances, the plastic surgeon may be the best person to perform the mastectomy.
- A second opinion should be sought before surgery is undertaken and should be given by a practitioner who is not involved in the patient's care.
- If a preventive mastectomy is considered because of histologic factors, such as LCIS, pathologic review of the biopsy material should be undertaken. Adequate biopsy material, usually from an open surgical procedure, must be available for review.
- Total (simple) mastectomy is the most effective procedure. Subcutaneous mastectomy should be reserved for women judged to be the best candidates by a surgeon who has experience with high-risk patients.
- Following prophylactic mastectomy, mammography is not generally necessary. Self-examination should continue, and an annual physician examination is recommended.

Preventive mastectomy should be reserved for high-risk women for whom the risk of breast cancer clearly exceeds that of the general population. In these women, risk of cancer death usually exceeds similar risks in screened populations. Some women may request mastectomy to avoid breast cancer occurrence and will not be persuaded by low estimates of cancer mortality. A range of risk estimates should be provided, based on best judgment and available risk models. When appropriate, genetic counseling and advice about *BRCA1* and *BRCA2* testing should be offered. Carriers of these susceptibility genes should be quoted risks determined by population-based studies, in addition to the highest estimates provided by initial linkage families. Women seeking prophylactic mastectomy should be counseled in depth about the negative effects on quality of life, the complications of preventive surgery, and the loss of normal breast functions. Despite these disadvantages, a small number of women may still be candidates for prophylactic mastectomy.

REFERENCES

1. Carlson GW. Skin sparing mastectomy: anatomic and technical considerations. *Am Surg* 1996;62:151.
2. Woods JE. Detailed technique of subcutaneous mastectomy with and without mastopexy. *Ann Plast Surg* 1987;18:51.
3. Goodnight JE Jr, Quagliana JM, Morton DL. Failure of subcutaneous mastectomy to prevent the development of breast cancer. *J Surg Oncol* 1984;26:198.
4. Schnitt SJ, Goldwyn RM, Slavin SA. Mammary ducts in the areola: implications for patients undergoing reconstructive surgery of the breast. *Plast Reconstr Surg* 1993;92:1290.
5. Bhatia S, Robison LL, Oberlin O, et al. Breast cancer and other second neoplasms after childhood Hodgkin's disease. *N Engl J Med* 1996;334:745.
6. Travis LB, Curtis RE, Boice JD. Late effects of treatment for childhood Hodgkin's disease. *N Engl J Med* 1996;335:352.
7. Easton DF, Ford D, Bishop DT. Breast and ovarian cancer incidence in BRCA1-mutation carriers. *Am J Hum Genet* 1995;56:265.
8. Ford D, Easton DF, Bishop DT, et al. Breast Cancer Linkage Consortium. Risks of cancer in BRCA1-mutation carriers. *Lancet* 1994;343:692.
9. Easton DF, Bishop DT, Ford D, Crockford GP. Breast Cancer Linkage Consortium. Genetic linkage analysis in familial breast and ovarian cancer: results from 214 families. *Am J Hum Genet* 1993;52:678.
10. Wooster R, Neuhausen SL, Mangion J, et al. Localization of a breast cancer susceptibility gene, BRCA2, to chromosome 13q12–13. *Science* 1994;265:2088.
11. Struewing JP, Hartge P, Wacholder S, et al. The risk of cancer associated with specific mutations of BRCA1 and BRCA2 among Ashkenazi Jews. *N Engl J Med* 1997;336:1401.
12. Whittemore AS, Gong G, Itnyre J. Prevalence and contribution of BRCA1 mutations in breast cancer and ovarian cancer: results from three U.S. population-based case-control studies of ovarian cancer. *Am J Hum Genet* 1997;60:496.
13. Whittemore AS. Risk of breast cancer in carriers of BRCA gene mutations (correspondence). *N Engl J Med* 1997;337:787.
14. Frank TS, Manley SA, Olopade OI, et al. Sequence analysis of BRCA1 and BRCA2: correlation of mutations with family history and ovarian cancer risk. *J Clin Oncol* 1998;16:2417.
15. Schubert EL, Lee MK, Mefford HC, et al. BRCA2 in American families with four or more cases of breast or ovarian cancer: recurrent and novel mutations, variable expression, penetrance, and the possibility of families whose cancer is not attributable to BRCA1 or BRCA2. *Am J Hum Genet* 1997;60:1031.
16. Phelan CM, Lancaster JM, Tonin P, et al. Mutation analysis of the BRCA2 gene in 49 site-specific breast cancer families. *Nat Genet* 1996;13:120.
17. Vehmanen P, Friedman LS, Eerola H, et al. Low proportion of BRCA1 and BRCA2 mutations in Finnish breast cancer families: evidence for additional susceptibility genes. *Hum Mol Genet* 1997;6:2309.
18. Berry DA, Parmigiani G, Sanchez J, Schildkraut J, Winer E. Probability of carrying a mutation of breast-ovarian cancer gene BRCA1 based on family history. *J Natl Cancer Inst* 1997;89:227.
19. Parmigiani G, Berry DA, Aguilar O. Determining carrier probabilities for breast cancer-susceptibility genes BRCA1 and BRCA2. *Am J Hum Genet* 1998;62:145.
20. Iglehart JD, Miron A, Rimer BK, et al. Overestimation of hereditary breast cancer risk. *Ann Surg* 1998;228:375.
21. Gail MH, Brinton LA, Byar DP, et al. Projecting individualized probabilities of developing breast cancer for white females who are being examined annually. *J Natl Cancer Inst* 1989;81:1879.
22. Claus EB, Risch N, Thompson WD. Autosomal dominant inheritance of early-onset breast cancer. Implications for risk prediction. *Cancer* 1994;73:643.
23. Fisher B, Costantino JP, Wickerham DL, et al. Tamoxifen for prevention of breast cancer: report of the National Surgical Adjuvant Breast and Bowel Project P-1 study. *J Natl Cancer Inst* 1998;90:1371.
24. Smart CR, Byrne C, Smith RA, et al. Twenty-year follow-up of the breast cancers diagnosed during the Breast Cancer Detection Demonstration Project. *CA Cancer J Clin* 1997;47:134.
25. Carter CL, Corle DK, Micozzi MS, et al. A prospective study of the development of breast cancer in 16,692 women with benign breast disease. *Am J Epidemiol* 1988;128:467.
26. Dupont WD, Page DL. Risk factors for breast cancer in women with proliferative breast disease. *N Engl J Med* 1985;312:146.

27. Dupont WD, Page DL. Breast cancer risk associated with proliferative disease, age at first birth, and a family history of breast cancer. *Am J Epidemiol* 1987;125:769.
28. Rosen PP, Lieberman PH, Braum DW, et al. Lobular carcinoma in situ of the breast. Detailed analysis of 99 patients with average follow-up of 24 years. *Am J Surg Pathol* 1978;2:225.
29. Wheeler JE, Enterline HT, Roseman JM, et al. Lobular carcinoma in situ of the breast. Long term follow-up. *Cancer* 1974;34:554.
30. Ottesen GL, Graversen HP, Blichert-Toft M, et al. Lobular carcinoma in situ of the female breast. Short-term results of a prospective study. The Danish Breast Cancer Cooperative Group. *Am J Surg Pathol* 1993;17:14.
31. Fisher ER, Costantino J, Fisher B, et al. Pathologic findings from the National Surgical Adjuvant Breast Project (NSABP) Protocol B-17. Five-year observations concerning lobular carcinoma in situ. *Cancer* 1996;78:1403.
32. Ciatto S, Cataliotti L, Cardona G, Bianchi S. Risk of infiltrating breast cancer subsequent to lobular carcinoma in situ. The Coordinating Center and Writing Committee of FONCAM (National Task Force for Breast Cancer). *Tumori* 1992;78:244.
33. Schell SR, Montague ED, Spanos WJ, et al. Bilateral breast cancer in patients with initial stage I and II disease. *Cancer* 1982;50:1191.
34. Robbins GF, Berg JW. Bilateral primary breast cancers: a prospective clinicopathological study. *Cancer* 1964;17:1501.
35. Strom HH, Jensen OM. Risk of contralateral breast cancer in Denmark 1943–80. *Int J Cancer* 1986;54:483.
36. Rosen PP, Groshen S, Kinne DW, Hellman S. Contralateral breast carcinoma: an assessment of risk and prognosis in stage I (T1N0M0) and stage II (T1N1M0) patients with 20-year follow-up. *Surgery* 1989;106:904.
37. Morrow M, Harris JR, Schnitt SJ. Local control following breast-conserving surgery for invasive cancer: results of clinical trials. *J Natl Cancer Inst* 1995;87:1669.
38. Fisher B, Redmond C. Lumpectomy for breast cancer: an update of the NSABP experience. *J Natl Cancer Inst Monogr* 1992;11:7.
39. Ashikari R, Huvos AG, Urban JA, Robbins GF. Infiltrating lobular carcinoma of the breast. *Cancer* 1973;31:110.
40. Dixon JM, Anderson TJ, Page DL, et al. Infiltrating lobular carcinoma of the breast: an evaluation of the incidence and consequence of bilateral disease. *Br J Surg* 1983;70:513.
41. Cody HS. Routine contralateral breast biopsy: helpful or irrelevant? Experience in 871 patients, 1979–1993. *Ann Surg* 1997;225:370.
42. Lee JS, Grant CS, Donohue JH, et al. Arguments against routine contralateral mastectomy or undirected biopsy for invasive lobular breast cancer. *Surgery* 1995:118:640.
43. Yeatman TJ, Lyman GH, Smith SK, et al. Bilaterality and recurrence rates for lobular breast cancer: considerations for treatment. *Ann Surg Oncol* 1997;4:198.
44. Webber BL, Heise H, Neifeld JP, Costa J. Risk of subsequent contralateral breast carcinoma in a population of patients with in-situ breast carcinoma. *Cancer* 1981;47:2928.
45. Belanger D, Moore M, Tannock I. How American oncologists treat breast cancer: an assessment of the influences of clinical trials. *J Clin Oncol* 1991;9:7.
46. Houn F, Helzlsouer KJ, Friedman NB, Stefanek ME. Prophylactic mastectomy: a survey of Maryland surgeons. *Am J Public Health* 1995;85:801.
47. Huggins C, Yang NC. Induction and extinction of mammary cancer. *Science* 1962;137:257.
48. Jackson CF, Palmquist M, Swanson J, et al. The effectiveness of prophylactic subcutaneous mastectomy in Sprague-Dawley rats induced with 7,12-dimethylbenzanthracene. *Plast Reconstr Surg* 1984;73:249.
49. Wong JH, Jackson CF, Swanson JS, et al. Analysis of the risk reduction of prophylactic partial mastectomy in Sprague-Dawley rats with 7,12-dimethylbenzanthracene-induced breast cancer. *Surgery* 1986;1986:67.
50. Jameson MB, Roberts E, Nixon J, et al. Metastatic breast cancer 42 years after bilateral subcutaneous mastectomies. *Clin Oncol (R Coll Radiol)*. 1997;9:119.
51. Willemsen HW, Kaas R, Peterse JH, Rutgers EJT. Breast carcinoma in residual breast tissue after prophylactic bilateral subcutaneous mastectomy. *Eur J Surg Oncol* 1998;24:331.
52. Pennisi VR, Capozzi A. Subcutaneous mastectomy data: a final statistical analysis of 1500 patients. *Aesth Plast Surg* 1989;13:15.
53. Hartmann LC, Schaid DJ, Woods JE, et al. Efficacy of bilateral prophylactic mastectomy in women with a family history of breast cancer. *N Engl J Med* 1999;340:77.
54. Schrag D, Kuntz KM, Garber JE, Weeks JC. Decision analysis—effects of prophylactic mastectomy and oophorectomy on life expectancy among women with BRCA1 or BRCA2 mutations. *N Engl J Med* 1997;336:1465.
55. Grann VR, Panageas KS, Whang W, et al. Decision analysis of prophylactic mastectomy and oophorectomy in BRCA1-positive or BRCA2-positive patients. *J Clin Oncol* 1998;16:979.
56. Eisen A, Weber BL. Prophylactic mastectomy—the price of fear [Editorial]. *N Engl J Med* 1999;340:137.
57. Gabriel SE, Woods JE, O'Fallon WM, et al. Complications leading to surgery after breast implantation. *N Engl J Med* 1997;336:677.
58. Unic I, Stalmeier PFM, Verhoef LCG, Van Daal WAJ. Assessment of the time-tradeoff values for prophylactic mastectomy of women with a suspected genetic predisposition to breast cancer. *Med Decis Making* 1998;18:268–277.
59. Borgen PI, Hill ADK, Tran KN, et al. Patient regrets after bilateral prophylactic mastectomy. *Ann Surg Oncol* 1998;5:603–606.
60. Stefanek ME, Helzlsouer KJ, Wilcox PM, Houn F. Predictors of and satisfaction with bilateral prophylactic mastectomy. *Prev Med* 1995;24:412–419.
61. Stefanek ME. Bilateral prophylactic mastectomy: issues and concerns. *J Natl Cancer Inst Monogr* 1995:17:37–42.

Diseases of the Breast, 2nd ed.,
edited by Jay R. Harris.
Lippincott Williams & Wilkins, Philadelphia © 2000.

CHAPTER 19

Chemoprevention

V. Craig Jordan and Alberto F. Costa

Strategies to prevent breast cancer are focused either on dietary changes based on epidemiologic studies or on endocrine changes based on both epidemiologic studies and a strong biological rationale developed from laboratory studies. The use of retinoids to prevent breast cancer draws on knowledge of both the endocrinology of receptors and concepts in nutrition. The dietary approach advocates trials with reduced fat intake designed to mimic the diets of countries with low breast cancer incidence. Opponents of this approach argue that only a lifetime dietary change can decrease the risk of breast cancer. If this is true, major dietary changes undertaken now may not alter breast cancer incidence for another generation. In contrast, endocrine dependency is a unique feature of breast cancer that can be manipulated to control growth[1] or prevent tumor development.[2,3] Unfortunately, the inability to predict precisely who will develop breast cancer has required broad, population-based strategies to prevent the disease. A successful strategy must be effective and acceptable to the majority of treated women who will not develop breast cancer. This goal has proved to be both difficult and controversial.

This chapter provides a synthesis of laboratory findings and clinical considerations to explain the biological rationale for current hormonal approaches to prevention of breast cancer. A fundamental issue in developing a strategy for breast cancer prevention is understanding when carcinogenesis occurs. In laboratory models of mammary cancer, the timing of the carcinogenic insult is critical, and tumor development is influenced by the hormonal milieu. A series of experiments performed over 20 years in different strains of rat using different carcinogens[4–6] have shown that mammary cancer can be induced only by carcinogen administration during the first few months of puberty (Fig. 1). Unfortunately, the nature and timing of the carcinogenic insult in women are not known. Progress in clarifying and cloning the *BRCA1* gene[7] may result in the identification of women who harbor germ-line breast cancer susceptibility. However, these women, who have early-onset disease, represent a minority (fewer than 10%) of all breast cancer cases. Most of the knowledge about carcinogenesis in the breast is based on small epidemiologic studies of known cancer-causing agents.

Data from women exposed to radiation suggest a long period of promotion after initiation at a young age. Among survivors of the atomic bombings, the greatest increase in breast cancer incidence was seen in women exposed during their early teens. Breast cancer development in these women did not occur at an early age, however.[8] Additional support for the concept of a long period of hormonal promotion after an early carcinogenic insult is found in the data for female infants undergoing thymic irradiation[9] and adolescent girls irradiated during fluoroscopy for tuberculosis.[10] In both groups, a significant increase in breast cancer incidence is observed.

STRATEGY TO PREVENT MAMMARY CANCER IN THE LABORATORY

Animal models of mammary carcinogenesis have been studied extensively. High-incidence strains of mice that are infected with the mouse mammary tumor virus spontaneously develop tumors. The mice are particularly sensitive to tumorigenesis through the activation of the integrated virus by progesterone. Thus, pregnancy enhances mammary carcinogenesis in this model. Early oophorectomy retards the development of mammary cancer.[11] This observation led Lacassagne to suggest in 1936 that, because breast cancer appears to be due to a special hereditary sensitivity to estrogen, perhaps a therapeutic agent to inhibit estrogen accumulation could be found to prevent breast cancer.[12] Unfortunately, no therapeutic inhibitor was available at that time, and all of Lacassagne's suggestions were based on the use of oophorectomy. In modern times, tamoxifen (tamoxifen citrate) has been studied in mouse models of carcinogenesis to provide a basis for clinical testing of the concept of prevention. Early, long-term tamoxifen therapy inhibits mouse mammary tumorigenesis,[13,14] and the therapy is

V. C. Jordan: Department of Cancer Pharmacology, Robert Lurie Cancer Center, Northwestern University Medical School, Chicago, Illinois

A. F. Costa: Breast Cancer Division, European Institute of Oncology, Milan, Italy

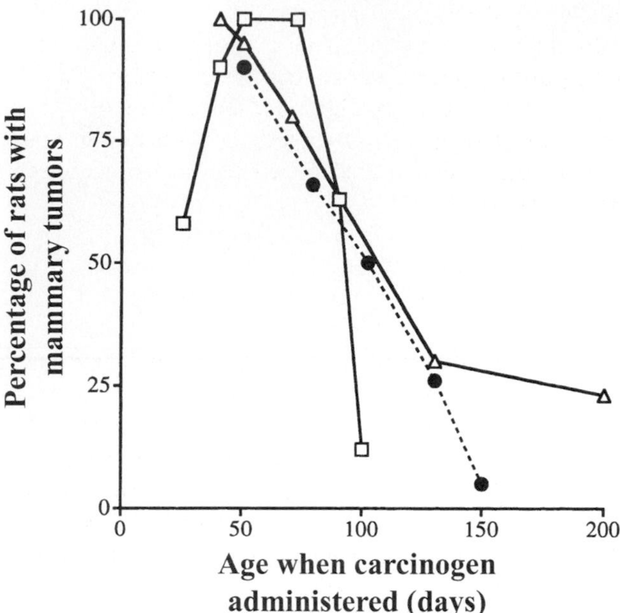

FIG. 1. Incidence of mammary cancer in groups of female rats given oral 3-methylcholanthrene (66 mg/100 g; *squares*),[4] intravenous 7,12-dimethylbenzanthracene (3 mg/100 g; *circles*),[5] or intravenous nitroso-*N*-methylurea (5 mg/100 g; *triangles*)[6] at different days of age. Tumor incidence was evaluated at least 180 days after each administration of carcinogen.

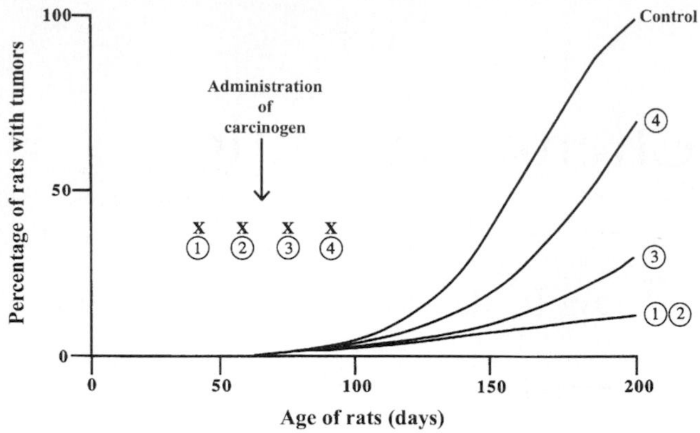

FIG. 2. Effect of oophorectomy (X) at different times on the appearance of rat mammary cancer. 7,12-dimethylbenzanthracene, 20 mg orally in 2 mL of peanut oil, was administered to groups of female Sprague-Dawley rats at 55 days of age.[20]

Overall, the animal model systems demonstrate that intervention soon after initiation of the carcinogenic insult is the most effective form of breast cancer prevention. In addition, changes in the hormonal milieu can affect the process of carcinogenesis, either by altering the receptivity of the epithelial tissue to carcinogens or by preventing the process of promotion to produce an invasive carcinoma.

superior to early oophorectomy. However, this is only one piece of laboratory evidence that can be used as a rationale to support the use of tamoxifen as a preventive treatment.

The administration of chemical carcinogens to sensitive strains of young female rats causes mammary tumorigenesis. Unlike in mice, pregnancy or the administration of a suitable combination of progesterone and estrogen can prevent mammary carcinogenesis in rats if this occurs at the time of the carcinogenic insult or soon after.[15–17] However, later pregnancy or progesterone administration can reduce the latency of rat mammary carcinogenesis and increase the growth rate of some tumors.[18,19] As in mice, oophorectomy can interfere with the process of chemical carcinogenesis in rats (Fig. 2). The earlier it is performed after the carcinogenic insult, the more effective is oophorectomy. Similarly, the administration of antiestrogens for different times around the time of carcinogen administration can alter carcinogenesis.[20–22] The coadministration of carcinogens and antiestrogens to female rats prevents mammary carcinogenesis.[21] Short-term (4-week) administration of tamoxifen a month after carcinogen administration only delays carcinogenesis, but it does reduce the number of mammary tumors produced.[23] In contrast, long-term treatment with low dosages of tamoxifen after the carcinogenic insult can almost completely prevent the development of mammary tumors.[24] Paradoxically, progesterone administration can reverse the antitumor action of tamoxifen.[25]

TARGET PROBLEMS

Potential agents for breast cancer prevention must have a strong scientific basis for action and minimal toxicity. Ideally, a true preventive agent would block the carcinogenic insult in readily identifiable individuals and would have minimal side effects. This goal is not possible now, however, and broad approaches are being suggested.

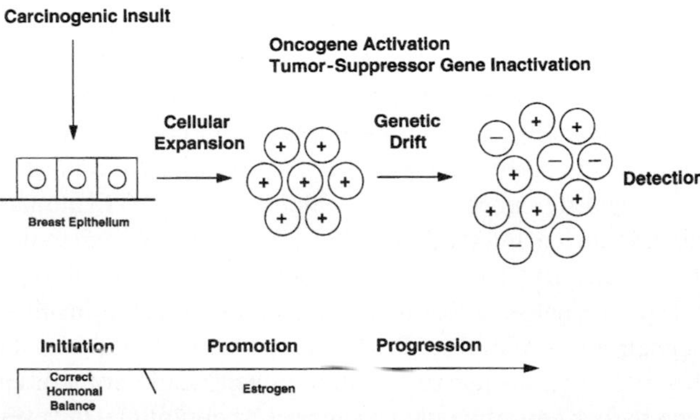

FIG. 3. Potential process of carcinogenesis in the breast. The carcinogenic insult causes genomic alterations in the receptive epithelial cells, and the insult is consolidated through promotion with estrogen. The estrogen receptor–positive cells then drift to become hormone independent and estrogen receptor–negative.

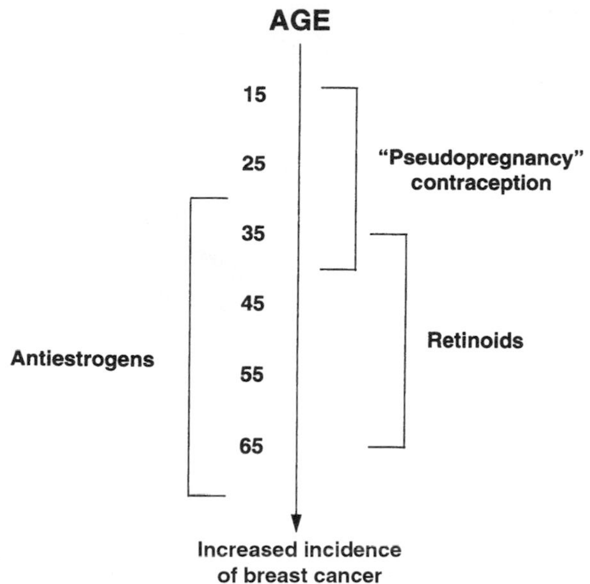

FIG. 4. Potential windows of opportunity to apply prevention strategies.

Figure 3 illustrates a sequence of events that can be exploited in a prevention strategy. In general, an intervention must be given over a prolonged period to protect the individual from repeated carcinogenic insults. The agent could either prevent metabolic activation of the carcinogen or change the hormonal balance necessary for the epithelium to be receptive to the carcinogen. Estrogen is key to consolidating the carcinogenic insult through promotion of the transformed cell. At this stage, the dividing cell population is directly or indirectly sensitive to estrogen stimulation through the estrogen receptor. As tumorigenesis progresses, however, the genetic instability of the transformed cells results in a mixed population of receptor-positive and receptor-negative breast cancer cells. To exploit this knowledge, a number of endocrine strategies have been proposed or studied in clinical trials (Fig. 4). The use of a contraceptive that could protect young women from pregnancy and breast cancer would be the most effective strategy because, based on all existing knowledge, it would be applied at the correct time during the process of tumorigenesis.

PSEUDOPREGNANCY

The repeated feeding of carcinogens to rats at the onset of pregnancy[15] or to other animals injected with large quantities of equine gonadotropins[26] seldom results in mammary tumors. This observation provided the basis for the rigorous investigations of Russo et al.[27] The administration of human chorionic gonadotropin can prevent the initiation and progression of rat mammary carcinogenesis.[28] Russo et al.[29] hypothesize that human chorionic gonadotropin initiates ovarian estrogen and progesterone synthesis to induce differentiation of the mammary epithelium.[30] Unfortunately, the dosing schedules used reduced rat mammary tumorigenesis by only 50%,[30] and an optimal treatment is needed. Although pregnancy at an early age is known to reduce the risk of breast cancer, the development of a prevention strategy in which gonadotropin is administered to teenage girls has major societal implications.

CONTRACEPTION

The finding is well established that women who use oral contraceptives, a combination of progestin and estrogen, have a reduced incidence of both endometrial and ovarian cancer.[31] In contrast, women who take oral contraceptives have either the same or a slightly higher relative risk of breast cancer compared to those who have never used birth control pills.[31] These findings may not be too surprising, because the breast responds to the administrated estrogen. What is surprising is the fact that the orally administered progestins, which cause differentiation of the proliferating endometrium, do not protect the breast. The explanation for this observation is obscure, but the report that the progestins have a proliferative effect on normal human breast tissue,[32] as well as the laboratory finding that many progestins used in oral contraceptives cause proliferation of breast cancer cells through an estrogen receptor–mediated mechanism,[33] suggest that these compounds have site-specific activity and may in fact promote breast cancer.

Clearly, a novel steroid could be devised to prevent breast cancer cell replication while also preventing ovulation. As yet, however, no progress has been made with this approach.

An alternate contraceptive strategy has been proposed by Pike et al.[34] Because early oophorectomy reduces breast cancer incidence, this strategy attempts to perform a "medical oophorectomy" by administering a luteinizing hormone–releasing hormone superagonist (leuprolide acetate, 7.5 mg every 28 days). To avoid the negative effects of a premature menopause on cardiovascular risk and bone density, conjugated estrogens (0.625 mg orally) are administered for 6 days every week, and medroxyprogesterone acetate (10 mg orally) is given for 13 days every fourth 28-day cycle.[35,36] This approach has the potential to reduce ovarian, endometrial, and breast cancer while maintaining bone density and a low cardiovascular risk.[37] It meets all the criteria for an effective preventive strategy. However, the precise dosage of estrogen that supports physiologic functions without supporting the developing breast tumor is unknown.

ANTIESTROGENS

The successful use of adjuvant tamoxifen therapy for all stages of breast cancer and the reported low incidence of side effects[38,39] initially prompted the evaluation of tamoxifen as a preventive agent in high-risk women. The biological rationale for testing tamoxifen was based on laboratory studies[21–23] and the clinical observation that tamoxifen prevents second primary breast cancers.[40]

Most important, tamoxifen does not act as an antiestrogen in all estrogen target tissues of a woman's body. Initially, concerns were raised that, if estrogen is important to prevent osteoporosis and coronary heart disease, then antiestrogens could be harmful, in the long term, for postmenopausal women's health. Tamoxifen maintains bone density in postmenopausal women,[41–44] however, and reduces the level of circulating cholesterol.[45] Tamoxifen could therefore potentially be beneficial to prevent osteoporosis and coronary heart disease. This hypothesis, however, has not been tested prospectively in high-risk groups.

The carcinogenic potential of tamoxifen is an important, but often overstated, concern regarding the use of tamoxifen as a chemopreventive. Tamoxifen induces liver tumors in rats,[46,47] and initially the concern was raised that tamoxifen had the potential to induce hepatocellular carcinoma in women. Studies demonstrate, however, that the metabolic pathways necessary to produce DNA adducts are unique to the rat.[48,49] No DNA adducts have been noted in human liver in patients receiving tamoxifen,[50] and no increase has been reported in hepatocellular carcinoma in patients taking tamoxifen.[40]

A threefold increase is seen, however, in the incidence of endometrial cancer in postmenopausal breast cancer patients taking tamoxifen.[40,51,52] Although this is a significant increase in relative risk, the absolute increase in risk is small. In a population of postmenopausal women, endometrial cancer would be detected at a rate of 1 per 1,000 women per year. In women taking tamoxifen, the endometrial cancer rate would be 3 per 1,000 women per year. This is consistent with an increase in the detection of occult disease, which is estimated from autopsy studies to be five times[53] the incidence of disease reported symptomatically. Although controversy exists regarding the precise mechanism of tamoxifen action in human carcinogenesis, DNA adducts are not routinely observed in human tissues,[54,55] and no genomic changes are noted in the human uterus.[56]

With this background regarding the rationale and safety evaluation of tamoxifen, the evidence to support the use of tamoxifen in breast cancer risk reduction is described. The National Surgical Adjuvant Breast and Bowel Project (NSABP) has completed the only prospective clinical trial to address the issue of chemoprevention,[57] but an interim report from the Royal Marsden Hospital[58] pilot study of high-risk women and a study of normal-risk women from an Italian trial[59] are discussed as well.

NATIONAL SURGICAL ADJUVANT BREAST AND BOWEL PROJECT BREAST CANCER PREVENTION TRIAL

The specific aim of NSABP Breast Cancer Prevention Trial P-1 was to test the value of tamoxifen as a preventive for breast cancer. This prospective clinical trial closed after accruing 13,388 women because of the exceptionally high-risk status of the participants, which made the projected events adequate to establish statistical significance. The study design is illustrated in Fig. 5. Those eligible for entry included any woman over the age of 60 and women between the ages of 35 and 59 whose 5-year risk of developing breast cancer, as predicted by the Gail model,[60] was equal to that of a 60-year-old woman. In addition, any woman older than 35 years with a diagnosis of lobular carcinoma *in situ* (LCIS) was eligible for entry into the study. In the absence of LCIS, the risk factors necessary to enter the study varied with age. A 35-year-old woman must have had a relative risk of 5.07, whereas the required relative risk for a 45-year-old woman was 1.79. Routine endometrial biopsies were also performed to evaluate the incidence of endometrial carcinoma in both arms of the study.

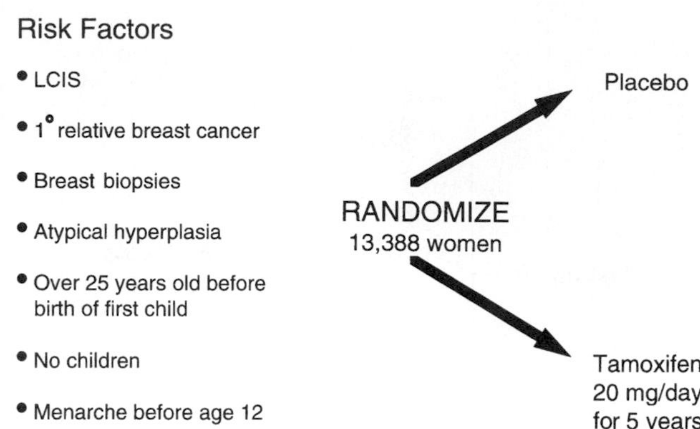

FIG. 5. Eligibility and design of the National Surgical Adjuvant Breast and Bowel Project tamoxifen breast cancer prevention trial. Originally, the recruitment goal was 16,000 volunteers, but the actual calculated risk of the recruited group was higher than anticipated and resulted in a change in recruitment goals. A total of 13,388 women were recruited by summer 1997, and the preliminary results were reported in April 1998. A full report was presented in September 1998.[57] LCIS, lobular carcinoma *in situ.*

The breast cancer risk of women enrolled in the study was extremely high; no age group, including the over-60 group, had a relative risk of less than 4. Recruitment was also balanced, with approximately one-third of participants younger than 50 years, one-third between 50 and 60 years, and one-third older than 60 years. Secondary end points of the study included the effect of tamoxifen on the incidence of fractures and cardiovascular deaths. Most important, the study will eventually provide the first prospective information about the role of genetic markers in the etiology of breast cancer. It will also establish whether tamoxifen therapy has a role to play in the treatment of women who are found to carry somatic mutations in the *BRCA1* or *BRCA2* gene. These data, however, are not yet available.

The first results of the NSABP study were reported after a mean follow-up of 47.7 months.[51] A total of 368 cases of inva-

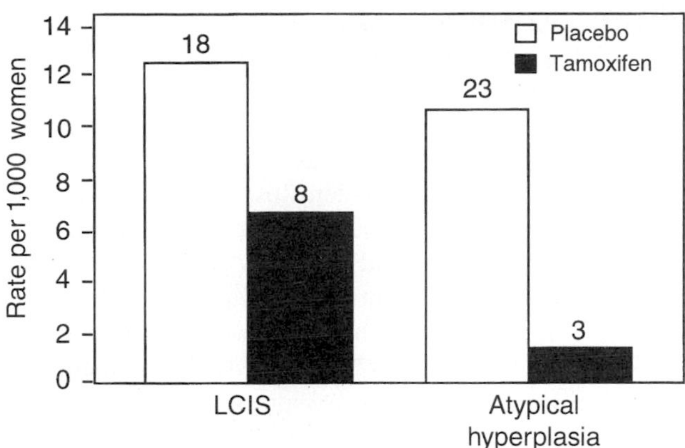

FIG. 6. Reduction in invasive breast cancer observed in the National Surgical Adjuvant Breast and Bowel Project tamoxifen breast cancer prevention trial (see Fig. 5) for women with a prior diagnosis of lobular carcinoma *in situ* (LCIS) or atypical hyperplasia.[57]

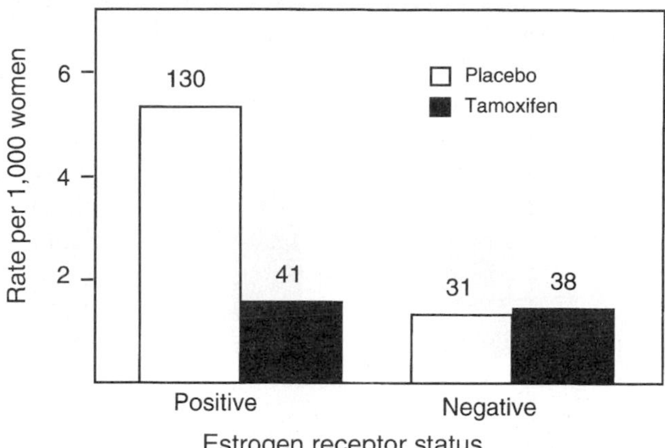

FIG. 8. Incidence of estrogen receptor (ER)–positive and ER-negative breast cancer in the placebo- and tamoxifen-treated groups of the National Surgical Adjuvant Breast and Bowel Project tamoxifen breast cancer prevention trial (see Fig. 5).[57] The antiestrogen reduced the risk of developing ER-positive breast cancer, but no change was seen in the incidence of ER-negative breast cancer. The number of invasive breast cancers is shown at the top of the histogram for each treatment group.

sive and noninvasive breast cancer occurred among the participants, 124 in the tamoxifen group and 244 in the placebo group. A 47% reduction in the risk of invasive breast cancer and a 50% reduction in the risk of noninvasive breast cancer were observed in women taking tamoxifen. A subset analysis of women at risk due to a diagnosis of LCIS demonstrated a 56% reduction in this group. The most dramatic reduction was seen in women at risk due to a diagnosis of atypical hyperplasia, for whom risk was reduced by 86% (Fig. 6).

The benefits of tamoxifen were observed in all age groups. The relative risk of breast cancer ranged from 0.45 in women aged 60 and older, to 0.49 for those in the 50- to 59-year age group, and to 0.56 for women aged 49 and younger. A benefit of tamoxifen was also observed for women with all levels of breast cancer risk within the study, a finding that indicates that the benefits of tamoxifen are not confined to a particular lower-risk or higher-risk subset (Fig. 7). Benefits were observed in women at risk on the basis of family history and those whose risk was due to other factors.

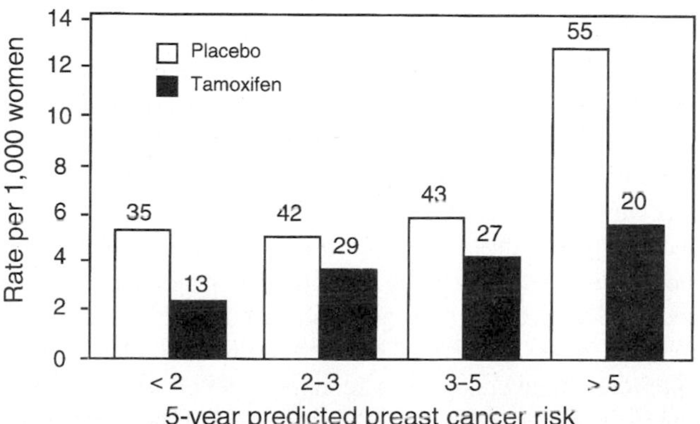

FIG. 7. Reduction in invasive breast cancer observed in the National Surgical Adjuvant Breast and Bowel Project tamoxifen breast cancer prevention trial (see Fig. 5) for groups of women with different relative risk of developing breast cancer.[57]

As expected, the effect found for tamoxifen was on the incidence of tumors positive for estrogen receptor (ER), which was reduced by 69% per year. The rate of ER-negative tumors in the tamoxifen group (1.46 per 1,000 women) did not significantly differ from the rate in the placebo group (1.20 per 1,000 women) (Fig. 8). Tamoxifen use reduced the rate of invasive cancers of all sizes, but the greatest differences were seen in the incidence of tumors 2.0 cm or less in size. Tamoxifen also reduced the incidence of both node-positive and node-negative breast cancers. The beneficial effects of tamoxifen were observed for each year of follow-up study. After year 1, the risk was reduced by 33%, and in year 5, it was reduced by 69%.

Tamoxifen also reduced the overall incidence of osteoporotic fractures of the hip, spine, and radius by 19%[57,58] (Fig. 9). This difference approached, but did not reach, statistical significance. Reduction was greatest in women aged 50 and older at study entry. No difference in the risk of myocardial infarction, angina, coronary artery bypass grafting, or angioplasty was noted between groups.[57] These were secondary end points monitored in low-risk populations, however, so a major benefit would not be anticipated.

This study confirmed the association between tamoxifen use and endometrial carcinoma.[40,51] The relative risk of endometrial cancer in the tamoxifen group was 2.5. The increased risk was seen in women aged 50 and older, whose relative risk was 4.01. All endometrial cancers in the tamoxifen group were grade 1, and none of the women on tamoxifen died of endometrial cancer. An endometrial cancer death occurred in the placebo group. Although no doubt exists that

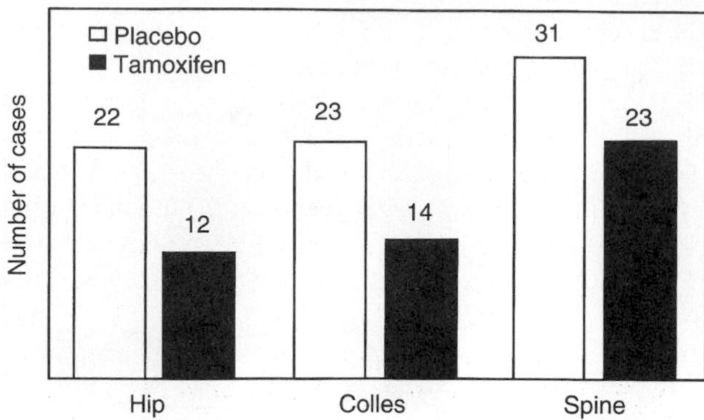

FIG. 9. Incidence of osteoporotic fractures of the hip, wrist, and spine observed in the placebo- and tamoxifen-treated groups of the National Surgical Adjuvant Breast and Bowel Project tamoxifen breast cancer prevention trial (see Fig. 5).[57] The number of fractures is shown at the top of the histogram for each treatment group.

tamoxifen increases the risk of endometrial cancer, one must recognize that this increase translates to an annual incidence of 2.3 women per 1,000 who develop endometrial carcinoma.

More women in the tamoxifen group than in the placebo group developed deep vein thrombosis.[57] Again, this excess risk was confined to women aged 50 and older. The relative risk of deep vein thrombosis in the older group was 1.71 (95% confidence interval, 0.85 to 3.58). An increase in the occurrence of pulmonary emboli was also seen in the older women taking tamoxifen, who had a relative risk of approximately 3. Three deaths from pulmonary emboli occurred in the tamoxifen arm of the study, but all were in women with significant comorbidities. An increased incidence of stroke (relative risk, 1.75) was also seen in the tamoxifen group, but this did not reach statistical significance.

An assessment of the incidence of cataract formation was made using patient self-reporting. A small increase in cataracts was noted in the tamoxifen group—a rate of 24.8 women per 1,000, compared with 21.7 per 1,000 in the placebo group. Risk of cataract surgery also increased in the women on tamoxifen. These differences were marginally statistically significant and were observed in the older patients in the study. These findings emphasize the need to assess the patient's overall health status before making a decision to use tamoxifen for breast cancer risk reduction.

An assessment of quality of life showed no difference in depression scores between groups. Hot flashes were noted in 81% of the women on tamoxifen compared with 69% of the placebo group; the tamoxifen-associated hot flashes appeared to be of no greater severity than those in the placebo group. Moderately bothersome or severe vaginal discharge was reported by 29% of the women in the tamoxifen group and by 13% of the women in the placebo group. No differences in the occurrence of irregular menses, nausea, fluid retention, skin changes, or weight gain or loss were reported.

ROYAL MARSDEN HOSPITAL AND ITALIAN STUDIES

Two other studies[58,59] have been published that suggest that tamoxifen does not reduce the risk of breast cancer. The stated goal of the Royal Marsden Hospital pilot study was to act as a vanguard for a 20,000-strong volunteer trial throughout the United Kingdom and Australia. The national study is still ongoing, but the recruitment goal has been cut to 12,000.

Powles et al.[61] recruited high-risk women aged 30 to 70 years for the Royal Marsden study, entering them in a placebo-controlled trial using 20 mg of tamoxifen daily for up to 8 years. Women were eligible if their risk of breast cancer was increased due to a family history of breast cancer. Each participant had at least one first-degree relative who had breast cancer before age 50, a first-degree relative affected at any age plus an additional affected first-degree or second-degree relative, or a first-degree relative with bilateral breast cancer. Women with a history of benign breast biopsy and an affected first-degree relative of any age were also eligible. Women with a history of venous thrombosis, any previous malignancy, or an estimated life expectancy of fewer than 10 years were excluded.[58,62] A total of 2,494 women consented to participate in the study; 23 were excluded from final analysis due to the presence of preexisting ductal carcinoma *in situ* (DCIS) or invasive breast carcinoma.[58]

Acute symptomatic toxicity was low for participants on tamoxifen or placebo in the pilot study, and compliance remained correspondingly high: 77% of women on placebo remained on medication at 5 years.[62] Compared with the placebo group, the group taking tamoxifen experienced a significant increase in hot flashes (34% versus 20%; $p < .005$); the increase was seen mostly among premenopausal women. Women in the tamoxifen group also experienced an increase in vaginal discharge (16% versus 4% for the placebo group; $p < .005$) and menstrual irregularities (14% versus 9%; $p < .005$). At the most recent follow-up, 320 women had discontinued tamoxifen and 176 had discontinued placebo before the study's completion ($p < .005$).[58]

In the years before their report in 1994,[62] the Marsden group observed no thromboembolic episodes; a detailed analysis of other coagulation parameters in a sequential subset of women also found no significant changes in the levels of protein S, protein C, or cross-linked fibrinogen degradation products. At 70 months, no significant difference in the incidence of deep vein thrombosis or pulmonary embolism was observed between groups.[63] This result is not unexpected, given the fact that most participants were premenopausal. A significant fall in total plasma cholesterol occurred within 3 months and was sustained for more than 5 years of treatment.[44,63,64] The decrease involved low-density lipoproteins; no change was seen in the levels of apolipoproteins A and B or high-density lipoprotein cholesterol.

Tamoxifen exerted antiestrogenic or estrogenic effects on bone density, depending on menopausal status. In premenopausal women, early findings demonstrated a small but significant ($p < .005$) loss of bone in both the lumbar spine and hip at 3 years.[44] Evaluating the results at 5 and 8 years of therapy is very important, as current indications suggest bone stabilization rather than continued loss. In contrast, treated postmenopausal women had increased bone mineral density in the spine ($p < .005$) and hip ($p < .001$) compared to untreated women.[44]

Finally, the Marsden group has made an extensive study of gynecologic complications associated with tamoxifen treatment in healthy women. Because ovarian and uterine assessment by transvaginal ultrasonography became available some time after the trial's start, many subjects did not have a baseline evaluation. Ovarian screening demonstrated a significantly greater risk ($p < .005$) of detection of benign ovarian cysts in premenopausal women who had received tamoxifen for more than 3 months than in control subjects. No changes were seen in ovarian appearance in postmenopausal women.[62] In women taking tamoxifen, a careful examination of the uterus with transvaginal ultrasonography using color Doppler imaging showed that the organ was usually large; moreover, women with sonographic abnormalities had significantly thicker endometria.[65] Of particular interest in this regard was the observation that the use of 20 mg of tamoxifen daily caused a time-dependent proliferation of the endometrium in premenopausal and early postmenopausal women.[65] This effect appeared to be mediated by the stromal component, because no cases of cancer or even of epithelial hyperplasia were observed among the 33 tamoxifen-treated women.[66]

An analysis of breast cancer incidence was reported at a median follow-up of 70 months, when 42% of the participants had completed therapy or had withdrawn from the study.[58] No difference in the incidence of breast cancer was observed between the group receiving tamoxifen and the control group. Thirty-four carcinomas were seen in the tamoxifen group and 36 in the placebo group—a relative risk of 0.98 for the women taking tamoxifen. Of the 70 cancers, only 8 were DCIS. An analysis of the subset of women on hormone replacement therapy did not demonstrate an interaction with tamoxifen treatment. No satisfactory explanation exists as to why the Marsden pilot study showed no decrease in breast cancer incidence among the group receiving tamoxifen. The authors suggested[58] that perhaps they have a high population of *BRCA1* and *BRCA2* carriers that are hormone-unresponsive, but this is unproven. In addition, the incidence of breast cancer among women in the placebo group of the Royal Marsden study is lower than that seen in the placebo group of the NSABP trial, which argues against the presence of a high number of *BRCA1* and *BRCA2* carriers in this study.

The third tamoxifen study, performed in Italy, randomized 5,408 women aged 35 to 70 years to 20 mg tamoxifen daily for 5 years or to placebo.[59] Originally, 20,000 volunteers without risk factors were to be recruited, but the study was stopped prematurely because of poor recruitment and poor compliance. Women were required to have had a hysterectomy for a nonneoplastic condition to obviate concerns about an increased risk of endometrial carcinoma. No requirement was made that participants be at risk for breast cancer development; in fact, those who underwent premenopausal oophorectomy with hysterectomy (47%) actually had a reduced risk of breast cancer development. Women with endometriosis, cardiac disease, and deep venous thrombosis were excluded from the study. Although 5,408 women (mean age, 51 years) were randomized into this study, 1,422 withdrew, and only 149 completed 5 years of treatment. A valid breast cancer prevention study would be possible only if more than 10,000 normal-risk women had completed 5 years of tamoxifen treatment and were compared with 10,000 women on placebo.

The incidence of breast cancer did not differ between groups, with 19 cases occurring in the tamoxifen group and 22 in the placebo group. Tumor characteristics, including size, lymph node status, and receptor status, also did not differ between groups.

The incidence of thrombophlebitis was increased in the tamoxifen group ($p = .0053$). Fifty-six women, including 38 women in the tamoxifen group and 18 women in the placebo group, experienced a total of 64 events. Forty-two of these cases, however, were superficial phlebitis. No difference between groups was observed in the incidence of cerebrovascular ischemic events.

CHEMOPREVENTION USING TAMOXIFEN

Given a single trial with a positive result and two with negative results, the role of tamoxifen in breast cancer prevention may seem at first glance to remain unresolved. Clinical characteristics of the study sample differ among these three studies, however (see study characteristics in Table 1).

The negative finding in the Italian study[59] is readily explained by the relatively low risk of breast cancer in the study population (47% had had an oophorectomy), the high dropout rate (25%), the fact that the volunteers were young women, and the small number of participants who completed 5 years of treatment (149 women). Despite these problems, the Italian study showed a trend toward a statistically significant benefit among women who took tamoxifen for more than 1 year; this suggests that, with further follow-up, the results of this study may demonstrate a benefit for women who took tamoxifen. The overview analysis of the Early Breast Cancer Trialists' Collaborative Group[40] demonstrated that at least 2 years of tamoxifen therapy are necessary to significantly reduce the risk of primary (contralateral) breast cancer (Fig. 10).

The Royal Marsden study was initially described as a pilot study to examine toxicity and compliance[61,62,64] that would serve as a feasibility assessment for a larger trial to determine whether tamoxifen prevents breast cancer. Although it was designed as a pilot study, the trial is now said to have a 90% power to detect a 50% reduction in breast cancer incidence, yet it shows no effect.[58] The authors suggest that the positive results of the NSABP trial at 3.5 years

TABLE 1. *Comparison of tamoxifen prevention studies*

Characteristic	NSABP	Royal Marsden Hospital	Italian study
Sample size	13,388	2,471	5,408
Woman-years of follow-up	46,858	12,355	5,408
Percentage of participants younger than age 50	40	62	36
Percentage of participants with first-degree relative with breast cancer	55	55	18
Percentage of participants with more than two first-degree relatives with breast cancer	13	17	2.5
Percentage of participants using hormone replacement therapy	0	42	8
Breast cancer incidence/1,000			
Placebo	6.7	5.5	2.3
Tamoxifen	3.4	4.7	2.1

NSABP, National Surgical Adjuvant Breast and Bowel Project.

of follow-up are most likely due to the treatment of clinically occult carcinoma rather than the prevention of new breast cancers. Of the 363 total cancers in the NSABP study,[57] however, 104 (26%) were DCIS, compared with 11% of the 70 cancers in the Royal Marsden study. The higher percentage of DCIS in the NSABP trial indicates that the cancers were not truly amenable to detection by currently available means. Whether occult carcinoma was treated or true prevention occurred, a significantly greater number of women were spared surgery, irradiation, and chemotherapy. The data of the Early Breast Cancer Trialists' Collaborative Group[40] do not support the contention that these cancers become clinically evident when tamoxifen is stopped, because the reduction in contralateral breast cancer persisted through 10 years, even though tamoxifen treatment was stopped at 5 years.

Overall, the results of the NSABP trial,[57] with its large study population, clearly support the benefit of tamoxifen for breast cancer prevention in high-risk women. These findings are consistent with laboratory observations and with the contralateral breast cancer risk reduction seen with 5 years of adjuvant tamoxifen therapy (see Fig. 10). Tamoxifen is approved for risk reduction in premenopausal and postmenopausal women whose breast cancer risk is elevated according to the Gail model.[60]

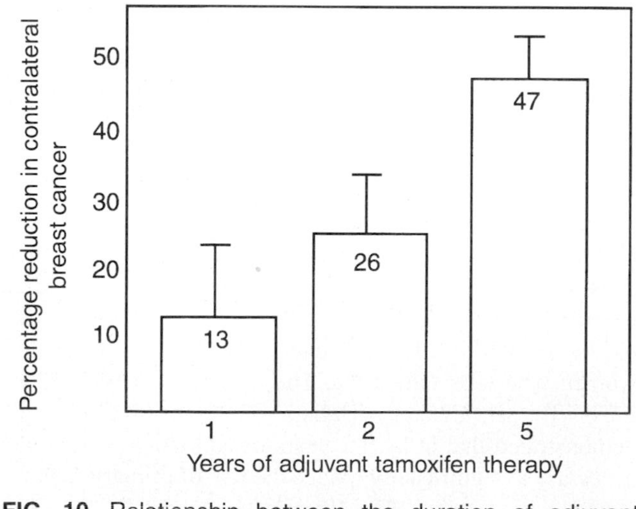

FIG. 10. Relationship between the duration of adjuvant tamoxifen and the reduction in contralateral breast cancer in the overview analysis of the Oxford Early Breast Cancer Trialists' Collaborative Group.[40] A longer duration of tamoxifen is superior to a short duration of tamoxifen in preventing primary breast cancer. The 5-year result that showed a 47% reduction in contralateral breast cancer is equivalent to the result observed in the National Surgical Adjuvant Breast and Bowel Project tamoxifen breast cancer prevention trial noted in Fig. 11.

RATIONALE FOR RALOXIFENE TESTING

Raloxifene (raloxifene hydrochloride), a tamoxifenlike compound, is being studied as a chemopreventive, primarily because it shows no evidence of rat liver carcinogenesis and has less estrogenlike action in the rodent uterus. These laboratory qualities possibly could translate into fewer endometrial cancers in women during raloxifene therapy, but this can be established only in large prospective clinical trials.

Raloxifene is an antiestrogen in the rodent uterus, and the compound has a high binding affinity for ER.[67] It shows antitumor activity in laboratory animals.[68–70] However, raloxifene has not been tested extensively in the treatment of breast cancer. Studies show modest activity for treatment with a 300-mg dose of raloxifene in ER-positive patients with advanced disease,[71] although one study of patients with heavily pretreated stage IV disease demonstrated no activity for the drug.[72] Raloxifene is classified as a selective ER modulator (SERM) because, like tamoxifen, the compound has estrogenlike effects on bone in animal studies[73–75] and human studies[76,77] and also lowers circulating cholesterol.[78] Raloxifene is currently approved for the prevention of osteoporosis and is being tested for risk reduction in coronary heart disease in a prospective placebo-controlled clinical trial referred to as *Raloxifene Use for the Heart* (*RUTH*). Ten thousand high-risk women are being randomized to 5

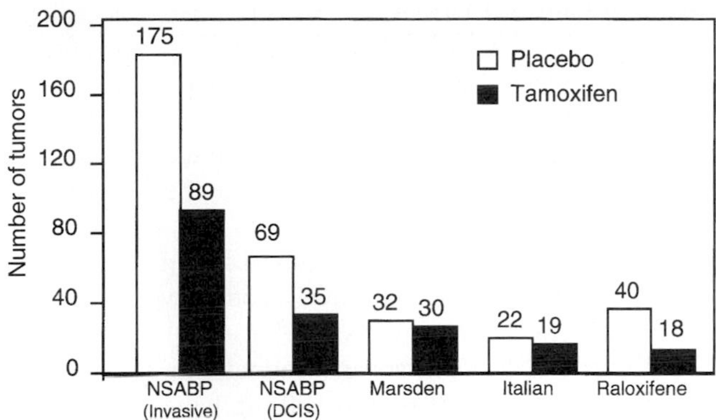

FIG. 11. Comparison of evaluable events observed in the studies of antiestrogen therapy to reduce the incidence of breast cancer. The National Surgical Adjuvant Breast and Bowel Project (NSABP) result is from the only prospective clinical trial designed to test the value of antiestrogen therapy to prevent breast cancer; it enrolled approximately 13,000 high-risk premenopausal and postmenopausal women.[57] The figure illustrates the effects of tamoxifen on both invasive and noninvasive [ductal carcinoma *in situ* (DCIS)] breast cancer. By contrast, the study of the Royal Marsden Hospital is a pilot project[61] originally designed to be a toxicity evaluation; the study enrolled approximately 2,000 predominantly premenopausal high-risk women. The Italian study reports data from the compliant original population of approximately 5,000 normal-risk postmenopausal women.[59] The figure shows only the number of invasive carcinomas for the Marsden[58] and Italian[59] studies. Finally, the raloxifene data, estimated from published abstracts, is a secondary end point from studies involving 10,533 postmenopausal women in osteoporosis trials.[80,81] The reported cases are invasive and noninvasive breast cancers.

years of placebo or 60 mg raloxifene daily (i.e., the recommended daily dose of raloxifene to prevent osteoporosis in some women). Results should be available in 2007.

Raloxifene is also being tested for use in risk reduction in breast cancer (see next section, Study of Tamoxifen and Raloxifene) based on preliminary data obtained as a secondary end point in clinical trials of osteoporosis.[79–81] The rationale behind this approach to drug development is that, because tamoxifen is able to maintain bone density and lower cholesterol, then perhaps another compound could be used to prevent osteoporosis but also reduce the risk of breast cancer as a beneficial side effect in normal-risk populations.[82] An overall evaluation of breast cancer incidence in a population of 10,355 postmenopausal women participating in placebo-controlled osteoporosis studies has confirmed a total of 67 invasive and noninvasive breast cancers. Raloxifene use resulted in a 54% decrease in the total number of breast cancers, with a selective reduction in the incidence of ER-positive breast cancers.[81] Figure 11 compares the number of cancers observed in the NSABP prospective clinical trial of tamoxifen in a high-risk population[57] with the events noted in the Royal Marsden[58] and Italian studies[59] of tamoxifen, as well as with the combined results obtained in osteoporosis trials with raloxifene at dosages of both 60 and 120 mg daily versus placebo.

STUDY OF TAMOXIFEN AND RALOXIFENE

The Study of Tamoxifen and Raloxifene (STAR) trial is a phase III, double-blind trial that will assign eligible postmenopausal women to daily therapy with either tamoxifen (20 mg orally) or raloxifene (60 mg orally) for 5 years. Trial participants will also complete a minimum of 2 additional years of follow-up after therapy is stopped. All women older than age 60 years are eligible for study entry, as are postmenopausal women aged 35 and older whose breast cancer risk, as determined by the Gail model,[60] is equal to that of a 60-year-old woman.

The primary aim of the STAR trial is to determine whether long-term raloxifene therapy is effective in preventing the occurrence of invasive breast cancer in postmenopausal women who are identified as being at high risk for the disease. The comparison is being made to the established drug, tamoxifen. The secondary aim of the study is to evaluate the net effect of raloxifene therapy by comparing cardiovascular data, fracture data, and general toxicities with those for tamoxifen.

The comparison of rates of endometrial cancer will be most instructive, because the standard of care (i.e., investigation of symptoms) will be used in the STAR trial rather than routine screening with annual biopsies. Raloxifene is not associated with an increase in endometrial hyperplasia,[77,83] but long-term follow-up in large populations is required to monitor the low event rates for endometrial cancer. Results from the STAR trial are anticipated in 2006.

Premenopausal women at risk for breast cancer are currently not eligible for the STAR trial. Although extensive information is available regarding the antitumor efficacy of tamoxifen use in premenopausal breast cancer patients[40] and women at risk for breast cancer,[57] clinical experience with raloxifene is confined to postmenopausal women. Raloxifene is classified as an antiestrogen with less estrogenlike actions than tamoxifen.[67] Tamoxifen has been shown to produce a small decrease in bone density in premenopausal women,[44] however, and concern exists that raloxifene might produce greater decreases in bone density. The National Cancer Institute is conducting a randomized study of raloxifene use (60 mg daily and 300 mg daily) in high-risk premenopausal women to address the issue of raloxifene and bone density. Short-term raloxifene treatment (5 days or 28 days) causes elevations in the level of circulating estradiol but does not prevent ovulation[84]; these effects are consistent with the known elevation of steroid hormones produced by tamoxifen in premenopausal breast cancer patients.[85] The changes in endocrine function produced by raloxifene will also be assessed as a prelude to the recruitment of premenopausal high-risk women to the STAR trial.

CLINICAL CONSIDERATIONS

The most important step required before tamoxifen can be considered for risk reduction is an evaluation of the patient's immediate and lifetime risk of developing breast cancer. This evaluation can be accomplished using the "risk disk" obtainable from the National Cancer Institute. This interactive computer program is based on the Gail model[60] used to select volunteers for the NSABP P-1 tamoxifen prevention trial.[57] In essence, the physician can obtain an estimate of risk for an individual based on her risk factors for the disease, so the benefit for the woman can be weighed against the risks of side effects. In general, the risks of thromboembolic events or endometrial cancer caused by tamoxifen are not important for premenopausal women. Concerns about pregnancy must be addressed, however. Premenopausal women who take tamoxifen are at risk for pregnancy and must use barrier contraceptive methods. A woman who finds herself pregnant should not take tamoxifen because of concerns about teratogenesis. In the premenopausal woman at increased risk of breast cancer, the major negative impact of tamoxifen may be on quality of life due to the occurrence of hot flashes and vaginal dryness.

Postmenopausal women who take tamoxifen are at risk for a modest increase in thromboembolic events, but the rate is small and is equivalent to that observed with either hormone replacement therapy or raloxifene therapy. Postmenopausal women without a uterus are not at risk for endometrial cancer, and when such women have breast cancer risk factors, the risk-benefit ratio for tamoxifen use tends to fall on the favorable side. Even women with a uterus, however, have only a modestly increased risk of low-grade, early stage endometrial cancer.

Raloxifene is not approved as a chemopreventive for breast cancer risk reduction in women, and its effect on high-risk women is unknown. Raloxifene has not been tested in premenopausal women and should not be used outside of a clinical trial in this population. Because raloxifene is still being evaluated for the reduction of risk in postmenopausal women, it cannot be said to be superior to tamoxifen. Appropriate women should be considered for participation in the STAR trial. Raloxifene has not been proven to reduce the incidence of endometrial cancer in postmenopausal women. Providing data to address this issue is one of the goals of the STAR trial. Raloxifene is an appropriate alternative for osteoporosis protection in postmenopausal women who do not wish to take estrogen and do not meet the risk levels suggested for the use of tamoxifen.

SYNTHETIC RETINOIDS

Natural retinoids play a crucial role in cellular proliferation and differentiation, but their poor clinical tolerability has prevented the use of these compounds as cancer preventive agents.[86] Toxic symptoms, which may be acceptable in treating established cancer, are not considered acceptable for reducing cancer risk. One of the less toxic vitamin A analogues studied for breast cancer chemoprevention is 4-HPR, a synthetic amide derivative of all-*trans*-retinoic acid.[87,88] The inhibition of chemically induced mammary carcinoma in rats by 4-HPR was first described by Moon et al.[89] Based on these results, 4-HPR was proposed for chemoprevention trials in human breast cancer.[90] This compound has been studied extensively and proved to be less toxic than many other retinoids.[87,88,91]

Early reports showing adverse retinal and dermatologic effects at daily doses of 600 to 800 mg halted the clinical development of this compound.[92,93] Subsequently, a phase I–II study identified a regimen of 200 mg per day with a monthly 3-day interruption as the best-tolerated schedule to allow partial retinol recovery and storage in the retina.[94,95] Studies demonstrated that, in contrast to retinoic acid, blood levels of 4-HPR remain constant during administration for as long as five years,[96,97] the drug selectively accumulates in the human breast,[98] and, finally, a significant decline of plasma retinol levels is responsible for the increased rod thresholds occurring in a certain proportion of subjects.[99] Research also showed that 4-HPR causes an early drop in plasma retinol concentrations[96] and that the plasma level of *N*-(4-methoxyphenyl)retinamide (the principal metabolite of 4-HPR) is also associated with the retinol decrease.[100]

Although 4-HPR was synthesized in the 1970s, only since the early 1990s has its mechanism of action been partially elucidated. This retinoid appears to be the prototype of a new class of selective ligands of the retinoic acid receptors, in which the transactivation function can be separated from the transrepression function.[101,102] This selective binding to the nuclear receptors is likely to be the basis for its specific biological activities and its favorable pharmaceutical properties.[102] Interestingly, 4-HPR is a potent inhibitor of the pivotal AP-1 transcription factor that regulates the *jun-fos* protooncogene-mediated cell growth signal.[101] Because the AP-1 motif is required for the estrogen proliferative stimulation mediated by insulinlike growth factor type I,[103] this may be an important pathway by which 4-HPR inhibits breast proliferation. Indeed, 4-HPR has been shown to inhibit two estrogen target genes, the pS2 and progesterone receptor genes, in breast cancer cell lines; these results provide further evidence for an interference with the ER signal transduction pathway.[104]

In recent years, 4-HPR has been shown to be active *in vitro* and *in vivo* against mammary, bladder, lung, ovary, and cervical tumors, neuroblastoma, leukemia, and prostate tumors in preclinical models (reviewed in Lotan[105]). A characteristic feature of 4-HPR is its ability to inhibit cell growth through the induction of apoptosis rather than differentiation, an effect that is strikingly different from that of the parent compound all-*trans*-retinoic acid and that may occur even in retinoic acid–resistant cell lines.[106,107]

Because of the selective accumulation of 4-HPR in the breast[89] and the good tolerability in humans,[94,95] a phase III trial aimed at reducing the incidence of contralateral breast cancer was started in 1987. The final results of this trial, after a median follow-up of 10 years, have been prepared (U. Veronesi, M.D., et al., *unpublished data*, 1999).

The study randomly assigned 2,972 women aged 30 to 70 years with operated stage I breast cancer to 5 years of therapy with fenretinide (4-HPR), 200 mg per day orally, or no treatment. The primary efficacy end point was the incidence of contralateral breast cancer. At a median observation time of 97 months, no significant difference was seen in contralateral breast cancer occurrence between the two groups (65 events occurred in the fenretinide group versus 71 in the control group; $p = .642$). A significant interaction was detected between treatment and menopausal status ($p = .045$), however. A beneficial effect was seen in premenopausal women (fenretinide group, 27 events; control group, 42 events; adjusted hazard ratio, 0.66; 95% confidence interval, 0.14 to 1.07), and an opposite trend was found in postmenopausal women (fenretinide group, 38 events; control group, 29 events; adjusted hazard ratio, 1.32; 95% confidence interval, 0.82 to 2.15). A similar pattern was observed with regard to ipsilateral breast cancer reappearance (premenopausal women: fenretinide group, 58 events; control group, 87 events; adjusted hazard ratio, 0.65; 95% confidence interval, 0.46 to 0.92; postmenopausal women: fenretinide group, 42 events; control group, 34 events; adjusted hazard ratio, 1.19; 95% confidence interval, 0.75 to 1.89; p value for the treatment × menopause interaction = .045). No difference was seen between groups in the incidence of distant metastasis and mortality from all causes. In addition, no difference was found between groups in the incidence of tumors in other organs, except that a protective effect for ovarian cancer was observed for the fenretinide group during treatment. Fenretinide was well tolerated, and treatment discontinuation due to severe adverse events was uncommon (4.4%).

The data indicate that treatment for 5 years with fenretinide reduces the incidence of contralateral breast cancer and the reappearance of ipsilateral breast cancer in premenopausal women with early breast cancer (U. Veronesi, M.D., et al., *unpublished data*, 1999).

COMBINATION OF TAMOXIFEN AND RETINOIDS

The concept of combining multiple agents with different mechanisms of action to enhance activity and minimize toxicity has been pursued for more than 20 years in cancer chemoprevention research.[108] Moreover, the rationale for combining an estrogen response modifier with a retinoid is supported by the structural homology at the nuclear receptor level, at which reciprocal interactions in the signal transduction pathways and shared modulation of cognate target genes has been shown.[109] Indeed, the dominant role played by the superfamily of steroid-thyroid-retinoid-vitamin D_3 receptors in the regulation of several physiologic functions, including development and homeostasis, has been a major focus of research in recent years.[110,111] This family of structurally related nuclear transcriptional factors provides the best-known example of a highly sophisticated cooperative network that maintains homeostasis through a complex pattern of activation or inhibition of overlapping target genes.[109] Despite the structural diversity among most of the ligands, the similarity of the hormone response elements in the promoter region of these genes, as well as between the receptors themselves, indicates conservation of a general strategy for the hormonal control of gene expression among vertebrate animals.[111] Importantly, this family of receptors interacts with distinct classes of transcription factors (e.g., AP-1/Jun-Fos) through recognition of common DNA regulatory sequences as a means of modulating the balance between the growth and differentiating factors, a mechanism referred to as *cross coupling*.[112]

In addition to a mechanistic rationale for this combination, synergistic efficacy has been observed *in vivo* in animal studies of tamoxifen/tamoxifen citrate in combination with 4-HPR at lower, less toxic dosages.[113–116] Tamoxifen and 4-HPR have some complementary chemopreventive activities (e.g., modulation of growth factors, inhibition of prostaglandin synthesis, decrease in polyamide levels), and synergistic activity has also been documented *in vitro*.[117] The dietary combination of 4-HPR with tamoxifen citrate (0.125 mg per kilogram of dietary intake, or approximately 0.011 nmol per kilogram of body weight per day) showed synergistic activity against nitroso-*N*-methylurea–induced mammary carcinogenesis in older rats. Interestingly, subcutaneously administered tamoxifen plus dietary 4-HPR was found to be even more effective in an adjuvant study in which the induction of subsequent mammary carcinomas after surgical removal of the first cancer was the end point (reviewed by Kelloff et al.[87,118]).

Subchronic (90-day) toxicity studies of tamoxifen citrate at 0.4 to 32.0 mg per kilogram of body weight per day by gavage alone and in combination with 4-HPR have been performed in two species. In female beagle dogs, no synergistic toxicity was observed with a combination of both agents. Moreover, subtoxic dosages of tamoxifen combined with 4-HPR have produced synergistic chemopreventive effects in rat mammary carcinogenesis models (reviewed in Kelloff et al.[87,118]).

FUTURE OF CHEMOPREVENTION

The concept of the chemoprevention of cancer was proposed in the mid-1970s by Sporn and colleagues.[119,120] Essentially, effective implementation of the strategy requires a target that allows prevention of either the initiation or the promotion (or both) of cancer cells. The key to success is therefore identification of a well-defined target so a selective action can be applied without general toxicity.

Retinoid action appears to be modulated by a large number of targets. The first clinical studies continue to show promise, and future drug discovery will provide new agents with increased target specificity. The clinical success of tamoxifen and raloxifene, however, now raises the question of whether additional benefit can accrue from drug combinations of retinoids and antiestrogens.[70] In addition, the use of reduced dosages of tamoxifen as a chemopreventive intervention is being studied.[121] The goal would be to maintain efficacy as a chemopreventive but to reduce side effects. Indeed, low-dose combined maintenance therapy might be a useful approach.

A major strategic problem for the current round of clinical trials in chemoprevention with antiestrogens is determining the optimal duration of the intervention. Five years of tamoxifen treatment are generally believed to be optimal in adjuvant therapy,[122] but this may not be true for the prevention of breast cancer. Unfortunately, resolution of this question requires a decade of clinical testing; alternatively, it may be resolved by future generations of epidemiologists, when the incidence of breast cancer is evaluated in women who elect to take raloxifene or another SERM indefinitely.

The potential of SERMs to prevent osteoporosis and reduce the risk of breast and endometrial cancer has resulted in the development of numerous analogues or structural derivatives of metabolites. Clinical studies are under way with idoxifene, droloxifene, LY353381, EM800, and EM652. Each of these compounds bears a structural similarity to either tamoxifen or raloxifene, but with alterations in the molecule that enhance bioavailability.[123–127] Although laboratory studies are extremely important to identify clear advantages of these compounds over existing molecules to justify clinical trials, only randomized clinical trials will establish their value to women over existing drugs.

Major advances in the development of targeted chemopreventives could accrue from novel drug design based on the emerging knowledge of the hormone receptor superfamily and the orphan receptors.[112] As an example, the crystallization of the ligand-binding domain of ERα with estradiol, raloxifene,[128] and 4-hydroxytamoxifen[129] has enhanced knowledge of the molecular mechanism of antihormone actions. However, the discovery of a second receptor for estrogen, ERβ, has introduced a new dimension in the targeting of drug molecules.[130] A menu of new medicines may be developed to become new hormone maintenance therapies. These could address a number of diseases associated with the menopause but with the beneficial side effect of preventing breast and endometrial cancer. The most important issue, however, will be the quality of life achieved with SERM therapy. At present, no agent can reduce the incidence of hot flashes and ameliorate the symptoms of the menopause. In addition, SERMs could change the natural history of breast cancer and radically alter treatment options decades from now. One intriguing observation[57,58] from the NSABP P-1 trial and the early data from the raloxifene osteoporosis trials is that the agents appear to reduce the occurrence of ER-positive cancer exclusively. That raloxifene is being used as a preventive for osteoporosis, however, and is being tested in high-risk populations for the prevention of coronary heart disease, points to a broader future application of this group of SERMs. As novel SERMs are developed and targeted for different diseases, one might speculate that the incidence of breast cancer will decrease. Nevertheless, with the aging of the population, the absolute numbers of breast cancers may remain the same. These tumors, however, may be refractory to traditional endocrine therapy because of antiestrogen drug resistance or ER negativity of the tumor. Second-line endocrine therapy, such as the use of aromatase inhibitors or pure antiestrogens, will become more important. The development of additional treatment strategies is the challenge for cancer pharmacology in the twenty-first century.

REFERENCES

1. Boyd, S. On oophorectomy in cancer of the breast. *BMJ* 1900;2:1161.
2. Feinleib M. Breast cancer and artificial menopause: a cohort study. *J Natl Cancer Inst* 1968;41:315.
3. Trichopoulos DB, MacMahon B, Cole P. Menopause and breast cancer risk. *J Natl Cancer Inst* 1972;48:605.
4. Huggins C, Grand LC, Brillantes FP. Mammary cancer induced by a single feeding of polynuclear hydrocarbons and their suppression. *Nature* 1961;189:204.
5. Dao TL. Mammary cancer induction by 7,12 dimethylbenzanthracene: relation to age. *Science* 1969;165:810.
6. Grubbs CJ, Peckham JC, Cato KD. Mammary carcinogenesis in rats in relation to age at time of nitroso-N-methyl urea administration. *J Natl Cancer Inst* 1983;70:209.
7. Bowcock AM. Molecular cloning of BRCA1: a gene for early onset familial breast and ovarian cancer. *Breast Cancer Res Treat* 1993;28:121.
8. Tokanaga M, Land CE, Yamamoto T, et al. Incidence of female breast cancer among atomic bomb survivors: Hiroshima and Nagasaki 1950–1980. *Radiat Res* 1987;112:243.
9. Hildreth N, Shore R, Dvukresteski P, et al. The risk of breast cancer after irradiation of the thymus in infancy. *N Engl J Med* 1989;321:1281.
10. Miller AB, How G, Sherman G, et al. The risk of breast cancer after irradiation during fluoroscopic examinations in patients being treated for tuberculosis. *N Engl J Med* 1989;321:1285.
11. Lathrop AEC, Loeb L. Further investigations on the origins of tumors in mice. III. On the part played by internal secretions in the spontaneous development of tumors. *J Cancer Res* 1916;1:1.
12. Lacassagne A. Hormonal pathogenesis of adenocarcinoma of the breast. *Am J Cancer* 1936;27:713.
13. Jordan VC, Lababidi MK, Mirecki DM. The antiestrogen and antitumor properties of prolonged tamoxifen therapy in C3H/OUJ mice. *Eur J Cancer* 1990;26:718.
14. Jordan VC, Lababidi MK, Langen-Fahey S. Suppression of mouse mammary tumorigenesis by long-term tamoxifen therapy. *J Natl Cancer Inst* 1991;83:492.
15. Dao TL, Sutherland H. Mammary carcinogenesis by 3-methylcholanthrene. 1. Hormonal aspects in tumor induction and growth. *J Natl Cancer Inst* 1959;23:567.
16. Dao TL, Bock FG, Greiner MJ. Mammary carcinogenesis by 3-methylcholanthrene. 2. Inhibitory effects of pregnancy and lactation on tumor induction. *J Natl Cancer Inst* 1959;23:567.
17. Huggins C, Moon R, Morii S. Extinction of experimental mammary cancer. 1. Estradiol-17 and progesterone. *Proc Natl Acad Sci U S A* 1962;48:379.
18. Jabara AC, Toyne PH, Harcourt AG. Effects of time and duration of progesterone administration on mammary tumors induced by 7,12-dimethylbenzanthracene in Sprague-Dawley rats. *Br J Cancer* 1973;27:63
19. Grubbs CJ, Hill DL, McDonough KC, et al. N-nitroso-N-methylurea–induced mammary carcinogenesis: effect of pregnancy on preneoplastic cells. *J Natl Cancer Inst* 1983;71:625.
20. Dao TL. The role of ovarian hormones in initiating the induction of mammary cancer in rats by polynuclear hydrocarbons. *Cancer Res* 1962;22:973.

21. Jordan VC. Effect of tamoxifen (ICI 46,474) on initiation and growth of DMBA-induced rat mammary carcinomata. *Eur J Cancer* 1976;12:419.
22. Tsai TLS, Katzenellenbogen BS. Antagonism of development and growth of 7,12 dimethylbenzanthracene–induced rat mammary tumors by the anti-estrogen U23,469 and effects on estrogen and progesterone receptors. *Cancer Res* 1977;37:1537.
23. Jordan VC, Allen KE. Evaluation of the antitumor activity of the non–steroidal antioestrogen monohydroxytamoxifen in the DMBA-induced rat mammary carcinoma model. *Eur J Cancer* 1980; 16:239.
24. Jordan VC, Allen KE, Dix CJ. Pharmacology of tamoxifen in laboratory animals. *Cancer Treat Rep* 1980;64:745.
25. Robinson SP, Jordan VC. Reversal of the antitumor effects of tamoxifen by progesterone in the 7,12-dimethylbenzanthracene-induced rat mammary carcinoma model. *Cancer Res* 1987;47:5386.
26. Huggins C, Grand LC, Brillantes F. Clinical significances of breast structure in the induction of mammary cancer in the rat. *Proc Natl Acad Sci U S A* 1959;45:1294.
27. Russo J, Gusterson BA, Rogers AE, et al. Comparative study of human and rat mammary tumorigenesis. *Lab Invest* 1990;62:244.
28. Russo IH, Koszalka M, Russo J. Human chorionic gonadotropin and rat mammary cancer prevention. *J Natl Cancer Inst* 1990;82:1286.
29. Russo IH, Koszalka M, Gimotty PA, et al. Protective effect of chorionic gonadotropin on DMBA-induced mammary carcinogenesis. *Br J Cancer* 1990;62:243.
30. Russo IH, Koszalka M, Russo J. Effect of gonadotropin on mammary gland differentiation and carcinogenesis. *Carcinogenesis* 1990;11:1849.
31. Prentis RL, Thomas DB. On the epidemiology of oral contraceptive and disease. *Adv Cancer Res* 1987;49:285.
32. Battersby S, Robertson BJ, Anderson TJ, et al. Influence of cycle parity and oral contraceptive use on steroid hormone in normal breast. *Br J Cancer* 1992;65:601.
33. Jeng MH, Parker C, Jordan VC. Estrogenic potential of progestins in oral contraceptives to stimulate human breast cancer cell proliferation. *Cancer Res* 1992;52:6539.
34. Pike MC, Ross RK, Lobo RA, et al. LHRH antagonists and the prevention of breast and ovarian cancer. *Br J Cancer* 1989;60:142.
35. Spicer DV, Shoupe D, Pike M. GnRH agonists as contraceptive agents: predicted significantly reduced risk of breast cancer. *Contraception* 1991;44:289.
36. Spicer DV, Pike MC, Pike A, et al. Pilot trial of a gonadotropin hormone agonist with replacement hormones as a prototype contraceptive to prevent breast cancer. *Contraception* 1993;45:427.
37. Spicer DV, Pike MC. Breast cancer prevention through modulation of endogenous hormones. *Breast Cancer Res Treat* 1993;28:179.
38. Jordan VC. Fourteenth Gaddum memorial lecture: a current view of tamoxifen for the treatment and prevention of breast cancer. *Br J Pharmacol* 1993;110:507.
39. Osborne CK. Tamoxifen in the treatment of breast cancer. *N Engl J Med* 1998;339:1609.
40. Early Breast Cancer Trialists Collaborative Group. Tamoxifen for early breast cancer: an overview of the randomized trials. *Lancet* 1998;351:1451.
41. Turken S, Siris E, Seldin D, et al. Effects of tamoxifen on spinal bone density in women with breast cancer. *J Natl Cancer Inst* 1989;81:1086.
42. Love RR, Mazess RB, Barden HS, et al. Effects of tamoxifen on bone mineral density in postmenopausal women with breast cancer. *N Engl J Med* 1992;326:852.
43. Kristensen B, Ejlertsen B, Dolgard P, et al. Tamoxifen and bone metabolism in postmenopausal low risk breast cancer patients: a randomized study. *J Clin Oncol* 1994;12:992.
44. Powles TJ, Hickish T, Kanis JA, et al. Effect of tamoxifen on bone mineral density measured by dual energy x-ray absorptiometry in healthy premenopausal and postmenopausal women. *J Clin Oncol* 1996;14:78.
45. Love RR, Weibe DA, Newcomb PA, et al. Effects of tamoxifen on cardiovascular risk factors in postmenopausal women. *Am Int Med* 1991;115:860.
46. Williams GM, Iatropoulos MJ, Djordjevic MV, et al. The triphenylethylene drug tamoxifen is a strong liver carcinogen in the rat. *Carcinogenesis* 1993;14:1993.
47. Greaves P, Goonetilleke R, Nunn G, et al. Two-year carcinogenicity study of tamoxifen in Alderley Park Wistar-derived rats. *Cancer Res* 1993;59:3919.
48. Phillips DH, Carmichael PL, Hewer A, et al. Activation of tamoxifen and its metabolite alpha-hydroxytamoxifen to DNA binding products: comparison between human, rat and mouse hepatocytes. *Carcinogenesis* 1996;14:89.
49. Glak H, Davis W, Meinl W, et al. Rat but not human sulphotransferase activates a tamoxifen metabolite to produce DNA adducts and gene mutation in bacteria and mammalian cells in culture. *Carcinogenesis* 1998;19:1708.
50. Martin EA, Rich KJ, White IN, et al. 32P-Postlabeled DNA adducts in liver obtained from women treated with tamoxifen. *Carcinogenesis* 1995;16:1651.
51. Fisher B, Costantino JP, Redmond CK, et al. Endometrial cancer in tamoxifen treated breast cancer patients. Findings from the National Surgical Adjuvant Breast and Bowel Project (NSABP) B-14. *J Natl Cancer Inst* 1994;86:527.
52. Assikis VJ, Neven P, Jordan VC, et al. A realistic clinical perspective of tamoxifen and endometrial carcinogenesis. *Eur J Cancer* 1996; 32A:1464.
53. Horwitz RI, Feinstein AR, Horwitz SM, et al. Necropsy diagnosis of endometrial cancer and detection-bias in case/control studies. *Lancet* 1981;ii:66.
54. Carmichael PL, Ugwaumadu AHN, Neven P, et al. Lack of genotoxicity of tamoxifen in human endometrium. *Cancer Res* 1996;56:1475.
55. Philips DH, Hewer A, Grover PL, et al. Tamoxifen does not form detectable DNA adducts in white blood cells of breast cancer patients. *Carcinogenesis* 1996;17:1149.
56. Dal Cin P, Timmerman D, Van den Berghe I, et al. Genomic changes in endometrial polyps associated with tamoxifen show no evidence for its actions as an external carcinogen. *Cancer Res* 1998;58:2278.
57. Fisher B, Costantino JP, Wickerham DL, et al. Tamoxifen for the prevention of breast cancer: report of the National Surgical Adjuvant Breast and Bowel Project P-1 study. *J Natl Cancer Inst* 1998; 90:1371.
58. Powles TJ, Eeles R, Ashley S, et al. Interim analysis of the incident breast cancer in the Royal Marsden Hospital tamoxifen randomized chemoprevention trial. *Lancet* 1998;362:98.
59. Veronesi U, Maisonneuve P, Costa A, et al. Prevention of breast cancer with tamoxifen: preliminary findings from the Italian randomized trial among hysterectomized women. *Lancet* 1998;362:93.
60. Gail MH, Brinton LA, Byar DP, et al. Projecting individualized probabilities of developing breast cancer for white females who are being examined annually. *J Natl Cancer Inst* 1989;81:1879.
61. Powles TJ, Hardy JR, Ashley SE, et al. A pilot trial to evaluate the acute toxicity and feasibility of tamoxifen for prevention of breast cancer. *Br J Cancer* 1989;60:126.
62. Powles TJ, Jones AL, Ashley SE, et al. The Royal Marsden Hospital pilot tamoxifen chemoprevention trial. *Breast Cancer Res Treat* 1994;31:73.
63. Jones AL, Powles TJ, Treleaven J, et al. Homeostatic changes and thromboembolic risk during tamoxifen therapy in normal women. *Br J Cancer* 1992;66:744.
64. Powles TJ, Tillyer CP, Jones AL, et al. Prevention of breast cancer with tamoxifen—an update on the Royal Marsden pilot program. *Eur J Cancer* 1990;26:680.
65. Kedar RP, Bourne TH, Powles TJ, et al. Effects of tamoxifen on uterus and ovaries of postmenopausal women in a randomized breast cancer prevention trial. *Lancet* 1994;342:1318.
66. Decensi A, Fontana V, Bruno S, et al. Effect of tamoxifen on endometrial proliferation. *J Clin Oncol* 1996;14:434.
67. Black LJ, Jones CD, Falcone JF. Antagonism of estrogen action with a new benzothiophene derived antiestrogen. *Life Sci* 1983;32:1031.
68. Clemens JA, Bennett DR, Black LJ, et al. Effects of new antiestrogen keoxifene LY156758 on growth of carcinogen-induced mammary tumors and on LH and prolactin levels. *Life Sci* 1983;32:2869.
69. Gottardis MM, Jordan VC. The antitumor actions of keoxifene (raloxifene) and tamoxifen in the N-nitrosomethylurea-induced rat mammary carcinoma model. *Cancer Res* 1987;47:4020.
70. Anzano MA, Peer CW, Smith JM, et al. Chemoprevention of mammary carcinogenesis in the rat: combined use of raloxifene and 9-cis-retinoic acid. *J Natl Cancer Inst* 1996;88:123.
71. Gradishar WJ, Glusman JE, Vogel CL, et al. Raloxifene HCl: a new endocrine agent is active in estrogen receptor positive metastatic breast cancer. *Breast Cancer Res Treat* 1997;46:53(abst no 209).
72. Buzdar AU, Marcus C, Holmes F, et al. Phase II evaluation of LY156758 in metastatic breast cancer. *Oncology* 1988;45:344.

73. Jordan VC, Phelps E, Lindgren JU. Effects of antiestrogens on bone in castrated and intact female rats. *Breast Cancer Res Treat* 1987;10:31.
74. Black LJ, Sato M, Rowley ER, et al. Raloxifene (LY139 481 HCl) prevents bone loss and reduces serum cholesterol without causing uterine hypertrophy in ovariectomized rats. *J Clin Invest* 1994;93:63.
75. Sato M, Kim J, Short LL, et al. Longitudinal and cross sectional analysis of raloxifene effects on tibiae from ovariectomized aged rats. *J Pharmacol Exp Ther* 1995;279:298.
76. Heaney RP, Draper MW. Raloxifene and estrogen: comparative bone remodeling kinetics. *J Clin Endocrinol Metab* 1997;82:3425.
77. Delmas PD, Bjarnason NH, Mitlak BH, et al. Effects of raloxifene on bone mineral density, serum cholesterol concentrations and uterine–endometrium in postmenopausal women. *N Engl J Med* 1997;337:1641.
78. Walsh BW, Kuller LH, Wild RA, et al. Effects of raloxifene on serum lipids and coagulation factors in healthy postmenopausal women. *JAMA* 1998;279:1445.
79. Cummings SR, Eckert S, Krueger KA, et al. The effect of raloxifene on risk of breast cancer in postmenopausal women. *JAMA* 1999;281:2189.
80. Jordan VC, Glusman JE, Eckert S, et al. Incident primary breast cancers are reduced by raloxifene: integrated data from multicenter double blind, randomized trials in 12,000 postmenopausal women. *Proc Am Soc Clin Oncol* 1998;122a(abst no 466).
81. Jordan VC, Glusman JE, Eckert S, et al. Raloxifene reduces incident primary breast cancers: integrated data from multicenter double blind placebo controlled, randomized trials in postmenopausal women. *Breast Cancer Res Treat* 1998;50:227(abst no 2).
82. Lerner LJ, Jordan VC. Development of antiestrogens and their use in breast cancer: eighth Cain memorial award lecture. *Cancer Res* 1990;50:4177.
83. Boss SM, Huster WJ, Neild JA, et al. Effect of raloxifene hydrochloride on the endometrium of postmenopausal women. *Am J Obstet Gynecol* 1997;177:1458.
84. Baker VL, Draper M, Paul S, et al. Reproductive endocrine and endometrial effects of raloxifene hydrochloride, a selective estrogen receptor modulator in women with regular menstrual cycles. *J Clin Endocrinol Metab* 1998;83:6.
85. Jordan VC, Fritz NF, Langan-Fahey S, et al. Alteration of endocrine parameters in premenopausal women with breast cancer during long term adjuvant therapy with tamoxifen as the single agent. *J Natl Cancer Inst* 1991;83:1488.
86. Sporn MB, Newton DL. Chemoprevention of cancer with retinoids. *Fed Proc* 1979;38:2528.
87. Kelloff GJ, Crowell JA, Boone CW, et al. Clinical development plan: N-(4-hydroxyphenyl)retinamide. *J Cell Biochem Suppl* 1994;20:176.
88. Costa A, Fornelli F, Chiesa F, et al. Prospects of chemoprevention of human cancers with the synthetic retinoid fenretinide. *Cancer Res Suppl* 1994;54:2032.
89. Moon RC, Thompson HJ, Becci PJ, et al. N-(4-hydroxyphenyl)retinamide, a new retinoid for prevention of breast cancer in the rat. *Cancer Res* 1979;39:1339.
90. Veronesi U, De Palo G, Costa A, et al. Chemoprevention of breast cancer with retinoids. *Monogr Natl Cancer Inst* 1992;12:93.
91. Naik HR, Kalemkerian G, Pienta KJ. 4-Hydroxyphenylretinamide in the chemoprevention of cancer. *Adv Pharmacol* 1995;33:315.
92. Kaiser Kupfer MI, Peck GL, Caruso RC, et al. Abnormal retinal function associated with fenretinide, a synthetic retinoid. *Arch Ophthalmol* 1986;104:69.
93. Kingstone TP, Lowe NJ, Winston J, et al. Visual and cutaneous toxicity which occurs during N-(4-hydroxyphenyl)retinamide therapy for psoriasis. *Clin Exp Dermatol* 1986;11:624.
94. Costa A, Malone W, Perloff M, et al. Tolerability of the synthetic retinoid fenretinide (HPR). *Eur J Clin Oncol* 1989;25:805.
95. Rotmensz N, De Palo G, Formelli F, et al. Long term tolerability of fenretinide (4-HPR) to breast cancer patients. *Eur J Cancer* 1991;2:1127.
96. Formelli F, Carsana R, Costa A, et al. Plasma retinol level reduction by the synthetic retinoid fenretinide: a one-year follow-up study of breast cancer patients. *Cancer Res* 1989;49:6149.
97. Formelli F, Clerici M, Campa T, et al. Five year administration of fenretinide: pharmacokinetics and effects on plasma retinol concentration. *J Clin Oncol* 1993;11:2036.
98. Metha RG, Moon RC, Hawthorne M, et al. A distribution of fenretinide in the mammary gland of breast cancer patient. *Eur J Cancer* 1991:27:138.
99. Decensi A, Torrisi R, Polizzi A, et al. Effect of the synthetic retinoid fenretinide on dark-adaptation and the ocular surface. *J Natl Cancer Inst* 1994;86:105.
100. Torrisi S, Parodi V, Fontana G, et al. Factor affecting plasma retinol decline during long-term administration of the synthetic retinoid fenretinide. *Cancer Epidemiol Biomarkers Prev* 1994;3:507.
101. Fanjul AN, Dawson MI, Hobbs PD, et al. A new class of retinoids with selective inhibition of AP-1 inhibits proliferation. *Nature* 1994;372:107.
102. Fanjul AN, Delia D, Pierotti D, et al. 4-Hydroxyphenyl retinamide is a highly selective activator of retinoid receptors. *J Biol Chem* 1996;271:22441.
103. Umayara Y, Kawamori R, Watada H, et al. Estrogen regulation of the insulin–like growth factor I gene transcription involves an AP-1 enhancer. *J Biol Chem* 1994;269:16433.
104. Kazmi SML, Plante RK, Visconti V, et al. Comparison of N-(4-hydroxyphenyl)retinamide and all-trans retinoic acid in the regulation of retinoid receptor-mediated gene expression in human breast cancer cell lines. *Cancer Res* 1996;56:1056.
105. Lotan R. Retinoids and apoptosis: implications for cancer chemoprevention and therapy. *J Natl Cancer Inst* 1995;87:1655.
106. Delia D, Aiello A, Lombardi L, et al. N-(4-hydroxyphenyl)retinamide induces apoptosis of malignant hemopoietic cell lines including those unresponsive to retinoic acid. *Cancer Res* 1993;53:6036.
107. Ponzoni M, Bocca P, Chiesa V, et al. Differential effects of N–(4–hydroxyphenyl)retinamide and retinoic acid on neuroblastoma cells: apoptosis versus differentiation. *Cancer Res* 1995;55:853.
108. Sporn MB. Combination of chemoprevention of cancer. *Nature* 1980;287:107.
109. Wahli W, Martinez E. Superfamily of steroid nuclear receptors: positive and negative regulators of gene expression. *FASEB J* 1991;5:2243.
110. Evans RM. The steroid and thyroid hormone receptor superfamily. *Science* 1988;240:889.
111. Mangelsdorf DJ, Thummel C, Beato M, et al. The nuclear receptor superfamily: the second decade. *Cell* 1995;83:835.
112. Beato M, Herrlich P, Schütz G. Steroid hormone receptors: many actors in search of a plot. *Cell* 1995;83:851.
113. McCormick DL, Metha RG, Thompson CA, et al. Enhanced inhibition of mammary carcinogenesis by combined treatment with N-(4-hydroxyphenyl)retinamide and ovariectomy. *Cancer Res* 1982; 42:508.
114. McCormick DL, Moon RC. Retinoid-tamoxifenoxifen interaction in mammary cancer chemoprevention. *Carcinogenesis* 1986;7:193.
115. Moon RC, Kelloff GJ, Detrisac CJ, et al. Chemoprevention of MNU–induced mammary tumors in the mature rat by 4-HPR and tamoxifen. *Anticancer Res* 1992;12:1147.
116. Ratko TA, Dentrisac CJ, Dinger NM, et al. Chemoprevention efficacy of combined retinoid and tamoxifen treatment following surgical excision of a primary mammary cancer in female rats. *Cancer Res* 1989; 49:4472.
117. Fontana JA. Interaction of retinoids and tamoxifen on the inhibition of human mammary carcinoma cell proliferation. *Exp Cell Biol* 1987;55:136.
118. Kelloff GJ, Crowell JA, Boone CW, et al. Clinical development plan: tamoxifen. *J Cell Biochem Suppl* 1994;20:252.
119. Sporn MB, Dunlop NM, Newton DL, Smith JM. Prevention of chemical carcinogenesis by vitamin A and its synthetic analogs (retinoids). *Fed Proc* 1976;35:1332
120. Sporn MB. Approaches to prevention of epithelial cancer during the preneoplastic period. *Cancer Res* 1976;36:2699.
121. Decensi A, Bonanni B, Guerrieri-Gonzaga A, et al. Biologic activity of tamoxifen at low doses in healthy women. *J Natl Cancer Inst* 1998;90:1461.
122. Fisher B, Dignam J, Bryant J, et al. Five years versus more than five years of tamoxifen therapy for breast cancer patients with negative lymph nodes and estrogen receptor–positive tumors. *J Natl Cancer Inst* 1996;88:1529.
123. Gradishar WJ, Jordan VC. The clinical potential of new antiestrogens. *J Clin Oncol* 1997;15:480.

124. MacGregor JI, Jordan VC. Basic guide to the mechanisms of antiestrogen action. *Pharmacol Rev* 1998;50:151.
125. Grese TA, Cho S, Finley DR, et al. Structure activity relationships of selective estrogen receptor modulators: modifications to the 2-arylbenzothiophene core of raloxifene. *J Med Chem* 1997;40:146.
126. Simard J, Sanchez R, Poirier D, et al. Blockade of the stimulatory effect of estrogens, OH-tamoxifen, OH-toremifene, droloxifene and raloxifene on alkaline phosphatase activity by the antiestrogen EM-800 in human endometrial adenocarcinoma Ishikawa cells. *Cancer Res* 1997;57:3494.
127. MacGregor JI, Liu H, Tonetti DA, et al. The interaction of raloxifene and the active metabolite of the antiestrogen EM-800 with the human estrogen receptor (ER). *Cancer Res (in press)*.
128. Brzozowski AM, Pike ACW, Dauter A, et al. Molecular basis of agonism and antagonism in the estrogen receptor. *Nature* 1995;389:753.
129. Shiau AK, Barstad D, Loria PM, et al. The structural basis of estrogen receptor/coactivator recognition and the antagonism of this interaction by tamoxifen. *Cell* 1998;95:927.
130. Kuiper GG, Enmark E, Pelto-Huikko M, et al. Cloning of a novel estrogen receptor expressed in rat prostate and ovary. *Proc Natl Acad Sci U S A* 1996;93:5925.

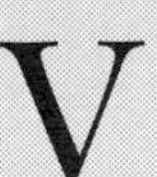

Diseases of the Breast, 2nd ed.,
edited by Jay R. Harris.
Lippincott Williams & Wilkins, Philadelphia © 2000.

Pathogenesis of Breast Cancer

CHAPTER 20

Oncogenes, Suppressor Genes, and Signal Transduction

Robert B. Dickson and Marc E. Lippman

GENETIC ALTERATIONS IN BREAST CANCER: GENERAL PRINCIPLES

The study of genetic alterations and gene expression in breast cancer underwent a revolution during the 1990s. Multiple lines of investigation—including detection of chromosomal abnormalities in breast tissue of women at high risk of the disease, evaluations of breast tumors in their early stages, and characterization of highly malignant stages of the disease—all contributed to the progress. The principal genetic lesions include gene amplifications, gene deletions, point mutations, loss of heterozygosity, chromosomal rearrangements, and overall aneuploidy. Microsatellite instability has also been reported in advanced disease. Some of the earliest hints at a genetic basis for the disease were recorded by the ancient Romans, who noticed that certain families were at high risk for the disease. Four genes have now been cloned (*BRCA1*, *BRCA2*, *TP53*, and *PTEN/MMAC1*) that are likely to function as tumor-suppressor genes for disease onset; when a mutant allele is inherited, subsequent loss of heterozygosity at the other allele then contributes to disease onset (in 5% to 10% of all breast cancer cases), with increased risk in both breasts and at an early age. The study of genetic changes during the progression of breast tumors now suggests that a progressive series of genomic and chromosomal alterations occur under the influence of multiple types of selective pressure; successive generations of tumor cells overtake the tissue, eventually giving rise to clonal or very nearly clonal metastatic disease.[1]

Although metastatic breast cancer can exhibit a tremendous range of genetic and chromosomal alterations, certain very specific, common lesions have been described. The genes involved in a high proportion of these lesions are now recognized as oncogenes [c-*myc*, c-*erb*-b2, and *cyclin* D_1 (*CCND1*)] and suppressor genes [*Rb-1, TP53, p16* (*CDKNZA*), and *E-cadherin* (*CDH1*)] that have been identified in many other can-

R. B. Dickson: Departments of Cell Biology and Pharmacology, Lombardi Cancer Center, Georgetown University Medical Center, Washington, D.C.
M. E. Lippman: Departments of Pharmacology and Medicine, Lombardi Cancer Center, Georgetown University Medical Center, Washington, D.C.

TABLE 1. *Oncoproteins and suppressor proteins in breast cancer*

A. Onset of familial breast cancer: suppressor proteins mutated or lost at the gene level	
p53 (Li-Fraumeni syndrome)	
PTEN (Cowden disease)	
BRCA1 (familial breast and ovarian cancer)	
BRCA2 (familial breast cancer)	
B. Progression of breast cancer	
Oncoproteins (gene amplified)	Oncoprotein candidates (overexpressed)
c-Erb-b_2	AIB1 (src-3)
c-myc	EGFR
cyclin D_1	FGFR1
	Telomerase
	ER
	Cyclin E
	β-catenin
	Life-promoting Bcl-2 family members
	Signal transduction proteins: c-ras^H, AKT, PI3K, PKC, Fak, Src
	α6β1 integrin
	CD44 variant
	Aromatase
Suppressor proteins (gene mutated, methylated, or lost)	Suppressor protein candidates (down-modulated)
Rb-1	IGF-II receptor
p53	TGFβRII—SMAD system
p16	Tsg 101
E-cadherin	p27
	PTEN
	nm23
	BARD-1
	BAP-1
	Death-promoting Bax family members
	α6β4 and α2β1 integrins
	KiSS-1
	KAI-1
	Mxi-1, Mad
	Maspin

cers. Functionally, very few activated oncogenes were first identified from breast cancer by their ability to transform rodent fibroblasts *in vitro* in the classical oncogene assay. Instead, most oncogenes in breast cancer have been identified by detailed study of amplified and translocated chromosomal regions using cytogenetics. So far, point mutation does not appear to be a common mechanism for oncogenic activation in breast cancer; gene amplification predominates. In contrast, tumor-suppressor genes in breast cancer are characterized primarily by inactivating point mutations, methylation, and loss of heterozygosity. In ongoing, evolving areas of study, multiple candidate oncogenes and suppressor genes have been proposed, primarily based on their up-regulation or down-regulation in the disease by nongenetic mechanisms. Although such nongenetic alterations of protooncogenes and suppressor genes have not classically been considered as important as genetic mechanisms, their roles in cancer progression deserve considerably more study.[2,3] Characterization of the major genetic changes in breast cancer (Table 1) requires many more years of study to complete.

In this chapter, the discussion of oncogenes and suppressor genes is organized according to their functional hierarchy within the pathways of growth-regulatory signals delivered to the nucleus from the cell surface. The reason for this organization is that the biochemical pathways of growth factor–dependent and adhesion-dependent signal transduction for cell cycle regulation and cell survival/death contain most of the defined protooncogenes and suppressor genes in breast cancer. However, an ever-increasing number of additional candidate protooncogenes and suppressor genes include other important regulatory pathways: steroid receptors and coactivating genes, differentiation-modulating genes, motility-controlling genes, and others.

EPIDERMAL GROWTH FACTOR, RELATED GROWTH FACTORS, AND THEIR RECEPTORS

Epidermal growth factor (EGF) was one of the first growth factors discovered. Stanley Cohen and colleagues made this discovery in 1962, while trying to isolate the component of mouse saliva that facilitated the opening of the eyelids and eruption of teeth in mouse pups. Due, again in part, to the pioneering work of Cohen and colleagues, the epidermal growth factor receptor (EGFR) has served as a prototype for the understanding of tyrosine kinase signaling, receptor dimerization, and signal transduction cascades. Most important to the current discussion is the fact that mutation, alternate splicing, or amplification of the *EGFR* gene and other members of its family can convert the receptor protein to forms that confer increased cancer risk on experimental animals and humans. Researchers have now known for many years that the genes for EGF and its receptor (EGFR) are expressed in breast tissue (and many other tissues), where they regulate mitogenesis, survival, and differentiation of multiple cell types. Knowledge of the EGF family of growth factors and receptors in the breast and other organ sites has expanded rapidly in the past few years and continues to command the attention of a large number of breast cancer researchers.[4,5]

The EGF family of factors now includes transforming growth factor α (TGF-α), amphiregulin (AR), heparin-binding EGF (HbEGF), β-cellulin, epiregulin, cripto-1, the neuregulin subfamily of three genes (with multiply spliced, expressed isoforms), and a number of viral-encoded members. The EGFR family is now known to contain three members, in addition to the well-known EGFR itself: c-*erb*-b2, c-*erb*-b3, and c-*erb*-b4. Study of this entire superfamily of factors and receptors has resulted in critical insights into regulation of the normal mammary gland, in identification of one of the most commonly activated oncogenes in the disease (c-*erb*-b2, also known as *HER-2/neu*), in recognition of critical mechanisms of breast tumor promotion, in identification of mechanisms of resistance of the disease to therapy, in understanding of mechanisms of immune surveillance of breast cancer, and in stimulation of new ideas for drug therapy for the disease. Although the *EGFR* itself has not generally been considered to be an oncogene in breast cancer (because its gene is not commonly amplified, as it is in many head and neck tumors, for example), this receptor has many oncogenelike characteristics. Understanding of its role is critical in evaluating both mechanisms of tumor promotion and the function of its close homologue, c-*erb*-b2, which, to date, has been considered the most important oncogene in this disease.[6,7]

Epidermal Growth Factor Receptor-Protooncogene

Numerous studies comparing hormone-dependent and hormone-independent breast cancer cell lines and primary tumors have noted that the absence of the estrogen receptor (ER) is often coupled with expression of high levels of EGFR and with more aggressive states of the disease.[8–10] Although coexpression of moderate levels of the EGFR with the estrogen receptors (ERs) and progesterone receptors (PgRs) is seldom observed in breast carcinoma, this is not the case in normal mammary luminal epithelial cells and fibroadenoma, in which coexpression of the three receptors is common.[11] EGFR is also commonly detected in normal myoepithelial cells and fibroblastic stroma of the breast.[11] However, paradoxically, in the normal gland the cells positive for ER and PgR appear to be proliferating only slowly, whereas the opposite is true in early cancers. This finding has led to the suggestion that hormone regulation of normal proliferation in the gland may involve the elaboration of paracrine-acting growth factors, such as those of the EGF family, which then act on steroid receptor–negative epithelial cells.[12]

The EGFR is a 170,000-d transmembrane glycoprotein that possesses intrinsic, ligand-regulable tyrosine kinase activity.[13] Binding of EGF (or other family members) to the EGFR leads to kinase activation, autophosphorylation of EGFR, phosphorylation of other intracellular substrates, internalization, and down-regulation of the receptor.[14,15] Molecular cloning of the *EGFR* gene has allowed exploration of its biological role by gene transfer methodology. Some of the earliest studies in this area explored the role of its overexpression in tumorigenic conversion of the cells. Overexpression of the EGFR was observed to result in EGF-dependent phenotypic transformation of immortalized rodent fibroblasts,[16,17] implicating this growth factor–receptor system in the process of cellular transformation. Independent studies documenting extensive homology between mammalian *EGFR* and the avian erythroblastosis-derived v-*erb*-b oncogene demonstrated that the *EGFR* is the cellular homologue of this oncogene.[18] Although the exact molecular defects of the v-*erb*-b oncogene (truncation and mutation) are seldom seen in the gene encoding the EGFR in human cancers, the gene encoding the EGFR is sometimes amplified (particularly in head and neck tumors) or overexpressed at the transcriptional and protein levels (in breast cancer). In both types of tumor, an activated, alternatively spliced variant of the receptor appears to be commonly expressed and is the subject of current study.[19,20]

The EGFR serves to regulate the proliferation of multiple tissues in fetal development, in nonreproductive aspects of adult life, and in many aspects of spermatogenesis and pregnancy.[4] The EGF and EGFR ligand–receptor superfamily system appears to be quite ancient. All of the EGF family of ligands described to date are structurally related to *Drosophila melanogaster grk, spi, vein*, and *argos* and to the *Caenorhabditis elegans lin-3* and *glp-1* genes,[4] whereas the EGFR family has only one homologue each in *Drosophila melanogaster* (*DER*) and in *C. elegans* (*let-23*). The growth factors that make up the EGF family are all thought to be synthesized from transmembrane precursors, which are cleaved by proteolytic enzymes to yield the fully processed, soluble forms. Although complete processing of the EGF family of growth factors to their soluble forms may predominate in many cell types, research has shown that the uncleaved precursors can act on the receptors of adjacent cells in a mode that has been termed *juxtacrine*.[21] All members of this growth factor family (except cripto-1) possess a consensus array of three characteristic disulfide linkages, which strongly define the three-dimensional structure of the protein and are required for growth factor action.[4,5]

The EGFR delivers its mitogenic, differentiation-modulatory, and survival-promoting signals to the cell, coincident with growth factor binding and receptor homodimerization or heterodimerization within the plane of the membrane (Fig. 1). Signal transduction itself is ultimately mediated through

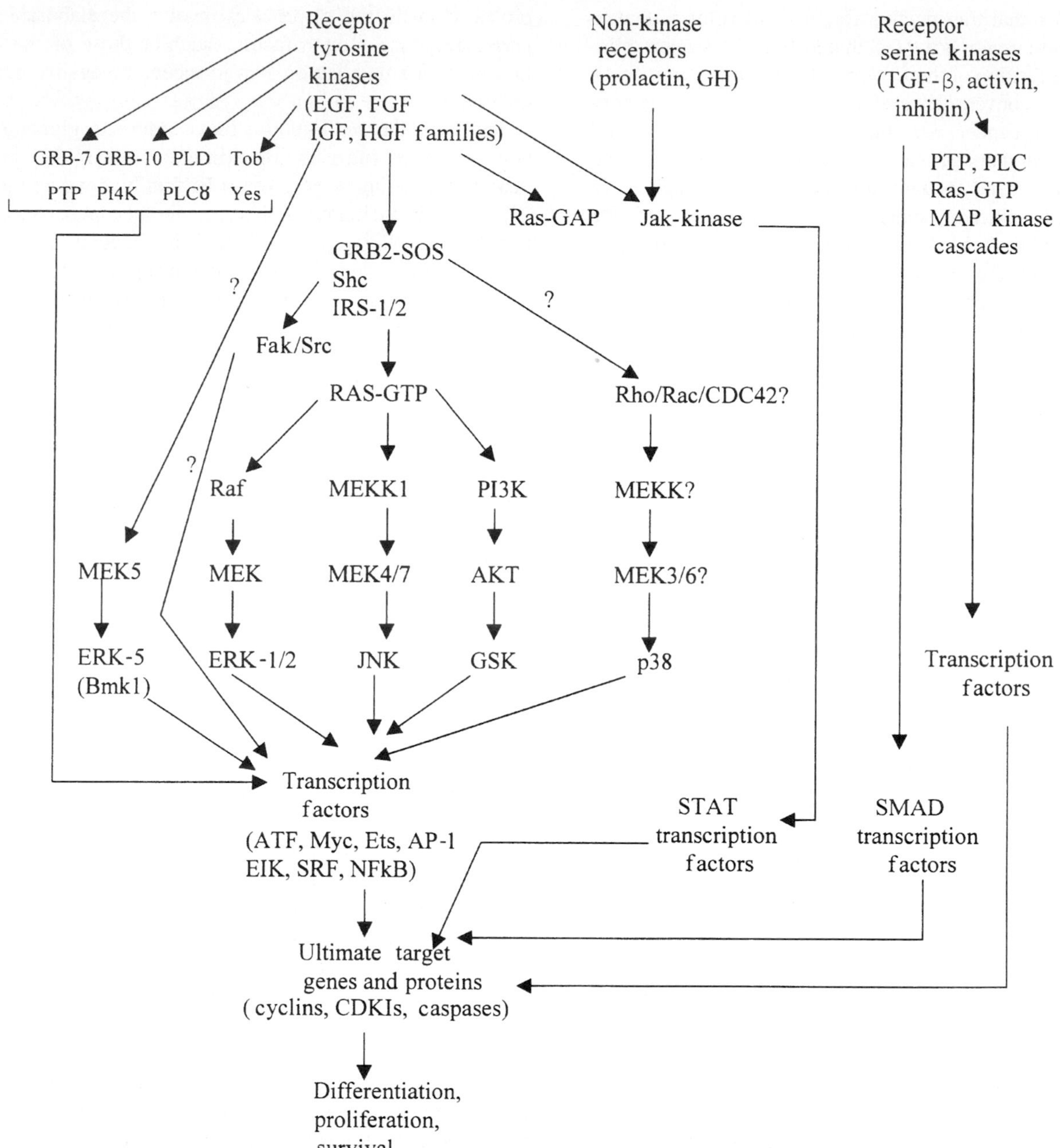

FIG. 1. Growth factors, cytokines, and peptide hormones signal cells to undergo differentiation, proliferation, and survival through a complex series of interconnected signal transduction pathways. Receptor tyrosine kinases signal through at least two primary protein interactions, growth factor receptor–binding protein 2 (GRB2) and associated protein SOS adapter, and the Jak kinase family. Multiple other proteins also interact with tyrosine kinase receptors, but their downstream effectors remain more obscure. Tyrosine kinase receptors are negatively regulated by interactions with the Ras-GAP protein. At least three major pathways emanate from GRB2-SOS; one of these, involving Ras–guanosine triphosphate (GTP), regulates at least three well-known subpathways, each of which controls a series of transcription factors determining cell physiology. The Jak kinase family is also of primary importance in delivering signals from the nonkinase, prolactin, and growth hormone receptors. The Jak kinases signal the cell through a very unique series of factors known as the signal transduction- and transcription-activating (STAT) factors. A third major series of receptors, the transforming growth factor β (TGF-β) family, signals through serine kinases; this family uses some of the same pathways as do tyrosine kinase receptors, but it also uses its own unique SMAD (Sma-Mad) transcription factor system. Dozens of known and suspected breast cancer cellular protooncogene and tumor-suppressor gene products reside within the complex network, including c-*erb*-b2, c-*myc*, the insulinlike growth factor type II receptor, and the TGF-β pathway. EGF, epidermal growth factor; FGF, fibroblast growth factor; HGF, hepatocyte growth factor; IGF, insulinlike growth factor; GH, growth hormone; TGF-β, transforming growth factor; other abbreviations defined in the text.

activation of a cytoplasmic domain of the receptor, which is homologous to the c-Src oncogenic kinase. Substrate specificity of the receptor kinase involves protein-protein structural recognition through additional cytoplasmic domains (*Src* homology 2, or SH2; and protein-tyrosine-binding, or PTB, types), which are located amino terminal to the kinase domain. Several primary kinase substrates, including growth factor receptor–binding protein 2 (GRB2) and an associated protein termed SOS, Shc, and IRS (inulin receptor substrate) have been identified, along with Ras-GAP (GTP-activated protein), Jak kinases, and several other kinases, phosphatases, and other enzymes. Many important signaling pathways are triggered through the GRB2-SOS, Shc, and IRS adapter proteins, including Src-Fak and Rho-Rac-CDC42 pathways, and at least three pathways dependent on Ras–guanosine triphosphate (GTP).[15,16,22] These pathways are discussed in more detail in the section Signal Transduction from Tyrosine Kinase Receptors.

Receptor function may be directly attenuated by means of cytoplasmic protein kinases. Examples of this mode of regulation in the EGFR pathway are an inhibitory phosphorylation of a submembranous EGFR threonine residue and a downstream, inhibitory phosphorylation of the Raf protein by a protein kinase dependent on cyclic adenosine monophosphate (cAMP).[19,23] Activated receptors are also internalized to attenuate their signaling through a mechanism involving another short cytoplasmic region amino terminal to the kinase. Recognition of the receptors by adaptan proteins, located on the cell surface in coated pits, results in their internalization into endosomes. Further routing of the EGFR for their destruction in lysosomes or their recycling back to the cell surface is regulated by other cellular mechanisms, including interaction with the CBL protein.[24]

How genetic alterations during the process of breast tumorigenesis interact with the EGFR signal transduction mechanisms is not fully clear. The function of the EGFR may change as a result of modulation of the kinetics of receptor turnover, heterodimeric coupling of the EGFR to other family members, aberrant modulation of phosphorylation of one or more EGFR kinase substrates, or more distal modulation of signal transduction targets. Specific examples of these circumstances are presented later in connection with discussions of EGFR interaction with c-Erb-b2, with c-Erb-b2 activation of c-Src, with c-Erb-b2 modulation of the function of the estrogen receptor, and with c-Myc modulation of EGFR action.[1]

In clinical studies of breast cancer, it has been suggested that high levels of EGFR in breast tumors (in striking contrast to the type I insulinlike growth factor, or IGF-I, receptor) correlate with a poor prognosis, even independent of ER status.[1,25] Although early EGFR studies on clinical specimens depended on a ligand-binding assay, using tumor membranes, more recent studies have used immunohistochemical approaches to quantify EGFR in paraffin-fixed, pathologic material. As noted earlier in this section, expression of high levels of EGFR is often accompanied by expression of very low levels or complete lack of ER.[1,5,26] This finding may suggest the existence of a mechanistic link between up-regulation of EGFR and hormone independence, or an incompatibility between overexpression of the growth factor system and overexpression of the steroid growth-control system. The basis for the variations in EGFR expression appears to lie in a transcription-enhancing element located in the first intron of the EGFR gene. This element is selectively stimulated in ER-negative breast cancer cells.[27,28] Most hormones and drugs that are capable of regulating the expression of EGFR and ER [e.g., estrogen and phorbol esters such as TPA (tumor promoting agent)] have opposing effects on these two types of receptors.[28–31]

c-*erb*-b2 Coreceptor-Protooncogene

The protein encoded by the c-*erb*-b2 coreceptor-protooncogene (also called p185, p185^{erbB-2}, p185^{neu}, HER-2/neu, p185^{HER-2}) has substantial homology to EGFR and is considered as one of its four family members. This protein was initially thought to be a receptor for a human TGF-α–related growth factor termed heregulin-1,[32] and for its rat homologue neu differentiating factor (NDF).[33] However, more recent studies have strongly suggested that, instead, the heregulin-1 and NDF (now known as neuregulins) bind with high affinity directly to two different EGFR family members, Erb-b4 and Erb-b3. Interestingly, Erb-b2 thus appears to have evolved as a heterodimeric, signal-transduction-involved partner of each of the other three ligand-binding family members.[4,5]

Estimates are that 20% to 30% of breast cancers overexpress the c-Erb-b2 gene product at a sufficiently high level that this protein serves as an oncogene; it can be easily detected using immunohistochemical staining of formalin-fixed and paraffin-embedded sections. Staining, when positive, is usually uniform for the entire tumor. These characteristics have facilitated the rapid development of assays of the Erb-b2 protein product as a tumor prognostic marker. Overexpression of the Erb-b2 protein has also been reported to commonly result from gene amplification in cancers involving many other organ systems, including adenocarcinomas of the lung, ovary, stomach, pancreas, and endometrium.[6] Although the gene encoding the Erb-b2 oncoprotein is usually amplified in connection with overexpression of the corresponding messenger RNA (mRNA) and protein product, this is not always the case; occasionally, protein overexpression may not correlate with gene amplification.

In contrast to c-*erb*-b2, the c-*erb*-b3 and c-*erb*-b4 genes are not commonly amplified in human cancer, but both possess transforming activity in fibroblast models *in vitro*. The function of the Erb-b2 protein in normal tissues is not completely known. However, data in the mouse mammary gland and in human breast cancer cells suggest that it is critically involved in lactational differentiation. Studies have also suggested its importance in neural and neuromuscular junction development.[4] The function of the structurally related Erb-b3 or Erb-b4 receptors in normal development and physiology is less certain. However, a complex picture has now emerged to implicate these additional family members at specific stages of mammary development. Gene knockout studies in mice have clearly demonstrated an essential role for the EGFR in ductal morphogenesis. During this period, the EGFR and Erb-b2 form homodimers whose activity is regulated by EGF family members, the synthesis of some of which are regulated by estrogen and progesterone.[34] In contrast, lobuloalveolar growth and lactational differentiation are controlled by heterodimers of all four EGFR family members and the multiple hormones of pregnancy.[35]

Overexpression of either EGFR or Erb-b2 in the mammary glands of transgenic mice can lead to the development of long-latency mammary tumors.[36] Evidence has been presented that an EGFR/Erb-b2 heterodimeric receptor form is critical for initiation of tumor formation in this type of model system. Additional transgenic and gene knockout studies have strongly supported the association with and activation of the c-Src protooncogene product by the c-Erb-b2 protein in this model as critical to the c-Erb-b2–induced tumorigenic pathway.[37–39] Because the Erb-b2 protein can heterodimerize with its other receptor family members, the status of each family member must be taken into account as future work in this area proceeds. So far, only Erb-b2 and EGFR family members are clearly associated with poor prognosis of the disease. Preliminary studies have suggested that expression of Erb-b4 and a neuregulin family member are both indicators of good prognosis, perhaps because of their association with lactational differentiation.[40–44]

Several other important tyrosine-kinase-encoding receptors (the fibroblast growth factor receptor, or FGFR, family; the insulin receptor and IGF receptor family; and the hepatocyte growth factor/scatter factor receptor, c-Met) may be considered as oncogenes in other types of cancer. Even in breast cancer, they may exhibit oncogene-like activity; however, among these, only FGFR1 is gene amplified in a few percent of cases. Conversely, the type II insulinlike growth factor (IGF-II) receptor, a non–kinase-binding/transport protein, is under active study as a possible tumor-suppressor protein in breast cancer and other malignancies.[1,25,45,46]

Signal Transduction from Tyrosine Kinase Receptors

A signal transduction cascade from the EGF receptor homodimer or heterodimers (see Fig. 1) begins with receptor occupancy by one of its cognate ligands (EGF, TGF-α, AR, HbEGF, etc.). Analogous cascades may be triggered from Erb-b3 and Erb-b4 homodimers or heterodimers by a neuregulin. As noted in the previous section, Erb-b2 does not appear to form high-affinity complexes with any ligand and appears to serve a coreceptor role, although it may take on special significance in cancer. Signal transduction results from an altered three-dimensional conformation of a receptor dimer in the plasma membrane, which activates receptor tyrosine kinase activity.[4,19,47] Kinase activation leads to receptor autophosphorylation and to further conformational change to allow binding and phosphorylation of intracellular substrates. As discussed in the previous three sections, one insight into function of the entire EGFR family is that heterodimerization among apparently all family members can occur; the nature of the dimer can determine the detailed nature of the signal pathways activated.[4,40] For example, the EGFR/Erb-b2 heterodimer can selectively stimulate transformed growth of mammary epithelial cells through interaction with the c-Src protein kinase,[41–43] and an EGFR/Erb-b3 heterodimer can selectively recruit the lipid signal transduction enzyme PI3K and stimulate its activity.[48] Receptor variants with dominant negative mutations of their cytoplasmic (kinase) domains have been used to interfere with this type of dimerization and kinase activation process. These mutated receptors can have powerful antiproliferative and antioncogenic activities.[49,50] As noted in the previous section, kinase activation initially results in autophosphorylation of several C-terminal tyrosine residues of the receptor cytoplasmic tail. This appears to allow a conformational change providing full exposure of the kinase active site for docking and for further interactions with multiple substrates. The formation of receptor-signaling complexes appears to mediate the major effects of EGF receptor-ligand binding on such diverse processes as ion fluxes, additional phosphorylation events, gene expression, DNA synthesis, and malignant growth.[4,5,19]

The next step in signal transduction (see Fig. 1) involves interaction of receptor tyrosine phosphorylated residues with SH2 and PTB domains on a variety of cellular proteins. GRB2 and SOS have been described as central for nucleating a receptor-binding protein complex in signal transduction.[51] GRB2 is a cytoplasmic protein that exists in a heterodimeric complex with a protein termed mammalian son of sevenless (mSOS). The derivation of this name is the homologous protein in *Drosophila*, which was discovered in the context of eye development. SOS is homologous to yeast protein kinase, which is also of central importance. When the EGF receptor is phosphorylated, the GRB2-SOS complex binds to the phosphotyrosine residues via its SH2 domains. Phosphotyrosine-binding domains allow other receptor docking proteins, such as insulin receptor substrate 1 (IRS-1) or insulin receptor substrate 2 (IRS-2), of particular importance for the insulin or IGF-I receptors, or the Shc protein (for the EGFR and for other cytoplasmic tyrosine kinases).[52,53] The receptor-GRB2-SOS complex then binds to the Fak-Src, the Rho-Rac-CDC42, or the Ras-GTP proteins.[4,19,51] Fak-Src are a pair of cytoplasmic tyrosine kinases that not only form a signal transduction complex noted earlier to be critical to Erb-b2–dependent breast tumorigenesis but also are important for cell-substrate adhesion-dependent signaling.[54] This kinase pair is further described in the section Adhesion-Dependent Signal Transduction. The proteins binding to Rac-Rho-CDC42 GTP are involved in both cell motility and cell survival and are also described in this section.[55] Ras-GTP is the best known of these signaling pathways.

Ras–guanosine diphosphate (GDP) is associated with the inner leaflet of the plasma membrane through a fatty acid residue incorporated in its structure (see Fig. 1). The formation of this high-order receptor complex serves to catalyze the Ras-activating exchange reaction of GTP for GDP.[56–58] Some G-protein–coupled, non–EGF-related, nontyrosine kinase receptors may also activate Ras in a similar manner.[59] Also, although older literature suggests that growth-inhibitory actions of TGF-β may serve to activate Ras,[60] a second signal transduction pathway of this growth factor family now is thought to be entirely different from, although interconnected with, that of tyrosine kinases; it involves SMAD proteins. The acronym for these signal transduction proteins stands for the Sma and Mad gene products, initially discovered in *Drosophila* and *C. elegans*.[61] A general mechanism of Ras deactivation involves the protein termed p120^{GAP}, which catalyzes the exchange of Ras-GDP for GTP to help end the signal transduction process.[62,63]

Other signal-transduction–related proteins also interact with receptor tyrosine kinases. They include the lipid signal transduction enzymes PI3K (Fig. 2) and PLCδ (which activates Ca^{++} flux and protein kinase C, or PKC),[64–66] protein-tyrosine-phosphatases (PTPs),[67,68] other tyrosine kinases (such as Yes and Jak), and other poorly understood proteins (such as Tob).[4,19] The Jak kinase, also critical for signal transduction from the prolactin and growth hormone receptors, signals gene transcription directly through signal transduction- and transcription-activating (STAT) transcription factors.[68]

The next step of the EGFR family pathway is the triggering of several mitogen-activated protein (MAP) kinase cascades.[69,70] The Raf-1 serine kinase mediates one of the best known of these signaling cascades. How the Ras-GTP complex formation serves to activate the Raf-1 kinase is still not fully defined, but association of Raf-1 with Ras probably serves to localize Raf-1 in the plane of the plasma membrane, where it can respond to activational signals from the receptor.[71] Separate activational mechanisms for Raf-1 also appear to exist that involve PKC and a family of proteins termed the 14-3-3 family.[72,73] The activated Raf-1 kinase triggers phosphorylation of an MAP kinase termed MEK. MEK-dependent phosphorylation of the ERK-1 and ERK-2 kinases leads to their nuclear translocation, where they modulate gene function by phosphorylation of transcription factors.[74,75]

The MAP kinase family is recognized as central to mitogenic signals and to other types of phosphorylation-dependent signal transduction pathways (see Fig. 1). A diverse series of phosphotyrosine, phosphoserine, and phosphothreonine kinase pathways, as well as some G-protein–mediated pathways from other receptor types, may mediate mitogenic signals in this manner.[75] Although the earliest described MAP kinase pathway was the Ras-Raf system, a second important pathway (termed a stress response MAP kinase pathway) is triggered by Ras-MEKK1 interactions. Ras-PI3K interactions trigger a third pathway, involving phospholipid-activated kinases.[76] Collectively, MAP kinases activate transcription or phosphorylation of the nuclear c-Myc, c-Fos/c-Jun, c-Ets, ATF, and NFkB transcription factors. Phosphorylation of these nuclear proteins regulates their transcription activity.[77–79] A general mechanism for control of transcription factor activity is through their heterodimer formation (exemplified by Myc-Max and Fos-Jun); regulation of the amount and the phosphorylation state of each heterodimeric partner serves a modulatory role.[77,80] Mitogen-inducible phosphatases are also thought to act in a regulatory fashion to attenuate MAP kinase pathways.[81] Members of this complex series of cascades, down to the level of the MAP kinases, have been demonstrated to have oncogenic potential in model systems or in various human cancers.[82] Specifically, MAP kinase activities are also elevated in hormone-independent breast cancers in comparison with hormone-dependent cancers.[83] Currently, a large body of work is also addressing the roles in breast cancer of the Fak, Src, Raf, and Ras^H gene products. For example, in human breast cancer, a high level of protooncogene polymorphism (rare alleles) occurs, which might suggest structural alterations in the Ras protein[84]; elevated levels of the three signaling kinases, Fak, Src, and Raf, also have been reported.[1] Of the transcription factors themselves, only c-Myc (described in more detail in the section c-Myc Nuclear Oncoproteins) has been clearly demonstrated to date to be a potentially important oncogene in breast cancer.[85]

A great deal of research is under way to make the final links in signal transduction from transcription factors to mitosis, cell differentiation, and cell survival (see Fig. 1). In yeast, the protein kinases at the end of the mitogenic pathways are CDC2 and CDC28; the mammalian homologue is termed p34^{cdc2} (or cyclin-dependent kinase 1, CDK1). Again, this family of kinases forms complexes with activating members of the cyclin family and with inhibitory proteins termed CDK inhibitors (CDKIs). As is discussed later (in the section Cyclins, Cyclin-Dependent Kinases, and Cyclin-Dependent Kinase Inhibitors) in breast cancer, one of the principal oncogenes (cyclin D_1) and a major suppressor gene (the CDKI termed p16) are found in this group. Cyclins are regulatory subunits of the kinases. Different cyclin-kinase complexes catalyze different phosphorylations required for the cell cycle; examples are histones (for mitotic condensation of chromatin), nuclear lamina (for mitotic dissolution of the nuclear membrane), and the retinoblastoma tumor-suppressor protein (for release of a G_1 mitotic blockade).[86] This entire system is discussed in greater detail in the later section of this chapter, Cyclins, Cyclin-Dependent Kinases, and Cyclin-Dependent Kinase Inhibitors.

A second class of genes downstream of growth factor–signaling pathways modulates differentiation. For example, prolactin, growth hormone, and EGFR family members (particularly Erb-b2) promote lactational differentiation, probably to a large degree through the Jak-STAT pathways.[68] Further downstream, CDKIs (such as p16 and p27) and c-Myc heterodimers with Mad or Mxi-l are thought to promote differentiation. In addition, the TGF-βR family elicits differentiation-promoting effects through the SMAD signal transduction/transcription factor system. Among these pathways, the TGF-β system may function in a powerful, tumor suppressor–like manner; however, inactivating mutations have not yet been commonly detected in the system in breast can-

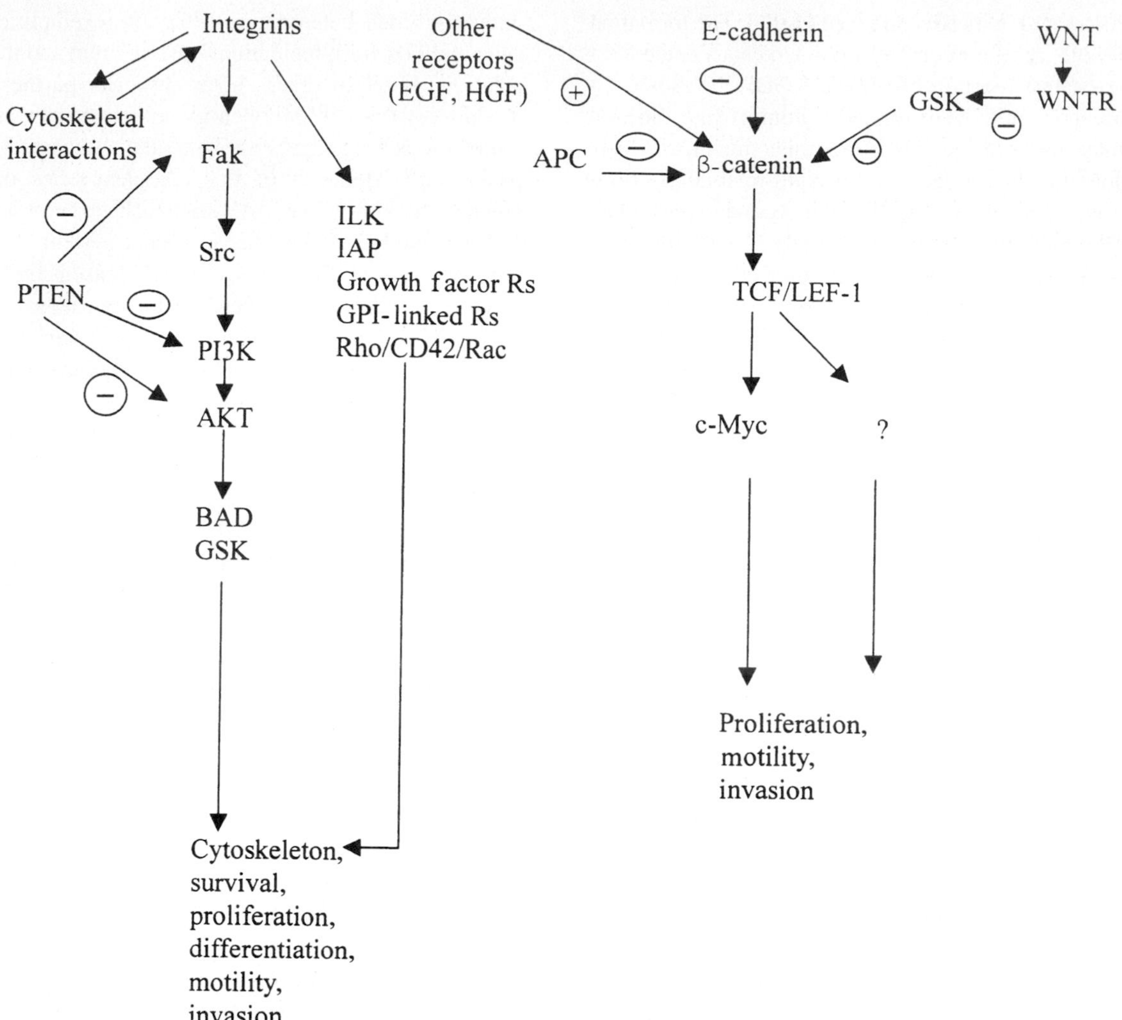

FIG. 2. Integrin and cadherin adhesion molecules also signal multiple cellular processes. Integrins carry signals from the extracellular matrix to the cell. Several kinase systems are activated by integrins, one pathway of which is attenuated by the tumor-suppressor phosphatase on chromosome ten (PTEN). Integrins also interact with multiple receptors and the cytoskeleton. In turn, the cytoskeleton can regulate the distribution and function of integrins on the cell surface. The transcription factor β-catenin serves as a nexus of control by E-cadherin–mediated cell-cell adhesion, several receptors, and the APC tumor-suppressor gene. β-Catenin regulates the TCF (T-cell factor) family of transcription factors and the transcription of *c-myc*. Thus, several oncoproteins and tumor-suppressor proteins also reside in these adhesion-dependent signal transduction pathways, including c-Myc, Fak, E-cadherin, and PTEN. EGF, epidermal growth factor; HGF, hyperglycemic-glycogenolytic factor.

cer, and TGF-β serves instead to promote tumor progression through aberrant tumor-host interactions (such as angiogenesis) as the disease proceeds.[87]

The third type of receptor-mediated influence, survival promotion, also contains many clues to mechanisms of oncogenesis and tumor suppression. The survival-promoting Bcl-2 and Bcl-X_L proteins are considered to be oncogene candidates, and the death-promoting Bax and Bcl-Xs are suppressor gene candidates in breast cancer; the former are induced by growth factor and sex steroid pathways, whereas the latter are induced by the multihormonal withdrawal of lactational involution of the gland. However, no common gene amplifications, mutations, or deletions have been observed to date for these gene families in breast cancer.[1]

Clinical Significance of Overexpression of Epidermal Growth Factor Receptor Family and Ligand Family Systems

As described in Chapter 2, EGFR, a tyrosine-kinase–associated receptor, and some of its ligands (EGF, TGF-α, and AR) are closely associated, probably in a causal fashion, with mammary epithelial development, proliferation, and survival. TGF-α mRNA and protein have been detected in 70% or more of human breast cancer biopsies, compared with 30% of benign breast lesion biopsies.[5,88,89] TGF-α has been detected by immunoassay both in fibroadenomas and in 25% to 50% of primary human mammary carcinomas.[5,90] An EGF-related protein of 43 kd has also been isolated from the urine of breast cancer patients.[91] Probably, detection of TGF-α/EGF in tumor biopsies, serum, or urine will eventually be found to be useful in determining prognosis or tumor burden, although this is not yet proven. Expression of AR and neuregulin-1 is also detected by immunohistochemistry in a significant proportion of primary breast tumors.[5,92,93] Other members of the EGF family of ligands (EGF itself, HbEGF, the neuregulins, and cripto-1) are also produced in breast cancer, but their prevalence and functions are less clear at present.[5]

The current data suggesting that EGFR is a clinical prognostic indicator and its inverse relationship with ER in both tumors and cell lines emphasize the need to understand the mechanisms of regulation of EGFR in breast cancer.[10,26,94–96] Human breast tumor lines exhibit substantial variation in their level of EGFR, and the mechanisms responsible for elevated EGFR differ.[97] Cell lines have been identified that contain EGFR gene amplifications with or without gene rearrangements and with or without overexpression of EGFR in the absence of gene amplification. Human cell lines expressing a nonrearranged EGFR gene contain two major species of EGFR mRNA (10 kb and 5.6 kb); the levels of these transcripts and EGFR protein are usually closely correlated. Differences in expression are controlled at least in part at the level of transcription; EGFR gene amplification appears to be a rare event in breast cancer (occurring in less than 5% of cases). Overexpression of the EGF receptor also appears to signal poor tumor prognosis and poor response to tamoxifen citrate therapy.[98,99]

Of the three other EGFR family members, c-Erb-b2, c-Erb-b3, and c-Erb-b4,[4,100] all of which have also been detected in breast cancer, the former appears to be the most critically involved in tumor growth, differentiation, and prognosis. Over a large number of studies, 20% to 30% of primary, invasive breast cancers overexpress c-Erb-b2 receptor protein; approximately 90% of these tumors overexpress the oncogene as a result of gene amplification. The c-Erb-b2 receptor protein is overexpressed in a larger proportion of cases of ductal carcinoma *in situ*[101,102] and in essentially 100% of comedo carcinomas at a very early stage of malignancy. However, it is poorly expressed in lobular carcinoma *in situ*. Thus, Erb-b2 seems to be correlated with an early transition to invasiveness selectively in the ductal morphotype. The expression of Erb-b2 is associated with a high cellular mitotic rate; it has been reported to correlate with poor clinical response to certain chemotherapeutic and antihormonal drugs (regimens containing 5-fluorouracil, methotrexate, cyclophosphamide, or tamoxifen citrate) and insensitivity to tamoxifen citrate and *cis*-platinum *in vitro*.[20,103–106] In contrast, Erb-b2 expression is also associated with a better patient response to therapy regimens containing doxorubicin.[107] Mechanisms of these effects may relate to an interference with DNA repair mechanisms,[108] an activational phosphorylation of the ER,[109] and promotion of cell survival mechanisms.[110] Another potentially interesting application of Erb-b2 expression is as a marker of tumor burden. Autoantibodies have been detected in the sera of tumor-bearing patients, and the shed extracellular domain of the Erb-b2 protein may represent an additional useful blood-borne marker of the disease.[111] Finally, the Erb-b2 protein, like the EGF receptor,[112] may be an effective target of cancer immunotherapy. Current clinical trials with the humanized anti-Erb-b2 antibody trastuzumab (Herceptin) are consistent with this possibility.[7,113] Active targeting of Erb-b2 protein for immunotherapy was also suggested by a study demonstrating that a lymphoplasmocytic infiltrate is indicative of good prognosis for an Erb-b2–positive subset of patients. In this study, the authors observed that tumor growth–inhibitory antibodies were produced by peripheral lymphocytes from these patients.[114] Because c-*erb*-b2 gene amplification predominates in breast tumors *in situ* and is associated with poor prognosis, it could hypothetically serve as a direct modulator of metastatic capacity. However, based on data with tumor models, any effect of Erb-b2 on metastasis would appear to be indirect and to require additional mutations.[115]

ADHESION-DEPENDENT SIGNAL TRANSDUCTION

Growth factor–dependent and hormone-dependent signaling are not the only important signal transduction pathways that derive from the cell surface (see Fig. 2). Two important classes of adhesion-dependent signals also play roles in cell growth, differentiation, and survival, as well as in motility and invasion of breast cancer.[116–118] Homotypic epithelial cell-cell junctions depend on the E-cadherin protein to form cell-cell bonds. A submembranous complex of cadherins and other proteins then assembles to engage the cytoskeleton. Thus, not only does E-cadherin serve to restrict cell motility, but it also diminishes the cytoplasmic pool of the important proliferation-modulating β-catenin transcription factor. Likewise, β-catenin function or degradation is modulated by its growth factor–dependent phosphorylation and its complexation with the APC (adenosis polyposis cell) protein. The tumor-suppressive E-cadherin gene is commonly silenced by methylation or mutation in breast cancer, releasing β-catenin to potentially up-regulate expression of the c-*myc* protooncogene.[119–120] The β-catenin pathway may also be up-regulated by growth factor pathways, such as EGF, hyperglycemic-glycogenolytic factor, and WNT (wingless) signaling.[121]

Epithelial cell–substrate adhesion is largely regulated by the complex integrin family of heterodimeric proteins. Integrins signal cells through many pathways, but one that has received considerable current interest is the Fak-Src pathway.

Activation of these two tyrosine-kinase–encoding oncoproteins activates the PI3K and AKT candidate oncoproteins, leading to multiple aspects of malignant behavior.[116–118] Of considerable interest, the tumor-suppressive phosphatase on chromosome ten, or PTEN (the gene that carries the mutation responsible for Cowden disease), acts on Fak, PI3P, and AKT as its substrates to suppress survival and induce apoptosis. However, mutations of *PTEN* do not appear to be particularly common in sporadic breast cancer.[122–124]

Drugs that target the mitogenic cascade could represent new classes of anticancer therapy. Current approaches involve tyrosine kinase inhibitors such as tyrophostins[82,125] and other classes, and inhibitors of Ras farnesylation, which may block its membrane localization.[126,127] Studies have also determined that a natural inhibitory pathway for the tyrosine kinase signal transduction cascade is regulated by cAMP; cAMP inhibits Ras activation of the Raf-1 kinase by means of inhibitory phosphorylations. Thus, drugs that activate protein kinase A may have potential as new anticancer therapeutics.[128–130] However, much work remains to define the principal hormonal regulators of cAMP in normal and malignant breast tissue.

Some work has also identified a separate signal transduction pathway shared by EGF, interferons, interleukins, prolactin, other cytokines, and growth hormone (see Fig. 1).[131] Receptor binding triggers autophosphorylation and activation of cytoplasmic TYK and Jak tyrosine kinases. The molecular mechanisms of receptor-Jak interaction are still under study. The activated Jak kinases phosphorylate STAT family proteins. Once phosphorylated, STAT proteins translocate to the nucleus and act as transcription factors to regulate genes containing GAS or ISRE sequences in their promoters.[132] Function of this pathway does not depend on the Ras protein.[133] The role of this pathway has not yet been defined in breast cancer. However, the pathway could conceivably be activated to mediate adverse responses of the tumor to cytokines of the immune system.

C-MYC NUCLEAR ONCOPROTEIN

Regulation of nuclear protooncogenes occurs by growth-promoting steroids, by growth factors, and by adhesion in many tissues. Nuclear protooncogenes may thus be regulated by convergent pathways of growth regulatory stimuli through direct steroid action, through growth factor–induced or adhesion-induced signal transduction, or through cytokine-induced Jak-STAT pathways.[68,133–135] For example, protooncogene products of the c-*fos*, c-*myc*, c-*myb*, and c-*jun* genes are commonly observed to be induced shortly after mitogenic treatment of cells. Many studies support a causal link between induction of this gene superfamily and proliferation processes. In breast cancer, the products of at least three nuclear protooncogenes (c-*myc*, c-*fos*, and c-*jun*) appear to be induced by both estrogen and progesterone.[85,134] Progestins have been shown to induce c-*jun*-b, a protooncogene related to c-*jun*.[134] Antihormonal therapy may also modulate these genes; tamoxifen citrate down-modulates c-*myc* expression during treatment-induced tumor regression in patient tumors.[136] In the context of proliferation of the normal gland, whether these nuclear protooncogenes are regulatory is not known. However, c-*myc*, c-*fos,* and c-*jun* induction have been shown to occur in the rat uterus in response to estrogen treatment.[109,137] The protein products of the c-*fos* and c-*jun* genes contain specific domains allowing them to form a heterodimeric complex that can interact with a gene-promoter consensus sequence termed AP-1. Similarly, the c-*myc* gene product dimerizes with another protein termed Max (or Myn in the mouse) to modulate genes through a different consensus sequence termed an E-box (and possibly through other sequences). The availability of Max for productive dimerization with Myc depends on the availability of other family members, termed Mad and Mxi-1. Max interaction with either of these proteins serves to reduce its availability for Myc interactions and possibly to exert negative transactivational effects through E-box sites. Myc-Max dimers are known to induce proliferation, apoptosis, and chromosomal instability, depending on the cellular context and degree of expression. One transactivational mechanism involves Myc-Max interaction with the TATA binding protein (TBP) to stimulate basal transcription. A specific transactivational mechanism involves E-box proteins, such as the CAD, DHFR, and ODC enzymes.[138] However, many Myc-regulated genes do not appear to possess E-boxes, and E-box-interactive sequences do not appear to be required for Myc effects on proliferation and apoptosis.[139] A handful of Myc-interactive proteins other than TBP and Max are found; they include TRRAP, Bin1, DAM, p107, YYI, Mizl, and TFII-1. Thus, multiple other potential mechanisms for transactivational and transcriptional suppressive effects of Myc may exist.[138] A primary effect of c-*myc* expression on the mammary epithelial cell cycle appears to be induction of both synthesis of cyclin E and degradation of p27, activating CDK2 and inhibiting Rb-1 by phosphorylation. A second primary effect appears to be induction of cyclin A, activating CDK2.[85,138,140]

Use of antisense oligonucleotides directed against the c-Myc mRNA has demonstrated that the estrogen-induced Myc protein is critical for estrogen induction of proliferation in breast cancer cells.[141] Two oncogenelike coactivators of the estrogen receptor in this process appear to be the AIB1/Src-3 protein and the cyclin D_1 protein.[142,143] Each of the oncogenes is amplified in approximately one-third of breast cancers.[1] Amplification of the c-*myc* gene is also one of the most common genetic alterations in breast cancer; approximately one-third of breast cancers contain this genetic change.[144–147] A putative (but currently unidentified) suppressor gene on 1p32-pter is proposed to control c-*myc* amplification in breast cancer. Study of the expression of the c-*myc* gene in breast cancer has been slow because of difficulties in measuring the protein in tumor biopsies. The protein has a very short half-life. In addition, suitable monoclonal antibodies capable of staining paraffin sections are lacking. Several studies focusing on gene amplification have shown that c-*myc* is associated with poor prognosis,[85,147–149] high S phase,[150] and postmenopausal disease,[151] although the latter has not been confirmed. A meta-analysis of the published data has confirmed the poor prognostic significance of c-*myc* gene amplification.[152] Studies of various epithelial malignancies, including those of the ovary and liver,[153] have shown that c-*myc* amplification is associated with TGF-α overexpression. Dual stimulation of the EGFR pathway and c-Myc may serve a general cooperative function in epithelial survival or transformation, or both.[85,153–155]

As noted, the Myc protein acts in multiple systems to regulate gene expression, to promote cell proliferation, to inhibit differentiation, to modulate cell adhesion, and to effect immune recognition.[85,138] Cellular proliferation is modulated because Myc regulates initiation of DNA replication. The most clearly defined gene regulatory activities of the protein[138] encompass both activation and suppression; cell cycle, apoptosis, DNA metabolism, DNA dynamics, energy metabolism, and macromolecular synthesis are all involved. The c-*myc* protooncogene product can be used to immortalize cells[156] and modulate their responsiveness to growth factors.[157,158] Another interesting feature of c-*myc* amplification is that it may so dysregulate the cell cycle that programmed cell death results.[85,138] This process depends on $p19^{ARF}$-mediated activation of the p53 tumor-suppressor gene, at least in fibroblasts[157–160]; however, this mechanism has not yet been demonstrated in mammary cancer.[161]

As studies have proceeded, a variety of other malignancy-associated biological consequences of c-*myc* amplification have been described. Reports have suggested that expression of the c-*myc* gene may allow amplification of other genes,[138] may alter cellular resistance to *cis*-platinum and other drugs inducing DNA strand scission,[162] and may act to suppress differentiation in association with the decrease of collagen gene transcription.[163] The Myc protein also inhibits transcription of the rat *neu* oncogene (c-*erb*-b2 homologue).[164] Although the importance of this interaction for human breast cancer is not yet known, the c-*myc* amplification appears not to be closely associated with c-*erb*-b2 amplification in primary breast cancer.[85] Another aspect of c-Myc function (discussed in more detail in the section Cell Senescence and Immortalization Controls) may relate to the aging and senescence process. Increased expression of the protooncogene product in multiple tissue types with aging may reflect cumulative proliferation-associated dysregulation and may contribute to aberrant mitogenic responses of the tissue in postmenopausal breast cancer.[165] However, increased expression of the Myc partner Mxi-1 is also enhanced during aging and may attenuate the effects of Myc.[166]

To study its role in transformation, the c-*myc* gene and other oncogenes have been introduced into immortalized human or mouse mammary epithelial cells using an amphotropic retroviral vector. It was observed that c-*myc* or *SV40T* nuclear oncogene (but not v-ras^H or v-*mos*) allowed the cells to grow in soft agar in response to fibroblast growth factor 1 (FGF-1), FGF-2, EGF, or TGF-α.[158,167] Because mammary fibroblasts produce EGF-related and FGF-related growth factors,[168] and because their conditioned media could support transforming growth of nuclear-oncogene–transfected mammary epithelial cells,[158] these observations have supported a role *in vivo* for stromal-epithelial interactions. This synergy has been observed *in vitro* in TGF-α/Myc bitransgenic mice. Expression of these two gene products allows rapid onset (10 weeks) of highly proliferative mammary tumors, independent of sex hormones in either sex.[154,155] These data suggest that an amplified c-*myc* gene may function in breast cancer to allow growth factors or hormones to drive aberrant, transformed growth.[85]

CYCLINS, CYCLIN-DEPENDENT KINASES, AND CYCLIN-DEPENDENT KINASE INHIBITORS

Stimulatory and inhibitory growth factors, sex steroids, and tumor suppressors primarily function in the G_1 phase of the cell cycle (see Fig. 2). The cell cycle is tightly controlled by a series of cyclin-dependent kinases (CDKs), their positive regulatory subunits (cyclins), and their inhibitors (cyclin-dependant kinase inhibitors, or CDKIs). The early G_1 phase is driven by cyclin Ds bound to CDK4 and CDK6, whereas the G_1-S transition is driven by cyclin E–CDK2. The S phase itself is driven by cyclin A-CDK2, and the G_2-M transition is driven by cyclin B/A–CDK2 (DDK1). Tyrosine-kinase–acting growth factors and sex steroids induce both c-Myc and cyclin D_1, whereas Myc itself may suppress D_1, induce degradation of the CDKI termed p27 (CDI1 and CIP2), induce the activational CDK phosphatase CDC25A, and induce cyclin E. The cyclin D_1–CDK4/CDK6 complexes are inhibited by several CDKIs, including p16 (or INKA, CDK4I, or MTS-1), p15 (or INK4B or MTS-2, which is induced by senescence and TGF-β), p18, and p19, all of which are structurally related proteins. Synthesis of CDK4 is thus inhibited by TGF-β; overexpression of this CDK leads to TGF-β resistance, at least in model systems. Estrogen and progesterone both stimulate the cell cycle, although their effects are not identical. Both steroids induce cyclin D_1 and c-Myc and then promote the redistribution of p21 from CDK2 to CDK4 to provide cycle directionality; however, only estrogen induces multiple cell cycles. Progesterone, in contrast, induces p27 and the related p21 CDKI to block subsequent cycles, as it promotes differentiation. Two other CDKIs, p21 and p57, are described later in this section and in the section on Cell Death and DNA Repair Controls in the context of DNA damage control and cellular senescence. To integrate all of these signals, Rb-1 is phosphorylated and inactivated by the cyclin D–CDK4/CDK6 and cyclin E–CDK2 kinases, leading to induction of genes (such as cyclin A) that are important in the S phase. As noted in the section on the C-Myc Nuclear Oncoprotein, cyclin A is also a direct transcriptional target of c-Myc.[138,140,169–174]

A major body of very exciting work has begun to implicate cyclins as oncogenes and CDKIs as tumor suppressors. Although studies involving breast cancer are just beginning, the cyclin D_1 gene appears to be commonly amplified[175,176] in this disease, and the cyclin E gene is also under study as a candidate oncogene (although it is seldom amplified). Both cyclins can function as mammary cancer–inducing oncogenes when driven by the MMTV promoter in the transgenic mouse.[36] Interestingly, cyclin D_1 is selectively required for lobuloalveolar development of the mammary gland, as described by gene knockout studies in the mouse.[177] Cyclin D_1 amplification in breast cancer may serve two separate oncogenic roles; both estrogen receptor coactivational and CDK activational mechanisms are evident. Probably because of its association with the estrogen receptor, amplification of the cyclin D_1 gene signifies favorable prognosis in breast cancer.[170,175] Whereas little doubt exists that cyclin D_1 serves an oncogenic role in human breast cancer, less certainty is found regarding cyclin E. Although the cyclin E gene is seldom amplified in breast cancer, it is commonly overexpressed and is associated with poor prognosis of the disease.[178,179]

Studies have also implicated the CDK inhibitor p16 as a major tumor suppressor, at least in cancer cell lines; the incidence of inactivation of this gene in primary tumors such as breast cancer is under current investigation, but it appears to involve both methylation to silence gene expression and mutation.[180–182] Interestingly, an alternate reading frame variant of this CDKI has been identified to additionally activate the function of the p53 protein by interacting with its MDM-2–binding protein. This results in induction of p21 and allows proliferative arrest by a second mechanism. Mutation of the p53 gene (often associated with accumulation of its protein) and expression of the p21 gene are under current study as possible indicators of poor and good prognosis, respectively.[183,184] Whereas p16 is clearly a tumor suppressor in breast cancer, p27 has also stimulated much additional interest in this regard, although the p27 gene is seldom mutated in the disease. This CDKI is apparently haplo-insufficient for tumor suppression, so that only its down-regulation is required to attenuate its tumor-suppressive abilities.[185–187]

Finally, Rb-1 has been recognized for many years as an important tumor-suppressor gene in breast cancer. However, multiple nongenetic mechanisms appear to exist for blockade of its function to allow aberrant cell cycle control.[188]

CELL DEATH AND DNA REPAIR CONTROLS

Breast cancer, like most other malignancies, is characterized by an instability in its genome and in its chromosomes. As noted earlier, most oncogenic mechanisms known to exist in the disease result from gene amplification. Gene amplification is thought to result from the combination of spindle defects (which also lead to aneuploidy) and defects in cell cycle checkpoint control (Fig. 3). In contrast, loss of tumor-suppressor gene function in breast cancer is thought to result from a combination of point mutagenesis, loss of heterozygosity, homozygous deletion, and gene silencing by methylation.[189] Some studies[190] have suggested that DNA synthesis itself is error prone in human breast cancer cell lines. In addition, the microsatellite type of genomic instability has been detected in metastatic breast cancer and in ductal carcinoma *in situ*, although this mechanism seems much less prevalent in breast cancer than in colon cancer.[191]

What mechanisms exist for cell cycle checkpoint control and DNA repair? The answers are rapidly emerging from clues in familial breast cancer. Broca[192] established in the previous century that breast cancer may have a pattern of high familial incidence in 5% to 10% of cases. Families showing a very high incidence of the disease sometimes have been noted to exhibit a high incidence of an additional cancer, such as ovarian cancer. Such families have been thought to inherit a defective or deleted allele encoding a tumor-suppressor gene. This supposition has been based largely on work by Knudson postulating the inactivation of two alleles of a gene in retinoblastoma[193] and work by Harris and coworkers demonstrating that certain chromosomes can suppress malignancy in cell-cell hybridization studies.[194]

The first tumor-suppressor gene shown to be associated with inherited breast cancer was termed *TP53* (on 17p13). Mutations in this locus were inherited in families with the rare breast cancer and sarcoma syndrome termed Li-Fraumeni syndrome[195]; the *TP53* gene encodes a multifunctional damage response protein. The larger group of patients with an inherited pattern of breast or ovarian cancer has also been characterized by more recent studies. The chromosomal locations of the two major genes responsible for the breast and ovarian cancer syndrome as well as the familial breast cancer only syndrome were reported in the early 1990s.[196,197] They are now known to be zinc finger–containing DNA-binding proteins whose genes, termed *BRCA1* and *BRCA2,* are located on 17q21 and 13q12-13, respectively.[198] The BRCA proteins also function in DNA repair. A third familial breast cancer locus, termed *PTEN,* was more recently localized to 10q23; its inherited mutation gives rise to Cowden disease.[3] *PTEN* encodes a tyrosine phosphatase that blocks cell survival signaling (discussed in this section).

The *TP53* gene is a tumor-suppressor gene, but when it is mutated in one of several sensitive regions, its conformation of the cognate protein changes, its stability increases, and it functions as an inhibitor of unmutated p53. In addition, gain of function mutations has been described.[199,200] The *TP53* gene may be mutated differently in African-American women with high mortality from the disease than in a corresponding white control population with breast cancer.[201] Although p53 is considered to be a nuclear protein, some have also proposed that p53 may be excluded from the cell nucleus by an unknown mechanism to prevent its func-

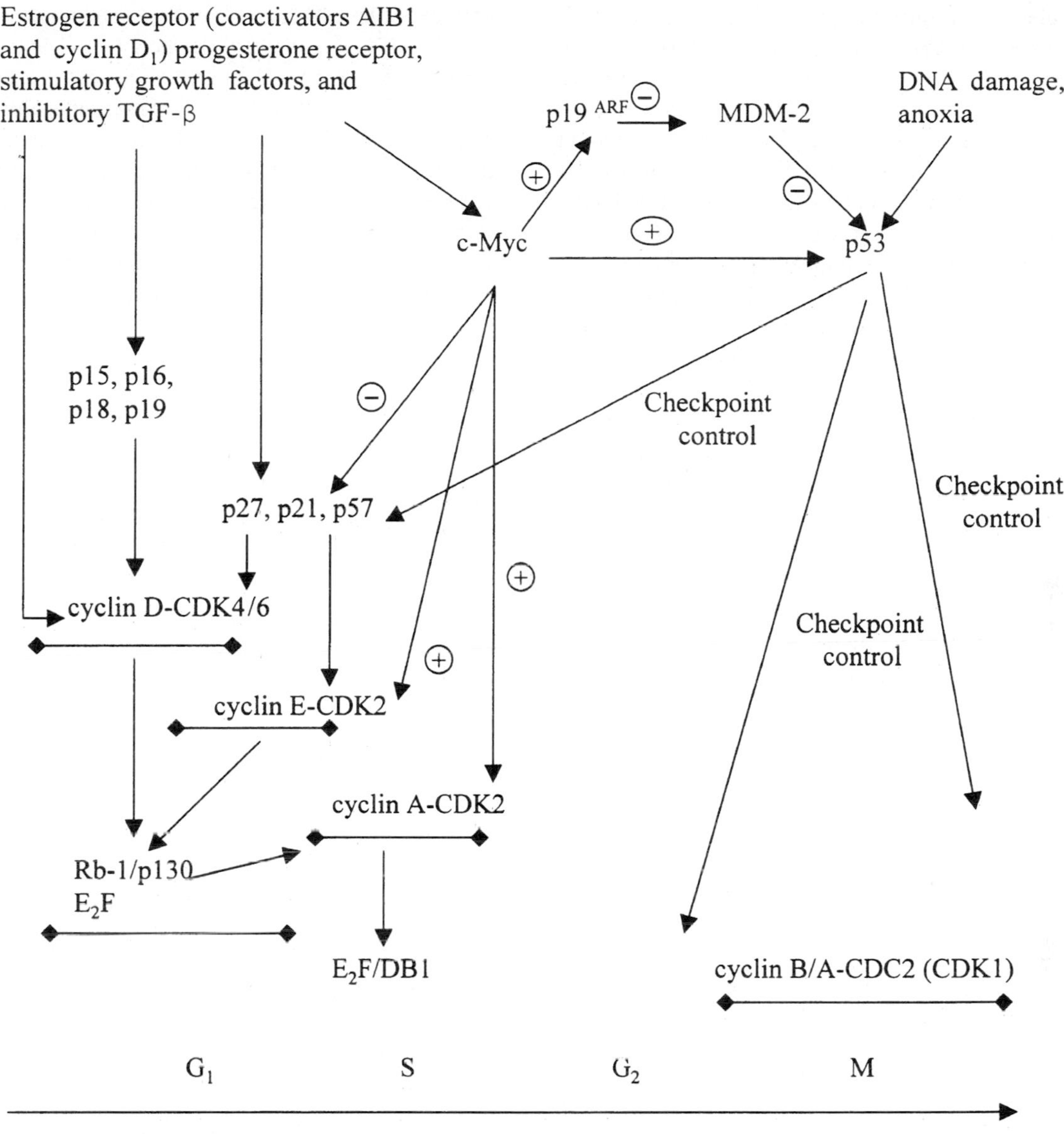

FIG. 3. The cell cycle is normally regulated by sex steroid and growth factor receptors, which primarily regulate G_1 and G_1-S through their actions on cyclin D_1, c-Myc, and the seven cyclin-dependent kinase inhibitors. The best-defined targets of G_1 and G_1-S cyclin-dependent kinases are Rb-1 and p130, which release E_2F to allow transactivation of genes involved in cell cycle progression. The major cell cycle checkpoint control molecule is p53; it is activated through c-Myc–induced derepression of MDM-2, and it is induced by c-Myc, DNA damage, and hypoxia. Important breast cancer oncogenes here are those for cyclin D_1, AIB1, and c-Myc, whereas those for p53, p16, and Rb-1 serve tumor suppressive roles. TGF-β, transforming growth factor β.

tion.[202] The p53 protein is known to be an oligomeric DNA-binding protein that regulates expression of DNA damage-response genes of MDM-2 (a p53-binding antagonist), the CDKI p21, the DNA replication–promoting PCNA, the apoptosis-inducing Bax, and the DNA repair proteins cyclin G, ERCC, and Gadd-45. The properties of p53, when transfected into cells, include cell cycle blockade at the G_1-S boundary, induction of apoptosis, and induction of differentiation. Thus, p53 appears to function in the context of DNA damage to slow cell growth and induce DNA repair. Loss of p53 function may thus importantly contribute to the genomic and chromosomal instability of cancer. However, some programmed cell death pathways do not depend on p53. Furthermore, overexpression of survival-promoting

Bcl-2 and related family members may suppress multiple types of apoptotic pathways in cancer.[202–206] Mutations in the *TP53* gene have been detected in approximately 30% of breast tumors, ranging from ductal carcinoma *in situ* to metastatic lesions; however, hyperplasias do not exhibit these mutations.[207] As noted earlier, a group of studies strongly implicates the p53 tumor-suppressor protein in cell cycle controls. This protein is induced by DNA damage and anoxia. The MDM-2 protein is induced by p53; it commonly serves in a negative-feedback autoregulatory loop unless countered by $p19^{ARF}$, a c-Myc-inducible protein.[208] The p53 protein then serves to induce p21, blocking the cell cycle in G_1; however, it also serves as a DNA/chromatin/spindle apparatus checkpoint controller at the G_2-M interface and at the exit of the M phase.[207,208] Two *TP53*-related genes termed *p73* and *p63* have been described; however, their roles in breast cancer are unknown.[209]

The *BRCA1* gene is probably the most prevalent familial risk gene for breast cancer. Mutations in this gene are particularly common in breast cancer among Ashkenazi Jewish women, some of whom belong, surprisingly, to families nearly devoid of multiple afflicted members. Although the *BRCA1* gene is mutated in familial breast and ovarian cancer patients, mutations have not been detected in sporadic breast cancers. These results suggest that BRCA1 may be a specialized tumor-suppressor gene of specific relevance to tumor onset.[198] Some studies, however, have reported that the BRCA1 protein, normally nuclear, has a cytoplasmic localization or decreased levels in breast cancer cell lines from sporadic tumors, suggesting that a nonclassical mode of functional inactivation is at work during the progression of this tumor type. Consistent with this hypothesis, antisense oligonucleotides directed against the BRCA1 mRNA can enhance the proliferation of breast cancer and mammary epithelial cells in culture *in vitro* and in nude mice *in vivo*.[210–212] The BRCA1 protein appears to induce growth arrest by inducing p21.[212] In addition, the BRCA1 protein binds to putative tumor-suppressor proteins termed Bap-1 and Bard-1. BRCA1 and BRCA2 are also thought to be involved in DNA repair through complex formation with the Rad51 protein.[198,213] The BRCA2 protein is strongly homologous to the BRCA1 protein and appears to be nearly indistinguishable in function. Nevertheless, the disease spectrum of the two is not identical; mutant BRCA1 predisposes to female breast and ovarian cancer, whereas mutant BRCA2 is closely associated with female and male breast cancer, independent of ovarian cancer. Interestingly, although BRCA-positive tumors are of rapid onset and aggressive histology, they are not characterized by particularly poor survival characteristics.[214,215] Genetic counseling of high-risk *BRCA* carriers is an active area of research. Preventive tamoxifen citrate regimens and prophylactic mastectomy both appear to be effective for risk reduction.[216,217]

Very exciting work has placed the BRCA1, BRCA2, and p53 proteins at the center of control of cell death (apoptosis) and DNA repair (Fig. 4). DNA damage at the onset or progression of breast cancer may be sensed by the ATM protein, by DNA-PK, or somehow by the BRCA1 and BRCA2 proteins. DNA-PK and ATM serve to induce p53, which forms a complex with the BRCA and Rad51 proteins (probably along with other DNA repair–related proteins). Although p53 may thus be involved in DNA repair, cell cycle arrest (through p21) or apoptosis (through Bax induction), may also occur. Bax is thought to act on the mitochondrion to form pores, which directly or indirectly lead to cytochrome C release. Adhesion, growth factor, and steroid survival factors may counter this effect by inducing or phosphorylating other Bcl family members. Cytochrome C release triggers activation of caspase 9, which activates other death-inducing caspases. Interestingly, cell death receptors at the cell surface mediated by tumor necrosis factor or FasL also have the same effect, but through a different mechanism involving caspase 8.[218–220] *PTEN*, a suppressor gene, also appears to modulate apoptosis by blocking survival pathways through its tyrosine phosphatase activity (see Fig. 2).[221]

INTEGRATION OF GENETIC CHANGES DURING TUMOR PROGRESSION

Cancer is a process involving not only proliferative factors and activation of oncogenes but also loss of suppressor gene function. The role of germ-line deletion or mutation of suppressor genes in familial breast cancer and somatic mutation or deletion during breast tumor progression has been emphasized. Although numerous studies have focused for several years on breast tumor oncogenes, identification of breast tumor suppressor genes is probably only in its infancy.[199]

Malignant progression of breast cancer involves a transition from nearly normal mechanisms of proliferation and apoptosis in its early stages to highly abnormal regulation in metastatic disease.[1,203,222,223] Proliferative and survival alterations early in the disease progression depend on systemic hormones (estrogen and progesterone) and local growth factors (such as TGF-α and the IGFs). Critical additional damage or repair error events may then occur to compound the problem. Early genetic damage in combination with proliferation is thought to trigger gene amplification.[224] Amplification of c-*erb*-b2, c-*myc,* and the *CCDN1* genes in breast cancer may be critical in this respect. Mutations of *TP53* and *Rb-1* suppressor genes and down-modulation of the expression of other proposed suppressor genes appear to be frequently associated with poorer prognosis.[225–227] Finally, response to therapy may critically depend on p21-mediated mechanisms of cycle checkpoint control.[228] A major unknown, however, is the determination of the stage of progression at which these genes become mutated or dysregulated. Mechanisms for mutations and genetic instability in other cancers have been proposed to depend on overexpression of mutator genes such as *MSH2*[229] and on a chromosome stability–regulating gene termed *telomerase* (discussed in the following section). However, these mechanisms for genetic instability have not been demonstrated to date. As multiple genetic alterations occur,

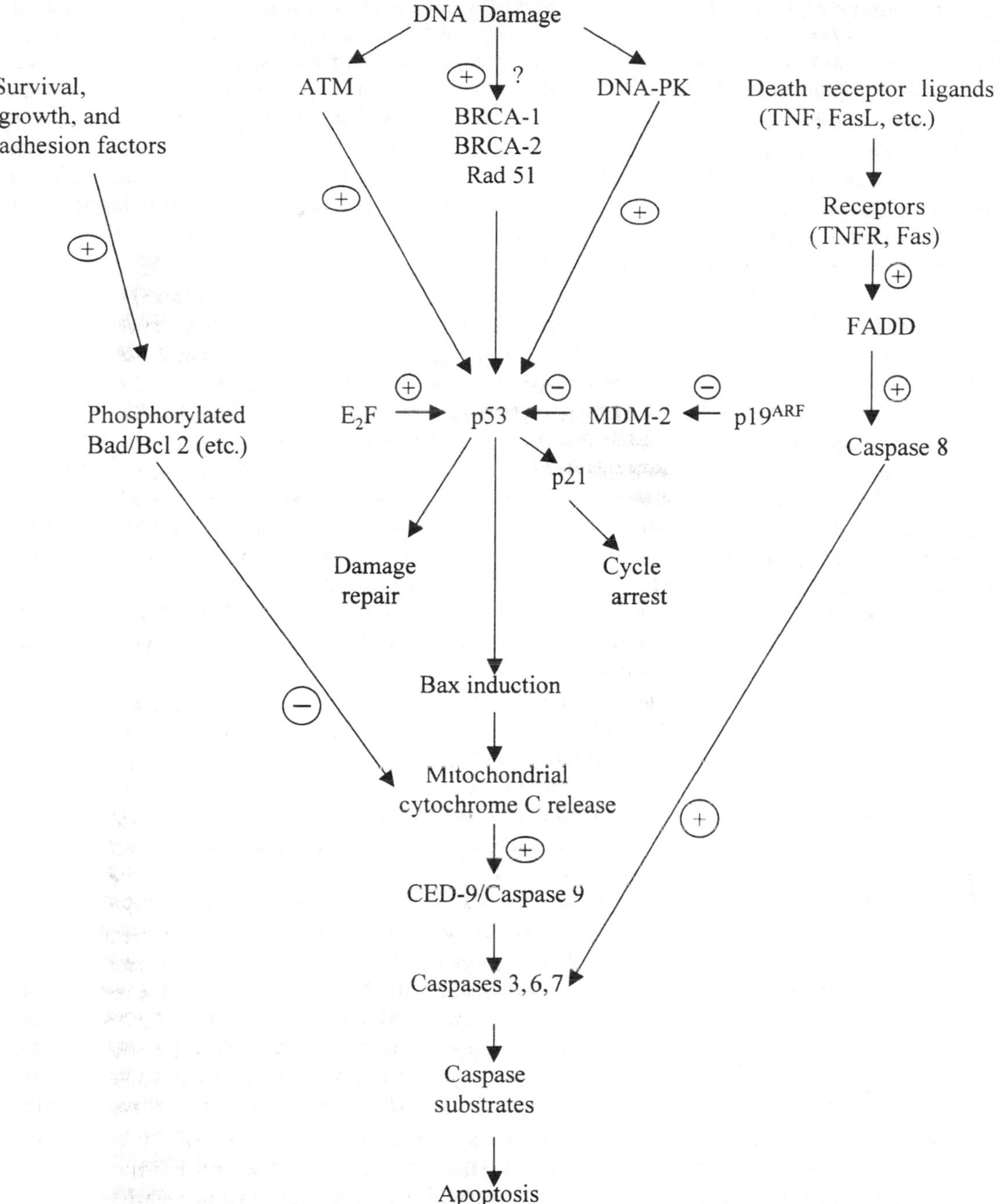

FIG. 4. Cell death is induced by DNA damage, by signaling through death receptors, and by withdrawal of survival-promoting hormones, growth factors, and adhesion signals. Multiple pathways mediate the detection of DNA damage, including the BRCA proteins; p53 is a major mediator of damage-induced cell cycle arrest, DNA repair, or apoptosis. Both p53 and survival factor pathways serve to regulate mitochondrial function to control cytochrome C release and caspase activation. In contrast, death receptors initiate caspase activation independent of mitochondrial involvement. The oncoprotein-like Bcl-2 and its family members function here, as do suppressorlike Bax and related proteins. The BRCA proteins and p53 are well-known tumor suppressors in breast cancer.

cancer cells with the greatest capacity for growth, invasion, and survival undergo positive selection.[230,231]

CELL SENESCENCE AND IMMORTALIZATION CONTROLS

A revolution has occurred in the past few years in the understanding of how cancer may prevent the senescence process and result in immortalization of a cell lineage. The process of aging has been considered to represent a gradual slowdown in the ability of the body to repair and renew itself. In the breast, this process has been connected, in particular, with the onset of menopause and associated arrest of reproductive cycles. However, at the cellular level, aging is considered to result from accumulated physiologic stresses, which lead to a decreased ability to proliferate, and from gradual loss of the enzyme telomerase. These two features are each thought to be associated with important mechanistic hypotheses. Physiologic stresses inhibit the cell cycle, largely through induction of p16 and inhibition of CDK4-CDK6. This mechanism is commonly abrogated in breast cancer, as described earlier. As far as telomerase is concerned, a decreased expression of the enzymatic hTERT component leads to a gradual shortening of telomeres with age and a resultant accumulation of damaged telomeric ends of chromosomes. Telomerase is often overexpressed in breast cancer, even in the earliest steps of the disease (Fig. 5).[232–242]

Research now indicates that amplification and dysregulation of the c-*myc* gene may provide a mechanism for overcoming both aging-associated pathways. Although slightly increased c-*myc* expression has been associated with aging in many tissues, age-dependent expression of its Mxi-1 partner normally would serve to counter its effects. However, in the case of dysregulated or amplified c-*myc*, both of which are common in breast cancer, *telomerase* (a gene regulated by c-Myc) would be induced, and CDK2–cyclin E would be induced (after Myc-dependent p27 degradation, cyclin E induction, and CDC25A induction), overcoming p16-mediated cell cycle arrest.[232,238]

GENE-GENE INTERACTIONS IN TUMOR PROGRESSION

Studies using breast cancer cell lines *in vitro* are currently attempting to sort out the potential biological roles and inter-

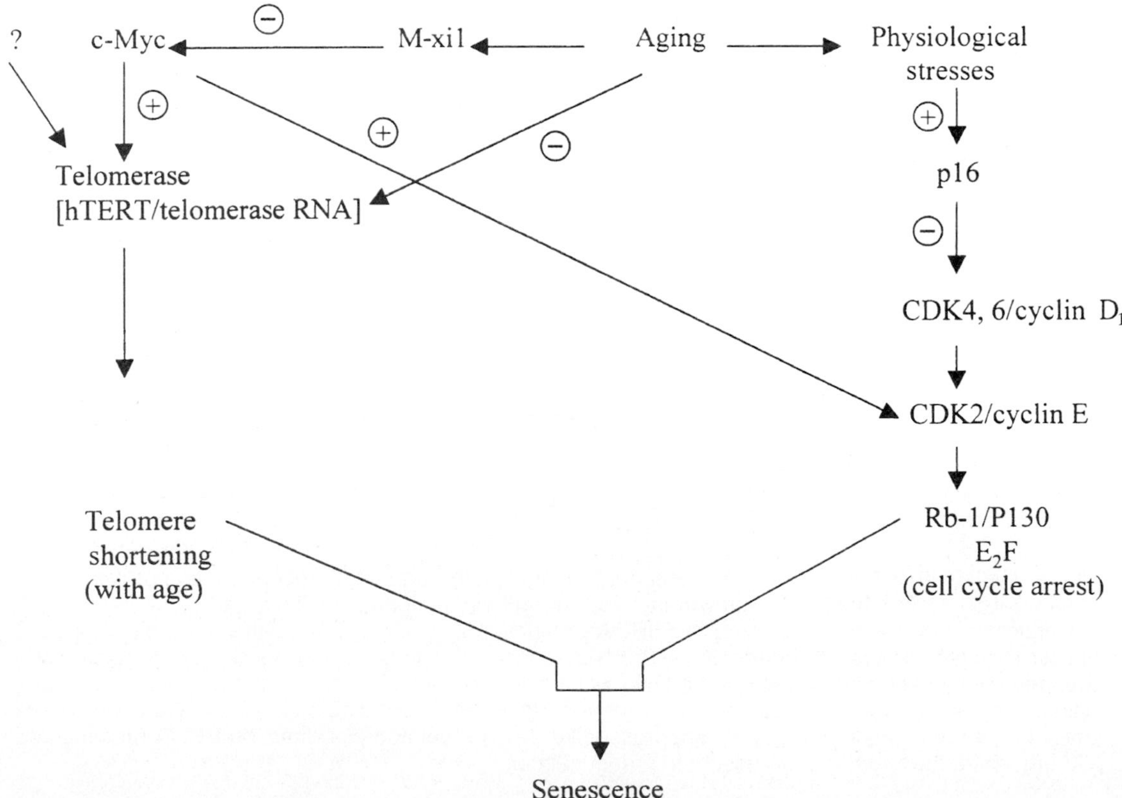

FIG. 5. Cell senescence and immortalization play important roles in breast cancer. Senescence results from the combined effects of age-dependent telomere shortening and cell cycle arrest. Telomerase controls the former; diminution in the levels of telomerase as a result of aging is countered by c-Myc, whose action itself is thought to be under age-dependent control by its antagonist Mxi-1. Aging also induces physiologic stresses, which lead to cell cycle arrest. Although c-Myc and cyclin D_1 are known oncoproteins here, telomerase may have oncogenelike properties. Both p16 and Rb-1 are known suppressors, but Mxi-1 may also have tumor-suppressive properties.

actions of a wide variety of potentially significant tumor prognostic factors. Certain common patterns of cytogenetic defects have also been described in breast tumors.[2,239] Examples were presented concerning the negative prognostic interaction of amplified c-*erb*-b2 or *myc* genes in the presence of an autocrine-activated or paracrine-activated EGF receptor system. Amplification of c-*erb*-b2 is also particularly unfavorable in association with c-ras^H overexpression[240] and mutation of the *TP53* gene.[241] Thus, the tyrosine kinase/ras/MAP kinase pathways are emerging as central in interaction with nuclear oncogenes *in vitro*, in transgenic mouse models of mammary cancer, and in patient prognosis of the disease.[242,243] Another type of interaction is also reported to occur with c-*myc* amplification. As noted previously, the Myc protein is known to simultaneously speed the cell cycle, abrogate checkpoint controls, and trigger apoptosis[138,242]; interactions of c-Myc with survival-promoting growth factors or other oncogenes may be critical for Myc oncogenicity.[154,244] Finally, AIB1 and cyclin D_1 may require expression of the ER gene for important aspects of their function.[170] Transgenic models have validated some of these proposed gene-gene interactions in tumor progression.[36,243,244]

During the malignant progression of breast cancer to its fully metastatic state, mutation, inactivation, loss, or down-regulated expression of tumor-suppressing genes may also occur. The *rb-1* and *TP53* genes are mutated in approximately 20% and 30% of cases, respectively.[245,246] Suppressor protein candidates include the cell-cell adhesion protein E-cadherin,[247] the α_6 integrin subunit,[248] and the IGF-II receptor.[249] The function of each of these appears to be quite different. For example, loss of E-cadherin may activate transcription of c-Myc,[250] whereas IGF-II receptor may sequester IGF-I away from the IGF-I receptor.[249]

METASTASIS-RELATED ONCOGENES AND SUPPRESSOR GENES?

Whether any specific oncogenes or suppressor genes are associated with the process of invasion and metastasis is not yet clear. The three major oncogene-encoded proteins (c-erb-b2, c-Myc, and cyclin D_1) and the four major suppressor gene–encoded proteins (Rb-1, p53, p16, and E-cadherin) are all associated with deregulated cell cycle, aberrant cell death regulation, cell immortalization, and genomic instability. However, none has been specifically implicated as a specific regulator of invasion and metastasis of the disease. Much current investigation is focusing on the roles of E-cadherin–mediated and integrin-mediated pathways in triggering cell motility, on the roles of adhesion and growth factor pathways in triggering protease and angiogenesis pathways, and on the roles of growth factors and adhesion in allowing survival of metastatic deposits in distant organs. In addition, several genes are under investigation as metastatic genes, but with poorly understood mechanisms of action; these include nm23, TSG101 (a signal transduction molecule), KAI-1 (a putative adhesion molecule), and KiSS-1 (a phosphoprotein). Clearly, much research remains to be done in this area of study. Finally, much work has focused on the roles of proteases as ultimate effectors of invasion. Although growth factor pathways acting through PKC and other signal transduction mechanisms are thought to play a role in protease mechanisms, complex stromal-epithelial interactions require much further study in this regard.[251–263]

SUMMARY AND FUTURE PROSPECTS

The study of interactions of growth-regulatory pathways with mutations in genes involved in signal transduction and cell cycle pathways is in its infancy. Almost certainly a major approach for the future understanding of these phenomenon is the transgenic and gene knockout mouse models, with the eventual hope of establishing likely patterns of malignant progressions. At present, however, few studies have focused on combinations of oncogenes, growth factors, and loss of suppressor genes that are thought to be important in the human disease. Future studies aimed at detailed characterization of the interaction of ERs, PgRs, growth factors, and protooncogenes in animal models are likely to shed much light on their interactive roles in the onset and progression of breast cancer. The future outlook is bright, as significant advances in risk assessment (*BRCA* screening), prevention (tamoxifen and mastectomy approaches), and therapy (Herceptin and c-Erb-b2 antibodies) were finally achieved in the late 1990s.[264,265]

REFERENCES

1. Dickson RB, Lippman ME. Molecular biology of breast cancer. In: DeVita VT, Hellman S, Rosenberg SA, eds. *Principles and practice of oncology*, 5th ed. Philadelphia: JP Lippincott Co, 1997:1541.
2. Heim S, Teixeira MR, Pandis N. Cytogenetic approaches to breast cancer. In: Bowcock AM, ed. *Breast cancer: molecular genetics, pathogenesis, and therapeutics*. Totowa, NJ: Humana Press, 1998:373.
3. Callahan R. The role of tumor suppressor genes in breast cancer progression. In: Manni A, ed. *Endocrinology of breast cancer*. Totowa, NJ: Humana Press, 1999:119.
4. Ben-Baruch N, Alroy I, Yarden Y. Developmental and physiologic roles of ErbB receptors and their ligands in mammals. In: Dickson RB, Salomon DS, eds. *Hormones and growth factors in development and neoplasia*. New York: Wiley-Liss, 1998:145.
5. Martinez-Lacaci I, Bianco C, De Santis M, Salomon DS. Epidermal growth factor-related peptides and their cognate receptors in breast cancer. In: Bowcock AM, ed. *Breast cancer: molecular genetics, pathogenesis, and therapeutics*. Totowa, NJ: Humana Press, 1998:31.
6. Esteva-Lorenzo FJ, Sastry L, King CR. The *erb*B-2 gene in human cancer: translation from research to application. In: Dickson RB, Salomon DS, eds. *Hormones and growth factors in development and neoplasia*. New York: Wiley-Liss, 1998:445.
7. Fan Z, Mendelsohn J. Breast cancer therapy using monoclonal antibodies against epidermal growth factor receptor and HER-2. In: Bowcock AM, ed. *Breast cancer: molecular genetics, pathogenesis, and therapeutics*. Totowa, NJ: Humana Press, 1998:419.
8. Fitzpatrick SL, Brightwell J, Wittliff J, Barrows GH, Schultz GS. Epidermal growth factor binding by breast tumor biopsies and relationship to estrogen and progestin receptor levels. *Cancer Res* 1984; 44:3448.

9. Sainsbury JRC, Farndon JR, Sherbert GV, Harris AL. Epidermal growth factor receptors and oestrogen receptors in human breast cancers. *Lancet* 1985;1:364.
10. Klijn JGM, Berns PMJJ, Schmitz PIM, Foekens JA. The clinical significance of epidermal growth factor receptor (EGF-R) in human breast cancer: a review on 5,232 patients. *Endoc Rev* 1992;13:3.
11. Van Agthoven T, Timmermans M, Foekens JA, Dorssers LCJ, Henzen-Logmans SC. Differential expression of estrogen, progesterone, and epidermal growth factor receptors in normal, benign and malignant human breast tissues using dual staining immunohistochemistry. *Am J Pathol* 1994;144:1.
12. Clarke RB, Howell A, Anderson E. Estrogen sensitivity of normal human breast tissue in vivo and implanted into athymic nude mice: analysis of the relationship between estrogen-induced proliferation and progesterone receptor expression. *Breast Cancer Res Treat* 1997;45:121.
13. Cohen S, Ushiro H, Stoscheck C, Chinkers M. A native 170,000 epidermal growth factor receptor-kinase complex from shed plasma membrane vesicles. *J Biol Chem* 1982;257:1523.
14. Ushiro H, Cohen S. Identification of phosphotyrosine as a product of epidermal growth factor-associated protein kinase in A-431 cell membranes. *J Biol Chem* 1980;255:8363.
15. Carpenter G, Cohen S. ^{125}I-labelled human epidermal growth factor (hEGF): binding, internalization, and degradation in human fibroblasts. *J Cell Biol* 1976;71:159.
16. Velu TJ, Beguinot L, Vass WC, et al. Epidermal growth factor dependent transformation by a human EGF receptor proto-oncogene. *Science* 1987;238:1408.
17. DiFiore PP, Pierce JH, Fleming TP, et al. Overexpression of the human EGF receptor confers an EGF-dependent transformed phenotype to NIH3T3 cells. *Cell* 1987;51:1063.
18. Downward J, Yarden Y, Mayes E, et al. Close similarity of epidermal growth factor receptor and v-*erb*B oncogene protein sequence. *Nature* 1984;307:521.
19. Gullick WJ. Type 1 growth factor receptors: current status and future work. In: Rudland PS, Fernig DG, Leinster S, Lunt GG, eds. *Mammary development and cancer.* London: The Biochemical Society, 1998:193.
20. Wikstrand CJ, Hale LP, Batra SK, et al. Monoclonal antibodies against EGFRvIII are tumor specific and react with breast and lung carcinomas and malignant gliomas. *Cancer Res* 1995;55:340.
21. Luetteke NC, Lee DC. Transforming growth factor alpha expression, regulation and biological action of its integral membrane precursor. *Semin Cancer Biol* 1990;1:265.
22. Hunter T, Cooper JA. Epidermal growth factor induces rapid tyrosine phosphorylation of proteins in A431 human tumor cells. *Cell* 1981;24:741.
23. Nishibe S, Carpenter G. Tyrosine phosphorylation and the regulation of cell growth: growth factor-stimulated tyrosine phosphorylation of phospholipase C. *Semin Cancer Biol* 1990;1:285.
24. Segatto O, Leonardo F, Wexler D, et al. The juxtamembrane regions of the EGF receptor and gp185erbB2 determine the specificity of signal transduction. *Mol Cell Biol* 1991;11:3191.
25. Ellis MJ. The insulin-like growth factor network and breast cancer. In: Bowcock AM, ed. *Breast cancer: molecular genetics, pathogenesis, and therapeutics*. Totowa, NJ: Humana Press, 1998:121.
26. Davidson NE, Gelmann EP, Lippman ME, Dickson RB. Epidermal growth factor receptor gene expression in estrogen receptor-positive and negative human breast cancer cell lines. *Mol Endocrinol* 1987;1:216.
27. Hudson LG, Santon JB, Gill GN. Regulation of epidermal growth factor receptor gene expression. *Mol Endocrinol* 1989;3:400.
28. Chrysogelos SA, Dickson RB. EGF receptor expression, regulation, and function in breast cancer. *Breast Cancer Res Treat* 1994;29:29.
29. Mukku VR, Stancel GM. Regulation of epidermal growth factor receptor by estrogen. *J Biol Chem* 1985;260:9820.
30. Lingham RB, Stancel GM, Loose-Mitchell DS. Estrogen regulation of epidermal growth factor receptor messenger ribonucleic acid. *Mol Endocrinol* 1988;2:230.
31. Saceda M, Lippman ME, Chambon P, Lindsey RK, Puente M, Martin MB. Regulation of the estrogen receptor in MCF-7 cells by estradiol. *Mol Endocrinol* 1988;2:1157.
32. Holmes WE, Sliwkowski MX, Akita RW, et al. Identification of heregulin, a specific activator of p185^{erbB2}. *Science* 1992;256:1205.
33. Wen D, Peles E, Cupples R, et al. Neu differentiation factor: a transmembrane glycoprotein containing and EGF domain and an immunoglobulin homology unit. *Cell* 1992;69:559.
34. Sebastian J, Richards RG, Walker MP, et al. Activation and function of the epidermal growth factor receptor and erbB-2 during mammary gland morphogenesis. *Cell Growth Differ* 1998;9:777.
35. Schroeder JA, Lee DC. Dynamic expression and activation of ERBB receptors in the developing mouse mammary gland. *Cell Growth Differ* 1998;9:451.
36. Amundadottir LT, Merlino GT, Dickson RB. Transgenic models of breast cancer. *Breast Cancer Res Treat* 1996;39:103.
37. Muthuswamy SK, Siegel PM, Dankort DL, Webster MA, Muller WJ. Mammary tumors expressing the *neu* proto-oncogene possess elevated c-Src tyrosine kinase activity. *Mol Cell Biol* 1994;14:735.
38. Siegel PM, Muller WJ. Tyrosine kinases and signal transduction in mouse mammary tumorigenesis. In: Dickson RB, Salomon DS, eds. *Hormones and growth factors in development and neoplasia.* New York: Wiley-Liss, 1998:397.
39. Muller WJ, Arteaga CL, Muthuswamy SK, et al. Synergistic interaction of the neu proto-oncogene product and transforming growth factor alpha in the mammary epithelium of transgenic mice. *Mol Cell Biol* 1996;16:5726.
40. Carraway KL, Cantley LC. A new acquaintance for $erbB_3$ and $erbB_4$: a role for receptor heterodimerization in growth signaling. *Cell* 1994;78:5.
41. Goldman R, Levy RB, Peles E, Yarden Y. Heterodimerization of the erbB-1 and erbB-2 receptors in human breast carcinoma cells: a mechanism for receptor transregulation. *J Biochem* 1990;29:11024.
42. Quian XL, Decker SJ, Greene MI. p185-c-neu and epidermal growth factor receptor associate into a structure composed of activated kinases. *Proc Natl Acad Sci U S A* 1992;89:1330.
43. Qian X, LeVea CM, Freeman JK, Dougall WC, Greene MI. Heterodimerization of epidermal growth factor receptor and wild-type or kinase-deficient Neu: a mechanism of interreceptor kinase activation and transphosphorylation. *Proc Natl Acad Sci U S A* 1994;91:1500.
44. Baens SS, Plowman G, Yardin Y. Expression of $erbB_2$ receptor family and their ligands: implication to breast cancer biological behavior. *Breast Cancer Res Treat* 1994;32[Suppl]:93.
45. Baserga R. The IGF-I receptor in normal and abnormal growth. In: Dickson RB, Salomon DS, eds. *Hormones and growth factors in development and neoplasia*. New York: Wiley-Liss, 1998:269.
46. Hankins GR, DeSousa AT, Bentley MR, et al. M6P/IGF2 receptor: a candidate breast tumor suppressor gene. *Oncogene* 1996;12:2003.
47. Segatto O, Leonardo F, Wexler D, et al. The juxtamembrane regions of the EGF receptor and gp185erbB2 determine the specificity of signal transduction. *Mol Cell Biol* 1991;11:3191.
48. Soltoff SP, Carraway KL, Prigent SA, Gullick WG, Cantley LC. $ErbB_3$ is involved in activating phosphatidylinositol 3-kinase by epidermal growth factor. *Mol Cell Biol* 1994;14:3550.
49. Quian X, Dougall WC, Hellma ME, Greene MI. Kinase-deficient neu proteins suppress epidermal growth factor receptor function and abolish cell transformation. *Oncogene* 1994;9:1507.
50. Honegger AM, Schmidt A, Ullrich A, Schlessinger J. Evidence for epidermal growth factor (EGF)-induced intermolecular antiphosphorylation of the TGF receptors in living cells. *Mol Cell Biol* 1990;10:4035.
51. McCormick F. How receptors turn Ras on. *Nature* 1993;363:15.
52. Batzer AG, Rotin B, Urena JM, Skolnik EY, Schlesinger J. Hierarchy of binding sites for Grb2 and Shc on the epidermal growth factor receptor. *Mol Cell Biol* 1994;14:5192.
53. Myers MG, Sun X-J, White MF. IRS-1 signaling system. *Trends Biochem Sci* 1994;19:289.
54. Rosfjord EC, Dickson RB. Growth factors, apoptosis, and survival of mammary epithelial cells. *J Mammary Gland Biol and Neoplasia* 1999; 4:229.
55. Keely PJ, Westwick JK, Whitehead IP, Der CJ, Parise LV. Cdc42 and rac1 induce integrin-mediated cell motility and invasiveness through pi(3)k. *Nature* 1997;390:632.
56. Medema RH, De Vries-Smits AMM, Van Der Zon GCM, Maassen JA, Bos JL. Ras activation by insulin and epidermal growth factor through enhanced exchange of guanine nucleotides on p21^{ras}. *Mol Cell Biol* 1993;13:155.
57. Bollag G, McCormick F. Regulators and effectors of *ras* proteins. *Ann Rev Cell Biol* 1991;7:601.
58. Chardin P, Camonis JH, Gale NW, et al. Human Sos 1: a guanine nucleotide exchange factor for Ras that binds to GRB2. *Science* 1993;260:1338.
59. Cresp P, Xu N, Simonds WF, Gutkind JS. Ras-dependent activation of MAP kinase pathway mediated by G-protein bg subunits. *Nature* 1994;369:418.

60. Yan Z, Winnwer S, Friedman E. Two different signal transduction pathways can be activated by transforming growth factor β_1 in epithelial cells. *J Biol Chem* 1994;269:13231.
61. Padgett RW, Das P, Krishna S. TGF-beta signaling, smads, and tumor suppressors. *Bioessays* 1998;20:382.
62. Liu X, Pawson T. The epidermal growth factor receptor phosphorylates GTPase-activating protein (GAP) at Tyr-460, adjacent to the GAP SH2 domains. *Mol Cell Biol* 1991;11:2511.
63. Ellis C, Moran M, McCormick F, Pawson T. Phosphorylation of GAP and GAP-associated proteins by transforming and mitogenic tyrosine kinases. *Nature* 1990;343:377.
64. Panayotou G, Waterfield MD. The assembly of signaling complexes by receptor tyrosine kinases. *Bioessays* 1993;15:171.
65. Davis RJ. The mitogen-activated protein kinase signal transduction pathway. *J Biol Chem* 1993;268:14553.
66. Karin M, Smeal T. Control of transcription factors by signal transduction pathways: the beginning of the end. *Trends Biochem Sci* 1992; 17:418.
67. Hubbara SR, Mohammadi M, Schlessinger J. Autoregulatory mechanisms in protein-tyrosine kinases. *J Biol Chem* 1998; 273:11987.
68. Hennighausen L. Signal networks in the mammary gland: lessons from animal models. In: Dickson RB, Salomon DS, eds. *Hormones and growth factors in development and neoplasia.* New York: Wiley-Liss, 1998:239.
69. Elion EA. Routing MAP kinase cascades. *Science* 1998;281:1625.
70. Avruch J, Zhang X-F, Kyriakis JM. Raf meets Ras: completing the framework of a signal transduction pathway. *Trends Biochem Sci* 1994;19:279.
71. Leevers SL, Paterson HF, Marshall CJ. Requirement for Ras in Raf activation is overcome by targeting Raf to the plasma membrane. *Nature* 1994;369:411.
72. Freed E, Symons M, Macdonald SG, McCormick F, Ruggieri R. Binding of 14-3-3 proteins to the protein kinase Raf and effects on its activation. *Science* 1994;265:1713.
73. Hafner S, Adler HS, Mischak H, et al. Mechanism of inhibition of Raf-1 by protein kinase C. *Mol Cell Biol* 1994,14.6696.
74. Hall A. A biochemical function for ras—at last. *Science* 1994; 264:1413.
75. Whitmarsh AJ, Davis RJ. Structural organization of MAP-kinase signaling modules by scaffold proteins in yeast and mammals. *Trends Biochem Sci* 1998;23:481.
76. Rodriguez-Viciana R, Warne PH, Dhand R, et al. Phosphatidylinositol-3-OH kinase as a direct target of Ras. *Nature* 1994;370:527.
77. Ransone LJ, Verma I. Nuclear proto-oncogenes FOS and JUN. *Annu Rev Cell Biol* 1990;6:539.
78. Kato GJ, Dang CV. Function of the c-Myc oncoprotein. *FASEB J* 1992;6:3065.
79. Franklin CC, Unlap T, AdlerV, Kraft AS. Multiple signal transduction pathways mediate *c*-Jun protein phosphorylation. *Cell Growth Differ* 1993;4:377.
80. Amati B, Dalton S, Brooks MW, Littlewood TD, Evan GI, Land H. Transcriptional activation by the human c Myc oncoprotein in yeast requires interaction with Max. *Nature* 1992;359:423.
81. Nebreda AR. Inactivation of MAP kinases. *Trends Biochem Sci* 1994;19:1.
82. Fry DW, Kraker AJ, McMichael A, et al. A specific inhibitor of the epidermal growth factor receptor tyrosine kinase. *Science* 1994;265:1093.
83. Murphy AS, Coutts LC. Elevated mitogen-activated protein kinase activity in estrogen-nonresponsive human breast cancer cells. *Cancer Res* 1998;58:4071.
84. Garrett PA, Hulka BS, Kim YL, Farber RA. HRAS protooncogenes polymorphism and breast cancer. *Cancer Epidemiol Biomarkers Prev* 1993;2:131.
85. Nass SJ, Dickson RB. Defining a role for c-myc in breast tumorigenesis. *Breast Cancer Res Treat* 1997;44:1.
86. Atherton-Fessler S, Parker LL, Geahlen R, Piwnica-Worms H. Mechanisms of $p34^{cdc2}$ regulation. *Mol Cell Biol* 1993;13:1675.
87. Koli KM, Arteaga CL. Transforming growth factor-β and breast cancer. In: Bowcock AM, ed. *Breast cancer: molecular genetics, pathogenesis, and therapeutics.* Totowa, NJ: Humana Press, 1998:95.
88. Gregory H, Thomas CE, Willshire IR, et al. Epidermal and transforming growth factor α in patients with breast tumors. *Br J Cancer* 1989;59:605.
89. Travers MR, Barrett-Lee PJ, Berger U, Luqmani YA, Gazet J-C, Powles TJ. Growth factor expression in normal, benign, and malignant breast tissue. *BMJ* 1988;296:1621.
90. Macias A, Perez R, HägerströmT, Skoog L. Identification of transforming growth factor alpha in human primary breast carcinomas. *Anticancer Res* 1987;7:1271.
91. Eckert K, Granetzny A, Fischer J, Nexo E, Grosse R. An Mr 43,000 epidermal growth-factor related protein purified from the urine of breast cancer patients. *Cancer Res* 1990;50:642.
92. Qi C-F, Liscia DS, Normanno N, et al. Expression of transforming growth factor α, amphiregulin and cripto-1 in human breast carcinomas. *Br J Cancer* 1994;69:903.
93. Le June S, Leak R, Horak E, Plowman G, Greenall M, Harris AL. Amphiregulin, epidermal growth factor receptor, and estrogen receptor expression in human primary breast cancer. *Cancer Res* 1993;53:3597.
94. Fitzpatrick SL, Brightwell J, Wittliff J, Barrows GH, Schultz GS. Epidermal growth factor binding by breast tumor biopsies and relationship to estrogen and progestin receptor levels. *Cancer Res* 1984;44:3448.
95. Sainsbury JRC, Farndon JR, Sherbert GV, Harris AL. Epidermal growth factor receptors and oestrogen receptors in human breast cancers. *Lancet* 1985;1:364.
96. Fox SB, Smith K, Hollyer J, Greenall M, Hastrich D, Harris AL. The epidermal growth factor receptor as a prognostic marker: results of 370 patients and a review of 3,009 patients. *Breast Cancer Res Treat* 1994;29:41.
97. Chrysogelos SA. Chromatin structure of the EGFR gene suggests a role for intron-1 sequences in its regulation in breast cancer cells. *Nucl Acids Res* 1993;21:5736.
98. Klijn JGM, Cook MP, Portengen H, Alexieva-Figusch J, Van Putten WLJ, Fochans JA. The prognostic value of epidermal growth factor receptor (EGF-R) in primary breast cancer: results of a 10-year follow-up study. *Breast Cancer Res Treat* 1994;29:73.
99. Toi M, Tominaga T, Osaki A, Toge T. Role of epidermal growth factor receptor expression in primary breast cancer: results of a biochemical and immunochemical study. *Breast Cancer Res Treat* 1994;29:51.
100. Bargmann CI, Hung MC, Weinberg RA. The neu oncogene encodes an epidermal growth factor receptor-related protein. *Nature* 1986;319:226.
101. Gusterson BA, Machin LG, Gullick WJ, et al. Immunohistochemical distribution of c-erbB-2 in infiltrating and *in situ* breast cancer. *Int J Cancer* 1988;42:842.
102. Paik S, Hazan R, Fisher ER, et al. Pathologic findings from the National Surgical Adjuvant Breast and Bowel Project: prognostic significance of *erb*B-2 protein overexpression in primary breast cancer. *J Clin Oncol* 1990;8:103.
103. Muss HB, Thor AD, Berry DA, et al. c-$ErbB_2$ expression and response to adjuvant therapy in women with node positive breast cancer. *N Engl J Med* 1994;330:1260.
104. Allred DC, Clark GM, Tandon AK, et al. *Her-2/neu* in node negative breast cancer: prognostic significance of overexpression influenced by the presence of *in situ* carcinoma. *J Clin Oncol* 1992;10:599.
105. Toikkanen S, Helin H, Isola J, Joensuu H. Prognostic significance of *HER-2* oncoprotein expression in breast cancer: a 30-year follow up. *J Clin Oncol* 1992;10:1044.
106. Hancock MC, Langton BC, Chan T, et al. A monoclonal antibody against the c-erbB-2 protein enhances the cytotoxicity of *cis*-diamminidi chloroplatinum against human breast and ovarian tumor cell lines. *Cancer Res* 1991;51:4575.
107. Paik S, Bryant J, Park C, et al. ErbB-2 and response to doxorubicin in patients with axillary lymph node-positive, hormone receptor-negative breast cancer. *J Natl Cancer Inst* 1998;90:1361.
108. Pietras RJ, Arboleda J, Reese DM, et al. Her-2 tyrosine kinase pathway targets estrogen receptor and promotes hormone-independent growth in human breast cancer cells. *Oncogene* 1995;10:2435.
109. Chiappetta C, Kirkland JL, Loose-Mitchell DS, Murthy L, Stancel GM. Estrogen regulates expression of the *jun* family of protooncogenes in the uterus. *J Steroid Biochem Mol Biol* 1992;41:113.
110. Kumar R, Mandal M, Lipton A, Harvey H, Thompson C. Overexpression of HER2 modulates Bcl-2, Bcl-XL, and tamoxifen-induced apoptosis in human MCF-7 breast cancer cells. *Clin Cancer Res* 1996;2:1215.
111. Willsher PC, Beaver J, Pinder S, et al. Prognostic significance of serum c-erbB2 protein in breast cancer patients. *Breast Cancer Res Treat* 1996;40:251.
112. Pastan I, Fitzgerald D. Recombinant toxins for cancer treatment *Science* 1992;254:1173.
113. Baselga J, Norton L, Albanell J, Kim YM, Mendelsohn J. Recombinant humanized anti-HER2 antibody (Herceptin) enhances the antitumor

activity of paclitaxel and doxorubicin against HER2/neu overexpressing human breast cancer xenografts. *Cancer Res* 1998;58:2825.
114. Pupa SM, Bufalino R, Invernizzi AM, et al. Macrophage infiltrate and prognosis in c-erbB2-overexpressing breast carcinomas. *J Clin Oncol* 1996;14:85.
115. Yu D, Shi D, Scanlon M, Hung M. Reexpression of *neu*-encoded oncoprotein counteracts the tumor-suppressing but not the metastasis-suppressing function E1A. *Cancer Res* 1993;53:5784.
116. Streuli CH, Edwards GM. Control of normal mammary epithelial phenotype by integrins. *J Mammary Gland Biol Neoplasia* 1998;3:151.
117. Zutter MM, Sun H, Santoro SA. Altered integrin expression and the malignant phenotype: the contribution of multiple integrated integrin receptors. *J Mammary Gland Biol Neoplasia* 1998;3:191.
118. Rosfjord EC, Dickson RB. Role of integrins in the development and malignancy of the breast. In: Bowcock AM, ed. *Breast cancer: molecular genetics, pathogenesis, and therapeutics*. Totowa, NJ: Humana Press, 1998:285.
119. Sommers CL. The role of cadherin-mediated adhesion in breast cancer. *J Mammary Gland Biol Neoplasia* 1996;1:219.
120. Pfeifer M. β-Catenin as oncogene: the smoking gun. *Science* 1997; 275:1752.
121. Jonsson M, Smith K, Harris AL. WNT and fibroblast growth factor gene expression during development of the mammary gland and role of WNTs in human cancer. In: Dickson RB, Salomon DS, eds. *Hormones and growth factors in development and neoplasia*. New York: Wiley-Liss, 1998:361.
122. Teng D, Hu R, Lin H, et al. MMACI/PTEN mutations in primary tumor specimens and tumor cell lines. *Cancer Res* 1997;57:5221.
123. Tamura M, Gu J, Matsumot K, Aota S, Parsons R, Yamada KM. Inhibition of cell migration, spreading, and focal adhesions by tumor suppressor PTEN. *Science* 1998;3:241.
124. Wu X, Senechal K, Neshat MS, Whang YE, Sawyers CL. The PTEN/MMAC1 tumor suppressor phosphatase functions as a negative regulator of the phosphoinositide 3-kinase/Akt pathway. *Proc Natl Acad Sci U S A* 1998;95:15587.
125. Levitzki A, Gazit A. Tyrosine kinase inhibition: an approach to drug development, *Science* 1995;267:1782.
126. James GL, Goldstein JL, Brown MS, et al. Benzodiazepine peptidomimetics: potent inhibitors of Ras farnesylation in animals cells. *Science* 1993;260:1937.
127. Kohl NE, Mosser SD, deSolms SJ, et al. Selective inhibition of ras-dependent transformation by a farnesyltransferase inhibitor. *Science* 1993;260:1934.
128. Wu J, Dent P, Jelinek T, Wolfman A, Weber MJ, Sturgill TW. Inhibition of the EGF-activated MAP kinase signaling pathway by adenosine 3',5'-monophosphate. *Science* 1993;262:1065.
129. Cho-Chung YS. Role of cyclic AMP receptor proteins in growth, differentiation, and suppression of malignancy: new approaches to therapy. *Cancer Res* 1990;50:7093.
130. Cook SJ, McCormick F. Inhibition by cAMP of Ras-dependent activation of raf. *Science* 1993;262:1069.
131. Sadowski HB, Shuai K, Darnell Jr JE, Gilman MZ. A common nuclear signal transduction pathway activated by growth factor and cytokine receptors. *Science* 1993;261:1739.
132. Darnell JE, Kerr IM, Starb GR. Jak-STAT pathways and transcriptional activation in response to IFNs and other extracellular signaling pathways. *Science* 1994;264:1415.
133. Sadowski HB, Shuai K, Darnell JE, Gilman MZ. A common nuclear signal transduction pathway activated by growth factor and cytokine receptors. *Science* 1993;261:1739.
134. Alkahalf M, Murphy LC. Regulation of c-*jun* and *jun* B by progestins in T47D human breast cancer cells. *Mol Endocrinol* 1992;6:1625.
135. Silvennoinen O, Schindler C, Schlessinger J, Levy DE. Ras-independent growth factor signaling by transcription factor tyrosine phosphorylation. *Science* 1993;261:1736.
136. LeRoy X, Escot C, Browillet JP, Theillet C, Maudelonde T, Simony-Lafontaine J. Decrease of c-erbB$_2$ and c-myc mRNA levels in tamoxifen-treated breast cancer. *Oncogene* 1992;6:431.
137. Murphy LJ. Estrogen induction of insulin-like growth factors and myc proto-oncogene expression in the uterus. *J Steroid Biochem Mol Biol* 1991;40:223.
138. Dang CV. c-Myc target genes involved in cell growth, apoptosis, and metabolism. *Mol Cell Biol* 1999;19:1.
139. Xiao Q, Claasses G, Shi J, Adachi S, Sedivy J, Hann SR. Transactivation-defective c-MycS retains the ability to regulate proliferation and apoptosis. *Genes Dev* 1998;12:3806.
140. Nass SJ, Dickson RB. Epidermal growth factor-dependent cell cycle progression is altered in mammary epithelial cells which overexpress c-myc. *Clin Cancer Res* 1998;4:1813.
141. Watson PH, Pon RT, Shiu RPC. Inhibition of c-myc expression by phosphorothioate antisense oligonucleotide identifies a critical role for c-myc in the growth of human breast cancer. *Cancer Res* 1991;51:3996.
142. Neuman E, Ladha MH, Lin N, et al. Cyclin D1 stimulation of estrogen receptor transcriptional activity independent of cdk4. *Mol Cell Biol* 1997:17:5338.
143. Anzick SL, Kononen J, Walker RL, et al. AIB1, a steroid receptor coactivator amplified in breast and ovarian cancer. *Science* 1997;277:965.
144. Escot C, Theillet C, Lidereau R, et al. Genetic alteration of the c-myc proto-oncogene in human primary breast carcinomas. *Proc Natl Acad Sci U S A* 1986:83:4834.
145. Bonilla M, Ramirez M, Lopez-Cuento J, Gariglio P. In vivo amplification and rearrangements of c-myc oncogene in human breast tumors. *J Natl Cancer Inst* 1988;80:665.
146. Cline M, Battifora H, Yokota JJ. Protooncogene abnormalities in human breast cancer: correlations with anatomic features and clinical course of diagnosis. *J Clin Oncol* 1987;5:999.
147. Varlay JM, Swallow JE, Brammer VJ, Wittaker JL, Waekor RA. Alterations to either c-erb$_2$ (neu) short term prognosis. *Oncogene* 1987;1:423.
148. Bieche I, Champeme M-H, Lidereau R. A tumor suppressor gene on chromosome 1p32-pter controls the amplification of MYC family genes in breast cancer. *Cancer Res* 1994;54:4274.
149. Berns EMJJ, Klijn JGM, Van Putten WLJ, Van Staveren IL, Portengen H, Foekens JA. c-Myc amplification is a better prognostic factor than HER2/neu amplification in primary breast cancer. *Cancer Res* 1992;52:1107.
150. Borg A, Baldetorp B, Ferno M, et al. c-Myc amplification is an independent prognostic factor in postmenopausal breast cancer. *Int J Cancer* 1992;51:687.
151. Escot C, Theillet C, Lideream R, et al. Genetic alterations of the c-myc protooncogene in human breast carcinomas. *Proc Natl Acad Sci U S A* 1986;83:4834.
152. Deming SL, Nass SJ, Dickson RB, Trock BJ. C-Myc amplification in breast cancer: a meta analysis of its frequency and association with risk factors. *Proc Annu Meet AACR* 1999:1358(abstr).
153. Lee LW, Raymond VW, Tsao MS, Lee DC, Earp HS, Grisham JW. Clonal cosegregation of tumorigenicity with overexpression of c-myc and transforming growth factor α genes in chemically transformed rat liver epithelial cells. *Cancer Res* 1991;51:5238.
154. Amundadottir LT, Nass S, Berchem G, Johnson MD, Dickson RB. Cooperation of TGF and c-myc in mouse mammary tumorigenesis: coordinated stimulation of growth and suppression of apoptosis. *Oncogene* 1996;13:757.
155. Amundadottir LT, Johnson MD, Merlino GT, Smith GH, Dickson RB. Synergistic interaction of transforming growth factor β and c-myc in mouse mammary and salivary gland tumorigenesis. *Cell Growth Differ* 1995;6:737.
156. Kelekar A, Cole MD. Immortalization by c-myc, H-ras, Ela oncogenes induces differential cellular gene expression and growth factor responses. *Mol Cell Biol* 1987;7:3899.
157. Stern DF, Roberts AB, Roche NS, Sporn MB, Weinberg RA. Differential responsiveness of myc- and ras-transfected cells to growth factors: selective stimulation of myc-transfected cells by epidermal growth factor. *Mol Cell Biol* 1986;6:870.
158. Valverius EM, Ciardiello F, Heldin NE, et al. Stromal influences on transformation of human mammary epithelial cells overexpressing c-myc and SV40T. *J Cell Physiol* 1990;145:207.
159. Hermeking H, Eick D. Mediation of c-Myc-induced apoptosis by p53. *Science* 1994;265:2091.
160. Zindy F, Eischen CM, Randle DH, et al. Myc signaling via the ARF tumor suppressor regulates p53-dependent apoptosis and immortalization. *Genes Dev* 1998;12:2424.
161. McCormack SJ, Weaver Z, Deming S, et al. Myc/p53 interactions in transgenic mouse mammary development, tumorigenesis, and chromosomal instability. *Oncogene* 1998;16:2755.
162. Sklar MD, Prochownik EV. Modulation of cis-platinum resistance in friend erythroleukemia cells by c-myc. *Cancer Res* 1991;51:2118.
163. Yang BS, Geddes TJ, Pogulis RJ, de Crombrugghe B, Freytag SO. Transcriptional suppression of cellular gene expression by c-myc. *Mol Cell Biol* 1991;11:2291.
164. Suen TC, Hung M-C. c-Myc reverse neu-induced transformed morphology by transcriptional repression. *Mol Cell Biol* 1991;11:354.

165. Semsei I, Ma S, Culter RG. Tissue and age specific expression of the myc protooncogene family throughout the lifespan of the C57BL/6J mouse strain. *Oncogene* 1989;4:465.
166. Schreiber-Agus N, Meng Y, Hoang T, et al. Role of Mxi1 in ageing organ systems and the regulation of normal and neoplastic growth. *Nature* 1998;393:483.
167. Telang NT, Osborne MP, Sweterlitsch LA, Tarayanan R. Neoplastic transformation of mouse mammary epithelial cells by deregulated myc expression. *Cell Regulation* 1990;1:863.
168. Cullen KJ, Lippman ME. Stromal-epithelial interactions in breast cancer. In: Lippman ME, Dickson RB, eds. *Genes, oncogenes and hormones*. Boston: Kluwer, 1992:413.
169. Prall OWJ, Rogan EM, Sutherland RL. Estrogen regulation of cell cycle progression in breast cancer cells. *J Steroid Biochem Mol Biol* 1998;65:169.
170. Hansen RK, Fuqua SAW. The estrogen receptor and breast cancer. In: Bowcock AM, ed. *Breast cancer: molecular genetics, pathogenesis, and therapeutics*. Totowa, NJ: Humana Press, 1998:1.
171. Russel P. Checkpoints on the road to mitosis. *Trends Biochem Sci* 1998;23:399.
172. Nakayama K-I, Nakayama K. Cip/Kip cyclin-dependent kinase inhibitors: brakes of the cell cycle engine during development. *Bioessays* 1998;20:1020.
173. Nevins JR. Toward an understanding of the functional complexity of the E2F and retinoblastoma families. *Cell Growth Differ* 1998: 9:585.
174. Koff A, Ohtsuki M, Polyak K, Roberts JM, Massagué J. Negative regulation of G1 in mammalian cells: inhibition of cyclin E-dependent kinase by TGF-β. *Science* 1993;260:536.
175. Barnes DM, Gillett GE. Cyclin D_1 in breast cancer. *Breast Cancer Res Treat* 1999;52:1.
176. Oyama T, Kashiwabara K, Yoshimoto K, Arnold A, Koerner F. Frequent overexpression of the cyclin D_1 oncogene in invasive lobular carcinoma of the breast. *Cancer Res* 1998;58:2876.
177. Sicinski P, Donaher JL, Parker SB, et al. Cyclin D_1 provides a link between development and oncogenesis in the retina and breast. *Cell* 1995;82:621.
178. Keyomarsi K, Conte D Jr, Toyofuku W, Fox MP. Deregulation of cyclin e in breast cancer. *Oncogene* 1995;11:941.
179. Nielsen NH, Arnerlov C, Emdin SO, Landberg G. Cyclin e overexpression, a negative prognostic factor in breast cancer with strong correlation to oestrogen receptor status. *Br J Cancer* 1996;74:874.
180. Brenner AJ, Aldaz CM. Chromosome 9p allelic loss and p16/cdkn2 in breast cancer and evidence of p16 inactivation in immortal breast epithelial cells. *Cancer Res* 1995;55:2892.
181. Kamb A, Gruis NA, Weaver-Feldhaus J, et al. A cell cycle regulator potentially involved in genesis of many tumor types. *Science* 1994; 264:436.
182. Xu L, Sgroi D, Sterner CJ, et al. Mutational analysis of CDKN2 (MTS1/p16^{ink4}) in human breast carcinomas. *Cancer Res* 1994;54:5262.
183. Chin L, Pomerantz J, DePinho RA. The INK4α/ARF tumor suppressor: one gene-two products-two pathways. *Trends Biochem Sci* 1998;23:291.
184. Bates S, Phillips AC, Clark PA, et al. p14ARF links the tumour suppressors RB and p53. *Nature* 1998;395:124.
185. Sgambato A, Zhang Y, Ciaparrone M, et al. Overexpression of p27kip1 inhibits the growth of both normal and transformed human mammary epithelial cells. *Cancer Res* 1998;58:3448.
186. Catzavelos C, Bhattacharya N, Ung YC, et al. Decreased levels of the cell-cycle inhibitor p27kip1 protein: prognostic implications in primary breast cancer. *Nat Med* 1997;3:227.
187. Fero ML, Randel E, Gurley KE, Roberts JM, Kemp CJ. The murine gene p27 kip1 is haplo-insufficient for tumour suppression. *Nature* 1998;396:177.
188. Pietilainen T, Lipponen P, Aaltomaa S, Eskelinen M, Kosma VM, Syrjanen K. Expression of retinoblastoma gene protein (rb) in breast cancer as related to established prognostic factors and survival. *Eur J Cancer* 1995;31A:329.
189. Lengauer C, Kinzler KW, Vogelstein B. Genetic instabilities in human cancers. *Nature* 1998;396:643.
190. Sekowski JW, Malkas LH, Schnaper L, Bechtel PE, Long BJ, Hickey RJ. Human breast cancer cells contain an error-prone DNA replication apparatus. *Cancer Res* 1998;58:3259.
191. Walsh T, Chappell SA, Shaw JA, Walker RA. Microsatellite instability in ductal carcinoma in situ of the breast. *J Pathol* 1998;185:18.
192. Broca P. *Traite des Tumeurs*. Paris: Asselin, 1866.
193. Knudson AG. Mutation and cancer: statistical study of retinoblastoma. *Proc Natl Acad Sci U S A* 1971;68:820.
194. Harris H, Miller OJ, Klein G, Worst P, Tachibana T. Suppression of malignancy by cell fusion. *Nature* 1969;223:368.
195. Malkin D, Li FP, Strong LC, et al. Germ line p53 mutations in a familial syndrome of breast cancer, sarcomas, and other neoplasms. *Science* 1990;250:1233.
196. Hall JM, Lee MK, Morrow J, et al. Linkage of early-onset familial breast cancer to chromosome 17q21. *Science* 1990;250:1684.
197. Wooster R, Neuhausen SL, Mangion J, et al. Localization of a breast cancer susceptibility gene, BRCA2, to chromosome 13q12-13. *Science* 1994;265:2088.
198. Bennett LB, Taurog JD, Bowcock AM. Hereditary breast cancer genes. In: Bowcock AM, ed. *Breast cancer: molecular genetics, pathogenesis, and therapeutics*. Totowa, NJ: Humana Press, 1998:199.
199. White RL. Tumor suppressing pathways. *Cell* 1998;92:591.
200. Cullotta E, Koshland DE. Molecules of the year: p53 sweeps through cancer research. *Science* 1993;262:1958.
201. Blaszyk H, Vaughn CB, Hartmann A, et al. Novel pattern of p53 gene mutations on an American black cohort with high mortality from breast cancer. *Lancet* 1994;343:1195.
202. Moll UM, Riou G, Levine AJ. Two distinct mechanisms alter p53 in breast cancer: mutation and nuclear exclusion. *Proc Natl Acad Sci U S A* 1992;89:7262.
203. Furth PA. Apoptosis and the development of breast cancer. In: Bowcock AM. *Breast cancer: molecular genetics, pathogenesis, and therapeutics*. Totowa, NJ: Humana Press, 1998:171.
204. Reed JC. Balancing cell life and death: bax, apoptosis, and breast cancer. *J Clin Invest* 1996;97:2403.
205. Gasparini G, Barbareschi M, Doglioni C, et al. Expression of bcl-2 protein predicts efficacy of adjuvant treatments in operable node-positive breast cancer. *Clin Cancer Res* 1995;2:189.
206. Sumantran VN, Ealovega MW, Nunez G, Clarke MF, Wicha MS. Overexpression of bcl-xs-sensitizes MCF-7 cells to chemotherapy-induced apoptosis. *Cancer Res* 1995;55:2507.
207. Done SJ, Arneson NC, Ozcelik H, Redston M, Andrulis I. p53 mutations in mammary ductal carcinoma in situ but not in epithelial hyperplasias. *Cancer Res* 1998;58:785.
208. Palmero I, Pantoja C, Serrano M. p19ARF links the tumour suppressor p53 to Ras. *Nature* 1998;395:125.
209. Kaghad M, Bonnet H, Yang A, et al. Monoallelically expressed gene related to p53 at 1p36, a region frequently deleted in neuroblastoma and other human cancers. *Cell* 1997;90:809.
210. ChenY, Chen C, Riley D, et al. Aberrant subcellular localization of BRCA-1 in breast cancer. *Science* 1995;270:789.
211. Holt JT, Thompson ME, Szabo C, et al. Growth retardation and tumour inhibition by BRCA1. *Nat Genet* 1996;12:298.
212. Somasundaram K, Zhang H, Zeng YX, et al. Arrest of the cell cycle by the tumour-suppressor brca1 requires the cdk-inhibitor p21waf1/cip1. *Nature* 1997;389:187.
213. Zhang H, Tombline G, Weber B. BRCA1, BRCA2, and DNA damage response: collision or collusion? *Cell* 1998;92:433.
214. Verhoog LC, Brekelmans CTM, Seynaeve C, et al. Survival and tumour characteristics of breast cancer patients with germline mutation of BRCA1. *Lancet* 1998;351:316.
215. Ranstam OT, Borg J, Johansson A, et al. Survival of BRCA1 breast and ovarian cancer patients: a population-based study from Southern Sweden. *J Clin Oncol* 1998;16:397.
216. Lynch HT, Lemon SJ, Marcus JN, Lerman C, Lynch J, Narod S. Breast cancer genetics. In: Copeland EM, ed. *The breast*, 2nd ed. Philadelphia: WB Saunders, 1998:370.
217. Lerman C, Peshkin BN. Psychosocial issues in BRCA1/2 testing. In: Bowcock AM, ed. *Breast cancer: molecular genetics, pathogenesis, and therapeutics*. Totowa, NJ: Humana Press, 1998:247.
218. Vorochovsky I, Rasido D, Luo L, et al. The ATM gene and susceptibility to breast cancer: analysis of 38 breast tumors reveals no evidence for mutation. *Cancer Res* 1996;56:2726.
219. Woo RA, McLure KG, Lees-Miller SP, Rancourt DE, Lee PWK. DNA-dependent protein kinase acts upstream of p53 in response to DNA damage. *Nature* 1998;394:700.
220. Salvesen GS, Dixit VM. Caspases: intracellular signaling by proteolysis. *Cell* 1997;91:443.
221. Li J, Yen C, Liaw D, et al. PTEN, a putative protein phosphatase gene mutated in human brain, breast, and prostate cancer. *Science* 1997; 275:1943.
222. Drake JW. Mutation rates. *Bioessays* 1992;2:137.
223. Cohen SM, Ellwein LB. Genetic errors, cell proliferation, and carcinogenesis. *Cancer Res* 1991;51:6493.

224. Tilsty TD, White AL, Sanchez J. Suppression of gene amplification in human cell hybrids. *Science*1992;256:1425.
225. Thompson AM, Steel CM, Chetty U, Hawkins RA, Miller WR, Carter DC. p53 gene mRNA expression and chromosome 17p allele loss in breast cancer. *Br J Cancer* 1990;61:74.
226. Davidoff AM, Kerns BJM, Pence JC, Marks JR, Iglehart JD. p53 alterations in all stages of breast cancer. *J Surg Oncol* 1991;48:260.
227. Elledge RM, Allred DC. Prognostic and predictive value of p53 and p21 in breast cancer. *Breast Cancer Res Treat* 1999;52:79.
228. Waldman T, Lengauer C, Kinzler K, Vogelstein B. Uncoupling of S-phase and mitosis induced by anticancer agents in cells lacking p21. *Nature* 1996;381:713.
229. Fishel R, Lescoe MK, Rao MRS, et al. The human mutator gene homolog MSH2 and its association with hereditary nonpolyposis colon cancer. *Cell* 1993;75:1027.
230. Moffett BF, Baban D, Bao L, Tarin D. Fate of clonal lineages during neoplasia and metastasis studied with an incorporated genetic marker. *Cancer Res* 1992;52:1737.
231. Sato T, Akiyama F, Sakamoto G, Kasami F, Nakamurai Y. Accumulation of genetic alterations and progression of primary breast cancer. *Cancer Res* 1991;51:5794.
232. Weinberg RA. Bumps on the road to immortality. *Nature* 1998; 396:23.
233. Faragher RGA, Kipling D. How might replicative senescence contribute to human ageing? *Bioessays* 1998;20:985.
234. Greider CW. Telomere length regulation. *Annu Rev Biochem* 1996; 65:337.
235. Greenberg RA, O'Hagan RC, Deng H, et al. Telomerase reverse transcriptase gene is a direct target of c-myc but is not functionally equivalent in cellular transformation. *Oncogene* 1999;18:1219.
236. Hiyama E, Gollahon L, Kataoka T, et al. Telomerase activity in human breast tumors. *J Natl Cancer Inst* 1996;88:116.
237. Yashima K, Gollahon S, Milchgrub LS, et al. Telomerase enzyme activity and RNA expression during the multistage pathogenesis of breast carcinoma. *Clin Cancer Res* 1998;4:229.
238. Kiyono T, Foster SA, Koop JI, Galloway JK, Klingelhutz DA, McDougall AJ. Both Rb/p16INK4a inactivation and telomerase activity are required to immortalize human epithelial cells. *Nature* 1998; 396:84.
239. Lundin C, Mertens F. Cytogenetics of benign breast lesions. *Breast Cancer Res Treat* 1998;51:1.
240. Dati C, Muraca R, Tazartes O, et al. c-ErbB-2 and ras expression levels in breast cancer are correlated and show a cooperative association with unfavorable clinical outcome. *Int J Cancer* 1991;47:833.
241. Horuck E, Smith K, Bromley L, et al. Mutant p53, EGF receptor, and c-erbB$_2$ expression in human breast cancer. *Oncogene* 1991;6:2277.
242. Kreipe H, Feist H, Fischer L, et al. Amplification of *c-myc* but not of c-*erb*B-2 is associated with high proliferative capacity in breast cancer. *Cancer Res* 1993;53:1956.
243. Li B, Rosen J, McMenamin-Balano J, Muller W, Perkins AS. neu/erbB2 cooperates with p53-172H during mammary tumorigenesis in transgenic mice. *Mol Cell Biol* 1997;17:3155.
244. Hundley JE, Koester SK, Troyer DA, Hilsenbeck SG, Barrington RE, Windle JJ. Differential regulation of cell cycle characteristics and apoptosis in mmtv-myc and mmtv-ras mouse mammary tumors. *Cancer Res* 1997;57:600.
245. Allred DC, Elledge R, Clark GM, Fuqua SAW. The p53 tumor-suppressor gene in human breast cancer. In: Dickson RB, Lippman ME, eds. *Mammary tumorigenesis and malignant progression*. Boston: Kluwer, 1994:63.
246. Fung YK, T'Ang A. The role of the retinoblastoma gene in breast cancer development. In: Dickson RB, Lippman ME, eds. *Genes, oncogenes and hormones*. Boston: Kluwer, 1992:59.
247. Gamillo C, Palacios J, Suarez A, et al. Correlation of E-cadherin expression with differentiation grade and histological type in breast carcinoma. *Am J Pathol* 1993;142:987.
248. Sager R, Anisowicz A, Neveu M, Liang P, Sotiropoulou G. Identification by differential display of alpha 6 integrin are a candidate tumor suppressor gene. *FASEB J* 1993;7:964.
249. Oats AJ, Schumaker LM, Jenkins SB, et al. The mannose-6-phosphate/insulin-like growth factor 2 receptor (M6P/IGF2R), a putative tumor suppressor gene. *Breast Cancer Res Treat* 1998;47:269.
250. He TC, Sparks AB, Rago C, et al. Identification of c-MYC as a target of the APC pathway. *Science* 1998;281:1509.
251. Tan M, Yu D. Overexpression of the c-erbB2 gene enhanced intrinsic metastasis potential in human breast cancer cells without increasing their transformation abilities. *Cancer Res* 1997;57:1199.
252. Heimann R, Ferguson DJF, Hellman S. The relationship between nm23, angiogenesis, and the metastatic proclivity of node-negative breast cancer. *Cancer Res* 1998:58:2766.
253. Welch DR, Wei LL. Genetic and epigenetic regulation of human breast cancer progression and metastasis. *Endocrine-Related Cancer* 1998;5:155.
254. Graeber TG, Osmanian C, Jacks T, et al. Hypoxia-mediated selection of cells with diminished apoptotic potential in solid tumours. *Nature* 1996;379:88.
255. Kuukasjarvi T, Karhu R, Tanner M, et al. Heterogeneity and clonal evolution underlying development of asynchronous metastasis in human breast cancer. *Cancer Res* 1997;57:1597.
256. Steeg PS, Hartsough MT, Clare SE. Nm23, breast differentiation, and cancer metastasis. In: Bowcock AM, ed. *Breast cancer: molecular genetics, pathogenesis, and therapeutics*. Totowa, NJ: Humana Press, 1998:267.
257. Freije JMP, MacDonald NJ, Steeg PS. Nm23 and tumour metastasis: basic and translational advances. *Biochem Soc Symp* 1996;63:261.
258. Li L, Cohen SN. Tsg101: a novel tumor susceptibility gene isolated by controlled homozygous functional knockout of allelic loci in mammalian cells. *Cell* 1996;85:319.
259. Tamura M, Gu J, Takino T, Yamada KM. Tumor suppressor PTEN inhibition of cell invasion, migration, and Growth: differential involvement of focal adhesion kinase and p130. *Cancer Res* 1999;59:442.
260. Ellis LM, Nicolson GL, Fidler IJ. Concepts and mechanisms of breast cancer metastasis. In: Bland KI, Copeland EM, eds. *The breast,* 2nd ed. Philadelphia: WB Saunders, 1998:564.
261. Davidson NE, Kennedy MJ.Protein kinase C and breast cancer. In: Dickson RB, Lippman ME, eds. *Mammary tumor cell cycle, differentiation and metastasis*. Boston: Kluwer, 1996:91.
262. Benaud C, Dickson RB, Thompson EW. Roles of matrix metalloproteases in mammary gland development and cancer. *Breast Cancer Res Treat* 1998;50:97.
263. Massova I, Kotra LP, Fridman R, Mobashery S. Matrix metalloproteinases: structures, evolution, and diversification. *FASEB J* 1998;1075.
264. Fisher B, Costantino JP, Wickerham L, et al. Tamoxifen for prevention of breast cancer: report of the national surgical adjuvant breast and bowel project P-1 study. *J Natl Cancer Inst* 1998;90:1371.
265. Nass SJ, Hahm HA, Davidson NE. Breast cancer biology blossoms in the clinic. *Nat Med* 1998;4:761.

Diseases of the Breast, 2nd ed.,
edited by Jay R. Harris.
Lippincott Williams & Wilkins, Philadelphia © 2000.

CHAPTER 21

Autocrine and Paracrine Growth Factors in the Normal and Neoplastic Breast

Robert B. Dickson and Marc E. Lippman

Studies during the last two decades of the twentieth century have begun to address the mechanisms of action of estrogen and progesterone at the local tissue level in the early promotion and later progression of malignancy of the breast. Tissue regulation by these hormones is modulated in a very complex fashion by locally acting polypeptide hormones (growth factors), by the stage of epithelial cellular differentiation, by epithelial cell–cell and cell-stromal adhesion, by various stromal cell types, and by additional, poorly understood serum factors.[1–4] Much research is focused on examining the interaction of growth factors with defective or overexpressed growth-regulatory genes (oncogenes or protooncogenes) in mediating or modulating endocrine steroid action in breast cancer. A second topic of concern is the possibility that an appropriate expression of positive-acting growth factors by fully or partially malignant cells may promote malignant progression in nearby tumor cells, which would benefit from an additive proliferation advantage. A third, very important area of research is examining defective tumor-host interactions, including stromal-epithelial communication to support estrogen-responsive growth, to induce aberrant stromal collagen synthesis (desmoplasia), to directly or indirectly regulate epithelial cell invasion, and to induce vascular infiltration (angiogenesis) to promote metastasis. Finally, certain growth factors may suppress the host immune response to the tumor and may compromise the tumor response to therapy (Table 1).

Early studies in the 1970s by Todaro, Sporn, Delarco, and others (reviewed in Reference 1) identified the transforming growth factors (TGFs) in conditioned media-transformed fibroblasts, in breast cancer, and in other cancers. In these pioneering studies, TGFs initially derived their name from their ability to reversibly induce the transformed phenotype (defined as the capacity for anchorage-independent or disordered focal growth of cellular monolayers) in certain rodent fibroblasts. This group of growth factors is now known to consist of several families of polypeptides that are synthesized and secreted by a wide variety of normal human and rodent cell lines as well as cell lines transformed by retroviruses, chemicals, radiation, or oncogenes. Growth factors have been proposed to have actions that are autocrine or intracrine (self-regulatory), paracrine or juxtacrine (regulatory of other local cells), and endocrine (regulatory of distant cells).[5–10]

R. B. Dickson: Departments of Cell Biology and Pharmacology, Lombardi Cancer Center, Georgetown University Medical Center, Washington, D.C.

M. E. Lippman: Departments of Pharmacology and Medicine, Lombardi Cancer Center, Georgetown University Medical Center, Washington, D.C.

MULTIPLE CLASSES OF GROWTH FACTORS

Epidermal Growth Factor Family

Two major classes of structurally and functionally distinct transforming growth factor families were initially characterized by the prototypes transforming growth factor α (TGF-α) and transforming growth factor β (TGF-β). TGF-α was closely homologous to epidermal growth factor (EGF), which had been described even earlier in salivary glands and placenta. Many factors of the TGF-α/EGF family compete with EGF for binding its cognate receptor (EGFR), promote EGFR dimerization, activate receptor tyrosine-kinase specific activity, and stimulate cellular proliferation, motility, survival, or differentiation.[11–13] These EGF-related growth factors are each single-chain polypeptides, nearly all with a consensus pattern of three intrachain disulfide bonds. The family members that bind to the EGF receptor include TGF-α, EGF, amphiregulin (AR, a heparin-binding factor), epiregulin, heparin-binding EGF (HbEGF), and β-cellulin.[13–15] A factor known as *cripto-1*[16] is related in structure but has an unknown, probably unrelated receptor. A set of related but virally encoded factors, including VGF (vaccinia growth factor) and others, has also been described to bind the EGF receptor.[13] More recently, a separate EGF-related, heparin-binding subfamily with members known as *heregulins* (from human) and *NDFs* (*neu* differentiating factor, from rat) were identified and cloned[17–20]; this three-gene EGF subfamily is now termed the *neuregulins*.

TABLE 1. *Autocrine and paracrine factors in progression of breast cancer*

Normal
Tight control of epithelial growth and regression cycles by steroids and growth factors
Strong compartmentalization of tissue function controlled by cell-cell and cell-substrate interactions
Expression of steroid receptors in nonproliferative luminal epithelial cells; likely paracrine control of proliferative cells

Early progression of breast cancer
Epithelial desensitization to inhibitory factors
Epithelial sensitization to stimulatory factors
Steroid regulation of growth factor synthesis in proliferative tumor cells
Stromal support of steroid effects

Later progression of breast cancer
Growth factor disruption of stromal architecture (desmoplasia)
Tumor cell motility and local invasion
Angiogenesis
Survival of distant metastases
Chemotherapeutic, radiation, and antihormonal drug resistance
Immune suppression

Neuregulin (heregulin α), a prototype member of a major subclass of EGF-related molecules, has a dominant form of 44 kDa in breast cancer. The rat and human neuregulin homologues have substantial regions of sequence identity and are representative of a large number of gene-splice variants, many of which are focused in neural and neuromuscular tissue.[21] This subfamily does not appear to bind directly to the EGF receptor, unlike most other EGF family members. Instead, neuregulin-1 was initially reported to bind to c-Erb-b2 (HER-2/neu), an EGFR family member and the best known oncoprotein in the disease. Knowledge of the EGFR family has expanded rapidly; in addition to EGFR and c-Erb-b2, the family is now known also to include c-Erb-b3, and c-Erb-b4, two other closely related tyrosine kinase-linked receptors.[22–24] Contrary to initial interpretations of data on the receptor-binding specificity of neuregulins, this growth factor subfamily is now known to bind directly to c-Erb-b4 and c-Erb-b3 receptors. These factors interact only indirectly with c-Erb-b2 by means of receptor heterodimerization.[24–28] All four members of the EGFR family and all of the EGF-related growth factors (except the viral family members epiregulin, and β-cellulin) have been widely detected in breast cancer. They are likely to play a central role in tumor growth as well as in interactions of the tumor with the surrounding host tissue.[29]

Transforming Growth Factor β Family

The TGF-β family of growth factors consists of at least three related gene products, each forming 25-kd homodimeric or heterodimeric species. These species are found in the normal mammary epithelium and in breast cancer. These TGF-β isoforms have a complex pattern of interaction with at least two different soluble binding proteins and with three different molecular weight classes of specific binding proteins.[30–34] Although one of these classes of binding proteins appears to represent a nonsignaling entity (type III receptors), the other two classes (types I and II receptors) are heterodimeric receptor subunits that deliver intracellular signals by means of their serine-threonine-specific kinase activities.[35–38] This entire multiple growth factor–receptor system is now known to be analogous to the receptor system for the related activin family of hormones (which regulate reproductive function).[39] Four type I receptors have been cloned; they each may associate with one of several type II receptors. The specific type II receptor used in a particular dimeric complex appears to recognize TGF-β directly and to determine relative affinity for each of the TGF-β species. The function of a given type II receptor is determined on the basis of which type I receptor is recruited into dimer formation.[40] Separate pathways appear to exist through SMAD (Sma-Mad) transcription factors for regulation of growth versus differentiation by TGF-β.[41] Growth-inhibitory effects of TGF-β on epithelial cells are now known to be mediated by multiple effects on cell cycle regulatory proteins; TGF-β signaling is attenuated by poorly understood mechanisms in the onset and progression of breast cancer.[42–44]

TGF-β (as well as TGF-α) family members have been found in many cancers, in the urine and pleural and peritoneal effusions of cancer patients, and in many normal tissues.[45–49] Initial studies *in vitro* suggested that TGF-β was inhibitory and differentiating in breast cancer cell lines, in normal mammary epithelial cells, and in most other normal and malignant epithelial cell types. However, TGF-β overexpression in breast tumor biopsies was associated with increased malignant progression of the clinical disease.[44,50,51] TGF-β is thus likely to have additional complex effects on breast cancer *in vivo*, including immune suppression and angiogenesis.[30,44,52] At least five other inhibitory factors may also be relevant to breast cancer: mammary-derived growth inhibitor (MDGI),[53] mammostatin,[54] α-lactalbumin,[55] whey acidic protein,[56] and lactoferrin.[57] Neither receptors for these additional factors nor their roles in cancer have been established at present. They are all unrelated to the TGF-β family and have not been thoroughly studied to date in clinical breast cancer.[1]

Other Families of Growth Factors

At least five other families of stimulatory growth factors are also found in breast cancer.[58] These are the insulinlike growth factors [types I and II (IGF-I and IGF-II), and at least six soluble binding proteins],[59] members of the WNT (wingless) growth factor–receptor family,[60] platelet-derived growth

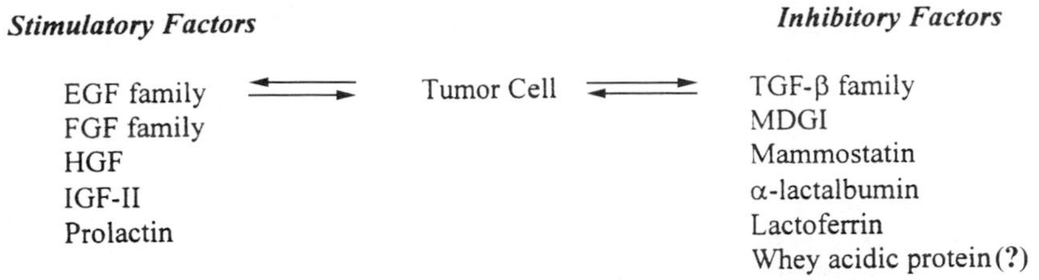

Stimulatory Factors				***Inhibitory Factors***
EGF family	⇄	Tumor Cell	⇄	TGF-β family
FGF family				MDGI
HGF				Mammostatin
IGF-II				α-lactalbumin
Prolactin				Lactoferrin
				Whey acidic protein(?)

FIG. 1. Proposed autocrine factors in breast cancer. Tumor cells release a wide variety of growth factors that have been proposed to play autocrine roles *in vivo* based largely on their activities *in vitro*. Many of the same factors are known to play paracrine and endocrine roles as well. EGF, epidermal growth factor; FGF, fibroblast growth factor; HGF, hepatocyte growth factor; IGF-II, insulinlike growth factor type II; MDGI, mammary-derived growth inhibitor; TGF-β, transforming growth factor β.

factors A and B,[61] and fibroblast growth factors (FGFs, a family of at least thirteen members and a soluble binding protein).[62] Each of these growth factor classes binds to one or more specific tyrosine kinase–encoding receptors. Vascular endothelial growth factor (VEGF, a member of a different family of tyrosine kinase receptor–binding factors),[63,64] pleiotrophin (a developmental, neurotropic factor),[65] and scatter factor (also called *HGF, hepatocyte growth factor*) and its tyrosine kinase–encoding receptor, Met,[66] are also produced by breast cancer, although the latter is synthesized largely by the tumor stroma. Finally, the hormone prolactin[67,68] and an incompletely characterized growth factor known as *mammary-derived growth factor 1 (MDGF-1)*[69] are produced by breast cancer cells. Thus, a widely diverse collection of growth factors is proposed to mediate a multitude of effects in breast cancer (Figs. 1, 2, and 3).

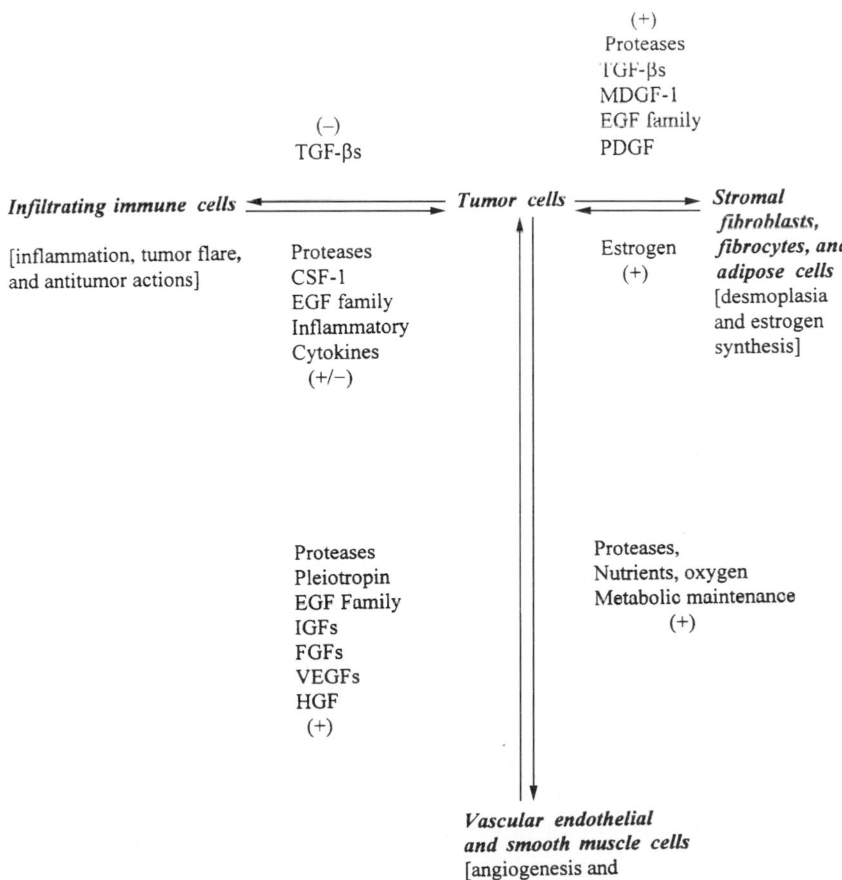

FIG. 2. A diverse group of growth factors and other molecules are thought to play paracrine roles in breast cancer. These interactions involve infiltration of immune cells, the tumor vasculature, and the stromal fibroblasts, fibrocytes, and adipocytes. CSF-1, colony-stimulating factor-1; EGF, epidermal growth factor; FGF, fibroblast growth factor; HGF, hepatocyte growth factor; IGF, insulinlike growth factor; MDGF-1, mammary-derived growth factor 1; PDGF, platelet-derived growth factor; TGF-β, transforming growth factor β; VEGF, vascular endothelial growth factor.

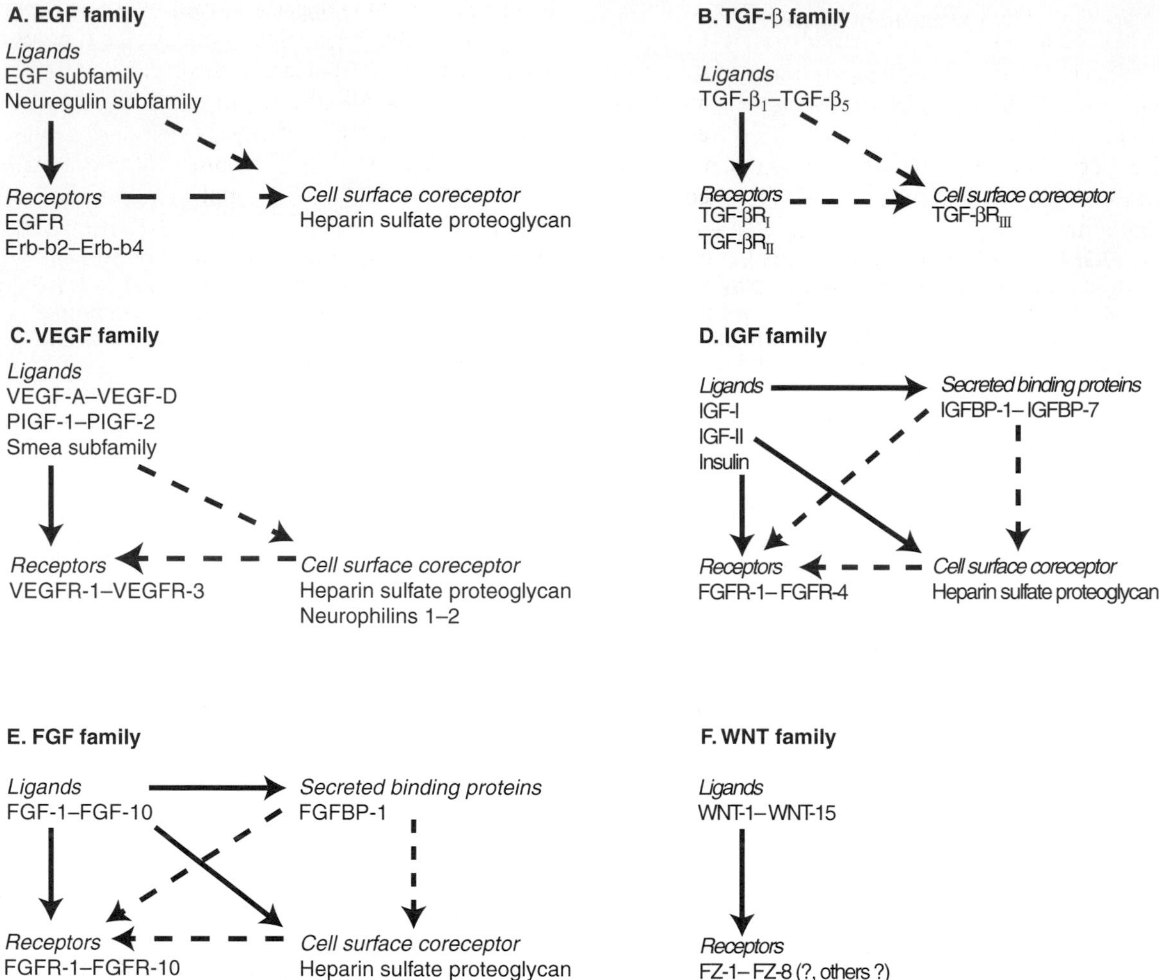

FIG. 3. Six of the major growth factor families are depicted in this figure. Each family contains a minimum of several related growth factors and receptors. Several families also contain cell surface coreceptors or ligand-binding proteins that contribute positively or negatively to receptor activation. Some systems also contain secreted ligand-binding proteins that can positively or negatively influence ligand presentation to its receptors and coreceptors. EGF, epidermal growth factor; EGFR, epidermal growth factor receptor; FGF, fibroblast growth factor; FGFBP, fibroblast growth factor binding protein; FGFR, fibroblast growth factor receptor; FZ, frizzled; IGF, insulinlike growth factor; IGFBP, insulinlike growth factor binding protein; PIGF, placental growth factor; Smea, semaphorins; TGF-β, transforming growth factor β; TGF-βR_I, transforming growth factor β_I receptor I; TGF-βR_{II}, transforming growth factor β_{II} receptor II; TGF-βR_{III}, transforming growth factor β_{III} receptor III; VEGF, vascular endothelial growth factor; VEGFR, vascular endothelial growth factor receptor; WNT, wingless.

ROLE OF GROWTH FACTORS IN TUMOR ONSET AND EARLY PROGRESSION

An early hypothesis in cancer biology was that transformation of cells from normal to malignant may indirectly or directly result from increased production of growth-stimulatory factors or decreased production of growth-inhibitory factors. A revision of this hypothesis has invoked, in addition, altered responsiveness to both negative-acting and positive-acting growth factors.[8,9] Testing of these hypotheses depends on an understanding of pathways of growth control both in neoplastic cells and in the normal cells from which the cancer derived. Three experimental approaches to this issue have been taken. First, primary cultures of mammary epithelial cells have been immortalized and transformed. Second, hormone-dependent and hormone-independent cell lines and tumor biopsies have been compared with normal ones. Finally, transgenic mouse and gene knockout mouse approaches have been used.[1,58]

Development of serum-free culture conditions has facilitated the study of growth regulation in normal human mammary epithelial cells.[70–72] The cellular outgrowths from such cultures possess characteristics suggestive of a basal epithelial "stem cell" relationship.[73] More recently, relatively nonproliferative, more differentiated luminal cells and basal cells have been isolated based on differential expression of antigenic markers; these cells have been immortalized with SV40T antigen.[74–76] Other studies involving primary mammary organoid-derived cultures and milk-derived, shed epithelial cultures have used benzopyrene, human papillomavirus, and prolonged culture in a low Ca^{2+} medium to achieve immortalization.[72,77,78] Further transformation of these basal epithelial cells to full malignancy is associated with conversion of epithelial to mesenchymal morphology and can occur in the presence of an overexpressed nuclear oncogene plus an activated kinase/signal transduction oncogene.[79–81] Transformation of more differentiated, luminal human mammary epithelial cells to a mesenchymal phenotype has been described after expression of a single oncogenic molecule; c-Erb-b2, Bcl-2, c-Ras^{H}, and c-Fos were all effective.[82] Although human mammary epithelial cells may be cultured *in vitro*, whether any of the cultured subtypes is of the lineage or differentiation type that gives rise to breast cancer in women is not yet clear. For example, receptors for estrogen and progesterone have not been demonstrated in normal mammary culture–derived cell types.

Steroid–growth factor interactions have been studied in human mammary tissue only in the context of malignant epithelium, although they are almost certainly crucial as well in the regulation of the normal gland and in its conversion to cancer. In hormone-responsive human breast cancer cells, estrogen-induced proliferation is accompanied by an increase in growth-stimulatory TGF-α, amphiregulin, and IGF-II, modulation of IGF-binding proteins, induction of EGF and IGF-I receptors, inhibition of IGF-II and c-Erb-b2 receptors, and inhibition of TGF-βs.[83–90] Antiestrogenic inhibition of proliferation of the same cell types *in vitro* and of primary breast tumors *in vivo* is paralleled by decreased levels of positive-acting growth factors and augmented secretion of growth-inhibitory TGF-β.[91] Effects that are similar but not identical to those of estrogen have been observed with progestins. Not surprisingly, antiprogestational drugs have an effect opposite to that of progestins.[92–96] Growth-stimulatory steroids and growth factors also exert similar or additive effects on certain other genes, such as those encoding the protooncogene c-*myc*, the secreted protein pS2, and the protease cathepsin D.[95] As one might expect, in hormone-independent breast cancer cell lines, most of the growth factors noted above are constitutively produced, although their levels of secretion may not significantly exceed those of the normal tissue (except possibly for TGF-β).[97,98] Sex hormone–regulated growth factor systems have also been observed in prostate and ovarian cancers.[99,100] As noted in Chapter 2, another level of steroid–growth factor interaction is related to the function of steroid receptors themselves. In addition, signal transduction pathways activated by growth factors and other hormones may directly modulate steroid receptor function at the level of the chromatin, further adding to the complexity of interactions.[101]

In cell lines *in vitro* and in experimental animal models *in vivo*, TGF-α has been directly implicated as a powerful, but incomplete, positive modulator of cellular transformation, probably due to the diversity of its effects to promote proliferation, survival, and motility, as well as to modulate differentiation. Transfection of a human TGF-α complementary DNA (cDNA) into the immortal but nontumorigenic mouse mammary epithelial cell line NOG-8 using a strong promoter-induced anchorage-independent growth but not full tumorigenicity.[102] A different study that used MCF-10A, a spontaneously immortalized human breast ductal epithelial cell line, as recipient for an expression vector containing the TGF-α gene obtained similar results.[103] In contrast, when fully malignant MCF-7 cells were used as a recipient for TGF-α transfection, no significant growth advantage to the cells was observed either in tumors grown *in vitro* or in the nude mouse *in vivo*.[104] Divergent results have also been obtained when fibroblasts are transfected with the TGF-α gene. In one study, when immortalized rodent fibroblasts were used as recipients for the human or rat TGF-α cDNA, transformation to full tumorigenicity was achieved.[105] The closely related factor EGF was also observed to act as an oncogene-like molecule when transfected and overexpressed in immortalized rodent fibroblasts.[106] In contrast, TGF-α transfection into other fibroblasts induced increased proliferation but not full malignant progression to tumorigenicity.[107] To add to the complexity of the situation, TGF-α can induce its own synthesis, and the relative levels of secretion of TGF-α by breast cancer and by rodent fibroblasts are associated with the degree of cellular transformation and levels of expression of other oncogenes or protooncogenes. For example, a clear correlation among TGF-α production, c-*ras*^{H} oncogene expression (after transfection of its cDNA), and malignant transformation has been demonstrated in MCF-10A mammary epithelial cells *in vitro*.[103] The oncogenic c-Erb-b2 receptor is also transforming in this system.[101] The functioning of TGF-α and other family members as oncogenic or tumor progression factors and the relationships among growth factor and oncogene expression depend on the mammary epithelial cell type in question, its level of EGF receptors, and its stage in malignant progression.[5] This type of complexity requires *in vivo* modeling to assess biological relevance more fully.

Several studies have addressed the effect of overexpression of TGF-α (and other EGF family members) in the mammary glands of transgenic mice. These studies have used multiple strategies of localized pellet release, retroviral expression of growth factors, and growth factor transgenic mice, with the gene of interest under general or mammary-specific promotion. The results clearly showed that proliferation of the gland induced by TGF-α, AR, and cripto-1 may be important in early stages of onset of mammary cancer.[108–112] Using TGF-α, under control of the metallothionein promoter, and an outbred mouse strain, one study found the mammary gland to be hyperproliferative and delayed in developmental penetration of the epithelial ducts into the stromal fat pad.[113] A similar block in glandular differentiation was previously observed with local mammary implants of EGF.[114] Other TGF-α transgenic mouse studies using inbred strains have further corroborated the TGF-α transgenic glands to be hyperproliferative and partially defective in postlactational involution, resulting in mammary cancer after multiple pregnancies.[115,116] A subsequent study also suggested that expression of a TGF-α transgene accelerates the progression of carcinogen-induced mouse mammary tumors.[117]

Evidence *in vitro* of very strong autocrine growth dependence on the TGF-α/EGF receptor system has been seen only with use of an EGF receptor–blocking antibody in the hormone-independent MDA-MB-468 cell line. This line has a uniquely high expression of TGF-α due to an amplified gene encoding the EGFR. The level of expression of EGF receptor in this line is so high (in excess of 10^6 per cell) that endogenous TGF-α is stimulatory, whereas even higher levels of exogenous EGF can have a growth-inhibitory effect *in vitro*[118] and lead to apoptosis. When antibody strategies, antisense oligonucleotides complementary to TGF-α, or tyrosine kinase inhibitors are used, estrogen-induced growth of hormone-dependent MCF-7 cells can also be attenuated.[119–121] Autocrine function of another EGF family, amphiregulin, has been demonstrated in nonimmortalized and carcinogen-immortalized human mammary epithelial cells in culture using antisense amphiregulin and heparin (which binds and blocks the factor).[121,122] These studies suggest that the TGF-α/amphiregulin/EGFR system may play multiple roles both in onset and in later proliferation of hormone-dependent and hormone-independent breast cancer. More recent work[123] has demonstrated the presence of HbEGF in human mammary cancer cells. HbEGF and other EGF family members are synthesized as a transmembrane form, which is released by proteolytic cleavage on activation of protein kinase C (PKC) in the cell.

Studies have also addressed the function of the erb-b3/erb-b4 ligand family and the neuregulins in breast cancer. This family of factors appears to act by growth stimulation at lower concentrations and by growth inhibition and differentiation at higher levels. Accordingly, neuregulins induce casein synthesis in breast cancer cells.[19] Neuregulin-1 can induce mammary hyperplasias and tumors after prolonged expression in the transgenic mouse mammary gland.[124] Not surprisingly, c-Erb-b2 overexpression in the transgenic mouse or in the transgenic mammary gland after retroviral transfer also leads to pregnancy-promoted mammary tumors.[110,112] Current strategies using EGF receptor ligands or antibodies coupled to toxins or other therapeutic drugs and directed to the EGF receptor or c-Erb-b2 also show promise for therapeutic use, as a large proportion of hormone-independent breast cancers express significant levels of these receptors.[125–130]

Another important family of growth-regulatory factors in the normal and malignant breast is the FGF family. This family of growth factors requires a heparan cofactor for proper presentation to receptors, and it accumulates in the extracellular matrix after its secretion. Some FGF family members do not possess a signal sequence; nonetheless, all forms appear to be released by cells. FGF-1, FGF-2, and FGF-7 have been detected in mouse mammary preneoplasias, tumors, and cell lines, but not at elevated levels. However, FGF-3 (int-2) is a well-known oncogenic growth factor activated by mouse mammary tumor virus (MMTV) insertional mutagenesis, and FGF-4 (also called *HST*, for human stomach tumor or *K-FGF*) has been associated with metastasis of the mouse mammary gland.[131] FGF-1 and FGF-2 have been detected in the human gland, but their levels are not elevated in human breast cancer. FGF-2 has been proposed as an autocrine growth factor in immortalized human mammary epithelial cells.[132] Although FGF-2 is expressed in breast cancer, it is apparently correlated with good prognosis. The biological roles of FGF-2 and FGF-1 in breast cancer are not fully known; however, they could contribute to inflammation and angiogenesis, as discussed later (see section Growth Factors, Hormone Response, Angiogenesis, and Metastasis). FGF-3 and FGF-4 are not detected in human breast cancer despite their importance in mouse mammary tumorigenesis. Receptors for FGF-1 through FGF-4 are expressed in human breast cancer cells; the FGF-1 receptor gene is occasionally amplified and possibly serves an oncogenic role.[133–136]

The epithelial inhibitory TGF-β family is also found in normal and malignant mammary epithelium and in human milk.[137] It clearly has a negative effect on ductal epithelial proliferation and lactation in mouse mammary glands *in vivo*.[138] As noted above, production of TGF-β increases as breast cancer progresses; its accumulation may be significant in the characteristic fibrous desmoplastic stroma of the disease[139] in immune suppression, and in tumor angiogenesis. Thus, although TGF-β clearly serves a growth-inhibitory role in the normal gland, in which the system may be tumor suppressive, as discussed below, overproduction of TGF-β may contribute to aberrant tumor-host interactions in the later progression of breast cancer.[137,140] In some breast cancer cell lines, TGF-β has even been observed to stimulate cell invasion *in vitro*.[141] The full significance of this observation *in vivo* awaits further study, however. TGF-β is down-regulated by transcriptional and posttranscriptional mechanisms by estrogens and progestins and is induced by antiestrogens and antiprogestins. The synthetic progestin gestodene inhibits anchorage-dependent growth of hormone-dependent breast cancer cells at least partially via TGF-β induction[142]; retinoids, acting through RAR and RXR receptors, can modulate TGF-β1 transcription.[143]

A complex regulatory system is also being revealed by studies of the insulinlike growth factors. IGF-II production, as well as cellular responsiveness to IGFs, is stimulated by estrogen and inhibited by antiestrogens in some hormone-dependent breast cancer cell lines. The cellular responsiveness to IGFs appears to be modulated by estrogens and antiestrogens as a result of regulation of both receptors (type I is induced and type II is repressed), IGF binding proteins

2, 4, and 5 (each of which is estrogen induced), and IGF binding protein 3 (which is estrogen inhibited).The biological functions of these binding proteins are not fully understood, although IGF binding protein 1 appears to inhibit the actions of IGF-I, even in *in vivo* models. Whereas expression of high levels of IGF binding proteins 3 and 4 and expression of high levels of the IGF-II receptor signify poor prognosis for breast cancer, the IGF-I receptor signifies good prognosis. A body of literature has been developing on the roles of steroid regulation of growth factors in the uterus and in the breast.[144–152]

The endocrine hormone prolactin has been observed to be synthesized in the mammary glands of rats, goats, and sheep and in T47D human breast cancer cells. Although its physiologic role as an endocrine hormone in the mammary gland has long been studied, the hormone may play an additional role as a positive stimulatory, locally acting factor, possibly even in breast cancer.[153–156]

Still other work has begun to implicate the WNT family of paracrine factors in breast cancer. This family was initially identified in connection with MMTV insertional transactivation of genes involved in mouse mammary cancer. Nearly a dozen WNT genes are now known, some of which can confer a transforming phenotype on cells. The WNT proteins are transmembrane cell surface factors that interact with the extracellular matrix and are thought to mediate epithelial-mesenchymal interactions. Among the family members, WNT-2, WNT-3, WNT-4, WNT-5a, and WNT-7b are expressed in the human mammary gland and in breast cancer.[157]

GROWTH FACTORS AND CELL ADHESION MOLECULES AS SURVIVAL FACTORS

As with most epithelial cancers, key features of breast cancer are its ability to undergo genomic changes and its ability to exist in hostile environments outside the mammary gland. Clearly, each of these characteristics requires partial or complete suppression of the cell machinery that would normally trigger programmed cell death (apoptosis) under such circumstances.[158] The best-known growth factors that signal survival of the mammary gland epithelial cells are TGF-α, FGFs, and the IGFs, whereas the TGF-βs, the cytokine Il-4, and the death factors tumor necrosis factor and Fas ligand (FasL) trigger the process.[158–160] The cellular mechanisms of regulation of apoptosis by these factors is an area of very active research, due to its obvious clinical translational importance.

Although estrogen and progesterone are known to promote growth and survival of the mammary epithelium, the role of growth factors in epithelial survival is not yet known. This may be particularly important in the context of c-*myc* oncogene amplification, in which cells appear to be sensitized to both growth-inducing and death-inducing stimuli. In fibroblasts, for example, several growth factor families can promote survival of cells overexpressing the c-*myc* oncogene.[161] Similar results have been observed in transgenic mouse models.[162] Some have proposed that growth factors can prevent apoptosis by inducing the *bcl*-2 gene[163,164] or its related family members. Accordingly, a dramatic cooperation has been observed between the proliferation- and survival-promoting TGF-α and c-Myc in the transgenic mouse mammary tumor model.[165–167] Future studies will address the relevance of this finding in primary human breast cancer.

In summary, local functions of growth factors in normal breast tissue may include stimulation of epithelial proliferation and survival by TGF-α, IGF, and FGF family members and inhibition of epithelial proliferation and survival by other factors, including TGF-β and tumor necrosis factor. In cancer, aberrant growth factor overproduction, perturbation of signal transduction mechanisms, and loss of tissue compartmentalization may lead to tumor progression. Effects of tumor factor overpopulation may encompass angiogenesis (TGF-β, FGF), desmoplasia, collagen deposition (MDGF-1, TGF-α, TGF-β), and immune suppression (TGF-β).

GROWTH FACTORS, HORMONE RESPONSE, ANGIOGENESIS, AND METASTASIS

Growth factor and receptor genes have been transfected into hormone-responsive breast cancer cell lines, such as MCF-7 and ZR-75-1, to assess their possible effects on the final steps in malignant progression, including loss of hormone response and metastasis. Although transfection of TGF-α or the EGF receptor had very little effect on MCF-7, partial growth-enhancing effects have been reported for overexpression of the IGF-II gene product and for the c-Erb-b2 protooncogene product.[168–170] In dramatic contrast, very strong enhancement of tumor growth and metastasis was observed after transfection of FGF-1, VEGF, and FGF-4 into MCF-7 cells.[171,172] One mechanism of enhancement of tumorigenesis by these growth factors appears to be promotion of angiogenesis (described later in this section).[173]

Studies consistent with these gene transfection experiments have noted that continuous infusion of EGF is capable of limited stimulation of MCF-7 tumor growth. Tumors grew briefly but regressed after several weeks.[174] In testing the effects of TGF-β on breast tumors, the TGF-β–inhibited MDA-MB-231 cell line was grown as tumors in the nude mouse and the factor was continuously infused. Unexpectedly in these experiments, tumor growth was unaffected by TGF-β *in vivo*, but the animals exhibited cachexia, multiple organ fibrosis, and splenic regression.[175] A later study further characterized the effects of release of endogenous TGF-β from hormone-independent breast tumors *in vivo* and observed that neutralizing anti–TGF-β antibodies suppressed tumor growth and enhanced natural killer cell immune function.[176] As noted earlier, TGF-β, like FGFs, may have additional tumor progression–associated effects on angiogenesis, immune suppression, and tumor invasion. Current studies have also demonstrated the importance of the IGF-I receptor for adhesion, invasion, and metastasis of human breast cancer cells.[177] These data are consistent with earlier observations that pegelated IGF binding protein 1 is capable of suppressing the growth of the highly aggressive MDA-MB-231 and MBA-MB-435 cell lines in nude mice, presumably by interfering with IGF-I.[150]

Growth factor transfection studies have also led to a greater appreciation of the multifaceted interactions of cell surface receptor signaling pathways with those of the sex steroids. For a number of years, both estrogen and growth factors have been known to serve as important mediators between the developing mammary tumor and the tumor stroma. The tumor and stroma both release factors that enhance local synthesis of estrogen through aromatization of steroid precursors[178,179]; this synthesis enhancement may facilitate estrogenic damage of epithelial cells[180] and allow the steroids to then function more effectively to drive epithelial proliferation[181] through regulation of growth factors, protooncogenes, and survival factors.[182–185] Although the growth factors mediating these effects in normal tissue are only beginning to be understood,[186] aberrant expression of TGF-βs, EGF receptor ligands, and FGF receptor ligands is emerging as central in the process of desensitizing the estrogen receptor (ER) system to the effects of antiestrogens in breast cancer.[187–189]

Regulation of local invasion and metastasis by breast cancer is not fully understood. Although some studies have suggested that identification of a specific, dominant, mutated gene or genes is central to the process, this is not yet certain.[190] For example, c-Erb-b2 is a protooncogene whose amplification is closely associated with poor prognosis for node-positive breast cancer, but as described earlier, its role at the cellular level may be complex and indirect. A tumor-suppressor protein whose loss may lead to metastasis is E-cadherin,[191] but tumor cell adhesion is also quite complex.[192,193] Cellular motility as well is almost certainly involved in the progression of breast cancer. Motility-promoting molecules that have been proposed to act in disease progression are the FGF family members,[194,195] HGF,[196] autotaxin,[197] TGF-β,[198] and the EGF family members.[199] Among these, the motility-enhancing effects of the latter are probably the best understood at the cellular level. Activation of the EGF receptor specifically enhances the accumulation of actin filament at the leading edge of the "lamellipod" of the advancing cell.[199] Metastasis also depends on the formation of a tumor vasculature (angiogenesis),[200,201] escape of cells into the vasculature (extravasation), formation of tumor cell emboli in the bloodstream, and their subsequent entrapment of cells in capillary networks of metastasis and organs. The latter process is thought to depend on platelet activation and adhesion of the embolus to endothelial cells by $\alpha_{IIb}\beta_3$ integrin. Because $\alpha_{IIb}\beta_3$ is under regulation by PKC and prostaglandin pathways, it may represent another target of growth factor enhancement of metastatic progression.[202,203]

The reconstituted basement membrane extract Matrigel has been used extensively in attempts to model the process of invasion *in vitro*. With this type of system, ER-negative cells have generally been observed to be more invasive than ER-positive ones, and estrogen has been found to increase invasiveness of ER-positive cell lines. Tamoxifen citrate was sufficiently estrogenic also to induce invasion of a breast cancer cell line in an *in vitro* model; the pure antiestrogen ICI 164,384 is suppressive.[204] The integrin $\alpha_2\beta_1$ appears to play a major role in adhesion and invasion of breast cancer cells. Although this integrin is a receptor for laminin and collagen in ER-positive breast cancer, it appears to bind only collagen in the ER-negative disease. In MCF-7 cells, PKC stimulation induces $\alpha_2\beta_1$-dependent adhesion, motility, and invasion.[205,206] So far, research has not clearly demonstrated that growth factors strongly regulate cellular invasion, although TGF-β may be a candidate, as noted earlier. TGF-β, like PKC, may modulate invasion through the NFkB transcription factor.[207] TGF-β may regulate both growth and adhesion through the cyclin inhibitor p27.[208] As noted earlier, blockade of IGF-I signaling may also suppress motility and invasion.[177] In addition, a protein termed BCSG1 (or SNC-γ), which is homologous to the synuclein protein related to Alzheimer's disease and is expressed in invasive breast cancer, stimulates breast tumor cell motility and invasion.[209]

Invasive breast cancer is marked by abnormal stromal-epithelial interaction and deposition of tenascin, an embryonic matrix component.[210] Aspects of this stromal dysfunction include increased motility of tumor fibroblasts and altered secretion of growth factor by fibroblasts in the area of the tumor. The growth factor IGF-II is expressed by breast tumor–derived fibroblasts, whereas IGF-I is expressed by normal breast fibroblasts.[211] Many other growth factors, including FGF-1, FGF-2, FGF-5, and possibly HGF, are also secreted by breast fibroblasts, regardless of whether the source was tumor or normal tissue.[211,212] Stromal fibroblastic production of the protease styromelysin III (matrix metalloprotease 11, or MMP-11) is also an early marker of invasive breast cancer[213]; the regulation of this and other proteases in the area of the tumor probably involve growth factors. The role of the local growth factor environment is emerging as critical to the regulation of proteases in invasive breast cancer. For example, both HGF and stromelysin III are strongly regulated by TGF-β.[214,215] The 72-kd gelatinase (MMP-2), as well as MMP-1 and MMP-3, are induced by a new factor known as *tumor cell–derived collagenase-stimulatory factor*.[216] In contrast, the 92-kd gelatinase (MMP-9) is induced by a different autocrine growth factor, although unidentified at the present time.[217] Although these proteases may be important in tissue invasion itself, they also may have critical roles in the processing of growth factors and cytokines (such as tumor necrosis factor α).[218,219] A further role for growth factors is proposed in the motility of tumor cell invasion. Although, as noted earlier, many growth factors may modulate motility, components of a more specific motility-inducing-factor pathway (the autocrine motility factor receptor and autotoxin) have been characterized.[197,220]

Angiogenesis (blood vessel invasion into the tumor area) is an important event required for tumor expansion and for full metastatic dissemination of breast cancer.[200,221,222] For many years, this process has been appreciated as necessary for tumor growth beyond a few millimeters in size due to tumor tissue requirements for a proper metabolic environment. FGFs, EGF-family factors, TGF-βs, HGF, pleiotrophin, and VEGF are all thought to have the capacity to mediate angiogenesis.[223,224] Emerging antiangiogenic therapies use compounds such as TNP 470 and thalidomide, which appear to directly block the endothelial cell cycle, as well as protease inhibitors.[224] In addition, endostatin and angiostatin, two naturally occurring fragments of plasminogen and collagen (respectively), have generated much interest as antiangiogenic drugs.[224] Chemotherapy is potentially synergistic with this type of therapy, and this interaction will be examined in future clinical trials.[225,226] Necrosis is the result of an improperly vascularized tissue, such as in the lumen of a large tumor.[200]

Studies show that the degree of tumor metastases is also directly proportional to the number of capillaries infiltrating the tumor (neoangiogenesis). At least two mechanisms might explain this effect. First, simple tumor size is known to be a poor prognostic indicator. The ability of a tumor to recruit a high degree of local microvasculature clearly contributes to its large size. Large tumor size then facilitates a greater diversity of mutational events and an increased likelihood that highly aggressive, metastatic cells will arise. A second angiogenic mechanism of tumor progression probably directly involves the vasculature (venous and lymphatic drainage) as a necessary escape route for tumor cells. Tumor cells preferentially accumulate very early in metastasis in local lymph nodes and in organ capillary beds. Thus, biopsy of the local lymph nodes is an accurate indicator of disease progression.[200] A close, perhaps causal relationship between breast tumor neoangiogenesis and metastases has been observed in breast cancer patients.[200,227–229] In some experimental models, the existence of a primary tumor is closely associated with increased proliferation of distant metastases, implying the possibility of continued growth factor communication among tumor colonies after dissemination.[230] However, potential growth factor mediators of such an effect have not yet been identified.

In vivo model systems of human breast cancer invasion have been developed. Hormone-independent breast cancer cells are generally more locally invasive than hormone-dependent cells in the nude mouse.[231] In particular, the MDA-MB-435 line has been developed into a model of hematogenous metastases in the nude mouse. This line is widely metastatic in 6 to 9 months.[232] The inoculation site and dietary fat content strongly modulate tumor growth and metastatic spread in experimental models of breast cancer.[233,234] The inoculation site effect may relate to local factor specificity in tumor progression; dietary fat may also modulate levels of estrogenic hormones. As noted above, angiogenesis and metastases may be strongly regulated by heparin-binding growth factors, such as FGFs, VEGF, and pleiotrophin. Accordingly, studies have shown that FGF-4, FGF-1, or VEGF transfection into human MCF-7 breast cancer cells strongly promotes tumor growth and lymphatic/hematogenous metastases.[171,172,235,236] These studies have been facilitated by cotransfecting cells with a gene encoding a chromogenic enzyme, lacZ, which renders cells easily stainable. LacZ staining of an MCF-7 line transfected with FGF-4 afforded clear indication of metastatic cells. Ipsilateral lymph nodes were 100% positive for metastases by 3 weeks; by 6 weeks, other more distant lymph nodes, lung, and kidney were positive; and by 12 weeks, multiple organs showed evidence of metastases.[171,172] Identification and mechanistic studies of the principal metastasis-inducing growth factors for breast cancer will continue to be a priority for breast cancer research in the foreseeable future.

Tumor cell invasion is thought to depend on a combination of proteolytic activities and enhanced capacity for carcinoma cell motility. The MMP class of enzymes has been widely studied from the point of view both of vascular invasion into the tumor site and of invasion of tumor cells out of the lesion. Although most of the known MMPs and their tissue inhibitors of metalloprotease (TIMPs) inhibitors are actually synthesized to a large degree in the stromal fibroblasts and vasculature, several, such as MMP-2 and MMP-9, can bind carcinoma-associated receptors (such as the integrin $\alpha_1\beta_3$) to allow their presentation by the developing tumor cells. An exception to this proposed model is MMP-7, whose synthesis may be more restricted to the carcinoma itself.[214,236,237] Current studies have reported that the presentation of MMP in breast tumor cells is linked closely to those cells that have undergone an epithelial-mesenchymal transition within the lesion.[238] Growth factors, acting through their signal transduction pathways, particularly PKC, are thought to play a role in the invasiveness and MMP up-regulation in this mechanism,[206,239] leading to increased levels of MMP in blood and urine of patients.[240] Inhibition of MMPs with anti-MMP drugs (Batimastat, Marimastat) in animal models and early clinical trials has suggested that these drugs suppress tumor growth and angiogeneses but may have little effect on tumor invasion itself.[241] A second, larger body of work has addressed the serine proteases in breast cancer. The urokinase-type plasminogen activator (uPA) system and its plasminogen activator inhibitors I and II (PAI-1, PAI-2) are also largely produced in the tumor stroma, with tumor presentation occurring mostly indirectly through tumor-associated uPA receptors. In contrast to the MMP system, detection of uPA and PAI-1 has clear prognostic significance in human breast cancer.[242,243] Other studies have focused on a novel, carcinoma-membrane-associated, trypsin-related serine protease that is produced directly in breast carcinoma cells.[244] Because broad-spectrum protease inhibitors, such as maspin, are found in breast cancer, in which they are thought to be tumor suppressive,[245] serine proteases and their inhibition are likely to be the subject of much future investigation.

SUMMARY AND FUTURE PROSPECTS

Progression of the normal breast through early stages of malignancy to metastasis almost certainly reflects a gross

TABLE 2. *Sex steroid regulation of growth factors*

Growth factor or binding protein	Effect of estrogen	Effect of progesterone
Transforming growth factor α	+	+
Epidermal growth factor	?	+
Amphiregulin	+	?
Insulinlike growth factor type II	+	?
Transforming growth factor β1	−	−
Transforming growth factor β2	−	?
Transforming growth factor β3	−	?
Insulinlike growth factor binding protein 2	+	?
Insulinlike growth factor binding protein 3	−	?
Insulinlike growth factor binding protein 4	+	?
Insulinlike growth factor binding protein 5	+	?

alteration in function of autocrine and paracrine factors. Whereas in mammary development these factors are under tight regulation, both quantitatively and regionally, in cancer, a progressive perturbation occurs in growth controls (see Table 1). One principal example is the altered regulation of cancer cell proliferation itself (see Fig. 1). The EGF receptor pathway is perturbed in the presence of an amplified c-*myc* or c-*erb*-b2 gene to enhance malignant progression dramatically through multiple mechanisms. In addition, the sex steroids regulate critical growth factor pathways and vice versa (Tables 2 and 3). Later progression appears to involve more changes in the epithelial cell that seem both to abrogate the need for exogenous growth factors to drive the cell cycle and to block the ability of TGF-β to attenuate proliferation. One aspect of this further series of perturbations is overproduction of growth factors and proteases. A good example is TGF-β, which may carry out multiple functions in advanced cancers to enhance angiogenesis, suppress immune function, and modulate the stromal environment (see Fig. 2). Better understanding of growth factor pathways will certainly enhance the chances for drug discovery in cancer. Indeed, secreted factors that compromise the host to the benefit of the tumor may represent an Achilles heel in the defenses of breast cancer. Blockade of these activities with kinase inhibitors and other pharmacologic agents should be a major goal for the future.

TABLE 3. *Sex steroid regulation of growth factor receptors*

Growth factor or binding protein	Effect of estrogen	Effect of progesterone
Epidermal growth factor receptor	+	+
c-Erb-b2 receptor	−	−
Insulinlike growth factor type I receptor	+	+
Insulinlike growth factor type II receptor	−	?
Insulin receptor	?	+

REFERENCES

1. Dickson RB, Lippman ME. Growth regulation of normal and malignant breast epithelium. In: Bland KI, Copeland EM, eds. *The breast*, 2nd ed. Philadelphia: WB Saunders, 1998:518.
2. Maemura M, Dickson RB. Are cellular adhesion molecules involved in the metastasis of breast cancer? *Breast Cancer Res Treat* 1994;32:239.
3. Van Der Burg B, Kulkhoven E, Isbruecken L, DeLaat SW. Effects of progestins on the proliferation of estrogen-dependent human breast cancer cells under growth factor-defined conditions. *J Steroid Biochem Molec Biol* 1992;42:457.
4. Zugmaier G, Knabbe C, Fritsch C, et al. Tissue culture conditions determine the effects of estrogen and growth factors on the anchorage independent growth of human breast cancer cell lines. *J Steroid Biochem Molec Biol* 1991;39:684.
5. Dickson RB, Lippman ME. Estrogenic regulation of growth and polypeptide growth factor secretion in humor breast carcinoma. *Endocrine Rev* 1987;8:29.
6. Paul D, Schmidt GH. Immortalization and malignant transformation of differentiated cells by oncogenes *in vitro* and in transgenic mice. *Crit Rev Oncog* 1989;1:307.
7. Heldin CH, Westermark B. Growth factors: mechanism of action and relations to oncogenes. *Cell* 1984;37:9.
8. Goustin AS, Leof EB, Shipley GD, Moses HL. Growth factors and cancer. *Cancer Res* 1986;46:1015.
9. Sporn MB, Roberts AB. Peptide growth factors and inflammation, tissue repair, and cancer. *J Clin Inv* 1986;78:329.
10. Basilico C, Moscatelli D. The FGF family of growth factors and oncogenes. *Adv Cancer Res* 1992;59:115.
11. Massague J. Epidermal growth factor–like transforming growth factor. *J Biol Chem* 1983;258:13606.
12. Derynck R. Transforming growth factor α. *Cell* 1988;54:593.
13. Todaro GJ, Rose TM, Spooner CE, Shoyab M, Plowman GD. Cellular and viral ligands that interact with the EGF receptor. *Semin Cancer Biol* 1990;1:257.
14. Higashigama S, Abraham JA, Miller J, Fiddles JC, Klagsbrun M. A heparin-binding growth factor secreted by macrophage-like cells that is related to EGF. *Science* 1991;251:936.
15. Bates SE, Davidson NE, Valverius EM, Dickson RB, Freter CE, Tam JP, et al. Expression of transforming growth factor alpha and its mRNA in human breast cancer: its regulation by estrogen and its possible functional significance. *Mol Endocrinol* 1988;2:543.
16. Normanno N, Qi C-F, Gullick WJ, Persico G, Yarden Y, Wen D, et al. Expression of amphiregulin, cripto-1, and heregulin α in human breast cancer cells. *Intl J Oncol* 1993;2:903.
17. Holmes WE, Sliwkowski MX, Akita RW, Henzel WJ, Lee J, Park JW. Identification of heregulin, a specific activator of $p185^{erbB2}$. *Science* 1992;256:1205.
18. Wen D, Peles E, Cupples R, Suggs SV, Bacus SS, Luo Y. Neu differentiation factor: a transmembrane glycoprotein containing an EGF domain and an immunoglobulin homology unit. *Cell* 1992;69:559.
19. Peles E, Bacus SS, Koski RA, Lu HS, Wen D, Ogden SG. Isolation of the neu/HER-2 stimulatory ligand: a 44 kd glycoprotein that induces differentiation of mammary tumor cells. *Cell* 1992;69:205.
20. Falls DL, Rosen KM, Corfas G, Lane WS, Fischbach GD. ARIA, a protein that stimulates acetylcholine receptor synthesis, is a member of the neu ligand family. *Cell* 1993;72:801.
21. Dickson R, Lippman ME. Growth factors in breast cancer. *Endocrine Rev* 1995;16:559.
22. Marchionni MA, Goodearl ADJ, Chen MS, Bermingham-McDonogh O, Kirk C, Hendricks M. A new acquaintance for $erbB_3$ and $erbB_4$: a role for receptor heterodimerization in growth signaling. *Cell* 1994;78:5.
23. Gullick WJ, Srinivasan R. The type 1 growth factor receptor family: new ligands and receptors and their role in breast cancer. *Breast Cancer Res Treat* 1998;52:43.
24. Plowman GD, Green JM, Culouscou JM, Carlton GW, Rothwell VM, Buckley S. Heregulin induces tyrosine phosphorylation of HER4/P180 ($erbB_4$). *Nature* 1993;366:473.
25. Carraway KL, Cantley LC. A new acquaintance for $erbB_3$ and $erbB_4$: a role for receptor heterodimerization in growth signalling. *Cell* 1994; 78:5.
26. Carraway KL, Slikowski MX, Akita R, Platko JV, Guy PM, Nuijens A. The $erbB_3$ gene product is a receptor for heregulin. *J Biol Chem* 1994;269:14303.

27. Slikowski MX, Schaefer G, Akita RW, Lofgren JA, Fitzpatrick VD, Nuijens A. Coexpression of $erbB_2$ and $erbB_3$ proteins reconstitutes a high affinity receptor for heregulin. *J Biol Chem* 1994;26:14661.
28. Pinkas-Kramarski R, Alroy I, Yarden Y. ErbB receptors and EGF-like ligands: cell lineage determination and oncogenesis through combinatorial signaling. *J Mammary Gland Biol and Neoplasia* 1997;2:97.
29. Martinez-Lacaci I, Bianco C, DeSantis M, Salomon DS. Epidermal growth factor-related peptides and their cognate receptors in breast cancer. In: Bowcock A, ed. *Breast cancer: molecular genetics, pathogenesis, and therapeutics*. Totowa, NJ: Humana Press, 1999:31.
30. Wakefield LM, Colletta AA, Maccune BK, Sporn MB. Roles for transforming growth factors β in the genesis, prevention, and treatment of breast cancer. In: Dickson RB, Lippman ME, eds. *Genes, oncogenes, and hormones*. Boston: Kluwer, 1992:97.
31. Liu X, Yue J, Frey RS, Zhu Q, Muldek KM. Transforming growth factor beta signaling through smad1 in human breast cancer cells. *Cancer Res* 1998;58:4752.
32. Alevizopouolos A, Mermod N. Transforming growth factor-β: the breaking open of a black box. *Bioessays* 1997;19:581.
33. Padgett RW, Das P, Krishna S. TGF-beta signaling, smads, and tumor suppressors. *Bioessays* 1998;20:382.
34. Helden CH, Miyazono K, Dijke PT. TGF β signalling from cell membrane to nucleus through SMAD proteins. *Nature* 1997;390:465.
35. Massague J. Receptors for the TGFβ family. *Cell* 1992;69:1067.
36. Ebner R, Chen R-H, Shum L, Lawler S, Zioncheck TF, Lee A. Cloning of a type 1 TGF-beta receptor and its effect on TGF-beta binding to the type 2 receptor. *Science* 1993;260:1344.
37. Attisamo L, Caracomo J, Ventura F, Weis FMB, Massague J, Wrana JL. Identification of human activin and TGFβ type I receptors that form heteromeric kinase complexes with type II receptors. *Cell* 1993;75:671.
38. Liu X, Yue J, Frey RS, Zhu Q, Mulder KM. Transforming growth factor beta signaling through smad1 in human breast cancer cells. *Cancer Research* 1998;58:4752.
39. Mathews LS. Activin receptors and cellular signaling by the receptor serine kinase family. *Endocrine Rev* 1994;15:310.
40. Wrana JL, Attisano L, Wieser R, Ventura F, Massague J. Mechanism of activation of the TGF-β receptor. *Nature* 1994;370:341.
41. Chen R-H, Ebner R, Derynck R. Inactivation of the type II receptor reveals two receptor pathways for the diverse TGF-β activities. *Science* 1993;260:1335.
42. Soriano JV, Pepper MS, Orci L, and Montesano R. Roles of hepatocyte growth factor/scatter factor and transforming growth factor-beta1 in mammary gland ductal morphogenesis. *J Mammary Gland Biol Neoplasia* 1998;3:133.
43. Brattain MG, Ko Y, Banerji SS, Wu G, Willson JKV. Defects of TGF-beta receptor signaling in mammary cell tumorigenesis. *J Mammary Gland Biol Neoplasia* 1996;1:365.
44. Koli KM, Arteaga CL. Transforming growth factor-beta and breast cancer. In: Bowcock A, ed. *Breast cancer: molecular genetics, pathogenesis, and therapeutics*. Totowa, NJ: Humana Press, 1999:95.
45. Stromberg K, Hudgins R, Orth DN. Urinary TGFα in neoplasia: immunoreactive TGF-α in the urine of patients with disseminated breast carcinoma. *Biochem Biophys Res Commun* 1987;144:1059.
46. Artega CL, Hanauske AR, Clark GM, Osborne CK, Hazarika P, Pardue RL. Immunoreactive alpha transforming growth factor (IraTGF) activity in effusions from cancer patients: a marker of tumor burden and patient prognosis. *Cancer Res* 1988;48:5023.
47. Sairenji M, Suzuki K, Murakami K, Motohashi H, Okamoto T, Umeda M. Transforming growth factor activity in pleural and peritoneal effusions from cancer and non-cancer patients. *Jpn J Cancer Res (Gann)* 1987;78:814.
48. Ohmura E, Tsushima T, Kamiya Y, et al. Epidermal growth factor and transforming growth factor α induce ascitic fluid in mice. *Cancer Res* 1990;50:4915.
49. Massaque J. The transforming growth factor β family. *Ann Rev Cell Biol* 1990;6:597.
50. Gorsch SM. Immunohistochemical staining for transforming growth factor beta associates with disease progression in human breast cancer. *Cancer Res* 1992;52:6949.
51. Samuel SK, Hurta RAR, Kondaiah P, Khalil N, Turley EA, Wright JA. Autocrine induction of tumor protease production and invasion by a metallothionein-regulated TGF-$β_1$. *EMBO J* 1992;11:1599.
52. Enenstein J, Walek NS, Kramer RH. Basic FGF and TGFβ differentially modulate integrin expression of human microvascular endothelial cells. *Exp Cell Res* 1992;203:499.
53. Grosse R, Bohmer FD, Binas B, et al. Mammary-derived growth inhibitor. In: Dickson RB, Lippman ME, eds. *Genes, oncogenes and hormones*. Boston: Kluwer, 1992:69.
54. Ervin PR, Kaminski M, Cody RL, Wicha MS. Production of mammostatin, a tissue-specific growth inhibitor, by normal human mammary cells. *Science* 1989;244:1585.
55. Thompson MP, Farrell HM, Mohanam S, Liu S, Kidwell WR, Bansal MP. Identification of human milk α-lactalbumin as a cell growth inhibitor. *Protoplasma* 1992;167:134.
56. McKnight RA, Burdon T, Parsel VG, et al. The whey acidic protein. In: Lippmann ME, Dickson RB, eds. *Genes, oncogenes, and hormones.* Boston: Kluwer, 1992,399.
57. Hurley WL. *In vitro* inhibition of mammary cell growth by lactoferrin: a comparative study. *Life Sci* 1994;55:1955.
58. Dickson RB, Lippman ME. Molecular biology of breast cancer. In: DeVita VT, Hellman S, Rosenberg SA, eds. *Principles and practice of oncology*, 5th ed. Philadelphia: JB Lippincott, 1997:1541.
59. Ellis MJ. The insulin-like growth factor network and breast cancer. In: Bowcock A, ed. *Breast cancer: molecular genetics, pathogenesis, and therapeutics*. Totowa, NJ: Humana Press, 1999:121.
60. Bergstein I, Brown AMC. WNT genes and breast cancer. In: Bowcock A, ed. *Breast cancer: molecular genetics, pathogenesis, and therapeutics*. Totowa, NJ: Humana Press, 1999:181.
61. Bronzert DA, Pantazis P, Antoniades HN, et al. Synthesis and secretion of PDGF by human breast cancer cell lines. *Proc Natl Acad Sci U S A* 1987;84:5763.
62. Kern FG. The role of fibroblast growth factors in breast cancer pathogenesis and progression. In: Bowcock A, ed. *Breast cancer: molecular genetics, pathogenesis, and therapeutics*. Totowa, NJ: Humana Press, 1999:59.
63. Ferrara N, Houck K, Jakeman L, Leung DW. Molecular and biological properties of the vascular endothelial growth factor family of proteins. *Endocrine Rev* 1992;13:18.
64. Neufeld G, Cohen T, Gengrinovitch, Poltorak Z. Vascular endothelial growth factor (VEGF) and its receptors. *FASEB J* 1999;13:9.
65. Wellstein A, Fang W, Khatri A, et al. A heparin-binding growth factor secreted from mammary epithelial cells is homologous to a developmentally regulated cytokine. *J Biol Chem* 1992;267:2582.
66. Rong S, Bodescot M, Blair D, Dunn J, Nakamura T, Mizuno K. Tumorigenicity of the met proto-oncogene and the gene for hepatocyte growth factor. *Mol Cell Biol* 1992;12:5152.
67. Clevenger CV, Chang WP, Ngo W, Pasha TL, Montone KT, Tomaszewski JE. Expression of prolactin and prolactin receptor in human breast carcinoma: evidence for an autocrine/paracrine loop. *Am J Pathol* 1995;146:695.
68. Vonderhaar BK. Prolactin and its receptors in human breast cancer. In: Manni A, ed. *Contemporary endocrinology: endocrinology of breast cancer.* Totowa, NJ: Humana Press, 1999:261.
69. Bano M, Kidwell WR, Dickson RB. MDGF-1: a multifunctional growth factor in human milk and human breast cancer. In: Dickson RB, Lippman ME, eds. *Mammary tumorigeneses and maligant progression*. Boston: Kluwer, 1994:193.
70. Kamalati T, Niranjan B, Atherton A, Anbazhagan R, Gusterson B. Differentiation antigens in stromal and epithelial cells of the breast. In: Dickson RB, Lippman ME, eds. *Mammary tumor cell cycle, differentiation, and metastasis*. Boston: Kluwer, 1996:227.
71. Hammond SL, Ham RG, Stampfer MR. Serum-free growth of human mammary epithelial cells: rapid clonal growth in defined medium and extended serial passage with pituitary extract. *Proc Natl Acad Sci U S A* 1984;81:5435.
72. Stampfer MR, Bartley JC. Induction of transformation and continuous cell lines from normal human mammary epithelial cells after exposure to benzo-*a*-pyrene. *Proc Natl Acad Sci U S A* 1985; 82:2394.
73. Chepko G, Smith GH. Mammary epithelial stem cells: our current view. *J Mammary Gland Biol Neoplasia* 1999;4:35.
74. Bartek J, Bartkova J, Kyprianou N, et al. Efficient immortalization of luminal epithelial cells from human mammary gland by introduction of simian virus 40 large tumor antigen with a recombinant retrovirus. *Proc Natl Acad Sci U S A* 1991;88:3520.
75. Dundas SR, Ormerod MG, Gusterson BA, O'Hare MJ. Characterization of luminal and basal cells flow-sorted from the adult rat mammary parenchyma. *J Cell Sci* 1991;100:459.

76. Gusterson BA, Monaghan P, Mahendran R, Ellis J, O'Hare MJ. Identification of myoepithelial cells in human and rat breasts by anti-common acute lymphoblastic leukemia antigen antibody. *J Natl Cancer Inst* 1986;77:81.
77. Band V, Zajchowski D, Kulesa V, Sager R. Human papilloma virus DNAs immortalize normal human mammary epithelial cells and reduce their growth factor requirements. *Proc Natl Acad Sci U S A* 1990;87:463.
78. Soule HD, McGrath A. Simplified method for passage and long-term growth of human mammary epithelial cells. *In Vitro Cell Dev Biol* 1986;22:6.
79. Clark R, Stampfer MR, Milley B, et al. Transformation of human mammary epithelial cells by oncogenic retroviruses. *Cancer Res* 1988;48:4689.
80. Valverius EM, Ciardiello F, Heldin NE, et al. Stromal influence on transformation of human mammary cells overexpressing c-myc and SV40 T. *J Cell Physiol* 1990;145:207.
81. Thompson EW, Torri J, Sabol M, et al. Oncogene cooperation in human mammary epithelial cells. *Clin Exp Metastasis* 1994;12:181.
82. Alford D, Pitha-Rowe P, Taylor-Papadimitriou J. Adhesion molecules in breast cancer: role of α_2 β_1 integrin. In: Rudland PS, Fernig DG, Leinster S, Lunt GG, eds. *Mammary development and cancer*. London: Portland Press, 1998:245.
83. Dickson RB, Huff KK, Spencer EM, Lippman ME. Induction of epidermal growth factor-related polypeptides by 17-beta estradiol in MCF-7 human breast cancer cells. *Endocrinol* 1986;118:138.
84. Liu SC, Sanfilippo B, Perroteau I, Derynch R, Salomon DS, Kidwell WR. Expression of transforming growth factor α (TGFα) in differentiated rat mammary tumors: estrogen induction of TGFα production. *Mol Endocrinol* 1987;1:683.
85. Knabbe C, Wakefield L, Flanders K, et al. Evidence that TGF beta is a hormonally regulated negative growth factor in human breast cancer. *Cell* 1987;48:417.
86. King RJB, Wang DY, Daley RJ, Darbre PD. Approaches to studying the role of growth factors in the progression of breast tumors from the steroid sensitive to insensitive state. *J Steroid Biochem* 1989;34:133.
87. Knabbe C, Zugmaier G, Schmal M, Dietel M, Lippman ME, Dickson RB. Induction of transforming growth factor beta by the antiestrogens droloxifen, tamoxifen, and toremifen in MCF-7 cells. *Am J Clin Oncol* 1991;14[Suppl 2]:515.
88. Arrick BA, Korc M, Derinck R. Differential regulation of expression of three transforming growth factor-β species in human breast cancer cell lines by estradiol. *Cancer Res* 1990;50:299.
89. Murphy LC, Dotzlau H. Regulation of transforming growth factor β messenger ribonucleic acid abundance in T47D human breast cancer cells. *Mol Endocrinol* 1989;3:611.
90. Stewart AJ, Johnson MD, May FEB, Westley BR. Role of insulin-like growth factors and the type I insulin-like growth factor receptor in the estrogen-stimulated proliferation of human breast cancer cells. *J Biol Chem* 1990;265:21172.
91. Butta A, MacLennan K, Flanders KC, Sacks NPM, Smith I, McKinna A. Induction of transforming growth factor β_1 in human breast cancer *in vivo* following tamoxifen treatment. *Cancer Res* 1992;52:4261.
92. Murphy LC, Murphy LJ, Dubik D, Bell GI, Shiu RPC. Epidermal growth factor gene expression in human breast cancer cells: regulation of expression by progestins. *Cancer Res* 1988;48:4555.
93. Murphy LC, Dotzlau H. Regulation of transforming growth factor α messenger ribonucleic acid abundance in T47D, human breast cancer cells. *Mol Endocrinol* 1989;3:611.
94. Musgrove EA, Lee CSL, Sutherland RL. Progestins both stimulate and inhibit breast cancer cell cycle progression while increasing expression of transforming growth factor α, epidermal growth factor receptor, c-*fos*, and c-*myc* genes. *Mol Cell Biol* 1991;11:5032.
95. Goldfine ID, Papa V, Vigneri R, Siiteri P, Rosenthal S. Progestin regulation of insulin and insulin-like growth factor I receptors in cultured human breast cancer cells. *Br Cancer Res Treat* 1992;22:69.
96. Bates SE, McManaway ME, Lippman ME, Dickson RB. Characterization of estrogen responsive transforming activity in human breast cancer cell lines. *Cancer Res* 1986;46:1707.
97. Arteaga CL, Tandon AK, Von Hoff DD, Osborne CK. Transforming growth factor β: potential autocrine growth inhibitor of estrogen receptor-negative human breast cancer cells. *Cancer Res* 1988;48:3898.
98. Dickson RB, Lippman ME. Control of human breast cancer by estrogen, growth factors, and oncogenes. In: Lippman ME, Dickson RB, eds. *Breast cancer: cellular and molecular biology*. Boston: Kluwer, 1988:119.
99. Lopez-Otin C, Diamardis EP. Breast and prostate cancer: an analysis of common epidemiological, genetic and biochemical features. *Endocrine Rev* 1998;19:365.
100. Simpson BJB, Langdon SP, GJ Rabiasz, et al. Estrogen regulation of transforming growth factor–alpha in ovarian cancer. *J Steroid Biochem Mol Biol* 1998;64:137.
101. Kenny NJ, Dickson RB. Growth factor and sex steroid interactions in breast cancer. *J Mammary Gland Biol Neoplasia* 1996;1:189.
102. Shankar V, Ciardiello F, Kim N, Derynck R, Liscia DS, Merlo G. Transformation of normal mouse mammary epithelial cells following transfection with a human transforming growth factor alpha cDNA. *Mol Carcinog* 1989;2:1.
103. Ciardiello F, McGready M, Kim N, et al. TGFα expression is enhanced in human mammary epithelial cells transformed by an activated c-Ha-ras but not by the c-neu protooncogene and overexpression of the TGFα cDNA leads to transformation. *Cell Growth Differ* 1990;1:407.
104. Clarke R, Brunner N, Katz D, et al. The effects of a constitutive production of TGFα on the growth of MCF-7 human breast cancer cells *in vitro* and *in vivo*. *Mol Endocrinol* 1989;3:372.
105. Rosenthal A, Lindquist PB, Bringman TS, Goeddel DV, Derynck R. Expression in rat fibroblasts of a human transforming growth factor-α cDNA results in transformation. *Cell* 1986;46:301.
106. Stern DF, Hare DL, Cecchini MA, Weinberg RA. Construction of a novel oncogene based on synthetic sequences encoding epidermal growth factor. *Science* 1987;235:321.
107. Finzi E, Fleming T, Segatto O, et al. The human transforming growth factor type α coding sequence is not a direct-acting oncogene when overexpressed in NIH3T3 cells. *Proc Natl Acad Sci U S A* 1987;84:3733.
108. Kenney NJ, Smith GH, Johnson MD, et al. Cripto-1 activity in the intact and ovariectomized virgin mouse mammary gland. *Pathogenesis* 1997;1:57.
109. Kenny NJ, Smith GH, Rosenberg K, Cutler ML, Dickson RB. Induction of ductal morphogenesis and lobular hyperplasia by amphiregulin in the mouse mammary gland. *Cell Growth Differ* 1996;7:1769.
110. Amundadottir LT, Merlino GT, Dickson RB. Transgenic models of breast cancer. *Breast Cancer Res Treat* 1996;39:119.
111. Schroeder JA, Lee DC. Transgenic mice reveal roles for TGF alpha and EGF receptor in mammary gland development and neoplasia. *J Mammary Gland Biol Neoplasia* 1997;2:119.
112. Edwards PAW. Control of the three dimensional growth pattern of mammary epithelium: role of genes of the WNT and erbB families studied using reconstituted epithelium. In: Rudland PS, Fernig DG, Leinster S, Lunt GG. *Mammary development and cancer*. London: Portland Press, 1998:21.
113. Jhappan C, Stahle C, Harkins RN, Fausto N, Smith GH, Merlino GT. TGFα overexpression in transgenic mice induces liver neoplasia and abnormal development of the mammary gland and pancreas. *Cell* 1990;61:1137.
114. Coleman S, Daniel CW. Inhibition of mouse mammary ductal morphogenesis and down regulation of the EGF receptor by epidermal growth factor. *Develop Biol* 1990;137:425.
115. Sandgren EP, Luetteke NC, Palmiter RD, Brinster RL, Lee DC. Overexpression of TGFα in transgenic mice: induction of epithelial hyperplasia, pancreatic metaplasia and carcinoma of the breast. *Cell* 1990;61:1121.
116. Matsui Y, Halter SA, Holt JT, Hogan BLM, Coffey RJ Jr. Development of mammary hyperplasia and neoplasia in MMTV-TGFα transgenic mice. *Cell* 1990;61:1147.
117. Coffey RJ Jr, Meise KS, Matsui Y, Hogan BLM, Dempsey PJ, Halter SA. Acceleration of mammary neoplasia in transforming growth factor α transgenic mice by 7,12-dimethylbenzanthracene. *Cancer Res* 1994;54:1678.
118. Ennis BW, Valverius EM, Lippman ME, et al. Anti EGF receptor antibodies inhibit the autocrine stimulated growth of MDA-MB-468 breast cancer cells. *Mol Endocrinol* 1989;3:1830.
119. Kenney N, Saeki T, Gottardis M, et al. Expression of transforming growth factor α (TGFα) antisense mRNA inhibits the estrogen-induced production of TGFα and estrogen-induced proliferation of estrogen-responsive human breast cancer cells. *J Cell Physiol* 1993;156:497.
120. Bates SE, Davidson NE, Valverius E, et al. Expression of transforming growth factor-alpha and its mRNA in human breast cancer: regulation by estrogen and evidence for a transforming role. *Mol Endocrinol* 1988;2:543.

121. Reddy KB, Mangold GL, Tandon AK, et al. Inhibition of breast cancer cell growth *in vitro* by a tyrosine kinase inhibitor. *Cancer Res* 1992;52:3636.
122. Kenney N, Johnson G, Selvam MP, et al. Transforming growth factor α (TGFα) and amphiregulin (AR) as autocrine growth factors in nontransformed immortalized 184AIN4 human mammary epithelial cells. *Mol Cell Differ* 1993;1:163.
123. Raab G, Higashiyama S, Hetelekidis S, et al. Biosynthesis and processing by phorbol ester of the cell surface-associated precursor form of heparin-binding egf-life growth factor. *Biochem Biophys Res Commun* 1994;204:592.
124. Krane IM, Leder P. NDF/heregulin induces persistence of terminal end buds and adenocarcinomas in the mammary glands of transgenic mice. *Oncogene* 1996;12:1781.
125. Pastan IH, Chaudhary V, Fitzgerald DJ. Recombinant toxins as novel therapeutic agents. *Ann Rev Biochem* 1992;61:331.
126. Fry DW, Kraker AJ, McMichael A, et al. A specific inhibitor of the epidermal growth factor receptor tyrosine kinase. *Science* 1994;265:1093.
127. Fan Z, Mendelsobn J. Breast cancer therapy using monoclonal antibodies against epidermal growth-factor receptor and Her-2. In: Bowcock AM, ed. *Breast cancer: molecular pathogenesis, and therapeutics*. Totowa, NJ: Humana Press, 1998:419.
128. Esteva-Lorenzo FJ, Sastry L, King CR. The erbB-2 gene in human cancer: translation from research to application. *Hormones and growth factors in development and neoplasia*. New York: Wiley-Liss, 1998:421.
129. Paik S, Bryant J, Park C, et al. *erb*-b-2 and response to doxorubicin in patients with axillary lymph node-positive, hormone receptor-negative breast cancer. *J Natl Cancer Inst* 1998;90:1361.
130. Fox S, Harris AL. The epidermal growth factor receptor in breast cancer. *J Mammary Gland Biol Neoplasia* 1997;2:131.
131. Coleman-Krnacik S, Rosen JM. Differential temporal and spatial gene expression of fibroblast growth factor family members during mouse mammary gland development. *Mol Endocrinol* 1994;8:218.
132. Soutton B, Hamelin R, Crepin M. FGF-2 as an autocrine growth factor for immortal human breast epithelial cells. *Cell Growth Differ* 1994;5:615.
133. McLeskey SW, Ding IYF, Lippman ME, Kern FG. MDA-MB-134 breast carcinoma cells overexpress fibroblast growth factor (FGF) receptors and are growth-inhibited by FGF ligands. *Cancer Res* 1994;54:523.
134. Wang H, Rubin M, Fenig E, et al. Basic fibroblast growth factor causes growth arrest in MCF-7 human breast cancer cells while inducing both mitogenic and inhibitory G1 events. *Cancer Res* 1997;57:1750.
135. Jouanneau J, Gavrilovic J, Caruelle D, et al. Secreted or nonsecreted forms of acidic fibroblast growth factor produced by transfected epithelial cells influence cell morphology, motility, and invasive potential. *Proc Natl Acad Sci U S A* 1991;88:2893.
136. Kern FG. The role of fibroblast growth factors in breast cancer pathogenesis and progression. In: Bowcock A, ed. *Breast cancer: molecular genetics, pathogenesis, and therapeutics*. Totowa, NJ: Humana Press, 1998:59.
137. McCure BK, Mullin BR, Flanders KC, Jaffurs WJ, Muller LT, Sporn MB. Localization of transforming growth factor–β isotypes in lesions of the human breast. *Hum Pathol* 1991;23:13.
138. Daniel CW, Silberstein GB. Developmental biology of the mammary gland. In: Neville MC, Daniel CW, eds. *The mammary gland*. New York: Plenum, 1987:3.
139. Stampfer MR, Yaswen P, Alhadeff M, Hosoda J. TGFβ induction of extracellular matrix associated proteins in normal and transformed human mammary epithelial cells in culture is independent of growth effects. *J Cell Physiol* 1993;155:21.
140. Travers MT, Barrett-Lee PJ, Berger U, et al. Growth factor expression in normal, benign, and malignant breast tissue. *BMJ* 1988;296:1621.
141. Welch DR, Fabra A, Nakajima M. Transforming growth factor β stimulates mammary adenocarcinoma cell invasion and metastatic potential. *Proc Natl Acad Sci U S A* 1990;87:7676.
142. Colleta AA, Wakefield LM, Howell FV, Danielpour D, Baum M, Sporn MB. The growth inhibition of human breast cancer cells by a novel synthetic progestin involves the induction of transforming growth factor beta. *J Clin Invest* 1991;87:277.
143. Salbert G, Fanjul F, Piedrafita J, et al. Retinoic acid receptors and retinoid X receptor-α down-regulate the transforming growth factor-β_1 promoter by antagonizing AP-1 activity. *Mol Endocrinol* 1993;7:1347.
144. Ellis M, Jenkins S, Hanfelt J, et al. Insulin-like growth factors in human breast cancer. *Breast Cancer Res Treat* 1998;52:175.
145. Surmacz E, Guvakova MA, Nolan MK, Nicosia RF, Sciacca L. Type I insulin-like growth factor receptor function in breast cancer. *Breast Cancer Res Treat* 1998;47:255.
146. Oates AJ, Schumaker LM, Jenkins SB, et al. The mannose 6-phosphate/insulin-like growth factor 2 receptor (M6P/IGF2R), a putative breast tumor suppressor gene. *Breast Cancer Res Treat* 1998;47:269.
147. Oh Y. IGF-independent regulation of breast cancer growth by IGF binding proteins. *Breast Cancer Res Treat* 1998;47:238.
148. Lee AV, Hilsenbeck SG, Yee D. IGF system components as prognostic markers in breast cancer. *Breast Cancer Res Treat* 1998;47:295.
149. Richert MM, Wood TL. Expression and regulation of insulin-like growth factors and their binding proteins in the normal breast. In: Manni A, ed. *Contemporary endocrinology: endocrinology of breast cancer*. Totowa, NJ: Humana Press, 1999:39.
150. Cullen KJ, Kaup SS, Rasmussen AA. Interactions between stroma and epithelium in breast cancer: implications for tumor genesis growth, and progression. In: Manni A, ed. *Contemporary endocrinology: endocrinology of breast cancer*. Totowa, NJ: Humana Press, 1999:155.
151. Lee AV, Yee D. Role of the IGF system in breast cancer proliferation and progression. In: Manni A, ed. *Contemporary endocrinology: endocrinology of breast cancer*. Totowa, NJ: Humana Press, 1999:187.
152. Baserga R. The IGF-I receptor in normal and abnormal growth. In: Dickson RB, Salomon DS, eds. *Hormones and growth factors in development and neoplasia*. New York: Wiley-Liss, 1998:269.
153. Forsyth I. Prolactin, growth hormones, and placental lactogens: an historical perspective. *J Mammary Gland Biol Neoplasia* 1997;2:3.
154. Goffin V, Kelly PA. The prolactin/growth hormone receptor family: structure/function relationships. *J Mammary Gland Biol Neoplasia* 1997;2:7.
155. Clevenger CV, Plank TL. Prolactin as an autocrine/paracrine factor in breast tissue. *J Mammary Gland Biol Neoplasia* 1997;2:59.
156. Vonderhaar BK. Prolactin in development of the mammary gland and reproductive tract. In: Dickson RB, Salomon DS, eds. *Hormones and growth factors in development and neoplasia*. New York: Wiley-Liss 1998:193.
157. Jonsson M, Smith K, Harris AL. WNT and fibroblast growth factor gene expression during development of the mammary gland and role of WNTs in human cancer. In: Dickson RB, Salomon DS, eds. *Hormones and growth factors in development and neoplasia*. New York: Wiley-Liss, 1998:361.
158. Rosfjord EC, Dickson RB. Growth factors, apoptosis, and survival of mammary epithelial cells. *J Mammary Gland Biol Neoplasia* 1999; 4:229.
159. Gooch JL, Lee AV, Yee D. Interleukin 4 inhibits growth and induces apoptosis in human breast cancer cells. *Cancer Res* 1998;58:4199.
160. Ashkenazi A, Dixit VM. Death receptors: signaling and modulation. *Science* 1998;281:1305.
161. Harrington EA, Bennett MR, Fanidi A, Evan GI. c-Myc-induced apoptosis in fibroblasts is inhibited by specific cytokines. *Biochem Cell Nucleus Lab* 1994;3286.
162. Christofori G, Nalk P, Hanahan D. A second signal supplied by insulin-like growth factor II in oncogene-induced tumorigenesis. *Nature* 1994;369:414.
163. Vaux DL, Cory S, Adams JM. Bcl-2 gene promotes hematopoietic cell survival and cooperation with c-myc to immortalize pre-B cells. *Nature* 1988;335:440.
164. Adams JM, Cory S. The Bcl-2 protein family: arbiters of cell survival. *Science* 1998;281:1322.
165. Evan G, Littlewood T. A matter of life and cell death. *Science* 1998;281:1317.
166. Amundadottir LT, Johnson MD, Merlino GT, Smith GH, Dickson RB. Synergistic interaction of transforming rowth factor alpha and c-myc in mouse mammary and salivary gland tumorigenesis. *Cell Growth Differ* 1995;6:737.
167. Amundadottir LT, Nass S, Berchem G, Johnson MD, Dickson RB. Cooperation of TGF alpha and c-myc in mouse mammary tumorigenesis: coordinated stimulation of growth and suppression of apoptosis. *Oncogene* 1996;13:757.
168. Daly RJ, Harris WH, Wang DY, Darbre PD. Autocrine production of insulin-like growth factor II using an inducible expression system results in reduced estrogen sensitivity of MCF-7 human breast cancer cells. *Cell Growth Differ* 1991;2:457.
169. Cullen KJ, Lippman ME, Chow D, Hill S, Rosen N, Zwiebel JA. Insulin-like growth factor-II overexpression in MCF-7 cells induces

phenotypic changes associated with malignant progression. *Mol Endocrinol* 1992;6:91.
170. Kern FG, Mcleskey SW, Zhang L, et al. Transfected MCF-7 cells as a model for breast cancer progression. *Breast Cancer Res Treat* 1994;31:153.
171. McLeskey SW, Kurebayashi J, Honig SF, et al. Development of an estrogen-independent, antiestrogen resistant, metastatic breast carcinoma line by transfection of MCF-7 cells with fibroblast growth factor-4. *Cancer Res* 1993;53:2168.
172. Kurebayashi J, McLeskey SW, Johnson MD, Lippman ME, Dickson RB, Kern FG. Spontaneous metastasis of MCF-7 human breast cancer cell line cotransfected with fibroblast growth factor-4 and bacterial lacZ genes. *Cancer Res* 1993;53:2178.
173. Mcleskey SW, Zhang L, Kharbanda S, et al. Fibroblast growth factor-overexpressing models of angiogenesis and metastasis in breast cancer. *Breast Cancer Res Treat* 1996;39:103.
174. Dickson RB, McManaway M, Lippman ME. Estrogen induced factors of breast cancer cells partially replace estrogen to promote tumor growth. *Science* 1986;232:1540.
175. Zugmaier G, Paik S, Wilding G, et al. Transforming growth factor beta 1 induces cachexia and systemic fibrosis without an antitumor effect in nude mice. *Cancer Res* 1991;51:3590.
176. Arteaga CL, Carty-Dugger T, Moses HL, Hurd SD, Pietenpol JA. Transforming growth factor β_1 can induce estrogen-independent tumorigenicity of human breast cancer cells in athymic mice. *Cell Growth Differ* 1993;4:193.
177. Dunn SE, M Ehrkich, NJH Sharp, et al. A dominant negative mutant of the insulin-like growth factor-I receptor inhibits the adhesion, invasion, and metastasis of breast cancer. *Cancer Res* 1998;58:3353.
178. Sasano H, Harada N. Intratumoral aromatase in human breast, endometrial, and ovarian malignancies. *Endocr Rev* 1998;19:593.
179. Tekmal RR, Santen RJ. Local estrogen production: is aromatase an oncogene? In: Manni A, ed. *Contemporary endocrinology: endocrinology of breast cancer*. Totowa, NJ: Humana Press, 1999:79.
180. Service RF. New role for estrogen in cancer? *Science* 1998;279:1631.
181. Woodward TL, Xie JX, Haslam SZ. The role of mammary stroma in modulating the proliferative response to ovarian hormones in the normal mammary land. *J Mammary Gland Biol Neoplasia* 1998;3:117.
182. El-Ashry D, Chrysogelos SA, Lippman ME, Kern FG. Estrogen induction of tgf-alpha is mediated by an estrogen response element composed of two imperfect palindromes. *J Steroid Biochem Mol Biol* 1996;59:261.
183. Leygue E, Gol-Winkler R, Gompel A, et al. Estradiol stimulates c-myc proto-oncogene expression in normal human breast epithelial cells in culture. *J Steroid Biochem Mol Biol* 1995;52:299.
184. Wang T, Phang J. Effects of estrogen on apoptotic pathways in human breast cancer cell line MCF-7. *Cancer Res* 1995;55:2487.
185. Streuli CH, Gilmore AP. Adhesion-mediated signaling in the regulation of mammary epithelial survival. *J Mammary Gland Biol Neoplasia* 1999;4:183.
186. Cunha GR, Hayward SW, Donjacour AA, Kurita T, Cooke PS, Lubahn DB. Growth factors as mediators of stromal-epithelial interactions in steroid hormone target organs. In: Dickson RB, Salomon DS, eds. *Hormones and growth factors in development and neoplasia*. New York: Wiley-Liss, 1998:207.
187. Mcleskey SW, Zhang L, Trock BJ, et al. Tamoxifen-resistant FGF-transfected MCF-7 cells are cross resistant in vivo to the antiestrogen ICI 182,780 and two aromatase inhibitors. *Clin Cancer Res* 1998;4:697.
188. Benson JR, Baum M, Collectta AA. Role of TGF beta in the anti-estrogen response/resistance of human breast cancer. *J Mammary Gland Biol Neoplasia* 1996;1:381.
189. De Bortoli M, Dati C. Hormonal regulation of type I receptor tyrosine kinase expression in the mammary gland. *J Mammary Gland Biol Neoplasia* 1997;2:175.
190. Barraclough R, Chen H-J, Davies BR, et al. Use of DNA transfer in the induction of metastasis in experimental mammary systems. In: Rudland PS, Fernig DG, Leinster S, Lunt GC, eds. *Mammary development and cancer*. London: Portland Press, 1998:273.
191. Christofori G, Semb H. The role of the cell-adhesion molecule E-cadherin as a tumor suppressor gene. *Trends Biochem Sci* 1999;24:73.
192. McCormick BA, Zetter BR. Adhesive interactions in angiogenesis and metastasis. *Pharmacol Ther* 1992;53:239.
193. Pishvain MJ, Feltes CM, Thompson P, Bussemakers MJ, Schalken JA, Byers-SW. Cadherin-11 is expressed in invasive breast cancer cell lines. *Cancer Res* 1999;59:947.
194. Valles AM, Tucker GC, Thiery JP, Boyer B. Alternative patterns of mitogenesis and cell scattering induced by acidic FGF as a function of cell density in a rat bladder carcinoma cell line. *Cell Regulat* 1990;1:975.
195. Jouanneau J, Gavrilovic J, Caruelle D, Jaye M, Moens G, Caruelle JP. Secreted or nonsecreted forms of acidic fibroblast growth factor produced by transfected epithelial cells influence cell morphology, motility, and invasive potential. *Proc Natl Acad Sci U S A* 1991;88:2893.
196. Rosen EM, Knesel J, Goldberg ID. Scatter factor and its relationship to hepatocyte growth factor and *met*. *Cell Growth Differ* 1991;2:603.
197. Stracke M, Clair T, Liotta LA. Autotaxin, tumor motility-stimulating exophosphodiesterase. *Adv Enzyme Regul England* 1997;37:135.
198. Koli KM, Arteaga CL. Complex role of tumor cell transforming growth factor (TGF)-βs on breast carcinoma progression. *J Mammary Gland Biol Neoplasia* 1996;1:373.
199. Chan AY, Ruft S, Bailly M, Wykoff TB, Segall JE, Condeelis JS. EGF stimulates an increase in actin nucleation and filament number at the leading edge of the lamellipod in mammary adenocarcinoma cells. *J Cell Sci* 1998;111:199.
200. Folkman J. Angiogenesis in breast cancer. In: Bland KI, Copeland EM, eds. *The breast*, 2nd ed. WB Saunders, 1998:586.
201. Kern FG. Role of angiogenesis in the transition to hormone independence and acquisition of the metastatic phenotype. In Manni A, ed. *Contemporary endocrinology: endocrinology of breast cancer*. Totowa, NJ: Humana Press, 1999:169.
202. Schneider MR, Schirner M. Antimetastatic prostacylin analogs. *Drugs Fut* 1993;18:29.
203. Schirner M, Schneider MR. The prostacyclin analogue cicaprost inhibits metastasis of tumours of R 3327 MAT Lu prostate carcinoma and SMT 2A mammary carcinoma. *J Cancer Res Clin Oncol* 1992; 118:497.
204. Thompson EW, Katz D, Shima TB, Wakeling AE, Lippman ME, Dickson RB. ICI 164,384: a pure antiestrogen for basement membrane invasiveness and proliferation of MCF-7 cells. *Cancer Res* 1989;49:6929.
205. Johnson MD, Torri J, Lippman ME, Dickson RB. Dual regulation of motility and protease expression in PKC-mediated induction of MCF-7 breast cancer cell invasiveness. *Exp Cell Res* 1999:247;1053.
206. Rosfjord E, Maemura M, Johnson MD, Akiyama S, Woods VC, Dickson RB. Protein kinase C modulates $\alpha_2\beta_1$ integrin on MCF-7 breast cancer cells. *Exp Cell Res* 1999;248:260.
207. Perez JR, Higgins-Sochaski KA, Maltese J-Y, Narayanan R. Regulation of adhesion and growth of fibrosarcoma cells by NfkB RelA involves transforming growth factor β. *Mol Cell Biol* 1994;14:5326.
208. Polyak K, Kato JY, Solomon MJ, et al. p27^{Kip1}, a cyclin-Cdk inhibitor, links transforming growth factor-beta and contact inhibition to cell cycle arrest. *Genes Dev* 1994;8:9.
209. Jia T, Liu YE, Liu J, Shi YE. Stimulation of breast cancer invasion and metastasis by synuclein gamma. *Cancer Res* 1999;59:742.
210. Sakakura T, Ishihara A, Yatani R. Tenascin in mammary gland development: from embryogenesis to carcinogenesis. In: Lippman ME, Dickson RB, eds. *Regulatory mechanisms in breast cancer*. Boston: Kluwer, 1991:365.
211. Cullen KJ, Smith HS, Hill S, Rosan N, Lippman ME. Growth factor mRNA expression by human breast fibroblasts from benign and malignant lesions. *Cancer Res* 1992;51:4978.
212. Sonnenberg E, Meyer D, Weidner KM, Birchmeier C. Scatter factor/hepatocyte growth factor and its receptor, the c-met tyrosine kinase, can mediate a signal exchange between mesechyme and epithelia during mouse development. *J Cell Biol* 1993;123:223.
213. Lamacher JM, Podhajcer OL, Chenard MP, Rio MC, Chambon P. A novel metalloproteinase gene specifically expressed in stromal cells of breast carcinomas. *Nature* 1990;348:699.
214. Benaud C, Dickson RB, Thompson EW. Roles of matrix metalloproteases in mammary gland development and cancer. *Cancer Res Treat* 1998;50:97.
215. Seslar SP, Nakamura T, Byers SW. Regulation of fibroblast hepatocyte growth factor/scatter factor expression by human breast carcinoma cell lines and peptide growth factors. *Cancer Res* 1993;53:1233.
216. Kataoka H, DeCastro R, Zucker S, Biswas C. Tumor cell-derived collagenase-stimulatory factor increases expression of interstitial collagenase, stromelysin and 72-kDa gelatinase. *Cancer Res* 1993; 53:3154.
217. Hyuga S, Nishikawa Y, Sakata K, et al. Autocrine factor enhancing the secretion of M_R 95,000 gelatinase (matrix metalloproteinase 9) in

serum-free medium conditioned with murine metastatic colon carcinoma cells. *Cancer Res* 1994;54:3611.

218. Gearing AJH, Beckett P, Christodoulou M, et al. Processing of tumour necrosis factor-α precursor by metalloproteinases. *Nature* 1994;370:555.
219. McGeehan GM, Becherer JD, Bast RC Jr, et al. Regulation of tumour necrosis factor-α processing by a metalloproteinase inhibitor. *Nature* 1994;370:558.
220. Murata J, Clair T, Lee A, et al. cDNA cloning of the autotaxin. *J Biol Chem* 1994;269:30479.
221. Liotta LA, Steeg PS, Stetler-Stevenson WG. Cancer metastasis and angiogenesis: an imbalance of positive and negative regulation. *Cell* 1991;64:327.
222. Gasparini G. Angiogenesis in breast cancer: role in biology, tumor progression, and prognosis. In: Bowcock A, ed. *Breast cancer: molecular genetics, pathogenesis, and therapeutics*. Totowa, NJ: Humana Press, 1999:347.
223. Relf M, LeJeune S, Scott PAE, et al. Expression of the angiogenic growth factors vascular endothelial growth factor, acidic and basic growth factor, tumor growth factor β-1 platelet-derived endothelial cell growth factor, placental growth factor, and pleiotropin in human primary breast cancer and its relation to angiogenesis. *Cancer Res* 1997;57:963.
224. Neufeld G, Cohen T, Gengrinovitch S, Poltorak Z. Vascular endothelial growth factor (VEGF) and its receptors. *FASEB J* 1999;13:9.
225. Teicher BA, Sotomayor EA, Huang ZD. Antiangiogenic agents potentiate cytotoxic cancer therapies against primary and metastatic disease. *Cancer Res* 1992;52:6702.
226. Boehm T, Folkman J, Browder T, O'Reilly MS. Antiangiogenic therapy of experimental cancer does not induce acquired drug resistance. *Nature* 1997;390:404.
227. Heimann R, Ferguson D, Gray S, Hellman S. Assessment of intratumoral vascularization (angiogenesis) in breast cancer prognosis. *Breast Cancer Res Treat* 1998;52:147.
228. Locopo N, Fanelli M, Gasparini G. Clinical significance of angiogenic factors in breast cancer. *Breast Cancer Res Treat* 1998;52:159.
229. Fox SB, Gatter KC, Bicknell R, et al. Relationship of endothelial cell proliferation to tumor vascularity in human breast cancer. *Cancer Res* 1993;53:4161.
230. Fisher B, Gunduz N, Coyle J, Rudoch C, Saffer E. Presence of a growth-stimulating factor in serum following primary tumor removal in mice. *Cancer Res* 1989;49:1996.
231. Thompson EW, Paik S, Brunner N, et al. Association of increased basement membrane-invasiveness with absence of estrogen receptor and expression of vimentin in human breast cancer cell lines. *J Cell Physiol* 1992;150:534.
232. Price JE, Polyzos A, Zhang RD, Daniels LM. Tumorigenicity and metastases of human breast carcinoma cell lines in nude mice. *Cancer Res* 1990;50:717.
233. Meschter CL, Connolly JM, Rose DP. Influence of regional location of the inoculation site and dietary fat on the pathology of MDA-MB-435 human breast cancer cell-derived tumors grown in nude mice. *Clin Exp Metastasis* 1992;10:167.
234. Naguchi M, Ohta N, Kifugawa H, Earashi M, Thomas M, Miyazaki I. Effects of switching from a high fat diet to a low fat diet on tumor proliferation and cell kinetics of DMBA-induced mammary carcinoma in rats. *Oncology* 1992;49:246.
235. Mcleskey SW, Tobias CA, Vezza PR, Filie A, Kern FG, Hanfelt J. Tumor growth of FGF or VEGF transfected MCF-7 breast carcinoma cells correlates with density of specific microvessels independent of the transfected angiogenic factor. *Am J Pathol* 1998; 153:1993.
236. MacDougall JR, Matrisian LM. Matrix metalloproteinases in the pathogenesis of breast cancer. In: Bowcock A, ed. *Breast cancer: molecular genetics, pathogenesis, and therapeutics*. Totowa, NJ: Humana Press, 1999:305.
237. Zhang L, Kharbanda S, Hanfelt J, Kern FG. Both autocrine and paracrine effects of transfected acidic fibroblast growth factor are involved in the estrogen-independent and antiestrogen-resistant growth of MCF-7 breast cancer cells. *Cancer Res* 1998;58:352.
238. Martorana AM, Zheng G, Crowe TC, O'Grady RL, Lyons JG. Epithelial cells up-regulative matrix metalloproteinases in cells within the same mammary carcinoma that have undergone an epithelial-mesenchymal transition. *Cancer Res* 1998;58:4970.
239. Welch DR, Wei LL. Genetic and epigenetic regulation of human breast cancer progression and metastasis. *Endocr Related Cancer* 1998;5:155.
240. Moses MA, Wiederschain D, Loughlin KR, Zurakowski D, Lamb CC, Freeman MR. Increased incidence of matrix metalloproteinases in urine of cancer patients. *Cancer Res* 1998;58:1395.
241. Wojtowicz-Praga SM, Dickson RB, Hawkins MJ. Matrix metalloproteinase inhibitors. *Invest New Drugs* 1997;15:61.
242. Stephens RW, Brunner N, Janicke F, Schmitt M. The urokinase plasminogen activator system as a target for prognostic studies in breast cancer. *Breast Cancer Res Treat* 1998;52:99.
243. Pedersen AN, Holst Hansen C, Frandsen TL, Nielsen BS, Stephens RW, Brunner N. The urokinase plasminogen activation system in breast cancer. In: Bowcock A, ed. *Breast cancer: molecular genetics, pathogenesis, and therapeutics*. Totowa, NJ: Humana Press, 1999:45.
244. Lin CY, Wang JK, Torri J, Dou L, Sang QX, Dickson RB. Characterization of a novel membrane-bound 80kDa matrix-degrading protease from human breast cancer cells. *J Biol Chem* 1997;272:9147.
245. Seftor RE, Seftor EA, Sheng S, Pemberton PA, Sager R, Hendrix MJC. Maspin suppresses the invasive phenotype in human breast carcinoma. *Cancer Res* 1998;58:5681.

CHAPTER 22

Diseases of the Breast, 2nd ed.,
edited by Jay R. Harris.
Lippincott Williams & Wilkins, Philadelphia © 2000.

Animal Models

Robert Clarke and Michael D. Johnson

GENERAL PRINCIPLES

Animal models of breast cancer have been widely used for many years and have contributed significantly to our understanding of breast cancer biology and to the development of several new therapeutic strategies. Because the number of species that develop spontaneous breast tumors is limited, there are few good animal models of spontaneous breast cancer. For example, in addition to rats and mice, mammary tumors also arise spontaneously in dogs,[1,2] but the cost of these models is generally prohibitive. The majority of experimental animal models of breast cancer are limited to the rodent species. However, several different groups of rodent models are available for experimental breast cancer research. These include chemically induced rat mammary carcinomas, virally induced mammary tumors, human tumor xenografts, and transgenic mouse models.

Many aspects of experimental breast cancer research require the use of an appropriate animal model. For example, reproducing the complexity of the endocrinologic environment of the pituitary-adrenal-ovarian axis is beyond the scope of current *in vitro* technologies. Tumor-host interactions, including immunologic, vascular, and stromal effects, and host-related pharmacologic-pharmacokinetic effects, also are relatively poorly modeled *in vitro*. However, even a well-justified requirement for the use of living animals imposes several ethical and scientific considerations. Investigators must give appropriate consideration to the health and welfare of experimental animals (e.g., by providing adequate diet, space, health monitoring, and hygiene).[3] Many of these concerns are of more importance than is often realized. For example, almost all mammary animal tumor models are sensitive to (i.e., inhibited by) caloric restriction.[4–6] Sufficient numbers of animals must be used to provide adequate statistical power and to ensure the validity of the study[7,8] but not such that there is unnecessary animal use.

Each of the rodent models has its own advantages and disadvantages, and a clear understanding of the limitations and use of each model is critical for its appropriate application. In general, the major models for spontaneous breast cancer are the mouse strains that are susceptible to mouse mammary tumor virus (MMTV)–induced mammary neoplasia and some transgenic mouse models. In these models, the mammary glands potentially express the transforming genes from early life onward (MMTV/neonatal; transgenics/fetal). For the chemically induced tumors, initiation events are induced by the carcinogen. The spontaneous and chemically induced models are particularly useful for chemoprevention studies, because full transformation of the gland has either not occurred (young transgenic and MMTV-infected mice) or occurs within a reproducible time after carcinogenic insult (chemically induced tumors). In the human tumor xenografts, the malignant tissue is directly inoculated into host tissues. Thus, effects on early events (i.e., initiation) are not amenable to study. However, these xenografts provide a good model for the study of malignant progression in the human disease and the screening of drugs and therapies against established human tumors. A major advantage of the xenografts is their human breast cancer origin, whereas a disadvantage of the rodent mammary models is their nonhuman origin. Choice of the appropriate model and a realistic assessment of its limitations are critical for adequate and appropriate experimental design. Siemann[9] made a simple but important observation when he stated that a critical consideration is to ". . . choose the model to address the question rather than force the question on the tumor model."

CHEMICALLY INDUCED RODENT MAMMARY TUMORS

The mammary glands of several rat strains are susceptible to transformation by chemical carcinogens, most notably Sprague-Dawley,[10] Buf/N,[11] Fischer 344,[12] Lewis,[13] and, to a lesser extent, Wistar-Furth.[12] Other strains are relatively resistant (e.g., the Copenhagen rat[14]). The genetic reasons for this resistance are unknown, but resistant strains appear to inherit a dominant autosomal allele on rat chromosome 2[15] that specifically inhibits the progression, but not initiation, of mammary

R. Clarke: Departments of Oncology and Physiology and Biophysics, Lombardi Cancer Center, Georgetown University Medical Center, Washington, D.C.
M. D. Johnson: Department of Oncology, Lombardi Cancer Center, Georgetown University Medical Center, Washington, D.C.

cells.[16] The primary end points measured with these models are changes in tumor latency, incidence, and multiplicity.[17]

These models appear to closely mimic several key components of the human disease. Rats that have completed a full-term pregnancy and lactation, or have been treated with estrogen and progesterone before carcinogen administration, exhibit a reduced incidence of mammary tumors.[10] Pregnancy at a young age also is known to reduce lifetime breast cancer risk in humans.[18] This may reflect an endocrine-induced differentiation that reduces the number of target undifferentiated stem cells.[19] For chemical carcinogens, the dose of carcinogen and age of the rats also are critical. The rats must be virgin, with the optimal age being 40 to 46 days. Chemically induced tumors also are initially estrogen responsive.[20] Progression to a hormone-unresponsive phenotype can occur rapidly in a significant proportion of tumors. Loss of hormone responsiveness also can occur in human breast tumors. Many of the mammary epithelial tumors that arise are well-differentiated adenocarcinomas. These are histologically similar to a significant proportion of the lesions that arise in the human breast. However, other tumors also can arise with 7,12-dimethylbenz[*a*]anthracene (DMBA) treatment, and it is important for investigators to confirm the origin of any tumors that arise in the mammary fat pad areas. Several excellent reviews are available that describe the comparative biology of these models.[10,21,22]

These mammary tumor models have been in constant use since their description by Huggins and associates in 1961,[23] and their use has provided critical insights into several aspects of breast cancer biology. For example, chemically induced tumors have been used to demonstrate the antitumor and chemopreventive effects of endocrine agents[24–26] and vitamins.[27] Perhaps the most notable example of the use of chemically induced rodent models is their role in the preclinical development of the antiestrogen tamoxifen.

Chemically induced mammary tumors exhibit a low metastatic potential.[28] Although some local invasion is apparent and occasional metastases have been reported, these are rarely sufficiently reproducible to provide a useful model of metastasis. The majority of tumors are initially prolactin dependent,[20] but a similar central role for prolactin in human breast cancer is not currently evident.[29] These characteristics and the high level of *ras* activation [e.g., *N*-nitrosomethylurea (NMU)-induced tumors] limit their applicability for some studies. In general, investigators should be cautious in designing experiments in which agents are coadministered with a chemical carcinogen, because effects on the carcinogen's pharmacokinetics can produce potentially artifactual observations that are specific for the carcinogen used.

The choice of carcinogen may depend to some degree on the study design. When coadministration of the test treatment or manipulation is required, NMU is likely to be a better choice, because it eliminates potentially confounding effects on metabolic activation. When cellular signaling is under investigation, DMBA may prove more useful, because the incidence of activate *ras* mutations is much lower. Interestingly, transformation of HBL100 cells (normal human breast epithelial-derived cells) by DMBA, but not NMU, is associated with an increased expression of basic fibroblast growth factor (FGF).[30] This suggests that cellular signaling is different in DMBA- than in NMU-induced mammary tumors. FGFs have been implicated in breast carcinogenesis.[31] For many studies, the choice of carcinogen is unlikely to significantly affect the outcome or interpretation of the studies.[32]

7,12-Dimethylbenz[*a*]anthracene

DMBA is a potent inducer of mammary carcinomas. It is generally administered by oral gavage, frequently as a solution in peanut oil. Generally within 10 to 15 weeks, 20 mg per animal produces a final incidence of 100% adenocarcinomas. The mammary tumors arise in the epithelium of the terminal end buds, which are comparable structures to the terminal ductal lobular unit in the human breast.[10] The tumors are generally ductal carcinomas, papillary carcinomas, and intraductal papillomas.[10] The comparative biology of DMBA-induced mammary carcinomas has been extensively reviewed by Russo and associates.[10,21]

DMBA is highly lipophilic and requires metabolic activation for its carcinogenicity.[32] Several tissues are capable of activating DMBA, and these include the mammary gland. However, there also is extensive hepatic activation, and some of the ultimate carcinogens may be systemically active. Both liver and mammary activation may be important in these models. The potential importance of hepatic metabolism is evident from the observation of reduced mammary tumorigenesis in animals in which glucuronidation is blocked.[33] Hepatic but not mammary DMBA activation is inhibited by dietary butylated hydroxytoluene, and this is sufficient to reduce DMBA binding to mammary gland DNA.[34] The ability of direct administration of DMBA to the mammary gland to induce mammary tumors provides clear evidence of the likely importance of its activation within the gland.[21,35] Primary cultures of rat mammary epithelial cells also are able to metabolize DMBA.[36]

Coadministration of agents that alter either its lipid biodisposition or its hepatic/mammary activation can influence subsequent tumor incidence. However, these apparent effects on tumorigenicity can be considered artifactual, because they are pharmacologic effects specific to the carcinogen. The potential for such artifacts requires careful experimental study design when DMBA is used, for example, in studies with agents that could alter hepatic function or in dietary studies that use high fat.[37] The metabolism of DMBA was reviewed in 1997.[32]

N-Nitrosomethylurea

The ability of NMU to produce mammary tumors was reported by Gullino and associates[38] in 1975. NMU induces mammary carcinomas in rodents when administered subcutaneously or intravenously at 50 mg per kg. Tumor incidence and latency are comparable to that observed with DMBA administration and also exhibit steroid hormone and prolactin responsiveness.[39] Because NMU does not require metabolic activation, there are fewer concerns regarding coadministration artifacts than for DMBA. However, approximately 75% of rodent mammary tumors induced by NMU exhibit altered *ras* expression/activation[11] that occurs during initiation.[40] The incidence of altered *ras* expression in human breast cancer is approximately 20% and represents rare alleles or slight overexpression, or both.[41] Furthermore, its role in human breast cancer initiation, promotion, progression, or a combination of the three remains unclear.[41,42] This contrasts with the high frequency of *ras* mutations observed in the NMU-induced rodent tumors.[11,40]

The high incidence of *ras* activation potentially reduces the use of NMU-induced tumors for signal transduction-mechanistic studies, because there is a high probability that *ras*/G protein–mediated pathways will predominate. The high incidence of activated *ras* increases the likelihood that data from such mechanistic studies could be heavily skewed. Although this also limits studies of the ability of agents (e.g., tumor promoters) to further increase the incidence of *ras* expression, it may prove to be a good model for studying treatments that could either reduce *ras* expression or use *ras*-mediated signal transduction pathways.

Activation of *ras* may not be the primary effect of NMU. It has been suggested that NMU-induced tumors arise in cells that already possess the activated *ras*.[43,44] One possible interpretation is that NMU either promotes the proliferation of these cells or it induces additional mutations that generate the fully transformed genotype, or both.

VIRALLY INDUCED RODENT MAMMARY TUMORS

Mouse Mammary Tumor Virus–Induced Tumors

Several mouse strains are susceptible to infections that subsequently produce mammary tumors (e.g., C3H, CD1, RIII, GR, SHN, BR6). Neonatal female mice are infected with MMTV through their mother's milk. Infected female mice of susceptible strains develop preneoplastic hyperplastic alveolar nodules that are generally apparent from 4 weeks of age. In C3H/OuJ[6] and C3H/HeJ mice,[45] mammary tumors begin to appear at 24 to 28 weeks of age. An approximately 50% incidence in mammary tumors is achieved in virgin mice by approximately 35 weeks of age.[6] Many of the MMTV models exhibit a strong pregnancy- or progesterone-dependent increase in incidence.[46] In common with the chemically induced rat mammary tumor models described previously, these models also exhibit a strong prolactin dependence[45] and are responsive to retinoids.[46] Both oophorectomy and treatment with tamoxifen also induce regression in these spontaneous mammary tumors.[46] However, the histology of many of these mammary tumors is not clearly comparable to that of the human disease. Atypical lobular type A lesions appear similar to the hypoplastic alveolar nodules that arise in susceptible, MMTV-infected mouse strains.[47] Metastasis occurs in many infected animals, with the lungs being a major metastatic site.[48]

The transforming potential of MMTV is almost certainly the result of virally induced mutational insertion.[49] MMTV proviral insertion can alter the expression of several genes. These include *int-1*/*Wnt-1* (mouse chromosome 15), *int-2*/FGF-3 (mouse chromosome 7), *int-3* (mouse chromosome 17; human 12q13), *HST/FGF4* (mouse chromosome; human 11q13), *Wnt-3* (mouse chromosome 11; human 17q21-22), *int-6* (mouse chromosome 15; human 8q22), *Wnt-10b* (mouse chromosome 15; human 12q13), and *FGF8* (mouse chromosome 19; human 10q).[48] The most common insertions are observed at the *int-1* and *int-2*/FGF-3 loci.[49] Different transcriptional/translational start sites and polyadenylation sites in different tissues can produce expression of various *int-2*/FGF-3 messenger RNA (mRNA) species. However, each of these mRNAs can produce the same protein (reviewed in reference 49). Although amplification of *int-2*/FGF-3 and *hst*/FGF-4 is observed in both human and mouse mammary tumors (e.g., approximately 30% of human breast tumors), their respective mRNAs and proteins are rarely expressed in the human disease.[50–52] MMTV-induced oncogene activation has been reviewed in detail.[48,49]

Polyoma-Induced Tumors

Mouse polyoma virus can induce mammary tumors when infection occurs neonatally and when infection is present in immunodeficient hosts. Mammary hyperplasia, dysplasia, and mammary tumors are observed in female mice infected with the polyoma WTA2 virus at 6 weeks of age.[53] Infected mammary glands exhibit an initial epithelial hyperplasia, followed by dysplasia 6 weeks *post inoculum*. Glands ultimately develop mammary adenocarcinomas of ductal origin (100% incidence) by 6 to 9 weeks *post inoculum*. The middle T antigen of the virus also has been successfully used to generate a transgenic mouse mammary tumor model. All of the polyoma virus–associated models produce tumors that are histologically comparable to mammary ductal adenocarcinomas in humans. Unlike the MMTV and chemically induced rodent models, the polyoma-induced tumors are ovarian independent.[53] Interested readers can find an excellent review of this model by Fluck and Haslam.[54]

Adenovirus-Induced Tumors

One-day-old Wistar-Furth rats (<24 hours of age) inoculated subcutaneously with human adenovirus type 9 develop benign mammary fibroadenomas, phyllodes-like tumors, and solid sarcomas.[55,56] Palpable mammary lesions develop by 3 to

5 months of age, with the benign lesions apparently of primarily mammary fibroblastic origin, as determined by expression of type IV collagen and vimentin. Unlike the other rodent mammary tumor models, the areas of neoplasia are of myoepithelial and not epithelial origin, as indicated by their continued expression of type IV collagen, vimentin, and muscle-specific actin. The tumors are estrogen responsive, as indicated by an oophorectomy-induced inhibition of tumor development, induction by diethylstilbestrol, and the presence of estrogen receptor (ER) mRNA.[55] The adenovirus tumors provide a novel and useful model of mammary fibroadenomas, which are relatively common benign human breast lesions. This model has been reviewed in detail by Javier and Shenk.[56]

HUMAN TUMOR XENOGRAFTS

The xenografting of human tumors into athymic nude mice has become almost routine. However, the nude mouse is not the only immune-compromised rodent available. Mutations at approximately 30 loci have been shown to produce reduced immune function in mice.[57] The major mutations used to generate hosts for xenografts are the nude (*nu*), beige (*bg*), severe combined immunodeficiency (*scid*), and X-linked immunodeficiency (*xid*). Of these, the *scid* mouse is generally considered to exhibit the greatest degree of immunosuppression. The combined *bg/nu/xid* mutation strain (e.g., NIH III) also produces severely immunocompromised animals but has received less attention, perhaps as a result of a clotting disorder that reduces their use in studies that require survival surgery.

Most investigators report a relatively low take rate when human breast tumor biopsies are xenografted directly into immune-compromised rodents. This low rate generally reflects the frequency with which cell lines or continuous xenografts can be established. For many purposes, slow-growing tumors are of limited value, and primary tumors with long doubling times have often been discarded. Sakakibara and associates[58] report that approximately 25% of primary breast tumors, when xenografted into *scid* mice, exhibited a sufficient growth rate to allow for repeated passage (i.e., tumors reached a 2- to 3-cm diameter within 6 months). Metastasis to lung or other sites, or both, was observed in 8 of 12 tumors. The generation of reproducibly metastatic models is an important goal, because relatively few well-characterized metastatic models are available. However, new models are occasionally reported. Mehta and colleagues[59] recently described an endocrine-responsive metastatic xenograft (UISO-BCA-NMT-18). It is hoped that the new metastasis models will be fully characterized and sufficiently distributed so that their uses will rapidly become apparent.

Human breast cancer cell lines inoculated into nude mice represent the majority of human breast tumor xenograft models. However, relatively few xenografts have been in regular and widespread use other than MCF-7 (endocrine-responsive) and MDA-MB-231 (endocrine-unresponsive) cells. In part, this reflects the low success rate for establishing human breast tumors either directly as xenografts or as stable established cell lines *in vitro*.

Despite the ability to apply selective pressures that result in variants with altered endocrine responsiveness,[60–62] the majority of endocrine-responsive xenografts are phenotypically stable, at least with respect to biologically important characteristics (e.g., tumorigenicity, steroid hormone receptor expression, hormone responsiveness). We have not observed any spontaneous loss of estrogen dependence in MCF-7 cells (estrogen receptor positive, estrogen dependent), gain of estrogen responsiveness in MDA-MB-435 cells (estrogen receptor negative, estrogen unresponsive), or alteration in estrogen responsiveness of MCF7/MIII cells (estrogen receptor positive, estrogen independent, estrogen responsive) maintained routinely in our laboratory in the absence of selective pressures. Indeed, the major phenotypic characteristics of hormone responsiveness, hormone receptor expression, antiestrogen responsiveness, tumorigenicity, and metastatic potential remain remarkably stable in the majority of human breast cancer cell lines. The stability of human tumor xenografts is widely reported (reviewed in reference 63). Some minor phenotypic diversity is observed between laboratories and is not surprising, because some of these cell lines have been in continuous culture for more than 15 years. Nevertheless, these models have the advantages of being human in origin and relatively reproducible with regard to their endocrine responsiveness and metastatic potential. A description of the characteristics of the major xenografts is provided in Table 1.

Many studies of endocrine agents, or of use of endocrine-responsive xenografts, are performed in oophorectomized mice. The levels of circulating estrogens in these animals are very low and approximate the levels found in postmenopausal women.[64–66] Because the major endocrine-responsive human breast cancer cell lines (e.g., MCF-7, ZR-75-1, T47D) were derived from tumors in postmenopausal women,[67] the endocrine environment of the oophorectomized mouse is appropriate. There also is increasing evidence that orthotopic implantation produces tumors with a more biologically relevant phenotype and greater tumor take rate.[68–71] Despite potential differences between the rodent mammary fat pad environment and the human breast,[10] the mammary fat pad provides an appropriate orthotopic site that is readily accessible. Although most human breast cancer cell lines grow adequately in almost any subcutaneous site (e.g., the flank is widely used), inoculation into the mammary fat pad is the preferred site. The incidence of metastasis from solid breast tumors is higher when the primary tumor is orthotopic rather than subcutaneous.

Endocrine-Responsive Xenografts

Relatively few human breast cancer xenografts exhibit an endocrine-responsive phenotype, and all are estrogen receptor

TABLE 1. *Characteristics of representative transplantable mammary tumor cells*

Cell line	Origin/derivation	Estrogen responsiveness	Invasive/metastatic	References
MCF-7	Human breast cancer cell line	Dependent	–/–	73,184
ZR-75-1	Human breast cancer cell line	Dependent	–/–	185,186
T47D	Human breast cancer cell line	Dependent	–/–	185,186
MCF7/MIII	MCF-7 variant	Independent/stimulated	+/±	60,73
MCF7/LCC1	MCF-7 variant	Independent/stimulated	+/±	73,79
MCF7/LCC2	MCF-7 variant	Independent/stimulated	ND	61
MCF7/LCC9	MCF-7 variant	Independent/stimulated	ND	187
MCF7/MKS-1	MCF-7 transfected with FGF-4	Independent/inhibited	+/+	183
MLα	MDA-MB-231 transfected with ER	Independent/inhibited	ND	87
T61	Human xenograft	Independent/inhibited	ND	188,189
NCI/ADR-RES (previously MCF-7ADR)	Selected for doxorubicin resistance. It is no longer clear that these cells are of MCF-7 origin	Independent/unresponsive	–/–	190,191
MDA-MB-435	Human breast cancer cell line	Independent/unresponsive	+/+	86
MDA-MB-231	Human breast cancer cell line	Independent/unresponsive	+/+	86
Hs578T	Human breast cancer cell line	Independent/unresponsive	+/±	185

ND, no data available; +, phenotype observed reproducibly; –, phenotype rare; ±, phenotype observed occasionally.

positive. There are two categories of endocrine-responsive cells, (a) estrogen dependent and (b) estrogen independent and estrogen responsive.[72] The estrogen-dependent xenografts do not form proliferating tumors in the mammary fat pads of oophorectomized immunodeficient mice without estrogen supplementation, generally in the form of a 60-day release, 0.72 mg 17β-estradiol pellet placed subcutaneously in the interclavicular region. Examples of estrogen-dependent xenografts include the MCF-7, ZR-75-1, and T47D cell lines. Most of the estrogen-responsive xenografts produce relatively well-differentiated adenocarcinomas,[73] are inhibited by tamoxifen,[74–78] and are poorly invasive and nonmetastatic.[73]

Several estrogen-independent and estrogen-responsive variants have been derived from estrogen-dependent cells in the authors'[60,61,79] and other laboratories.[62] These variants form proliferating tumors in oophorectomized immunodeficient mice without estrogen supplementation. However, they grow more rapidly in the presence of an estrogen pellet.[60,79] Examples of estrogen-independent and estrogen-responsive xenografts derived from MCF-7 cells include MCF7/MIII,[60] BSK-3,[60,62] MCF7/LCC1,[79] and MCF7/LCC2 (tamoxifen resistant).[61]

Analysis of the growth and endocrine responsiveness of the various endocrine-responsive xenografts has provided useful information on the biology of malignant progression[80,81] and cross-resistance among antiestrogen therapies.[61,72] For example, the ability to isolate estrogen-independent cells from estrogen-dependent cells indicates a possible progression pathway to acquired estrogen independence in breast tumors that arise in postmenopausal women.[72,80,82]

MCF7/LCC2 cells are resistant to the inhibitory effects of 4-hydroxytamoxifen when growing both *in vitro* and *in vivo*.[61] However, MCF7/LCC2 cells are not cross-resistant to the steroidal antiestrogens ICI 182,780[61] and ICI 164,384.[83] These data would predict that patients in whom tamoxifen has induced a response but subsequently failed would respond to a steroidal antiestrogen. Preliminary data from a phase I trial of ICI 182,780 now demonstrate responses in patients in whom tamoxifen has failed.[84] Thus, the pattern of antiestrogen responsiveness exhibited by the MCF7/LCC2 cells accurately predicted for a previously unknown pattern of clinical response.

MCF-7 human breast cancer cells transfected with an expression vector directing a high constitutive expression of FGF-4/kFGF produce highly vascular tumors that are inhibited by physiologic doses of estrogen and stimulated by pharmacologic doses of tamoxifen.[31,85] The inverse response is exhibited by the parental MCF-7 cells.[77,78] However, these tumors produce a high incidence of lung and lymphatic metastases. Estrogen receptor–negative (estrogen unresponsive) and metastatic MDA-MB-231 cells[86] transfected with the estrogen-receptor gene also exhibit an estrogen-inhibited phenotype.[87] These cells may provide potentially novel breast cancer metastasis models. MCF-7 tumors selected *in vivo* for resistance to tamoxifen also exhibit a tamoxifen-stimulated/estrogen-inhibited response pattern.[74,78]

The relevance of the inverted endocrine responsiveness of these models to the human disease is not immediately apparent. Tumors inhibited by physiologic estrogen concentrations may not arise frequently, because most breast tumors appear to contain physiologic concentrations of estrogens, irrespective of menopausal status.[88] Pharmacologic doses of estrogens produce remissions in hormone-responsive breast tumors,[89,90] and there is no clear evidence that either physiologic estrogen doses or hormone replacement therapy produces remissions in postmenopausal patients with breast cancer. Indeed, hormone replacement therapy is associated with a modest increase in the risk of breast cancer.[18] However, these models do suggest that withdrawal responses to tamoxifen may occur more frequently than has been previously reported. Despite the estimation that the total exposure to tamoxifen between 1971 and 1988 was more than 1.5 million patient-years,[91] and is now in excess of 8 million patient-years, reports of tamoxifen withdrawal responses are relatively rare[89,92,93] and often represent individual case histories.[94–96] This issue will remain controversial until sufficient clinical trials are conducted to specifically address the actual frequency of withdrawal responses to tamoxifen.

Endocrine-Unresponsive Xenografts

The majority of human breast tumor xenografts are estrogen receptor negative and therefore are estrogen unresponsive. These xenografts also tend to be more locally aggressive and exhibit a significantly increased metastatic potential. Two estrogen-unresponsive xenograft models (MDA-MB-231 and MDA-MB-435) are capable of producing distant metastases in an apparently reproducible manner and with a sufficient incidence to be of use in the study of spontaneous metastasis.[86] The MDA-MB-435 model is sensitive to dietary manipulations.[97,98] We have isolated an ascites variant of these cells (MDA435/LCC6), which is sensitive to a variety of cytotoxic drugs with proven efficacy in the human disease.[99] More recently, we have isolated an estrogen-unresponsive cell line (LCC15-MB) from a bone metastasis.[100,101] Most endocrine-unresponsive xenografts produce poorly differentiated tumors. The MDA-MB-231, MDA-MB-435, MDA435/LCC6, and LCC15-MB cell lines can produce metastases in immunodeficient mice.

Immunodeficient Mouse Models

We have previously reviewed the immunodeficiencies of the most widely used xenograft hosts.[102] These are discussed only briefly here. Mice that are homozygous for the nude (*nu*) mutation are athymic[103] and exhibit a defect in thymic-dependent B-cell maturation but possess apparently normal virgin B cells.[104] Primary responses to T-dependent antigens are low[105] and may be reversed by reconstitution of the mice with T cells.[106–108] Serum immunoglobulin M (IgM) levels are similar to those of their heterozygote littermates.[109] However, there is a significant decrease in the number of cells making IgG and IgA.[107] Despite their ability to maintain human tumor xenografts, nude mice retain considerable immunity. For example, they possess substantially *greater* numbers of natural killer (NK) cells than comparable heterozygotes, and this may contribute to the relatively low incidence of metastases from human tumor xenografts.[110,111] Nude mice possess a relatively normal primary response to T cell–independent antigens,[109] and their splenocytes generate lymphocyte-activated killer (LAK) cells at levels similar to those observed in normal mice.[112] The levels of macrophages are equivalent in *nu/nu* and *nu/+* mice and frequently exhibit tumoricidal properties.[113]

The *scid* mutation is one of the few single mutations that produce viable severely immunodeficient mice. It causes a deficiency in the rearrangement of genes coding for antigen-specific receptors on B and T cells.[114] Pre-B and B cells are absent, and the remaining T cells are nonfunctional. However, myeloid lineage cells appear normal.[115,116] Homozygotes generally have no detectable levels of IgGs 2a, 2b, and 3a[57] and IgA.[117] Some individual animals produce detectable levels of two or more IgG isotypes or IgM, or both.[117] NK cells, macrophages,[118] and LAK activity are comparable to those of normal mice.[112]

Several immunodeficiency mutations have been combined to produce severely immunodeficient animals. The most widely used to date are mice that bear the combined *bg/nu/xid* mutations (e.g., NIH III).[119] The *bg* mutation produces a significant block in NK function.[120,121] This is in marked contrast to the increased NK activity observed in mice that are homozygous for the *nu* mutation.[110,111] The *bg* mutation also produces functional defects in T cells, macrophages, and granulocytes.[57] The *xid* mutation in males (*xid*/Y) and homozygous females produces mice that cannot generate a humoral response to thymus-independent type-II antigens.[57,122] In the *bg/nu/xid* combination, the *nu* mutation produces mice that are deficient in mature T cells; the *xid* mutation produces a deficiency in mature B cells[123,124]; and the *bg* mutation reduces the elevated NK activity conferred by the *nu* mutation.[120,121] However, some NK activity remains detectable.[78,119] The *bg/nu/xid* strain is deficient in B-cell and T-cell activities and cannot produce detectable LAK activity.[119] Mice that are homozygous for *bg* also exhibit a clotting deficiency due to a platelet disorder. This latter characteristic can be problematic in the *bg/nu/xid* mice if the experimental design requires survival surgery (e.g., oophorectomy).

Endocrine Effects on Immune Function

Endocrine treatments are known to modulate immune function both in immunodeficient mice and in humans. Estrogen receptors have been demonstrated on peripheral blood mononuclear cells, splenic cells, thymic cells,[125] and $CD8^+$ T cells.[126,127] Estrogens can alter B-cell function and increase IgM secretion.[128] Inhibition of T-suppressor function and T-helper maturation also have been reported.[129,130] Physiologic concentrations of estrogen stimulate pokeweed mitogen–induced Ig synthesis of B lymphocytes.[129,131] Pharmacologic administration of the progestin medroxyprogesterone acetate results in a reduced $T4^+/T8^+$ ratio, perhaps as a result of its glucocorticoid activity.[132] The progestagen lynestrenol has been reported to stimulate active T rosetting and phagocytosis by monocytes.[133]

The number of macrophages does not appear to be significantly modulated by E2 in nude mice,[134] but there are several reports of altered NK cell activity. Pharmacologic but not physiologic concentrations of E2 inhibit NK activity in athymic nude mice.[134–137] The effect of pharmacologic concentrations of E2 is biphasic; a stimulation of NK activity occurs within the first 30 days, with inhibition being observed thereafter.[135] The delay in detecting an E2-induced suppression of NK activity has been widely reported.[134–137] E2-induced effects on NK activity are unlikely to be responsible for E2's effects on breast tumor cell growth *in vivo*. The majority of breast tumor xenografts produce readily palpable tumors within 10 to 14 days, during which time the already high NK activity in nude mice is further elevated.[135] Furthermore, the concentrations of estrogens reported to suppress NK activity appear to exceed the physiologic concentrations used to stimulate MCF-7 hormone-dependent breast tumor growth in nude mice.[60,64,138–140]

Tamoxifen stimulates NK activity both *in vitro*[141] and *in vivo*.[78] Other antiestrogens can increase pokeweed mitogen–induced Ig synthesis of B lymphocytes.[142] The aromatase inhibitor aminoglutethimide reduces serum estrogens and increases NK activity in patients with breast cancer.[143] Clearly, there are significant interactions between endocrine agents and effectors of cell-mediated immunity. The isolation of breast cancer cell variants with differing responsiveness to both hormonal manipulations and immune response effectors will greatly improve our ability to determine the nature of these interactions and how they can be manipulated to therapeutic advantage. In 1998, we observed that the tamoxifen resistance of the MCF7/LCC2 cell line can be affected *in vivo* by the administration of blocking transforming growth factor (TGF)-β antibodies, which appears to reflect up-regulated secretion of TGF-β sufficient to block NK cell lysis.[144] This suggests that the endocrinologic effects of some agents may have important immunologic consequences for some breast cancers.

The ability of endocrine agents to perturb several effectors of cell-mediated immunity requires careful consideration for study design. For example, the ultimate reduction in NK activity by estrogens (at 30 or more days) depends on the dose of estrogen used and the length of the analysis. Long-term *in vivo* experiments of both more than 6 weeks' duration and using pharmacologic doses of estrogens could be influenced by perturbations in immunologic function. Although there is little direct evidence to the contrary, the relatively low estrogen levels (~300 pg/mL estradiol)[145] released from the widely used 60-day release, 0.72-mg estrogen pellets (Innovative Research of America, Toledo, OH) are probably insufficient to suppress NK activity to a level at which tumorigenicity data would be markedly influenced.

Use of Animal Models in Drug Screening

A major use of the human xenograft models described previously is for the identification of new drugs or evaluation of new drug combinations, or both. In general, relatively few breast cancer models have the characteristics most widely sought, such as rapid and reproducible tumor doubling time. Nonetheless, several models are included in the current National Cancer Institute *in vivo* screen and appear useful in this context. MCF-7 xenografts are often relatively slow growing (compared with the P388 or L1210 mouse models) and generally do not produce lethality within an acceptable time frame. These are among the most widely used xenografts and are particularly helpful in assessing antiestrogenic compounds. Other models in use include the T47D (also endocrine responsive) and the HS578T, BT-549, MDA-MB-231, and MDA-MB-435 models (all endocrine unresponsive).

There are several important considerations in the use of animal models for drug screening, including the choice of xenograft, host, end point, and data analysis. Several of these have recently been described in detail.[7,8] An appropriate experimental design requires some consideration of the nature and quality of the data that are likely to be obtained. One of the more important, but often overlooked, areas is in the choice of numbers of animals per experimental group. Most institutional animal care and use committees now require investigators to provide a realistic estimate of their predicted animal usage before initiation of experimentation. The most effective means to this end is to perform an appropriate statistical power estimation. Group size must be sufficient to enable statistical analysis of the data, and the power estimate should ensure that power is maintained should some animals die from unrelated causes. This issue is discussed in some detail by Hanfelt.[7]

The major end points for assessing drug activity include percentage increased life span and tumor growth delay. Whereas survival studies were a mainstay of anticancer drug evaluation for decades, they are becoming less common, largely due to restrictions in the use of death as an experimental end point. In some cases, it may be possible to substitute morbidity, particularly when the characteristics of the tumor model are well defined and the animals experience reproducible and predictable morbidity before death. This approach can still allow for survival studies while substantially reducing suffering. The most common approach for data analysis is the use of standard survival analyses (e.g., using a Kaplan-Meier approach with the log rank test).

Generally, tumor growth delay studies are much less stressful for the animals but provide essentially comparable estimates of activity to other types of studies. For these studies, tumors are grown to a predetermined size, and animals are randomized into groups so that the mean tumor size is effectively the same in each group. Only proliferating tumors are used, and all selected tumors should have similar tumor doubling times. In principle, growth delay is the difference, among treated and untreated groups, in the times needed for tumors to reach a predetermined size. There are several ways to approach data analysis from such studies. Survival analysis can be used, because these are essentially time-to-event analyses. Repeated measures of analyses of variance also can be used, particularly if a larger than expected number of treated tumors fail to reach the predetermined size.[7,8] For cytostatic treatments, tumor doubling times can be estimated and compared by analysis of variance or multivariate analysis of variance.[146]

TRANSGENIC AND TARGETED MUTANT MOUSE MODELS

The development of transgenic and targeted mutant mouse technologies has, over the last few years, led to the development of a number of new animal models of breast cancer. The nature of this technology makes these models particularly useful for studying the impact of specific genetic lesions on normal mammary development, carcinogenesis, and tumor progression, and often a single model can be used to study all three processes.

In a typical transgenic model, the mice have been genetically altered so that the expression of a particular gene—c-*myc*, for example—has been altered in some way. This might include increasing the expression of the gene, altering the temporal aspects of its normal regulation, or both. A new strain of transgenic mice is often generated as follows: A DNA expression construct is prepared in which sequences that code for the protein of interest are ligated next to other sequences (the promoter) that will drive the expression of the gene in the manner desired. This DNA construct is then injected into one of the pronuclei of single-cell mouse embryos. The embryos are implanted into the reproductive tract of pseudopregnant female mice that then carry the embryos to term. In a proportion of the resultant pups (approximately 5%), the injected DNA will have become integrated into the genome and be passed to subsequent generations.[147] If the DNA construct has not been rearranged, otherwise damaged during this integration event, or integrated into a part of the genome where expression is suppressed, the promoter drives the expression of the introduced gene. The choice of promoter used to prepare the construct to a large extent determines the level, site, and timing of transgene expression. Various different promoters have been used, and they fall into three basic classes: those that exhibit marked tissue specificity, those that do not, and those in which expression can be regulated by external manipulation.

Although there are transgenic models with mammary phenotypes that have used nontissue-specific promoters,[148] many investigators interested in breast cancer have chosen to use promoters that predominantly direct expression to the mammary tissue. There are a number of such promoters, of which two have proved particularly useful. The first is MMTV, which consists of a portion of the MMTV long terminal repeat (LTR) that directs expression in the adult mouse to the mammary glands, salivary glands, and several other secretory tissues. Studies with MMTV-Cre mice have shown that there can be widespread low-level expression from this promoter, however.[149] The second promoter is the whey acidic protein (WAP) promoter, which directs expression to the mammary gland in a pregnancy- and lactation-dependent manner. High levels of expression are achieved by day 16 of pregnancy, although it can be detected by approximately day 10.[150] Despite this dependence on pregnancy and lactation for maximal promoter activity, in some models there is sufficient expression in virgin animals for a phenotype to develop.[151] Studies with WAP-Cre mice suggest that there is much less low-level expression in nonmammary tissues than is found with MMTV.[149]

Other promoters that have been used include the ovine beta-lactoglobulin promoter, which is expressed predominantly in the mammary gland during lactation, and the rat prostatic steroid-binding protein C3(1) promoter, which directs expression to the prostate and mammary gland.[152] Substantial research is being conducted to develop other mammary-specific promoters, largely with the goal of being able to produce valuable proteins in the milk of farm animals. As these promoters are developed further, they may be useful for making transgenic models of breast cancer.[153] Inducible promoters have also been used in transgenic model systems, specifically a system based around the tetracycline operator protein and a system based on the receptor for the insect hormone ecdysone.[154,155] In both systems, the gene of interest is placed under the control of a promoter that depends for function on the presence of an activator protein (the tetracycline transactivator protein or the ecdysone receptor). In the ecdysone receptor system, expression is then induced by administering a ligand for the receptor. The tetracycline system can be engineered such that administration of tetracycline either induces or represses expression. By placing the gene for the activator protein under the control of a mammary-directed promoter, such as the MMTV promoter, it is possible to obtain inducible expression of the gene of interest in the salivary gland.[156] Although few models thus far have made use of this potentially very useful technology, a study in which the SV40 large T antigen was inducibly expressed in the mammary gland has clearly demonstrated the possibilities of this approach, although expression in the mammary gland has been problematic.[157]

In a targeted mutant mouse model, a specific genetic lesion has been introduced into the genome of the mice. This could include the deletion of a gene (knockout mouse), the introduction of a specific mutation, or the substitution of the mouse gene for the human gene, producing a "humanized" mouse. These models are created by use of pluripotent embryonic stem cell cultures. These cells, when introduced into a mouse embryo, become integrated, resulting in a mosaic animal in which some of the cells are of embryonic stem (ES) cell origin. If the ES cells make up the gametes of the mouse, then any genetic changes within the ES cells are passed on to the next generation. This means that the powerful genetic techniques (e.g., gene deletion, mutation, substitution, or a combination, mediated by homologous recombination) that are only practicable in tissue culture systems can be applied to animal models. Thus far, the majority of such models have been ones in which a gene had been knocked out, although several humanized models have been created that may prove useful in the study of breast cancer. One problem with the majority of the knockout mice made so far is that the gene is disrupted in all cells from the time of conception. This can lead to problems with embryonic lethality, as is the case with BRCA-1 and -2 knockout mice,[158] or with difficulty in seeing a mammary phenotype, due to the rapid death of the animals caused by another malignancy.[159] The use of the Cre-Lox recombinase system to make genetic alterations *in vivo* that are specific to the mammary gland by expressing Cre using a WAP or beta-lactoglobulin promoter may alleviate both problems in the next few years.[149,160]

Transgenic models have several advantages and disadvantages when compared with other animal models of breast cancer. One of the principal advantages is that these models allow the study of oncogenes and other proteins that are believed to be important in human mammary carcinogenesis. In many transgenic models that use oncogenes relevant to human mammary cancer, the tumors that result are histologically similar to human cancers.[161,162] One feature of some transgenic mammary tumor models can be seen both as a technical advantage and as a potential deficit in terms of relevance to the human disease. In some models, all animals develop tumors with almost exactly the same latency.[163,164] Clearly, this is quite different than the natural history of the disease in humans but can be extremely helpful when these mice are used in cancer prevention studies to assess the impact of some anticancer strategy. Another feature of transgenic systems that has been used very effectively is the ability to cross two transgenic strains, allowing the impact of two defined genetic insults to be examined.[164]

Transgenic models can assist in bridging the gap between *in vivo* and *in vitro* studies, because they can be used as a source of mammary epithelial and mammary cancer cell lines that can then be further studied and indeed reimplanted to form transgenic mammary glands.[165] Transgenic systems can also be used in combination with carcinogens to study the impact of a specific genetic change on the timing and biology of the tumors that are produced. For example, this method has been used to investigate the impact of the presence of mutant p53 on the effects of carcinogen insult.[166]

It has been known for some time that the genetic background of the transgenic strain can have a significant effect on the latency, penetrance, and aggressiveness of the phenotype that a given transgene produces. For example, dramatic differences in the latency of tumor formation are seen when the MMTV-polyoma middle T transgene is bred onto different inbred mouse backgrounds. These systems are being used in attempts to clone modifier genes that may be relevant to the penetrance issues seen in human disease and are simplified by the relative ease of doing genetic studies in mouse models.

Transgenic models of breast cancer are not without their disadvantages. Some of the mammary tissue–specific promoters currently available require parity for expression. However, the endocrine environment of pregnancy and lactation, and the resulting physiologic and morphologic changes that concurrently occur in the mammary gland, can affect phenotype in a manner that does not directly reflect the activity of the expressed gene in nonpregnant or nonlactating mammary tissues. Although expression of some genes can be restricted to the mammary gland, it can be difficult to differentiate among endocrine versus local effects (e.g., autocrine, paracrine) when the transgene is a secreted factor. In many systems, expression of the transgene *in utero* can adversely impact the normal development of the gland. We have previously alluded to the importance of the *in utero* environment in affecting subsequent breast cancer risk. Some transgenes may affect normal gland development, producing a deformed gland from an early age.[167] This is likely to be different than most sporadic human breast cancers, in which oncogene activation presumably occurs as the result of some insult after normal mammary development. The transgenic models may more closely reflect the pattern of familial breast cancer. These gland abnormalities also can present a technical problem, with some female mice being unable to suckle their pups.[152,167] It is likely that the increasing use of regulable transgenic models will circumvent this problem.

An important issue to consider when evaluating a transgenic system is the possibility that the integration of the transgene into the mouse genome may have resulted in some form of insertional mutagenesis. This could be considered analogous to the insertional mutagenesis that is responsible for MMTV-induced neoplasia. This issue is usually addressed by assessing the phenotype of several strains bearing the same transgene in an attempt to ensure that the pathology seen is truly the result of transgene expression.

A further significant difference between most transgenic models and human disease is that the transgene is usually expressed in most or all of the mammary epithelial cells, whereas it is usual to think of the oncogenic event as occurring in one or only a few cells. Tumors can be multifocal, polyclonal, or both. Polyclonality is rare in human breast tumors.[82] However, this also may apply to some of the virus- and chemical-induced models, in which it is likely that many cells are infected or exposed, but not all give rise to tumors.

The concept of these models relies to some extent on the ability of a single gene to produce a fully neoplastic phenotype that would include initiation, promotion, and progression events. It is not clear that cancer is a single-gene/single-hit phenomenon in humans. Thus, these models perhaps more accurately indicate what overexpression of a single specific gene *can do* rather than what this gene *does* in normal versus malignant tissues. The basic assumption is that, in most cases, these two are the same. Despite the potential limitations inherent in transgenic mouse models, the ability to express an oncogene in the glandular or stromal tissues, or both, of otherwise normal breast tissues provides a unique and powerful technique to address the transforming potential of individual genes.

TABLE 2. *Characteristics of several transgenic models that affect the mammary gland*

Transgene	Promoter	Background	Phenotype	References
c-*myc*	MMTV	FVB	50% of virgin female mice develop tumors in 9–12 mo. Incidence increased and latency reduced with parity. Mice do not lactate well. When crossed with MT-TGF-α, latency was reduced to 66 days in both males and virgin females.	167 164
c-*myc*	WAP	FVB	80% of mice develop tumors after pregnancy (mean latency, 7 mo). Some metastasize to lungs.	151
TGF-α	MT	FVB	64% of multiparous women develop adenomas and adenocarcinomas that are preceded by hypoplastic lesions. Tumors are rare in virgin mice.	148
TGF-α	WAP	FVB	100% of parous mice develop tumors with variable latency. Latency reduced and tumors seen in virgin and male mice when crossed with WAP–c-*myc* mice.	151
TGF-α	MMTV	C57BL/DBA	Females develop hyperplasia throughout the mammary glands. Sporadic tumors in multiparous animals. No abnormalities in males.	196
Middle T	MMTV	FVB	*In situ* carcinoma seen at 3 wk. All male and female mice develop tumors that metastasize to lungs. Metastasis greatly reduced when mice crossed onto plasminogen knockout background.	163 198
ras	MMTV	CD1/C57BL	20% of animals have hyperplasia of the Harderian glands. Sporadic mammary tumors in females and a few males.	199
neu	MMTV	FVB	8-wk-old virgin females have hyperplastic nodules through entire gland. By 89 days 50% of females have tumors and 50% of males by 114 days. Multiple tumors arise synchronously.	200
Mutant p53	WAP	FVB	Mice show normal mammary development, rates of proliferation, and apoptosis. When treated with DMBA, latency of tumor formation is significantly reduced.	166
SV40T	C3(1)	FVB	Mammary hyperplasia seen at 8 wk progressing through a DCIS-like stage to cancer by approximately 16 wk. Homozygous mice lactate poorly.	152

DCIS, ductal carcinoma *in situ*; DMBA, 7,12-dimethylbenz[*a*]anthracene; MMTV, mouse mammary tumor virus; MT, metallothionein; WAP, whey acidic protein.

Table 2 summarizes many of the best-characterized transgenic models of mammary carcinogenesis. It is not intended to provide an exhaustive list or to give a complete description of the models listed. Rather, it is meant to provide some idea of the diversity of mammary phenotypes that have been produced and to give a feel for the classes of transgene that have been used. Further information regarding transgenic models of breast cancer can be found at the Biology of the Mammary Gland web site (http://www.mammary.nih.gov/).

USE OF ANIMAL MODELS FOR OTHER ASPECTS OF BREAST CANCER RESEARCH

These animal models have uses that go beyond studies of biology and therapeutic evaluation. Diet has been widely implicated as a possible contributor to breast cancer risk. The chemically induced models have been most widely applied to these studies and have contributed to considerable controversy in several areas. Perhaps most notable has been the evaluation of dietary fat intake as a risk factor for breast cancer. The DMBA and NMU models have consistently demonstrated sensitivity to the promotional effects of diets high in ω-6 polyunsaturated fatty acids. This effect was further confirmed in two metaanalyses of the numerous animal studies in this field.[168,169] Rose and Connolly[170] have demonstrated the ability of these fatty acids to increase the metastatic potential of human breast cancer xenografts. Data from human studies have been less consistent. Most migrant, international, and case control studies have produced data consistent with the modest effects seen in the animal models.[171,172] Cohort studies have been less consistent, with the majority failing to find such an association. In our rodent studies, we found that *in utero* exposure to the ω-6 polyunsaturated fatty acids can significantly affect breast cancer risk in female offspring.[173] This suggests that the timing of exposure may be critical. In contrast to the potentially promotional effects of the ω-6, there is evidence that the ω-3 polyunsaturated fats may reduce breast cancer risk.[174] Consumption of a diet higher in the ω-3 versus the ω-6 polyunsaturated fatty acids is more common in Eastern than in Western populations.

Other dietary components that have received significant attention include soy and several vitamins and analogues thereof. Soy contains several potentially active components, including the isoflavones (e.g., genistein), Bowman-Birk protease inhibitor, and a relatively beneficial balance of ω-3 to ω-6 fatty acids. The isoflavones have received the most attention. These data suggest that dose and timing are critical. Exposure in xenograft models of postmenopausal breast cancer suggests an estrogenic effect that increases the risk of breast cancer.[175] A similar effect has been reported for *in utero* exposure.[176] In contrast, exposure in the normal prepubertal gland[177] and exposure in the chemically induced models (probably reflective of relatively early neoplastic disease) can reduce breast cancer risk.[178] Several studies have suggested that the Bowman-Birk protease inhibitor may be the active component against breast and other cancers (reviewed by Kennedy[179]). However, Barnes and associates[180] report that soy retains its chemopreventive activity after autoclaving, a process that was expected to inactivate soy protease inhibitors but not the isoflavones.[180]

Retinoids and analogues of vitamin A continue to attract increasing attention, both as chemopreventive strategies and as new therapeutic modalities for breast cancer. When administered in the diet, both retinyl acetate and *N*-(4-hydroxyphenyl)retinamide reduce chemically induced mammary carcinogenesis.[181] This latter compound is currently under evaluation as a chemopreventive agent for breast cancer in a large study in Italy.

CONCLUSION

Many models for the study of breast cancer are available to the interested investigator. Each has its own advantages and disadvantages, and these should be clearly weighed and evaluated before their use. Because none of the models accurately reflects every aspect of the human disease, some studies may require the use of more than one model.

There are two areas in which more models are needed. Currently, there are relatively few human xenograft models that are ER positive and E2 dependent. Because this represents an early phenotype, the ability to study malignant progression is restricted. There also are few reproducible metastatic models of breast cancer, particularly ER positive and E2 dependent. The MDA-MB-231 and MDA-MB-435 xenografts are ER negative,[182] and the MCF7/FGF4 transfectants are E2 inhibited and tamoxifen stimulated.[183] We described a model derived from a bone metastasis that has a preference for metastasis to bone when inoculated into the heart.[100,101] However, additional metastasis models are required.

Although relatively new in terms of their use in breast cancer research, the polyoma and adenovirus models may provide us with new and important models for breast cancer research. Their further evaluation as models and their similarities and differences to the human disease should be clearly defined. If appropriate, they also could become an important component of our collection of animal models of breast cancer.

ACKNOWLEDGMENT

This work was funded in part by Public Health Service grants R01-CA/AG58022, P30-CA51008, and P50-CA58185.

REFERENCES

1. Nerurkar VR, Chitale AR, Jalnapurkar BV, Naik SN, Lalitha VS. Comparative pathology of canine mammary tumours. *J Comp Pathol* 1989;101:389.
2. Bartnitzke S, Motzko H, Caselitz J, Kornberg M, Bullerdiek J, Schloot W. A recurrent marker chromosome involving chromosome 1 in two mammary tumors of the dog. *Cytogenet Cell Genet* 1992;60:135.
3. Schiffer SP. Animal welfare and colony management in cancer research. *Breast Cancer Res Treat* 1997;46:313.
4. Kritchevesky D, Weber MM, Klurfeld DM. Dietary fat versus caloric intake in initiation and promotion of 7,12-dimethylbenz(a)anthracene-induced mammary tumorigenesis in rats. *Cancer Res* 1984;44:3174.
5. Welsch CW. Enhancement of mammary tumorigenesis by dietary fat: review of potential mechanisms. *Am J Clin Nutr* 1987;45:192.
6. Engelman RW, Day NK, Chen R-F, et al. Calorie consumption level influences development of C3H/Ou breast adenocarcinoma with indifference to calorie source. *Proc Soc Exp Biol Med* 1990;193:23.
7. Hanfelt J. Statistical approaches to experimental design and data analysis of in vivo studies. *Breast Cancer Res Treat* 1997;46:279.
8. Clarke R. Issues in experimental design and endpoint analysis in the study of experimental cytotoxic agents in vivo in breast cancer and other models. *Breast Cancer Res Treat* 1997;46:255.
9. Siemann DW. Rodent tumor models in experimental cancer therapy. In: Kallman RF, ed. *Rodent tumor models in experimental cancer therapy*. New York: Pergamon, 1987:12.
10. Russo J, Gusterson BA, Rogers AE, Russo IH, Wellings SR, van Zwieten MJ. Biology of disease: comparative study of human and rat mammary tumorigenesis. *Lab Invest* 1990;62:244.
11. Sukumar S, Notario V, Martin-Zanca D, Barbacid M. Induction of mammary carcinomas in rats by nitroso-methylurea involves malignant activation of Ha-ras-1 locus by single point mutations. *Nature* 1983;306:658.
12. Gould MN. Inheritance and site of expression of genes controlling susceptibility to mammary cancer in an inbred rat model. *Cancer Res* 1986;46:1995.
13. Rivera EM, Vijayaraghavan S. Proliferation of ductal outgrowths by carcinogen-induced rat mammary tumors in gland-free mammary fat pads. *J Natl Cancer Inst* 1982;69:517.
14. Gould MN, Zhang R. Genetic regulation of mammary carcinogenesis in the rat by susceptibility and suppressor genes. *Environ Health Perspect* 1991;93:161.
15. Hsu L-C, Kennan WS, Shepel LA, et al. Genetic identification of Mcs-1, a rat mammary carcinoma suppressor gene. *Cancer Res* 1994;54:2765.
16. Isaacs JT. A mammary cancer suppressor gene and its site of action in the rat. *Cancer Res* 1991;51:1591.
17. Rogers AE. Considerations in the design of studies of dietary influences on mammary carcinogenesis in rats and mice. *Breast Cancer Res Treat* 1997;46:247.
18. Hulka BS, Stark AT. Breast cancer: cause and prevention. *Lancet* 1995;346:883.
19. Raynaud A. Observations sur les modifications provoquees pas les hormones oestrogenes, du mode de developpement des mamelons des foetus de souris. *C R Acad Sci* 1955;240:674.
20. Manni A, Rainieri J, Arafah BM, Finegan HM, Pearson OH. Role of estrogen and prolactin in the growth and receptor levels of N-nitrosomethylurea-induced rat mammary tumors. *Cancer Res* 1982;42:3492.
21. Russo J, Russo IH. Experimentally induced mammary tumors in rats. *Breast Cancer Res Treat* 1996;39:7.
22. Russo J, Russo I. Role of differentiation in the pathogenesis and prevention of breast cancer. *Endocr Related Cancer* 1997;4:7.
23. Huggins C, Grand LC, Brillantes FP. Mammary cancer induced by a single feeding of polynuclear hydrocarbons, and its suppression. *Nature* 1961;189:204.
24. Chan PC, Cohen LA. Effect of dietary fat, antiestrogen and antiprolactin on the development of mammary tumors in rats. *J Natl Cancer Inst* 1974;52:25.
25. Ip C, Ip MM. Serum estrogens and estrogen responsiveness in 7,12-dimethylbenz(a)anthracene-induced mammary tumors as influenced by dietary fat. *J Natl Cancer Inst* 1981;66:291.
26. Jordan VC, Allen K. Evaluation of the antitumor activity of the non-steroidal antioestrogen monohydroxytamoxifen in the DMBA-induced rat mammary carcinoma model. *Eur J Cancer* 1980;16:239.

27. Lacroix A, Doskas C, Bhat PV. Inhibition of growth of established N-methyl-N-nitrosourea-induced mammary cancer in rats by retinoic acid and ovariectomy. *Cancer Res* 1990;50:5731.
28. Briand P. Hormone-dependent mammary tumors in mice and rats as a model for human breast cancer. *Anticancer Res* 1983;3:273.
29. L'Hermite M, L'Hermite-Baleriaux M. Prolactin and breast cancer. *Eur J Cancer Clin Oncol* 1988;24:955.
30. Lazzaro G, Mehta R, Shilkaitis A, Gupta TKD. Transformation of human breast epithelial cells by 7,12, dimethylbenz(a)anthracene, but not by N-methyl-N-nitrosourea, is accompanied by up-regulation of basic fibroblast growth factor. *Oncol Rep* 1997;4:1175.
31. McLeskey SW, Zhang L, Kharbanda S, et al. Fibroblast growth factor overexpressing breast carcinoma cells as models for angiogenesis and metastasis. *Breast Cancer Res Treat* 1995;39:103.
32. Clarke R. Animal models of breast cancer: experimental design and their use in nutrition and psychosocial research. *Breast Cancer Res Treat* 1997;46:117.
33. Walaszek Z, Hanausek-Walaszek M, Webb TE. Inhibition of 7,12-dimethylbenzanthracene-induced rat mammary tumorigenesis by 2,5-di-O-acetyl-D-glucaro-1,4:6,3-dilactone, an in vivo glucuronidase inhibitor. *Carcinogenesis* 1984;5:767.
34. Singletary KW. Effect of butylated hydroxytoluene on the in vivo distribution, metabolism and DNA-binding of 7,12-dimethylbenz[a]anthracene. *Cancer Lett* 1990;49:187.
35. Russo J, Tay LK, Russo IH. Differentiation of the mammary gland and susceptibility to carcinogenesis. *Breast Cancer Res Treat* 1982;2:5.
36. Richards J, Nandi S. Primary culture of rat mammary epithelial cells. II. Cytotoxic effects and metabolism of 7,12-dimethylbenz[a]anthracene and N-nitroso-N-methylurea. *J Natl Cancer Inst* 1978;61:772.
37. Lee SY, Walsh CT, Ng SF, Rogers AE. Toxicokinetics of 7,12-dimethylbenz(a)anthracene (DMBA) in rats fed high lard or control diets. *J Nutr Growth Cancer* 1986;3:167.
38. Gullino PM, Pettigrew HM, Grantham FH. N-Nitrosomethylurea as a mammary gland carcinogen in rats. *J Natl Cancer Inst* 1975;54:401.
39. Gottardis MM, Jordan VC. Antitumor actions of keoxifene and tamoxifen in the N-nitrosomethylurea-induced rat mammary carcinoma model. *Cancer Res* 1987;47:4020.
40. Zarbl H, Sukumar S, Arthur AV, Martin-Zanca D, Barbacid M. Direct mutagenesis of H-ras-1 oncogenes by N-nitroso-N-methylurea during initiation of mammary carcinogenesis in rats. *Nature* 1985;315:382.
41. Bos JL. ras Oncogenes in human cancer: a review. *Cancer Res* 1989;49:4682.
42. Rochlitz CF, Scott GK, Dodson JM, et al. Incidence of activating ras oncogene mutations associated with primary and metastatic human breast cancer. *Cancer Res* 1989;49:357.
43. Cha RS, Thilly WG, Zarbl H. N-nitroso-N-methylurea-induced rat mammary tumors arise from cells with preexisting oncogenic Hras1 gene mutations. *Proc Natl Acad Sci U S A* 1994;91:3749.
44. Jin Z, Houle B, Mikheev AM, Cha RS, Zarbl H. Alterations in H-ras-1 promoter conformation during N-nitroso-N-methylurea-induced mammary carcinogenesis and pregnancy. *Cancer Res* 1996;56:4927.
45. Welsch CW, Gribler C. Prophylaxis of spontaneously developing mammary carcinoma in C3H/HeJ female mice by prolactin. *Cancer Res* 1973;33:2939.
46. Osborne MP, Telang NT, Kaur S, Bradlow HL. Influence of chemopreventive agents on estradiol metabolism and mammary preneoplasia in the C3H mouse. *Steroids* 1990;55:114.
47. Wellings SR. A hypothesis of the origin of human breast cancer from the terminal ductal lobular unit. *Path Res Pract* 1980;166:515.
48. Callahan R. MMTV induced mutations in mouse mammary tumors: their potential relevance to human breast cancer. *Breast Cancer Res Treat* 1995;39:33.
49. Nusse R. Insertional mutagenesis in mouse mammary tumorigenesis. *Curr Top Microbiol Immunobiol* 1991;171:43.
50. Theillet C, Le Roy X, De Lapeyriere O, et al. Amplification of FGF-related genes in human tumors: possible involvement of HST in breast carcinomas. *Oncogene* 1989;4:915.
51. Lidereau R, Callaghan R, Dickson C, Peters G, Escot C, Ali IU. Amplification of the int-2 proto-oncogene in DNA from primary breast carcinomas. *Oncogene Res* 1988;2:285.
52. Zhou DJ, Casey G, Cline MJ. Amplification of human int-2 in breast cancers and squamous carcinomas. *Oncogene* 1988;2:279.
53. Haslam SZ, Wirth JJ, Counterman LJ, Fluck MM. Characterization of the mammary hyperplasia, dysplasia and neoplasia induced in athymic female adult mice by polyomavirus. *Oncogene* 1992;7:1295.
54. Fluck MM, Haslam SZ. Mammary tumors induced by polyoma virus. *Breast Cancer Res Treat* 1995;45.
55. Javier R, Raska K, MacDonald GJ, Shenk T. Human adenovirus type 9-induced rat mammary tumors. *J Virol* 1991;65:3192.
56. Javier R, Shenk T. Mammary tumors induced by adenovirus type-9: a role for the viral early region 4 gene. *Breast Cancer Res Treat* 1995;39:57.
57. Shultz LD. Single gene models of immunodeficiency diseases. In: Wu B, Zheng J, eds. *Immune-deficient animals in experimental medicine*. Basel: Karger, 1989:19.
58. Sakakibara T, Xu Y, Bumpers HL, et al. Growth and metastasis of surgical specimens of human breast carcinomas in SCID mice. *Cancer J Sci Am* 1996;2:291.
59. Mehta RR, Graves JM, Shilkaitis A, Gupta TKD. Development of a new metastatic human breast carcinoma xenograft line. *Br J Cancer* 1998;77:595.
60. Clarke R, Brünner N, Katzenellenbogen BS, et al. Progression from hormone dependent to hormone independent growth in MCF-7 human breast cancer cells. *Proc Natl Acad Sci U S A* 1989;86:3649.
61. Brünner N, Frandsen TL, Holst-Hansen C, et al. MCF7/LCC2: a 4-hydroxytamoxifen resistant human breast cancer variant which retains sensitivity to the steroidal antiestrogen ICI 182,780. *Cancer Res* 1993;53:3229.
62. Katzenellenbogen BS, Kendra KL, Norman MJ, Berthois Y. Proliferation, hormonal responsiveness, and estrogen receptor content of MCF-7 human breast cancer cells grown in the short-term and long-term absence of estrogens. *Cancer Res* 1987;47:4355.
63. Fodstad Ø. Limitations for studies in human tumor biology. In: Boven E, Winograd B, eds. *The nude mouse in oncology research*. Boca Raton, FL: CRC Press, 1991:277.
64. Seibert K, Shafie SM, Triche TJ, et al. Clonal variation of MCF-7 breast cancer cells in vitro and in athymic nude mice. *Cancer Res* 1983;43:2223.
65. van Steenbrugge GJ, Groen M, van Kreuningen A, De Jong FH, Gallee MWP, Schroeder FH. Transplantable human prostatic carcinoma (PC-82) in athymic nude mice (III). Effects of estrogens on the growth of the tumor. *Prostate* 1988;12:157.
66. Brünner N, Svenstrup B, Spang-Thompsen M, Bennet P, Nielsen A, Nielsen JJ. Serum steroid levels in intact and endocrine ablated Balb/c nude mice and their intact litter mates. *J Steroid Biochem* 1986; 25:429.
67. Clarke R, Leonessa F, Brunner N, Thompson EW. In vitro models of human breast cancer. In: Harris JR, Hellman S, Lippman ME, Morrow M, eds. *Diseases of the breast*. Philadelphia: JB Lippincott, 1996:245.
68. Meyvisch C. Influence of implantation site on formation of metastases. *Cancer Metastasis Rev* 1983;2:295.
69. Morikawa K, Walker SM, Nakajima M, Pathak S, Jessup JM, Fidler IJ. Influence of organ environment on the growth, selection, and metastasis of human colon carcinoma cells in nude mice. *Cancer Res* 1988;48:6863.
70. Volpe JPG, Milas L. Influence of tumor transplantation methods on tumor growth rate amd metastatic potential of solitary tumors derived from metastases. *Clin Exp Metastasis* 1990;8:381.
71. Kozlowski JM, Fidler IJ, Campbell D, Xu Z-L, Kaighn ME, Hart IR. Metastatic behavior of human tumor cell lines grown in the nude mouse. *Cancer Res* 1984;44:3522.
72. Clarke R, Thompson EW, Leonessa F, Lippman J, McGarvey M, Brünner N. Hormone resistance, invasiveness and metastatic potential in human breast cancer. *Breast Cancer Res Treat* 1993;24:227.
73. Thompson EW, Brünner N, Torri J, et al. The invasive and metastatic properties of hormone-independent and hormone-responsive variants of MCF-7 human breast cancer cells. *Clin Exp Metastasis* 1993;11:15.
74. Osborne CK, Coronado EB, Robinson JP. Human breast cancer in athymic nude mice: cytostatic effects of long-term antiestrogen therapy. *Eur J Cancer Clin Oncol* 1987;23:1189.
75. Gottardis MM, Jordan VC. Development of tamoxifen-stimulated growth of MCF-7 tumors in athymic mice after long-term antiestrogen administration. *Cancer Res* 1988;48:5183.
76. Gottardis MM, Robinson SP, Satyaswaroop PG, Jordan VC. Contrasting actions of tamoxifen on endometrial and breast tumor growth in the athymic nude mouse. *Cancer Res* 1988;48:812.
77. Brunner N, Bronzert D, Vindelov LL, Rygaard K, Spang-Thomsen M, Lippman ME. Effect of growth and cell cycle kinetics of estradiol and tamoxifen on MCF-7 human breast cancer cells grown in vitro in nude mice. *Cancer Res* 1989;49:1515.

78. Gottardis MM, Wagner RJ, Borden EC, Jordan VC. Differential ability of antiestrogens to stimulate breast cancer cell (MCF-7) growth in vivo and in vitro. *Cancer Res* 1989;49:4765.
79. Brünner N, Boulay V, Fojo A, Freter C, Lippman ME, Clarke R. Acquisition of hormone-independent growth in MCF-7 cells is accompanied by increased expression of estrogen-regulated genes but without detectable DNA amplifications. *Cancer Res* 1993;53:283.
80. Clarke R, Dickson RB, Brünner N. The process of malignant progression in human breast cancer. *Ann Oncol* 1990;1:401.
81. Leonessa F, Boulay V, Wright A, Thompson EW, Brünner N, Clarke R. The biology of breast tumor progression: acquisition of hormone-independence and resistance to cytotoxic drugs. *Acta Oncol* 1991;31:115.
82. Clarke R, Skaar T, Baumann K, et al. Hormonal carcinogenesis in breast cancer: cellular and molecular studies of malignant progression. *Breast Cancer Res Treat* 1994;31:237.
83. Coopman P, Garcia M, Brünner N, Derocq D, Clarke R, Rochefort H. Antiproliferative and antiestrogenic effects of ICI 164,384 in 4-OH-tamoxifen-resistant human breast cancer cells. *Int J Cancer* 1994;56:295.
84. Nicholson RI, Gee JMW, Anderson E, et al. Phase I study of a new pure antiestrogen ICI 182,780 in women with primary breast cancer: immunohistochemical analysis. *Breast Cancer Res Treat* 1993;27:135.
85. McLeskey SW, Honig S, Lippman ME, Kern FG. MCF-7 cells transfected with an expression vector for fibroblast growth factor 4 exhibit opposite responses to tamoxifen in vivo and in vitro. *Proc Am Assoc Cancer Res* 1992;33:269.
86. Price JE, Polyzos A, Zhang RD, Daniels LM. Tumorigenicity and metastasis of human breast carcinoma cell lines in nude mice. *Cancer Res* 1990;50:717.
87. Jiang S-Y, Jordan VC. Growth regulation of estrogen receptor negative breast cancer cells transfected with estrogen receptor cDNAs. *J Natl Cancer Inst* 1992;84:580.
88. Pasqualini JR, Chetrite G, Nestour EL. Control and expression of oestrone sulphatase activities in human breast cancer. *J Endocrinol* 1996;150:S99.
89. Gockerman JP, Spremulli EN, Raney M, Logan T. Randomized comparison of tamoxifen versus diethylstilbestrol in estrogen receptor-positive or -unknown metastatic breast cancer: a southeastern cancer study group trial. *Cancer Treat Rep* 1986;70:1199.
90. Kennedy BJ. Hormonal therapies in breast cancer. *Semin Oncol* 1974;1:119.
91. Litherland S, Jackson IM. Antioestrogens in the management of hormone-dependent cancer. *Cancer Treat Rev* 1988;15:183.
92. Vogel CL, East DR, Voigt W, Thomsen S. Response to tamoxifen in estrogen receptor-poor metastatic breast cancer. *Cancer* 1987;60:1184.
93. Howell A, Dodwell DJ, Anderson H, Redford J. Response after withdrawal of tamoxifen and progestogens in advanced breast cancer [see comments]. *Ann Oncol* 1992;3:611.
94. Belani CP, Pearl P, Whitley NO, Aisner J. Tamoxifen withdrawal response. Report of a case. *Arch Intern Med* 1989;149:449.
95. Stein W, Hortobagyi GN, Blumenschein GR. Response of metastatic breast cancer to tamoxifen withdrawal: report of a case. *J Surg Oncol* 1983;22:45.
96. McIntosh IH, Thynne GS. Tumour stimulation by anti-oestrogens. *Br J Surg* 1977;64:900.
97. Meschter CL, Connolly JM, Rose DP. Influence of regional location of the inoculation site and dietary fat on the pathology of MDA-MB-435 human breast cancer cell-derived tumors growing in nude mice. *Clin Exp Metastasis* 1992;10:167.
98. Rose DP, Hatala MA, Connolly JM, Rayburn J. Effect of diets containing different levels of linoleic acid on human breast cancer growth and lung metastasis in nude mice. *Cancer Res* 1993;53:4686.
99. Leonessa F, Green D, Licht T, et al. MDA435/LCC6 and MDA435/LCC6^{MDR1}: ascites models of human breast cancer. *Br J Cancer* 1996;73:154.
100. Thompson EW, Sung V, Lavigne M, et al. LCC15-MB: a human breast cancer cell line from a femoral bone metastasis. *Clin Exp Metastasis* 1999;17:193.
101. Sung V, Gilles C, Murray A, et al. The LCC15-MB human breast cancer cell line expresses osteopontin and exhibits an invasive and metastatic phenotype. *Exp Cell Res* 1998;241:273.
102. Clarke R. Human breast cancer cell line xenografts as models of breast cancer: the immunobiologies of recipient mice and the characteristics of several tumorigenic cell lines. *Breast Cancer Res Treat* 1996;39:69.
103. Pantelouris EM. Absence of thymus in a mutant mouse. *Nature* 1968;217:370.
104. Weisz-Carrington P, Schrater AF, Lamm ME, Thorbecke GJ. Immunoglobulin isotypes in plasma cells of normal and athymic mice. *Cell Immunol* 1979;44:343.
105. Kindred B. The inception of the response to SRBC by nude mice injected with various doses of congenic or allogeneic thymus cells. *Cell Immunol* 1975;17:277.
106. Jacobson EB, Caporale LH, Thorbecke GJ. Effect of thymus cell injections on germinal center formation in lymphoid tissues of nude (thymusless) mice. *Cell Immunol* 1974;13:416.
107. Guy-Grand D, Griscelli C, Vassalli P. Peyer's patches, gut IgA, plasma cells and thymic function: study in nude mice bearing thymic grafts. *J Immunol* 1975;115:361.
108. De Sousa M, Pritchard H. The cellular basis of immunological recovery in nude mice after thymus grafting. *Immunology* 1974;26:769.
109. Manning JK, Reed ND, Jutila JW. Antibody response to Escherichia coli lipopolysaccharide by congenitally thymusless (nude) mice. *J Immunol* 1972;108:1470.
110. Herberman RB, Nunn ME, Holden HT, Staal S, Djeu JY. Augmentation of natural cytotoxic reactivity of mouse lymphoid cells against syngeneic and allogeneic tumors. *Int J Cancer* 1977;19:555.
111. Kiessling R, Klein E, Wagzell H. "Natural" killer cells in the mouse. I. Cytotoxic cells with specificity for mouse Moloney leukemia cells. Specificity and distribution according to phenotype. *Eur J Immunol* 1975;72:2130.
112. Hasui M, Saikawa Y, Miura M, et al. Effector and precursor phenotypes of lymphokine-activated killer cells in mice with severe combined immunodeficiency (Scid) and athymic (Nude) mice. *Cell Immunol* 1989;120:230.
113. Johnson WJ, Balish E. Macrophage function in germ-free, athymic (nu/nu) mice and conventional flora (nu/+) mice. *J Reticuloendothel Soc* 1980;28:55.
114. Schuler W, Weiler IJ, Schuler A, et al. Rearrangement of antigen receptor genes is defective in mice with severe combined immune deficiency. *Cell* 1986;46:963.
115. Dorshkind K, Keller GM, Phillips RA, et al. Functional status of cells from lymphoid and myeloid tissues in mice with severe combined immunodeficiency disease. *J Immunol* 1984;132:1804.
116. Custer RP, Bosma GC, Bosma MJ. Severe combined immunodeficiency (scid) in the mouse. Pathology, reconstitution, neoplasms. *Am J Pathol* 1985;120:464.
117. Bosma GC, Custer RP, Bosma MJ. A severe combined immunodeficiency mutation in the mouse. *Nature* 1983;301:527.
118. Quimby FW. *Immunodeficient rodents. A guide to their immunobiology, husbandry, and use*. Washington, DC: National Academy Press, 1989.
119. Andriole GL, Mule JJ, Hansen CT, Linehan WM, Rosenberg SA. Evidence that lymphokine-activated killer cells and natural killer cells are distinct based on an analysis of congenitally immunodeficient mice. *J Immunol* 1985;135:2911.
120. Roder JC. The beige mutation in the mouse. I. A stem cell predetermined impairment in natural killer cell function. *J Immunol* 1979;123:2168.
121. Roder JC, Duwe AK. The beige mutation in the mouse selectively impairs natural killer cell function. *Nature* 1979;278:451.
122. Ahmed A, Scher I, Sharrow SO, et al. B-lymphocyte heterogeneity: development and characterization of an alloantiserum which distinguishes B-lymphocyte differentiation alloantigens. *J Exp Med* 1977;145:101.
123. Azar HA, Hansen CT, Costa J. N:NIH(S)II-nu/nu mice with combined immunodeficiency: a new model for human tumor heterotransplantation. *J Natl Cancer Inst* 1980;65:421.
124. Karagogeos D, Rosenberg N, Wortis HH. Early arrest of B cell development in nude, X-linked immune-deficient mice. *Eur J Immunol* 1986;16:1125.
125. Danel L, Souweine G, Monier JC, Saez S. Specific estrogen binding sites in human lymphoid cells and thymic cells. *J Steroid Biochem* 1983;18:559.
126. Cohen JHM, Danel L, Gordier G, Saez S, Revillard JP. Sex steroid receptors in peripheral T cells: absence of androgen receptors and restriction of estrogen receptors to OKT 8 positive cells. *J Immunol* 1983;131:2767.
127. Stimson WH. Oestrogen and human T cell lymphocytes: presence of specific receptors in the T-suppressor/cytotoxic subset. *Scand J Immunol* 1980;28:345.
128. Myers MJ, Peterson BH. Estradiol induced alterations in the immune system. I. Enhancement of IgM production. *Int J Immunopharmacol* 1985;7:207.

129. Paavonen T, Andersson LC, Adlercreutz H. Sex hormone regulation of in vitro immune response. Estradiol enhances human B cell maturation via inhibition of suppressor T cells in pokeweed mitogen stimulated cultures. *J Exp Med* 1981;154:1935.
130. Ahmed AS, Dauphinee MJ, Talal N. Effects of short term administration of sex hormones on normal and autoimmune mice. *J Immunol* 1985;134:204.
131. Sthoeger ZM, Chiorazzi N, Lahita RG. Regulation of the immune response by sex steroids. I. In vitro effects of estradiol and testosterone on pokeweed mitogen-induced human B cell differentiation. *J Immunol* 1988;141:91.
132. Scambia G, Panci PB, Maccio A, Castelli P, Serri F, Mantovani G, Massidda B, Iacobelli S, Del Giacco S, Mancuso S. Effects of antiestrogen and progestin on immune functions in breast cancer patients. *Cancer* 1988;61:2214.
133. Wyban J, Govaerts A, van Dam D, Appelbloom T. Stimulating properties of lynestrenol on normal human blood T-lymphocytes and other leucocytes. *Int J Immunopharmacol* 1979;1:151.
134. Seaman WE, Talal N. The effect of 17β-estradiol on natural killing in the mouse. In: Herberman RB, ed. *Natural cell-mediated immunity against tumors*. New York: Academic, 1980:765.
135. Screpanti I, Santoni A, Gulino A, Herberman RB, Frati L. Estrogen and antiestrogen modulation of mouse natural killer activity and large granular lymphocytes. *Cell Immunol* 1987;106:191.
136. Seaman WE, Blackman MA, Gindhart TD, Roubinian JR, Loeb JM, Talal N. β-Estradiol reduces natural killer cells in mice. *J Immunol* 1978;121:2193.
137. Hanna N, Schneider M. Enhancement of tumor metastases and suppression of natural killer cell activity by β-estradiol treatment. *J Immunol* 1983;130:974.
138. Shafie SM, Grantham FH. Role of hormones in the growth and regression of human breast cancer cells (MCF-7) transplanted into athymic nude mice. *J Natl Cancer Inst* 1981;67:51.
139. Welsch CW, Swim EL, McManus MJ, White AC, McGrath CM. Estrogen induced growth of human breast cancer cells (MCF-7) in athymic nude mice is enhanced by secretions from transplantable pituitary tumor. *Cancer Lett* 1981;14:309.
140. Clarke R, Brünner N, Thompson EW, et al. The inter-relationships between ovarian-independent growth, antiestrogen resistance and invasiveness in the malignant progression of human breast cancer. *J Endocrinol* 1989;122:331.
141. Mandeville R, Ghali SS, Chausseau JP. In vitro stimulation of NK activity by an estrogen antagonist (Tamoxifen). *Eur J Cancer Clin Oncol* 1984;20:983.
142. Paavonen T, Andersson LC. The oestrogen antagonists tamoxifen, FC-1157a display oestrogen like effects on human lymphocyte functions in vitro. *Clin Exp Immunol* 1985;61:467.
143. Berry J, Green BJ, Matheson DS. Modulation of natural killer cell activity in stage I postmenopausal breast cancer patients on low-dose aminogluthemide. *Cancer Immunol Immunother* 1987;24:72.
144. Arteaga CL, Koli KM, Dugger TC, Clarke R. Reversal of tamoxifen resistance of human breast carcinomas in vivo with neutralizing anti-transforming growth factor (TGF)-β antibodies involves paracrine mechanisms. *J Natl Cancer Inst* 1999;91:46.
145. Blumenthal RD, Jordan JJ, McLaughlin WH, Bloomer WD. Animal modeling of human breast tumors: limitations in the use of estrogen pellet implants. *Breast Cancer Res Treat* 1988;11:77.
146. Heitjan DF, Manni A, Santen RJ. Statistical analysis of in vivo tumor growth experiments. *Cancer Res* 1993;53:6042.
147. Hogan B, Beddington R, Costantini F, Lacy E. *Manipulating the mouse embryo, a laboratory manual*. Cold Spring Harbor, NY: Cold Spring Harbor Laboratory Press, 1994;1.
148. Smith GH, Sharp R, Kordon EC, Jhappan C, Merlino G. Transforming growth factor-alpha promotes mammary tumorigenesis through selective survival and growth of secretory epithelial cells. *Am J Pathol* 1995;147:1081.
149. Wagner KU, Wall RJ, St-Onge L, et al. Cre-mediated gene deletion in the mammary gland. *Nucleic Acids Res* 1997;25:4323.
150. Robinson GW, McKnight RA, Smith GH, Hennighausen L. Mammary epithelial cells undergo secretory differentiation in cycling virgins but require pregnancy for the establishment of terminal differentiation. *Development* 1995;121:2079.
151. Sandgren EP, Schroeder JA, Qui TH, Palmiter RD, Brinster RL, Lee DC. Inhibition of mammary gland involution is associated with transforming growth factor alpha but not c-myc-induced tumorigenesis in transgenic mice. *Cancer Res* 1995;55:3915.
152. Maroulakou IG, Anver M, Garrett L, Green JE. Prostate and mammary adenocarcinoma in transgenic mice carrying a rat c3(1) simian virus 40 large tumor antigen fusion gene. *Proc Natl Acad Sci U S A* 1994;91:11236.
153. Yarus S, Hadsell D, Rosen JM. Engineering transgenes for use in the mammary gland. *Genet Eng* 1996;18:57.
154. Furth PA, St Onge L, Boger H, et al. Temporal control of gene expression in transgenic mice by a tetracycline-responsive promoter. *Proc Natl Acad Sci U S A* 1994;91:9302.
155. No D, Yao TP, Evans RM. Ecdysone-inducible gene expression in mammalian cells and transgenic mice. *Proc Natl Acad Sci U S A* 1996;93:3346.
156. Hennighausen L, Wall RJ, Tillmann U, Li M, Furth PA. Conditional gene expression in secretory tissues and skin of transgenic mice using the mmtv–ltr and the tetracycline responsive system. *J Cell Biochem* 1995;59:463.
157. Ewald D, Li M, Efrat S, et al. Time-sensitive reversal of hyperplasia in transgenic mice expressing sv40 t antigen. *Science* 1996;273:1384.
158. Ludwig T, Chapman DL, Papaioannou VE, Efstratiadis A. Targeted mutations of breast cancer susceptibility gene homologs in mice: lethal phenotypes of brca1, brca2, brca1/brca2, brca1/p53, and brca2/p53 nullizygous embryos. *Genes Dev* 1997;11:1226.
159. McCormack SJ, Weaver Z, Deming S, et al. Myc/p53 interactions in transgenic mouse mammary development, tumorigenesis and chromosomal instability. *Oncogene* 1998;16:2755.
160. Selbert S, Bentley DB, Melton DW, et al. Efficient BLG-CRE mediated gene deletion in the mammary gland. *Transgenic Research* 1998;7:387.
161. Munn RJ, Webster M, Muller WJ, Cardiff RD. Histopathology of transgenic mouse mammary tumors (a short atlas). *Semin Cancer Biol* 1995;6:153.
162. Cardiff RD, Munn RJ. Comparative pathology of mammary tumorigenesis in transgenic mice. *Cancer Lett* 1995;90:13.
163. Guy CT, Cardiff RD, Muller WJ. Induction of mammary tumors by expression of polyomavirus middle t oncogene: a transgenic mouse model for metastatic disease. *Mol Cell Biol* 1992;12:954.
164. Amundadottir LT, Johnson MD, Merlino G, Smith GH, Dickson RB. Synergistic interaction of transforming growth factor alpha and c-myc in mouse mammary and salivary gland tumorigenesis. *Cell Growth Differ* 1995;6:737.
165. Nass SJ, Dickson RB. Epidermal growth factor-dependent cell cycle progression is altered in mammary epithelial cells that overexpress c-myc. *Clin Cancer Res* 1998;4:1813.
166. Li B, Murphy KL, Laucirica R, Kittrell F, Medina D, Rosen JM. A transgenic mouse model for mammary carcinogenesis. *Oncogene* 1998;16:997.
167. Stewart TA, Pattengale PK, Leader P. Spontaneous mammary adenocarcinoma in transgenic mice that carry and express mtv/myc fusion genes. *Cell* 1984;38:627.
168. Fay MP, Freedman LS. Meta-analyses of dietary fats and mammary neoplasms in rodent experiments. *Breast Cancer Res Treat* 1997;46:215.
169. Fay MP, Freedman LS, Clifford CK, Midthune DN. Effect of different types and amounts of fat on the development of mammary tumors in rodents: a review. *Cancer Res* 1997;57:3979.
170. Rose DP, Connolly JM. Dietary fat and breast cancer metastasis by human tumor xenografts. *Breast Cancer Res Treat* 1997;46:225.
171. Carroll KK, Khor HT. Dietary fat in relation to tumorigenesis. *Prog Biochem Pharmacol* 1975;10:308.
172. Howe GR, Hirohata T, Hislop G, et al. Dietary factors and risk of breast cancer: combined analysis of 12 case-control studies. *J Natl Cancer Inst* 1990;82:561.
173. Hilakivi-Clarke LA, Clarke R, Onojafe I, Raygada M, Cho E, Lippman ME. A high fat diet during pregnancy increases mammary epithelial density and breast cancer risk among female rat offspring. *Proc Natl Acad Sci U S A* 1997;94:9372.
174. Cave WT. Omega-3 polyunsaturated fatty acids in rodent models of breast cancer. *Breast Cancer Res Treat* 1997;46:239.
175. Hsieh C-Y, Santell RC, Haslam SZ, Helferich WG. Estrogenic effects of genistein on the growth of estrogen receptor-positive human breast cancer (MCF-7) cells in vitro and in vivo. *Cancer Res* 1998;58:3833.
176. Hilakivi-Clarke LA, Cho E, Raygada M, Onojafe I, Clarke R. Maternal genistein exposure during pregnancy increases breast cancer risk,

prostate weight, and alters aggressive behavior among offspring. *Proc Am Assoc Cancer Res* 1998;39:20.

177. Murrill WB, Brown NM, Zhang JX, Manzolillo PA, Barnes S, Lamartiniere CA. Prepubertal genistein exposure suppresses mammary cancer and enhances gland differentiation in rats. *Carcinogenesis* 1996;17:1451.
178. Barnes S. The chemopreventive properties of soy isoflavonoids in animal models of breast cancer. *Breast Cancer Res Treat* 1997;46:169.
179. Kennedy AR. The evidence for soybean products as cancer preventive agents. *J Nutr* 1995;125:733s.
180. Barnes S, Grubbs C, Setchell KD, Carlson J. Soybeans inhibit mammary tumors in models of breast cancer. *Prog Clin Biol Res* 1990;347:239.
181. Moon RC, Constantinou A. Dietary retinoids and carotenoids in rodent models of mammary tumorigenesis. *Breast Cancer Res Treat* 1997;46:181.
182. Price JE, Zhang RD. Studies of human breast cancer metastasis using nude mice. *Cancer Metastasis Rev* 1990;8:285.
183. Kurebayashi J, McLeskey SW, Johnson MD, Lippman ME, Dickson RB, Kern FG. Quantitative demonstration of spontaneous metastasis by MCF-7 human breast cancer cells cotransfected with fibroblast growth factor 4 and LacZ. *Cancer Res* 1993;53:2178.
184. Soule HD, Vasquez J, Long A, Albert S, Brennan M. A human cell line from a pleural effusion derived from a human breast carcinoma. *J Natl Cancer Inst* 1973;51:1409.
185. Thompson EW, Paik S, Brünner N, et al. Association of increased basement membrane-invasiveness with absence of estrogen receptor and expression of vimentin in human breast cancer cell lines. *J Cell Physiol* 1992;150:534.
186. Engel LW, Young NA. Human breast carcinoma cells in continuous culture: a review. *Cancer Res* 1978;38:4327.
187. Brünner N, Boysen B, Jirus S, et al. MCF7/LCC9: an antiestrogen resistant MCF-7 variant where acquired resistance to the steroidal antiestrogen ICI 182,780 confers an early crossresistance to the nonsteroidal antiestrogen tamoxifen. *Cancer Res* 1997;57:3486.
188. Brunner N, Bastert GB, Poulsen HS, Spang-Thomsen M. Characterization of the T61 human breast carcinoma established in nude mice. *Eur J Cancer Clin Oncol* 1985;21:833.
189. Brunner N, Spang-Thomsen M, Vindelov L, Wolff J, Engelholm SA. Effect of tamoxifen on the receptor-positive T61 and the receptor negative T60 human breast carcinomas grown in nude mice. *Eur J Cancer Clin Oncol* 1985;21:1349.
190. Vickers PJ, Dickson RB, Shoemaker R, Cowan KH. A multidrug-resistant MCF-7 human breast cancer cell line which exhibits cross-resistance to antiestrogens and hormone independent tumor growth. *Mol Endocrinol* 1988;2:886.
191. Scudiero DA, Monks A, Sausville EA. Cell line designation change: multidrug-resistant cell line in the NCI anticancer screen. *J Natl Cancer Inst* 1998;90:862.
192. Bronzert DA, Pantazis P, Antoniades HN, et al. Synthesis and secretion of platelet-derived growth factor by human breast cancer cell lines. *Proc Natl Acad Sci U S A* 1987;84:5763.
193. Nelson J, Clarke R, Dickson GR, van den Berg HW, Murphy RF. The effects of Mg^{++} ions on nuclear integrity and subcellular distribution of unoccupied oestrogen receptor in breast cancer cells. *J Steroid Biochem* 1986;25:619.
194. Carpenter G, Stoschech CM, Preston YA, De Larco LE. Antibodies to the epidermal growth factor receptor block the biological activities of sarcoma growth factor. *Proc Natl Acad Sci U S A* 1983;80:4684.
195. Campbell FC, Blamey RW, Elston CW, Nicholson RI, Griffiths FC, Haybittle JL. Oestrogen-receptor status and sites of metastasis in breast cancer. *Br J Cancer* 1981;44:456.
196. Matsui Y, Halter SA, Holt JT, Hogan BL, Coffey RJ. Development of mammary hyperplasia and neoplasia in MMTV-TGF alpha transgenic mice. *Cell* 1990;61:1147.
197. Bronson FH, Dagg CP, Snell GD. Biology of the laboratory mouse. *Reproduction* 1975:187.
198. Bugge TH, Lund LR, Kombrinck KK, et al. Reduced metastasis of polyoma virus middle T antigen-induced mammary cancer in plasminogen-deficient mice. *Oncogene* 1998;16:3097.
199. Sinn E, Muller W, Pattengale P, Tepler I, Wallace R, Leder P. Coexpression of MMTV/v-Haras and MMTV-c-myc genes in transgenic mice: synergistic action of oncogenes *in vivo*. *Cell* 1987;49:465.
200. Muller MJ, Sinn E, Pattengale P, Tepler I, Wallace R, Leder P. Single-step induction of mammary adenocarcinoma in transgenic mice bearing the activated c-neu oncogene. *Cell* 1988;54:105

Diseases of the Breast, 2nd ed.,
edited by Jay R. Harris.
Lippincott Williams & Wilkins, Philadelphia © 2000.

CHAPTER 23

In Vitro Models

Robert Clarke, Fabio Leonessa, W. Nils Brünner, and Erik W. Thompson

Breast cancer cells that grow *in vitro* represent one of the most widely used experimental models of breast cancer. For many studies, these models provide the only means to address a specific hypothesis. Most breast cancer cell lines can easily be maintained and studied *in vitro*, and are generally stable with respect to their endocrine responsiveness *in vitro* and *in vivo*. The current understanding of how breast cancer cells respond to estrogenic stimuli is, in no small part, the direct result of *in vitro* studies with human breast cancer cell lines.

Breast cancer cell lines are generally considered in terms of their estrogen-receptor (ER) content—that is, whether they are estrogen receptor–positive (ER+) or estrogen receptor–negative (ER–). This classification largely reflects the clinical value of steroid hormone expression in predicting response to endocrine therapy. However, other characteristics of human breast tumors that tend to follow ER status are frequently exhibited in a similar pattern by cell lines growing *in vitro* and *in vivo*.[1]

A detailed and inclusive review of all breast cancer cell lines and their origins, characteristics, and uses is beyond the scope of this chapter. Consequently, the chapter focuses primarily on the most widely used cell lines, some of their variants, and those models expressing characteristics that closely reflect many of the properties of breast tumors in patients. Also included is a brief description of cell lines that have more unique properties or that are best suited to specific studies, such as endocrine regulation or expression of growth factors or oncogenes. The parental cell lines are readily available (e.g., several are available through the American Type Culture Collection in Rockville, Maryland), and the variants can generally be obtained from their respective originators. For a more detailed description of the characteristics of several of these cell lines, the reader is referred to the review by Engel and Young.[2] Although more than two decades old, this review provides valuable information on the origin and characteristics of 22 breast cancer cell lines. The inclusion of the original citations for almost all of these cell lines provides a valuable reference for the interested reader.

R. Clarke: Departments of Oncology and Physiology and Biophysics, Lombardi Cancer Center, Georgetown University Medical Center, Washington, D.C.

F. Leonessa: Department of Physiology and Biophysics, Georgetown University Medical Center, Washington D.C.

W. N. Brünner: Finsen Laboratory, Copenhagen, Denmark

E. W. Thompson: Department of Surgery, University of Melbourne, Melbourne, Australia; VBCRC Invasion and Metastasis Unit, St. Vincent's Institute of Medical Research, Victoria, Australia

ESTROGEN-DEPENDENT (ER+/PR+) BREAST CANCER CELL LINES

Approximately 30% of all breast cancer patients respond to endocrine manipulation. The overall response rate to antiestrogens increases to 70% or more in patients whose tumors express both the estrogen receptor (ERs) and progesterone receptor (PR).[3–5] To define the mechanism of action of endocrine therapies and to develop and screen new agents and therapies require models that exhibit an endocrine response profile comparable to that found in breast cancer patients. In this regard, the steroid-dependent breast cancer cell lines have been most useful in studying the growth-inhibitory effects of estrogens, antiestrogens, progestins, and antiprogestins. These cell lines are characterized by a dependence on estrogens for growth *in vitro* or *in vivo* and by sensitivity to the growth-inhibitory effects of antiestrogenic and progestational drugs. In general, steroid-dependent cell lines are poorly invasive and nonmetastatic in athymic nude mice.

MCF-7

The MCF-7 cell line is the most widely used and best characterized of all the human breast cancer cell lines. The mitogenic effects of 17β-estradiol (E2) in human breast cancer cells *in vitro* were initially defined in these cells, as were the *in vitro* inhibitory effects of antiestrogens.[6,7] MCF-7 cells also are growth inhibited by luteinizing hormone–releasing hormone (LHRH) analogues[8] and retinoids.[9–11] The now widely reported E2 dependence for exponential growth both *in vitro* and *in vivo* has provided this cell line with a central role in the study of endocrine responsiveness and malignant progression *in vitro*. Much of the current understanding of the mechanism of action of estrogens and antiestrogens and their role in regulating the proliferation of hormone-dependent breast cancer cells has been derived from work performed using this cellular model. Consequently, a full and detailed discussion of all the data generated using MCF-7 cells alone is beyond the scope of this chapter.

MCF-7 cells were established from a pleural effusion arising in a postmenopausal woman with breast cancer. The patient had received radiotherapy and endocrine therapy before the appearance of the effusion.[12] In addition to the expression of ER,[12,13] MCF-7 cells express an E2-inducible PR[13,14] and cellular receptors for androgens,[13] LHRH,[8,15] glucocorticoids,[13] insulin,[16] retinoic acid receptors (RAR-α and RAR-γ),[17] and prolactin.[18] The expression/secretion of several growth factors and their receptors also has been described in detail, including the insulinlike growth factors (IGFs),[19–22] type I and type II IGF receptors,[22–24] and several IGF binding proteins[25–27]; transforming growth factor α (TGF-α) and epidermal growth factor receptor (EGFR)[28–30]; several fibroblast growth factors (FGFs)[31] and FGF receptors[32]; and platelet-derived growth factor (PDGF) but not PDGF receptors.[33] The expression of many of these growth factors, and their respective receptors, is strongly E2 regulated in MCF-7 cells.[34] The expression, secretion, and regulation of this wide variety of receptors and ligands has made the MCF-7 cells a valuable model for the study of the role of growth factor and growth factor receptor expression in the proliferation of breast cancer cells.

The E2 dependence for growth, antiestrogen sensitivity, and low metastatic potential of MCF-7 cells has led to the hypothesis that they represent an "early" breast cancer phenotype.[35,36] MCF-7 cells are an excellent model in which to study the process of malignant progression, because they can be subjected to appropriate endocrinologic and physiologic selective pressures for the derivation of variants with more progressed phenotypes. For example, the estrogenic requirement for tumorigenicity in immunocompromised mice has been used to select for E2-independent MCF-7 variants (see below and Chapter 22). Variants have also been selected for antiestrogen resistance, and the extent of induced cross-resistance among structurally diverse antiestrogens has been determined.

T47D

T47D cells were established by Keydar et al. from a 54-year-old patient with an infiltrating ductal carcinoma.[37] The cells express ER, PR, androgen, glucocorticoid,[37] and insulin receptors.[38] Approximately 60% of the original cell line expressed casein.[37,39] The T47D cells are perhaps most notable for their high levels of PR and their remarkable genetic and phenotypic instability.[40–43] Furthermore, these cells exhibit significant growth-regulatory responses to progestational agents.[44,45] Not surprisingly, T47D cells, and several T47D variants that have been obtained, represent the major *in vitro* human breast cancer models for the study of the antiproliferative effects of progestins and antiprogestins and the regulation of PR expression.[42–46] T47D cells also express RAR-α and RAR-γ[17] and are sensitive to the growth-inhibitory effects of retinoids and antiestrogens.[9,10]

The remarkable genetic instability of the T47D cells stands in contrast to the other ER+/PR+ human breast cancer cell lines. Subtle differences in the phenotypic characteristics of all of the ER+/PR+ cell lines are observed from laboratory to laboratory. However, these differences rarely extend to the pattern of expression of steroid hormone receptors, metastatic potential, antiestrogen responsiveness, the estrogen supplementation required for *in vivo* tumorigenicity, or metastatic potential. These are the major phenotypic characteristics of hormone-responsive breast cancer cells.[34–36] In cases in which significant divergent phenotypic responses in other ER+/PR+ cell lines are observed, these divergences are almost always the result of an imposed selective pressure (i.e., *in vivo* or *in vitro* growth in the absence of E2, selection for cytotoxic drug resistance). For example, no bona fide spontaneous ER– or PR– MCF-7 or ZR-75-1 cell lines have been described in detail, other than those generated by the imposition of selective pressures. In marked contrast, simple dilution cloning can produce T47D variants with fundamentally altered endocrine responsiveness, (e.g., ER–/PR+, estrogen unresponsiveness, and antiestrogen resistance).[40–42] Many of these variants are unstable and readily revert to the wild-type phenotype.[40,43] Other T47D variants (e.g., the ER–/PR+ $T47D_{CO}$) have been stable for many years.

ZR-75-1

ZR-75-1 cells were first described by Engel et al. in 1978.[47] They were established from an ascites that developed in a 63-year-old woman with an infiltrating ductal breast carcinoma. This patient had been receiving tamoxifen (tamoxifen citrate) for 3 months before the time when cells were removed to establish the ZR-75-1 cell line.[47] Although the ZR-75-1 cells are ER+/PR+ cells[47,48] and are growth stimulated by estrogens and inhibited by antiestrogens *in vitro*,[47,49] the patient did not respond to tamoxifen.[47] The expression of ER is up-regulated by interferons in these cells, and treatment with interferon 2α can increase sensitivity to tamoxifen.[48] ZR-75-1 cells exhibit an eightfold overexpression of c-*erb*-b2 messenger RNA (mRNA) relative to normal fibroblasts.[50] This overexpression is E2 regulated in ZR-75-1 cells, a down-regulation being associated with E2-induced cell proliferation.[51] Tamoxifen-resistant and hormone-independent ZR-75-1 variants have been described.[49,52,53]

ZR-75-1 cells also express androgen and glucocorticoid receptors[54] and are growth inhibited *in vitro* by progestins[54,55] and somatostatin analogues.[56] They express the RAR-α and RAR-γ retinoic acid isoforms[17] and are growth inhibited by several retinoids.[9,10] ZR-75-1 cells also express low levels of EGFR; altered EGFR expression is associated with tamoxifen resistance and hormone independence.[52,53] The ZR-75-1 cells appear to possess several steroid metabolism pathways.[57–59]

ESTROGEN-INDEPENDENT (ER+/PR+) AND ESTROGEN-RESPONSIVE BREAST CANCER CELL LINES

The estrogenic requirement of the MCF-7, T47D, and ZR-75-1 cells for growth *in vitro* or *in vivo* may not adequately reflect the endocrine environment of many breast tumors in postmenopausal women. Several breast cancer cell lines and variants of the MCF-7, ZR-75-1, and T47D cell lines have been generated that no longer require estrogenic supplementation for growth. These continue to express ER, PR, or both, and many also retain responsiveness to endocrine agents. Several steroid-independent and steroid-responsive cell lines or variants exhibit properties that more closely resemble those of breast tumors in patients than do the steroid-dependent cell lines.

MCF-7/MIII, MCF-7/LCC1: Cells Selected for Estrogen Independence *in Vivo*

Several aspects of the MCF-7 phenotype could be considered potentially inconsistent with the human disease. For example, these cells generally do not proliferate in cell culture media devoid of estrogens and do not form proliferating tumors when orthotopically transplanted into oophorectomized immunodeficient mice. If this dependence on estrogens for growth were to exist in a tumor cell in a postmenopausal woman, the source from which the MCF-7 cells were originally obtained,[12] the cells would not give rise to detectable disease. Despite their apparent metastatic site of origin, MCF-7 cells exhibit few characteristics associated with an invasive/metastatic phenotype. Thus, we have previously suggested that the MCF-7 phenotype represents an early hypothetical breast cancer cell.[35,36]

We wished to determine if, by applying appropriate physiologic and endocrinologic selective pressures, we could obtain cells more representative of many of the ER+/PR+ cells apparent in the breast tumors of postmenopausal women. Thus, we selected MCF-7 cells by xenotransplantation into the mammary fat pads of oophorectomized, athymic, nude mice. After approximately 6 months, we obtained cells (MCF-7/MIII) that were readily reestablished *in vitro*. MCF-7/MIII cells were determined to be of MCF-7 origin by karyotype and isozyme profile analyses.[14] A further selection of MCF-7/MIII cells produced a variant designated MCF-7/LCC1, which exhibits increased metastatic potential and a shorter lag time to tumor appearance compared with MCF-7/MIII.[60,61]

We studied these cells for their respective responses to estrogens and antiestrogens both *in vitro* and *in vivo*. MCF-7/MIII and MCF-7/LCC1 cells proliferate *in vivo* and *in vitro* without estrogen supplementation[14,60] and are responsive to drugs representing each of the major classes of antiestrogens.[60,62] MCF-7/MIII cells also are inhibited by LHRH analogues.[63] Both these variants exhibit an increased metastatic potential *in vivo* and *in vitro*,[14,61] although at a much lower level than ER– cell lines.[1,64] We interpret these observations as indicating that MCF-7/MIII and MCF-7/LCC1 cells exhibit a phenotype representative of many ER+/PR+ cells present in the tumors of postmenopausal breast cancer patients. The phenotype of these cells has been reviewed in detail.[35,36,65]

MCF-7 K3: Cells Selected for Estrogen Independence *in Vitro*

MCF-7 cells also can be selected *in vitro* for their ability to proliferate in the absence of estrogenic stimulation. For example, Katzenellenbogen et al.[66] selected MCF-7 cells in cell culture media devoid of estrogens. The resultant cells (MCF-7 K3) have a phenotype that is generally similar to the MCF-7/MIII cells.[14] In our studies, these cells also form tumors in oophorectomized nude mice, but with a longer doubling time[14] and without an apparently increased metastatic potential (R. Clarke, *unpublished data*, 1992). Other, perhaps more subtle differences appear to exist. For example, the estrogen-induced gene *pS2* is constitutively expressed in MCF-7/LCC1 cells *in vitro* but retains some estrogen-inducible expression *in vivo*.[60] In the MCF-7 K3 cells, pS2 mRNA expression appears to be inhibited by E2.[67] Some evidence exists that MCF-7 K3 cells may be estrogen supersensitive,[67] and estrogen supersensitive MCF-7 cells have been previously reported by others.[68] We have no data for the cells selected *in vivo* (MCF-7/MIII, MCF-7/LCC1) that would clearly suggest that they have a supersensitive phenotype. The biological significance of the apparent differences between cells selected *in vivo* (e.g., MCF-7/MIII) and *in vitro* (e.g., MCF-7 K3) remains to be established.

MCF-7 MKS: Cells Transfected with Fibroblast Growth Factor 4

The FGFs are potent angiogenic growth factors, and several appear to be present in or secreted by human breast cancer cells, or both. Transfection of cells with FGF-4 produces cells (MCF-7 MKS) that are able to generate proliferating tumors in the absence of estrogenic stimulation.[69,70] Whereas MCF-7 cells are generally nonmetastatic, MCF-7 MKS cells produce highly vascular tumors, from which both lymphatic and lung metastases arise with a high frequency. Unlike MCF-7 cells selected for an ability to grow in a low-estrogen environment, MCF-7 MKS cells are stimulated by tamoxifen and inhibited by physiologic concentrations of estrogen.[69] The extent to which this endocrine-inverted phenotype reflects a specific phenotype in the human disease is unclear. However, these cells exhibit an endocrine response pattern similar to that of MCF-7 cells selected for *in vivo* resistance to tamoxifen (see below).

ESTROGEN-INDEPENDENT (ER±/PR±) AND ESTROGEN-UNRESPONSIVE BREAST CANCER CELL LINES

BT 20 (Mutant ER)

The BT 20 cell line is one of the older breast cancer cell lines and was established in 1958 by Lasfargues and Ozzello.[71] The cell line was obtained from a breast cancer patient with an infiltrating ductal carcinoma.[71] BT 20 cells were initially described as being ER–/PR–,[72] but subsequently ER mRNA was detected.[73] More recently, these cells have been shown to express a novel ER mutant with an exon 5 deletion.[74] This mutation produces a protein that does not bind E2 and would appear ER– by ligand binding. Because some evidence exists that exon 5 mutant ER proteins can be transcriptionally active,[75] BT 20 cells could be considered to be ER+, hormone independent, and hormone unresponsive. These cells also express glucocorticoid receptor (GR),[72] and they have a 16-fold elevation in the mRNA levels of EGFR expression resulting from a fourfold to eightfold amplification.[50,76] BT 20 cells are tumorigenic but nonmetastatic when grown in athymic nude mice.[77]

BT474 (ER–/PR+)

BT474 cells were obtained from a solid primary infiltrating ductal carcinoma of the breast in a 60-year-old woman.[78] The cells express PR but not ER *in vitro*[78] and significantly overexpress c-Erb-b2 due to an amplification in the c-*erb*-b2 gene.[50] The level of c-Erb-b2 mRNA expression in BT474 cells is 128-fold that of normal fibroblasts, whereas EGFR is not overexpressed.[50]

T47D$_{CO}$ (ER–/PR+)

T47D$_{CO}$ cells are a variant of the ER+/PR+ T47D cells[37] and were originally described by Horwitz et al.[79] The most notable feature of these cells is their loss of ER but elevated and constitutive expression of PR.[38,45,79] The cells grow *in vitro* without E2 supplementation and are antiestrogen resistant.[79] Whereas the PR in T47D$_{CO}$ cells is E2 independent, insulin receptor expression is up-regulated by progestins, despite their growth-inhibitory effects.[45] The constitutive expression of PR in the absence of ER makes this an excellent *in vitro* model for screening progestins and antiprogestins, because no complicating requirement for E2 supplementation exists. For example, the antiproliferative effects of the progestin R5020 in T47D cells were initially thought to reflect an antiestrogenic effect.[44] Subsequent data obtained in the T47D$_{CO}$ cells demonstrated that progestins and antiprogestins exert direct growth-inhibitory effects independent of ER-mediated events.[45]

ESTROGEN-UNRESPONSIVE (ER–/PR–) BREAST CANCER CELL LINES

The majority of human breast cancer cell lines are ER–. Just as the ER+ cell lines tend to reflect the nature of ER+ tumors in breast cancer patients, the ER– cell lines exhibit characteristics similar to those of ER– breast tumors. For example, ER– tumors are generally more rapidly growing,[80] more aggressive, and exhibit a poorer prognosis[81–83]; similarly, the ER– cell lines tend to produce rapidly growing tumors in nude mice, several of which are highly invasive and some of which can produce distant metastases.[1,64] None of these cell lines responds to the antiproliferative effects of estrogens and antiestrogens unless exposed to suprapharmacologic doses. However, the absence of response to steroids does not preclude response to other noncytotoxic agents. Several ER– cell lines express retinoic acid receptors[17] and are growth inhibited by retinoids.[11,84]

MDA-MB-231 and MDA-MB-435

The MDA-MB-231 cell line is among the most widely used of the ER– human breast cancer cell lines and is frequently used as a negative control in many laboratories studying the endocrine regulation of breast cancer cell growth. The MDA-MB-231 cells were established from a 51-year-old woman with breast cancer who developed a pleural effusion. The patient had received prior endocrine therapy (oophorectomy) and cytotoxic chemotherapy (initially 5-fluorouracil and then a combination of cyclophosphamide, methotrexate, and adriamycin). She had received the combination regimen 3 weeks before removal of the fluid from which the MDA-MB-231 cell line was isolated.[85] The MDA-MB-231 cells are highly tumorigenic and can produce lung metastases from mammary fat pad tumors in nude mice.[64]

The MDA-MB-435 cells were established from a pleural effusion in a 31-year-old white woman with metastatic breast cancer.[39,85] Unlike many other patients from whom breast cancer cell lines have been obtained, this patient had received no prior systemic therapy.[86] Despite being initially described as nontumorigenic,[87] MDA-MB-435 is generally reported to be highly tumorigenic and is one of the few human breast cancer cell lines that produce lung metastases from solid tumors.[64,88] When growing as xenografts, the growth and metastases of these cells also appear responsive to several dietary manipulations.[89–91] The study of metastasis from the MDA-MB-435 cell line has been greatly simplified by the introduction of a marker (β-galactosidase) that can facilitate visualization of micrometastases.[92]

We have established an ascites variant of the MDA-MB-435 cells (MDA435/LCC6). We have routinely maintained these cells as ascites for several years and assessed their sensitivity to a series of cytotoxic drugs.[86] The ascites has a pattern of responsiveness to single agents that closely reflects the activity of these agents in breast cancer patients. The cells are also easily maintained *in vitro* and can be successfully reestablished as solid tumors or ascites in nude mice. The MDA435/LCC6 cells may provide an alternative to the L1210/P388 murine ascites (leukemia) for the screening of new agents for activity in breast cancer. The MDA435/LCC6 cells also respond to nanomolar concentrations of all-*trans*-retinoic acid, fenretinimide, and 9-*cis*-retinoic acid[11]; this response perhaps reflects the expression of the RAR-α, RAR-β, and RAR-γ isoforms by the parental MDA-MB-435 cells.[17]

Other MDA-MB Cell Lines

Up to 19 cell lines bear the MDA-MB designation; most were derived by Cailleau et al. at the M. D. Anderson Hospital and

Tumor Institute.[39] The basic characteristics and isozyme and karyotype patterns have been previously reported in some detail.[39,93] Most cell lines are ER–, with the notable exception of the MDA-MB-134 and MDA-MB-175 cell lines, which are ER+.[94] Several of these lines are of specific interest. The MDA-MB-468 cells overexpress EGFR[50]; in contrast to other breast cancer cell lines, their growth is inhibited by exogenous EGF.[95] FGF receptors are overexpressed by MDA-MB-175 cells, which are growth inhibited by FGF.[96] The MDA-MB-175 cells also exhibit an eightfold overexpression of c-*erb*-b2 relative to normal fibroblasts.[50] The MDA-MB-361 cells, which were obtained from a brain metastasis,[39] and the MDA-MB-453 cells exhibit a twofold to fourfold amplification of the c-*erb*-b2 gene, overexpressing the gene product by approximately 64-fold.[50] The external domain of c-Erb-b2 is shed from MDA-MB-361 cells and can be detected in the serum of nude mice bearing these xenografts.[97] The MDA-MB-436 cell line was derived from a 43-year-old woman with metastatic breast cancer.[39] These cells are ER– and are sensitive to several cytotoxic drugs. The MDA-MB-436 cells have been used to investigate the effects of insulin and cell-seeding density on methotrexate metabolism[98,99] and the non–ER-mediated effects of estrogens and antiestrogens on both the cytotoxicity of methotrexate[100,101] and cell membrane structure and function.[102]

SkBr3

SkBr3 cells were obtained from a pleural effusion that developed in a 43-year-old patient with a breast adenocarcinoma.[103] These cells have been widely used in the study of c-Erb-b2 expression, because they overexpress c-Erb-b2 128-fold relative to normal fibroblasts owing to a fourfold to eightfold amplification of this gene.[50] SkBr3 cells also secrete a truncated c-Erb-b2 into their cell culture medium.[104] The coexpression of EGFR and c-Erb-b2 has enabled studies into the mechanisms of EGF-induced heterodimerization.[105]

NEW BREAST CANCER CELL LINES

The following section is not intended to be exhaustive but includes several new cell lines with some novel or unusual characteristics. The methods of isolation vary across studies, but all cell lines have been confirmed to be of breast origin. When the information is available, tumorigenicity, oncogene expression, and other potentially relevant information is described.

The establishment of new cell lines is a difficult and time-consuming process. Primary cultures can be initiated with a relatively high success rate.[106,107] Biopsy material can be cultured in a manner that allows for the preferential growth of neoplastic rather than normal epithelial cells.[108] However, the proportion of these cultures that spontaneously develop into established cell lines—for example, lines that can be maintained successfully for over 50 passages—is relatively low. In a study of 135 primary breast cancers, only 10 produced cell lines. All were negative for ER.[109] The success rate appears similar when the material for culture is derived from lymph node metastases. Thus, tumor stage would not seem to be a particularly good predictor for *in vitro* establishment.[106] The very poor success rate in establishing ER+ cell lines remains problematic.

Although ER can be overexpressed in ER– breast cancer cells by transfection, the resulting cells are almost exclusively growth inhibited by physiologic concentrations of estrogens.[110] A similar phenotype is reported for overexpression of ER in the normal human breast epithelial cell line MCF10A,[111] although the antiproliferative responses to estrogens appear relatively small. Breast tumors generally contain these levels of intratumor estrogens, regardless of the patient's menopausal status.[112] Such tumors might not arise if these intratumor estrogens were growth inhibitory, or at least would not arise until this signaling was eliminated or overcome. Furthermore, the administration of exogenous estrogens—for example, estrogen-based hormone replacement therapy—generally increases breast cancer risk.[113] This is consistent with the mitogenic effects of estrogens in cells that "normally" express ER, such as MCF-7 cells, and the growth-inhibitory effects of antiestrogens. Thus, the phenotypic relevance of these transfected cells is difficult to determine. Some transfectants can regulate estrogen-responsive element (ERE)–regulated gene expression in transient transfection assays but do not regulate endogenous genes, such as the genes for PR, pS2, and cathepsin D, in response to estrogens.[111] Thus, the function of some estrogen-regulated genes may be unaffected by expression of ER.

Some breast cancers possibly may arise from cells that were normally negative for ER,[114] and cellular signaling within these populations may be different from that in cells that normally express ER and require estrogens for proliferation. Some critical genes may be regulated in a direction not seen in cells that normally express ER, perhaps accounting for the inverted—that is, estrogen-inhibited—phenotype. If the ER function is significantly different than that in cells which normally express ER, the use of these models to study signaling to estrogenic/antiestrogenic responses may require careful consideration.

One cell population has been studied that is naturally inhibited by estrogens—namely, vascular smooth muscle cells.[115–117] These cells are naturally growth inhibited by estrogens, a finding that is not surprising, as estrogen is known to reduce the risk of cardiovascular disease. One mechanism might be through the inhibition of vascular smooth muscle cell proliferation after vascular injury.[117] Although an estrogen-inhibited phenotype is not physiologically unimportant in other tissues, the extent to which it applies to breast cancer is unclear.

BRC-230

The patient from whom cells for this line were obtained was a 79-year-old woman with a metastatic, infiltrating ductal carcinoma. The primary tumor was ER–/PR– and exhibited a high thymidine (TdR)-labeling index.[118] The cell line, designated BRC-230, was established from surgical material obtained from the primary tumor. The cells are ER–/PR– and show no evidence of amplification or rearrangement of c-*erb*-b2, c-*myc,* or *mdr*-1. BRC-30 cells are tumorigenic in nude mice and produce carcinoembryonic antigen, CA15-3, CA19-9, and CA125.[118] Of potential interest is the pattern of chemosensitivity, which closely reflects that seen in the patient. BRC-230 cells exhibit a multiple drug–resistant phenotype and are resistant to doxorubicin hydrochloride, etoposide, idarubicin hydrochloride, mitoxantrone hydrochloride, 4'-epidoxorubicin, and 4-idroperoxy-cyclophosphamide.[118] BRC-20 cells may be useful in studying non–*MDR1*-mediated multiple drug resistance.

HMT-3909S1 and HMT-3909S8

Petersen et al.[119] have described two cell lines derived from the same primary tumor. The primary tumor was an infiltrating ductal carcinoma that arose in a 61-year-old white woman. The patient had received no prior therapy. The cell lines were established in serum-free media.[119] HMT-3909 is nontumorigenic, whereas the HMT-3909S8 line forms tumors in athymic nude mice. HMT-3909S8 cells are aneuploid and express the mesenchymal glycoprotein vimentin, keratins 8 and 18, and the MAM-6 glycoprotein. HMT-3909S1 cells express vimentin and several keratins, including keratin 18, but MAM-6 reactivity is weak and keratin 8 staining is not detected.[119] The cells are not entirely ER–, but expression appears very low. The presence of two phenotypically distinct cell lines, each derived from a single hypothetical stem cell, may provide a novel means to study progression and acquisition of phenotypic diversity in tumors.

KPL-3C

KPL-3C cells were derived from a 37-year-old Japanese woman with invasive ductal carcinoma. The patient was initially treated by radical mastectomy and subsequently received radiotherapy to the locally recurrent lesions and systemic chemoendocrine therapy. Liver metastasis and a pleural effusion were subsequently diagnosed. The cell line was established from the pleural fluid.[120] The resulting cell line (KPL-3C) is tumorigenic in athymic nude mice, with a doubling time of approximately 7 days, and produces tumors reminiscent of comedo-type intraductal neoplasms. The tumors often exhibit an area of central necrosis characterized by microcalcification. The cells express cytokeratin, epithelial membrane antigen, carcinoembryonic antigen, and CA15-3, but do not express either vimentin or c-Erb-b2. Expression of ER and PR is low, with the levels reported as approximately 15 fmol per mg protein and 14 fmol per mg protein, respectively.[120] The cell population doubling time *in vitro* is approximately 72 hours. A potentially unusual characteristic of this cell line is its secretion of parathyroid hormone–related protein. Interestingly, the patient from whom these cells were derived required treatment for humoral hypercalcemia. This cell line may be useful for studying the role of tumor-derived parathyroid hormone–related protein in humoral hypercalcemia of malignancy.[120]

LCC15-MB

The LCC15-MB cell line was established from a femoral bone metastasis. The patient was a 29-year-old woman initially diagnosed with an infiltrating ductal mammary adenocarcinoma.[121] Approximately 3 years after the initial primary tumor was diagnosed, the patient presented with acute bone metastasis. Material from the bone metastasis, a poorly differentiated adenocarcinoma lacking ER, PR, and *erb*-b2 expression, was used to establish the cell culture. The LCC15-MB cells exhibit these characteristics, although ER can be reexpressed by treatment of the LCC15-MB cells for 5 days with 5-aza-2'-deoxycytidine. LCC15-MB cells are tumorigenic in athymic nude mice and produce long-bone metastases after intracardiac injection.[121] These cells strongly express vimentin. The presence of keratin 18 mRNA has been demonstrated using assay by polymerase chain reaction, but the low overall levels of keratin protein and the lack of keratin 19 mRNA suggest that these cells have selectively lost epithelial characteristics while gaining a more mesenchymal phenotype, consistent with the epithelial to mesenchymal transition that can occur during malignant progression in breast cancer.[121] The cells are invasive in the *in vitro* Boyden chamber assay and activate matrix metalloprotease 2 after treatment with concanavalin A.[122] Significantly, LCC15-MB cells express the bone matrix protein osteopontin, and this expression is retained by subcutaneous xenografts and intraosseous metastases.[122] The LCC15-MB cells provide a unique model in which to study bone metastasis and the role of osteopontin in this process.

MFM-233

The MFM-233 cell line was derived from a pleural effusion that arose in a postmenopausal patient. The patient had not received any prior treatment and presented with a widespread grade 3 ductal carcinoma. The established cell line was designated MFM-223.[123] These cells are tumorigenic in nude mice, producing moderate to poorly differentiated adenocarcinomas. MFM-233 cells express cytokeratins 8 and 18, epithelial membrane antigen, and milk fat globulins 1 and 2. Relatively low levels of ER (5 to 10 fmol/mg protein) are expressed, but PR is not detected in the cultures and is not induced by estradiol treatment. In contrast, expression of androgen receptors is high (160 fmol/mg protein), and proliferation of the cells is inhibited by more than 0.01 nanomolar dihydrotestosterone.[123] This cell line may prove useful in the study of androgen responsiveness and signaling.

MODELS OF ACQUIRED ANTIESTROGEN RESISTANCE (ER+ CELLS)

Although acquired resistance to antiestrogens is one of the more pressing clinical problems in breast cancer, few *in vitro* models exist for the analysis of this aspect of malignant progression. The most common approaches to the isolation of antiestrogen-resistant cells use an *in vitro* selection of hormone-dependent cells against either a high single dose of antiestrogen[124] or a stepwise increase in concentrations of drug. These approaches have been widely used to generate variants of cell lines resistant to many antineoplastic agents. Several problems are encountered when this approach is applied to generate antiestrogen-resistant variants of estrogen-dependent breast cancer cells. For example, isolation of resistant clones that retain stability for several years has often been difficult. Several laboratories have reported resistant variants that revert to a sensitive phenotype with a high frequency.[49,125–127] Some cell lines alter other critical aspects of their phenotypes. The MCF-7 variant LY-2 has become nontumorigenic.[62] MCF-7 cells selected *in vivo* can become dependent on or stimulated by tamoxifen.[128,129] Cells transfected with FGFs also reverse their endocrine responsiveness, becoming stimulated by tamoxifen and inhibited by physiologic concentrations of estrogens.[70] These models may reflect a tamoxifen-withdrawal effect, although the prevalence of this response in humans is difficult to determine.

LY-2: MCF-7 Cells Selected against a Benzothiophene (LY117018) *in Vitro*

The MCF-7 variant LY-2[124] is perhaps the most stable antiestrogen-resistant variant and was generated in 1985. These cells were selected *in vitro* in an anchorage-independent (soft agar) colony assay for resistance against LY117018.[124] LY-2 cells have been demonstrated to be cross-resistant to drugs representative of the major structural classes of antiestrogens, including nafoxidine, 4-hydroxytamoxifen, and ICI 164,384.[62] In addition to exhibiting a significant shift in their dose-response relationship for antiestrogens, LY-2 cells exhibit a blunted mitogenic response to E2.[124] However, LY-2 cells have lost their ability to form proliferating tumors in oophorectomized or E2-supplemented nude mice,[62] limiting their use to *in vitro* studies.

Although the precise resistance mechanism in the LY-2 cells is unclear, these cells express ER levels approximately one-third those of their parental MCF-7 cells and have become negative for PR.[124] A reduced level of ER expression would be expected to induce resistance to all antiestrogens, because interaction with ER is likely to be the most important early event in antiestrogen function. Thus, the altered ER levels or the reduced ability to mount an estrogenic response in the LY-2 cells may explain their antiestrogen-resistance pattern. LY-2 cells still express levels of ER that would be considered high in a breast tumor biopsy.[124] Furthermore, the remaining ER appears normal—that is, it is not mutated or altered.[130] The LY-2 cells may mimic some aspects of the antiestrogen-resistance profile in patients with ER+/PR– tumors.

MCF-7 Cells Selected against Tamoxifen *in Vivo*

Several groups have generated resistance models by selecting MCF-7 xenografts growing in nude mice against tamoxifen, an approach that would appear to more closely mimic the human disease than *in vitro* selection. However, MCF-7 cells do not form proliferating tumors in castrated female mice, which have an endocrine environment similar to that of postmenopausal women.[131–133] Because the xenografts would not be proliferating, their growth could not be further suppressed; tamoxifen is generally considered a cytostatic, not cytotoxic, drug. Consequently, it might be predicted that the most efficient response to such a selective pressure would be a change in the cell's perception of tamoxifen from inhibition to the widely documented partial agonist (growth promotion at low concentrations) properties of tamoxifen.[134] Indeed, the resultant tumors exhibit a tamoxifen-stimulated/tamoxifen-dependent phenotype,[128,129] suggesting that this "inverted" phenotype reflects a sensitization to the partial agonist (estrogenic) effects of the triphenylethylenes.[134] Tamoxifen dependence is evidenced by withdrawal responses to tamoxifen that induce regression of the xenografts.[128] More recently, an ER variant has been identified that may explain these changes in responses to antiestrogens.[135,136] Jiang et al. have identified a glycine-to-valine mutation at amino acid position 400 in the ER protein. When transfected into breast cancer cells, this mutation confers a growth-inhibitory response to estrogens and a growth-stimulatory response to antiestrogens.[135,136]

A breast tumor in a patient that possessed a tamoxifen-dependent phenotype could respond to removal of tamoxifen by exhibiting a tamoxifen-withdrawal response. Withdrawal responses have been widely reported for other endocrine therapies, including high-dose estrogen and progestin treatment.[137] Whether this occurs for antiestrogens is unclear, because the incidence of tamoxifen withdrawal responses has not been clearly defined and documented. Several anecdotal and single case reports of tamoxifen withdrawal responses have been published.[138–143] Several larger studies indicate a low incidence of tamoxifen withdrawal responses.[144,145] Thus, the data from these models may be predicting a response yet to be clearly demonstrated in the clinic or demonstrating an experimental artifact. Should these models be correct, the potential for a significant incidence of tamoxifen withdrawal responses could indicate an important, and potentially underestimated, clinical response pattern.

Selection of Hormone-Independent but Hormone-Responsive Cells against 4-Hydroxytamoxifen

Rather than use hormone-dependent cells and risk a loss of tumorigenicity (e.g., the LY-2 phenotype) or select *in vivo* using hormone-dependent cells and obtain a tamoxifen-stimulated phenotype, we hypothesized that cells already hormone independent and responsive might provide a more appropriate starting point for the generation of resistant variants. These cells already proliferate in the absence of estrogenic stimulation both *in vivo* and *in vitro*. To eliminate species-specific metabolic differences between rodents and humans, we chose to perform a stepwise selection of the MCF-7/LCC1 cells *in vitro* against the potent tamoxifen metabolite 4-hydroxytamoxifen. We obtained a stable resistant population designated MCF-7/LCC2. These cells are resistant to tamoxifen when growing either *in vitro* or as xenografts in nude mice[146] and have remained stably resistant in the absence of selective pressure.

We determined the likely cross-resistance profile of these cells by assessing their *in vitro* growth response to steroidal antiestrogens. Although resistant to tamoxifen, MCF-7/LCC2 cells are not cross-resistant to either ICI 182,780 or ICI 164,384.[146,147] This response pattern suggested that some patients who initially respond to tamoxifen but ultimately relapse may retain the ability to respond to a steroidal antiestrogen. Subsequently, this resistance pattern has been observed in preliminary data from a Phase I trial of ICI 182,780 in heavily tamoxifen pretreated patients.[148] These data indicate that, as predicted by the MCF-7/LCC2 phenotype, patients that ultimately relapse on tamoxifen can obtain responses to a subsequent steroidal antiestrogen treatment. Thus, an *in vitro* observation correctly predicted a subsequent pattern of response in breast cancer patients. These data suggest that the clinical responses to ICI 182,780 probably represent a genuine direct antitumor effect, rather than a possible tamoxifen withdrawal response, and suggest that the MCF-7/LCC2 phenotype is not merely an *in vitro* artifact. The relevance of these cells and their phenotypes has been reviewed.[36,65]

Cells Selected for Resistance to Steroidal Antiestrogens

MCF-7/LCC1 cells selected against the steroidal antiestrogen ICI 182,780 have been isolated and characterized. An *in vitro* stepwise selection was used similar to that used to generate the MCF-7/LCC2 cells. The stable ICI 182,780–resistant population was designated MCF-7/LCC9. MCF-7/LCC9 cells are resistant to ICI 182,780 *in vitro* and *in vivo*.[149] Our data indicate that these cells exhibit cross-resistance to tamoxifen, even though the cells have not been exposed to a triphenylethylene antiestrogen. If correct, this pattern of *in vitro* resistance would suggest that patients may be better served if treated initially with tamoxifen and subsequently with a steroidal antiestrogen, rather than vice versa. The validity of this prediction remains to be tested in patients.

MODELS FOR STUDYING MULTIPLE-DRUG RESISTANCE (*MDR1*/GP170)

Many breast tumors are often initially responsive to cytotoxic chemotherapy. Almost all develop a multiple drug–resistant phenotype, however, and this is ultimately responsible for the failure of current cytotoxic regimens.[34] Acquired resistance is frequently associated with expression of the *MDR1* gene and its gp170 glycoprotein product. The level and incidence of detectable *MDR1*/gp170 expression is significantly higher in the tumors of treated versus untreated breast cancer patients[150–152] and correlates with *in vitro* resistance to cytotoxic drugs.[152–154] Several *in vitro* models have been established with which to screen for new agents that can reverse this form of multiple drug resistance.

Cells Selected for Resistance against Adriamycin

Cell lines selected *in vitro* for resistance to adriamycin frequently overexpress gp170, often as a result of amplification of the *MDR1* gene. Among the most widely used cell lines are the MCF-7^{ADR} line[155] and the HeLa (ovarian carcinoma) variant KbV series.[156] The origin of the MCF-7^{ADR} cells, as used in the current National Institutes of Health (NIH) drug-screening program, has been questioned. The MCF-7 origin of these cells could not readily be determined, and the cell line has been redesignated NCI/ADR-RES.[157] The extent to which these cells can be used as a specific model of multiple drug–resistant breast cancer is unclear.

One problem with cells selected *in vitro* is that they frequently acquire multiple drug–resistance mechanisms. For example, we have demonstrated that NCI/ADR-RES (MCF-7^{ADR}) cells, but not *MDR1*-transduced MCF-7 cells (CL 10.3), are cross-resistant to tumor necrosis factor.[158] Because both adriamycin and tumor necrosis factor can inhibit cells by the generation of free radicals,[159,160] this cross-resistance in NCI/ADR-RES cells strongly suggests the presence of adriamycin-resistant mechanisms in addition to gp170, including altered expression of manganous superoxide dismutase.[158] Indeed, NCI/ADR-RES cells also exhibit increased glutathione transferase and topoisomerase II activities[161,162] and have become estrogen independent and antiestrogen resistant due to their loss of steroid hormone receptor expression.[155]

The complexity of the resistance phenotype in these cells may explain why the gp170-reversing potency of isomers of flupenthixol identified in NCI/ADR-RES (MCF-7^{ADR}) cells could not be confirmed in *MDR1*-transfected NIH 3T3 cells,[163] which suggests a non–gp170-mediated mechanism. Although NCI/ADR-RES cells are clearly of considerable use for screening new resistance-modifying agents and combinations, their use for detailed mechanistic studies of resistance reversal may be limited. These cells are widely used and very well characterized, however, and they provide an important benchmark for comparing data among different studies.

Cells Transduced with the *MDR1* Gene

To obtain cells in cases in which gp170 is the major multiple drug–resistance mechanism, a cloned, E2-dependent, MCF-7 human breast cancer subline was transduced with a retroviral vector directing the constitutive expression of the *MDR1* gene.[164] After selection in the presence of the gp170 substrate colchicine, cell populations (MCF-7^{MDR1}) were isolated, and their ability to produce gp170 was determined by radioimmunoprecipitation.[164] In this study, one of the MCF-7^{MDR1} clones designated CL 10.3 was used. Transduced cells express high levels of a 170-kd glycoprotein exhibiting immunoreactivity with specific anti-gp170 antibodies. Immunoreactivity is not detected in either the parental MCF-7 cells or MCF-7 cells transduced with a control pSV2neo vector. The level of expression of MCF-7^{MDR1} cells is estimated to be within twofold to threefold of that expressed by the adriamycin-selected NCI/ADR-RES cells.[163] The function of the expressed glycoprotein was confirmed by determining the sensitivity of parental and MCF-7^{MDR1} cells to a gp170 substrate (adriamycin) and to a non-gp170 substrate (gossypol).[164,165] Transduced cells have a tenfold greater IC_{50} for adriamycin, whereas sensitivity to gossypol is equivalent in both parental and transduced cells.[164] A similar relationship has been observed for colchicine and the non-gp170 substrate methotrexate (R. Clarke and F. Leonessa, *unpublished observations*, 1990).

The increase in resistance exhibited by the transduced MCF-7^{MDR1} cells would be expected to be sufficient to induce clinical resistance in tumors. Perturbations in energy metabolism in the MCF-7^{MDR1} cells have also been observed that are not present in the parental cells.[165] *MDR1*-transduced cells retain ER and PR expression and sensitivity to the triphenylethylene antiestrogen 4-hydroxytamoxifen.[164] Expression of the estrogen-inducible pS2 and EGFR genes are similar in parental and MCF-7^{MDR1} cells.[164] EGFR is upregulated, and pS2 expression is lost in NCI/ADR-RES cells.[155,164] The data indicate that overexpression of the *MDR1* gene alone confers a multiple drug–resistance phenotype but does not result in either cross-resistance to antiestrogens or a loss of steroid hormone receptor expression.[164]

The ascites variant MDA435/LCC6 of the ER– breast cancer cell line MDA-MB-435 has been transduced with the *MDR1* complementary DNA. The MDA435/LCC6 cells appear to retain the major characteristics of their parental cells; that is, they are ER–, highly tumorigenic, invasive, and metastatic.[166] When the cells are grown as an ascites, the mice become moribund within a reproducible time (approximately 30 days) and exhibit a pattern of responses to established cytotoxic drugs that closely reflects the activity of the agents when administered as single agents to previously untreated breast cancer patients.[166] The *MDR1*-transduced cells (MDA435/LCC6^{MDR1}) provide an ER– model for comparison with the ER+ MCF-7^{MDR1} CL 10.3 cells. The ascites variants provide an alternative to the murine leukemia ascites models (e.g., L1210, P388) for screening gp170-reversing agents.[166]

NORMAL BREAST EPITHELIAL CELLS AND THEIR DERIVATIVES

Culturing Normal Breast Epithelial Cells *in Vitro*

Major advances have been made in the culture of normal mammary cells from both humans and rodents. Not all of the approaches can be discussed in detail here, but several excellent reviews are available.[167,168] Of particular importance are models that allow for the coculturing of stromal and epithelial cells, because the interactions among these populations appear critical for normal glandular development and function. The approaches reviewed by Ip and Darcy[167] demonstrate the ability of cells maintained *in vitro* to complete a phenotypically normal lobuloalveolar development. These structures secrete milk proteins in response to appropriate hormonal stimuli and undergo an apparent involution on hormone withdrawal.[167] The culture techniques have been optimized for, and widely applied to, both human and rodent mammary cells.[167,168] For example, normal human epithelial cells proliferate and differentiate in a three-dimensional sponge-gel matrix culture system.[169]

These approaches require the isolation of viable epithelial or stromal cells from solid tissues. Many investigators appear to use one of several collagenase-based disaggregation methods,[167,170] but explant, organ culture, and organoid approaches also are successful.[106,167,171] The most effective approaches generally differ from the standard cell culture techniques used to propagate and study breast cancer cells, primarily in the provision of a three dimensional environment and the inclusion of stromal cells.[167,168] The success rate in establishing primary cultures of both normal and neoplastic mammary tissues has increased significantly. Even relatively simple approaches can produce short-term cultures on plastic with good reproducibility. For example, Volpi et al. have reported success rates of 83% for primary human breast cancers and 78% for normal breast tissue.[106]

Several specialized cell culture media have been generated that have greatly increased the success rate for establishing primary cultures. In general, these are semi-synthetic media that contain little or no serum, have low levels of Ca^{2+}, and are supplemented with various hormones, growth factors, and chemically undefined ingredients, such as conditioned cell culture media and bovine pituitary extract.[106,172–175]

Although these cells represent primary cultures—that is, they have a finite life span *in vitro*—they may be immortalized by treating them with carcinogens and transformed by inducing an overexpression of several oncogenes. As with the neoplastic breast cell lines, several caveats should be borne in mind. For example, the primary and immortalized cells are adapted to *in vitro* growth, and some of their expressed (or repressed) characteristics may be more closely associated with this adaptation than their normal *in vivo* function. However, this concern most likely is minimized when three-dimensional culture matrices are used and stromal cells are included. Immortalized cells are continually proliferating, a state quite different from the resting tissues from which their parental cells were derived.

All the available cell lines established from normal mammary cells are ER–. ER has been introduced into several normal human breast epithelial cell lines. However, the resultant phenotype is growth inhibited by estradiol.[176] A similar phenotype occurs when breast cancer cells are transfected with ER.[110] This E2-inhibited phenotype appears counterintuitive, because estrogens are generally considered mitogens in both normal and neoplastic breast tissues. Nevertheless, these potentially "normal" cells are important models that provide the opportunity to study aspects of the biology of normal mammary epithelial cells, to identify agents that may contribute to the malignant transformation of normal mammary cells, and to determine phenotypic and genotypic perturbations associated with this process.

Benzo(*a*)Pyrene-Immortalized 184 and B5 Lineages from Reduction Mammoplasties

Stampfer and Bartley[173] have successfully established primary organoid cultures from normal reduction mammoplasty tissues. The source tissues for these cultures were essentially resting, in that they were not obtained during a functional or active period, such as early pregnancy, lactation, or involution.[173] These cells can readily be immortalized by treatment with benzo(*a*)pyrene (e.g., 184 cells). Immortalized normal mammary epithelial cells can exhibit evidence of their breast epithelial origin. For example, the cells are clearly epithelial,[172] express several human milk fat globulin antigens, and synthesize α-lactalbumin and β-casein.[173] Although immortalized—that is, they can be maintained continuously *in vitro*—these cells are not considered transformed according to several criteria, including their inability to form tumors in nude mice or significant anchorage-independent growth.[173]

Transformation of Immortalized Human Mammary Epithelial Cells with Oncogenes

The introduction of viral or cellular oncogenes into benzo(*a*)pyrene-immortalized human mammary epithelial cell lines results in a stepwise progression from a normal to a malignant phenotype.[173,177–179] Two distinct immortalized lineages (184AIN4 and 184B5) have been characterized after transformation by several viral oncogenes. Tumorigenicity in nude mice is observed after infection of the benzo(*a*)pyrene-immortalized 184A1N4 subline with v-Ha-*ras* (A1N4-H), but not v-*mos* (A1N4-M), c-*myc* (A1N4-myc), or *SV40T* (A1N4-T; after limited passaging of cells).[177] Although they are nontumorigenic, v-*mos*-, c-*myc*-, and *SV40T*-transformed cells do exhibit phenotypic transformation and autonomy from growth factors *in vitro* to varying degrees. Combination of v-Ha-*ras* with v-*mos* (A1N4-MH) or *SV40T* (A1N4-TH) resulted in highly malignant and metastatic tumors in the nude mouse.[177,178] Consistent with the effects of v-Ha-*ras* on the A1N4 cell line, infection of the 184B5 subline with v-Ki-*ras* (B5kTu cells) also confers tumorigenicity in nude mice.[173]

MCF-10A, MCF10AT, and MCF10AT1

Soule et al.[175] have described a spontaneously immortalized "normal" human breast epithelial cell line (MCF-10). The cells were isolated from mastectomy tissue obtained from a 36-year-old premenopausal woman with benign fibrocystic disease. After 849 days in culture, a population designated MCF-10A was established. These cells exhibit a stable t(3;9)(3p13;9p22) translocation.[175] The MCF-10A cells resemble luminal epithelial cells rather than myoepithelial cells, and express antigens for several keratins and epithelial sialomucins.[180] The cells are nontumorigenic in nude mice and do not exhibit anchorage-independent growth.[175] These cells have also been used to assess the transforming ability of several oncogenes. Transfection with the ER gene was not sufficient to produce transformation.[111] MCF-10 cells cotransfected with the *erb*-b2 and Ha-*ras* oncogenes (MCF-10A HE) exhibited a substantial increase in soft agar clonogenicity but lacked significant tumorigenicity in nude mice.[181]

Transformation with the Ha-*ras* oncogene alone (MCF10AT) caused an increase in clonogenicity chemotaxis and degradation of basement membrane *in vitro*.[182] However, the cells are poorly tumorigenic in nude mice. Small, palpable nodules do arise, and these can persist.[183] Sporadic progression to carcinoma was observed, and cells from one of these was reestablished *in vitro* (MCF10AT1). MCF10T1 cells can produce simple ducts when embedded in Matrigel and transplanted into immunodeficient mice.[183,184] Up to 25% progress to invasive carcinoma.[184] Expression of c-*erb*-b2 was detected in 50% of the atypical hyperplasias and 78% of the invasive adenocarcinomas.[185] These cells provide an important and unique model for the progression from atypical hyperplasia to carcinoma.

HBL-100

The HBL-100 cell line is comprised of cells obtained from an early lactation sample.[186] The cells have been described as being of myoepithelial origin.[187] The donor was an apparently healthy woman and had no evidence of breast lesions.[186,188] The cells can form colonies in soft agar, however, and are aneuploid.[186] Although early passage cells are nontumorigenic, HBL-100 cells become tumorigenic after repeated passage *in vitro*, generally around passage 70.[187,189–191] This appears to be associated with the acquisition of specific marker chromosomes[192] and alterations in microfilament and microtubules,[189] and overexpression of an 89-kd heat shock protein in late passage.[193] Although some HBL-100 cell stocks contain Mason-Pfizer monkey virus,[194] the ability to acquire a transformed phenotype appears to be related to the incorporation of *SV40* sequences into the genome.[188,190,195,196] The cells bind and respond to glucocorticoids and EGF,[197] and express functional β-adrenergic receptors[198] and the IGF-I receptor.[199] Although HBL-100 cells are negative for ER and prolactin receptors,[200] they may require activity of their FGF-2 autocrine loop for maximal proliferation.[201]

Although these cells are derived from an apparently normal donor, it is not entirely clear that they can be considered to represent normal mammary cells. Care must be exercised when selecting HBL-100 cells as a model of normal breast cells. For such a model, their use should probably be restricted to cultures of as early a passage as possible, and almost certainly to cells of passages earlier than 70. Under other circumstances, HBL-100 cells provide a potentially useful model in which to study transformation and progression.

IN VITRO MODELS FOR STUDYING INVASION AND METASTASIS

To metastasize effectively, cells must accomplish a complex compendium of activities, including escape from the primary lesion, avoidance of immune surveillance, and penetration into normal tissue at distant sites.[202] Invasion of extracellular matrices occurs repeatedly in this process, and basement membrane invasion, in particular, has received considerable attention.[203] The loss of basement membrane at the parenchymal-mesenchymal interface of locally invasive tumors has been closely associated with metastatic dissemination.[204–206] The uniformity of basement membrane composition and structure suggests that the molecular mechanisms involved in basement membrane recognition, attachment, degradation, and traversal may yield novel targets for cancer therapy. Several *in vitro* models have been used to study the process of basement membrane invasion and its relationship to malignant progression.

In Vitro Assays for Invasive Potential

The development of Matrigel, a reconstituted basement membrane extract from the EHS (Engelbreth-Holm-Swarm) sarcoma,[207] has been instrumental in facilitating compositional and functional analyses of basement membranes. Matrigel is liquid at 4°C, so that various manipulations are possible before it sets into a homogeneous gel at 37°C. Matrigel contains the major basement membrane components, including laminin, collagen type IV, and heparan sulfate proteoglycan. Matrigel has been used in two different assays to examine *in vitro* invasiveness of breast cancer cells.[208]

The Boyden chamber chemoinvasion assay[209] compares the ability of cells to traverse a Matrigel-coated polycarbonate filter as they migrate toward different chemical attractants. Invasive cells, stained on the lower filter surface, can be quantitated either by image analysis or crystal violet staining.[210] Although the assay was originally developed in modified blind-well Boyden chambers, two-compartment chamber systems, such as Transwell from Gibco (Rockville, MD) and Bio-Coat wells from Collaborative Research/Beckton Dickinson Labware (Franklin Lakes, NJ), have been used successfully. Other adaptations include prelabeling of the cells with either a nontoxic fluorescent dye or radioactive agent to facilitate quantitation of invaded cells.

The ability of cells to form invasive colonies when embedded in a three-dimensional gel of Matrigel is compared qualitatively in the Matrigel-outgrowth assay.[209,210] Cells dispersed in a three-dimensional layer of Matrigel are examined after culture for 2 to 10 days. Although dispersal of single cells throughout the upper layer of Matrigel provides the most stringent test for invasive outgrowth, characteristic morphologies can be achieved more rapidly with cells sandwiched between two layers of Matrigel or simply plated on top of Matrigel.

The presence or lack of ER is an important determinant of both prognosis and choice of treatment of breast cancer. The hormone-responsive or hormone-dependent breast cancer cell lines represent a model system for the analysis of hormonal influences on the invasive process. Effects of estrogens, antiestrogens, and progestins on the *in vitro* invasiveness of steroid-dependent and steroid-responsive human breast cancer cells have been reviewed.[211–214] In addition, progression to hormone independence has implications for invasiveness and metastasis. For example, MCF-7/MIII and MCF-7/LCC1 cells have been shown to acquire an increased metastatic potential as they become estrogen independent.[61] This increased metastatic potential is reflected in increased activity in the Boyden chamber[62] (but not in Matrigel outgrowth assays), increased local invasiveness *in vivo*, and an ability to produce occasional distant metastases in nude mice.[61]

To examine the hypothesis that ER– human breast cancer cell lines are constitutively more invasive than their ER+ counterparts, a large number of the human breast cancer cell lines described above have been examined for invasiveness in the Boyden chamber assay *in vitro* and for metastatic potential in the nude mouse. These studies clearly indicate that the majority of ER– cell lines are inherently more aggressive than ER+ cells both *in vitro* and *in vivo*.[1,208] Because the incidence of distant metastases is significantly lower and less reproducible than that observed in the MDA-MB-435 cells, the MCF-7/MIII and MCF-7/LCC1 cells appear to represent a phenotype intermediate between the poorly invasive MCF-7 and the metastatic MDA-MB-435.[61]

Cell Lines and the Epithelial-to-Mesenchymal Transition

An emerging development in progression studies for breast carcinoma is the immunocytochemical analysis of markers characteristic of epithelial or mesenchymal phenotypes. The mesenchymal intermediate filament glycoprotein vimentin (VIM) has been associated with lack of ER, high growth fraction, and poor nuclear grade in human breast cancer.[215–219] VIM expression in the tumor component is indicative of an epithelial-to-mesenchymal transition, which may occur during the process of malignant progression. Consistent with this notion, the epithelial marker E-cadherin, a homotypic cell adhesion molecule, is lost from more aggressive tumors.[220–222] Loss of E-cadherin and acquisition of VIM expression are events that characterize the epithelial-to-mesenchymal transition that occurs during embryogenesis.[223]

To begin to address this hypothesis, the invasiveness of epithelial-like (VIM–) and mesenchymal-like (VIM+) human breast cancer cells has been compared in the Boyden chamber and Matrigel outgrowth assays. Irrespective of hormone responsiveness, VIM+ cells exhibited significantly higher levels of both *in vitro* invasiveness and metastatic potential than did the VIM– negative group.[1,208] VIM expression was not detected in cells containing ER and was present in only some of the cell lines lacking ER, whereas E-cadherin was expressed functionally in all cell lines expressing ER as well as some that had lost ER expression and did not express VIM. These data suggest that the loss of E-cadherin expression is not linked to hormone independence but occurs earlier than VIM expression in the progression cascade. VIM expression also appears to be downstream of hormone independence.

E-cadherin expression, indicative of an epithelial phenotype, is associated with a compacted spherical morphology in VIM– cell lines when cultured in Matrigel.[224] E-cadherin is not present in any VIM+ cell lines. Absence of both E-cadherin and VIM is associated with a noninvasive cluster-type morphology. The NCI/ADR-RES cell line, derived from the MCF-7 cells by stepwise selection for increasing resistance to the drug adriamycin (see the previous section, Cells Selected for Resistance against Adriamycin), is interesting in this regard. Thought to be derived from the E-cadherin+/ER+/VIM– MCF-7 phenotype, this subline has lost ER and E-cadherin, gained VIM expression, and become significantly more invasive. Examination of additional adriamycin-resistant and vinblastine sulfate–resistant variants of the MCF-7 and ZR-75-1B cell lines shows that most, but not all, drug-resistant sublines expressed VIM.[225] Understanding of the relationships among drug resistance, VIM expression, and invasiveness may provide important clues for the optimization of chemotherapy for breast tumors.

The MCF-7/MIII and MCF-7/LCC1 variants retain ER and uvomorulin (UVO) expression, generally lack VIM expression, and exhibit somewhat lower levels of invasiveness than the VIM+ human breast cancer cells.[1,208] These observations support the hypothesis that these MCF-7 variants represent an intermediate point in the metastatic progression of breast cancer. The metastatic potential of the MCF-7/MIII and MCF-7/LCC1 cells, compared with the ER–/VIM– cell lines (e.g., MDA-MB-468),[61] however, suggests that metastatic potential may also develop independently of an event similar to the epithelial-to-mesenchymal transition.[226]

Oncogene Expression and *in Vitro* Metastatic Potential

The effects of oncogenes on mammary cell invasiveness have been examined. The *ras* oncogene is perhaps best studied and can induce the invasive phenotype in a variety of both human and rodent epithelial systems. Transfection of human bronchial epithelial cells transfected with v-Ha-*ras* increased both invasiveness *in vitro* and metastatic potential in the nude mouse.[227,228] In NIH/3T3 cells, transfection with either v-Ha-*ras* or genomic DNA containing various forms of activated *ras* also resulted in increased invasiveness across the amniotic membrane *in vitro* and metastatic dissemination *in vivo*.[229]

MCF-7 cells transfected with v-Ha-*ras* show increased *in vitro* invasiveness of Matrigel, increased migration potential, and increased recognition of laminin,[230] but no apparent increases in metastatic potential in nude mice.[231,232] Although both of the 184 sublines (A1N4 and B5) are transformed to a tumorigenic phenotype by expression of *ras* alone, only the initially more invasive A1N4 cells respond to *ras* transformation with increased invasiveness. The refractory nature of the 184B5 cells to *ras*-induced effects on invasiveness, despite the induction of tumorigenicity, suggests a possible lineage specificity for this response and begins to dissociate *ras* effects on tumorigenicity from invasiveness.

Differential induction of metastatic potential by v-Ha-*ras* has been previously reported.[182,231–233] Detailed analysis of a highly stable rat mammary subclone after *ras* transduction implicated rapid phenotypic diversification rather than direct effects on a cascade of metastasis-effector genes.[234] No changes similar to the epithelial-to-mesenchymal transition were seen after *ras* transformation of the A1N4 or B5 cells[213] or in the *ras*-transfected MCF-7 cells.[211] In contrast, combined transformation of 184A1N4–immortalized human mammary epithelial cells with v-Ha-*ras* and either *SV40T* or v-*mos* induces a VIM+, invasive phenotype indicative of the epithelial-to-mesenchymal transition event.[213]

The chemotactic activity and invasive property of the MCF-10A cells cotransfected with both Ha-*ras* and *erb*-b2 (MCF-10 HE cells) has also been further investigated using the Matrigel-based assays. MCF-10A HE cells showed tenfold higher invasiveness than the nontransfected cells, formed branching colonies in Matrigel, and showed a high cloning efficiency in soft agar (Thompson et al., *unpublished data*, 1999). These attributes are indicative of a VIM+ phenotype resulting from an event similar to the epithelial-to-mesenchymal transition.

CONCLUDING COMMENTS ON *IN VITRO* MODELS

Human breast cancer cell lines growing *in vitro* and as human xenografts *in vivo* have a central role in most basic and preclinical breast cancer research. They have been widely used to investigate the cellular and molecular events associated with endocrine responsiveness, malignant progression, invasiveness, and metastatic potential. With the increasing restrictions being imposed on the use of vertebrate animals, and the relatively limited number of species that develop spontaneous mammary carcinomas, the emphasis on the *in vitro* use of human breast cancer cell lines seems likely to increase in the coming decades. Consequently, the introduction of additional representative human breast cancer cell lines, particularly hormone-responsive lines, and the realistic assessment and acknowledgment of the caveats associated with the use of *in vitro* models are critical.

Some Caveats Regarding the Use of *in Vitro* Models

Despite their widespread use and the considerable data arising from it, *in vitro* models have several potential limitations. Relatively few well-characterized ER+ cell lines exist. Although these cell lines tend to exhibit comparable estrogenic responses in the end points most widely applied, the extent to which these observations may be applied to all ER+ human breast tumors is unclear. Certainly, many of the most important attributes, such as growth inhibition by antiestrogens, are likely to closely reflect the human disease. In cases in which responses differ markedly from predicted or observed responses in humans, such as growth inhibition by physiologic levels of E2, a greater degree of caution is clearly warranted. A clear deficit in the range of breast cancer cell lines currently available is the relatively small number of ER+ and E2-responsive cell lines.

The majority of steroid-responsive cell lines have been established, not from solid tumors, but from malignant effusions. Although such effusions can occur with a 26% to 49% frequency in breast cancer patients,[235,236] they may not be fully representative of all solid tumors. Despite the likely metastatic origin of these cells, the ER+ cell lines from these sites are rarely metastatic *in vivo*, even in severely immunocompromised animals (see Chapter 22).

The most widely used cell lines have now been in use since the 1970s. Subtle changes may have been acquired during this period, and these may not adequately reflect changes that occur in human tumors in patients. Because the cells are clearly adapted to grow *in vitro*, the perturbations that have conferred this ability also may not occur in patients' tumors. Human breast tumors are highly heterogeneous and contain many subpopulations of cells with different phenotypic characteristics, including both ER+ and ER– cells.[237] In contrast, breast cancer cell lines are relatively homogeneous. This can be viewed either as an advantage or as a disadvantage. Although responses in a cell line may not fully reflect the response of a complex human tumor, they do provide the ability to study, in considerable detail and complexity, the responses of cells representative of tumor subpopulations.

In principle, cell lines are like any other experimental model. When their limitations are openly acknowledged and appropriately considered in experimental design and data analysis, they can provide useful and important tools. Otherwise, the risk exists of overinterpretation of data or the pursuit of a potential *in vitro* artifact. As a generalization, those observations from *in vitro* models that clearly reflect the human disease are more likely to reflect real events and lead to new insights into mechanistic processes. When these models are used to generate hypotheses for future testing in humans, the validity of the observation awaits completion of the human trials. Thus, major strengths of *in vitro* models include the ability (a) to study a specific cell type and elucidate the mechanism of its response to agents at the cellular and molecular level, (b) to identify mechanistic processes by comparing related cells with different phenotypic characteristics, (c) to facilitate further hypothesis generation and testing *in vivo* when cells are grown as xenografts, and (d) to generate hypotheses for testing in the ultimate model, the human being.

Establishment and Characterization of New Breast Cancer Cell Lines and Variants

Despite the presence of a number of breast cancer cell lines[2] and the emergence of new cell lines,[238] only three of those that are in common or widespread usage (the parental MCF-7, T47D, and ZR-75-1) are clearly estrogen dependent or estrogen responsive. Few of the established cell lines are metastatic in nude mice, and those that metastasize with a high frequency are generally ER–. Thus, new breast cell lines from malignant, solid metastatic (e.g., bone, lung), and normal tissues—specifically, steroid-hormone-responsive cell lines—are needed. Unfortunately, breast cancer cells from patients' tumors are notoriously difficult to establish *in vitro*.[239–241] The take rate for xenografts of tumor tissue in immunocompromised rodents also is relatively poor, although it is generally higher than that for direct *in vitro* growth.[242] Also, a well-characterized panel of nonmalignant breast epithelial cell lines that could be used for comparative studies is notably absent. Of those "normal" cell lines available, none is steroid hormone responsive.[172,173]

New breast cancer cell lines require careful description and characterization. When possible, the characteristics and history of the patient (e.g., age, sex, race, treatment) and the known characteristics of the tumor (e.g., histopathologic diagnosis, tumor grade, nodal status, ER and PR expression, S-phase/proliferativeness, and any other pertinent information) should be provided. The human origin of the tissues should be confirmed, and a karyotype and isoenzyme profile should be reported. Typical polymorphic enzymes analyzed include lactate dehydrogenase, glucose-6-phosphate dehydrogenase (EC 1.1.1.49), phosphoglucomutase-1 (EC 2.7.5.1), phosphoglucomutase-3 (EC 2.7.5.1), esterase D (EC 3.1.1.1), mitochondrial malic enzyme (EC 1.1.1.40), adenylate kinase (EC 2.7.4.3), and glyoxalase (EC 4.4.1.5).[14] These data are particularly useful in confirming the origin of a variant as being derived from its parent and in excluding contamination of a new cell line with cells of an established cell line. To this end, we have routinely used the services currently provided by Dr. Joseph Kaplan through the Cell Culture Laboratory of the Children's Hospital of Michigan in Detroit. This facility is currently maintained under National Cancer Institute contract to provide these services.

The general characteristics of the new cell line or variant should be clearly provided. This includes *in vitro* growth characteristics (e.g., culture conditions, cell doubling time, split ratio, and the passage number at which these data were obtained) and the hormone-receptor profile and endocrine responsiveness. A description of the morphology of the cells (e.g., ultrastructural analyses), particularly one that addresses tissue origin or evidence of differentiated function (e.g., secretory activity, production of milk proteins), is strongly encouraged.[2]

The tumorigenicity of a new cell line should be determined in at least one immunocompromised rodent model (preferably several) and reported. Different immunocompromised mice strains can exhibit different abilities to support xenografts, and the model in which tumorigenicity is assessed should be clearly indicated. The inability to form tumors in athymic nude mice may not indicate that the cells are nontumorigenic in other strains (e.g., *scid*; see Chapter 22). The histology of any arising tumors should be compared with that of the original tumor when possible. The presence of any metastases and their histology also should be documented. When available, any other pertinent data (e.g., oncogene expression or amplification) should also be provided.

The designation of a cell line or variant should follow the guidelines of the Tissue Culture Association and should reflect both the tissue of origin and the laboratory in which it was established.[243] For our variant cells, we have chosen to use a designation that appends our institution to that of the original (parental) cell line (e.g., MCF-7/LCC1).

Cell Culture Conditions

The choice of culture conditions often can inadvertently influence the experimental outcome. For example, for many years, insulin was routinely added to the cell culture media used to maintain breast cancer cells. Although insulin is a potent mitogen for many of these cells, it does not appear to be required for growth *in vitro* in serum-supplemented media for most human breast cancer cell lines. Insulin can down-regulate ER expression, however.[244] Insulin and EGF have been added to serum-free media for breast cancer cells,[245] and both can influence the growth-inhibitory effects of antiestrogens.[246,247] Phenol red is widely used as a pH indicator in cell culture media. A contaminant in phenol red is known to be estrogenic, and this activity can alter both the growth and antiestrogen responsiveness.[248,249]

Serum contains various growth factors and steroid hormones. The steroids can be readily removed by treatment with charcoal-coated dextran.[250] MCF-7 cells also can use the steroid sulfates present in serum.[251] These steroid sulfates can be removed by prior treatment with sulfatase.[250] The growth factors and other proteins can be chemically inactivated to produce a growth factor–free serum.[252] The concentration of serum used also can be important. The dose-response relationship for antiestrogens is altered significantly by serum concentration.[253] We have found a final concentration of either 5% fetal calf serum or 5% charcoal/dextran-stripped serum to provide appropriate *in vitro* growth characteristics for most human breast cancer cell lines. The concentrations of steroids, growth factors, and other constituents in serum may vary considerably from batch to batch.

Estrogens remain within cells for several days,[254] and when stripping cells of endogenous estrogens, one must often thoroughly wash cell monolayers and maintain cells for several days in the absence of estrogens. We routinely wash cells at least three times with phenol red–free media supplemented with 5% dextran/charcoal-stripped serum and maintain the washed monolayers in this medium for a further 3 to 5 days to ensure adequate removal of endogenous steroids.[14,62]

The cell-seeding density also can have considerable effects on cellular growth and metabolism. Cells seeded at different densities have previously been demonstrated to exhibit both different cell population doubling times and differences in methotrexate poly-γ-glutamate formation.[99] In many instances, one must closely control for seeding density, proliferative capacity, confluence, and serum batch. The handling of cells, including duration of trypsinization and time at room temperature during passage or treatment, may also be important. For some cell lines, a trypsinized cell suspension must be passed through a sterile needle to generate a single cell suspension.

These examples indicate the general importance of closely controlling cell culture conditions. The reader is referred to several excellent books on tissue culture techniques for a more detailed description of cell culture procedures.[255–257]

SUMMARY

The development of stable cell lines derived from malignant and normal human breast tissue has been of considerable use in breast cancer research, and such cell lines continue to occupy a central position in basic breast cancer research. These cell lines provide the ability to conduct studies that could not easily be performed in experimental animals or human beings. The ease of use, relatively low cost of maintenance, general reproducibility of phenotype, and ability to mimic properties seen in tumors in patients are considerable advantages. However, the use and applicability of cell lines are not without limitations. For example, cell lines cannot be used to reliably predict *in vivo* toxicity or to assess the toxicologic properties of new agents. Cell lines also may be ineffective in establishing mechanisms of drug metabolism or in elucidating critical tumor-host interactions. Their metabolic adaptations to *in vitro* growth may not reflect adaptations that occur *in vivo*. Nevertheless, breast cancer cell lines have been used successfully for many years to generate new hypotheses, screen new agents, and study the biology of breast cancer. Many cell lines have the advantage of being tumorigenic and thus can facilitate further studies *in vivo* in experimental animals. Provided their limitations are freely acknowledged, human breast cancer cell lines will continue to provide one of the most powerful tools in breast cancer research.

ACKNOWLEDGMENTS

This work was supported in part by grants NIH R01-CA/AG58022, NIH P30-CA51008, and NIH P50-CA58185 (Public Health Service) and USAMRMC (Department of Defense) BC980629 and BC980586.

REFERENCES

1. Thompson EW, Paik S, Brünner N, et al. Association of increased basement membrane-invasiveness with absence of estrogen receptor and expression of vimentin in human breast cancer cell lines. *J Cell Physiol* 1992;150:534.
2. Engel LW, Young NA. Human breast carcinoma cells in continuous culture: a review. *Cancer Res* 1978;38:4327.
3. Magdelenat H, Pouillart P. Steroid hormone receptors in breast cancer. In: Sheridan PJ, Blum K, Trachtenberg MC, eds. *Steroid receptors and disease: cancer autoimmune, bone and circulatory disorders*. New York: Marcel Dekker, 1988:435.
4. McGuire WL, Clark GM. The prognostic role of progesterone receptor in human breast cancer. *Semin Oncol* 1983;10:2.
5. Ravdin PM, Green S, Dorr TM, et al. Prognostic significance of progesterone receptor levels in estrogen receptor–positive patients with metastatic breast cancer treated with tamoxifen: results of a prospective Southwest Oncology Group study. *J Clin Oncol* 1992;10:1284.
6. Lippman ME, Bolan G, Huff K. The effects of estrogens and antiestrogens on hormone responsive human breast cancer cells in long term tissue culture. *Cancer Res* 1976;36:4595.
7. Lippman ME, Bolan G, Huff K. Interactions of antiestrogens with human breast cancer in long-term tissue culture. *Cancer Treat Rep* 1976;60:1421.
8. Yano T, Korkut E, Pinski J, et al. Inhibition of growth of MCF-7 MIII human breast carcinoma in nude mice by treatment with agonists or antagonists of LH-RH. *Breast Cancer Res Treat* 1992;21:35.
9. Fontana JA, Hobbs PD, Dawson MI. Inhibition of mammary carcinoma growth by retinoidal benzoic acid derivatives. *Exp Cell Biol* 1988;56:254.
10. Fontana JA. Interaction of retinoids and tamoxifen on the inhibition of human mammary carcinoma cell proliferation. *Exp Cell Biol* 1987;55:136.
11. Baumann K, Clarke R. Effects of all-*trans*-retinoic acid on proliferation and gene expression of human breast cancer cells *in vitro*. *Proc Am Assoc Cancer Res* 1994;35:275.
12. Soule HD, Vasquez J, Long A, Albert S, Brennan M. A human cell line from a pleural effusion derived from a human breast carcinoma. *J Natl Cancer Inst* 1973;51:1409.
13. Horwitz KB, Costlow ME, McGuire WL. MCF-7: a human breast cancer cell line with estrogen, androgen, progesterone and glucocorticoid receptors. *Steroids* 1975;26:785.
14. Clarke R, Brünner N, Katzenellenbogen BS, et al. Progression from hormone dependent to hormone independent growth in MCF-7 human breast cancer cells. *Proc Natl Acad Sci U S A* 1989;86:3649.
15. Eidne KA, Flanagan CA, Harris NS, Millar RP. Gonadotropin-releasing hormone (GnRH)-binding sites in human breast cancer cell lines and inhibitory effects of GnRH antagonists. *J Clin Endocrinol Metab* 1987;64:425.
16. Monaco ME, Lippman ME. Insulin stimulation of fatty acid synthesis in human breast cancer cells in long term tissue culture. *Endocrinology* 1977;101:1238.
17. Swisshelm K, Ryan K, Lee X, Tsou HC, Peacocke M, Sager R. Down regulation of retinoic acid receptor β in mammary carcinoma cell lines and its upregulation in senescing normal mammary epithelial cells. *Cell Growth Differ* 1994;5:133.
18. Shafie SM, Brooks SC. Effect of prolactin on growth and estrogen receptor levels of human breast cancer cells (MCF-7). *Cancer Res* 1977;37:792.
19. Huff KK, Kaufman D, Gabbay KH, Spencer EM, Lippman ME, Dickson RB. Secretion of an insulin-like growth factor-I-related protein by human breast cancer cells. *Cancer Res* 1986;46:4613.
20. Huff KK, Knabbe C, Lindsey R, et al. Multihormonal regulation of insulin-like growth factor-I-related protein in MCF-7 human breast cancer cells. *Mol Endocrinol* 1988;2:200.
21. van der Burg B, Isbrucker L, van Selm-Miltenburg AJ, de Laat SW, van Zoelen EJ. Role of estrogen-induced insulin-like growth factors in the proliferation of human breast cancer cells. *Cancer Res* 1990;50:7770.
22. Stewart A, Johnson MD, May FEB, Westley BR. Role of insulin-like growth factors and the type I insulin-like growth factor receptor in the estrogen-stimulated proliferation of human breast cancer cells. *J Biol Chem* 1990;265:21172.
23. Furlanetto RW, DiCarlo JN. Somatomedin C receptors and growth effects in human breast cancer cells maintained in long term tissue culture. *Cancer Res* 1984;44:2122.
24. Arteaga CL, Osborne CK. Growth inhibition of human breast cancer cells in vitro with an antibody aganst the Type I somatomedin receptor. *Cancer Res* 1989;49:6237.
25. Yee D, Cullen KJ, Paik S, et al. Insulin-like growth factor-II mRNA expression in human breast cancer. *Cancer Res* 1988;48:6691.
26. Clemmons DR, Camacho-Hubner C, Coronado E, Osborne CK. Insulin-like growth factor binding protein secretion by breast carcinoma cell lines: correlation with estrogen receptor status. *Endocrinology* 1990;127:2679.
27. Yee D, Favoni R, Lupu R, et al. The insulin-like growth factor binding protein BP-25 is expressed by human breast cancer cells. *Biochem Biophys Res Commun* 1989;158:38.
28. Davidson NE, Gelmann EP, Lippman ME, Dickson RB. Epidermal growth factor receptor gene expression in estrogen receptor-positive and negative human breast cancer cell lines. *Mol Endocrinol* 1987;1:216.
29. Bates SE, Davidson NE, Valverius EM, et al. Expression of transforming growth factor-α and its mRNA in human breast cancer: its regulation by estrogen and its possible functional significance. *Mol Endocrinol* 1988;2:543.
30. Clarke R, Brünner N, Katz D, et al. The effects of a constitutive production of TGF-α on the growth of MCF-7 human breast cancer cells in vitro and in vivo. *Mol Endocrinol* 1989;3:372.
31. Kern FG, Wellstein A, Flamm S, et al. Secretion of heparin binding growth factors by breast cancer cells and their role in promoting cancer cell growth. *Cancer Chemother* 1990;5:167.
32. Lehtola L, Partanen J, Sistonen L, et al. Analysis of tyrosine kinase mRNAs including four FGF receptors expressed in the MCF-7 breast cancer cells. *Int J Cancer* 1992;50:598.
33. Bronzert DA, Pantazis P, Antoniades HN, et al. Synthesis and secretion of platelet-derived growth factor by human breast cancer cell lines. *Proc Natl Acad Sci U S A* 1987;84:5763.
34. Clarke R, Dickson RB, Lippman ME. Hormonal aspects of breast cancer: growth factors, drugs and stromal interactions. *Crit Rev Oncol Hematol* 1992;12:1.
35. Clarke R, Dickson RB, Brünner N. The process of malignant progression in human breast cancer. *Ann Oncol* 1990;1:401.
36. Clarke R, Skaar T, Baumann K, et al. Hormonal carcinogenesis in breast cancer: cellular and molecular studies of malignant progression. *Breast Cancer Res Treat* 1994;31:237.
37. Keydar I, Chen L, Karby S, et al. Establishment and characterization of a cell line of human carcinoma origin. *Eur J Cancer* 1979;15:659.
38. Horwitz KB, Friedenberg GR. Growth inhibition and increase of insulin receptors in antiestrogen-resistant T47Dco human breast cancer cells by progestins: implications for endocrine therapies. *Cancer Res* 1985;45:167.
39. Cailleau R, Olive M, Cruciger QVA. Long-term human breast carcinoma cell lines of metastatic origin: preliminary characterization. *In Vitro* 1978;14:911.
40. Reddel RR, Alexander IE, Koga M, Shine J, Sutherland RL. Genetic instability and the development of steroid hormone insensitivity in cultured T 47D human breast cancer cells. *Cancer Res* 1988;48:4340.
41. Graham ML, Smith JA, Jewett PB, Horwitz KB. Heterogeneity of progesterone receptor content and remodelling by tamoxifen characterize subpopulations of cultured human breast cancer cells: analysis by quantitative dual parameter flow cytometry. *Cancer Res* 1992;52:593.
42. Sartorius CA, Groshong SD, Miller LA, et al. New T47D breast cancer cell lines for the independent study of progesterone B- and A-receptors: only antiprogestin-occupied B-receptors are switched to transcriptional agonists by cAMP. *Cancer Res* 1994;54:3868.
43. Graham ML, Dalquist KE, Horwitz KB. Simultaneous measurement of progesterone receptors and DNA indices by flow cytometry: analysis of breast cancer cell mixtures and genetic instability of the T47D line. *Cancer Res* 1989;49:3943.

44. Vignon F, Bardon S, Chalbos D, Rochefort H. Antiestrogenic effect of R5020, a synthetic progestin in human breast cancer cells in culture. *J Clin Endocrinol Metab* 1983;56:1124.
45. Horwitz KB. The antiprogestin RU38 486: receptor-mediated progestin versus antiprogestin actins screened in estrogen-insensitive T47Dco human breast cancer cells. *Endocrinology* 1985;116:2236.
46. Mockus MB, Lessey BA, Bower MA, Horwitz KB. Estrogen-insensitive progesterone receptors in a human breast cancer cell line: characterization of receptors and of a ligand exchange assay. *Endocrinology* 1982;110:1564.
47. Engel LW, Young NA, Tralka TS, Lippman ME, O'Brien SJ, Joyce MJ. Establishment and characterization of three new continuous cell lines derived from human breast carcinomas. *Cancer Res* 1978;38:3352.
48. van den Berg HW, Leahey WJ, Lynch M, Clarke R, Nelson J. Recombinant human interferon alpha increases oestrogen receptor expression in human breast cancer cells (ZR-75-1) and sensitises them to the anti-proliferative effects of tamoxifen. *Br J Cancer* 1987;55:255.
49. van den Berg HW, Lynch M, Martin J, Nelson J, Dickson GR, Crockard AD. Characterization of a tamoxifen-resistant variant of the ZR-75-1 human breast cancer cell line (ZR-75-9a1) and stability of the resistant phenotype. *Br J Cancer* 1989;59:522.
50. Kraus MH, Popescu NC, Amsbaugh SC, King CR. Overexpression of the EGF receptor-related proto-oncogene erbB-2 in human mammary tumor cell lines by different molecular mechanisms. *EMBO J* 1987;6:605.
51. Warri AM, Laine AM, Majasuo KE, Alitalo KK, Harkonen PL. Estrogen suppression of erbB2 expression is associated with increased growth rate of ZR-75-1 human breast cancer cells in vitro and in nude mice. *Int J Cancer* 1991;49:616.
52. Long B, McKibben BM, Lynch M, van den Berg HW. Changes in epidermal growth factor receptor expression and response to ligand associated with acquired tamoxifen resistance or oestrogen independence in the ZR-75-1 human breast cancer cell line. *Br J Cancer* 1992;65:865.
53. van Agthoven T, van Agthoven TL, Portengen H, Foekens JA, Dorssers LC. Ectopic expression of epidermal growth factor receptors induces hormone independence in ZR-75-1 human breast cancer cells. *Cancer Res* 1992;52:5082.
54. Poulin R, Baker D, Poirier D, Labrie F. Androgen and glucocorticoid receptor-mediated inhibition of cell proliferation by medroxyprogesterone acetate in ZR-75-1 human breast cancer cells. *Breast Cancer Res Treat* 1989;13:161.
55. Poulin R, Baker D, Poirier D, Labrie F. Multiple actions of synthetic "progestins" on the growth of ZR-75-1 human breast cancer cells: an in vitro model for the simultaneous assay of androgen, progestin, estrogen, and glucocorticoid agonistic and antagonistic activities of steroids. *Breast Cancer Res Treat* 1991;17:197.
56. Weckbecker G, Liu R, Tolcsvai L, Bruns C. Antiproliferative effects of the somatostatin analogue octreotide (SMS 201-995) on ZR-75-1 human breast cancer cells in vivo and in vitro. *Cancer Res* 1992;52:4973.
57. Theriault C, Labrie F. Multiple steroid metabolic pathways in ZR-75-1 human breast cancer cells. *J Steroid Biochem Mol Biol* 1991;38:155.
58. Poulin R, Poirier D, Merand Y, Theriault C, Belanger A, Labrie F. Extensive esterification of adrenal C19-delta 5-sex steroids to long-chain fatty acids in the ZR-75-1 human breast cancer cell line. *J Biol Chem* 1989;264:9335.
59. Roy R, Belanger A. ZR-75-1 breast cancer cells generate nonconjugated steroids from low density lipoprotein-incorporated lipoidal dehydroepiandrosterone. *Endocrinology* 1993;133:683.
60. Brünner N, Boulay V, Fojo A, Freter C, Lippman ME, Clarke R. Acquisition of hormone-independent growth in MCF-7 cells is accompanied by increased expression of estrogen-regulated genes but without detectable DNA amplifications. *Cancer Res* 1993;53:283.
61. Thompson EW, Brünner N, Torri J, et al. The invasive and metastatic properties of hormone-independent and hormone-responsive variants of MCF-7 human breast cancer cells. *Clin Exp Metastasis* 1993;11:15.
62. Clarke R, Brünner N, Thompson EW, et al. The inter-relationships between ovarian-independent growth, antiestrogen resistance and invasiveness in the malignant progression of human breast cancer. *J Endocrinol* 1989;122:331.
63. Jones DY, Schatzkin A, Green SB, et al. Dietary fat and breast cancer in the National Health and Nutrition Examination Survey I epidemiologic follow-up study. *J Natl Cancer Inst* 1987;79:465.
64. Price JE, Polyzos A, Zhang RD, Daniels LM. Tumorigenicity and metastasis of human breast carcinoma cell lines in nude mice. *Cancer Res* 1990;50:717.
65. Clarke R, Thompson EW, Leonessa F, Lippman J, McGarvey M, Brünner N. Hormone resistance, invasiveness and metastatic potential in human breast cancer. *Breast Cancer Res Treat* 1993;24:227.
66. Katzenellenbogen BS, Kendra KL, Norman MJ, Berthois Y. Proliferation, hormonal responsiveness, and estrogen receptor content of MCF-7 human breast cancer cells grown in the short-term and long-term absence of estrogens. *Cancer Res* 1987;47:4355.
67. Cho H, Ng PA, Katzenellenbogen BS. Differential regulation of gene expression by estrogen in estrogen growth-independent and -dependent MCF-7 human breast cancer cell sublines. *Mol Endocrinol* 1991; 5:1323.
68. Natoli C, Sica G, Natoli V, Serra A, Iacobelli S. Two new estrogen-supersensitive variants of the mcf-7 human breast cancer cell line. *Breast Cancer Res Treat* 1983;3:23.
69. McLeskey SW, Kurebayashi J, Honig SF, et al. Fibroblast growth factor 4 transfection of MCF-7 cells produces cell lines that are tumorigenic and metastatic in ovariectomized or tamoxifen-treated athymic nude mice. *Cancer Res* 1993;53:2168.
70. Kurebayashi J, McLeskey SW, Johnson MD, Lippman ME, Dickson RB, Kern FG. Quantitative demonstration of spontaneous metastasis by MCF-7 human breast cancer cells cotransfected with fibroblast growth factor 4 and LacZ. *Cancer Res* 1993;53:2178.
71. Lasfargues EY, Ozzello L. Cultivation of human breast carcinomas. *J Natl Cancer Inst* 1958;21:1131.
72. Horwitz KB, Zava DT, Thilagar AK, Jensen EM, McGuire WL. Steroid receptor analyses of nine human breast cancer cell lines. *Cancer Res* 1978;38:2434.
73. Hall RE, Lee CSL, Alexander IE, Shine J, Clark CL, Sutherland RL. Steroid hormone receptor gene expression in human breast cancer cells: inverse relationship between oestrogen and glucocorticoid receptor messenger RNA levels. *Int J Cancer* 1990;46:1081.
74. Castles CG, Fuqua SA, Klotz DM, Hill SM. Expression of a constitutively active estrogen receptor variant in the estrogen receptor-negative BT-20 human breast cancer cell line. *Cancer Res* 1993;53:5934.
75. Fuqua SAW, Fitzgerald SD, Chamness GC, et al. Variant human breast tumor estrogen receptor with constitutive transcriptional activity. *Cancer Res* 1991;51:105.
76. Kurokawa M, Michelangeli VP, Findlay DM. Induction of calcitonin receptor expression by glucocorticoids in T47D human breast cancer cells. *J Endocrinol* 1991;130:321.
77. Ozzello L, Sordat B, Merenda C, Carrel S, Hurlimann J, Mach JP. Transplantation of a human mammary carcinoma cell line (BT 20) into nude mice. *J Natl Cancer Inst* 1974;52:1669.
78. Lasfargues EY, Coutinho WG, Redfield ES. Isolation of two human tumor epithelial cell lines from solid breast carcinomas. *J Natl Cancer Inst* 1978;61:967.
79. Horwitz KB, Mockus MB, Lessey BA. Variant T47D human breast cancer cells with high progesterone-receptor levels despite estrogen and antiestrogen resistance. *Cell* 1982;28:633.
80. Ballare C, Bravo AI, Laucella S, et al. DNA synthesis in estrogen receptor positive human breast cancer takes place preferentially in estrogen receptor-negative cells. *Cancer* 1989;64:842.
81. Shek LL, Godlophin W. Survival with breast cancer: the importance of estrogen receptor quantity. *Eur J Cancer Clin Oncol* 1989;25:243.
82. Clark GM, McGuire WL. Steroid receptors and other prognostic factors in primary breast cancer. *Semin Oncol* 1988;15:20.
83. Skoog L, Humla S, Axelsson M, et al. Estrogen receptor levels and survival of breast cancer patients. *Acta Oncol* 1987;26:95.
84. Halter SA, Fraker LD, Adcock D, Vick S. Effect of retinoids on xenotransplanted human mammary carcinoma cells in athymic mice. *Cancer Res* 1988;48:3733.
85. Cailleau R, Young R, Olive M, Reeves WJ. Breast tumor cell lines from pleural effusions. *J Natl Cancer Inst* 1974;53:661.
86. Leonessa F, Green D, Licht T, et al. MDA435/LCC6 and MDA435/LCC6MDRI: ascites models of human breast cancer. *Br J Cancer* 1996;73:154.
87. Osborne CK, Coronado E, Allred DC, Wiebe V, DeGregorio M. Acquired tamoxifen resistance: correlation with reduced breast tumor levels of tamoxifen and isomerization of trans-4-hydroxytamoxifen. *J Natl Cancer Inst* 1991;83:1477.
88. Meschter CL, Connolly JM, Rose DP. Influence of regional location of the inoculation site and dietary fat on the pathology of MDA-MB-435 human breast cancer cell-derived tumors growing in nude mice. *Clin Exp Metastasis* 1992;10:167.

89. Rose DP, Connolly JM, Meschter CL. Effect of dietary fat on human breast cancer growth and lung metastasis in nude mice. *J Natl Cancer Inst* 1991;83:1491.
90. Rose DP, Hatala MA, Connolly JM, Rayburn J. Effect of diets containing different levels of linoleic acid on human breast cancer growth and lung metastasis in nude mice. *Cancer Res* 1993;53:4686.
91. Rose DP, Connolly JM. Influence of dietary fat intake on local recurrence and progression of metastases arising from MDA-MB-435 human breast cancer cells in nude mice after excision of the primary tumor. *Nutr Cancer* 1992;18:113.
92. Brünner N, Thompson EW, Spang-Thomsen M, Rygaard J, Dano K, Zwiebel JA. LacZ transduced human breast cancer xenografts as an in vivo model for the study of invasion and metastasis. *Eur J Cancer* 1992;28A:1989.
93. Siciliano MJ, Barker PE, Cailleau R. Mutually exclusive genetic signatures of human breast tumor cell lines with a common chromosomal marker. *Cancer Res* 1979;39:919.
94. Osborne CK, Lippman ME. Human breast cancer in tissue culture. In: McGuire WL, ed. *Breast cancer advances in research and treatment*. New York: Plenum, 1978:103.
95. Kaplan O, Jaroszewski JW, Faustino PJ, et al. Toxicity and effects of epidermal growth factor on the glucose metabolism of MDA-468 human breast cancer cells. *J Biol Chem* 1990;265:13641.
96. McLeskey SW, Ding IY, Lippman ME, Kern FG. MDA-MB-134 breast carcinoma cells overexpress fibroblast growth factor (FGF) receptors and are growth-inhibited by FGF ligands. *Cancer Res* 1994;54:523.
97. Langton BC, Crenshaw MC, Chao LA, Stuart SG, Akita RW, Jackson JE. An antigen immunologically related to the external domain of gp185 is shed from nude mouse tumors overexpressing the c-erbB2 (HER-2/neu) oncogene. *Cancer Res* 1991;51:2593.
98. Kennedy DG, Clarke R, van den Berg HW, Murphy RF. The kinetics of methotrexate polyglutamate formation and efflux in a human breast cancer cell line (MDA-MB-436): the effect of insulin. *Biochem Pharmacol* 1983;32:41.
99. Kennedy DG, van den Berg HW, Clarke R, Murphy RF. The effect of the rate of cell proliferation on the synthesis of methotrexate poly-τ-glutamates in two human breast cancer cell lines. *Biochem Pharmacol* 1985;34:3087.
100. Clarke R, van den Berg HW, Kennedy DG, Murphy RF. Reduction of the antimetabolic and antiproliferative effects of methotrexate by 17β-estradiol in a human breast carcimoma cell line (MDA-MB-436). *Eur J Cancer Clin Oncol* 1983;19:19.
101. Clarke R, van den Berg HW, Kennedy DG, Murphy RF. Oestrogen receptor status and the response of human breast cancer cells to a combination of methotrexate and 17β-estradiol. *Br J Cancer* 1985;51:365.
102. Clarke R, van den Berg HW, Murphy RF. Tamoxifen and 17β-estradiol reduce the membrane fluidity of human breast cancer cells. *J Natl Cancer Inst* 1990;82:1702.
103. Fogh J. Cell lines established from human tumors. In: Fogh J, ed. *Human tumor cell lines in vitro*. New York: Plenum, 1975:115.
104. Alpet O, Yamaguchi K, Hitomi J, Honda S, Matsushima T, Abe K. The presence of c-erbB-2 gene product-related protein in culture medium conditioned by breast cancer cell line SK-BR-3. *Cell Growth Differ* 1990;1:591.
105. Goldman R, Levy MB, Peles E, Yarden Y. Heterodimerization of the erbB-1 and erbB-2 receptors in human breast carcinoma cells: a mechanism for receptor transregulation. *Biochemistry* 1990;29:11024.
106. Volpi A, Savini S, Zoli W, et al. An efficient method for culturing human breast epithelium: analysis of results. *Tumori* 1991;77:460.
107. Zoli W, Volpi A, Bonaguri C, et al. An efficient method for culturing human breast carcinoma to evaluate antiblastic drug activity in vitro: experience on 136 primary cancers and 116 recurrences. *Breast Cancer Res Treat* 1990;17:231.
108. Dairkee SH, Deng G, Stampfer MR, Waldman FM, Smith HS. Selective cell culture of primary breast carcinoma. *Cancer Res* 1995; 55:2516.
109. McCallum HM, Lowther GW. Long-term culture of primary breast cancer in defined medium. *Breast Cancer Res Treat* 1996;39:247.
110. Jiang S-Y, Jordan VC. Growth regulation of estrogen receptor negative breast cancer cells transfected with estrogen receptor cDNAs. *J Natl Cancer Inst* 1992;84:580.
111. Pilat MJ, Christman JK, Brooks SC. Characterization of the estrogen receptor transfected MCF10A breast line 139B6. *Breast Cancer Res Treat* 1996;37:253.
112. Pasqualini JR, Chetrite G, Nestour EL. Control and expression of oestrone sulphatase activities in human breast cancer. *J Endocrinol* 1996;150:S99.
113. Hulka BS, Stark AT. Breast cancer: cause and prevention. *Lancet* 1995;346:883.
114. Brunner N, Zugmaier G, Bano M, et al. Endocrine therapy of human breast cancer cells: the role of secreted polypeptide growth factors. *Cancer Cells* 1989;1:81.
115. Bei M, Foegh M, Ramwell PR, Clarke R. Specific high affinity binding sites for 17β-estradiol in rat heart smooth muscle cells. *J Steroid Biochem Mol Biol* 1996;58:83.
116. Lavigne MC, Ramwell PW, Clarke R. Growth and phenotypic characterization of porcine coronary artery smooth muscle cells. *In Vitro Cell Dev Biol* 1999;35:136.
117. Lavigne MC, Ramwell PW, Clarke R. Inhibition of estrogen receptor function promotes porcine coronary artery smooth muscle cell proliferation. *Steroids* 1999;64:472.
118. Amadori D, Bertoni L, Flamigni A, et al. Establishment and characterization of a new cell line from primary human breast carcinoma. *Breast Cancer Res Treat* 1993;28:251.
119. Petersen OW, van Deurs B, Nielsen KV, et al. Differential tumorigenicity of two autologous human breast carcinoma cell lines, HMT-3939S1 and HMT-3939S8, established in serum-free medium. *Cancer Res* 1990;50:1257.
120. Kurebayashi J, Kurosumi M, Sonoo H. A new human breast cancer cell line, KPL-3C, secretes parathyroid hormone-related protein and produces tumors associated with microcalcifications in nude mice. *Br J Cancer* 1996;74:200.
121. Thompson EW, Sung V, Lavigne M, et al. LCC15-MB: a human breast cancer cell line from a femoral bone metastasis. *Clin Exp Metastasis* 1999;17:193.
122. Sung V, Gilles C, Murray A, et al. The LCC15-MB human breast cancer cell line expresses osteopontin and exhibits an invasive and metastatic phenotype. *Exp Cell Res* 1998;241:273.
123. Hackenberg R, Lüttchens S, Hofmann J, Kunzmann R, Holzel F, Schulz K-D. Androgen sensitivity of the new breast cancer cell line MFM-233. *Cancer Res* 1991;51:5722.
124. Bronzert DA, Greene GL, Lippman ME. Selection and characterization of a breast cancer cell line resistant to the antiestrogen LY 117018. *Endocrinology* 1985;117:1409.
125. Nawata H, Chang MJ, Bronzert D, Lippman ME. Estradiol independent growth of a subline of MCF-7 human breast cancer cells in culture. *J Biol Chem* 1981;256:6895.
126. Nawata H, Bronzert D, Lippman ME. Isolation and characterization of a tamoxifen resistant cell line derived from MCF-7 human breast cancer cells. *J Biol Chem* 1981;256:5016.
127. van den Berg HW, Clarke R. Preliminary characterization of a tamoxifen resistant variant of the oestrogen responsive human breast cancer cell line ZR-75-1. *Br J Cancer* 1985;52:421.
128. Gottardis MM, Jordan VC. Development of tamoxifen-stimulated growth of MCF-7 tumors in athymic mice after long-term antiestrogen administration. *Cancer Res* 1988;48:5183.
129. Osborne CK, Coronado EB, Robinson JP. Human breast cancer in athymic nude mice: cytostatic effects of long-term antiestrogen therapy. *Eur J Cancer Clin Oncol* 1987;23:1189.
130. Mullick A, Chambon P. Characterization of the estrogen receptor in two antiestrogen-resistant cell lines, LY2 and T47D. *Cancer Res* 1990;50:333.
131. Seibert K, Shafie SM, Triche TJ, et al. Clonal variation of MCF-7 breast cancer cells in vitro and in athymic nude mice. *Cancer Res* 1983;43:2223.
132. van Steenbrugge GJ, Groen M, van Kreuningen A, De Jong FH, Gallee MWP, Schroeder FH. Transplantable human prostatic carcinoma (PC-82) in athymic nude mice (III). Effects of estrogens on the growth of the tumor. *Prostate* 1988;12:157.
133. Brünner N, Svenstrup B, Spang-Thompsen M, Bennet P, Nielsen A, Nielsen JJ. Serum steroid levels in intact and endocrine ablated Balb\c nude mice and their intact litter mates. *J Steroid Biochem* 1986;25:429.
134. Clarke R, Lippman ME. Antiestrogen resistance: mechanisms and reversal. In: Teicher BA, ed. *Drug resistance in oncology*. New York: Marcel Dekker, 1992:501.
135. Jiang SY, Parker CJ, Jordan VC. A model to describe how a point mutation of the estrogen receptor alters the structure-function relationship of antiestrogens. *Breast Cancer Res Treat* 1993;26:139.

136. Jiang SY, Langan-Fahey SM, Stella AL, McCague R, Jordan VC. Point mutation of estrogen receptor (ER) in the ligand-binding domain changes the pharmacology of antiestrogens in ER-negative breast cancer cells stably expressing complementary DNAs for ER. *Mol Endocrinol* 1992;6:2167.
137. Engelsman E. Therapy of advanced breast cancer; a review. *Eur J Cancer Clin Oncol* 1983;19:1775.
138. Gockerman JP, Spremulli EN, Raney M, Logan T. Randomized comparison of tamoxifen versus diethylstilbestrol in estrogen receptor-positive or -unknown metastatic breast cancer: a southeastern cancer study group trial. *Cancer Treat Rep* 1986;70:1199.
139. Vogel CL, East DR, Voigt W, Thomsen S. Response to tamoxifen in estrogen receptor-poor metastatic breast cancer. *Cancer* 1987; 60:1184.
140. Howell A, Dodwell DJ, Anderson H, Redford J. Response after withdrawal of tamoxifen and progestogens in advanced breast cancer [See comments]. *Ann Oncol* 1992;3:611.
141. Belani CP, Pearl P, Whitley NO, Aisner J. Tamoxifen withdrawal response. Report of a case. *Arch Intern Med* 1989;149:449.
142. Stein W, Hortobagyi GN, Blumenschein GR. Response of metastatic breast cancer to tamoxifen withdrawal: report of a case. *J Surg Oncol* 1983;22:45.
143. McIntosh IH, Thynne GS. Tumour stimulation by anti-oestrogens. *Br J Surg* 1977;64:900.
144. Canney PA, Griffiths T, Latief TN, Priestman TJ. Clinical significance of tamoxifen withdrawal response. *Lancet* 1989;1:36.
145. Beex LVAM, Pieters GFFM, Smals AGH, Koenders AJM, Benraad TJ, Kloppenborg PWC. Diethylstilbestrol versus tamoxifen in advanced breast cancer. *N Engl J Med* 1981;304:1041.
146. Brünner N, Frandsen TL, Holst-Hansen C, et al. MCF7/LCC2: A 4-hydroxytamoxifen resistant human breast cancer variant which retains sensitivity to the steroidal antiestrogen ICI 182,780. *Cancer Res* 1993;53:3229.
147. Coopman P, Garcia M, Brünner N, Derocq D, Clarke R, Rochefort H. Antiproliferative and antiestrogenic effects of ICI 164,384 in 4-OH-tamoxifen-resistant human breast cancer cells. *Int J Cancer* 1994;56:295.
148. Nicholson RI, Gee JMW, Anderson E, et al. Phase I study of a new pure antiestrogen ICI 182,780 in women with primary breast cancer: immunohistochemical analysis. *Breast Cancer Res Treat* 1993;27:135.
149. Brünner N, Boysen B, Jirus S, et al. MCF7/LCC9: An antiestrogen-resistant MCF-7 variant in which acquired resistance to the steroidal antiestrogen ICI 182,780 confers an early cross-resistance to the non-steroidal antiestrogen tamoxifen. *Cancer Res* 1997;57:3486.
150. Schneider J, Bak M, Efferth T, Kaufmann M, Mattern J, Volm M. P-glycoprotein expression in treated and untreated human breast cancer. *Br J Cancer* 1989;60:815.
151. Trock BJ, Leonesa F, Clarke R. Multidrug resistance in breast cancer: a meta analysis of MDR1/gp170 expression and its possible functional significance. *J Natl Cancer Inst* 1997;89:917.
152. Sanfilippo O, Ronchi E, De Marco C, Di Fronzo G, Silvestrini R. Expression of P-glycoprotein in breast cancer tissue and in vitro resistance to doxorubicin and vincristine. *Eur J Cancer* 1991;27:155.
153. Salmon SE, Grogan TM, Miller T, Scheper R, Dalton WS. Prediction of doxorubicin resistance in vitro in myeloma, lymphoma and breast cancer by P-glycoprotein staining. *J Natl Cancer Inst* 1989;81:696.
154. Veneroni S, Zaffaroni N, Daidone MG, Benini E, Villa R, Silvestrini R. Expression of P-glycoprotein and in vitro or in vivo resistance to doxorubicin and cisplatin in breast and ovarian cancers. *Eur J Cancer* 1994;30A:1002.
155. Vickers PJ, Dickson RB, Shoemaker R, Cowan KH. A multidrug-resistant MCF-7 human breast cancer cell line which exhibits cross-resistance to antiestrogens and hormone independent tumor growth. *Mol Endocrinol* 1988;2:886.
156. Willingham MC, Cornwell MM, Cardarelli CO, Gottesman MM, Pastan I. Single cell analysis of daunomycin uptake and efflux in multidrug resistant and sensitive KB cells: effects of verapamil and other drugs. *Cancer Res* 1986;46:5941.
157. Scudiero DA, Monks A, Sausville EA. Cell line designation change: multidrug-resistant cell line in the NCI anticancer screen. *J Natl Cancer Inst* 1998;90:862.
158. Zyad A, Bernard J, Clarke R, Tursz T, Brockhaus M, Chouaib S. Human breast cancer cross-resistance to TNF and adriamycin: relationship to MDR1, MnSOD and TNF gene expression. *Cancer Res* 1994;54:825.
159. Doroshow JH, Akman S, Esworthy S, Chu FF, Burke T. Doxorubicin resistance is conferred by selective enhancement of intracellular glutathione peroxidase or superoxide dismutase content in human MCF-7 breast cancer cells. *Free Radic Res Commun* 1991;12–13, part 2:779.
160. Iwamoto S, Takeda K. Possible cytotoxic mechanisms of TNF in vitro. *Hum Cell* 1990;3:107.
161. Batist G, Tuple A, Sinha BK, Katki AG, Myers CE, Cowan KH. Overexpression of a novel anionic glutathione transferase in multidrug-resistant human breast cancer cells. *J Biol Chem* 1986;261:15544.
162. Sinha BK, Mimnaugh EG, Rajagopalan S, Myers CE. Adriamycin activation and oxygen free radical formation in human breast tumor cells: protective role of glutathione peroxidase in adriamycin resistance. *Cancer Res* 1989;49:3844.
163. Ford JM, Bruggemann EP, Pastan I, Gottesman MM, Hait WN. Cellular and biochemical characterization of thioxanthenes for reversal of multidrug resistance in human and murine cell lines. *Cancer Res* 1990;50:1748.
164. Clarke R, Currier S, Kaplan O, et al. Effect of P-glycoprotein expression on sensitivity to hormones in MCF-7 human breast cancer cells. *J Natl Cancer Inst* 1992;84:1506.
165. Kaplan O, Jaroszewski JW, Clarke R, et al. The multidrug resistance phenotype: 31P NMR characterization and 2-deoxyglucose toxicity. *Cancer Res* 1991;51:1638.
166. Leonessa F, Green D, Licht T, et al. MDA435/LCC6 and MDA435/LCC6^{MDR1}: ascites models of human breast cancer. *Br J Cancer* 1996;73:154.
167. Ip MM, Darcy KM. Three-dimensional mammary culture model systems. *J Mammary Gland Biol Neoplasia* 1996;1:91.
168. Petersen OW, Ronnov L, Bissell MJ. The microenvironment of the breast: three-dimensional models to study the roles of the stroma and the extracellular matrix in function and dysfunction. *Breast J* 1995;1:22.
169. Baibakov BA, Chipisheva TA, Guelsheva VI, et al. Organotypic growth and differentiation of human mammary gland in sponge-gel matrix supported histoculture. *In Vitro Cell Dev Biol* 1994;30A:490.
170. Dairkee SH, Heid HW. Cytokeratin profile of immunomagnetically separated epithelial subsets of the mammary gland. *In Vitro Cell Dev Biol* 1993;29A:427.
171. Speirs V, Green AR, Walton DS, et al. Short-term primary culture of epithelial cells derived from human breast tumours. *Br J Cancer* 1998;78:1421.
172. Stampfer M, Hallowes RC, Hackett AJ. Growth of normal human mammary cells in culture. *In Vitro* 1980;16:415.
173. Stampfer MR, Bartley JC. Human mammary epithelial cells in culture: differentiation and transformation. In: Lippman ME, Dickson RB, eds. *Breast cancer: cellular and molecular biology*. Boston: Kluwer Academic, 1988:1.
174. Smith HS. In vitro models in human breast cancer. In: Harris J, Hellman S, Henderson IC, Kinne D, eds. *Breast diseases*. New York: Lippincott–Raven, 1994.
175. Soule HD, Maloney TM, Wolman SR, et al. Isolation and characterization of a spontaneously immortalized human breast epithelial cell line, MCF-10. *Cancer Res* 1990;50:6075.
176. Lundholt BK, Madsen MW, Lykkesfeldt AE, Petersen OW, Briand P. Characterization of a nontumorigenic human breast epithelial cell line stably transfected with the human estrogen receptor (ER) cDNA. *Mol Cell Endocrinol* 1996;119:47.
177. Clark R, Stampfer MR, Milley R, et al. Transformation of human mammary epithelial cells with oncogenic viruses. *Cancer Res* 1988;48:4689.
178. Valverius EM, Ciardiello F, Heldin NE, et al. Stromal influences on transformation of human mammary epithelial cells overexpressing c-myc and sv40t. *J Cell Physiol* 1990;145:207.
179. Pierce JH, Arnstein P, DiMarco E, et al. Oncogenic potential of erbb-2 in human mammary epithelial cells. *Oncogene* 1991;6:1189.
180. Tait L, Soule H, Russo J. Ultrastructural and immunocytochemical characterization of an immortalized human breast epithelial cell line, MCF-10. *Cancer Res* 1990;50:6087.
181. Ciardello F, Gottardis M, Basolo F, et al. Additive effects of c-erbB-2, c-Ha-ras, and transforming growth factor-α genes on in vitro transformation of human mammary epithelial cells. *Mol Carcinog* 1992; 6:43.
182. Ochieng J, Basolo F, Albini A, et al. Increased invasive, chemotactic and locomotive abilities of c-Ha-ras-transformed human breast epithelial cells. *Invasion Metastasis* 1991;11:38.
183. Miller FR, Soule HD, Tait L, et al. Xenograft model of progressive human proliferative disease. *J Natl Cancer Inst* 1993;85:1725.

184. Dawson PJ, Wolman SR, Tait L, Heppner GH, Miller FR. MCF10-AT: a model for the evolution of cancer from proliferative breast disease. *Am J Pathol* 1996;148:313.
185. Iravani S, Mora L, Miller FR, Dawson PJ. Altered expression of c-*erbb*B-2, DF3, B72.3, p53 and Ki-67 with progression and differentiation to two distinct histologic types of invasive carcinoma in the MCF10AT human xenograft model of proliferative breast disease. *Int J Oncol* 1998;12:369.
186. Gaffney EV. A cell line (HBL-100) established from human breast milk. *Cell Tissue Res* 1982;227(3):563.
187. Krief P, Saint-Ruf C, Bracke M, et al. Acquisition of tumorigenic potential in the human myoepithelial HBL100 cell line is associated with decreased expression of HLA class I, class II and integrin beta 3 and increased expression of c-myc. *Int J Cancer* 1989;43:658.
188. Caron de Fromentel C, Nardeux PC, Soussi T, et al. Epithelial HBL-100 cell line derived from milk of an apparently healthy woman harbours SV40 genetic information. *Exp Cell Res* 1985;160:83.
189. Decloitre F, Cassingena R, Estrade S, Martin M. Concomitant alterations of microfilaments and microtubules in human epithelial cells (HBL-100) in relation to their malignant conversion. *Tumour Biol* 1991;12:111.
190. Marlhens F, Saint-Ruf C, Nardeux P, et al. Karyotype evolution of the human HBL-100 cell line and mapping of the integration site of SV40 DNA. *Ann Genet* 1988;31:81.
191. Saint-Ruf C, Nardeux P, Estrade S, et al. Accelerated malignant conversion of human HBL-100 cells by the v-Ki-ras oncogene. *Exp Cell Res* 1988;176:60.
192. Dhaliwal MK, Giovanella BC, Pathak S. Cytogenetic characterization of two human milk-derived cell line (HBL-100) passages differing in tumorigenicity. *Anticancer Res* 1990;10:113.
193. Lebeau J, Le Chalony C, Prosperi MT, Goubin G. Constitutive overexpression of a 89 kDa heat shock protein gene in the HBL100 human mammary cell line converted to a tumorigenic phenotype by the EJ/T24 Harvey-ras oncogene. *Oncogene* 1991;6:1125.
194. Robert-Guroff M, Stern TL, Richardson ES, Giovanella BC, Michaels FH. Presence of Mason-Pfizer monkey virus in some stocks of the human HBL-100 mammary epithelial cell line. *J Natl Cancer Inst* 1996;88:372.
195. Vanhamme L, Szpirer C. Transforming activity of the human mammary line HBL100 DNA is associated with SV40 large T antigen genetic information integrated in its genome. *Carcinogenesis* 1988;9:653.
196. Saint-Ruf C, Nardeux P, Cebrian J, Lacasa M, Lavialle C, Cassingena R. Molecular cloning and characterization of endogenous SV40 DNA from human HBL-100 cells. *Int J Cancer* 1989;44:367.
197. Rao KV, Williams RE, Fox CF. Altered glucocorticoid binding and action in response to epidermal growth factor in HBL100 cells. *Cancer Res* 1987;47:5888.
198. Wellner RB, He XJ, Marmary Y, Baum BJ. Functional beta-adrenergic receptors in a human mammary cell line (HBL-100). *Biochem Pharmacol* 1988;37:3035.
199. Peyrat JP, Bonneterre J. Type I IGF receptor in human breast diseases. *Breast Cancer Res Treat* 1992;22:59.
200. Laherty RF, Balcavage WX, Goff C, et al. HBL-100 cells do not secrete casein and lack prolactin and estradiol receptors. *In Vitro Cell Dev Biol* 1990;26:933.
201. Bagheri-Yarmand R, Liu JF, Ledoux D, Morere JF, Crepin M. Inhibition of human breast epithelial HBL100 cell proliferation by a dextran derivative (CMDB7): interference with the FGF2 autocrine loop. *Biochem Biophys Res Commun* 1997;239:424.
202. Schirrmacher V. Cancer metastasis: experimental approaches, theroetical concepts and impacts for treatment strategies. *Adv Cancer Res* 1985;43:1.
203. Terranova VP, Hujanen ES, Martin GR. Basement membrane and the invasive activity of metastatic tumor cells. *J Natl Cancer Inst* 1986; 77:311.
204. Barsky SH, Siegal GP, Jannotta F, Liotta LA. Loss of basement membrane components by invasive tumors but not by their benign counterparts. *Lab Invest* 1994;49:140.
205. Liotta LA, Rao CN, Barsky SH. Tumor invasion and the extracellular matrix. *Lab Invest* 1994;49:636.
206. Barsky SH, Togo S, Garbisa S, Liotta LA. Type IV collagenase immunoreactivity in invasive breast carcinoma. *Lancet* 1994;1:296.
207. Kleinman HK, McGarvey ML, Hassell JR, et al. Basement membrane complexes with biological activity. *Biochemistry* 1986;25:312.
208. Bae S-N, Arand G, Azzam H, et al. Molecular and cellular analysis of basement membrane invasion by human breast cancer cells in Matrigel-based in vitro assays. *Breast Cancer Res Treat* 1993;24:241.
209. Albini A, Iwamoto Y, Kleinman HK, et al. A rapid in vitro assay for quantitating the invasive potential of tumor cells. *Cancer Res* 1987;47:3239.
210. Frandsen TL, Boysen BE, Jirus S, et al. Experimental models for the study of human cancer cell invasion and metastasis. *Fibrinolysis* 1992;6[Suppl 4]:71.
211. Noel CT, Reed MJ, Jacobs HS, James VHT. The plasma concentration of oestrone sulphate in postmenopausal women: lack of diurnal variation, effect of ovariectomy, age and weight. *J Steroid Biochem* 1981;14:1101.
212. Thompson EW, Katz D, Shima TB, Wakeling AE, Lippman ME, Dickson RB. ICI 164,384: a pure antagonist of estrogen-stimulated MCF-7 cell proliferation and invasiveness. *Cancer Res* 1989;49:6929.
213. Thompson EW, Torri J, Sabol M, et al. Oncogene-induced basement membrane invasiveness in human mammary epithelial cells. *Clin Exp Metastasis* 1994;12:181.
214. Shi YE, Torri J, Yieh L, et al. Expression of 67 kDa laminin receptor in human breast cancer cells: regulation by progestins. *Clin Exp Metastasis* 1993;11:251.
215. Cattoretti G, Andreola S, Clemente C, D'Amato L, Rilke F. Vimentin and P53 expression in epidermal growth factor receptor-positive oestrogen receptor-negative breast carcinomas. *Br J Cancer* 1988;57:353.
216. Raymond WA, Leong AS-Y. Co-expression of cytokeratin and vimentin intermediate filament proteins in benign and neoplastic breast epithelium. *J Pathol* 1989;157:299.
217. Raymond WA, Leong AS-Y. A new prognostic parameter in breast carcinoma? *J Pathol* 1989;158:107.
218. Domagala W, Lasota J, Bartowiak J, Weber K, Osborne M. Vimentin is preferentially expressed in human breast carcinomas with low estrogen receptor and high Ki67 growth fraction. *Am J Pathol* 1994;136:219.
219. Domagala W, Leszek W, Lasota J, Weber K, Osborne M. Vimentin is preferentially expressed in high grade ductal and medullary, but not in lobular breast carcinomas. *Am J Pathol* 1994;137:1059.
220. Gamallo C, Palacios J, Suarez A, et al. Correlation of E-cadherin expression with differentiation grade and histological type in breast carcinoma. *Am J Pathol* 1993;142:987.
221. Rasbridge SA, Gillett CE, Sampson SA, Walsh FS, Millis RR. Epithelial (E-) and placental (P-) cadherin cell adhesion molecule expression in breast carcinoma. *J Pathol* 1993;169:245.
222. Oka H, Shiozaki H, Kobayashi K, et al. Expression of E-cadherin cell adhesion molecule in human breast cancer tissues and its relationship to metastases. *Cancer Res* 1993;53:1696.
223. Thiery J-P, Boyer B, Tucker G, Gavrilovic J, Valles AM. Adhesion mechanisms in embryogenesis and in cancer invasion and metastasis. *Ciba Found Symp* 1988;141:48.
224. Sommers SL, Byers SW, Thompson EW, Torri JA, Gelmann EP. Differentiation state and invasiveness of human breast cancer cell lines. *Breast Cancer Res Treat* 1994;325.
225. Sommers CL, Heckford SE, Skerker JM, et al. Loss of epithelial markers and acquisition of vimentin expression in adriamycin- and vinblastine resistant human breast cancer cells. *Cancer Res* 1992;52:5190.
226. Brünner N, Johnson MD, Holst-Hansen C, Kiilgaard JF, Thompson EW, Clarke R. Acquisition of estrogen independence and antiestrogen resistance in breast cancer: association with the invasive and metastatic phenotype. *Endocr Related Cancer* 1995;2:27.
227. Ura H, Bonfil RD, Reich R, Reddel RR, Pfeifer A, Harris CC. Expression of type IV collagenase and procollagen genes and its correlation with the tumorigenic, invasive and metastatic abilities of oncogene-transformed human bronchial epithelial cells. *Cancer Res* 1989;49:4615.
228. Bonfil DR, Reddel RR, Ura H, et al. Invasive and metastatic potential of a v-Ha-ras transformed human bronchial epithelial cell line. *J Natl Cancer Inst* 1989;81:587.
229. Thorgeirsson UP, Turpeenniemi-Hujanen T, Williams JE, et al. NIH/3T3 cells transfected with human tumor cDNA containing activated ras oncogenes express the metastatic phenotype in nude mice. *Mol Cell Biol* 1985;5:259.
230. Albini A, Graf J, Kitten GT, et al. 17β-estradiol regulates and V-Ha-ras transfection constitutively enhances MCF-7 breast cancer cell interactions with basement membrane. *Proc Natl Acad Sci U S A* 1986;83:8182.
231. Sommers CL, Papageorge A, Wilding G, Gelmann EP. Growth properties and tumorigenesis of MCF-7 cells transfected with isogenic mutants of rasH. *Cancer Res* 1990;50:67.
232. Van Roy F, Mareel M, Vleminckx K, et al. Hormone sensitivity in vitro and in vivo of v-ras-transfected MCF-7 cell derivatives. *Int J Cancer* 1990;46:522.

233. Muschel RJ, Williams JE, Lowy DR, Liotta LA. Harvey ras induction of metastatic potential depends upon oncogene activation and type of recipient cell. *Am J Pathol* 1985;121:1.
234. Nicholson GL, Gallick GE, Sphon WH, Lembo TM, Tainsky MA. Transfection of activated c-Ha-rasEJ/pSV2neo genes into rat mammary cells: rapid stimulation of clonal diversification of spontaneous metastatic and cell surface properties. *Oncogene* 1992;7:1127.
235. De Vita VT. Principles of chemotherapy. In: De Vita VT, Hellman S, Rosenberg SA, eds. *Cancer principles and practice of oncology,* 3rd ed. Philadelphia: JB Lippincott, 1989:276.
236. Fracchia AA, Knapper WH, Carey JT, Farrow JH. Intrapleural chemotherapy for effusion from metastatic breast cancer. *Cancer* 1970; 26:626.
237. Van Netten JP, Armstrong JB, Carlyle SS, et al. Estrogen receptor distribution in the peripheral, intermediate and central regions of breast cancers. *Eur J Cancer Clin Oncol* 1988;24:1885.
238. Meltzer P, Leibovitz A, Dalton W, et al. Establishment of two new cell lines derived from human breast carcinomas with HER2/neu amplification. *Br J Cancer* 1991;63:727.
239. Whitescarver J. Problems of in vitro culture of human mammary tumor cells. *J Invest Dermatol* 1974;63:58.
240. Foley JF, Aftonomos BT. Growth of human breast neoplasms in cell culture. *J Natl Cancer Inst* 1965;34:217.
241. Bastert G, Fortmeyer HP, Eichholz H, Michel RT, Huck R, Schmidt-Matthiesen H. Human breast cancer in thymus aplastic nude mice. In: Bastert GB, ed. *Thymus-aplastic nude mice and rats in clinical oncology*. New York: Verlag, 1981:157.
242. Berger DP, Winterhalter BR, Fiebig HH. Establishment and characterization of human tumor xenografts in thymus-aplastic nude mice. In: Fiebig HH, Berger DP, eds. *Immunodeficient mice in oncology*. Basel: Karger, 1992:23.
243. Federoff S, Evans VJ, Perry VP, Vincent MM, eds. *Manual of the Tissue Culture Association.* 1975:53.
244. Gibson SL, Hilf R. Regulation of estrogen-binding capacity by insulin in 7,12-dimethylbenz(*a*)anthracene-induced mammary tumors in rats. *Cancer Res* 1980;40:2343.
245. Barnes D, Sato G. Growth of a human mammary tumor cell line in a serum free medium. *Nature* 1978;281:388.
246. Vignon F, Bouton MM, Rochefort H. Antiestrogens inhibit the mitogenic effect of growth factors on breast cancer cells in the total absence of estrogens. *Biochem Biophys Res Commun* 1987; 146:1502.
247. Koga M, Sutherland RL. Epidermal growth factor partially reverses the inhibitory effects of antiestrogens on T47D human breast cancer cell growth. *Biochem Biophys Res Commun* 1987;146:738.
248. Berthois Y, Katzenellenbogen JA, Katzenellenbogen BS. Phenol red in tissue culture is a weak estrogen: implications concerning the study of estrogen-responsive cells in culture. *Proc Natl Acad Sci U S A* 1986;83:2496.
249. Bindal RD, Carlson KE, Katzenellenbogen BS, Katzenellenbogen JA. Lipophylic impurities, not phenolsulfonphthalein, account for the estrogenic properties in commercial preparations of phenol red. *J Steroid Biochem* 1988;31:287.
250. Darbre P, Yates J, Curtis S, King RJB. Effect of estradiol on human breast cancer cells in culture. *Cancer Res* 1983;43:349.
251. Vignon F, Terqui M, Westley B, Derocq D, Rochefort H. Effects of plasma estrogen sulfates in mammary cancer cells. *Endocrinology* 1980;106:1079.
252. van der Burg B, Ruterman GR, Blankenstein MA, DeLaat SW, van Zoelen EJJ. Mitogenic stimulation of human breast cancer cells in a growth factor-defined medium: synergistic action of insulin and estrogen. *J Cell Physiol* 1988;134:101.
253. Reddel RR, Murphy LC, Sutherland RL. Factors affecting the sensitivity of T-47D human breast cancer cells to tamoxifen. *Cancer Res* 1984;44:2398.
254. Strobl JS, Lippman ME. Prolonged retention of estradiol by human breast cancer cells in tissue culture. *Cancer Res* 1979;39:3319.
255. Freshney RI, Freshey I, eds. *Culture of animal cells. A manual of basic technique*. New York: Wiley-Liss, 1991.
256. Hayflick L. *Tissue culture*. New York: Academic, 1973:220.
257. *Methods in enzymology LVIII: cell culture methods.* New York: Academic, 1979.

Diseases of the Breast, 2nd ed.,
edited by Jay R. Harris.
Lippincott Williams & Wilkins, Philadelphia © 2000.

CHAPTER 24

Biological Features of Human Premalignant Breast Disease

D. Craig Allred and Syed K. Mohsin

Invasive breast cancers (IBCs) are thought to arise from preexisting benign breast lesions. Benign breast lesions are very common, and many different types are seen, not all of which have premalignant potential. Those recognized as premalignant include usual ductal hyperplasia (UDH), atypical ductal hyperplasia (ADH), atypical lobular hyperplasia (ALH), ductal carcinoma *in situ* (DCIS), and lobular carcinoma *in situ* (LCIS) (Fig. 1). Although DCIS and LCIS possess some malignant properties (e.g., loss of growth control), they lack the ability to invade and metastasize and, in this sense, may be considered as premalignant. The currently favored working hypothesis of human breast cancer evolution, based on many types of direct and indirect evidence, proposes a nonobligatory serial progression from usual hyperplasia, to atypical hyperplasia, to *in situ* carcinoma, to IBC. This model is similar to the model proposed for colon cancer[1]; usual hyperplasias of the breast are analogous to benign colonic polyps, atypical hyperplasias to dysplastic polyps, *in situ* carcinomas to the same arising in dysplastic polyps, and invasive carcinomas arising from *in situ* carcinomas to the same in the colonic setting. Although most investigators consider this theory of breast cancer evolution to be imperfect and oversimplified, particularly for early stages of tumor progression, some elements of the model are almost certainly relevant. The model has been very useful in designing experimental studies into the biological mechanisms of breast cancer evolution, which are still in their infancy.

The idea that benign breast lesions might be precursors of IBC was suggested by historic studies as far back as the early nineteenth century, which noted that certain types of benign lesions appeared to lie on a histologic continuum with IBC[2–8] and were more common in cancerous than noncancerous breasts.[9–28] Additional evidence came from more recent epidemiologic studies showing that women with a history of benign breast disease had an increased relative risk of developing IBC.[29–52] The most enlightening of these epidemiologic studies was reported in a series of articles by Page et al. based on a large prospective study that assigned risk to specific types of benign epithelial lesions (those named above) and set forth reproducible histologic criteria for identifying them.[33,42–44,53] These findings have been confirmed by others,[46,49,50] and the combined results indicate that women with usual hyperplasias, atypical hyperplasias, and *in situ* carcinoma have approximately a twofold, fivefold, and tenfold increased relative risk, respectively, of eventually developing IBC compared with age-matched controls.

The elevated risks associated with UDH, ADH, ALH, and LCIS are bilateral, suggesting that these conditions may be only markers, rather than precursors, of the development of IBC.[42,43,46,49,50] However, the epidemiologic studies defining the magnitude and laterality of these risks were limited in the sense that they examined women with previously resected benign lesions whose evolutionary fate was unknowable. In fact, UDH, ADH, ALH, and LCIS are often multifocal and bilateral,[9,18,19,54,55] and the results from these epidemiologic studies do not exclude the possibility that these lesions can be both precursors and risk factors if similar residual disease in one or the other breast progressed to IBC in a subset of patients, which seems likely. Some of these lesions are also morphologically similar to unequivocally premalignant lesions in certain animal models of breast cancer evolution,[56–58] and they share important features with well-established precursors in other human malignancies, such as colon cancer.[1] Perhaps the strongest evidence that they may be precursors comes from genetic studies showing that they share identical genetic abnormalities with synchronous ipsilateral IBC.[59–62]

DCIS is less likely to be multifocal or bilateral than the other premalignant breast lesions, and the elevated risk for developing IBC associated with DCIS is primarily ipsilateral, consistent with the idea that DCIS is a relatively committed precursor lesion.[53,54,63] In microscopic examination, IBC is frequently observed to extend

D. C. Allred: Department of Pathology, Breast Center, Baylor College of Medicine, Houston, Texas
S. K. Mohsin: Breast Center, Baylor College of Medicine, Houston, Texas

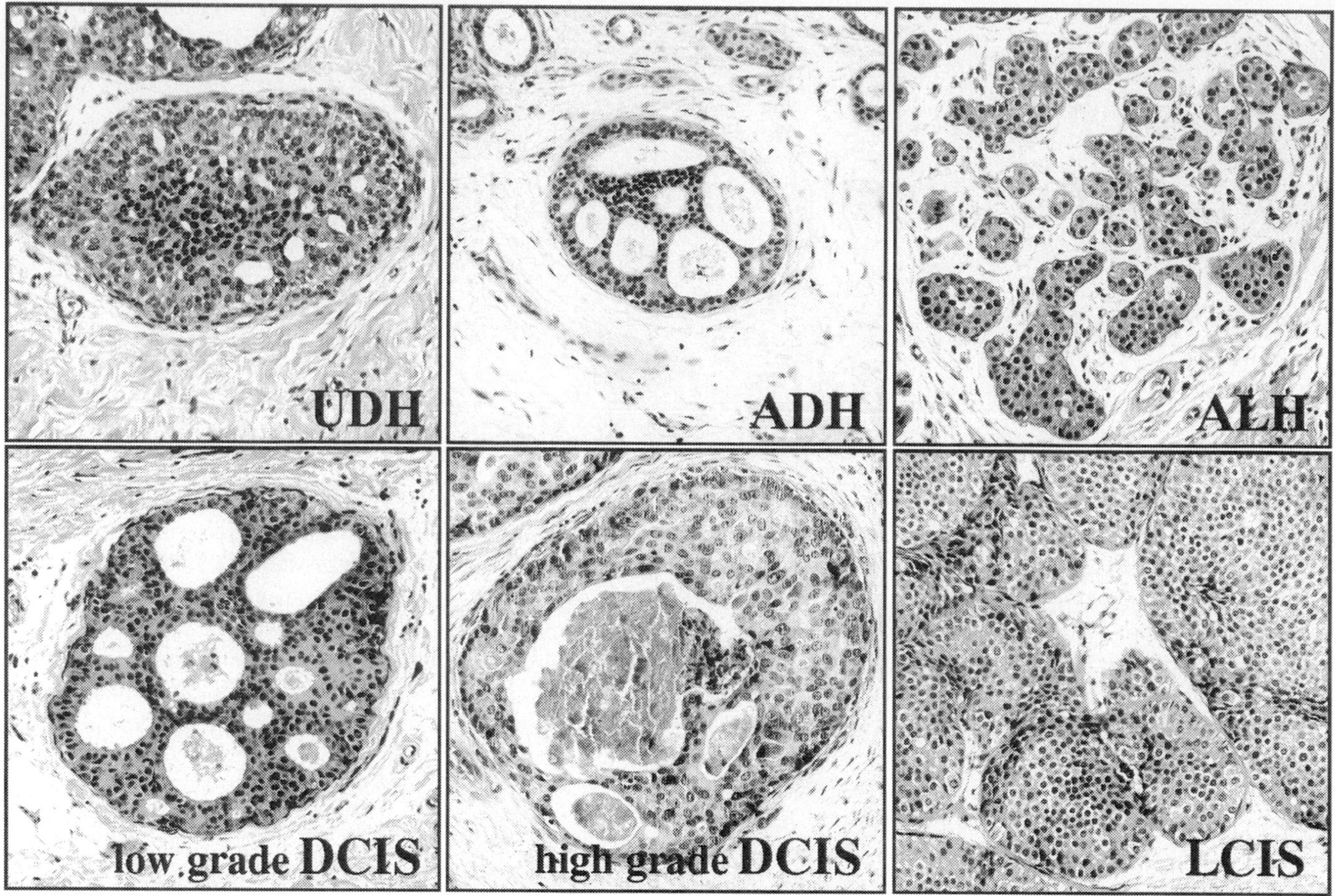

FIG. 1. Representative photomicrographs of the major types of premalignant breast lesions recognized today, including usual ductal hyperplasia (UDH), atypical ductal hyperplasia (ADH), atypical lobular hyperplasia (ALH), low-grade (noncomedo) ductal carcinoma *in situ* (DCIS), high-grade (comedo) DCIS, and lobular carcinoma *in situ* (LCIS) (hematoxylin-eosin stained; ×200 magnification).

directly from ducts containing DCIS, providing commonsense evidence that one evolved from the other. In addition, DCIS nearly always shares multiple clonal genetic alterations with coexistent IBC, which is the most compelling evidence of a precursor-product relationship between them.[60]

Premalignant breast lesions are common, and they are being diagnosed more frequently because of screening mammography. They are currently defined by their histologic features, and their prognosis is imprecisely estimated based on indirect epidemiologic evidence. Although lesions within the various categories are histologically similar, they must possess biological differences motivating some of them to progress to IBC. Understanding more about their biology may lead to safe and effective strategies for preventing their development and progression. Unfortunately, relatively little is known about the biological characteristics of premalignant breast disease. One hopes this will change as research in this area gains momentum.[64,65] Although several hundred articles have been published on many biological factors in premalignant breast disease, only a handful of these factors have been studied in a relatively comprehensive manner. These factors are reviewed in this chapter.

CELLULAR PROLIFERATION

Premalignant breast lesions are thought to arise primarily from stem cells in normal terminal duct lobular units (TDLUs).[66] On a microscopic scale, they are mass lesions that expand TDLUs and proximal subsegmental ducts to many times their normal size (Fig. 2). Abnormal proliferation contributes to this overall growth imbalance through alterations of several normal growth-regulating mechanisms. Many studies, using a variety of techniques, have measured the magnitude of proliferation in TDLUs and premalignant breast lesions (Table 1).

All studies evaluating histologically normal TDLUs reported low rates of proliferation, averaging only approximately 2%.[67–77] In premenopausal women, the rate fluctuates and is approximately twice as high in the luteal than in the fol-

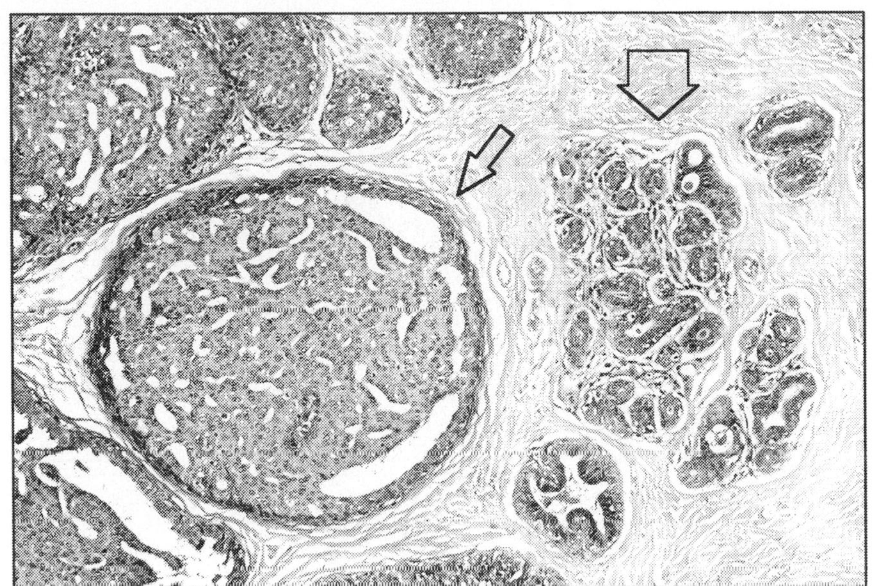

FIG. 2. Premalignant breast lesions are thought to arise from stem cells in normal terminal duct lobular units (TDLUs), expanding them and proximal subsegmental ducts to many times their normal size. This example shows a TDLU (*wide arrow*) adjacent to a focus of usual ductal hyperplasia (*narrow arrow*), which occupies a space originally as small as a single acinus in the TDLU (hematoxylin-eosin stained; ×200 magnification).

licular phase of the menstrual cycle.[67,68,70,72,73,78–83] In postmenopausal women, the proliferation rate is somewhat lower and relatively stable.[84,85] The association between menstrual status and proliferation emphasizes the importance of sex hormones, such as estrogen and progesterone, as mitogens for normal breast epithelium[81,86–89]; this relationship has been demonstrated experimentally in cell lines and animal models.[89,90]

A few studies have evaluated proliferation in UDH (Fig. 3) and ADH and have shown that the average rate in both is approximately 5%,[75–77,91,92] which is two to three times higher than the rate in normal TDLUs. No published studies exist of proliferation in ALH. Proliferation has been studied most extensively in DCIS. An unfortunate consensus has existed for many years to dichotomize these histologically diverse lesions into high-grade (also referred to as "comedo") and low-grade ("noncomedo") subtypes, and the results of most biologic studies of DCIS, including those evaluating proliferation, have been presented in this oversimplified manner. Studies assessing proliferation in DCIS reported rates averaging approximately 5% in low-grade lesions compared with 15% in high-grade lesions[77,93–99]; both rates are substantially higher than in normal TDLUs. A few studies have used more comprehensive grading systems to convey more accurately the histologic diversity of DCIS and have found a strong direct correlation between grade and proliferation rate; rates range from less than 1% in the lowest grade to more than 70% in the highest grade lesions,[77,95–97,99] depending on the assay used to measure proliferation. Proliferation rates in LCIS appear to be very low, averaging only approximately 2%,[100–102] similar to the rate observed in normal breast epithelium.

A few studies have observed substantially higher rates of proliferation in premalignant lesions from cancerous breasts than in those from noncancerous breasts,[91,103] suggesting that some measurement of proliferation in premalignant lesions may be a useful prognostic indicator for the development of IBC.

TABLE 1. *Summary of results from studies evaluating proliferation rate, estrogen-receptor expression, c-*erb*-b2 amplification or overexpression, and p53 mutation or protein accumulation in normal terminal duct lobular units and premalignant breast lesions*

Characteristic	TDLU	UDH	ADH	Low-grade (noncomedo) DCIS	High-grade (comedo) DCIS	LCIS
Proliferation rate (% positive cells)	2%	5%	5%	5%	15%	2%
Estrogen receptor (% positive cases)	70%	60%	80%	75%	30%	80%
c-*erb*-b2 (% positive cases)	0%	0%	2%	10%	70%	2%
p53 (% positive cases)	0%	0%	0%	5%	45%	5%

ADH, atypical ductal hyperplasias; DCIS, ductal carcinoma *in situ*; LCIS, lobular carcinoma *in situ*; TDLU, terminal duct lobular units; UDH, usual ductal hyperplasias.
Data are averages calculated from published studies using diverse methodologies, which were considered equivalent for the purposes of compiling this table (see text for references).

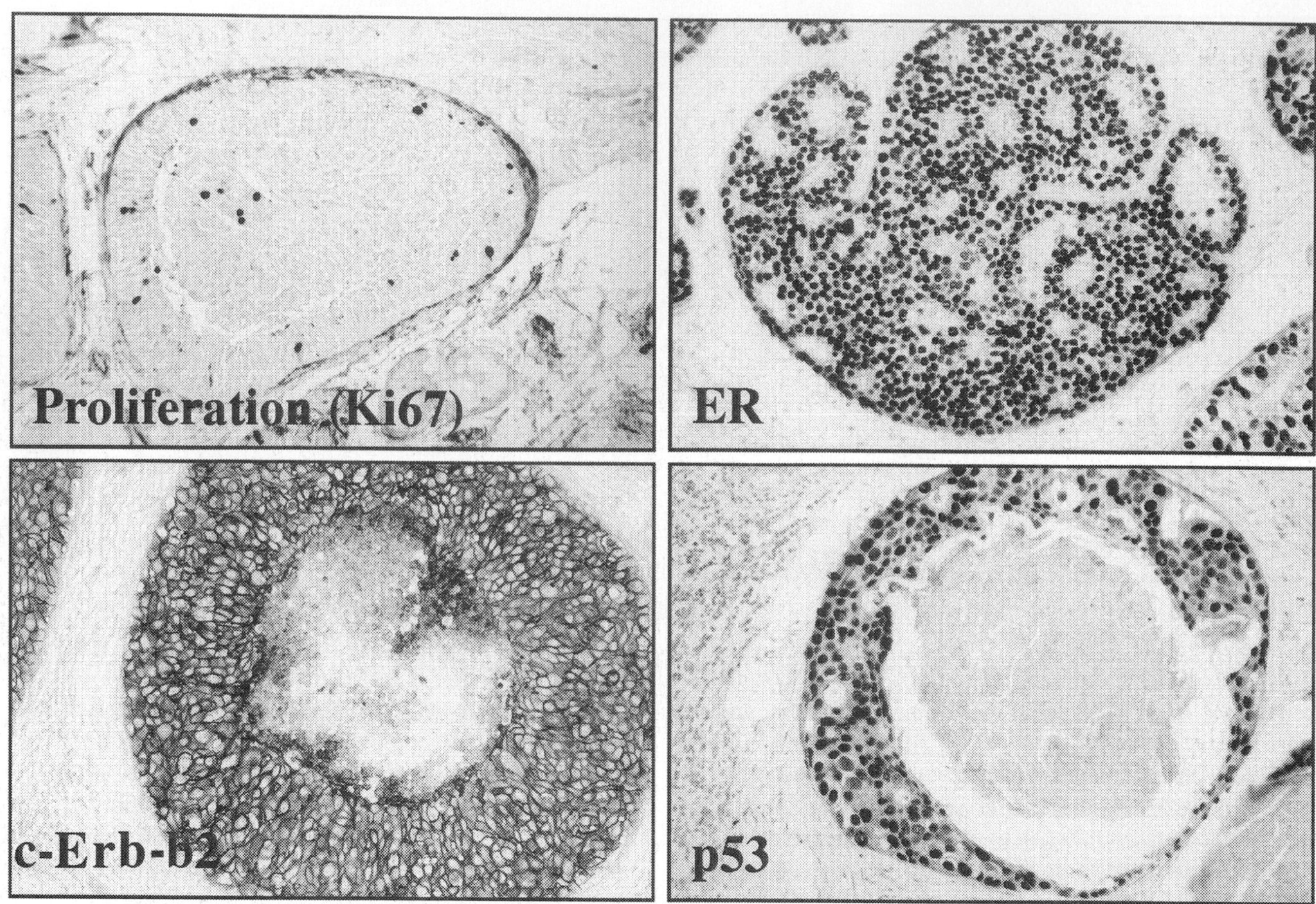

FIG. 3. Representative photomicrographs of premalignant breast lesions immunostained to illustrate some of the biological phenotypes reviewed in this chapter. Usual ductal hyperplasias show very low proliferation rates, as illustrated in this example immunostained with the cell cycle–associated Ki67 antibody (dark nuclei indicate actively dividing cells). Low-grade ductal carcinoma *in situ* (DCIS) nearly always expresses very high levels of nuclear estrogen receptor (ER) (dark nuclei indicate cells expressing ER). High-grade DCIS are commonly positive for membrane overexpression of the c-*erb*-b2 oncoprotein, and approximately one-half show nuclear accumulation of mutated p53 (×200 magnification).

HORMONES AND RECEPTORS

Estrogen plays a central role in regulating the growth and differentiation of normal breast epithelium.[89,90,104,105] By interacting with estrogen receptors (ERs), it stimulates cellular proliferation and induces the expression of many other gene products, including the progesterone receptor (PR). The PR then mediates the mitogenic effect of progesterone, further stimulating proliferation in normal breast epithelium.[89,90,104,105] Many additional factors, collectively referred to as *coactivators* and *corepressors*, have been discovered that appear to modulate the functions of these hormones and receptors, including their mitogenic activity.[106]

Several studies have evaluated ER expression in normal breast epithelium and premalignant breast lesions (see Table 1), primarily by immunohistochemistry. Studies assessing ER expression in normal TDLUs observed that a majority express the receptor, but generally at low levels averaging only approximately 10% of positive cells.[75,107–109] The level of positivity fluctuates with the menstrual cycle and is highest during the follicular phase.[109–112] This pattern is in contrast to peak proliferation, which occurs during the luteal phase[67,68,70,72,73,78–83]; these findings suggest that the growth stimulation by estrogen is partially delayed or is indirect and mediated by other downstream interactions, such as that between progesterone and the PR.

Of the few studies assessing ER expression in hyperplastic breast lesions,[75,113,114] most observed significant overexpression relative to normal epithelium. On average, approximately 60% of UDH and 80% of ADH lesions express ER, usually in a large proportion of cells. Many studies have evaluated ER expression in DCIS.[97–99,113–121] Approximately 75% of low-grade DCIS lesions express ER, frequently at very high levels in a majority of cells (see Fig. 3). In comparison, only 30% of high-grade DCIS lesions appear to express ER, often at relatively low levels involving a small minority of cells.

Approximately 80% of LCIS lesions appear to have a high level of ER expression[100,102,113,122]; the situation is probably similar in ALH.

Prolonged estrogen exposure is an important risk factor for developing IBC,[89,90,104,105] perhaps because it allows random genetic alterations to accumulate in cells stimulated to replicate.[90] Excess estrogen may contribute to the progression of premalignant breast lesions by similar mechanisms,[75] but this view may be an oversimplification. For example, in one study,[77] proliferation was measured in TDLUs and premalignant lesions from the same breasts in a large number of patients dichotomized by menstrual status. Proliferation rates in TDLUs were significantly higher in premenopausal than in postmenopausal women; this finding is consistent with the well-known mitogenic effect of estrogen in normal cells. In contrast, although proliferation was substantially higher in premalignant lesions than in TDLUs, no significant difference was found in the proliferation of premalignant lesions in premenopausal and in postmenopausal women, suggesting that the hormonal regulation of proliferation in these lesions is abnormal. Consistent with this observation, a study of premalignant lesions by Fuqua et al.[123] found a common somatic mutation in the region of the ER gene encoding the hormone-binding domain that, when transfected into breast cell lines, stimulated high levels of proliferation at very low concentrations of estrogen. This hypersensitivity to estrogen may stimulate proliferation and contribute to the development and progression of premalignant lesions, even in postmenopausal women with low circulating levels of estrogen.

Assessing ER status may eventually be important in the clinical management of patients with premalignant breast disease. Its most promising role may be in identifying patients with high-risk premalignant disease who are likely to benefit from antihormonal drugs used as chemopreventive agents. For example, in the National Surgical Adjuvant Breast and Bowel Project P-1 prevention trial,[124] patients with a history of ADH or LCIS who received tamoxifen experienced a dramatic decrease in breast cancer incidence compared with those receiving placebo. ADH and LCIS lesions nearly always express ER at very high levels, suggesting that ER-positive premalignant lesions may be particularly susceptible to suppression by tamoxifen and perhaps other antihormonal compounds as well.

C-*ERB*-B2 ONCOGENE

The c-*erb*-b2 oncogene is the most thoroughly studied biological factor in premalignant breast disease (see Table 1). In fully developed IBC, c-*erb*-b2 is amplified or overexpressed in 20% to 30% of cases, and these abnormalities are associated with poor clinical outcome and altered response to adjuvant therapy.[125,126] Several studies have observed strong associations between amplified or overexpressed c-*erb*-b2 and high proliferation rates in IBC, consistent with its hypothesized function as a growth factor receptor.[127–130] In addition, c-*erb*-b2 may promote cell motility, perhaps contributing to the ability of cells overexpressing it to become invasive and metastasize.[131]

Nearly all studies of c-*erb*-b2 in premalignant breast disease have used immunohistochemical analysis to detect overexpression of the oncoprotein, which is highly correlated with gene amplification.[132] Studies assessing normal TDLUs and UDH lesions found no evidence of c-*erb*-b2 overexpression,[133–135] and it has been rarely detected in ADH lesions.[133–136] Many studies have evaluated c-*erb*-b2 in DCIS.[95–99,119,130,135–147] The average incidence of amplification or overexpression was approximately 10% in low-grade DCIS compared with 70% in high-grade DCIS lesions (see Fig. 3). Alterations of c-*erb*-b2 are very rare in LCIS, occurring in less than 2% of cases.[100–102,133,136,139,142,143,148,149] Abnormalities of c-*erb*-b2 are also probably very rare in ALH, although formal studies are unavailable.

Just how alterations of c-*erb*-b2 lead to the development and progression of premalignant breast disease is unknown, although the increased proliferation and cell motility associated with amplification and overexpression may both contribute. Whatever the mechanism, the absence of overexpression in normal breast epithelium and hyperplasias, compared with the high rate in DCIS, suggests that alteration of c-*erb*-b2 is a very important event in early malignant transformation, leading to a substantial proportion of *in situ* disease. Furthermore, the incidence of c-*erb*-b2 overexpression is much lower in IBC than in pure DCIS,[125,130,144] suggesting that expression discontinues in a significant proportion of DCIS lesions as they progress to invasive disease or, alternatively, that a subset of IBC arises *de novo* by mechanisms that are independent of c-*erb*-b2.

Evaluation of c-*erb*-b2 status may become a useful prognostic factor in managing patients with premalignant breast disease. Its usefulness was suggested by a study finding that overexpression of c-*erb*-b2 in breast epithelial cells from random fine-needle aspirates of high-risk women, some with a history of ADH or DCIS, was associated with additionally elevated risk for developing IBC.[150] However, another similar study failed to confirm this finding,[151] and a clinical role for c-*erb*-b2 in premalignant disease remains to be defined.

P53 TUMOR-SUPPRESSOR GENE

The p53 tumor-suppressor gene has also been studied in a relatively comprehensive manner in human premalignant breast disease (see Table 1). Located on 17p13, the p53 gene encodes a 53 kd nuclear transcription factor with several important functions, including down-regulation of the cell cycle, facilitation of DNA repair, and promotion of programmed cell death.[152] In many types of cancer, the p53 gene is commonly mutated[153,154]; most mutations are missense point mutations resulting in an inactivated protein with a prolonged half-life, which accumulates to very high levels in the cell nucleus.[155,156] Thus, measurement of protein levels is a relatively easy and accurate surrogate assay for detecting mutations, and most studies of clinical tissue samples have used immunohistochemistry to assess levels of p53 protein. Up to 50% of IBCs contain mutated or accumulated p53, which is associated with generally aggressive biological features and poor clinical outcome.[157–159]

Except in morphologically "normal" breast epithelium in patients with Li-Fraumeni syndrome who have inherited mutations,[160,161] p53 is not mutated or significantly overexpressed in normal breast epithelium.[155,162–164] In UDH and ADH, p53 also appears to be normal.[155,165–167] No published studies exist regarding the expression of p53 in ALH. Many studies have assessed p53 expression in DCIS.[96–99,119,121,140,146,163,166–171] Approximately 5% of low-grade DCIS lesions contain mutated or overexpressed p53, compared with 45% of high-grade DCIS lesions (see Fig. 3); levels for the latter rival those observed in IBC. Alterations of p53 appear to be very rare in LCIS, occurring in an average of approximately 5% of cases.[101,102,171–173]

Mutations of the p53 gene may contribute to the development and progression of premalignant breast disease by several mechanisms. These include increased proliferation; interference with DNA repair through loss of an important G_1 cell-cycle checkpoint, leading to replication of a damaged DNA template and genetic instability; and also perhaps clonal expansion through inhibition of programmed cell death.[152]

Assessment of p53 status may become a useful prognostic tool in the clinical management of patients with premalignant breast disease, as suggested by studies finding a slightly increased risk of IBC among patients with normal or hyperplastic breast epithelium showing mildly elevated levels of p53 protein.[150,151,174]

OTHER GENETIC ALTERATIONS

Most of the biological abnormalities responsible for the development and progression of human premalignant breast lesions are almost certainly still unknown. Genetic studies demonstrate that their evolution is biologically very complex. These include studies evaluating loss of heterozygosity of polymorphic microsatellite markers to identify inactivated tumor-suppressor genes or, more rarely, amplified oncogenes. The majority of loss-of-heterozygosity studies have assessed genetic loci showing losses in previous studies of IBC, which is a reasonable strategy in the sense that precursor lesions should contain some of the same defects.

Loss of heterozygosity has not been observed in normal breast epithelium, with a few important exceptions. Deng et al.[175] noted that a subset of histologically normal TDLUs occasionally shared loss of heterozygosity for a marker on 3p with closely adjacent IBC, whereas TDLUs farther away in the same breast did not. The same study reported similar findings involving loci on 11p and 17p, although these were not as frequent as 3p losses. These findings suggest that histologically normal–appearing epithelium may have an abnormal genetic phenotype that may be associated with an elevated risk for developing breast cancer.

Several reports have been published of loss of heterozygosity in premalignant lesions from noncancerous breasts, a setting emphasizing alterations that may be important in the early development of such lesions (Table 2). In these studies, approximately 30% of UDH lesions and 40% of ADH lesions showed one or more losses of heterozygosity among the nearly 30 loci distributed over 10 chromosomes that were examined.[59,60,62,176–179] Whereas the cumulative rates of loss of heterozygosity were relatively high in UDH and ADH, they were generally less than 10% at individual loci, and most lesions contained only one or two losses. These loss-of-heterozygosity data, and results from earlier studies showing nonrandom inactivation of the X chromosome[180] and aneuploid DNA content,[181] emphasize that "hyperplasias" are actually misnamed clonal neoplasms. Loss of heterozygosity was more common in DCIS than in hyperplasias, consistent with the notion that DCIS represents a later stage of evolution. Up to 80% of both noncomedo and comedo DCIS showed at least one loss of heterozygosity among the more than 100 loci on 17 chromosomes that have been examined.[59,60,182–190] In contrast to hyperplasias, most DCIS lesions, especially comedo subtypes, show multiple losses of heterozygosity, with as many as eight in a single lesion in one study.[60] The highest rates of loss in DCIS involved loci on 16q, 17p, and 17q; the rates approached 60% to 80% in some studies,[189,191] suggesting that suppressor genes in these regions may be particularly important in the development of DCIS. Candidate genes for these regions include the gene for E-cadherin on 16q,[192] the gene for p53 on 17p,[193] *NF1*[194] on 17q, and *BRCA1* on 17q.[195] No candidate genes are known for most of the other loci showing loss of heterozygosity in DCIS, or in any other type of premalignant lesion for that matter. Studies evaluating loss of heterozygosity in LCIS have demonstrated that losses are also very common in these lesions, especially involving loci on 11q, 16q, and 17q.[61,196]

A few studies have evaluated loss of heterozygosity in premalignant lesions from cancerous breasts and compared it to that in histologically identical lesions from noncancerous breasts as a strategy to identify alterations that might be important in the progression to IBC.[60,62,186,187,197–200] From these preliminary studies, the overall rates of loss of heterozygosity involving most loci appear to be only slightly higher in premalignant lesions from cancerous breasts than in those from noncancerous breasts. However, a few loci show large increases, which suggests that genetic alterations in these regions may be particularly important in the progression to invasive disease. For example, in one study,[60] loss of heterozygosity at a marker on 11p (D11S988) increased from 10% to 20% in UDH, from 10% to 40% in ADH, and from 20% to 70% in DCIS in lesions taken from noncancerous breasts and from cancerous breasts, respectively. The gene for cyclin D_1 resides near this locus,[201] and alterations of cyclin D_1 might be providing the selection

TABLE 2. *Summary of results from published studies assessing loss of heterozygosity in various categories of premalignant breast lesions*

	Chromosomal location of loss of heterozygosity																							
	1p	1q	2p	2q	3p	3q	4p	4q	5p	5q	6p	6q	7p	7q	8p	8q	9p	9q	10p	10q	11p	11q	12p	12q
UDH			x	x				x				x			x		x				x	x		
ADH		x	x									x					x				x	x		
ALH																						x		
DCIS	x	x	x	x	x	x		x			x	x	x	x	x	x	x				x	x	x	
LCIS																						x		

	13p	13q	14p	14q	15p	15q	16p	16q	17p	17q	18p	18q	19p	19q	20p	20q	21p	21q	22p	22q	Xp	Xq	Yp	Yq
UDH		x		x				x	x	x														
ADH		x		x				x	x	x												x		
ALH																								
DCIS		x		x		x	x	x	x	x	x	x						x						
LCIS		x						x	x	x														

Note: x indicates that loss of heterozygosity was found (see text for references).
ADH, atypical ductal hyperplasia; ALH, atypical lobular hyperplasia; DCIS, ductal carcinoma *in situ;* LCIS, lobular carcinoma *in situ*; UDH, usual ductal hyperplasia.

pressure for this alteration, although other as yet unknown genes may also be involved. In the same study, comedo DCIS showed increasing losses at several other loci, including D2S362 on 2q (10% to 40%), D13S137 on 13q (10% to 40%), and D17S597 on 17q (5% to 40%); these findings suggest that this precursor lesion is particularly unstable and likely to acquire multiple genetic defects, leading to an invasive phenotype. Known genes that may be playing a role in some of these escalating losses in comedo DCIS include *RB*[202] on 13q, *BRCA2* on 13q,[203] and *BRCA1* on 17q.[195]

Allelic imbalance has also been assessed in DCIS lesions using fluorescent *in situ* hybridization and comparative genomic hybridization.[204–208] Studies using these techniques have demonstrated segmental gains and losses involving more than ten chromosomes. Amplification of the c-*erb*-b2 locus was particularly common in comedo DCIS evaluated by these methods,[204,205] a finding consistent with those of earlier studies showing overexpression of the c-*erb*-b2 oncoprotein.[125] Nearly all DCIS lesions are aneuploid at the relatively high resolutions of fluorescent *in situ* hybridization and comparative genomic hybridization, and most appear to have a large number of independent gains and losses. The genetic diversity of DCIS assessed by loss of heterozygosity, fluorescent *in situ* hybridization, and comparative genomic hybridization rivals the complexity observed in IBC.

Study of allelic imbalance in premalignant lesions from cancerous breasts also provides an opportunity to look for shared alterations between synchronous lesions as an indication of their genetic and perhaps evolutionary relatedness. In a study by O'Connell et al.[60] evaluating loss of heterozygosity at 15 genetic loci in a large number of premalignant lesions, 40% of UDH and 50% of ADH lesions shared one or more losses of heterozygosity with synchronous ipsilateral breast cancer; these findings provide the first genetic evidence that hyperplasias may be direct precursors of malignant disease. Many studies have shown that up to 80% of DCIS and LCIS lesions share from one to several independent losses of heterozygosity with synchronous IBC, providing compelling, if not surprising, evidence that they are genetically related.[59,61,185–187,196–200] Studies using comparative genomic hybridization have also shown that DCIS and IBC lesions from the same breasts share multiple genetic gains and losses.[205] Interestingly, synchronous DCIS and IBC occasionally both show distinct allelic imbalances, suggesting that there may also be divergent aspects to their evolution.[187,205]

Studies of allelic imbalance through examination of loss of heterozygosity, fluorescent *in situ* hybridization, and comparative genomic hybridization provide compelling but crude evidence that IBC evolves from premalignant breast lesions by diverse genetic mechanisms. During the 1990s, many other types of studies into the biology of premalignant breast disease were conducted, revealing a multitude of genetic and epigenetic alterations. Although potentially important, most of these alterations have been studied in a relatively preliminary fashion. Future studies must provide more detailed information about specific genes and biological interactions. Progress has been hampered by a reliance on correlative studies of small, difficult to obtain, archival samples of human premalignant lesions, and a paucity of appropriate cell lines or truly representative animal models to support mechanistic studies. A few innovations have the potential to overcome some of these limitations and stimulate progress. For example, laser-capture microdissection technology (Fig. 4) allows the efficient collection of large numbers of samples that are sufficiently enriched in target cells to support precise genetic evaluations, such as direct sequencing of DNA to find mutations, something that

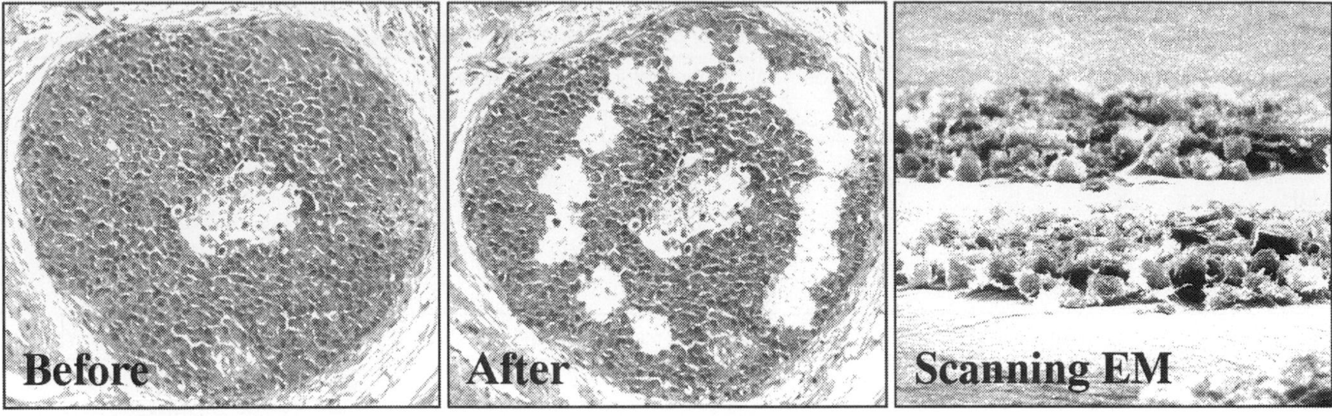

FIG. 4. Using laser capture microdissection (LCM), samples composed of pure populations of cells can be harvested from very small lesions within heterogeneous tissues on routine histologic slides, enabling precise molecular analysis, which was previously impossible. This representative example shows a human ductal carcinoma *in situ* before (left) and after (center) LCM. The tissue from the "holes" (right) has been adhered to a thermoplastic film laid over the slide with a pulse of laser energy applied under direct microscopic visualization. The film is transferred to a microcentrifuge tube for harvesting DNA, RNA, or protein.

was previously impossible.[209] In addition, stable cell lines, such as MCF10AT,[58,210] have been established from human premalignant lesions that can be studied *in vitro* or studied *in vivo* using xenograft models derived from them. Other animal models of premalignant and malignant breast disease have been developed that have mammary-specific inducible genetic defects with the ability to support very detailed mechanistic studies. These and similar innovations should greatly accelerate the understanding of human premalignant breast disease and the ability to prevent its development and progression, thereby helping to prevent invasive breast cancer.

ACKNOWLEDGMENT

This work was supported by National Institutes of Health grants P01-CA30195, P30-CA54174, and P50-CA58183.

REFERENCES

1. Feron ER, Vogelstein B. A genetic model for colorectal tumorigenesis. *Cell* 1990;61:759.
2. Cooper AP. *Illustrations of the diseases of the breast*. London: Longman, Rees, 1829.
3. MacCarty WC. The histogenesis of cancer (carcinoma) of the breast and its clinical significance. *Surg Gynecol Obstet* 1913;17:441.
4. MacCarty WC, Mensing EH. The relation between chronic mastitis and carcinoma of the breast. *Coll Papers Mayo Clin* 1915;7:918.
5. Cheatle GL. Desquamative and dysgenetic epithelial hyperplasias in the breast: their situation and characteristics: their likeness to lesions induced by tar. *Br J Surg* 1926;13:509.
6. Fraser J. The breast in health and disease. *Edinb Med J* 1929;36:217.
7. Muir R. The evolution of carcinoma of the mamma. *J Pathol Bacteriol* 1941;52:155.
8. Dawson EK. Premalignant conditions in breast carcinoma. In: Severi L, ed. *The morphological precursors of cancer*. Perugia, Italy: Perugia University Press, 1962:383.
9. Foote FW, Stewart FW. Comparative studies of cancerous versus noncancerous breasts. *Ann Surg* 1945;121:6,197.
10. Frantz VK, Pickren JW, Melcher GW, Auchincloss H. Incidence of chronic cystic disease in so-called "normal breasts." *Cancer* 1951;4:762.
11. Sloss PT, Bennett WA, Clagett OT. Incidence in normal breasts of features associated with chronic cystic mastitis. *Am J Pathol* 1957;33:1181.
12. Sandison AT. An autopsy study of the adult human breast: with special reference to proliferative epithelial changes of importance in the pathology of the breast. *National Cancer Institute monograph*, vol. 8. Washington: US Department of Health, Education, and Welfare, 1962:1.
13. Humphrey LJ, Swerdlow M. Relationship of benign breast disease to carcinoma of the breast. *Surgery* 1962;52:84.
14. Tellem M, Prive L, Meranze DR. Four-quadrant study of breasts removed for carcinoma. *Cancer* 1962;15:10.
15. Ryan JA, Coady CJ. Intraductal epithelial proliferation in the human breast—a comparative study. *Can J Surg* 1962;5:12.
16. Karpas CM, Leis HP, Oppenheim A, Merscheimer WL. Relationship of fibrocystic disease to carcinoma of the breast. *Ann Surg* 1965;162:1.
17. Humphrey LJ, Swerdlow M. Histologic changes in clinically normal breasts at postmortem examination. *Arch Surg* 1966;92:192.
18. Wellings RR, Jensen HM. On the origin and progression of ductal carcinoma in the human breast. *J Natl Cancer Inst* 1973;50:1111.
19. Wellings SR, Jensen HM, Marcum RG. An atlas of subgross pathology of the human breast with special reference to possible precancerous lesions. *J Natl Cancer Inst* 1975;55:231.
20. Simpson HW, Mutch F, Halberg F, Griffiths K, Wilson D. Bimodal age-frequency distribution of epitheliosis in cancer mastectomies. Relevance to preneoplasia. *Cancer* 1982;50:2417.
21. Mutch F, Simpson HW, Wilson D, Griffiths K, Halberg F. Age distribution of epitheliosis in cancer mastectomies: possible relevance to "false-positive" thermograms. In: *Biomedical thermology*. New York: Alan R. Liss, 1982:313.
22. Bhathal PS, Brown RW, Lesueur GC, Russell IS. Frequency of benign and malignant breast lesions in 207 consecutive autopsies in Australian women. *Br J Cancer* 1985;51:271.
23. Nielsen M, Jensen J, Andersen J. Precancerous and cancerous breast lesions during lifetime and at autopsy. A study of 83 women. *Cancer* 1984;54:612.
24. Nielsen M, Thomsen JL, Primdahl S, Dyreborg U, Andersen JA. Breast cancer and atypia among young and middle-aged women: a study of 110 medicolegal autopsies. *Br J Cancer* 1987;56:814.
25. Alpers CE, Wellings SR. The prevalence of carcinoma in situ in normal and cancer-associated breasts. *Hum Pathol* 1985;16:796.
26. Bartow SA, Pathak DR, Black WC, Key CR, Teaf SR. Prevalence of benign, atypical, and malignant breast lesions in populations at different risk for breast cancer. A forensic autopsy study. *Cancer* 1987;60:2751.

27. Lampejo OT, Barnes DM, Smith P, Millis RR. Evaluation of infiltrating ductal carcinomas with a DCIS component: correlation of the histologic type of the in situ component with grade of the infiltrating component. *Semin Diagn Pathol* 1994;11:215.
28. Wazer DE, Gage I, Horner MJ, Krosnick SH, Schmid C. Age-related differences in patients with nonpalpable breast carcinomas. *Cancer* 1996;78:1432.
29. Davis HH, Simons M, Davis BD. Cystic disease of the breast: relationship to carcinoma. *Cancer* 1964;17:957.
30. Shapiro S, Strax P, Venet L, Fink R. The search for risk factors in breast cancer. *Am J Public Health* 1968;58:820.
31. Black MM, Barclay THC, Cutler SJ, Hankey BF, Asire AJ. Association of atypical characteristics of benign breast lesions with subsequent risk of breast cancer. *Cancer* 1972;29:338.
32. Kodlin D, Winger EE, Morgenstern ML, Chen U. Chronic mastopathy and breast cancer: a follow-up study. *Cancer* 1977;39:2603.
33. Page DL, Zwaag RV, Rogers LW, Williams LT, Walker WE, Hartmann WH. Relation between component parts of fibrocystic disease complex and breast cancer. *J Natl Cancer Inst* 1978;61:1055.
34. Wynder EL, MacCormack FA, Stellman SD. The epidemiology of breast cancer in 785 U.S. Caucasian women. *Cancer* 1978;41:2341.
35. Vessey MP, Doll R, Jones K, McPherson K, Yeates D. An epidemiological study of oral contraceptives and breast cancer. *BMJ* 1979;i: 1755.
36. Brinton LA, Williams RR, Hoover RN, et al. Breast cancer risk factors among screening program participants. *J Natl Cancer Inst* 1979;62:37.
37. Coombs LJ, Lilienfeld AM, Bross IDJ, Burnett WS. A prospective study of the relationship between benign breast diseases and breast carcinoma. *Prev Med* 1979;8:40.
38. Hutchinson WB, Thomas DB, Hamlin WB, Roth GJ, Peterson AV, Williams B. Risk of breast cancer in women with benign breast disease. *J Natl Cancer Inst* 1980;65:13.
39. Paffenbarger RS, Kampert JB, Chang HG. Characteristics that predict risk of breast cancer before and after the menopause. *Am J Epidemiol* 1980;112:258.
40. Lubin JH, Burns PE, Blot WJ. Risk factors for breast cancer in women in Northern Alberta, Canada, as related to age at diagnosis. *J Natl Cancer Inst* 1982;68:211.
41. Roberts MM, Jones V, Elton RA, Fortt RW, Williams S, Gravelle IH. Risk of breast cancer in women with history of benign disease of the breast. *BMJ* 1984;288:275.
42. Dupont WD, Page DL. Risk factors for breast cancer in women with proliferative breast disease. *N Engl J Med* 1985;312:146.
43. Page DL, Dupont WD, Rogers LW, Rados MS. Atypical hyperplastic lesions of the female breast. A long-term follow-up study. *Cancer* 1985;55:2698.
44. Page DL, Dupont WD, Rogers LW. Breast cancer risk of lobular-based hyperplasia after biopsy: "ductal" pattern lesions. *Cancer Detect Prev* 1986;9:441.
45. Carter CL, Corle DK, Micozzi MS, Schatzkin A, Taylor PR. A prospective study of the development of breast cancer in 16,692 women with benign breast disease. *Am J Epidemiol* 1988;128:467.
46. Palli D, del Turco MR, Simoncini R, Bianchi S. Benign breast disease and breast cancer: a case-control study in a cohort in Italy. *Int J Cancer* 1991;47:703.
47. Krieger N, Hiatt RA. Risk of breast cancer after biopsy of benign breast diseases. *Am J Epidemiol* 1992;135:619.
48. McDivitt RW, Stevens JA, Lee NC, Wingo PA, Rubin GL. Histologic types of benign breast disease and the risk for breast cancer. *Cancer* 1992;69:1408–1414.
49. London SJ, Connolly JL, Schnitt SJ, Solditz GA. A prospective study of benign breast disease and the risk of breast cancer. *JAMA* 1992;267:941.
50. Dupont WD, Parl FF, Hartmann WH, et al. Breast cancer risk associated with proliferative breast disease and atypical hyperplasia. *Cancer* 1993;71:1258.
51. Bodian CA, Perzin KH, Lattes R, Hoffmann P, Abernathy G. Prognostic significance of benign proliferative breast disease. *Cancer* 1993;71:3896.
52. Marshall LM, Hunter DJ, Connolly JL, et al. Risk of breast cancer associated with atypical hyperplasia of lobular and ductal types. *Cancer Epidemiol Biomarkers Prev* 1997;6:297.
53. Page DL, Dupont WD, Rogers LW, Landenberger M. Intraductal carcinoma of the breast: follow-up after biopsy only. *Cancer* 1982; 49:751.
54. Rosen PP, Braun DW Jr, Kinne DE. The clinical significance of preinvasive breast carcinomas. *Cancer* 1980;46:919.
55. Haagensen CD. Lobular neoplasia (lobular carcinoma in situ). *Diseases of the breast*, 3rd ed. Philadelphia: WB Saunders, 1986:192.
56. Medina D. Mammary tumors. In: Foster HL, Small DS, Fox JG, eds. *The mouse in biomedical research*. New York: Academic Press, 1982:373.
57. Russo J, Gusterson BA, Rogers AE, Russo IH, Wellings SR, van Zwieten MJ. Comparative study of human and rat mammary tumorigenesis. *Lab Invest* 1990;62:244.
58. Miller FR, Soule HD, Tait L, et al. Xenograft model of progressive human proliferative breast disease. *J Natl Cancer Inst* 1993;85:1725.
59. O'Connell P, Pekkel V, Fuqua S, Osborne CK, Allred DC. Molecular genetic studies of early breast cancer evolution. *Breast Cancer Res Treat* 1994;32:5.
60. O'Connell P, Pekkel V, Fuqua SAW, Osborne CK, Allred DC. Analysis of loss of heterozygosity in 399 premalignant breast lesions at 15 genetic loci. *J Natl Cancer Inst* 1998;90:697.
61. Lakhani SR, Collins N, Sloane JP, Stratton MR. Loss of heterozygosity in lobular carcinoma in situ. *J Clin Pathol* 1995;48:M74.
62. Rosenberg CL, Larson PS, Romo JD, De Las Morenas A, Faller DV. Microsatellite alterations indicating monoclonality in atypical hyperplasias associated with breast cancer. *Hum Pathol* 1997;28:214.
63. Bestill WL Jr, Rosen PP, Lieberman PH, Robbins GF. Intraductal carcinoma. Long-term follow-up after treatment by biopsy alone. *JAMA* 1978;239:1863.
64. Berardo MD, O'Connell POC, Allred DC. Biologic characteristics of premalignant and preinvasive breast disease. In: Pasqualini JR, Katzenellenbogen BS, eds. *Hormone-dependent cancer*. New York: Marcel Dekker, 1996:1.
65. Allred DC, Berardo DM, Prosser J, O'Connell P. Biologic and genetic features of in situ breast cancer. In: Silverstein MJ, ed. *Ductal carcinoma in situ of the breast*. Williams & Wilkins, 1997:37.
66. Rudland PS. Epithelial stem cells and their possible role in the development of the normal and diseased breast. *Histol Histopathol* 1993; 8:385.
67. Meyer JS. Cell proliferation in normal human breast ducts, fibroadenomas, and other ductal hyperplasias measured by nuclear labeling with tritiated thymidine. *Hum Pathol* 1977;8:67.
68. Ferguson DJP, Anderson TJ. Morphological evaluation of cell turnover in relation to the menstrual cycle in the "resting" human breast. *Br J Cancer* 1981;44:177.
69. Joshi K, Smith JA, Perusinghe N, Monoghan P. Cell proliferation in the human mammary epithelium: differential contribution by epithelial and myoepithelial cells. *Am J Pathol* 1986;124:199.
70. Longacre TA, Bartow SA. A correlative morphologic study of human breast and endometrium in the menstrual cycle. *Am J Surg Pathol* 1986;10:382.
71. Russo J, Calaf GRL, Russo IH. Influence of age and gland topography on cell kinetics of normal breast tissue. *J Natl Cancer Inst* 1987; 78:413.
72. Going JJ, Anderson TJ, Battersby S, Macintyre CCA. Proliferative and secretory activity in human breast during natural and artificial cycles. *Am J Pathol* 1988;130:193.
73. Potten CS, Watson RJ, Williams GT, et al. The effect of age and menstrual cycle upon proliferative activity of the normal human breast. *Br J Cancer* 1988;58:163.
74. Kamel OW, Franklin WA, Ringus JC, Meyer JS. Thymidine labeling index and Ki-67 growth fraction in lesions of the breast. *Am J Pathol* 1989;134:107.
75. Schmitt FC. Multistep progression from an oestrogen-dependent growth towards an autonomous growth in breast carcinogenesis. *Eur J Cancer* 1995;31A:2049.
76. Visscher DW, Gingrich DS, Buckley J, Tabaczka P, Crissman JD. Cell cycle analysis of normal, atrophic, and hyperplastic breast epithelium using two-color multiparametric flow cytometry. *Anal Cell Pathol* 1996;12:115.
77. Prosser J, Hilsenbeck SG, Fuqua SAW, O'Connell P, Osborne CK, Allred DC. Cell turnover (proliferation and apoptosis) in normal epithelium and premalignant lesions in the same breast. *Lab Invest* 1997;76:119(abst).
78. Meyer JS, Bauer WC. Tritiated thymidine labeling index of benign and malignant human breast epithelium. *J Surg Oncol* 1976;8:165.
79. Masters JRW, Drife JO, Scarisbrick JJ. Cyclic variation of DNA synthesis in human breast epithelium. *J Natl Cancer Inst* 1977;58:1263.

80. Anderson TJ, Ferguson DJP, Raab GM. Cell turnover in the "resting" human breast: influence of parity, contraceptive pill, age and laterality. *Br J Cancer* 1982;46:376.
81. Anderson TJ, Battersby S, King RJB, McPherson K, Going JJ. Oral contraceptive use influences resting breast proliferation. *Hum Pathol* 1989;20:1139.
82. Olsson H, Jernstrom H, Alm P, et al. Proliferation of the breast epithelium in relation to menstrual cycle phase, hormonal use, and reproductive factors. *Breast Cancer Res Treat* 1996;40:187.
83. Soderqvist G, Isaksson E, Von Schoultz B, Carlstrom K, Tani E, Skoog L. Proliferation of breast epithelial cells in healthy women during the menstrual cycle. *Am J Obstet Gynecol* 1997;176:123.
84. Lelle RJ, Heidenreich W, Stauch G, Wecke I, Gerdes J. Determination of growth fractions in benign breast disease (BBD) with monoclonal antibody Ki-67. *J Cancer Res Clin Oncol* 1987;113:73.
85. Meyer JS, Connor RE. Cell proliferation in fibrocystic disease and postmenopausal breast ducts measured by thymidine labeling. *Cancer* 1982;50:746.
86. Thomas DB. Do hormones cause cancer? *Cancer* 1984;53:595.
87. King RJB. A discussion of the roles of oestrogen and progestin in human mammary carcinogenesis. *J Steroid Biochem Mol Biol* 1991;39:811.
88. King RJB. Estrogen and progestin effects in human breast carcinogenesis. *Breast Cancer Res Treat* 1993;27:3.
89. Pike MC, Spicer DV, Dahmoush L, Press MF. Estrogens, progestins, normal breast cell proliferation, and breast cancer risk. *Epidemiol Rev* 1993;15:17.
90. Henderson BE, Ross R, Bernstein L. Estrogens as a cause of human cancer: the Richard and Hindau Rosenthal Foundation Award Lecture. *Cancer Res* 1988;48:246.
91. De Potter CR, Praet MM, Slavin RE, Verbeeck P, Roels HJ. Feulgen DNA content and mitotic activity in proliferative breast disease: a comparison with ductal carcinoma in situ. *Histopathology* 1987;7:1307
92. Hoshi K, Tokunaga M, Mochizuki M, et al. Pathological characterization of atypical ductal hyperplasia of the breast. *Jpn J Cancer Chemotherapy* 1995;22[Suppl 1]:36.
93. Meyer JS. Cell kinetics of histologic variants of in situ breast carcinoma. *Breast Cancer Res Treat* 1986;7:171.
94. Locker AP, Horrocks C, Gilmour AS, et al. Flow cytometric and histological analysis of ductal carcinoma in situ of the breast. *Br J Surg* 1990;77:564.
95. Poller DN, Silverstein MJ, Galea M, et al. Ductal carcinoma in situ of the breast: a proposal for a new simplified histological classification association between cellular proliferation and c-erbB-2 protein expression. *Mod Pathol* 1994;7:257.
96. Bobrow LG, Happerfield LC, Gregory WM, Springall RD, Millis RR. The classification of ductal carcinoma in situ and its association with biological markers. *Semin Diagn Pathol* 1994;11:199.
97. Zafrani B, Leroyer A, Fourquet A, et al. Mammographically detected ductal in situ carcinoma of the breast analyzed with a new classification. A study of 127 cases: correlation with estrogen and progesterone receptors, p53, and c-erbB-2 proteins, and proliferative activity. *Semin Diagn Pathol* 1994;11:208.
98. Albonico G, Querzoli P, Feretti S, Magri E, Nenci I. Biophenotypes of breast carcinoma in situ defined by image analysis of biological parameters. *Pathol Res Pract* 1996;192:117.
99. Berardo M, Hilsenbeck SG, Allred DC. Histological grading of noninvasive breast cancer and its relationship to biological features. *Lab Invest* 1996;74:68.
100. Fisher ER, Costantino J, Fisher B, et al. Pathologic findings from the National Surgical Adjuvant Breast Project (NSABP) protocol B-17. *Cancer* 1996;78:1403.
101. Rudas M, Neumayer R, Gnant M, Mittelbock M, Jakesz R, Reiner A. p53 protein expression, cell proliferation and steroid hormone receptors in ductal and lobular in situ carcinomas of the breast. *Eur J Cancer* 1997;33:39.
102. Libby AL, O'Connell P, Allred DC. Lobular carcinoma in situ: biologic features including loss of heterozygosity. *Mod Pathol* 1998;11:22A.
103. Kobayashi S, Iwase H, Itoh Y, et al. Estrogen receptor, c-erB-2 and nm23/NDP kinase expression in the intraductal and invasive components of human breast cancers. *Jpn J Cancer Res* 1992;83:859.
104. Osborne CK. Receptors. In: Harris JR, Hellman S, Henderson IC, Kinne DW, eds. *Breast diseases*. Philadelphia: JB Lippincott, 1991:301.
105. Fuqua SAW. Estrogen and progesterone receptors and breast cancer. In: Harris JR, Lippman ME, Morrow M, Hellman S, eds. *Diseases of the breast*. Philadelphia: Lippincott-Raven, 1996:301.
106. Horwitz KB, Jackson TA, Bain DL, Richer JK, Takimoto GS, Tung L. Nuclear receptor coactivators and corepressors. *Mol Endocrinol* 1996;10:1167.
107. Allegra JC, Lippman ME, Green L, et al. Estrogen receptor values in patients with benign breast disease. *Cancer* 1979;44:228.
108. Peterson OW, Hoyer PE, van Deurs B. Frequency and distribution of estrogen receptor-positive cells in normal, nonlactating human breast tissue. *J Natl Cancer Inst* 1986;77:343.
109. Ricketts D, Turnbull L, Tyall G, et al. Estrogen and progesterone receptors in the normal female breast. *Cancer Res* 1991;51:1817.
110. Markopoulos C, Berder U, Wilson P, Gazet JC, Coombes RC. Oestrogen receptor content of normal breast cells and breast carcinoma throughout the menstrual cycle. *BMJ* 1988;296:1149.
111. Williams G, Anderson E, Howell A, et al. Oral contraceptive (OCP) use increases proliferation and decreases oestrogen receptor content of epithelial cells in the normal human breast. *Int J Cancer* 1991;48:206.
112. Battersby S, Robertson BJ, Anderson TJ, King RJB, McPherson K. Influence of menstrual cycle, parity, and oral contraceptive use on steroid hormone receptors in normal breast. *Br J Cancer* 1992;65:601.
113. Giri DD, Dundas AC, Nottingham JF, Underwood JCE. Oestrogen receptors in benign epithelial lesions and intraduct carcinomas of the breast: an immunohistological study. *Histopathology* 1989;15:575.
114. Barnes R, Masood S. Potential value of hormone receptor assay in carcinoma in situ of breast. *Am J Clin Pathol* 1990;94:533.
115. Helin HJ, Helle MJ, Kallioneimi OP, Isona JJ. Immunohistochemical determination of estrogen and progesterone receptors in human breast carcinoma: correlation with histopathology and DNA flow cytometry. *Cancer* 1989;63:1761.
116. Pallis L, Wilking N, Cedermark B, Rutqvist LE, Skoog L. Receptors for estrogen and progesterone in breast carcinoma in situ. *Anticancer Res* 1992;12:2113.
117. Poller DN, Snead DRJ, Roberts EC, et al. Oestrogen receptor expression in ductal carcinoma in situ of the breast: relationship to flow cytometric analysis of DNA and expression of the c-erbB-2 oncoprotein. *Br J Cancer* 1993;68:156.
118. Chaudhuri B, Crist KA, Mucci S, Malafa M, Chaudhuri PK. Distribution of estrogen receptor in ductal carcinoma in situ of the breast. *Surgery* 1993;113:134.
119. Leal CB, Schmitt FC, Bento MJ, Maia NC, Lopes CS. Ductal carcinoma in situ of the breast. Histologic categorization and its relationship to ploidy and immunohistochemical expression of hormone receptors, p53, and c-erbB-2 protein. *Cancer* 1995;75:2123.
120. Karayiannakis AJ, Bastounis EA, Chatzigianni EB, Makri GG, Alexiou D, Karamanakos P. Immunohistochemical detection of oestrogen receptors in ductal carcinoma in situ of the breast. *Eur J Surg Oncol* 1996;22:578.
121. Bose S, Lesser ML, Norton L, Rosen PP. Immunophenotype of intraductal carcinoma. *Arch Pathol Lab Med* 1996;120:81.
122. Pertschuk LP, Kim DS, Nayer K, et al. Immunocytochemical estrogen and progestin receptor assays in breast cancer with monoclonal antibodies. *Cancer* 1990;66:1663.
123. Fuqua SAW, Wiltschke C, Lemieux P, et al. A "hyperactive" estrogen receptor variant in hyperplastic breast lesions. *Lab Invest* 1996;74:15A.
124. Fisher B, Costantino JP, Wickerham DL, et al. Tamoxifen for prevention of breast cancer: report of the National Surgical Adjuvant Breast and Bowel Project P-1 study. *J Natl Cancer Inst* 1998;90:1371.
125. De Potter CR, Schelfheut AM. The neu-protein and breast cancer. *Virchows Arch* 1995;426:107.
126. Ravdin PM, Chamness GC. The c-erbB-2 proto-oncogene as a prognostic and predictive marker in breast cancer: a paradigm for the development of other macromolecular markers—a review. *Gene* 1995;159:19.
127. Borg A, Baldetorp B, Ferno M, Killander D, Olsson H, Sigurdsson H. ERBB2 amplification in breast cancer with a high rate of proliferation. *Oncogene* 1991;6:137.
128. Kallioniemi OP, Holli K, Visakorpi T, Koivula T, Helin HH, Isola JJ. Association of c-erbB-2 protein over-expression with high rate of cell proliferation, increased risk of visceral metastasis, and poor long-term survival in breast cancer. *Int J Cancer* 1991;49:650.
129. Tommasi S, Paradiso A, Mangia A, et al. Biological correlation between HER-2/neu and proliferative activity in human breast cancer. *Anticancer Res* 1991;11:1395.

130. Allred DC, Clark GM, Tandon AK, et al. HER-2/neu in node-negative breast cancer: prognostic significance of overexpression influenced by the presence of in situ carcinoma. *J Clin Oncol* 1992;10:599.
131. De Potter CR. The neu-oncogene: more than a prognostic factor? *Hum Pathol* 1994;25:1264.
132. Venter DJ, Tuzi NL, Kumar S, Gullick WJ. Overexpression of the c-erbB-2 oncoprotein in human breast carcinomas: immunohistological assessment correlates with gene amplification. *Lancet* 1987;2:69.
133. Gusterson BA, Machin LG, Gullick WJ, et al. c-erbB-2 expression in benign and malignant breast disease. *Br J Cancer* 1988;58:453.
134. De Potter CR, van Daele S, van de Vijer MJ, et al. The expression of the neu oncogene product in breast lesions and in normal fetal and adult human tissues. *Histopathology* 1989;15:351.
135. Allred DC, Clark GM, Molina R, et al. Overexpression of HER-2/neu and its relationship with other prognostic factors change during the progression of in situ to invasive breast cancer. *Hum Pathol* 1992;23:974.
136. Lodato RF, Maguire HC Jr, Greene MI, Weiner DB, LeVolsi VA. Immunohistochemical evaluation of c-erbB-2 oncogene expression in ductal carcinoma in situ and atypical ductal hyperplasia of the breast. *Mod Pathol* 1990;3:449.
137. van de Vijer MJ, Peterse JL, Mooi WJ, et al. neu-Protein overexpression in breast cancer. Association with comedo-type ductal carcinoma in situ and limited prognostic value in stage II breast cancer. *N Engl J Med* 1988;319:1239.
138. Bartkova J, Barnes DM, Millis RR, Gullick WJ. Immunohistochemical demonstration of c-erbB-2 protein in mammary ductal carcinoma in situ. *Hum Pathol* 1990;21:1164.
139. Ramachandra S, Machin L, Ashley S, Monaghan P, Gusterson BA. Immunohistochemical distribution of c-erbB-2 in in situ breast carcinoma: a detailed morphological analysis. *J Pathol* 1990;161:7.
140. Walker RA, Dearing SJ, Lane DP, Varley JM. Expression of p53 protein in infiltrating and in-situ breast carcinomas. *J Pathol* 1991;165:203.
141. Barnes DM, Meyer JS, Gonzalez JG, Gullick WJ, Millis RR. Relationship between c-erbB-2 immunoreactivity and thymidine labelling index in breast carcinoma in situ. *Breast Cancer Res Treat* 1991;18:11.
142. Schimmelpenning H, Eriksson ET, Pallis L, Skoog L, Cedermark B, Auer GU. Immunohistochemical c-erbB-2 proto-oncogene expression and nuclear DNA content in human mammary carcinoma in situ. *Am J Clin Pathol* 1992;97[Suppl]:S48.
143. Somerville JE, Clarke LA, Biggart JD. c-erbB-2 overexpression and histological type of in situ and invasive breast carcinomas. *J Clin Pathol* 1992;45:16.
144. Barnes DM, Bartkova J, Camplejohn RS, Gullick WJ, Smith PJ, Millis RR. Overexpression of the c-erbB-2 oncoprotein: Why does this occur more frequently in ductal carcinoma in situ than in invasive mammary carcinoma and is this of prognostic significance? *Eur J Cancer* 1992;28:644.
145. De Potter CR, Foschini MP, Schelfhout AM, Schroeter CA, Eusebi V. Immunohistochemical study of neu protein overexpression in clinging in situ duct carcinoma of the breast. *Virchows Arch* 1993;422:375.
146. Tsuda H, Iwaya K, Fukutomi T, Hiroshashi S. p53 Mutations and c-erbB-2 amplification in intraductal and invasive breast carcinomas of high histologic grade. *Jpn J Cancer Res* 1993;84:394.
147. De Potter CR, Schelfhout AM, Verbeeck P, et al. neu-Overexpression correlates with extent of disease in large cell ductal carcinoma in situ of the breast. *Hum Pathol* 1995;26:601.
148. Porter PL, Garcia R, Moe R, Corwin DJ, Gown AM. c-erbB-2 oncogene protein in in situ and invasive lobular breast neoplasia. *Cancer* 1991;68:331.
149. Midulla C, Giovagnoli MR, Valli C, Vecchione A. Correlation between ploidy status, ERB-B2 and P53 immunohistochemical expression in primary breast carcinoma. *Anal Quant Cytol Histol* 1995;17:157.
150. Fabian CJ, Zalles C, Kamel S, Zeiger S, Simon C, Kimler BF. Breast cytology and biomarkers obtained by random fine needle aspiration: use in risk assessment and early chemoprevention trials. *J Cell Biochem Suppl* 1997;28:29.
151. Rohan TE, Hartwick W, Miller AB, Kandel RA. Immunohistochemical detection of c-erbB-2 and p53 in benign breast disease and breast cancer risk. *J Natl Cancer Inst* 1998;90:1262.
152. Levine AJ. p53, the cellular gatekeeper for growth and division. *Cell* 1997;88:323.
153. Harris CC, Hollstein M. Clinical implications of the p53 tumor-suppressor gene. *N Engl J Med* 1993;329:1318.
154. Chang F, Syrjanen S, Syrjanen K. Implications of the p53 tumor-suppressor gene in clinical oncology. *J Clin Oncol* 1995;13:1009.
155. Bartek J, Bartkova J, Vojtesek B, et al. Patterns of expression of the p53 tumor suppressor in human breast tissues and tumors in situ and in vitro. *Int J Cancer* 1990;46:839.
156. Davidoff AM, Humphrey PA, Iglehart JD, Marks JR. Genetic basis for p53 overexpression in human breast cancer. *Proc Natl Acad Sci U S A* 1991;88:5006.
157. Elledge RM, Allred DC. The p53 tumor suppressor gene in breast cancer. *Breast Cancer Res Treat* 1994;32:39.
158. Soussi T, Legros Y, Lubin R, Ory K, Schlichthols B. Multifactorial analysis of p53 alteration in human breast cancer: a review. *Int J Cancer* 1994;57:1.
159. Allred DC, Elledge R, Clark GM, Fuqua SAW. The p53 tumor suppressor gene in human breast cancer. In: Dickson RB, Lippman ME, eds. *Mammary tumorigenesis and malignant progression.* Boston: Kluwer Academic, 1994:63.
160. Barnes DM, Hanby AM, Gillett CE, et al. Abnormal expression of wild type p53 protein in normal cells of a cancer family patient. *Lancet* 1992;340:259.
161. Thor AD, Moore DHI, Edgerton SM, et al. Accumulation of p53 tumor suppressor gene protein: an independent marker of prognosis in breast cancers. *J Natl Cancer Inst* 1992;34:345.
162. Davidoff AM, Kerns B-JM, Pence JC, Marks JR, Iglehart JD. p53 alterations in all stages of breast cancer. *J Surg Oncol* 1991;48:260.
163. Eriksson ET, Schmmelpenning H, Aspenblad U, Zetterberg A, Auer GU. Immunohistochemical expression of the mutant p53 protein and nuclear DNA content during the transition from benign to malignant breast disease. *Hum Pathol* 1994;25:1228.
164. Allred DC, Clark GC, Elledge R, et al. Association of p53 protein expression with tumor proliferation rate and clinical outcome in node-negative breast cancer. *J Natl Cancer Inst* 1993;35:200.
165. Umekita Y, Takasaki T, Yoshida H. Expression of p53 protein in benign epithelial hyperplasia, atypical ductal hyperplasia, non-invasive and invasive mammary carcinoma: an immunohistochemical study. *Virchows Arch* 1994;424:491.
166. Chitemere M, Andersen TI, Hom R, Karlsen F, Borresen A-L, Nesland JM. TP53 alterations atypical ductal hyperplasia and ductal carcinoma in situ of the breast. *Breast Cancer Res Treat* 1996;41:103.
167. Rajan PB, Scott DJ, Perry RH, Griffith CDM. p53 protein expression in ductal carcinoma in situ (DCIS) of the breast. *Breast Cancer Res Treat* 1997;42:283.
168. Poller DN, Roberts EC, Bell JA, Elston CW, Blamey RW, Ellis IO. p53 protein expression in mammary ductal carcinoma in situ: relationship to immunohistochemical expression of estrogen receptor and c-erbB-2 protein. *Hum Pathol* 1993;24:463.
169. O'Malley FP, Vnencak-Jones CL, Dupont WD, Parl F, Manning S, Page DL. p53 mutations are confined to the comedo type ductal carcinoma in situ of the breast: immunohistochemical and sequencing data. *Lab Invest* 1994;71:67.
170. Schmitt FC, Leal D, Lopes C. p53 protein expression and nuclear DNA content in breast intraductal proliferations. *J Pathol* 1995;176:233.
171. Siziopikou KP, Prioleau JE, Harris JR, Schnitt SJ. Bcl-2 expression in the spectrum of preinvasive breast lesions. *Cancer* 1996;77:499.
172. Domagala W, Markiewski M, Kubiak R, Bartkowiak J, Osborn M. Immunohistochemical profile of invasive lobular carcinoma of the breast: predominantly vimentin and p53 protein negative, cathepsin D and oestrogen receptor positive. *Virchows Arch* 1993;423:497.
173. Querzoli P, Albonico G, Ferretti S, et al. Modulation of biomarkers in minimal breast carcinoma: a model for human breast carcinoma progression. *Cancer* 1998;83:89.
174. Allred DC, Hilsenbeck SG. Biomarkers in benign breast disease: risk factors for breast cancer. *J Natl Cancer Inst* 1998;90:1247–1248.
175. Deng G, Lu Y, Zlotnikov G, Thor AD, Smith HS. Loss of heterozygosity in normal tissue adjacent to breast carcinomas. *Science* 1996; 274:2057.
176. Lakhani SR, Collins N, Stratton MR, Sloane JP. Atypical ductal hyperplasia of the breast: clonal proliferation with loss of heterozygosity on chromosomes 16q and 17p. *J Clin Pathol* 1995;48:611.
177. Lakhani SR, Slack DN, Hamoudi RA, Collins N, Stratton MR, Sloane JP. Detection of allelic imbalance indicates that a proportion of mammary hyperplasia of usual type are clonal neoplastic proliferations. *Lab Invest* 1996;74:129.
178. Kasami M, Vnencak-Jones CL, Manning S, Dupont WD, Page DL. Loss of heterozygosity and microsatellite instability in breast hyper-

plasia. No obligate correlation of these genetic alterations with subsequent malignancy. *Am J Pathol* 1997;150:1925.
179. Chauqui RF, Zhuang Z, Emmert-Buck MR, Liotta LA, Merino MJ. Analysis of loss of heterozygosity on chromosome 11q13 in atypical ductal hyperplasia and in situ carcinoma of the breast. *Am J Pathol* 1997;150:297.
180. Noguchi S, Aihara T, Koyama H, Motomura K, Inaji H, Imaoka S. Clonal analysis of benign and malignant human breast tumors by means of polymerase chain reaction. *Cancer Lett* 1995;90:57.
181. Carpenter R, Gibbs N, Matthews J, Cooke T. Importance of cellular DNA content in premalignant breast disease and pre-invasive carcinoma of the female breast. *Br J Surg* 1987;74:905.
182. Radford DM, Fair K, Thompson AM, et al. Allelic loss on chromosome 17 in ductal carcinoma in situ of the breast. *Cancer Res* 1993;53:2947.
183. Radford DM, Fair KL, Phillips NJ, Ritter JH, Steinbrueck T, Holt MS. Allelotyping of ductal carcinoma in situ of the breast: deletion of loci on 8p, 13q, 16q, 17p and 17q. *Cancer Res* 1995;55:3399.
184. Aldaz CM, Chen T, Sahin A, Cunningham J, Bondy M. Comparative allelotype of in situ and invasive human breast cancer: high frequency of microsatellite instability in lobular breast carcinomas. *Cancer Res* 1995;55:3976.
185. Munn KE, Walker RA, Varley JM. Frequent alterations of chromosome 1 in ductal carcinoma in situ of the breast. *Oncogene* 1995;10:1653.
186. Stratton MR, Collins N, Lakhani SR, Sloane JP. Loss of heterozygosity in ductal carcinoma in situ of the breast. *J Pathol* 1995;175:195.
187. Fujii H, Marsh C, Cairns P, Sidransky D, Gabrielson E. Genetic divergence in the clonal evolution of breast cancer. *Cancer Res* 1996;56:1493.
188. Man S, Ellis IO, Sibbering M, Blamey RW, Brook JD. High levels of allele loss at the FHIT and ATM genes in non-comedo ductal carcinoma in situ and grade I tubular invasive breast cancers. *Cancer Res* 1996;56:5484.
189. Chen T, Sahin A, Aldaz CM. Deletion map of chromosome 16q in ductal carcinoma in situ of the breast: refining a putative tumor suppressor gene region. *Cancer Res* 1996;56:5605.
190. Chappell SA, Walsh T, Walker RA, Shaw JA. Loss of heterozygosity at chromosome 6q in preinvasive and early invasive breast carcinomas. *Br J Cancer* 1997;75:1324.
191. Fujii H, Szumel R, Marsh C, Zhou W, Gabrielson E. Genetic progression, histologic grade, and allelic loss in ductal carcinoma in situ of the breast. *Cancer Res* 1996;56:5260.
192. Berx G, Cleton-Jansen A-M, Nollet F, et al. E-cadherin is a tumour/invasion suppressor gene mutated in human lobular breast cancers. *EMBO J* 1995;14:6107.
193. Levine AJ, Mamand J, Finlay CA. The p53 tumor suppressor gene. *Nature* 1991;351:453.
194. Gutmann D, Wood D, Collins F. Identification of the neurofibromatosis type 1 gene product. *Proc Natl Acad Sci U S A* 1991;88:9658.
195. Friedman LS, Ostermeyer EA, Lynch ED, et al. The search for BRCA1. *Cancer Res* 1994;54:6374.
196. Nayar R, Zhuang Z, Merino MJ, Silverberg SG. Loss of heterozygosity on chromosome 11q13 in lobular lesions of the breast using tissue microdissection and polymerase chain reaction. *Hum Pathol* 1997;28:277.
197. Radford DM, Phillips NJ, Fair KL, Ritter JH, Holt M, Donis-Keller H. Allelic loss and the progression of breast cancer. *Cancer Res* 1995;55:5180.
198. Zhuang Z, Merino MJ, Chuaqua R, Liotta LA, Emmert-Buck MR. Identical allelic loss on chromosome 11q13 in microdissected in situ and invasive human breast cancer. *Cancer Res* 1995;55:467.
199. Ahmadian M, Wistuba II, Fong KM, et al. Analysis of the FHIT gene and FRA3B regions in sporadic breast cancer, preneoplastic lesions, and familial breast cancer probands. *Cancer Res* 1997;57:3664.
200. Dillon EK, de Boer WB, Papadimitrious JM, Turbett GR. Microsatellite instability and loss of heterozygosity in mammary carcinoma and its probable precursors. *Br J Cancer* 1997;76:156.
201. Peters G, Fantl V, Smith R, Brookes S, Dickson C. Chromosome 11q13 markers and D-type cyclins in breast cancer. *Breast Cancer Res Treat* 1995;33:125.
202. Lee W-H, Bookstein R, Hong F, Young L-J, Shew J-Y, Lee EY-H. Human retinoblastoma susceptibility gene: cloning, identification, and sequence. *Science* 1987;235:1394.
203. Wooster R, Neuhausen SL, Magnion J. Localization of a breast cancer susceptibility gene, BRCA2, to chromosome 13q12-13. *Science* 1994;265:2088.
204. Murphy DS, McHardy P, Coutts J, et al. Interphase cytogenetic analysis of cerB2 and topoII-alpha co-amplification in invasive breast cancer and polysomy of chromosome 17 in ductal carcinoma in situ. *Int J Cancer* 1995;64:18.
205. Murphy DS, Hoare SF, Going JJ, et al. Characterization of extensive genetic alterations in ductal carcinoma in situ by fluorescence in situ hybridization and molecular analysis. *J Natl Cancer Inst* 1995; 87:1694.
206. Visscher DW, Wallis TL, Crissman JD. Evaluation of chromosome aneuploidy in tissue sections of preinvasive breast carcinomas using interphase cytogenetics. *Cancer* 1996;77:315.
207. Kuukasjarvi T, Minna T, Pennanen S, Karhu R, Kallioniemi O-P, Isola J. Genetic changes in intraductal breast cancer detected by comparative genomic hybridization. *Am J Pathol* 1997;150:1465.
208. James LA, Mitchell ELD, Menasce L, Varley JM. Comparative genomic hybridisation of ductal carcinoma in situ of the breast: identification of regions of DNA amplification and deletion in common with invasive breast carcinoma. *Oncogene* 1997;14:1059.
209. Bonner RF, Emmert-Buck M, Cole K, et al. Laser capture microdissection: molecular analysis of tissue. *Science* 1977;278:1481.
210. Dawson PJ, Wolman SR, Tait L, Heppner GH, Miller FR. MCF10AT: a model for the evolution of cancer from proliferative breast disease. *Am J Pathol* 1996;148:313.

Diseases of the Breast, 2nd ed.,
edited by Jay R. Harris.
Lippincott Williams & Wilkins, Philadelphia © 2000.

CHAPTER 25

Control of Invasion and Metastasis

W. Nils Brünner, Ross W. Stephens, and Keld Danø

The extracellular matrix, including the basement membranes, is essential for the architecture of the organism as a whole, as well as for individual organs and tissues. Throughout life, a number of physiologic and pathologic events involve degradation of the extracellular matrix. One example is embryo implantation, in which the placental trophoblasts actively invade the uterine wall. Several studies have shown that the expression of matrix-degrading protease systems during trophoblast invasion closely resembles that seen during cancer cell invasion,[1,2] including the expression of related components in different cell types—for example, urokinase plasminogen activator (uPA) and gelatinase B (Gel B) in trophoblasts—whereas plasminogen activator inhibitor (PAI-1) and tissue inhibitor of metalloproteinase (TIMP-1) are found in decidual cells. Another example of nonmalignant tissue remodeling is involution of the mammary gland after lactation.[3] The major difference between nonmalignant and malignant tissue remodeling appears not to be in the proteolytic mechanisms as such, but in a lack of normal regulation of this process in cancer, resulting in a continuous and self-perpetuating tissue destruction.

During the process of invasion, cancer cells degrade and traverse the first barrier represented by the basement membrane, and it is thus a prerequisite that cancers arising in epithelial tissues either acquire the ability themselves to secrete proteolytic enzymes that can cleave basement membrane proteins or induce production of the required proteases in the normal tissue cells that are progressively recruited into the tumor stroma. Thus, certain proteases are highly expressed in tumor tissue, including members of the serine protease family (e.g., uPA), the metalloprotease family (matrix metalloproteases, MMPs), and a number of cysteine proteases.

The level of expression of components of the different protease systems and the cellular pattern of their expression are important in the invasive process. Increased expression of serine proteases and metalloproteases has been demonstrated to be responsible for tumor invasion in several *in vivo* models. It is also significant that both classes of enzymes are often expressed in the same cells in tumor tissue *in vivo*, even in cases such as breast cancer, in which the stromal cells are the main source of proteases.[4] Furthermore, the level of uPA and some MMPs in human tumors has been shown to have significant prognostic value in predicting which patients will fare worse from the progress of their cancer,[5,6] apparently because the levels of both types of proteases are related to the invasive capacity of the tumor *in vivo*. However, the relative importance and relationship between the various proteases in tumor-directed tissue remodeling remain unclear. The task becomes even more complex with the discovery of an increasing number of MMPs—for example, the membrane-type MMPs. Studies of protease-deficient transgenic mice (see Serine Proteases) suggest that a certain degree of functional overlap exists between different protease systems.

A detailed and comprehensive review of all studies on matrix-degrading protease systems in breast cancer is beyond the scope of this chapter. For a full and detailed discussion of all the biological and clinical aspects of proteases in breast cancer, the reader is referred to specific reviews.[6–8] This chapter focuses on protease systems involved in breast cancer progression, with special emphasis on the value of these molecules as prognostic markers.

PROTEASE SYSTEMS INVOLVED IN INVASION AND METASTASIS

The role of proteases in cancer invasion can be described as a deregulated version of the role that they would normally perform in physiologic remodeling processes in the corresponding normal tissue (reviewed elsewhere[9]). Thus, it is proposed that the involvement of proteases in breast cancer invasion is not unlike the concerted action they perform in breast involution subsequent to cessation of lactation.[3] The types of proteases involved in the two processes are closely similar. In cancer tissue, their expression may be found in the nonneoplastic stromal cells as well as the cancer cells (see

W. N. Brünner: Finsen Laboratory, Copenhagen, Denmark
R. W. Stephens: Finsen Laboratory, Copenhagen, Denmark
K. Danø: Finsen Laboratory, Copenhagen, Denmark

Cellular Localization of Proteases, Their Receptors, and Inhibitors in Breast Cancer), and in both processes a certain component is often expressed by the same cell type—that is, in both cases in epithelial cells or in both cases in fibroblasts.

The classes of matrix-degrading proteases expressed in breast cancer tissue are the following:

1. Serine proteases, particularly the uPA/plasmin system[7,10]
2. MMPs, particularly MMP-9 and MMP-3[6]
3. Cysteine proteases, particularly cathepsin B[8]
4. Aspartic acid proteases, such as cathepsin D[11]

Although each of these types of proteases has a preferred substrate, such as plasmin-degrading fibrin, it is becoming apparent that there may be considerable overlap in function between the different classes so that, for example, fibrin may also be degraded by MMPs,[12] including the membrane-type MMPs.[13] The activation of cytokines and growth factors, the release of such molecules from the cell surface[14] or the extracellular matrix,[15] or both, also represents important functions of some of these proteases.

Serine Proteases

Serine proteases are a class of enzymes from which the highly specific plasminogen activators and their broad-spectrum protease plasmin product have long been implicated in the tissue degradation of tumor invasion.[16] Although it is the tissue-type plasminogen activator that functions mainly in intravascular surveillance of sites of thrombosis, uPA appears to be the principal extravascular activator, which is often overexpressed in cancer tissue and during nonneoplastic tissue remodeling.

The important role of the plasminogen activation system in tissue remodeling has been directly demonstrated by wound-healing experiments in mice that were rendered plasminogen deficient by targeted gene inactivation.[17] Wound healing is delayed in these mice, which indicates that keratinocytes migrating to cover the wound need to proteolytically dissect their way through the fibrin-rich wound site. The healing is not stopped altogether, however, suggesting that other proteases can carry out the same function(s) as plasmin. A similar delay in tissue remodeling has now been found in breast involution in plasminogen-deficient mice (L. R. Lund, *personal communication*, 1999) In these mice there is also reduced metastasis of a genetically induced breast tumor. Mice that carry the polyoma middle T oncogene under control of the mouse mammary tumor virus promoter all develop mammary cancer, which in all cases metastasizes to the lung. In plasminogen-deficient mice, lung metastasis is substantially delayed but does eventually occur. In contrast, growth of the primary tumor is independent of the plasminogen status of the host animals, and the delay in metastasis is probably caused by a delay in invasion.[18]

The urokinase receptor (uPAR) is a 55-kd, three-domain glycoprotein attached to the cell membrane by a glycolipid anchor extending from the carboxy terminal of domain 3.[10,19] uPAR binds uPA, and its inactive proenzyme form with high affinity (k_d approximately 1 nM), thus localizing them at the interface of the cell surface with adhesion proteins of the extracellular matrix, particularly vitronectin, which also binds to uPAR.[19–21] At this location, uPAR also positions uPA and pro-uPA in close proximity to plasmin(ogen), which is bound to the cell surface and matrix proteins by low-affinity lysine-binding sites in the kringle domains. This produces an acceleration of both the plasmin activation of bound pro-uPA and the uPA-catalyzed activation of bound plasminogen.[19–22] A notable feature of this assembly of bound enzyme components is that the bound plasmin is protected from inhibition by antiplasmins[22] and thus is able to facilitate cell detachment and migration by cleaving a broad spectrum of adhesion proteins, proteoglycans, and glycoproteins in the pericellular matrix.

Two fast-acting endogenous inhibitors, PAI-1 and PAI-2, regulate plasminogen activation. PAI-1 is the most abundant in breast cancer as well as other types of cancer. Both inhibitors are able to inactivate uPA, which is bound to uPAR. PAI-1 is secreted in an active but unstable form whose inhibitory activity is stabilized through binding to vitronectin.[23] The interaction between vitronectin, PAI-1, and the cell surface uPA system may also be involved in a modulation of cell adhesion and migration.[24] Based on the pattern of expression of PAI-1 in experimental and human tumors, it has been proposed that this inhibitor protects the cancer tissue against undue uPA-mediated degradation.[25] Consistent with this assumption, a large number of clinical studies have shown that high tumor tissue levels of PAI-1 are associated with short survival of cancer patients.[5] In 1998, a promoting role of PAI-1 in cancer progression was directly demonstrated by experimental studies that showed arrest of angiogenesis and invasion when transformed keratinocytes were transplanted to transgenic mice deficient in PAI-1.[26]

Matrix Metalloproteases

The list of specific members of the class of MMPs continues to grow, and 16 are now included. They can be divided into the collagenases (MMPs 1, 8, and 13), the gelatinases (MMPs 2 and 9), the stromelysins (MMPs 3, 10, and 11), the metalloelastases (MMPs 12, 18, and 19), and the membrane-type metalloproteinases (MMPs 14 to 17); matrilysin (MMP 7) is unique as the smallest member of the class. Functionally, they are able to degrade a wide spectrum of extracellular matrix proteins, including fibrillar collagen, proteoglycans, laminin, fibronectin, elastin, and collagen type IV, as well as fibrin. The MMPs are most typically secreted as inactive proenzymes, and plasmin may be involved in the activation of some of the most important MMPs in cancer invasion, either directly or through the activation of membrane-type MMPs.[27] All of the metalloproteinases share an active site dependence on zinc and thus are susceptible in varying degrees to the hydroxamate class of inhibitors, which are under clinical development for cancer treatment.[28] The role of the metalloproteases in cancer invasion is thus best exemplified in the animal tumor models, in which the hydroxamates give clear inhibition of tumor growth and metastasis.[29] It should be noted that a certain group of membrane-bound metalloproteases, the ADAMS, which are structurally distinct from the MMPs, function in release of cytokine precursors as well as the ectodomains of several other cell surface proteins.[14,30]

The naturally occurring inhibitors of MMPs, TIMP 1–4, form tight stoichiometric complexes with the activated forms of the MMPs, thereby inhibiting the catalytic activity of these enzymes. However, TIMPs have more complex roles than only enzyme inhibition and also function in activation of MMP proenzymes.[27]

Cysteine Proteases

Cysteine proteases include cathepsin B, H, and L, with cathepsin B being the best studied of this class in cancer invasion. Cathepsin B, unlike most cathepsins, is proteolytically active at neutral pH[31] and is also found extracellularly, where it is active in degradation of several matrix proteins, including laminin, elastin, fibronectin, proteoglycans, and collagen.[32] Under normal physiologic conditions, cathepsin B is localized mostly in lysosomes, whereas in tumors, alterations in expression, processing, translocation pathways, or a combination of these may provoke increased secretion and uncontrolled extracellular proteolysis.[33] Cathepsin B has also been shown to activate pro-uPA and may thereby enhance plasmin formation.[34]

Cysteine proteases are regulated by endogenous cysteine protease inhibitors (CPIs).[35] The CPIs consist of at least four families of closely related proteins, such as stefins, cystatins, kininogens, and various structurally related but noninhibitory proteins.[36] Of all known CPIs, cystatin C is the most potent inhibitor of cysteine proteases.[37]

Aspartic Proteases

The class of aspartic proteases is primarily located intracellularly in the lysosomal compartment, which has a low pH and is the site of degradation of many proteins by enzymes with optima near pH 4.0. However, it has been proposed that such enzymes may have some extracellular degradative action on matrix proteins if pericellular compartments are formed that may be continuous with the lysosomal system or a defect arises in enzyme processing that causes oversecretion, or both.[38] As discussed in the section Prognostic Impact of Proteases, Their Receptors, and Inhibitors in Breast Cancer, high levels of one member of this class of proteases, cathepsin D, in breast cancer tissue are associated with poor prognosis. Conclusive studies have, however, not been conducted to test the hypothesis that elevated tissue levels of cathepsin D are directly related to a function in invasion, as established for the neutral proteases, or to determine whether higher levels actually reflect other features—for example, an increased intracellular protein turnover caused by the higher level of tissue remodeling associated with tumor tissue.

CELLULAR LOCALIZATION OF PROTEASES, THEIR RECEPTORS, AND INHIBITORS IN BREAST CANCER

Breast cancer tissue consists of the epithelial cancer cells and infiltrating nonmalignant stromal cells, such as fibroblasts (including myofibroblasts), endothelial cells, and other vascular cells, macrophages, and neutrophils. Many of the proteases, their receptors, and inhibitors are not expressed by the epithelial cancer cells but, rather, by the infiltrating stromal cells. For example, uPA messenger ribonucleic acid (mRNA) is located in stromal fibroblast-like cells that have been identified as myofibroblasts, whereas the cancer cells in virtually all cases lack any detectable uPA mRNA.[39] The uPA receptor protein is found mainly in tumor-infiltrating macrophages, and only in 10% to 20% of the cases can it also be detected in some cancer cells.[40,41]

PAI-1 immunostaining of breast cancer tissue was associated with fibroblasts, cancer cells, and also capillaries at the periphery of the tumor.[42,43] An *in situ* hybridization study showed that PAI-1 mRNA particularly was expressed at the invasion front, located in some cancer cells, but also in stromal cells including fibroblasts, macrophages, and endothelial cells.

The localization studies of MMPs in breast cancer tissue have from the beginning indicated stromal recruitment of matrix-degrading enzymes by tumor cells. Thus, the gene for stromelysin-3 (MMP 11) was the first found to be expressed specifically in the stromal cells surrounding invasive breast carcinomas.[44] Since then, mRNAs for a number of MMPs, including MMP 1,[45,46] MMP 2,[47] MMP 3,[46] and MMP 14,[48] have all been found to be expressed in stromal cells in breast cancer tissue, but with differing patterns. Although RNAs for MMPs 1 to 3, 11, and 14 were found in fibroblasts of tumor stroma, MMPs 9, 12, and 13 were more focalized in vascular structures, macrophages, and tumor cells, respectively. A 1997 study has further localized MMP 9 mRNA to macrophages and vascular pericytes,[49] whereas only MMP 7 mRNA has shown a strict localization to epithelial cells,[45,46] both neoplastic and normal.

The expression patterns of mRNAs for TIMP-1,[50–52] -2,[53] and -3[54] have been investigated in breast cancer tissue, and the findings indicate expression primarily in the stromal compartment, with only weak staining in the cancer cells. TIMP-1 expression in small vessels at the tumor invasion front, reminiscent of that seen with PAI-1 probes, has also been observed.[51,52]

PROGNOSTIC IMPACT OF PROTEASES, THEIR RECEPTORS, AND INHIBITORS IN BREAST CANCER

Because approximately 70% of lymph node–negative breast cancer patients are cured by the primary surgery, whether to expose this group as a whole to the side effects of adjuvant treatment modalities is controversial. Therefore, strong prognostic markers are urgently needed to identify lymph node–negative patients at high risk of relapse.

New prognostic biochemical markers must be reproducible with respect to the involved assay and the prognostic impact; they should be compared with the already used clinical, histopathologic, and biochemical parameters and possess significantly independent, prognostic impact. New markers that have a known role in cancer progression are particularly valuable, because they can provide the basis for identification of even better markers and give an insight in human cancer biology that can be useful for development of new therapeutic approaches. Components of protease systems involved in tumor invasion and metastasis are therefore attractive as potential prognostic markers.

The following section is not intended to be exhaustive but includes a more general overview of published studies on the clinical value of measuring proteases, their receptors, and inhibitors in patients with breast cancer. It is not possible to discuss all of the different approaches—for example, activity assays, Western blotting, zymography, and immunohistochemistry—that have been used; rather, this chapter focuses on studies performed with the most common and reliable quantitation method, enzyme-linked immunosorbent assay (ELISA). As with the other assay techniques, the use of ELISA involves several caveats that should be borne in mind. ELISAs should be specific, sensitive, and reproducible. Specificity is particularly important for biologically relevant markers. Lack of specificity means introduction of a random noise factor that decreases the prognostic impact of the measured values. The sensitivity should ideally be less than one-half of the lowest values found for any patient. The intraassay variation should as a rule be less than 10%. The difference between the highest and lowest values obtained from the same sample should not substantially influence the predicted risk. When a new assay is introduced, a careful description and characterization are required. Information on epitopes recognized by the antibodies used in the assay, analytical sensitivity, measurement range, intra- and interassay variation, recovery, and immunoabsorption should be provided. Extraction procedures should be optimized for the molecule in question and described in detail. Cooperative quality control protocols may be useful to obtain reproducibility of the data obtained in different laboratories.[55]

When starting clinical studies, the marker in question should be correlated to the clinical course of the disease, and the value of the new factor should be validated by performing multivariate analysis, including all well-established prognostic factors. Ultimately, validation of the results should be performed with an independent set of patients.

The aspartic protease cathepsin D was the first protease to be related to prognosis in breast cancer. Several reports have established that a high tumor tissue level of cathepsin D is associated with a short relapse-free survival (RFS) and short overall survival (OS).[56–58] This association has been quantitatively established from ELISA antigen measurement of tissue extracts, verifying earlier indications from histochemistry.[59] It has been proposed that higher cathepsin D levels may be associated with chemoresistant tumors,[60] whereas low tissue levels of this enzyme, together with low PAI-1 levels, could be useful in defining a low-risk group of node-negative patients.[61] The literature on the prognostic value of cathepsin D in breast cancer has been extensively reviewed.[62]

The extensive literature on the prognostic significance of the uPA system in breast cancer was reviewed in 1998.[5,63] Table 1 gives a selected overview of the literature relating to prognostic studies using ELISA measurements of the respective enzyme, inhibitor, and receptor proteins in extracts of tumor tissue.[65–88] As seen from Table 1, almost all studies concur that the measured levels of uPA are related to prognosis, generally relevant to most patients with breast cancer. High tumor tissue levels of uPA in most studies are associated with short RFS and short OS, in agreement with the previously discussed role of uPA in cancer invasion. The main exception relates to a study of low-risk patients,[83] in which the number of patients and events may have been too low to reveal a relationship.

It is also evident from Table 1 that the level of PAI-1 measured in extracts of breast tumor tissue is consistently a strong prognostic variable, being equally predictive for node-positive and node-negative patients and also retaining predictive value over a long period of follow-up.[81] High PAI-1 levels are consistently associated with a short RFS and OS. At first sight, this may seem surprising, given the ability of PAI-1 to rapidly and effectively inactivate uPA. As discussed in the section Serine Proteases, however, this result is consistent with the hypothesis made from earlier expression studies,[25,64] namely that PAI-1 has a role in protection of the tumor tissue. It is also consistent with a 1998 study of tumor-directed neoangiogenesis in transgenic mice that lack expression of the PAI-1 gene.[26]

The level of uPAR in breast cancer tissue has also been found to have a prognostic significance; high levels, as with uPA, are generally associated with poor prognosis.[61,76,77] Once again, this significance may not always be found in subgroups with low risk and therefore relatively few events.[83] The prognostic significance of uPAR is in good agreement with the strong enhancement of cell surface plasminogen activation produced consequent to binding of uPA to uPAR. It is noteworthy that the results obtained so far indicate that the majority of the uPAR measured may be present on tumor-infiltrating macrophages.[40,41] The prognostic information gained so far from uPAR in extracts of tumor tissue is, however, not as strong in its predictive value as that obtained for uPA and PAI-1. The most predictive relationship was found for uPAR in cytosols (i.e., nondetergent extracts) of breast cancer tissue,[76] representing a soluble form of uPAR (suPAR) released from cell membranes. This is particularly noteworthy because of a strong prognostic relationship found for suPAR measured in preoperative blood from patients with colorectal cancer in 1999.

TABLE 1. *Studies on the prognostic significance of urokinase plasminogen activation type 1 and urokinase receptor levels in primary breast cancer tissue*[a]

Reference	No. of patients[b]	Median follow-up time (mo)	Prognostic significance of uPA	Prognostic significance of PAI-1	Prognostic significance of uPAR
Jänicke et al., 1989[65]	115	125	Yes	nd	nd
Duffy et al., 1990[66]	166	35	Yes	nd	nd
Jänicke et al., 1991[67]	113	25	Yes	Yes	nd
Spyratos et al., 1992[68]	319	72	Yes	nd	nd
Foekens et al., 1994, 1992[69,70c]	657	48	Yes	Yes	nd
Grøndahl-Hansen et al., 1993[71]	191	102	Yes	Yes	nd
Jänicke et al., 1993[72]	247	30	Yes	Yes	nd
Duffy et al., 1994[73]	149	58	Yes	nd	nd
Bouchet et al., 1994[74]	314	84	Yes	Yes	nd
Foekens et al., 1995[75]	1,012	71	Yes	Yes	nd
Grøndahl-Hansen et al., 1995[76]	505	54	nd	nd	Yes
Duggan et al., 1995[77]	134	59	Yes	nd	Yes
Mayerhofer et al., 1996[78]	268	32	nd	Yes	nd
Fersis et al., 1996[79]	155	46	Yes	Yes	nd
Fernö et al., 1996[80]	688	42	Yes	nd	nd
Schmitt et al., 1997[81]	314	58	Yes	Yes	nd
Grøndahl-Hansen et al., 1997[82]	250[d]	80	Yes	Yes	nd
Grøndahl-Hansen et al., 1997[83]	195[e]	72	No	Yes	No
Shiba et al., 1997[84]	226	60	Yes	nd	nd
Knoop et al., 1998[85]	429	61	Yes	Yes	nd
Kute et al., 1998[61]	162[f]	58	Yes	Yes	Yes
Eppenberger et al., 1998[86]	305	37	Yes	Yes	nd
Kim et al., 1998[87]	130[f]	52	Yes	Yes	nd
Harbeck et al., 1999[88]	316	77	Yes	Yes	nd

nd, not determined; PAI-1, plasminogen activator inhibitor 1; uPA, urokinase plasminogen activator; uPAR, urokinase receptor.
[a]Only studies using enzyme-linked immunosorbent assay measurements of the respective proteins are included.
[b]Patients unselected unless marked.
[c]Same patients in both studies.
[d]All node positive.
[e]All low risk.
[f]All node negative.

In 1997, we investigated the prognostic impact of PAI-1 levels in tumor extracts in a total of 432 node-negative patients, none of whom received any adjuvant therapy ([83] and unpublished results). In agreement with previous studies,[69,81,83] we find the PAI-1 level to be a very strong prognostic parameter for RFS and OS in node-negative patients. Figure 1 shows the univariate survival curves from these patients when PAI-1 is dichotomized according to the median PAI-1 value (ng/mg protein). These results demonstrate that PAI-1 may potentially be a valuable parameter for selection of node-negative patients, who have a relatively high risk and therefore should be offered adjuvant therapy.

The findings reported to date on the prognostic relevance of the MMPs in breast cancer are considerably fewer in number than those on the uPA system. A few reports have appeared using semiquantification with immunostaining of tissue sections,[89,90] which suggests that high tumor tissue levels of MMP 2 and MMP 11 are associated with poor prognosis of patients with breast cancer. Only one study has been reported using ELISA quantification of MMPs in tumor tissue extracts.[91] Although this study included only 84 patients with breast cancer, it is noteworthy that of these only 12% of the extracts had detectable levels of MMP 1, and MMP 3 was found in only 2% of the samples. Neither MMP 2 nor MMP 9 levels correlated with patient outcome. These latter results could indicate that the ELISAs for MMPs are not yet sufficiently optimized to achieve specificity and sensitivity when applied to tissue extracts or that the MMPs evaluated in this study are not those most expressed or used in invasive breast cancer. In the light of the mRNA and immunostaining results reported for MMP 11 in breast cancer tissue, it would seem that a careful ELISA study of MMP 11 in tumor extracts could yield a clearer relationship between the tissue concentration of an MMP and patient prognosis.

The regulators of MMPs have received even less attention than MMPs in prognostic studies of breast cancers. The first prognostic study using ELISA measurements of TIMP-1 in tumor tissue extracts was in 1999 reported to show that high tissue levels of TIMP-1 predicted shorter survival of patients.[92] This result, although paradoxic from a consideration of TIMP-1 as an inhibitor of MMP-mediated matrix

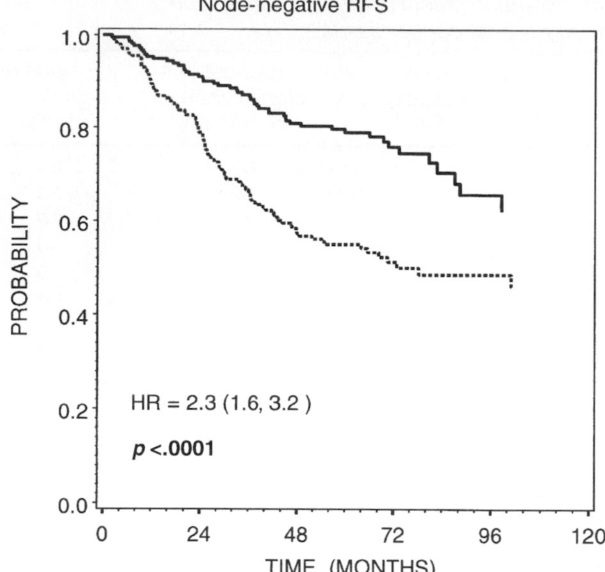

EVENTS	PATIENTS AT RISK				
51	224	186	146	61	———— LOW
92	208	148	101	43	·········· HIGH

FIG. 1. Impact of plasminogen activator inhibitor (PAI)-1 level in tumor extracts on relapse-free survival (RFS) and overall survival in 432 patients with node-negative breast cancer. Patients were divided into two groups with PAI-1 levels below (*solid line*) and above (*dashed line*) the median level. *p* values were calculated by the log rank test. Hazard ratio risks (HR) with 95% confidence intervals (indicated in parentheses) were calculated by the Cox regression model. The number of patients at risk are indicated below the figure. (From ref. 83 and unpublished results.)

degradation, is reminiscent of those obtained for PAI-1 and suggests that the role of protease inhibitors in the tissue remodeling process associated with breast cancer invasion is more complex than previously thought.

Three studies on the prognostic impact of biochemically quantitated cysteine proteases in breast cancer have been published[93–95]; these agree that high levels of cathepsin B or L are associated with poor prognosis. No studies on the prognostic value of CPIs in breast cancer exist. The reader is referred to a review by Kos and Lah[8] on cysteine proteases and cancer.

In a study by Foekens et al.,[69] the prognostic values of several individual markers were weighed against each other by multivariate analysis. Breast cancer extracts from 657 patients were analyzed for uPA, PAI-1, estrogen and progesterone receptors (ER/PR), the estrogen regulation protein pS2, and cathepsin D. For RFS, PAI-1 was the strongest parameter, and of the biochemical parameters mentioned, only PAI-1 and uPA were retained as independent parameters in the multivariate analysis. For OS, ER/PR was the strongest biochemical parameter, and ER/PR and PAI-1 were the only ones retained in the multivariate analysis. These data are consistent with findings in our laboratory.[71,83]

The mentioned studies used ELISAs for antigen determination. These assays usually have been developed with the purpose of measuring all forms of a given component, including inactive proforms, degraded forms, and free as well as complex-bound forms. However, a selective quantitation of the active forms of a component may more precisely reflect the net tumor proteolytic activity, which in turn may be more closely related to prognosis. For example, because only the active forms of uPA and PAI-1 can form a complex, we have developed a specific and highly sensitive uPA:PAI-1 complex assay.[96] Breast tumor extracts contain significant amounts of preformed complexes,[96] and we are studying their prognostic value.

The large majority of the studies published on the prognostic value of proteases, their receptors, and inhibitors in breast cancer have been based on measurements of the analytes in tumor tissue extracts. However, for an increasing number of patients such extracts are not available, mainly because of the use of mammography, which has resulted in smaller tumors at time of diagnosis. It would therefore be desirable if prognostic information similar to that obtained from the tumor tissue could be obtained from a blood sample. Additional advantages would be an easier sample collection and the facts that an extraction procedure would not be needed, inherent problems of tissue heterogeneity would not apply, and blood sampling would allow for repeated measurements during clinical follow-up after the primary surgery. In a study by Grøndahl-Hansen et al.,[97] uPA was measured in plasma from patients with breast cancer, and a positive correlation was found to the extent of disease. In 1997, von Tempelhof et al.[98] showed that PAI-1 activity, as measured in plasma obtained preoperatively from 183 patients with primary breast cancer, was associated with both RFS and OS—that is, patients with high plasma PAI-1 activity had a significantly shorter survival. These findings are supported by a 1998 study in which high plasma PAI-1 antigen levels were found to be associated with short survival in patients with colorectal cancer.[99]

We have previously found that high breast tumor tissue levels of soluble uPAR (but not total uPAR) were associated with poor prognosis.[76] suPAR can be found in blood from healthy blood donors.[100] With the aim of studying plasma and serum levels of suPAR in patients with cancer, we developed a kinetic ELISA specifically evaluated for measurements of suPAR in blood.[100] We have now found that patients with lung,[101] colorectal,[100] ovarian,[102] and breast cancers[100] have elevated levels of suPAR in their blood. Although we showed that in patients with colorectal cancer there is a highly significant association between elevated plasma suPAR levels and shorter survival,[103] a potential prognostic value of plasma suPAR in breast cancer patients has not yet been established.

We have developed a highly sensitive and specific ELISA for the determination of TIMP-1 in blood samples and have shown that patients with metastatic breast cancer have highly significantly elevated plasma TIMP-1 levels as compared to levels found in healthy blood donors.[104] The prognostic value of such measurements have still to be studied.

SUMMARY

Enzymatic degradation of the extracellular matrix, including the basement membranes, plays a crucial role in breast cancer progression. In human breast cancer, the components of matrix-degrading protease systems are expressed mainly by the nonneoplastic stromal cells, a finding that represents a new paradigm with important implications not only for our understanding of breast cancer pathophysiology but also for the development of antiinvasive and antimetastatic cancer therapy. Studies on the prognostic impact of proteases, their receptors, and inhibitors have not only supported the assumption that proteases promote cancer progression, but some of these studies have also reached a point at which the clinical value of these molecules has been thoroughly documented, providing the basis for the use of such determinations as an aid in the clinical management of patients with breast cancer.

Several pharmaceutical companies have developed synthetic MMP inhibitors, and many of these are now in early clinical testing. Because of redundancy or functional overlap between the different proteolytic systems, studies may reveal a need for a combination of inhibitors with specificities for different classes of protease systems to effectively control the progression of cancer.

REFERENCES

1. Cross JC, Werb Z, Fisher SJ. Implantation and the placenta: key pieces of the development puzzle. *Science* 1994;266:1508.
2. Rinkenberger JL, Cross JC, Werb Z. Molecular genetics of implantation in the mouse. *Dev Genet* 1997;21:6.
3. Lund LR, Rømer J, Thomasset N, et al. Two distinct phases of apoptosis in mammary gland involution: proteinase-independent and -dependent pathways. *Development* 1996;122:181.
4. Hewitt R, Danø K. Stromal cell expression of components of matrix-degrading systems in human cancer. *Enzyme Protein* 1996;49:163.
5. Stephens RW, Brünner N, Jänicke F, Schmitt M. The urokinase plasminogen activator system as a target for prognostic studies in breast cancer. *Breast Cancer Res Treat* 1998;52:99.
6. Duffy MJ, McCarthy K. Matrix metalloproteinases in cancer: prognostic markers and targets for therapy. *Int J Cancer* 1998;12:1343.
7. Andreasen PA, Kjøller L, Christensen L, Duffy MJ. The urokinase-type plasminogen activator system in cancer metastasis: a review. *Int J Cancer* 1997;72:1.
8. Kos J, Lah TT. Cysteine proteases and their endogenous inhibitors: target proteins for prognosis, diagnosis and therapy in cancer. *Oncol Rep* 1998;5:1349.
9. Johnsen M, Lund LR, Rømer J, Almholt K, Danø K. Cancer invasion and tissue remodeling: common themes in proteolytic matrix degradation. *Curr Opin Cell Biol* 1998;10:667.
10. Behrendt N, Stephens RW. The urokinase receptor. *Fibrinol Proteol* 1998;12:191.
11. Ren WP, Sloane BF. Cathepsins D and B in breast cancer. *Cancer Treat Res* 1996; 83:325.
12. Bini A, Itoh Y, Kudryk B, Nagase H. Degradation of cross-linked fibrin by matrix metalloproteinase 3 (stromelysin 1): hydrolysis of the gamma Gly 404–Ala 405 peptide bond. *Biochemistry* 1996;35:13056.
13. Hiraoka N, Allen E, Apel IJ, Gyetko MR, Weiss SJ. Matrix metalloproteases regulate neovascularization by acting as pericellular fibrinolysins. *Cell* 1998;95:365.
14. Peschon JJ, Slack JL, Reddy P, et al. An essential role for ectodomain shedding in mammalian development. *Science* 1998;292:1281.
15. Saksela O, Rifkin DB. Release of basic fibroblast growth factor–heparan sulfate complexes from endothelial cells by plasminogen activator–mediated proteolytic activity. *J Cell Biol* 1990;110:767.
16. Danø K, Andreasen PA, Grøndahl Hansen J, Kristensen P, Nielsen LS, Skriver L. Plasminogen activators, tissue degradation, and cancer. *Adv Cancer Res* 1985;44:139.
17. Rømer J, Bugge TH, Pyke C, et al. Impaired wound healing in mice with a disrupted plasminogen gene. *Nature Med* 1996;2:287.
18. Bugge TH, Lund LR, Kombrinck KK, et al. Reduced metastasis of polyoma virus middle T antigen–induced mammary cancer in plasminogen-deficient mice. *Oncogene* 1998;16:3097.
19. Danø K, Behrendt N, Brünner N, Ellis V, Ploug M, Pyke C. The urokinase receptor: protein structure and role in plasminogen activation and cancer invasion. *Fibrinolysis* 1994;8:189.
20. Pöllanen J, Stephens RW, Vaheri A. Directed plasminogen activation at the surface of normal and malignant cells. *Adv Cancer Res* 1991;57:273.
21. Wei Y, Waltz DA, Rao N, Drummond RJ, Rosenberg S, Chapman HA. Identification of the urokinase receptor as an adhesion receptor for vitronectin. *J Biol Chem* 1994;269:32380.
22. Stephens RW, Pöllanen J, Tapiovaara H, et al. Activation of pro-urokinase and plasminogen on human sarcoma cells: a proteolytic system with surface-bound reactants. *J Cell Biol* 1989;108:1987.
23. Seiffert D, Loskutoff DJ. Kinetic analysis of the interaction between type 1 plasminogen activator inhibitor and vitronectin and evidence that bovine inhibitor binds to a thrombin-derived amino-terminal fragment of bovine vitronectin. *Biochem Biophys Acta* 1991;1078:23.
24. Deng G, Curriden SA, Wang SJ, Rosenberg S, Loskutoff DJ. Is plasminogen activator inhibitor-1 the molecular switch that governs urokinase receptor-mediated cell adhesion and migration? *J Cell Biol* 1996;134:1563.
25. Kristensen P, Pyke C, Lund LR, Andreasen PA, Danø K. Plasminogen activator inhibitor type 1 in Lewis lung carcinoma. *Histochemistry* 1990;93:559.
26. Bajou K, Noel A, Gerard RD, et al. Absence of host plasminogen activator inhibitor-1 prevents cancer invasion and vascularization. *Nature Med* 1998;4:923.
27. Strongin AY, Collier I, Bannikov G, Marmer BL, Grant GA, Goldberg GI. Mechanism of cell surface activation of 72-kDa type IV collagenase: isolation of the activated form of the membrane metalloprotease. *J Biol Chem* 1995;270:5331.
28. Brown PD. Matrix metalloproteinase inhibitors in the treatment of cancer. *Med Oncol* 1997;14:1.
29. Wang X, Fu X, Brown PD, Crimmin MJ, Hoffman RM. Matrix metalloproteinase inhibitor BB-94 (batimastat) inhibits human colon tumor growth and spread in a patient-like orthotopic model in nude mice. *Cancer Res* 1994;54:4726.
30. Black RA, Rauch CY, Kozlosky CJ, et al. A metalloproteinase disintegrin that releases tumor necrosis factor alpha from cells. *Nature* 1997;385:729.
31. Werle B, Julke B, Lah T, Spiess E, Ebert W. Cathepsin B fraction active at physiological pH of 7.5 is of prognostic significance in squamous cell carcinoma of human lung. *Br J Cancer* 1997;75:1137.
32. Lah TT, Buck MR, Honn KV, et al. Degradation of laminin by human tumour cathepsin B. *Clin Exp Metastasis* 1989;7:461.
33. Uchiyama Y, Waguri S, Sato N, Watanabe T, Ishido K, Kominami E. Cell and tissue distribution of lysosomal cysteine proteinases, cathepsin B, H and L, and their biological roles. *Acta Histochem Cytochem* 1994;27:287.
34. Kobayashi H, Schmitt M, Goretzki L, et al. Cathepsin B efficiently activates the soluble and the tumor cell receptor bound form of the proenzyme urokinase-type plasminogen activator (pro-uPA). *J Biol Chem* 1990;266:5147.
35. Turk V, Bode W. The cystatins: protein inhibitors of cysteine proteinases. *FEBS Lett* 1991;285:213.
36. Rawling ND, Barrett AJ. Evolution of proteins of the cystatin superfamily. *J Mol Evol* 1990;30:60.
37. Lindahl P, Nycander M, Ylienjarvi K, Pol E, Bjork I. Characterization by rapid-kinetic and equilibrium methods of the reaction between N-

terminally truncated forms of chicken cystatin and the cysteine proteinases papain and actinidin. *Biochem J* 1992;286:165.
38. Mathieu M, Vignon F, Capony F, Rochefort H. Estradiol down-regulated the mannose-6-phosphate/insulin-like growth factor-II receptor gene and induces cathepsin-D in breast cancer cells: a receptor saturation mechanism to increase the secretion of lysosomal proenzymes. *Mol Endocrinol* 1991;5:815.
39. Nielsen BS, Sehested M, Thimshel S, Pyke C, Danø K. Messenger RNA for urokinase plasminogen activator is expressed in myofibroblasts adjacent to cancer cells in human breast cancer. *Lab Invest* 1996;74:168.
40. Pyke C, Grœm N, Ralfkiœr E, et al. Receptor for urokinase is present in tumor-associated macrophages in ductal breast carcinoma. *Cancer Res* 1993;53:1911.
41. Bianchi E, Cohen RL, Thor AT, et al. The urokinase receptor is expressed in invasive breast cancer but not in normal breast tissue. *Cancer Res* 1994;54:861.
42. Bianchi E, Cohen RL, Dai A, Thor AT, Shuman MA, Smith HS. Immunohistochemical localization of the plasminogen activator inhibitor-1 in breast cancer. *Int J Cancer* 1995;60:597.
43. Christensen L, Wiborg Simonsen AC, Heegaard CW, Moestrup SK, Andersen JA, Andreasen PA. Immunohistochemical localization of urokinase-type plasminogen activator, type-1 plasminogen-activator inhibitor, urokinase receptor and alpha(2)-macroglobulin receptor in human breast carcinomas. *Int J Cancer* 1996;66: 441.
44. Basset P, Bellocq JP, Wolf C, et al. A novel metalloproteinase gene specifically expressed in stromal cells of breast carcinomas. *Nature* 1990;348:699.
45. Wolf C, Rouyer N, Lutz Y, et al. Stromelysin 3 belongs to a subgroup of proteinases expressed in breast carcinoma fibroblastic cells and possibly implicated in tumor progression. *Proc Natl Acad Sci U S A* 1993;90:1843.
46. Heppner KJ, Matrisian LM, Jensen RA, Rodgers WH. Expression of most matrix metalloproteinase family members in breast cancer represents a tumor-induced host response. *Am J Pathol* 1996;149:273.
47. Polette M, Gilbert N, Stas I, et al. Gelatinase A expression and localization in human breast cancers. An in situ hybridization study and immunohistochemical detection using confocal microscopy. *Virchows Arch* 1994;424:641.
48. Okada A, Bellocq JP, Rouyer N, et al. Membrane-type matrix metalloproteinase (MT-MMP) gene is expressed in stromal cells of human colon, breast, and head and neck carcinomas. *Proc Natl Acad Sci U S A* 1995;92:2730.
49. Nielsen BS, Sehested M, Kjeldsen L, Borregaard N, Danø K. Expression of the matrix metalloprotease-9 in vascular pericytes in human breast cancer. *Lab Invest* 1997;77:345.
50. Polette M, Clavel C, Cockett M, et al. Detection and localization of mRNAs encoding matrix metalloproteinases and their tissue inhibitor in human breast pathology. *Invasion Metastasis* 1993;13:31.
51. Lindsay CK, Thorgeirsson UP, Tsuda H, Hirohashi S. Expression of tissue inhibitor of metalloproteinase-1 and type IV collagenase/gelatinase messenger RNAs in human breast cancer. *Hum Pathol* 1997;28:359.
52. Ree AH, Florenes VA, Berg JP, Maelandsmo GM, Nesland JM, Fodstad O. High levels of messenger RNAs for tissue inhibitors of metalloproteinases (TIMP-1 and TIMP-2) in primary breast carcinomas are associated with development of distant metastases. *Clin Cancer Res* 1997;3:1623.
53. Poulsom R, Hanby AM, Pignatelli M, et al. Expression of gelatinase A and TIMP-2 mRNAs in desmoplastic fibroblasts in both mammary carcinomas and basal cell carcinomas of the skin. *J Clin Pathol* 1993;46:429.
54. Byrne JA, Tomasetto C, Rouyer N, Bellocq JP, Rio MC, Basset P. The tissue inhibitor of metalloproteinases-3 gene in breast carcinoma: identification of multiple polyadenylation sites and a stromal pattern of expression. *Mol Med* 1995;1:418.
55. Sweep CGJ, Geurts-Moespot J, Grebenschikov N, et al. External quality assessment of trans-European multicentre antigen determinations (ELISA) of urokinase-type plasminogen activator (uPA) and its type-1 inhibitor (PAI-1) in human breast cancer tissue extracts. *Br J Cancer* 1998;78:1434.
56. Thorpe SM, Rochefort H, Garcia M, et al. Association between high concentrations of Mr 52,000 cathepsin D and poor prognosis in primary human breast cancer. *Cancer Res* 1989;49:6008.
57. Spyratos F, Maudelode T, Brouillet JP, et al. Cathepsin D: an independent prognostic factor for metastasis of breast cancer. *Lancet* 1989;334:1115.
58. Tandon AK, Clark GM, Chamness GC, Chirgwin JM, McGuire WL. Cathepsin D and prognosis in breast cancer. *N Engl J Med* 1990;322:297.
59. Rochefort H, Capoy F, Augereau P, et al. The estrogen-regulated 52K-cathepsin-D in breast cancer: from biology to clinical applications. *Int J Rad Appl Instrum* 1987;14:377.
60. Namer M, Ramaioli A, Fontana X, et al. Prognostic value of total cathepsin D in breast tumors: a possible role in selection of chemoresistant patients. *Breast Cancer Res Treat* 1991;19:85.
61. Kute TE, Grøndahl-Hansen J, Shao SM, Long R, Russell G, Brünner N. Low cathepsin D and low plasminogen activator type 1 inhibitor in tumor cytosols defines a group of node negative breast cancer patients with low risk of recurrence. *Breast Cancer Res Treat* 1998;47:9.
62. Garcia M, Platet N, Liaudet E, et al. Biological and clinical significance of cathepsin D in breast cancer metastasis. *Stem Cells* 1996;14:642.
63. Harbeck N, Graeff H, Höfler H, Brünner N, Schmitt M. Plasminogen activator system in breast cancer tissue and blood: clinical relevance and methodological considerations. *J Tumor Marker Oncol* 1998;13:19.
64. Pyke C, Kristensen P, Ralfkiœr E, Eriksen J, Danø K. The plasminogen activation system in human colon cancer: messenger RNA for the inhibitor PAI-1 is located in endothelial cells in the tumor stroma. *Cancer Res* 1991;51:4067.
65. Jänicke F, Schmitt M, Ulm K, Gössner W, Graeff H. Urokinase-type plasminogen activator antigen and early relapse in breast cancer. *Lancet* 1989;8670:1049.
66. Duffy MJ, Reilly D, O'Sullivan C, O'Higgins N, Fenelly JN, Andreasen P. Urokinase-plasminogen activator, a new and independent prognostic marker in breast cancer. *Cancer Res* 1990;50:6827.
67. Jänicke F, Schmitt M, Graeff H. Clinical relevance of the urokinase-type and tissue-type plasminogen activators and of their type 1 inhibitor in breast cancer. *Semin Thromb Hemost* 1991;17:303.
68. Spyratos F, Martin PM, Hacene K, et al. Multiparametric prognostic evaluation of biological factors in primary breast cancer. *J Natl Cancer Inst* 1992;84:1266.
69. Foekens JA, Schmitt M, van Putts WL, et al. Plasminogen activator inhibitor-1 and prognosis in primary breast cancer. *J Clin Oncol* 1994;12:1648.
70. Foekens JA, Schmitt M, van Putts WL, et al. Prognostic value of urokinase-type plasminogen activator in 671 primary breast cancer patients. *Cancer Res* 1992;52:6101.
71. Grøndahl-Hansen J, Christensen IJ, Rosenquist C, et al. High levels of urokinase-type plasminogen activator and its inhibitor PAI-1 in cytosolic extracts of breast carcinomas are associated with poor prognosis. *Cancer Res* 1993;53:2513.
72. Jänicke F, Schmitt M, Pache L, et al. Urokinase (uPA) and its inhibitor PAI-1 are strong, independent prognostic factors in node-negative breast cancer. *Breast Cancer Res Treat* 1993;24:195.
73. Duffy MJ, Reilly D, McDermott E, O'Higgins N, Fenelly JJ, Andreasen PA. Urokinase plasminogen activator as a prognostic marker in different subgroups of patients with breast cancer. Cancer 1994;74:2276.
74. Bouchet C, Spyratos F, Martin PM, Hacne K, Gentile A, Oglobine J. Prognostic value of urokinase-type plasminogen activator (uPA) and plasminogen activator inhibitors PAI-1 and PAI-2 in breast carcinomas. *Bull Cancer* 1994;81:77.
75. Foekens JA, Bussecker F, Peters HA, et al. Plasminogen activator inhibitor-2: prognostic relevance in 1012 patients with primary breast cancer. *Cancer Res* 1995;55:1423.
76. Grøndahl-Hansen J, Peters HA, van Putts WL, et al. Prognostic significance of the receptor for urokinase plasminogen activator in breast cancer. *Clin Cancer Res* 1995;1:1079.
77. Duggan C, Maguire T, McDermott E, O'Higgins N, Fenelly JJ, Duffy MJ. Urokinase plasminogen activator and urokinase plasminogen activator receptor in breast cancer. *Int J Cancer* 1995;29:597.
78. Mayerhofer K, Stolzlechner J, Yildiz S, et al. Plasminogenaktivator Inhibitor 1 und Prognose beim Mammakarzinom. *Geburtshilfe Frauenheilkunde* 1996;56:23.
79. Fersis N, Kaufmann M, Kramer MD, Wittmann G, Wallwiener D, Bastert G. Prognostische Bedeutung des Plasminogenaktivator

Inhibitor-1 (PAI-1) beim primären Mammakarzinom. *Geburtshilfe Frauenheilkunde* 1996;56:28.

80. Fernö M, Bendahl PO, Borg A, et al. Urokinase plasminogen activator, a strong independent prognostic factor in breast cancer, analysed in steroid receptor cytosols with a luminometric immunoassay. *Eur J Cancer* 1996;32A:793.
81. Schmitt M, Thomssen C, Ulm K, et al. Time-varying prognostic impact of tumor biological factors urokinase (uPA), PAI-1, and steroid hormone receptor status in primary breast cancer. *Br J Cancer* 1997;76:306.
82. Grøndahl-Hansen J, Hilsenbeck SG, Christensen IJ, Clark GM, Osborne CK, Brünner N. Prognostic significance of PAI-1 and uPA in cytosolic extracts obtained from node-positive breast cancer patients. *Breast Cancer Res Treat* 1997;43:153.
83. Grøndahl-Hansen J, Christensen IJ, Briand P, et al. Plasminogen activator inhibitor type 1 in cytosolic tumor extracts predicts prognosis in low-risk breast cancer patients. *Clin Cancer Res* 1997;3:233.
84. Shiba E, Kim SJ, Taguchi T, et al. A prospective study on the prognostic significance of urokinase-type plasminogen activator levels in breast cancer patients. *J Cancer Res Clin Oncol* 1997;123:555.
85. Knoop A, Andreasen PA, Andersen JA, et al. Prognostic significance of urokinase plasminogen activator and plasminogen activator inhibitor 1 in primary breast cancer. *Br J Cancer* 1998;77:932.
86. Eppenberger U, Kueng W, Schlaeppi J-M, et al. Markers of tumor angiogenesis and proteolysis independently define high- and low-risk subsets of node-negative breast cancer patients. *J Clin Oncol* 1998;16:3129.
87. Kim SJ, Shiba E, Kobayashi T, et al. Impact of urokinase-type plasminogen activator (PA), PA inhibitor type-1, and tissue-type PA antigen levels in node-negative breast cancer: a prospective study on multicentre basis. *Clin Cancer Res* 1998;4:177.
88. Harbeck N, Thomssen C, Berger U, et al. Invasion marker PAI-1 remains a strong prognostic factor after long-term follow-up both for primary breast cancer and following first relapse. *Breast Cancer Res Treat* 1999;54:147.
89. Talvensaari-Mattila A, Paakko P, Hoyhtya M, Blanco-Sequeiros G, Turpeenniemi Hujanen T. Matrix metalloproteinase 2 immunoreactive protein. A marker of aggressiveness in breast carcinoma. *Cancer* 1998;83:1153.
90. Ahmad A, Hanby A, Dublin E, et al. Stromelysin 3: an independent prognostic factor for relapse-free survival in node-positive breast cancer and demonstration of novel breast carcinoma cell expression. *Am J Pathol* 1998;152:721.
91. Remacle AG, Noel A, Duggan C, et al. Assay of matrix metalloproteinases types 1, 2, 3 and 9 in breast cancer. *Br J Cancer* 1998;77:926.
92. McCarthy K, Maguire T, McGreal G, McDermott E, O'Higgins N, Duffy MJ. High levels of tissue inhibitor of metalloproteinase-1 predict poor outcome in patients with breast cancer. *Int J Cancer* 1999;84:44.
93. Thomssen C, Schmitt M, Goretzki L, et al. Prognostic values of the cysteine protease cathepsin B and L in human breast cancer. *Clin Cancer Res* 1995;1:741.
94. Budihna M, Skrk J, Zakotnik B, Gabrijelcic D, Lindner J. Prognostic value of total cathepsin B in invasive ductal carcinoma of the breast. *Eur J Cancer* 1995;31:661.
95. Foekens JA, Kos J, Peters IJA, et al. Prognostic significance of cathepsin B and L in primary human breast cancer. *J Clin Oncol* 1998;16:1013.
96. Pedersen AN, Høyer-Hansen G, Brünner N, et al. The complex between urokinase plasminogen activator and its type-1 inhibitor in breast cancer extracts quantitated by ELISA. *J Immunol Methods* 1997;203:55.
97. Grøndahl-Hansen J, Agerlin N, Munkholm-Larsen P, et al. Sensitive and specific enzyme-linked immunosorbent assay for urokinase-type plasminogen activator and its application to plasma from patients with breast cancer. *J Lab Clin Med* 1988;111:42.
98. Von Tempelhof GF, Heilmann L, Dietrich M, Schneider D, Niemann F, Hommel G. Plasmatic plasminogen activator inhibitor activity in patients with primary breast cancer. *Thromb Haemost* 1997;77:600.
99. Nielsen HJ, Pappot H, Christensen IJ, et al. Association between plasma concentration of plasminogen activator inhibitor-1 and survival in patients with colorectal cancer. *BMJ* 1998;316:829.
100. Stephens RW, Pedersen AN, Nielsen HJ, et al. ELISA determination of soluble urokinase receptor in blood from healthy donors and cancer patients. *Clin Chem* 1997;43:1868.
101. Pappot H, Høyer-Hansen G, Rønne E, et al. Elevated plasma levels of urokinase plasminogen activator receptor in non-small cell lung cancer patients. *Eur J Cancer* 1997;33:867.
102. Sier CFM, Stephens R, Bizik J, et al. The level of urokinase plasminogen activator receptor is increased in serum of ovarian cancer patients. *Cancer Res* 1998;58:1843.
103. Stephens RW, Nielsen HJ, Christensen IJ, et al. Plasma urokinase receptor in colorectal cancer patients: relation to prognosis. *J Natl Cancer Inst* 1999;91:869.
104. Holten-Andersen MN, Murphy G, Nielsen HJ, et al. Quantitation of TIMP-1 in plasma of healthy blood donors and patients with advanced cancer. *Br J Cancer* 1999;80:495.

VI

Diseases of the Breast, 2nd ed.,
edited by Jay R. Harris.
Lippincott Williams & Wilkins, Philadelphia © 2000.

In Situ *Carcinoma*

CHAPTER 26

Lobular Carcinoma *in Situ*

Monica Morrow and Stuart J. Schnitt

In 1941, Foote and Stewart[1] described a noninvasive lesion arising from the lobules and terminal ducts of the breast that they called *lobular carcinoma* in situ (*LCIS*). A review of 300 mastectomy specimens at Memorial Hospital in New York City resulted in only two examples of pure LCIS; in 12 additional cases, LCIS was identified in association with infiltrating carcinoma, leading Foote and Stewart to conclude that LCIS was a rare entity. Despite the limited number of cases examined, their initial report identified three important features of LCIS: (a) the lesion is an incidental microscopic finding that cannot be identified clinically or by gross pathologic examination, (b) the lesion is multicentric in the breast, and (c) the invasive carcinomas that develop after LCIS may be infiltrating ductal or infiltrating lobular tumors. Based on these observations, Foote and Stewart concluded that simple mastectomy was the appropriate treatment for LCIS. Additional information about LCIS gained since 1941 suggests that the lesion does not invariably progress to carcinoma and that the risk of subsequent cancer is roughly equal in both breasts. The uncertainties about the biological significance of a diagnosis of LCIS have caused considerable confusion regarding its management.

M. Morrow: Department of Surgery, Northwestern University Medical School, Chicago, Illinois; Lynn Sage Comprehensive Breast Program, Northwestern Memorial Hospital, Chicago, Illinois

S. J. Schnitt: Department of Pathology, Harvard Medical School, Brigham and Women's Hospital, Dana-Farber Cancer Institute, Boston, Massachusetts; Department of Surgical Pathology, Beth Israel Deaconess Medical Center, Boston, Massachusetts

INCIDENCE

The true incidence of LCIS in the general population is unknown because of the lack of both clinical and mammographic signs. Page et al.[2] reviewed 10,542 benign breast biopsies performed for clinical abnormalities and found only 48 cases (0.5%) that met strict diagnostic criteria for LCIS. In contrast, Haagensen et al.[3] reviewed results from 5,000 patients who had breast biopsies between 1930 and 1972 and observed that 3.6% of the benign breast lesions were LCIS. Page et al.,[2] however, commented that some of the lesions in this series would not meet their diagnostic criteria for LCIS and would be classified as *atypical lobular hyperplasia*. This illustrates a further problem in determining the incidence of LCIS. Wheeler et al.[4] noted LCIS in 0.8% of 3,570 benign

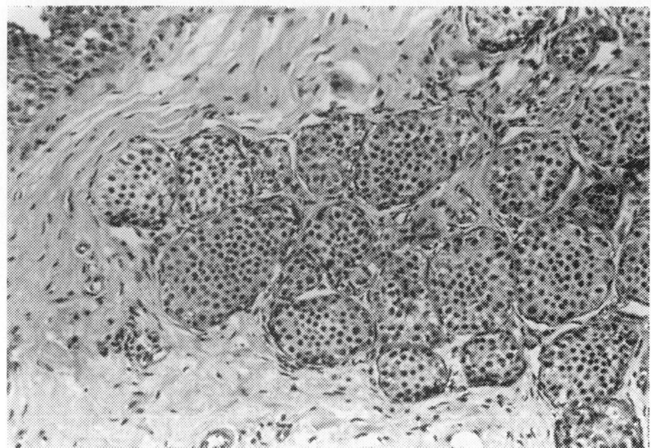

FIG. 1. This example shows the most typical appearance of lobular carcinoma *in situ*. The acini of this lobule are filled with and distended by a population of small cells with uniform round to oval nuclei.

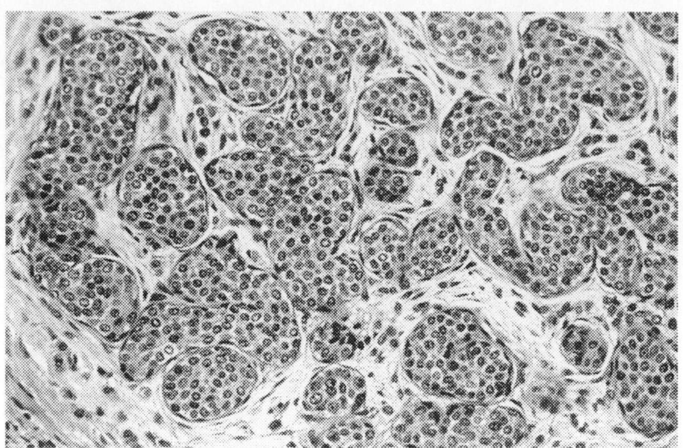

FIG. 2. In this example of lobular carcinoma *in situ* (LCIS), the lesion is composed of slightly larger tumor cells that have larger nuclei than the LCIS lesion shown in Fig. 1.

biopsies performed for clinical problems, and Andersen[5] found a 1.5% incidence of LCIS in 3,299 specimens. The variable incidence of LCIS reported in these series reflects differences in diagnostic criteria, differences in the amount of normal breast tissue removed and examined, and differences in the patient populations undergoing biopsy. Although the exact incidence of LCIS varies, agreement exists that LCIS is an uncommon finding. Autopsy studies also suggest a low incidence of LCIS. Frantz et al.[6] found no cases of LCIS in a study of the breasts of 225 women with a median age of 45 years. Alpers and Wellings[7] and Kramer and Rush[8] also found no evidence of LCIS in detailed autopsy studies. Nielsen et al.[9] examined 110 younger women and identified only four cases of LCIS, confirming that LCIS is uncommon in the general population. In all reports, LCIS is noted to be more common in younger women. The mean age at diagnosis usually is reported to be between 44 and 46 years,[2–5,10–12] and 80% to 90% of cases of LCIS occur in premenopausal women.[2–5,10–12] This age distribution may be due to regression of LCIS in the absence of estrogen or may simply reflect the fact that benign breast abnormalities requiring biopsy are more common in premenopausal women, resulting in more frequent identification of LCIS in this group. LCIS is reported to occur approximately 10 times more frequently in white women than in African-American women in the United States.[13–15]

The frequency with which LCIS is diagnosed is increasing. One series[16] reported a 15% rise in the number of cases seen from 1973 to 1988. Although some of this increase is due to greater recognition of LCIS as a pathologic entity, the major factor responsible is the increasing use of screening mammography. A review of 6,287 mammographically generated biopsies showed that LCIS was present in 2.3% of total cases, accounting for 9.8% of mammographically detected lesions classified as malignancies.[17] No specific mammographic findings are associated with LCIS.[18,19] Calcifications have frequently been the indication for surgery in cases in which LCIS has been identified, but histologically the calcifications are located in normal epithelial cells adjacent to areas of LCIS, rather than in the involved lobules.[18]

Several studies have examined the distribution of LCIS in an involved breast and the contralateral breast. Foote and Stewart[1] recognized the multicentric nature of LCIS in their original report, and subsequent reports[20–24] confirmed that multicentric LCIS is identified in 60% to 80% of mastectomy specimens. In addition, LCIS is frequently noted to be bilateral. Haagensen et al.[3] found bilateral LCIS in 19 of 73 women (26%) for whom bilateral breast tissue was available. Mirror-image biopsies done in patients with LCIS also provide an estimate of the incidence of bilateral disease. Newman[23] found contralateral LCIS in 6 of 26 women (23%) undergoing mirror image biopsy, and Urban[25] noted a 35% incidence of bilateral LCIS in 26 women. The incidence of bilaterality of LCIS has minimal clinical relevance, however, because the cancer risk associated with LCIS is bilateral, regardless of the presence of LCIS in the contralateral breast.

PATHOLOGY

LCIS is not detectable on macroscopic examination and is always an incidental microscopic finding in breast tissue removed for another reason. In contrast with ductal carcinoma *in situ* (DCIS), which is highly heterogeneous in its histologic appearance, the histologic features of LCIS show little variation and are usually easily recognized.[26–31] LCIS is most often characterized by a solid proliferation of small cells, with small, uniform, round-to-oval nuclei and variably distinct cell borders (Fig. 1). The cells often show loss of cohesion. The cytoplasm is clear to lightly eosinophilic; occasionally, the cells contain intracytoplasmic vacuoles that may be large enough to produce signet-ring cell forms. This description refers to the type of LCIS described by Haagensen as *type A*, or *classical type*. Some cases of LCIS, however, are characterized by larger cells with larger nuclei that show some degree of pleomorphism; these were referred to by Haagensen as *type B cells*[32] (Fig. 2). LCIS is typically present in the terminal duct lobular units and distends and distorts the involved spaces. In some instances, LCIS cells involve extralobular ducts. The growth within these ducts may be either solid or pagetoid (i.e., the LCIS cells are insinuated between the duct basement membrane and the native ductal epithelial cells). Although some authors previously recognized a cribriform pattern of involvement of extralobular ducts by LCIS,[33] *in situ* lesions with a cribriform pattern are probably best categorized as DCIS.

Cell kinetic studies have shown that LCIS has a low proliferative rate.[34–36] The cells of LCIS are also typically estrogen-receptor positive[35–37] and rarely, if ever, show overexpression of the c-*erb*-b2 (*HER-2/neu*) oncogene[35,36,38,39] or accumulation of the p53 protein.[35,36] In addition, studies have indicated that the cells of LCIS are characterized by loss of expression of the adhesion molecule E-cadherin.[40]

TABLE 1. *Follow-up of patients diagnosed with lobular carcinoma* in situ

Study	*n*	Invasive cancer (%)	Follow-up (yr)	Relative risk
Haagensen et al.[3]	287	18	16.3	6.9
Rosen et al.[12]	99	34.5[a]	24	9.0
Wheeler et al.[4]	32	12.5	17.5	—
Andersen[5]	47	26.4[b]	15	12.0
Page et al.[2]	44	23	18	9.0
Salvadori et al.[47]	80	6.3	5	10.3
Ottesen et al.[48]	69	11.6	5	11.0
Bodian et al.[46]	236	26[c]	18	5.4
Fisher et al.[45]	182	3.3	5	—

[a]Percentage calculated for 85 patients with follow-up.
[b]Includes two patients with bilateral cancers counted separately.
[c]Includes ductal carcinoma *in situ* and invasive carcinoma.

DIFFERENTIAL DIAGNOSIS

The cells composing atypical lobular hyperplasia are similar to those that characterize LCIS, but in atypical lobular hyperplasia the degree of involvement of the terminal ducts and lobules is less extensive. Unfortunately, no sharp dividing line exists between atypical lobular hyperplasia and LCIS, and diagnostic criteria for this distinction vary among experts. Some authors require that at least 50% of the spaces in a given lobule be filled with and distended by the characteristic cells to warrant a diagnosis of LCIS,[27] whereas others do not consider lobular distention and enlargement an essential feature for the diagnosis of LCIS.[28] In some patients, LCIS may involve areas of breast tissue that have preexisting benign alterations; for example, LCIS may involve foci of sclerosing adenosis and produce a pattern that mimics invasive carcinoma.[41] However, low-power examination of such specimens usually reveals the lobulocentric configuration characteristic of adenosis. Finally, as discussed in Chapter 27, in the section dealing with the pathology of DCIS, sometimes the distinction between LCIS and DCIS is problematic.[42–45]

NATURAL HISTORY AND TREATMENT

The major issue in the management of LCIS is the risk of invasive carcinoma after a diagnosis of LCIS. Treatment strategies have varied, depending on whether LCIS was considered to be the anatomic precursor of invasive carcinoma, an obligate premalignant lesion, or simply a marker for an increased risk of breast cancer development. Six series[2–5,12,46] with long-term follow-up address the malignant potential of LCIS after biopsy alone (Table 1). Patients with LCIS and without associated invasive carcinoma were studied, although women who had contralateral invasive carcinoma before receiving a diagnosis of LCIS were included in some reports, making calculation of the incidence of invasive carcinoma difficult. The largest series, reported by Haagensen et al.,[3] included 287 women monitored for a mean of 16.3 years, with only 2 patients lost to follow-up. Breast cancer developed in 63 patients (21% of those in the series). If the 10 patients whose LCIS diagnosis followed treatment for contralateral invasive breast cancer are excluded, 18% of the women developed carcinoma, a ratio of observed to expected cases of 6.9 to 1.0. In a similar study from Memorial Hospital, Rosen et al.[12] identified 99 patients with LCIS who were monitored for a mean of 24 years, although complete follow up was available for only 84 women. Twenty-nine women subsequently developed invasive carcinoma (34.5%); however, if all the patients lost to follow-up are considered free of disease, this figure falls to 29.2%. The relative risk of breast cancer development in this series was 9, the same level of risk observed by Page et al.[2] in a report of 44 cases of LCIS followed for 18 years. Page's group, however, observed that the risk of developing infiltrating carcinoma was greatest during the first 15 years after biopsy (relative risk, 10.8) and decreased to 4.2 for those women remaining free of carcinoma for 15 years. In contrast, Rosen et al.[12] observed no decrease in the risk of development of invasive carcinoma during their 24-year follow-up period. Wheeler et al.[4] and Andersen[5] reported the development of invasive carcinoma in 12.5% and 26.4% of women monitored for 17.5 and 15 years, respectively. In two other studies,[47,48] similar levels of risk associated with LCIS were noted. Salvadori et al.[47] reported on 80 women with LCIS who were monitored for a median of 58 months. Five cases of invasive carcinoma (6.3%) were noted, a ratio of observed to expected cases of 10.3 to 1.0. Sixty-nine cases of LCIS were identified in a prospective study by the Danish Breast Cancer Cooperative Group[48]; at a median follow-up of 61 months, 8 infiltrating carcinomas had occurred (11.6%). The relative risk of cancer development among women with LCIS in this study was 11.

In contrast, a study of 182 women with LCIS reported by Fisher et al.[45] noted only a 3.3% incidence of invasive carcinoma after 5 years of follow-up. The authors note that these lesions were excised to negative margins because they were initially diagnosed as DCIS and suggest that this may be the factor responsible for the low incidence of invasive carcinoma. This seems somewhat counterintuitive, given the excess of cancers observed in both breasts and the known multicentricity of LCIS.[45] With this exception, the studies discussed agree that LCIS is associated with an increased risk of development of breast carcinoma that is 7 to 10 times that of the index population. In addition, the five studies with long-term follow-up periods agree that the risk of subsequent cancer development is equal in both breasts. Most carcinomas that develop in women with LCIS are infiltrating ductal, not infiltrating lobular, carcinoma. Infiltrating lobular carcinomas accounted for 25% to 37% of subsequent cancers in four of the six studies for which this information is available.[3,4,12,47] Page et al.[2] observed that 70% of the infiltrating carcinomas in their series that occurred after a diagnosis of LCIS were of lobular histology, whereas none of the five cancers in the report of Salvadori et al.[47] had infiltrating lobular histology. Although most cancers occurring after a diagnosis of LCIS are infiltrating ductal carcinomas, the incidence of infiltrating lobular carcinoma in this group of patients is significantly elevated, compared with the 5% to 10% incidence observed among breast cancer patients in general. Wheeler et al.[4] estimated that invasive lobular carcinomas occur at 18 times the expected rate, whereas infiltrating ductal carcinomas occur at only 4 times the expected rate.

More recent information about invasive cancer risk associated with a diagnosis of LCIS comes from the National Surgical Adjuvant Breast and Bowel Project tamoxifen prevention trial.[49] This study included 826 women with LCIS. The rate of invasive carcinoma development was 12.99 per 1,000 women. The use of tamoxifen (tamoxifen citrate) reduced this risk to 5.69, a relative risk of 0.44. This level of risk reduction was slightly higher than that seen in women at risk on the basis of other factors.

The observations that most women with LCIS do not develop breast cancer, that the risk of breast cancer is bilateral, and that most tumors that develop are infiltrating ductal carcinomas give credence to the hypothesis that LCIS is a risk factor for cancer development. One management option for women with LCIS is careful observation, as would be done for any woman known to be at increased risk of developing breast cancer due to a positive family history or prior personal history of breast cancer. The use of tamoxifen in women opting for observation is worthy of serious consideration. An alternative for women unwilling to accept a risk of breast cancer development of approximately 1% per year associated with a policy of careful observation is bilateral simple mastectomy, usually with immediate reconstruction. Treatment strategies addressing one breast, such as unilateral simple mastectomy with contralateral biopsy, would seem illogical, because the risk of LCIS is bilateral regardless of the findings of the contralateral biopsy. The effectiveness of a program of careful follow-up in detecting potentially curable carcinoma in a population of high-risk women is uncertain. A meta-analysis of 389 reported cases of LCIS followed for a mean of 10.9 years reported a breast cancer mortality rate of 2.8%, although 16.4% of the group developed carcinoma.[50] In contrast, of 391 women treated initially with mastectomy, the breast cancer mortality rate was 0.9%. Frykberg and Bland,[17] analyzing data on 515 patients with LCIS treated with observation, reported a 7% breast cancer mortality rate. Many of these series antedate the use of modern mammography, however, and uniform clinical follow-up was not used.

Wide surgical excision and histologically negative margins are not needed when follow-up is chosen, given that LCIS is known to be a multicentric lesion. Similarly, radiation therapy has no role in the management of LCIS. The authors examine women with LCIS at 4- to 6-month intervals and obtain annual diagnostic mammograms. When observation is elected, it must last for the patient's lifetime, because the increased risk of breast cancer persists indefinitely. Carson et al.[51] reported that 12 of 51 women (24%) monitored after a diagnosis of LCIS had a subsequent breast biopsy, although only 3 were found to have infiltrating carcinoma. Efforts to identify features of LCIS associated with a higher likelihood of the development of malignancy have been largely unsuccessful. Haagensen et al.[3] noted that the combination of LCIS and a family history of breast cancer increased the relative risk of breast cancer development to 8.5 (compared with 5.7 for women with LCIS alone). In an analysis of Haagensen's patient cohort, however, Bodian et al.[46] found that a family history of breast cancer increased the risk beyond that seen with LCIS alone only for women younger than age 40 when LCIS was diagnosed. Page et al.[2] did not find that a positive family history further increased risk in women with LCIS. Rosen et al.[12] extensively reviewed the histologic features of LCIS, including the amount of LCIS present, and were unable to identify any factors predictive of the subsequent development of invasive carcinoma, an observation similar to that made by Haagensen et al.[3] Research using the tools of molecular biology to further define risk will provide critically important information for women with LCIS.

The choice between careful observation with or without tamoxifen treatment and bilateral prophylactic mastectomy can be made only by the patient who thoroughly understands the risk she assumes. Surgical treatment of LCIS is not an emergency, and detailed discussions of treatment options are important for patients to overcome the confusion often associated with this diagnosis. The use of mastectomy to treat LCIS appears to be decreasing.[11] In light of the increasing use of breast-preserving approaches for invasive carcinoma and the significant reduction in breast cancer risk seen with tamoxifen treatment, this trend is probably appropriate.

MANAGEMENT SUMMARY

LCIS, which lacks clinical or mammographic signs, is a risk factor for bilateral breast cancer development.

Careful clinical follow-up is appropriate for most women with LCIS and carries a risk of breast cancer development of approximately 1% per year. This risk persists indefinitely.

Treatment with tamoxifen citrate at 20 mg daily for 5 years reduces the risk of breast cancer development by 55%.

Bilateral prophylactic mastectomy, usually with reconstruction, is an alternative approach for women unwilling to undergo follow-up, with or without tamoxifen treatment.

Excision to negative margins, radiation therapy, and chemotherapy have no role in treatment of women with LCIS.

REFERENCES

1. Foote FW Jr, Stewart FW. Lobular carcinoma in situ: a rare form of mammary carcinoma. *Am J Pathol* 1941;17:491.
2. Page DL, Kidd TE Jr, Dupont WD, et al. Lobular neoplasia of the breast: higher risk for subsequent invasive cancer predicted by more extensive disease. *Hum Pathol* 1991;22:1232.
3. Haagensen CD, Bodian C, Haagensen DE. *Lobular neoplasia (lobular carcinoma in situ) breast carcinoma: risk and detection*. Philadelphia: WB Saunders, 1981:238.
4. Wheeler JE, Enterline HT, Roseman JM, et al. Lobular carcinoma in situ of the breast: long-term follow-up. *Cancer* 1974;34:554.
5. Andersen JA. Lobular carcinoma in situ of the breast: an approach to rational treatment. *Cancer* 1977;39:2597.
6. Frantz VK, Pickren JW, Melcher GW, et al. Incidence of chronic cystic disease in so-called normal breasts: a study based on 225 post mortem examinations. *Cancer* 1951;4:762.
7. Alpers CE, Wellings SR. The prevalence of carcinoma in situ in normal and cancer associated breasts. *Hum Pathol* 1985;16:796.
8. Kramer WM, Rush BF Jr. Mammary duct proliferation in the elderly. A histopathologic study. *Cancer* 1973;31:130.
9. Nielsen M, Thomsen JL, Primdahl L, Dyreborg U, Andersen JA. Breast cancer and atypia among young and middle aged women: a study of 100 medicolegal autopsies. *Br J Cancer* 1987;56:814.
10. Singletary SE. Lobular carcinoma in situ of the breast: a 31-year experience at the University of Texas, M. D. Anderson Cancer Center. *Breast Dis* 1994;7:157.
11. Walt AJ, Simon M, Swanson GM. The continuing dilemma of lobular carcinoma in situ. *Arch Surg* 1992;127:904.
12. Rosen PP, Kosloff C, Lieberman PH, Adair F, Braun DW Jr. Lobular carcinoma in situ of the breast. Detailed analysis of 99 patients with average follow-up of 24 years. *Am J Surg Pathol* 1978;2:225.
13. Farrow JH. Current concepts in the detection and treatment of the earliest of early breast cancers. *Cancer* 1970;25:468.
14. Newman W. In situ lobular carcinoma of the breast: report of 26 women with 32 cancers. *Ann Surg* 1963;57:591.
15. Rosner D, Bedwani RN, Vana J, Baker HW, Murphy GP. Noninvasive breast carcinoma: results of a national survey by the American College of Surgeons. *Ann Surg* 1980;192:139.
16. Lemanne D, Simon M, Martino S, et al. Breast carcinoma in situ: greater rise in ductal carcinoma in situ vs lobular carcinoma in situ. *Proc Am Soc Clin Oncol* 1991;10:45.
17. Frykberg ER, Bland KI. In situ breast carcinoma. *Adv Surg* 1993;26:29.
18. Hutter RVP, Snyder RE, Lucas JC, Foote FW Jr, Farrow JH. Clinical and pathologic correlation with mammographic findings in lobular carcinoma in situ. *Cancer* 1969;23:826.
19. Pope TL Jr, Fechner RE, Wilhelm MC, Wanebo HJ, de Paredes ES. Lobular carcinoma in situ of the breast: mammographic features. *Radiology* 1988;168:63.
20. Lewison EF, Finney GG Jr. Lobular carcinoma in situ of the breast. *Surg Gynecol Obstet* 1968;126:1280.
21. Donegan W, Perez-Mesa CM. Lobular carcinoma: an indication for elective biopsy of the second breast. *Ann Surg* 1972;176:178.
22. Carter D, Smith RL. Carcinoma in situ of the breast. *Cancer* 1977;40:1189.
23. Newman W. In situ lobular carcinoma of the breast: report of 26 women and 32 cancers. *Ann Surg* 1963;157:591.
24. Lambird PA, Shelley WM. The spatial distribution of lobular in situ mammary carcinoma. Implications for size and site of breast biopsy. *JAMA* 1969;210:689.
25. Urban JA. Bilaterality of cancer of the breast: biopsy of the opposite breast. *Cancer* 1967;11:1867.
26. Azzopardi JG. *Problems in breast pathology*. Philadelphia: WB Saunders, 1983.
27. Page DL, Anderson TJ. *Diagnostic histopathology of the breast*. Edinburgh, UK: Churchill Livingstone, 1987.
28. Rosen PP, Oberman H. *Tumors of the mammary gland*. Washington, DC: Armed Forces Institute of Pathology, 1993.
29. Wheeler JE, Enterline HT. Lobular carcinoma of the breast in situ and infiltrating. *Pathol Annu* 1976;11:161.
30. Frykberg ER, Santiago F, Betsill WL Jr, O'Brien PH. Lobular carcinoma in situ of the breast. *Surg Gynecol Obstet* 1987;164:285.
31. Goldschmidt RA, Victor TA. Lobular carcinoma in situ of the breast. *Semin Surg Oncol* 1996;12:314.
32. Haagensen CD, Lane N, Lattes R, Bodian CA. Lobular neoplasia (so-called lobular carcinoma in situ of the breast. *Cancer* 1978;42:737.
33. Fechner RE. Epithelial alterations in the extralobular ducts of breasts with lobular carcinoma. *Arch Pathol* 1972;93:164.
34. Meyer JS. Cell kinetics of histologic variants of in situ breast carcinoma. *Breast Cancer Res Treat* 1986;7:171.
35. Albonico G, Querzoli P, Ferretti S, Rinaldi R, Nenci I: Biological profile of in situ breast cancer investigated by immunohistochemical technique. *Cancer Detect Prev* 1998;22:313.
36. Rudas M, Neumayer R, Gnant MF, Mittelbock M, Jakesz R, Reiner A. p53 protein expression, cell proliferation and steroid hormone receptors in ductal and lobular in situ carcinomas of the breast. *Eur J Cancer* 1997;33:39.
37. Bur ME, Zimarowski MJ, Schnitt SJ, Baker S, Lew R. Estrogen receptor immunohistochemistry in carcinoma in situ of the breast. *Cancer* 1992;69:1174.
38. Ramachandra S, Machin L, Ashley S, Monaghan P, Gusterson BA. Immunohistochemical distribution of c-erbB-2 in in situ breast carcinoma: a detailed morphological analysis. *J Pathol* 1990;161:7.
39. Porter PL, Garcia R, Moe R, Corwin DJ, Gown AM. c-erbB-2 oncogene protein in in situ and invasive lobular breast neoplasia. *Cancer* 1991;68:331.
40. Vos CB, Cleton-Jansen AM, Berx G, et al. E-cadherin inactivation in lobular carcinoma in situ of the breast; an early event in tumorigenesis. *Br J Cancer* 1997;76:1131.
41. Fechner RE. Lobular carcinoma in situ in sclerosing adenosis: a potential source of confusion with invasive carcinoma. *Am J Surg Pathol* 1981;5:233.
42. Fechner RE. Ductal carcinoma involving the lobule of the breast: a source of confusion with lobular carcinoma in situ. *Cancer* 1971;28:274.
43. Kerner H, Lichtig C. Lobular cancerization: incidence and differential diagnosis with lobular carcinoma in situ of the breast. *Histopathology* 1986;10:621.
44. Rosen PP. Coexistent lobular carcinoma in situ and intraductal carcinoma in a single lobular-duct unit. *Am J Surg Pathol* 1980;4:241.
45. Fisher ER, Costantino J, Fisher B, et al. Pathologic findings from the National Surgical Adjuvant Breast Project (NSABP) protocol B-17. Five-year observations concerning lobular carcinoma in situ. *Cancer* 1996;78:1403.
46. Bodian CA, Perzin KH, Lattes R. Lobular neoplasia. Long-term risk of breast cancer and relation to other factors. *Cancer* 1996;78:1024.
47. Salvadori B, Bartolic C, Zurrida S, et al. Risk of invasive cancer in women with lobular carcinoma in situ of the breast. *Eur J Cancer* 1991;27:35.
48. Ottesen GL, Graversen HP, Blichert-Toft M, Zedeler K, Andersen JA. Lobular carcinoma in situ of the female breast: short-term results of a prospective nationwide study. *Am J Surg Pathol* 1993;17:14.
49. Fisher B, Costantino JP, Wickerham DL, et al. Tamoxifen for prevention of breast cancer: report of the National Surgical Adjuvant Breast and Bowel Project P-1 study. *J Natl Cancer Inst* 1998;90:1371.
50. Bradley SJ, Weaver DW, Bouwman DL. Alternatives in the surgical management of in situ breast cancer: a meta-analysis of outcome. *Am Surg* 1990;58:428.
51. Carson W, Sanchez-Forgach E, Stomper P, Penetrante R, Tsangaris TN, Edge SB. Lobular carcinoma in situ: observation without surgery as an appropriate therapy. *Ann Surg Oncol* 1994;1:141.

Diseases of the Breast, 2nd ed.,
edited by Jay R. Harris.
Lippincott Williams & Wilkins, Philadelphia © 2000.

CHAPTER 27

Ductal Carcinoma *in Situ* and Microinvasive Carcinoma

Monica Morrow, Stuart J. Schnitt, and Jay R. Harris

DUCTAL CARCINOMA *IN SITU*

Ductal carcinoma *in situ* (DCIS), also known as *intraductal carcinoma,* is an entity distinct in both its clinical presentation and its biological potential from lobular carcinoma *in situ* (LCIS), the other lesion classified as noninvasive carcinoma. Previously, DCIS was an uncommon lesion that was routinely cured by mastectomy, and little attention was given to defining its natural history or exploring alternative local treatments. The widespread use of screening mammography has resulted in a significant increase in the rate of detection of DCIS, and the acceptance of breast-conserving therapy for the treatment of invasive carcinoma has raised questions about the routine need for mastectomy for a lesion that may only be precancerous. The proportion of women with mammographically detected DCIS who will develop invasive carcinoma within their lifetimes is uncertain. This uncertainty has led to debate as to whether all DCIS should be regarded as early-stage carcinoma and treated with either mastectomy or lumpectomy and irradiation or whether excision and observation can be used to treat some DCIS.

Presentation

DCIS has various clinical presentations. In the past, most DCIS was gross or palpable. Gross DCIS accounts for only a small percentage of palpable breast cancers. An American College of Surgeons survey found that only 2% of 10,000 ductal and lobular cancers reported in 1980 were DCIS.[1] DCIS also presents as pathologic nipple discharge, with or without a mass, and may be identified as an incidental finding in a breast biopsy performed to treat or diagnose another abnormality. Today, an abnormal mammographic result is the most common presentation of DCIS. DCIS usually appears as clustered microcalcifications, although nonpalpable masses may also represent DCIS. In many reports of mammographically directed biopsies, DCIS accounts for one-half or more of the malignancies identified.[2–5] However, clinical presentations of DCIS accounted for 23% of 202 cases seen between 1988 and 1996 in the series of Brenin and Morrow.[6] Pandya et al.[7] compared the features of DCIS lesions treated from 1969 to 1985 to those treated from 1986 to 1990. During this time, clinical presentations of DCIS fell from 81% of cases to 20% of cases, and grade 3 lesions increased from 24% to 33% of cases.

The use of screening mammography has resulted in a remarkable increase in the incidence (or detection rate) of DCIS. Between 1973 and 1992, age-adjusted DCIS incidence rates rose from 2.3 to 15.8 per 100,000 women, a 587% increase. In comparison, the incidence of invasive breast cancer increased by 34.3% in the same time period.[8] This increase in the incidence of DCIS was observed for women both younger and older than 50 years, and for both white and African-American women.

The dramatic increase in the number of DCIS cases seen in recent years has led some authors to suggest that screening results in the detection of biologically indolent DCIS that is unlikely to become clinically significant during a woman's lifetime. The data discussed earlier, indicating a higher frequency of grade 3 lesions in the screen-detected patients, argues against this interpretation. A number of studies have also examined risk factors for DCIS and invasive carcinoma to see if these are similar. Gapstur et al.[9] examined prospectively collected risk factor data from the 37,105 women in the Iowa Women's Health Study. After a follow-up of 11 years, 1,520 carcinomas have developed in this cohort, including 175 cases of DCIS. No differences in risk factors for DCIS and infiltrating carcinoma were observed. Similar findings have been reported in case-control studies that have addressed this issue.[10,11]

M. Morrow: Department of Surgery, Northwestern University Medical School, Chicago, Illinois; Lynn Sage Comprehensive Breast Program, Northwestern Memorial Hospital, Chicago, Illinois

S. J. Schnitt: Department of Pathology, Harvard Medical School, Brigham and Women's Hospital, Dana-Farber Cancer Institute, Boston, Massachusetts; Department of Surgical Pathology, Beth Israel Deaconess Medical Center, Boston, Massachusetts

J. R. Harris: Department of Radiation Oncology, Harvard Medical School, Brigham and Women's Hospital, Dana-Farber Cancer Institute, Boston, Massachusetts

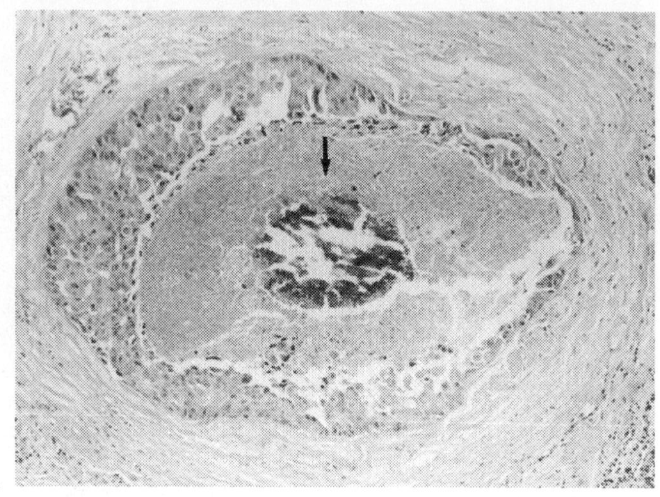

A

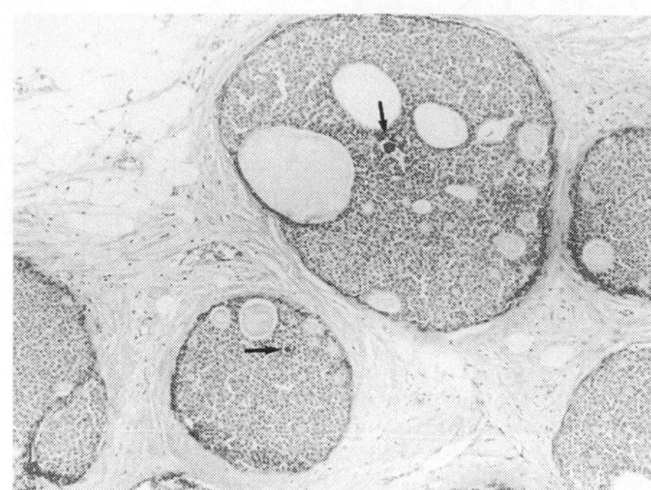

B

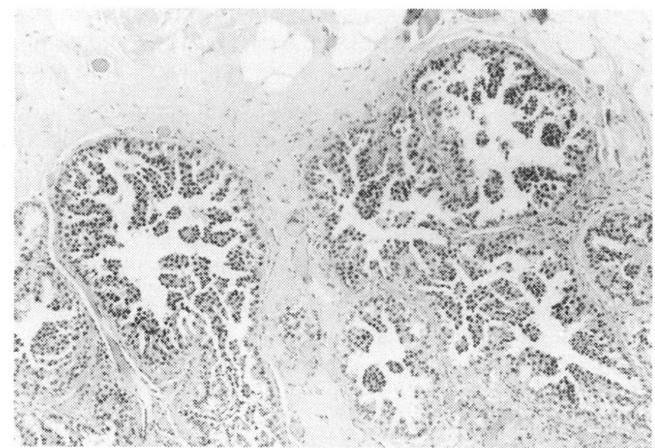

C

FIG. 1. Comedo pattern ductal carcinoma *in situ.* **A:** Prominent central necrosis and an area of coarse calcification (*arrow*) in this involved space are seen. **B:** Cribriform pattern ductal carcinoma *in situ.* The cells comprising this lesion grow in a fenestrated, sievelike pattern. Scattered, fine calcifications are present (*arrows*). **C:** Micropapillary pattern ductal carcinoma *in situ.* The tumor cells form tufts that project into the lumens of the involved spaces. These tufts lack fibrovascular cores. (*Continued*)

Pathology

DCIS is characterized by a proliferation of presumably malignant epithelial cells within the mammary ductal-lobular system without light-microscopic evidence of invasion into the surrounding stroma.

Classification

The term *ductal carcinoma in situ* encompasses a pathologically heterogeneous group of lesions that differ in their growth patterns and cytologic features. Although the diversity of DCIS lesions is well recognized, no universal agreement exists as to how best to subclassify these lesions. Proposed classification schemes for DCIS have variously emphasized architectural features or growth pattern of the neoplastic cells within the ductal-lobular system, cytologic features of the neoplastic cells, and cellular necrosis, singly and in combination.

The traditional system for classifying DCIS was based primarily on the architectural pattern of the lesion and recognized five major subtypes: comedo, cribriform, micropapillary, papillary, and solid.[12–14] The hallmark of the *comedo* pattern is the presence of prominent necrosis in the involved spaces. This necrosis can often be appreciated on macroscopic examination as cords of pasty material exuding from the cut surface of the specimen or readily expressed from involved ducts by palpation. Microscopically, the cells comprising lesions with a comedo pattern are most often large and show nuclear pleomorphism. Mitotic figures, including abnormal mitoses, are usually evident and are often numerous. Many of the involved spaces contain necrotic cellular debris within their centers. This necrotic material frequently becomes calcified, and these calcifications may be detected mammographically, characteristically as linear, branching ("casting") calcifications (Fig. 1A). The *cribriform* pattern is characterized by a fenestrated, sievelike proliferation of neoplastic cells (Fig. 1B). The *micropapillary* pattern features small tufts of cells that are oriented perpendicular to the basement membrane of the involved spaces and project into the lumina. The apical region of these small papillations is frequently broader than the base, imparting a club-shaped appearance. The micropapillae lack fibrovascular cores (Fig. 1C). The cells comprising lesions with cribriform and micropapillary patterns are most often small to medium in size, and the nuclei are usually monomorphic. The *papillary* pattern shows intraluminal projections of tumor cells that, in contrast with the micropapillary variant, demonstrate fibrovascular cores and thus constitute true papillations

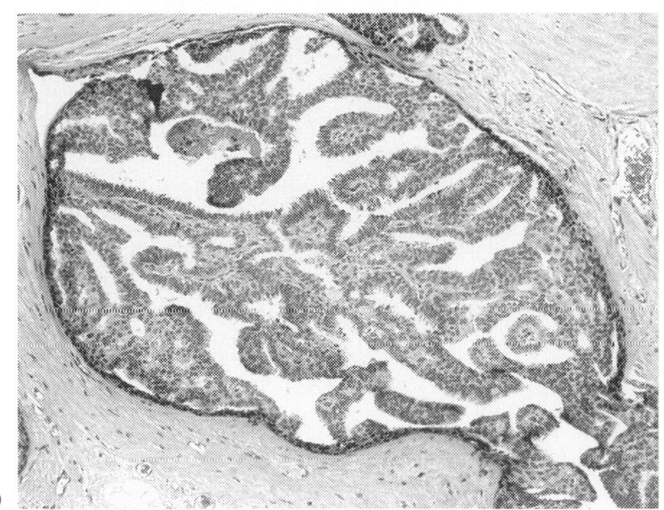

D

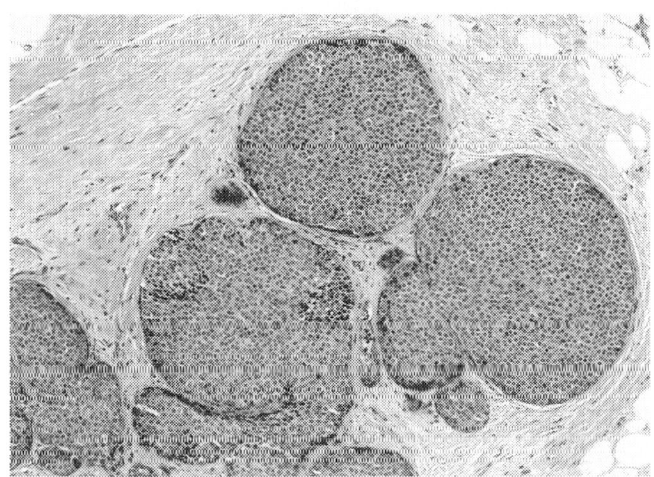

E

FIG. 1. *Continued.* **D:** Papillary pattern ductal carcinoma *in situ.* The neoplastic cells cover fingerlike projections that contain fibrovascular cores. **E:** Solid pattern ductal carcinoma *in situ.* In this lesion, the tumor cells grow in a solid pattern without evidence of necrosis, fenestrations, or papillations.

(Fig. 1D). In one variant of papillary DCIS, the tumor cells are primarily or exclusively present in a single cystically dilated space (intracystic or encysted papillary carcinoma).[15–17] In the *solid* pattern, the tumor cells fill and distend the involved spaces and lack significant necrosis, fenestrations, or papillations (Fig. 1E). As is the case for comedo lesions, other variants of DCIS may show calcifications that can be detected mammographically. However, the mammographic appearance of the microcalcifications associated with other DCIS patterns is less distinctive than the appearance of the calcifications seen in comedo lesions and overlaps with that of a number of benign processes.

Less common variants of DCIS are also recognized. Some of these variants are defined by the cytologic characteristics of the cells comprising the lesion. For example, certain DCIS lesions are composed of cells that have apocrine features (apocrine DCIS).[18,19] Others are comprised of cells that have a signet-ring configuration (intraductal signet-ring cell carcinoma).[20] Still other variants of DCIS are composed of cells that exhibit neuroendocrine differentiation (endocrine DCIS and solid papillary carcinoma).[21,22] Some of the less frequent DCIS types are defined by their architectural features. Cystic hypersecretory carcinoma is characterized by neoplastic cells that line dilatated spaces filled with eosinophilic secretion, resembling the colloid seen in thyroid follicles.[23,24] The term *clinging carcinoma* has been used to describe two different types of lesions. One is characterized by a single layer of cytologically malignant cells lining the involved spaces; general agreement exists that such lesions should be categorized as DCIS. In the other variant, ductal-lobular spaces are lined by a layer of cells with low-grade nuclear features. Whereas some authors consider such lesions to represent variants of DCIS, others regard them as atypical ductal hyperplasia.[12,25,26]

Some authors believe it useful to subdivide DCIS into two subgroups: the comedo type and the noncomedo type (which encompasses the other variants). This subdivision is based on the observations that the comedo type usually appears more malignant cytologically[12–14] and is more often associated with invasion[27–29] than are the other DCIS types. Another difference reported for these two groups is in regard to the relationship between the extent of microcalcifications on the mammogram and the histologic extent of the lesion. When standard two-view mammography is used, the histologic extent of comedo-type DCIS is highly correlated with the extent of the calcifications on the mammogram in most cases. In contrast, the extent of the calcifications associated with noncomedo DCIS on mammography frequently underestimates the pathologic extent of the lesion.[30] A subsequent study, however, has indicated that when standard mammographic images are supplemented with magnification views, a much better correlation is found between the extent of mammographic calcifications and the histologic extent of the lesion, even for DCIS lesions of the noncomedo type.[31]

These classification systems based primarily on architecture have a number of important limitations. First, DCIS lesions may be difficult to classify using architecture alone, because many display a mixture of patterns, particularly when the lesion is large.[27] For example, in one study of 100 consecutive cases of DCIS reviewed in a consultation practice, 23 of 76 noncomedo lesions (30%) showed a mixture of histologic patterns, the most common being cribriform and micropapillary. Among 24 comedo lesions, 10 (42%) also contained areas with noncomedo patterns.[32] In another study of 121 cases of DCIS, mixtures of architectural patterns were identified in 62% of cases.[33] Second, although DCIS lesions with a comedo pattern are most often composed of malignant-appearing cells with high-grade nuclei, whereas noncomedo lesions are usually composed of cells with low-grade to intermediate-grade nuclei, the correlation between architecture and nuclear grade is far from absolute. For example, some DCIS lesions with small, uniform, low-grade nuclei display central comedo-type necrosis in the involved spaces (Fig. 2), whereas others with cribriform, micropapillary, or papillary architectural patterns may be composed of cytologically malignant cells exhibiting large,

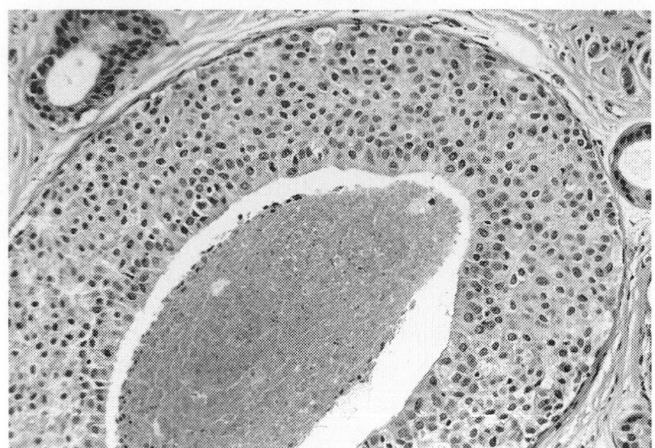

FIG. 2. Comedo pattern ductal carcinoma *in situ* with low nuclear grade.

high-grade nuclei (Fig. 3). In addition, interobserver reproducibility in the categorization of DCIS lesions by architectural pattern is poor, even if a simplified, dichotomous comedo/noncomedo classification scheme is used.[34] Finally, although the architectural classification scheme was perfectly acceptable in an era in which all cases of DCIS were treated by mastectomy, a pressing clinical need now exists to develop a classification system that has prognostic significance for patients considered for treatment with breast conservation.

A number of alternative classification schemes for DCIS have been proposed in an attempt to overcome the limitations of the traditional, primarily architectural classification system. These newer classification systems stratify DCIS lesions largely on the basis of nuclear grade or necrosis, with architectural pattern given secondary or no consideration (Fig. 4). Lagios et al. were the first to propose a system based primarily on nuclear grade and necrosis, rather than on architecture.[35] A modification of this system recognizes three major categories of DCIS: high, intermediate, and low grade.[26] Investigators in Nottingham, England, have developed a classification system based primarily on the presence or absence of necrosis.[36] This group divides DCIS into three categories: pure comedo (lesions in which involved spaces show centrally necrotic debris surrounded by large, pleomorphic tumor cells in solid masses); DCIS with necrosis, also called nonpure comedo (lesions with necrotic neoplastic cells but with a cribriform or micropapillary pattern); and DCIS without necrosis (lesions with a cribriform, papillary, micropapillary, or solid pattern and no necrosis). The classification scheme proposed by Silverstein et al.[37] is essentially a modification of the Nottingham system in which DCIS lesions are classified based on nuclear grade as either high-grade or non–high-grade. The non–high-grade lesions are further stratified by the presence or absence of comedo-type necrosis. Thus, this is a three-tiered system in which DCIS is classified as either high-grade, non–high-grade with necrosis, or non–high-grade without necrosis. A group of European pathologists have proposed classifying DCIS as well differentiated, intermediately differentiated, or poorly differentiated, based primarily on cytonuclear differentiation and cell polarization.[38] Pathologists associated with the United Kingdom National Breast Cancer Screening Program use a classification scheme for DCIS based solely on nuclear grade, recognizing high-grade, intermediate-grade, and low-grade types.[34] Other classification systems have been proposed by other authors as well.[39–43]

To attain widespread clinical use, a classification system not only must be clinically relevant but also must be able to be applied reliably by different observers. The clinical importance of classifying DCIS using these various approaches is discussed below. Although some authors have claimed that their systems are or should be easy to use, few studies have been conducted to assess interobserver agreement in the classification of DCIS using these newer categorization schemes. In one study, two pathologists classified the DCIS component associated with 180 invasive cancers using six different classification systems. These investigators found that the highest level of agreement was obtained using the Silverstein system.[44] Another study found a 94% level of agreement among six observers using the Lagios classification system.[26] More sobering results were reported by the European Commission Working Group on Breast Screening Pathology.[34] In that study, 33 cases of DCIS were categorized by 23 pathologists using five classification systems. The level of interobserver agreement, as defined by kappa statistics, was only fair to moderate for each of the classification schemes evaluated.

In 1997, a consensus conference was convened in an attempt to reach agreement on the classification of DCIS.[45] Although the panel did not endorse any one system of classification, agreement was reached that certain features be routinely documented in pathology reports of DCIS lesions. These include nuclear grade (low, intermediate, or high), the presence of necrosis (comedo or punctate), cell polarization, and architectural pattern. In fact, if these individual features are recorded, sufficient information is then available to per-

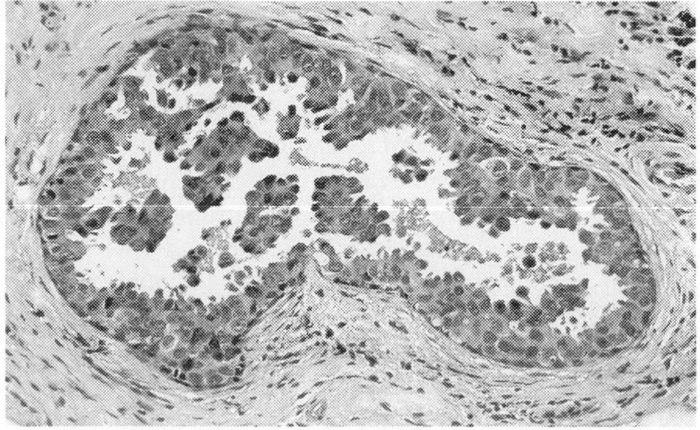

FIG. 3. Micropapillary pattern ductal carcinoma *in situ* with high nuclear grade.

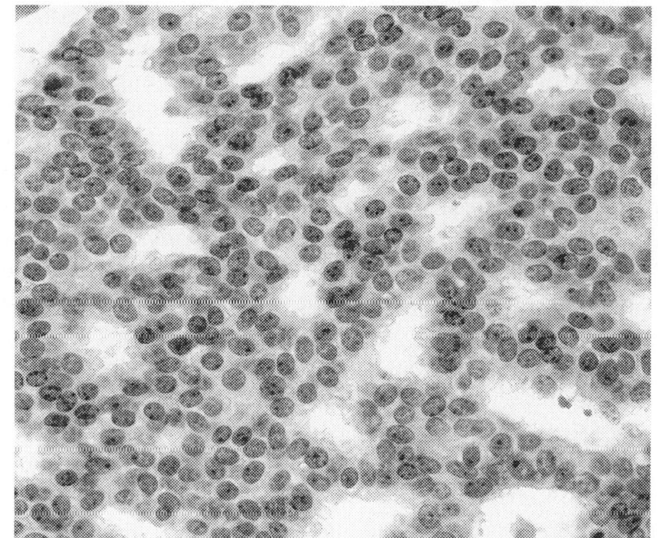

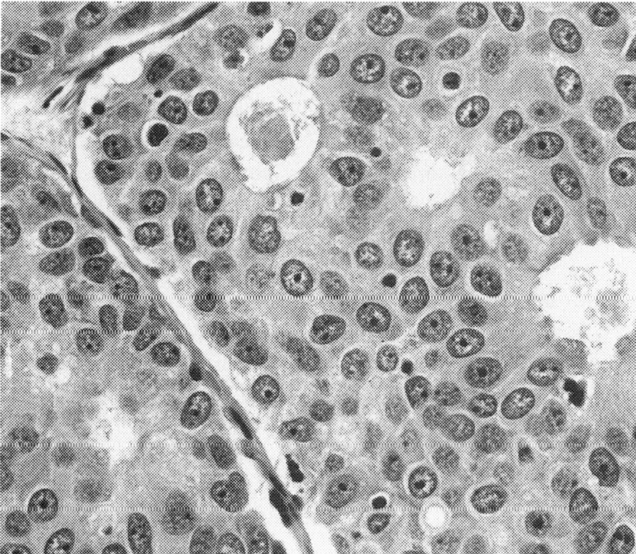

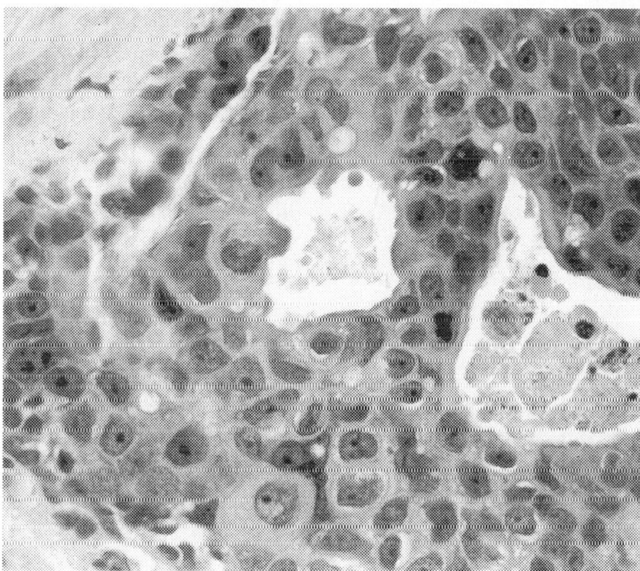

FIG. 4. Nuclear grading in ductal carcinoma *in situ*. **A:** Low nuclear grade. **B:** Intermediate nuclear grade. **C:** High nuclear grade.

mit the categorization of a DCIS lesion according to virtually all of the newly proposed classification schemes.

Biological Markers

The study of tumor markers in DCIS lesions to provide a better understanding of the biology of these lesions and to aid in their classification has provoked considerable interest. The results of studies of these markers are somewhat difficult to compare due to differences in the classification used for the DCIS lesions, patient populations, and methodology; however, a number of trends have emerged. These studies have generally shown that lesions demonstrating a comedo pattern or high nuclear grade exhibit a profile of biological markers that has been associated with aggressive clinical behavior in invasive cancers more often than do noncomedo or low-nuclear-grade lesions. For example, comedo or high-grade lesions are more likely than noncomedo or low-grade lesions to lack estrogen and progesterone receptors,[46–50] to have a high proliferative rate,[48–52] and to exhibit aneuploidy,[53] overexpression of the HER-2/neu (c-*erb*-b2) oncogene,[47–51,54–56] mutations of the p53 tumor-suppressor gene with accumulation of its protein product,[47–51,57,58] and angiogenesis in the surrounding stroma.[59,60]

In addition, genetic analyses have indicated that loss of heterozygosity at various chromosomal loci may differ according to DCIS pattern and grade.[61]

Distribution of Tumor in the Breast and Axillary Lymph Node Involvement

The distribution of tumor in the breast, the incidence of unsuspected invasive carcinoma, and the incidence of axillary lymph node metastases are all important considerations in selecting appropriate therapy for patients with DCIS.

The reported incidence of multicentricity in mastectomy specimens from patients with DCIS varies considerably and has ranged from 0% to 47%.[50,62] A number of factors have contributed to this variability, including differences in the definition of multicentricity and differences in the methods and extent of specimen sampling. Most authors define *multicentricity* as the presence of DCIS foci in breast quadrants other than the one harboring the index lesion (in contrast to *multifocality*, which denotes foci of DCIS in the same quadrant as the index lesion). Others define foci as multicentric if they are a specified distance from the index lesion (e.g., 5 cm), regardless of the quadrant.[63] These studies of multicentricity were conducted before the widespread use of screening mammography, and these data probably cannot be extrapolated to the small (often less than 1 cm), mammographically detected lesions commonly seen today. In these studies, the frequency of multicentricity appeared to be related to the size of the index lesion. In one study, multicentricity was much more common in DCIS lesions larger than 2.5 cm (13 of 25 cases, 52%) than in smaller lesions (4 of 29, 14%).[63] In another study, the frequency of multicentricity also correlated with the size of the lesion as determined by the number of involved ducts in the index lesion.[28] These investigators also noted a higher frequency of multicentricity in micropapillary lesions (8 of 10 cases, 80%) than in other types of DCIS (16 of 45, 36%).[27] A similar association between micropapillary DCIS and frequent multiple-quadrant involvement has also been recognized by others.[40] Because of the sampling methods used, however, it is not possible to determine if the foci of DCIS characterized as multicentric in these studies were truly independent lesions or if they represented tumor that was, in fact, contiguous with the index lesion.

More recent studies suggest that, in most cases, true multicentricity in DCIS is rare. Holland and Hendriks studied 119 mastectomy specimens containing DCIS by a subgross pathologic-mammographic technique.[31] In all but one case, the tumor was confined to a single "segment" of the breast. Clear-cut multicentric distribution (defined in this study as foci of DCIS separated by 4 cm or more of uninvolved breast tissue) was seen in only one patient. Faverly et al., using stereomicroscopic three-dimensional analysis to define the growth pattern of DCIS within the mammary duct system, studied 60 mastectomy specimens containing DCIS.[64] They found that within the segment of breast involved by DCIS, growth was continuous in some cases and discontinuous in others. Overall, 50% of cases showed a continuous growth pattern and 50% showed a discontinuous pattern, characterized by uninvolved breast tissue between foci of DCIS ("gaps"). In most instances, these gaps were small (less than 5 mm in 82% of cases), and the likelihood of finding such gaps was related to the histologic type of the lesion. Whereas 90% of the cases of poorly differentiated DCIS grew in a continuous manner without gaps, only 30% of well-differentiated lesions and 45% of intermediately differentiated lesions were continuous. The findings in these two studies indicate that, in most cases, DCIS involves the breast in a segmental distribution, and truly multicentric disease is uncommon. In some cases, however, the segment involved by DCIS may be quite large. For example, in the study of Holland and Hendriks, although 86% of the DCIS lesions were nonpalpable and were detected mammographically, 46% were larger than 3 cm. One study of clonality in DCIS supports the contention that most DCIS is unifocal, at least with regard to comedo lesions.[65] In that study, clonality was assessed in widely separated sites of comedo-type DCIS in the same breast. Each of these widely separated sites was found to be monoclonal, and each showed inactivation of the same X chromosome–linked phosphoglycerokinase allele, suggesting an origin from the same clone.

The incidence of nipple involvement in patients with DCIS has been evaluated in a few studies and appears to be related to the method of detection of the lesion. For example, Contesso et al. found nipple involvement in 49% of 117 mastectomy specimens from patients in whom DCIS presented primarily with a palpable mass, nipple discharge, or Paget's disease.[66] In contrast, Lagios et al. found involvement of the nipple in 8 of 40 mastectomy specimens (20%) from patients with DCIS, the majority of whom presented with mammographic calcifications or had DCIS as an incidental finding. Of these eight cases, five were Paget's disease and three had lactiferous duct involvement.[63]

The incidence of occult invasion, either near the primary tumor or in other parts of the breast, has also been examined in mastectomy series. The reported incidence of occult invasion ranges from 0% to 26%.[62] However, these series are difficult to interpret for several reasons. The completeness of initial biopsy varies, which affects the likelihood of finding residual cancer with invasion at mastectomy if the initial biopsy shows only "noninvasive" disease. Also, the extent of sampling of the initial biopsy specimen and of the remainder of the breast also differs substantially from series to series. The likelihood of finding occult invasion appears to be related to the size of the index lesion. In one series, patients with lesions larger than 2.5 cm were more likely to have occult invasion (16 of 55, 29%) than were patients with smaller tumors (1 of 60, 2%).[63] However, all four invasive tumors in the 90 patients with lesions 4.5 cm or smaller were found after inadequate initial excision. The frequency of occult invasion is also related to the method of detection of the DCIS. In one series, invasive cancer was identified in the mastectomy specimen in 6 of 54 patients (11%) with DCIS who presented with a palpable mass, nipple discharge, or Paget's disease and in none of 16 patients who presented with mammographic microcalcifications or in whom DCIS was an incidental finding.[67] In another series, 6 of 41 tumors (15%) from patients that presented with a mass showed occult invasion, compared with only 1 of 21 tumors (5%) detected only on mammography.[68] The incidence of occult invasion also appears to be correlated with the histologic type of DCIS and is much more common in comedo lesions. For example, Patchefsky et al. noted microinvasion in 12 of 19 cases (63%) of comedo DCIS and in only 4 of 36 (11%) noncomedo lesions.[27]

Incidence rates reported for axillary nodal involvement in patients given the diagnosis of DCIS range from 0% to 7%,[12] with the higher rates noted in studies performed in the premammography era, when most patients with DCIS presented with a palpable mass. In such cases, invasion is undoubtedly present but is either not recognized by the pathologist or is undetected due to sampling error. Axillary lymph node involvement in patients with DCIS detected by mammography is a rare event. In one series of 189 patients with DCIS, most of whose tumors were detected by mammography alone, none showed metastases on axillary dissection.[69]

In a National Cancer Data Base review of 10,946 patients with DCIS who had an axillary dissection between 1985 and 1991, only 406 (3.6%) were found to have axillary metastases.[70]

Differential Diagnosis

In most instances, the pathologic diagnosis of DCIS is straightforward. However, occasional cases present diagnostic difficulties. At one end of the spectrum, distinguishing low-grade (noncomedo) DCIS from atypical ductal hyperplasia is sometimes difficult. Although a number of authors have published criteria useful in making this distinction, some cases are subject to considerable interobserver variability in diagnosis, even with use of standardized criteria.[71,72]

At the other end of the spectrum, distinguishing examples of pure DCIS from DCIS with focal stromal invasion (microinvasion) may sometimes be difficult.[73] This distinction is discussed in detail below.

DCIS may also be difficult to distinguish from frankly invasive breast cancer in certain instances, because some breast cancers (e.g., invasive cribriform carcinoma) invade the stroma in rounded nests simulating DCIS.[74,75] Another diagnostic problem occasionally encountered is distinguishing nests of tumor cells in lymphatic or vascular spaces from DCIS.

Finally, although the distinction between DCIS and lobular carcinoma *in situ* (LCIS) is usually not difficult to make, areas of overlap exist between these two lesions. DCIS may extend into recognizable lobules,[76,77] LCIS may involve extralobular ducts,[78] and some lesions have cytologic features intermediate between the two disorders.[13,14,79] Furthermore, DCIS and LCIS may coexist in the same breast and even in the same ductal-lobular unit.[80] For example, in the National Surgical Adjuvant Breast and Bowel Project (NSABP) Protocol B-17 study of patients with DCIS treated with either conservative surgery alone or conservative surgery and radiation therapy, approximately 7% of patients had LCIS in addition to DCIS.[81]

Microinvasive Carcinoma

One of the most important goals in the histologic examination of DCIS lesions is the identification of foci of stromal invasion, because in general the therapeutic algorithm for patients with pure DCIS differs from that for patients with DCIS and associated invasive breast cancer. A frequently encountered problem in the examination of such specimens is the identification of the smallest foci of invasive carcinoma, or *microinvasion*. Although this diagnosis often appears in surgical pathology reports, this term has not been applied in a consistent, standardized manner, and the histologic diagnosis of microinvasion is not straightforward and is often problematic for the pathologist.

In the 1997 edition of the American Joint Committee on Cancer (AJCC) *Cancer Staging Manual*,[82] microinvasion is defined as "the extension of cancer cells beyond the basement membrane into the adjacent tissues with no focus more than 0.1 cm in greatest dimension." Lesions that fulfill this definition are staged as T1mic, a subset of T1 breast cancer. The staging manual further states that "when there are multiple foci of microinvasion, the size of only the largest focus is used to classify the microinvasion" and that the size of the individual foci should not be added together. This is the first edition of the AJCC staging manual that recognizes a specific T substage for microinvasion. Unfortunately, widely varying definitions of microinvasion have been used in the past, and some of these definitions differ substantially from that offered in the AJCC staging manual. For example, microinvasion has been variously defined as: (a) DCIS with "evidence of stromal invasion"[83]; (b) "DCIS with limited microscopic stromal invasion below the basement membrane, but not invading more than 10% of the surface of the histologic sections examined"[84]; and (c) "breast cancer cells confined to the duct system of the breast with only a microscopic focus of malignant cells invading beyond the basement membrane of the duct as determined by light microscopy."[85] This lack of a uniform definition for microinvasion has clearly contributed to the confusion regarding this entity.

The identification of microinvasion in a lesion that is primarily DCIS can be difficult for the pathologist, because a variety of patterns in DCIS may be misconstrued as stromal invasion. Lesions that are commonly mistaken for microinvasion include: (a) DCIS involving lobules ("cancerization of lobules"), (b) branching of ducts, (c) distortion or entrapment of involved ducts or acini by fibrosis, (d) inflammation present in association with and obscuring involved ducts or acini, (e) crush artifact, (f) cautery effect, (g) artifactual displacement of DCIS cells into the surrounding stroma or adipose tissue due to tissue manipulation or a prior needling procedure, and (h) DCIS involving benign sclerosing processes, such as radial scars, complete sclerosing lesions, and sclerosing adenosis.[77,86–91]

What, then, are the minimum criteria for identifying bona fide stromal invasion in the setting of DCIS? Remarkably, few guidelines have been published in this regard. Page and Anderson require "more than a single collection of cells outside the lobular unit or immediate periductal area."[13] Fisher indicates that the suspicious focus should be comprised of a "recognized type of invasive cancer."[86] Elston and Ellis state that "only when unequivocal invasion is seen outside the spe-

TABLE 1. *Incidence of axillary lymph node involvement in patients with microinvasion*

Study	No. of patients	No. (%) node positive
Wong et al.[85]	33	0
Silverstein[95]	17	0
Akhtar et al.[96]	25	0
Silver and Tavassoli[93]	38	0
Rosner et al.[84]	34	1 (3)
Solin et al.[94]	39	2 (5)
Penault-Llorca et al.[97]	58	3 (5)
Patchefsky et al.[27]	16	2 (12)
Prasad et al.[98]	11	2 (18)
Schuh et al.[83]	30	6 (20)

cialized lobular stroma should microinvasive carcinoma be diagnosed."[92] The definition offered by Silver and Tavassoli seems to be less restrictive, because they consider invasive tumor cells singly and in clusters in the periductal stroma to represent microinvasion.[93] In the authors' view, for a diagnosis of unequivocal stromal invasion or microinvasion in the setting of DCIS, the worrisome area should be present clearly beyond the immediate periductal and perilobular region and should consist of a recognized type of invasive cancer. Furthermore, the suspicious area should clearly not be in a benign sclerosing lesion. The clinical significance of a few single tumor cells or tumor cell clusters admixed with inflammatory cells in the immediate periductal region is unclear. In such cases, the authors note the presence of such foci, but indicate uncertainty about their clinical importance. Although the presence of stromal desmoplasia and inflammation should heighten the suspicion of invasion, these phenomena are so often present in association with high-grade DCIS without demonstrable invasion that their presence cannot be depended on to make this distinction.

Another potential problem with the pathologic diagnosis of microinvasion relates to tissue sampling. Previous published studies of microinvasion have generally failed to indicate how much of a given specimen was submitted for microscopic evaluation. Thus, some lesions categorized as microinvasive based on limited tissue sampling could in truth represent frankly invasive carcinomas in which the largest area of invasion was not submitted for histologic evaluation or was not represented on the slides because the cancer was deeper in the blocks. Even when an entire specimen is submitted for histologic evaluation, only a fraction of the tissue is ultimately examined microscopically. For example, if a 6-cm excision specimen is sectioned grossly at 3-mm intervals (producing 20 slices), each of these slices is embedded in a separate paraffin block, and one 5-μm section is cut from each block, less than 1% of the entire specimen will be examined microscopically.

Given the problems with the definition and pathologic diagnosis of microinvasion, the controversy surrounding the clinical significance of this lesion should not be surprising. The reported incidence of axillary lymph node involvement in patients given the diagnosis of microinvasion ranges from 0% to 20%[27,83–85,93–98] (Table 1).

Ideally, the term *microinvasion* should be used with regard to the breast in the same way it is used with regard to the cervix—that is, to identify those invasive lesions of limited extent that have virtually no risk of metastasis. Unfortunately, the available data are inadequate to permit the reproducible identification of such a subset due to differences among studies with regard to the definition of microinvasion, variations in the extent of tissue sampling, small patient numbers, and limited follow-up. Additional clinicopathologic studies using a standardized definition of microinvasion are clearly needed to address this important question. Although the definition of microinvasion in the current edition of the AJCC *Cancer Staging Manual* may ultimately be modified, it represents an important step toward standardization, and its use in both clinical research and clinical practice should be encouraged.

Natural History

The major issue in the management of DCIS is the risk of progression to invasive carcinoma. Few clinically relevant data are available to address this question, primarily because DCIS has traditionally been treated with mastectomy. In addition, most DCIS cases treated in the past for which long-term follow-up is available were gross DCIS, a form that may not be equivalent to the mammographic DCIS more commonly seen today.

Long-term follow-up data are available for several small series of women found to have DCIS on review of biopsy specimens that were originally classified as benign. No attempt was made to assess margin status in these studies, lesion size was unknown, and the completeness of excision remains uncertain. Page et al.[99] identified 25 such cases in a review of 11,760 breast biopsies. Invasive carcinoma developed in seven women (28%) at intervals of 3 to 10 years (mean of 6.1 years) postbiopsy. This incidence of carcinoma represents a relative risk of 11 compared with that of age-matched controls from the Third National Cancer Survey for white women in Atlanta. An update of this series with follow-up extended to 24 years demonstrated that the relative risk of carcinoma remained constant.[100] In a similar study, Rosen et al.[101] described 30 women with untreated DCIS; complete follow-up was available only for 15. Seven invasive cancers occurred at a mean of 9.7 years after the diagnosis of DCIS—an incidence of 27% if all cases are included or 53% if only patients with complete follow-up are considered. In both the reports, all carcinomas were in the index breast, usually in the vicinity of the biopsy site. In a similar report, Eusebi et al.[25] described 28 cases of DCIS with an 11% incidence of invasive carcinoma at a median follow-up of 16.7 years. Eusebi et al.[102] subsequently reported on 80 cases of DCIS followed for a mean of 17.5 years, only two of which

TABLE 2. *Results of treatment of ductal carcinoma* in situ *with simple mastectomy*

Study	Dates	No. of patients	Follow-up (absolute no. of yr)	Nonpalpable tumor (%)	Recurrence (absolute no.)
Von Rueden and Wilson[106]	1960–1981	45	—	7	0
Sunshine et al.[107]	1960–1980	70	10.0	—	3
Schuh et al.[83]	1965–1984	52	5.5	33	1
Silverstein[108]	1979–1996	228	6.7	72	2
Kinne et al.[109]	1970–1976	82	11.5	—	1
Cataliotti et al.[110]	1975–1995	129	10.4	—	2
Ward et al.[111]	1979–1983	123	10.0	20	1

were high grade. Eleven patients developed invasive carcinoma and five had recurrent DCIS, for a total recurrence rate of 20%. The risk of invasive carcinoma was twice that of the general population. In all these studies, most cases included were low-grade, noncomedo lesions, representing one extreme of the histologic spectrum of DCIS.

Further information on the natural history of DCIS can be obtained from autopsy studies. Alpers and Wellings[103] assessed a series of 185 randomly selected breasts from 101 women examined by a subgross sampling technique. One or more foci of DCIS were found in 11 cases (6%). This finding was unrelated to age; DCIS was identified in 3 of 56 women (5%) 49 years of age or younger, in 7 of 70 women (10%) between the ages of 50 and 69, and in 1 of 59 women older than 70 years. In a study with similar methodology, Bartow et al.[104] examined the breasts of 519 women aged 14 years or older. Only one case of DCIS was identified; five occult invasive carcinomas were found. An autopsy study from Denmark reported by Andersen et al.[105] found DCIS in 11 of 86 breasts examined (13%). As a group, these studies indicate that many, but not all, cases of DCIS progress to invasive carcinoma within a woman's lifetime.

Treatment

Treatment Options

The uncertainty regarding the natural history of DCIS has resulted in a wide range of treatment practices, ranging from excision alone to mastectomy. Making comparisons among reports is difficult because of differences in patient populations, lack of standardization of surgical and radiotherapeutic techniques, and changes in treatment practice over time.

Mastectomy is a curative treatment for approximately 98% of patients with DCIS, whether gross or mammographic.[83,106–111] Representative studies are summarized in Table 2. Patients whose initial biopsies showed DCIS but for whom invasive carcinoma was later identified in the mastectomy specimens were excluded from these reports. This consideration is important when comparing survival after different methods of local therapy.

Although many of the initial reports assessing mastectomy for the treatment for DCIS contained small numbers of patients,[83,106,107] more recent, larger studies confirm the finding that treatment failure after mastectomy is rare.[108,110,111] Recurrences are almost all invasive carcinomas and may present as local failure or distant metastases without evidence of local recurrence. Treatment failure after mastectomy for DCIS may be due to unsampled or unrecognized invasive carcinoma that results in local recurrence or distant metastases, or it may be due to incomplete removal of breast tissue. Residual breast tissue has the potential to develop a new carcinoma that would be manifested as a "local recurrence." The failure of recurrence rates after mastectomy to increase with longer follow-up intervals, however, suggests that the majority of recurrences are due to undiagnosed invasive carcinoma rather than the malignant transformation of residual breast tissue.

Mastectomy is a highly effective treatment for DCIS, but it is a radical approach to a lesion that may not progress to invasive carcinoma during the patient's lifetime. It seems somewhat paradoxical that a woman with a palpable invasive carcinoma should be able to preserve her breast, whereas the "reward" for screening and early detection of DCIS is a mastectomy. The acceptance of breast-conserving therapy for the treatment of invasive carcinoma has led to its use as a treatment for DCIS. No randomized trial has ever compared the treatment of DCIS by mastectomy to treatment by excision and irradiation. In many cases, the assumption has been made that, because these two treatments result in equivalent survival for patients with invasive carcinoma, the same is true for patients with DCIS. This assumption is flawed, due to the fundamental difference in the risk of metastatic disease for patients with invasive carcinoma and those with DCIS. In patients with invasive carcinoma, the risk of metastatic disease is present at diagnosis and is not altered by local recurrence in the breast. In DCIS, the risk of metastases at diagnosis is negligible, and an invasive local recurrence carries with it the potential risk of breast cancer mortality. The suitability of excision and irradiation as a treatment for DCIS should be determined by the incidence of invasive recurrence and the results of salvage therapy. A number of nonrandomized studies have addressed this issue (Table 3).[108,110,112–118] Solin et al.[112] reported the results for 268 women in whom 271 breasts were treated with excision and irradiation at ten institutions in Europe and the United States. At a median follow-up of

TABLE 3. *Results of treatment of ductal carcinoma* in situ *with excision and radiation therapy*

Study	No. of patients	Median follow-up (yr)	No. (%) of recurrences	Invasive recurrences (%)
Hiramatsu et al.[114]	76	6.2	7 (9)	57
McCormick et al.[115]	54	3	10 (18)	30
Ray et al.[116]	56	5	5 (9)	20
Silverstein[108]	185	7.5	30 (15)	53
Cataliotti et al.[110]	83	6.6	6 (7.2)	100
Solin et al.[112,113]	268	10.3	46 (17)	53
Fisher et al. (NSABP Protocol B-06)[117]	27	6.9	2 (7)	50
Fisher et al. (NSABP Protocol B-17)[118]	399	7.5	51 (12)	44

NSABP, National Surgical Adjuvant Breast and Bowel Project.

10.3 years (range, 0.9 to 26.8), 46 failures were observed. These included 43 local failures, 1 combined local and regional, 1 local and distant, and 1 distant-only failure. The 15-year actuarial rate of local failure was 19%, and the median time to failure was 5.2 years. Noteworthy is the fact that, although the local failure rate in this study was relatively high, the 15-year cause-specific survival was 96%[113] (Fig. 5). The methods of evaluation and the extent of surgical resection used in this study would probably not be considered adequate today. Gross excision of the tumor was performed in all cases, but only 15% underwent reexcision, and margin status was unknown in 120 cases (46%). The median whole-breast radiation dose delivered was 5,000 cGy, and 164 of 261 cases (63%) received a boost to the primary tumor site. In spite of these caveats, this study is noteworthy for the large number of patients and relatively long duration of follow-up, and the low cause-specific mortality is reassuring. An examination of the subset of patients with mammographically detected lesions from this series (n = 110) did not reveal a significantly lower rate of local failure than that seen in the group as a whole,[119] a finding also reported by Hiramatsu et al.[114]

Because one-half of the local failures seen after breast-conserving therapy for intraductal carcinoma are invasive carcinoma, the outcome of salvage treatment of these recurrences is important. Solin et al.[120] described 42 cases of local failure in 274 cases of DCIS treated with excision plus irradiation. The median time to local failure was 5.1 years, and the median follow-up after salvage treatment was 3.7 years. Nineteen of the recurrences (45%) were intraductal carcinoma, and 14 of these were detected with mammographic findings alone. All of the women with intraductal recurrences remained free of disease after mastectomy with a median follow-up of 4.7 years. Five patients with invasive recurrence developed distant metastases, either simultaneously with the recurrence (one patient) or subsequently (four patients). Chest wall recurrences were seen in three patients who had salvage mastectomy for an invasive recurrence, and all of these women developed distant metastases. Of the entire group of 42 women with recurrence, 36 patients

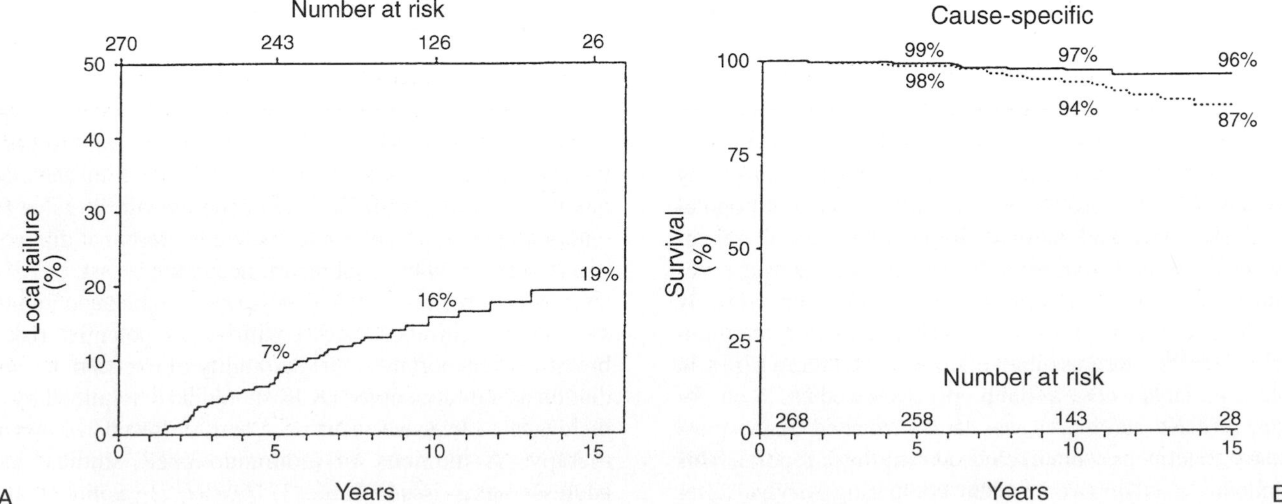

FIG. 5. A: Actuarial risk of local failure in 270 cases of ductal carcinoma *in situ* treated with excision and radiation therapy. The number at risk is the number of treated breasts at risk by 5-year intervals. **B:** Actuarial overall and cause-specific survival of 268 patients treated with excision and radiation therapy.

TABLE 4. *Results of treatment of ductal carcinoma* in situ *with excision alone*

Study	No. of patients	Follow-up (mo)	No. (%) of recurrences	Invasive recurrences (%)
Arnesson & Olsen[123]	169	80[a]	25 (14.8)	36
Carpenter et al.[124]	28	38[b]	5 (18)	20
Lagios et al.[35]	79	124[b]	15 (19.2)	56
Schwartz et al.[122]	191	55[a]	28 (14.4)	18
Silverstein[108]	130	45[a]	18 (14)	33
Fisher et al. (NSABP Protocol B-06)[117]	21	83[b]	9 (43)	56
Fisher et al. (NSABP Protocol B-17)[118]	391	90	109 (27.9)	53

NSABP, National Surgical Adjuvant Breast and Bowel Project.
[a]Median.
[b]Mean.

(86%) were alive and free of disease, 4 patients (10%) died of disease, 1 patient was alive with disease, and 1 patient died of other causes. Similarly high rates of salvage have been reported in other studies[117,118,121]; however, the ultimate breast cancer mortality resulting from breast-preserving treatment cannot yet be assessed. The 42 cases of recurrence reported by Solin et al.[120] occurred in a study population with a median follow-up of 78 months. Forty percent of the recurrences reported were seen between 5 and 10 years after treatment, and an additional 12% occurred after 10 years, indicating that a significant risk of further local recurrence exists among these women. In addition, the median follow-up after salvage therapy was only 3.7 years, too short an interval to determine the eventual risk of distant metastases.

Uncertainty about the biological significance of DCIS has led a number of investigators to examine the use of excision alone as a treatment (Table 4). In general, patients treated with this approach are highly selected and are usually chosen on the basis of low histologic grade or small size of the tumor. The percentage of patients with DCIS in the study population who meet these selection criteria is usually not stated, so that the number of women with DCIS who are candidates for this type of treatment is unclear. Lagios et al.[35] described 79 women with DCIS lesions 25 mm or smaller (mean size, less than 8 mm) who were treated with wide excision alone. Fifteen local recurrences (19%) were noted at a mean follow-up of 124 months. Eight of the recurrences were invasive carcinoma and seven were DCIS.[66] No breast cancer deaths occurred; ten deaths occurred from other causes. Schwartz et al.[122] reported on 191 women in whom 194 breasts were treated by excision alone and who were followed for a mean of 55 months. Approximately two-thirds of the cases were detected as mammographic calcifications, and one-third as incidental findings. The crude rate of recurrence was 14.4%, and the 10-year actuarial rate of recurrence was 24.6%. Only 18% of the recurrences were invasive carcinoma, a much lower rate of invasive recurrence than reported in other studies, and no breast cancer deaths have occurred. The patients were accrued between 1978 and 1996, which indicates the highly selected nature of the population. All of the tumors measured less than 2.5 cm in greatest dimension, and reexcision was routinely used. In contrast, a 43% recurrence rate was noted at a mean follow-up of 85 months for 22 patients treated by local excision alone as part of Protocol B-06.[117] These women were initially diagnosed as having invasive carcinoma and were later reclassified as having DCIS. Only one of these cases was nonpalpable cancer, and tumor size averaged 2.2 cm. These wide variations in local failure rates emphasize the importance of patient selection when attempting to treat women with DCIS by excision alone. In general, studies of the management of DCIS with excision alone show that, when local failure occurs, DCIS is present in approximately one-half of the cases and invasive carcinoma in the other one-half.[35,108,117,118,123–125] The time course to local failure is prolonged; studies with longer follow-up show higher local failure rates. In the report of Gallagher et al.,[126] the median time to local failure was 47 months; four of eight patients monitored for more than 9 years had recurrent disease, a finding that emphasizes the importance of long-term follow-up.

Two studies from the NSABP have described treatment outcomes in women with DCIS who were randomized to receive excision alone or excision plus radiation therapy.[81,117,118] Protocol B-06[117] (discussed in Chapter 33) was designed to evaluate the local therapy of invasive carcinoma. On review of pathologic material, 78 patients with DCIS alone were identified. At a follow-up of 83 months, 12 of the 27 patients (7%) treated with irradiation and 9 of the 21 patients (43%) treated with lumpectomy alone had local failures. No local failures occurred in the 28 women treated with mastectomy. The NSABP has also reported the results of a prospective study designed to evaluate the role of radiation therapy in DCIS.[81,118] In this study, 818 women were randomized to excision alone or excision plus 5,000 cGy of irradiation to the breast. Histologically negative surgical margins, defined as no contact between tumor-filled ducts

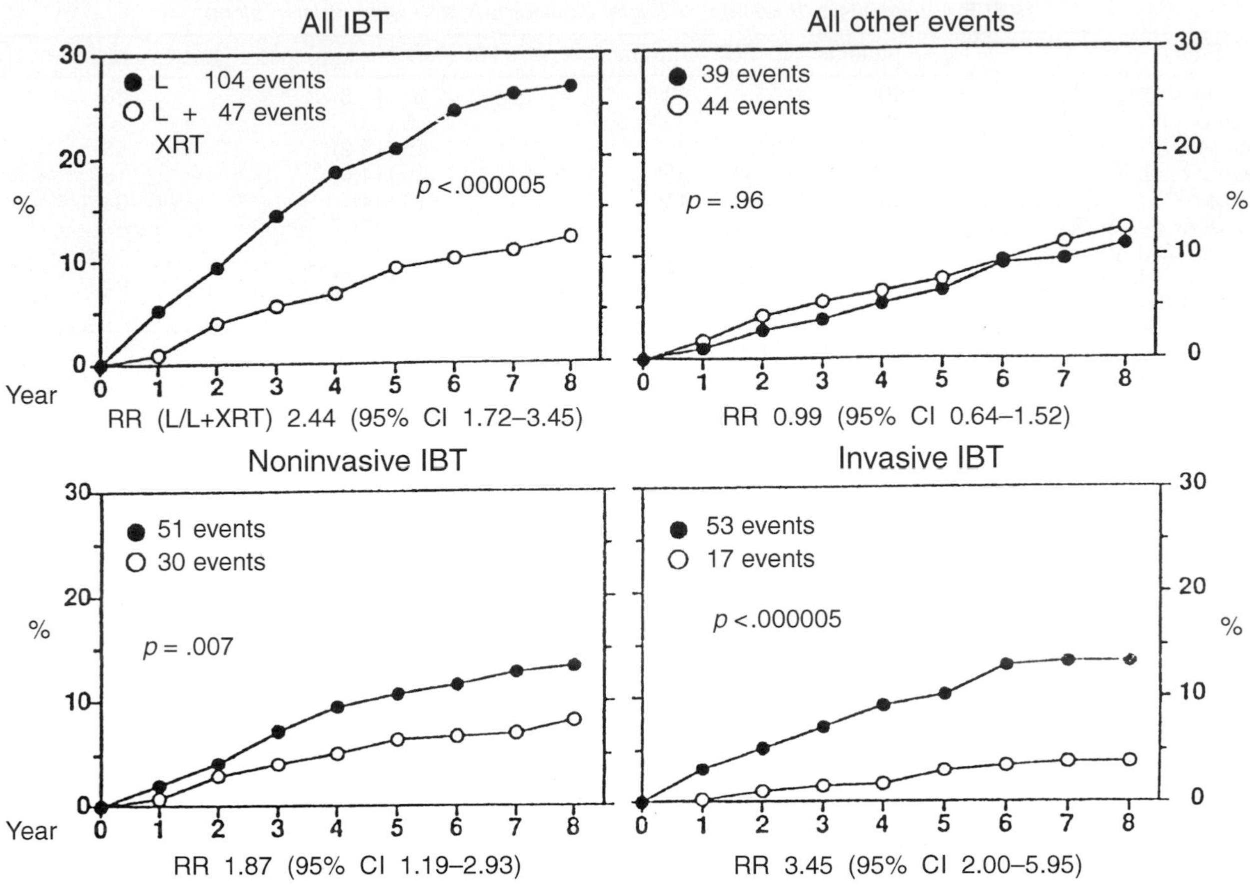

FIG. 6. Cumulative incidence of all ipsilateral breast tumor recurrences, of noninvasive and invasive ipsilateral breast tumor recurrences, and of all other first events in women treated by lumpectomy or lumpectomy and radiation therapy in National Surgical Adjuvant Breast Project Protocol B-17. *p* values are comparisons of average annual rates of failure. CI, confidence interval; IBT, ipsilateral breast tumor; L, lumpectomy; RR, relative risk; XRT, radiation therapy. (Reprinted with permission.)

and an inked surface, were required in both groups. Eighty percent of the women in the study had tumors detected by mammographic screening. The study was first reported at a median follow-up of 43 months, at which time a 58.8% reduction in the annual incidence of ipsilateral breast recurrence was observed in the irradiated group relative to the nonirradiated group. At 90 months of follow-up, the incidence of invasive recurrence was reduced from 13.4% in the nonirradiated group to 3.9% ($p = .000005$) in the irradiated group.[118] The incidence of recurrent DCIS was also significantly reduced, from 13.4% in the group without radiation to 8.2% in the group with radiation (Fig. 6). The continued benefit of radiation therapy in reducing the risk of both invasive and noninvasive recurrences over time strongly suggests that its benefit is not due solely to the control of clinically occult invasive carcinoma, as was suggested after the initial publication of this study. The overall survival does not differ between the two groups. Thirteen deaths have occurred in the 814 evaluable patients; overall survival rate is 94% for patients treated by lumpectomy alone and 95% for those receiving radiation therapy.

Prognostic Factors for Treatment Selection

As is apparent from the preceding discussion, identification of women with a high risk of developing invasive carcinoma after breast-conserving therapy for apparently localized DCIS would be extremely helpful. Physicians are presently unable to differentiate tumors that will recur as invasive carcinoma from those that will recur as DCIS. Some studies have suggested, however, that infiltrating carcinoma that develops after high-grade DCIS is more likely to be poorly differentiated and associated with poor prognosis than infiltrating carcinoma that develops after low-grade DCIS.[102,127] Histologic subtype and grade of DCIS have generally been the most widely studied predictive factors for recurrence. The limitations of histologic subtyping are discussed in detail in the section on Pathology. Despite these limitations, evidence suggests that histologic subtype and nuclear grade, alone or in combination, may be prognostic factors for local failure after treatment with excision alone or excision plus radiation therapy. In the study of Lagios et al.[35] of women treated with wide excision alone, a 33%

recurrence rate (12 of 36 cases) for patients with high-grade DCIS containing comedo-type necrosis was noted, compared with a rate of 2% (1 of 43) for patients with intermediate-grade or low-grade DCIS. Similar findings were reported by Schwartz et al.[28] After wide excision alone, 32% of patients with comedo histology experienced local recurrence, whereas only 3% of those with noncomedo histology had recurrent disease. Eusebi et al.[102] observed that local failure occurs earlier with high-grade DCIS than with low-grade DCIS. Long-term follow-up is needed to see whether these differences persist. However, other studies have observed no relationship between grade and failure.[123]

High nuclear grade and comedo-type histology have also been found to be prognostic for local recurrence when radiation is added to excision. Silverstein et al.[29] reported an 11% rate of local recurrence in women with comedo DCIS compared with a 2% failure rate in those with noncomedo DCIS among 96 women studied; median follow-up was 45 months. An update of this study with a longer follow-up (median of 62 months), however, showed no difference in the rate of local failure based on histologic subtype.[128] Pathology slides were available for review for 172 women from the multicenter study reported by Solin et al.[112,120,129] Sixteen local recurrences occurred in the 172 patients studied.[129] A comparison of recurrence rates for women with the comedo and noncomedo subtypes showed no significant differences (14% compared with 6%, respectively). However, recurrence rates were significantly higher for patients with a tumor of the comedo subtype and a nuclear grade of 3 than for any other groups (20% compared with 5%; $p = .009$). Forty-four of the 172 patients studied had this combination of factors, and one-half of the observed local recurrences occurred in this group. A multivariate analysis, including histologic subtype of the primary tumor, nuclear grade, amount of necrosis, final pathology margin, and the combination of histologic subtype of comedo carcinoma plus nuclear grade 3, found that only the combination of comedo carcinoma plus nuclear grade 3 correlated significantly with local control method. These patients also had a shorter time to treatment failure (median of 38 months) than did patients without the combination of comedo subtype and nuclear grade 3 (median of 78 months). With additional follow-up, however, the combination of comedo subtype and grade 3 no longer identified a group at increased risk for recurrence.[119] This finding, combined with the Silverstein data discussed earlier,[29,128] suggests that the importance of the comedo subtype in predicting local recurrence may be overemphasized in studies with short-term follow-up. The pathologic predictors studied had no impact on overall survival or freedom from distant metastases. The NSABP has reported the results of two analyses of the pathologic features of 623 of the 824 patients enrolled in Protocol B-17.[130,131] In the initial report, moderate or marked comedo necrosis and uncertain or involved margins were associated with an increased risk of local failure. Although radiation therapy reduced the risk of failure in all subgroups, the benefits were greatest in those patients at highest risk for recurrence.[130] In their second report, multivariate analysis of nine histologic features, including margins, histologic type, nuclear grade, tumor size, and comedo necrosis, demonstrated that only comedo necrosis significantly predicted an increased risk of ipsilateral breast recurrence after 8 years. A breast recurrence was seen in 23% of patients with absent or slight comedo necrosis who did not receive radiation therapy. The addition of radiation therapy eliminated most of the risk associated with this factor; 13% of those with absent or slight comedo necrosis and 14% of those with moderate or marked comedo necrosis experienced recurrence after radiation therapy.[131]

Several studies have suggested that age may influence the risk of local recurrence after breast-conserving therapy. Solin et al.[113] noted a 25% incidence of local failure in patients aged 50 or younger who were treated with excision and irradiation compared with 2% in patients older than age 50, in spite of the fact that nuclear grade, tumor size, and margin status did not differ between groups. The median time to local failure was also shorter in the younger patients (4.9 years versus 8.7 years). Van Zee et al.[132] also observed higher rates of local failure in women younger than age 40 than in their older counterparts after treatment with excision and irradiation or excision alone. Fourquet et al.[133] noted an actuarial 10-year recurrence rate of 30% for women aged 40 and younger treated with excision and irradiation, compared with 14% for those older than age 40. One possible explanation for these results may be the presence of higher circulating levels of estrogen in the younger patients, because estrogen is known to have promotional effects in breast cancer cell lines.

Other studies have suggested that a family history of breast cancer may influence the risk of local failure after excision and irradiation. Hiramatsu et al.[114] observed a 37% failure rate in patients with a family history of breast cancer compared with a 9% failure rate in those without a family history. McCormick et al.[115] reported that 40% of patients who experienced local-control failure had a first-degree relative with breast cancer compared with 11.4% of patients in whom local control was maintained.

Use of Tamoxifen

Data from the NSABP Breast Cancer Prevention trial[134] demonstrating that tamoxifen (tamoxifen citrate) therapy reduces the risk of both invasive and intraductal carcinoma in women at increased risk for breast cancer development (see Chapter 19), coupled with data from tamoxifen treatment trials demonstrating a reduction in contralateral breast cancer incidence,[135] strongly suggests that tamoxifen therapy would be beneficial in DCIS. The initial results of NSABP Protocol B-24, in which 1,804 patients with DCIS treated by lumpectomy and radiation therapy were randomized to tamoxifen 20 mg daily for 5 years or placebo, have been reported after a mean follow-up of 62 months.[136] The addition of tamoxifen reduced the average annual rate of invasive breast recurrence

TABLE 5. *Results of NSABP Protocol B-24: Addition of tamoxifen to lumpectomy and radiation therapy*

	Placebo *n* = 899			Tamoxifen *n* = 899				
	No. of events	Annual rate per 100 patients	Cumulative 5-year incidence (%)	No. of events	Annual rate per 100 patients	Cumulative 5-year incidence (%)	Relative risk	*p* Value
Recurrent invasive breast carcinoma	40	0.90	4.2	23	0.50	2.1	0.56	.03
Recurrent noninvasive breast carcinoma	47	1.10	5.1	40	0.87	3.9	0.82	.43
All first breast cancer events (ipsilateral, contralateral, and distant)	130	2.93	13.4	84	1.83	8.2	0.63	.0009

NSABP, National Surgical Adjuvant Breast and Bowel Project.
From ref. 136, with permission.

from 0.90 per 100 patients to 0.50 per 100 patients (relative risk, 0.56; $p = .03$) and reduced the rate of recurrent DCIS from 1.10 to 0.87 per 100 patients (relative risk, 0.82; $p = .43$). Overall, the risk of ipsilateral recurrence of any type (invasive or noninvasive) or of new contralateral breast cancers, or distant disease was reduced from 13.4% to 8.2% at 5 years, a highly significant reduction. These results are summarized in Table 5. As discussed in the section Treatment Options, because invasive recurrence has the potential to impact mortality, these results provide a strong rationale for the use of tamoxifen in patients with DCIS treated with a breast-conserving approach. These benefits must be weighed against the potential risks of treatment, which are lowest in patients younger than age 50 years and in those with a prior hysterectomy.

Treatment Selection

The available information on DCIS suggests that, although all patients can be treated with mastectomy, many are candidates for treatment with excision and irradiation, and a smaller group may be appropriately treated with excision alone. In treatment selection, it is useful to consider the risk of breast cancer recurrence, the risk of invasive breast cancer, and the risk of dying of breast cancer associated with breast-conserving treatment.

The available data on breast-conserving treatment combined with radiation therapy generally show recurrence rates of 10% to 15% at 10 years. Approximately one-half of these recurrences are invasive carcinoma, a risk of 5% to 7%. The risk of dying of breast cancer is approximately one-third the risk of developing the disease, so the risk of breast cancer death is 2% to 3% at 10 years. The risk of death 10 years after a mastectomy for DCIS is 1% to 2%. The major force of breast cancer mortality after mastectomy is likely to be evident in the first 10 years after treatment, however, given that death is presumably due to occult invasive disease present at the time of diagnosis. Local recurrences in DCIS continue to occur after 10 years, with additional breast cancer–associated mortality. Comparisons of breast cancer mortality rates 30 years after treatment could show greater differences in survival between women treated with mastectomy and those treated with excision and radiation therapy than the 1% to 2% estimated here. However, the use of tamoxifen significantly reduces the risk of invasive recurrence, eliminating most of the potential survival difference between treatment with excision and radiation therapy, and mastectomy. Whether radiation is necessary for all patients with DCIS treated with a breast-sparing approach remains uncertain. Retrospective data indicate that highly selected patients, usually with small, low-grade DCIS, have a very low local failure rate after excision alone. The only results available from a prospective study are those from NSABP Protocol B-17.[118] Although this study indicates that radiation therapy reduces the risk of local recurrence in all subgroups of patients with DCIS, Page and Lagios[137] have questioned whether a more detailed mammographic and pathologic evaluation would allow the identification of a subgroup of patients who will do well without radiation therapy. In addition, the impact of tamoxifen therapy on recurrence when radiation therapy is not given is uncertain.

That DCIS, rather than being a single entity, represents a spectrum of diseases of differing biological potential is becoming increasingly clear. This clinical observation is supported by studies of biological markers,[48–60] which indicate that characteristics of the malignant phenotype are more likely to be expressed in high-grade DCIS. Until developments in molecular biology allow more precise prediction of which tumors progress to invasive carcinoma, efforts must be directed toward minimizing local recurrence in women treated with a breast-conserving approach. The initial step in the evaluation of patients with DCIS is the determination of the extent of the lesion. Because most patients with DCIS have nonpalpable mammographic lesions, careful mammographic evaluation before treatment selection is critical. Holland et al.[30] have previously reported that the extent of poorly differentiated DCIS assessed by microscopy correlated well with the extent of the lesion evaluated radiologically, but the mammographic appearance of well-differentiated tumors substantially underestimated the microscopic extent. However, the routine use of magnification views as part of the mammographic evaluation allowed the detection of additional calcifications that reduced the discrepancy between the pathologically and mammographically determined extent of well-differentiated DCIS.[31] Needle localization should be used to guide the biopsy; if the calcifications are extensive, bracketing wires are useful to aid in complete excision. Specimen mammography is essential to confirm the excision of calcifications. In cases in which calcifications are extensive or approach the edge of the surgical specimen, postexcision mammograms are useful to confirm the removal of all suspicious calcifications. Gluck et al.[138] performed postexcision mammograms, including spot compression views, on 43 women who required reexcision due to positive or unknown margins after a diagnosis of breast carcinoma. Twenty-eight patients had DCIS; the positive predictive value of residual calcifications as an indicator of residual tumor was 0.67 and increased to 0.9 when more than five calcifications were present. Even when the margins are negative, postexcision mammography can demonstrate residual calcifications indicative of the need for further resection.[139] Although DCIS lesions are not clinically detectable, they may be quite large. Morrow et al.[140] found that contraindications to breast-preservation methods were present in 33% of patients with DCIS compared with only 10% of patients with stage I invasive carcinoma. Extensive disease that could not be encompassed with a cosmetic resection was the major contraindication to breast-conserving therapy in patients with DCIS.

A detailed pathologic evaluation is also needed and should include orientation marking, inking of the specimen, and measurement of both specimen and tumor size before sectioning. Because accurate measurement of microscopic DCIS is often difficult, reporting the number of blocks in which DCIS is present, as well as its largest single extent in any one slide, is often useful. The correlation of microcalcifications with DCIS (i.e., whether DCIS is present only in areas of calcification or in calcification and adjacent breast tissue) as well as the margin status should be noted. If margins are involved, the extent of involvement should be stated; when margins are negative, proximity of the lesion to the margin should be noted.

Attempts have been made to incorporate the size of the lesion, its histologic features, and the extent of the surgical excision into a prognostic index that would direct treatment selection. One such index is the Van Nuys Prognostic Index (VNPI), which assigns scores of 1, 2, or 3 for histologic type, width of the surgical margin, and size of the lesion.[141] Lesions with low VNPI scores are said to be suitable for excision alone; those with intermediate scores (5 to 7) require the addition of radiation therapy; and those with high scores require mastectomy. Although such a simplification of the decision-making process is attractive, this index has a number of limitations. The index was developed using retrospective data on 254 patients and was validated using retrospective data on 79 patients from another institution. The use of the classification system is dependent on the reproducibility of the individual components. Because the histologic classification scheme and method of tumor measurement are not in universal or even routine use, this is a significant issue. The potential problems in duplicating these elements have been discussed in detail by Schnitt et al.[142] Equally important is the fact that the patients used to develop this index were treated over a large time span from 1972 and 1995. However, treatment with excision alone was used in more recent years, whereas treatment with excision and irradiation was more common in the past. This suggests that the low rate of local recurrence seen after excision alone may be due to improvements in mammographic and pathologic evaluation. Hiramatsu et al.[114] reported that the incidence of local recurrence 6.5 years after excision and irradiation decreased from 12% to 2% when patients treated between 1976 and 1985 were compared with those treated between 1985 and 1995, although radiation technique did not change. Finally, although the VNPI is based on factors that most clinicians would consider important in predicting the behavior of DCIS, whether these are the most important factors in determining outcome is not clear. In a subsequent report,[143] the authors of the VNPI noted that, when DCIS was widely excised to negative margins, nuclear grade was not a predictor of recurrence in patients treated with excision alone or excision and radiation therapy. As noted previously, age and a family history of breast carcinoma have been suggested to influence the risk of local recurrence in retrospective studies. For these reasons, the authors do not believe that the VNPI is an appropriate substitute for an individualized assessment of the risks and benefits of the available treatment options for DCIS.

The lack of a single appropriate treatment option for all patients with DCIS is reflected in national patterns of care. A review of 39,010 patients with DCIS reported to the National Cancer Data Base between 1985 and 1993 demonstrated that the use of breast-preserving techniques increased from 31% to 54% in that 8-year interval. Overall, only 45% of the patients treated with breast-preserving techniques received radiation therapy, although the use of this modality increased from 38% of cases to 54% during the study period. Smaller tumors and low-grade lesions were most likely to be treated with breast-preserving surgery alone.[144]

MICROINVASIVE CARCINOMA

Microinvasive carcinoma is a poorly defined pathologic entity. As with DCIS, it is being diagnosed more frequently because of the increased use of screening mammography. To properly treat patients with microinvasive carcinoma, one must know whether this lesion behaves like DCIS, invasive carcinoma, or something in between. The behavior of microinvasive carcinoma is difficult to determine because of the variety of definitions used in the past.

As illustrated in Table 1, axillary lymph node metastases are infrequent in microinvasive carcinoma.

The limited available long-term follow-up data on patients with microinvasive carcinoma suggest that the prognosis after surgical treatment is excellent. Rosner et al.[84] reported on 36 cases of DCIS with microinvasion treated between 1976 and 1987. Thirty-three patients underwent mastectomy. At a mean follow-up time of 57 months, all patients remained free of disease. Wong et al.[85] also observed no treatment failures at a median follow-up of 47 months, and Kinne et al.[109] reported a 94% disease-free survival rate at a median follow-up of 11.5 years. Most patients in these reports were treated with mastectomy. Solin et al.[94] reported on the outcome of 39 patients treated with breast-conserving surgery and radiation therapy. With a median follow-up time of 55 months, the overall survival rate was 97%. However, nine patients (23%) developed a recurrence in the breast. Outcome was compared for patients with microinvasive carcinoma, patients with DCIS, and patients with node-negative invasive carcinoma treated during the same period. Patients with microinvasive carcinoma were found to have a higher local recurrence rate than those with pure DCIS or those with invasive carcinoma, and a survival rate intermediate between the two groups. In a retrospective study, Silverstein[95] compared 21 patients with microinvasion to 622 patients with pure DCIS and observed no difference in local recurrence, disease-free survival, or overall survival.

From the limited information available on microinvasive carcinoma, several tentative conclusions may be drawn. First, because of variability in the definition of microinvasion, results from the literature are applicable to an individual patient only if microinvasion is defined in the same way. The incidence of axillary node metastases is low, and axillary dissection is not routinely indicated. Survival of patients with microinvasive carcinoma seems to be intermediate between that of patients with DCIS and that of patients with small invasive carcinomas. The use of breast-conserving treatment in these patients should follow the same guidelines for careful mammographic and pathologic evaluation and the requirement for negative margins of resection as for patients with an extensive intraductal component–positive invasive carcinoma.

MANAGEMENT SUMMARY

DCIS represents a heterogeneous group of lesions of varying malignant potential. Total (simple) mastectomy is associated with a cure rate of 98% to 99% for all types of DCIS.

Patients with localized DCIS are candidates for breast-sparing surgery and irradiation. Detailed mammography and careful pathologic evaluation are essential to confirm the localized nature of the lesion and to judge the adequacy of resection. The goals of surgery are to remove all suspicious microcalcifications and to achieve negative margins of resection.

Excision alone may be an appropriate treatment for selected women with small (less than 1-cm to 2-cm) low-grade DCIS lesions with clearly negative margins.

Axillary dissection is not indicated in DCIS. In women with large high-grade lesions undergoing mastectomy, a low axillary sampling obviates the need for reoperation if invasion is identified.

The use of tamoxifen should be considered to reduce the risk of ipsilateral breast tumor recurrence after breast-sparing surgery and to reduce the risk of contralateral breast cancer in all patients.

A detailed discussion of the risks and benefits of the various options must be undertaken to allow each woman with DCIS to make an informed treatment choice.

REFERENCES

1. Rosner D, Bedwani RN, Vana J, Baker HW, Murphy GP. Noninvasive breast carcinoma: results of a national survey by the American College of Surgeons. *Ann Surg* 1980;192:139.
2. Morrow M, Schmidt R, Cregger B, Hassett C, Cox S. Preoperative evaluation of abnormal mammographic findings to avoid unnecessary breast biopsy. *Arch Surg* 1994;129:1091.
3. Alexander HR, Candela F, Dershaw D. Needle localized mammographic lesions: results and evolving treatment strategy. *Arch Surg* 1990;125:1441.
4. Silverstein M, Gamagami P, Colburn W, et al. Non-palpable breast lesions: diagnosis with slightly over-penetrated screen-film mammography and hook wire-directed biopsy in 1014 cases. *Radiology* 1989;171:633.
5. Wilhelm MC, Edge S, Cole D, de Paredes E, Frierson HF Jr. Nonpalpable invasive breast cancer. *Ann Surg* 1991;213:600.
6. Brenin D, Morrow M. Is mastectomy over-treatment for ductal carcinoma in situ? *Breast Cancer Res Treat* 1998;50:250.
7. Pandya S, Mackarem G, Lee AKC, McLellan R, Heatley GJ, Hughes KS. Ductal carcinoma in situ: the impact of screening on clinical presentation and pathologic features. *Breast J* 1998;4:146.
8. Ernster VL, Barclay J, Kerlikowske K, Grady D, Henderson IC. Incidence and treatment for ductal carcinoma in situ of the breast. *JAMA* 1996;275:913.
9. Gapstur S, Morrow M, Sellers TA. Hormone replacement therapy and risk of breast cancer with a favorable histology. Results of the Iowa Women's Health Study. *JAMA* 1999;281:2091.
10. Weiss HA, Brinton LA, Brognan D, et al. Epidemiology of in situ and invasive breast cancer in women aged under 45. *Br J Cancer* 1996; 73:1298.
11. Kerlikowske K, Barclay J, Grady D, Sickles EA, Ernster VL. Risk factors for ductal carcinoma in situ. *J Natl Cancer Inst* 1997;89:76.
12. Azzopardi JG. *Problems in breast pathology*. Philadelphia: WB Saunders, 1983.
13. Page DL, Anderson TJ. *Diagnostic histopathology of the breast*. Edinburgh, UK: Churchill Livingstone, 1987.
14. Rosen PP, Oberman H. *Tumors of the mammary gland*. Washington, DC: Armed Forces Institute of Pathology, 1993.
15. Carter D, Orr SL, Merino MJ. Intracystic papillary carcinoma of the breast after mastectomy, radiotherapy, or excision alone. *Cancer* 1983;52:14.
16. Lefkowitz M, Lefkowitz W, Wargotz ES. Intraductal (intracystic) papillary carcinoma of the breast and its variants: a clinico-pathological study of 77 cases. *Hum Pathol* 1994;25:802.
17. Leal C, Costa I, Fonseca D, Lopes P, Bento MJ, Lopes C. Intracystic (encysted) papillary carcinoma of the breast: a clinical, pathological, and immunohistochemical study. *Hum Pathol* 1998;29:1097.
18. Tavassoli FA, Norris HJ. Intraductal apocrine carcinoma: a clinicopathologic study of 37 cases. *Mod Pathol* 1994;7:813.
19. O'Malley FP, Page DL, Nelson EH, Dupont WD. Ductal carcinoma in situ of the breast with apocrine cytology: definition of a borderline category. *Hum Pathol* 1994;25:164.
20. Fisher ER, Brown R. Intraductal signet ring cell carcinoma. A hitherto undescribed form of intraductal carcinoma of the breast. *Cancer* 1985;55:2533.
21. Tsang WYW, Chan JKC. Endocrine ductal carcinoma in situ (E-DCIS) of the breast. A form of low-grade DCIS with distinctive clinicopathologic and biologic characteristics. *Am J Surg Pathol* 1996; 20:921.
22. Maluf HM, Koerner FC. Solid papillary carcinoma of the breast. A form of intraductal carcinoma with endocrine differentiation frequently associated with mucinous carcinoma. *Am J Surg Pathol* 1995;19:1237.

23. Rosen PP, Scott M. Cystic hypersecretory duct carcinoma of the breast. *Am J Surg Pathol* 1984;8:31.
24. Guerry P, Erlandson RA, Rosen PP. Cystic hypersecretory hyperplasia and cystic hypersecretory duct carcinoma of the breast: pathology, therapy, and follow-up of 39 patients. *Cancer* 1988;61:1611.
25. Eusebi V, Foschini M, Cook M, Berrino F, Azzopardi JG. Long term follow-up of in situ carcinoma of the breast with special emphasis on clinging carcinoma. *Semin Diagn Pathol* 1989;6:165.
26. Scott MA, Lagios MD, Axelsson K, Rogers LW, Anderson TJ, Page DL. Ductal carcinoma in situ of the breast: reproducibility of histologic subtype analysis. *Hum Pathol* 1997;28:967.
27. Patchefsky AS, Schwartz GF, Finkelstein SD, et al. Heterogeneity of intraductal carcinoma of the breast. *Cancer* 1989;63:731.
28. Schwartz GF, Patchefsky AS, Finkelstein SD, et al. Nonpalpable in situ ductal carcinoma of the breast: predictors of multicentricity and microinvasion and implications for treatment. *Arch Surg* 1989; 124:29.
29. Silverstein MJ, Waisman JR, Gamagami P, et al. Intraductal carcinoma of the breast (208 cases): clinical factors influencing treatment choice. *Cancer* 1990;66:102.
30. Holland R, Hendricks JH, Verbeek AL, Mravunac M, Schuurmans Stekhoven JH. Extent, distribution, and mammographic/histological correlations of breast ductal carcinoma in situ. *Lancet* 1990;335:519.
31. Holland R, Hendriks J. Microcalcifications associated with ductal carcinoma in situ: mammographic-pathologic correlation. *Semin Diagn Pathol* 1994;11:181.
32. Lennington WJ, Jensen RA, Dalton LW, Page DL. Ductal carcinoma in situ of the breast. Heterogeneity of individual lesions. *Cancer* 1994;73:118.
33. Quinn CM, Ostrowski JL, Parkin GJS, Horgan K, Benson EA. Ductal carcinoma in situ of the breast: the clinical significance of histological classification. *Histopathology* 1997;30:113.
34. European Commission Working Group on Breast Screening Pathology. Consistency achieved by 23 European pathologists in categorizing ductal carcinoma in situ of the breast using five classifications. *Hum Pathol* 1998;9:1056.
35. Lagios MD, Margolin FR, Westdahl PR, Rose MR. Mammographically detected duct carcinoma in situ: frequency of local recurrence following tylectomy and prognostic effect of nuclear grade on local recurrence. *Cancer* 1989;63:618.
36. Poller DN, Silverstein MJ, Galea M, et al. Ductal carcinoma in situ of the breast: a proposal for a new simplified histological classification association between cellular proliferation and c-erbB-2 protein expression. *Mod Pathol* 1994;7:257.
37. Silverstein MJ, Poller DN, Waisman JR, et al. Prognostic classification of breast ductal carcinoma in situ. *Lancet* 1995;345:1154.
38. Holland R, Peterse JL, Millis RR, et al. Ductal carcinoma in situ: a proposal for a new classification. *Semin Diagn Pathol* 1994;11:167.
39. Ottesen GL, Graversen HP, Blichert-Toft M, Zedeler K, Andersen JA. Ductal carcinoma in situ of the female breast. Short-term results of a prospective nationwide study. *Am J Surg Pathol* 1992;16:1183.
40. Bellamy CO, McDonald C, Salter DM, Chetty U, Anderson TJ. Noninvasive ductal carcinoma of the breast: the relevance of histologic categorization. *Hum Pathol* 1993;24:16.
41. Tavassoli FA, Man Y. Morphofunctional features of intraductal hyperplasia, atypical intraductal hyperplasia, and various grades of intraductal carcinoma. *Breast J* 1995;1:155.
42. Schnitt SJ, Connolly JL. Classification of ductal carcinoma in situ: striving for clinical relevance in the era of breast conserving therapy. *Hum Pathol* 1997;28:877.
43. Millis RR. Classification of ductal carcinoma in situ. *Adv Anat Pathol* 1996;3:114.
44. Douglas-Jones AG, Gupta SK, Attanoos RL, Morgan JM, Mansel RE. A critical appraisal of six modern classifications of ductal carcinoma in situ of the breast (DCIS): correlation with grade of associated invasive cancer. *Histopathology* 1996;29:397.
45. Consensus Conference Committee. Consensus conference of the classification of ductal carcinoma in situ. *Cancer* 1997;80:1798.
46. Bur ME, Zimarowski MJ, Schnitt SJ, Baker S, Lew R. Estrogen receptor immunohistochemistry in carcinoma in situ of the breast. *Cancer* 1992;69:1174.
47. Bose S, Lesser ML, Norton L, Rosen PP. Immunophenotype of intraductal carcinoma. *Arch Pathol Lab Med* 1996;120:81.
48. Bobrow LG, Happerfield LC, Gregory WM, Springalll RD, Millis RR. The classification of ductal carcinoma in situ and its association with biological markers. *Semin Diagn Pathol* 1994;11:199.
49. Albonico G, Querzoli P, Ferretti S, Rinaldi R, Nenci I. Biological profile of in situ breast cancer investigated by immunohistochemical technique. *Cancer Detect Prev* 1998;22:313.
50. Rudas M, Neumayer R, Gnant MF, Mittelbock M, Jakesz R, Reiner A. p53 protein expression, cell proliferation, and steroid hormone receptors in ductal and lobular in situ carcinomas of the breast. *Eur J Cancer* 1997;33:39.
51. Mack L, Kerkvliet, Doig G, O'Malley FP. Relationship of a new histological categorization of ductal carcinoma in situ of the breast with size and the immunohistochemical expression of p53, c-erbB-2, bcl-2 and ki-67. *Hum Pathol* 1997;28:974.
52. Meyer JS. Cell kinetics of histologic variants of in situ breast carcinoma. *Breast Cancer Res Treat* 1986;7:171.
53. Killeen JL, Namiki H. DNA analysis of ductal carcinoma in situ of the breast. A comparison with histologic features. *Cancer* 1991;68:2602.
54. van de Vijver MJ, Peterse JL, Mooi WJ, et al. Neu-protein overexpression in breast cancer: association with comedo-type ductal carcinoma in situ and limited prognostic value in stage II breast cancer. *N Engl J Med* 1988;319:1239.
55. Bartkova J, Barnes DM, Millis RR, Gullock WJ. Immunohistochemical demonstration of c-erbB-2 protein in mammary ductal carcinoma in situ. *Hum Pathol* 1990;21:1164.
56. Lodato RF, Maguire HC Jr, Greene MI, Weiner DB, LiVolsi VA. Immunohistochemical evaluation of c-erbB-2 oncogene expression in ductal carcinoma in situ and atypical ductal hyperplasia of the breast. *Mod Pathol* 1990;3:449.
57. Poller DN, Roberts EC, Bell JA, Elston CW, Blamey RW, Ellis IO. p53 protein expression in mammary ductal carcinoma in situ: relationship to immunohistochemical expression of estrogen receptor c-erbB-2 protein. *Hum Pathol* 1993;24:463.
58. O'Malley FP, Vnencak-Jones CL, Dupont WD. p53 mutations are confined to comedo type ductal carcinoma in situ of the breast: immunohistochemical and sequencing data. *Lab Invest* 1994;71:67.
59. Guidi AJ, Fischer L, Harris JR, Schnitt SJ. Microvessel density and distribution in ductal carcinoma in situ of the breast. *J Natl Cancer Inst* 1994;85:614.
60. Engels K, Fox SB, Whitehouse RM, Gatter, KC, Harris AL. Distinct angiogenic patterns are associated with high grade in situ ductal carcinomas of the breast. *J Pathol* 1997;181:207.
61. Tsuda H, Fukutomi T, Hirohasi S. Pattern of gene alteration in intraductal breast neoplasms associated with histological type and grade. *Clin Cancer Res* 1995;1:261.
62. Fowble B. In situ breast cancer. In: Fowble B, Goodman RL, Glick JH, Rosato EF, eds. *Breast cancer treatment. A comprehensive guide to management*. St. Louis: Mosby–Year Book, 1991.
63. Lagios MD, Westdahl PR, Margolin FR, Rose MR. Duct carcinoma in situ: relationship of extent of noninvasive disease to the frequency of occult invasion, multicentricity, lymph node metastases, and short-term treatment failures. *Cancer* 1982;50:1309.
64. Faverly DRG, Burgers L, Bult P, Holland R. Three dimensional imaging of mammary ductal carcinoma in situ: clinical implications. *Semin Diagn Pathol* 1994;11:193.
65. Noguchi S, Motomura K, Inaji H, Imaoka S, Koyama H. Clonal analysis of predominantly intraductal carcinoma and precancerous lesions of the breast by means of polymerase chain reaction. *Cancer Res* 1994;54:1849.
66. Contesso G, Mouriesse H, Petit JY. *Intraductal carcinoma studies on mastectomy specimens: preferential localization of DCIS: the nipple*. Castle Marquette, The Netherlands: Proc EORTC In Situ Breast Cancer Workshop, 1988.
67. Gump FE, Jicha DL, Ozello L. Ductal carcinoma in situ (DCIS): a revised concept. *Surgery* 1987;102:790.
68. Fentiman IS, Fagg N, Millis RR, Hayward JL. In situ ductal carcinoma of the breast: implications of disease pattern and treatment. *Eur J Surg Oncol* 1986;12:261.
69. Silverstein MJ, Gierson ED, Waisman JR, Senofsky GM, Colburn WJ, Gamagami P. Axillary lymph node dissection for T1a breast carcinoma. Is it indicated? *Cancer* 1994;73:664.
70. Winchester DP, Menck HR, Osteen RT, Kraybill W. Treatment trends for ductal carcinoma in situ of the breast. *Ann Surg Oncol* 1995;2:207.

71. Rosai J. Borderline epithelial lesions of the breast. *Am J Surg Pathol* 1991;15:209.
72. Schnitt SJ, Connolly JL, Tavassoli FA, et al. Interobserver reproducibility in the diagnosis of ductal proliferative breast lesions using standardized criteria. *Am J Surg Pathol* 1992;16:1133.
73. Schnitt SJ. Microinvasive carcinoma of the breast. *Int J Surg Pathol* 1998;6:183.
74. Page DL, Dixon JM, Anderson TJ, Lee D, Stewart HJ. Invasive cribriform carcinoma of the breast. *Histopathology* 1983;7:525.
75. Venable JG, Schwartz AM, Silverberg SG. Infiltrating cribriform carcinoma of the breast: a distinctive clinico-pathologic entity. *Hum Pathol* 1990;21:333.
76. Fechner RE. Ductal carcinoma involving the lobule of the breast. A source of confusion with lobular carcinoma in situ. *Cancer* 1971;28:274.
77. Kerner H, Lichtig C. Lobular cancerization: incidence and differential diagnosis with lobular carcinoma in situ of the breast. *Histopathology* 1986;10:621.
78. Fechner RE. Epithelial alterations in the extralobular ducts of breasts with lobular carcinoma. *Arch Pathol* 1972;93:164.
79. Fisher ER, Costantino J, Fisher B, et al. Pathologic findings from the National Surgical Adjuvant Breast Project (NSABP) protocol 17. Five-year observations concerning lobular carcinoma in situ. *Cancer* 1996;78:1403.
80. Rosen PP. Coexistent lobular carcinoma in situ and intraductal carcinoma in a single lobular-duct unit. *Am J Surg Pathol* 1980;4:241.
81. Fisher B, Costantino J, Redmond C, et al. Lumpectomy compared with lumpectomy and radiation therapy for the treatment of intraductal breast cancer. *N Engl J Med* 1993;328:1581.
82. American Joint Committee on Cancer. *AJCC cancer staging manual*. Philadelphia: Lippincott–Raven, 1997:172.
83. Schuh ME, Nemoto T, Penetrante R, Rosner D, Dao TL. Intraductal carcinoma. Analysis of presentation, pathologic findings, and outcome of disease. *Arch Surg* 1986;121:1303.
84. Rosner D, Lane WW, Penetrante R. Ductal carcinoma in situ with microinvasion. A curable entity using surgery alone without need for adjuvant therapy. *Cancer* 1991;67:1498.
85. Wong JH, Kopald KH, Morton DL. The impact of microinvasion on axillary node metastases and survival in patients with intraductal breast cancer. *Arch Surg* 1990;125:1298.
86. Fisher ER. Pathobiological considerations relating to the treatment of intraductal carcinoma (ductal carcinoma in situ) of the breast. *CA Cancer J Clin* 1996;47:52.
87. Eusebi V, Collina G, Bussolati G. Carcinoma in situ in sclerosing adenosis of the breast. An immunocytochemical study. *Semin Diagn Pathol* 1989;6:146.
88. Oberman HA, Markey BA. Noninvasive carcinoma of the breast presenting in adenosis. *Mod Pathol* 1991;4:31.
89. Youngson BJ, Cranor M, Powell C, Rosen PP. Epithelial displacement in surgical breast specimens following needling procedures. *Am J Surg Pathol* 1994;18:896.
90. Youngson BJ, Liberman L, Rosen PP. Displacement of carcinomatous epithelium in surgical breast specimens following stereotaxic core biopsy. *Am J Clin Pathol* 1995;103:598.
91. Lagios MD. Microinvasion in ductal carcinoma in situ. In: Silverstein MJ, ed. *Carcinoma in situ of the breast*. Baltimore: Williams & Wilkins, 1997:241.
92. Elston CW, Ellis IO, eds. *Diagnostic histopathology of the breast*. Edinburgh, UK: Churchill Livingstone, 1998:242.
93. Silver SA, Tavassoli FA. Mammary ductal carcinoma in situ with microinvasion. *Cancer* 1998;82:2382.
94. Solin LJ, Fowble BL, Yeh I-T, et al. Microinvasive ductal carcinoma of the breast treated with breast-conserving surgery and definitive irradiation. *Int J Radiat Oncol Biol Phys* 1992;23:961.
95. Silverstein MJ. Ductal carcinoma in situ with microinvasion. In: Silverstein MJ, ed. *Ductal carcinoma in situ of the breast*. Baltimore: Williams & Wilkins, 1997:557.
96. Akhtar S, Zablow A, Michaelson RA, Hutter RVP, Leitner SP. Predictors of axillary lymph node metastases in small (one centimeter or less) T1a,b primary breast cancer. *J Clin Oncol* 1998;17:120a(abst).
97. Penault-Llorca F, Le Bouedec G, Pomel C, Feillel V, Dauplat J, de Latour M. Microinvasive carcinoma of the breast: is axillary lymph node dissection indicated? *Lab Invest* 1998;78:25A(abst).
98. Prasad ML, Giri G, Hoda S. Clinicopathologic features of microinvasive (<1mm) carcinoma of the breast. *Lab Invest* 1998;78:25A(abst).
99. Page DL, Dupont WD, Rogers LW, Landenberger M. Intraductal carcinoma of the breast: follow-up after biopsy only. *Cancer* 1982; 49:751.
100. Page DL, Dupont WD, Rogers LW, Jensen RA, Schuyler PA. Continued local recurrence of carcinoma 15–25 years after a diagnosis of low grade ductal carcinoma in situ of the breast treated only by biopsy. *Cancer* 1995;76:1197.
101. Rosen PP, Braun D, Kinne D. The clinical significance of pre-invasive breast carcinoma. *Cancer* 1980;46:919.
102. Eusebi V, Feudale E, Foschini M, et al. Long term follow-up of in situ carcinoma of the breast. *Semin Diagn Pathol* 1994;11:223.
103. Alpers C, Wellings S. The prevalence of carcinoma in situ in normal and cancer associated breast. *Hum Pathol* 1985;16:796.
104. Bartow S, Pathak D, Black W, Key CR, Teaf SR. Prevalence of benign, atypical, and malignant breast lesions in populations at different risk for breast cancer. *Cancer* 1987;60:2751.
105. Andersen J, Nielsen M, Christensen L. New aspects of the natural history of in situ and invasive carcinoma in the female breast: results from autopsy investigations. *Verh Dtsch Ges Pathol* 1985;69:88.
106. Von Rueden DG, Wilson RE. Intraductal carcinoma of the breast. *Surg Gynecol Obstet* 1984;158:105.
107. Sunshine JA, Moseley MS, Fletcher WS, Krippaehne WW. Breast carcinoma in situ: a retrospective review of 112 cases with a minimum 10 year follow-up. *Am J Surg* 1985;150:44.
108. Silverstein MJ. Van Nuys experience by treatment. In: Silverstein MJ, ed. *Ductal carcinoma in situ of the breast*. Baltimore: Williams & Wilkins, 1997:443.
109. Kinne DW, Petrek JA, Osborne MP, Fracchia AA, DePalo AA, Rosen PP. Breast carcinoma in situ. *Arch Surg* 1989;124:33.
110. Cataliotti L, Distante V, Pacini P. Florence experience. In: Silverstein MJ, ed. *Ductal carcinoma in situ of the breast*. Baltimore: Williams & Wilkins, 1997:449.
111. Ward BA, McKhann CF, Ravikumar TS. Ten year follow-up of breast carcinoma in situ in Connecticut. *Arch Surg* 1992;127:1392.
112. Solin LJ, Recht A, Fourquet A, et al. Ten-year results of breast-conserving surgery and definitive irradiation for intraductal carcinoma (ductal carcinoma in situ) of the breast. *Cancer* 1991;68:2337.
113. Solin LJ, Kurtz J, Fourquet A, et al. Fifteen year results of breast-conserving surgery and definitive breast irradiation for the treatment of ductal carcinoma in situ of the breast. *J Clin Oncol* 1996;14:754.
114. Hiramatsu H, Bornstein BA, Recht A, et al. Local recurrence after conservative surgery and radiation therapy for ductal carcinoma in situ: possible importance of family history. *Cancer J Sci Am* 1995;1:55.
115. McCormick B, Rosen PP, Kinne D, Cox L, Yahalom J. Duct carcinoma in situ of the breast: an analysis of local control after conservation surgery and radiotherapy. *Int J Radiat Oncol Biol Phys* 1991;21:289.
116. Ray GR, Adelson J, Hayhurst E, et al. Ductal carcinoma in situ of the breast: results of treatment by conservative surgery and definitive irradiation. *Int J Radiat Oncol Biol Phys* 1993;28:105.
117. Fisher E, Leeming R, Anderson S, Redmond C, Fisher B. Conservative management of intraductal carcinoma (DCIS) of the breast. *J Surg Oncol* 1991;47:139.
118. Fisher B, Dignam J, Wolmark N, et al. Lumpectomy and radiation therapy for the treatment of intraductal breast cancer: findings from National Surgical Adjuvant Breast and Bowel Project B-17. *J Clin Oncol* 1998;16:441.
119. Solin LJ, McCormick B, Recht A, et al. Mammographically detected clinically occult ductal carcinoma in situ (intraductal carcinoma) treated with breast-conserving surgery and definitive breast irradiation. *Cancer J Sci Am* 1996;2:158.
120. Solin LJ, Fourquet A, McCormick B, et al. Salvage treatment for local recurrence following breast conserving surgery and definitive irradiation for ductal carcinoma in situ (intraductal carcinoma) of the breast. *Int J Radiat Oncol Biol Phys* 1994;30:3.
121. Kuske RR, Bean JM, Garcia DM, et al. Breast conservation therapy for intraductal carcinoma of the breast. *Int J Radiat Oncol Biol Phys* 1993;26:391.
122. Schwartz GF. Treatment of subclinical ductal carcinoma in situ by local excision and surveillance: a personal experience. In: Silverstein MJ, ed. *Ductal carcinoma in situ of the breast*. Baltimore: Williams & Wilkins, 1997:353.
123. Miller NA, Chapman JW, Fish EB, et al. In situ duct carcinoma of the breast: clinical and histopathologic factors and association with recurrent cancer. *Breast Cancer Res Treat* 1998;50:251.

124. Arnesson LG, Olsen K. Linköping experience. In: Silverstein MJ, ed. *Ductal carcinoma in situ of the breast.* Baltimore: Williams & Wilkins, 1997:373.
125. Carpenter R, Boulter PS, Cooke T, et al. Management of screen detected ductal carcinoma in situ of the female breast. *Br J Surg* 1989;76:564.
126. Gallagher WJ, Koerner FC, Wood WC. Treatment of intraductal carcinoma with limited surgery: long-term follow-up. *J Clin Oncol* 1989; 7:376.
127. Lampejo OT, Barnes DM, Smith P, Millis RR. Evaluation of infiltrating ductal carcinomas with a DCIS component: correlation of the histologic type of the in situ component with grade of the infiltrating component. *Semin Diagn Pathol* 1994;11:215.
128. Silverstein MJ, Cohlan BF, Gierson ED, et al. Duct carcinoma in situ: 227 cases without microinvasion. *Eur J Cancer* 1992;28:630.
129. Solin LJ, Yeh IT, Kurtz J, et al. Ductal carcinoma in situ (intraductal carcinoma) of the breast treated with breast-conserving surgery and definitive irradiation: correlation of pathologic parameters with outcome of treatment. *Cancer* 1993;71:2532.
130. Fisher ER, Costantino J, Fisher B, Palekar AS, Redmond C, Mamounas E. Pathologic findings from the National Surgical Adjuvant Breast Project (NSABP) Protocol B-17. Intraductal carcinoma (ductal carcinoma in situ). *Cancer* 1995;75:1310.
131. Fisher ER, Dignam J, Tan-Chiu E, et al. Pathologic findings from the National Surgical Adjuvant Breast Project (NSABP) eight-year update of Protocol B-17. *Cancer* 1999;86:492.
132. Van Zee K, Borgen PI. Memorial Sloan Kettering Cancer Center Experience. In: Silverstein MJ, ed. *Ductal carcinoma in situ of the breast.* Baltimore: Williams & Wilkins, 1997:455.
133. Fourquet A, Zafrani B, Campana F, Clough KB. Institut Curie experience. In: Silverstein MJ, ed. *Ductal carcinoma in situ of the breast.* Baltimore: Williams & Wilkins, 1997:391.
134. Fisher B, Costantino JP, Wickerham DL, et al. Tamoxifen for prevention of breast cancer: report of the National Surgical Adjuvant Breast and Bowel Project P-1 Study. *J Natl Cancer Inst* 1998;90:1371.
135. Mamounas EP, Bryant J, Fisher B, Wickerham DL, Wolmark N. Primary breast cancer (PBC) as a risk factor for subsequent contralateral breast cancer (CBC): NSABP experience from nine randomized adjuvant trials. *Breast Cancer Res Treat* 1998;50:230.
136. Fisher B, Dignam J, Wolmark N, et al. Tamoxifen in treatment of intraductal breast cancer: National Surgical Adjuvant Breast and Bowel Project B24 randomised controlled trial. *Lancet* 1999;353:1993.
137. Page DL, Lagios MD. Pathologic analysis of the National Surgical Adjuvant Breast Project (NSABP) B17 trial: unanswered questions remaining unanswered considering current concepts of ductal carcinoma in situ. *Cancer* 1995;75:1219.
138. Gluck BS, Dershaw DD, Liberman L, Deutsch BM. Microcalcifications on postoperative mammograms as an indicator of adequacy of tumor excision. *Radiology* 1993;188:469.
139. Aref A, Yousse PE, Washington T, et al. The value of postlumpectomy mammogram in the management of breast cancer patients presenting with suspicious microcalcifications. *Int J Radiat Oncol Biol* 1998;42:256.
140. Morrow M, Bucci C, Rademaker A. Medical contraindications are not the major factor in the underutilization of breast conserving therapy. *J Am Coll Surg* 1998;186:269.
141. Silverstein MJ, Lagios MD, Craig PH, et al. A prognostic index for ductal carcinoma in situ of the breast. *Cancer* 1996;77:2267.
142. Schnitt SJ, Harris JR, Smith BL. Developing a prognostic index for ductal carcinoma in situ of the breast. Are we there yet? *Cancer* 1996;77:2189.
143. Silverstein MJ, Lagios M, Lewinsky BS, et al. Breast irradiation is unnecessary for widely excised ductal carcinoma in situ (DCIS). *Breast Cancer Res Treat* 1997;46:23.
144. Winchester DJ, Menck HR, Winchester DP. National treatment trends for ductal carcinoma in situ of the breast. *Arch Surg* 1997;132:660.

VII

Diseases of the Breast, 2nd ed.,
edited by Jay R. Harris.
Lippincott Williams & Wilkins, Philadelphia © 2000.

Staging and Natural History of Breast Cancer

CHAPTER 28

Staging of Breast Cancer

Jay R. Harris

Staging refers to the grouping of patients according to the extent of their disease. Staging is useful in (a) determining the choice of treatment for individual patients, (b) estimating their prognosis, and (c) comparing the results of different treatment programs. Staging can be based on either clinical or pathologic findings. The first clinical staging system widely used in the United States was the Columbia Clinical Classification. This system was developed by Dr. Cushman Haagensen and coworkers and was based primarily on patients treated by radical mastectomy between 1915 and 1942 at Columbia-Presbyterian Hospital.[1,2]

Currently, the staging of cancer is determined by the American Joint Committee on Cancer (AJCC), which is jointly sponsored by the American Cancer Society and the American College of Surgeons. The AJCC system is a clinical and pathologic staging system and is based on the TNM system, in which *T* refers to tumor, *N* to nodes, and *M* to metastasis. The fifth edition of the system, published in 1997,[3] is provided in this chapter. It details rules for classification, definition of the anatomy, and stage groupings. Of particular note in the new classification are (a) the designation of T1mic for invasive cancers with microinvasion measuring 0.1 cm or smaller in greatest dimension, and (b) the designation of pN1a for nodal micrometastasis (none larger than 0.2 cm).

The many changes in the AJCC system over time and its complexity have limited its use and usefulness. In addition, the current system does not address present-day issues, such as a patient's suitability for breast-conserving treatment or the risk of distant relapse with and without systemic therapy. In practice, most clinicians simply use the tumor size and the histologic findings of axillary dissection, often grouped for convenience into negative, 1 to 3 positive nodes, 4 to 9 positive nodes, and ten or more positive nodes.

AMERICAN JOINT COMMITTEE ON CANCER RULES FOR CLASSIFICATION

Clinical Staging

Clinical staging is based on physical examination, with careful inspection and palpation of the skin, mammary glands,

J. R. Harris: Department of Radiation Oncology, Harvard Medical School, Dana-Farber Cancer Institute, Brigham and Women's Hospital, Boston, Massachusetts

and lymph nodes (axillary, supraclavicular, and cervical); imaging; and pathologic examination of the breast or other tissues to establish the diagnosis of breast carcinoma. The extent of tissue examined pathologically for clinical staging is less than that required for pathologic staging. Appropriate operative findings are elements of clinical staging, including the size of the primary tumor and chest wall invasion, and the presence or absence of regional or distant metastasis.

Pathologic Staging

Pathologic staging relies on all data used for clinical staging, surgical exploration, and resection, as well as pathologic examination of the primary carcinoma, including no less than excision of the primary carcinoma with no macroscopic tumor in any margin of resection as determined by pathologic examination. A case can be classified pT for pathologic stage grouping if only microscopic, but not macroscopic, involvement is found at the margin. If tumor is found in the margin of resection by macroscopic examination, the case is coded TX, because the extent of the primary tumor cannot be assessed. If no clinical evidence of axillary metastasis is found, resection of at least the low axillary lymph nodes (level 1)—that is, those lymph nodes located lateral to the lateral border of the pectoralis minor muscle—should be performed for pathologic (pN) classification. Such a resection ordinarily includes six or more lymph nodes. Metastatic nodules in the fat adjacent to the mammary carcinoma within the breast, without evidence of residual lymph node metastases, are classified as regional lymph node metastases (N). Pathologic stage grouping includes any of the three following combinations: pT pN pM, pT pN cM, or cT cN pM.

ANATOMY

Primary Site

The mammary gland, situated on the anterior chest wall, is composed of glandular tissue within a dense fibroareolar stroma. The glandular tissue consists of approximately 20 lobes, each of which terminates in a separate excretory duct in the nipple.

Regional Lymph Nodes

The breast lymphatics drain by way of three major routes: axillary, transpectoral, and internal mammary. Intramammary lymph nodes are considered with, and coded as, axillary lymph nodes for staging purposes; metastasis to any other lymph node, including supraclavicular, cervical, or contralateral internal mammary, is considered distant (M1). The following are the regional lymph nodes:

1. Axillary (ipsilateral): interpectoral (Rotter's) nodes and lymph nodes along the axillary vein and its tributaries, which may be (but are not required to be) divided into the following levels:
   (a) Level I (low axilla): lymph nodes lateral to the lateral border of the pectoralis minor muscle.
   (b) Level II (mid axilla): lymph nodes between the medial and lateral borders of the pectoralis minor muscle and the interpectoral (Rotter's) lymph nodes.
   (c) Level III (apical axilla): lymph nodes medial to the medial margin of the pectoralis minor muscle, including those designated as subclavicular, infraclavicular, or apical.
   Note: Intramammary lymph nodes are coded as axillary lymph nodes.
2. Internal mammary (ipsilateral): lymph nodes in the intercostal spaces along the edge of the sternum in the endothoracic fascia.

Any other lymph node metastasis, including in supraclavicular, cervical, or contralateral internal mammary lymph nodes, is coded as a distant metastasis (M1).

Metastatic Sites

All distant visceral sites are potential sites of metastasis. The four major sites of involvement are bone, lung, brain, and liver, but this widely metastasizing disease has been found in many other sites.

TNM CLASSIFICATION

Primary Tumor

The clinical assessment used for classifying the primary tumor (T) is the one judged to be most accurate for that particular case (e.g., physical examination or imaging, such as a mammogram). The pathologic tumor size for classification (T) is a measurement of *only the invasive component*. For example, if a 4.0-cm intraductal component and a 0.3-cm invasive component are found, the tumor is classified T1a. The size of the primary tumor is measured for T classification before any tissue is removed for special studies, such as testing for estrogen receptors.

Microinvasion of Breast Carcinoma

Microinvasion is the extension of cancer cells beyond the basement membrane into the adjacent tissues, with no focus larger than 0.1 cm in greatest dimension. When multiple foci of microinvasion are seen, the size of only the largest focus is used to classify the microinvasion. (The sum of all the individual foci should not be used.) The presence of multiple foci of microinvasion should be noted, as it is with multiple larger invasive carcinomas.

Multiple Simultaneous Ipsilateral Primary Carcinomas

The following guidelines are used when classifying multiple simultaneous ipsilateral primary (infiltrating, macroscopically measurable) carcinomas. These criteria do not apply to one macroscopic carcinoma associated with multiple separate microscopic foci.

1. Use the largest primary carcinoma to classify T.
2. Enter into the record that this is a case of multiple simultaneous ipsilateral primary carcinomas. Such cases should be analyzed separately.

Simultaneous Bilateral Breast Carcinomas

Each carcinoma is staged as a separate primary carcinoma in a separate organ.

Inflammatory Carcinoma

Inflammatory carcinoma is a clinicopathologic entity characterized by diffuse brawny induration of the skin of the breast with an erysipeloid edge, usually without an underlying palpable mass. Radiologic evaluation may show a detectable mass and characteristic thickening of the skin over the breast. This clinical presentation is because of tumor embolization of dermal lymphatics. The tumor of inflammatory carcinoma is classified T4d.

Paget's Disease of the Nipple

Paget's disease of the nipple without an associated tumor mass (clinical) or invasive carcinoma (pathologic) is classified Tis. Paget's disease with a demonstrable mass (clinical) or an invasive component (pathologic) is classified according to the size of the tumor mass or invasive component.

Skin of Breast

Dimpling of the skin, nipple retraction, or any other skin change except those described under T4b and T4d may occur in T1, T2, or T3 without changing the classification.

Chest Wall

The chest wall includes the ribs, intercostal muscles, and serratus anterior muscle but not pectoral muscle.

DEFINITION OF TUMOR, NODE, METASTASIS

Definitions for classifying the primary tumor (T) are the same for clinical and for pathologic classification. The telescoping method of classification can be applied. If the measurement is made by physical examination, the examiner uses the major headings (T1, T2, or T3). If other measurements, such as mammographic or pathologic measurements, are used, the telescoped subsets of T1 can be used.

Primary Tumor (T)

TX	Primary tumor cannot be assessed
T0	No evidence of primary tumor
Tis	Carcinoma *in situ*: intraductal carcinoma, lobular carcinoma *in situ*, or Paget's disease of the nipple with no tumor
T1	Tumor 2 cm or smaller in greatest dimension
T1mic	Microinvasion 0.1 cm or smaller in greatest dimension
T1a	Tumor larger than 0.1 cm but not larger than 0.5 cm in greatest dimension
T1b	Tumor larger than 0.5 cm but not larger than 1 cm in greatest dimension
T1c	Tumor larger than 1 cm but not larger than 2 cm in greatest dimension
T2	Tumor larger than 2 cm but not larger than 5 cm in greatest dimension
T3	Tumor larger than 5 cm in greatest dimension
T4	Tumor of any size with direct extension to (a) chest wall or (b) skin, only as described below
T4a	Extension to chest wall
T4b	Edema (including *peau d'orange*) or ulceration of the skin of the breast or satellite skin nodules confined to the same breast
T4c	Both (T4a and T4b)
T4d	Inflammatory carcinoma (see previous definition)

Note: Paget's disease associated with a tumor is classified according to the size of the tumor.

Regional Lymph Nodes (N)

NX	Regional lymph nodes cannot be assessed (e.g., previously removed)
N0	No regional lymph node metastasis
N1	Metastasis to movable ipsilateral axillary lymph node(s)
N2	Metastasis to ipsilateral axillary lymph node(s) fixed to one another or to other structures
N3	Metastasis to ipsilateral internal mammary lymph node(s)

Pathologic Classification (pN)

pN0	No regional lymph node metastasis
pN1	Metastasis to movable ipsilateral axillary lymph node(s)
pN1a	Only micrometastasis (none larger than 0.2 cm)
pN1b	Metastasis to lymph node(s), any larger than 0.2 cm

pN1bi Metastasis in one to three lymph nodes, any larger than 0.2 cm and smaller than 2 cm in greatest dimension
pN1bii Metastasis to four or more lymph nodes, any larger than 0.2 cm and smaller than 2 cm in greatest dimension
pN1biii Extension of tumor beyond the capsule of a lymph node metastasis smaller than 2 cm in greatest dimension
pN1biv Metastasis to a lymph node 2 cm or larger in greatest dimension

pN2 Metastasis to ipsilateral axillary lymph nodes that are fixed to one another or to other structures

pN3 Metastasis to ipsilateral internal mammary lymph node(s)

Distant Metastasis (M)

MX Distant metastasis cannot be assessed
M0 No distant metastasis
M1 Distant metastasis (includes metastasis to one or more ipsilateral supraclavicular lymph nodes)

STAGE GROUPING

Stage 0	Tis	N0	M0
Stage I	T1*	N0	M0
Stage IIA	T0	N1	M0
	T1*	N1†	M0
	T2	N0	M0
Stage IIB	T2	N1	M0
	T3	N0	M0
Stage IIIA	T0	N2	M0
	T1*	N2	M0
	T2	N2	M0
	T3	N1	M0
	T3	N2	M0
Stage IIIB	T4	Any N	M0
	Any T	N3	M0
Stage IV	Any T	Any N	M1

*T1 includes T1mic.
†The prognosis of patients with N1a is similar to that of patients with pN0.

HISTOPATHOLOGIC TYPE

The histologic types are the following:

Carcinoma, not otherwise specified (NOS)
Ductal
- Intraductal (*in situ*)
- Invasive with predominant intraductal component
- Invasive, NOS
- Comedo
- Inflammatory
- Medullary with lymphocytic infiltrate
- Mucinous (colloid)
- Papillary
- Scirrhous
- Tubular
- Other

Lobular
- *In situ*
- Invasive with predominant *in situ* component
- Invasive

Nipple
- Paget's disease, NOS
- Paget's disease with intraductal carcinoma
- Paget's disease with invasive ductal carcinoma

Other
- Undifferentiated carcinoma

HISTOPATHOLOGIC GRADE (G)

GX Grade cannot be assessed
G1 Well-differentiated
G2 Moderately differentiated
G3 Poorly differentiated
G4 Undifferentiated

REFERENCES

1. Haagensen C. *Diseases of the breast*, 3rd ed. Philadelphia: WB Saunders, 1986:852.
2. Haagensen CD, Stout AP. Carcinoma of the breast: results of treatment. *Ann Surg* 1942;116:801.
3. American Joint Committee on Cancer. Breast. In: *AJCC cancer staging manual*, 5th ed. Philadelphia: Lippincott–Raven, 1997:171.

Diseases of the Breast, 2nd ed.
edited by Jay R. Harris.
Lippincott Williams & Wilkins, Philadelphia © 2000.

CHAPTER 29

Natural History of Breast Cancer

Samuel Hellman and Jay R. Harris

The clinical behavior of breast cancer is characterized by a long natural history and by heterogeneity among patients in its clinical course. The prognosis of patients with breast cancer has been well documented in terms of the size of the tumor and the presence and extent of involvement of regional lymph nodes. Patients diagnosed with breast cancer, however, are at risk for metastases for extended time periods, and the definition of cure in this disease is problematic. Models to describe the growth of breast cancer have been described, but they remain controversial. The treatment of breast cancer has been directed at the breast and regional lymph nodes locally and at sites of metastases systemically, but the importance of local treatment has been debated. This chapter reviews information related to these important aspects of the disease.

PLOTTING SURVIVAL IN UNTREATED AND TREATED BREAST CANCER

By documenting the natural history of untreated breast cancer, one can establish a baseline by which to judge the effects of treatment. Because breast cancer has been considered a treatable disease for at least the last several hundred years, series of untreated but well-documented patients are uncommon. One such series is from Middlesex Hospital in England, where one of the first cancer wards was established in 1792. Bloom et al.[1] reported on a group of 250 patients seen at Middlesex Hospital between 1805 and 1933. Patients generally were admitted to the hospital with locally advanced breast cancer. Seventy-four percent were in stage IV, 23% were in stage III, and only 2% were in stage II. Patients were not admitted to the hospital at the clinical onset of the disease but were for terminal care. No patient was treated with any form of surgery, radiation therapy (RT), or hormone therapy. Because of the meticulous medical records kept, it was possible to estimate the onset of the disease with a fair degree of accuracy. Only 7% of the patients presented within 6 months of the initial symptom of the disease and only 39% within 1 year. Figure 1 shows the percentage of patients surviving, plotted from the time of the first onset of symptoms. The median survival time from the onset of symptoms was 2.7 years. Eighteen percent of untreated patients survived 5 years, and 4% survived 10 years. These figures indicate that survival of breast cancer patients can be lengthy, even with advanced disease and even if the disease is untreated.

Figure 1B shows the usefulness of plotting survival curves semilogarithmically. In this figure, the same survival data from the Middlesex Hospital given in Fig. 1A are shown, with survival plotted semilogarithmically. The approximately straight line in this figure indicates that the annual hazard or force of mortality (i.e., the percentage of remaining patients who die each year) is constant. In this group of patients, approximately 25% of the patients at the start of any year died by the end of that year.

Compare the results in the Middlesex Hospital with results seen in modern times. Figure 2 shows the survival results collected by the End Results Section of the Biometry Branch of the National Cancer Institute (NCI) on a large group of patients with histologically confirmed breast cancer.[2] The results apply to patients who were treated for their cancer and are corrected for causes of death other than breast cancer. The biphasic shape of this survival curve has been interpreted as indicating that there are two subgroups of breast cancer patients. One subgroup is manifested by the curve past 10 years and represents patients who have a force of mortality rate of 2.5% per year. By backward extrapolation of this portion of the curve to time zero, one can estimate that this subgroup represents approximately 60% of the total group. The other subgroup has more aggressive disease, with a force of mortality rate of 25% per year, similar to that observed for untreated patients seen at Middlesex Hospital. There are, however, potential problems in making such a comparison. The Middlesex Hospital experience represents a highly selected group of patients because only 250 patients were collected over 128 years, or approximately two per year. These patients were identified for inclusion in the series only if a postmortem examination had been per-

S. Hellman: Department of Radiation and Cellular Oncology, Center for Advanced Medicine, University of Chicago Medical Center, Chicago, Illinois

J. R. Harris: Department of Radiation Oncology, Harvard Medical School, Dana-Farber Cancer Institute, Brigham and Women's Hospital, Boston, Massachusetts

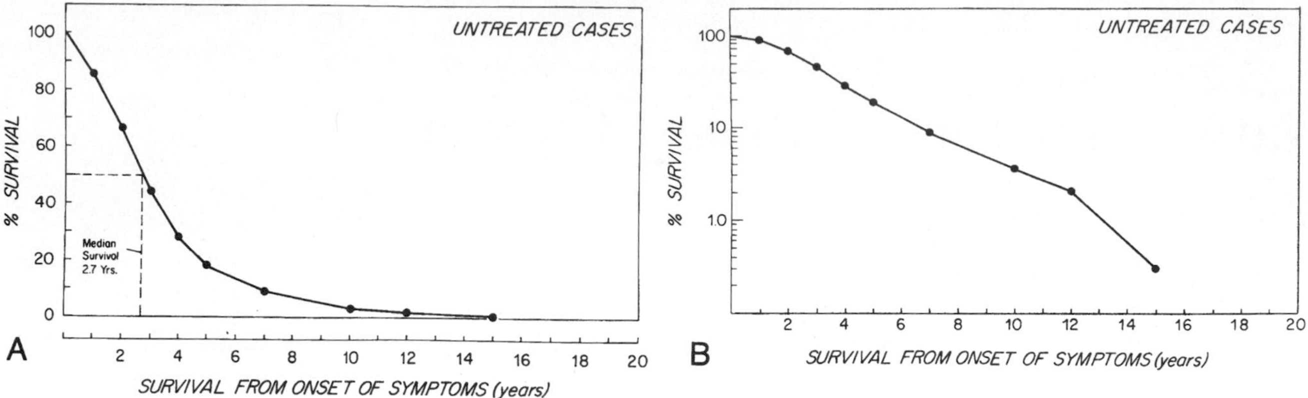

FIG. 1. Survival of 250 untreated breast cancer patients from Middlesex Hospital plotted linearly (**A**) and semilogarithmically (**B**). (From ref. 1, with permission.)

formed, not at the onset of their disease. Given these caveats, the results seen in the NCI data indicate that breast cancer is a heterogeneous disease and that its natural history is even more protracted than was apparent in the Middlesex series. These data also suggest that there are clinically definable subsets of patients with a high annual hazard of death (>25%) and other subsets with a low annual hazard of death (<2%). The cause of the second slope is complicated by competing mortality from other causes. This is not completely accounted for by considering relative mortality compared with a peer population.

An understanding of the survival curve for breast cancer patients is important in assessing prognosis in patient subgroups and in assessing new therapies.[3] For most populations, the slope of the survival curve of treated patients becomes more shallow at 10 years. The demonstration of a "cured" subgroup therefore requires follow-up of longer than 10 years. (Whether such patients are actually cured is discussed in the next section, Curability of Breast Cancer.) With long-term follow-up, it is possible to distinguish the disease's virulence and metastagenicity.[4–6] *Virulence* is the pace, or rate, of appearance of metastases or mortality, whereas *metastagenicity* is the ultimate likelihood of metastases. We[3] have also stressed elsewhere that improvements in the early portion of the survival curve by new therapies do not always result in an improvement in the survival curve past the inflection point. Conversely, in some cases, an early detrimental effect may obscure a benefit in long-term outcome. These considerations emphasize that effects seen on the early portion of survival curves may be premature and also misleading.

CURABILITY OF BREAST CANCER

The protracted nature of the survival curve shown in Fig. 2 raises the question of whether a patient with breast cancer is ever truly cured of the disease. Given that breast cancer has a relatively late age of onset and a long natural history, a large group of patients must be followed for a long time to address this question. Furthermore, the definition of "cure" is not straightforward, and a number of definitions have been proposed.[7] The most commonly used definition of cure is referred to as *statistical cure*. A group of treated patients can be considered statistically cured if the group's subsequent death rate from all causes is similar to that of a normal population group with the same age and sex distribution. *Clinical cure* for an individual refers to the apparent complete eradication of the disease. Clinical cure for a group occurs when long-term follow-up of the causes of death for the group shows that the risk of dying from breast cancer is the same as for women of the same

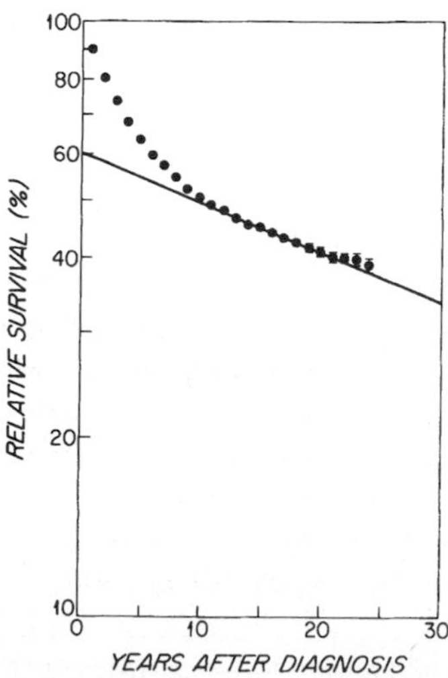

FIG. 2. Relative survival rates of breast cancer patients (all stages) from the End Results Section, Biometry Branch, National Cancer Institute, 1977. (From ref. 2, with permission.)

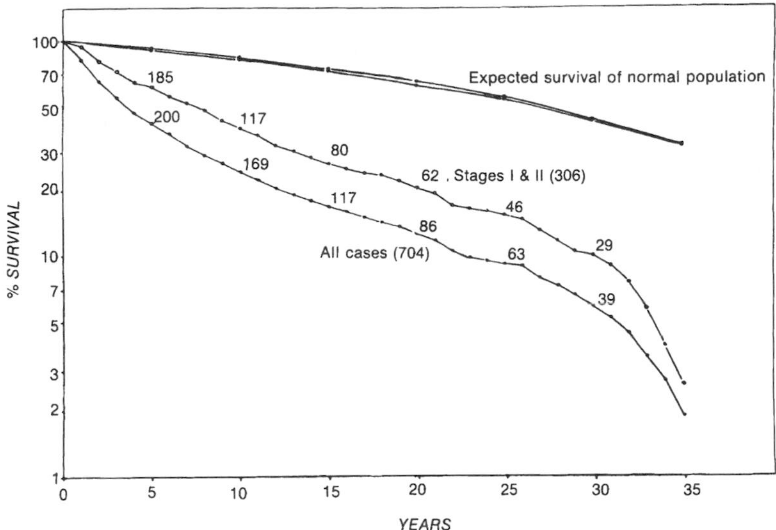

FIG. 3. Survival rate curve for 704 breast cancer patients treated between 1947 and 1950 and observed for at least 31 years, compared with survival curve of the normal population. (From ref. 8, with permission.)

age in the general population. An assessment of the likelihood of clinical cure involves determining the cause of death for treated patients. Inaccuracies in the information recorded on death certificates, however, limits the usefulness of this definition of cure. *Personal cure* for an individual refers to a patient living symptom-free from breast cancer and dying of other causes.

Attempts to assess statistical cure in breast cancer patients have all indicated a persistent excess risk of mortality. Brinkley and Haybittle[8] reported on a group of 704 breast cancer patients from the Cambridge, England, area in whom the first diagnosis was made between 1947 and 1950. The minimum follow-up period for survivors was 31 years. Figure 3 shows the survival curves calculated by the life-table method and the expected curves for the normal population of the region with the same age distribution. The survival curves for breast cancer patients never become parallel with those for the normal population. Eight deaths from breast cancer occurred more than 25 years after treatment, which is 15 times the number that would be expected. Hibberd and associates[9] followed 2,019 cases for 30 years and found a small excess of observed over expected deaths, even between 25 and 30 years. Rutqvist and Wallgren[10] presented follow-up on 458 patients 40 years of age or younger at diagnosis and found an excess mortality that persisted for at least 40 years. These studies indicate a persistent excess risk of mortality after treatment for breast cancer. This finding was not confirmed in southeast Finland, where the relative survival became flat and no further cancer deaths occurred after 27 years.[11]

Despite the lack of evidence for a statistical cure, a considerable percentage of patients experience a personal cure, as defined earlier. In the Brinkley and Haybittle report,[8] 176 (26%) of the 683 patients fell into this category. In the experience from Memorial Sloan-Kettering Cancer Center reported by Adair and coworkers,[12] 300 of the 1,458 patients (21%) with operable breast cancer had a personal cure of their disease. In a more recent report from Memorial Sloan-Kettering Cancer Center, Rosen and associates[13] reported on 382 patients with breast cancer 2 cm or smaller and axillary nodes negative for metastasis who were treated with radical mastectomy and followed for a median of 18.2 years. Although recurrences were observed during the entire 20-year follow-up period, it was estimated that 80% of patients with tumors 1 cm or smaller had personal cures, and 70% of patients with tumors 1.1 cm to 2.0 cm had personal cures. This means that many patients treated for breast cancer will live out their normal life expectancy free of further evidence of the disease. Similar findings were seen in the long-term follow-up of node-negative breast cancer patients from the University of Chicago.[4,5,14] Overall survival is compared with metastasis-free survival in Fig. 4. The flattening of the distant metastasis–free curve is evidence of a sizable group of patients cured with regional treatment only. This does not mean that there are no patients with metastases first appearing long after the primary treatment; there are, but they are small in number. Only 1.3% of the failures in this series occurred after 20 years. Put differently, this represented 3.7% of the 20-year survivors. Breast cancer requires long-term follow-up to determine outcome. Such observation reveals significant numbers of patients cured by only local-regional treatment, although there is a continuing small risk of failure. Five-year survival is influenced primarily by tumor virulence, whereas 10-year survival is influenced by both virulence and metastagenicity. Only 20-year survival measures metastagenicity alone.

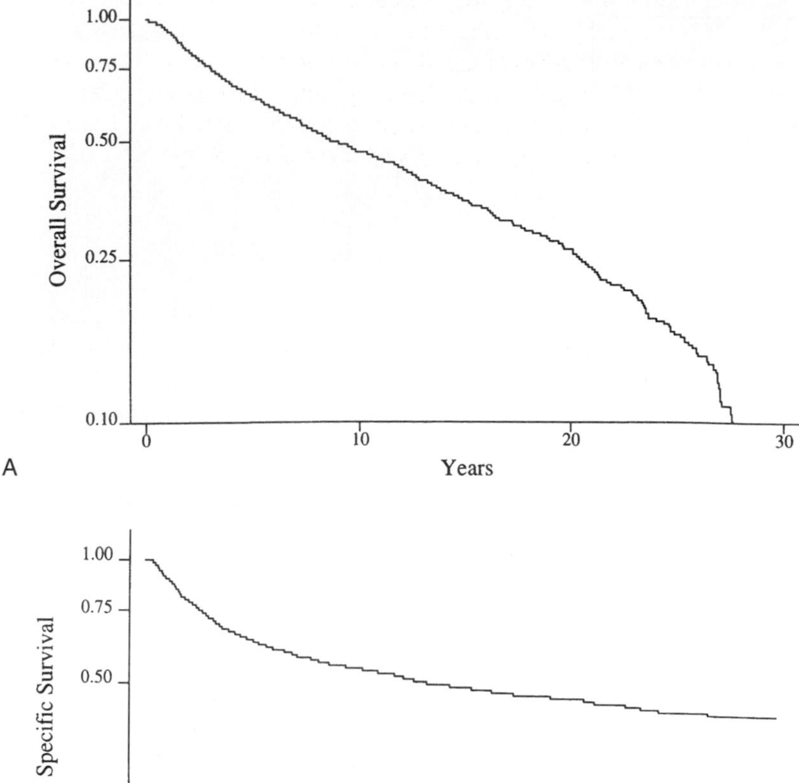

FIG. 4. A: Overall survival of patients treated with local-regional treatment only from 1927 to 1987. **B:** Distant disease–free survival of this same patient population.

GROWTH RATE OF BREAST CANCER

The long natural history of breast cancer has been evaluated in terms of the clinical growth rate of the disease. The determination of clinical growth rate can provide information on the heterogeneity of the disease and has been used to estimate the time from oncogenesis to clinical presentation.

One of the ways in which the growth rate of breast cancer has been assessed is by the time required for a tumor to double its diameter, an amount equivalent to an eightfold increase in volume. In 1956, Collins and colleagues[15] described the clinical growth rates of several human tumors, including carcinoma of the breast. They assumed an exponential model for tumor growth—that is, tumor cells divide at a constant rate over time. According to this model, a single cancer cell will grow to a nodule 1 mm in diameter in 20 doublings. Another 10 doublings would produce approximately 1 kg of tumor tissue, an amount commonly observed at the time of death from the disease. Collins and associates plotted the clinical doubling time for a group of 24 patients with metastatic cancer involving the lungs in whom measurements of tumor size could be performed on serial chest radiographs. The observed doubling times ranged from 28 to 164 days for patients with tumors of epithelial origin. The median volume doubling time for this group was 78 days. This study established the heterogeneity of clinical growth rates for human tumors and was used to estimate the duration of the preclinical phases of the disease. If one assumes this exponential model, a doubling time of 100 days, and that a primary tumor and metastatic tumor have similar growth rates, then the time required for a single malignant cell to grow to a clinically detectable 1-cm mass would be slightly more than 8 years. Other investigators have noticed similar findings.[16–19] This model of exponential tumor growth provided the first theoretic basis for the use of cancer chemotherapy.[20,21]

It is also possible to estimate the interval between mammographic detectability and clinical detectability from data obtained from mammographic screening programs.[22] Using the data from the Health Insurance Plan of Greater New York study, the mean interval was estimated to be 1.7 years. Other estimates of the interval that used different mathematic models vary from 1.3 to 2.4 years.[23,24]

Deficiencies exist, however, in the concept of exponential tumor growth. In fact, for breast cancer and other epithelial malignancies, a Gompertzian model rather than an exponential model better describes tumor growth.[25] In a Gompertzian model, the growth constant is exponentially slowing. Therefore, although the tumor mass increases in size, its doubling time becomes progressively longer. *In vitro* and *in vivo* studies have indicated that the human tumor cell cycle time is on the order of 2 days, not 100 days.[26] Gross tumor doubling times, in fact, represent a complex relationship between cell cycle time, the percentage of cells cycling (growth fraction), and the likelihood that a newly divided cell will not contribute to the tumor mass (cell loss factor). For breast cancer, the growth fraction is approximately 5%, and the cell loss factor is approximately 75%. Thus, most of a tumor is made of cells that are not cycling. Furthermore, each cell that is cycling does so at a very rapid rate, but most of its progeny do not survive. In this light, it is necessary to interpret volume-doubling times as only a rough index of the aggressiveness of the tumor and as not valid for estimating the time from oncogenesis to clinical presentation.

The observed clinical growth rate of breast cancer ultimately needs to account for the evolving information on the molecular and genetic biology of the disease. Breast cancer, similar to other malignancies for which more precise information is known, results from a series of mutations in growth-regulatory genes, DNA repair, and other genes. It is unknown, however, whether these mutations need to occur in any particular order or how many separate pathways involving different genetic changes may eventually lead to the phenotype of breast cancer.[27] The heterogeneity in the clinical behavior of breast cancer suggests that the genetic basis for the disease may be variable. These genetic changes result in growth under conditions that would be limiting for normal cells, and it is presumed that additional genetic changes favoring the survival of this clone, its uncontrolled growth, and its ability to change (genetic instability) are selected over time. Although this model of oncogenesis (clonal selection) was developed in the 1970s,[28] the details are just becoming available. By the time of clinical presentation, it is estimated that the extent of genetic change is large, as evidenced by the common finding of aneuploidy. A large variety of genetic changes have been described in the human breast cancers, although their pathogenetic significance has not been fully elucidated.

Even more complicated models of breast cancer growth have been proposed. In a model proposed by Speer et al.[29] and Demicheli et al.,[30] tumor growth occurs in spurts (dormancy), during which Gompertzian growth pertains, separated by periods of little or no growth for varying lengths of time. It is possible to select specific values for the time between growth spurts and for their growth rates that are consistent with well-described clinical data sets. These authors[30] have argued that their theory of tumor growth is consistent with tumor growth by clonal selection. They have hypothesized that additional genetic changes (e.g., for the ability to obtain new blood vessels for additional growth) can provide incremental spurts in tumor growth.

PRIMARY CANCER IN THE BREAST

The spread of primary cancer through the breast occurs (a) by direct infiltration into the breast parenchyma, (b) along mammary ducts, and (c) by way of breast lymphatics. Direct infiltration of the cancer tends to occur by ramifying projections that give a characteristic stellate appearance on gross examination and on mammography. If untreated, direct involvement of overlying skin or deep pectoral fascia can occur. Involvement along ducts is observed frequently and may involve an entire segment of the breast. It is unclear, however, whether this intraductal involvement represents spread of a primary cancer along previously uninvolved ducts or the development of an invasive cancer or cancers from a diffuse area of ductal carcinoma *in situ*. Spread also can occur by the extensive network of breast lymphatics. Investigators have emphasized lymphatic spread vertically down to the lymphatic plexus in the deep pectoral fascia underlying the breast. In addition, spread to the central subareolar region has been described. These multiple mechanisms of spread through the breast emphasize the likelihood for cancer to be present in the breast wall beyond the palpable primary mass.

Holland and colleagues[31] performed a detailed study of the distribution of cancer in a breast containing a localized tumor. They examined 264 specimens from patients with clinically unifocal breast cancer measuring 4 cm or smaller. In only 40% of cases was the cancer in the breast restricted to the palpable tumor. Nineteen percent of the cases had additional foci of cancer but restricted to the immediate 2 cm around the tumor. Forty-one percent of the cases showed cancer foci further than 2 cm from the reference tumor, including 27% in which the additional foci were entirely intraductal and 14% in which they were invasive and intraductal. This study and its implications for breast-conserving treatment are further discussed in Chapter 33.

The primary site of breast cancer usually is described by its location by quadrant in the breast. In one series of 696 cases, 48% were located in the upper outer quadrant, 15% in the upper inner quadrant, 11% in the lower outer quadrant, 6% in the lower inner quadrant, and 17% in the central region (designated as within 1 cm of the areola).[32] An additional 3% were termed diffuse because of multicentric or massive involvement of the breast. The reason for the increased frequency of breast cancer in the upper outer quadrant is thought to be simply the greater amount of breast tissue in that quadrant. In this series of patients, no differences in survival based on quadrant location were observed. The relationship between the location of the pri-

TABLE 1. *Five-year recurrence rates (RRs) related to tumor size, tumor location, and involvement of axillary nodes*

	Negative nodes				Positive nodes			
	Medial		Lateral		Medial		Lateral	
Tumor size (cm)	N	RR (%)	N	RR (%)	N	RR (%)	N	RR (%)
0.1–1.0	141	12	408	10	19	32	83	21
1.1–2.0	471	16	1,357	12	102	41	411	34
2.1–3.0	347	19	1,034	13	114	43	424	36
3.1–5.0	227	20	721	17	102	47	406	45
≥5.1	54	34	191	21	46	33	166	57
All	1,240	18	8,711	14	383	42	1,490	39

N, number.
Nemoto T, Natarajan N, Bedwani R, et al. Breast cancer in the medial half: results of the 1978 National Survey of the American College of Surgeons. *Cancer* 1983;51:1333.

mary tumor in the breast and prognosis has also been examined in a large series of patients from the 1978 National Survey of the American College of Surgeons (ACS)[33] and by the National Surgical Adjuvant Breast and Bowel Project (NSABP).[34] In the ACS study, outcome in 9,401 patients was examined in relation to the size of the primary tumor, its location, and involvement of axillary nodes. Patients were treated with mastectomy without RT; the 5-year results are shown in Table 1. The distribution of tumor size for patients with medial and lateral tumors was nearly identical. Patients with medial tumors and node-negative breast cancer, however, did somewhat worse than patients with lateral tumors and node-negative disease (recurrence rates, 18% versus 14%, p <.005). The results for patients with node-positive breast cancer were not statistically different, based on tumor location. The results obtained in the NSABP study were similar. Patients with medial tumors and node-negative disease also did slightly worse than patients with lateral tumors and node-negative disease (recurrence rates, 24% versus 19%). The number of patients in this study, however, was smaller, and the results did not reach statistical significance. Patients with node-positive disease had the same prognosis, regardless of location. The results from the ACS and NSABP studies suggest that patients with inner-half tumors and node-negative disease have a worse prognosis than patients with outer-half tumors and negative nodes. This is likely related to preferential involvement of internal mammary nodes (IMNs) with medial tumors, which is discussed further in the section Internal Mammary Node Involvement.

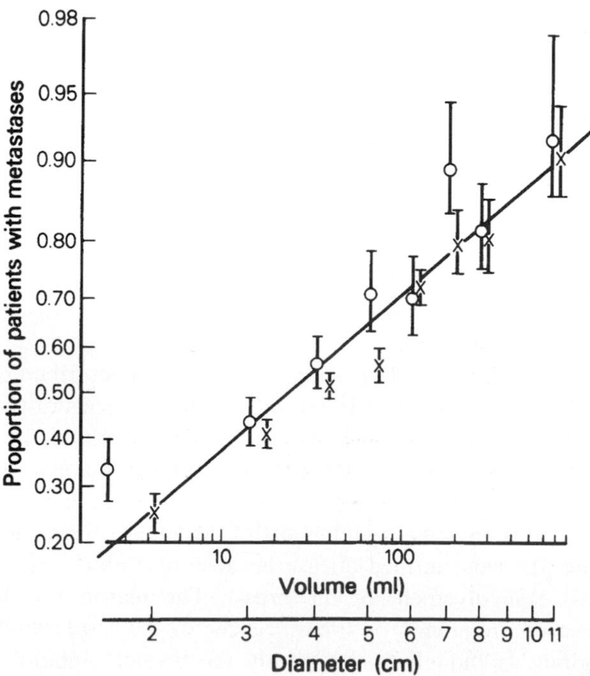

FIG. 5. Relation between clinical size of the tumor and the likelihood of distant metastasis for patients treated from 1954 to 1958 (O) and 1959 to 1972 (X). (From ref. 35, with permission.)

The clinical size of the primary tumor is highly correlated with prognosis. The data from Koscielny et al.,[35,36] of the Institut Gustave-Roussy, illustrates this point. They examined the relationship between the size of the primary tumor and the likelihood of distant metastasis in 2,648 patients with breast cancer treated at their institution between 1954 and 1972 (Fig. 5). The data, which were plotted using a log-probit coordinate system, indicate a direct relation between tumor size and the probability of metastasis. Similar findings have been reported in other studies.[12,37–40] The data

TABLE 2. *Metastagenicity (M) and virulence (V) of breast cancer as a function of size and nodal involvement*

Size (cm)	Nodes	M	V (%)
≤1	0	0.15	1
1.1–2.0	0	0.20	1.5
≤2	1–3	0.36	5
≤2	≥4	0.79	9
>2	0	0.38	5
>2	1–3	0.70	18
>2	≥4	0.89	21

M, (100 – plateau of distant disease–free survival)/100; V, initial slope of the semilog plot of distant disease–free survival. The rate of distant disease per year. (From ref. 14, with permission.)

from the University of Chicago[14] are shown in Table 2. Both virulence and metastagenicity increase with tumor size and nodal involvement, but in all groups of operable breast cancer patients, there is a cured population—that is, metastagenicity is not 1.0.

REGIONAL NODE INVOLVEMENT

The most common sites of regional involvement of breast cancer are the axillary node, IMN, and supraclavicular lymph node regions. Knowledge of the likelihood of involvement of these sites and their significance is important for the staging and planning of treatment for patients with breast cancer.

Axillary Node Involvement

The axillary lymph node region is the major regional drainage site for the breast. Approximately 50% of patients with breast cancer that is evident on physical examination have histologic evidence of axillary node involvement. The likelihood of axillary nodal involvement is directly related to the size of the primary tumor. This was shown in studies by Nemoto and coworkers,[33] Haagensen,[40] and Fisher and associates[39] and documented in greater detail in the report from the Surveillance, Epidemiology and End Results (SEER) Program of the NCI[41] (Table 3). The SEER data examined the relationship between tumor size, axillary lymph node involvement, and 5-year relative survival in 24,740 patients with breast cancer. The data were taken from the nine SEER population-based tumor registries for patients diagnosed between 1977 and 1982 whose pathologic or operative tumor size was recorded and who had at least eight lymph nodes examined. Patients with distant metastases at diagnosis, carcinoma *in situ*, or prior cancer were excluded. The larger the primary tumor, the greater the risk of axillary node involvement. As discussed in Chapter 37, patients with microinvasive breast cancer are the only subgroup in whom the risk of axillary nodal involvement is consistently reported to be less than 5%.

TABLE 3. *Frequency of axillary node involvement related to tumor size*

Frequency of axillary node involvement (%)	Tumor size (cm)
<0.5	20.6
0.5–0.9	20.6
1.0–1.9	33.2
2.0–2.9	44.9
3.0–3.9	52.1
4.0–4.9	60.0
>5.0	70.1

From ref. 41, with permission.

TABLE 4. *Incidence of positive axillary nodes relative to the location and size of the primary tumor*

	Medial		Lateral	
Tumor size (cm)	Patients	Positive (%)	Patients	Positive (%)
0.1–1.0	219	18	578	25
1.1–2.0	820	28	2,212	35
2.1–3.0	691	35	1,951	43
3.1–5.0	522	44	1,651	53
>5.1	165	58	592	63
Total	**2,417**	**35**	**6,984**	**43**

From ref. 33, with permission.

Evidence supports the theory that the location of the primary tumor in the breast influences the likelihood of axillary node involvement. Several studies have indicated that axillary nodes are more commonly involved when tumors are located in the lateral portion of the breast than when they are in the medial portion. In the 1978 National Survey of the ACS, 43% of patients with lateral-half tumors had node-positive node disease, compared with 35% of patients with medial-half tumors.[33] Haagensen[40] described similar results on the frequency of axillary node metastasis from his personal series of 917 patients treated with radical mastectomy. In this series, positive nodes were found in 47% of patients with upper outer-quadrant tumors, 38% with lower outer-quadrant tumors, 30% with upper inner-quadrant tumors, and 23% with lower inner-quadrant tumors. Similarly, Fisher and associates[34] had similar results. In the previously noted ACS study, the results were examined in relation to tumor size and location (Table 4). In each category of tumor size, patients with medial tumors were less likely to have positive axillary nodes, compared with patients with lateral tumors. The increased likelihood of axillary involvement for lateral compared with medial tumors is most likely related to preferential drainage of some medial tumors to IMNs. As a result, regional lymph node involvement (either axillary nodes or IMNs) is similar for medial and lateral tumors.

The reported incidence of histologic involvement of axillary nodes depends, to some degree, on the extent of the axillary dissection performed and on the thoroughness of the pathologic evaluation of the specimen. Radical mastectomy permits the most complete dissection of the axillary contents and yields the greatest number of axillary nodes. Lesser surgical procedures, such as the modified radical mastectomy, typically give a less complete axillary dissection and fewer axillary nodes. As a result of this variable extent of axillary dissection, the likelihood of histologic involvement must be viewed in terms of the surgical procedure performed. In one pathologic study of axillary specimens, it was observed that axillary node involvement after complete dissection would have been reduced by 29% if the axillary dissection had been extended only to the lateral border of the pectoralis

TABLE 5. *Accuracy of physical examination in predicting histologic involvement of axillary nodes*

Results	Bucalossi et al.[39]	Butcher[43]	Haagensen[46]	Schottenfeld et al.[37]
False-positive (%)	25	31	26	29
False-negative (%)	32	28	27	29

minor muscle.[42] Interest in using sentinel node biopsy to avoid the need for an axillary dissection in patients with uninvolved sentinel nodes is discussed in Chapter 33.

Detection of axillary involvement by physical examination has both a high false-positive and false-negative rate (Table 5).[37,40,43,44] When axillary lymph nodes are palpable and suspect for cancer, histologic evidence of metastatic disease is found in approximately 70% of cases. Conversely, when axillary nodes are not palpable, histologic involvement is detected in approximately 30% of cases. These figures indicate the shortcomings of clinical evaluation in predicting histologic involvement.

Histologic involvement of axillary nodes has a high correlation with prognosis. Table 6 shows 10-year survival figures related to axillary involvement from seven separate series of patients treated with radical mastectomy.[37,45–50] Patients with histologically negative axillary nodes have markedly better survival rates than do patients with histologic involvement. Furthermore, patients with one to three nodes positive for metastasis do better than patients with four or more positive nodes. In fact, prognosis is directly related to the number of axillary nodes positive for disease. This is illustrated in the results obtained in the ACS survey[38] (Table 7). These data suggest that any comparison of prognosis that is based on dividing patients by a certain number of positive nodes is artificial because there are no clear dividing lines. However, such a division is practical. Many groups now divide patients into groups having one to three positive nodes, four to nine positive nodes, or 10 or more positive nodes.

The axilla is commonly divided into three levels: level I, or proximal, defined as tissue inferior and lateral to the lower border of the pectoralis minor muscle; level II, or middle, tissue directly beneath the pectoralis minor; and level III, or distal, tissue superior and medial to the pectoralis minor. Prognosis has been shown to be related to the level of axillary involvement.[37] Involvement of the distal-level nodes carries a worse prognosis than involvement of the proximal-level nodes. In a study of 182 mastectomy specimens in which the axillary contents were completely examined (or cleared), involvement of nodes in the distal portion of the axilla was found in 15.[51] All 15 were associated with involvement of many nodes in the axilla (mean number of involved nodes was 16.2). In another study, axillary node involvement and survival were examined in 385 patients to determine whether the total number of involved nodes or the level of axillary node involvement was a better indicator of prognosis.[42] Researchers found that for any given number of involved nodes, survival was independent of the level of involvement, and they concluded that prognosis was related more directly to the total number of nodes involved.

Involvement of the axilla is generally orderly relative to levels. This was examined in two large series of patients treated with radical mastectomy[52,53] and in other smaller series of patients treated with modified radical mastectomy.[54–57] These results are discussed in greater detail in Chapter 33.

The axillary nodes also can be subclassified into the following: (a) external mammary, (b) central, (c) scapular, (d) axillary vein, (e) apical or subclavicular, and (f) interpectoral (Rotter) lymph nodes. Haagensen[58] documented sites of involvement by cancer in the axilla using this classification. He found that the most common site of involvement was the central group of nodes. When only one node was involved, in nearly all cases it was in the central group. The next most common site of involvement was the axillary vein group, followed by the scapular, interpectoral, and subclavicular groups.

TABLE 6. *Ten-year survival rate by axillary node status for patients treated with radical mastectomy*

	Survival rate (%)			
Study	Negative nodes	Positive nodes	1–3 Positive nodes	4 or More positive nodes
Valagussa et al.[45]	80	38	50	24
Haagensen[51]	76	48	63	27
Schottenfeld et al.[37]	72	43	—	—
Fisher et al.[47]	65	25	38	13
Spratt and Donegan[48]	68	27	—	—
Payne et al.[49]	76	35	—	—
Ferguson et al.[50]	72	39	52	27

TABLE 7. *Five-year results related to the number of axillary nodes pathologically positive*

Positive axillary nodes	Patients	Survival rate (%)	Recurrence rate (%)
0	12,299	72	19
1	2,012	63	33
2	1,338	62	40
3	842	59	43
4	615	52	44
5	478	47	54
6–10	1,261	41	63
11–15	562	29	72
16–20	301	29	75
≥21	225	22	82

From ref. 33, with permission.

TABLE 8. *Five-year breast cancer survival rates according to the size of the tumor and axillary node involvement*

	Patients surviving 5 years		
Tumor size (cm)	Negative nodes	1–3 Positive nodes	4 or More positive nodes
<0.5	269 (99.2%)	53 (95.3%)	17 (59.0%)
0.5–0.9	791 (98.3%)	140 (94.0%)	65 (54.2%)
1.0–1.9	4,668 (95.8%)	1,574 (86.6%)	742 (67.2%)
2.0–2.9	4,010 (92.3%)	1,897 (83.4%)	1,375 (63.4%)
3.0–3.9	2,072 (86.2%)	1,185 (79.0%)	1,072 (56.9%)
4.0–4.9	845 (84.6%)	540 (69.8%)	727 (52.6%)
≥5.0	809 (82.2%)	630 (73.0%)	1,259 (45.5%)

From ref. 41, with permission.

The question of whether the size of the primary tumor and the number of involved axillary nodes independently predict for prognosis has been addressed in several institutional studies and documented in greater detail in the SEER data (Table 8). The results indicate that these two factors are of independent prognostic value. Survival declines with increasing size when the nodes are negative or when less than four are involved. Patients with more extensive nodal involvement have a worse prognosis regardless of primary size. Even patients with limited nodal involvement are at greater risk than those without any regional node spread. Adair and others[12] reported that for patients with node-negative disease, the 30-year relative survival rate was 61% when the primary tumor was 2 cm or smaller, 46% for tumors between 2 cm and 5 cm, and 50% for tumors larger than 5 cm. For patients with involvement of level I axillary nodes, the 30-year relative survival rate was 40% when the tumor was 2 cm or smaller, 31% for tumors between 2 cm and 5 cm, and 14% for tumors larger than 5 cm. Table 2, from the University of Chicago, indicates that even within nodal groups, size remains an important determinant of eventual distant metastasis.[14] The results seen at the Institut Gustave-Roussy also are in general agreement.[35,36] This study population consisted of 2,408 patients treated at the Institut Gustave-Roussy using initial radical or modified radical mastectomy between 1954 and 1979. For each patient, they systematically assessed the primary tumor size and the number of axillary nodes positive for metastasis. The authors used a probit analysis to estimate the distribution of tumor sizes at the times of axillary node involvement and distant metastases. As shown in other studies, they found that increasing tumor size was associated with an increasing likelihood and extent of axillary nodal involvement. Among all subsets of patients, a strong correlation was observed between the propensity for axillary nodal involvement and for distant metastasis (indicating that both reflect the biologic aggressiveness of a tumor). However, the capacity for nodal involvement was acquired at a smaller tumor size than the capacity for distant metastasis. For any group of patients, prognosis was better assessed using both tumor size and extent of axillary node involvement rather than by one of these alone. These results stress that both tumor size and number of involved axillary nodes are useful in estimating prognosis and that a significant percentage of patients with involved axillary nodes have prolonged survival, without evidence of distant metastasis.

Approximately 20% to 30% of patients with negative axillary nodes develop distant metastases within 10 years (see Table 6). This observation has important implications regarding the natural history of the disease. It suggests that metastases can travel directly from the primary tumor in the breast to distant sites by way of the bloodstream without first involving the regional lymph nodes. A possible alternative explanation is that nodes that are called negative are in fact involved with metastases but are undetected. There is known to be a sampling error in the detection of axillary metastases. It is possible to miss axillary nodes in the axillary dissection specimen unless a meticulous clearing method is used, and it is possible to miss microscopic evidence of metastases in a given node unless it is thoroughly sectioned. In the United States, the routine method for detection of axillary nodal metastases does not involve clearing of the specimen and involves only a limited number of sections (typically only one per node). In 1948, Saphir and Amromin[59] reported that serial sectioning of the axillary nodes in 30 cases discovered metastases in 10 (33%) in which previous single-level sections had not shown metastases. This procedure, however, does not necessarily identify those node-negative patients who have a recurrence. In one study by Pickren,[60] of 51 patients reported to be node-negative cases by routine sectioning, 11 (22%) were positive on serial sectioning. The 5-year survival rate of these 11 patients was 91%. This was similar to that for patients without occult metastases on serial sectioning, and both were better than the 5-year survival rate of 53% for patients with metastases seen on routine sectioning. Similar results were found in studies by Fisher and coworkers[61] and by Wilkinson and associates.[62] In a more recent study, however, of 1,680 breast cancers reported to be node negative by routine sectioning, serial sectioning of axillary nodes revealed a single micrometastasis (defined as measuring 2 mm or less) in 120 cases (7%) and a single macrometastasis in 216 cases (13%).[63] With a median follow-up of 7 years, patients with either micrometastatic or macrometastatic involvement had a statistically significant worse disease-free and overall survival, although the magnitude of the differences was not large. In a multivariate analysis, the presence of macrometastatic involvement, but not micrometastatic involvement, remained in the final model for recurrence. Similar findings were seen in a study by the International (Ludwig) Breast Cancer Study Group.[64] These results indicate (a) that histologic involvement of axillary nodes can be detected by serial sectioning in 10% to 20% of cases judged to be node negative by routine sectioning; (b) that such involvement suggests a slightly worse prognosis compared with patients without involvement; and (c) that even in patients with negative nodes evaluated by serial sectioning, the 10-year recurrence rate is still 20% to 30%.

Attempts have been made to identify involvement in axillary nodes by the use of immunohistochemical techniques. Using a variety of monoclonal antibodies directed against epithelial cell antigens, a number of investigators[63,65–69] have reported detection of metastases in 10% to 20% of allegedly negative nodes. Similar to the findings with serial sectioning, the results using immunohistochemical staining indicate (a) that histologic involvement in axillary nodes can be detected in 10% to 30% of cases of invasive ductal carcinoma judged to be node negative by routine staining with hematoxylin and eosin[70]; (b) that such involvement suggests a slightly worse prognosis compared with patients without involvement; and (c) that even in patients with negative nodes evaluated by immunohistochemical staining, the 10-year recurrence rate is still 20% to 30%. This technique is still limited, however, by the sensitivity and specificity of currently available monoclonal antibodies, and its usefulness may change with the availability of better antibodies. It may also be possible to detect micrometastases by even more sensitive techniques of molecular biological examination.[71,72]

A related issue is the prognostic significance of minimal axillary involvement, variously called *micrometastases* (involvement of less than 2 mm) or *clandestine metastases* (involvement of small emboli of tumor cells in the sinuses of axillary nodes), detected by routine evaluation of axillary nodes. Information on this subject is available from two series with long follow-up. Investigators from Memorial Sloan-Kettering Cancer Center reported on 147 patients with T1 or T2 breast cancers and a single involved axillary lymph node followed for 10 years after treatment.[73] Overall, the 70 patients with micrometastases had fewer recurrences (24%) than did 77 patients with macrometastases (39%). In patients with T2 tumors and a micrometastasis, prognosis was similar to patients without involvement but worse than in patients with a macrometastasis. Friedman and others[74] from the Institut Gustave-Roussy compared the rate of distant metastases among 41 patients with one node involved with a clandestine metastasis, 205 patients with one node involved with a parenchymal metastasis, and 637 patients without nodal metastases (median follow-up time, 118 months). The authors found that clandestine and parenchymal involvement of a single lymph node had similar prognostic value and conferred a worse prognosis than negative node results (relative risk, 1.7). The results of these two studies are limited by small numbers, which is probably responsible for the inconsistencies seen.

Internal Mammary Node Involvement

The second major nodal site of involvement in carcinoma of the breast is the IMN chain, which lies at the anterior end of the intercostal spaces by the side of the internal thoracic artery. Because of their intrathoracic location and their uncommon clinical presentation, the frequency of IMN involvement was not appreciated as early as axillary node involvement. One of the first to document this second route of spread was Handley,[75] who reported his results of IMN biopsy in 1,000 patients in 1975 (Table 9). These results indicated (a) that, overall, axillary lymph node involvement is more likely to occur than IMN involvement (54% versus 22%); (b) that IMN involvement is more common when axillary nodes are involved than when uninvolved (35% versus

TABLE 9. *Internal mammary node involvement relative to location of the primary tumor and axillary node involvement*

	Location of primary tumor					
Axillary node status	UIQ	LIQ	Central	UOQ	LOQ	All
Negative	10/143 14%	2/36 6%	5/76 7%	7/170 4%	2/40 5%	8%
Positive	47/105 45%	18/25 72%	65/140 46%	47/212 22%	10/53 19%	35%
All	27%	33%	32%	14%	13%	22%

LIQ, lower internal quadrant; LOQ, lower outer quadrant; UIQ, upper internal quadrant; UOQ, upper outer quadrant.
From Handley R. Carcinoma of the breast. *Ann R Coll Surg Engl* 1975;57:59. With permission.

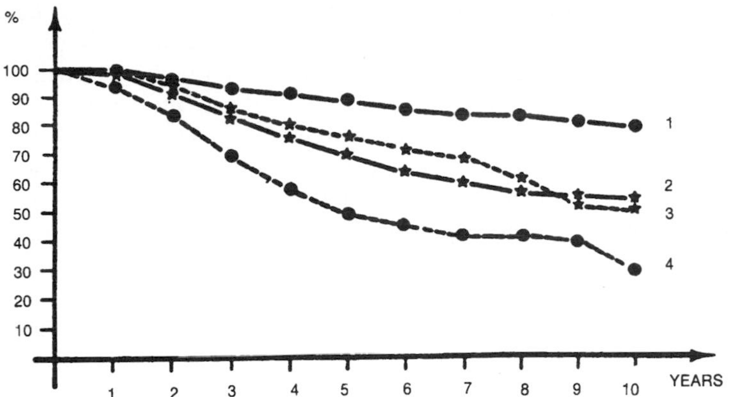

FIG. 6. Ten-year overall survival rates in patients without node metastases (1), with axillary node metastases only (2), with internal mammary node metastases only (3), and with both groups involved (4) ($p = 10^{-9}$). (From ref. 76, with permission.)

8%); and (c) that IMN involvement is more common for inner-quadrant or central primaries than for outer-quadrant primaries. Even in patients with inner or central tumors, however, axillary involvement was more common than IMN involvement (42% versus 28%). Furthermore, when axillary nodes were uninvolved, IMN involvement was uncommon, even with inner-quadrant or central tumors.

Veronesi and colleagues[76] have reported another large series of patients treated with IMN biopsy. In this series of 1,119 patients, axillary involvement was seen in 50% of patients, and IMN involvement was seen in 19%. They found that the likelihood of IMN involvement was related to axillary involvement (29% axillary node positive versus 9% node negative, $p < .01$), and to patient age (age 40 years or younger, 28%; age 41 to 50 years, 20%; older than 50 years of age, 16%; $p = .01$). Unlike the findings of Handley,[75] however, IMN involvement was not related to the location of the primary tumor in the breast (19% inner versus 18% outer). Veronesi and associates[76] found that axillary involvement, tumor size, and patient age all influence the likelihood of IMN involvement. For a patient younger than age 40 years with positive axillary node results and a primary tumor larger than 2 cm, the risk of IMN involvement was 44%. For a patient older than 50 years with negative axillary node results and a primary tumor smaller than 2 cm, the risk of IMN involvement was only 7%. In this study, the prognostic implication of IMN involvement was similar to that for axillary node involvement (Fig. 6). The 10-year disease-free survival rate was 73% when both axillary and IMNs tested negative, 47% when axillary nodes alone tested positive, 52% when IMNs alone tested positive, and 25% when both areas tested positive.

Other investigators have examined the relationship between tumor location and IMN involvement and, like Handley, have found that IMN involvement is more common for medial or central tumors. Haagensen[77] performed IMN biopsy in 1,007 patients and found IMN involvement in 29% of patients with medial tumors, compared with 17% of patients with lateral tumors. Patients with central tumors and positive axillary nodes had a 43% risk of IMN involvement. Similarly, LaCour and colleagues[78] studied a group of 703 patients and reported IMN involvement in 24% of patients with medial or central tumors and 16% of patients with lateral tumors.

Overall, roughly 50% of patients have axillary node involvement, and 20% of patients have IMN involvement. The most consistent finding in IMN involvement is its relation to axillary node involvement. When axillary nodes test negative, IMN involvement is uncommon (approximately 10%). When axillary nodes test positive, IMN involvement is approximately 30%. Furthermore, the greater the extent of axillary node involvement, the greater the likelihood of IMN involvement. The prognostic significance of IMN involvement is still apparent, however, even when adjusted for the extent of axillary node involvement.

Supraclavicular Lymph Node Involvement

Supraclavicular lymph node involvement is associated with extensive axillary node involvement. In one series of patients undergoing routine supraclavicular dissection, involvement of the supraclavicular region was found in 23 (18%) of 125 patients who had positive axillary nodes and in none of 149 patients whose axillary nodes did not test positive.[79] The significance of supraclavicular node involvement was first shown by Halsted,[80] who performed supraclavicular dissections in 119 patients: 44 patients were found to have involvement of these nodes, of whom only two were free of cancer at 5 years. Supraclavicular node involvement represents a late stage of axillary node involvement and carries a grave prognosis. Based on this, more recent staging systems categorize supraclavicular node involvement as M1 or distant metastatic.

THE INFLUENCE OF LOCAL TREATMENT ON SURVIVAL

The treatment of breast cancer has been directed both at the breast and regional lymph nodes and at sites of systemic metastases, but the importance of such treatment has been debated. It is useful to examine this debate from a historical perspective.[81] Perhaps no other disease or its treatment has evoked such strong feelings as breast cancer. The reasons for this can be found both in our culture in general and in medicine in particular. The breast, in certain contexts, is the symbol of motherhood, nourishment, and security, whereas in others it represents beauty and femininity. Equally compelling medical connotations have made supporters of certain therapeutic alternatives act like religious zealots.[82] Strongly held beliefs as well as the need for long-term follow-up have provided the ingredients for animated debate concerning the disease and its treatment.

In the middle of the nineteenth century, women with breast cancer typically were first seen by their physicians with locally advanced disease, not simply with an asymptomatic lump in the breast. No effective local therapy or any useful systemic anticancer treatment was available at that time. Attempts at surgical extirpation generally resulted in a prompt return of the disease locally. The futility of therapy only reinforced the nihilistic attitude of the population toward the advisability of prompt treatment for suspicious breast masses.

The introduction of the radical mastectomy by Meyer[83] and Halsted[84] at the end of the nineteenth century was an important therapeutic advance and provided the first important therapeutic paradigm for the disease. The use of radical mastectomy was based on a model of cancer spread that was centrifugal. According to this view, a tumor started locally, infiltrated by way of the lymphatics in a direct and contiguous fashion to the regional lymph nodes, and only then spread to distant sites. In its most doctrinaire presentation, espoused by Halsted,[84] even distant metastases occurred by contiguous extension. This notion of the disease provided a rational basis for a radical operation designed to resect widely the tumor and contiguous tissues, including the overlying skin, both of the underlying pectoral muscles, and all of the ipsilateral axillary lymph nodes. The rapid and widespread use of radical mastectomy was a result of the acceptance of this theory of disease spread and of improvements in surgical and anesthetic techniques that were required for the operation to be feasible.

The radical mastectomy was later expanded to extended radical and superradical operations, including dissections of the IMNs and supraclavicular lymph nodes. RT was advocated as a further regional treatment to augment surgery in certain cases. Although these techniques may have improved the results for some patients, physicians became frustrated by the frequent appearance of distant metastasis despite proper application of this comprehensive regional treatment. Laboratory studies performed on mastectomy specimens by Gray[85] demonstrated that lymphatics surrounding a primary tumor did not always show involvement, thereby weakening the concept of permeative spread of the disease. Such clinical and biologic observations suggested that, in many patients, metastases were present, but occult, at the time of a patient's initial presentation and were unaffected by local management.[86] This led to a new paradigm that hypothesized that there are two types of cancer: (a) one that remains local and rarely spreads and (b) one in which occult micrometastases are already present when the patient is first seen.[87] In either of these circumstances, local therapy does not alter outcome. If the patient is in the former group, only minimal local therapy is needed. For the patient who already has micrometastases at original diagnosis, local therapy has no effect on the distant metastases already present.

This new paradigm, taken to its logical conclusion, denies the existence of a circumstance in which effective treatment to the local and regional area is important to survival. It suggests that metastatic spread never occurs during the clinical phase of disease evolution. The acceptance of this paradigm leads to less aggressive local treatment. It encourages the development of methods to separate patients who already have occult metastases from those for whom breast cancer is a local condition. The pioneers of this new viewpoint were courageous surgeons who were anxious to move away from the mutilation of radical mastectomy and whose views were considered by many to be heresy.[87–89] Fisher[90] most clearly articulated the differences between these two views of breast cancer biology and provided strong support for the newer paradigm.

It is generally acknowledged that the Halstedian view of breast cancer does not apply to all patients. The simple observation that 20% to 30% of node-negative patients develop metastases demonstrates that lymph node involvement is not a necessary precedent to more distant spread and that blood-borne dissemination occurs in at least some patients. Proponents of the importance of local therapy have replaced the Halstedian model with a Spectrum model of breast cancer spread, in which the disease is not viewed as systemic at its inception in all patients and therefore early diagnosis and effective local-regional treatment can affect survival in some patients.[4,81] The basis of this hypothesis is that metastases occur as a function of tumor growth and progression. This Spectrum view, however, stresses the importance of both local and systemic therapy. The contrasting elements of the Halsted and Systemic views are presented along with those for the Spectrum paradigm in Table 10.

The most important piece of evidence supporting the Spectrum view of breast cancer spread is the information derived from the randomized clinical trials testing the value of screening mammography. If metastases occur at the inception of a breast cancer, earlier detection will not be effective in preventing metastases or decreasing breast cancer mortality. A number of screening trials have been performed and are reviewed in detail in Chapter 11. Overall, mammographic screening of asymptomatic women has been shown to result in a decrease in mortality from breast cancer of approximately 25%.[91–93] In the two-county Swedish trial,[92] the mean diameter of mammographically detected tumors was 1.4 cm and of clinically detected tumors, 2.2 cm. This is approximately a fourfold volume increase that is

TABLE 10. *Comparisons of the various models of breast cancer spread*

Halsted[84]	Systemic[90]	Spectrum[81]
Tumor spreads in an orderly manner based on mechanical considerations.	There is no orderly pattern of tumor cell dissemination.	In most patients, axillary nodal involvement precedes distant metastases.
The positive lymph node is an indicator of tumor spread and is the instigator of distant metastases.	The positive lymph node is an indicator of a host-tumor relationship that permits development of metastases, rather than the instigator of distant metastases.	The positive lymph node is an indicator of a host-tumor relationship that is correlated with the subsequent appearance of distant disease.
RLNs are barriers to passage of tumor cells.	RLNs are ineffective as barriers to tumor cell spread.	RLNs are ineffective as barriers to tumor spread, but involvement of RLNs is not always associated with distant metastases.
The bloodstream is of little significance as a route of tumor dissemination.	The bloodstream is of considerable importance in tumor dissemination.	The bloodstream is of considerable importance in tumor dissemination.
Operable breast cancer is a local-regional disease.	Operable breast cancer is a systemic disease.	Operable breast cancer is a systemic disease in many but not all cases.
The extent and nuances of the operations are the dominant factors influencing a patient's outcome.	Variations in local-regional therapy are unlikely to affect survival.	Variations in local-regional therapy are unlikely to have a major influence on survival but are of significance in some patients.

RLNs, regional lymph nodes.

associated with a 30% reduction in breast cancer deaths. This observation provides compelling evidence that breast cancer can metastasize during its clinical evolution.

A second, but less direct, support for the Spectrum view comes from clinical studies that demonstrate that, as tumor size increases, the likelihood of metastases increases. As presented earlier in this chapter, the likelihood of metastasis increases with a sigmoid distribution when plotted against the logarithm of tumor volume.[35,94]

A third prima facie argument supporting the Spectrum paradigm is that 30% of the long-term survivors of radical mastectomy have had positive nodes. Because regional treatment was sufficient, some tumors have the capacity for lymph node spread but have not acquired facility in metastasizing distantly.[12,50] This is particularly true for small tumors measuring 2 cm or less, even when a limited number of axillary lymph nodes are involved.[4] Given the general level of awareness about breast cancer in the population and the widespread use of screening mammography, patients increasingly are being diagnosed with early-stage breast cancers.

Another important point in evaluating these views of breast cancer spread is to determine whether variations in local-regional treatment affect outcome. If variations in local-regional treatment do not affect survival, then the case for breast cancer as a systemic disease is strengthened. The trials testing variations in local and regional treatment are discussed in Chapter 37. The ideal trial to evaluate these competing views is one that is properly conducted and accrues a large number of patients (approximately 1,000 in each arm), with early-stage breast cancer randomly assigned to receive either effective local-regional treatment or to receive no or highly ineffective local-regional treatment without an opportunity for salvage treatment in the event of a local-regional failure. Such a trial would rightly be viewed as unethical. Virtually all available studies compare treatments with similar levels of effectiveness in obtaining local-regional control, allow for salvage, or have insufficient numbers of patients to eliminate small differences. As a result, these trials are inconclusive and have been used by advocates of both views as evidence in their favor.

The NSABP B-0488 and B-0689 trials are two of the major studies on the importance of local-regional treatment. The B-04 trial tested the value of axillary treatment. A total of 1,159 breast cancer patients with clinically negative axillary nodes were randomly assigned to receive (a) radical mastectomy, (b) total mastectomy and RT to the axilla and other draining lymph nodes (TMR), or (c) total mastectomy alone, without any axillary treatment. The 10-year results of this trial do not show a statistically significant survival advantage for any of the treatment arms. This study does provide a clear comparison of effective axillary treatment to no axillary treatment (axillary recurrence rates were <5% for radical mastectomy and TMR). The trial, however, allowed for salvage, and by 10 years, 18% of the total mastectomy group developed recurrence in the axilla and underwent delayed axillary dissection. There were also difficulties in the conduct of the trial, such that 35% of the patients assigned to total mastectomy, in fact, had a limited axillary dissection.[95] Also, it must be asked whether enough patients were included in the study to eliminate the possibility that axillary treatment has a small effect on survival.[96] It is possible to estimate the possible benefit of axillary treatment, given the data presented in this chapter. Some 360 patients were assigned to each treatment arm, and axillary metastases were found in 38.6% of patients undergoing radical mastectomy. Because the value of axillary treatment is restricted to patients who have positive nodes, the critical population would be the 137 patients (38.6% of 360) presumed to have positive axillary nodes. Axillary treatment is also not of value in patients who have occult disease at the time of presentation. Overall, approximately one-third of patients with positive axillary nodes are estimated to be free of occult distant disease. Therefore, the critical population is further restricted to the 48 patients (one-third of 137) who have positive nodes and no occult distant spread, and could therefore possibly benefit from axillary treatment. In addition, one must consider the salvage potential of delayed axillary treatment. If one estimates that one-third of patients initially treated by total mastectomy alone, who subsequently develop axillary adenopathy, are curable, then delayed axillary dissection is effective in an additional 16 patients. This leaves 32 patients who could possibly have benefited from initial axillary treatment, or 9% of the total group. To have a 90% chance of detecting a 9% difference between two treatment arms in a clinical trial at a statistically significant level of $p = .05$, approximately 1,000 patients would be required. This analysis suggests that the results obtained in the NSABP B-04 trial do not prove that axillary treatment is of no value, but rather that the benefit, if present, must be small. The most recent report of this trial indicates a 10-year survival rate of 58% for the radical mastectomy group and 59% for the TMR group, compared with 54% for the total mastectomy group, yielding a difference of 4% to 5%, which was not statistically significant.[97] This degree of benefit is roughly equivalent to a 10% reduction in mortality for axillary treatment. If this degree of benefit were shown to be valid and were applied to the general population of breast cancer patients, the absolute number of patients who benefit would be large. The case for effective axillary treatment is also supported by the results of the Guy's Hospital trial, in which inadequate axillary treatment was associated with an increased rate of metastases and a decreased survival (see Chapter 37).

Similar considerations apply to effective control of the primary tumor, as analyzed in the NSABP B-06 trial.[98,99] In this trial, 1,843 evaluable patients with early-stage breast cancer were randomly assigned to undergo total mastectomy, lumpectomy, or lumpectomy and RT. All patients underwent axillary dissection. The trial demonstrated a clear difference in control of the primary tumor [recurrence in the breast was 39% for the lumpectomy group and 10% for the lumpectomy and RT group ($p <.001$)], but no statistically significant difference in survival was observed. It is similarly possible to estimate the potential effect on survival by maximizing local tumor control. In approximately 60% of patients treated by lumpectomy, the use of RT is not of value because no residual disease is present in the breast. In addition, approximately one-third of patients who have a recurrence in the breast are estimated to have had occult metastases at presentation and thus were incurable by local treatment from the onset. Also, one would anticipate that approximately 50% of the patients would be cured by mastectomy performed at the time of local recurrence. Given these estimates, the possible adverse effect on survival of the ineffective local tumor control would be only 5%. The 8-year results of the B-06 trial, in fact, show a 5.3% difference in survival among node-negative patients in favor of lumpectomy plus RT compared with lumpectomy alone, but this was not statistically significant. In reporting the 12-year results, the authors state, "Significantly or nearly significantly higher percentages of patients with node-negative cancer treated by total mastectomy or lumpectomy and breast irradiation remained free of disease and free of distant disease than of patients with node-negative cancer treated by lumpectomy."[99]

Evidence to support the view that persistent tumor in the breast or lymph nodes can be the cause of distant metastases is reported by Fortin et al.,[100] who studied the hazard rate for distant metastases in patients treated with lumpectomy and radiation. The hazard rate was higher in those with local failure, with the major increase between 4 and 8 years, a time when the hazard rate in those patients locally controlled was decreasing. The source of these metastases is suggested to be persistent local disease.

The acceptance of the use of adjuvant systemic therapy for all but the earliest-stage disease has posed new natural history questions. What are the consequences of the limited effectiveness of adjuvant chemotherapy on distant metastases and survival? Can these be modified by postmastectomy RT? Overgaard et al.[101,102] and Ragaz et al.,[103] performing randomized trials, both found a decrease in local recurrences in irradiated patients, with an associated decrease in metastases and an improvement in survival. Thus, the natural history of breast cancer is altered by chemotherapy by primarily affecting distant metastasis likelihood. In these circumstances, persistent regional disease becomes a source of new metastases.[104]

DISTANT METASTASES

Metastases from carcinoma of the breast can be seen in a variety of organs. The likelihood of organ involvement has been studied in a number of autopsy series[77,105,106] (Table 11). The most common sites of metastatic spread are bone, lung, and liver.

The time course to the appearance of clinically detected distant metastases can be extremely long. It is common for metastases to become manifest 10 years or more after initial diagnosis. Koscielny and colleagues[35] showed that the time course to distant metastases is influenced by the size of the primary tumor (Fig. 7). For patients with the smallest tumors (1.0 to 2.5 cm), the time course to the appearance of distant disease was the greatest. The cumulative proportion of patients with metastases reached one-half its ultimate value (median delay or median interval) 42 months after initial treatment. In contrast, the median interval was only 4

TABLE 11. *Sites of metastases from breast cancer in three collected series*

Organ	160 Cases[105] (%)	43 Cases[106] (%)	100 Cases[77] (%)
Lung	59	65	69
Liver	58	56	65
Bone	44	—	71
Pleura	37	23	51
Adrenal glands	31	41	49
Kidneys	—	14	17
Spleen	14	23	17
Pancreas	—	11	17
Ovaries	9	16	20
Brain	—	9	22
Thyroid	—	—	24
Heart	—	—	11
Diaphragm	—	—	11
Pericardium	—	21	19
Intestine	—	—	18
Peritoneum	12	9	13
Uterus	—	—	15
Skin	39	7	30

months for patients with tumors 8.5 cm or larger. The median interval between diagnosis and detection of first distant metastasis was 69 months for patients with axillary node–negative disease, 43 months when one to three axillary nodes were positive for metastasis, and 30 months when four or more axillary nodes were positive. Similarly, the median interval was 65 months for patients with histologic grade I tumors, 44 months for grade II tumors, and 21 months for grade III tumors. This inverse relation between initial stage and time to the appearance of distant metastases is also reflected in mortality statistics, as seen in the Edinburgh study[107] and in the study from the End Results Program of the NCI.[108] The risk of distant metastases was

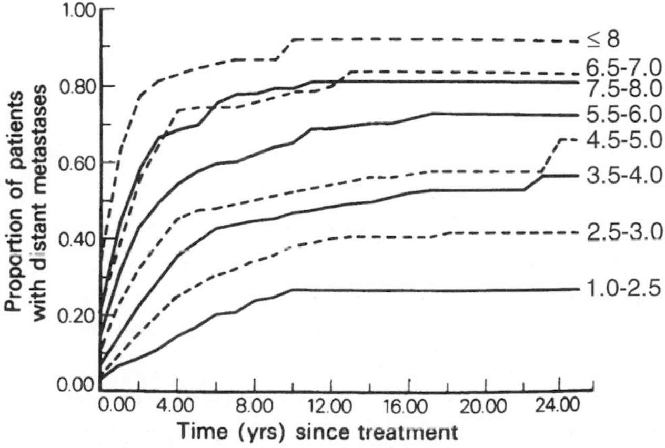

FIG. 7. The cumulated proportions of patients with metastases as a function of the time after treatment in the different groups of patients defined by the clinical size of the tumor in centimeters. (From ref. 35, with permission.)

studied using the University of Chicago Series 6. The likelihood of metastases increased with lymph node involvement, and these metastases were seen sooner. T1, N0 breast cancer had a 20% metastatic frequency, but less than one-half of these were seen before 5 years, whereas large tumors with involved nodes had an 89% likelihood of metastases, with three-fourths of these seen within 5 years.

CONCLUSION

The data presented in this chapter demonstrate that breast cancer is a heterogeneous disease that has a propensity for systemic involvement and commonly has a long natural history. Because of this long natural history and its onset typically at middle age, it is difficult to demonstrate, in a strict sense, that breast cancer is a curable disease. It is clear, however, that a considerable percentage of patients with treated breast cancer (particularly when detected at an early stage) live their lives without further evidence of the disease.

The axilla is the principal site of regional node involvement, and the likelihood of axillary involvement is directly related to tumor size. Both tumor size and the presence and extent of axillary involvement are highly associated with survival. The proper view of breast cancer spread remains controversial. Although some have argued that all breast cancer is a systemic disease at its inception, implying that local treatment does not influence survival, the paradigm most consistent with the clinical evidence is that breast cancer comprises a heterogeneous spectrum of malignant capacities resulting from tumor progression. Thus, on average, large tumors are more likely to have metastasized, but for any size there are some that have not acquired that facility.

REFERENCES

1. Bloom H, Richardson W, Harrier E. Natural history of untreated breast cancer (1805–1933). *BMJ* 1962;2:213.
2. Fox M. On the diagnosis and treatment of breast cancer. *JAMA* 1979; 241:489.
3. Harris J, Hellman S. Observations on survival curve analysis with particular reference to breast cancer treatment. *Cancer* 1986;57:925.
4. Hellman S. The natural history of small breast cancers. David A. Karnofsky memorial lecture. *J Clin Oncol* 1994;12:2229.
5. Quiet CA, Ferguson DJ, Weichselbaum RR, et al. Natural history of node-negative breast cancer: a study of 826 patients with long term follow up. *J Clin Oncol* 1995;13:1144.
6. Quiet CA, Ferguson DJ, Weichselbaum RR, et al. Natural history of node-positive breast cancer: the curability of small cancers with a limited number of positive nodes. *J Clin Oncol* 1996;14:3105.
7. Haybittle J. The evidence for cure in female breast cancer. *Comment Res Breast Dis* 1983;3:181.
8. Brinkley D, Haybittle J. Long-term survival of women with breast cancer. *Lancet* 1984;1:1118.
9. Hibberd A, Harwood L, Well J. Long-term prognosis of women with breast cancer in New Zealand: study of survival to 30 years. *BMJ* 1983;286:1777.
10. Rutqvist L, Wallgren A. Long-term survival of 458 young breast cancer patients. *Cancer* 1985;55:658.
11. Joensuu H, Toikkanen S. Cured of breast cancer? *J Clin Oncol* 1995;13:62.

12. Adair F, Berg J, Joubert L. Long term follow-up of breast cancer patients: the thirty-year report. *Cancer* 1974;33:1145.
13. Rosen P, Groshen S, Siago P, et al. A long-term follow-up study of survival in stage I (T1N0M0) and stage II (T1N1M0) breast carcinoma. *J Clin Oncol* 1989;7:355.
14. Heimann R, Hellman S. The clinical progression of breast cancer malignant behavior: what to expect and when to expect it. (*in press*)
15. Collins V, Loeffler R, Tivey H. Observations on growth rates of human tumors. *AJR Am J Roentgenol* 1956;76:988.
16. Gershon Cohen J, Berger S, Klickstein H. Roentgenography of breast cancer moderating concept of "biological predeterminism." *Cancer* 1963;16:961.
17. Fournier D, Weber E, Hoeffken W, et al. Growth rate of 147 mammary carcinomas. *Cancer* 1980;45:2198.
18. Kusama S, Spratt J, Donegan W, et al. The gross rates of growth of human mammary carcinoma. *Cancer* 1972;30:594.
19. Pearlman A. Breast cancer: influence of growth rate on prognosis and treatment evaluation. *Cancer* 1976;38:1826.
20. Laird A. Dynamics of growth in tumors and in normal organisms. *J Natl Cancer Inst Monogr* 1969;30:15.
21. Skipper H, Schnabel F Jr, Lloyd H. Dose-response and tumor cell repopulation rate in chemotherapeutic trials. *Adv Cancer Chemother* 1979;1:205.
22. Walter S, Day N. Estimation of the duration of a preclinical disease state using screening data. *Am J Epidemiol* 1983;118:865.
23. Zelen M, Feinleib M. On the theory of screening for chronic diseases. *Biometrika* 1969;56:601.
24. Shapiro S, Goldbert J, Hutchinson G. Lead time in breast cancer detection and implications for periodicity of screening. *Am J Epidemiol* 1974;100:357.
25. Norton L. A Gompertzian model of human breast cancer growth. *Cancer Res* 1988;48:7067.
26. Tubiana M, Malaise E. Growth rate and cell kinetics in human tumors. In: Symington T, Carter RL, eds. *On scientific functions of oncology*. Chicago: Year Book, 1976:126.
27. Hellman S. Darwin's clinical relevance. *Cancer* 1997;79:2275.
28. Nowell P. The clonal evolution of tumor cell populations. *Science* 1976;194:23.
29. Speer J, Petrosky V, Retsky M, et al. A stochastic numerical model of breast cancer growth that simulates clinical data. *Cancer Res* 1984;44:4124.
30. Demicheli R, Retsky M, Schwartzenbruber D, et al. Proposal for a new model of breast cancer metastatic development. *Ann Oncol* 1997;8:1075.
31. Holland R, Veling S, Mravunac M, et al. Histologic multifocality of Tis, T1-2 breast carcinomas. *Cancer* 1985;56:979.
32. Spratt J, Donegan W. *Cancer of the breast*. Philadelphia: WB Saunders, 1971:133.
33. Nemoto T, Natarajan N, Bedwani R, et al. Breast cancer in the medial half: results of the 1978 national survey of the American College of Surgeons. *Cancer* 1983;51:1333.
34. Fisher B, Slack N, Ausman R, et al. Location of breast carcinoma and prognosis. *Surg Gynecol Obstet* 1969;129:705.
35. Koscielny S, Tubiana M, Le M, et al. Breast cancer: relationship between the size of the primary tumor and the probability of metastatic dissemination. *Br J Cancer* 1984;49:709.
36. Koscielny S, Le M, Tubiana M. The natural history of human breast cancer: the relationship between involvement of axillary lymph nodes and the initiation of distant metastases. *Br J Cancer* 1989;59:775.
37. Schottenfeld D, Nash A, Robbins G, et al. Ten-year results of the treatment of primary operable breast carcinoma. *Cancer* 1976;38:1001.
38. Nemoto T, Vana J, Bedwani R, et al. Management and survival of female breast cancer: results of a national survey by the American College of Surgeons. *Cancer* 1980;45:2917.
39. Fisher B, Slack N, Bross I, et al. Cancer of the breast: size of neoplasm and prognosis. *Cancer* 1969;24:1071.
40. Haagensen C. *Diseases of the breast*, 3rd ed. Philadelphia: WB Saunders, 1986:656.
41. Carter C, Allen C, Henson D. Relation of tumor size, lymph node status, and survival in 24,740 breast cancer cases. *Cancer* 1989;63:181.
42. Smith J, Gamez-Araujo J, Gallager H, et al. Carcinoma of the breast: analysis of total lymph node involvement versus level of metastasis. *Cancer* 1977;39:527.
43. Butcher H. Radical mastectomy for mammary carcinoma. *Ann Surg* 1969;170:833.
44. Bucalossi P, Veronesi U, Zingo L, et al. Enlarged mastectomy for breast cancer: review of 1213 cases. *Am J Roentgenol Radium Ther Nucl Med* 1971;111:119.
45. Valagussa P, Bonadonna G, Veronesi V. Patterns of relapse and survival following radical mastectomy. *Cancer* 1978;41:1170.
46. Haagensen C. Treatment of curable carcinoma of the breast. *Int J Radiat Oncol Biol Phys* 1977;2:975.
47. Fisher B, Slack N, Katrych D, et al. Ten-year followup results of patients with carcinoma of the breast in a cooperative clinical trial evaluating surgical adjuvant chemotherapy. *Surg Gynecol Obstet* 1975;140:528.
48. Spratt J, Donegan W. *Carcinoma of the breast*. Philadelphia: WB Saunders, 1971.
49. Payne W, Taylor W, Khonsari S, et al. Surgical treatment of breast cancer: trends and factors affecting survival. *Arch Surg* 1970;101:105.
50. Ferguson D, Meier P, Karrison T, et al. Staging of breast cancer and survival rates: an assessment based on 50 years of experience with radical mastectomy. *JAMA* 1982;248:1337.
51. Haagensen C. *Diseases of the breast*, 3rd ed. Philadelphia: WB Saunders, 1986:663.
52. Veronesi U, Rilke F, Luini A, et al. Distribution of axillary node metastases by level of invasion: an analysis of 539 cases. *Cancer* 1987;59:682.
53. Rosen P, Martin L, Kinne D, et al. Discontinuous or "skip" metastases in breast carcinoma: analysis of 1228 axillary dissections. *Ann Surg* 1983;197:276.
54. Pigott J, Nicols R, Maddox W, et al. Metastases to the upper levels of the axillary nodes in carcinoma of the breast and its implications for nodal sampling procedures. *Surg Gynecol Obstet* 1984;158:255.
55. Boova R, Bonanni R, Rosato F. Patterns of axillary nodal involvement in breast cancer: predictability of level one dissection. *Ann Surg* 1982;196:642.
56. Danforth DJ, Findlay P, McDonald H, et al. Complete axillary lymph node dissection for stage I–II carcinoma of the breast. *J Clin Oncol* 1986;4:655.
57. Schwartz G, D'Ugo D, Rosenberg A. Extent of axillary dissection preceding irradiation for carcinoma of the breast. *Arch Surg* 1986;121:1395.
58. Haagensen C. *Diseases of the breast*, 3rd ed. Philadelphia: WB Saunders, 1986:656.
59. Saphir O, Amromin G. Obscure axillary lymph metastasis in carcinoma of the breast. *Cancer* 1948;1:238.
60. Pickren J. Significance of occult metastases. *Cancer* 1961;14:1266.
61. Fisher E, Swamidoss S, Lee C, et al. Detection and significance of occult axillary node metastases in patients with invasive breast cancer. *Cancer* 1978;42:2025.
62. Wilkinson EJ, Hause LL, Kuzma JF, et al. Occult axillary lymph node metastasis in patients with invasive breast cancer. *Lab Invest* 1984;44,83(abstr).
63. de Mascarel I, Bonichon F, Coindre J, et al. Prognostic significance of breast cancer axillary lymph node micrometastases assessed by two special techniques: reevaluation with longer follow-up. *Br J Cancer* 1992;66:523.
64. International (Ludwig) Breast Cancer Study Group. Prognostic importance of occult axillary lymph node micrometastases from breast cancers. *Lancet* 1990;335:1565.
65. Trojani M, de Mascarel I, Bonichon F, et al. Micrometastases to axillary lymph nodes from carcinoma of breast: detection by immunohistochemistry and prognostic significance. *Br J Cancer* 1983;55:303.
66. Wells C, Heryet A, Brochier J, et al. The immunocytochemical detection of axillary micrometastases in breast cancer. *Br J Cancer* 1984;50:193.
67. Elson C, Kuf D, Scholm J, et al. Detection of occult foci of metastatic breast carcinoma in axillary lymph nodes using monoclonal antibodies B72.3 and DF3. *Lab Invest* 1988;58:27(abst).
68. Sedmak D, Meineke T, Knechtges D, et al. Prognostic significance of cytokeratin-positive breast cancer metastases. *Mod Pathol* 1989;3:516.
69. Nasser I, Lee A, Bosari S, et al. Occult axillary lymph node metastases in "node-negative" breast carcinoma. *Hum Pathol* 1993;24:950.
70. McGucken M, Cummings M, Walsh M, et al. Occult axillary node metastases in breast cancer: their detection and prognostic significance. *Br J Cancer* 1996;73:88.

71. Noguchi S, Aihara T, Nakamori S, et al. The detection of breast cancer micrometastases in axillary lymph nodes by means of reverse transcriptase—polymerase chain reaction. *Cancer* 1994;74:1595.
72. Schoenfeld A, Luqmani Y, Smith D, et al. Detection of breast cancer micrometastases in axillary lymph nodes by using polymerase chain reaction. *Cancer Res* 1994;54:2986.
73. Rosen P, Saigo P, Braun D, et al. Axillary micro- and macro-metastases in breast cancer: prognostic significance of tumor size. *Ann Surg* 1981;194:585.
74. Friedman S, Bertin F, Mouriesse H, et al. Importance of tumor cells in axillary node sinus margins ("clandestine" metastases) discovered by serial sectioning in operable breast cancer. *Acta Oncol* 1988;27:483.
75. Handley R. Carcinoma of the breast. *Ann R Coll Surg Engl* 1975;57:59.
76. Veronesi U, Cascinelli N, Greco M, et al. Prognosis of breast cancer patients after mastectomy and dissection of internal mammary nodes. *Ann Surg* 1985;202:702.
77. Haagensen C. *Diseases of the breast*, 3rd ed. Philadelphia, WB Saunders, 1986:686.
78. LaCour J, Le M, Caceres E, et al. Radical mastectomy versus radical mastectomy plus internal mammary dissection. *Cancer* 1983; 51:1941.
79. Dahl Iversen E. Recherches sur les metastases microscopiques des cancers du sein dans les ganglions lymphatiques parasternaux et sus-claviculaires. *Mem Acad Clin* 1952;78:651.
80. Halsted W. The results of radical operations for the cure of cancer of the breast. *Ann Surg* 1907;46:1.
81. Hellman S, Harris J. The appropriate breast carcinoma paradigm. *Cancer Res* 1987;2:339.
82. Hellman, S. Dogma and inquisition in medicine: breast cancer as a case study. *Cancer* 1993;71:2430.
83. Meyer W. An improved method of the radical operation for carcinoma of the breast. *Med Rec* 1894;46:746.
84. Halsted W. The results of operations for the cure of cancer of the breast performed at the Johns Hopkins Hospital from June 1889 to January 1894. *Johns Hopkins Hosp Bull* 1895;4:297.
85. Gray J. The relation of lymphatic vessels to the spread of cancer. *Br J Surg* 1939;26:462.
86. Park W, Lee V. The absolute curability of cancer of the breast. *Surg Gynecol Obstet* 1951;93:129.
87. Fisher B. Breast cancer management: alternatives to radical mastectomy. *N Engl J Med* 1979;301:326.
88. Crile GJ. *A biological consideration of the treatment of breast cancer*. Springfield, IL: Charles C Thomas, 1967.
89. Keynes G. Carcinoma of the breast, the unorthodox view. *Proc Cardiff Med Soc* 1953–1954:40.
90. Fisher B. A commentary on the role of the surgeon in primary breast cancer. *Breast Cancer Res Treat* 1981;1:17.
91. Shapiro S. Determining the efficacy of breast cancer screening. *Cancer* 1989;63:1873.
92. Tabar L, Fagerberg C, Duffy S, et al. Update of the Swedish two-county program of mammographic screening for breast cancer. *Radiol Clin North Am* 1992;30:187.
93. Wald N, Frost C, Cuckle H. Breast cancer screening: the current position. *BMJ* 1991;302:845.
94. Tubiana M, Koscielny S. Natural history of human breast cancer: recent data and clinical implications. *Breast Cancer Res Treat* 1991;18:125.
95. Fisher B, Wolmark N, Bauer M, et al. The accuracy of clinical nodal staging and of limited axillary dissection as a determinant of histologic nodal status in carcinoma of the breast. *Surg Gynecol Obstet* 1981;152:765.
96. Harris J, Osteen R. Patients with early breast cancer benefit from effective axillary treatment. *Breast Cancer Res Treat* 1985;5:17.
97. Fisher B, Redmond C, Fisher E, et al. Ten-year results of a randomized clinical trial comparing radical mastectomy and total mastectomy with or without radiation. *N Engl J Med* 1985;312:674.
98. Fisher B, Redmond C, Poisson R, et al. Eight-year results of a randomized clinical trial comparing total mastectomy and lumpectomy with or without irradiation in the treatment of breast cancer. *N Engl J Med* 1989;320:822.
99. Fisher B, Anderson S, Redmond C, et al. Reanalysis and results after 12 years of follow-up in a randomized clinical trial comparing total mastectomy with lumpectomy with or without irradiation in the treatment of breast cancer. *N Engl J Med* 1995;333:1456.
100. Fortin A, Larochelle M, Laverdiere J, et al. Local failure is responsible for the decrease in survival for patients with breast cancer treated with conservative surgery and postoperative radiotherapy. *J Clin Oncol* 1999;17:101.
101. Overgaard M, Hanson PS, Overgaard J, et al. Postoperative radiotherapy in high risk premenopausal women with breast cancer who receive adjuvant chemotherapy. *N Engl J Med* 1997;337:949.
102. Overgaard M, Jensen M-B, Overgaard J, et al. Randomized controlled trial evaluating postoperative radiotherapy in high-risk postmenopausal breast cancer patients given tamoxifen: report from the Danish Breast Cancer Cooperative Group DBCG 82c trial. *Lancet* 1999 (*in press*).
103. Ragaz J, Jackson SM, Le N, et al. Adjuvant radiotherapy and chemotherapy in node-positive premenopausal women with breast cancer. *N Engl J Med* 1997;337:956.
104. Hellman S. Stopping metastases at their source. *N Engl J Med* 1997;337:996.
105. Warren S, Witham E. Studies on tumor metastases: the distribution of metastases in cancer of the breast. *Surg Gynecol Obstet* 1933;57:81.
106. Saphir O, Parker M. Metastases of primary carcinoma of the breast with special reference to spleen, adrenal glands and ovaries. *Arch Surg* 1941;42:1003.
107. Langlands A, Pocock S, Kerr G, et al. Long-term survival of patients with breast cancer: a study of the curability of the disease. *BMJ* 1979;2:1247.
108. Hankey B, Steinhorn S. Long-term patient survival for some of the more frequently occurring cancers. *Cancer* 1982;50:1904.

VIII

Diseases of the Breast, 2nd ed.,
edited by Jay R. Harris.
Lippincott Williams & Wilkins, Philadelphia © 2000.

Pathology and Biological Markers of Invasive Breast Cancer

CHAPTER 30

Pathology of Invasive Breast Cancer

Stuart J. Schnitt and Anthony J. Guidi

Invasive breast cancers constitute a heterogeneous group of lesions that differ with regard to their clinical presentation, radiographic characteristics, pathologic features, and biological potential. Despite these differences, however, these tumors have in common infiltration of neoplastic cells into the breast stroma and at least the potential for invasion of surrounding structures and distant metastasis. The most widely used classification of invasive breast cancers, and the one used in this chapter (with minor modifications), is that of the World Health Organization.[1] This classification scheme is based on the growth pattern and cytologic features of the invasive tumor cells and does not imply histogenesis or site of origin within the mammary duct system. For example, although the classification system recognizes invasive carcinomas designated *ductal* and *lobular*, this categorization is not meant to indicate that the former originates in extralobular ducts and the latter in lobules. In fact, subgross whole-organ sectioning has demonstrated that most invasive breast cancers arise in the terminal duct lobular unit, regardless of histologic type.[2]

The most common histologic type of invasive breast cancer by far is invasive (infiltrating) ductal carcinoma.[3–6] In fact, the diagnosis of invasive ductal carcinoma is a diagnosis by default, because this tumor type is defined as a type of cancer "not classified into any of the other categories of invasive mammary carcinoma."[1] To further emphasize this point, and to distinguish these tumors from invasive breast cancers with specific or special histologic features (e.g., invasive lobular, tubular, mucinous, medullary, and other rare types), some authorities prefer the term *infiltrating ductal carcinoma, not otherwise specified* (*NOS*)[3] or *infiltrating carcinoma of no special type* (*NST*).[5] In this chapter, the terms *invasive ductal carcinoma, infiltrating ductal carcinoma*, and *infiltrating or invasive carcinoma of no special type* are used interchangeably.

The distribution of histologic types of invasive breast cancer has varied among published series (Table 1). These differences may be related to a number of factors, including

S. J. Schnitt: Department of Pathology, Harvard Medical School, Brigham and Women's Hospital, Dana-Farber Cancer Institute, Boston, Massachusetts; Department of Surgical Pathology, Beth Israel Deaconess Medical Center, Boston, Massachusetts

A. J. Guidi: Department of Pathology, North Shore Medical Center, Salem, Massachusetts

TABLE 1. *Histologic types of invasive breast cancer in four large series before the widespread use of mammographic screening*

Study	No. of cancers	Histologic type (%)							
		Ductal[a]	Lobular	Medullary	Mucinous	Tubular	Tubular mixed	Mixed	Other
Fisher et al.[3]	1,000	53	5	6	2	1	—	32	—
Rosen[4]	857	75	10	9	2	2	—	—	—
Ellis et al.[6]	1,547	49	16	3	1	2	14	14	2
Edinburgh[5]	Not stated	70	10	5	2	3	—	2	8

[a]In some series, designated "not otherwise specified" (NOS) or "no special type" (NST).

the nature of the patient population and variability in the definitions for the different histologic types. In general, special-type cancers comprise 20% to 30% of invasive carcinomas, and at least 90% of a tumor should demonstrate the defining histologic characteristics of a special-type cancer for the tumor to be designated as that histologic type.[5,6]

The widespread use of screening mammography has had a dramatic impact on the nature of invasive breast cancers encountered in clinical practice.[7] The value of mammography in detecting more cases of ductal carcinoma *in situ* (DCIS), smaller invasive breast cancers, and fewer cancers with axillary lymph node involvement is well recognized. Mammography, however, has also resulted in a change in the distribution of the histologic features of the invasive breast cancers detected. In particular, special-type cancers (especially tubular carcinomas)[8–12] and cancers of lower histologic grade[13–15] have been more frequently observed in mammographically screened populations than in patients who present with a palpable mass, particularly in the prevalent round of screening.[16,17]

Most invasive breast cancers have an associated component of *in situ* carcinoma, although the extent of the *in situ* component varies considerably.[18] The prevailing view has long been that the invasive carcinomas derive from the *in situ* component. This view is based not only on the frequent coexistence of the two lesions, but also on the histologic similarities between the invasive and *in situ* components within the same lesion. For example, a number of studies have clearly documented that low-grade invasive cancers are most often associated with low-grade DCIS, and high-grade invasive cancers with high-grade *in situ* lesions.[19–21] In addition, studies evaluating profiles of biological markers and genetic abnormalities have shown that coexisting invasive and *in situ* carcinomas often share the same immunophenotype and genetic alterations.[22–24]

The routine pathologic examination of invasive breast cancers has now extended beyond simply determining and reporting the histologic type of the tumor. Although histologic typing provides important prognostic information in and of itself,[25] other morphologic features that are evaluable on routine histologic sections are also of prognostic value. In this chapter, the various histologic types of invasive breast cancer are discussed, as are pathologic features important in the assessment of prognosis (prognostic factors) and, possibly, response to therapy (predictive factors).

INVASIVE (INFILTRATING) DUCTAL CARCINOMA

As noted, invasive ductal carcinomas represent the single largest group of invasive breast cancers. Although these tumors are most commonly encountered in pure form, a substantial minority exhibit admixed foci of other histologic types. In one series examining 1,000 invasive breast cancers, such combinations of invasive ductal carcinoma and other types were seen in 28% of cases.[3] The classification of tumors composed primarily of invasive ductal carcinoma with a minor component consisting of one or more other histologic types is problematic. Some authorities categorize such lesions as invasive ductal carcinomas (or invasive carcinomas of no special type) and simply note the presence of the other types,[5] whereas others classify them as "mixed."[6]

Clinical Presentation

Invasive ductal carcinomas most often present as a palpable mass or mammographic abnormality. No specific clinical or mammographic characteristics distinguish invasive ductal carcinomas from other histologic types of invasive cancer. Rarely, patients with these lesions present with Paget's disease of the nipple.

Gross Pathology

The classic macroscopic appearance of invasive ductal carcinoma is that of a scirrhous carcinoma, characterized by a firm, sometimes rock-hard mass that has a grey-white, gritty surface on cut section (Fig. 1). This consistency and appearance are due to the desmoplastic tumor stroma and not to the neoplastic cells themselves. Some invasive ductal carcinomas are composed primarily of tumor cells with little desmoplastic stromal reaction, and such lesions are tan and soft on gross examination. Although most invasive ductal cancers have a stellate or spiculated contour with irregular peripheral mar-

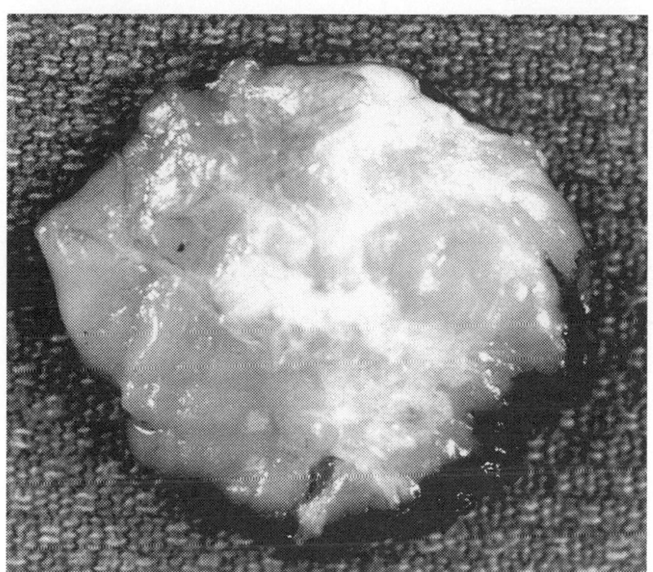

FIG. 1. Cut surface of an excision specimen containing an invasive ductal carcinoma. The tumor appears as an irregular area of whitish tissue.

gins, some lesions have rounded, pushing margins, and still others are grossly well circumscribed.

Histopathology

The microscopic appearance of invasive ductal carcinomas is highly heterogeneous with regard to growth pattern, cytologic features, mitotic activity, stromal desmoplasia, extent of the associated DCIS component, and contour. Variability in histologic features may even be seen within a single case. The tumor cells may be arranged as glandular structures; as nests, cords, or trabeculae of various sizes; or as solid sheets. Foci of necrosis are evident in some cases and may be extensive. Cytologically, the tumor cells range from those showing little deviation from normal breast epithelial cells to those exhibiting marked cellular pleomorphism and nuclear atypia. Mitotic activity can range from imperceptible to marked. Stromal desmoplasia is inapparent to minimal in some cases. At the other end of the spectrum, some tumors show such prominent stromal desmoplasia that the tumor cells constitute only a minor component of the lesion. Similarly, some invasive ductal carcinomas have no identifiable component of DCIS, whereas in others, the *in situ* carcinoma is the predominant component of the tumor. Finally, the microscopic margins of these cancers may be infiltrating, pushing, circumscribed, or mixed.

Recognizing that invasive ductal carcinomas are a histologically diverse group of lesions, many investigators have attempted to stratify them based on certain microscopic features. The most common method for subclassifying invasive ductal carcinomas is grading, which may be based solely on nuclear features (*nuclear grading*) or on a combination of architectural and nuclear characteristics (*histologic grading*). In nuclear grading, the appearance of the tumor cell nuclei is

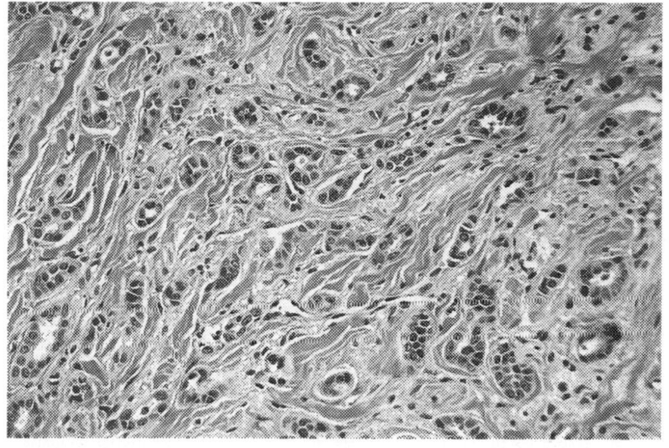

A

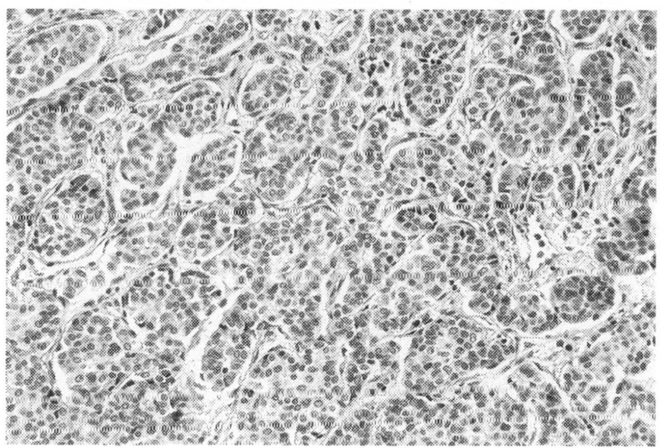

B

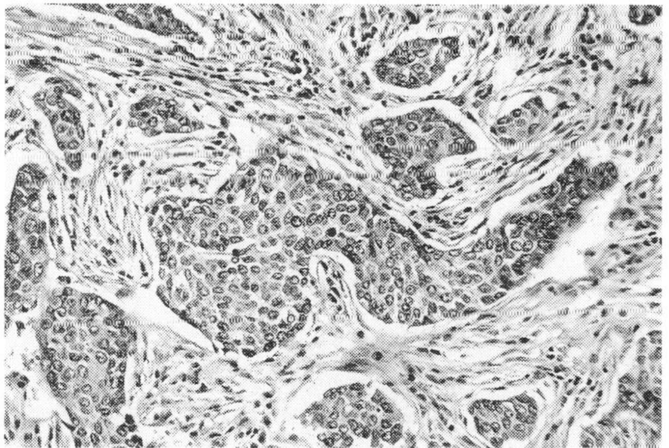

C

FIG. 2. Invasive ductal carcinoma. **A:** Histologic grade 1. **B:** Histologic grade 2. **C:** Histologic grade 3.

compared with those of normal breast epithelial cells. The nuclear grading system most commonly used is that of Black et al.[26,27] In this system, nuclei are classified as well differentiated, intermediately differentiated, and poorly differentiated. That the numeric designations used for these three grades are the opposite of those used for histologic grading (i.e., well-differentiated nuclei are considered grade 3 and poorly differentiated nuclei are considered grade 1) is unfortunate. In current practice, however, histologic grading is the method of grading most often used. In histologic grading,

TABLE 2. *Histologic grading system for invasive breast cancers (Elston and Ellis modification of Bloom and Richardson grading system)*

Components of grade	Score
Tubules	
>75% of tumor composed of tubules	1 point
10–75% of tumor composed of tubules	2 points
<10% of tumor composed of tubules	3 points
Nuclear grade	
Nuclei small and uniform	1 point
Moderate variation in nuclear size and shape	2 points
Marked nuclear pleomorphism	3 points
Mitotic rate	
Dependent on microscope field area	1–3 points
Histologic grade	**Total points**
1 (well differentiated)	3–5
2 (moderately differentiated)	6–7
3 (poorly differentiated)	8–9

Adapted from ref. 28.

breast carcinomas are categorized based on the evaluation of three features: tubule formation, nuclear pleomorphism, and mitotic activity. The histologic grading system currently in most widespread use is that described in detail by Elston and Ellis.[28] This system is a modification of the grading system proposed by Bloom and Richardson in 1957, but provides strictly defined criteria that are lacking in the original description. Tubule formation, nuclear pleomorphism, and mitotic activity are each scored on a scale of 1 to 3. The sum of the scores for these three parameters provides the overall histologic grade; thus, tumors for which the sum of the scores is 3 to 5 are designated grade 1 (well differentiated), those with summed scores of 6 and 7 are designated grade 2 (moderately differentiated), and those with summed scores of 8 and 9 are designated grade 3 (poorly differentiated) (Fig. 2; Table 2). The prognostic significance of histologic grading is discussed in the section Pathologic Factors Useful in Assessing Prognosis).

The expression of biological markers, such as estrogen and progesterone receptors, growth factors, oncogene and tumor-suppressor gene products, and other markers, is highly variable in invasive ductal carcinomas, as might be anticipated from their histologic heterogeneity. The clinical significance of the expression of such markers by these tumors is discussed in detail in Chapters 24 and 32.

Clinical Course and Prognosis

Although invasive ductal carcinomas have the poorest prognosis of all invasive breast cancers, even within this group prognostically favorable subsets can be identified, as discussed in the section Pathologic Factors Useful in Assessing Prognosis. The role of conservative surgery and radiation therapy for the local management of patients with invasive ductal carcinoma is discussed in Chapter 33.

INVASIVE (INFILTRATING) LOBULAR CARCINOMA

Invasive lobular carcinomas constitute the second most frequent type of invasive breast cancer. In most series, these tumors account for 5% to 10% of invasive breast carcinomas.[3–6,29,30] However, the reported incidence of this tumor type has ranged from under 1% to as high as 20%.[25] Some of this difference may be related to differences in patient populations. Most of this variability, however, appears to be related to differences in diagnostic criteria. In particular, since the time the classic form of invasive lobular carcinoma was described by Foote and Stewart,[31] a variety of authors have described invasive breast cancers that they consider variants of invasive lobular carcinoma,[30,32–41] thereby expanding the spectrum of this histologic type and accounting for a higher incidence of invasive lobular carcinoma in more recent series than in the past.

Invasive lobular carcinomas are characterized by multifocality in the ipsilateral breast and appear to be more often bilateral than other types of invasive breast cancer, although the reported range of bilaterality has been broad (6% to 47%).[3,29,42–46] In two clinical follow-up studies of patients with invasive lobular carcinoma, however, the incidence of subsequent contralateral breast cancer among patients with invasive lobular carcinoma was similar to that of patients with invasive ductal carcinoma.[47,48]

Lobular carcinoma *in situ* coexists with invasive lobular carcinoma in the majority of cases.[29,30,35,37,49–51] Overall, 70% to 80% of cases of invasive lobular carcinoma contain foci of lobular carcinoma *in situ*.[52]

Clinical Presentation

Invasive lobular carcinoma may present as a palpable mass or a mammographic abnormality with characteristics similar to those of invasive ductal carcinomas (i.e., discrete, firm mass on palpation; spiculated mass on mammogram). The findings on physical examination and the mammographic appearance in some cases of invasive lobular carcinomas may be quite subtle, however. Physical examination may reveal only a vague area of thickening or induration, without definable margins. Mammographic findings may be equally subtle, with many invasive lobular carcinomas appearing as poorly defined areas of asymmetric density with architectural distortion, and others revealing no mammographic abnormalities, even in the presence of a palpable mass.[53–58] In fact, the extent of the tumor may be substantially underestimated by both physical examination and mammography.

Gross Pathology

Some invasive lobular carcinomas appear as firm, gritty, grey-white masses, indistinguishable from invasive ductal carcinomas. In other cases, however, no mass is grossly evident, and the breast tissue may have only a rubbery consistency. In

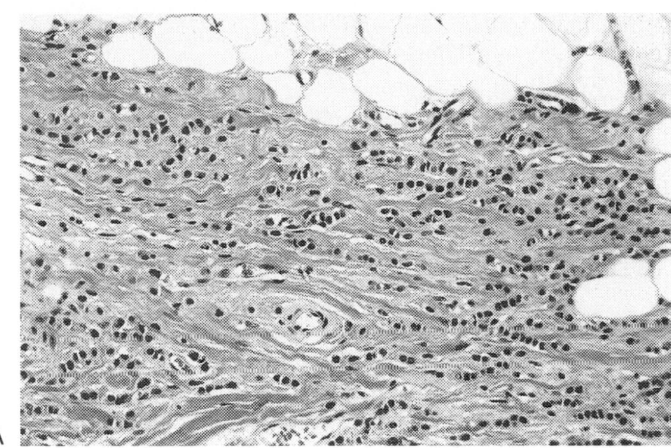

A

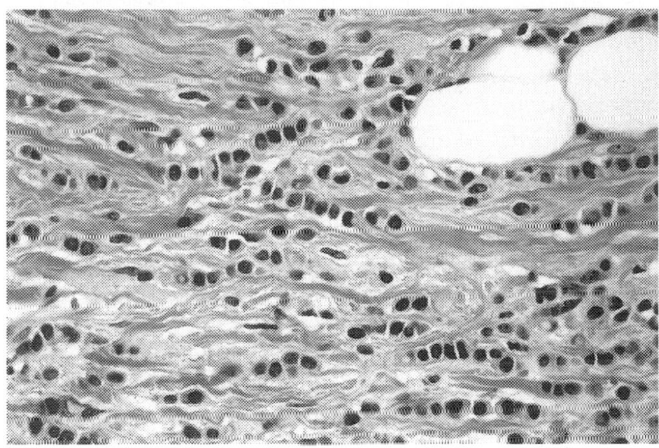

B

FIG. 3. Invasive lobular carcinoma, classic type. **A:** Linear strands of tumor cells infiltrate the stroma. **B:** Higher-power view to demonstrate cytologic detail. The tumor cells have small, relatively uniform nuclei.

still other cases, no abnormality is evident on visual inspection or on palpation of the involved breast tissue, and the presence of carcinoma is revealed only on microscopic examination.

Histopathology

Invasive lobular carcinomas as a group show distinctive cytologic features and patterns of tumor cell infiltration of the stroma. The *classic form* is characterized by small, relatively uniform neoplastic cells that invade the stroma singly and in a single-file pattern that results in the formation of linear strands (Fig. 3).[1,29–31,37–38] These cells frequently encircle mammary ducts in a targetoid manner. Furthermore, the tumor cells may infiltrate the breast stroma and adipose tissue in an insidious fashion, invoking little or no desmoplastic stromal reaction. This feature accounts for the difficulty in detecting some invasive lobular carcinomas on physical examination, mammography, and gross pathologic examination. The nuclei of the neoplastic cells are small, show little variation in size, and are often eccentric. Mitotic figures are infrequent. The cells may contain intracytoplasmic vacuoles that, in some, may be large enough to impart a

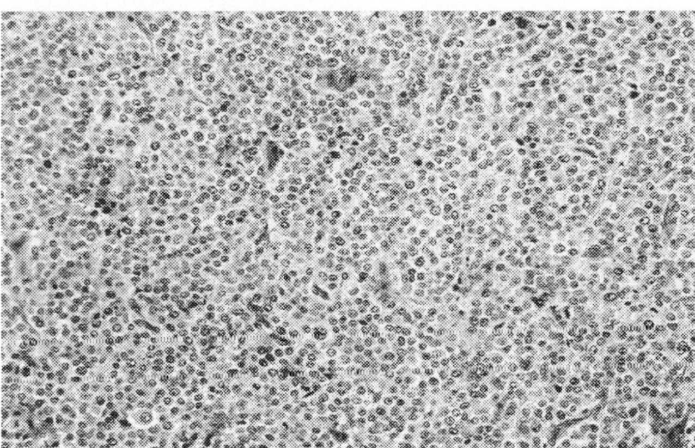

FIG. 4. Invasive lobular carcinoma, solid type. The tumor cells grow in a confluent sheet with little intervening stroma.

signet-ring cell appearance. In the classic form of invasive lobular carcinoma, however, cells with a signet-ring configuration comprise only a small proportion of the tumor cell population. Many examples of invasive lobular carcinoma (as well as lobular carcinoma *in situ*) are characterized histologically by tumor cells that are loosely cohesive. This phenotype may be related at least partly to the fact that both *in situ* and invasive lobular carcinomas typically show loss of expression of the adhesion molecule E-cadherin,[59–62] due in many cases to mutations in the gene encoding this protein.[62,63] This feature distinguishes lobular carcinomas from ductal-type carcinomas, which characteristically exhibit E cadherin protein expression, albeit to a variable degree.[59–61]

Variant forms of invasive lobular carcinoma differ from the classic form with regard to architectural and cytologic features. In the solid, alveolar, and tubulolobular variants, the cells comprising the lesion have features characteristic of the classic form of invasive lobular carcinoma but differ from the classic form with regard to the growth pattern of the tumor cells.[30,32,34,35,38,64] In the *solid form*, the neoplastic cells grow in large confluent sheets with little intervening stroma (Fig. 4).[30,32,37,38,51] The *alveolar form* is characterized by tumor cells that grow in groups of 20 or more cells. These cellular aggregates are separated from one another by a delicate fibrovascular stroma (Fig. 5).[30,32,37,38,51] Although a *trabecular variant* has also been described,[30] considerable overlap exists between this pattern and that seen in the classic form of invasive lobular carcinoma. In the *tubulolobular variant*, some of the tumor cells invade in the linear strands, characteristic of the classic form of invasive lobular carcinoma, whereas others form small tubules that tend to have rounded to ovoid contours.[34,64] These tubules are smaller and less angulated than those found in tubular carcinoma (see Tubular Carcinoma). In other variants, the invasive pattern is similar to that seen in the classic form of invasive lobular carcinoma, but the cytologic features differ. In the *pleomorphic variant*, the neoplastic cells are larger and exhibit more nuclear variation than that seen in the classic form of invasive lobular carcinoma (Fig. 6).[37,39–41] Although signet-ring cell forms can be seen in the classic type of invasive lobular carcinoma and in some examples of invasive duc-

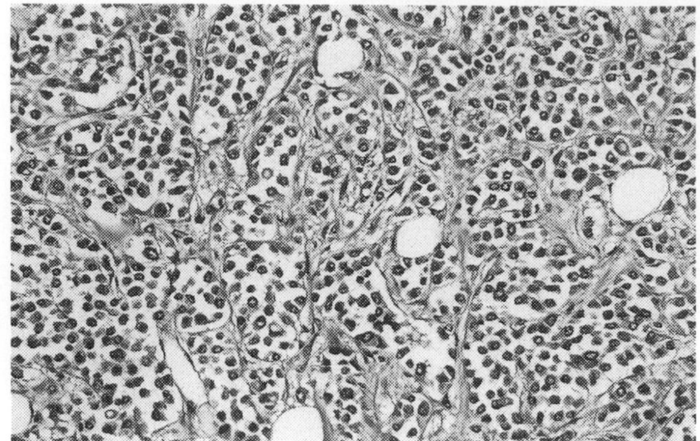

FIG. 5. Invasive lobular carcinoma, alveolar type. Loosely cohesive tumor cell aggregates are separated by delicate fibrous septa.

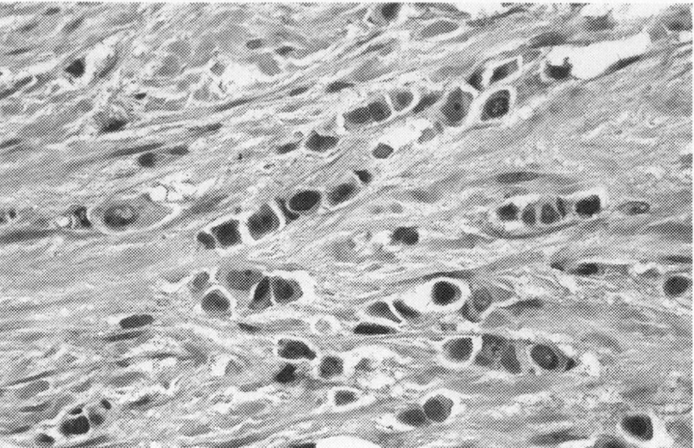

FIG. 6. Invasive lobular carcinoma, pleomorphic type. The tumor cells infiltrate the stroma in linear strands, similar to those seen in the classic type of invasive lobular carcinoma. However, the cells in this lobular variant show considerable nuclear pleomorphism, in contrast to the small, monomorphic nuclei characteristic of the classic type of invasive lobular carcinoma (compare with Fig. 3B).

tal carcinoma,[36,65] tumors that are composed of a prominent component of signet-ring cells that otherwise have the characteristic features of invasive lobular carcinoma are considered to represent the *signet-ring cell variant* of invasive lobular carcinoma.[33,36,66–68] Some authors also regard as lobular variants neoplasms composed of cells with a histiocyte-like appearance that show a single-file pattern of infiltration and contain intracytoplasmic vacuoles (*histiocytoid variant*).[69–71] Finally, several authors have recognized a *mixed* category of invasive lobular carcinomas. This term is generally used to designate lesions in which no single pattern comprises more than 80% to 85% of the lesion.[5,51,72] However, Dixon et al. also included in their "mixed" group the pleomorphic variant.[46]

The relative frequency of these various lobular subtypes is difficult to discern, because not all subtypes have been recognized in all series. In addition, patient selection criteria varied among these studies. In the series of Dixon et al., among 103 invasive lobular carcinomas, 30% were of the classic type, 22% were solid, 19% were alveolar, and 29% were mixed lesions.[46] In the experience of Ellis et al., 40% of invasive lobular carcinomas were of the classic type, 10% were solid type, 4% were alveolar, 6% were tubulolobular, and 40% were mixed.[6] In contrast, in a study from Memorial Sloan-Kettering Cancer Center, 176 of 230 invasive lobular carcinomas (77%) were of the classic type, and the remainder were variants: 10 (4%) solid, 14 (6%) alveolar, and 30 (13%) mixed[51] (Table 3). The pleomorphic variant is particularly uncommon, with only 9 cases identified among 843 invasive carcinomas in one series.[41]

The results of studies of biological markers in invasive lobular carcinoma largely reflect the profile seen in the classic type of this tumor. Invasive lobular carcinomas typically show expression of estrogen and progesterone receptors and rarely show expression of the HER-2/neu oncoprotein[73] or accumulation of the p53 gene product.[74] Gross cystic disease fluid protein is seen in approximately one-third of all invasive lobular carcinomas but is present in the majority of lesions that show prominent signet-ring cell features.[75]

Clinical Course and Prognosis

Several aspects of the clinical course of invasive lobular carcinomas merit consideration. First, a number of studies have noted differences in the pattern of metastatic spread between invasive lobular and invasive ductal carcinomas. In particular, metastases to the lungs, liver, and brain parenchyma appear to be less common, and metastases to bone more common, in patients with lobular cancers than in those with ductal cancers.[76–79] Furthermore, lobular carcinomas have a greater propensity to metastasize to the leptomeninges, peritoneal surfaces, retroperitoneum, gastrointestinal tract, and reproductive organs. In fact, the majority of cases of carcinomatous meningitis in patients

TABLE 3. *Frequency of invasive lobular carcinoma subtypes in series with more than 100 patients*

Study	No. invasive lobular carcinomas	Subtypes				
		Classic	Solid	Alveolar	Tubulolobular	Mixed
Dixon et al.[37]	103	30	22	19	Not included	29
Ellis et al.[6]	243	40	10	4	6	40
DiCostanzo et al.[51]	230	77	4	6	Not included	13

with metastatic breast cancer occur in patients with lobular cancers.[76,77,79–81] Peritoneal metastases may appear as numerous small nodules studding the peritoneal surfaces in a manner similar to that seen in ovarian carcinoma.[36,76,77,79] Metastases to the stomach can produce an appearance that simulates an infiltrative (*linitis plastica*) type of primary gastric carcinoma.[82,83] Involvement of the uterus may result in vaginal bleeding,[84] whereas a metastatic tumor in the ovary may produce ovarian enlargement and the appearance of Krukenberg's tumor.

Whether invasive lobular carcinomas differ in overall prognosis from invasive ductal carcinomas is difficult to determine, due in large part to variations in the application of histologic criteria for the diagnosis of invasive lobular carcinoma. However, the prognosis of patients with invasive lobular carcinoma as a group has not consistently been shown to differ from that of patients with invasive ductal carcinoma.[85] Several studies have suggested that the prognosis for the classic form of invasive lobular carcinoma is better than that for the solid variant,[6,46,51] and that the tubulolobular variant has a particularly favorable prognosis.[6] However, attempts to assess prognostic differences between classic and variant forms of invasive lobular carcinoma have been limited by the small numbers of patients in the variant subgroups in virtually all of the published series and by the failure in some series to stratify patients by stage, and the results across studies have been inconsistent. Some studies have suggested that the classic form of invasive lobular carcinoma is associated with a more favorable prognosis than is invasive ductal carcinoma.[6,51,86] In the study of DiCostanzo et al., however, a prognostic advantage for invasive lobular carcinomas over invasive ductal cancers was seen only among patients with stage I disease.[51] Available evidence suggests that the pleomorphic variant[39–41] and the signet-ring cell variant (when defined as lesions in which more than 10% of the neoplastic cells are of the signet-ring cell type)[68] appear to be associated with a particularly poor clinical outcome.

Numerous clinical follow-up studies have indicated that patients with invasive lobular carcinoma can be adequately treated with conservative surgery and radiation therapy after a complete gross excision of the tumor; local recurrence rates are comparable to those seen in patients with invasive ductal carcinoma (reviewed in Schnitt[87]).

INVASIVE CARCINOMAS WITH DUCTAL AND LOBULAR FEATURES

A small proportion of invasive breast cancers are not readily classifiable as either ductal or lobular. This was acknowledged by Azzopardi, who noted that "infiltrating ductal and infiltrating lobular carcinoma cannot be separated quite as easily as is implied by much of the literature."[88] In his experience, such tumors accounted for approximately 4% of invasive breast cancers.[88] Tumors with such indeterminate histologic features were noted in 2.2% of 11,036 cancers studied by Sastre-Garau et al.,[47] 2.6% of the 879 cancers in a study by Weiss et al.,[89] and 4.4% of 1,337 invasive cancers reviewed by Peiro et al.[48] Ellis et al. noted that 4.7% of 1,536 invasive cancers had mixed ductal and lobular features.[6] In the authors' experience, invasive cancers may be difficult to categorize definitively as either ductal or lobular for a variety of reasons. First, some cancers show distinct areas of invasive ductal carcinoma and invasive lobular carcinoma but also exhibit foci that appear to represent a transition between those two patterns. Although such lesions may be categorized as mixed, this designation ignores the transitional component. Second, some lesions are composed of cells that have cytologic features of invasive lobular carcinoma but infiltrate the stroma in a manner that more closely resembles invasive ductal carcinoma than any of the described lobular variants. Third, some lesions have cytologic features that are more typical of invasive ductal carcinomas but invade the stroma in a single-file pattern. Although some such lesions represent the pleomorphic variant of invasive lobular carcinoma,[39–41] others do not show the degree of nuclear variability required for that diagnosis. Finally, some invasive cancers have both cytologic and architectural features that are intermediate between those of invasive ductal and invasive lobular carcinomas. Given the heterogeneous nature of the lesions included in this group, data on clinical features and outcome are difficult to interpret. In three series, however, lesions designated as having both ductal and lobular features were not distinctive in their rate of local recurrence or distant failure when compared with patients with invasive ductal or invasive lobular carcinomas.[47,48,89]

TUBULAR CARCINOMA

Tubular carcinoma is a special-type cancer that is typically associated with limited metastatic potential and an excellent prognosis. The reported incidence of tubular carcinoma varies depending on the histologic definition and the method of cancer detection used in the study population. In most studies performed before the widespread use of screening mammography, tubular carcinomas accounted for less than 1% to 4% of all breast cancers.[3,90–94] These tumors account for a much higher proportion of cancers detected in mammographically screened populations, however, with incidence rates ranging from 7.7% to 27%.[8–12,95–98]

CLINICAL PRESENTATION

The mean age at presentation for patients with tubular carcinoma is in the early sixth decade (range, 23 to 89 years).[90–94,99–114] Historically, the majority of tubular carcinomas were detected as palpable lesions.[107] Now, however, the majority (60% to 70%) present as nonpalpable mammographic abnormalities.[94,110,111] Not infrequently, tubular carcinomas are discovered incidentally in biopsies performed for unrelated reasons. Lagios et al. reported that 40% of patients with tubular carcinoma have a positive family history of breast cancer in a first-degree relative, a significantly higher rate than that observed among patients with other types of breast cancer.[103] However, this strong association with family history has not been observed by others.[115] Rare examples of tubular carcinoma have been reported in men.[99,116]

Mammographic abnormalities have been reported in the majority (80%) of patients with tubular carcinomas, most often in the absence of palpable abnormalities. However, mammographically occult tubular carcinomas are not infrequent.[110] When a mammographic abnormality is present, it is usually a mass lesion and is only occasionally associated with microcalcifications. The mass may be irregular, round, oval, or lobulated. The mammographic characteristics of the majority of tubular carcinomas were described as "highly suggestive of malignant tumor" in one study. However, 10% were interpreted as having "low to moderate probability" of being a malignant tumor.[110] The majority of tubular carcinomas have spiculated margins and cannot be distinguished radiologically from infiltrating ductal carcinomas.

Gross Pathology

Pure tubular carcinomas are typically small, with an average diameter of less than 1.0 cm in most series.[95,101,102,106,112–114] Tubular carcinomas detected by screening mammography are typically smaller than palpable lesions,[94,103,111] and pure tumors are smaller, on average, than tumors comprised of mixtures of tubular carcinoma and other histologic types.[107] In gross appearance, tubular carcinomas are firm, spiculated lesions that are indistinguishable from infiltrating ductal carcinomas.

Histopathology

Tubular carcinomas are characterized by a proliferation of well-formed glands or tubules formed by a single layer of epithelial cells without a myoepithelial cell component. These tubules tend to be ovoid in shape and have sharply angular contours with tapering ends. The cells comprising the tubules are characterized by low-grade nuclear features and often exhibit apical cytoplasmic "snouting" (Fig. 7). Tubular carcinomas should not be confused with invasive ductal carcinomas with glandlike structures, in which the cells are typically less well differentiated.[1] The stroma of tubular carcinomas usually has desmoplastic features, and prominent elastosis may be present in some cases.[117] General agreement now exists that more than 90% of the tumor should exhibit this characteristic morphology to be categorized as a pure tubular carcinoma[5,6]; tumors with less than 90% tubular elements are generally referred to as *mixed tubular carcinomas*. In published studies, however, the proportion required for the diagnosis of tubular carcinoma has varied from 75% to 100%.

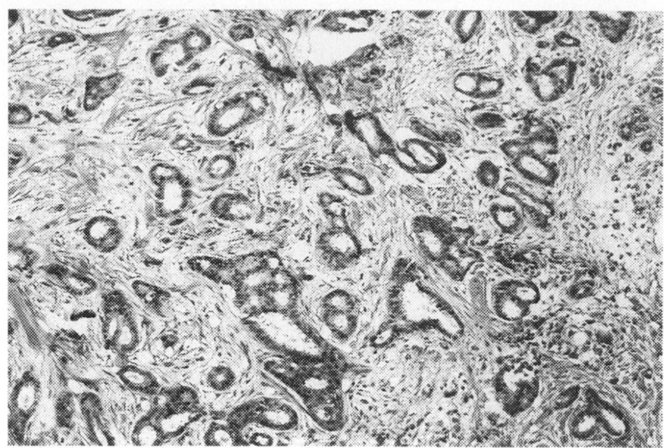
A

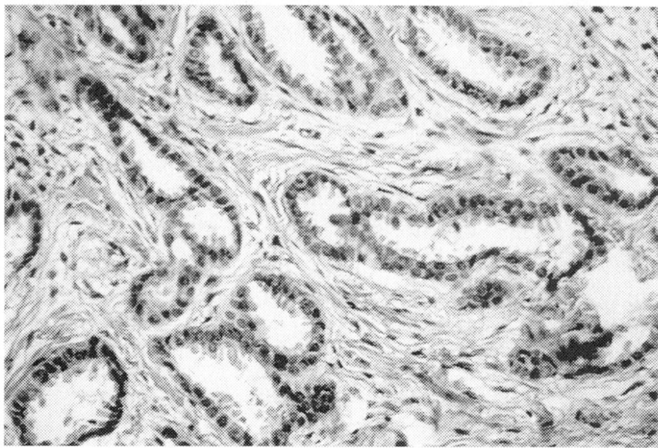
B

FIG. 7. Tubular carcinoma. **A:** This tumor is composed of well-formed glandular structures within a desmoplastic stroma. **B:** The glands, or tubules, are elongated, and some have tapering ends. Numerous cytoplasmic "snouts" are evident at the luminal aspect of the tumor cells.

The majority of tubular carcinomas have an associated component of DCIS.[94,100,101,106,107,110] The DCIS seen in association with tubular carcinoma is usually of low nuclear grade, with cribriform, micropapillary, papillary, or solid patterns, and does not typically comprise a large proportion of the tumor mass. Lobular carcinoma *in situ* is also observed in association with tubular carcinoma, but only in a minority of cases.[91,93,101,103,107,110] The frequency of multifocality and multicentricity in tubular carcinoma is difficult to determine due to the variations in definition and methods of specimen sampling used by different investigators. In one report, in which 17 mastectomy specimens with tubular carcinomas were examined using the Egan serial subgross method,[118] Lagios et al. found a 56% incidence of multicentricity, defined in that study as carcinoma of any type present 5 cm from the index lesion. This incidence was significantly greater than a control group comprised of mastectomy specimens containing breast cancers of other types.[103] The incidence of contralateral breast cancers in patients with tubular carcinomas ranges from 4.5% to 38.0%.[92,94,100,101,103,104,107,112,119] The 38% incidence of contralateral breast cancers reported in one study was significantly higher than that seen in patients with other types of breast cancer.[103]

Because tubular carcinomas are composed of tumor cells with low-grade nuclei, they may be associated with false-negative fine-needle aspiration results.[120] In addition, because these lesions are extremely well differentiated, several benign entities, such as sclerosing adenosis, radial scars, complex sclerosing lesions, and microglandular adenosis, may enter into the differential diagnosis. In such cases, the use of adjunctive immunohistochemical stains may be necessary to arrive at the correct diagnosis.[121–124] Although stains for myoepithelial cells such as actin are useful for distinguishing between tubular carcinomas and benign sclerosing lesions (i.e., sclerosing adenosis, radial scars, and complex sclerosing lesions), they do not permit a distinction to be made between tubular carcinoma and microglandular adenosis.

The expression of various biological markers in tubular carcinomas generally reflects the well-differentiated nature and good prognosis associated with these lesions. Estrogen-receptor positivity has been reported in 70% to 100% of tubular carcinomas and progesterone-receptor positivity in 60% to 83%.[94,112,113,125–127] DNA studies of 18 examples of tubular carcinoma revealed that 13 (72%) were diploid, 4 (22%) were aneuploid, and 1 (6%) was tetraploid.[113] A review of the karyotypic analysis of six tubular carcinomas revealed that all but one were associated with uncomplicated cytogenetic abnormalities, rather than the complex abnormalities exhibited by most breast cancers of no special type.[128] In addition, tubular carcinomas do not typically overexpress the protein products of the HER-2/neu[129,130] or p53 genes[131] as determined by immunohistochemical methods.

Clinical Course and Prognosis

The reported incidence of axillary lymph node metastases in patients with tubular carcinomas ranges from 0% to 30%.[90–95,100–114,119,132] A number of reasons exist for this wide range. Perhaps most important is variation in the histologic definition used in different studies. Many studies have shown an inverse relationship between the degree of tubular differentiation and the incidence of lymph node metastases.[91,93,100,103,104,107,109,113] Nevertheless, even patients with pure tubular carcinomas have nodal metastases in up to 15% of cases.[112] As with other types of breast cancer, however, the size of the tumor strongly influences the likelihood of axillary metastases. Winchester et al. reported that 67% of tubular carcinomas associated with nodal metastases were larger than the median size of 1.0 cm.[112] The relative infrequency of nodal disease in patients with small tubular carcinomas has led some investigators to advocate abandoning axillary lymph node dissection in these patients.[94,113]

With regard to survival, all studies suggest that patients with tubular carcinoma have a good prognosis, albeit to a variable degree.[6,90–95,100–114,119,132–135] In the randomized prospective trial National Surgical Adjuvant Breast and Bowel Project (NSABP) Protocol B-06, 1,090 node-negative and 651 node-positive patients were classified with regard to histologic type; the "favorable" category included 120 patients with tubular carcinoma.[135] Both node-negative and node-positive patients in the "favorable" category experienced significantly greater overall survival at 10 years compared with other patients in a univariate analysis. "Favorable" histology also proved to be an independent predictor of survival in node-negative patients by multivariate analysis.[135] Similar improved survival rates in patients with tubular carcinoma were reported in a series of 1,621 patients, although these patients were not stratified by node status.[6] In this latter study, even patients with "tubular mixed" tumors (which were defined as stellate cancers composed of cells typical of invasive ductal carcinoma but with central tubules identical to those of tubular carcinoma) experienced significantly better overall survival compared with patients with invasive ductal carcinoma.[6] Two additional series—one examining node-negative early-stage breast cancer patients treated with mastectomy, and the other examining early-stage patients treated with breast-conserving therapy—both reported that patients with tubular carcinoma had significantly lower rates of distant recurrences compared with patients with invasive ductal carcinoma.[133,134]

Other investigators have suggested that even patients with node-positive tubular carcinomas have a relatively good prognosis. When tubular carcinoma does metastasize to axillary lymph nodes, usually one and seldom more than three level I nodes are involved.[93,94,103,106,110,112] Furthermore, several investigators have concluded that the presence of nodal disease in patients with tubular carcinoma does not affect disease-free or overall survival rates in these patients.[91,112]

Two reports examined the use of conservative surgery and radiation therapy in a total of 39 patients with tubular carcinoma. In these studies, no significant differences were found in local recurrence rates when patients with tubular carcinomas were compared with patients with invasive ductal carcinoma.[89,134] Although one is tempted to speculate that at least some patients with tubular carcinoma can be treated adequately with local excision alone (i.e., without radiation therapy), insufficient data currently exist regarding this point.

MUCINOUS CARCINOMA

Mucinous carcinoma (also known as *colloid carcinoma*) is another special-type cancer that is associated with a relatively favorable prognosis. The reported incidence of mucinous carcinoma varies depending on the histologic criteria. Most studies have indicated that fewer than 5% of invasive breast carcinomas have a mucinous component, and of these, fewer than one-half represent pure mucinous carcinomas.[136–139]

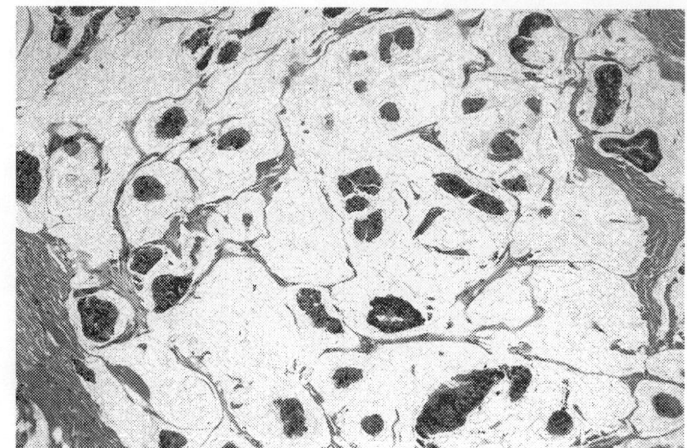
A

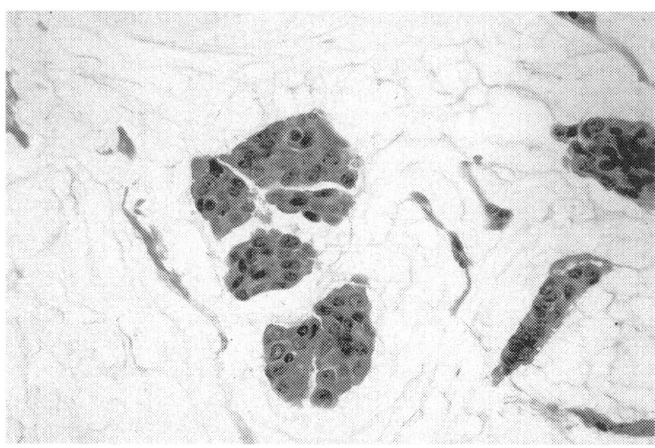
B

FIG. 8. Mucinous carcinoma. **A:** The tumor is composed of clusters of neoplastic cells dispersed within mucous pools. **B:** In this specimen, the neoplastic cells have intermediate-grade nuclei.

Clinical Presentation

The mean age at presentation for patients with mucinous carcinoma is in the seventh decade in most studies (range, 21 to 94 years) and is older than that for patients with breast cancers of no special type.[136,137,140–147] Most patients with mucinous carcinoma included in published reports presented with palpable tumors. Some reports, however, suggest that a substantial proportion of patients with mucinous carcinoma (30% to 70%) present with nonpalpable mammographic abnormalities.[148,149]

On mammography, mucinous carcinomas are most often poorly defined or lobulated mass lesions that are rarely associated with calcification.[148–151] Wilson et al. reported that pure mucinous carcinomas were more often associated with a circumscribed, lobulated contour than with the irregular borders characteristic of tumors with a mixture of mucinous and nonmucinous components (mixed mucinous tumors).[148] In addition, mammographically occult mucinous carcinomas are not infrequent, accounting for 4 of 23 cases (17%) in one study.[150] On ultrasonography, mucinous carcinomas are typically hypoechoic mass lesions.[151]

Gross Pathology

Mucinous carcinomas average approximately 3 cm in size, with a wide range reported in the literature.[152] In some studies, tumors composed exclusively of mucinous features are smaller, on average, than mixed tumors.[145,148] Mucinous carcinomas have a distinctive gross appearance. These lesions are typically circumscribed and have a variably soft, gelatinous consistency, and a glistening cut surface. Lesions with a greater amount of fibrous stroma may have a firmer consistency, however.

Histopathology

The hallmark of mucinous carcinomas is extracellular mucin production. The extent of extracellular mucin varies from tumor to tumor, however. Typically, tumor cells in small clusters, sheets, or papillary configurations are dispersed within pools of extracellular mucin (Fig. 8). This characteristic histology should comprise at least 90% of the tumor (or 100%, according to some)[6] for the tumor to qualify for the diagnosis of mucinous carcinoma. Mucinous neoplasms intermixed with other nonmucinous histologic features are classified as mixed mucinous tumors. The cellularity of mucinous carcinomas is variable. Some tumors are relatively paucicellular; in these cases, the differential diagnosis includes mucocele-like lesions, which are benign lesions characterized by cystically dilated ducts associated with rupture and extravasation of mucin into the stroma.[153,154] The cells comprising mucinous carcinomas are usually of low or intermediate nuclear grade. Many studies have documented the presence of cytoplasmic argyrophilic granules in a significant subset of lesions, although this finding does not appear to be clinically meaningful.[139] Mucinous carcinomas are often accompanied by a DCIS component, which may have a papillary, micropapillary, cribriform, or even comedo pattern. In some cases, the DCIS may also exhibit prominent extracellular mucin production.[152]

The expression of various biological markers in mucinous carcinomas generally reflects the good prognosis associated with these lesions. Estrogen-receptor positivity has been reported in 86% to 90% of tumors[125,127,146] and progesterone-receptor positivity in 63% to 67%.[126,127] DNA studies of 26 pure mucinous carcinomas revealed that 25 (96%) were diploid, compared with only 8 of 19 mixed tumors (42%). The rate of diploidy among the mixed tumors was comparable to that seen in breast cancers of no special type.[155] In a review examining the karyotypic analysis of 20 mucinous carcinomas, 17 exhibited chromosomal aberrations that were simple in comparison with the complex aberrations typically associated with breast cancers of no special type.[128] In addition, mucinous carcinomas usually do not overexpress the

HER-2/neu oncoprotein (0% to 4% of cases) or show p53 protein accumulation (18% of cases).[129–131]

Clinical Course and Prognosis

The incidence of axillary lymph node metastases in pure mucinous carcinomas, although variable (range, 4% to 39%; average, 15%), is significantly less than the incidence of node positivity seen in mixed mucinous tumors (38% to 59%) or in breast cancers of no special type (43% to 63%).[136–138,140–146] Some investigators have questioned the necessity of performing lymph node dissections in patients with mucinous carcinoma, particularly if 100% of the tumor shows typical mucinous histology.[144,145]

With regard to survival, 38 patients with mucinous carcinoma were enrolled in the NSABP B-06 trial, and they experienced the same significantly increased survival rate as patients with tubular carcinoma, particularly those in the node-negative group.[135] Similar results were reported by Ellis et al. in their retrospective series; however, the patients in their study were not stratified by nodal status.[6] Survival data reported in most other retrospective reports suggest that, to a variable degree, patients with mucinous carcinoma experience lower recurrence rates and greater short- and long-term survival than patients with mixed mucinous carcinomas and breast cancers of no special type.[136–146,156] Several studies have noted that a significant number of late recurrences are seen in patients with mucinous carcinoma[138,143,157]; one report documented a recurrence 30 years after initial treatment.[157] Results from the SEER database were published comparing 20-year survival data from 3,356 patients with mucinous carcinoma and 117,163 patients with invasive ductal carcinoma diagnosed between 1973 and 1990.[147] Similar to the studies cited earlier, this report indicated that patients with mucinous carcinoma present with localized disease more commonly than patients with invasive ductal carcinoma (78.1% versus 53.1%). In addition, even after prolonged follow-up, only 25.1% of patients with mucinous carcinoma died as a consequence of breast cancer, compared with 58.3% of patients with invasive ductal carcinoma. These results were highly statistically significant, even after correction for potentially confounding variables, such as age, year of diagnosis, race, stage, and grade.[147] In addition, two series—one examining node-negative early-stage breast cancer patients treated with mastectomy (with a 20-year follow-up) and the other examining early-stage patients treated with breast-conserving therapy (with a 10-year follow-up)—reported that patients with mucinous carcinoma had significantly lower rates of distant recurrences compared with patients with invasive ductal carcinoma.[133,134]

Three studies have examined the use of conservative surgery and radiation therapy in a total of 38 patients with mucinous carcinoma and report no significant differences in local recurrence rates for these patients compared with patients with invasive ductal carcinoma.[89,134,158] Given the relatively good prognosis of patients with mucinous carcinoma, some authors have raised the question of whether radiation therapy can be safely omitted after breast-conserving surgery in patients with this tumor type.[145] At this time, however, not enough data exist to support such a recommendation.

Mucinous carcinomas have rarely been associated with unusual metastatic manifestations, including mucin embolism resulting in fatal cerebral infarcts[159,160] and pseudomyxoma peritonei.[161]

MEDULLARY CARCINOMA

Medullary carcinomas account for fewer than 5% to 7% of all invasive breast cancers.[152] Some studies have indicated that this type of breast cancer has a favorable prognosis, despite its aggressive histologic appearance.[162–169] However, considerable controversy exists regarding the appropriate histologic definition of medullary carcinoma, as well as the reproducibility of this diagnosis among pathologists. As a result, the prognostic implications of this diagnosis are uncertain.[162–176]

Clinical Presentation

Patients with medullary carcinoma usually present at a relatively younger age than patients with other breast cancers; the mean age at presentation is in the late fifth and early sixth decades, with a wide age range reported.[162–169] The majority of patients with medullary carcinoma present with a palpable mass, usually in the upper outer quadrant.[169] Of interest, some patients with this tumor type exhibit axillary lymphadenopathy at the time of presentation, suggesting the presence of metastatic disease. Histologic examination of the lymph nodes in such cases, however, typically reveals benign reactive changes.[177,178] Rare examples of medullary carcinoma have been reported in men.[165]

To some degree, the mammographic features of medullary carcinoma reflect the pathologic features, although they are not specific. Most lesions are associated with a moderately well defined mass unassociated with calcifications.[178,179] However, a significant proportion of cases of medullary carcinoma show an ill-defined margin. Moreover, the majority of mammographically well-circumscribed cancers are infiltrating ductal carcinomas rather than medullary carcinomas.[180] On ultrasonographic examination, medullary carcinomas are generally well circumscribed, frequently lobulated, and hypoechoic.[179,180]

Gross Pathology

The mean size of medullary carcinomas is similar to that of breast cancers of no special type.[152] In gross appearance, these lesions are well-circumscribed, soft, tan-brown to grey tumors that bulge above the cut surface of the specimen. A

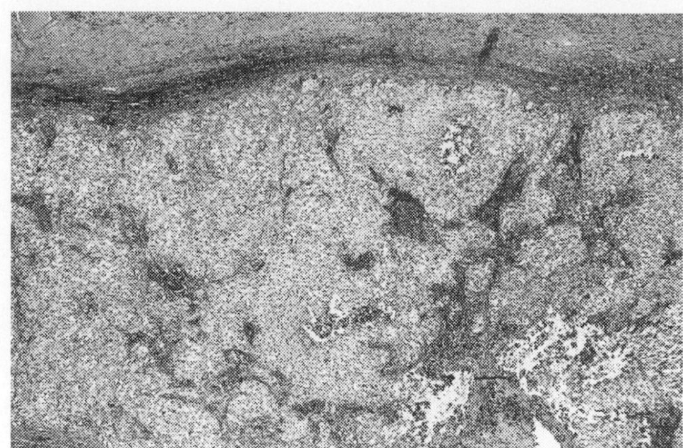

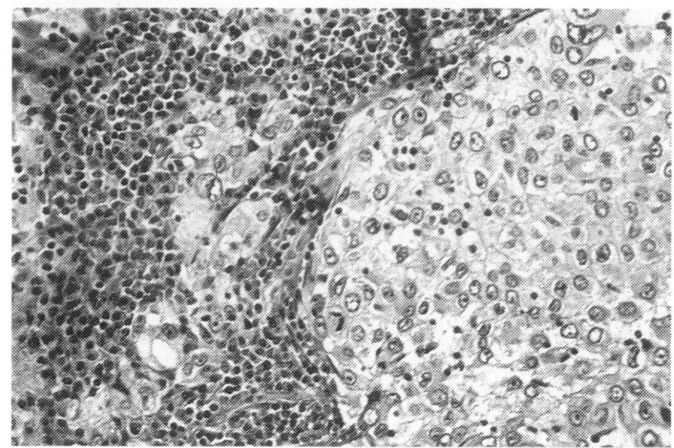

FIG. 9. Medullary carcinoma. **A:** Low-power photomicrograph demonstrating the well-circumscribed border of the tumor. **B:** The tumor cells show high-grade nuclear features, and a prominent admixture of lymphocytes and plasma cells is seen.

multinodular appearance may be appreciated in some cases. Areas of hemorrhage, necrosis, or cystic degeneration may be present in tumors of any size, but prominent necrosis is usually seen in larger tumors.

Histopathology

Three similar but distinct classification systems for the histologic diagnosis of medullary carcinomas have been proposed by Ridolfi et al.,[164] Wargotz and Silverberg,[167] and Pedersen et al.[168] All three classification schemes recognize the following attributes of medullary carcinomas, but the relative importance and the mandatory nature of each are stressed to different degrees: (a) syncytial growth pattern of the tumor cells in more than 75% of the tumor, (b) admixed lymphoplasmacytic infiltrate, (c) microscopic circumscription, (d) grade 2 or grade 3 nuclei, and (e) absence of glandular differentiation (Fig. 9). Tumors that lack a variable number of these characteristics (depending on the system used) are classified either as *atypical medullary carcinoma* or *invasive ductal carcinoma.* The Ridolfi system[164] has the most stringent and the Pedersen system[168] the least stringent criteria. Regardless of the classification system used, however, medullary carcinoma is frequently overdiagnosed.[174,181] Studies assessing the reproducibility and prognostic implications of the various classification systems have yielded conflicting results and are summarized below.

In addition to the histologic features listed earlier, medullary carcinomas may be associated with a DCIS component (usually comprised of cells that are morphologically similar to the invasive component), hemorrhage, tumor necrosis, cystic degeneration, and various types of metaplasia of the tumor cells, most often squamous metaplasia.[152] Patients with medullary carcinoma do not appear to have an increased incidence of multicentricity or contralateral cancers.[166]

The expression of various biological markers in medullary carcinomas is more reflective of the aggressive histologic features of these tumors than of the favorable prognosis reported by some investigators.[162–169] Estrogen-receptor positivity has been reported in 0% to 33% of medullary carcinomas[125–127,169,172] and progesterone-receptor positivity in 0% to 36%.[125–127,169] DNA studies performed in conjunction with various NSABP protocols demonstrated that 85% of medullary carcinomas are aneuploid.[172] A review of the karyotypic analysis of 14 examples of medullary carcinoma revealed complex chromosomal alterations in 9 (64%), which was a significantly greater proportion than that seen in tubular and mucinous carcinomas.[128] In addition, medullary carcinomas are associated with p53 protein accumulation in the majority of cases,[131] and HER-2/neu overexpression has been reported in 0% to 14% of lesions.[129,130]

Clinical Course and Prognosis

Although studies have differed in the histologic criteria used, most studies indicate that the incidence of axillary lymph node metastases is lower in patients with medullary carcinomas (19% to 46%) than in those with atypical medullary carcinomas (30% to 52%) or invasive ductal carcinomas (29% to 65%).[164–167,169]

Data regarding survival rates in patients with medullary carcinoma must be interpreted with an understanding of the histologic criteria used for diagnosis. Most pathologists currently use the histologic criteria set forth by Ridolfi et al.,[164] who reported a significantly better 10-year survival rate for 57 patients with medullary carcinoma (84%) than for 79 patients with atypical medullary carcinomas (74%) and 56 patients with nonmedullary carcinomas (63%). A later study by Wargotz and Silverberg, using slightly modified criteria, reported 5-year survival rates of 95% for 24 patients with medullary carcinoma, 80% for 16 patients with atypical medullary carcinoma, and 70% for 10 patients with breast cancers of no special type.[167] A subsequent study using the Ridolfi criteria confirmed these findings and reported 10-year survival rates of 92% for 26 patients with medullary carcinoma, 53% for 23 patients with atypical medullary carcinoma, and 51% for 46 patients with breast cancers other than medullary carcinoma.[166] Several other reports have called these earlier findings into question, however. Pedersen et al.[171] examined the prognostic implications of each of the criteria put forth by Ridolfi and found many to be poorly reproducible or to lack prognostic significance. Furthermore, the authors could not demonstrate a survival advantage in patients with medullary carcinoma as defined using these criteria.[171] These authors proposed their own classification and suggested that it yielded superior prognostic information.[168,169] Similarly, using Ridolfi's criteria, Ellis et al. could not demonstrate a significant difference in the 10-year survival rate for patients with medullary carcinoma (51%) compared with patients with atypical medullary carcinoma (55%) and patients with carcinoma of no special type (47%); patients with medullary carcinoma did demonstrate a more favorable survival rate than did patients with grade 3 tumors of no special type.[6] Moreover, in a review of the NSABP experience, Fisher analyzed survival data for 198 patients with medullary carcinomas and 149 patients with atypical medullary carcinomas enrolled in multiple trials and reported that node-negative patients with medullary carcinoma and node-positive patients with medullary carcinoma treated with chemotherapy (melphalan and 5-fluorouracil) experienced modestly improved survival rates compared with control patients with breast cancers of no special type. This improved survival was not observed, however, in untreated node-positive patients, although the sample sizes in this group were small.[172] The authors concluded that "the prognosis of typical medullary cancer is not as 'good' as previously perceived."[172]

In addition to the clinical follow-up studies that question a favorable prognosis for medullary carcinoma, several studies have also questioned the practical applicability of the diagnostic criteria. Specifically, several studies have been published in which a number of pathologists (including those with expertise in breast pathology) failed to attain acceptable consensus in diagnosing medullary carcinomas using the criteria of Ridolfi.[170,173,174] In one of these studies,[174] a direct comparison was made between the criteria advocated by Ridolfi et al.,[164] Wargotz and Silverberg,[167] and Pedersen et al.[168] In that study, the criteria of Pedersen were the most reproducible. None of the three classification systems, however, was related to axillary lymph node status or overall survival.[174] In contrast, a clinical follow-up study examining a relatively small number of patients with medullary carcinoma suggested that the Ridolfi classification system is superior to the Pedersen classification system in predicting improved survival.[182]

In summary, although some patients with medullary carcinoma may have improved survival compared with patients with breast cancers of no special type, the ability of pathologists to reliably and reproducibly identify this subset of patients is suboptimal. Clinicians must be aware of these limitations when confronted with a pathology report suggesting the diagnosis of medullary carcinoma. Given the difficulty in diagnosing these lesions, one could argue that treatment decisions, particularly those related to the use of adjuvant chemotherapy, should not rest solely on assumptions regarding the prognostic implications of medullary carcinoma.

The results of the use of breast-conserving therapy in patients with medullary carcinoma have been reported in three studies with a total of 72 patients.[89,134,158] The local recurrence rates in the two studies with a median follow-up of approximately 5 years were 4%[158] and 7%.[89] In one study with a 10-year median follow-up, however, local recurrences were observed in 5 of 17 patients (29%).[134] In all three studies, no significant differences were seen in local recurrence rates among patients with medullary carcinoma and patients with invasive ductal carcinoma. Thus, the available limited data suggest that conservative surgery and radiation therapy are an appropriate local treatment for patients with medullary carcinoma.

INVASIVE CRIBRIFORM CARCINOMA

Invasive cribriform carcinoma is a well-differentiated cancer that shares some morphologic features with tubular carcinoma and is also associated with a favorable prognosis. Five percent to 6% of invasive breast cancers show at least a partial invasive cribriform component.[183,184]

Clinical Presentation

The majority of patients with invasive cribriform carcinoma present in the sixth decade of life (range, 19 to 86 years).[183,184] A significant proportion of invasive cribriform carcinomas were mammographically occult in one study.[185] The remaining lesions showed nonspecific mammographic findings, usually spiculated masses with or without calcification.[185]

Gross Pathology

No distinctive gross features of invasive cribriform carcinoma have been described.

Histopathology

Invasive cribriform carcinomas are characterized by tumor cells that invade the stroma in a cribriform or fenestrated growth pattern similar to that seen in the cribriform pattern of DCIS (Fig. 10). These tumors often show admixtures of other histologic patterns of invasive breast cancer, particularly tubular carcinoma, which is seen in 17% to 23% of cases. The classic variant of invasive cribriform carcinoma, described by Page et al.,[183] is defined as a tumor composed of an exclusively invasive cribriform pattern or a tumor with more than 50% invasive cribriform features, in which the remainder of the tumor exhibits features of tubular carcinoma. Tumors with any component of nontubular carcinoma

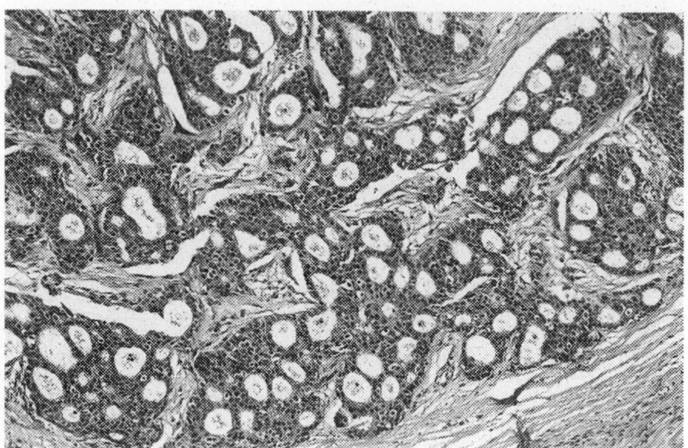

FIG. 10. Invasive cribriform carcinoma. The tumor cells invade the stroma in nests that have a fenestrated growth pattern, similar to that seen in the cribriform pattern of ductal carcinoma *in situ.*

were described as "mixed" in that study. Venable et al.[184] subdivided 62 cases studied into pure invasive cribriform carcinoma (12 of 62), lesions with 50% to 99% cribriform features (20 of 62), and lesions with less than 50% cribriform features (30 of 62).[184] The cribriform component of these lesions was associated with low-grade or intermediate-grade nuclear features. Significant nuclear pleomorphism, when present, was seen only in the noncribriform component. In both studies, most invasive cribriform carcinomas were associated with DCIS, usually of the cribriform type. The average size of these tumors was relatively large and varied from 3.1 cm (range, 1 to 14 cm) for the classic variant of cribriform carcinoma to 4.2 cm (range, 2 to 9 cm) for tumors of mixed histology.[183]

Venable et al. reported that all 16 tumors in which the cribriform component constituted more than 50% of the tumor were positive for estrogen receptor; 11 of 16 (69%) were also positive for progesterone receptor.[184] In the six examples of invasive cribriform carcinoma examined in one study, none was associated with the overexpression of the HER-2/neu oncoprotein.[129] Little is known regarding the expression of other biological markers in invasive cribriform carcinoma.

Clinical Course and Prognosis

In the series of Page et al.,[183] none of the 35 lesions categorized as the classic variant of invasive cribriform carcinoma exhibited lymphatic and vascular space invasion, compared with 3 of 16 tumors (19%) with mixed histology. In that study, axillary lymph node metastases were seen in 14% of patients with classic cribriform carcinoma and 16% of patients with tumors of mixed histology.[183] In the series of Venable et al., 37% of patients with pure invasive cribriform carcinoma had axillary lymph node metastases, compared with 48% to 50% of patients with tumors of mixed histology.[184] In a study with a median follow-up interval of 14.5 years, Page et al. reported no deaths related to invasive cribriform carcinoma in patients with the classic variant (although 1 patient had recurrence in axillary and supraclavicular lymph nodes), but 38% (6 of 16) patients with tumors of mixed histology died of their disease.[183] Similarly, Venable et al. reported that after 5 years of follow-up, no patient with tumors comprised of 50% or greater cribriform features died of disease, whereas the death rate was 7% (2 of 30) for patients with tumors with less than 50% cribriform features.[184] The authors of both studies stated that, although patients with pure or classic lesions did better than patients with mixed tumors, even the latter group experienced significantly better overall survival compared with control groups that included patients with tumors without a cribriform component.

The relatively good prognosis for invasive cribriform carcinoma was confirmed by Ellis et al.,[6] who reported a 10-year survival of 91% for 13 patients, compared with a 47% 10-year survival for patients with invasive carcinoma of no special type.

INVASIVE PAPILLARY CARCINOMA

Most of the published literature concerning papillary carcinomas of the breast includes both invasive and *in situ* papillary lesions.[186–192] In this section, however, only data concerning invasive papillary carcinomas are reviewed. Invasive papillary carcinomas comprise less than 1% to 2% of invasive breast cancers and are characterized by a relatively good prognosis.[193,194]

Clinical Presentation

Invasive papillary carcinomas are diagnosed predominantly in postmenopausal patients. Fisher et al.[193] noted a disproportionate number of cases in nonwhite women. As with medullary carcinomas, Fisher et al. noted that a significant proportion of patients with invasive papillary carcinoma exhibit axillary lymphadenopathy that is suggestive of metastatic disease but that on pathologic examination is seen to be due to benign reactive changes.[193]

On mammography, invasive papillary carcinoma is usually characterized by nodular densities that may be multiple and are frequently lobulated.[194–196] These lesions are often hypoechoic on ultrasonography.[196] One study noted the difficulty in distinguishing between intracystic papillary carcinoma, intracystic papillary carcinoma with invasion, and invasive papillary carcinoma.[196]

Gross Pathology

Fisher et al. reported that invasive papillary carcinoma is grossly circumscribed in two-thirds of cases.[193] Other invasive papillary carcinomas are grossly indistinguishable from invasive breast cancers of no special type.

Histopathology

Of the 1,603 breast cancers reviewed in the NSABP B-04 study, 38 had papillary features, and all but 3 of these were pure, without an admixture of other invasive histologic types. Microscopically, invasive papillary carcinomas are characteristically circumscribed, show delicate or blunt papillae, and exhibit focal solid areas of tumor growth (Fig. 11). The cells typically show amphophilic cytoplasm but may have apocrine features and also may exhibit apical "snouting" of cytoplasm similar to that in tubular carcinoma. The nuclei of tumor cells are typically intermediate grade, and most tumors are histologic grade 2.[193] Tumor stroma is not abundant in most cases, and occasional cases show prominent extracellular mucin production. Calcifications, although not usually evident mammographically, are commonly seen histologically but usually are present in associated DCIS. DCIS is present in more than 75% of cases and usually, but not exclusively, has a papillary pattern. In some lesions in which both the invasive and *in situ* components have papillary features, determining the relative proportion of each may be difficult. Lymphatic vessel invasion has been noted in one-third of cases. Microscopic involvement of skin or nipple was present in 8 of 35 cases (23%) in one study, but Paget's disease of the nipple was not observed.[193]

Estrogen-receptor positivity was observed in all five cases of invasive papillary carcinoma examined in one study, and progesterone-receptor positivity was seen in four of five (80%).[125] In a review of cytogenetic findings in five examples of invasive papillary carcinoma, three (60%) exhibited relatively simple cytogenetic abnormalities.[128] In addition, none of the four examples of papillary carcinomas examined in two reports was associated with p53 protein accumulation or HER-2/neu oncoprotein overexpression.[129,131]

Clinical Course and Prognosis

Only limited data exist on the prognostic significance of a diagnosis of invasive papillary carcinoma.[135,193,197] Among 35 patients with this tumor in the NSABP B-04 trial, after a median follow-up of 5 years, only 3 treatment failures occurred, including 1 patient who died from metastatic papillary carcinoma. These survival data were similar to those reported in patients with pure tubular and mucinous carcinomas in this study.[193] A later publication updating the NSABP B-04 results at 15 years revealed that patients with tumors classified histologically as "favorable" (including invasive papillary carcinomas) still had significantly better survival in univariate analysis, but tumor histology was not an independent predictor of survival in multivariate analysis.[197] Node-negative patients with invasive papillary carcinomas enrolled in the NSABP B-06 trial, however, experienced higher rates of survival after a 10-year follow-up than did patients with carcinomas of no special type, and tumor histology was an independent predictor of survival in multivariate analysis.[135]

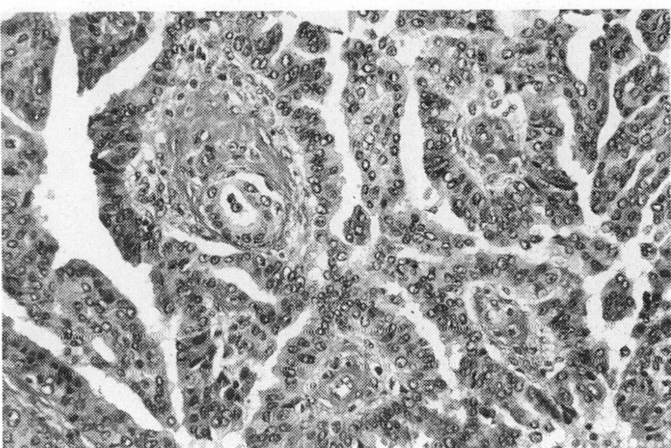

FIG. 11. Invasive papillary carcinoma. The tumor cells are organized around fibrovascular cores.

INVASIVE MICROPAPILLARY CARCINOMA

Invasive micropapillary carcinoma is an entity that, unlike invasive papillary carcinoma, appears to be associated with a relatively poor prognosis.[198,199] This tumor comprised 2.7% of breast cancers in one study.[199]

Clinical Presentation

The mean age at presentation for patients with invasive micropapillary carcinoma is 54 to 62 years (range 36 to 81 years).[198,199] In one study, seven of nine patients (78%) presented with a palpable mass; two of nine (22%) lesions were mammographically detected.[198] As with carcinomas of no special type, these lesions most frequently arise in the upper outer quadrant of the breast.[198]

The mammographic features of this tumor type have not been well defined. Of two mammographically detected lesions in one study, one was described as a "suspicious soft-tissue lesion" and the other as "suspicious microcalcifications."[198]

Gross Pathology

In a report describing nine examples of invasive micropapillary carcinoma, seven were solitary, one was "multifocal," and two were not grossly apparent.[198] No distinguishing gross features have been described. The median size was reported as 1.5 cm in one study (range, 0.8 to 3.0 cm) and 4.9 cm in a second study,[198,199] significantly larger than invasive carcinomas of no special type.[199]

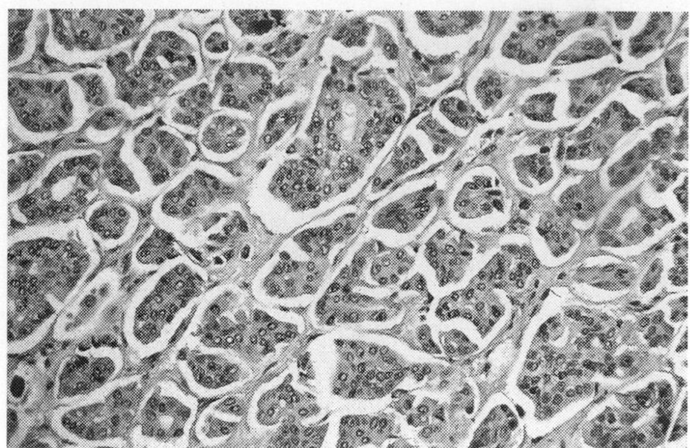

FIG. 12. Invasive micropapillary carcinoma. Clusters of neoplastic cells, some forming glands, are present within clear spaces separated by fibrovascular tissue.

Histopathology

In most reported cases, invasive micropapillary carcinomas have been admixed to a variable degree with invasive carcinomas of no special type or, in a minority of cases, with mucinous carcinoma. Unlike other special-type carcinomas, however, the prognostic implications appear to be the same whether the micropapillary component is present focally or diffusely within the tumor.[199] The lesions are characterized by clusters of cells in a micropapillary or tubular-alveolar arrangement that appear to be suspended in a clear space, or in some cases in a mucinous or aqueous-type fluid. These micropapillary clusters, unlike "true" papillary lesions, lack fibrovascular cores (Fig. 12). The overall appearance of invasive micropapillary carcinoma may mimic serous papillary carcinomas of the ovary or may simulate lymphatic and vascular space invasion.[198] True lymphatic and vascular space invasion has been reported in 33% to 67% of cases and may be extensive.[198,199] Cytologically, the cells comprising the invasive micropapillary carcinoma usually have low-grade to intermediate-grade nuclei. The majority of tumors (67% to 70%) are associated with a DCIS component with micropapillary and cribriform patterns.[198,199] A minority of cases (33%) have shown calcifications histologically.[198]

An immunohistochemical study evaluating 33 examples of invasive micropapillary carcinoma reported that 72% were positive for estrogen receptor and 45% were positive for progesterone receptor. HER-2/neu overexpression was observed in 36% of cases, and p53 protein accumulation was seen in 12% of cases.[200]

Clinical Course and Prognosis

The two published studies describing patients with invasive micropapillary carcinoma differ with regard to their conclusions concerning the prognostic implications of this entity.[198,199] In one report describing nine patients with invasive micropapillary carcinoma, only three (33%) had metastases to regional lymph nodes, and only one experienced a chest wall recurrence after mastectomy. The authors felt that, based on these results, no firm conclusions could be made regarding the prognostic significance of this histologic subtype.[198] In contrast, in a study of 27 patients with invasive micropapillary carcinoma, axillary lymph node metastases were seen in all 27 patients, compared with 66% of patients with invasive carcinoma of no special type.[199] Furthermore, four or more lymph nodes were involved in 82% of cases, and on average, nine lymph nodes were positive for metastatic carcinoma. Follow-up information was available for 12 patients; of these, 6 died at an average of 22 months after their initial treatment.[199]

Available data appear to indicate that patients with carcinomas having an invasive micropapillary component typically present at a higher disease stage than patients with invasive carcinoma of no special type and appear to have a poor prognosis. However, further information is needed to confirm these observations.

METAPLASTIC CARCINOMA

Metaplastic carcinomas represent a morphologically heterogeneous group of invasive breast cancers in which a variable portion of the glandular epithelial cells comprising the tumor have undergone transformation into an alternate cell type—either a nonglandular epithelial cell type (e.g., squamous) or a mesenchymal cell type (e.g., spindle, chondroid, osseous, myoid). Many reports have been published describing various aspects of metaplastic carcinomas, and many names have been applied to the various tumors comprising this group.[201–230] No uniformly agreed upon classification scheme exists for these tumors, however. Metaplastic carcinomas are uncommon lesions, representing fewer than 5% of all breast cancers. The prognostic implications of a diagnosis of metaplastic carcinoma is difficult to define and may relate to some degree to the type of metaplasia present, as discussed below.

Clinical Presentation

Patients with metaplastic carcinoma are similar to patients with invasive carcinoma of no special type with regard to age at presentation, the manner in which the tumors are detected, and the location within the breast at which these tumors arise.[218,219] Most patients present with a single palpable lesion that not infrequently is associated with rapid growth of short duration.[219] In one study, skin fixation was noted in 9 of 26 patients (35%), and fixation to deep tissues was noted in 6 of 26 patients (23%).[218]

The mammographic appearance of metaplastic carcinoma is not specific. Most are fairly circumscribed, noncalcified lesions, which in some cases appear benign.[228] Some show

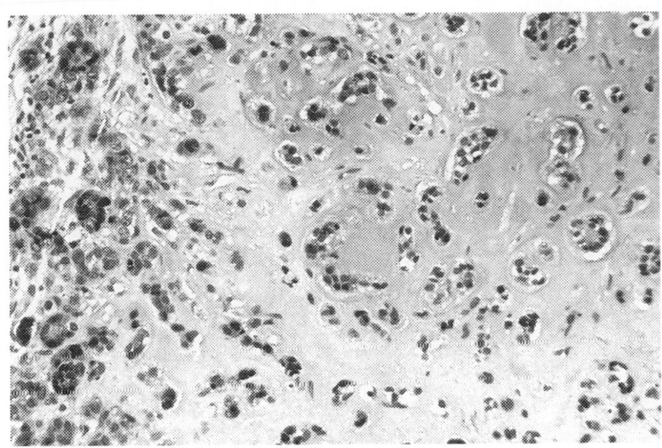

FIG. 13. Metaplastic carcinoma with chondroid metaplasia. A small area of conventional invasive ductal carcinoma is present at the left side of this photomicrograph. The major portion of this tumor, however, is composed of neoplastic cells within a chondroid matrix.

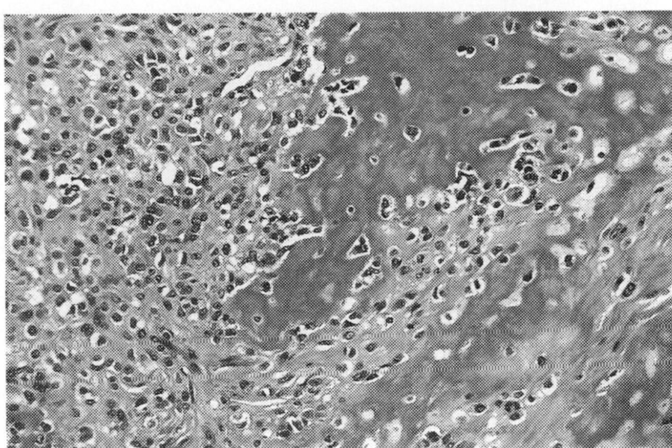

FIG. 14. Metaplastic carcinoma with osseous metaplasia. Although some of this neoplasm shows features of invasive ductal carcinoma (*left*), foci of osteoid formation are evident.

both a circumscribed portion and a spiculated portion, which in one study correlated with the metaplastic and invasive epithelial components, respectively.[228] Foci of osseous metaplasia may be detected mammographically in a subset of cases.

Gross Pathology

The gross appearance of metaplastic carcinomas is not distinctive, and these tumors can either be well circumscribed or show an indistinct or irregular border. Cystic degenerative changes are not infrequent, particularly in lesions with squamous differentiation. In general, metaplastic carcinomas tend to be relatively large tumors compared with invasive carcinomas of no special type, with a mean size of 3.9 cm (range 1.2 to 10 cm) reported in one study.[226]

Histopathology

Microscopically, metaplastic carcinomas are highly distinctive but vary in the types and extent of metaplastic changes. Most reports divide metaplastic carcinomas into two broad categories: those that show squamous differentiation[201–208] and those that feature heterologous elements, such as cartilage, bone, muscle, adipose tissue, vascular elements, and even melanocytes, among others (Figs. 13–15).[217–228] Investigators at the Armed Forces Institute of Pathology place metaplastic carcinomas into five categories: squamous cell carcinomas,[208] spindle cell carcinomas,[212] carcinosarcomas,[221] matrix-producing carcinomas,[220] and carcinomas with osteoclastlike giant cells,[224] although others consider this last group a separate entity.

Squamous differentiation can range from well to poorly differentiated. In some tumors composed primarily of squamous cells, cystic degeneration is prominent. In such cases, parts of the tumor may be composed of squamous epithelial–lined cysts resembling benign epidermal inclusion cysts. Spindle cell differentiation is common in metaplastic carcinomas and is frequently seen in association with squamous differentiation. The term *spindle cell carcinoma* has been used by some investigators to describe metaplastic carcinomas in which the majority of the tumor shows this growth pattern.[209–212]

The most common heterologous types of metaplastic carcinoma show chondroid or osseous differentiation (Figs. 13 and 14). In these tumors, the cartilage and bone may appear histologically benign or frankly malignant, resembling chondrosarcoma and osteosarcoma, respectively. If the heterologous metaplastic component of a particular tumor predominates, the differential diagnosis must include a sarcoma, either primary or metastatic. Determining the correct diagnosis in such cases may require extensive tissue sampling to demonstrate epithelial elements. In some cases, immunohistochemical staining for epithelial markers such as keratin may be required for proper diagnosis. Although this is often helpful in tumors with spindle cell differentiation (see Fig. 15), not all metaplastic carcinomas show expression of epithelial markers, particularly those with heterologous differentiation. The results of immunohistochemical staining for other markers have been even more variable, and this subject has been reviewed in detail.[229] Finally, ultrastructural analysis may be of value to demonstrate epithelial features that may not be evident on routine examination by light microscope.[229]

One unusual subtype of metaplastic carcinoma, low-grade adenosquamous carcinoma, appears to represent a distinct clinicopathologic entity.[213–215] These tumors are typically smaller than other metaplastic carcinomas, with a median size between 2.0 and 2.8 cm (range, 0.5 to 8.6 cm).[213,214] They exhibit a firm yellow cut surface with

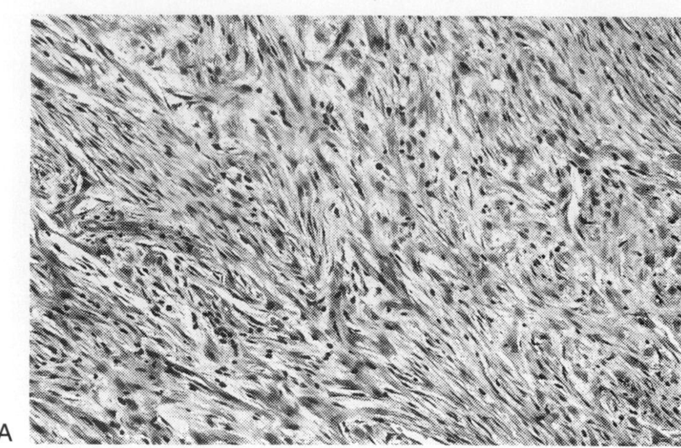

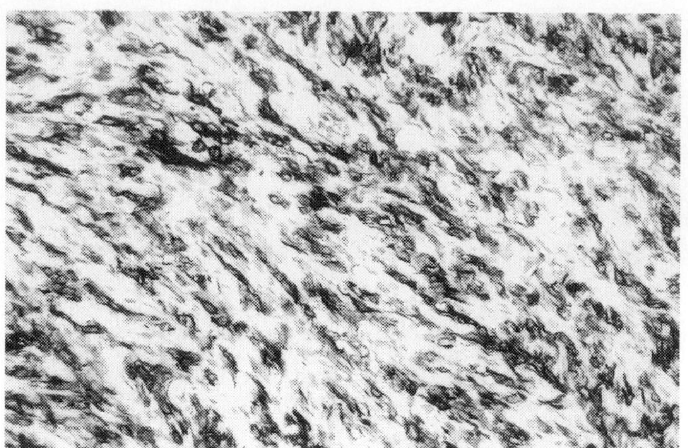

FIG. 15. Metaplastic carcinoma, spindle cell type. **A:** Hematoxylin-eosin–stained sections reveal interlacing fascicles of spindle cells without evidence of epithelial differentiation. **B:** Immunoperoxidase stain for keratin reveals that the majority of tumor cells show immunoreactivity for this protein, characteristic of cells with an epithelial phenotype.

irregular borders. Histologically, these tumors are well differentiated and show a peculiar collagenized, lamellated stroma. In most tumors, areas of squamous differentiation are admixed with areas of glandular differentiation (Fig. 16). However, in some tumors, squamous differentiation can be quite limited in extent. The glands often show elongated, compressed lumens, which may suggest syringomatous differentiation. Microcysts filled with keratinaceous material may be present. DCIS is usually not seen. As discussed below, these lesions may be locally aggressive but have a relatively good prognosis when compared with other metaplastic carcinomas (see section Clinical Course and Prognosis).[213–215]

The frequency of DCIS seen in association with metaplastic carcinoma varies among published reports. In lesions characterized by a prominent mesenchymal component in which a true sarcoma is in the differential diagnosis, the presence of DCIS argues in favor of metaplastic carcinoma.

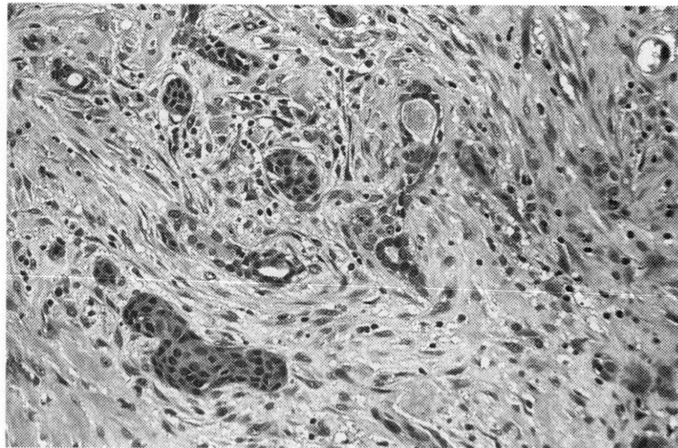

FIG. 16. Low-grade adenosquamous carcinoma. The tumor shows foci of glandular and squamous differentiation. The neoplastic cells have low-grade nuclear features.

Estrogen-receptor and progesterone-receptor studies in metaplastic carcinomas are typically negative, regardless of the histologic subtype examined. A review of the literature shows that only 13 of 115 metaplastic carcinomas (11%) were positive for estrogen receptors, and only 5 of 77 (6%) were positive for progesterone receptors.[208,210–212,215,219–222,226,227] Using flow cytometry, Pitts et al. reported that six of eight metaplastic carcinomas (75%) were aneuploid or tetraploid.[222] Similarly, using Feulgen-stained sections from 12 examples of metaplastic carcinoma, Flint et al. reported that the epithelial component demonstrated aneuploidy in all cases, and the mesenchymal elements were aneuploid in 11 of 12 (92%).[230] In another study, 61% of metaplastic carcinomas with heterologous elements demonstrated p53 protein accumulation, and 11% demonstrated HER-2/neu overexpression.[226] Drudis et al. reported that 46% of low-grade adenosquamous carcinomas overexpressed HER-2/neu, and 13% showed p53 protein accumulation.[215]

Clonality in metaplastic carcinomas has been assessed using microdissection techniques and evaluation of loss of heterozygosity at multiple chromosomal loci.[231] In that study, all six cases of metaplastic carcinoma demonstrated identical clonality of the epithelial and mesenchymal components, and the same clone was also identified in nearby DCIS in one case. The authors concluded that the mesenchymal component of these lesions arose from mutation of the epithelial component.[231]

Clinical Course and Prognosis

The reported frequency of axillary lymph node metastases in patients with squamous or spindle cell carcinomas ranges from 6% to 54% of cases.[208,212,216,219] In patients with metaplastic carcinoma with heterologous elements, lymph node metastases have been noted in 6% to 31% of cases.[216,218–220,222,226]

In most cases, the routes of metastatic dissemination in metaplastic carcinomas are similar to those seen in breast cancers of no special type, including lymphatic spread to axillary lymph nodes rather than the hematogenous spread characteristic of mammary sarcoma. Metastatic lesions may demonstrate an epithelial phenotype, the metaplastic phenotype, or both.

Survival data reported in various studies are difficult to compare due to the relatively small numbers of patients included in the studies, differences in tumor types, differences in treatment and follow-up intervals, differences in the use of appropriate control groups, and paucity of studies that stratify patients by stage. Nevertheless, in patients with squamous or spindle cell carcinomas, reported overall survival rates have ranged from 43% to 86%.[208,212,216,219] In patients with metaplastic carcinomas with heterologous elements, the reported overall survival rates range from 38% to 69%.[216,218,220,222,226] One of these studies stratified patients by stage and reported that the overall survival rate at 5 years was 56% for stage I patients, 26% for stage II patients, and 18% for stage III patients.[218] Chhieng et al. evaluated 32 patients with metaplastic carcinoma with heterologous elements, and follow-up information was available in 29 of these patients.[226] The authors reported that metastases developed in six patients (21%) after an average follow-up of 6.25 years. The 5-year survival rate was 60%. The authors compared these patients with a control group of 112 patients with invasive ductal carcinoma matched for age at diagnosis, tumor size, and nodal status. Although patients with metaplastic carcinoma experienced a longer time to recurrence and a relatively better 5-year survival, the difference was not statistically significant.[226]

In summary, the available data suggest that the prognosis for patients with metaplastic carcinoma is not appreciably different from that for patients with invasive carcinomas of no special type when tumor size and stage are taken into consideration. The one exception among the variants of metaplastic carcinoma that does appear to have prognostic implications is low-grade adenosquamous carcinoma. Among 16 patients with low-grade adenosquamous carcinoma who had lymph node dissections performed, only 1 (6%) had evidence of metastatic disease (in a single lymph node).[213,214] Only 1 of the 43 patients included in both studies experienced distant metastases. In one study, however, four of eight patients treated with excision alone developed a local recurrence.[213] In a second study, local recurrence after excision alone was seen in 5 of 19 (26%) patients.[214] Unfortunately, details regarding the margin status in these lesions are not provided. Although it is possible that these lesions may be adequately treated with wide excision alone, the use of conventional local therapy for these patients until further data become available seems most prudent. The use of conservative surgery and radiation therapy for patients with other types of metaplastic carcinoma should also follow the same guidelines used for patients with conventional types of invasive breast cancer.

INVASIVE CARCINOMA WITH NEUROENDOCRINE DIFFERENTIATION

Some invasive breast cancers show evidence of neuroendocrine differentiation at the morphologic level, histochemical level, immunohistochemical level, or some combination of these. In addition, in rare instances, breast carcinomas can secrete hormonal products that cause clinical symptoms.

Clinical Presentation

With the exception of the very rare functioning neuroendocrine tumor that results in clinical manifestations due to hormone production and secretion,[232–236] carcinomas with neuroendocrine differentiation do not demonstrate unique clinical manifestations.[237–250] Most of these tumors have been diagnosed in women, but neuroendocrine tumors have also been reported in men,[240,241,243] and some types may be proportionally more common in men than in women.[243,244] In most studies, the median age of patients at presentation and the location in which these tumors arise in the breast are found to be similar to those seen in invasive cancers of no special type; in one study, however, the most common tumor location was subareolar.[248]

No distinctive mammographic or ultrasonographic characteristics of invasive carcinomas with neuroendocrine differentiation have been reported.

Gross Pathology

Invasive carcinomas with neuroendocrine differentiation are not associated with distinctive gross characteristics, and the reported mean size in most studies is similar to that of invasive cancers of no special type.

Histopathology

Carcinomas with neuroendocrine differentiation represent a heterogeneous group of neoplasms. This is related to the fact that neuroendocrine differentiation is defined differently in various studies. Most reports refer to "argyrophilic" carcinomas, which are defined as lesions that demonstrate distinctive granular material in the cytoplasm of tumor cells (argyrophilic granules) when stained with histochemical stains, such as the Grimelius' argyrophil method. However, argyrophilic granules reflect neuroendocrine differentiation in some but not all cases.[237–244] Argyrophilic carcinomas have been reported to comprise from 3.3% to as many as 52% of all breast carcinomas. This wide range of estimates is probably related to methodologic differences in histochemical staining and interpretation and possibly differences in patient selection.[237–240,247] Argyrophilic carcinomas can be associated with a variety of histologic appearances, including tumors with no overt morphologic evidence of neuroen-

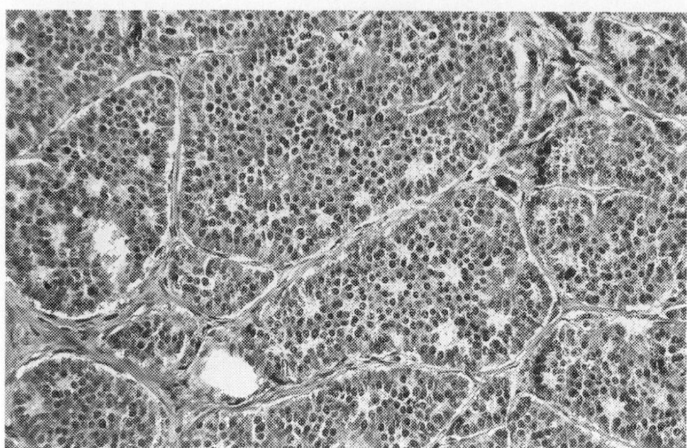

FIG. 17. Carcinoid tumor. This tumor is composed of nests of cells that focally form acinar structures. The nuclei are small and uniform, and the cytoplasm is eosinophilic and granular. This histologic appearance is identical to that seen in carcinoid tumors in other sites.

docrine differentiation (usually invasive ductal carcinoma or mucinous carcinoma), tumors with histologic features suggestive but not diagnostic of neuroendocrine differentiation, and tumors showing the organoid growth pattern with uniform epithelioid or spindle cells arranged in trabeculae and ribbonlike configurations that is diagnostic of carcinoid tumors.[237–250] However, tumors with typical neuroendocrine morphology may fail to demonstrate histochemical evidence of argyrophilia.[246] Furthermore, although most tumors with morphologic evidence of neuroendocrine differentiation also demonstrate immunoreactivity for one or more specific neuroendocrine markers, such as chromogranin or synaptophysin, many "argyrophilic" tumors are negative for these markers by immunohistochemical analysis.[241,244,249] Therefore, argyrophilic carcinomas clearly represent a heterogeneous group of tumors, only some of which should be considered as showing true neuroendocrine differentiation.

Among tumors that show histologic evidence of neuroendocrine differentiation by routine light microscopy, several distinct morphologic subtypes have been recognized. Although the histogenesis of such lesions is debated, primary tumors that are morphologically indistinguishable from carcinoid tumors occurring elsewhere in the body can arise in the breast; these tumors comprise fewer than 1% of all breast cancers (Fig. 17).[246] These tumors must be distinguished from metastatic carcinoids, which occasionally involve the breast[251–256] and may even initially present as breast masses.[255] In some cases, the presence of DCIS in the region of the tumor can assist with this differential diagnosis. In equivocal cases, a clinical evaluation to rule out an alternate primary site may be required.

At the other end of the neuroendocrine spectrum are primary breast carcinomas that are indistinguishable from small cell neuroendocrine (oat cell) carcinomas in other sites.[239,257–262] Again, these tumors must be distinguished from metastatic small cell neuroendocrine carcinoma involving the breast, and a clinical evaluation to rule out an alternate primary site, such as the lung, may be required.[263,264]

Only limited information exists regarding the expression of biological markers in invasive carcinomas with neuroendocrine differentiation. Of 20 tumors from four studies in which estrogen-receptor and progesterone-receptor data were provided, 19 (95%) were positive for estrogen receptors, and 15 (75%) were positive for progesterone receptors.[238,242,250,265] Jablon et al. performed flow cytometric DNA studies on two carcinoid tumors and reported diploidy in one and aneuploidy in the other.[250] Wilander et al. performed DNA studies on four examples of argyrophilic carcinoma unassociated with morphologic evidence of neuroendocrine differentiation and reported that all four cases were diploid.[266]

Clinical Course and Prognosis

The incidence of axillary lymph node metastases does not appear to be significantly different in patients with invasive carcinoma with neuroendocrine differentiation than in patients with invasive carcinoma of no special type.

With regard to survival data, some of the retrospective reports provide limited follow-up data, but reaching firm conclusions regarding the prognostic implications of neuroendocrine differentiation in invasive breast cancer is difficult due to the relatively small numbers of patients included in the studies, differences in the definition of neuroendocrine differentiation, differences in treatment and follow-up intervals, the lack of appropriately matched control groups, and the lack of studies that stratify patients by stage. Nevertheless, the available data do not point to any differences in prognosis for patients with argyrophilic tumors and carcinoid tumors and for patients with invasive cancers of no special type. On the other hand, as may be expected, based on the behavior of small cell carcinoma arising from other sites, most[258–262] but not all case reports indicate an aggressive clinical course in patients with primary small cell carcinoma of the breast.

Only one study has examined the use of breast-conserving treatment for patients with neuroendocrine carcinomas. In that study, three patients with node-negative carcinoid tumors were treated by excision alone and followed for 15 months to 7 years[250]; no recurrences were observed. Firm conclusions cannot be drawn from these anecdotal data, however, and patients with invasive breast cancers with neuroendocrine differentiation should be treated in a manner appropriate for the size and stage of the lesion.

ADENOID CYSTIC CARCINOMA

Adenoid cystic carcinoma is a rare and morphologically distinct form of invasive carcinoma that has been the subject of numerous published reports.[267–292] These tumors comprise 0.1% of all breast cancers[274,283] and are associated with an excellent prognosis.

Clinical Presentation

The median age of patients with adenoid cystic carcinoma varies among studies but is usually in the sixth or early seventh decade, with a wide age range reported. In most reports, these tumors present as a palpable mass; the majority of lesions are discovered in the subareolar or central region of the breast.[270,274,284,292] Skin involvement has been reported in rare cases.[280] These lesions are rarely multicentric, and the incidence of contralateral breast cancers does not appear increased. Rarely, this tumor has been reported in males.[273,276,288,292]

On mammography, these tumors can appear as well-defined lobulated masses, ill-defined masses, or spiculated lesions.[180] Some adenoid cystic carcinomas present with mammographic microcalcifications, whereas others are mammographically occult.[286]

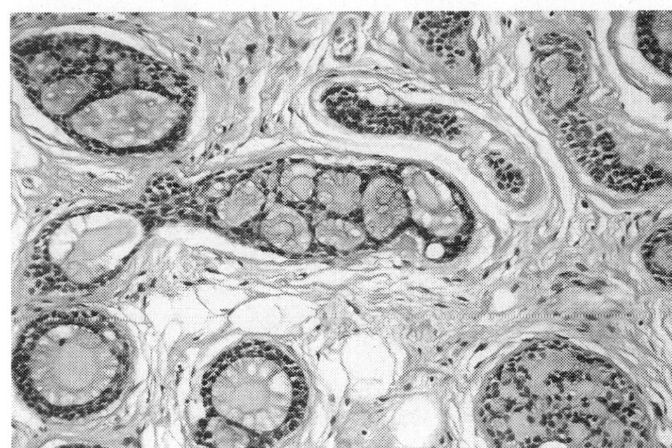

FIG. 18. Adenoid cystic carcinoma. In this specimen, the invasive tumor cells grow in a cribriform pattern. Intraluminal aggregates of basement membrane material are present.

Gross Pathology

The reported size range of adenoid cystic carcinomas is broad. In one study, the mean size was 1.8 cm.[292] In gross appearance, these tumors are usually circumscribed and nodular; however, the microscopic extent of the lesion is appreciably larger than the grossly evident lesion in 50% to 65% of cases.[286–292]

Histopathology

Histologically, these tumors are similar to adenoid cystic carcinomas that arise in the salivary glands and are composed of epithelial cells with variable degrees of glandular, squamous, and sebaceous differentiation, myoepithelial cells, and characteristic collections of acellular basement membrane material (Fig. 18).[281,286] The epithelial component can assume variable architectural patterns, including solid, cribriform, tubular, and trabecular configurations. Some of these patterns may raise the differential diagnosis of *in situ* or invasive cribriform carcinoma, or benign conditions such as collagenous spherulosis.[293,294] Immunohistochemical studies have documented the presence of true lumens in the glandular component, lined by cytokeratin-positive cells with intact polarity, as well as of pseudolumens surrounded by cells immunohistochemically consistent with myoepithelial cells.[291] Associated DCIS is seen in a minority of cases. Perineural invasion is also seen in some cases and may be prominent. Lymphatic vessel invasion is only rarely identified.[286]

Scattered reports indicate that these tumors are usually estrogen receptor– and progesterone receptor–negative.[125,279,285–287,290] Kleer and Oberman, however, reported that 26% (5 of 19) of the tumors they studied were estrogen receptor–positive.[292] In addition, DNA studies by image analysis were reported in four examples of adenoid cystic carcinoma; in all cases, the tumors were diploid.[290] Only one of four tumors demonstrated p53 mutations using polymerase chain reaction testing.[290]

Clinical Course and Prognosis

Patients with adenoid cystic carcinoma usually have an excellent prognosis. Only rare instances of axillary lymph node metastases have been reported.[271,273,284,290] Distant metastases are also infrequent,[267,277,279,282,284,289] and death due to adenoid cystic carcinoma is exceedingly rare.[284] Nevertheless, Ro et al. proposed applying the same histologic grading system used for adenoid cystic carcinomas of the salivary glands and reported that the grading system provided prognostically helpful information.[284] The prognostic usefulness of this grading system has been disputed, however.[290,292]

Only sporadic reports exist of the use of breast-conserving treatment for patients with adenoid cystic carcinoma. Although local recurrences after excision alone have been described,[269,275,277,278,284,292] details regarding microscopic margin status are rarely provided. At present, treatment of patients with adenoid cystic carcinoma should follow the same guidelines as for treatment of other invasive breast cancers.

INVASIVE APOCRINE CARCINOMA

Although many invasive breast cancers of various types show some evidence of apocrine differentiation, fewer than 1% of invasive breast carcinomas demonstrate pure apocrine features (i.e., exhibit cytologic characteristics that resemble those of apocrine sweat glands).[295] Although the morphologic features of these tumors are distinctive, available evidence suggests that patients with these tumors have the same prognosis as patients with invasive breast cancers of no special type.

Clinical Presentation

Patients with apocrine carcinomas are similar in age and mode of presentation to patients with invasive carcinoma of no special type. As an exception, one study reported that 7 of 34 patients (21%) demonstrated skin involvement by tumor.[296] Only rare examples of apocrine carcinoma have been reported in males.[297] A low incidence of multifocal lesions and contralateral tumors is reported.[297,298]

The mammographic characteristics of apocrine carcinomas are not distinctive.[180,199] Most tumors present as masses with ill-defined margins, and microcalcifications are infrequent.[299] In addition, the ultrasonographic findings associated with these tumors are nonspecific.[180]

Gross Pathology

No distinctive gross findings are associated with apocrine carcinoma, and the size distribution is similar to that of invasive carcinomas of no special type.[297,298]

Histopathology

The histologic features of apocrine carcinoma, in contrast, are highly distinctive.[295–305] The invasive patterns are usually those seen in invasive ductal carcinoma, but in some cases, lesions with apocrine cytology can exhibit a pattern of invasion more characteristic of invasive lobular carcinomas.[304] One variant with a distinctive dyshesive and diffusely infiltrative pattern has been designated as having "myoblastoid" or "histiocytoid" features,[305] and in some cases, this lesion may mimic a granular cell tumor. Cytologically, the tumor cells have cytoplasm that is abundant and eosinophilic, with obvious granularity in some cases. The nuclei vary in grade, but typically show prominent nucleoli (Fig. 19). DCIS is frequently associated and may have apocrine features. Extensive lymphatic vessel invasion, including dermal lymphatic involvement, was identified in 4 of 34 cases (12%) in one study.[296]

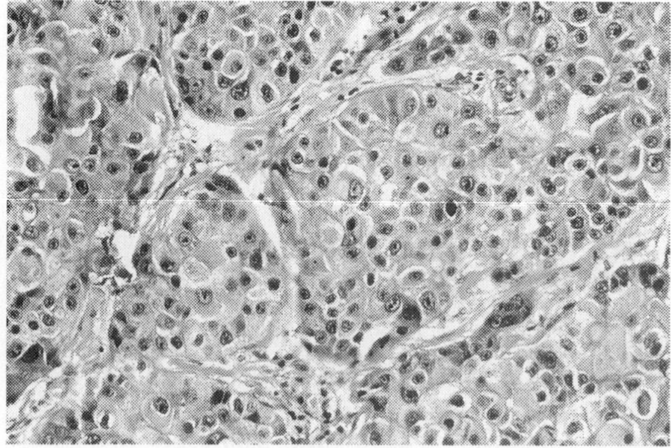

FIG. 19. Apocrine carcinoma. The tumor cells show abundant eosinophilic granular cytoplasm.

Apocrine carcinomas characteristically show immunostaining for gross cystic disease fluid protein.[75] Five of 18 apocrine carcinomas (28%) described in three studies were positive for estrogen receptors.[126,295,298] DNA studies using Feulgen-stained tissue sections demonstrated that 14 of 17 apocrine carcinomas were aneuploid, and the remainder were diploid.[304] These data may be skewed, however, because all but two of the tumors analyzed were high grade. In addition, only 1 of 5 apocrine carcinomas (20%) exhibited p53 protein accumulation by immunohistochemistry.[131]

Clinical Course and Prognosis

Patients with apocrine carcinoma do not appear to have a significantly different incidence of axillary lymph node involvement at presentation than patients with invasive carcinoma of no special type. Furthermore, a number of studies have compared patients with apocrine carcinoma with control patients with invasive carcinomas of no special type, matched for stage, and have observed no appreciable differences in disease-free or overall survival.[296,298,300] These observations have led some to conclude that apocrine carcinomas are more a morphologic curiosity than a distinct clinicopathologic entity.

SECRETORY CARCINOMA

Secretory carcinoma is an exceedingly rare form of invasive breast carcinoma that accounts for fewer than 0.01% of all breast cancers.[306] Although secretory carcinomas occur over a wide age range, they account for a substantial number of primary breast cancers diagnosed in childhood and thus have also been referred to as *juvenile carcinomas*. In most cases, secretory carcinomas are associated with an indolent clinical course.

Clinical Presentation

Secretory carcinomas present over a wide age range (3 to 73 years) with a median age in the third decade.[306–326] The majority of reported cases have been in women, but rare cases have occurred in men,[306,318,319,324,325] including several examples occurring in association with gynecomastia.[318,325] Most lesions are detected as palpable masses; these can arise anywhere in the breast, with no obvious site predilection. No association has been documented with underlying medical conditions or hormonal abnormalities. In addition, no increased incidence of a positive family history of breast cancer has been reported in patients with secretory carcinoma. Only rare cases have been reported to be multicentric,[320] and incidence of contralateral breast cancer does not appear to be increased in these patients.

Mammographic abnormalities associated with secretory carcinoma in adults have not been described in detail. On ultrasonography, these lesions sometimes appear as hypoechoic lesions with heterogeneous internal echo texture and posterior acoustic enhancement, similar to a fibroadenoma.[180]

Gross Pathology

Secretory carcinomas are typically grossly circumscribed. A broad size range has been reported, with a median size of 3 cm noted in one relatively large series.[311]

Histopathology

Histologically, these lesions are characterized by a proliferation of relatively low-grade tumor cells that form glandular structures and microcystic spaces filled with a vacuolated, lightly eosinophilic secretion (Fig. 20). The tumor cells have abundant eosinophilic or clear cytoplasm. DCIS is frequently present in association with the invasive component and can be of the solid, cribriform, or papillary patterns, most often with low-grade nuclear features.

Sporadic reports regarding hormone-receptor status in secretory carcinoma indicate that approximately one-third of cases are estrogen receptor–positive, and three-fourths are progesterone receptor–positive.[306,316,317,321,323] In addition, DNA studies indicate that virtually all secretory carcinomas are diploid or near diploid.[306,323,324]

Clinical Course and Prognosis

The majority of patients with secretory carcinoma have stage I disease and an indolent clinical course. Nevertheless, one-fourth to one-third of the reported cases of secretory carcinoma have been associated with axillary lymph node metastases, and this ratio holds true in both younger and older age groups.[306,309,311,313,314,319,325] The vast majority of axillary metastases involve three lymph nodes or less.

Most of the case reports do not provide adequate follow-up data, so that estimating the recurrence rates of patients with secretory carcinoma is difficult. Local recurrences in the breast[307,308,310,311,313,319] and chest wall[323] have been reported, and the interval between initial treatment and recurrence can be quite prolonged. Some of these recurrences were seen in patients treated with excision alone.

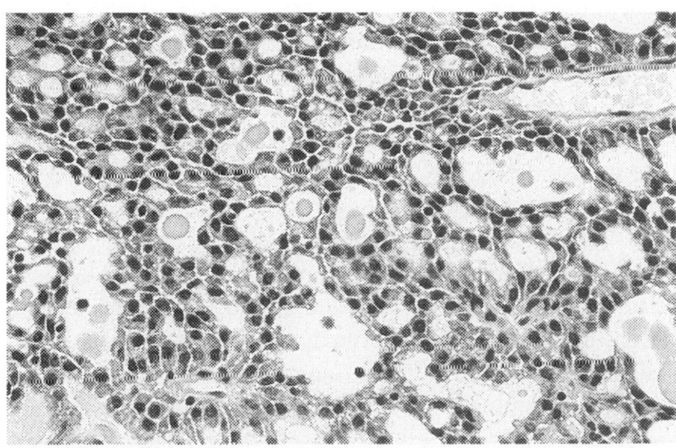

FIG. 20. Secretory carcinoma. The tumor cells form glandular spaces, many of which contain eosinophilic secretions.

Distant metastases are rare but do occur in patients with secretory carcinoma and have resulted in patient deaths in rare instances.[311,319] Neither the efficacy of conservative surgery and radiation therapy nor the role of adjuvant chemotherapy in patients with secretory carcinoma has been defined.

MISCELLANEOUS RARE INVASIVE BREAST CANCERS

Invasive Carcinoma with Osteoclastlike Giant Cells

Invasive carcinoma with osteoclastlike giant cells is characterized by an invasive epithelial component with admixed giant cells that morphologically resemble osteoclasts and have the phenotypic features of histiocytes on immunohistochemical and ultrastructural analysis.[327–339] The clinical features of these tumors and their location within the breast are similar to those of invasive carcinomas of no special type. Invasive carcinoma with osteoclastlike giant cells is associated with a benign appearance both mammographically[331,338] and grossly, due to the presence of circumscribed borders. On macroscopic examination, these lesions are typically circumscribed, fleshy, and brown due to recent and remote hemorrhage and benign vascular proliferation. The epithelial component of the tumor is usually moderately to poorly differentiated invasive ductal carcinoma (Fig. 21), but osteoclastlike giant cells have been reported in invasive lobular carcinomas and most other special-type cancers.[224,328,330,332,334,335,339] The giant cell component can be, but is not invariably, present in metastatic lesions.[335] Although the prognostic significance of this unusual lesion is not known with certainty, available evidence suggests that these tumors do not appear to be any more or less aggressive than breast cancers of no special type.

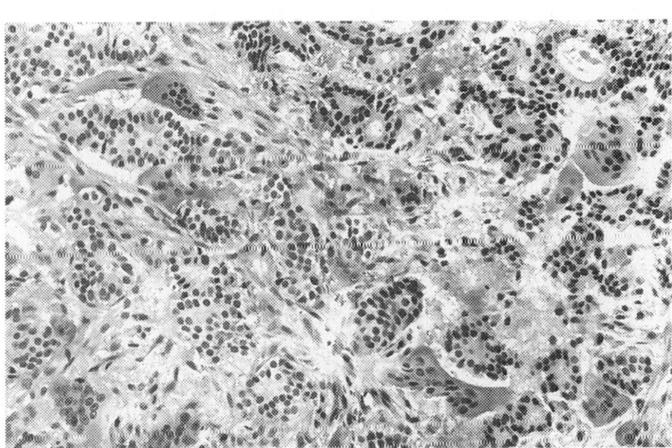

FIG. 21. Invasive carcinoma with osteoclastlike giant cells. The epithelial component of this tumor forms solid nests and glands and has low-grade nuclear features. Numerous multinucleated giant cells resembling osteoclasts are admixed with the neoplastic epithelial cells.

Invasive Carcinoma with Choriocarcinomatous Features

Invasive carcinoma with choriocarcinomatous features is an exceedingly rare form of breast cancer. Only two reports have described the presence of choriocarcinomatous elements (i.e., trophoblastic differentiation) admixed with conventional breast carcinomas.[340,341] The choriocarcinomatous component was associated with invasive ductal carcinoma in one case[340] and with metastatic mucinous carcinoma in the second.[341] The choriocarcinomatous elements in these tumors produce human chorionic gonadotropin.[340] If choriocarcinomatous features are encountered in a breast tumor, the differential diagnosis should include choriocarcinoma metastatic to the breast, as several such cases have been reported.[342,343]

Lipid-Rich Carcinoma

Lipid is commonly present in the cytoplasm of breast cancer cells. Lipid-rich carcinoma, however, is a rare type of invasive breast carcinoma that is characterized by tumor cells containing abundant lipid within their cytoplasm.[344–348] On routine light microscopy, the tumor cells comprising these lesions show vacuolated, clear-cell cytoplasmic features, due to the fact that the lipid is dissolved during tissue processing. The importance of recognizing this tumor lies in the fact that it may mimic other forms of malignancy that may have metastasized to the breast, such as renal cell carcinoma. The prognostic significance of a diagnosis of lipid-rich carcinoma is not currently known.

Glycogen-Rich Carcinoma

Glycogen-rich carcinoma is a rare variant of invasive breast carcinoma characterized by tumor cells that contain abundant glycogen within their cytoplasm.[348–355] As with lipid-rich carcinoma, the intracytoplasmic glycogen is often dissolved during specimen processing, imparting a vacuolated or clear-cell appearance to the tumor cells. Glycogen-rich carcinomas not infrequently are associated with DCIS, and the presence of DCIS may help in distinguishing these lesions from metastatic tumors involving the breast. Although relatively few cases have been reported, some have suggested that these tumors are associated with a more aggressive clinical course than invasive breast cancers of no special type.[355]

Mucinous Cystadenocarcinoma

Mucinous cystadenocarcinoma is a variant of invasive breast carcinoma that is morphologically indistinguishable from mucinous cystadenocarcinoma of the ovary or pancreas.[356] Although these tumors may be associated with the extravasation of mucin, they are otherwise morphologically distinct from conventional mucinous carcinoma of the breast and are therefore considered separately. The importance of recognizing these tumors is that they must be distinguished from metastatic lesions in the breast, particularly those of ovarian origin.[357] The prognostic significance of a diagnosis of primary mucinous cystadenocarcinoma of the breast is currently unknown.

Extramammary Malignancies Metastatic to the Breast

Numerous reports exist of metastatic tumors involving the breast. Secondary tumor deposits in the breast may emanate from the contralateral breast[358] or from virtually any nonmammary site. In one series, metastases to the breast from nonmammary malignancies comprised 1.2% of all malignancies diagnosed in the breast.[264] Because many nonmammary malignancies mimic the features of usual or unusual types of primary breast tumors, distinguishing between the two in a subset of cases can be very difficult, particularly when no history of a prior nonmammary malignancy exists. Nevertheless, this distinction is critical for appropriate patient management.

Metastatic lesions involving the breast almost never occur in the absence of metastases to other sites, even when the breast metastasis is the first clinically detected site. When metastases are detected in the breast, a solitary unilateral lesion is present in 85% of cases; multiple lesions are present in 10% of cases; and diffuse involvement of the breast occurs in 5% of cases.[359] The presence of tumor in ipsilateral axillary lymph nodes does not necessarily imply that the malignancy is a primary breast tumor, as metastatic deposits simultaneously involving the breast and axillary lymph nodes are not infrequent.[359]

Although on mammography, metastatic lesions in the breast can mimic the appearance of primary breast cancers, they are more likely to be multiple, to be bilateral, and to exhibit well-defined margins without evidence of spiculation.[180,357,359] Mammographic microcalcifications associated with metastatic lesions are rare, but have been reported in association with metastatic ovarian tumors.[357,360–364] On ultrasonographic examination, metastatic tumors involving the breast are usually round or ovoid masses with some degree of lobulation and variable internal echoes.[180]

Metastatic tumors to the breast have a variable gross appearance, depending on the type of metastasis. In general, however, these lesions may be single or multiple and are generally well demarcated from the surrounding breast parenchyma. The histologic appearance of these neoplasms is related to the site of origin of the primary tumor. Metastatic lesions most frequently described in the breast include malignant melanoma,[264,358,359,365–369] lung carcinoma,[263,264,359,370–372] prostate carcinoma,[369,370,373–380] and carcinoid tumors from a variety of primary sites.[251–256,381–386] Less frequent metastases to the breast include ovarian carcinoma,[357,360–364] gastric carcinoma,[358,387] renal cell carcinoma,[358,369,387,388] thyroid carcinoma,[369,389] various malignant tumors from the head and neck,[359,390] various types of sarcoma,[357–359,367,391,392] colorectal carcinoma,[393] medulloblastoma,[394] neuroblastoma,[366] malignant mesothelioma,[371] carcinoma of the urinary bladder,[358] endometrial carcinoma,[369] cervical carcinoma,[395] chloroma,[358] and choriocarcinoma.[342,343]

To a variable degree, many of the aforementioned tumors may mimic unusual primary breast carcinomas. Therefore, the pathologist must consider the possibility of metastasis, particularly in a case associated with unusual clinical, mammographic, or pathologic features. Relevant information (e.g., a history of prior malignancy or simultaneous unexplained masses occurring elsewhere) must also be relayed to the pathologist. If a tumor displays unusual histologic findings that raise the possibility of metastases, the pathologist may opt to additionally sample the tumor to look for areas more typical of primary breast carcinoma, as well as associated DCIS. In addition, immunohistochemical stains for a variety of markers may be helpful to provide adjunctive evidence of mammary or nonmammary derivation in a subset of cases.

PATHOLOGIC FEATURES OF BREAST CANCER IN PATIENTS WITH *BRCA1* AND *BRCA2* MUTATIONS

The pathology of the breast cancers that develop in women with a genetic predisposition to this disease as a result of mutations in the breast cancer susceptibility genes *BRCA1* and *BRCA2* has generated considerable interest. Recognition of histologic features that may indicate a genetic predisposition might be useful for providing insight into the function of these genes and for aiding identification of patients in whom screening for these genetic abnormalities might provide a high yield. General agreement exists that *BRCA1*-related cancers are more frequently medullary carcinomas, atypical medullary carcinomas, and high-grade invasive ductal carcinomas than are cancers in patients without this genetic alteration. With regard to individual histologic features, cancers associated with *BRCA1* mutations have a significantly higher mitotic rate, a larger proportion of the tumor with a continuous pushing margin, and more lymphocytic infiltration than sporadic breast cancers. In addition, *BRCA1*-related cancers are less often positive for estrogen and progesterone receptors, are more often aneuploid, more often have a high S-phase fraction, and more often show accumulation of the p53 protein than do sporadic breast cancers.[396–406] However, none of these features, singly or in combination, uniquely identifies a cancer as being related to *BRCA1* mutation.[407] Despite this constellation of adverse features, most studies have indicated that the clinical outcome of patients with *BRCA1*-related cancers appears to be similar to that of patients with sporadic breast cancer.[396,397,399,401,402,408,409]

The histologic features reported in *BRCA2*-related breast cancers have been less consistent. One study noted a significantly higher proportion of tubular-lobular-group cancers (including tubular, lobular, tubulolobular, and invasive cribriform carcinomas) in *BRCA2* mutation carriers than in other patients.[396,397] However, another group found tubular carcinomas to be less common in *BRCA2* mutation carriers.[398] In another small study, the pleomorphic variant of invasive lobular carcinoma was found to be related to *BRCA2* mutation.[406] Some investigators have reported that *BRCA2*-related cancers tend to be of high histologic grade,[398,410] whereas others have not noted a significant difference in histologic grade when *BRCA2*-related cancers are compared with controls.[411]

PATHOLOGIC FACTORS USEFUL IN ASSESSING PROGNOSIS

Considerable interest exists in identifying biological, molecular, and genetic markers that may useful to help assess the prognosis of patients with invasive breast cancer; these are discussed in Chapter 32. However, a considerable amount of useful prognostic information can be obtained from routine pathologic examination of specimens containing breast cancer, without the need for special diagnostic procedures, equipment, or reagents. Clinical follow-up studies have repeatedly demonstrated that features such as axillary lymph node status, tumor size, histologic type, histologic grade, and lymphatic vessel invasion represent powerful and independent prognostic indicators. Other factors have also been shown to provide important prognostic information in many studies.[412–414] In fact, these traditional prognostic factors should be considered the standard against which any new prognostic factors are measured.

The status of the axillary lymph nodes remains the most important prognostic factor for patients with breast cancer, and this is discussed in detail in Chapter 32. This section focuses on pathologic features of the primary tumor that provide important information regarding patient prognosis.

Tumor Size

Numerous studies have demonstrated that the size of an invasive breast cancer is one of the most powerful prognostic factors for both axillary lymph node involvement and clinical outcome.[133,412–424] In a study of almost 25,000 breast cancer cases, Carter et al. demonstrated a linear relationship between tumor size and axillary nodal involvement and between tumor size and survival.[418] The prognostic significance of tumor size is independent of axillary lymph node status and is a particularly valuable prognostic indicator in women with node-negative disease[418,419,423] (Tables 4 and 5). A number of studies have suggested that, even among patients with breast cancers 2 cm and smaller (T1), assessment of tumor size permits further stratification of patients with regard to the likelihood of axillary lymph node involvement and outcome.

TABLE 4. *Five-year survival rates (in percent) according to tumor size and axillary lymph node status*

	Lymph node status		
Tumor size (cm)	Negative	1–3 Positive	≥4 Positive
<2	96.3	87.4	66.0
2–5	89.4	79.9	58.7
>5	82.2	73.0	45.5

Adapted from ref. 418.

TABLE 5. *Five-year survival rates according to tumor size in patients with axillary node–negative breast cancer*

Tumor size (cm)	No. patients	5-year survival (%)
<0.5	269	99.2
0.5–0.9	791	98.3
1.0–1.9	4,668	92.3
2.0–2.9	4,010	90.6
3.0–3.9	2,072	86.2
4.0–4.9	845	84.6
>5.0	809	82.2

Adapted from ref. 418.

In a study of 644 patients with T1 breast cancer from Memorial Sloan-Kettering Cancer Center, the likelihood of axillary nodal involvement was 11% for tumors 0.1 to 0.5 cm, 15% for lesions 0.6 to 1.0 cm, 25% for tumors 1.1 to 1.3 cm, 34% for tumors 1.4 to 1.6 cm, and 43% for cancers 1.7 to 2.0 cm.[420] Furthermore, among node-negative patients treated by mastectomy without adjuvant systemic therapy, those with cancers 1 cm or smaller had a 20-year recurrence-free survival rate of 88%, significantly higher than the 72% recurrence-free survival rate observed for patients with tumors 1.1 to 2.0 cm in size.[133] Substantial variation is seen in the reported rates of axillary node involvement and clinical outcome for patients with small tumors, however, particularly for those with tumors that are 1 cm and smaller[425,426]; not all investigators have observed that patients with tumors 1 cm and smaller have significantly lower rates of axillary node involvement and disease recurrence than those with tumors between 1 and 2 cm.[424,427] Nonetheless, most studies have reported a very favorable clinical outcome for node-negative patients with tumors 1 cm and smaller, with 5- to 10-year disease-free survival rates of 90% or higher.[426]

Accurate measurement of breast cancer size is essential to provide the most clinically meaningful information. Studies of the significance of tumor size in breast cancer have used various methods to determine size, however, including clinical measurement, mammographic assessment, gross measurement, microscopic measurement of the entire lesion, and microscopic measurement of only the invasive component. In some studies, the method used to measure the tumor is not stated. This may at least partially explain differences in observed rates of axillary node involvement and clinical outcome in various studies. General agreement now exists that the most clinically significant measure of tumor size is the size of the invasive component of the lesion as determined from microscopic evaluation. In fact, the 1997 edition of the American Joint Committee on Cancer *Cancer Staging Manual* states that "the pathologic tumor size for classification (T) is a measurement of only the invasive component."[433] This approach appears to be justified, because several studies have indicated that, in many cases, substantial differences exist in the size of the lesion as determined from gross pathologic examination and the size as determined from microscopic measurement of the invasive component, particularly for small lesions. For example, in one series of 118 patients in whom the gross tumor size was measured as 2 cm or smaller, the gross tumor size was smaller than the microscopic size in 31% of cases, larger in 46%, and the same in only 22%.[425] In 35% of these cases, the gross and microscopic tumor sizes differed by more than 3 mm. Similar discrepancies between gross and microscopic size were seen when the analysis was limited to those lesions in which the gross tumor size was measured as smaller than 1 cm.[434] Of greatest importance, however, is the observation that the microscopic size of the invasive component of the tumor is the one that is most closely correlated with prognosis.[425,434,435]

One important but unresolved issue for both pathologists and clinicians is how to assess and report the tumor size in lesions that have more than one focus of invasive cancer, because whether the prognosis is related to the largest single focus or to the cumulative volume of invasive cancer is not known. The results of one study suggested that tubular and tubulolobular carcinomas with multiple foci of invasion were more likely to show axillary lymph node involvement than those lesions characterized by a single focus of invasion.[64] Whether these results can be generalized to other types of invasive breast cancer remains to be determined, however, and additional studies are needed to address this question. At the time of this writing, it seems most prudent for the pathologist to measure microscopically the size of each focus of invasive cancer and to report the individual sizes rather than adding them together.

Histologic Type

As noted in the discussion of the individual histologic types of invasive breast cancer, some special-type lesions are associated with a particularly favorable clinical outcome. Special-type tumors that have consistently been shown to have an excellent prognosis include tubular, invasive cribriform, mucinous, and adenoid cystic carcinomas. Some authors also place tubulolobular carcinomas and papillary carcinomas in this group.[6,193] Moreover, Rosen et al. have shown that the 20-year recurrence-free survival of patients with special-type tumors 1.1 to 3.0 cm in size is similar to that of patients with invasive ductal carcinomas 1

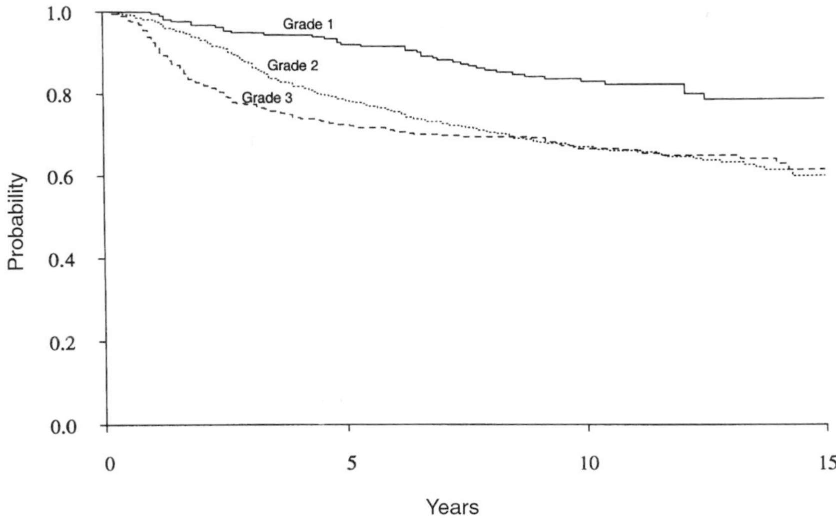

FIG. 22. Kaplan-Meier curves indicating time to distant failure for 1,081 patients with invasive breast cancer according to histologic grade.

cm and smaller (87% and 86%, respectively).[133] Strict diagnostic criteria must be used to observe the favorable outcomes reported for these lesions, however. For example, cancers in which the special type of interest comprises between 75% and 90% of the tumor ("variant types") have a prognosis more favorable than invasive ductal carcinomas, but do not have the same excellent prognosis as special-type lesions that are more homogeneous (i.e., those in which the special type of interest comprises more than 90% of the tumor).[436,437]

Histologic Grade

The importance of tumor grading as a prognostic factor in breast cancer has been clearly demonstrated in numerous clinical-outcome studies. These studies have repeatedly shown higher rates of distant metastasis and poorer survival in patients with higher grade (poorly differentiated) tumors, independent of lymph node status and tumor size.[28,135,413,438–446] In fact, tumor grading has been shown to be of prognostic value even in patients with breast cancers 1 cm and smaller.[426] Although a variety of methods of nuclear and histologic grading have been used in these studies, as noted earlier, the grading method in most widespread clinical use is the histologic grading system of Elston and Ellis (see Table 2).[28,443] These authors advocate the use of histologic grading for all types of invasive breast cancer, although they acknowledge that histologic grade partially defines some of these histologic types (for example, tubular carcinomas are by definition grade 1 and medullary carcinomas are grade 3 lesions). However, these authors have also pointed out that the combination of histologic type and grade provides a more accurate assessment of prognosis than histologic type alone.[447]

The results of a study of 1,081 invasive breast cancers from patients treated with conservative surgery and radiation therapy at the Joint Center for Radiation Therapy in Boston illustrate the value of this histologic grading system and also point up some important caveats in the interpretation of grading data. In that study, time to distant recurrence was greatest for grade 1 cancers and least for grade 3 tumors (Fig. 22). Furthermore, in a polychotomous logistic regression analysis, increasing tumor grade was associated with a significantly increased risk of distant metastasis at 10 years.[445] The hazard ratios for distant failure among the three grades were not constant over time, however. In particular, the risk of distant metastasis was highest for grade 3 tumors only within the first 3 years of follow-up. Beyond that time, the risk of metastasis associated with grade 2 tumors was actually higher than the risk associated with grade 3 cancers (Fig. 23). These observations emphasize that the length of follow-up must be taken into consideration in interpreting data relating histologic grade to clinical outcome. They further suggest that grade may best be viewed as an indicator of time to recurrence rather than as an indicator of absolute rate of recurrence.

Histologic grade also appears to provide useful information with regard to response to chemotherapy and may therefore be of value as a predictive factor. The results of several studies have suggested that the presence of high histologic grade is associated with a better response to certain chemotherapy regimens than the presence of low histologic grade.[448,449]

A frequent criticism of the use of histologic grading is that this assessment is subjective and, as a consequence, prone to considerable interobserver variability.[450–453] Most of the studies that have suggested this shortcoming have used grading systems that lack precisely defined criteria or did not attempt to educate the participating pathologists in the use of the system evaluated. Studies have indicated that the use of strict criteria and guidelines for histologic grading can result in acceptable levels of interobserver agreement and also identify areas that might benefit from refinement. In one of these studies, six pathologists graded 75 invasive

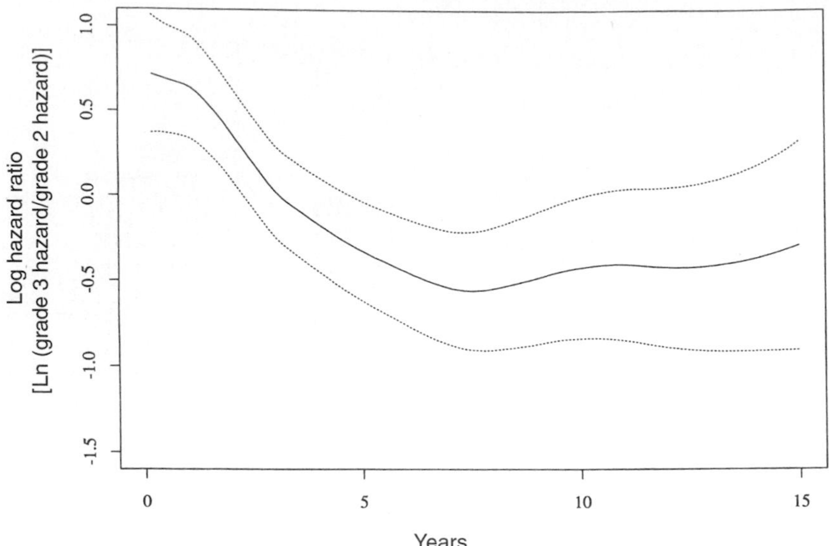

FIG. 23. Hazard ratio for distant recurrence for patients with histologic grade 3 tumors compared with those with grade 2 tumors. Distant recurrence is greater for patients with grade 3 tumors than for those with grade 2 tumors when the curve is above zero, and less for those with grade 3 than for those with grade 2 when the curve is below zero (*dotted lines* represent 95% confidence limits).

ductal carcinomas using the Elston and Ellis grading system.[454] Moderate to substantial agreement was found with regard to overall histologic grade. Substantial agreement existed on tubule formation, moderate agreement on mitotic count, and near-moderate agreement on nuclear pleomorphism as determined by generalized kappa statistics. These authors concluded that this grading system is suitable for use in clinical practice and suggested that efforts to improve agreement on nuclear grading would be of value in further fostering agreement in histologic grading. In another study, a substantial level of agreement (kappa statistic, 0.70) was found among 25 pathologists who used the Elston and Ellis grading system, albeit on a small number of cases.[455]

Lymphatic Vessel Invasion

The presence of tumor emboli within small, thin-walled vascular spaces in the breast is most often interpreted as lymphatic vessel invasion. In fact, some of the structures categorized as lymphatic vessels using these criteria actually represent blood capillaries and postcapillary venules. Although some authors have advocated use of the term *vascular invasion* without further qualification to circumvent this issue,[456] the term *lymphatic vessel invasion* has become entrenched in both the pathology and clinical literature and is likely to remain in common use.

In patients with breast cancer, lymphatic vessel invasion has been shown in numerous studies to be an important and independent prognostic factor. Its major clinical value is in identifying node-negative patients at increased risk for axillary lymph node involvement[429,456–463] and adverse outcome.[441,458,459,464–472] The identification of lymphatic vessel invasion may be of particular importance in patients with T1 node-negative breast cancers, because this finding may permit the identification of a subset of patients at increased risk for axillary lymph node involvement and distant metastasis in this group with an otherwise favorable prognosis. For example, in one study, lymphatic vessel invasion was the only clinical or pathologic factor associated with lymph node metastasis in patients with tumors 1 cm and smaller (T1a, T1b). In that study, lymph node involvement was present in 4 of 7 patients whose tumors showed lymphatic vessel invasion (57%) compared with only 1 of 100 patients without lymphatic vessel invasion.[426] In another study of 461 patients with T1 node-negative breast cancer, patients with tumors lacking lymphatic vessel invasion had a 20-year survival rate of 81%, compared with a rate of 64% for those whose tumors exhibited lymphatic vessel invasion.[441] Similar findings have been reported by others,[432,466,467] even when the analysis is restricted to the subset of T1 breast cancers that are 1 cm and smaller.[432,472]

As with histologic grade, the ability of pathologists to reproducibly identify lymphatic vessel invasion has been challenged. For example, in one study, three pathologists concurred on the presence or absence of lymphatic vessel invasion in only 12 of 35 cases.[473] A higher level of interobserver agreement has been noted in other studies, however.[456–459,467] In one of these studies, in which stringent criteria were used, an 85% level of overall agreement between two pathologists was found for the presence or absence of lymphatic vessel invasion.[456] The use of strict criteria for the identification of lymphatic vessel invasion is therefore imperative. Lymphatic vessels are thin-walled vascular spaces that have an endothelial lining and lack mural smooth muscle and elastic fibers (Fig. 24). Artifactual retraction of the stroma is commonly present around tumor cell nests within invasive breast cancers and in ducts harboring DCIS, and this can be difficult or impossible to distinguish from true lymphatic vessel invasion (Fig. 25).[456–458,473] For this reason, the identification of lymphatic vessel invasion is best performed in the peritumoral

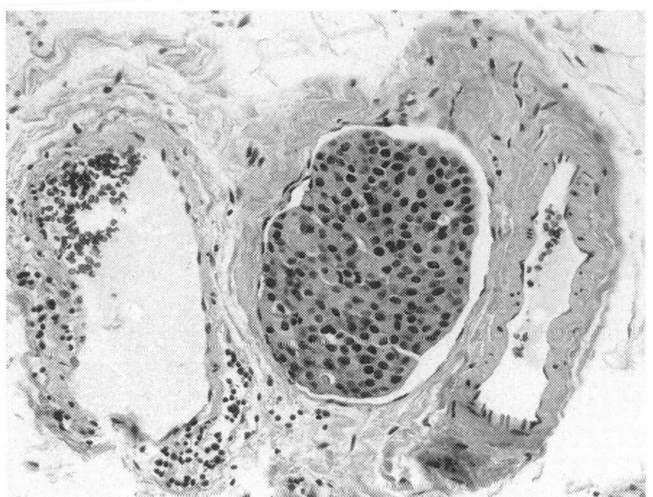

FIG. 24. Lymphatic vessel invasion. A tumor embolus is present within a thin-walled, endothelial-lined space.

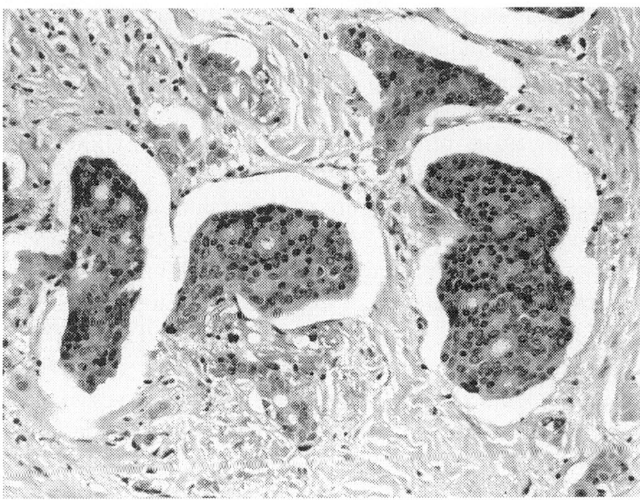

FIG. 25. Retraction artifact. Tumor cells are present within artifactual tissue spaces, created by retraction of the surrounding stroma. These spaces lack an endothelial lining.

region.[458] Unequivocal lymphatic vessel invasion within the tumor is clinically significant, however, and should not be disregarded.[457] Attention to the topographic pattern of presumed lymphatic spaces is also helpful in distinguishing between true lymphatic vessel invasion and artifact.[457] Lymphatic spaces are often present in close proximity to other vascular structures that have well-defined muscular walls and are present in the interlobular stroma.

A number of investigators have evaluated the use of immunohistochemical stains for endothelial cells (including stains for factor VIII–related antigen, CD34, *Ulex europaeus* agglutinin I, and blood group isoantigens) and basement membrane components as an aid in the identification of lymphatic vessel invasion.[471,474–480] These stains have been of limited value in this context, however. In particular, immunostains for blood group isoantigens and *Ulex* are not specific for endothelial cells and show reactivity with normal and malignant mammary epithelial cells in some cases. False-negative staining is not infrequently seen with the vascular endothelial markers, particularly factor VIII–related antigen.[471,480] CD34 is not specific for endothelial cells, as anti-CD34 antibodies can stain stromal cells around tumor cell nests and blood vessels.[480] Immunostains for the basement membrane components laminin and type IV collagen are unable to distinguish between vascular structures and mammary ducts and lobules.[471] Therefore, lymphatic vessel invasion is best assessed on routine hematoxylin-eosin–stained sections using strict diagnostic criteria.

In some cases, determining whether a collection of tumor cells within a given space represents unequivocal lymphatic vessel invasion may be difficult or impossible, even with the application of stringent guidelines. The significance of such indeterminate foci is not clear at this time. Pinder et al. analyzed the clinical implications of "probable vascular invasion," defined as the presence of tumor cells "in a space with the appearances of a vessel but without a clear endothelial layer."[456] In their study, the prognosis of patients whose tumors exhibited probable vascular invasion was intermediate between that of patients with and without vascular invasion. Node-negative and node-positive patients were included in the analysis, however, and the significance of "probable vascular invasion" in node-negative patients is not reported. In an analysis of 746 node-negative patients treated at the Joint Center for Radiation Therapy, the 10-year actuarial distant failure rate for patients with definite lymphatic vessel invasion was 34%, significantly higher than for patients without lymphatic vessel invasion (20%). Of note, patients whose tumors were categorized as indeterminate for lymphatic vessel invasion had a 23% distant failure rate, similar to that of patients without lymphatic invasion and significantly better than that of patients with definite lymphatic vessel invasion.

Other Factors

A number of other histologic factors have been reported to have prognostic value in patients with invasive breast cancer. The presence of blood vessel invasion (i.e., invasion of veins and arteries) has been reported to have an adverse effect on clinical outcome. Broad variation is found in the reported incidence of blood vessel invasion, however, ranging from less than 5% to almost 50%.[3,460,466,467,481–485] This disparity is due to a variety of factors, including the nature of the patient population, the criteria and methodology used to determine the presence of blood vessel invasion, and the occasional difficulty in distinguishing blood vessels from mammary ducts. Some studies use the term *blood vessel invasion* to denote those vascular structures that possess a muscular or elastic tissue component in their walls, whereas others also include thin-walled vessels of capillary caliber, many of which probably represent lymphatic spaces. Furthermore, some studies have based the evaluation for blood vessel invasion on examination of hematoxylin-eosin–stained sections, whereas others have used elastic tissue stains. In the authors' experience, invasion of arterial- and venous-caliber vascular structures is uncommon. In the long-term follow-up study performed at Memorial Sloan-Kettering Cancer Center, blood vessel invasion was identified in 14% of patients with T1 N0 cancers and in 22% with T1 N1 lesions using elastic tissue stains.[441] A significantly worse outcome was seen for patients with blood vessel invasion than for those without in both groups in that study.

The prognostic significance of tumor necrosis has also been investigated in a number of studies.[467,486–489] In most studies, the presence of necrosis has been associated with an adverse clinical outcome,[486–489] although in one of these studies, necrosis was associated with a worse prognosis only within the first 2 years after diagnosis.[488]

A number of issues must be addressed before tumor necrosis is accepted as an important prognostic factor. First, the extent of necrosis that must be present to be considered clinically significant requires more precise definition. Second, the presence of necrosis is highly correlated with other features associated with a poor prognosis, such as larger tumor size and high histologic grade,[445,486] and whether the adverse prognostic influence of necrosis is independent of these other factors is not clear. Additional studies using multivariate analysis are needed to address this question.

The relationship between clinical outcome and the extent of mononuclear inflammatory cell infiltrate in association with invasive breast cancers has also been investigated. The presence of a prominent mononuclear cell infiltrate has been correlated in some studies with high histologic grade.[445] The prognostic significance of this finding is controversial, however; some studies note an adverse effect of a prominent mononuclear cell infiltrate on clinical outcome,[490–494] and others observe either no significant effect or a beneficial effect.[440,466,490,495]

The presence of perineural invasion is sometimes observed in invasive breast cancers. This phenomenon is often seen in association with lymphatic vessel invasion, but it has not been shown to be an independent prognostic factor.[496]

The extent of DCIS associated with invasive cancers has also been studied as a potential prognostic factor. Numerous investigators have shown that the presence of an extensive intraductal component is a prognostic factor for local recurrence in the breast in patients treated with conservative surgery and radiation therapy when the status of the excision margins is unknown. More recent studies, however, have indicated that this factor is not an independent predictor of local recurrence after conservative surgery and radiation therapy when the microscopic margin status is taken into consideration (reviewed in Schnitt[87]). Silverberg and Chitale reported an inverse relationship between the amount of DCIS and both the risk of axillary lymph node metastasis and the 5-year survival rate in a series of patients with invasive ductal carcinoma treated by mastectomy.[18] In another series of 573 patients with invasive ductal carcinoma treated by mastectomy, however, no significant relationship was seen between the extent of intraductal involvement and either recurrence or survival.[497] Similarly, among 533 patients with invasive carcinoma treated with conservative surgery and radiation therapy, the presence of an extensive intraductal component was not associated with the risk of distant metastasis, according to a multiple logistic regression analysis.[498] Therefore, although the extent of associated DCIS is a consideration in the local management of patients treated with breast-conserving therapy, it does not appear to be a significant prognostic factor with regard to distant metastasis or survival.

Combination of Prognostic Factors

Although a variety of prognostic factors have been reported for patients with invasive breast cancer, how best to integrate these factors to assess patient outcome and formulate therapeutic decisions is an unresolved issue.[499] Several authors have developed prognostic indices for this purpose that take into account various combinations of factors. One of these, the Nottingham Prognostic Index, considers tumor size, lymph node status, and histologic grade. This index has been used to stratify patients with breast cancer into good, moderate, and poor prognostic groups with annual mortality rates of 3%, 7%, and 30%, respectively.[500] Another group of investigators has proposed a prognostic index that combines tumor size, lymph node status, and mitotic index (Morphometric Prognostic Index).[501] This index has been shown to be a useful prognostic discriminator for premenopausal patients with both node-negative and node-positive disease. Although prognostic indices such as these have not yet been widely accepted into clinical practice, they represent important attempts to refine prognostication in patients with invasive breast cancer.

SPECIMEN PROCESSING

A variety of types of breast specimens are encountered by the surgical pathologist in daily practice. Appropriate processing of these specimens is necessary to obtain the maximum clinically relevant information from them.

Core-Needle Biopsy

In contrast to fine-needle aspiration, which provides material for cytologic evaluation, core-needle biopsy yields tissue fragments suitable for routine histologic examination. Core-needle biopsy has been used for many years for the evaluation of palpable breast lesions. Core-needle biopsy using image-directed guidance methods (i.e., stereotactic mammography and ultrasonography) has been used increasingly for the evaluation of nonpalpable breast lesions. Core-needle biopsy is discussed in detail in Chapter 13. With regard to pathologic processing, core-needle biopsy specimens should be submitted for microscopic evaluation in their entirety, and drying and distortion of the specimens should be avoided. In most practices, several levels are cut from each paraffin block to ensure adequate sampling. Immunohistochemical evaluation of hormone receptors and a wide variety of other biological markers can be readily performed on core-needle biopsy specimens.[502] Immediate diagnosis is rarely needed, and the use of frozen sections is discouraged because of the small size of these specimens. If an immediate evaluation is needed, however, touch-imprint cytology can provide highly accurate results without compromising the specimen.[503]

Incisional Biopsy

Incisional biopsies should be submitted completely for histopathologic examination. As for core-needle biopsy specimens, these specimens are suitable for the evaluation of hormone-receptor status and other biological markers.

Excisional Biopsy (Lumpectomy, Partial Mastectomy) Performed for a Palpable Mass

Careful macroscopic examination of excisional biopsy specimens is an essential component of their evaluation. At a minimum, every breast excision should be measured in three dimensions. If a palpable tumor is present, it should also be measured in three dimensions, and its relationship to overlying skin or underlying fascia or skeletal muscle, if present, should be noted. The distance of any macroscopically evident tumor from the margins of excision should also be recorded.

Numerous studies have now demonstrated that the presence of carcinoma at the final microscopic margins of breast excision specimens is a significant and independent risk factor for local recurrence in patients with invasive breast cancer treated with conservative surgery and radiation therapy.[504–512] Therefore, the status of the microscopic margins is one of the major factors considered in determining patient suitability for this treatment approach. In view of the importance of margin assessment, an understanding of technical and interpretive issues that may influence the categorization of the margin status is in order.

Methods of Margin Evaluation

Accurate assessment of the microscopic margins of a specimen requires that the specimen be presented to the pathologist as a single, intact tissue fragment. The pathologist may find it difficult or impossible to evaluate the margins of specimens that have been previously incised or that arrive in the pathology laboratory in more than one fragment. Ideally, the intact specimen should be oriented by the surgeon by means of sutures, clips, or a diagram. Specimen orientation is of value in the event that a positive margin is identified, because this information can be used to direct further surgery to a particular area of margin involvement rather than reexcising the entire biopsy site. In this way, the amount of tissue removed can be minimized, thereby optimizing the cosmetic result. Furthermore, knowledge that a positive margin is the deep margin abutting pectoral fascia is valuable, because even mastectomy may not improve the margin of concern in such instances.

A number of methods are available for microscopic margin evaluation.[513] In the method most commonly used, the specimen surface is painted with an insoluble ink or dye before sectioning. If the specimen has been oriented by the surgeon, the margins may be inked in different colors to retain orientation and to permit the identification of specific margins on histopathologic examination. After inking, the specimen is sectioned through the equatorial plane ("bread-loafed"), and sections perpendicular to the inked tissue edges are obtained and submitted for microscopic evaluation. With this method, the precise distance between cancer cells and the inked margin can be determined histologically. Several technical difficulties exist in the evaluation of inked margins, however. First, ink placed on the surface of the specimen tends to track down into the substance of the specimen through defects in the surface. This may create difficulties in defining the true margin of excision on microscopic examination. In addition, the surfaces of breast excisions are highly complex and irregular, and the surface area of some specimens is quite large. Therefore, margin assessment using the inked margin method is highly subject to sampling error. For example, some have estimated that, using this method, complete examination of a spherical 2-cm specimen would require in excess of 3,000 sections.[514] A further problem in the evaluation of margins is the lack of uniformly accepted definitions of "positive," "negative," and "close" margins. Pathologists generally agree that tumor present at an inked surface of the specimen represents a positive margin. The definition of a negative margin is more variable, however. Some authors believe that unless tumor is identified directly at the inked surface, the margin should be considered negative. For example, in the NSABP B-06 protocol, the presence of a few adipocytes or collagen fibers between the tumor and the inked surface was sufficient for a margin to be classified as negative.[515] Others require that the edge of the tumor be some arbitrary minimum distance (e.g., 5 mm) from the inked surface for the margin to be categorized as negative. At the authors' institution, a margin is regarded as positive when tumor cells are present directly at the inked tissue edge. If the cancer cells do not reach the tissue edge, the closest distance of the tumor to the margin is reported in millimeters or fractions thereof. In an analysis of data from the Joint Center for Radiation Therapy, patients with tumor cells 1 mm or less from the inked surface ("close" margins) were found to have a local recurrence rate similar to patients with tumor cells more than 1 mm from the inked surface ("negative" margins). In that study, the 5-year crude local recurrence rates were 2% for patients with close margins and 3% for those with negative margins. In contrast, patients with positive margins had a 5-year crude local recurrence rate of 16%.[504,505]

To overcome the limitations of the inked margin method, some authors have proposed an alternative method of margin evaluation, in which some or all of the surface of the specimen is peeled or shaved and these tangentially obtained (*en face*) sections are submitted for histologic examination.[514,516] In this method, a margin is considered positive when cancer cells are present anywhere on the histologic sections of these margins. The advantage of this method is that it permits examination of a large proportion of the specimen's surface with relatively few sections. In a study in which shaved margins and inked margins were simultaneously examined in the same breast excision specimens, however, tumor cells were present at the inked margin in only 55% of cases in which the shaved margins were considered positive.[516] Thus, if the inked margin method is considered the gold standard, the shaved margin method results in the categorization of a large number of patients as having positive margins when, in fact, no cancer exists at the inked surface of the specimen (false-positives). These findings have several important implications. The finding of a negative shaved margin is likely to be associated with a very low risk of local recurrence, given the known low risk of local recurrence in patients with negative inked margins and the extensive sampling with the use of the shaved margin technique. The significance of a positive shaved margin is less certain, because the cancer in a shaved margin section could be as far as 2 to 3 mm from the inked tissue edge, depending on the thickness of the shaved margin. Such tumors would therefore have been categorized as having close or negative margins by the standard inked margin method. As noted above, at our institution, patients having tumors with either close or negative inked margins have a very low rate of local recurrence.[504,505] Thus, categorizing the margins of these patients as positive using the shaved margin method could result in their being considered poor candidates for conservative surgery and radiation therapy, when in truth they may be good candidates. This could result in unnecessary additional surgery or even mastectomy in these patients.

A third method of margin evaluation has been proposed. In this method, the surgeon removes arcs of additional tissue from the medial, lateral, inferior, superior, and deep walls of the biopsy cavity immediately after the surgical specimen has been excised. These are then submitted to the pathologist as separate specimens and processed individually.[517] The purported advantage of this method is that the marginal tissue is obtained from the patient rather than the specimen. These are shaved margins, however, and are subject to the problems regarding shaved margin evaluation cited above, as well as to sampling error.

Virtually all of the clinical studies in which margin status has been related to local recurrence risk are based on evaluation of inked margins. Generalizing these results to patients who have margins evaluated in a different manner may not be appropriate. Therefore, clinicians formulating therapeutic options for patients with breast cancer must understand how the margins from that patient were evaluated, particularly if the patient had her surgery at another institution.

Intraoperative Evaluation of Margins

Given the clinical importance of microscopic margin evaluation, some authors have suggested that margins of breast specimens should be evaluated intraoperatively with frozen sections or by cytologic evaluation using touch preparations or scrapings from the surface of the specimen.[518–523] The theoretical advantage of this intraoperative approach is that it could reduce the need for a second surgical procedure in patients with positive margins in the initial excision specimen. Although frozen sections may be of value in evaluating a grossly close margin of particular concern to the surgeon, routinely performing intraoperative margin assessment of grossly negative margins is more problematic. A few studies have suggested that accurate frozen section results can be obtained on margins of breast specimens.[518,519] However, these studies probably underestimated the false-negative rate for frozen sections due to the limited permanent section evaluation of margins considered negative on frozen section. Several potential problems exist with the routine use of frozen sections for margin evaluation. First, performing frozen sections on grossly negative margins of breast specimens is technically problematic, because these margins are typically composed primarily of fat. Obtaining satisfactory frozen sections of fatty tissue is extremely difficult. Furthermore, certain lesions, such as intraductal proliferative lesions, may be difficult to categorize definitively on frozen section, and freezing may create artifacts and distortion that may preclude accurate evaluation of these lesions, even on the subsequent permanent sections. For this reason, frozen section evaluation has largely been abandoned for nonpalpable, mammographically detected breast lesions and for grossly benign breast biopsies. Finally, frozen section evaluation of margins represents more limited sampling than is feasible by permanent section evaluation. Cytologic evaluation of margins is also problematic. First, interpretation of such specimens requires expertise in breast cytopathology, and this expertise may not be available at all institutions or among all pathologists at a given institution. Second, limitations exist even for experienced cytopathologists. For example, reliably distinguishing between atypical ductal hyperplasia and low-grade ductal carcinoma on cytologic material is impossible.

The premise underlying the use of intraoperative margin evaluation is that the surgeon excises more tissue if one or more margins are involved. The ultimate consequence of this endeavor could well be mastectomy. In fact, in one study evaluating the use of frozen sections, 7 of 21 patients who had positive margins on frozen section underwent mastectomy at the time of operation.[519] Conversion to mastectomy while under anesthesia would not be acceptable to many patients. In current practice, the majority of women prefer to have time to discuss their therapeutic choices, including the possibility of immediate reconstruction should mastectomy be deemed necessary by the surgeon. Furthermore, many women for whom mastectomy is recommended seek additional opinions regarding their treatment options.

Another argument against the routine use of intraoperative margin evaluation is related to the fact that, although margin status is clearly important, it should not be considered in isolation and needs to be interpreted in light of other clinical and pathologic information. One consideration in evaluating the significance of a positive margin relates to the overall prognosis of the patient. For example, focal margin involvement may be of less concern in patients with multiple positive lymph nodes. In such patients, the risk of distant metastasis is substantial and may well outweigh the risk of local recurrence. Furthermore, most patients with multiple positive nodes receive adjuvant systemic therapy, and this has been shown to further reduce the risk of local recurrence in patients treated with conservative surgery and radiation therapy.[524,525] Determination of the nodal status requires thorough permanent section evaluation of the lymph nodes. In addition, among node-negative patients, pathologic characteristics of the primary tumor as determined from permanent section evaluation (e.g., size, histologic grade, and presence of lymphatic vessel invasion) help determine the need for adjuvant systemic therapy.

Finally, the need for intraoperative evaluation of margins may become less of an issue with the increasing use of core-needle biopsy as the initial procedure to diagnose breast cancer. Several studies have shown that, among patients who have a core biopsy diagnosis of carcinoma, the likelihood is increased that the surgeon can perform a complete excision of the lesion in a single surgical procedure without the need for intraoperative margin assessment.[526,527]

Unresolved Issues

A number of issues regarding microscopic margin evaluation remain to be resolved. First, the results of one study suggested that some patients with only limited microscopic margin involvement have a lower risk of local recurrence after conservative surgery and radiation therapy than patients with more extensive margin involvement.[504,505] Additional studies are needed, however, to further evaluate the relationship between the extent of margin involvement and the risk of local recurrence. This research, in turn, will help to determine if some patients with only limited margin involvement can be safely treated with conservative surgery and radiation therapy. Second, the relative importance of invasive cancer and DCIS at the margins needs to be evaluated. Third, given the limitations of current methods for margin assessment, alternative methods to assess the extent of the lesion and adequacy of excision need to be developed. These may include newer radiologic imaging modalities, such as digital mammography, magnetic resonance imaging, and positron emission tomography.[528] In addition, alternative methods for pathologic evaluation of the margins need to be explored. One approach may be the use of molecular markers to analyze microscopically normal–appearing breast tissue adjacent to the cancer. In one study, loss of heterozygosity at several chromosomal loci was identified in benign breast tissue adjacent to breast cancers.[529] The authors of this study postulated that these chromosomal abnormalities may define an area of increased risk for the development of cancer and may account for some local recurrences in patients with margins categorized as negative by conventional pathologic examination.

Needle-Localization Breast Biopsy for Nonpalpable Lesions

With the increasing use of mammographic screening, a growing number of breast biopsies are performed because of an abnormality detected by mammography in the absence of a palpable mass. In most cases, the needle-localization technique is used to guide the surgeon to the area of mammographic abnormality. Communication among the radiologist, surgeon, and pathologist is essential to ensure proper processing and evaluation of such specimens.[513,530]

The most frequent mammographic abnormalities prompting biopsy are microcalcifications, a soft-tissue density, or a combination of the two. Specimen radiography is a crucial component in the evaluation of these specimens both to document the presence of the lesion detected by mammography and to localize the suspicious area for histologic examination. Although the specimen radiograph may also be of some value in assessing the margins of excision, the overall accuracy of this procedure was only 62% in one study.[531,532]

Several aspects of specimen radiography merit comment. First, the value of magnification views cannot be overemphasized. Such views frequently permit the identification of mammographic abnormalities (particularly microcalcifications) that are not well demonstrated using standard nonmagnified radiographs. Second, many radiologists consider specimen compression to be an essential component of specimen radiography, because this enhances image resolution. Finally, specimen radiographs should always be compared with the preoperative mammograms to be certain that the lesion of concern has been excised. Note, however, that if the biopsy has been performed for a soft-tissue density without calcifications, the lesion may be difficult or impossible to detect on the specimen radiograph, unless it has a well-defined configuration (i.e., a stellate mass or a sharply circumscribed nodule).

After radiography of the intact specimen has demonstrated that the lesion of interest is present within the specimen, this area must be identified by the pathologist. Some specimens contain a grossly evident tumor, in which case further efforts to demonstrate the lesion are not necessary. If no lesion is grossly evident, however, a number of methods can be used to identify the lesion within the specimen. One simple method consists of comparing the gross specimen with the specimen radiograph and placing a pin or needle into the specimen at the site of the mammographic lesion to permit the identification of its location by the prosector. Another method consists of performing the initial specimen radiograph after placing the tissue in a specimen holder that incorporates a grid visible on the radiograph. The holder containing the specimen and the specimen radiograph are then compared to precisely locate the target lesion using the X and Y coordinates of the grid. The preferred method at our institution involves slicing the specimen at 3- to 5-mm intervals and obtaining a radiograph of the sliced specimen. The slices on the radiograph can then be labeled and the tissue slices placed in correspondingly labeled tissue cassettes to permit correlation between the histologic sections and the radiograph of the sliced specimen. In any case, as for biopsies performed for palpable lesions, the specimen should not be incised before the surface is painted with ink, so the surgical margins can be evaluated on the permanent sections.

Once the breast tissue containing the mammographically detected lesion is submitted, the extent to which the remaining breast tissue is sampled for microscopic evaluation varies among different institutions, particularly in cases in which no grossly apparent abnormality is noted. Although submitting such specimens for histologic evaluation in their entirety would permit the highest level of detection of clinically significant lesions, such exhaustive examination often is not feasible. In a study of 157 consecutive breast biopsies performed because of the mammographic finding of microcalcifications,[533] 49 of 50 cancers (98%) and 14 of 19 atypical hyperplasias (74%) were associated with the radiographic calcifications. If histologic examination had been restricted to the areas of the specimen containing the radiographic microcalcifications, 38% fewer tissue blocks would have been processed, but one case of noncomedo DCIS and five cases of atypical hyperplasia would have gone undetected. If microscopic evaluation had also included all additional tissue consisting of fibrous parenchyma, all 50 carcinomas and 17 of the 19 atypical hyperplasias would have been detected, and 20% fewer tissue blocks would have been processed. These findings indicate that, for breast biopsies containing microcalcifications, restricting histologic examination to the areas of radiographic calcifications results in a high level of detection of clinically significant lesions and a considerable reduction in the amount of tissue processed. In addition, submitting the fibrous parenchymal tissue component of the specimen further improves the likelihood of detecting such lesions.

In some cases, the initial histologic sections of breast specimens containing radiographic calcifications fail to reveal microscopic calcifications, even when the specimen radiograph clearly indicated that the calcifications are contained within the specimen. Several explanations for this are possible. First, the calcifications may be composed of calcium oxalate rather than the usual calcium phosphate.[534–536] Both types of calcium deposits produce the mammographic appearance of microcalcifications, but they appear different histologically. The basophilic nature of calcium phosphate deposits is well known and easily recognized by pathologists. In contrast, in hematoxylin-eosin–stained sections, calcium oxalate deposits are pale and refractile and may be difficult to identify using routine microscopy. Examination of such specimens under polarized light readily demonstrates this type of calcification, however. If examination under polarized light still reveals no microscopic evidence of calcifications, other possibilities must be considered. For example, the paraffin blocks may not have been cut deeply enough to provide histologic sections that demonstrate the calcifications. To investigate this possibility, the blocks may themselves be radiographed; any blocks containing radiographic calcifications should be cut more deeply, until the calcifications are microscopically identified. Finally, in some cases, larger calcifications may shatter out of the block during sectioning and therefore are not demonstrable on histologic sections. The pathologist must make every effort to identify histologically the lesion for which the surgical excision was performed.

Several potential pitfalls exist in the histologic examination of needle-localization breast biopsies. Although some authors have reported that frozen section diagnosis can be performed on nonpalpable breast lesions with a high degree of accuracy,[537,538] the routine use of frozen sections to examine such lesions should be discouraged.[539,540] Many of these lesions are small, and it may not be possible both to perform a frozen section and to retain a sufficient amount of lesional tissue for permanent sections. Moreover, artifacts resulting from freezing the specimen may make it extremely difficult or impossible to accurately evaluate the permanent sections. Finally, at many institutions, the results of the frozen section analysis do not alter the immediate management of the patient. For these reasons, nonpalpable breast lesions are usually best evaluated on permanent sections only.

Calcifications are commonly identified in histologic sections of breast tissue, even in breast biopsies performed for indications other than mammographic microcalcifications. Therefore, to ensure accurate mammographic-pathologic correlation, the calcifications identified histologically should correspond to the mammographic calcifications. For example, the histologic identification of a few small calcifications in normal lobules is not sufficient to explain the presence of linear, branching calcifications on a mammogram. In such a case, additional effort should be made to identify microscopically calcifications that more closely correspond to those seen mammographically. Finally, a few studies[541–544] have indicated that needling procedures, such as fine-needle aspiration, core-needle biopsy, and wire localization, can induce a number of artifacts in subsequent breast excision specimens, including displacement of benign ductal epithelium or DCIS cells into the stroma or into vascular spaces. This can result in an erroneous diagnosis of invasive or intralymphatic or intravascular cancer in a patient with benign disease or DCIS. Pathologists must therefore be aware of this potential diagnostic pitfall.

Reexcision Specimens

Some patients with breast cancer who are considered candidates for conservative surgery and radiotherapy require a reexcision of the initial tumor site. The size of the reexcision specimens is quite variable and at the authors' institution has ranged from 2 cm to larger than 20 cm in greatest dimension; the average size is approximately 6 cm. This variation depends on the location of the primary site (obtaining a wide margin around a very superficial or a very deep tumor is difficult), the ease with which the surgeon can identify the tumor site, and the size of the breast. As for primary excision specimens, the surgeon should present the reexcision specimen to the pathologist intact, and sutures may be used by the surgeon to orient the specimen. The surface of the specimen should be examined for defects that might suggest that the previous biopsy site has been cut across and therefore has not been entirely removed. Before incising the specimen, as for primary excisions, the outer surface of the reexcision should be inked. Subsequent processing is similar to that described for primary excisions and depends on the size of the specimen. In most cases, hemorrhage, fat necrosis, and fibrosis in the vicinity of the tumor site render accurate gross evaluation for the presence or absence of residual neoplasm extremely difficult, if not impossible. This judgment is best deferred to examination of the permanent sections. Frozen sections on reexcision specimens are usually not necessary and should be performed only on the rare occasion when a margin of excision is grossly suspicious for involvement by malignancy.

Only limited data exist on the most cost-effective method of sampling reexcision specimens, which are often large and rarely exhibit grossly identifiable areas of carcinoma. One study suggested that, for grossly benign reexcisions, submitting two tissue blocks for each centimeter of the largest specimen diameter is sufficient in most cases to provide the clinically essential information needed from these specimens.[545]

Mastectomy Specimens

The methods used to examine a mastectomy specimen and the extent of sampling depend, in part, on the type of surgical procedure and the reasons for which the procedure was performed. Nonetheless, several aspects of the examination apply to all mastectomy specimens. Ideally, the specimen should be oriented for the pathologist by the surgeon, particularly for mastectomy specimens that do not have a contiguous axillary tail. The following features should be recorded before any mastectomy specimen is incised: the specimen weight; the overall dimensions; descriptions and measurements of the skin, areola, nipple, and any incisions or scars; composition of the deep margin (i.e., presence of fascia or muscle); description of the axillary tail (if present); and the location and size of any palpable tumor, with careful attention paid to its relationship to the overlying skin and deep margin.

Before the specimen is incised, the deep margin should be painted with ink to facilitate its identification on histologic sections. Superficial margins should not be inked, because no clinical studies have evaluated the significance of tumor involvement of these surfaces of the specimen. Further examination of the specimen is best performed by placing the specimen skin side down and making multiple parallel incisions through the deep aspect 1 to 2 cm apart, leaving the skin intact. The cut surfaces of each slice should be examined carefully for the presence of grossly evident tumor or biopsy site.

Sampling for histologic examination should include sections of any grossly apparent tumor or biopsy site, the deep margin, the overlying skin (including scars), the nipple, and random sections of the grossly unremarkable quadrants of breast tissue. If the specimen is a radical mastectomy (which is uncommon in current practice), the interpectoral fascia should be examined for the presence of Rotter's nodes.

In a number of situations, more extensive examination of a mastectomy specimen may be required. In patients with DCIS, particularly those with larger lesions, many sections may be required to determine the presence of stromal invasion, a finding of clinical importance. Similarly, extensive sampling may be required to identify a carcinoma in the breast in patients who have Paget's disease of the nipple and in patients who present with metastatic carcinoma in an axillary lymph node and an "occult" primary tumor. In these situations, radiography of the mastectomy specimen (either intact or after it has been sectioned) may be of value in directing histologic sampling. Finally, some patients with locally advanced breast cancer undergo chemotherapy or radiation therapy before mastectomy. The pathologist must carefully examine the mastectomy specimen to assess the therapeutic response and to document the morphologic effects of treatment on the tumor and on the nontumorous breast tissue.[546]

Axillary Lymph Nodes

Pathologic evaluation of axillary lymph nodes is used to assess prognosis and to determine the need for adjuvant systemic therapy. Traditionally, axillary lymph nodes have been submitted to the pathologist either as part of a mastectomy specimen (usually in contiguity with the breast) or as a separate axillary dissection specimen. In either case, initial pathologic examination should include gross inspection and palpation for lymph nodes. A variety of methods are available for further examination of these specimens. The simplest method consists of careful dissection of the adipose tissue in the fresh state to retrieve the excised lymph nodes. The number, size range, and gross appearance of the identified nodes should be recorded. An alternative method consists of immersing the axillary adipose tissue in Bouin's solution for several hours before attempting to locate the lymph nodes. When this method is used, the lymph nodes appear white and stand out against the surrounding adipose tissue, which stains yellow. Some investigators have advocated radiographic imaging of the axillary dissection specimen[547,548] or clearing of the axillary adipose tissue with substances such as methyl salicylate[549] to assist in the identification of lymph nodes. Although these methods do increase the number of nodes identified, the additional information obtained is of questionable clinical value. For example, Morrow et al.[550] found that clearing the fat in 42 axillary dissections led to a 30% increase in the number of lymph nodes identified. Among 31 patients considered to be node negative after routine manual dissection, however, none of the additional nodes identified by specimen clearing contained metastases. The only patients in whom clearing the axillary fat yielded lymph nodes containing metastases were those already categorized as node positive by routine nodal dissection. Similar results have been obtained by others.[551] In contrast, in a study of 13 selected axillary dissection specimens in which fewer than 10 lymph nodes were found by routine manual dissection, the use of a "lymph node–revealing solution" composed of a mixture of ethanol, ether, acetic acid, and formalin resulted in a change in the lymph node status in four of the cases evaluated.[552] Nevertheless, the time and expense required to clear the axillary adipose tissue as a matter of routine are difficult to justify.

Once lymph nodes have been grossly identified, the pathologist must decide to what extent they should be sampled for microscopic evaluation. Despite the acknowledged importance of the axillary lymph node status in patients with breast cancer, wide variation exists among pathologists with regard to the extent of lymph node examination. Although a number of studies have clearly shown that more thorough gross and microscopic sampling results in an increase in the detection of positive lymph nodes and a change in the lymph node status from negative to positive in some patients,[553–555] no consensus exists regarding the optimal means for the routine pathologic examination of axillary lymph nodes.

Sentinel lymph node biopsy has been proposed as an alternative to axillary dissection for the assessment of axillary lymph node status in patients with breast cancer,[556] as discussed in Chapter 33. At some institutions, frozen sections or touch imprints are performed to provide an intraoperative evaluation of these nodes. Regardless of whether intraoperative assessment is performed, general agreement exists that sentinel nodes should be submitted in their entirety for permanent sections. Considerable variation is seen among institutions, however, with regard to the number of levels cut from each paraffin block and the use of immunohistochemical stains to detect occult micrometastatic foci in nodes that are negative on routine hematoxylin-eosin–stained sections.

CONTENTS OF THE FINAL SURGICAL PATHOLOGY REPORT

The final surgical pathology report for specimens containing invasive breast cancer should include, in addition to the diagnosis, information needed for staging and therapeutic decision making.[557,558] The information used by clinicians in determining treatment options varies among different institutions. At a minimum, however, every surgical pathology report for specimens containing an invasive breast cancer should include the type of specimen submitted, laterality, specimen size, tumor size, histologic type, histologic grade, presence or absence of lymphatic vessel invasion, presence or absence of an extensive intraductal component, the status of the microscopic margins, and lymph node status (if applicable). In addition, for specimens removed because of the presence of mammographically detected microcalcifications, the location of the calcifications (i.e., in association with invasive cancer, carcinoma *in situ*, benign breast ducts and lobules, stroma, or blood vessels) must be noted. If ancillary studies are in progress (e.g., hormone-receptor assays and tests for prognostic markers), this should also be documented in the final report. The use of a standardized, synoptic report, either in addition to or in place of a narrative report, should also be considered.[557,558]

REFERENCES

1. Azzopardi JG, Chepick OF, Hartmann WH, et al. The World Health Organization histological typing of breast tumors, second edition. *Am J Clin Pathol* 1982;78:806.
2. Wellings SR, Jensen HM, Marcum RG. An atlas of subgross pathology of the human breast with special reference to possible precancerous lesions. *J Natl Cancer Inst* 1975;55:231.
3. Fisher ER, Gregorio R, Fisher B, et al. The pathology of invasive breast cancer. A syllabus derived from findings of the National Surgical Adjuvant Breast Project (Protocol No. 4). *Cancer* 1975;36:1.
4. Rosen PP. The pathological classification of human mammary carcinoma: past, present and future. *Ann Clin Lab Sci* 1979;9:144.
5. Page DL, Anderson TJ. *Diagnostic histopathology of the breast.* Edinburgh, UK: Churchill Livingstone, 1987:193.
6. Ellis IO, Galea M, Broughton N, et al. Pathological prognostic factors in breast cancer II. Histological type. Relationship with survival in a large study with long-term follow-up. *Histopathology* 1992;20:479.
7. Cady B, Stone MD, Shuler JG, et al. The new era in breast cancer. Invasion, size and nodal involvement dramatically decreasing as a result of mammographic screening. *Arch Surg* 1996;131:301.
8. Stierer M, Rosen HR, Weber R, Marczell A, Kornek GV, Czerwenka E. Long term analysis of factors influencing the outcome in carcinoma of the breast smaller than one centimeter. *Surg Gynecol Obstet* 1992;175:151.
9. Cowan WK, Kelly P, Sawan A, et al. The pathological and biological nature of screen-detected breast carcinomas: a morphological and immunohistochemical study. *J Pathol* 1997;182:29.

10. Mustafa IA, Cole B, Wanebo HJ, Bland KI, Chang HR. The impact of histopathology on nodal metastases in minimal breast cancer. *Arch Surg* 1997;132:384.
11. Tan P, Cady B, Wanner M, et al. The cell cycle inhibitor p27 is an independent prognostic marker in small (T1a,b) invasive breast carcinomas. *Cancer Res* 1997;57:1259.
12. Chen YY, Connolly J, Harris J, Schnitt S. Predictors of axillary lymph node metastases (ALNM) in patients with breast cancers 1 cm or smaller (T1a,b): implications for axillary dissection. *Mod Pathol* 1998;78:17A(abst).
13. Henson DE, Ries L, Freedman LS, Carriaga M. Relationship among outcome, stage of disease, and histologic grade for 22,616 cases of breast cancer: the basis for a prognostic index. *Cancer* 1991;68:2142.
14. Rosner D, Lane WW. Should all patients with node-negative breast cancer receive adjuvant therapy? Identifying additional subsets of low-risk patients who are highly curable by surgery alone. *Cancer* 1991;68:1482.
15. Tabar L, Fagerberg G, Duffy SW, Day NE, Gad A, Grontoft O. Update of the Swedish two-county program of mammographic screening for breast cancer. *Radiol Clin North Am* 1992;30:187.
16. Anderson TJ, Lamb J, Donnan P, et al. Comparative pathology of breast cancer in a randomized trial of screening. *Br J Cancer* 1991;64:108.
17. Ellis IO, Galea MH, Locker A. Early experience in breast cancer screening: emphasis on development of protocols for triple assessment. *Breast* 1993;2:148.
18. Silverberg SG, Chitale AR. Assessment of significance of proportions of intraductal and infiltrating tumor growth in ductal carcinoma of the breast. *Cancer* 1973;32:830.
19. Lampejo OT, Barnes DM, Smith P, Millis RR. Evaluation of infiltrating ductal carcinoma with a DCIS component: Correlation of the histologic type of the in situ component with grade of the infiltrating component. *Semin Diagn Pathol* 1994;11:215.
20. Moriya T, Silverberg SG. Intraductal carcinoma (ductal carcinoma in situ) of the breast. A comparison of pure noninvasive tumors with those including different proportions of infiltrating carcinoma. *Cancer* 1994;74:2972.
21. Gupta SK, Douglas-Jones AG, Fenn N, et al. The clinical behavior of breast carcinoma is probably determined at the preinvasive stage (ductal carcinoma in situ). *Cancer* 1997;80:1740.
22. Ravdin PM. Biomarkers. In: Silverstein MJ, ed. *Ductal carcinoma in situ of the breast.* Baltimore: Williams & Wilkins, 1997:51.
23. Lakhani SR, Stratton MR, Poller DN. Cytogenetics and molecular biology. In Silverstein MJ, ed. *Ductal carcinoma in situ of the breast.* Baltimore: Williams & Wilkins, 1997:77.
24. O'Conell P, Pekkel V, Fuqua SAW, et al. Analysis of loss of heterozygosity in 399 premalignant breast lesions at 15 genetic loci. *J Natl Cancer Inst* 1998;90:697.
25. Simpson JF. Predictive utility of the histopathologic analysis of carcinoma of the breast. *Adv Pathol Lab Med* 1994;7:107.
26. Black MM, Speer FD. Nuclear structure in cancer tissues. *Surg Gynecol Obstet* 1957;105:97.
27. Cutler SJ, Black MM, Mork T, et al. Further observations on prognostic factors in cancer of the female breast. *Cancer* 1969;24:653.
28. Elston CW, Ellis IO. *The breast.* Edinburgh, UK: Churchill Livingstone, 1998:365.
29. Wheeler JE, Enterline HT. Lobular carcinoma of the breast in situ and infiltrating. *Pathol Annu* 1976;11:161.
30. Martinez V, Azzopardi JG. Invasive lobular carcinoma of the breast: incidence and variants. *Histopathology* 1979;3:467.
31. Foote FW Jr, Stewart FW. A histologic classification of carcinoma of the breast. *Surgery* 1946;19:74.
32. Fechner RE. Histologic variants of infiltrating lobular carcinoma of the breast. *Hum Pathol* 1975;6:373.
33. Steinbrecher JS, Silverberg SG. Signet-ring cell carcinoma of the breast. The mucinous variant of infiltrating lobular carcinoma? *Cancer* 1976;37:828,
34. Fisher ER, Gregorio RM, Redmond C, Fisher B. Tubulolobular invasive breast cancer: a variant of lobular invasive cancer. *Hum Pathol* 1977;8:679.
35. Van Bogaert L-J, Maldague P. Infiltrating lobular carcinoma of the female breast. Deviations from the usual histopathologic appearance. *Cancer* 1980;45:979.
36. Merino MJ, Livolsi VA. Signet ring cell carcinoma of the female breast: a clinicopathologic analysis of 24 cases. *Cancer* 1981;48:1830.
37. Dixon JM, Anderson TJ, Page DL, et al. Infiltrating lobular carcinoma of the breast. *Histopathology* 1982;6:149.
38. du Toit RS, Locker AP, Ellis IO, et al. Invasive lobular carcinomas of the breast—the prognosis of histopathologic subtypes. *Br J Cancer* 1989;60:605.
39. Eusebi V, Magalhaes F, Azzopardi JG. Pleomorphic lobular carcinoma of the breast: an aggressive tumor showing apocrine differentiation. *Hum Pathol* 1992;23:655.
40. Weidner N, Semple JP. Pleomorphic variant of invasive lobular carcinoma of the breast. *Hum Pathol* 1992;23:1167.
41. Bentz JS, Yassa N, Clayton F. Pleomorphic lobular carcinoma of the breast: clinicopathologic features of 12 cases. *Mod Pathol* 1998;11:814.
42. Ashikari R, Huvos A, Urban JA, Robbins GF. Infiltrating lobular carcinoma of the breast. *Cancer* 1973;31:110.
43. Lesser M, Rosen PP, Kinne D. Multicentricity and bilaterality in invasive breast carcinoma. *Surgery* 1982;91:234.
44. Tinnemans JGM, Wobbes T, vander Sluis RF, et al. Multicentricity in nonpalpable breast carcinoma and its implications for treatment. *Am J Surg* 1986;151:334.
45. Gump FE, Shikora S, Habif DV, et al. The extent and distribution of cancer in breasts with palpable primary tumors. *Ann Surg* 1986;204:384.
46. Dixon JM, Anderson TJ, Page DL, et al. Infiltrating lobular carcinoma of the breast: an evaluation of the incidence and consequence of bilateral disease. *Br J Surg* 1983;70:513.
47. Sastre-Garau X, Jouve M, Asselain B, et al. Infiltrating lobular carcinoma of the breast. Clinicopathologic analysis of 975 cases with reference to data on conservative therapy and metastatic patterns. *Cancer* 1996;77:113.
48. Peiro G, Schnitt S, Gage I, et al. Treatment outcome following conservative surgery and radiation therapy (CS + RT) for infiltrating carcinoma with mixed ductal and lobular features (IMC): comparison with infiltrating ductal (IDC) and infiltrating lobular carcinoma (ILC). *Lab Invest* 1995;72:32A(abst).
49. Newman W. Lobular carcinoma of the female breast. Report of 73 cases. *Ann Surg* 1966;164:305.
50. Davis RP, Nora PF, Kooy RG, Hines JR. Experience with lobular carcinoma of the breast. Emphasis on recent aspects of management. *Arch Surg* 1979;114:485.
51. DiCostanzo D, Rosen PP, Gareen I, et al. Prognosis in infiltrating lobular carcinoma. An analysis of "classical" and variant tumors. *Am J Surg Pathol* 1990;14:12.
52. Azzopardi JG. *Problems in breast pathology.* Philadelphia: WB Saunders, 1979:243.
53. Mendelson EB, Harris KM, Tobon H. Infiltrating lobular carcinoma: mammographic patterns with pathologic correlation. *AJR Am J Roentgenol* 1989;153:265.
54. Hilleren DJ, Andersson IT, Lindholm K, Linnell FS. Invasive lobular carcinoma: mammographic findings in a 10-year experience. *Radiology* 1991;178:149.
55. Le Gal M, Ollivier L, Asselain B, et al. Mammographic features of 455 invasive lobular carcinomas. *Radiology* 1992;185:705.
56. Helvie MA, Paramagul C, Oberman HA, Adler DD. Invasive lobular carcinoma: imaging features and clinical detection. *Invest Radiol* 1993;28:202.
57. Krecke KN, Gisvold JJ. Invasive lobular carcinoma of the breast: mammographic findings and extent of disease at diagnosis in 183 patients. *AJR Am J Roentgenol* 19931;61:957.
58. White JR, Gustafson GS, Wimbish K, et al. Conservative surgery and radiation therapy for infiltrating lobular carcinoma of the breast. The role of preoperative mammograms in guiding treatment. *Cancer* 1994;74:640.
59. Moll R, Mitze M, Frixen UH, Birchmeier W. Differential loss of E-cadherin expression in infiltrating ductal and lobular breast carcinomas. *Am J Pathol* 1993;143:1731.
60. Rasbridge SA, Gillette CE, Sampson SA, et al. Epithelial (E-) and placental (P-) cadherin cell adhesion molecule expression in breast carcinoma. *J Pathol* 1993;169:245.
61. Palacios J, Benito N, Pizarro A, et al. Anomalous expression of P-cadherin in breast carcinoma. Correlation with E-cadherin expression and pathological features. *Am J Pathol* 1995;146:605.
62. De Leeuw WJF, Berx G, Vos CBJ, et al. Simultaneous loss of expression of e-cadherin and catenins in invasive lobular breast cancer and lobular carcinoma in situ. *J Pathol* 1997;183:404.
63. Berx G, Cleton-Jansen AM, Strumane K, et al. E-cadherin is inactivated in a majority of invasive human lobular breast cancers by trun-

cation mutations throughout its extracellular domain. *Oncogene* 1996;13:1919.
64. Green I, McCormick B, Cranor M, Rosen PP. A comparative study of tubular and tubulolobular carcinoma of the breast. *Am J Surg Pathol* 1997;21:653.
65. Hull MT, Seo IS, Battersby JS, Csicsko JF. Signet-ring cell carcinoma of the breast. A clinicopathologic study of 24 cases. *Am J Clin Pathol* 1980;73:31.
66. Raju U, Ma CK, Shaw A. Signet ring cell variant of lobular carcinoma of the breast: a clinicopathologic and immunohistochemical study. *Mod Pathol* 1993;6:516.
67. Eltorky M, Hall C, Osborne PT, El Zeky F. Signet ring cell variant of invasive lobular carcinoma of the breast. A clinicopathologic study of 11 cases. *Arch Pathol Lab Med* 1994;118:245.
68. Frost AR, Terahata S, Yeh I-T, et al. The significance of signet ring cells in infiltrating lobular carcinoma of the breast. *Arch Pathol Lab Med* 1995;119:64.
69. Azzopardi JG. *Problems in breast pathology*. Philadelphia: WB Saunders, 1979:301.
70. Allenby PA, Chowdhury LN. Histiocytic appearance of metastastic lobular breast carcinoma. *Arch Pathol Lab Med* 1986;110:759.
71. Walford N, Ten Velden J. Histiocytoid breast carcinoma: an apocrine variant of lobular carcinoma. *Histopathology* 1989;14:515.
72. Elston CS, Ellis IO. *The breast*. Edinburgh, UK: Churchill Livingstone, 1998:291.
73. Porter PL, Garcia R, Moe R, et al. C-erbB-2 oncogene protein in in situ and invasive lobular breast neoplasia. *Cancer* 1991;68:331.
74. Domagala W, Markiewski M, Kubiak R, et al. Immunohistochemical profile of invasive lobular carcinoma of the breast: predominantly vimentin and p53 protein negative cathepsin D and oestrogen receptor positive. *Virchows Arch [A]* 1993;423:497.
75. Mazoujian G, Bodian C, Haagensen DE Jr, Haagensen CD. Expression of GCDFP-15 in breast carcinomas. Relationship to pathologic and clinical features. *Am J Pathol* 1983;110:105.
76. Harris M, Howell A, Chrissohou M, et al. A comparison of the metastatic pattern of infiltrating lobular carcinoma and infiltrating duct carcinoma of the breast. *Br J Cancer* 1984;50:23.
77. Lamovec J, Bracko M. Metastatic pattern of infiltrating lobular carcinoma of the breast: an autopsy study. *J Surg Oncol* 1991;48:28.
78. Borst MJ, Ingvold MA. Metastatic patterns of invasive lobular versus invasive ductal carcinoma of the breast. *Surgery* 1993;114:637.
79. Dixon AR, Ellis IO, Elston CW, Blamey RW. A comparison of the clinical metastatic pattern of infiltrating lobular and ductal carcinomas of the breast. *Br J Cancer* 1991;63:634.
80. Smith DB, Howell A, Harris M, et al. Carcinomatous meningitis associated with infiltrating lobular carcinoma of the breast. *Eur J Surg Oncol* 1985;11:33.
81. Lamovec J, Zidar A. Association of leptomeningeal carcinomatosis in carcinoma of the breast with infiltrating lobular carcinoma. An autopsy study. *Arch Pathol Lab Med* 1991;115:507.
82. Cormier WJ, Gaffey TA, Welch TA, et al. Linitis plastica caused by metastatic lobular carcinoma of the breast. *Mayo Clinic Proc* 1980;55:747.
83. Battifora H. Metastatic breast carcinoma to the stomach simulating linitis plastica. *Appl Immunohistochem* 1994;2:225.
84. Kumar NB, Hart WR. Metastases to the uterine corpus from extragenital cancers. *Cancer* 1982;50:2163.
85. Rosen PP. *Rosen's breast pathology*. Philadelphia: Lippincott–Raven, 1997:560.
86. Silverstein MJ, Lewinsky BS, Waisman JR, et al. Infiltrating lobular carcinoma. Is it different from infiltrating duct carcinoma? *Cancer* 1994;73:1673.
87. Schnitt SJ. Morphologic risk factors for local recurrence in patients with invasive breast cancer treated with conservative surgery and radiation therapy. *Breast J* 1997;3:261.
88. Azzopardi JG. *Problems in breast pathology*. Philadelphia: WB Saunders, 1979:279.
89. Weiss M, Fowble B, Solin LF, et al. Outcome of conservative therapy for invasive breast cancer by histologic type. *Int J Radiat Oncol Biol Phys* 1992;23:94.
90. Tobon H, Salazar H. Tubular carcinoma of the breast. Clinical, histological, and ultrastructural observations. *Arch Pathol Lab Med* 1977;101:310.
91. Cooper HS, Patchefsky AS, Krall RA. Tubular carcinoma of the breast. *Cancer* 1978;42:2334.
92. Carstens PHB. Tubular carcinoma of the breast. A study of frequency. *Am J Clin Pathol* 1982;70:204.
93. Parl FF, Richardson LD. The histologic and biologic spectrum of tubular carcinoma of the breast. *Hum Pathol* 1983;14:694.
94. McBoyle MF, Razek HA, Carter JL, et al. Tubular carcinoma of the breast: an institutional review. *Am Surg* 1997;63:639.
95. Patchefsky AS, Shaberm GS, Schwartz GF, et al. The pathology of breast cancer detected by mass pathology screening. *Cancer* 1977;40:1659.
96. Beahrs OH, Shapiro S, Smart C. Report of the working group to review the National Cancer Institute–American Cancer Society Breast Cancer Detection Demonstration Projects. *J Natl Cancer Inst* 1979;62:640.
97. Rajakariar R, Walker RA. Pathological and biological features of mammographically detected invasive breast cancer. *Br J Cancer* 1995;71:150.
98. Feig SF, Shaber GS, Patchefsky A, et al. Analysis of clinically occult and mammographically occult breast tumors. *AJR Am J Roentgenol* 1977;128:403.
99. Taxy JB. Tubular carcinoma of the male breast. *Cancer* 1975;36:462.
100. Carstens PHB, Huvos AG, Foote FW, et al. Tubular carcinoma of the breast: a clinicopathologic study of 35 cases. *Am J Clin Pathol* 1972;58:231.
101. Oberman, HA, Fidler WJ. Tubular carcinoma of the breast. *Am J Surg Pathol* 1979;13:387.
102. Eusebi V, Betts CM, Bussolati G. Tubular carcinoma: a variant of secretory breast carcinoma. *Histopathology* 1979;3:407.
103. Lagios MD, Rose MR, Margolin FR. Tubular carcinoma of the breast. association with multicentricity, bilaterality, and family history of mammary carcinoma. *Am J Clin Pathol* 1980;73:25.
104. Peters GN, Wolff M, Haagensen CD. Tubular carcinoma of the breast. Clinical pathologic correlations based on 100 cases. *Ann Surg* 1981; 193:138.
105. Bogaert LJ. Clinicopathologic hallmarks of mammary tubular carcinoma. *Hum Pathol* 1982;13:558.
106. McDivitt RW, Boyce W, Gersell D. Tubular carcinoma of the breast. Clinical and pathological observations concerning 135 cases. *Am J Surg Pathol* 1982;6:401.
107. Deos PH, Norris HJ. Well-differentiated (tubular) carcinoma of the breast. A clinicopathologic study of 145 pure and mixed cases. *Am J Clin Pathol* 1982;78:1.
108. Carstens PHB, Greenberg RA, Francis D, et al. Tubular carcinoma of the breast. A long-term follow-up. *Histopathology* 1985;9:271.
109. Gadaleanu V, Galatar N, Tzortzi E. Tubular carcinoma of the breast. *Morphol Embryol* 1985;31:197.
110. Elson BC, Helvie MA, Frank TS, et al. Tubular carcinoma of the breast: mode of presentation, mammographic appearance, and frequency of nodal metastases. *AJR Am J Roentgenol* 1993;161:1173.
111. Leibman AJ, Lewis M, Kruse B. Tubular carcinoma of the breast: mammographic appearance. *AJR Am J Roentgenol* 1993;160:263.
112. Winchester DJ, Sahin AA,Tucker S, et al. Tubular carcinoma of the breast. Predicting axillary nodal metastases and recurrence. *Ann Surg* 1996;223:342.
113. Berger AC, Miller SM, Harris MN, et al. Axillary dissection for tubular carcinoma of the breast. *Breast J* 1996;2:204.
114. Feig SA, Shaver GS, Patchefsky AS. Tubular carcinoma of the breast: mode of presentation, mammographic appearance and pathologic correlation. *Diagn Radiol* 1993;129:311.
115. Claus EB, Risch N, Thompson WD, et al. Relationship between histopathology and family history of breast cancer. *Cancer* 1993;71:147.
116. Visfeldt J, Schieke O. Male breast cancer: I. Histologic typing and grading of 187 Danish cases. *Cancer* 1973;32:985.
117. Tremblay G. Elastosis in tubular carcinoma of the breast. *Arch Pathol* 1974;98:302.
118. Egan RL, Ellis JT, Powell RW. Team approach to the study of diseases of the breast. *Cancer* 1969;23:847.
119. Taylor HB, Norris HJ. Well-differentiated carcinoma of the breast. *Cancer* 1970;25:687.
120. Lamb J, Anderson TJ. Influence of cancer histology on the success of fine needle aspiration of the breast. *J Clin Pathol* 1989;42:733.
121. Flotte TJ, Bell DA, Greco MA. Tubular carcinoma and sclerosing adenosis. The use of basal lamina as a differential feature. *Am J Surg Pathol* 1980;4:75.
122. Ekblom P, Miettinen M, Forsman L, et al. Basement membrane and apocrine epithelial antigens in differential diagnosis between tubular

carcinoma and sclerosing adenosis of the breast. *J Clin Pathol* 1984;37:357.

123. O'Leary TJ, Mikel UV, Becker RL. Computer-assisted image interpretation: use of neural network to differentiate tubular carcinoma from sclerosing adenosis. *Mod Pathol* 1992;5:402.
124. Eusebi V, Foschini MP, Betts CM, et al. Microglandular adenosis, apocrine adenosis, and tubular carcinoma of the breast. An immunohistochemical comparison. *Am J Surg Pathol* 1993;17:99.
125. Reiner A, Reiner G, Spona J, et al. Histopathologic characterization of human breast cancer in correlation with estrogen receptor status. A comparison of immunocytochemical and biochemical analysis. *Cancer* 1988;61:1149.
126. Helin HJ, Helle MJ, Kallioniemi O, et al. Immunohistochemical determination of estrogen and progesterone receptors in human breast carcinoma. Correlation with histopathology and DNA flow cytology. *Cancer* 1989;63:1761.
127. Stierer M, Rosen H, Weber R, et al. Immunohistochemical and biochemical measurement of estrogen and progesterone receptors in primary breast cancer. Correlation of histopathology and prognostic factors. *Ann Surg* 1993;218:13.
128. Adeyinka A, Mertens F, Idvall I, et al. Cytogenetic findings in invasive breast carcinomas with prognostically favorable histology: a less complex karyotypic pattern? *Int J Cancer* 1998;79:361.
129. Soomro S, Shousa S, Taylor P, et al. c-erbB-2 expression in different histologic types of invasive breast carcinoma. *J Clin Pathol* 1991;44:211.
130. Somerville JE, Clarke LA, Biggart JD. c-erbB-2 overexpression and histologic type of in situ and invasive breast carcinoma. *J Clin Pathol* 1992;45:16.
131. Rosen PP, Lesser ML, Arroyo CD, et al. p53 in node-negative breast carcinoma: an immunohistochemical study of epidemiologic risk factors, histologic features, and prognosis. *J Clin Oncol* 1995;13:821.
132. Kouchoukos NT, Ackerman LV, Butcher HR. Prediction of axillary nodal metastases from the morphology of primary mammary carcinomas. *Cancer* 1967;20:948.
133. Rosen PP, Groshen S, Kinne D, et al. Factors influencing prognosis in node-negative breast carcinoma: analysis of 767 T1N0M0/T2N0M0 patients with long-term follow-up. *J Clin Oncol* 1993;11:2090.
134. Haffty BG, Perrotta PL, Ward B, et al. Conservatively treated breast cancer: outcome by histologic subtype. *Breast J* 1997;3:7.
135. Fisher ER, Anderson S, Redmond C, et al. Pathologic findings from the National Surgical Adjuvant breast project protocol B-06. 10-year pathologic and clinical prognostic discriminants. *Cancer* 1993;71:2507.
136. Norris HJ, Taylor HB. Prognosis of mucinous (gelatinous) carcinoma of the breast. *Cancer* 1965;18:879.
137. Silverberg SG, Kay S, Chitale AR, et al. Colloid carcinoma of the breast. *Am J Clin Pathol* 1971;55:355.
138. Rosen PP, Wang TY. Colloid carcinoma of the breast. Analysis of 64 patients with long term follow up. *Am J Clin Pathol* 1980;73:304.
139. Rasmussen BB. Human mucinous breast carcinomas and their lymph node metastases. A histological review of 247 cases. *Pathol Res Pract* 1985;180:377.
140. Clayton F. Pure mucinous carcinoma of the breast: morphological features and prognostic correlates. *Hum Pathol* 1986;17:34.
141. Rasmussen BB, Rose C, Christensen I. Prognostic factors in primary mucinous carcinoma. *Am J Clin Pathol* 1987;87:155.
142. Komaki K, Sakamoto G, Sugano H, et al. Mucinous carcinoma of the breast in Japan. A prognostic analysis based on morphologic features. *Cancer* 1988;61:989.
143. Toikkanen S, Kujari H. Pure and mixed mucinous carcinomas of the breast: a clinicopathologic analysis of 61 cases with long term follow up. *Hum Pathol* 1989;20:758.
144. Andre S, Cunha F, Bernardo M, et al. Mucinous carcinoma of the breast. A pathologic study of 82 cases. *J Surg Oncol* 1995;58:162.
145. Fentiman IS, Millis RR, Smith P, et al. Mucoid carcinoma of the breast: histology and prognosis. *Br J Cancer* 1997;75:1061.
146. Avisar E, Khan AK, Axelrod D, et al. Pure mucinous carcinoma of the breast: a clinicopathologic correlation study. *Ann Surg Oncol* 1998; 5:447.
147. Northridge ME, Rhoads GG, Wartenberg D, et al. The importance of histologic type on breast cancer survival. *J Clin Epidemiol* 1997;50:283.
148. Wilson TE, Helvie MA, Oberman HA, et al. Pure and mixed mucinous carcinoma of the breast: pathologic basis for differences in mammographic appearance. *AJR Am J Roentgenol* 1995;165:285.
149. Cardenosa G, Doudna C, Eklund GW. Mucinous (colloid) breast cancer: clinical and mammographic findings in 10 patients. *AJR Am J Roentgenol* 1994;162:1077.
150. Goodman DN, Boutross-Tadross O, Jong RA. Mammographic features of pure mucinous carcinoma of the breast with pathologic correlation. *Can Assoc Radiol* 1995;46:296.
151. Chopra S, Evans AJ, Pinder SE, et al. Pure mucinous breast cancer—mammographic and ultrasound findings. *Clin Radiol* 1996;51:421.
152. Rosen PP, Oberman HA. *Tumors of the mammary gland. Atlas of tumor pathology*, 3rd series, Fascicle 7. Washington: Armed Forces Institute of Pathology, 1993.
153. Rosen PP. Mucocele-like tumors of the breast. *Am J Surg Pathol* 1986;10:464.
154. Ro JY, Sniege N, Sahin AA, et al. Mucocele-like tumor of the breast associated with atypical ductal hyperplasia or mucinous carcinoma. A clinicopathologic study of seven cases. *Arch Pathol Lab Med* 1991;115:137.
155. Toikkanen S, Eerola E, Ekfors T. Pure and mixed mucinous breast carcinomas: DNA stemline and prognosis. *J Clin Pathol* 1988;41:300.
156. Scopsi L, Andreola S, Pilotti S, et al. Mucinous carcinoma of the breast. A clinicopathologic, histochemical and immunohistochemical study with special reference to neuroendocrine differentiation. *Am J Surg Pathol* 1994;18:702.
157. Sharnhorst D, Huntrakoon M. Mucinous carcinoma of the breast: recurrence 30 years after mastectomy. *South Med J* 1988;81:656.
158. Kurtz JM, Jacquemier J, Torhorst J, et al. Conservation therapy for breast carcinomas other than infiltrating ductal carcinoma. *Cancer* 1989;63:1630.
159. Deck JHN, Lee MA. Mucin embolism to cerebral arteries: a fatal complication of carcinoma of breast. *Can J Neurol Sci* 1978;5:327.
160. Towfighi J, Simmonds MA, Davidson EA. Mucin and fat emboli in mucinous carcinoma: cause of hemorrhagic cerebral infarcts. *Arch Pathol Lab Med* 1983;107:646.
161. Hawes D, Robinson R, Wina R. Pseudomyxoma peritonei from metastatic colloid carcinoma of the breast. *Gastrointest Radiol* 1991;16:80.
162. Richardson WW. Medullary carcinoma of the breast. A distinctive tumor type with a relatively good prognosis following radical mastectomy. *Br J Cancer* 1956;10:415.
163. Bloom HJG, Richardson WW, Fields JR. Host resistance and survival in carcinoma of the breast: a study of 104 cases of medullary carcinoma in a series of 1411 cases of breast cancer followed for 20 years. *BMJ* 1970;3:181.
164. Ridolfi RL, Rosen PP, Port A, et al. Medullary carcinoma of the breast—a clinicopathological study with a 10 year follow up. *Cancer* 1977;40:1365.
165. Maier WP, Rosemond GP, Goldman LI, et al. A ten year study of medullary carcinoma of the breast. *Surg Gynecol Obstet* 1977;144:695.
166. Rapin V, Contesso G, Mouriesse H, et al. Medullary breast carcinoma. A re-evaluation of 95 cases of breast cancer with inflammatory stroma. *Cancer* 1988;61:1149.
167. Wargotz ES, Silverberg SG. Medullary carcinoma of the breast: a clinicopathologic study with appraisal of current diagnostic criteria. *Hum Pathol* 1988;19:1340.
168. Pedersen L, Holck S, Shiodt T, et al. Medullary carcinoma of the breast, prognostic importance of characteristic histopathological features evaluated in a multivariate cox analysis. *Eur J Cancer* 1994;30A:1792.
169. Pedersen L, Zedeler K, Holck S, et al. Medullary carcinoma of the breast. Prevalence and prognostic importance of classical risk factors in breast cancer. *Eur J Cancer* 1995;31A:2289.
170. Pedersen L, Holck S, Schiodt T, et al. Inter- and intraobserver variability in the histopathological diagnosis of medullary carcinoma of the breast, and its prognostic implications. *Breast Cancer Res Treat* 1989;14:91.
171. Pedersen L, Zedeler K, Holck S, et al. Medullary carcinoma of the breast, proposal for a new simplified histopathological definition. *Br J Cancer* 1991;63:591.
172. Fisher ER, Kenny JP, Sass R, et al. Medullary cancer of the breast revisited. *Breast Cancer Res Treat* 1990;16:215.
173. Rigaud C, Theobald S, Noel P, et al. Medullary carcinoma of the breast. A multicenter study of its diagnostic consistency. *Arch Pathol Lab Med* 1993;117:1005.
174. Gaffey MJ, Mills SE, Frierson HF, et al. Medullary carcinoma of the breast: interobserver variability in histopathologic diagnosis. *Mod Pathol* 1995;8:31.

175. Crotty TB. Medullary carcinoma: is it a reproducible and prognostically significant type of mammary carcinoma? *Adv Anat Pathol* 1996;3:179.
176. Jensen ML, Kiaer H, Anderson J, et al. Prognostic comparison of three classifications for medullary carcinoma of the breast. *Histopathology* 1977;30:523.
177. Schwartz GF. Solid circumscribed carcinoma of the breast. *Ann Surg* 1969;169:165.
178. Neuman ML, Homer MJ. Association of medullary carcinoma with reactive axillary adenopathy. *AJR Am J Roentgenol* 1996;167:185.
179. Meyer JE, Amin E, Lindfors KK, et al. Medullary carcinoma of the breast: mammographic and US appearance. *Radiology* 1989;170:79.
180. Kopans DB. *Breast imaging*, 2nd ed. Philadelphia: Lippincott–Raven, 1998.
181. Rubens JR, Lewandrowski KP, Kopans DB, et al. Medullary carcinoma of the breast. Overdiagnosis of a prognostically favorable neoplasm. *Arch Surg* 1990;125:601.
182. Jensen ML, Kiaer H, Anderson H, et al. Prognostic comparison of 3 classifications for medullary carcinomas of the breast. *Histopathology* 1997;30:523.
183. Page DL, Dixon JM, Anderson TJ, et al. Invasive cribriform carcinoma of the breast. *Histopathology* 1983;7:525.
184. Venable JG, Schwartz AM, Silverberg SG. Infiltrating cribriform carcinoma of the breast: a distinctive clinicopathologic entity. *Hum Pathol* 1990;21:333.
185. Stutz JA, Evans AJ, Pinder S, et al. The radiologic appearances of invasive cribriform carcinoma of the breast. *Clin Radiol* 1994;49:693.
186. Gatchell FG, Dockerty MB, Clagett OT. Intracystic carcinoma of the breast. *Surg Gynecol Obstet* 1958;106:347.
187. Czernobilsky B. Intracystic carcinoma of the female breast. *Surg Gynecol Obstet* 1967;124:93.
188. McKittrick JE, Doane WA, Failing RM. Intracystic papillary carcinoma of the breast. *Am Surg* 1969;35:195.
189. Hunter CE, Sawyers JL. Intracystic papillary carcinoma of the breast. *South Med J* 1980;73:1484.
190. Carter D, Orr SL, Merino MJ. Intracystic papillary carcinoma of the breast after mastectomy, radiotherapy or excisional biopsy alone. *Cancer* 1983;52:14.
191. Lefkowitz M, Lefkowitz W, Wargotz ES. Intraductal (intracystic) papillary carcinoma of the breast: a clinicopathological study of 77 cases. *Hum Pathol* 1994;25:802.
192. Leal C, Costa I, Fonseca, et al. Intracystic (encysted) papillary carcinoma of the breast: a clinical, pathological, and immunohistochemical study. *Hum Pathol* 1998;29:1097.
193. Fisher ER, Palekar A, Redmond C, et al. Pathologic findings from the National Surgical Adjuvant Breast Project (Protocol no. 4). VI. Invasive papillary cancer. *Am J Clin Pathol* 1980;73:313.
194. Schneider JA. Invasive papillary breast carcinoma: mammographic and sonographic appearance. *Radiology* 1989;171:377.
195. Mitnick JS, Vazquez MF, Harris MN, et al. Invasive papillary carcinoma of the breast: mammographic appearance. *Radiology* 1990;177:83.
196. McCulloch GL, Evans AJ, Yeoman L, et al. Radiological features of papillary carcinoma of the breast. *Clin Radiol* 1997;52:865.
197. Fisher ER, Constantino J, Fisher B, et al. Pathologic findings from the National Surgical Adjuvant Breast Project (Protocol 4). Discriminants for 15-year survival. *Cancer* 1993;71:2141.
198. Siriaunkgul S, Tavassoli FA. Invasive micropapillary carcinoma of the breast. *Mod Pathol* 1993;6:660.
199. Luna-More S, Gonzalez B, Acedo C, et al. Invasive micropapillary carcinoma of the breast. A new special type of invasive mammary carcinoma. *Pathol Res Pract* 1994;190:668.
200. Luna-More S, de los Santos F, Breton JJ, et al. Estrogen and progesterone receptors, c-erbB-2, p53, and Bcl-2 in thirty-three invasive micropapillary breast carcinomas. *Pathol Res Pract* 1996;192:27.
201. Cornog JL, Mobini J, Steiger E, et al. Squamous carcinoma of the breast. *Am J Clin Pathol* 1971;55:410.
202. Hasleton PS, Misch KA, Vasudev KS, et al. Squamous carcinoma of the breast. *J Clin Pathol* 1978;31:116.
203. Toikkanen S. Primary squamous cell carcinoma of the breast. *Cancer* 1981;48:1629.
204. Bogomoletz WV. Pure squamous cell carcinoma of the breast. *Arch Pathol Lab Med* 1982;106:57.
205. Eggers JW, Chesney TM. Squamous cell carcinoma of the breast: a clinicopathologic analysis of eight cases and review of the literature. *Hum Pathol* 1984;15:526.
206. Shousa S, James AH, Fernandez D, et al. Squamous cell carcinoma of the breast. *Arch Pathol Lab Med* 1984;108:893.
207. Eusebi V, Lamovec J, Cattani MG, et al. Acantholytic variant of squamous-cell carcinoma of the breast. *Am J Surg Pathol* 1986;10:855.
208. Wargotz ES, Norris HJ. Metaplastic carcinomas of the breast. IV. Squamous cell carcinoma of ductal origin. *Cancer* 1990;65:272.
209. Gersell DJ, Katzenstein AL. Spindle cell carcinoma of the breast. A clinicopathologic and ultrastructural study. *Hum Pathol* 1981;12:550.
210. Merino MJ, LiVolsi VA, Kennedy S, et al. Spindle-cell carcinoma of the breast: a clinicopathologic, ultrastructural, and immunohistochemical study of eight cases. *Surg Pathol* 1988;1:193.
211. Bauer TW, Rostock RA, Eggleston JC, et al. Spindle cell carcinoma of the breast: four cases and review of the literature. *Hum Pathol* 1984;15:147.
212. Wargotz ES, Deos PH, Norris HJ. Metaplastic carcinomas of the breast. II. Spindle cell carcinoma. *Hum Pathol* 1989;20:732.
213. Rosen PP, Ernsberger D. Low-grade adenosquamous carcinoma. A variant of metaplastic mammary carcinoma. *Am J Surg Pathol* 1987;11:351.
214. Van Hoeven KH, Drudis T, Cranor ML, et al. Low-grade adenosquamous carcinoma of the breast. A clinicopathologic study of 32 cases with ultrastructural analysis. *Am J Surg Pathol* 1993;17:248.
215. Drudis T, Arroyo C, Van Hoeven K, et al. The pathology of low-grade adenosquamous carcinoma of the breast. An immunohistochemical study. *Pathol Ann* 1994;29:181.
216. Huvos AG, Lucas JC, Foote FW. Metaplastic breast carcinoma. *NY State J Med* 1973;73:1078.
217. Kahn LB, Uys CJ, Dale J, et al. Carcinoma of the breast with metaplasia to chondrosarcoma: a light and electron microscopic study *Histopathology* 1978;2:93.
218. Kaufman MW, Marti JR, Gallagher HS, et al. Carcinoma of the breast with pseudosarcomatous metaplasia. *Cancer* 1984;53:1908.
219. Oberman HA. Metaplastic carcinoma of the breast. A clinicopathologic study of 29 patients. *Am J Surg Pathol* 1987;11:918.
220. Wargotz ES, Norris HJ. Metaplastic carcinomas of the breast. I. Matrix-producing carcinoma. *Hum Pathol* 1989;20:628.
221. Wargotz ES, Norris HJ. Metaplastic carcinomas of the breast. III. Carcinosarcoma. *Cancer* 1989;64:1490.
222. Pitts WC, Rojas V, Gaffey MJ, et al. Carcinomas with metaplasia and sarcomas of the breast. *Am J Clin Pathol* 1991;95:623.
223. Foschini MP, Dina RE, Eusebi V. Sarcomatoid neoplasms of the breast: proposed definitions for biphasic and monophasic sarcomatoid mammary carcinomas. *Semin Diagn Pathol* 1993;10:128.
224. Wargotz ES, Norris HJ. Metaplastic carcinomas of the breast: V. Metaplastic carcinoma with osteoclastic giant cells. *Hum Pathol* 1990;21:1142.
225. Ruffolo EF, Koerner FC, Maluf HM. Metaplastic carcinoma of the breast with melanocytic differentiation. *Mod Pathol* 1997;10:592.
226. Chhieng C, Cranor ML, Lesser ME, et al. Metaplastic carcinoma of the breast with osteocartilaginous heterologous elements. *Am J Surg Pathol* 1998;22:188.
227. Brenner RJ, Turner RR, Schiller V, et al. Metaplastic carcinoma of the breast. Report of 3 cases. *Cancer* 1998;82:1082.
228. Patterson SK, Tworek JA, Robidoux MA, et al. Metaplastic carcinoma of the breast: mammographic appearance with pathologic correlation. *AJR Am J Roentgenol* 1997;169:709.
229. Rosen PP. *Rosen's breast pathology*. Philadelphia: Lippincott–Raven, 1997:375.
230. Flint A, Oberman HA, Davenport RD. Cytophotometric measurements of metaplastic carcinoma of the breast: correlation with pathologic features and clinical behavior. *Mod Pathol* 1988;1:193.
231. Zhuang Z, Lininger RA, Yan-gao M, et al. Identical clonality of both components of mammary carcinosarcoma with differential loss of heterozygosity. *Mod Pathol* 1997;10:354.
232. Mavligit GM, Cohen JL, Sherwood LM. Ectopic production of parathyroid hormone by carcinoma of the breast. *N Engl J Med* 1971;285:154.
233. Coombes RC, Easty GC, Detre SI, et al. Secretion of immunoreactive calcitonin by human breast carcinomas. *Br Med J* 1975;4:197.
234. Kaneko H, Hojo H, Ishikawa S, et al. Norepinephrine-producing tumors of bilateral breasts. A case report. *Cancer* 1978;41:2002.
235. Cohle SD, Tschen JA, Smith FE, et al. ACTH-secreting carcinoma of the breast. *Cancer* 1979;43:2370.
236. Woodard BH, Eisenbarth G, Wallace NR, et al. Adrenocorticotropin-production by a mammary carcinoma. *Cancer* 1981;47:1823.

237. Partanen S, Syrjanen K. Argyrophilic cells in carcinoma of the female breast. *Virchows Arch [A] Pathol Anat Histol* 1981;391:45.
238. Clayton F, Sibley RK, Ordonez NG, et al. Argyrophilic breast carcinomas. Evidence of lactational differentiation. *Am J Surg Pathol* 1982;6:323.
239. Toyoshima S. Mammary carcinoma with argyrophil cells. *Cancer* 1983;52:2129.
240. Festissof F, Dubois MP, Arbeille-Brassart B, et al. Argyrophil cells in mammary carcinoma. *Hum Pathol* 1983;14:127.
241. Bussolati G, Papotti M, Sapino A, et al. Endocrine markers in argyrophilic carcinomas of the breast. *Am J Surg Pathol* 1987;11:248.
242. Maluf H, Zukerberg LR, Dickersin GR, et al. Spindle-cell argyrophilic mucin-producing carcinoma of the breast. Histological, ultrastructural, and immunohistochemical studies of two cases. *Am J Surg Pathol* 1991;15:677.
243. Scopsi L, Andreola S, Saccozzi R, et al. Argyrophilic carcinoma of the male breast. A neuroendocrine tumor containing predominantly chromogranin B (secretogranin I). *Am J Surg Pathol* 1991;15:1063.
244. Scopsi L, Andreola S, Pilotti S, et al. Argyrophilia and granin (chromogranin/secretogranin) expression in female breast carcinomas. Their relationship to survival and other disease parameters. *Am J Surg Pathol* 1992;16:561.
245. Cubilla AL, Woddruff JM. Primary carcinoid tumor of the breast. *Am J Surg Pathol* 1977;1:283.
246. Fisher ER, Palekar AS. Solid and mucinous varieties of so-called mammary carcinoid tumors. *Am J Clin Pathol* 1979;72:909.
247. Taxy JB, Tischler AS, Insalaco, et al. "Carcinoid" tumour of the breast. A variant of conventional breast cancer? *Hum Pathol* 1981;12:170.
248. Azzopardi JG, Muretto P, Goddeeris P, et al. "Carcinoid" tumours of the breast: the morphological spectrum of argyrophil carcinomas. *Histopathology* 1982;6:549.
249. Bussolati G, Gugliotta P, Sapino A, et al. Chromogranin-reactive endocrine cells in argyrophilic carcinomas ("carcinoids") and normal tissue of the breast. *Am J Pathol* 1985;120:186.
250. Jablon LK, Somers R, Kim PY. Carcinoid tumor of the breast: treatment with breast conservation in three patients. *Ann Surg Oncol* 1998;5:261.
251. Kashlan RB, Powell RW, Nolting SF. Carcinoid and other tumors metastatic to the breast. *J Surg Oncol* 1982;20:25.
252. Ordonez NG, Manning JT, Raymond K. Argentaffin endocrine carcinoma (carcinoid) of the pancreas wih concomitant metastasis: an immunohistochemical and electron microscopic study. *Hum Pathol* 1985;16:746.
253. Fishman A, Kim HS, Girtanner RE, et al. Solitary breast metastasis as a first manifestation of ovarian carcinoid tumor. *Gynecol Oncol* 1994; 54:222.
254. Moreno A, Gonzalo MA, Sarasa JL, et al. Bilateral breast metastases as the first manifestations of an occult ileal carcinoid. *Med Clin (Barc)* 1995;104:515.
255. Wozniak TC, Naunheim KS. Bronchial carcinoid metastatic to the breast. *Ann Thorac Surg* 1998;65:1148.
256. Rubio IT, Korourian S, Brown H, et al. Carcinoid tumor metastatic to the breast. *Arch Surg* 1998;133:1117.
257. Yogore MG, Sagal S. Small cell carcinoma of the male breast. Report of a case. *Cancer* 1977;39:1748.
258. Wade PM, Mills SE, Read M, et al. Small cell neuroendocrine (oat cell) carcinoma of the breast. *Cancer* 1983;52:121.
259. Jundt G, Shultz A, Heitz P, et al. Small cell neuroendocrine (oat cell) carcinoma of the male breast. Immunocytochemical and ultrastructural investigations. *Virchows Arch [A] Pathol Anat Histol* 1984;404:213.
260. Papotti M, Gherardi G, Eusebi V, et al Primary oat cell (neuroendocrine) carcinoma of the breast. Report of four cases. *Virchows Arch [A] Pathol Anat Histol* 1992;420:103.
261. Francois A, Chatikhine VA, Chevallier B, et al. Neuroendocrine primary small cell carcinoma of the breast. Report of a case and review of the literature. *Am J Clin Oncol* 1995;18:133.
262. Carlson HJ, Trujillo YP, Taxy JB. Prolonged survival in a case of small cell carcinoma of the breast. *Breast J* 1996;2:160.
263. Deeley TJ. Secondary deposits in the breast. *Br J Cancer* 1965; 19:738.
264. Hadju SI, Urban JA. Cancers metastatic to the breast. *Cancer* 1972; 29:1691.
265. Birsak CA, Janssen PJ, van Vrannhoven CL, et al. Sex steroid receptor expression in "carcinoid" tumors of the breast. *Breast Cancer Res Treat* 1996;40:243.
266. Wilander E, Lindgren A, Nister N, et al. Nuclear DNA and endocrine activity in carcinomas of the breast. *Cancer* 1984;54:1016.
267. Nayer HR. Cylindroma of the breast with pulmonary metastases. *Dis Chest* 1957;31:324.
268. Wilson WB, Spell JP. Adenoid cystic carcinoma of the breast. A case with recurrence and regional metastases. *Ann Surg* 1967;166:861.
269. Cavanzo FJ, Taylor HB. Adenoid cystic carcinoma of the breast. An analysis of 21 cases. *Cancer* 1969;24:740.
270. Friedman BA, Oberman HA. Adenoid cystic carcinoma of the breast. *Am J Clin Pathol* 1970;54:1.
271. Lusted D. Structural and growth patterns of adenoid cystic carcinoma of breast. *Am J Clin Pathol* 1970;54:419.
272. Eisner B. Adenoid cystic carcinoma of the breast. *Pathol Euro* 1970;3:357.
273. Verani RR, van der Bel-Kahn J. Mammary adenoid cystic carcinoma with unusual features. *Am J Clin Pathol* 1973;59:653.
274. Anthony PP, James PD. Adenoid cystic carcinoma of the breast: prevalence, diagnostic criteria, and histogenesis. *J Clin Pathol* 1977;28:647.
275. Qizilbash AH, Patterson MC, Oliveira KF. Adenoid cystic carcinoma of the breast. Light and electron microscopy and a brief review of the literature. *Arch Pathol Lab Med* 1977;101:302.
276. Hjorth S, Magnusson PH, Blomquist P. Adenoid cystic carcinoma of the breast. Report of a case in a male and review of the literature. *Acta Chir Scand* 1977;143:155.
277. Lim SK, Kovi J, Warner OG. Adenoid cystic carcinoma of the breast with metastasis: a case report and review of the literature. *J Natl Med Assoc* 1979;71:329.
278. Peters GN, Wolff M. Adenoid cystic carcinoma of the breast. Report of 11 new cases: review of the literature and discussion of biological behavior. *Cancer* 1982;52:680.
279. Zaloudek C, Oertel YC, Orenstein JM. Adenoid cystic carcinoma of the breast. *Am J Clin Pathol* 1984;81:297.
280. Wells CA, Nicoll S, Ferguson DJP. Adenoid cystic carcinoma of the breast: a case with axillary lymph node metastases. *Histopathology* 1986;10:415.
281. Tavassoli FA, Norris HJ. Mammary adenoid cystic carcinoma with sebaceous differentiation. A morphologic study of cell types. *Arch Pathol Lab Med* 1986;110:1045.
282. Koller M, Ram Z, Findler G, et al. Brain metastasis: a rare manifestation of adenoid cystic carcinoma of the breast. *Surg Neurol* 1986;70:470.
283. Sumpio BE, Jennings TA, Sullivan PD, et al. Adenoid cystic carcinoma of the breast. Data from the Connecticut Tumor registry and a review of the literature. *Ann Surg* 1987;205:295.
284. Ro JY, Silva EG, Gallagher HS. Adenoid cystic carcinoma of the breast. *Hum Pathol* 1987;18:1276.
285. Lamovec J, Us-Krasovec M, Zidar A, et al. Adenoid cystic carcinoma of the breast: a histologic, cytologic, and immunocytochemical study. *Semin Diagn Pathol* 1989;6:153.
286. Rosen PP. Adenoid cystic carcinoma of the breast. A morphologically heterogeneous neoplasm. *Pathol Ann* 1989;24:237.
287. Due W, Herbst H, Loy V, et al Characterization of adenoid cystic carcinoma of the breast by immunohistology. *J Clin Pathol* 1989;42:470.
288. Miliauskas JR, Leong AS. Adenoid cystic carcinoma in a juvenile male breast. *Pathology* 1991;23:298.
289. Herzberg AJ, Bossen EH, Walter PJ. Adenoid cystic carcinoma of the breast metastatic to the kidney. A clinically symptomatic lesion requiring surgical management. *Cancer* 1991;68:1015.
290. Pastolero G, Hanna W, Zbieranowski I, et al. Proliferative activity and p53 expression in adenoid cystic carcinoma of the breast. *Mod Pathol* 1996;9.215.
291. Kasami M, Olson SJ, Simpson JF, et al. Maintenance of polarity and a dual cell population in adenoid cystic carcinoma of the breast. *Histopathology* 1998;32:232.
292. Kleer CG, Oberman HA. Adenoid cystic carcinoma of the breast. Value of histologic grading and proliferative activity. *Am J Surg Pathol* 1998;22:569.
293. Clement PB, Young RH, Azzopardi JG. Collagenous spherulosis of the breast. *Am J Surg Pathol* 1987;11:411.
294. Harris M. Pseudoadenoid cystic carcinoma of the breast. *Arch Pathol Lab Med* 1977;101:307.
295. Mossler JA, Barton TK, Brinkhous AD, et al. Apocrine differentiation in human mammary carcinoma. *Cancer* 1980;46:2463.

296. d'Amore ESG, Terrier-Lacombe MJ, Travagli JP, et al. Invasive apocrine carcinoma of the breast: a long-term follow-up study of 34 cases. *Breast Cancer Res Treat* 1988;12:37.
297. Bryant J. Male breast cancer: a case of apocrine carcinoma with psammoma bodies. *Hum Pathol* 1981;12:751.
298. Abati AD, Kimmel M, Rosen PP. Apocrine mammary carcinoma. A clinicopathologic study of 72 cases. *Am J Clin Pathol* 1990;94:371.
299. Gilles R, Lesnik A, Guinebretiere JM, et al. Apocrine carcinoma: clinical and mammographic features. *Radiology* 1994;190:495.
300. Frable WJ, Kay S. Carcinoma of the breast: histological and clinical features of apocrine tumors. *Cancer* 1968;21:756.
301. Yates AJ, Ahmed A. Apocrine carcinoma and apocrine metaplasia. *Histopathology* 1988;13:228.
302. Lee BJ, Pack GT, Scharnagel I. Sweat gland cancer of the breast. *Surg Gynecol Obstet* 1933;54:975.
303. Eusebi V, Millis RR, Cattani MG, et al. Apocrine carcinoma of the breast. A morphologic and immunocytochemical study. *Am J Pathol* 1986;123:532.
304. Raju U, Zarbo RJ, Kubus J, et al. The histologic spectrum of apocrine breast proliferations: a comparative study of morphology and DNA content by image analysis. *Hum Pathol* 1993;24:173.
305. Eusebi V, Foschini MP, Bussolati G, et al. Myoblastoid (histiocytoid) carcinoma of the breast. A type of apocrine carcinoma. *Am J Surg Pathol* 1995;19:553.
306. Lamovec J, Bracko M. Secretory carcinoma of the breast: light microscopical, immunohistochemical, and flow cytometric data. *Mod Pathol* 1994;7:475.
307. McDivitt RW, Stewart FW. Breast carcinoma in children. *J Am Med Assoc* 1966;195:388.
308. Oberman HA, Stephens PJ. Carcinoma of the breast in childhood. *Cancer* 1972;30:470.
309. Byrne MP, Fahey MM, Gooselaw GG, et al. Breast cancer with axillary metastasis in an 8-1/2 year old girl. *Cancer* 1972;31:726.
310. Sullivan JJ, Magee JJ, Donald KJ. Secretory (juvenile) carcinoma of the breast. *Pathology* 1977;9:341.
311. Tavassoli FA, Norris HJ. Secretory carcinoma of the breast. *Cancer* 1980;45:2404.
312. Masse SR, Rioux A, Beauchesne C. Juvenile carcinoma of the breast. *Hum Pathol* 1981;12:1044.
313. Botta G, Fessia L, Ghiringhello B. Juvenile milk protein secreting carcinoma. *Virchows Arch (A)* 1982;395:145.
314. Karl SR, Ballantine TVN, Zaino R. Juvenile secretory carcinoma of the breast. *J Pediatr Surg* 1985;20:368.
315. d'Amore ESG, Maisto L, Gatteschi MB, et al. Secretory carcinoma of the breast. Report of a case with fine needle aspiration biopsy. *Acta Cytol* 1986;30:309.
316. Abe R, Masuda T. Secretory carcinoma of the breast in a Japanese woman. *Jpn J Surg* 1986;16:52.
317. Ferguson TB, McCarty KS, Filston HC. Juvenile secretory carcinoma and juvenile papillomatosis: diagnosis and treatment. *J Pediatr Surg* 1987;22:637.
318. Roth JA, Discafini C, O'Malley M. Secretory breast carcinoma in a man. *Am J Surg Pathol* 1988;12:150.
319. Krausz T, Jenkins D, Grontoft O, et al. Secretory carcinoma of the breast in adults: emphasis on late recurrence and metastases. *Histopathology* 1989;14:25.
320. Richard G, Hawk JC, Baker AS, et al. Multicentric adult secretory carcinoma: DNA flow cytometric findings, prognostic features, and review of the world literature. *J Surg Oncol* 1990;44:238.
321. Dominguez F, Riera JR, Junco P, et al. Secretory carcinoma of the breast. Report of a case with diagnosis by fine needle aspiration. *Acta Cytol* 1992;36:507.
322. Serour F, Gilad A, Kopolovic J, et al. Secretory breast cancer in childhood and adolescence: report of a case and review of the literature. *Med Pediatr Oncol* 1992;20:341.
323. Mies C. Recurrent secretory carcinoma in residual mammary tissue after mastectomy. *Am J Surg Pathol* 1993;17:715.
324. Pohar-Marinsek Z, Golouh R. Secretory breast carcinoma in a man diagnosed by fine needle aspiration biopsy. A case report. *Acta Cytol* 1994;38:446.
325. Kuwabara H, Yamane M, Okada S. Secretory breast carcinoma in a 66 year old man. *J Clin Pathol* 1998;51:545.
326. Furugaki K, Nagai E, Shinohara M, et al. Secretory carcinoma of the breast in an elderly woman: report of a case. *Surg Today* 1998;28:219.
327. Factor FM, Biempica L, Ratner I, et al. Carcinoma of the breast with multinucleated reactive stromal giant cells. A light and electron microscopic study of two cases. *Virchows Arch (A)* 1977;374:1.
328. Agnantis NT, Rosen PP. Mammary carcinoma with osteoclast-like giant cells. *Am J Clin Pathol* 1979;72:383.
329. Sugano I, Nagao K, Kondo Y, et al. Cytologic and ultrastructural studies of a rare breast carcinoma with osteoclast-like giant cells. *Cancer* 1983;52:74.
330. Fisher ER, Gregorio RM, Palekar AS, et al. Mucoepidermoid and squamous cell carcinoma of the breast with reference to squamous metaplasia and giant cell tumors. *Am J Surg Pathol* 1983;7:15.
331. Holland R, Van Haelst VJGM. Mammary carcinoma with osteoclast-like giant cells. Additional observations on six cases. *Cancer* 1984; 53:1963.
332. Nielsen BB, Kiaer HW. Carcinoma of the breast with stromal multinucleated giant cells. *Histopathology* 1985;9:183.
333. McMahon RFT, Ahmed A, Connolly CF. Breast carcinoma with stromal multinucleated giant cells. A light microscopic, histochemical, and ultrastructural study. *J Pathol* 1986;150:175.
334. Ichijima K, Kobashi Y, Ueda Y, et al. Breast cancer with reactive multinucleated giant cells: report of three cases. *Acta Pathol Jpn* 1986; 36:449.
335. Tavassoli FA, Norris HJ. Breast carcinoma with osteoclast-like giant cells. *Arch Pathol Lab Med* 1986;110:636.
336. Athanasou NA, Wells CA, Quinn J, et al. The origin and nature of stromal osteoclast-like multinucleated giant cells in breast carcinoma: implications for tumor osteolysis and macrophage biology. *Br J Cancer* 1989;59:491.
337. Philipson J, Ostrzega N. Fine needle of invasive cribriform carcinoma with benign osteoclastlike giant cells of histiocytic origin. A case report. *Acta Cytol* 1994;38:479.
338. Viacava P, Naccarato AG, Nardini V, et al. Breast carcinoma with osteoclast-like giant cells: immunohistochemical and ultrastructural study of a case and review of the literature. *Tumori* 1995; 81:135.
339. Takahashi T, Moriki T, Hiroi M, et al. Invasive lobular carcinoma of the breast with osteoclast-like giant cells. A case report. *Acta Cytol* 1998;42:734.
340. Saigo PE, Rosen PP. Mammary carcinoma with "choriocarcinomatous" features. *Am J Surg Pathol* 1981;5:773.
341. Green DM. Mucoid carcinoma of the breast with choriocarcinoma in its metastasis. *Histopathology* 1990;16:504.
342. Alvarez RD, Gleason BP, Gore H, et al. Co-existing intraductal breast carcinoma and metastatic choriocarcinoma presenting as a breast mass. *Gynecol Oncol* 1991;43:295.
343. Fowler CA, Nicholson S, Lott M, et al. Choriocarcinoma presenting as a breast lump. *Eur J Surg Oncol* 1995;21:576.
344. Aboumrad MH, Horn RC, Fine G. Lipid-secreting mammary carcinoma: report of a case associated with Paget's disease of the nipple. *Cancer* 1963;16:521.
345. Ramos CV, Taylor HB. Lipid-rich carcinoma of the breast. A clinicopathologic analysis of 13 examples. *Cancer* 1974;33:812.
346. Van Bogaert LJ, Maldague P. Histologic variants of lipid-secreting carcinoma of the breast. *Virchows Arch [A] Pathol Anat Histol* 1977;375:345.
347. Lapey JD. Lipid-rich mammary carcinoma: diagnosis by cytology. Case report. *Acta Cytol* 1977;21:120.
348. Dina R, Eusebi V. Clear cell tumors of the breast. *Semin Diagn Pathol* 1997;14:175.
349. Hull MT, Priest JB, Broadie TA, et al. Glycogen-rich clear cell carcinoma of the breast. A light and electron microscopic study. *Cancer* 1981;48:2003.
350. Benisch B, Peison B, Newman R, et al. Solid glycogen-rich clear cell carcinoma of the breast (a light and ultrastructural study). *Am J Clin Pathol* 1983;79:243.
351. Fisher ER, Tavares J, Bulatao IS, et al. Glycogen-rich clear cell breast cancer: with comments concerning other clear cell variants. *Hum Pathol* 1985;16:1085.
352. Hull MT, Warfel KA. Glycogen-rich clear cell carcinomas of the breast. A clinicopathologic and ultrastructural study. *Am J Surg Pathol* 1986;10:553.
353. Sorensen FB, Paulsen SM. Glycogen-rich clear cell carcinoma of the breast: a solid variant with mucus. A light microscopic, immunohistochemical and ultrastructural study of a case. *Histopathology* 1987; 11:857.

354. Toikkanen S, Joensuu H. Glycogen-rich clear cell carcinoma of the breast: a clinicopathologic and flow cytometric study. *Hum Pathol* 1991;22:81.
355. Hayes MMM, Seidman JD, Ashton MA. Glycogen-rich clear cell carcinoma of the breast: a clinicopathologic study of 21 cases. *Am J Surg Pathol* 1995;19:904.
356. Koenig C, Tavassoli FA. Mucinous cystadenocarcinoma of the breast. *Am J Surg Pathol* 1998;22:698.
357. Bohman LG, Bassett LW, Gold RH, et al. Breast metastases from extramammary malignancies. *Radiology* 1982;144:309.
358. Sandison AT. Metastatic tumors in the breast. *Br J Surg* 1959;47:54.
359. Toombs BD, Kalisher L. Metastatic disease in the breast: clinical, pathologic and radiologic features. *AJR Am J Roentgenol* 1977:129:673.
360. Moncada R, Cooper RA, Garces M, et al. Calcified metastasis from metastatic ovarian neoplasm. *Radiology* 1977;113:31.
361. Laifer S, Buscema J, Parmley TH, et al. Ovarian carcinoma metastatic to the breast. *Gynecol Oncol* 1986; 24:97.
362. Duda RB, August CZ, Schink JC. Ovarian carcinoma metastatic to the breast and axillary node. *Surgery* 1991;110:552.
363. Yamasaki H, Saw D, Zdanowitz J, et al. Ovarian carcinoma metastasis to the breast. Case report and review of the literature. *Am J Surg Pathol* 1993;17:193.
364. Elit LM, Cunnane MF. Breast metastasis from ovarian carcinoma: report of two cases and literature review. *J Surg Pathol* 1995;1:69.
365. Pressman PI. Malignant melanoma and the breast. *Cancer* 1973; 31:784.
366. Silverman JF, Feldman PS, Covell JL, et al. Fine needle aspiration cytology of neoplasms metastatic to the breast. *Acta Cytol* 1987;31:291.
367. Sneige N, Zachariah S, Fanning TV, et al. Fine needle aspiration cytology of metastatic neoplasms in the breast. *Am J Clin Pathol* 1989;92:27.
368. Cangiarella J, Symmans WF, Cohen JM, et al. Malignant melanoma metastatic to the breast: a report of seven cases diagnosed by fine needle aspiration cytology. *Cancer* 1998;84:160.
369. Charache H. Metastatic tumors in the breast with a report of ten cases. *Surgery* 1953;33:385.
370. Kelly C, Henderson D, Corris P. Breast lumps: rare presentation of oat cell carcinoma of lung. *J Clin Pathol* 1988;41:171.
371. McCrea ES, Johnston C, Haney PJ, Metastases to the breast. *AJR Am J Roentgenol* 1983;141:685.
372. Nielsen M, Andersen JA, Henriksen FW, et al. Metastases to the breast from extramammary carcinomas. *Acta Pathol Microbiol Scand [A]* 1981;89:251.
373. Pribe WA. Prostatic metastasis to the breast and the role of estrogens. *J Urol* 1963;11:891.
374. Pribe WA, Ockuly EA. Prostatic metastasis to the breast and the role of estrogens: case report and review. *J Am Geriatr Soc* 1963;11:891.
375. Salyer WR, Salyer DC. Metastases of prostatic carcinoma to the breast. *J Urol* 1973;109:671.
376. Hartley LCJ, Little JH. Bilateral mammary metastases from carcinoma of the prostate during oestrogen therapy. *Med J Aust* 1971;I:434.
377. Scott J, Robb-Smith AHT, Burns I. Bilateral breast metastases from carcinoma of the prostate. *Br J Urol* 1974;46:209.
378. Benson WR. Carcinoma of the prostate with metastases to the breast and testes. *Cancer* 1957;10:1235.
379. Malek GA, Madsen PO. Carcinoma of the prostate with unusual metastases. *Cancer* 1969;24:194.
380. Wilson SE, Hutchinson WB. Breast masses in males with carcinoma of the prostate. *J Surg Oncol* 1976;8:105
381. Harrist TJ, Kalisher L. Breast metastasis: an unusual manifestation of a malignant carcinoid tumor. *Cancer* 1977; 40:3102.
382. Turner M, Gallagher HS. Occult appendiceal carcinoid. Report of a case with fatal metastases. *Arch Pathol* 1959;88:188.
383. Schurch W, Lamoureux E, Lefebre R, et al. Solitary breast metastasis: first manifestation of an occult carcinoid of the ileum. *Virchows Arch [A] Pathol Anat Histol* 1980;386:117.
384. Hawley PP. A case of secondary carcinoid tumors in both breasts following excision of primary carcinoid of the duodenum. *Br J Surg* 1966;53:818.
385. Landon D, Sneige N, Ordonez NG, et al. Carcinoid metastatic to breast diagnosed by fine-needle aspiration biopsy. *Diagn Cytopathol* 1987;3:230.
386. Lozowski MS, Faegenberg D, Mishriki Y, et al. Carcinoid tumor metastatic to breast diagnosed by fine needle aspiration. Case report and literature review. *Acta Cytol* 1989;33:191.
387. Silverman EM, Oberman HA. Metastatic neoplasms in the breast. *Surg Gynecol Obstet* 1974;138:26.
388. Chica GA, Johnson DE, Ayala AG. Renal cell carcinoma presenting as breast carcinoma. *J Urol* 1980;15:389.
389. Ascani S, Nati S, Liberati F, et al. Breast metastasis of thyroid follicular carcinoma. *Acta Oncol* 1994;33:71.
390. Nunez DA, Sutherland CGC, Sood RK. Breast metastasis from a pharyngeal carcinoma. *J Laryngol Otol* 1989;103:227.
391. Breitbart AS, Harris MN, Vazquez M, et al. Metastatic hemangiopericytoma of the breast. *NY State J Med* 1992; 92:158.
392. Howarth GB, Cases JN, Pratt CB. Breast metastases in children with rhabdomyosarcoma. *Cancer* 1980;46:2520.
393. Alexander HR, Turnbull AD, Rosen PP. Isolated breast metastases from gastrointestinal carcinomas. *J Surg Oncol* 1989;42:264.
394. Baliga M, Holmquist MD, Espinoza CJ. Medulloblastoma metastatic to breast diagnosed by fine-needle aspiration biopsy. *Diagn Cytopathol* 1994;10:33.
395. Speert H, Greeley AV. Cervical cancer with metastasis to the breast. *Am J Obstet Gynecol* 1948;55:894.
396. Marcus JN, Watson P, Page DL, et al. Hereditary breast cancer. Pathobiology, prognosis, and BRCA1 and BRCA2 gene linkage. *Cancer* 1996;77:697.
397. Marcus JN, Page DL, Watson P, et al. BRCA1 and BRCA2 hereditary breast carcinoma phenotypes. *Cancer* 1997;80:543.
398. Breast Cancer Linkage Consortium. Pathology of familial breast cancer: differences between breast cancer in carriers of BRCA1 or BRCA2 mutations and sporadic cases. *Lancet* 1997;349:1505.
399. Robson M, Gilewski T, Haas B, et al. BRCA-associated breast cancer in young women. *J Clin Oncol* 1998;16:1642.
400. Karp SE, Tonin PN, Begin LR, et al. Influence of BRCA1 mutations on nuclear grade and estrogen receptor status of breast carcinoma in Ashkenazi Jewish women. *Cancer* 1997;80:435.
401. Verhoog LC, Brekelmans CET, Seynaeve C, et al. Survival and tumor characteristics of breast-cancer patients with germline mutations of BRCA1. *Lancet* 1998;351:316.
402. Johansson OT, Idvall I, Anderson C, et al. Tumor biological features of BRCA1-induced breast and ovarian carcinoma. *Eur J Cancer* 1997;33:372.
403. Eisinger F, Stoppa-Lyonnet D, Longy M, et al. Germ line mutation at BRCA1 affects the histoprognostic grade in hereditary breast cancer. *Cancer Res* 1996;56:471.
404. Lynch BJ, Holden JA, Buys SS, et al. Pathobiologic characteristics of hereditary breast cancer. *Hum Pathol* 1998;29:1140.
405. Lakhani SR, Jacquemier J, Sloane JP, et al. Multifactorial analysis of differences between sporadic breast cancers and cancers involving BRCA1 and BRCA2 mutations. *J Natl Cancer Inst* 1998; 90:1138.
406. Armes JE, Egan AJM, Southey MC, et al. The histologic phenotypes of breast carcinoma occurring before age 40 years in women with and without BRCA1 or BRCA2 germline mutations. *Cancer* 1998; 83:2335.
407. Henderson IC, Patek AJ. Are breast cancers in young women qualitatively distinct? *Lancet* 1997;349:1488.
408. Lynch HT, Watson P. BRCA1, pathology, and survival. *J Clin Oncol* 1998;16:395.
409. Watson P, Marcus JN, Lynch HT. Prognosis of BRCA1 hereditary breast cancer. *Lancet* 1998;351:304.
410. Agnarsson BA, Jonasson JG, Bjornsdottir IB, et al. Inherited BRCA2 mutation associated with high grade breast cancer. *Breast Cancer Res Treat* 1998;47:121.
411. Marcus JN, Watson P, Page DL, et al. BRCA2 hereditary breast cancer phenotype. *Breast Cancer Res Treat* 1997;44:275.
412. Mansour EG, Ravdin PM, Dressler L. Prognostic factors in early breast carcinoma. *Cancer* 1994;74:381.
413. Weidner N, Cady B, Goodson WH. Pathologic prognostic factors for patients with breast carcinoma. Which factors are important? *Surg Oncol Clin N Am* 1997;6:415.
414. Donnegan WL. Tumor-related prognostic factors for breast cancer. *CA Cancer J Clin* 1997;47:28.
415. Fisher B, Slack NH, Bross IDJ, et al. Cancer of the breast: size of the neoplasm and prognosis. *Cancer* 1969;24:1071.
416. Say CC, Donegan WL. Invasive carcinoma of the breast: prognostic significance of tumor size and involved axillary lymph nodes. *Cancer* 1974;34:468.

417. Valagussa P, Bonnadona G, Veronesi U. Patterns of relapse and survival following radical mastectomy. Analysis of 716 consecutive patients. *Cancer* 1978;41:1170.
418. Carter CL, Allen C, Henson DE. Relation of tumor size, lymph node status, and survival in 24,740 breast cancer cases. *Cancer* 1989; 63:181.
419. McGuire WL, Tandon AK, Allred DC, et al. How to use prognostic factors in axillary node-negative breast cancer patients. *J Natl Cancer Inst* 1990;82:1007.
420. Rosen PP, Groshen S. Factors influencing survival and prognosis in early breast carcinoma (T1N0M1-T1N1M0). Assessment of 644 patients with median follow-up of 18 years. *Surg Clin N Am* 1990;70:937.
421. Rosen PP, Groshen S, Saigo PE, et al. A long-term follow-up study of survival in stage I (T1N0M0) and stage II (T1N1M0) breast carcinoma. *J Clin Oncol* 1989;7:355.
422. Rosen PP, Groshen S, Kinne DW. Prognosis in T2N0M0 stage I breast carcinoma: a 20-year follow-up study. *J Clin Oncol* 1991;9:1650.
423. Koscielny S, Tubiana M, Le MG, et al. Breast cancer: relationship between the size of the primary tumour and the probability of metastatic dissemination. *Br J Cancer* 1984;49:709.
424. Quiet CA, Ferguson DJ, Weichselbaum RR, Hellman S. Natural history of node-negative breast cancer: a study of 826 patients with long-term follow-up. *J Clin Oncol* 1995;13:1144.
425. Abner AL, Collins L, Peiro G, et al. Correlation of tumor size and axillary lymph node involvement with prognosis in patients with T1 breast carcinoma. *Cancer* 1998;82:2502.
426. Chen Y-Y, Schnitt SJ. Prognostic factors for patients with breast cancers 1 cm and smaller. *Breast Cancer Res Treat* 1998;51:209.
427. Fisher B, Redmond C. Systemic therapy in node-negative patients: updated findings from NSABP clinical trials. *J Natl Cancer Inst Monogr* 1992;11:159.
428. Silverstein MJ, Gierson E, Waisman JR, Colburn WJ, Gamagami P. Predicting axillary node positivity in patients with invasive carcinoma of the breast by using a combination of T category and palpability. *J Am Coll Surg* 1995;180:700.
429. Barth AM, Craig PH, Silverstein MJ. Predictors of axillary lymph node metastases in patients with T1 breast carcinoma. *Cancer* 1997; 79:1918.
430. Arnesson L-G, Smeds S, Fagerberg G. Recurrence-free survival in patients with small breast cancers. *Eur J Surg* 1994;160:271.
431. Halverson K, Taylor ME, Perez CA, et al. Management of the axilla in patients with breast cancers one centimeter or smaller. *Am J Clin Oncol* 1994;17:461.
432. Lee AKC, Loda M, Mackarem G, et al. Lymph node negative invasive breast carcinoma 1 centimeter or less in size: clinicopathologic features and outcome. *Cancer* 1997;79:761.
433. American Joint Committee on Cancer. *AJCC cancer staging manual.* Philadelphia: Lippincott–Raven, 1997:172.
434. Peiro G, Abner A, Silver B, Connolly J, Harris J, Schnitt S. Discrepancies between gross and microscopic size of small breast cancers and their prognostic significance. *Mod Pathol* 1995;8:23A(abst).
435. Seidman JD, Schnaper LA, Aisner SC. Relationship of the size of the invasive component of the primary breast carcinoma to axillary lymph node metastasis. *Cancer* 1995;75:65.
436. Simpson JF, Page DL. Status of breast cancer prognostication based on histopathologic data. *Am J Clin Pathol* 1994;102[Suppl1]:S3.
437. Dixon JM, Page DL, Anderson TJ, et al. Long term survivors after breast cancer. *Br J Surg* 1985;72:445.
438. Davis BW, Gelber RD, Goldhirsch A, et al. Prognostic significance of tumor grade in clinical trials of adjuvant therapy for breast cancer with axillary lymph node metastasis. *Cancer* 1986;58:2662.
439. Contesso G, Mouriesse H, Friedman S, et al. The importance of histologic grade in long-term prognosis of breast cancer: a study of 1,010 patients, uniformly treated at the Institut Gustave-Roussy. *J Clin Oncol* 1987;5:1378.
440. Le Doussal V, Tubiana-Hulin M, Friedman S, et al. Prognostic value of histologic grade nuclear components of Scarff-Bloom Richardson (SBR). An improved score modification based on multivariate analysis of 1262 invasive ductal breast carcinomas. *Cancer* 1989; 64:1914.
441. Rosen PP, Groshen S, Saigo PE, et al. Pathological prognostic factors in stage I (T1N0M0) and stage II (T1N1M0) breast carcinoma: a study of 644 patients with median follow-up of 18 years. *J Clin Oncol* 1989;7:1239.
442. Henson DE, Ries L, Freedman LS, Carriaga M. Relationship among outcome, stage of disease, and histologic grade for 22,616 cases of breast cancer. The basis for a prognostic index. *Cancer* 1991;68:2142.
443. Elston CW, Ellis IO. Pathological prognostic factors in breast cancer. I. The value of histological grade in breast cancer: experience from a large study with long-term follow-up. *Histopathology* 1991;19:403.
444. Page DL. Prognosis and breast cancer. Recognition of lethal and favorable prognostic types. *Am J Surg Pathol* 1991;15:334.
445. Nixon AJ, Schnitt SJ, Gelman R, et al. Relationship of tumor grade to other pathologic features and to treatment outcome of patients with early stage breast carcinoma treated with breast-conserving therapy. *Cancer* 1996;78:1426.
446. Roberti NE. The role of histologic grading in the prognosis of patients with carcinoma of the breast. Is this a neglected opportunity? *Cancer* 1997;80:1708.
447. Pereira H, Pinder SE, Sibbering DM, et al. Pathologic prognostic factors in breast cancer. IV: Should you be a typer or a grader? A comparative study of two histological prognostic features in operable breast carcinoma. *Histopathology* 1995;27:219.
448. Fisher ER, Redmond C, Fisher B, et al. Pathologic findings from the National Surgical Adjuvant Breast Project. VIII. Relationship of chemotherapeutic responsiveness to tumor differentiation. *Cancer* 1983;51:181.
449. Pinder SE, Murray S, Ellis I, et al. The importance of the histologic grade of invasive breast carcinoma and response to chemotherapy. *Cancer* 1998;83:1529.
450. Delides G, Garas G, Georgouli G, et al. Intralaboratory variations in the grading of breast carcinoma. *Arch Pathol Lab Med* 1982;106:126.
451. Stenkvist B, Westman-Naeser S, Vegelius J, et al. Analysis of reproducibility of subjective grading systems for breast carcinoma. *J Clin Pathol* 1979;32:979.
452. Gilchrist KW, Kalish L, Gould VE, et al. Interobserver reproducibility of histopathological features in stage II breast cancer. *Breast Cancer Res Treat* 1985;5:3.
453. Harvey JM, deKlerk NH, Sterrett GT. Histological grading in breast cancer: interobserver agreement and relation to other prognostic factors and to ploidy. *Pathology* 1992;24:63.
454. Frierson HF, Wober RA, Berean KW, et al. Interobserver reproducibility of the Nottingham modification of the Bloom and Richardson histologic grading scheme for infiltrating ductal carcinoma. *Am J Clin Pathol* 1995;103:195.
455. Dalton LW, Page DL, Dupont WD. Histologic grading of breast carcinoma. A reproducibility study. *Cancer* 1994;73:2765.
456. Pinder S, Ellis IO, O'Rourke S, et al. Pathological prognostic factors in breast cancer. III. Vascular invasion: relationship to recurrence and survival in a large series with long-term follow-up. *Histopathology* 1994;24:41.
457. Orbo A, Stalsberg H, Kunde D. Topographic criteria in the diagnosis of tumor emboli in intramammary lymphatics. *Cancer* 1990;66:972.
458. Rosen PP. Tumor emboli in intramammary lymphatics in breast carcinoma: pathological criteria for diagnosis and clinical significance. *Pathol Annu* 1993;18:215.
459. Davis BW, Gelber R, Goldhirsch A, et al. Prognostic significance of peritumoral vessel invasion in clinical trials of adjuvant therapy for breast cancer with axillary node metastases. *Hum Pathol* 1985;16:1212.
460. Lauria R, Perrone F, Carlomagno C, et al. The prognostic value of lymphatic and blood vessel invasion in operable breast cancer. *Cancer* 1995;76:1772.
461. Chen Y-Y, Connolly JL, Harris J, Schnitt S. Predictors of axillary lymph node metastases (ALNM) in patients with breast cancers 1 cm and smaller (T1a,b): implications for axillary dissection. *Mod Pathol* 1998;78:17A.
462. Fein DA, Fowble BL, Hanlon AL, et al. Identification of women with T1-T2 breast cancer at low risk of positive axillary nodes. *J Surg Oncol* 1997;65:34.
463. Chadha M, Chabon AB, Friedmann P, Vikrum B. Predictors of axillary lymph node metastases in patients with T1 breast carcinoma. *Cancer* 1994;73:350.
464. Nealon Jr TF, Nkongho A, Grossi C, Gillooley J. Pathologic identification of poor prognosis stage I (T1N0M0) cancer of the breast. *Ann Surg* 1979;190:129.
465. Nealon Jr TF, Nkongho A, Grossi CE, et al. Treatment of early cancer of the breast (T1N0M0 and T2N0M0) on the basis of histologic characteristics. *Surgery* 1981;89:279.

466. Rosen PP, Saigo PE, Braun DW, et al. Predictors of recurrence in stage I (T1N0M0) breast carcinoma. *Ann Surg* 1981;193:15.
467. Roses DF, Bell DA, Flotte TJ, et al. Pathologic predictors of recurrence in stage 1 (T1N0M0) breast cancer. *Am J Clin Pathol* 1982;78:817.
468. Bettleheim R, Penman HG, Thornton-Jones H, Neville AM. Prognostic significance of peritumoral vascular invasion in breast cancer. *Br J Cancer* 1984;50:771.
469. Clayton F. Pathologic correlates of survival in 378 lymph node-negative breast carcinomas. Mitotic count is the best single predictor. *Cancer* 1991;68:1309.
470. Clemente CG, Boracchi P, Andreola S, et al. Peritumoral lymphatic invasion in patients with node-negative mammary duct carcinoma. *Cancer* 1992;69:1396.
471. Lee AKC, DeLellis RA, Silverman ML, Wolfe HJ. Lymphatic and blood vessel invasion in breast carcinoma: a useful prognostic indicator? *Hum Pathol* 1986;17:984.
472. Leitner SP, Swern AS, Weinberger D, et al. Predictors of recurrence for patients with small (one centimeter or less) localized breast cancer (T1a,bN0M0). *Cancer* 1995;76:2266.
473. Gilchrist KW, Gould VE, Hirschl S, et al. Interobserver variation in the identification of breast carcinoma in intramammary lymphatics. *Hum Pathol* 1982;13:170.
474. Bettleheim R, Mitchell D, Gusterson B. Immunocytochemistry in the identification of vascular invasion in breast cancer. *J Clin Pathol* 1984;37:364.
475. Lee AKC, DeLellis RA, Rosen PP, et al. ABH blood group isoantigen expression in breast carcinomas—an immunohistochemical evaluation using monoclonal antibodies. *Am J Clin Pathol* 1985;83:308.
476. Lee AKC, DeLellis RA, Wolfe HJ. Intramammary lymphatic invasion in breast carcinomas. Evaluation using ABH isoantigens as endothelial markers. *Am J Surg Pathol* 1986;10:589.
477. Martin SA, Perez-Reyes N, Mendelsohn G. Angioinvasion in breast carcinoma. An immunohistochemical study of factor VIII-related antigen. *Cancer* 1987;59:1918.
478. Saigo PE, Rosen PP. The application of immunohistochemical stains to identify endothelial lined channels in mammary carcinoma. *Cancer* 1987;59:51.
479. Ordonez NG, Brooks T, Thompson S, Batsakis JG. Use of ulex europaeus agglutinin I in the identification of lymphatic and blood vessel invasion in previously stained microscopic slides. *Am J Surg Pathol* 1987;11:543.
480. Hanau CA, Machera H, Miettinen M. Immunohistochemical evaluation of vascular invasion in carcinomas with five different markers. *Appl Immunohistochem* 1993;1:46.
481. Rosen PP, Saigo PE, Braun DW, et al. Prognosis in stage II (T1N1M0) breast cancer. *Ann Surg* 1981;194:576.
482. Bell JR, Friedell GH, Goldberg IS. Prognostic significance of pathologic findings in human breast carcinoma. *Surg Gynecol Obstet* 1969;129:258.
483. Kister SJ, Sommers SC, Haagensen CD, Cooley E. Reevaluation of blood vessel invasion and lymphocytic infiltrates in breast carcinoma. *Cancer* 1966;19:1213.
484. Sampat MB, Sirsat MV, Gangadharan P. Prognostic significance of blood vessel invasion in carcinoma of the breast in women. *J Surg Oncol* 1977; 9:623.
485. Weigand RA, Isenberg WM, Russo J, et al. Blood vessel invasion and axillary lymph node involvement as prognostic indicators for human breast cancer. *Cancer* 1982;50:962.
486. Fisher ER, Palekar AD, Gregorio RM, et al. Pathological findings from the National Surgical Adjuvant Breast Project (Protocol No. 4). IV. Significance of tumor necrosis. *Hum Pathol* 1978;9:523.
487. Carter D, Pipkin RD, Shepard RH, et al. Relationship of necrosis and tumor border to lymph node metastases and 10-year survival in carcinoma of the breast. *Am J Surg Pathol* 1978;2:39.
488. Gilchrist KW, Gray R, Fowble B, et al. Tumor necrosis is a prognostic predictor of recurrence and death in lymph node-positive breast cancer: a 10-year follow-up study of 728 Eastern Cooperative Oncology Group patients. *J Clin Oncol* 1993;11:1929.
489. Parham DM, Hagen N, Brown RA. Simplified method of grading primary carcinomas of the breast. *J Clin Pathol* 1992;45:517.
490. Stenkvist B, Bengtsson E, Dahlqvist B, et al. Predicting breast cancer recurrence. *Cancer* 1982;50:2884.
491. Cutler SJ, Black MM, Mork T, et al. Further observations on prognostic factors in cancer of the female breast. *Cancer* 1969;24:653.
492. Black MM, Barclay THC, Hankey BF. Prognosis in breast cancer utilizing histologic characteristics of the primary tumor. *Cancer* 1975;36:2048.
493. Alderson MR, Hamlin E, Staunton MD. The relative significance of prognostic factors in breast carcinoma. *Br J Cancer* 1971;25:646.
494. Berg JW. Morphological evidence for immune response to cancer—an historical review. *Cancer* 1971;28:1453.
495. Dawson PJ, Ferguson DJ, Karrison T. The pathologic findings of breast cancer in patients surviving 25 years after radical mastectomy. *Cancer* 1982;50:2131.
496. Rosen PP. *Rosen's breast pathology*. Philadelphia: Lippincott–Raven, 1997:287.
497. Rosen PP, Kinne DW, Lesser M, Hellman S. Are prognostic factors for local control of breast cancer treated by primary radiotherapy significant for patients treated by mastectomy? *Cancer* 1986;57:1415.
498. Park C, Misumori M, Recht A, et al. The relationship between pathologic margin status and outcome after breast conserving therapy. *Int J Radiat Oncol Biol Phys* 1998;42[Suppl]:125.
499. McGuire WL, Clark GM. Prognostic factors and treatment decisions in axillary node-negative breast cancer. *N Engl J Med* 1992;326:1756.
500. Galea MH, Blamey RW, Elston CW, et al. The Nottingham Prognostic Index in primary breast cancer. *Breast Cancer Res Treat* 1992; 22:187.
501. van Diest PJ, Baak JPA. The morphometric prognostic index is the strongest prognosticator in premenopausal lymph node-negative and lymph node-positive breast cancer patients. *Hum Pathol* 1991;22:326.
502. Jacobs TW, Siziopikou KP, Prioleau JE, et al. Do prognostic marker studies on core needle biopsy specimens of breast carcinoma accurately reflect the marker status of the tumor? *Mod Pathol* 1998; 11:259.
503. Jacobs TW, Silverman JF, Schroeder B, et al. Accuracy of touch-imprint cytology of image-directed breast core needle biopsies. *Acta Cytol* 1999;43:169.
504. Schnitt SJ, Abner A, Gelman R, et al. The relationship between microscopic margins of resection and the risk of local recurrence in patients with breast cancer treated with breast-conserving surgery and radiation therapy. *Cancer* 1994;74:1746.
505. Gage I, Schnitt SJ, Nixon A, et al. Pathologic margin involvement and the risk of local recurrence in patients treated with breast-conserving therapy. *Cancer* 1996;78:1821.
506. Smitt MC, Nowels KW, Zdeblick MJ, et al. The importance of lumpectomy surgical margin status in long term results of breast conservation. *Cancer* 1995;76:259.
507. Solin LJ, Fowble BL, Schultz DJ, et al. The significance of the pathology margins of the tumor excision on the outcome of patients treated with definitive irradiation for early stage breast cancer. *Int J Radiat Oncol Biol Phys* 1991;21:279.
508. Borger J, Kemperman H, Hart A, et al. Risk factors in breast conservation therapy. *J Clin Oncol* 1994;12:653.
509. Kurtz JM, Jacquemier J, Amalric R, et al. Risk factors for breast recurrence in premenopausal and postmenopausal patients with ductal cancers treated by conservation therapy. *Cancer* 1990;65:1867.
510. Anscher MS, Jones P, Prosnitz LR, et al. Local failure and margin status in early-stage breast carcinoma treated with conservation surgery and radiation therapy. *Ann Surg* 1993;218:22.
511. Spivack B, Khanna MM, Tafra L, Juillard G, Giuliano AE . Margin status and local recurrence after breast-conserving surgery. *Arch Surg* 1994;129:952.
512. Heimann R, Powers C, Halpern HJ, et al. Breast preservation in stage I and II carcinoma of the breast. The University of Chicago experience. *Cancer* 1996;78:1722.
513. Schnitt SJ, Connolly JL. Processing and evaluation of breast excision specimens. A clinically oriented approach. *Am J Clin Pathol* 1992; 98:125.
514. Carter D. Margins of "lumpectomy" for breast cancer. *Hum Pathol* 1986;17:330.
515. Fisher ER, Sass R, Fisher B, et al. Pathologic findings from the National Surgical Adjuvant Breast Project (Protocol 6). II. Relation of local breast recurrence to multicentricity. *Cancer* 1986;57:1717.
516. Guidi AJ, Connolly JL, Harris JR, Schnitt SJ. The relationship between shaved margin and inked margin status in breast excision specimens. *Cancer* 1997;79:1568.
517. The Consensus Conference Committee. Consensus conference on the classification of ductal carcinoma in situ. *Cancer* 1997;80:1798.

518. Sauter ER, Hoffman JP, Ottery FD, et al. Is frozen section analysis of reexcision lumpectomy margins worthwhile? *Cancer* 1994;73:2607.
519. Weber S, Storm FK, Stitt J, Mahvi DM. The role of frozen section analysis of margins during breast conservation surgery. *Cancer J Sci Am* 1997;3:273.
520. Cox CE, Ku NN, Reintgen DS, et al. Touch preparation cytology of breast lumpectomy margins with histologic correlation. *Arch Surg* 1991;126:490.
521. Gal R. Scrape cytology assessment of margins of lumpectomy specimens in breast cancer. *Acta Cytol* 1988;32:838.
522. England DW, Chan SY, Stonelake PS, Lee MJ. Assessment of excision margins following wide local excision for breast carcinoma using specimen scrape cytology and tumor bed biopsy. *Eur J Surg Oncol* 1994;20:425.
523. Klimberg VS, Westbrook KC, Korourian S. Use of touch preps for diagnosis and evaluation of surgical margins in breast cancer. *Ann Surg Oncol* 1998;5:220.
524. Fisher B, Anderson S, Redmond C, et al. Reanalysis and results of follow-up in a randomized clinical trial comparing total mastectomy with lumpectomy with or without irradiation in the treatment of breast cancer. *N Engl J Med* 1995;333:1456.
525. Forrest AP, Stewart HJ, Everington D, et al. Randomised controlled trial of conservation therapy for breast cancer: 6-year analysis of the Scottish trial. *Lancet* 1996;348:708.
526. Liberman L, LaTrenta LR, Dershaw DD, et al. Impact of core biopsy on the surgical management of impalpable breast cancer. *AJR Am J Roentgenol* 1997;168:495.
527. Smith DN, Christian R, Meyer JE. Large-core needle biopsy of nonpalpable breast cancers. The impact on subsequent surgical excisions. *Arch Surg* 1997;132:256.
528. Adler DD, Wahl RL. New methods for imaging the breast: techniques, findings, and potential. *AJR Am J Roentgenol* 1997;164:19.
529. Deng G, Lu Y, Zlotnikov G, et al. Loss of heterozygosity in normal tissue adjacent to breast carcinomas. *Science* 1996;274:2057.
530. Bennington JL, Lagios MD (eds). *The mammographically directed biopsy*. Philadelphia: Hanley and Belfus, 1992.
531. Graham RA, Homer MJ, Sigler CJ, et al. The efficacy of specimen radiography in evaluating the surgical margins of impalpable breast carcinoma. *AJR Am J Roentgenol* 1994;162:33.
532. Lee CH, Carter D. Detecting residual tumor after excisional biopsy of impalpable breast carcinoma: efficacy of comparing preoperative mammograms with radiographs of the biopsy specimen. *AJR Am J Roentgenol* 1995;164:81.
533. Owings DV, Hann L, Schnitt SJ. How thoroughly should needle localization breast biopsies be sampled for microscopic examination? A prospective mammographic-pathologic correlative study. *Am J Surg Pathol* 1990;14:578.
534. Radi MJ. Calcium oxalate crystals in breast biopsies. An overlooked form of microcalcification associated with benign breast disease. *Arch Pathol Lab Med* 1989;113:1367.
535. Tornos C, Silva E, El-Naggar A, Pritzker KPH. Calcium oxalate crystals in breast biopsies. The missing microcalcifications. *Am J Surg Pathol* 1990;14:961.
536. Gonzalez JEG, Caldwell RG, Valaitis J. Calcium oxalate crystals in the breast. Pathology and significance. *Am J Surg Pathol* 1991;15:586.
537. Bianchi S, Palli D, Ciatto S, et al. Accuracy and reliability of frozen section diagnosis in a series of 672 nonpalpable breast lesions. *Am J Clin Pathol* 1995;103:199.
538. Ferreiro JA, Gisvold JJ, Bostwick DG. Accuracy of frozen-section diagnosis of mammographically directed breast biopsies. Results of 1490 consecutive cases. *Am J Surg Pathol* 1995;19:1267.
539. Oberman HA. A modest proposal. *Am J Surg Pathol* 1992;16:69.
540. Association of Directors of Anatomic and Surgical Pathology. Immediate management of mammographically detected breast lesions. *Am J Surg Pathol* 1993;17:850.
541. Lee KC, Chan JKC, Ho LC. Histologic changes in the breast after fine-needle aspiration. *Am J Surg Pathol* 1994;18:1039.
542. Youngson BJ, Cranor M, Rosen PP. Epithelial displacement in surgical breast specimens following needling procedures. *Am J Surg Pathol* 1994;18:896.
543. Youngson BJ, Liberman L, Rosen PP. Displacement of carcinomatous epithelium in surgical breast specimens following stereotaxic core biopsy. *Am J Clin Pathol* 1995;103:598.
544. Tavassoli FA, Pestaner JP. Pseudoinvasion in intraductal carcinoma. *Mod Pathol* 1995;8:380.
545. Abraham S, Fox K, Fraker D, et al. Sampling of grossly benign breast re-excisions: a multidisciplinary approach to assessing adequacy. *Am J Surg Pathol* 1999;23:316.
546. Kennedy S, Merino MJ, Swain SM, et al. The effects of hormonal and chemotherapy on tumoral and nonneoplastic breast tissue. *Hum Pathol* 1990;21:192.
547. Andersen J, Jensen J. Lymph node identification. Specimen radiography of tissue predominated by fat. *Am J Clin Pathol* 1977;68:511.
548. Groote AD, Oosterhuis JW, Molenar WM, et al. Radiographic imaging of lymph nodes in lymph node dissection specimens. *Lab Invest* 1985;52:326.
549. Durkin K, Haagensen CD. An improved technique for the study of lymph nodes in surgical specimens. *Ann Surg* 1980;191:419.
550. Morrow M, Evans J, Rosen PP, Kinne DW. Does clearing of axillary lymph nodes contribute to accurate staging of breast carcinoma? *Cancer* 1984;53:1329.
551. Kingsley WB, Peters GN, Cheek JH. What constitutes adequate study of axillary lymph nodes in breast cancer? *Ann Surg* 1985;301:311.
552. Koren R, Kyzer S, Paz A, et al. Lymph node revealing solution: A new method for detection of minute axillary lymph nodes in breast cancer specimens. *Am J Surg Pathol* 1997;21:1387.
553. de Mascarel I, Bonichon F, Coindre JM, Trojani M. Prognostic significance of breast cancer axillary node micrometastases assessed by two special techniques: re-evaluation with longer follow up. *Br J Cancer* 1992;66:523.
554. Neimann TH, Yilmaz AG, Marsh Jr. WL, Lucas JG. A half a node or a whole node. A comparison of methods for submitting lymph nodes. *Am J Clin Pathol* 1998;109:571.
555. Zhang PJ, Reisner RM, Nangia R, et al. Effectiveness of multiple-level sectioning in detecting axillary nodal micrometastasis in breast cancer. A retrospective study with immunohistochemical analysis. *Arch Pathol Lab Med* 1998;122:687.
556. Hansen NM. Current status of sentinel node biopsy. *Semin Breast Dis* 1998;1:146.
557. Association of Directors of Anatomic and Surgical Pathology. Recommendations for the reporting of breast carcinoma. *Am J Clin Pathol* 1995;104:614.
558. Henson DE, Oberman HA, Hutter RVP, et al. Practice protocol for the examination of specimens removed from patients with cancer of the breast. A publication of the Cancer Committee, College of American Pathologists. *Arch Pathol Lab Med* 1997;121:27.

CHAPTER 31

Diseases of the Breast, 2nd ed.,
edited by Jay R. Harris.
Lippincott Williams & Wilkins, Philadelphia © 2000.

Estrogen and Progesterone Receptors

Richard M. Elledge and Suzanne A. W. Fuqua

The powerful, probing tools of molecular biology now enable us to see further and deeper into the cellular universe of breast cancer, greatly expanding the horizons of knowledge and understanding. Still, in the center of this complex and vast molecular space, steroid receptors remain, playing important and crucial roles in the basic biology of the disease and also illuminating the pathways involved in the clinical management and treatment of women with breast cancer.

In the early 1960s, radiolabeled estrogens were first observed to be preferentially concentrated in the estrogen target organs of animals and also in human breast cancers—observations that gave rise to the concept of an "estrogen receptor."[1–3] Since then, it has become clear that human breast cancers are dependent on estrogen or progesterone, or both, for growth. This stimulatory effect is mediated through the estrogen receptor (ER) and progesterone receptor (PR). Probably not coincidentally, both are found relatively overexpressed in most malignant breast tissue. The concept of targeting therapy toward molecular components preferentially overexpressed by breast cancer cells has become a popular one[4,5]; more than 100 years ago, however, the ER was the therapeutic target for the first breast cancer systemic therapy, hormonal manipulation.[6] The usefulness of targeting the receptor has clearly stood the test of time,[7] something that cannot yet be said of the most recent contenders.

New insights into the biology of the ER and the wide array of coregulatory proteins that can modify its function have already begun to lead to better therapies. In the clinic, the number of available drugs that interact with the receptor, drugs that are sometimes called *selective estrogen-receptor modulators* (*SERMs*), grows steadily each year. Along with this, methods for assaying receptor proteins have led to less expensive, simpler, and possibly more accurate measurements of ER and PR for clinical use. This chapter reviews the structural and mechanistic biology of ER and PR, especially as it relates to therapy, discusses current methods for measuring ER and PR for clinical use, and presents evidence that supports the usefulness of ER and PR in assessing clinical outcome and selecting therapy.

R. M. Elledge: Breast Care Center, Departments of Medicine and Oncology, Baylor College of Medicine, Houston, Texas

S. A. W. Fuqua: Department of Medicine, Baylor College of Medicine, Houston, Texas

ORGANIZATIONAL STRUCTURE

The ER and PR belong to a superfamily of nuclear hormone receptors that, in addition to several other steroid hormone receptors, also includes thyroid hormone, vitamin D, and retinoic acid receptors. These receptor proteins function as transcription factors when they are bound to their respective ligands. Since the original cloning of complementary DNAs (cDNAs) for ER[8,9] and PR,[10] an explosion of information has occurred in the field of steroid hormone action. These receptors share a common structural and functional organization; their functional domains have been designated A through F (Fig. 1). Classic ER (now called *ERα*) contains 595 amino acids with a central DNA-binding domain, along with a carboxy-terminal hormone-binding domain. Binding of hormone to the ER facilitates the activation of the receptor with the coincident disassociation of chaperone proteins, such as heat shock protein 90. Hormone-bound ER then dimerizes and binds to the estrogen response elements present in the promoter of estrogen-responsive genes. ER is also complexed with a number of coregulatory proteins that coordinately act to influence the transcription of estrogen-responsive genes.

STRUCTURE-FUNCTION RELATIONSHIP

On estrogen binding, the ER forms homodimers and binds to DNA through its DNA-binding domain (DBD) (see Fig. 1, region C) with high affinity at specific sites termed *estrogen-responsive elements* (*ERE*s).[11,12] The DNA-binding domain contains eight cysteine residues that are arranged in two zinc-finger motifs, each of which is followed by an extended α helix.[13] EREs have classically been viewed as two inverted, palindromic half-sites of the sequence GGTCA separated by three variant nucleotides. Of interest is the discovery that novel sequences containing restricted homology to the canonical ERE half-site can function as EREs in mammalian cells,[14] thus enlarging the number of

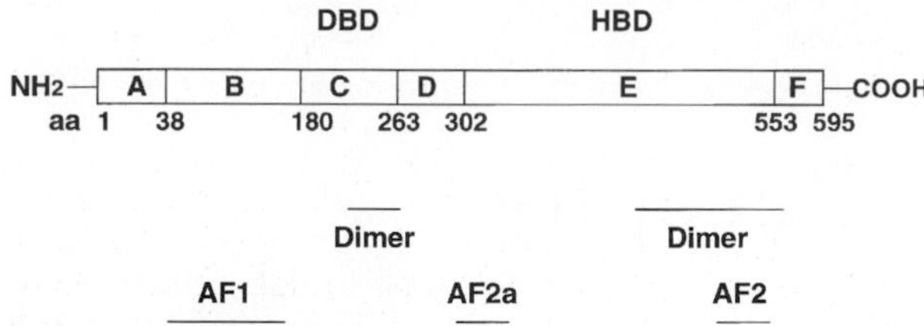

FIG. 1. Schematic diagram of estrogen receptor α functional domains. The ER contains 595 amino acids (aa) with the functional domains labeled A through F and a central DNA-binding domain (DBD) and hormone-binding domain (HBD). The regions important for dimerization (Dimer) and transactivation functions (AF-1, AF-2a, AF-2) are shown. Region A/B is important for hormone-independent ER transcription; region C is the DBD; region D is the hinge domain; region E is the HBD responsible for hormone-dependent transcription; region F is important for modulation of ER activity.

genes that potentially are regulated by estrogen. The crystal structure of the ER has also been solved as a complex with DNA,[15] and this structure confirmed the models of the DNA-binding domain developed from models predicted from mutational analysis.[12,16]

Through DNA binding, the ER influences the expression of estrogen-responsive genes, such as the PR, which are important in mitogenic signaling, and their transcription is stimulated through at least two distinct transactivation domains located in the amino-terminal A/B region (AF-1) and the carboxy-terminal E region of the receptor (AF-2).[17–19] These two ER regions appear to act in concert to promote full transcriptional activation of estrogen-responsive genes. The genomic organization of the human ER gene is quite complex; eight exons span more than 140 kilobase pairs of DNA.[20] The two ER transcriptional activation domains are not encoded within single exons but rather encompass large regions of the receptor. A hormone-independent, amino-terminal ER activation domain is contained within exons 1 and 2 and is termed *AF-1*. A hormone-dependent, carboxy-terminal activation domain is contained within portions of exons 4 through 8 and is termed *AF-2*.[21] A region exists within AF-2 that is highly conserved among nuclear hormone receptors and is composed of hydrophobic and charged residues critically important for hormone-dependent transcriptional activation.[22]

A third activation domain has been identified in the human ER within the amino-terminal part of AF-2 that has been designated *AF-2a*[23] (see Fig. 1). This region has either a constitutive transcriptional activating function or, alternatively, a stimulatory effect on AF-1. In addition, just downstream of the AF-2a domain is a negatively acting domain.[23] This region is also involved in binding of heat shock protein 90, a process that modulates receptor activation.[24] Similarly, a third potential activation domain has been mapped within the amino-terminus of the B form of the PR.[25] Thus, the steroid receptor transactivation domains appear numerous and more complex than previously appreciated, and further work is required to completely delineate the various regions important for different transcriptional activating functions on specific genes.

Both AF-1 and AF-2 are required for maximal ER transcriptional activity in most cellular environments[26]; both cellular and promoter contexts are important for determining transcriptional activity.[27] On certain promoters, AF-1 and AF-2 can function independently.[26] Research has now determined that, when AF-2 is required for ER transcriptional activity, antiestrogens such as tamoxifen (tamoxifen citrate) function as pure antagonists. However, in cellular contexts in which AF-2 is not required and AF-1 is sufficient for ER transcriptional activity, then tamoxifen can function as a partial agonist.[26,28] Therefore, antiestrogens can behave as AF-2 antagonists and AF-1 agonists. The fact that antiestrogens interact differentially with these two transactivational domains depending on the cellular environment may explain why, in the clinic, these molecules can function both as antagonists in breast tissue and as ER agonists in the uterus, bone, and cardiovascular system.

NEW ESTROGEN RECEPTOR SUBTYPE—ESTROGEN RECEPTOR β

An important discovery is the identification of another ER subtype, now termed *ERβ*[29,30] (Fig. 2). It is localized to a different chromosome (chromosome 14)[31] than ERα (chromosome 6). It is somewhat smaller than ERα and contains 530 amino acids.[32] The region of highest homology (95%) between ERα and ERβ is in the DNA-binding domain, which encompasses the functional C region of the receptor. Less conservation is found in the ERβ A/B and hinge domains (16% and 29%, respectively, compared with ERα; see Fig. 2). The high degree of homology in the DNA-binding domain suggests that both ER subtypes can bind EREs, and conservation in regions within the DNA-binding domain required for dimerization suggests that the two receptors may heterodimerize. This prediction has been proved true,[33,34] which implies that the heterodimer may be functionally active in tissues that coexpress both ER subtypes. Evidence from research with the ERα knockout mouse also suggests that the biological function of ERβ may be dependent on the

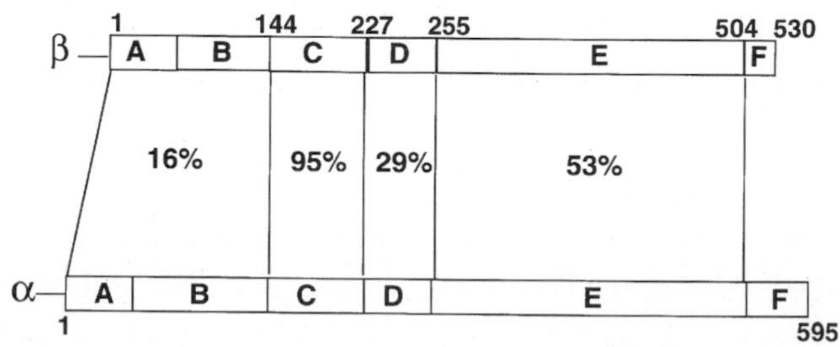

FIG. 2. Comparison of estrogen receptor β (ERβ) and estrogen receptor α functional domains. The amino acid residues of ERβ are shown above domains A–F, and the degree of homology between them is shown as percentages.

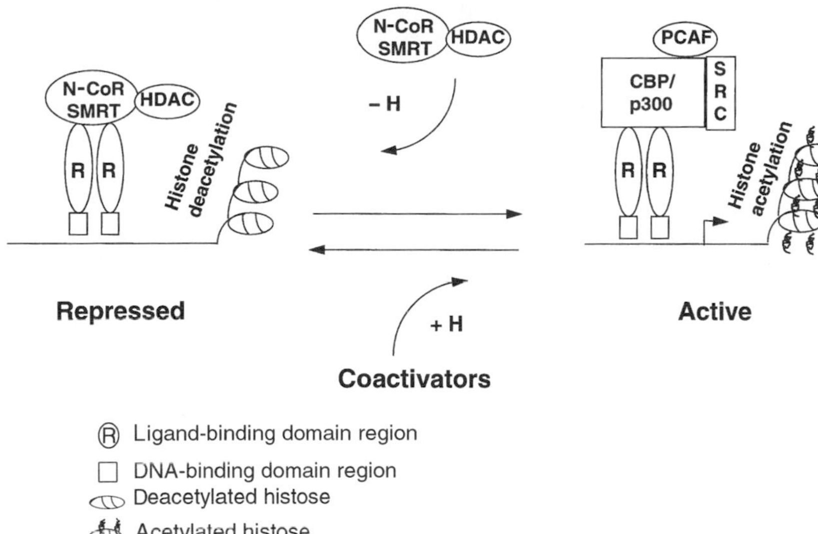

FIG. 3. Regulation of receptor-initiated gene transcription by receptor coregulatory proteins. In the inactivated state, DNA-bound histone deacetylase results in tight coiling of DNA, and corepressor proteins bound to receptor inhibit receptor function. When hormone (ligand) binds receptor, corepressor proteins are replaced by coactivators, some of which contain acetylase activity; the coactivators relax DNA and facilitate the recruitment of transcription factors to the complex, all of which serves to enhance transcription. H, hormone; HDAC, histone deacetylase activity; R, steroid receptor; N-CoR and SMRT are corepressors; CBP, p300, SRC, and PCAF are coactivators.

coexpression of ERα in certain tissues—for example, in the ovary, in which both ER types are required for proper cell and gene regulation during folliculogenesis.[35]

The degree of homology of ERβ with ERα within the ligand-binding domain (53%; see Fig. 2), along with their different tissue distribution,[36] also suggests that the two receptors may have distinct physiologic roles. Indeed, certain ligands, such as 16β,17α-epiestriol along with the phytoestrogen genistein, are ERβ-selective agonists.[37,38] In addition, because their transactivation domains are not identical, ERα and ERβ may potentially activate different genes, as has been suggested by research using receptor chimeras.[39] Furthermore, ERβ appears to lack a large portion of the carboxy-terminal F domain,[30] which influences the agonist-antagonist balance of antiestrogens such as tamoxifen.[40] In certain cells, antiestrogens are less effective if ER is lacking the F domain. Thus, ERβ might contribute to clinical tamoxifen resistance by interfering with antiestrogen inhibition of tumor growth.

A pivotal discovery was the finding that differential ligand activation of the two receptor subtypes can occur at AP-1 sites.[41] Thus, a second way that ER can mediate gene transcription is through binding to AP-1 protein complexes at AP-1 enhancer sites. Activation requires both ligand and the AP-1 transcription factors Fos and Jun.[42] Tamoxifen activates the transcription of genes that are under the control of an AP-1 element when ERα or ERβ is expressed, but estradiol does not activate genes containing AP-1 when ERβ alone is expressed.[41] Further experiments should be focused on which genes are differentially activated by the two receptor subtypes.

ERβ expression may also enhance tumor aggressiveness. ERβ messenger RNA (mRNA) had been shown to be coexpressed with ERα mRNA in some breast tumors,[43,44] and ERβ mRNA expression is inversely associated with PR expression in breast tumors.[45] One report suggests that coexpression of both receptor subtypes is associated with poor prognostic factors in breast cancer.[46] Thus, ERβ expression in tumors might prove to be an important biomarker for tumor progression or spread.

NUCLEAR RECEPTOR COREGULATORY PROTEINS

The list of additional coregulatory proteins that function as signaling intermediaries between the ER and the general transcriptional machinery is growing. The coregulatory proteins are components in a complex of proteins bound to the ER, and their presence or absence can help determine whether ER acts as a transcriptional repressor or activator. Numerous factors that associate with ligand-bound ER have been identified using *in vitro* and *in vivo* protein interaction assays, yeast two-hybrid systems, or protein interaction library screening. These include CBP/p300; coactivators, such as members of the p160 family (SRC-1, TIF2/GRIP-1 and AIB-1/ACTR/RAC3/pCIP); and corepressors, such as N-CoR and SMRT (for a review, see Horwitz et al.[47]). One protein identified, NSD1, exhibits bifunctional transcription activation properties of both a coactivator and a corepressor.[48] The function of these various coregulatory proteins is just beginning to be appreciated. For instance, CREB-binding protein (CBP)[49] also interacts with components of the basal transcriptional machinery, RNA polymerase II and TFIIB, as well as a number of other proteins (reviewed in Chrivia et al.[49]). CBP and the closely related protein p300 associate with and stimulate the transcriptional activity of the ER.[50] Because CBP and p300 are coactivators for a number of different transcription factors, some have proposed that they function as coordinators or cointegrators for nuclear receptors with other signaling pathways.[51]

A working model of steroid hormone action, as suggested from work with the retinoic acid receptor, is shown schematically in Fig. 3. In the absence of hormone, histone deacety-

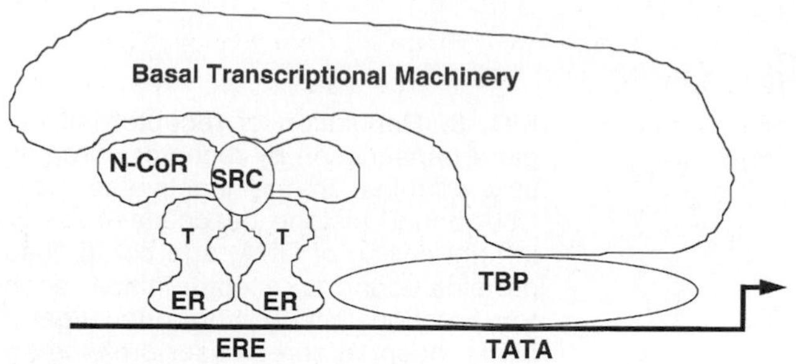

FIG. 4. Hypothetical model of agonist activity of estrogen receptor (ER) when bound to tamoxifen (T). T-bound ER promotes the simultaneous binding of the corepressor and coactivator molecules, N-CoR and SRC, respectively, thereby influencing interactions with the basal transcriptional machinery and subsequent complexes with TATA-binding protein (TBP) at its TATA binding site. The relative amount of corepressor and coactivator in a given tissue may determine whether tamoxifen acts as an agonist or an antagonist. ERE, estrogen-responsive element.

lase (HDAC) and the corepressors N-CoR and SMRT are bound to the receptor. Histone deacetylation silences or inhibits transcription by causing DNA to wrap more tightly around the core histone proteins. When hormone then binds to the receptor, the activated receptor complex displaces the repressor proteins, and the acetyltransferases CBP/p300 and PCAF are recruited to the complex, along with coactivator proteins, such as the SRC family. The acetyltransferases add acetyl groups to histones, loosening their interaction with DNA, which exposes important residues to the basal transcriptional machinery. Therefore, a complex array of proteins is present on the promoter, many of which are involved in chromatin remodeling; these coordinately contribute to the hormonal regulation of gene expression. The precise mechanism by which coactivators modulate ER transactivation function, however, remains to be determined.

Like the ER, the SRC-1 family of coactivators also has a complex structure. The amino-terminal region of the SRC-1 family of proteins contains a PAS A/helix-loop-helix domain, which is a dimerization interface that has been identified in several other nuclear proteins, including period (PER), the aryl hydrocarbon receptor (AHR), and single-minded (SIM).[52] SRC-1 contains two activation domains and multiple receptor-interacting domains that cooperatively enhance the receptor AF-1 and AF-2 domains.[53] The receptor-interacting motif LXXLL has been identified within nearly all coregulators and is indispensable for receptor interaction with coactivators.

Initially, the view was that coactivators enhanced estrogen-stimulated transcription and that corepressors simply suppressed this signal. But the situation is much more complex than first thought. In certain cells in which antiestrogens are agonists, SRC-1 enhances its agonist activity.[54] Conversely, N-CoR and SMRT can repress the partial agonist activity of tamoxifen,[55] but they have no effect on estrogen-stimulated gene expression. Overexpression of SRC-1 cannot overcome SMRT's repression of tamoxifen's agonist activity either.[54] This suggests that full agonists enable the ER to overcome corepressor function, but that partial agonists, such as tamoxifen, cannot overcome this repression. Because distinct steady-state nuclear receptor coregulator complexes exist *in vivo*,[56] the composition of these large, transcriptional complexes is dependent on the unique cellular distribution of individual members. Agonist activity may manifest itself in tissues in which corepressor expression is low, or perhaps mixed antiestrogens such as tamoxifen enable the receptor to interact with both corepressors and coactivators simultaneously (Fig. 4). Thus, it may be the relative balance of bound coregulators that ultimately determines ER's signal to the basal transcriptional machinery.

SELECTIVE ESTROGEN-RECEPTOR MODULATORS

Discoveries in understanding the structure and function of the ER have paved the way for the development of new classes of selective estrogen-receptor modulators (SERMs), agents that behave like estrogen in some tissues (bone and cardiovascular tissues) but block its action in others (e.g., the breast). Tamoxifen is considered one of the first SERMs; it exhibits antagonist activity in the breast but undesired agonist activity in the uterus. The identification of tamoxifen as a SERM suggested that additional SERMs with unique and perhaps more desirable tissue selectivity could be developed. This prediction proved correct with the development of raloxifene (raloxifene hydrochloride), which has similar properties in the breast[54] and bone but lacks significant uterotropic activity.[57] One molecular explanation lies in the fact that the ER undergoes extensive conformational changes on ligand binding. Crystal structures of the ER ligand-binding domain demonstrate that its conformation is determined by the nature of the bound ligand.[58] In the ER-ligand complex, helix 12 within the ligand-binding domain of the receptor sits snugly over the ligand-binding cavity, forming a secure "lid" over the ligand. The repositioning of helix 12 over the ligand-binding cavity is prevented by raloxifene. Thus, the precise positioning of helix 12 is a prerequisite for transcriptional activation. The crystal structure of the ER ligand-binding domain bound to both the agonist diethylstilbestrol (DES) and a peptide corresponding to the GRIP-1 coactivator has been obtained.[59] GRIP-1 binds to a hydrophobic groove on the surface of the DES-bound ER, whereas the repositioning of helix 12 in tamoxifen-bound ER occludes the coactivator recognition groove in the ligand-binding domain, preventing transcriptional activity. One could envision the development of designer SERMs that have different effects on ER structure, influencing the controlled recruitment of specific coregulators. When clinical trials with the SERMs idoxifene,[60] droloxifene,[61] GW5638,[61] EM652,[62] and LY353381[63] are complete, clinicians will have additional choices for endocrine therapy, perhaps ones with greater safety, additional health-promoting effects, or modestly improved antitumor efficiency.

ALTERNATIVE SIGNALING OF THE ESTROGEN RECEPTOR AND ESTROGEN INDEPENDENCE

An active area of current research is alternative pathways of steroid-receptor activation. Cross talk between the ER and the protein kinase A (PKA) pathway has been observed,[64–66] and stimulation of the PKA pathway has been found to activate the agonist activity of antiestrogens.[67] This finding has potential clinical importance in tamoxifen-resistant breast cancer if fluctuations in PKA activators, such as cyclic adenosine monophosphate (cAMP), are found to accompany the development of resistance. Similar results have been observed with antagonist-occupied PR[68]; one study suggested that this agonist-to-antagonist switch is specific only for the β form of the PR.[69] Certain growth factors, such as insulinlike growth factor type I, have also been shown to stimulate ER activity.[70] Another element involved in the acquisition of hormone independence could be the deregulated expression of downstream growth-regulatory pathways that liberate the cell cycle from normal steroid control. For example, cyclin D_1 overexpression activates ER-mediated gene transcription directly, independent of the cyclin-dependent kinases,[71,72] and the suggestion has been made that cyclin D_1 manifests its oncogenic potential in part through its activation of the ER pathway.

GENOMIC ALTERATIONS OF ESTROGEN RECEPTOR α IN BREAST CANCER

As soon as cDNAs to the human ERα became available for use, several groups investigated whether genomic ERα structure was altered in breast cancer, a likely possibility given the extensive cytogenetic changes that have been documented in breast tumors. One of the central questions in all of these studies was whether genomic deletion or rearrangement was the basis for the failure of some tumors to express ERα. In a series of 188 primary breast tumor biopsies, no gross structural rearrangements of the ERα gene could be detected using Southern hybridization analysis.[73] Subsequent studies have confirmed that large deletions, rearrangements, or gene amplification in the ERα are infrequent in breast cancer.[74,75]

Another plausible explanation for the absence of ERα expression in ER negative (ER–) breast cancer cells is gene methylation. Studies examining this question again have reached conflicting conclusions, with some studies finding no relationship between ERα gene methylation patterns and ERα expression in breast tumors[74,76,77] and other studies concluding that extensive methylation in the 5' ERα promoter region is associated with ER-negativity in breast cancer cell lines[78] and tumors.[79] These latter studies examined a region known to be important for transcriptional control of gene expression, the cytosine-rich CpG islands. These data, along with data demonstrating the ability to reactivate ERα expression in ER– cell lines with inhibitors of DNA methylation,[80] suggest that further work should be directed at determining whether abnormal methylation could indeed account for transcriptional inactivation of the ERα and ERβ.

The lack of ERα protein expression in tumors appears to be due to a lack of gene transcription, because the majority of tumors negative for ERα are devoid of ERα mRNA.[81] Accordingly, several groups have begun to delineate the elements within the 5' ERα region that are responsible for promoter activity and ERα expression in breast tumors.[82,83] A negative element with strong silencing activity has been identified in the chicken ER promoter.[84] One is tempted to speculate that such negative elements may be involved in the transcriptional down-regulation of ERα in human tumors; however, no such element has been reported. Positive regulatory elements have also been delineated in the ERα promoter[85–87]; however, little evidence exists at this time to support their role in the *in vivo* regulation of ERα expression. ERα expression is also modulated by estrogen, both by use of classic EREs within the ERα promoter[88] and by as yet unknown mechanisms in the proximal promoter region.[89] Thus, understanding of the details of transcriptional control of the ER may prove very useful clinically in modulating ER expression for therapeutic benefit. Further work on the human promoter is in progress in several laboratories.

POTENTIAL RELEVANCE OF VARIANT ESTROGEN RECEPTOR α ISOFORMS

The early 1990s brought the first demonstration that alternative RNA splicing of ERα potentially generated truncated forms of the receptor protein and that this was a common event in breast tumors.[90–92] A large body of evidence now exists in support of the expression of variant and mutant ERα mRNA species. Essentially, transcripts containing precise or multiple exon deletions of each of the eight exons in ERα have been reported, and these are invariably coexpressed along with wild-type ERα RNA. A number of reviews are available detailing the structure and potential role of most of the variants,[93–96] and this subject is not reviewed exhaustively here. Instead, the focus is on those variants or mutations with potential important roles in breast tumor biology, and those for which some evidence exists that the variant mRNAs are actually translated *in vivo*.

One potentially important ERα variant has a deletion of exon 5, which involves the hormone-binding domain and results in a receptor with constitutive, hormone-independent activity.[90] This variant appears to result from alternative splicing and produces a frame shift in the coding sequence, leading to a receptor protein with only the amino-terminal AF-1 and DNA-binding regions.[97] The transcriptional activity of the exon 5 ER deletion variant appears to be highly dependent on the cellular environment in which it is expressed. For instance, it has very low transcriptional activity in yeast[90] and higher activity in the ER– MDA-MB-231 cell line[92] but is a dominant-negative receptor in another ER– cell line, HMT-3522S1.[98] In U2-OS osteosarcoma cells, the variant has no effect on basal or estrogen-mediated activity but very strongly increases the activity of wild-type ERα.[99] These seemingly conflicting data are perhaps not surprising, given the available information on the transcriptional activity of AF-1 in different cell systems and the differential expression of receptor coactivators and corepressors that influence ER signaling.

Some have hypothesized that the exon 5 deletion variant might play a role in hormone resistance because its overexpression confers resistance to tamoxifen *in vitro*[92]; however, another group has not been able to find similar results.[100] This discrepancy is not presently understood but again may relate to the cellular complement of coregulators present in the cell lines used by the investigators. *In vivo* evidence is now accumulating, however, that the exon 5 ER variant may play a role in clinical endocrine resistance.[101,102] One provocative study showed that significantly higher levels of the exon 5 variant were seen in relapse tissues of tamoxifen-resistant patients than in the respective primary tumors.[103] Tamoxifen treatment may favor the selection for or remodeling of cell clones expressing higher levels of the exon 5 variant ER,[92] conferring a growth advantage to some tumors. The development of antibodies specific for this variant that can be used for immunohistochemical assessment of its expression in tumors[104] will facilitate the exploration of this hypothesis.

Some of the ERα variants have been reported to be associated with various clinical parameters in breast tumors. For instance, a variant with exon 4 deletion is preferentially detected in tumors with low histologic grade or high PR levels, whereas variants deleted in exons 2 to 4 or exons 3 to 7 are associated with tumors of higher grade and high ER levels.[105] Some evidence also exists that a number of these truncated variant ERα mRNAs are stably translated *in vivo*. For instance, a group of human breast tumors was analyzed immunohistochemically for ERα expression using antibodies to either the amino terminus or carboxy terminus, and the antibody to the carboxy terminus was found to correlate better with ligand-binding assays.[106] The tumors exhibiting higher staining with the amino terminus antibody and discordant ligand-binding data were then shown to contain a number of truncated ERα variants[107]; these findings thus demonstrate indirect evidence for translation of variant proteins *in vivo*.

In comparison with reports of alternative splicing, reports of missense mutations within ERα in primary breast cancers have been rare. Missense mutations are estimated to be present in only approximately 1% of primary tumors[108]; however, the frequency may be higher in metastatic lesions. Karnik et al.[109] examined five primary and metastatic breast tumor pairs for ER alterations. They found that one of the five metastatic lesions, but not the primary tumor from the same patient, contained a single nucleotide deletion in the ER. This deletion generates a frame shift and a translation termination codon in the hormone-binding domain and would potentially result in a carboxy-truncated receptor. Functional analysis of this ER variant has not yet been reported, however. Another study reported that 3 of 30 metastatic lesions had missense mutations in ERα.[110] One of these, a tyrosine-to-asparagine substitution at amino acid residue 537 at the end of the hormone-binding domain, contains a remarkable increase in its constitutive activity. Similar mutations at the corresponding site in ERβ result in a constitutive receptor.[111] Furthermore, the constitutive activity of the tyrosine 537-mutated receptor has been hypothesized to be due to its ability to bind coactivators such as SRC-1 in a ligand-independent manner,[111,112] because alterations at amino acid 537 facilitate the shift of helix 12 of ERα into an active conformation. The clinical significance of this variant in other metastatic breast tumors is currently under study.

VARIANT ESTROGEN RECEPTOR β ISOFORMS

Reports suggest that variant isoforms of human ERβ also exist. A number of alternatively spliced ERβ transcripts have been reported in tissues, including breast cancer cell lines. These variants include ERβ1 through ERβ5, which contain carboxy-terminal–truncated sequences.[113] A functional analysis of ERβ2 (also called *ERβcx*) suggests that, although this variant does not bind ligand, it can interfere with the activity of ERα, because it preferentially forms heterodimers with ERα as opposed to ERβ homodimers.[114] Thus, these investigators hypothesized that this isoform, if indeed it is translated *in vivo*, might inhibit ERα-mediated estrogen action. Another isoform has been reported, also called *ERβ2*, which contains an in-frame inserted exon of 54 nucleotides that results in an insertion of 18 amino acids within the hormone-binding domain, which reduces its ability to bind ligand.[115] This variant appears to be expressed in only a minority of cell lines tested, however, and the relevance of its expression in breast cancer is speculative. In summary, as with ERα, the ERβ gene appears to be subject to frequent alternative splicing and the generation of potential isoforms. As antibodies specific for human ERβ become available, the significance of these isoforms can be evaluated.

IMPORTANCE OF RECEPTORS IN CLINICAL BREAST CANCER

The laboratory discovery and subsequent measurement of ER and PR in tumors has given the clinician useful and powerful tools to aid in the management of women with breast cancer. Overall, 30% to 40% of patients with metastatic breast cancer objectively respond to hormone therapy.[116–118] A substantial fraction of patients also exists whose disease becomes stable, neither progressing nor regressing, for a clinically significant period of time. With first-line cytotoxic chemotherapy, the response rate is 50% to 60%. Although the response rate is higher than the objective response rate to hormone therapy, with chemotherapy, the toxicity is much greater, and the likelihood of a sustained response is low. Hormone therapy, on the other hand, is relatively nontoxic, and responses can sometimes last for years. Thus, hormone treatment offers several significant advantages to particular subsets of patients. It is now well established that measurement of ER levels, as well as PR levels, can distinguish those patients most likely to benefit from hormone therapy from those unlikely to respond, so the latter group may receive other more effective and appropriate management strategies, such as cytotoxic chemotherapy.

METHODS OF MEASURING ESTROGEN AND PROGESTERONE RECEPTORS

Although a multitude of assay methods are available that differ in detail, at present all clinically practical methods for quantitating ER and PR are based on two distinct and mechanically different strategies. The first strategy involves the competitive binding of radiolabeled steroid ligand to detect the receptor, whereas the second relies on the recognition of the receptor protein by specific antibodies.

Ligand-Binding Methods

The prototype for ligand-binding methods, and the one that remains most in use, is the dextran-coated charcoal (DCC) assay. With this assay, radiolabeled steroid (ligand) is first added to homogenized breast tumor cytosol and is incubated, allowing the labeled steroid to bind all available receptor protein.[119] For simultaneous determination of ER and PR, estradiol labeled with iodine[125] and progestin labeled with tritium (^{3}H) are used. DCC, which has the property of adsorbing unbound steroid, is added to the homogenate; the charcoal with adherent unbound steroid is then separated by centrifugation. Because the receptor-bound portion remains in the supernatant and the free fraction is found in the charcoal precipitate, the bound and unbound fractions can then be quantified and the results used to create a Scatchard plot. When the DCC assay is used to measure receptor levels, a range of ^{3}H-tagged steroid is used to generate this multipoint plot. From the Scatchard plot, total concentration of receptor protein in the cytosol is obtained and is usually expressed as femtomoles of receptor protein per milligram of total cytosol protein. Various cutoff values for separating ER+ from ER– samples are used in different laboratories; usually, the cutoff is between 3 and 20 fmol/mg. Unfortunately, this variation in definition can sometimes result in the same tumor's being defined as ER– by one laboratory and ER positive (ER+) by another. This discrepancy may help explain why some apparently ER– tumors respond to hormone therapy. This issue is addressed in more detail in the sections Definition of Cutoffs for Receptor Status and Responses in Patients with ER-Negative Tumors later in this chapter.

The DCC method has a number of advantages. It gives a specific and objective quantitation of ER or PR that is reproducible under conditions of good quality control.[120] Very low values, between 3 and 10 fmol, show the greatest variability. This has caused some labs to choose 10 fmol as a cutoff for a positive classification. Because results are objectively quantified, interobserver variability is not a significant problem; however, it can be with other assay types discussed below.

When the DCC assay is used for clinical purposes, a number of points should be kept in mind. To ensure the highest likelihood of accurate and reproducible results, specimens must be immediately fixed in liquid nitrogen at –70°C and shipped in dry ice to prevent protein degradation. Portions of tumor specimens should be reviewed to make sure that the submitted portion of the tumor contains representative malignant epithelial cells, the only component of a breast tumor that contains receptor protein. Other constituents, such as fibroblasts, fat, and inflammatory cells, do not. An adequate portion of tumor should be submitted, at least 0.5 to 1.0 cm in diameter, to avoid sampling error and to ensure sufficient material for the assay. If the patient is pregnant[121] or is being treated with high-dose estrogens or tamoxifen,[122] all receptor sites may be saturated, and a false-negative result could occur.

Variability in assay results can occur for a number of reasons. The tumor is usually divided into several portions, each to be used for different purposes. Tumor cellularity may be variable, with some regions being more necrotic or having a high proportion of connective or inflammatory tissue. Variation is also seen in the receptor content of the malignant epithelial component; areas of clonal proliferation may be found that are relatively richer or poorer in receptor protein. As mentioned above, treatment with ligands that bind ER or PR could influence the assay.

DCC assay also has certain disadvantages. It requires a relatively complex and sophisticated laboratory and involves the use of low-level radioactive materials. This complexity usually necessitates centralization, so that performing the assay in community hospitals or in less developed countries is difficult or impossible. Because of the complexity of the task, with the resulting opportunity for variability, strong quality control is essential. Specimens must be transported quickly and efficiently under very low temperatures to prevent degradation. The assay cannot be performed on fixed archival specimens, needle biopsy specimens, or small tumors. Finally, because of the dilutional effect resulting from homogenization of the whole tumor, very fibrotic or necrotic tumors with small malignant epithelial components can be reported as falsely low or negative.

Assays Using Monoclonal Antibodies

The second general strategy for detection of ER and PR uses antibodies specifically directed against epitopes unique

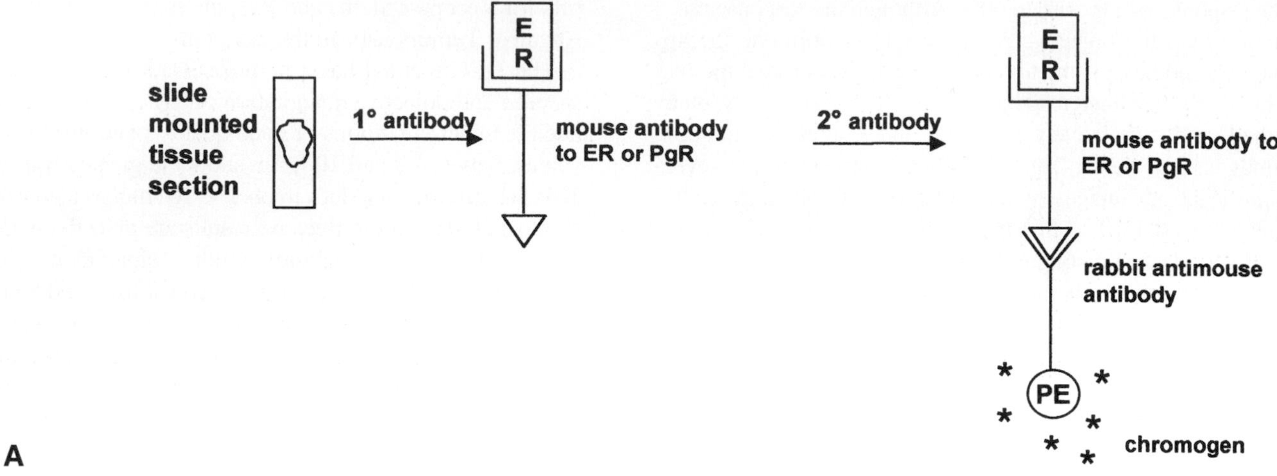

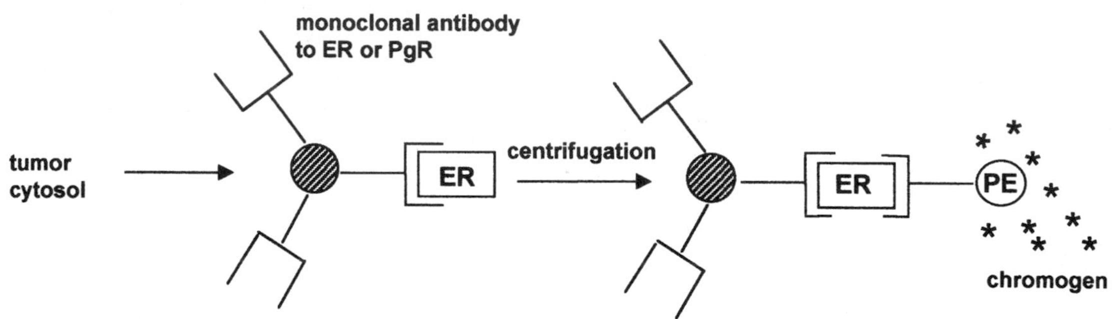

FIG. 5. Antibody assays for estrogen receptor (ER) or progesterone receptor (PgR). **A:** Immunohistochemical assay. Thin sections of fixed, paraffin-imbedded or frozen tissue are placed on a glass slide. The sections are then incubated with an antibody to ER or PgR and subsequently with a secondary antibody linked to an enzyme such as horseradish peroxidase (PE) that converts a substrate to a colorized molecule. **B:** Enzyme immunoassay. A monoclonal antibody to ER or PgR is fixed to polystyrene beads (*filled circles*) or a solid-state matrix. Tumor cytosol is added, incubated with the bead-antibody complex, then centrifuged, and the supernatant is removed. A second monoclonal antibody recognizing a separate receptor epitope and linked to an enzyme is added, along with a choleragenic substrate. The color intensity is then measured with a spectrophotometer. (* Indicates a chromogen such as 3',3' diaminobenzidine.)

to each receptor protein.[123] These antibodies may be monoclonal or polyclonal. At least two methodologic variations on this general strategy are commonly performed: immunohistochemical (IHC) analysis[124,125] and enzyme immunoassay (EIA).[126] IHC analysis can be performed on thin sections of tumor cut from formalin-fixed, paraffin-embedded or frozen biopsy specimens. Initially, 4- to 5-μm sections are cut and mounted on protein-coated glass slides. To increase detection sensitivity, the sections are sometimes first heated to uncover protein epitopes lost in the fixation process or from the passage of time.[127] The sections are exposed to a primary antibody directed against ER or PR, and then a secondary antibody that recognizes the first is added to amplify the subsequent signal (Fig. 5). Attached to these secondary antibodies are enzymes, such as horseradish peroxidase that convert substrates like diaminobenzidine into colorized molecules on exposure to a developer. The sections are counterstained and can then be viewed to semiquantitate the amount of protein present (Fig. 6). For ER and PR, the staining produces distinct nuclear signals,[123] and heterogeneity of staining of malignant epithelium is frequently seen.

IHC analysis offers several advantages. It can be performed on fine-needle aspirates, core biopsies, small tumors, and cell blocks from body fluids, such as pleural effusions. It can be done on either frozen or fixed, paraffin-embedded archival tissue. It measures the total receptor protein present, not just the unbound fraction, and is not affected by very high levels of

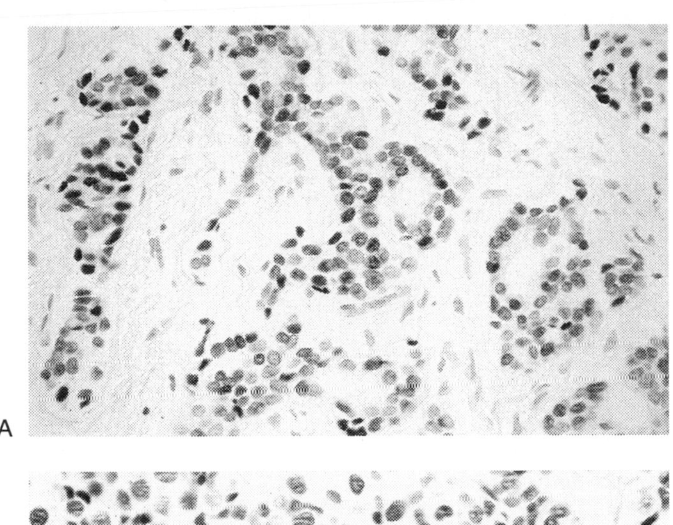

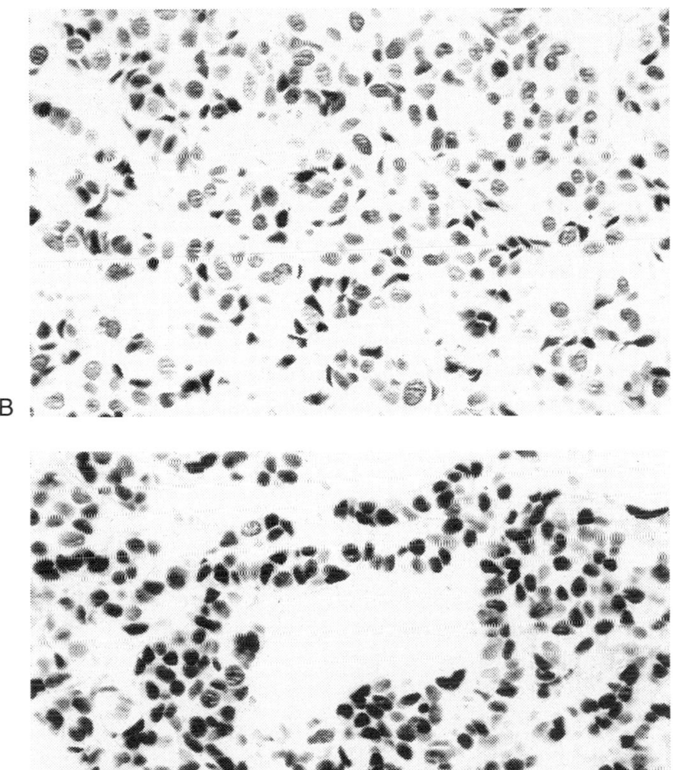

FIG. 6. Estrogen-receptor (ER) determination by immunohistochemical assay. Dark discrete staining nuclei represent the presence of ER. Note the heterogeneous staining of nuclei in the panels. **A:** Low ER, with only a small portion of cells staining weakly positive. **B:** Intermediate ER. **C:** High ER, with intense staining of virtually all nuclei.

endogenous or exogenous steroids or tamoxifen treatment. It allows the direct quantification of receptor protein in the malignant cell fraction. Due to the reasons outlined above and its relative simplicity and lack of requirements for specialized equipment, it is rapidly becoming the predominant method for measuring ER and PR in clinical practice.

IHC analysis has a number of drawbacks, however. Results can vary substantially because of differences in tissue fixation, procedural changes, type of antibody used,[128] and treatment of the antigen.[129] Depending on the epitope recognized, different antibodies may detect only certain forms of the receptor, such as the α or β form of ER, or conversely may not detect a specific isoform or variant. The method is semisubjective, and quantitation can definitely vary with the observer.[130] Scoring and evaluation systems and cut points separating positive and negative are different for individual laboratories, sometimes making direct comparison of results difficult. The semisubjective nature and lack of standardization of technique and scoring are the main limiting factors in the application of IHC analysis of ER and PR in the clinic. Consensus agreements on methods and procedures and computer image analysis to quantify results more objectively[131] could help to address these difficult issues.

The other antibody-based ER and PR assay in common clinical use is EIA.[126,132] In this technique, cytosols from tumor homogenates are incubated with a monoclonal antibody to ER or PR that is attached to a polystyrene bead or solid-state matrix (see Fig. 5). The receptor protein becomes bound to the antibody-bead complex and is separated from the cytosol by centrifugation. The cytosol is aspirated, and the remaining precipitated fraction is then exposed to a second monoclonal antibody that recognizes a separate receptor epitope. As with IHC analysis, this secondary antibody is linked to an enzyme, commonly horseradish peroxidase, that colorizes a developing substance. The intensity of the color is then quantified by a spectrophotometer, and the receptor level is determined by comparison with a standard curve of receptor. Objectivity, specific quantification, and the ability to measure total receptor protein are advantages for this technique. It does require fresh frozen tumor, however, and it cannot be performed on very small samples.

Comparison of Assay Methods

Many comparative studies of DCC and IHC assay methods have been carried out. Table 1 highlights a number of the largest and most representative. In summary, for ER, correlation between the two methods is high, in the 80% to 90% range. Discordances may occur for a number of reasons. Because an IHC assay measures total receptor protein, it may be positive in the face of a negative DCC test if all receptor sites are occupied by a ligand. Also, if the tumor contains only a small portion of malignant epithelium, this may be detected by IHC analysis, but due to dilution by other tumor elements, average receptor level in the homogenate may fall below a quantity detectable by the DCC method. Poor preservation of the specimen can cause false-negatives with either assay. Lastly, results of the DCC assay may be positive and those of the IHC assay negative if nonmalignant or noninvasive epithelial components contain receptor, whereas the malignant invasive component has

TABLE 1. *Agreement in determination of receptor status by ligand-binding assay and by immunohistochemical analysis*

Study	*n*	Agreement (%)
Estrogen receptor		
Stierer et al.[170]	299	87
Allred et al.[171]	130	91
Molino et al.[172]	405	82
Remmele et al.[173]	156	93
Reiner et al.[174]	192	80
Charpin et al.[175]	425	93
Hanna and Mobbs[176]	225	77
Elledge et al.[143]	205	90
Progesterone receptor		
Pertschuk et al.[136]	449	75
Helin et al.[177]	185	71
Gasparini et al.[178]	152	78
Reiner et al.[179]	426	74
Elledge et al.[143]	204	73

TABLE 2. *Cumulative data on response to endocrine therapy by tumor estrogen-receptor status*

Treatment	Estrogen receptor (responders/ total)–positive	Estrogen receptor (responders/ total)–negative
Ablative	59/107 (55%)	8/94 (8%)
Adrenalectomy	32/66	4/33
Oophorectomy	25/33	4/53
Hypophysectomy	2/8	0/8
Additive	51/85 (60%)	7/82 (8%)
Androgen	12/26	2/24
Estrogen	37/57	5/58
Glucocorticoid	2/2	—
Antiestrogen	8/20 (40%)	5/27 (18%)

Note: Response defined as 50% reduction in size or healing of lytic bone lesions.
Adapted from McGuire WL, Vollmer ER, Carbone PP, eds. *Receptors in human breast cancer.* New York: Raven Press, 1975.

evolved into a receptor-negative phenotype. Concordance of PR results by these two methods is somewhat lower than seen with ER, 70% to 80% (see Table 1).

EIA has been less extensively compared with other methods, although correlations appear generally high. One group found ER protein levels to be approximately two times higher with EIA than with DCC assay.[133] Concordance was approximately 80%, with all discordances being DCC negative and EIA positive. Others have also found a tight correlation between results of EIA and DCC assay.[134,135]

For clinical use, with respect to accuracy and, more importantly, correlation with outcome and response to therapy, none of the three methods has any clear or substantial advantage, although some have suggested that IHC analysis may have a slight edge in this regard.[136,137] If any one method has a true advantage, it is likely to be small. Simply because of the practical advantages discussed previously and because only a small amount of tissue is required, IHC analysis is likely to be the method used most often in the future. Perhaps the crucial issue facing the clinician is not really determining which methodology is "better," but finding a laboratory with high standards, meticulous quality control, experienced personnel, and a validation of results. This ensures greater reliability and reproducibility of any given assay, which is more important than any average subtle differences between assay types.

ESTROGEN AND PROGESTERONE RECEPTORS IN THE CLINICAL MANAGEMENT OF BREAST CANCER PATIENTS

ER and PR can be used as both predictive and prognostic factors. A *predictive factor* indicates the likelihood of a response (or no response) to a particular treatment—in the case of ER and PR, to hormone therapy. Study designs assessing a predictive factor are complex because of the additional variables involved. A *prognostic factor* is indicative of the inherent biological aggressiveness of a tumor, reflecting the natural history of the disease after local therapy. An example is nodal status. Prognostic factors are therefore most accurately assessed in systemically untreated patients, although in reality, most studies of prognostic factors contain a mixture of treated and untreated patients. Prognostic and predictive factors are not mutually exclusive—a given factor can be both prognostic and predictive, as is seen in the case of ER and PR, discussed in the following section.

Use of Estrogen-Receptor and Progesterone-Receptor Status to Predict Response to Hormone Therapy in Advanced Disease

By the late 1960s and early 1970s, several investigators, most prominently Elwood Jensen and William McGuire, observed that ER status might be a predictor of response to hormone therapy in advanced breast cancer. To bring these initial ideas into clearer focus, a consensus conference met in 1974 to study and analyze the predictive value of the ER. The cumulative results of this conference are shown in Table 2. Although these results are now more than 25 years old, they stand essentially unchanged, and many subsequent larger and better-controlled studies have confirmed the accuracy and validity of these original observations.[116,117,138,139] Overall, results indicate that 50% to 60% of all patients with ER+ tumors can benefit from first-line hormone therapy, whereas at most only 5% to 10% of patients with ER– tumors benefit. ER status is also important in predicting benefit from second-line and subsequent hormone manipulations; although response rates become progressively lower, they remain in the 20% to 40% range,[140,141] and treatment provides clinical benefit that is humanly worthwhile. Very few ER– patients respond to second-line therapy.

TABLE 3. *Relationship of estrogen-receptor and progesterone-receptor level to clinical benefit from hormone therapy in advanced disease*

Estrogen-receptor level, by ligand-binding assay (fmol/mg)	*n*	Response rate (%)	
<3.0	22	5	
3.0–10.0	76	18	
10.1–30.0	219	37	
30.1–300.0	63	78	
>300.0	35	77	
Total	**415**		
Progesterone-receptor level, by immunohistochemical analysis	***n***	**Response rate (%)**	**Time to treatment failure (mo)**
Negative	69	46	5
Intermediate	78	55	7
High	57	70	10
Total	**204**		

From ref. 116 (estrogen-receptor data) and ref. 143 (progesterone-receptor data), with permission.

ER status of metastases may not always correlate with ER status of the primary tumor. Approximately 20% of ER+ primary tumors have ER– metastases.[142] Indeed, the receptor status of the metastases may be more predictive of response. In one small study, only 12% of patients with ER+ primaries and ER– metastases responded to endocrine therapy, compared with 74% of patients whose recurrent tumor retained ER expression.[142] Truly ER– primaries rarely, if ever, give rise to ER+ metastases.

Once the probability of response is demonstrated to be related to the presence or absence of ER, it can then be asked whether the probability of this response is associated with how much ER is present in the tumor. Although for conceptual purposes and clinical convenience, tumors are frequently described as being simply ER– or ER+, ER concentration is a continuous variable, ranging from 0 in some tumors to more than 1,000 fmol/mg in others. Therefore, that response rates to endocrine therapies are also continuous and are directly related to the level of protein is not surprising. Tumors with a higher level of ER have a greater response rate than those with lower, albeit "positive," amounts[116,139,143] (Table 3).

In addition to the quantity of ER, other tumor factors can be used to further refine the ability to identify those patients who respond best. Response to hormone therapy requires functioning ER, so a marker that reflects the functional integrity of the pathway, rather than simply the presence or absence of receptor protein, could help to separate patients with ER+ tumors who respond from patients with ER+ tumors who do not. PR is a protein whose synthesis is positively regulated by ER and whose presence may therefore indicate a functionally intact ER response pathway. Therefore, tumors expressing PR in addition to ER might be expected to have a higher response rate to tamoxifen and other endocrine therapies.[144] Large clinical studies have supported this hypothesis. Higher PR levels are associated with better response, longer time to treatment failure, and longer survival (see Table 3).[116,139,145] Although ER and PR are correlated, PR status does seem to provide some useful information independent of ER status.[139] Compared with ER+ tumors, a higher proportion of PR+ tumors—approximately 40%—lose PR expression in their metastases. Whether this event is associated with a lower response rate to therapy is uncertain; however, it is correlated with a worse outcome.[146]

A small group of tumors are ER–/PR+; these comprise approximately 5% of all breast cancers. This phenomenon could be due to a false-negative in determining ER status or could reflect the existence of pathways that can induce PR expression independently of ER. In any event, these tumors have response rates that are not substantially different from those of the ER+ phenotype,[147] although some evidence exists that they may have a somewhat worse clinical outcome.[148]

Use of Estrogen-Receptor and Progesterone-Receptor Status to Predict Response to Adjuvant Therapy

Clearly, both ER and PR status predict treatment response in advanced or metastatic disease. Today, however, 80% to 90% of breast cancer patients present with localized disease that can be visibly removed by surgery. Although these patients have no clinically evident disease after primary local therapy, at least one-half already have microscopic distant spread of their disease. Because these microscopic seeds are ultimately responsible for the lethal aspect of breast cancer, knowing whether the steroid receptor status of the primary breast tumor predicts the efficacy of hormone therapy is important. An overview of trials of women with early-stage breast cancer who were randomized to adjuvant tamoxifen therapy versus no adjuvant tamoxifen therapy provides the best data for examining the relationship of ER and PR status to benefit from adjuvant hormone therapy.[7] This meta-analysis involved more than 37,000 women in 55 trials; in general, follow-up is at least 10 years. The results clearly and unequivocally demonstrate that women with ER+ tumors derive significant benefit from 5 years of tamoxifen treatment in terms of reduction in the odds of recurrence and death, whereas those with ER– tumors do not (Fig. 7). In addition, just as in advanced disease, the benefit of tamoxifen therapy is also directly related to the amount of ER protein present (Table 4). Women with tumors having more than 100 fmol/mg of protein experience greater risk reduction from 5 years of tamoxifen treatment than patients with lower amounts of ER. Unlike in advanced disease, however, knowing PR status does not provide much additional information in assessing the benefit of adjuvant therapy, except possibly for the small subgroup of patients whose tumors are ER–/PR+ (Table 5). This group did experience risk reduction from treatment, whereas patients with ER–/PR– tumors did not. Because of the small number of

	Recurrence as First Event						Mortality (Death from Any Cause)					
	Events/Patients		Tamoxifen events		Ratio of recurrence rates		Deaths/Patients		Tamoxifen deaths		Ratio of death rates	
Hormone receptor (ER) status	Allocated tamoxifen	Allocated control	O-E	Variance of O-E	Ratio Tamoxifen : control	Reduction (% and SD)	Allocated tamoxifen	Allocated control	O-E	Variance of O-E	Ratio tamoxifen : control	Reduction (% and SD)
(a) Tamoxifen ~1 yr												
ER poor	326/779 (41.8%)	348/812 (42.9%)	-8.9	144.5		6% SD 8	312/779 (40.1%)	342/812 (42.1%)	-9.0	146.4		6% SD 8
ER unknown ~ 69% ER+	944/2058 (45.9%)	1111/2127 (52.2%)	-97.8	448.7		20% SD 4	1073/2058 (52.1%)	1163/2127 (54.7%)	-51.9	498.7		10% SD 4
ER+	719/1706 (42.1%)	797/1646 (48.4%)	-78.7	336.3		21% SD 5	681/1706 (39.9%)	743/1646 (45.1%)	-49.8	325.0		14% SD 5
(a) subtotal ~ 69% ER+	1989/4543	2256/4585	-185.4	929.6		18% SD 3 (2*p* < .00001)	2066/4543 (45.5%)	2248/4585 (49.0%)	-110.7	970.1		11% SD 3 (2*p* = .0004)
Difference between tamoxifen effects in ER poor and ER+: $\chi^2_1 = 3.0$; 2p = .08							**$\chi^2_1 = 0.8$; 2p > .1; NS**					
(b) Tamoxifen ~2 yrs												
ER poor	887/2527 (35.1%)	980/2618 (37.4%)	-53.4	393.3		13% SD 5	859/2527 (34.0%)	904/2618 (34.5%)	-29.0	388.2		7% SD 5
ER unknown ~ 68% ER+	1051/2932 (35.8%)	1268/2910 (43.6%)	-167.5	510.0		28% SD 4	1093/2932 (37.3%)	1205/2910 41.4%)	-85.2	522.0		15% SD 4
ER+	1434/4379 (32.7%)	1715/4526 (40.3%)	-221.0	670.4		28% SD 3	1272/4379 (29.0%)	1428/4256 (33.6%)	-114.6	593.3		18% SD 4
(b) subtotal ~65% ER+	3372/9838 (34.3%)	3963/9784 (40.5%)	-441.8	1573.6		24% SD 2 (2*p* < .00001	3224/9838 (32.8%)	3538/9784 (36.2%)	-228.8	1503.6		14% SD 2 (2*p*<.00001)
Difference between tamoxifen effects in ER poor and ER+: $\chi^2_1 = 9.3$; 2p = .002							**$\chi^2_1 = 3.3$; 2p = .07**					
(c) Tamoxifen ~5 yrs												
ER poor	191/446 (42.8%)	210/476 (44.1%)	-5.4	83.3		6% SD 11	182/446 (40.8%)	178/476 (37.4%)	2.3	78.0		−3% SD 11
ER unknown ~72% ER+	200/772 (25.9%)	273/786 (34.7%)	-49.3	107.4		37% SD 8	219/772 (28.4%)	254/786 (32.3%)	-26.0	108.4		21% SD 9
ER+	692/2966 (23.3%)	1110/2903 (38.2%)	-281.7	412.2		50% SD 4	655/2966 (22.1%)	812/2903 (28.0%)	-111.5	343.5		28% SD 5
(c) subtotal ~ 81% ER+	1083/4184 (25.9%)	1593/4165 (38.2%)	-336.4	602.9		43% SD 3 (2*p* <.00001)	1056/4184 (25.2%)	1244/4165 (29.9%)	-135.2	529.9		23% SD 4 (2*p* <.00001)
Difference between tamoxifen effects in ER poor and ER+: $\chi^2_1 = 26.5$; 2p < .00001							**$\chi^2_1 = 8.0$; 2p = .005**					

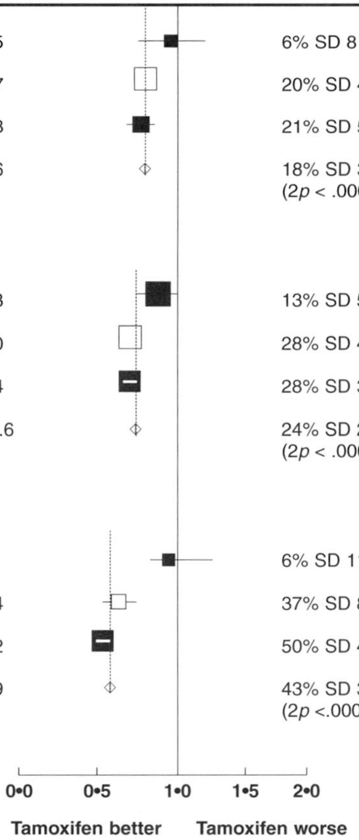

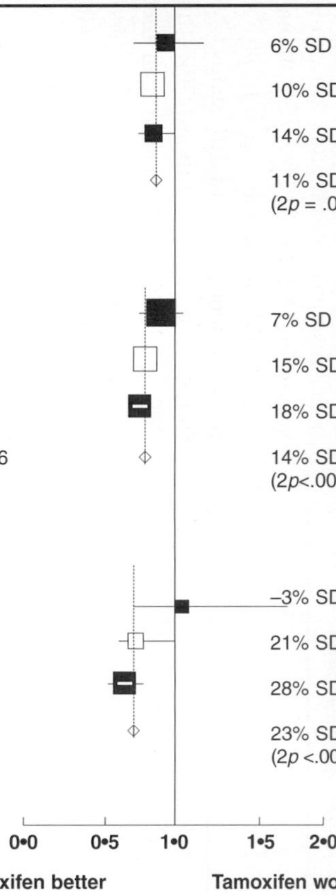

FIG. 7. Results of a meta-analysis assessing the proportional risk reduction associated with 5 years of adjuvant tamoxifen therapy, according to estrogen-receptor (ER) status. The size of the squares reflects the relative size of the sample, and the horizontal lines extending from each square reflect the 99% confidence interval for the effect. The vertical dashed line within the diamond is the point estimate of the meta-analysis, and the ends of the diamond represent the 95% confidence intervals. Patients were randomized to receive adjuvant tamoxifen or no adjuvant tamoxifen. Women with ER-positive tumors received substantial benefit from 5 years of tamoxifen treatment. Con., control; E, expected; NS, not significant; O, observed; SD, standard deviation. (From Early Breast Cancer Trialist Collaborative Group. Tamoxifen for early breast cancer: an overview of the Randomized Trials. *Lancet* 1998;351:1451–1467. With permission.)

TABLE 4. *Relative reduction in recurrence and mortality associated with 5 years of adjuvant tamoxifen therapy by level of estrogen receptor*

	Reduction in recurrence (%)	Reduction in mortality (%)
Estrogen receptor + (10–100 fmol/mg)	43 (±10)	23 (±12)
Estrogen receptor ++ (>100 fmol/mg)	60 (±12)	36 (±14)

Values in parentheses are 95% confidence intervals.
From ref. 7, with permission.

TABLE 5. *Relative reduction in recurrence and mortality associated with adjuvant tamoxifen therapy (any length) by estrogen-receptor and progesterone-receptor status*

	n	Reduction in recurrence (%)	Reduction in mortality (%)
ER+/PR+	7,000	37 (± 6)	16 (± 8)
ER+/PR–	2,000	32 (± 12)	18 (± 14)
ER–/PR+	602	23 (± 24)	9 (± 28)
ER–/PR–	2,000	1 (± 14)	1 (± 14)

ER, estrogen receptor; PR, progesterone receptor.
Values in parentheses are 95% confidence intervals.
From ref. 7, with permission.

patients in this particular analysis, results are somewhat tentative, and it should be noted that some of the 95% confidence intervals include 0% reduction.

Whereas ER negativity indicates lack of benefit from endocrine therapy, it conversely is associated with a modestly increased benefit from chemotherapy. Patients younger than 50 years with ER– tumors were found to have a 35% relative reduction in risk of death when treated with chemotherapy, compared with a 20% reduction for patients with ER+ tumors.[149] A similar pattern was also seen for women 50 years of age or older. ER– tumors on average have a higher S-phase fraction and more genetic abnormalities, and this theoretically could explain their increased sensitivity to chemotherapy. Because patients with ER– tumors are more responsive to chemotherapy and benefit little from tamoxifen, treatment with chemotherapy is the preferred option for this subgroup.

Taken together, these data indicate that quantitative measurement of both ER and PR is useful in the management of women with early-stage breast cancer and should represent a minimum standard of care.[150]

Responses in Patients with Estrogen Receptor–Negative Tumors

ER positivity is a good predictor of response both in the adjuvant setting and for metastatic disease. Thus, it is somewhat surprising that 5% to 10% of women with ER– metastatic breast cancer respond to hormone therapy and that, in an earlier meta-analysis, some ER– postmenopausal women treated with adjuvant tamoxifen therapy appeared to experience a slight increase in survival.[151] Two possibilities could explain these unexpected findings. First, endocrine therapy may exert an effect not mediated through the tumor ER or PR. For example, tamoxifen treatment lowers the serum concentration of type I insulinlike growth factor, a potent stimulator of breast cancer cell proliferation. A more likely explanation for the response observed in nominally ER– breast cancer, though, is that at least some of these tumors do contain ER, but the assay used failed to detect it. Such false-negatives might occur for a number of reasons. The proportion of malignant cells in the tumor may be low, so that receptor protein is diluted beneath the level of detectability when the tumor is processed. Breast tumors are heterogeneous, and the biopsy specimen is divided for various analyses after removal, with only a small portion being sent for receptor assay. The submitted portion may therefore contain little, if any, tumor. Specimen preservation may also be poor, with resultant protein degradation. The patient may be on estrogen replacement therapy or adjuvant tamoxifen, which could lead to a saturation of the ER hormone-binding sites, leading to a false-negative binding assay. Finally, some laboratories define a breast tumor as ER– even when low, but perhaps clinically significant amounts of ER are present. Routine clinical use of IHC analyses might help to obviate many of these false-negative results, because receptor antibodies recognize both occupied and unoccupied ER and because the signal produced by the malignant component of the tumor can be accurately assessed.

Definition of Cutoffs for Receptor Status

Like most biological phenomena, endocrine responsiveness is a continuous variable dependent on levels of ER and, to a lesser extent, PR. Establishing a threshold or lower range in which the likelihood of response is very low or nil is still important, however. In the past, cutoff points as high as 20 fmol/mg of protein were used to define ER negativity, perhaps with the notion of giving patients with the remaining "ER+" tumors the highest probability of responding. Because evidence indicates that tumors with even a small amount of measurable protein, 3 to 10 fmol/mg, have response rates in the 20% to 30% range,[152] classifying them as negative has two deleterious consequences. First, patients may be denied a trial of hormone therapy, from which they have a good chance of benefiting; second, as discussed, such classification can lead to the clinically erroneous impression that a substantial number of patients with ER– tumors benefit from hormone therapy. To avoid these pitfalls, stringently low cut points should be adopted. For example, evidence suggests that setting a cutoff for ER negativity of 3 fmol or less[152] of ER protein per milligram of cytosol protein by ligand assay and 1% of positively stained cells by IHC analysis[137] best separates patients who do not derive benefit from endocrine treatment from those who do. When stringently low cut points are adopted, special attention to quality control is crucial to avoid variability and false-positive results.

Estrogen-Receptor and Progesterone-Receptor Status as Prognostic Factors

Although ER status is clinically most valuable as a predictive factor, it can also be used as a prognostic factor. Women with ER+ tumors who do not receive any systemic therapy after surgery have a chance of recurrence by 5 years that is 5% to 10% lower than patients with ER– tumors.[153–155] ER status, however, may be a time-dependent variable; as follow-up time lengthens, the advantage of ER positivity in terms of relapse and death grows smaller and ultimately disappears.[156–158] Because ER status is not associated with nodal metastases and its prognostic significance diminishes over time, it is probably a marker more of growth rate than of metastatic potential. In addition to being a prognostic factor itself, ER status is also associated with a number of other established prognostic factors. ER+ tumors are more likely to be from older women,[159] to be well-differentiated histologically,[160] to have a lower fraction of dividing cells,[161] and to be diploid,[161] and are less likely to exhibit a mutation, loss, or amplification of breast cancer–related genes, such as the p53,[162,163] HER-2/neu,[164,165] and epidermal growth factor receptor genes.[166] ER status is also prognostic for the site of gross metastatic spread. For reasons that are unknown, ER+ tumors are more likely to initially manifest clinically apparent metastases in bone, soft tissue, or the reproductive and genital tracts, whereas ER– tumors more commonly metastasize to brain and liver. That ER status is associated with such a host of other good biological features further supports the rationale that it is associated with a better short-term prognosis. Because the benefit of systemic therapy is proportional to the risk of relapse, ER status may be particularly useful for further defining the prognosis of lower-risk patients—for example, node-negative patients with tumor size of 1 to 2 cm. Because of the relatively small benefits of systemic therapy for women with tumors in this range, ER status can help patients weigh the relative risks and benefits of systemic treatment.

The usefulness of PR status as a prognostic factor is not as clear; some evidence supports its usefulness,[154,167,168] whereas other data do not.[169] Unlike ER, PR is more likely to be higher or positive in young or premenopausal women, probably as a result of greater estrogen stimulation. PR status probably is a weak prognostic factor, even weaker than ER status, and this probably accounts for the variability in study results. Also, because of this weakness, it has not achieved any clinical usefulness based solely on its prognostic value. A more extensive discussion of ER status and PR status as prognostic factors can be found in Chapter 32.

CONCLUSION

ER and PR status have established usefulness in the clinical management of women with breast cancer. They should be obtained on all breast tumor specimens. Assays have become simpler and less costly, a development that should make them more readily available for all patients. Further progress remains to be made in the area of standardization of assay technique, objective quantification, and better reproducibility. A better functionally based assay could help to refine and improve the clinical use. Elucidation of downstream effector genes of hormone receptors could lead to inclusion of these genes in high-density oligonucleotide array panels to better test the endocrine response pathways in human tumors. More important, an understanding of receptor function and coregulatory molecules will lead to improved therapies, fewer side effects, and greater potential for cure or for the conversion of an otherwise lethal disease to one that can be managed more as a chronic condition, much like ischemic heart disease, hypertension, or tuberculosis. Perhaps most significantly, because breast cancer is a disease promoted by estrogen and progesterone, and their action is mediated through their cognate receptors, one of the most compelling opportunities for achieving the holy grail of breast oncology—prevention or eradication of the disease itself—lies in understanding and modifying receptor interaction and function.

It is ironic that steroid receptors create fertile ground for breast cancer yet can be used as an effective offensive platform for striking against the disease. These strikes have met with success. The application of laboratory and basic scientific knowledge of hormone receptor biology to complementary clinical study has proved to be a fruitful paradigm of translational research that is directly helpful to women with breast cancer—past, present, and future.

REFERENCES

1. Jensen EV, DeSombre ER. Mechanism of action of the female sex hormones. *Ann Rev Biochem* 1972;41:203.
2. Jensen EV, Jacobson HI. Basic guides to the mechanism of estrogen action. *Recent Prog Horm Res* 1962;18:387.
3. Folca PJ, Glascock RF, Irvine WT. Studies with tritium-labeled hexoestrol in advanced breast cancer. *Lancet* 1961;2:796.
4. Slamon D, Leyland-Jones B, Shak S, et al. Addition of Herceptin (humanized anti-Her2 antibody) to first line chemotherapy for Her2 overexpressing metastatic breast cancer (Her2+/MBC) markedly increases anticancer activity: a randomized, multinational controlled phase III trial. *Proceedings of the American Society of Clinical Oncology, Los Angeles, California, May 1998*, Los Angeles, CA. Vol. 17.
5. Cobleigh MA, Vogel CL, Tripathy D, et al. Efficacy and safety of Herceptin (humanized anti-her2 antibody) as a single agent in 222 women with her2 overexpression who relapsed following chemotherapy for metastatic breast cancer. *Proceedings of the American Society of Clinical Oncology, Los Angeles, California, May 1998*, Los Angeles, CA, 1998. Vol. 17.
6. Beatson GT. On the treatment of inoperable cases of carcinoma of the mamma: suggestions for a new method of treatment, with illustrative cases. *Lancet* 1896;2:104
7. Group EBCTC. Tamoxifen for early breast cancer: an overview of the randomised trials. *Lancet* 1998;351:1451.

8. Greene GL, Gilna P, Walterfield M, Baker A, Hort Y, Shine J. Sequence and expression of human estrogen receptor cDNA. *Science* 1986;231: 1150.
9. Walter P, Green S, Greene G, et al. Cloning of the human estrogen receptor cDNA. *Proc Natl Acad Sci U S A* 1985;82:7889.
10. Beato M, Arnemann J, Chalepakis G, Slater E, Willmann T. Gene regulation by steroid hormones. *J Steroid Biochem* 1987;27:9.
11. Klein-Hitpass L, Ryffel GU, Heitlinger E, Cato ACB. A 13bp palindrome is a functional estrogen responsive element and interacts specifically with estrogen receptor. *Nucleic Acids Res* 1988;16:647.
12. Kumar V, Chambon P. The estrogen receptor binds tightly to its responsive element as a ligand-induced homodimer. *Cell* 1988;55:145.
13. Freedman LP, Luisi BF, Korszun ZR, Basavappa R, Sigler PB, Yamamoto KR. The function and structure of the metal coordination sites within the glucocorticoid receptor DNA binding domain. *Nature* 1988;334:543.
14. Dana SL, Hoener PA, Wheeler DA, Lawrence CB, McDonnell DP. Novel estrogen response elements identified by genetic selection in yeast are differentially responsive to estrogens and antiestrogens in mammalian cells. *Mol Endocrinol* 1994;8:1193.
15. Schwabe J, Chapman L, Finch J, Rhodes D. The crystal structure of the estrogen receptor DNA-binding domain bound to DNA: how receptors discriminate between their response elements. *Cell* 1993;75:567.
16. Mader S, Kumar V, de Verneuil H, Chambon P. Three amino acids of the oestrogen receptor are essential to its ability to distinguish an oestrogen from a glucocorticoid-responsive element. *Nature* 1989;338:271.
17. Kumar V, Green S, Staub A, Chambon P. Localisation of the oestradiol-binding and putative DNA-binding domains of the human oestrogen receptor. *EMBO J* 1986;5:2231.
18. Kumar V, Green S, Stack G, Berry M, Jin J-R, Chambon P. Functional domains of the human estrogen receptor. *Cell* 1987;51:941.
19. Tora L, White J, Brou C, et al. The human estrogen receptor has two independent nonacidic transcriptional activation functions. *Cell* 1989;59:477.
20. Ponglikitmongkol M, Green S, Chambon P. Genomic organization for the human oestrogen receptor gene. *EMBO J* 1988;7:3385.
21. Webster NJG, Green S, Tasset D, Ponglikitmongkol M, Chambon P. The transcription activation function located in the hormone-binding domain of the human oestrogen receptor is not encoded by a single exon. *EMBO J* 1989;8:1441.
22. Danielian PS, White R, Lees JA, Parker MG. Identification of a conserved region required for hormone dependent transcriptional activation by steroid hormone receptor. *EMBO J* 1992;11:1025.
23. Pierrat B, Heery DM, Chambon P, Losson R. A highly conserved region in the hormone-binding domain of the human estrogen receptor functions as an efficient transactivation domain in yeast. *Gene* 1994;143:193.
24. Chambraud B, Berry M, Redeuilh G, Chambon P, Balieu EE. Several regions of human estrogen receptor are involved in the formation of receptor-heat shock protein 90 complexes. *J Biol Chem* 1990;265: 20686.
25. Sartorius CA, Melville MY, Hovland AR, Tung L, Takimoto GS, Horwitz KB. A third transactivation function (AF3) of human progesterone receptors located in the unique N-terminal segment of the B-isoform. *Mol Endocrinol* 1994;8:1347.
26. Tzukerman MT, Esty A, Santisomere D, et al. Human estrogen receptor transactivational capacity is determined by both cellular and promoter context and mediated by two functionally distinct intramolecular regions. *Mol Endocrinol* 1994;8:21.
27. Bocquel MT, Kumar V, Stricker C, Chambon P, Gronemeyer H. The contribution of the N- and C-terminal regions of steroid receptors in activation of transcription is both receptor and cell-specific. *Nucleic Acids Res* 1989;17:2581.
28. McDonnell D, Clemm D, Hermann T, Goldman M, Pike J. Analysis of estrogen receptor function in vitro reveals distinct classes of antiestrogens. *Mol Endocrinol* 1995;9:659.
29. Kuiper G, Enmark E, Pelto-Huikko M, Nilsson S, Gustafsson J-A. Cloning of a novel estrogen receptor expressed in rat prostate and ovary. *Proc Natl Acad Sci U S A* 1996;93:5925.
30. Mosselman S, Polman J, Kijkema R. Identification and characterization of a novel human estrogen receptor. *FEBS Lett* 1996;392:49.
31. Enmark E, Pelto-Huikko M, Grandien K, et al. Human estrogen receptor b-gene structure, chromosomal localization, and expression pattern. *J Clin Endocrinol* 1997;82:4258.
32. Ogawa S, Inoue S, Watanabe T, et al. The complete primary structure of human estrogen receptor β (hERβ) and its heterodimerization with ERα in vivo and in vitro. *Biochem Biophys Res Commun* 1998;243:122.
33. Pettersson K, Grandien K, Kuiper G, Gustafsson J-A. Mouse estrogen receptor β forms estrogen response element-binding heterodimers with estrogen receptor α. *Mol Endocrinol* 1997;11:1486.
34. Cowley S, Hoare S, Mosselman S, Parker M. Estrogen receptors α and β form heterodimers on DNA. *J Biol Chem* 1997;272:19858.
35. Couse J, Lindzey J, Grandien K, Gustafsson J-A, Korach K. Tissue distribution and quantitative analysis of estrogen receptor-α (ERα) and estrogen receptor-β (ERβ) messenger ribonucleic acid in the wild-type and ERα-knockout mouse. *Endocrinology* 1997;138:4613.
36. Kuiper G, Carlsson B, Grandien K, et al. Comparison of the ligand binding specificity and transcript tissue distribution of estrogen receptors α and β. *Endocrinology* 1997;138:863.
37. Barkhem T, Carlsson B, Nilsson Y, Enmark E, Gustafsson J, Nilsson S. Differential response of estrogen receptor alpha and estrogen receptor beta to partial estrogen agonists/antagonist. *Mol Pharmacol* 1998;54:105.
38. Kuiper G, Lemmen J, Carlsson B, et al. Interaction of estrogenic chemical and phytoestrogens with estrogen receptor beta. *Endocrinology* 1998;139:4252.
39. McInerney E, Weis K, Sun J, Mosselman S, Katzenellenbogen B. Transcription activation by the human estrogen receptor subtype β (ERβ) studied with ERβ and ERα receptor chimeras. *Endocrinology* 1998;139:4513.
40. Montano M, Muller V, Trobaugh A, Katzenellenbogen B. The carboxy-terminal F domain of the human estrogen receptor: role in the transcriptional activity of the receptor and the effectiveness of antiestrogens as estrogen antagonists. *Mol Endocrinol* 1995;9:814.
41. Paech K, Webb P, Kuiper GG, et al. Differential ligand activation of estrogen receptors ERalpha and ERbeta at AP1 sites [See comments]. *Science* 1997;277:1508.
42. Webb P, Lopez GN, Uht RM, Kushner PJ. Tamoxifen activation of the estrogen receptor/AP-1 pathway: potential origin for the cell-specific estrogen like effects of antiestrogens. *Mol Endocrinol* 1995;9:443.
43. Dotzlaw H, Leygue E, Watson P, Murphy L. Expression of estrogen receptor-beta in human breast tumors. *J Clin Endocrinol Metab* 1996;82:2371.
44. Vladusic E, Hornby A, Guerra Vladusic F, Lupu R. Expression of estrogen receptor β messenger RNA variant in breast cancer. *Cancer Res* 1998;58:210.
45. Dotzlaw H, Leygue E, Watson P, Murphy L. Estrogen receptor-β RNA expression in human breast tumor biopsies: relationship to steroid receptor status and regulation by progestins. *Cancer Res* 1999; 59:529.
46. Speirs V, Parkes A, Kerin M, et al. Coexpression of estrogen receptor α and β: poor prognostic factors in human breast cancer? *Cancer Res* 1999;59:525.
47. Horwitz KB, Jackson TA, Bain DL, Richer JK, Takimoto GS, Tung L. Nuclear receptor coactivators and corepressors. *Mol Endocrinol* 1996;10:1167.
48. Huang N, vomBaur E, Garnier J-M, et al. Two distinct nuclear receptor interaction domains in NSD1, a novel SET protein that exhibits characteristics of both corepressors and coactivators. *EMBO J* 1998;17:3398.
49. Chrivia J, Kwok R, Lamb N, Hagiwara M, Montminy M, Goodman R. Phosphorylated CREB binds specifically to the nuclear protein CBP. *Nature* 1993;365:855.
50. Smith C, Onate S, Tsai M, O'Malley B. CREB binding protein acts synergistically with steroid receptor coactivator-1 to enhance steroid receptor-dependent transcription. *Proc Natl Acad Sci U S A* 1996;93:8884.
51. Kamei Y, Xu L, Heinzel T, et al. A CBP integrator complex mediates transcriptional activation and AP-1 inhibition by nuclear receptors. *Cell* 1996;85:403.
52. Hankinson O. The aryl hydrocarbon receptor complex. *Annu Rev Pharmacol Toxicol* 1995;35:397.
53. Onate S, Boonyaratanakornkit V, Spencer T, et al. The steroid receptor coactivator-1 contains multiple receptor interacting and activation domains that cooperatively enhance the activation function 1 (AF1) and AF2 domains of steroid receptors. *J Biol Chem* 1998;273:12101.
54. Smith CL, Nawaz Z, O'Malley BW. Coactivator and corepressor regulation of the agonist/antagonist activity of the mixed antiestrogen, 4-Hydroxytamoxifen. *Mol Endocrinol* 1997;11:657.

55. Jackson TA, Richer JK, Bain DL, Takimoto GS, Tung, L, Horwitz KB. The partial agonist activity of antagonist-occupied steroid receptors is controlled by a novel hinge domain-binding coactivator L7/SPA and the corepressors N/CoR or SMRT. *Mol Endocrinol* 1997;11:693.
56. McKenna N, Nawaz Z, Tsai S, Tsai M-J, O'Malley B. Distinct steady-state nuclear receptor coregulator complexes exist in vivo. *Proc Natl Acad Sci U S A* 1998;95:11697.
57. Black L, Sato M, Rowley E, et al. Raloxifene (LY139481 HCl) prevents bone loss and reduces serum cholesterol without causing uterine hypertrophy in ovariectomized rats. *J Clin Invest* 1994;93:63.
58. Beekman J, Allan G, Tsai S, Tsai M-J, O'Malley B. Transcriptional activation by the estrogen receptor requires a conformational change in the ligand binding domain. *Mol Endocrinol* 1993;7:1266.
59. Shiau A, Barstad D, Loria P, et al. The structural basis of estrogen receptor/coactivator recognition and the antagonism of this interaction by tamoxifen. *Cell* 1998;95:927.
60. Johnston S, Riddler S, Haynes B, et al. The novel anti-oestrogen idoxifene inhibits the growth of human MCF-7 breast cancer xenografts and reduces the frequency of acquired anti-oestrogen resistance. *Br J Cancer* 1997;75:804.
61. Rauschning W, Pritchard KI. Droloxifene, a new antiestrogen: its role in metastatic breast cancer. *Breast Cancer Res Treat* 1994;31:83.
62. Tremblay A, Tremblay G, Labrie C, Labrie F, Giguere V. EM-800, a novel antiestrogen, acts as a pure antagonist of the transcriptional function of estrogen receptors alpha and beta. *Endocrinology* 1998;139:111.
63. Sato M, Turner C, Wang T, Adrian M, Rowley E, Bryant H. LY353381: a novel raloxifene analog with improved SERM potency and efficacy *in vivo*. *J Pharmacol Exper Ther* 1998;287:1.
64. Cho H, Katzenellenbogen BS. Synergistic activation of estrogen receptor-mediated transcription by estradiol and protein kinase activators. *Mol Endocrinol* 1993;7:441.
65. Aronica SM, Kraus WL, Katzenellenbogen BS. Estrogen action via the cAMP signaling pathway: stimulation of adenylate cyclase and cAMP-regulated gene transcription. *Proc Natl Acad Sci U S A* 1994;91:8517.
66. Ince BA, Montano MM, Katzenellenbogen BS. Activation of transcriptionally inactive human estrogen receptors by cyclic adenosine 3',5'-monophosphate and ligands including antiestrogens. *Mol Endocrinol* 1994;8:1397.
67. Fujimoto N, Katzenellenbogen BS. Alteration in the agonist/antagonist balance of antiestrogens by activation of protein kinase A signaling pathways in breast cancer cells: antiestrogen selectivity and promoter dependence. *Mol Endocrinol* 1994;8:296.
68. Sartorius CA, Tung L, Takimoto GS, Horwitz KB. Antagonist-occupied human progesterone receptors bound to DNA are functionally switched to transcriptional agonists by cAMP. *J Biol Chem* 1993;268:9262.
69. Sartorius CA, Groshong SD, Miller LA, et al. New T47D breast cancer cell lines for the independent study of progesterone β- and α-receptors: only antiprogestin-occupied β-receptors are switched to transcriptional agonists by cAMP. *Cancer Res* 1994;54:3868.
70. Aronica SM, Katzenellenbogen BS. Stimulation of estrogen receptor-mediated transcription and alteration in the phosphorylation state of the rat uterine estrogen receptor by estrogen, cyclic adenosine monophosphate, and insulin-like growth factor-I. *Mol Endocrinol* 1993;7:743.
71. Neuman E, Ladha MH, Lin N, et al. Cyclin D1 stimulation of estrogen receptor transcriptional activity independent of cdk4. *Mol Cell Biol* 1997;17:5338.
72. Zwijsen RM, Wientjens E, Klompmaker R, van der Sman J, Bernards R, Michalides RJ. CDK-independent activation of estrogen receptor by cyclin D1. *Cell* 1997;88:405.
73. Hill SM, Fuqua SAW, Chamness GC, Greene GL, McGuire WL. Estrogen receptor expression in human breast cancer associated with an estrogen receptor gene restriction fragment length polymorphism. *Cancer Res* 1989;49:145.
74. Watts CKW, Handel ML, King RJD, Sutherland RL. Oestrogen receptor gene structure and function in breast cancer. *J Steroid Biochem Mol Biol* 1992;41:529.
75. Yaich L, Dupont WD, Cavener DR. Analysis of the PvuII restriction fragment-length polymorphism and exon structure of the estrogen receptor gene in breast cancer and peripheral blood. *Cancer Res* 1994;52:77.
76. Piva R, Rimondi AP, Hanau S, et al. Different methylation of oestrogen receptor DNA in human breast carcinomas with and without oestrogen receptor. *Br J Cancer* 1990;61:270.
77. Kay P, Hahnel R, Gunn H, Harmon D, Song J. Hypermethylation of HpaII recognition sequences within the 5' coding region of the estrogen receptor gene is not associated with estrogen receptor negativity in primary breast tumours. *Anticancer Res* 1998;18:1709.
78. Ottaviano YL, Issa J-P, Parl FF, Smith HS, Baylin SB, Davidson NE. Methylation of the estrogen receptor gene CpG island marks loss of estrogen receptor expression in human breast cancer cells. *Cancer Res* 1994;54.
79. Lapidus R, Ferguson A, Ottaviano Y, et al. Methylation of estrogen and progesterone receptor gene 5' CpG islands correlates with lack of estrogen and progesterone receptor gene expression in breast tumors. *Clin Cancer Res* 1996;2:805.
80. Ferguson AT, Lapidus RG, Baylin SB, Davidson NE. Demethylation of the estrogen receptor gene in estrogen receptor–negative breast cancer cells can reactivate estrogen receptor gene expression. *Cancer Res* 1995;55:2279.
81. Weigel RJ, deConinck EC. Transcriptional control of estrogen receptor in estrogen receptor–negative breast carcinoma. *Cancer Res* 1993;53:3472.
82. Grandien KFH, Berkenstam A, Nilsson S, Gustafsson J-Å. Localization of DNase I hypersensitive sites in the human oestrogen receptor gene correlates with the transcriptional activity of two differentially used promoters. *J Mol Endocrinol* 1993;10:269.
83. Grandien K. Determination of transcription start sites in the human estrogen receptor gene and identification of a novel, tissue-specific, estrogen receptor-mRNA isoform. *Mol Cell Endocrinol* 1996; 116:207.
84. Nestor PV, Forde RC, Webb P, Gannon F. The genomic organisation, sequence and functional analysis of the 5' flanking region of the chicken estrogen receptor gene. *J Steroid Biochem Mol Biol* 1994; 50:121.
85. Weigel RJ, Crooks DL, Iglehart JD, deConinck EC. Quantitative analysis of the transcriptional start sites of estrogen receptor in breast carcinoma. *Cell Growth Differ* 1995;6:707.
86. deConinck EC, McPherson LA, Weigel RJ. Transcriptional regulation of estrogen receptor in breast carcinomas. *Mol Cell Biol* 1995; 15:2191.
87. Tang Z, Treilleux I, Brown M. A transcriptional enhancer required for the differential expression of the human estrogen receptor in breast cancers. *Mol Cell Biol* 1997;17:1274.
88. Treilleux, Peloux N, Brown M, Sergeant A. Human estrogen receptor (ER) gene promoter-P1: estradiol-independent activity and estradiol inducibility in ER+ and ER– cells. *Mol Endocrinol* 1997;11:1319.
89. Castles CG, Oesterreich S, Hansen R, Fuqua SA. Auto-regulation of the estrogen receptor promoter. *J Steroid Biochem Mol Biol* 1997;62:155.
90. Fuqua SAW, Fitzgerald SD, Chamness GC, et al. Variant human breast tumor estrogen receptor with constitutive transcriptional activity. *Cancer Res* 1991;51:105.
91. Fuqua SAW, Fitzgerald SD, Allred DC, et al. Inhibition of estrogen receptor action by a naturally occurring variant in human breast tumors. *Cancer Res* 1992;52:483.
92. Fuqua SAW, Wiltschke C, Castles C, Wolf D, Allred DC. A role for estrogen receptor variants in endocrine resistance. *Endocrine-Related Cancer* 1995;2:19.
93. Hopp T, Fuqua S. The estrogen receptor and breast cancer. *J Mammary Gland Neoplasia* 1999;3:73.
94. Fuqua S, Wolf D. Molecular aspects of estrogen receptor variants in breast cancer. *Breast Cancer Res Treat* 1995;35:233.
95. Murphy L, Dotzlaw H, Leygue E, Douglas D, Coutts A, Watson P. Estrogen receptor variants and mutations: minireview. *J Steroid Biochem Mol Biol* 1997;62:363.
96. Murphy L, Dotzlaw H, Leygue E, Coutts A, Watson P. The pathophysiological role of estrogen receptor variants in human breast cancer. *J Steroid Biochem Mol Biol* 1997;65:1.
97. Castles CG, Fuqua SAW, Klotz DM, Hill SM. Expression of a constitutively active estrogen receptor variant in the estrogen receptor–negative BT-20 human breast cancer cell line. *Cancer Res* 1993;53:5934.
98. Ohlsson H, Lykkesfeldt A, Madsen M, Briand P. The estrogen receptor variant lacking exon 5 has dominant negative activity in the human breast epithelial cell line HMT-3522S1. *Cancer Res* 1998;58:4264.
99. Chaidarun S, Alexander J. A tumor-specific truncated estrogen receptor splice variant enhances estrogen-stimulated gene expression. *Mol Endocrinol* 1998;12:1355.

100. Rea D, Parker MG. Effects of an exon 5 variant of the estrogen receptor in MCF-7 breast cancer cells. *Cancer Res* 1996;56:1556.
101. Villa E, Dugani A, Fantoni E, et al. Type of estrogen receptor determines response to antiestrogen therapy. *Cancer Res* 1996;56:3883.
102. Daffada AA, Johnston SR, Smith IE, Detre S, King N, Dowsett M. Exon 5 deletion variant estrogen receptor messenger RNA expression in relation to tamoxifen resistance and progesterone receptor/pS2 status in human breast cancer. *Cancer Res* 1995;55:288.
103. Gallacchi P, Schoumacher F, Eppenberger-Castori S, et al. Increased expression of estrogen-receptor exon-5-deletion variant in relapse tissues of human breast cancer. *Int J Cancer* 1998;79:44.
104. Desai A, Luqmani Y, Walter J, et al. Presence of exon5-deleted oestrogen receptor in human breast cancer:" functional analysis and clinical significance. *Br J Cancer* 1997;75:1173.
105. Leygue E, Huang A, Murphy L, Watson P. Prevalence of estrogen receptor variant messenger RNAs in human breast cancer. *Cancer Res* 1996;56:4324.
106. Huang A, Pettigrew N, Watson P. Immunohistochemical assay for oestrogen receptors in paraffin wax sections of breast carcinoma using a new monoclonal antibody. *J Pathol* 1996;180:223.
107. Huang A, Leygue E, Snell L, Murphy L, Watson P. Expression of estrogen receptor variant mRNAs and determination of estrogen receptor status in human breast cancer. *Am J Pathol* 1997;150.
108. Roodi N, Bailey LR, Kao WY, et al. Estrogen receptor gene analysis in estrogen receptor-positive and receptor-negative primary breast cancer. *J Natl Cancer Inst* 1995;87:446.
109. Karnik PS, Kulkarni S, Liu X-P, Budd GT, Bukowski RM. Estrogen receptor mutations in tamoxifen-resistant breast cancer. *Cancer Res* 1994;54:349.
110. Zhang QX, Borg A, Wolf DM, Oesterreich S, Fuqua SA. An estrogen receptor mutant with strong hormone-independent activity from a metastatic breast cancer. *Cancer Res* 1997;57:1244.
111. Tremblay G, Tremblay A, Labrie F, Giguère V. Ligand-independent activation of the estrogen receptors α and β by mutations of a conserved tyrosine can be abolished by antiestrogens. *Cancer Res* 1998;58:877.
112. Weis KE, Ekena K, Thomas JA, Lazennec G, Katzenellenbogen BS. Constitutively active human estrogen receptors containing amino acid substitutions for tyrosine 537 in the receptor protein. *Mol Endocrinol* 1996;10:1388.
113. Moore J, McKee D, Slentz-Kesler K, et al. Cloning and characterization of human estrogen receptor β isoforms. *Biochem Biophys Res Commun* 1998;247:75.
114. Ogawa S, Inoue S, Watanabe T, et al. Molecular cloning and characterization of human estrogen receptor bcx: a potential inhibitor of estrogen action in human. *Nucleic Acids Res* 1998;26:3505.
115. Hanstein B, Liu H, Yancisin M, Brown M. Functional analysis of a novel estrogen receptor-β isoform. *Mol Endocrinol* 1999;13.129.
116. Bezwoda WR, Esser JD, Dansey R, Kessel I, Lang M. The value of estrogen and progesterone receptor determinations in advanced breast cancer. *Cancer* 1991;68:867.
117. Manni A, Arafah B, Pearson OH. Estrogen and progesterone receptors in the prediction of response of breast cancer to endocrine therapy. *Cancer* 1980;46:2838.
118. McClelland RA, Berger U, Miller LS, Powles TJ, Jensen EV, Coombes RC. Immunocytochemical assay for estrogen receptor: relationship to outcome of therapy in patients with advanced breast cancer. *Cancer Res* 1986;46:4241s.
119. McGuire WL, De La Garza M, Chamness GC. Evaluation of estrogen receptor assays in human breast cancer tissue. *Cancer Res* 1977;37:637.
120. Hull DFI, Clark GM, Osborne CK, Chamness GC, Knight WAI, McGuire WL. Multiple estrogen receptor assays in human breast cancer. *Cancer Res* 1983;43:413.
121. Elledge RM, Ciocca DR, Langone G, McGuire WL. Estrogen receptor, progesterone receptor, and her-2/neu protein in breast cancers from pregnant patients. *Cancer* 1993;71:2499.
122. Encarnacion CA, Ciocca DR, McGuire WL, Clark GM, Fuqua SAW, Osborne CK. Measurement of steroid hormone receptors in breast cancer patients on tamoxifen. *Breast Cancer Res Treat* 1993;26:237.
123. King WJ, Greene GL. Monoclonal antibodies localize oestrogen receptor in the nuclei of target cells. *Nature* 1984;307:745.
124. Taylor CR. The current role of immunohistochemistry in diagnostic pathology. *Adv Pathol Lab Med* 1994;7:59.
125. Greene GL, Sobel NB, King WJ, Jensen EV. Immunochemical studies of estrogen receptors. *J Steroid Biochem* 1984;20:51.
126. Leclercq G, Bojar H, Goussard J, et al. Abbott monoclonal enzyme immunoassay measurement of estrogen receptors in human breast cancer: a European multicenter study. *Cancer Res* 1986;46:4233s.
127. Shi S-R, Cote RJ, Taylor CR. Antigen retrieval immunohistochemistry: past, present, and future. *J Histochem Cytochem* 1997;45:327.
128. Elledge RM, Clark GM, Fuqua SAW, Yu Y-Y, Allred DC. p53 protein accumulation detected by five different antibodies: relationship to prognosis and heat shock protein 70 in breast cancer. *Cancer Res* 1994;54:3752.
129. Jacobs TW, Prioleau JE, Stillman IE, Schnitt SJ. Loss of tumor marker-immunostaining intensity on stored paraffin slides of breast cancer. *J Natl Cancer Inst* 1996;88:1054.
130. Biesterfeld S, Veuskens U, Schmitz F-J, Amo-Takyl B, Bocking A. Interobserver reproducibility of immunocytochemical estrogen and progesterone receptor status assessment in breast cancer. *Anticancer Res* 1996;16:2497.
131. Cavaliere A, Bucciarelli E, Sidoni A, et al. Estrogen and progesterone receptors in breast cancer: comparison between enzyme immunoassay and computer-assisted image analysis of immunocytochemical assay. *Cytometry* 1996;26:204.
132. Jordan VC, Jacobson HI, Keenan EJ. Determination of estrogen receptor in breast cancer using monoclonal antibody technology: results of a multicenter study in the United States. *Cancer Res* 1986;46[Suppl]:4237s.
133. Heubner A, Beck T, Grill H-J, Pollow K. Comparison of immunocytochemical estrogen receptor assay, estrogen receptor enzyme immunoassay, and radioligand-labeled estrogen receptor assay in human breast cancer and uterine tissue. *Cancer Res* 1988; 46[Suppl]:4291s.
134. Dittadi R, Meo S, Amoroso B, Gion M. Detection of different estrogen receptor forms in breast cancer cytosol by enzyme immunoassay. *Cancer Res* 1997;57:1066.
135. Goussard J, Lechevrel C, Martin P-M, Roussel G. Comparison of monoclonal antibodies and tritiated ligands for estrogen receptor assays in 241 breast cancer cytosols. *Cancer Res* 1986;46[Suppl]: 4282s.
136. Pertschuk L, Kim D, Nayer K, et al. Immunocytochemical estrogen and progestin receptor assays in breast cancer with monoclonal antibodies. *Cancer* 1990;66:1663.
137. Harvey JM, Clark GM, Osborne CK, Allred DC. Estrogen receptor status by immunohistochemistry is superior to the ligand-binding assay for predicting response to adjuvant endocrine therapy in breast cancer. *J Clin Oncol* 1999;17:1474.
138. Robertson J, Bates K, Pearson D, Blkamey R, Nicholson R. Comparison of two oestrogen receptor assays in the prediction of the clinical course of patients with advanced breast cancer. *Br J Cancer* 1992;65:727.
139. Ravdin PM, Green S, Dorr TM, et al. Prognostic significance of progesterone receptor levels in estrogen receptor-positive patients with metastatic breast cancer treated with tamoxifen: results of a prospective Southwest Oncology Group study. *J Clin Oncol* 1992;10:1284.
140. Dombernowsky P, Smith I, Falkson G, et al. Letrozole, a new oral aromatase inhibitor for advanced breast cancer: double-blind randomized trial showing a dose effect and improved efficacy and tolerability compared with megestrol acetate. *J Clin Oncol* 1998;16:453.
141. Buzdar A, Jonat W, Howell A, et al. Anastrozole, a potent and selective aromatase inhibitor, versus megestrol acetate in postmenopausal women with advanced breast cancer: results of overview analysis of two phase III trials. *J Clin Oncol* 1996;14:2000.
142. Kuukasjarvi T, Kononen J, Helin H, Holli K, Isola J. Loss of estrogen receptor in recurrent breast cancer is associated with poor response to endocrine therapy. *J Clin Oncol* 1996;14:2584.
143. Elledge RM, Green S, Pugh R, et al. ER and PgR by ligand binding assay compared with ER, PgR, and pS2 by immunohistochemistry in predicting response to tamoxifen in metastatic breast cancer: a Southwest Oncology Group study. *Int J Cancer* 1999 (*in press*).
144. Horwitz K, McGuire W, Pearson O, Segaloff A. Predicting response to endocrine therapy in human breast cancer: a hypothesis. *Science* 1975;189:726.
145. Pertschuk L, Feldman J, Eisenberg K, et al. Immunocytochemical detection of progesterone receptor in breast cancer with monoclonal antibody. *Cancer* 1988;62:342.
146. Gross G, Clark G, Chamness G, McGuire W. Multiple progesterone receptor assays in human breast cancer. *Cancer Res* 1984;44:836.

147. Osborne C, Yochmowitz M, Knight W, McGuire W. The value of estrogen and progesterone receptors in the treatment of breast cancer. *Cancer* 1980;46:2884.
148. Keshgegian A, Cnaan A. Estrogen receptor–negative, progesterone receptor–positive breast carcinoma. *Arch Pathol Lab Med* 1996;120:970.
149. Group EBCTC. Polychemotherapy for early breast cancer: an overview of the randomised trials. *Lancet* 1998;352:930.
150. ASCO. Clinical practice guidelines for the use of tumor markers in breast and colorectal cancer. *J Clin Oncol* 1996;14:2843.
151. Group EBCTC. Systemic treatment of early breast cancer by hormonal, cytotoxic, or immune therapy. *Lancet* 1992;339:1.
152. Knight W, Osborne C, McGuire W. Hormone receptors in primary and advanced breast cancer. *Clin Endocrinol Metab* 1980;9:361.
153. Crowe JP, Hubay CA, Pearson OH, et al. Estrogen receptor status as a prognostic indicator for stage I breast cancer patients. *Breast Cancer Res Treat* 1982;2:171.
154. Fisher B, Redmond C, Fisher ER, Caplan R. Relative worth of estrogen or progesterone receptor and pathologic characteristics of differentiation as indicators of prognosis in node negative breast cancer patients: findings from National Surgical Adjuvant Breast and Bowel Project Protocol B-06. *J Clin Oncol* 1988;6:1076.
155. McGuire WL, Tandon AK, Allred DC, Chamness GC, Clark GM. How to use prognostic factors in axillary node-negative breast cancer patients. *J Natl Cancer Inst* 1990;82:1006.
156. Adami H-O, Graffman S, Lindgren A, Sällström J. Prognostic implication of estrogen receptor content in breast cancer. *Breast Cancer Res Treat* 1985;5:293.
157. Hilsenbeck S, Ravdin P, de Moor C, Chamness G, Osborne C, Clark GM. Time-dependence of hazard ratios for prognostic factors in primary breast cancer. *Breast Cancer Res Treat* 1998;52:227.
158. Schmitt M, Thomssen C, Ulm K, et al. Time-varying prognostic impact of tumour biological factors urokinase (uPA), PAI-1 and steroid hormone receptor status in primary breast cancer. *Br J Cancer* 1997; 76:306.
159. Clark G, Osborne C, McGuire W. Correlations between estrogen receptor, progesterone receptor, and patient characteristics in human breast cancer. *J Clin Oncol* 1984;2:1102.
160. Fisher E, Osborne CK, McGuire W, et al. Correlation of primary breast cancer histopathology and estrogen receptor content. *Breast Cancer Res Treat* 1981;1:37.
161. Wenger C, Beardslee S, Owens M, et al. DNA ploidy, S-phase, and steroid receptors in more than 127,000 breast cancer patients. *Breast Cancer Res Treat* 1993;28:9.
162. Falette N, Paperin M-P, Treilleux I, et al. Prognostic value of p53 gene mutations in a large series of node-negative breast cancer patients. *Cancer Res* 1998;58:1451.
163. Elledge RM, Fuqua SAW, Clark GM, Pujol P, Allred DC, McGuire WL. Prognostic significance of p53 gene alterations in node-negative breast cancer. *Breast Cancer Res Treat* 1993;26:225.
164. Andrulis I, Bull S, Blackstein M, et al. neu/erbB-2 amplification identifies a poor-prognosis group of women with node-negative breast cancer. *J Clin Oncol* 1998;16:1340.
165. Tandon AK, Clark GM, Chamness GC, Ullrich A, McGuire WL. HER-2/neu oncogene protein and prognosis in breast cancer. *J Clin Oncol* 1989;7:1120.
166. Bolla M, Chedin M, Souvignet C, Marron J, Arnould C, Chambaz E. Estimation of epidermal growth factor receptor in 177 breast cancers: correlation with prognostic factors. *Breast Cancer Res Treat* 1990;16:97.
167. Clark G, McGuire W, Hubay C, Pearson O, Marshall J. Progesterone receptors as a prognostic factor in stage II breast cancer. *N Engl J Med* 1983;309:1343.
168. Huseby R, Ownby H, Brooks S, Russo J, Associates BCPS. Evaluation of the predictive power of progesterone receptor levels in primary breast cancer: a comparison with other criteria in 559 cases with a mean follow-up of 74.8 months. *Henry Ford Hosp Med J* 1990;38:79.
169. Stierer M, Rosen H, Weber R, et al. A prospective analysis of immunohistochemically determined hormone receptors and nuclear features as predictors of early recurrence in primary breast cancer. *Breast Cancer Res Treat* 1995;36:11.
170. Stierer M, Rosen H, Weber R, Hanak H, Spona J, Tuchler H. Immunohistochemical and biochemical measurement of estrogen and progesterone receptors in primary breast cancer. *Ann Surg* 1993;218:13.
171. Allred DC, Bustamante MA, Daniel CO, Gaskill HV, Cruz AB Jr. Immunocytochemical analysis of estrogen receptors in human breast carcinomas. *Arch Surg* 1990;125:107.
172. Molino A, Micciolo R, Turassa M, et al. Prognostic significance of estrogen receptors in 405 primary breast cancers: a comparison of immunohistochemical and biochemical methods. *Breast Cancer Res Treat* 1997;45:241.
173. Remmele W, Hildebrand U, Hienz H, et al. Comparative histological, histochemical, immunohistochemical and biochemical studies on oestrogen receptors, lectin receptors, and Barr bodies in human breast cancer. *Virchows Arch* (*Pathol Anat*) 1986;409:127.
174. Reiner A, Sponza J, Reiner G. Estrogen receptor analysis on biopsies and fine-needle aspirates from breast carcinoma. *Am J Pathol* 1986;125:443.
175. Charpin C, Martin P, De Victor B, et al. Multiparametric study (SAMBA 200) of estrogen receptor immunocytochemical assay in 400 human breast carcinomas: analysis of estrogen receptor distribution heterogeneity in tissues and correlations with dextran coated charcoal assays and morphological data. *Cancer Res* 1988;48:1578.
176. Hanna W, Mobbs B. Comparative evaluation of ER-ICA and enzyme immunoassay for the quantitation of estrogen receptors in breast cancer. *Am J Clin Pathol* 1989;91:182.
177. Helin H, Isola J, Helle M, Koivula T. Discordant results between radioligand and immunohistochemical assays for steroid receptors in breast carcinoma. *Br J Cancer* 1990;62:109.
178. Gasparini G, Pozza F, Dittadi R, Meli S, Cazzavillan S, Bevilacqua P. Progesterone receptor determined by immunocytochemical and biochemical methods in human breast cancer. *J Cancer Res Clin Oncol* 1992;118:557.
179. Reiner A, Neumeister B, Spona J, Reiner G, Schemper M, Jakesz R. Immunocytochemical localization of estrogen and progesterone receptor and prognosis in human primary breast cancer. *Cancer Res* 1990;50:7057.

Diseases of the Breast, 2nd ed.,
edited by Jay R. Harris.
Lippincott Williams & Wilkins, Philadelphia © 2000.

CHAPTER 32

Prognostic and Predictive Factors

Gary M. Clark

The diagnosis of breast cancer presents several dilemmas for the patient and the physician. What type of surgery should be performed? Is radiation therapy necessary? Should additional systemic adjuvant therapy be used? If so, which therapy is best for this particular patient? To address these questions, one must first determine the likelihood that this patient will have a recurrence of the disease in the future if no additional therapy is administered. Then, the efficacy of the available therapies must be estimated and weighed against the potential side effects to determine the probable benefit for this patient. Unfortunately, the clinical course of primary breast cancer varies from patient to patient. Some patients have long disease-free survival times, whereas others experience a rapid deterioration with early recurrence of breast cancer, followed shortly by death. Some of this variability is undoubtedly explained by differences in tumor growth rates, invasiveness, metastatic potential, and other mechanisms that are not yet fully understand. Knowledge of biomarkers that could measure these functions, either directly or indirectly, would obviously be useful so individual patients could be classified into subsets with varying risks of disease recurrence.

Throughout this chapter, the terms *prognostic factor* and *predictive factor* are used. A *prognostic factor* is defined as any measurement available at the time of diagnosis or surgery that is associated with disease-free or overall survival in the absence of systemic adjuvant therapy. Potential prognostic factors include demographic characteristics (e.g., age, menopausal status, ethnicity), tumor characteristics (e.g., lymph node status, tumor size, pathologic subtype), biomarkers that measure or are associated with biological processes purportedly involved in tumor progression (e.g., altered oncogenes, tumor-suppressor genes, growth factors, measures of proliferation), and other factors. Prognostic factors can be used to predict the natural history of the tumor. A *predictive factor* is defined as any measurement associated with response or lack of response to a particular therapy. An example of a predictive factor is the estrogen receptor (ER) status of a tumor, which predicts response to hormonal therapy in the adjuvant setting and in metastatic disease.

This chapter describes the current standard prognostic and predictive factors for primary breast cancer and details several newer markers that are still being evaluated but have the potential for becoming standard factors in the future. Pitfalls to be considered when evaluating these new markers are also described.

HISTORICAL PERSPECTIVE

The role of prognostic factors in optimizing treatment for breast cancer patients has clearly changed with the trend toward general use of systemic adjuvant therapy. Several years ago, patients with axillary node–negative breast cancer were considered to have a relatively good prognosis, and few received adjuvant therapy after local surgery. In 1985, a National Cancer Institute (NCI) consensus development conference concluded that no standard therapy existed for patients with node-negative breast cancer.[1] Some of these patients were destined to have early recurrences of their disease, but despite attempts by several groups to identify subsets of patients at an increased risk of disease recurrence and death using prognostic factors, a consensus could not be reached concerning the identity of such high-risk patients. With the publication of early results from several randomized clinical trials showing a benefit from adjuvant therapy for patients with node-negative breast cancer[2–5] and the publication of the overview analysis by the Early Breast Cancer Trialists' Collaborative Group,[6] however, many clinicians began to adopt the treatment strategy of administering systemic adjuvant therapy to all breast cancer patients regardless of prognostic factors. A subsequent NCI consensus development conference[7] in 1991 recognized that clinical outcomes varied among patients with primary breast cancer, but the panelists generally concluded that, aside from the standard factors of nodal status, tumor size, and histopathologic subtype, none of the newer prognostic factors had been proved to have clinical use. Thus, one might question whether any new prognostic factors for breast cancer are really needed.

G. M. Clark: Breast Care Center, Baylor College of Medicine, Houston, Texas

Today, prognostic or predictive factors are useful in at least three clinical situations.[8] The first is to identify patients whose prognosis is so good after local surgery that the addition of systemic adjuvant therapy would not be cost-effective. The second is to identify patients whose prognosis is so poor with conventional treatment that other forms of more aggressive therapy might be warranted. The third is to ascertain which patients are or are not likely to benefit from specific therapies. As more is learned about the biology of breast tumors, these characteristics might be therapeutic targets for new treatments for patients with breast cancer.

The standard prognostic factors currently applied in cases of primary breast cancer include the following:

- Axillary lymph node status
- Histologic subtype
- Tumor size
- Nuclear or histologic grade
- Estrogen and progesterone receptor status
- Measure of proliferation

Unfortunately, none of these factors, alone or in combination, completely separates patients who are cured by local therapy from those whose cancer is destined to recur and who will die without intervention. Therefore, to accomplish this objective, newer markers that have not yet been fully evaluated must be considered. Special issues of the journal *Breast Cancer Research and Treatment* (1998, vol. 51, no. 3; 1998, vol. 52, nos. 1–3) have been published that describe many new prognostic and predictive factors. Caution must be exercised when interpreting results of published studies that have evaluated potential prognostic and predictive factors. McGuire[9] proposed guidelines for the design and conduct of prognostic factor studies, and Gasparini et al.[10] gave more details on evaluation of these factors. Hayes et al. created a tumor marker use grading system to evaluate the clinical use of tumor markers[11] and described a process for assessing the clinical impact of prognostic factors.[12]

Statistical p values, especially those from univariate analyses, can be misleading, because they depend on the number of patients included in the study and, more importantly, on the number of events. In this chapter, whenever possible, other statistics, including relative risks and absolute survival or recurrence rates, are presented to give the reader some estimates of the magnitude of the effects that have been observed for the various factors. In addition, emphasis is placed on multivariate analyses that at least partially take into account the prognostic significance of established factors and often of newer putative prognostic factors.

HISTOPATHOLOGIC FEATURES

Histologic Type

Infiltrating ductal and infiltrating lobular carcinomas, either in their pure form or in combination with other tumor types, are the most common types of breast cancer. When cells of two or more histologic types are present, the tumor is usually evaluated according to its most malignant-appearing elements, although Fisher et al.[13] have questioned the appropriateness of this practice. Patients with infiltrating ductal tumors generally have a higher incidence of positive axillary lymph nodes and poorer clinical outcomes than patients with the less common types of infiltrating tumors. With increased use of mammography and other screening programs, more and more noninvasive breast tumors are diagnosed. Although these tumors generally portend a favorable clinical outcome, some do recur as invasive carcinomas. Considerable interest exists in identifying prognostic factors for these noninvasive tumors. Because of the low relapse rates and relatively long disease-free survival times, however, large studies must be conducted to address this question, and such studies are currently being performed. The remainder of this chapter focuses on invasive, infiltrating ductal carcinomas.

Axillary Lymph Nodes

The presence or absence of metastatic involvement in the axillary lymph nodes is the most powerful prognostic factor available for patients with primary breast cancer. Although most clinical trials stratify patients into three nodal groups (those with negative nodes, those with one to three positive nodes, and those with four or more positive nodes), several groups have demonstrated a direct relationship between the number of involved nodes and clinical outcome.[14–16] Figure 1 displays disease-free survival time as a function of the number of positive lymph nodes for patients in the San Antonio Database. Although lymph node involvement is associated with larger tumors, it is relatively independent of other biomarkers, including presence of steroid receptors and measures of proliferation; for this reason, the conjecture has been put forward that axillary node status may merely reflect the relative chronologic age of the tumor and that the various biological prognostic factors might influence prognosis through other mechanisms.[17]

Although axillary lymph node dissection provides important prognostic information, debate exists about its therapeutic use for local and regional control. Some studies have found a modest benefit, whereas others have not. Consensus has been reached, however, that not all patients need undergo this procedure. Patients with small, pure, noninvasive ductal carcinoma *in situ* derive little benefit from an axillary dissection because their incidence of axillary involvement is low and their clinical prognosis is good. The value of axillary dissection in patients who present with systemic, metastatic disease is also questionable.

Several investigators have conducted studies to determine whether available prognostic factors could be used to replace axillary dissection in subsets of patients with primary breast cancer.[18–20] Ravdin et al.[20] showed that, in addition to tumor size, other factors—such as the patient's age, S-phase fraction by flow cytometry, and ER concentration—refined the prediction of nodal status from tumor size alone, but they could

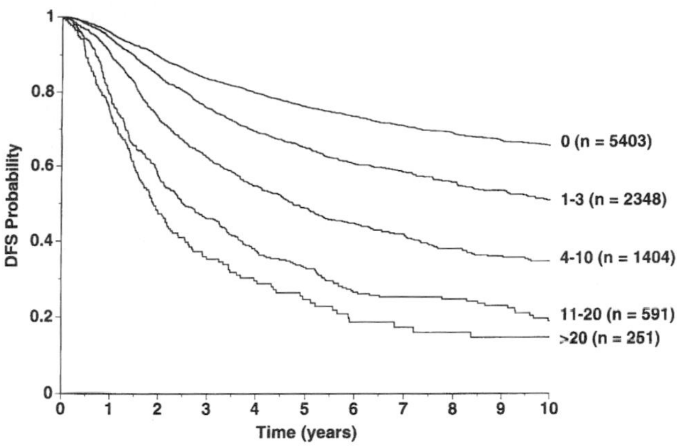

FIG. 1. Disease-free survival (DFS) by number of positive axillary lymph nodes. Data from San Antonio Database; median follow-up, 51 months.

not identify any patient subsets with at least a 95% chance of being node negative or node positive. Possibly, incorporation of some of the newer factors discussed in this chapter might permit the creation of more powerful multivariate prediction models. If ongoing clinical trials of neoadjuvant therapies suggest advantages of systemic therapy before surgery, then information regarding the number of involved lymph nodes and tumor size will no longer be available, and other factors may have to be reexamined to replace the loss of prognostic information provided by these two powerful factors.

Another area of considerable interest is the identification of micrometastases in bone marrow and evaluation of their prognostic significance. A meta-analysis of 20 published studies, which included 2,494 patients, concluded that micrometastases are not yet proven to contribute independent prognostic information for patients with breast cancer.[21] Braun and Pantel[22] do not disagree with this conclusion but argue that concerted international activities, not meta-analyses, are required to develop standardized procedures to address the question of the clinical significance of micrometastases in bone marrow.

Standard practice is to administer systemic adjuvant therapy to all patients with node-positive breast cancer unless otherwise contraindicated. Thus, little need exists for new prognostic factors for this subset of patients. Indeed, evaluation of new markers prospectively in untreated node-positive patients is nearly impossible. Therefore, this chapter concentrates on prognostic factors for patients with node-negative breast cancer. A great need remains to identify new predictive markers for all patients with primary breast cancer, however, and this discussion includes predictive factors for both node-negative and node-positive patients.

Tumor Size

Within the subset of patients with node-negative breast cancer, tumor size is the most powerful and consistent predictor of breast cancer recurrence. Several large studies have examined the relationship between tumor size and clinical outcome.[23–31] Disease recurrence generally increases as the tumor size increases, but some studies have found that patients with extremely large tumors tend to have better outcomes than those with tumors of intermediate size.[25] One might hypothesize that tumors that have grown to a large size without killing the patient or resulting in nodal involvement might have a lower potential for metastatic spread. Data from the San Antonio Data Base, however, suggest a plateau in the risk of recurrence for tumors between 3 and 6 cm in diameter, and a significant decrease in disease-free survival for node-negative patients with tumors larger than 6 cm (Table 1).

TABLE 1. *Actuarial 5-year disease-free survival by tumor size for node-negative patients*

Tumor size (cm)	*n*	5-yr disease-free survival (%± standard deviation)
1–2	2,014	79±1
2–3	1,162	77±1
3–4	536	72±2
4–5	276	74±3
5–6	134	72±5
>6	144	57±5

Data from San Antonio Database; median follow-up, 3.8 years.

McGuire and Clark[32] suggested that tumor size and histopathologic subtype might be used to make treatment decisions for up to 50% of all node-negative patients. Table 2 outlines criteria for adjuvant therapy in node negative breast cancer, including tumor size. Data from Memorial Sloan-Kettering Cancer Center indicate that patients with tumors smaller than 1 cm in diameter have a 20-year relapse rate of only 12%.[30,31] A study from the National Surgical Adjuvant Breast and Bowel Project (NSABP), however, reported a 25% recurrence rate among untreated node-negative patients with ER-negative tumors.[33] These results underscore the necessity to examine several factors before estimating disease recurrence probabilities for individual patients.

Although retrospective studies consistently confirm the excellent prognosis of patients with tumors smaller than 1 cm

TABLE 2. *Frequency of adjuvant therapy in node-negative breast cancer, according to various criteria*

Variable	Adjuvant therapy		
	Unlikely[a]	Possible	Probable
Percentage of patients	25	50	25
Patients per year	30,500	61,000	30,500
Tumor size (cm)	<1	1–3	>3
Eventual recurrence rate (%)	1–10	~30	>50
Patients receiving adjuvant therapy	Few	Unknown	Most or all

[a]Therapy is also unlikely if the tumor is ductal carcinoma *in situ*, pure tubular, papillary, or typical medullary.
From ref. 32, with permission.

in diameter, the increased use of mammography and other early detection systems has already changed the distribution of tumor sizes at diagnosis. Whether a 1-cm tumor detected mammographically has the same natural history as a 1-cm tumor detected on physical examination is unclear. Some of the small tumors detected by early screening intrinsically may have high proliferative capacity and metastatic potential, and other factors may have to be measured before the prognostic significance of small tumor size can be determined.

Tumor Grade

Tumor grade is a standard component of the pathology report, and several investigators have proposed that it is a powerful predictor of the course of a breast cancer. Indeed, when tumor grading is performed at single institutions by trained pathologists, most grading systems do correlate well with clinical outcomes. The primary difficulties with tumor grading are poor reproducibility and lack of agreement among different observers.[34–38] Some grading systems use only nuclear features and produce a nuclear grade. Others combine nuclear features with assessments of the architecture of the tumor and report a histologic grade. The most widely used grading systems for breast cancer are the Scarff-Bloom-Richardson (SBR) classification[39,40] and Fisher's nuclear grading system,[41] although both systems are frequently used in modified versions.

The SBR grading system consists of three components (degree of differentiation, extent of pleomorphism, and mitotic index), each scored on a scale from 1 to 3. The *degree of differentiation* is evaluated according to the ability of the tumor to form tubular, glandular, or papillary formations. *Pleomorphism* describes the shape of the nuclei, with particular attention to irregular cells distorted in size. The *mitotic index* evaluates the number of mitoses found in the tumor specimen. The scores for the three components are summed and categorized as grade 1 (well differentiated), grade 2 (moderately differentiated), or grade 3 (poorly differentiated). A modified SBR (MSBR) system considers only the extent of pleomorphism and the mitotic index, and rearranges the scoring system to yield five classifications of nuclear grade.[42]

Fisher's grading system includes a combined assessment of nuclear grade and the presence of tubule or gland formation. Nuclear grade considers nuclear size, shape, nucleolar content, chromatin pattern, and mitotic rate. Although histologic grading is only applicable to the invasive component of ductal carcinomas, the nuclear grade can be determined on all components of all histologic types of breast cancer.

Many published studies demonstrate the prognostic significance of individual grading systems.[42–52] Despite these observations, the Surveillance, Epidemiology, and End Results (SEER) Program of the NCI reported that only 25.1% of breast tumors in the SEER registry were graded.[53] Even though several different types of grading systems were used, survival analyses of the 29,642 patients in the SEER registry with graded tumors revealed that, within each stage of disease, grade provided additional prognostic information.

A standardized grading system likely could be one of the most powerful prognostic factors for breast cancer. Reproducibility of breast cancer grading probably can be achieved using grading schemes with specific guidelines.[38]

Other Histologic Factors

Several other histologic factors, including the presence of an extensive intraductal component, lymphatic vessel invasion, tumor necrosis, and mononuclear inflammatory cell reaction, have been associated with clinical outcome in one or more studies. A biological hypothesis supports the use of each of these factors, but no factor has yet been fully validated as prognostic or predictive.

PATIENT CHARACTERISTICS

Age at Diagnosis

The influence of age and menopausal status at diagnosis on the prognosis of patients with primary breast cancer remains controversial. Some studies have found that younger patients have worse clinical outcomes than older patients.[54–63] Others have reported that younger patients have a more favorable outcome.[64–67] Still others have found no relation between outcome and age.[68–70] Explanations for these conflicting results have included small numbers of patients in the studies, differences in patient selection, and differences in the age groupings used in the analyses.

Two large studies carefully analyzed the clinical outcomes of young patients with breast cancer.[62,63] Both concluded that breast cancer patients younger than 35 years of age have a worse prognosis than older patients. Nixon et al.[62] found highly significant trends for the prevalence of poor prognostic features (grade 3 histology, extensive intraductal component, lymphatic vessel invasion, necrosis, mononuclear inflammatory cell reaction) to decrease with increasing age. Albain et al.[63] also observed increases in lymph node involvement, tumor size, steroid receptor negativity, S-phase fractions, and p53 abnormalities in patients younger than 30 to 35 years. Multivariate analyses were performed in each study, and both concluded that young age remained a significant predictor of recurrence and death after adjustment for other prognostic factors. This might suggest that breast cancer in some young women is biologically different from breast cancer in older women. The identification of the *BRCA1* and *BRCA2* genes implicated in some forms of familial breast cancer may help to establish the biological basis of the disease in relation to age at diagnosis.[71–73]

At the other end of the age spectrum, controversy also exists about the appropriate therapy for older women with breast cancer. The meta-analysis by the Early Breast Cancer

Trialists' Collaborative Group provided some guidance on the efficacy of hormonal therapy and chemotherapy within menopausal groups.[6] In older, postmenopausal women, use of tamoxifen (tamoxifen citrate) significantly decreased mortality, and the magnitude of the effect generally grew with increasing concentrations of ER in the tumor. Chemotherapy is much less effective than tamoxifen treatment in this age group. Because of the effectiveness of tamoxifen and its relatively few side effects, some physicians have questioned whether it could be used as primary treatment with only minimal local and regional therapy in elderly breast cancer patients. Rubens[74] summarized the results of a series of studies that addressed this issue and described several disadvantages of this approach, including increased rates of local recurrence, the need for frequent monitoring, and the possibility that patients may not be fit for surgery or that the tumor may have become inoperable. He concluded that, irrespective of age, the treatment of breast cancer should be designed to give the best chance of both local and distant control of the disease in the long term.

Ethnicity

Survival after the diagnosis of breast cancer is poorer among African-American and Hispanic women than among white women.[75–80] Minorities tend to present with higher-stage or more advanced disease. An analysis of more than 100,000 women in the SEER program found significant increases in the incidence of early-stage breast cancers between 1983 and 1989.[81] Although increases were observed for both white and African-American women, African-American women had substantially lower rates of the least extensive breast cancers; this finding led the investigators to conclude that a major explanation for the increase might be the increased prevalence of breast cancer screening among women in the United States. Other researchers found, however, that even after adjusting for stage of disease, survival rates were lower for African-Americans[82,83] but not for Hispanics.[79] Differences in treatment might account for a portion of the poorer survival, but evidence indicates that African-American patients who receive the same or similar therapy still have a worse outcome.[82] Other factors, such as the lower socioeconomic status of minority women, are also associated with a worse prognosis; however, the precise cause of this association is unknown.[84,85] A delay in diagnosis related to lack of access to medical care or to cultural beliefs about cancer might contribute to a worse survival, but at least one study found no clinically significant interval between symptom recognition and medical consultation among African-Americans as compared with whites.[86]

Elledge et al.[80] compared several prognostic factors among 4,885 white, 1,016 African-American, and 777 Hispanic women. White women were older, presented with smaller tumors, had less lymph node involvement, had higher incidences of steroid receptor positivity, and had lower S-phase fractions than Hispanic or African-American women. No clinically important differences in DNA ploidy, histologic type, and HER-2/neu and p53 expression were found among the three groups. After adjustment for these poor prognostic factors, no significant differences were seen in disease-free survival or overall survival for node-negative patients, although African-Americans tended to have a worse prognosis. For node-positive or locally advanced disease and for metastatic disease, however, African-Americans had significantly worse disease-free and overall survival times than white or Hispanic women.

MEASURES OF PROLIFERATION

Growth fraction, or proliferative capacity, is important in the evolution of breast cancer. This has led many investigators to develop new techniques for evaluating potential markers of tumor cell proliferation that are expressed in various phases of the cell cycle (Table 3). Mitotic index (MI) has been an important component of all histologic grading systems. Newer methods, such as the thymidine-labeling index (TLI) and bromodeoxyuridine assay, have been applied to fresh breast cancer tissue, and flow cytometry has been used to determine the fraction of cells in various phases of the cell cycle in fresh, frozen, and paraffin-embedded tumor specimens. Several antibodies now available recognize specific cell cycle–associated antigens.

Rather than measure cell proliferation directly, many investigators have evaluated factors that may regulate cell proliferation. One such factor is the p53 tumor-suppressor gene, described in more detail later in this chapter in the section Tumor-Suppressor Genes. Studies designed to evaluate its prognostic significance have also demonstrated a strong relationship between expression of aberrant p53 protein and tumor proliferation rates. *In vitro* experiments have now demonstrated that other markers, such as p21 and p16, are positively regulated by p53. Cell proliferation during various phases of the cell cycle appears to be controlled by a series of multiprotein complexes that involve several cyclin-dependent kinases, p21, p16, D-type cyclins, and other factors, including the

TABLE 3. *Measures of proliferation*

Marker	G_0	G_1	S	G_2	M
Mitotic index	–	–	–	–	+
Thymidine labeling—BRdU	–	–	+	+	+
S-phase fraction	–	–	+	–	–
Ki67/MIB1	–	±	+	+	+
Mitosin	–	–	–	±	+
Histones (H2, H3)	–	–	+	±	–
Topoisomerase II	–	–	±	+	+
DNA polymerases (α, δ)	–	±	+	+	±
Cyclins (PCNA, A, D, E)	–	±	+	±	±

BRdU, bromodeoxyuridine; PCNA, proliferating cell nuclear antigen.

TABLE 4. *Technical considerations in the measurement of proliferation*

Method	Markers	Advantages	Disadvantages
Flow cytometry	S-phase	Specific for S-phase Quickly analyzes large numbers of cells	Expensive Admixture of stromal elements Variable reproducibility
Autoradiography	TLI BRdU	Specific for S+G_2M	Viable tissue required Exposure to radioactivity Slow
IHC frozen	Ki67	Requires only one slide Sensitive Specific for S+G_2M in tumor cells	Logistics (difficult shipping, handling, storage) Tedious scoring How to score?
IHC permanent	MIB1	Requires only one slide Specific for S+G_2M in tumor cells Logistics (easy shipping, handling, storage)	Variable immunostaining sensitivity Tedious scoring How to score?

BRdU, bromodeoxyuridine; IHC, immunohistochemical analysis; TLI, thymidine-labeling index.

retinoblastoma protein. Classic prognostic factor studies can be used to help elucidate some of these complex pathways.

One of the criticisms of measures of proliferation is the lack of standardization of the various methods. For some markers, multiple antibodies are available, each with its own sensitivity and specificity. In addition, different techniques, such as immunohistochemical analysis (IHC), immunoblotting, and measurement of enzymatic activity, have been used. Table 4 presents some technical considerations for some of these techniques. IHC can reliably be performed on small amounts of archival material. This becomes increasingly important as smaller and smaller tumors are diagnosed by mammography or other early detection methods. IHC has several disadvantages, however, including variability in the fixation of the tissue, which can lead to differences in staining, and the subjectivity of the interpretation of the staining. Table 5 lists some of the advantages and disadvantages of various scoring systems that have been used to measure tumor proliferation by IHC.

Mitotic Index

The MI is determined by using light microscopy on paraffin-embedded tumor specimens stained with hematoxylin and eosin to count mitotic figures. It has been described as the oldest, easiest, fastest, and cheapest way of assessing proliferation.[87] Mitotic activity is usually expressed as the number of mitoses per high-power field; however, other scoring systems have been suggested, such as relating the number of mitoses to tumor cellularity, tumor volume index, and area in square millimeters. Each of these systems has been correlated with clinical outcome, at least in univariate analyses. Expressing mitotic activity as the number of mitoses divided by the number of cancer cells eliminates variability in the size of high-power fields from one microscope to another, variation in tumor cellularity, and variation in tumor size. Reproducibility of the MI was demonstrated in the Multicenter Morphometric Mammary Carcinoma Project,[88] which included 14 pathology laboratories throughout the Netherlands. Correlation coefficients between 0.81 and 0.96 were obtained on tissue specimens from 2,469 patients with invasive breast cancer.

TABLE 5. *Immunohistochemical scoring systems*

Method	Advantages	Disadvantages
Absolute counting (light microscopy)	Sensitivity Specificity Reproducibility	Extreme slowness
Point counting (light microscopy)	Sensitivity Specificity	Slowness Variable reproducibility
Semiquantitative (light microscopy)	Sensitivity Specificity Speed	Variable reproducibility
Image analysis (computer)	Sensitivity	Slowness Variable specificity Variable reproducibility

Only a few studies have included the MI in multivariate analyses of clinical outcome and have reported multivariate relative risks. Russo et al.[89] reported relative risks of 1.59 and 2.12 for disease recurrence and death, respectively, for patients with higher mitotic grades. Clayton[90] found that patients with more than 4.5 mitotic figures per 10 high-power fields had a 2.8-fold increased risk of death in multivariate analyses. Aaltomaa et al.[91] found that volume-corrected MI is a more powerful predictor of clinical outcome than uncorrected MI. The MI, in combination with other histopathologic features, is a component of several prognostic indices. For example, both the Nottingham Prognostic Index[92] and the Multivariate Prognostic Index of Baak et al.[93] combine the MI with lymph node status and tumor size. Both indices have been shown to have more powerful prognostic value than any of the individual components.

Thymidine-Labeling Index

The TLI is determined autoradiographically by counting the number of labeled nuclei on autoradiographed microsec-

TABLE 6. *Prognostic significance of thymidine-labeling index (TLI) in node-negative patients*

Study	*n*	Follow-up (mo)	Cutoff point	High TLI (%)	Univariate *p* value		Multivariate *p* value	
					DFS	OS	DFS	OS
Héry et al.[95]	76	74	1.14	50	.02	<.001	—	—
Meyer and Province[96a]	148	49	3.0/8.0	67/33	.001	.001	—	—
Silvestrini et al.[97]	354	62	2.8	48	<.0001	.0005	.0009	.0098
Tubiana et al.[98a]	125	>180	0.25/3.84	67/17	<.01	<.01	.01	<.05
Courdi et al.[99]	167	—	2.14	50	.01	—	.37	—
Cooke et al.[100]	185	>93	7.25	50	.11	—	NS	—
Silvestrini et al.[101]	340	48	2.8	?	.00	—	.009	—

DFS, disease-free survival; NS, not significant; OS, overall survival.
[a]Used two cutoff points that produced three subsets of patients.

tions after incubation of the tumor specimen with tritiated thymidine. The TLI is independent of extent of disease at the time of diagnosis, axillary involvement, and tumor size but is inversely correlated with steroid receptor levels.[94–101] Silvestrini[94] reviewed the clinical use of cell kinetics, with particular emphasis on the TLI in node-negative patients. Most of the studies cited found an advantage in relapse-free survival for patients with slowly proliferating tumors. Table 6 presents an updated list of correlative studies in node-negative breast cancer. The relative risk of relapse based on multivariate analyses reported in these studies is approximately 2.

As with any new assay, methodologic standardization and reproducibility of results have been criticisms of the TLI. Initially, the requirement for fresh tumor material was a limitation of the technique. The availability of a kit for *in vitro* incubation with tritiated thymidine and histologic fixation of solid tumor specimens has contributed to the methodologic simplification and standardization of the technical procedure, however.[102] In addition, Silvestrini et al. have conducted quality-control studies throughout Italy. Despite the need for relatively labor-intensive counting of labeled nuclei on autoradiographed microsections, correlation coefficients ranging from 0.78 to 0.99 within and among laboratories have been reported.[94]

The role of the TLI as a predictive factor is being evaluated. Zambetti et al.[103] used the TLI as a stratification factor in a randomized clinical trial of high-risk node-negative patients. One might hypothesize that adjuvant chemotherapy would be more effective against tumors with a high TLI; however, a benefit from adjuvant therapy with cyclophosphamide, methotrexate (methotrexate sodium), and 5-fluorouracil (CMF therapy) was observed in all subgroups. In another study of cytoreductive chemotherapy before surgery in patients with locally advanced breast cancer, no correlation was noted between pretreatment TLI and objective clinical response, which was inversely related to posttreatment cell kinetics.[104] Amadori et al.[105] have reported a fourfold increase in response rate in women with highly proliferating metastatic breast cancer compared with those with tumors with a low TLI. Thus, the role of the TLI as a predictive factor remains to be determined.

S-Phase Fraction by Flow Cytometry

DNA flow cytometry can be performed on fresh tissue specimens, frozen biopsy samples, needle aspirates taken directly from the tumor, or paraffin-embedded tissues. This technique produces a DNA histogram from which a measure of DNA content (DNA ploidy) and cell cycle components can be estimated. Traditionally, the cell populations are classified into three cell cycle compartments. Theoretically, the G_0-G_1 compartment consists of normal nondividing (G_0) or quiescent cells (G_1); the S-phase fraction is composed of cells undergoing replication or cell synthesis; and the G_2-M compartment includes cells in the postsynthetic phase (G_2) and cells in mitosis (M).

A strong correlation exists between high S-phase fraction and other prognostic factors, including poor histologic or cytologic grade. Wenger et al.[106] reported correlations among S-phase fractions, DNA ploidy, and steroid receptor status in more than 127,000 patients with breast cancer. They also found correlations with the number of positive lymph nodes, tumor size, and age of the patient (Table 7).

The clinical use of DNA cytometry in carcinoma of the breast was the topic of a consensus conference that reviewed 43 published papers.[107] Despite the lack of standardized methods and suboptimal measurement of S-phase fraction, that literature clearly supported an association between high S-phase fraction and increased risk of recurrence and mortality for patients with both node-negative and node-positive invasive breast cancer. The investigators noted that S-phase fraction is a continuous biological variable, rather than a dichotomous function, and each laboratory must validate the prognostic significance of its own S-phase values. At a minimum, each laboratory should establish its own distribution of S-phase values and interpret individual results in the context of these distributions rather than by comparison with published cutoff points established by other laboratories. The optimal separation of patients into different risk groups by S-phase fraction has not been established, but the use of three rather than two risk groups may lessen the chance of misclassifying tumors with near-borderline values.

TABLE 7. *Correlation of S-phase fraction with other prognostic factors*

	Diploid and near-diploid tumors		Aneuploid tumors	
	n	Median S-phase fraction	*n*	Median S-phase fraction
Steroid receptors				
ER+/PR+	37,173	3.1	23,289	6.5
ER+/PR–	14,107	3.7	12,492	11.4
ER–/PR+	1,712	3.9	1,756	13.0
ER–/PR–	6,175	5.1	9,560	15.3
Positive nodes				
0	6,611	3.2	4,686	10.0
1–3	2,043	3.8	1,898	10.7
4–10	927	4.0	1,076	10.8
>10	475	4.4	583	11.6
Tumor size (cm)				
≤1	1,734	3.1	827	8.1
1–2	4,448	3.2	3,159	9.7
2–5	3,640	3.8	3,990	11.2
>5	531	3.9	614	12.2
Age (yr)				
<35	280	4.9	305	14.4
35–65	5,864	3.6	5,260	11.4
>65	5,248	3.2	3,631	8.8

ER, estrogen receptor; PR, progesterone receptor.
Adapted from ref. 106.

Wenger and Clark[108] reviewed a decade of experience with S-phase fraction determined by flow cytometry. They concluded that it does have clinical use in evaluating patients with breast cancer, but that standardization and quality control must be improved before it can be routinely used in community settings.

Herman et al.[109] reviewed some of the limitations of single-parameter DNA flow cytometry. A major limitation is the variable admixture of stromal elements in clinical samples. This produces DNA histograms that are composites of normal and malignant cells. This problem is greatest with DNA diploid tumors when, because of complete overlap between the two populations, the measured S-phase fraction is highly dependent on the percentage of normal host cells in the sample, in addition to the proliferation kinetics of the tumor cells. Combined staining with fluorescein-labeled anticytokeratin antibodies allows the DNA content of epithelial cells to be separated from that of other elements. Although definitive studies have not yet been published, this will probably further improve the prognostic significance of the S-phase fraction in breast cancer.

One is tempted to conclude that cell cycle–specific cytotoxic agents might work best against tumors with high S-phase fractions. Indeed, Remvikos et al.[110] noted that tumor responsiveness to neoadjuvant chemotherapy was directly related to S-phase fractions in 50 premenopausal women. In studies of adjuvant therapies, however, S-phase fractions have not been predictive of response to chemotherapy. Dressler et al.[111] performed flow cytometry on tumor specimens from node-negative patients enrolled in a large randomized Intergroup study comparing CMF therapy and observation. The chemotherapy was equally effective for patients with low and high S-phase fractions. Muss et al.[112] evaluated S-phase fractions on tumors from node-positive patients enrolled in a Cancer and Leukemia Group B study designed to study dose intensification of cyclophosphamide, doxorubicin [doxorubicin hydrochloride (adriamycin)], and 5-fluorouracil (CAF). Although the dose-intensity hypothesis was confirmed in this study, S-phase fraction did not predict response to therapy either alone or in combination with other predictive factors. An Intergroup study of patients with node-negative breast cancer used S-phase fraction as a stratification factor. Patients with high S-phase fractions were randomized to receive CMF or CAF therapy. This study will help to establish whether S-phase fraction is indeed a predictive factor for these patients. Additional retrospective and prospective clinical trials with well-defined treatment regimens that also measure S-phase fraction will be required to address this issue.

Ki67 Staining

Ki67 is a monoclonal antibody developed by Gerdes et al.[113] that is specific for a nuclear antigen expressed only in proliferating cells (late G_1, S, M, and G_2 phases of the cell cycle). This antibody can be used with fresh or frozen sections of breast tissue and can be detected by a rapid IHC assay. Newer antibodies, polyclonal Ki67 and MIB1, have been raised against peptides from recombinant fragments of the gene for the Ki67 antigen and are effective in fixed, archival sections after microwave irradiation.[114,115] Ki67 staining correlates directly with tumor size, histologic grade, vascular invasion, and axillary lymph node status and inversely with the presence of steroid receptors.[116–119] High levels of Ki67 correlate well with the TLI[120–122] but poorly with high levels of proliferating cell nuclear antigen (PCNA).[123–126] Strong correlations with S-phase fraction have been reported by some investigators[127,128] but not by others.[129–131]

Several studies investigated the prognostic significance of Ki67 staining, and most found a correlation with clinical outcome in univariate analyses.[94,125,130,132–140] Most studies had relatively few patients and were composed of heterogeneous groups of node-negative and node-positive patients who received a variety of treatments and had short follow-up intervals. Table 8 presents the results of studies that either focused on node-negative patients or reported a subset analysis within this group of patients. Although few studies reported relative risks of disease recurrence or death, inspection of the survival curves presented suggests that the increased risk of disease recurrence in patients with high Ki67 levels may be in the same range as for patients with a high TLI or increased S-phase fraction. Additional studies with multivariate analyses are needed to define the role of Ki67 as a prognostic factor.

TABLE 8. *Prognostic significance of high Ki67 in node-negative patients*

Study	*n*	Follow-up (mo)	Cutoff point	High Ki67 (%)	Univariate *p* value		Multivariate *p* value	
					DFS	OS	DFS	OS
Brown et al.[130]	673	52	7	21	.005	NS	<.05	NS
Bouzubar et al.[132]	77	88	4/13	71/33	<.01	—	—	—
Weikel et al.[133]	76	24	10/20	76/45	<.01	—	—	—
Sahin et al.[135]	42	20	20	25	.01	—	—	—
Veronese et al.[138]	71	42	20	25	.01	—	—	—
Gaglia et al.[140]	197	31	9	50	.01	—	—	—

DFS, disease-free survival; NS, not significant; OS, overall survival.

Proliferating Cell Nuclear Antigen

PCNA is a nuclear protein associated with DNA polymerase α, which is present throughout the cell cycle in proliferating cells. The monoclonal antibody PC10 recognizes an epitope of human PCNA in fixed breast cancer tissue. Most studies have found only weak correlations with other prognostic factors,[94,141–144] and associations with clinical outcomes have been disappointingly poor, especially in node-negative patients.

Comparison of Measures of Proliferation

Relatively few studies have compared different measures of proliferation in head-to-head prognostic studies. Rose et al.[145] compared five antibodies for IHC assessment of growth fraction in formalin-fixed, paraffin-embedded tissues (MIB1, polyclonal Ki67, monoclonal Ki67, PC10, JC1). Based on evaluations of the staining performance of the different antibodies, these researchers concluded that MIB1 and polyclonal Ki67 are the best proliferation markers in conventional histologic preparations and that the other markers could not be recommended for routine use. Gasparini et al.[125] directly compared the prognostic significance of S-phase fraction, Ki67 level, and PCNA level in a series of 168 breast cancer patients and concluded that S-phase fraction was the strongest prognostic factor. Neither Ki67 nor PCNA was an independent prognosticator in their study. Similar results have been published by other investigators.[126,131] Brown et al.[130] reported that S-phase fraction and Ki67 staining are significant predictors of disease recurrence, and they can be combined in a complex manner, depending on tumor size, to provide additional prognostic information. Clark et al.[146] compared S-phase fraction and level of mitosin, a new proliferation marker that is expressed in the late G_1, S, G_2, and M phases of the cell cycle but not in G_0; mitosin was found to be a better predictor of disease-free survival in multivariate analyses. They cautioned, however, that these results were preliminary and that additional studies would be necessary to validate these findings.

STEROID RECEPTORS AND ESTROGEN-REGULATED FACTORS

Estrogen and Progesterone Receptors

Steroid receptor status determined by ligand-binding assays has been used to make treatment decisions for patients with advanced breast cancer for many years. The first report on the prognostic significance of the ER was published in 1977.[147] Although conflicting results have appeared in the literature, the larger studies with longer follow-up have consistently demonstrated that patients with ER-positive tumors have longer disease-free intervals than patients with ER-negative tumors. Data from San Antonio and the NSABP indicate that the disease-free survival advantage is approximately 10% at 5 years.[148] The additional knowledge gained by measuring progesterone receptors (PRs) in patients with node-negative disease is not clear. Theoretically, the presence of PR is an indicator of an intact estrogen-response pathway, because it is produced by estrogen stimulation.[149] In multivariate analyses of node-negative patients, however, either ER status or PR status, but seldom both, is a significant predictor of clinical outcome. Often, ER status is a stronger predictor of disease-free survival, whereas PR status is more closely associated with overall survival, perhaps because it is a better indicator of response to endocrine therapy after disease recurrence.

Some studies have reported that disease-free survival curves tend to merge with longer follow-up,[150,151] which suggests that ER status is a reflection of proliferative capacity rather than metastatic potential. Figure 2 demonstrates a similar phenomenon for both ER and PR in untreated, node-negative patients from the San Antonio Data Base. ER and PR levels are strongly inversely correlated with measures of proliferation,[94,106] and they are directly related to histologic grade. ER concentrations increase almost linearly with increasing age, whereas PR levels depend more on menopausal status.[152]

A large Danish study of 952 untreated postmenopausal women with breast cancer found an unusual relationship between ER levels and clinical outcome.[153] Patients with extremely high ER levels had as poor a prognosis as ER-

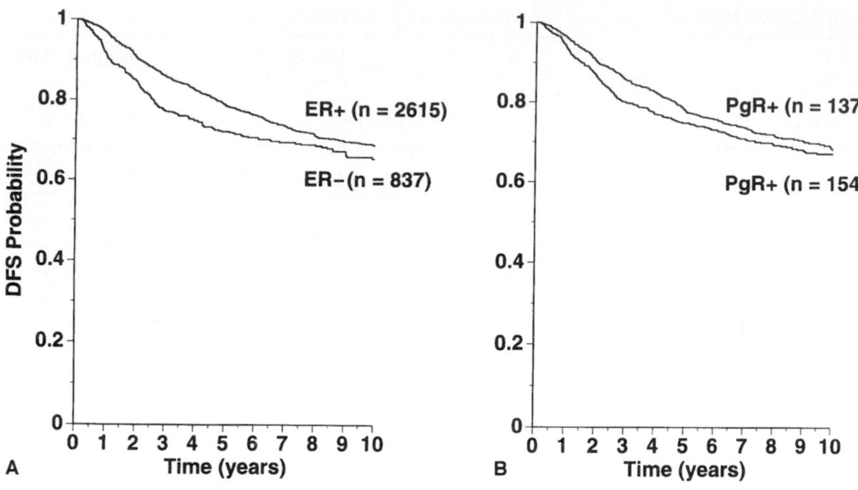

FIG. 2. Disease-free survival (DFS) by estrogen receptor (ER) **(A)** and progesterone receptor (PgR) **(B)** status. Data from San Antonio Data Base; median follow-up, 62 months. Relative risks of recurrence were the following (95% confidence intervals are given in parentheses): for negative ERs, 1.31 (1.12 to 1.53), p = .0008; for negative PgRs, 1.17 (1.00 to 1.37), p = .04.

negative patients, whereas patients with intermediate ER levels had the longest disease-free intervals. The investigators hypothesized that overexpression of ER might signify the progression of the tumor from a fully hormone-dependent to a hormone-independent state via a hormone-responsive state. Although patients with extremely high ER levels have poor disease-free survival if they do not receive adjuvant therapy, this group derives the greatest benefit from adjuvant treatment with hormonal therapies.

Because of the decreasing size of newly diagnosed breast cancers and the inability of biochemical assays to assess intratumoral heterogeneity, histochemical techniques have been proposed for determining steroid receptor levels. Despite the growing popularity of histochemical assays, few comparative studies have been performed. Kinsel et al.[154] reported a correlation of 0.63 between biochemical and histochemical ER levels in a series of 257 breast cancer patients. ER level as measured by both techniques correlated with disease-free and overall survival, but only the immunochemical values remained significant after 5 years of follow-up. Berger et al.[155] reported a correlation of 0.78 between PR levels determined by biochemical and immunocytochemical techniques, but they did not assess the prognostic significance of PR levels measured by either assay. Foekens et al.[156] compared ER and PR levels as determined by biochemical and enzyme immunoassay in 205 patients and reported correlations of 0.94 and 0.88, respectively, for ER and PR when the assays were performed on the same cytosols. Survival analyses showed that both methods were equally useful for predicting disease-free and overall survival. A limitation of this study is that the cutoffs used to define assay positivity were derived from the same data used to compare the assays. Andersen et al.[157] compared biochemical ER values with IHC assays on frozen and paraffin-embedded tissue from 130 postmenopausal high-risk breast cancer patients with a median follow-up of 75 months. The biochemical assay was slightly more sensitive (80% positive) than the IHC assay on frozen tissue (73% positive), which was more sensitive than the assay on paraffin-embedded tissue (60% positive). Correlations among the three assays ranged from 0.61 to 0.85. The relative risks of relapse for patients with ER-negative tumors determined by biochemical assay, IHC assay on frozen section, and IHC assay on paraffin-embedded tissue were 3.12, 2.90, and 1.94, respectively.

The cutoffs used to define ER positivity depend on the objective of the assay. If the intent is to identify patients who are likely to benefit from hormonal therapy, then high cutoffs that result in lower percentages of ER-positive patients would be preferred. On the other hand, if the intent is to identify patients who do not benefit from hormonal therapy, then lower cutoffs might be optimal. Indeed, Harvey et al.[158] demonstrated that patients whose tumors show as few as 1% of tumor cells expressing ER benefit from adjuvant endocrine therapy. The general tendency for IHC assays to be less sensitive than biochemical assays suggests that they might be more useful as predictive factors for response to endocrine therapies than as markers of resistance. Additional studies with standardized methods and definitions of receptor positivity are needed to adequately address this question.

pS2

The pS2 gene was first identified in a human breast cancer cell line in response to estrogen stimulation.[159] The pS2 protein is a small (6,450 kd), secreted protein of unknown function. The gene has been cloned and isolated to 21q. Sequencing has revealed homologies with a porcine pancreatic protein known to inhibit gastrointestinal mobility and secretion[160] and with human insulinlike growth factors I and II.[161] Investigators have suggested that pS2 expression could reflect the functional status of the ER, and it might be both a prognostic factor and predictive factor in primary breast cancer.[162]

Several studies have demonstrated strong associations between pS2 concentrations in human breast tumors and ER and PR status. Most studies have found no significant relation with nodal status or tumor size, however.

An initial study by Foekens et al.[162] found that patients whose tumors expressed high levels of pS2 as determined by radioimmunoassay had significantly better disease-free and overall survival in both univariate and multivariate analyses. When a data-derived cutoff point was used, 27% of patients were classified as pS2 positive. Subsequent studies by the same group, however, found that the prognostic significance disappeared when newer cytosolic factors, including cathepsin D, urokinase-type plasminogen activator (uPA), and plasminogen activator inhibitor 1 (PAI-1) were measured simultaneously. Other studies using radioimmunoassays have produced conflicting results. Predine et al.[163] reported increased risks of relapse (relative risk, 1.80) and death (relative risk, 2.56) for patients whose tumors had absent or low pS2 concentrations (15% of all patients). Attempts to validate the higher cutoff point used by Foekens et al.[162] failed to achieve statistical significance. A study by Gion et al.[164] did find strong prognostic significance for both disease-free and overall survival, however; a study by Spyratos et al.[165] reported that pS2 positivity was associated with longer overall survival, particularly in patients who received hormone therapy, but was not related to disease-free survival.

Four studies determined pS2 status by IHC techniques.[166–169] Even though similar rates of pS2 positivity were observed compared with studies using radioimmunoassays, none of these studies found associations between pS2 status and clinical outcome. In some studies, trends were found for better overall survival for pS2-positive patients, findings suggesting that these patients might be responding to hormonal therapy after disease recurrence. Investigators have hypothesized that expression of pS2 is not related to the ability of breast tumors to recur or to form metastases but rather to the aggressiveness of recurrences and metastases, perhaps through their stage of differentiation.[165]

Measurement of pS2 status is probably most useful as a predictor of response to hormone therapy for both primary and advanced breast cancer, especially when used in concert with ER and PR status.

Heat Shock Proteins

Heat shock proteins (HSPs) are produced in response to environmental stresses (e.g., exposure to heat, heavy metals, or oxidants) and physiologic stresses (e.g., viral and microbial infections, inflammation, ischemia, exposure to certain antineoplastic agents).[170] Several different HSPs are normally expressed in cells and are differentially expressed or regulated during the cell cycle by hormones at different stages of development and differentiation. Members of the HSP family are usually identified by their molecular weights (e.g., HSP27, HSP60, HSP70, HSP90, HSP100).

Initial studies by Chamness et al.[171] and Tandon et al.[172] suggested that HSP27, HSP70, and HSP90 might be prognostic factors, especially for time to recurrence for node-negative breast cancer patients. A follow-up study by Ciocca et al.,[173] however, which attempted to confirm the original findings in 345 node-negative patients, was unable to do so for HSP27 and HSP90. Nonetheless, HSP70 status continued to be an independent predictor of disease recurrence in multivariate analyses.

Thor et al.[174] found striking associations between HSP27 overexpression and ER content, nodal metastases, large tumor size, and lymphatic or vascular invasion. In univariate analyses, HSP27 status correlated with shorter disease-free survival, but in multivariate analyses, it was not a statistically significant independent prognostic factor for clinical outcome. Love and King[175] measured HSP27 in 361 patients with primary breast cancer and found a strong correlation with ER, but not PR, status. It was also unrelated to age, menstrual status, and tumor size. In univariate analyses, HSP27 status predicted a short disease-free interval, but longer survival from first relapse. In multivariate analyses, however, HSP27 status was not an independent predictor of clinical outcome.

Data reported by Ciocca et al.[176] suggest that HSP27 may be involved in cellular resistance to cytotoxic drugs, particularly doxorubicin. When cancer cell lines were exposed to heat shock treatment, significant elevations of HSP27 were observed. Subsequent treatment with doxorubicin showed increased resistance among the cells compared with control cells. This resistance, however, was not seen with other drugs, such as colchicine and methotrexate. Oesterreich et al.[177] conducted a series of experiments to determine whether HSP27 expression is *directly* involved in heat-induced doxorubicin resistance. They introduced HSP27 expression vectors into cells that express low levels of HSP27 and cells that express high levels of HSP27 as a result of gene amplification. When the cells with low HSP27 expression were then transfected with a full-length complementary DNA (cDNA), the cells displayed a threefold elevated resistance to doxorubicin. When the cells with high HSP27 expression were transfected with an antisense HSP27 construct, they became threefold more sensitive to doxorubicin. These results suggest that HSP27 specifically confers doxorubicin resistance in human breast cancer cells, and manipulation of HSP27 levels, either genetically or pharmacologically, may be useful in reversing this drug resistance in breast cancer patients.

Thus, although the HSPs may not be powerful prognostic factors, they may eventually have clinical use for predicting response to therapy. In addition, they may provide targets of opportunity for new therapeutic strategies.

GROWTH FACTORS AND RECEPTORS

The epithelial cells of the breast are under the influence of a variety of hormones and growth factors. The tyrosine kinase growth factor receptors are among the best studied,

TABLE 9. *Type I growth factor receptor families and their known ligands*

Growth factor receptor	Ligands
EGFR	EGF, TGF-α, amphiregulin, heparin-binding EGF, viral growth factors, β cellulin
HER-2/neu	Unknown
c-Erb-b3	Heregulin (?)
c-Erb-b4	Heparin-binding c-erb-b4 stimulatory factor, heregulin
Unknown	Cripto (?)

EGF, epidermal growth factor; EGFR, epidermal growth factor receptor; TGF-α, transforming growth factor α.
Adapted from ref. 178.

and they have been subclassified into nine different families based on the structure of their extracellular ligand-binding and intracellular kinase domains and the nature of their activating ligands.[178] The type I growth factor receptors include the epidermal growth factor receptor (EGFR) family, which contains several polypeptides that are expressed in the breast and are involved in the development of breast cancer. Members of this family are EGFR (also known as c-Erb-b1), HER-2/neu (also known as c-Erb-b2), HER-3 (also known as c-Erb-b3), and HER-4 (also known as c-Erb-b4). The specific ligands have yet to be identified for some of these receptors, but Table 9 displays what is presently known.

HER-3 and HER-4 have only recently been discovered, and definitive information is not yet available concerning the prognostic or predictive significance of either of these receptors. One study reported that patients whose tumors showed moderate to strong immunoreactivity to HER-3 were more likely to develop local recurrence, but no association was found with survival in any analysis performed.[179] Several studies have been conducted to evaluate EGFR and HER-2/neu, however, and these factors are discussed in more detail in the following two sections.

Epidermal Growth Factor Receptor

The EGFR is a 170-kd transmembrane glycoprotein translated from messenger RNAs (mRNAs) of 6 and 10 kb encoded by a gene on 7q21. EGFR has been identified by several methods, including radioligand-binding assays, autoradiography, immunocytohistochemical analysis, immunoenzymatic assays, and measurement of EGFR transcripts. An entire issue of the journal *Breast Cancer Research and Treatment* (1994, vol. 29, no. 1) was devoted to the biological, prognostic, and therapeutic roles of EGFR in breast cancer. EGFR is present at low levels on normal breast epithelial cells and in other tissues, including the liver. Thirty-five percent to 60% of primary breast cancers overexpress EGFR. No clear differences in EGFR positivity are seen among the various assay techniques, although EGFR positivity tends to be lowest when measured by immunologic methods. Nearly all studies have reported a negative relation between EGFR and steroid receptor status, with EGFR positivity twice as high in ER negativity or PR negativity. Most published reports have found statistically significant associations or trends for direct relation to worse tumor grade and increased proliferation indices. Only a few published studies have reported associations with age, menopausal status, histologic type, tumor size, or axillary nodal status. Studies suggest that EGFR positivity may be correlated with overexpression of abnormal p53 and angiogenesis factors.

The relation between EGFR status and clinical outcome remains controversial. Several reviews have summarized the results of many studies with more than 3,000 patients.[180–182] Care must be taken when summarizing these studies, because several publications are updated analyses of previously published studies. Most of the studies show a significant relation between EGFR status and disease-free or overall survival using univariate analyses. In some studies, however, the results apply only to node-negative or node-positive patients. In studies with longer follow-up, the initial significant separation of disease-free or overall survival curves tends to diminish with time. Multivariate analyses have been performed in few of the published studies. Another confounding factor is the variable systemic adjuvant therapies that the patients have received.

In summary, EGFR status is probably an important prognostic factor for primary breast cancer, but the lack of standardization of the assay methods, the small numbers of patients and short follow-up intervals in most of the studies, and the general lack of multivariate analyses make it impossible to draw firm conclusions about the optimal role of EGFR status in determining prognosis for the individual breast cancer patient.

On the other hand, the role of EGFR status as a predictive factor for hormone resistance or responsiveness is better defined. Several groups have clearly shown that tumors expressing EGFR are more likely to be resistant to endocrine therapy. Conversely, EGFR-negative tumors, especially if they are also ER positive, tend to have high response rates. Nicholson et al.[183] reported an 80% response rate for patients with EGFR-negative/ER-positive tumors, with 45% achieving complete or partial remission.

Perhaps the most exciting use of EGFR is as a target for new therapies. Baselga and Mendelsohn[184] have been the leaders in this area and have developed several monoclonal antibodies directed against EGFR. Some of these antibodies have been evaluated in clinical trials, and novel combinations of chemotherapeutic agents and anti-EGFR monoclonal antibodies are being evaluated.

HER-2/neu

The HER-2/neu gene is located on 17q21 and is transcribed into a 4.5-kb mRNA, which is translated into a 185-kd glycoprotein. The HER-2/neu protein is expressed at low

TABLE 10. *Prognostic significance of HER-2/neu overexpression as determined by immunohistochemical analysis in node-negative patients: studies with more than 3 years of follow-up and more than 100 patients*

Study	*n*	Follow-up (mo)	Univariate *p* value		Multivariate *p* value	
			DFS	OS	DFS	OS
Thor et al.[196]	141	102	NS	NS	—	—
Lovekin et al.[199]	250	~60	—	NS	—	—
McCann et al.[200]	113	48	—	NS	—	—
Kallioniemi et al.[201]	174	118	—	.01	—	.03
Tanner et al.[202]	105	36	NS	NS	—	—
Yuan et al.[203]	101	>120	.002	.003	NS	NS
Allred et al.[204]	453	61	NS	NS	—	—
Noguchi et al.[205]	151	~60	NS	NS	NS	NS
Gusterson et al.[206]	760	42	.22	.0	NS	.08
Press et al.[207]	210	108	.0004	—	—	—
Bianchi et al.[208]	230	>84	.03	.0007	NS	NS

DFS, disease-free survival; NS, not significant; OS, overall survival.
Adapted from ref. 186.

levels in the epithelial and myoepithelial cells of normal breast tissue. It is overexpressed in comedo, large-cell, ductal carcinoma *in situ*, but relatively low levels are found in papillary and cribriform *in situ* tumors.

The initial study of the prognostic value of HER-2/neu expression in breast cancer was published in 1985,[185] and its role is still being defined. Ravdin and Chamness[186] reviewed the published literature concerning HER-2/neu and concluded that the interpretation of studies on the use of this gene and its protein product in prognostic and predictive tests for breast cancer is complicated by multiple methods and inherent difficulties in many of the studies. The work has moved beyond the stage at which small studies with short follow-up (useful for hypothesis generation) are of value, to the stage in which large studies with sufficient statistical power to find significant correlations are central. These larger studies do not lend support to the use of HER-2/neu in the evaluation of patients with negative axillary lymph nodes, the group of breast cancer patients for whom refinement of prognostic estimates is now most important.

The first studies addressing the possible prognostic significance of HER-2/neu measured gene amplification. HER-2/neu amplification was generally found to be predictive of poorer disease-free and overall survival in node-positive patients but seldom in the node-negative subgroups.[185,187–195] Later studies measured expression of the HER-2/neu protein product rather than gene amplification. Protein expression correlates well with gene amplification,[188,190,196,197] but one might hypothesize that gene expression would more directly relate to tumor cell behavior. Both immunoblotting and IHC have been used to measure HER-2/neu protein levels; most of the work has been done with IHC, however, because if appropriate antibodies are used, this technique can be performed on paraffin-embedded archived material. Immunoblotting is more technically involved, requires fresh or frozen material, and is far less feasible for most centers. The two methods have been compared in a large series of patients with 95% concordance.[198]

Most of the published studies have used IHC, and this test is commercially available from several reference laboratories. Ravdin and Chamness[186] summarized the results from 18 studies, each of which had more than 100 patients with at least 3 years of follow-up. Some studies found that overexpression of HER-2/neu had prognostic use, although others did not. Not surprisingly, the univariate analyses were more positive than the multivariate analyses. Two of the studies that appeared to show positive results in univariate analyses had negative results in multivariate analyses, perhaps because of the inclusion of other uncommon prognostic variables. The reviewers concluded that overexpression of HER-2/neu as measured by IHC adds little to the prediction of disease-free survival but may add to the prediction of overall survival. Examination of 11 studies of node-negative patients (Table 10) suggests little clinical use for this group.[196,199–208] Only 1 of these 11 studies notes a positive finding in multivariate analysis. Even in the univariate analyses, the correlations appear weak. Thus, little support seems to exist for the application of HER-2/neu status in evaluating node-negative patients, the group for which prognostic factors are most important for making adjuvant treatment decisions.

Assay method is a major problem in this field. Different studies have used different antibody preparations for HER-2/neu detection. Different definitions have also been used for scoring HER-2/neu positivity, ranging from continuous scoring of the percentage of positively stained cells to simply scoring a case as positive if any staining was detectable. Use of different antibodies or tissue preparations (fresh or frozen versus fixed) may explain some of the variations among studies.[195,207] The number of different antibody preparations used complicates assessment of whether a particular antibody can be used with more valid prognostic results. Certainly, particularly in cases of node-negative disease, no consistent pattern emerges in these studies to support use of a given antibody or tissue preparation protocol.

The inconsistencies among studies suggest that method may be important, and the prognostic significance of HER-2/neu has not yet been adequately validated.

No validated predictive factors exist for response to chemotherapy. Evidence is accumulating, however, that HER-2/neu may be the first to make the list. The first studies that examined the potential role of HER-2/neu status for predicting response to adjuvant chemotherapy concentrated on regimens that contained CMF.[204,206] The general trend reported in these and subsequent studies is that patients whose tumors have little or no detectable levels of HER-2/neu derive considerable benefit from CMF regimens, but patients whose tumors have amplified HER-2/neu genes or overexpress HER-2/neu protein do not benefit from these therapies. These conclusions, however, are based on retrospective analyses and have not been validated in prospective studies with sufficient statistical power to detect interactions between treatment and HER-2/neu status.

In 1994, Muss et al.[112] published the first analysis of an interaction between expression of HER-2/neu and adjuvant therapy with doxorubicin-containing regimens. The finding that tumors with high expression of HER-2/neu responded better to dose-intensive treatment with CAF was contrary to the previous results with CMF regimens and spurred international efforts to validate or refute the published data and to understand the biological mechanisms that might explain such findings. Results from retrospective analyses of randomized clinical trials conducted by the Cancer and Acute Leukemia Group B,[209] the National Surgical Adjuvant Breast and Bowel Project (NSABP),[210] and the Southwest Oncology Group[211] have been reported regarding relationships between HER-2/neu status and node-positive breast cancer.

The Cancer and Acute Leukemia Group B study[209] was designed as a validation of the group's previous published results.[112] The original trial randomly assigned women to receive one of three regimens of adjuvant CAF to address questions about the efficacy of dose intensity. The hypothesized interaction between HER-2/neu expression and dose of CAF was not statistically significant, although the trend was in the same direction as reported previously. Subsequent subset analyses that adjusted for an apparent failure of randomization did produce the hypothesized result.

The NSABP study[210] was a retrospective analysis of patients enrolled in B-11, a trial originally designed to compare treatment with L-phenylalanine mustard plus 5-fluorouracil and treatment with L-phenylalanine mustard plus doxorubicin plus 5-fluorouracil. Unlike the Cancer and Acute Leukemia Group B study, this trial provided a comparison of a treatment regimen plus or minus doxorubicin and, therefore, a direct test of an interaction between doxorubicin and HER-2/neu expression. The results clearly indicated that patients with tumors negative for HER-2/neu have the same clinical outcomes with and without the use of doxorubicin. Patients with tumors positive for HER-2/neu who did not receive doxorubicin had significantly worse prognoses; the addition of doxorubicin improved clinical outcomes so that they were equivalent to those experienced by patients with tumors negative for HER-2/neu.

The Southwest Oncology Group study[211] examined treatment with tamoxifen plus or minus CAF. The results were very similar to those reported by the NSABP. Patients whose tumors expressed low levels of HER-2/neu did not benefit from the CAF treatment, but CAF significantly improved disease-free survival of patients whose tumors overexpressed HER-2/neu.

These studies, together with other results that have been presented at national and international meetings and preclinical data, strongly suggest that the hypothesized interaction between HER-2/neu expression and adjuvant doxorubicin therapy is real. Before selection of adjuvant chemotherapy for patients with breast cancer based on HER-2/neu status can become routine, however, a consensus must be reached about the most reliable, most reproducible, and most predictive method to determine HER-2/neu status.[212]

Some have suggested that HER-2/neu status may also predict response to endocrine therapy.[213] Several studies reported that patients with advanced breast cancer whose tumors overexpress HER-2/neu have lower response rates when treated with tamoxifen than patients whose tumors have low HER-2/neu levels.[214–217] At least one study, however, found no relationship between HER-2/neu status and response to tamoxifen.[218] High serum HER-2/neu levels have been associated with decreased response to droloxifene[219] and megestrol acetate or fadrazole[220] in advanced breast cancer. In the adjuvant setting, patients with tumors positive for HER-2/neu tend to have shorter disease-free and overall survival when treated with tamoxifen than do patients with low HER-2/neu levels.[221–224]

One is tempted to suggest that patients whose tumors overexpress HER-2/neu should not receive endocrine therapy even if the tumors are ER positive. With only one exception,[223] however, the results described above are from small, nonrandomized series of patients. In addition, although it may be true that the benefit from endocrine therapies for ER-positive patients with tumors overexpressing HER-2/neu may be reduced, the benefit may be better than might be expected with alternative therapies. Clearly, additional well-controlled and well-designed studies must be conducted before HER-2/neu status can be used to decide whether to administer or withhold endocrine therapy.

TUMOR-SUPPRESSOR GENES

p53

The p53 tumor-suppressor gene is located on 17p13 and encodes a 53-kd nuclear phosphoprotein. Alterations in this gene are the most frequent genetic changes found in many malignant diseases, including breast cancer.[225] The entire coding regions of the p53 gene can be sequenced,[226] but this is a tedious process with several unresolved issues, and sequencing does not detect inactivation of p53 by mechanisms other than mutation. The most commonly used technique to assess p53 alterations is IHC. Mutations are most prevalent in five conserved exons, resulting in a conformationally altered and nonfunctional, but apparently more stable, nuclear protein. Mutant protein accumulates to high concentrations that can be detected by IHC staining. IHC is relatively easy, inexpensive, and readily performed on a large number of specimens in a short period of time. It can detect nearly all missense mutations in the core domain, but its sensitivity is lower for mutations that produce protein truncation or for mutations that lie outside the core domain. IHC staining may be present in the absence of a mutation for several reasons. The major drawback of IHC is the lack of standardization of antibodies and scoring systems. Mutations can also be detected by DNA-based methods, such as single-strand conformation polymorphism (SSCP) or constant denaturing gel electrophoresis, or by RNA-based techniques.

Overexpression of p53 as determined by IHC is relatively independent of axillary lymph node status and menopausal status, is weakly related to tumor size, and is strongly associated with DNA ploidy and measures of proliferation, steroid receptors, and nuclear grade.[227–234] The incidence of p53 mutations detected by SSCP is significantly less than the overexpression rates measured by immunochemical analysis,[235,236] and studies that use paraffin-embedded tissue generally report lower rates of p53 abnormalities than studies that use frozen material.[237] Not all tumors that exhibit positive staining with the various p53 antibodies have mutations of the p53 gene,[238] nor are all mutations likely to contribute equally to the aggressiveness of breast tumors.[239]

At least 13 different monoclonal antibodies induced by the product of the human p53 gene are available.[240] Two studies compared panels of antibodies. Elledge et al.[241] evaluated five different antibodies (240, 1801, 421, BP53-12, CM1) and mutations as detected by SSCP in 169 node-negative patients. The staining rates for the different antibodies ranged from 18% to 36%. A cocktail of both 1801 and 240 produced a p53-positive rate of 45% and was the only technique that yielded results associated with worse clinical outcome. Jacquermier et al.[242] compared staining for four antibodies (240, 1801, DO7, DO1) and SSCP detection of mutations in 106 tumors from a heterogeneous group of primary breast tumors. Staining was observed in 17% to 30% of the tumors, depending on the antibody. Unfortunately, the median follow-up was only 10.7 months, so correlations with clinical outcomes were not observed for any of the antibodies. The investigators did not draw any conclusions regarding which antibody or combination of antibodies might be most useful in a clinical setting.

Assessing the clinical use of p53 as a prognostic or predictive marker for breast cancer based on published reports is difficult, because the majority of studies include heterogeneous patient populations undergoing a variety of treatments. Elledge and Allred[237] reviewed 57 studies involving more than 13,000 patients and concluded that inactivation of p53 appears to be associated with a poor outcome as measured by disease-free or overall survival, but that its prognostic significance is not powerful enough to allow it to be used alone in clinical decision making. Table 11, which summarizes results from seven studies that included only node-negative patients who received no systemic adjuvant therapy,[229,230,232,234,243–245] suggests that the true prognostic impact of p53 abnormalities in untreated patients is modest. Because the p53 gene is just one gene in a complex pathway that controls both proliferation and apoptosis, other factors in this pathway will probably have to be measured, including the Bcl-2 and Bax families, cyclins, and cyclin-dependent kinases to make accurate predictions about the course of an individual tumor.

Suggestions are found in the literature that p53 abnormalities may be associated with response or resistance to specific therapies. Most of these studies, however, were not designed to definitively address questions about the predictive value of p53 abnormalities, and few included a statistical test of interaction between p53 status and response to treatment.

Two groups reported improved response to radiation therapy among node-negative patients whose tumors had p53 abnormalities,[246,247] but one of these groups[248] also reported that radiation therapy was of less value for p53-mutated,

TABLE 11. *Prognostic significance of p53 abnormalities in node-negative patients*

Study	Antibodies	*n*	Follow-up (mo)	High p53 (%)	DFS		OS	
					RR	*p* value	RR	*p* value
Immunohistochemical analysis								
Thor et al.[228]	1081	127	84	24	2.7	.018	2.8	.057
Isola et al.[229]	CM1/Tab250	127	102	14	—	—	2.7	<.0001
Allred et al.[230]	1081/240	70	54	52	2.5	.002	1.7	.03
Barnes et al.[231]	CM1	103	120	19	—	.009	—	<.001
Silvestrini et al.[232]	1081	256	72	44	3.95	<.0001	3.10	.0001
Marks et al.[233]	1081	147	61	27	—	.03	—	.01
Gasparini et al.[234]	1081	254	62	28	3.08	.004	NS	.024
SSCP								
Elledge et al.[235]		200	71	14	2.2	.01	—	
Caleffi et al.[236]		78	48	15	—		—	NS

DFS, disease-free survival; NS, not significant; OS, overall survival; RR, relative risk; SSCP, single-strand conformation polymorphism.

node-positive tumors. A randomized trial of preoperative FAC (5-fluorouracil, adriamycin, cytoxan) chemotherapy versus preoperative radiotherapy demonstrated no relationship between p53 and tumor response for either treatment.[249] Patients whose tumors overexpress p53 may benefit from CMF chemotherapy,[250,251] but not all studies have confirmed this observation.[252] Other studies have suggested that these tumors may have increased resistance to doxorubicin-containing regimens,[253,254] although this may not be the case in locally advanced breast cancer.[255] Another report suggested that patients whose tumors overexpress both p53 and HER-2/neu may have increased survival if treated with high-dose CAF.[209] Relationships between p53 abnormalities and response to other chemotherapy regimens have also been examined. No relationships were found with epirubicin (epirubicin hydrochloride),[256] VCF (vincristine sulfate, cyclophosphamide, 5-fluorouracil) or MCF (mitoxantrone hydrochloride, cyclophosphamide, 5-fluorouracil),[257] or with EVM (epirubicin, vincristine sulfate, methotrexate sodium) followed by MTB (mitomycin C, thiotepa, vindesine sulfate).[258] Some studies have reported an association between p53 abnormalities and resistance to endocrine therapy,[259] but others have not.[260–262]

The associations observed between p53 abnormalities and clinical outcomes are exciting, and one might be tempted to add p53 to the list of biomarkers that should be routinely assessed in making treatment decisions. Much remains to be learned about the function of p53 and its interactions with other genes and their products, however. Standardized assays and guidelines for interpretation of the results must be developed, and interlaboratory studies need to be conducted before one can be confident of the clinical use of measuring p53 in breast cancers.

nm23

The nm23 gene was originally identified by Steeg et al.[263] by screening cDNA libraries from murine melanoma cell lines of varying metastatic potential. Investigators proposed that nm23 may function as a suppressor gene for tumor metastasis. The product of the nm23-H1 gene has been identified as the nucleoside diphosphate (NDP) kinase A.[264] Contradictory findings have been reported regarding correlations with other prognostic factors, especially lymph node status and tumor grade. Several small studies have reported a significant relation between expression of nm23 mRNA and longer disease-free or overall survival in patients with primary breast cancer,[265–269] whereas some have found no relation between nm23 activity and clinical outcome.[270,271] None of these studies performed multivariate analyses among node-negative patients, however. Heimann et al.[272] performed a multivariate analysis of 163 node-negative patients who received no adjuvant therapy and reported a hazard ratio of 0.38 ($p = .03$) for patients with high nm23 with respect to disease-free survival.

Perhaps NDP kinase activity of nm23 protein does not correlate well with nm23 protein levels, and the biochemical mechanism of nm23-suppressive activity is not due to its NDP kinase activity, association with guanosine triphosphatase–activating proteins, or secretion from cells.[273] Additional studies must be conducted to understand the biological significance and prognostic use of nm23.

MEASURES OF INVASIVENESS

Cancer invasion and metastasis are multifactorial processes involving complex interactions of a variety of proteolytic enzymes, growth factors, and cell-cell and cell-substrate adhesion molecules. A special issue of the journal *Breast Cancer Research and Treatment* (1993, vol. 23, no. 3) reviewed several invasion-related and metastasis-related factors in breast cancer. Several factors have been studied using *in vitro* and *in vivo* model systems to gain a better understanding of some of these interactions. Few have been evaluated as potential prognostic factors for primary breast cancer, however.

Cathepsin D

Cathepsin D is a glycoprotein that is originally translated and glycosylated to produce a 52-kd form, which is then processed into a 48-kd form that, on further processing, produces a 34-kd and a 14-kd protein. The 52-kd proenzyme and the processed 48- and 34-kd forms are all enzymatically active at acidic pHs (a pH of 3.5 is optimal) but have little or no enzymatic activity at physiologic pH. Cathepsin D has been proposed to be a marker of estrogenic activity, to act as a growth factor through the type II insulin receptor, and to play a role in tumor invasion as a protease by degrading the basement membrane and enhancing the processing or release of peptide growth factors. Thus, it is an attractive candidate to serve as a prognostic marker for invasion and metastasis.

Ravdin[274] reviewed many of the studies conducted to evaluate its prognostic use in breast cancer. Interpretation of these studies is hampered by their use of different antibodies and different assay techniques and by the use of optimized cutoff points that were obtained from the same data sets without validation in subsequent studies. Four different types of assays have been used in published studies: enzyme-linked immunoassay, Western blotting, enzymatic assay, and IHC. Although most studies were declared to show positive results by their authors, nearly all found statistical significance only in specific subsets of patients after optimizing the cutoff point for the particular group of patients. Ravdin concluded that cathepsin D is a potentially important prognostic marker whose clinical application awaits further definition.

Subsequent to this review, results from a number of other studies were published.[164,275–281] None of the studies that used IHC techniques found any relation between tumor staining and clinical outcome.[276–278,280,281] Têtu et al.[277] reported that, although cancer cell immunostaining was not associated with prognosis, positive staining of stromal elements was related to shorter metastasis-free survival. These researchers suggested that stromal cells may play a key role in local invasion and metastatic dissemination of the tumor. The discrepancy between results from immunostaining and those from other techniques has been noted by others. It is consistent with the findings of Johnson et al.,[282] whose work with cell lines also suggested that the poor prognosis of some tumors with high levels of cathepsin D is probably due to high levels of cathepsin D in the stromal components of the tumor, such as infiltrating inflammatory cells. If this is the case, then additional work must be carried out before the prognostic role of cathepsin D will be clear.

Plasminogen Activators and Inhibitors

Several teams of investigators have studied the uPA pathway of plasminogen activation in breast cancer and its involvement in the process of tumor cell invasion.[275,279,283–290] Urokinase-type plasminogen activator is a serine protease that catalyzes the conversion of plasminogen into the active enzyme plasmin. Plasmin can activate type IV collagenase, which then degrades collagen and proteins of the basement membranes. The uPA binds to its receptor, uPAR, which is a glycolipid-anchored cell surface protein. The uPA is controlled by two specific, naturally occurring inhibitors, plasminogen activator inhibitor 1 (PAI-1) and plasminogen activator inhibitor 2 (PAI-2). Inhibition of uPA activity leads to inhibition of invasion in several experimental systems, and PAI-1 inhibits receptor-bound uPA nearly as well as uPA in solution.

Studies have evaluated uPA, uPAR, PAI-1, and PAI-2 as potential prognostic markers in primary breast cancer. As with other new prognostic markers, slightly different assays with different antibodies have been used in these studies. Consequently, the median levels of activity have varied, different cutoff points have been used to define assay positivity, and the percentage of positive assays differs among studies. Published results of studies of uPA and PAI-1 are shown in Table 12.

Duffy et al.[286] reported a significant relation between uPA status and both disease-free and overall survival in univariate analyses of 166 patients with more than 5 years of median follow-up. Similar results were found for the 75 patients with node-negative disease ($p < .05$ for disease-free survival; $p = .055$ for overall survival).

Jänicke et al.[285] performed multivariate analyses of the results of uPA and PAI-1 positivity in 229 patients followed for a median of 30 months. Using optimized cutoff points of 2.97 and 2.18 ng per milligram of protein for uPA and PAI-1, respectively, these researchers found 39% of all tumors to be positive for uPA and 17% to be positive for PAI-1. Strong statistical significance of uPA positivity and a weaker relation to PAI-1 positivity were reported. Subset analyses of 101 node-negative patients, however, revealed that the multivariate relative risks of relapse were 5.5 and 4.9 for patients with tumors positive for uPA and PAI-1, respectively. Using these factors in combination permitted the identification of a subset of node-negative patients with less than a 10% probability of relapse at 3 years.

Grøndahl-Hansen et al.[284] measured uPA and PAI-1 in international and interim units, respectively, by calibration with standard preparations and defined assay positivity as values above the median. Studying 191 high-risk breast cancer patients with a median observation time of 8.5 years, they found both factors to correlate with relapse-free and overall survival. Because all patients were participants in clinical trials and randomization was based on menopausal status, separate multivariate analyses were reported by menopausal status. Positivity for uPA was an independent predictor of overall survival in premenopausal patients (relative risk, 2.0), and PAI-1 positivity was an independent predictor in postmenopausal women (relative risk, 2.9).

Foekens et al.[279,283] measured uPA and PAI-1 levels in nearly 700 breast cancer patients with a 48-month median follow-up. When optimally determined cutoffs of 1.15 ng per milligram of protein and 17 ng per milligram of protein were used for uPA and PAI-1, respectively, 32% of their patients were found to have tumors positive for uPA, and 44% were found to have tumors positive for PAI-1. Both factors were significant predictors of relapse-free and overall survival for both node-negative and node-positive patients. In multivariate analyses, the estimated relative risks of relapse for patients with uPA-positive and PAI-1-positive tumors were 1.47 and 3.10, respectively, for node-negative patients, and 1.50 and 1.80 for node-positive patients. No effect of menopausal status was observed.

TABLE 12. *Percentage of patients with high levels of urokinase-type plasminogen activator or plasminogen activator inhibitor 1*

	All patients		Node-negative patients		Node-positive patients	
Study	*n*	High uPA/PAI-1 (%)	*n*	High uPA/PAI-1 (%)	*n*	High uPA/PAI-1 (%)
Foekens et al.[279,283]	657	32/44	273	32/43	379	31/45
Grøndahl-Hansen et al.[284]	191	50/50	23	—/—	168	—/—
Jänicke et al.[285]	229	39/17	101	40/16	128	38/19
Duffy et al.[286]	166	50/—	75	40/—	74	58/—
Bouchet et al.[287]	314	32/26	146	34/30	168	31/23

PAI-1, plasminogen activator inhibitor 1; uPA, urokinase-type plasminogen activator.

Bouchet et al.[287] measured uPA, PAI-1 and PAI-2 levels in tumor specimens from 314 patients with primary breast cancer. Using a clustering technique that is independent of clinical outcome, they set cutoff points of 0.52, 3.0, and 14.5 ng per milligram protein for uPA, PAI-1, and PAI-2, respectively, which yielded positivity rates of 32%, 26%, and 14%. None of these factors was related to clinical outcome for node-positive patients. In multivariate analyses of 146 node-negative patients, both PAI-1 and PAI-2 status, but not uPA status, were predictive of disease-free and metastasis-free survival. High PAI-1 levels were associated with worse outcomes (relative risks, 2.0 and 4.8 for disease-free and metastasis-free survival), but high PAI-2 levels were associated with prolonged survival (relative risk, 0.1 for both clinical outcomes). The authors concluded that PAI-1 status provided prognostic information similar to that of uPA status, and PAI-1 does not appear to play a role as an inhibitor. In contrast, consideration of PAI-2 status enhanced the prognostic value of PAI-1 status for node-negative women. Subsequently, Foekens et al.[288] failed to find any significant association between PAI-2 status and prognosis in recurrent breast cancer but did report a strong correlation between high PAI-2 levels and better prognosis in patients whose tumors had a high uPA content.

Grøndahl-Hansen et al.[289] demonstrated an association between high uPAR levels and shorter survival in 505 patients with primary breast cancer. This finding was confirmed by Duggan et al.[290] in a study of 141 patients.

Measurement of complexes such as uPA:PAI-1 or uPA:PAI-2 may provide better prognostication than measurements of the individual analytes of the uPA system. The prognostic significance of uPA and PAI-1 has also been shown to change with time[290]; this finding indicates that more sophisticated data integration may be necessary to use these factors in the clinical management of patients with breast cancer.

These results are promising, but additional validation studies must be performed that use the same assay methods and the same cutoff points before the role of these biomarkers as prognostic factors for breast cancer is known.

Possibly, the uPA pathway of plasminogen activation might provide new therapeutic approaches. For example, the proteolytic activity of the tumor cell might be modified by blockade of uPA or uPA receptor or inhibition of uPA–uPA receptor synthesis.[291] Thus, these factors might become useful predictive indicators regardless of their eventual role as prognostic factors.

Laminin Receptors

The laminin receptor is a 67-kd cell surface protein that has been hypothesized to be involved in invasion and penetration of cancer cells through the basement membranes of endothelial vessels.[292] Expression of laminin receptors is associated with involved lymph nodes and young patient age, and a weak relation to tumor size may exist. Steroid receptor status and proliferative rate appear to be unrelated to laminin receptor levels, but *in vitro* experiments suggest that expression of the laminin receptor may be modulated by estrogen and progestins.[293]

Several studies have examined the prognostic significance of laminin receptors with mixed results. Marques et al.[294] measured laminin receptor expression in 235 consecutive patients with primary breast cancer and found that patients whose tumors expressed laminin receptors had a 40% lower risk of recurrence than those with no expression of these receptors. Daidone et al.[295] reported no associations between laminin receptor expression and disease-free or overall survival in a series studying 187 node-negative patients, but they did find that high levels were strong indicators of local and regional diffusion of the disease. Martignone et al.[296] measured laminin receptor expression in 1,160 tumor specimens from patients with node-negative disease who received no systemic adjuvant therapy. They found a small but statistically significant increased relative risk of death (1.33) among patients whose tumors expressed laminin receptors. Patients whose tumors expressed both laminin and its receptor had a particularly poor survival, suggesting that both factors might be important in determining the aggressiveness of the tumor.[297] Gasparini et al.[298] demonstrated that knowledge of laminin receptor expression adds prognostic information to determinations of intratumoral microvessel density in node-negative breast cancer, especially among patients that have low vascularization. Laminin receptors probably play a role in the metastatic process and may provide some prognostic information for some breast tumors. If new treatment strategies are developed that would decrease expression of these receptors, laminin receptors might be ideal therapeutic targets for decreasing tumor aggressiveness.

ANGIOGENESIS

Considerable experimental evidence indicates that tumor growth depends on the induction of new capillary blood vessels, or *angiogenesis*.[299] After a new tumor has grown to a few millimeters in diameter, further expansion of the tumor cell population requires neovascularization. Although endothelial cells are actively proliferating within the tumor, intratumoral microvessel density and intratumoral endothelial cell proliferation are independent of each other and of tumor cell proliferation.[300] Investigators have proposed that counting microvessel formation in tumors might provide prognostic information for predicting distant disease recurrence. Investigators have detected tumor-associated neovascularization by different methods, including staining with a polyclonal antiserum against factor VIII–related antigen and immunoperoxidase staining with a monoclonal antibody that recognizes the cell adhesion molecule CD31.

Several studies have reported correlations with clinical outcomes in primary breast cancer, and several of these have been reviewed by Craft and Harris.[301] Weidner et al.[302] originally demonstrated a correlation between the number of microvessel counts per 200× field and distant metastasis in 49 patients. In a follow-up study of 165 patients, these investigators found that microvessel count was an independent predictor of disease-free and overall survival when compared with lymph node status, tumor size, ER status, S-phase fraction, c-Erb-b2 expression, Ki67 status, EGFR expression, and cathepsin D status. Bosari et al.[303] studied 120 patients and found associations among microvessel count, axillary metastasis, and disease-free and overall survival.

Horak et al.[304] reported a strong correlation between tumor-associated vascular counts and axillary lymph node metastasis in 103 patients; however, they found no association between vascular counts and ER status or expression of EGFR, c-Erb-b2, or p53. Despite the small number of patients and relatively short follow-up, these investigators found a significant relationship with overall survival. Toi et al.[305] evaluated 220 tumors from Japanese women by immunostaining to factor VIII antigen. A multivariate analysis demonstrated that vessel density was an independent prognostic factor that was as potent as nodal status.

Two studies have focused on node-negative breast cancer. Gasparini et al.[234] reported that microvessel density was the strongest independent predictor of disease-free survival in 254 node-negative patients, and that high microvessel density was associated with a relative risk of relapse of 5.78 after a median follow-up of 62 months. Other significant factors in their multivariate analysis included peritumoral lymphatic vessel invasion, p53 mutation, and tumor size. When the cut-off for high microvessel density was changed from 80 vessels to 70 vessels per 200× field (0.74 mm^2 area), it was also a strong predictor of overall survival and was associated with a relative risk of death of 3.27. Fox et al.[306] studied 109 node-negative patients with a short median follow-up of only 25 months. Despite the short follow-up, the multivariate relative risks of relapse and survival for patients with high microvessel density were found to be 3.5 and 6.6, respectively.

The results of these studies are impressive, but the number of patients was small, and the follow-up interval was relatively short for determining the precise clinical use of angiogenesis as a prognostic factor. Tumor-associated angiogenesis is a particularly appealing putative prognostic factor because it appears to be a marker of invasion rather than of differentiation or proliferation, as are most of the other currently available biomarkers.[307]

Rather than counting microvessels, it may be more practical to measure angiogenic peptides, such as vascular endothelial growth factors, thymidine phosphorylase, hepatocyte growth factor, fibroblast growth factors, endogenous inhibitors of angiogenesis, and endothelial cell adhesion molecules and receptors. Locopo et al.[308] have reviewed several of these factors. They note that more than 25 angiogenic peptides have now been discovered and sequenced, but few have been evaluated in human breast cancer. Preliminary data suggest that some of these factors might be clinically useful and may be prognostic or predictive factors, but most of the results from these studies must be considered preliminary and inclusive.

An attractive feature of angiogenesis is that it offers a target for novel therapeutic interventions. Several antiangiogenic agents have been developed and evaluated in a variety of systems. Classes of antiangiogenic agents include the following[307]:

- Polysulfated glycosamines, peptidoglycans, polyglycosylated lipids
- Enzymes that control the vascularization process
- Steroids and steroid-related substances
- Antibiotics and synthetic antibiotic derivatives
- Specific immunotherapeutics
- Nonspecific biological response modifiers

Clinical trials are being designed to test these agents singly and in combination. Successful regimens may have their greatest efficacy early in the course of the disease, most likely in the adjuvant setting.

MICROARRAY TECHNOLOGY

Most published evaluations of prognostic or predictive factors have considered one factor at a time or a small panel of markers. The emerging technologies of microarray-based high-throughput analysis open the door for the simultaneous measurement of thousands of genes and gene products. Initial studies used cDNA arrays,[309] but microarrays also provide targets for parallel *in situ* detection of DNA, RNA, and protein targets.[310,311] Newer techniques combine other methods, such as suppression subtractive hybridization, to generate cDNA clones.[312]

Management, analysis, and interpretation of the vast amount of information generated by these techniques present new and unresolved challenges.[313] Analysis of the data is difficult because the number of samples in most experiments is much less than the number of variables (genes or gene products), often by an order of magnitude. Pairwise *t* tests have been proposed for interpreting profiles produced by comparative genomic hybridization.[314] Cluster analysis[315] and principal components analysis[316] have also been applied to data generated by expression arrays.

High-throughput microarray technology is still developing, but it may provide the tools needed to construct molecular fingerprints of individual tumors and eventually provide novel targets that can be used to individualize treatment decisions for patients with breast cancer.

MODELS OF PROGNOSTIC FACTORS

Given the number and diversity of the potential prognostic factors, physicians and patients have difficulty synthesizing and integrating the information that they provide. A special issue of the journal *Breast Cancer Research and Treatment* (1992, vol. 22, no. 3) was devoted to prognostic factor integration. Factor integration techniques include simple addition of points for each adverse factor (e.g., histologic grading systems) and the use of multiple regression equations, usually from Cox survival models (e.g., the Nottingham Prognostic Index); decision trees[317]; and neural networks.[318] No matter how sophisticated the model, however, it is only as good as the data used to construct and validate it.

Most of the information in this chapter is derived from retrospective studies that have included relatively few factors. Some of these studies involved large numbers of patients, but most had small to modest sample sizes with relatively short follow-up. Small studies that include patients who have received heterogeneous treatments are unlikely to answer any of the questions about new prognostic factors. Definitive studies of node-negative breast cancer, in which only approximately 30% of patients have a recurrence, must include large numbers of patients who are followed for long periods to evaluate new prognostic factors adequately. Each study has its own particular selection biases, and all the usual precautions concerning the interpretation of retrospective analyses pertain to most of these studies. A particular concern is the lack of multivariate analyses in the evaluation of potential prognostic factors. Many of these factors are related to each other and may in fact be alternative representations of the same biological phenomena. Without adjustments for these statistical correlations, the results of univariate correlative analyses may be misleading. One should always ask whether the new factor adds any information to what can be learned from the standard prognostic factors.

Another problem is lack of standardization of assay methods, scoring systems, and antibodies used to measure new biomarkers. Even though many of the new potential prognostic factors have been evaluated in several studies, few studies have been conducted under standardized conditions that would permit a true validation of previous results. Particularly worrisome is the use of different cutoff points to define assay positivity, especially when these cutoffs are derived from the same patients used to evaluate the new factor. Hilsenbeck et al.[319] demonstrated that performing multiple analyses on the same data set to find the optimal cutoff point for a new prognostic factor results in substantial type I errors. Validation of results on a truly independent, external population of patients using standardized methods is a necessity before any new factor can be considered ready for clinical application.[320] Another area of concern is the frequent violation of assumptions underlying many of the statistical modeling techniques widely used to create prognostic indices. For example, it is becoming clear that the hazard ratios for most prognostic factors change with time,[321–323] a condition that violates a basic assumption of Cox models. More care and creativity is required to create clinically useful prognostic models.

On the one hand, the field of prognostic factors might appear discouraging. Despite the plethora of potential prognostic factors, the list of established factors is short and has been unchanged for more than a decade. On the other hand, many studies have shed new light on the complex system of pathways that regulate human breast cancer. New therapeutic approaches are beginning to evolve that have become possible as a by-product of the search for new biomarkers. The goal of the future is to determine not only which patients should receive adjuvant therapy, but, more importantly, what specific therapy is optimal for each individual patient.

MANAGEMENT SUMMARY

Accurate diagnosis of breast cancer is critical before treatment and management decisions can be made. The diagnosis should clearly differentiate between invasive and noninvasive breast tumors, and it should include a description of the histologic subtype. The prognosis of the patient can then be estimated based on axillary lymph node status, pathologic tumor size, nuclear or histologic grade, and rate of proliferation. ER and PR status can be used to determine the likelihood of response to endocrine therapy. Even if a decision is made not to administer adjuvant endocrine therapy, determination of ER and PR status at the time of diagnosis provides valuable information in the event that the patient subsequently has a recurrence of breast cancer. If trastuzumab (Herceptin) or another anti–HER-2/neu antibody therapy is among the potential treatment options, determination of HER-2/neu status is also recommended.

REFERENCES

1. Consensus conference [No authors]. Adjuvant chemotherapy for breast cancer. *JAMA* 1985;254:3461.
2. Fisher B, Redmond C, Dimitrov NV, et al. A randomized clinical trial evaluating sequential methotrexate and fluorouracil in the treatment of patients with node-negative breast cancer who have estrogen-receptor-negative tumors. *N Engl J Med* 1989;320:473.
3. Fisher B, Constantino J, Redmond C, et al. A randomized clinical trial evaluating tamoxifen in the treatment of patients with node-negative breast cancer who have estrogen-receptor-positive tumors. *N Engl J Med* 1989;320:479.
4. Mansour EG, Gray R, Shatila AH, et al. Efficacy of adjuvant chemotherapy in high-risk node-negative breast cancer: an Intergroup study. *N Engl J Med* 1989;320:485.
5. The Ludwig Breast Cancer Study Group. Prolonged disease-free survival after one course of perioperative adjuvant chemotherapy for node-negative breast cancer. *N Engl J Med* 1989;320:491.
6. Early Breast Cancer Trialists' Collaborative Group. Systemic treatment of early breast cancer by hormonal, cytotoxic, or immune therapy. *Lancet* 1992;339:1.
7. National Institutes of Health Consensus Development Panel. Consensus statement: treatment of early-stage breast cancer. *J Natl Cancer Inst Monographs* 1992;11:1.
8. Clark GM. Do we really need prognostic factors for breast cancer? *Breast Cancer Res Treat* 1994;30:117.
9. McGuire WL. Breast cancer prognostic factors: evaluation guidelines. *J Natl Cancer Inst* 1991;83:154.
10. Gasparini G, Pozza F, Harris AL. Evaluating the potential usefulness of new prognostic and predictive indicators in node-negative breast cancer patients. *J Natl Cancer Inst* 1993;85:1206.
11. Hayes DF, Bast RC, Desch CE, et al. Tumor marker utility grading system: a framework to evaluate clinical utility of tumor markers. *J Natl Cancer Inst* 1996;88:1456.
12. Hayes DF, Trock B, Harris AL. Assessing the clinical impact of prognostic factors: when is "statistically significant" clinically useful? *Breast Cancer Res Treat* 1998;52:305.

13. Fisher ER, Gregorio RM, Fisher B, et al. The pathology of invasive breast cancer. *Cancer* 1975;36:1.
14. Berg JW, Robbins GF. Factors influencing short and long-term survival of breast cancer patients. *Surg Gynecol Obstet* 1966;122:1311.
15. Fisher B, Bauer M, Wickerham DL, et al. Relation of number of positive axillary nodes to the prognosis of patients with primary breast cancer: an NSABP update. *Cancer* 1983;52:1551.
16. Saez RA, McGuire WL, Clark GM. Prognostic factors in breast cancer. *Semin Surg Oncol* 1989;5:102.
17. Mittra I, MacRae KD. A meta-analysis of reported correlations between prognostic factors in breast cancer: does axillary lymph node metastasis represent biology or chronology? *Eur J Cancer* 1991;27:1574.
18. Chadha M, Chabon AB, Friedmann P, et al. Predictors of axillary lymph node metastases in patients with T1 breast cancer: a multivariate analysis. *Cancer* 1994;73:350.
19. Silverstein MJ, Gierson ED, Waisman JR, et al. Axillary lymph node dissection for T1a breast carcinoma. Is it indicated? *Cancer* 1994;73:664.
20. Ravdin PM, De Laurentiis M, Vendely T, et al. Prediction of axillary lymph node status in breast cancer patients by use of prognostic indicators. *J Natl Cancer Inst* 1994;86:1771.
21. Funke I, Schraut W. Meta-analysis of studies on bone marrow micrometastases: an independent prognostic impact remains to be substantiated. *J Clin Oncol* 1998;16:557.
22. Braun S, Pantel K. Prognostic significance of micrometastatic bone marrow involvement. *Breast Cancer Res Treat* 1998;52:201.
23. Carter CL, Allen C, Henson D. Five year survival of breast cancer by histology, tumor size, and extent of axillary lymph node involvement. *Proc 14th Int Cancer Congress* 1986;3:53.
24. Fisher B, Slack NH, Bross IDJ, et al. Cancer of the breast: size of neoplasm and prognosis. *Cancer* 1969;24:1071.
25. Adair F, Berg J, Joubert L, et al. Long-term followup of breast cancer patients: the 30-year report. *Cancer* 1974;33:1145.
26. Nemoto T, Vana J, Bedwani RN, et al. Management and survival of female breast cancer. Results of a national survey by the American College of Surgeons. *Cancer* 1980;45:2917.
27. Koscielny S, Tubiana M, Le MG, et al. Breast cancer: relationship between the size of the primary tumour and the probability of metastatic dissemination. *Br J Cancer* 1984;49:709.
28. Moon TE, Jones SE, Bonadonna G, et al. Development and use of a natural history data base of breast cancer studies. *Am J Clin Oncol* 1987;10:396.
29. Carter CL, Allen C, Henson DE. Relation of tumor size, lymph node status, and survival in 24,740 breast cancer cases. *Cancer* 1989;63:181.
30. Rosen PP, Groshen S, Saigo PE, et al. Pathological prognostic factors in stage I (T1N0M0) and stage II (T1N1M0) breast carcinoma: a study of 644 patients with median follow-up of 18 years. *J Clin Oncol* 1989;7:1239.
31. Rosen PP, Groshen S, Saigo PE, et al. A long-term follow-up study of survival in stage I (T1N0M0) and stage II (T1N1M0) breast carcinoma. *J Clin Oncol* 1989;7:355.
32. McGuire WL, Clark GM. Prognostic factors and treatment decisions in axillary-node-negative breast cancer. *N Engl J Med* 1992;326:1756.
33. Fisher B, Redmond C, Wickerham DL, et al. Systemic therapy in patients with node-negative breast cancer. *Ann Int Med* 1989;111:703.
34. Delides GS, Garas G, Georgouli G, et al. Intralaboratory variations in the grading of breast carcinoma. *Arch Pathol Lab Med* 1982;106:126.
35. Gilchrist KW, Kalish L, Gould VE, et al. Interobserver reproducibility of histopathological features in stage II breast cancer: an ECOG study. *Breast Cancer Res Treat* 1985;5:3.
36. Theissig F, Kunze KD, Haroske G, et al. Histological grading of breast cancer. Interobserver, reproducibility and prognostic significance. *Path Res Pract* 1990;186:732.
37. Harvey JM, de Klerk NH, Sterrett GF. Histological grading in breast cancer: interobserver agreement, and relation to other prognostic factors including ploidy. *Pathology* 1992;24:63.
38. Dalton LW, Page DL, Dupont WD. Histologic grading of breast carcinoma. A reproducibility study. *Cancer* 1994;73:2765.
39. Bloom HJG, Richardson WW. Histological grading and prognosis in breast cancer: a study of 1409 cases of which 359 have been followed for 15 years. *Br J Cancer* 1957;11:359.
40. Scarff RW, Torioni H. Histological typing of breast tumors. In: *International histological classification of tumors*, no. 2. Geneva, Switzerland: World Health Organization, 1968:13–20.
41. Fisher ER, Redmond C, Fisher B. Histologic grading of breast cancer. *Pathol Ann* 1980;15:239.
42. le Doussal V, Tubiana-Hulin M, Friedman S, et al. Prognostic value of histologic grade nuclear components of Scarff-Bloom-Richardson (SBR): an improved score modification based on a multivariate analysis of 1262 invasive ductal breast carcinomas. *Cancer* 1989;64:1914.
43. Davis BW, Gelber RD, Goldhirsch A, et al. Prognostic significance of tumor grade in clinical trials of adjuvant therapy for breast cancer with axillary lymph node metastasis. *Cancer* 1986;58:2662.
44. Contesso G, Mouriesse H, Friedman S, et al. The importance of histologic grade in long-term prognosis of breast cancer: a study of 1,010 patients, uniformly treated at the Institut Gustave-Roussy. *J Clin Oncol* 1987;5:1378.
45. Rank F, Dombernowsky P, Jespersen NCB, et al. Histologic malignancy grading of invasive ductal breast carcinoma: a regression analysis of prognostic factors in low-risk carcinomas from a multicenter trial. *Cancer* 1987;60:1299.
46. le Doussal V, Tubiana-Hulin M, Hacène K, et al. Nuclear characteristics as indicators of prognosis in node negative breast cancer patients. *Breast Cancer Res Treat* 1989;14:207.
47. Fisher B, Redmond C, Fisher ER, et al. Relative worth of estrogen or progesterone receptor and pathologic characteristics of differentiation as indicators of prognosis in node negative breast cancer patients: findings from National Surgical Adjuvant Breast and Bowel Project Protocol B-06. *J Clin Oncol* 1988;6:1076.
48. Chevallier B, Mosseri V, Dauce JP, et al. A prognostic score in histological node negative breast cancer. *Br J Cancer* 1989;61:436.
49. Elston CW, Ellis IO. Pathological prognostic factors in breast cancer. I. The value of histological grade in breast cancer: experience from a large study with long-term follow-up. *Histopathology* 1991;19:403.
50. Dawson AE, Austin RE Jr, Weinberg DS. Nuclear grading of breast carcinoma by image analysis. Classification by multivariate and neural network analysis. *Am J Clin Pathol* 1991;95[Suppl 1]:S29.
51. Henson DE, Ries L, Freedman LS, et al. Relationship among outcome, stage of disease, and histologic grade for 22,616 cases of breast cancer. The basis for a prognostic index. *Cancer* 1991;68:2142.
52. Schumacher M, Schmoor C, Sauerbrei W, et al. The prognostic effect of histological tumor grade in node-negative breast cancer patients. *Breast Cancer Res Treat* 1993;25:235.
53. Henson DE. The histological grading of neoplasms. *Arch Pathol Lab Med* 1988;112:1091.
54. Crosby CH, Barclay THC. Carcinoma of the breast: surgical management of patients with special conditions. *Cancer* 1971;28:1628.
55. Stoll BA. Does the malignancy of breast cancer vary with age? *Clin Oncol* 1976;2:73.
56. Ribeiro GG, Swindell R. The prognosis of breast carcinoma in women aged less than 40 years. *Clin Radiol* 1981;32:231.
57. Noyes RD, Spanos WJ Jr, Montague ED. Breast cancer in women aged 30 and under. *Cancer* 1982;49:1302.
58. Adami H-O, Malker B, Meirik O, et al. Age as a prognostic factor in breast cancer. *Cancer* 1985;56:898.
59. Host H, Lund E. Age as a prognostic factor in breast cancer. *Cancer* 1986;57:2217.
60. de la Rochefordiere A, Asselain B, Campana F, et al. Age as prognostic factor in premenopausal breast carcinoma. *Lancet* 1993;341:1039.
61. Fowble BL, Schultz DJ, Overmoyer B, et al. The influence of young age on outcome in early stage breast cancer. *Int J Radiation Oncology Biol Phys* 1994;30:23.
62. Nixon AJ, Neuberg D, Hayes DF, et al. Relationship of patient age to pathologic features of the tumor and prognosis for patients with stage I or II breast cancer. *J Clin Oncol* 1994;12:888.
63. Albain KS, Allred DC, Clark GM. Breast cancer outcome and predictors of outcome: are there age differentials? *J Natl Cancer Inst Mongr* 1994;16:35.
64. Hakama M, Riihimäki H. End results of breast cancer patients in Finland 1953–1968. *Ann Clin Res* 1974;6:115.
65. Langlands AO, Pocock SJ, Kerr GR, et al. Long-term survival of patients with breast cancer: a study of the curability of the disease. *BMJ* 1979;2:1247.
66. Rutqvist LE, Wallgren A. The influence of age on outcome in breast carcinoma. *Acta Radiol Oncol* 1983;22:289.
67. Mueller CB, Ames F, Anderson GD. Breast cancer in 3,558 women: age as a significant determinant in the rate of dying and causes of death. *Surgery* 1978;83:123.
68. Cutler SJ, Axtell LM, Schottenfeld D. Adjustment of long-term survival rates for deaths due to intercurrent disease. *J Chron Dis* 1969;22:485.

69. Wallgren A, Silfverswärd C, Hultborn A. Carcinoma of the breast in women under 30 years of age: a clinical and histopathological study of all cases reported as carcinoma to the Swedish Cancer Registry 1958–1968. *Cancer* 1977;40:916.
70. Hibberd AD, Horwood LJ, Wells JE. Long term prognosis of women with breast cancer in New Zealand: study of survival to 30 years. *BMJ* 1983;286:1777.
71. Miki Y, Swensen J, Shattuck-Eidens D, et al. A strong candidate for the breast and ovarian cancer susceptibility gene BRCA-1. *Science* 1994;266:66.
72. Futreal PA, Liu Q, Shattuck-Eidens D, et al. BRCA1 mutations in primary breast and ovarian carcinomas. *Science* 1994;266:120.
73. Wooster R, Neuhausen SL, Mangion J, et al. Localization of a breast cancer susceptibility gene, BRCA2, to chromosome 13q12-13. *Science* 1994;265:2088.
74. Rubens RD. Age and the treatment of breast cancer. *J Clin Oncol* 1993;11:3.
75. Freeman HP, Wasfie TJ. Cancer of the breast in poor black women. *Cancer* 1989;63:2562.
76. Bain RP, Greenberg RS, Whitaker JP. Racial differences in survival of women with breast cancer. *J Chron Dis* 1986;39:631.
77. Westbrook KC, Brown BW, McBride CM. Breast cancer: a critical review of a patient sample with a ten-year follow-up. *South Med J* 1975;68:543.
78. National Cancer Institute. Five-year relative survival rates by primary site and racial/ethnic group, SEER Program, 1973–81. In: *Cancer among blacks and other minorities statistical profiles.* DHEW Publ No. (NCI) 86-278S. Bethesda: National Cancer Institute, 1986.
79. Daly MB, Clark GM, McGuire WL. Breast cancer prognosis in a mixed Caucasian-Hispanic population. *J Natl Cancer Inst* 1985;74:753.
80. Elledge RM, Clark GM, Chamness GC, et al. Tumor biologic factors and breast cancer prognosis among white, Hispanic and black women in the United States. *J Natl Cancer Inst* 1994;86:705.
81. Swanson GM, Ragheb NE, Lin C-S, et al. Breast cancer among black and white women in the 1980s. *Cancer* 1993;72:788.
82. Pierce L, Fowble B, Solin LJ, et al. Conservative surgery and radiation therapy in black women with early stage breast cancer. Patterns of failure and analysis of outcome. *Cancer* 1992;69:2831.
83. National Cancer Institute. *Annual cancer statistics review, including cancer trends: 1950–1985.* Washington, DC: U.S. Govt Printing Office, 1988.
84. Vernon SW, Tilley BC, Neale AV, et al. Ethnicity, survival, and delay in seeking treatment for symptoms of breast cancer. *Cancer* 1985; 55:1563.
85. Gordon NH, Crowe JP, Brumberg DJ, et al. Socioeconomic factors and race in breast cancer recurrence and survival. *Am J Epidemiol* 1992;135:609.
86. Coates RJ, Bransfield DD, Wesley M, et al. Differences between black and white women with breast cancer in time from symptom recognition to medical consultation. *J Natl Cancer Inst* 1992;84:938.
87. Baak JPA. Mitosis counting in tumors. *Hum Pathol* 1990;21:683.
88. van Diest PJ, Baak JPA, Matze-Cok P, et al. Reproducibility of mitosis counting in 2,469 breast cancer specimens: results from the Multicenter Morphometric Mammary Carcinoma Project. *Hum Pathol* 1992;23:603.
89. Russo J, Frederick J, Ownby HE, et al. Predictors of recurrence and survival of patients with breast cancer. *Am J Clin Pathol* 1987;88:123.
90. Clayton F. Pathologic correlates of survival in 378 lymph node-negative infiltrating ductal breast carcinomas. Mitotic count is the best single predictor. *Cancer* 1991;68:1309.
91. Aaltomaa S, Lipponen P, Eskelinen M, et al. Predictive value of a morphometric prognostic index in female breast cancer. *Oncology* 1993;50:57.
92. Galea MH, Blamey RW, Elston CE, et al. The Nottingham Prognostic Index in primary breast cancer. *Breast Cancer Res Treat* 1992;22:207.
93. van der Linden JC, Lindeman J, Baak JPA, et al. The Multivariate Prognostic Index and nuclear DNA content are independent prognostic factors in primary breast cancer patients. *Cytometry* 1989;10:56.
94. Silvestrini R. Cell kinetics: prognostic and therapeutic implications in human tumours. *Cell Prolif* 1994;27:579.
95. Héry M, Gioanni J, Lalanne C-M, et al. The DNA labelling index: a prognostic factor in node-negative breast cancer. *Breast Cancer Res Treat* 1987;9:207.
96. Meyer JS, Province M. Proliferative index of breast carcinoma by thymidine labeling: prognostic power independent of stage, estrogen and progesterone receptors. *Breast Cancer Res Treat* 1988;12:191.
97. Silvestrini R, Daidone MG, Valagussa P, et al. Cell kinetics as a prognostic indicator in node-negative breast cancer. *Eur J Cancer Clin Oncol* 1989;25:1165.
98. Tubiana M, Pejovic MH, Koscielny S, et al. Growth rate, kinetics of tumor cell proliferation and long-term outcome in human breast cancer. *Int J Cancer* 1989;44:17.
99. Courdi A, Héry M, Dahan E, et al. Factors affecting relapse in node-negative breast cancer. A multivariate analysis including the labeling index. *Eur J Clin Oncol* 1989;25:351.
100. Cooke TG, Stanton PD, Winstanley J, et al. Long-term prognostic significance of thymidine labelling index in primary breast cancer. *Eur J Cancer* 1992;28:424.
101. Silvestrini R, Daidone MG, Del Bino G, et al. Prognostic significance of proliferative activity and ploidy in node-negative breast cancers. *Ann Oncol* 1993;4:213.
102. Silvestrini R. Feasibility and reproducibility of the [3H]-thymidine labelling index in breast cancer. *Cell Prolif* 1991;24:437.
103. Zambetti M, Bonadonna G, Valagussa P, et al. Adjuvant CMF for node-negative and estrogen receptor-negative breast cancer patients. *J Natl Cancer Inst Monogr* 1992;11:77.
104. Daidone MG, Silvestrini R, Valentinis B, et al. Changes in cell kinetics induced by primary chemotherapy in breast cancer. *Int J Cancer* 1991;47:380.
105. Amadori D, Volpi A, Maltoni R, et al. Cell proliferation as a predictor of response to chemotherapy in metastatic breast cancer: a prospective study. *Breast Cancer Res Treat* 1997;43:7.
106. Wenger CR, Beardslee S, Owens MA, et al. DNA ploidy, S-phase, and steroid receptors in more than 127,000 breast cancer patients. *Breast Cancer Res Treat* 1993;28:9.
107. Hedley DW, Clark GM, Cornelisse CJ, et al. Consensus review of the clinical utility of DNA cytometry in carcinoma of the breast. *Cytometry* 1993;14:482.
108. Wenger CR, Clark GM. S-phase fraction and breast cancer, a decade of experience. *Breast Cancer Res* 1998;51:255.
109. Herman CJ, Duque RE, Hedley D, et al. DNA cytometry in cancer prognosis. *Prin Pract Oncol PPO Updates* 1993;7:1.
110. Remvikos Y, Beuzeboc P, Zajdela A, et al. Correlation of pretreatment proliferative activity of breast cancer with the response to cytotoxic chemotherapy. *J Natl Cancer Inst* 1989;81:1383.
111. Dressler LG, Eudey L, Gray R, et al. Prognostic potential of DNA flow cytometry measurement in node-negative breast cancer patients: preliminary analysis of an Intergroup study (INT0076). *J Natl Cancer Inst Monogr* 1992;11:167.
112. Muss HB, Thor AD, Berry DA, et al. c-erbB-2 expression and response to adjuvant therapy in women with node-positive early breast cancer. *N Engl J Med* 1994;330:1260.
113. Gerdes J, Schwab U, Lemke H, et al. Production of mouse monoclonal antibody reactive with a human nuclear antigen associated with cell proliferation. *Int J Cancer* 1983;31:13.
114. Key G, Petersen JL, Becker MHG, et al. New antiserum against Ki-67 antigen suitable for double immunostaining of paraffin wax sections. *J Clin Pathol* 1993;46:1080.
115. Cattoretti G, Becker MHG, Key G, et al. Monoclonal antibodies against recombinant parts of the Ki-67 antigen (MIB1 and MIB3) detect proliferating cells in microwave-processed formalin-fixed paraffin sections. *J Pathol* 1992;168:357.
116. Charpin C, Andrac L, Vacheret H, et al. Multiparametric evaluation (SAMBA) of growth fraction (monoclonal Ki67) in breast carcinoma tissue sections. *Cancer Res* 1988;48:4368.
117. Walker RA, Camplejohn RS. Comparison of monoclonal antibody Ki-67 reactivity with grade and DNA flow cytometry of breast carcinomas. *Br J Cancer* 1988;57:281.
118. Gasparini G, Dal Fior S, Pozza F, et al. Correlation of growth fraction by Ki-67 immunohistochemistry with histologic factors and hormone receptors in operable breast carcinoma. *Breast Cancer Res Treat* 1989;14:329.
119. Brown RW, Allred DC, Clark GM, et al. Prognostic significance and clinical-pathological correlations of cell-cycle kinetics measured by Ki-67 immunocytochemistry in axillary node-negative carcinoma of the breast. *Breast Cancer Res Treat* 1990;16:192(abst).
120. Gerdes J, Lemke H, Baisch H, et al. Cell cycle analysis of a cell proliferation-associated human nuclear antigen defined by the monoclonal antibody Ki-67. *J Immunol* 1984;133:1710.
121. Kamel OW, Franklin WA, Ringus JC, et al. Thymidine labeling index and Ki-67 growth fraction in lesions of the breast. *Am J Pathol* 1989;134:107.

122. Rudas M, Gnant MF, Mittlböck M, et al. Thymidine labeling index and Ki-67 growth fraction in breast cancer: comparison and correlation with prognosis. *Breast Cancer Res Treat* 1994;32:165.
123. Leonardi E, Girlando S, Serio G, et al. PCNA and Ki67 expression in breast carcinoma: correlations with clinical and biological variables. *J Clin Pathol* 1992;45:416.
124. Sullivan RP, Mortimer G, Muircheartaigh IO. Cell proliferation in breast tumours: analysis of histological parameters Ki67 and PCNA expression. *Ir J Med Sci* 1993;162:343.
125. Gasparini G, Boracchi P, Verderio P, et al. Cell kinetics in human breast cancer: comparison between the prognostic value of the cytofluorimetric S-phase fraction and that of the antibodies to Ki-67 and PCNA antigens detected by immunocytochemistry. *Int J Cancer* 1994;57:822.
126. Keshgegian AA, Cnaan A. Proliferation markers in breast carcinoma. Mitotic figure count, S-phase fraction, proliferating cell nuclear antigen, Ki-67 and MIB-1. *Am J Clin Pathol* 1995;104:42.
127. Ellis PA, Makris A, Burton SA, et al. Comparison of MIB-1 proliferation index with S-phase fraction in human breast carcinomas. *Br J Cancer* 1996;73:640.
128. MacGrogan G, Jollet I, Huet S, et al. Comparison of quantitative and semiquantitative methods of assessing MIB-1 with the S-phase fraction in breast carcinoma. *Mod Pathol* 1997;10:769.
129. Vielh P, Chevillard S, Mosseri V, et al. Ki67 index and S-phase fraction in human breast carcinomas. Comparison and correlations with prognostic factors. *Am J Clin Pathol* 1990;94:681.
130. Brown RW, Allred DC, Clark GM, et al. Prognostic value of Ki-67 compared to S-phase fraction in axillary node-negative breast cancer. *Clin Cancer Res* 1996;2:585.
131. Dettmar P, Harbeck N, Thomssen C, et al. Prognostic impact of proliferation-associated factors MIB1 (Ki-67) and S-phase in node-negative breast cancer. *Br J Cancer* 1997;75:1525.
132. Bouzubar N, Walker KJ, Griffiths K, et al. Ki67 immunostaining in primary breast cancer: pathological and clinical associations. *Br J Cancer* 1989;59:943.
133. Weikel W, Beck T, Mitze M, et al. Immunohistochemical evaluation of growth fractions in human breast cancers using monoclonal antibody Ki-67. *Breast Cancer Res Treat* 1991;18:149.
134. Wintzer H-O, Zipfel I, Schulte-Mönting J, et al. Ki-67 immunostaining in human breast tumors and its relationship to prognosis. *Cancer* 1991;67:421.
135. Sahin AA, Ro J, Ro JY, et al. Ki-67 immunostaining in node-negative stage I/II breast carcinoma. Significant correlation with prognosis. *Cancer* 1991;68:549.
136. Gasparini G, Pozza F, Bevilacqua P, et al. Growth fraction (Ki-67 antibody) determination in early-stage breast carcinoma: histologic, clinical and prognostic correlations. *Breast* 1992;1:92.
137. Gottardi O, Scanzi F, Zurrida S, et al. Clinical and prognostic usefulness of immunohistochemical determination of Ki67 in early breast cancer. *Breast* 1993;2:33.
138. Veronese SM, Gambacorta M, Gottardi O, et al. Proliferation index as a prognostic marker in breast cancer. *Cancer* 1993;71:3926.
139. Railo M, Nordling S, von Boguslawsky K, et al. Prognostic value of Ki-67 immunolabelling in primary operable breast cancer. *Br J Cancer* 1993;68:579.
140. Gaglia P, Bernardi A, Venesio T, et al. Cell proliferation of breast cancer evaluated by anti-BrdU and anti-Ki-67 antibodies: its prognostic value on short-term recurrences. *Eur J Cancer* 1993;29A :1509.
141. Bianchi S, Paglierani M, Zampi G, et al. Prognostic value of proliferating cell nuclear antigen in lymph node–negative breast cancer patients. *Cancer* 1993;72:120.
142. Thomas M, Noguchi M, Kitagawa H, et al. Poor prognostic value of proliferating cell nuclear antigen labelling index in breast carcinoma. *J Clin Pathol* 1993;46:525.
143. Cummings MC, Furnival CM, Parsons PG, et al. PCNA immunostaining in breast cancer. *Aust N Z J Surg* 1993;63:630.
144. Aaltomaa S, Lipponen P, Syrjänen K. Proliferating cell nuclear antigen (PCNA) immunolabeling as a prognostic factor in axillary lymph node negative breast cancer. *Anticancer Res* 1993;13:533.
145. Rose DSC, Maddox PH, Brown DC. Which proliferation markers for routine immunohistology? A comparison of five antibodies. *J Clin Pathol* 1994;47:1010.
146. Clark GM, Allred DC, Hilsenbeck SG, et al. Mitosin (a new proliferation marker) correlates with clinical outcome in node-negative breast cancer. *Cancer Res* 1997;57:5505.
147. Knight WAI, Livingston RB, Gregory EJ, et al. Estrogen receptor as an independent prognostic factor for early recurrence in breast cancer. *Cancer Res* 1977;37:4669.
148. Clark GM, McGuire WL. Steroid receptors and other prognostic factors in primary breast cancer. *Semin Oncol* 1988;15:20.
149. Horowitz KB, McGuire WL, Pearson OH, et al. Predicting response to endocrine therapy in human breast cancer: a hypothesis. *Science* 1975;189:726.
150. Adami H-O, Graffman S, Lindgren A, et al. Prognostic implication of estrogen receptor content in breast cancer. *Breast Cancer Res Treat* 1985;5:293.
151. Mason BH, Holdaway IM, Mullins PR, et al. Progesterone and estrogen receptors as prognostic variables in breast cancer. *Cancer Res* 1983;43:2985.
152. Clark GM, Osborne CK, McGuire WL. Correlations between estrogen receptor, progesterone receptor, and patient characteristics in human breast cancer. *J Clin Oncol* 1984;2:1102.
153. Thorpe SM, Christensen IJ, Rasmussen BB, et al. Short recurrence-free survival associated with high oestrogen receptor levels in the natural history of postmenopausal, primary breast cancer. *Eur J Cancer* 1993;29A:971.
154. Kinsel LB, Szabo E, Greene GL, et al. Immunocytochemical analysis of estrogen receptors as a predictor of prognosis in breast cancer patients: comparison with quantitative biochemical methods. *Cancer Res* 1989;49:1052.
155. Berger U, Wilson P, Thethi S, et al. Comparison of an immunocytochemical assay for progesterone receptor with a biochemical method of measurement and immunocytochemical examination of the relationship between progesterone and estrogen receptors. *Cancer Res* 1989;49:5176.
156. Foekens JA, Portengen H, van Putten WLJ, et al. Prognostic value of estrogen and progesterone receptors measured by enzyme immunoassays in human breast tumor cytosols. *Cancer Res* 1989;49:5823.
157. Andersen J, Thorpe SM, King WJ, et al. The prognostic value of immunohistochemical estrogen receptor analysis in paraffin-embedded and frozen sections versus that of steroid-binding assays. *Eur J Cancer* 1990;26:442.
158. Harvey JM, Clark GM, Osborne CK, et al. Estrogen receptor status by immunohistochemistry is superior to ligand binding assay for predicting response to adjuvant endocrine therapy in breast cancer. *J Clin Oncol* 1999 (*in press*).
159. Masiakowski P, Breathnach R, Bloch J, et al. Cloning of cDNA sequences of hormone-regulated genes from the MCF-7 human breast cancer cell line. *Nucleic Acids Res* 1982;10:7895.
160. Rio MC, Bellocq JP, Daniel JY, et al. Breast cancer-associated pS2 protein: synthesis and secretion by normal stomach mucosa. *Science* 1988;241:705.
161. Jakowlew SB, Breathnach R, Jeltsch J-M, et al. Sequence of the pS2 mRNA induced by estrogen in the human breast cancer cell line MCF-7. *Nucleic Acids Res* 1984;12:2861.
162. Foekens JA, Rio M-C, Seguin P, et al. Prediction of relapse and survival in breast cancer patients by pS2 protein status. *Cancer Res* 1990;50:3832.
163. Predine J, Spyratos F, Prud'homme JF, et al. Enzyme-linked immunosorbent assay of pS2 in breast cancers, benign tumors, and normal breast tissues. *Cancer* 1992;69:2116.
164. Gion M, Mione R, Pappagallo GL, et al. PS2 in breast cancer—alternative or complementary tool to steroid receptor status? Evaluation of 446 cases. *Br J Cancer* 1993;68:374.
165. Spyratos F, Andrieu C, Hacène K, et al. pS2 and response to adjuvant hormone therapy in primary breast cancer. *Br J Cancer* 1994;68:394.
166. Henry JA, Piggott NH, Mallick UK, et al. pNR-2/pS2 immunohistochemical staining in breast cancer: correlation with prognostic factors and endocrine response. *Br J Cancer* 1991;63:615.
167. Thor AD, Koerner FC, Edgerton SM, et al. pS2 expression in primary breast carcinomas: relationship to clinical and histological features and survival. *Breast Cancer Res Treat* 1992;21:111.
168. Cappelletti V, Coradini D, Scanziani E, et al. Prognostic relevance of pS2 status in association with steroid receptor status and proliferative activity in node-negative breast cancer. *Eur J Cancer* 1992;28A:1315.
169. Soubeyran I, Wafflart J, Bonichon F, et al. Immunohistochemical determination of pS2 in invasive breast carcinomas: a study on 942 cases. *Breast Cancer Res Treat* 1995;34:119.
170. Ciocca DR, Oesterreich S, Chamness GC, et al. Biological and clinical implications of heat shock protein 27000 (Hsp27): a review. *J Natl Cancer Inst* 1993;85:1558.

171. Chamness GC, Ruiz A, Fulcher L, et al. Estrogen-inducible heat shock protein hsp27 predicts recurrence in node negative breast cancer. *Proc Am Assoc Cancer Res* 1989;30:252(abst).
172. Tandon AK, Clark GM, Chamness GC, et al. Clinical significance of heat-shock/stress-response proteins in breast cancer. *Breast Cancer Res Treat* 1990;16:146(abst).
173. Ciocca DR, Clark GM, Tandon AK, et al. Heat shock protein hsp70 in patients with axillary lymph node-negative breast cancer: prognostic implications. *J Natl Cancer Inst* 1993;85:570.
174. Thor A, Benz C, Moore DI, et al. Stress response protein (srp-27) determination in primary human breast carcinomas: clinical, histologic, and prognostic correlations. *J Natl Cancer Inst* 1991;83:170.
175. Love S, King RJB. A 27 kDa heat shock protein that has anomalous prognostic powers in early and advanced breast cancer. *Br J Cancer* 1994;69:743.
176. Ciocca DR, Fuqua SAW, Lock-Lim S, et al. Response of human breast cancer cells to heat shock and chemotherapeutic drugs. *Cancer Res* 1992;52:3648.
177. Oesterreich S, Weng C-N, Qiu M, et al. The small heat shock protein hsp27 is correlated with growth and drug resistance in human breast cancer cell lines. *Cancer Res* 1993;53:4443.
178. Rajkumar T, Gullick WJ. The Type I growth factor receptors in human breast cancer. *Breast Cancer Res Treat* 1994;29:3.
179. Travis A, Pinder SE, Robertson JFR, et al. C-erbB-3 in human breast carcinoma: expression and relation to prognosis and established prognostic indicators. *Br J Cancer* 1996;74:229.
180. Klijn JGM, Berns PMJJ, Schmitz PIM, et al. The clinical significance of epidermal growth factor receptor (EGF-R) in human breast cancer: a review on 5232 patients. *Endocr Rev* 1992;13:3.
181. Klijn JGM, Berns PMJJ, Schmitz PIM, et al. Epidermal growth factor receptor (EGF-R) in clinical breast cancer: update 1993. *Endocr Rev* 1993;1:171.
182. Fox SB, Smith K, Hollyer J, et al. The epidermal growth factor receptor as a prognostic marker: results of 370 patients and review of 3009 patients. *Breast Cancer Res Treat* 1994;29:41.
183. Nicholson RI, McClelland RA, Gee JMW, et al. Epidermal growth factor receptor expression in breast cancer: association with response to endocrine therapy. *Breast Cancer Res Treat* 1994;29:117.
184. Baselga J, Mendelsohn J. The epidermal growth factor receptor as a target for therapy in breast carcinoma. *Breast Cancer Res Treat* 1994;29:127.
185. Slamon DJ, Clark GM, Wong SG, et al. Human breast cancer: correlation of relapse and survival with amplification of the HER-2/neu oncogene. *Science* 1987;235:177.
186. Ravdin PM, Chamness GC. The c-erbB-2 proto-oncogene as a prognostic and predictive marker in breast cancer: a paradigm for the development of other macromolecular markers—a review. *Gene* 1995;159:19.
187. Ali IU, Campbell G, Lidereau R, et al. Lack of evidence for the prognostic significance of c-erbB-2 amplification. *Oncogene Res* 1988;3:139.
188. Slamon DJ, Godolphin W, Jones LA, et al. Studies of the HER-2/neu proto-oncogene in human breast and ovarian cancer. *Science* 1989;244:707.
189. Tsuda H, Hirohashi S, Shimosato Y, et al. Immunohistochemical study on overexpression of c-erbB-2 protein in human breast cancer: its correlation with gene amplification and long-term survival of patients. *Jap J Cancer Res* 1990;81:327.
190. Borg Å, Tandon AK, Sigurdsson H, et al. HER-2/neu amplification predicts poor survival in node-positive breast cancer. *Cancer Res* 1990;50:4332.
191. Winstanley J, Cooke T, Murray GD, et al. The long term prognostic significance of c-erbB-2 in primary breast cancer. *Br J Cancer* 1991;63:447.
192. Paterson MC, Dietrich KD, Danyluk J, et al. Correlation between c-erbB-2 amplification and risk of recurrent disease in node-negative breast cancer. *Cancer Res* 1991;51:556.
193. Clark GM, McGuire WL. Follow-up study of HER-2/neu amplification in primary breast cancer. *Cancer Res* 1991;51:944.
194. Berns EMJJ, Klijn JGM, van Putten WLJ, et al. c-myc amplification is a better prognostic factor than HER2/neu amplification in primary breast cancer. *Cancer Res* 1992;52:1107.
195. Press MF, Pike MC, Chazin VR, et al. Her-2/neu expression in node-negative breast cancer: direct tissue quantitation by computerized image analysis and association of overexpression with increased risk of recurrent disease. *Cancer Res* 1993;53:4960.
196. Thor AD, Schwartz LH, Koerner FC, et al. Analysis of c-erbB-2 expression in breast carcinomas with clinical follow-up. *Cancer Res* 1989;49:7147.
197. Ciocca DR, Fujimura FK, Tandon AK, et al. Correlation of HER-2/neu amplification with expression and with other prognostic factors in 1103 breast cancers. *J Natl Cancer Inst* 1992;84:1279.
198. Molina R, Ciocca DR, Tandon AK, et al. Expression of HER-2/neu oncoprotein in human breast cancer: a comparison of immunohistochemical and western blot techniques. *Anticancer Res* 1992;12:1965.
199. Lovekin C, Ellis IO, Locker A, et al. c-erbB-2 oncoprotein expression in primary and advanced breast cancer. *Br J Cancer* 1991;63:439.
200. McCann AH, Dervan PA, O'Regan M, et al. Prognostic significance of c-erbB-2 and estrogen receptor status in human breast cancer. *Cancer Res* 1991;51:3296.
201. Kallioniemi O-P, Holli K, Visakorpi T, et al. Association of c-erbB-2 protein over-expression with high rate of cell proliferation, increased risk of visceral metastasis and poor long-term survival in breast cancer. *Int J Cancer* 1991;49:650.
202. Tanner B, Friedberg T, Mitze M, et al. C-erbB-2-oncogene expression in breast carcinoma: analysis by S1 nuclease protection assay and immunohistochemistry in relation to clinical parameters. *Gynecol Oncol* 1992;47:228.
203. Yuan J, Hennessy C, Givan AL, et al. Predicting outcome for patients with node negative breast cancer: a comparative study of the value of flow cytometry and cell image analysis for determination of DNA ploidy. *Br J Cancer* 1992;65:461.
204. Allred DC, Clark GM, Tandon AK, et al. HER-2/neu in node-negative breast cancer: prognostic significance of overexpression influenced by the presence of in situ carcinoma. *J Clin Oncol* 1992;10:599.
205. Noguchi M, Koyasaki N, Ohta N, et al. C-erbB-2 oncoprotein expression versus internal mammary lymph node metastases as additional prognostic factors in patients with axillary lymph node-positive breast cancer. *Cancer* 1992;69:2953.
206. Gusterson BA, Gelber RD, Goldhirsch A, et al. Prognostic importance of c-erbB-2 expression in breast cancer. International (Ludwig) Breast Cancer Study Group. *J Clin Oncol* 1992;10:1049.
207. Press MF, Hung G, Godolphin W, et al. Sensitivity of HER-2/neu antibodies in archival tissue samples: potential source of error in immunohistochemical studies of oncogene expression. *Cancer Res* 1994; 54:2771.
208. Bianchi S, Paglierani M, Zampi G, et al. Prognostic significance of c-erbB-2 expression in node negative breast cancer. *Br J Cancer* 1993; 67:625.
209. Thor AD, Berry DA, Budman DR, et al. erbB-2, p53, and efficacy of adjuvant therapy in lymph node-positive breast cancer. *J Natl Cancer Inst* 1998;90:1346.
210. Paik S, Bryant J, Park C, et al. erbB-2 and response to doxorubicin in patients with axillary lymph node-positive, hormone receptor-negative breast cancer. *J Natl Cancer Inst* 1998;90:1361.
211. Ravdin PM, Green S, Albain KS, et al. Initial report of the SWOG biological correlative study of c-erbB-2 expression as a predictor of outcome in a trial comparing adjuvant CAF T with tamoxifen (T) alone. *Proc Am Soc Clin Oncol* 1998;17:97a(abst).
212. Clark GM. Should selection of adjuvant chemotherapy for patients with breast cancer be based on erbB-2 status? [Editorial] *J Natl Cancer Inst* 1998;90:1320.
213. De Placido S, Carlomagno C, De Laurentiis M, et al. C-erbB2 expression predicts tamoxifen efficacy in breast cancer patients. *Breast Cancer Res Treat* 1998;52:55.
214. Nicholson S, Wright C, Sainsbury JC, et al. Epidermal growth factor receptor (EGFr) as a marker for poor prognosis in node-negative breast cancer patients: neu and tamoxifen failure. *J Steroid Biochem Mol Biol* 1990;37:811.
215. Klijn JGM, Berns EMJJ, Bontenbal M, et al. Cell biological factors associated with the response of breast cancer to systemic treatment. *Cancer Treat Rev* 1993;19[Suppl B]:45.
216. Berns EMJJ, Foekens JA, van Staveren IL, et al. Oncogene amplification and prognosis in breast cancer: relationship with systemic treatment. *Gene* 1995;159:11.
217. Wright C, Nicholson S, Angus B, et al. Relationship between c-erbB-2 protein product expression and response to endocrine therapy in advanced breast cancer. *Br J Cancer* 1992;65:118.
218. Elledge RM, Green S, Ciocca D, et al. HER-2 expression and response to tamoxifen in estrogen receptor-positive breast cancer: a Southwest Oncology Group study. *Clin Cancer Res* 1998;4:7.
219. Yamauchi H, O'Neill A, Gelman R, et al. Prediction of response to antiestrogen therapy in advanced breast cancer patients by pretreatment circulating levels of extracellular domain of the HER-2/c-neu protein. *J Clin Oncol* 1997;15:2518.
220. Leitzel K, Teramoto Y, Konrad K, et al. Elevated serum c-erbB2 antigen levels and decreased response to hormone therapy of breast cancer. *J Clin Oncol* 1995;13:1129.

221. Borg Å, Baldetorp B, Fernö M, et al. ERBB2 amplification is associated with tamoxifen resistance in steroid-receptor positive breast cancer. *Cancer Lett* 1994;81:137.
222. Têtu B, Brisson J. Prognostic significance of HER-2/neu oncoprotein expression in node-positive breast cancer. The influence of the pattern of immunostaining and adjuvant therapy. *Cancer* 1994;73:2359.
223. Carlomagno C, Perrone F, Gallo C, et al. C-erbB2 overexpression decreases the benefit of adjuvant tamoxifen in early stage breast cancer without axillary lymph node metastases. *J Clin Oncol* 1996;14:2702.
224. Sjögren S, Inganäs M, Lindgren A, et al. Prognostic and predictive value of c-erbB-2 overexpression in primary breast cancer, alone and in combination with other prognostic markers. *J Clin Oncol* 1998;16:462.
225. Hollstein M, Sidransky D, Vogelstein B, et al. p53 mutations in human cancers. *Science* 1991;253:49.
226. Sjögren S, Inganäs M, Norberg T, et al. The p53 gene in breast cancer: prognostic value of complementary DNA sequencing versus immunohistochemistry. *J Natl Cancer Inst* 1996;88:173.
227. Elledge RM, Fuqua SAW, Clark GM, et al. The role and prognostic significance of p53 gene alterations in breast cancer. *Breast Cancer Res Treat* 1993;27:95.
228. Thor AD, Moore DHI, Edgerton SM, et al. Accumulation of p53 tumor suppressor gene protein: an independent marker of prognosis in breast cancers. *J Natl Cancer Inst* 1992;84:845.
229. Isola J, Visakorpi T, Holli K, et al. Association of overexpression of tumor suppressor protein p53 with rapid cell proliferation and poor prognosis in node-negative breast cancer patients. *J Natl Cancer Inst* 1992;84:1109.
230. Allred DC, Clark GM, Elledge R, et al. Association of p53 protein expression with tumor cell proliferation rate and clinical outcome in node-negative breast cancer. *J Natl Cancer Inst* 1993;85:200.
231. Barnes DM, Dublin EA, Fisher CJ, et al. Immunohistochemical detection of p53 protein in mammary carcinoma: an important new independent indicator of prognosis? *Hum Pathol* 1993;24:469.
232. Silvestrini R, Benini E, Daidone MG, et al. p53 as an independent prognostic marker in lymph node-negative breast cancer patients. *J Natl Cancer Inst* 1993;85:965.
233. Marks JR, Humphrey PA, Wu K, et al. Overexpression of p53 and HER-2/neu proteins as prognostic markers in early stage breast cancer. *Ann Surg* 1994;219:332.
234. Gasparini G, Weidner N, Bevilacqua P, et al. Tumor microvessel density, p53 expression, tumor size, and peritumoral lymphatic vessel invasion are relevant prognostic markers in node negative breast carcinoma. *J Clin Oncol* 1994;12:454.
235. Elledge RM, Fuqua SAW, Clark GM, et al. Prognostic significance of p53 gene alterations in node-negative breast cancer. *Breast Cancer Res Treat* 1993;26:225.
236. Caleffi M, Teague MW, Jensen RA, et al. P53 gene mutations and steroid receptor status in breast cancer: clinicopathologic correlations and prognostic assessment. *Cancer* 1994;73:2147.
237. Elledge RM, Allred DC. Prognostic and predictive value of p53 and p21 in breast cancer. *Breast Cancer Res Treat* 1998;52:79.
238. Battifora H. p53 immunohistochemistry: a word of caution. *Hum Pathol* 1994;25:435.
239. Callahan R. p53 mutations, another breast cancer prognostic factor. *J Natl Cancer Inst* 1992;84:826.
240. Legros Y, Lacabanne V, d'Agay MF, et al. Production of human p53 specific monoclonal antibodies and their use in immunohistochemical studies of tumor cells. *Bull Cancer* 1993;80:102.
241. Elledge RM, Clark GM, Fuqua SAW, et al. p53 protein accumulation detected by five different antibodies: relationship to prognosis and heat shock protein 70 in breast cancer. *Cancer Res* 1994;54:3752.
242. Jacquemier J, Molès JP, Penault-Llorca F, et al. p53 immunohistochemical analysis in breast cancer with four monoclonal antibodies: comparison of staining and PCR-SSCP results. *Br J Cancer* 1994;69:846.
243. Rosen PP, Lesser ML, Arroyo CD, et al. p53 in node-negative breast carcinoma: an immunohistochemical study of epidemiologic risk factors, histologic features, and prognosis. *J Clin Oncol* 1995;13:821.
244. Lampe B, Hantschmann P, Dimpfl TH. Prognostic relevance of immunohistology, tumor size and vascular space involvement in axillary node negative breast cancer. *Arch Gynecol Obstet* 1998;261:139.
245. Peyrat J-P, Vanlemmens L, Fournier J, et al. Prognostic value of p53 and urokinase-type plasminogen activator in node-negative human breast cancers. *Clin Cancer Res* 1998;4:189.
246. Jansson T, Inganäs M, Sjögren S, et al. p53 status predicts survival in breast cancer patients treated with or without postoperative radiotherapy: a novel hypothesis based on clinical findings. *J Clin Oncol* 1995;13:2745.
247. Silvestrini R, Veneroni S, Benini E, et al. Expression of p53, glutathione S-transferase-π, and bcl-2 proteins and benefit from adjuvant radiotherapy in breast cancer. *J Natl Cancer Inst* 1997;89:63.
248. Bergh J, Norberg T, Sjögren S, et al. Complete sequencing of the p53 gene provides prognostic information in breast cancer patients, particularly in relation to adjuvant systemic therapy and radiotherapy. *Nature Med* 1995;1:1029.
249. Rozan S, Vincent-Salomon A, Zafrani B, et al. No significant predictive value of c-erbB-2 or p53 expression regarding sensitivity to primary chemotherapy or radiotherapy in breast cancer. *Int J Cancer* 1998;79:27.
250. Elledge RM, Gray R, Mansour E, et al. Accumulation of p53 protein as a possible predictor of response to adjuvant combination chemotherapy with cyclophosphamide, methotrexate, fluorouracil, and prednisone for breast cancer. *J Natl Cancer Inst* 1995;87:1254.
251. Stål O, Askmalm MS, Wingren, S, et al. p53 expression and the result of adjuvant therapy of breast cancer. *Acta Oncologica* 1995;34:767.
252. Degeorges A, de Roquancourt A, Extra JM, et al. Is p53 a protein that predicts the response to chemotherapy in node negative breast cancer? *Breast Cancer Res Treat* 1998;47:47.
253. Aas T, Borresen A-L, Geisler S, et al. Specific p53 mutations are associated with de novo resistance to doxorubicin in breast cancer patients. *Nature Med* 1996;2:811.
254. Clahsen PC, van de Velde CJH, Duval C, et al. p53 protein accumulation and response to adjuvant chemotherapy in premenopausal women with node-negative early breast cancer. *J Clin Oncol* 1998;16:470.
255. Resnick JM, Sneige N, Kemp BL, et al. p53 and c-erbB-2 expression and response to preoperative chemotherapy in locally advanced breast cancer. *Breast Dis* 1995;8:149.
256. Järvinen TAH, Holli K, Kuukasjärvi T, et al. Predictive value of topoisomerase IIa and other prognostic factors for epirubicin chemotherapy in advanced breast cancer. *Br J Cancer* 1998;77:2267.
257. Jacquemier J, Penault-Llorca F, Viens P, et al. Breast cancer response to adjuvant chemotherapy in correlation with erbB2 and p53 expression. *Anticancer Res* 1994;14:2773.
258. MacGrogan G, Mauriac L, Durand M, et al. Primary chemotherapy in breast invasive carcinoma: predictive value of the immunohistochemical detection of hormonal receptors, p53, c-erbB-2, MiB1, pS2 and GSTπ. *Br J Cancer* 1996;74:1458.
259. Berns EMJJ, Klijn JGM, van Putten WLJ, et al. p53 protein accumulation predicts poor response to tamoxifen therapy of patients with recurrent breast cancer. *J Clin Oncol* 1998;16:121.
260. Archer SG, Eliopoulos A, Spandidos D, et al. Expression of ras p21, p53 and c-erbB-2 in advanced breast cancer and response to first line hormonal therapy. *Br J Cancer* 1995;72:1259.
261. Makris A, Powles TJ, Dowsett M, et al. Prediction of response to neoadjuvant chemoendocrine therapy in primary breast carcinomas. *Clin Cancer Res* 1997;3:593.
262. Elledge R, Green S, Howes L, et al. bcl-2, p53, and response to tamoxifen in estrogen receptor–positive metastatic breast cancer: a Southwest Oncology Group study. *J Clin Oncol* 1997;15:1916.
263. Steeg PS, Bevilacqua G, Kopper L, et al. Evidence for a novel gene associated with low tumor metastatic potential. *J Natl Cancer Inst* 1988;80:200.
264. Gilles A-M, Presecan E, Vonica A, et al. Nucleoside diphosphate kinase from human erythrocytes. *J Biol Chem* 1991;266:8784.
265. Hennessy C, Henry JA, May FEB, et al. Expression of the antimetastatic gene nm23 in human breast cancer: an association with good prognosis. *J Natl Cancer Inst* 1991;83:281.
266. Barnes R, Masood S, Barker E, et al. Low nm23 protein expression in infiltrating ductal breast carcinomas correlates with reduced patient survival. *Am J Pathol* 1991;139:245.
267. Tokunaga Y, Urano T, Furukawa K, et al. Reduced expression of nm23-H1, but not of nm23-H2, is concordant with the frequency of lymph-node metastasis of human breast cancer. *Int J Cancer* 1993;55:66.
268. Cropp CS, Lidereau R, Leone A, et al. NME1 protein expression and loss of heterozygosity mutations in primary human breast tumors. *J Natl Cancer Inst* 1994;86:1167.
269. Toulas C, Mihura J, de Balincourt C, et al. Potential prognostic value in human breast cancer on cytosolic Nme1 protein detection using an original hen specific antibody. *Br J Cancer* 1996;73:630.
270. Sawan A, Lascu I, Veron M, et al. NDP-K/nm23 expression in human breast cancer in relation to relapse, survival, and other prognostic factors: an immunohistochemical study. *J Pathol* 1994;172:27.
271. Kapranos N, Karaiossifidi H, Kouri E, et al. Nm23 expression in breast ductal carcinomas: a ten year follow-up in a uniform group of node-negative breast cancer patients. *Anticancer Res* 1996;16:3987.

272. Heimann R, Ferguson DJ, Hellman S. The relationship between nm23, angiogenesis, and the metastatic proclivity of node-negative breast cancer. *Cancer Res* 1998;58:2766.
273. Steeg PS, De La Rosa A, Flatow U, et al. Nm23 and breast cancer metastasis. *Breast Cancer Res Treat* 1993;25:175.
274. Ravdin PM. Evaluation of cathepsin D as a prognostic factor in breast cancer. *Breast Cancer Res Treat* 1993;24:219.
275. Spyratos F, Martin P-M, Hacène K, et al. Multiparametric prognostic evaluation of biological factors in primary breast cancer. *J Natl Cancer Inst* 1992;84:1266.
276. Remmele W, Sauer-Manthey J. Comparative biochemical and immunohistochemical studies on the cathepsin D content of human breast cancer. *Virchows Arch A Pathol Anat Histopathol* 1993;422:467.
277. Têtu B, Brisson J, Côté C, et al. Prognostic significance of cathepsin-D expression in node-positive breast carcinoma: an immunohistochemical study. *Int J Cancer* 1993;55:429.
278. Armas OA, Gerald WL, Lesser ML, et al. Immunohistochemical detection of cathepsin D in T2N0M0 breast carcinoma. *Am J Surg Pathol* 1994;18:158.
279. Foekens JA, Schmitt M, van Putten WLJ, et al. Plasminogen activator inhibitor-1 and prognosis in primary breast cancer. *J Clin Oncol* 1994;12:1648.
280. Gasparini G, Boracchi P, Bevilacqua P, et al. A multiparametric study on the prognostic value of epidermal growth factor receptor in operable breast carcinoma. *Breast Cancer Res Treat* 1994;29:59.
281. Ravdin PM, Tandon AK, Allred DC, et al. Cathepsin D by western blotting and immunohistochemistry: failure to confirm correlations with prognosis in node-negative breast cancer. *J Clin Oncol* 1994;12:467.
282. Johnson MD, Torri JA, Lippman ME, et al. The role of cathepsin D in the invasiveness of human breast cancer cells. *Cancer Res* 1993;53:873.
283. Foekens JA, Schmitt M, van Putten WLJ, et al. Prognostic value of urokinase-type plasminogen activator in 671 primary breast cancer patients. *Cancer Res* 1992;52:6101.
284. Grøndahl-Hansen J, Christensen IJ, Rosenquist C, et al. High levels of urokinase-type plasminogen activator and its inhibitor PAI-1 in cytosolic extracts of breast carcinomas are associated with prognosis. *Cancer Res* 1993;53:2513.
285. Jänicke F, Schmitt M, Pache L, et al. Urokinase (uPA) and its inhibitor PAI-1 are strong and independent prognostic factors in node-negative breast cancer. *Breast Cancer Res Treat* 1993;24:195.
286. Duffy MJ, Reilly D, McDermott E, et al. Urokinase plasminogen activator as a prognostic marker in different subgroups of patients with breast cancer. *Cancer* 1994;74:2276.
287. Bouchet C, Spyratos F, Martin PM, et al. Prognostic value of urokinase-type plasminogen activator (uPA) and plasminogen activator inhibitors PAI-1 and PAI-2 in breast carcinomas. *Br J Cancer* 1994;69:398.
288. Foekens JA, Look MP, Peters HA, et al. Urokinase-type plasminogen activator and its inhibitor PAI-1: predictors of poor response to tamoxifen therapy in recurrent breast cancer. *J Natl Cancer Inst* 1995;87:755.
289. Grøndahl-Hansen J, Peters HA, van Putten WLJ, et al. Prognostic significance of the receptor for urokinase plasminogen activator in breast cancer. *Clin Cancer Res* 1995;1:1079.
290. Duggan C, Maguire T, McDermott E, et al. Urokinase plasminogen activator and urokinase plasminogen activator receptor in breast cancer. *Int J Cancer* 1995;61:597.
291. Graeff H, Harbeck N, Pache L, et al. Prognostic impact and clinical relevance of tumor-associated proteases in breast cancer. *Fibrinolysis* 1992;6:45.
292. Hand PH, Thor A, Schlom J, et al. Expression of laminin receptor in normal and carcinomatous human tissues as defined by a monoclonal antibody. *Cancer Res* 1985;45:2713.
293. Castronovo V, Taraboletti G, Liotta LA, et al. Modulation of laminin receptor expression by estrogen and progestins in human breast cancer cell lines. *J Natl Cancer Inst* 1989;81:781.
294. Marques LA, Franco ELF, Torloni H, et al. Independent prognostic value of laminin receptor expression in breast cancer survival. *Cancer Res* 1990;50:1479.
295. Daidone MG, Silvestrini R, D'Errico A, et al. Laminin receptors, collagenase IV and prognosis in node-negative breast cancers. *Int J Cancer* 1991;48:529.
296. Martignone S, Ménard S, Bufalino R, et al. Prognostic significance of the 67-kilodalton laminin receptor expression in human breast carcinomas. *J Natl Cancer Inst* 1993;85:398.
297. Pellegrini R, Martignone S, Tagliabue E, et al. Prognostic significance of laminin production in relation with its receptor expression in human breast carcinomas. *Breast Cancer Res Treat* 1995;35:195.
298. Gasparini G, Barbareschi M, Boracchi P, et al. 67-kDa laminin-receptor expression adds prognostic information to intra-tumoral microvessel density in node-negative breast cancer. *Int J Cancer* 1995;60:604.
299. Folkman J. What is the evidence that tumors are angiogenesis dependent? *J Natl Cancer Inst* 1990;82:4.
300. Vartanian RK, Weidner N. Correlation of intratumoral endothelial cell proliferation with microvessel density (tumor angiogenesis) and tumor cell proliferation in breast carcinoma. *Am J Pathol* 1994;144:1188.
301. Craft PS, Harris AL. Clinical prognostic significance of tumour angiogenesis. *Ann Oncol* 1994;5:305.
302. Weidner N, Semple J, Welch WR, et al. Tumor angiogenesis and metastasis—correlation in invasive breast carcinoma. *N Engl J Med* 1991;324:1.
303. Bosari S, Lee AKC, DeLellis RA, et al. Microvessel quantitation and prognosis in invasive breast carcinoma. *Hum Pathol* 1992;23:755.
304. Horak ER, Leek R, Klenk N, et al. Angiogenesis, assessed by platelet/endothelial cell adhesion molecule antibodies, as indicator of node metastases and survival in breast cancer. *Lancet* 1992;340:1120.
305. Toi M, Hoshina S, Yamamoto Y, et al. Tumor angiogenesis in breast cancer: significance of vessel density as a prognostic indicator. *Gan To Kagaku Ryoho* 1994;21:178.
306. Fox SB, Leek RD, Smith K, et al. Tumor angiogenesis in node-negative breast carcinomas—relationship with epidermal growth factor receptor, estrogen receptor, and survival. *Breast Cancer Res Treat* 1994;29:109.
307. Hayes DF. Angiogenesis and breast cancer. *Hematol Oncol Clin North Am* 1994;8:51.
308. Locopo N, Fanelli M, Gasparini G. Clinical significance of angiogenic factors in breast cancer. *Breast Cancer Res Treat* 1998;52:159.
309. Schena M, Shalon D, Davis RW, et al. Quantitative monitoring of gene expression patterns with a complementary DNA microarray. *Science* 1995;270:467.
310. Kononen J, Bubendorf L, Kallioniemi A, et al. Tissue microarrays for high-throughput molecular profiling of tumor specimens. *Nature Med* 1998;4:844.
311. Osin P, Shipley J, Lu YJ, et al. Experimental pathology and breast cancer genetics: new technologies. *Recent Results Cancer Res* 1998;152:35.
312. Yang GP, Ross DT, Kuang WW, et al. Combining SSH and cDNA microarrays for rapid identification of differentially expressed genes. *Nucleic Acids Res* 1999;27:1517.
313. Ermolaeva O, Rastogi M, Pruitt KD, et al. Data management and analysis for gene expression arrays. *Nat Genet* 1998;20:19.
314. Moore DH III, Pallavicini M, Cher ML, et al. A t-statistic for objective interpretation of comparative genomic hybridization (CGH) profiles. *Cytometry* 1997;28:183.
315. Eisen MB, Spellman PT, Brown PO, et al. Cluster analysis and display of genome-wide expression patterns. *Proc Natl Acad Sci U S A* 1998;95:14863.
316. Hilsenbeck SG, Friedrichs WE, Schiff R, et al. Statistical analysis of array expression data as applied to the problem of tamoxifen resistence. *J Natl Cancer Inst* 1999;91:453.
317. Albain KS, Green S, LeBlanc M, et al. Proportional hazards and recursive partitioning and amalgamation analyses of the Southwest Oncology Group node-positive adjuvant CMFVP breast cancer data base: a pilot study. *Breast Cancer Res Treat* 1992;22:273.
318. Ravdin PM, Clark GM. A practical application of neural network analysis for predicting outcome of individual breast cancer patients. *Breast Cancer Res Treat* 1992;22:285.
319. Hilsenbeck SG, Clark GM, McGuire WL. Why do so many prognostic factors fail to pan out? *Breast Cancer Res Treat* 1992;22:197.
320. Altman DG, Lyman GH. Methodological challenges in the evaluation of prognostic factors in breast cancer. *Breast Cancer Res Treat* 1998;52:289.
321. Schmitt M, Thomssen C, Ulm K, et al. Time-varying prognostic impact of tumor biological factors urokinase (uPA), PAI-1 and steroid hormone receptor status in primary breast cancer. *Br J Cancer* 1997; 76:306.
322. Bryant J, Fisher B, Gündüz N, et al. S-phase fraction combined with other patient and tumor characteristics for the prognosis of node-negative, estrogen-receptor-positive breast cancer. *Breast Cancer Res Treat* 1998;51:239.
323. Hilsenbeck SG, Ravdin PM, de Moor CA, et al. Time-dependence of hazard ratios for prognostic factors in primary breast cancer. *Breast Cancer Res Treat* 1998;52:227.

IX

Diseases of the Breast, 2nd ed.,
edited by Jay R. Harris.
Lippincott Williams & Wilkins, Philadelphia © 2000.

Primary Treatment of Invasive Breast Cancer

CHAPTER 33

Local Management of Invasive Breast Cancer

Monica Morrow and Jay R. Harris

The local treatment of breast cancer has long been a source of controversy. For many years, it was considered the domain of the surgeon. However, changes in our understanding of the biology of the disease, the detection of smaller tumors over time, an increasing emphasis on systemic therapy, and greater patient participation in the decision-making process have radically changed our approach to the local treatment of breast cancer since the 1970s. Local treatment of breast cancer involves a collaborative effort between surgeons, reconstructive surgeons, radiologists, pathologists, radiation oncologists, and medical oncologists. This chapter reflects this multimodality approach by addressing the use of surgery and radiation therapy (RT) in a coordinated fashion and considering the integration of local and systemic treatment. We provide a brief history of the local treatment of breast cancer and the rationale for the current approach to management of the primary tumor, and we discuss studies that support this approach. The evolution of our approach to the management of the regional lymph nodes is described, including the alternatives of sentinel lymph node biopsy and axillary irradiation. The emerging data on postmastectomy radiotherapy and its impact on survival are discussed. In addition to providing the theoretical basis for local treatment, this chapter addresses practical issues in the local treatment of breast cancer, including the following:

- Guidelines for patient selection
- Timing of surgery
- Breast conservation after neoadjuvant chemotherapy
- Sequencing of RT and systemic therapy
- Breast-conserving surgery without RT
- Complications of breast-conserving surgery and modified radical mastectomy
- Oncologic considerations in the use of immediate breast reconstruction
- Complications of RT

Detailed information on surgical and radiation techniques can be found in Chapters 35 and 36.

M. Morrow: Department of Surgery, Northwestern University Medical School, Chicago, Illinois; Lynn Sage Comprehensive Breast Program, Northwestern Memorial Hospital, Chicago, Illinois

J. R. Harris: Department of Radiation Oncology, Harvard Medical School, Brigham and Women's Hospital, Dana-Farber Cancer Institute, Boston, Massachusetts

The modern era of breast cancer surgery began with the popularization of the radical mastectomy by William Halsted in 1894.[1,2] The development of the radical mastectomy was based on a theory of breast cancer spread that emphasized the local spread of the disease, particularly through the lymphatics. Radical mastectomy, an *en bloc* resection of the breast, the overlying skin, the pectoral muscles, and the entirety of the axillary contents, had two major advantages. It was technically possible in most women with breast cancer, even in the advanced cancers seen in the first half of the 1900s, and it was a relatively effective means of obtaining local control of the primary tumor. Of 1,640 women seen at Memorial Hospital[3] in New York, New York from 1940 to 1943, 89% were considered candidates for radical mastectomy. However, of the 1,458 patients who underwent radical mastectomy, only 13% survived 30 years free of cancer, with 57% of patients dying of breast cancer, 24% dying of other causes, and 6% lost to follow-up.

The failure of radical mastectomy to cure many patients with breast cancer was initially thought by some surgeons to be because of its failure to extirpate all of the draining lymphatics of the breast.[4] To address this, the extended radical mastectomy was developed. This procedure is a radical mastectomy combined with *en bloc* removal of the internal mammary nodes (IMNs). Nonrandomized studies suggested that survival might be improved in selected patients by this more radical procedure.[5,6] However, a prospective randomized trial comparing radical and extended radical mastectomy failed to show any difference in disease-free or overall survival between the two treatment groups.[7] The failure of this more extensive procedure to improve survival cast doubt on the validity of Halstedian principles and the need for radical mastectomy itself.

Modified radical mastectomy is the most commonly performed operative treatment for patients with invasive breast cancer in the United States.[8–10] The term *modified radical mastectomy* is used to describe a variety of surgical procedures, but all involve complete removal of the breast and some of the axillary nodes. Although the modified radical mastectomy may not seem to differ significantly from the radical mastectomy, it represented a major departure from Halstedian principles of *en bloc* cancer surgery. The switch to modified radical mastectomy occurred when it became recognized that treatment failure after breast cancer surgery usually is because of the systemic dissemination of cancer cells before surgery rather than an inadequate operative procedure. In addition, by the 1970s, fewer patients with large tumors with fixation to the pectoral muscle were being seen, making modified radical mastectomy feasible for most women. Several retrospective studies[11,12] demonstrated no difference in survival between patients treated with modified radical and radical mastectomy. These findings were confirmed in two prospective randomized trials.[13,14] Although only two randomized studies directly compared radical and modified radical mastectomy, further evidence that radical *en bloc* surgery did not prolong survival came from several randomized trials comparing radical mastectomy with simple mastectomy and RT. An overview analysis[15,16] of patients treated in four randomized trials demonstrated equivalent survival for patients treated with radical mastectomy and those who underwent simple mastectomy combined with RT. Perhaps the most influential of these studies was the National Surgical Adjuvant Breast and Bowel Project's (NSABP) B-04 trial, in which clinically node-negative patients were randomized to radical mastectomy, simple mastectomy and nodal irradiation, or simple mastectomy with axillary observation and delayed dissection if positive nodes developed.[17] The failure of this trial to demonstrate a difference in survival between groups was the final proof that the Halstedian concept of breast cancer did not apply to the majority of patients and was a landmark in our understanding of the local therapy of breast cancer.

Today there are few, if any, indications for radical mastectomy. If the pectoral fascia has been violated at the time of biopsy or if the tumor abuts the pectoral fascia or even invades a small portion of the pectoral muscle, it is preferable to resect a small portion of the muscle directly beneath the tumor to obtain a negative deep margin of resection. Large tumors that involve greater amounts of the pectoral muscle are best treated with systemic therapy, not radical surgery, as the initial approach. After a response to the initial therapy, a standard modified radical mastectomy with primary skin closure frequently can be done in these cases.

Some of the same principles that led to the use of the modified radical mastectomy contributed to the development of breast-conserving treatment (BCT). These included recognition that adherence to the Halstedian principle of *en bloc* extirpation of the breast and its draining lymphatics failed to cure many patients with breast cancer, the increasingly frequent identification of small breast cancers by mammography, and the success of moderate-dose RT in eliminating subclinical foci of breast cancer after mastectomy. An initial objection to the use of BCT was the known multicentricity of breast carcinoma. The reported incidence of multicentricity ranged from 9% to 75%, depending on the definition used, the extent of tissue sampling, and the techniques of pathologic examination used.[18–20] These studies were used to argue against anything less than complete mastectomy as optimal local treatment for breast cancer.

The strategy behind BCT is to remove the bulk of the tumor surgically and to use moderate doses of radiation to eradicate any residual cancer. A key element in the successful application of this approach is the preservation of a good cosmetic appearance of the treated breast. The application of this strategy requires an understanding of the extent and distribution of cancer in a breast with an apparently localized tumor. Considerable clarification of this issue has occurred as a result of the work of Holland et al.[21,22] In their initial study,[21] mastectomy specimens with primary tumors of 4 cm or less in size were studied. In all cases, the tumors were considered unicentric based on clinical and radiographic assessment. Detailed evaluation of the breast was carried out using 5-mm sections, radiography of these thin slices, and an average of 20 blocks per specimen for histologic evaluation. This technique allowed precise mapping of the extent and distribution of residual carcinoma in relation to the primary (or reference) tumor. Only 39% of specimens showed no evidence of cancer

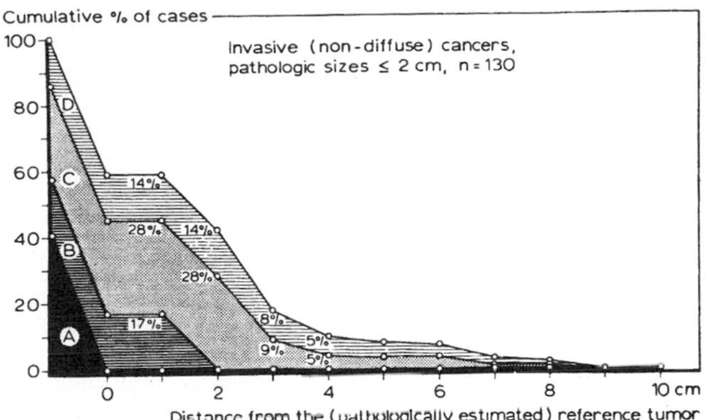

FIG. 1. Frequency of additional cancer foci at increasing distance from a clinically unifocal reference tumor. Two hundred sixty-four mastectomy specimens were studied from patients with breast cancers measuring 4 cm or smaller and judged to be unifocal based on clinical findings. Thirty-nine percent of cases (group A) showed no additional cancer foci beyond the reference tumor. In 20% of cases (group B), additional foci were found but were restricted to within 2 cm of the reference tumor. Forty-one percent of the cases showed cancer foci farther than 2 cm from the reference tumor, including 27% in which the additional foci were entirely intraductal (group C) and 14% in which they were invasive and intraductal (group D).

beyond the reference tumor. In 20%, additional cancer was found, but it was confined to within 2 cm of the reference tumor. Forty-one percent of patients had residual cancer more than 2 cm from the reference tumor; of these, two-thirds had pure intraductal carcinoma, and one-third had mixed intraductal and invasive carcinoma (Fig. 1). The percentage of patients with residual cancer more than 2 cm from the reference tumor corresponds well to the rate of local failure reported in patients treated with excision of the primary tumor alone.[23–27] In these series, local recurrence in the breast occurs at or near the site of the primary tumor in most cases, also emphasizing that multifocal breast cancer commonly remains after an excision of the tumor and that this multifocal involvement is biologically important. This is true even if the margins of surgical resection are assessed to be negative.

In a subsequent study, Holland et al.[22] quantitated the amount of residual intraductal carcinoma at various distances from the primary tumor. Prominent intraductal carcinoma was defined as a total of six or more low-power fields of intraductal carcinoma measured using a 6-mm field and a 2.5× objective. Approximately 10% of patients had prominent intraductal carcinoma that extended more than 2 cm from the reference tumor, and approximately 5% of patients had prominent intraductal carcinoma extending more than 3 cm. These studies of Holland et al. indicate that the extent and amount of microscopic cancer in the vicinity of a primary tumor, known as *multifocality*, is variable. Some patients seem to have minimal multifocal involvement, whereas others have extensive intraductal disease. However, multifocality clearly occurs more frequently than *multicentricity*, which is defined as additional foci of tumor geographically distant from the primary lesion, usually in separate quadrants of the breast. These results imply that the extent of surgical resection required in BCT varies from patient to patient. These issues are considered in more detail later in the sections Extent of Resection and Techniques and Complications of Breast-Conserving Surgery.

The ability to safely and effectively deliver RT to the breast was a crucial element in the development of BCT. The use of RT for breast cancer began at nearly the same time as surgical treatment. In 1895, Wilhelm Roentgen, using a primitive cathode-ray tube, discovered a new form of radiation that was able to penetrate various materials and darken photographic plates. To distinguish this new form of radiation from others, he chose to call it *x-rays*.

Within 1 year after Roentgen reported his discovery, patients with cancer were treated with x-rays. Early practitioners of this modality demonstrated the ability of x-rays to shrink and, in some cases, to eliminate cancerous growths completely. These practitioners were limited, however, by the rudimentary equipment available at that time and by the absence of a technique and treatment schedule able to deliver RT to the tumor while sparing normal tissues.

It was soon realized that the optimal use of RT depends on extending the course of treatment over time. Large single exposures to radiation result in significant and progressive adverse effects on normal tissues. Careful observation of treated patients determined that best results were achieved by delivering relatively small doses of radiation daily over an extended period. This fractionation and protraction of treatment allows greater recovery of normal tissues and still permits killing of tumor cells. Worldwide experience since then has generally established that a dose in the range of 1.8 to 2.0 Gy given once a day provides optimal results. [The current official unit of radiation dose absorbed in tissue is the *grey* (*Gy*); 1 Gy = 100 cGy (centigrey) = 100 rads (the previous unit of absorbed dose). The *roentgen* (*R*) is a unit of "exposure" or ionization induced in air and generally corresponds to less than 1 cGy.]

Among the first to document the dose of radiation required to achieve local tumor control of breast cancer was Gilbert Fletcher.[28] He examined the incidence of supraclavicular node relapse in patients with positive axillary nodes treated with radical mastectomy. Prior retrospective reports had indicated a relapse rate of 20% to 25% when no postoperative RT was given. Fletcher found that the rate of supraclavicular relapse was 3% when 30 to 35 Gy was delivered in 4 weeks and was only 1.3% when 50 to 55 Gy in 4 weeks was used. These inferential data provide support for the use of 45 to 50 Gy in 4.5 to 5.0 weeks to eradicate "subclinical" deposits of breast cancer in a high percentage of cases. In a test of this concept, a trial of historic importance was conducted in Copenhagen from 1951 to 1957. In this trial, 559 patients were randomly assigned to undergo either an extended radical mastectomy or a total mastectomy and postoperative RT. Despite the limitations of the RT techniques available at that time, long-term results reported by Kaae and Johansen[29] revealed equivalent local tumor control and survival for the two treatments. This trial was the first to

TABLE 1. *Prospective randomized trials comparing conservative surgery and radiation with mastectomy for early-stage breast cancer*

Trial	Years	No. of patients	Stage	Surgery for the primary	RT boost
Institut Gustave-Roussy[37]	1972–84	179	1	2-cm gross margin	15 Gy
Milan I[32,33]	1973–80	701	1	Quadrantectomy	10 Gy
NSABP B-06[34]	1976–84	1,219	1 and 2	Lumpectomy	None
NCI[35]	1979–87	237	1 and 2	Gross excision	15–20 Gy
EORTC[36,38]	1980–86	874	1 and 2	1-cm gross margin	25 Gy
Danish[39]	1983–89	904	1, 2, and 3	Wide excision	10–25 Gy

EORTC, European Organization for Research and Treatment of Cancer; NCI, National Cancer Institute; NSABP, National Surgical Adjuvant Breast and Bowel Project; RT, radiation therapy.

demonstrate the effectiveness of RT in treating areas of subclinical involvement.

The concept of combining conservative surgery (CS) with RT as a substitute for mastectomy is not new. Geoffrey Keynes[30] in London and M. Vera Peters[31] in Toronto were early proponents of this approach before supervoltage irradiation was available. Keynes,[30] a surgeon at St. Bartholomew's Hospital in London, began to treat patients with operable carcinoma of the breast in this manner as early as 1924. Peters, a radiation oncologist at the Princess Margaret Hospital in Toronto, began her large series in 1939.[31] With the development of supervoltage irradiation, it became feasible to pursue BCT with the goal of preserving highly satisfactory cosmetic results. Developers of this approach were Robert Calle of the Institut Curie in Paris, France; Bernard Pierquin of the Henri Mondor Hospital in Creteil, France; J.M. Spitalier of the Marseilles Cancer Institute in Marseilles, France; Eleanor Montague of M. D. Anderson Cancer Center in Houston, Texas; and Samuel Hellman at the Harvard Joint Center for Radiation Therapy (JCRT), Boston, Massachusetts. Formalized clinical trials to evaluate the effectiveness of this approach in comparison with mastectomy were initiated by Umberto Veronesi at the National Cancer Institute of Italy in Milan and Bernard Fisher of the NSABP.

RESULTS OF BREAST-CONSERVING THERAPY

The goal of BCT using CS and RT is to provide the survival equivalent to mastectomy with preservation of the cosmetic outcome and a low rate of recurrence in the treated breast. Because of the almost universal acceptance of the Halstedian dogma regarding breast cancer, a relatively large number of randomized clinical trials were conducted to determine whether survival after BCT equaled survival after mastectomy. The results of six modern, prospective, randomized clinical trials have been published comparing CS and RT and mastectomy[32–39] (Tables 1 and 2). All of these trials have shown equivalent survival between the two treatment approaches, and an overview of all the trials (including an unpublished one) has also demonstrated comparable survival (Fig. 2).[40] These data demonstrate that survival for most breast cancer patients is not dependent on their choice of local therapy.

In addition to the results of these trials, numerous reports from centers in Europe and North America on the use of CS and RT have demonstrated high rates of local tumor control with satisfactory cosmetic results.[41–49] The long follow-up available for many of these retrospective studies has helped to document the time course and pattern of recurrence in the breast, factors that may be associated with an increased risk of recurrence in the breast and information regarding cosmetic outcomes after BCT. This information is useful in determining the optimal approach to CS and RT, in providing guidelines for patient selection, and in providing patients treated with CS and RT with important information on their expected outcome.

Despite the consistency of the evidence, the use of BCT in the United States has shown relatively slow acceptance, with considerable geographic variation.[8–10,50] Studies indicate that fewer than 50% of women with stages I and II breast carcinoma are treated with BCT.[8] Potential explanations for this finding include (a) large numbers of patients

TABLE 2. *Comparison of survival after conservative surgery and radiation with that after mastectomy in prospective randomized trials*

Trial	Follow-up (yr)	Overall survival		Local recurrence	
		CS + RT (%)	Mastectomy (%)	CS + RT (%)	Mastectomy (%)
Institut Gustave-Roussy[37]	15	73	65	9	14
Milan I[32,33]	18	65	65	7	4
NSABP B-06[34]	12	63	59	10	8
NCI[35]	10	77	75	19	6
EORTC[36,38]	8	54	61	17	14
Danish[39]	6	79	82	3	4

CS + RT, conservative therapy and radiation therapy; EORTC, European Organization for Research and Treatment of Cancer; NCI, National Cancer Institute; NSABP, National Surgical Adjuvant Breast and Bowel Project.

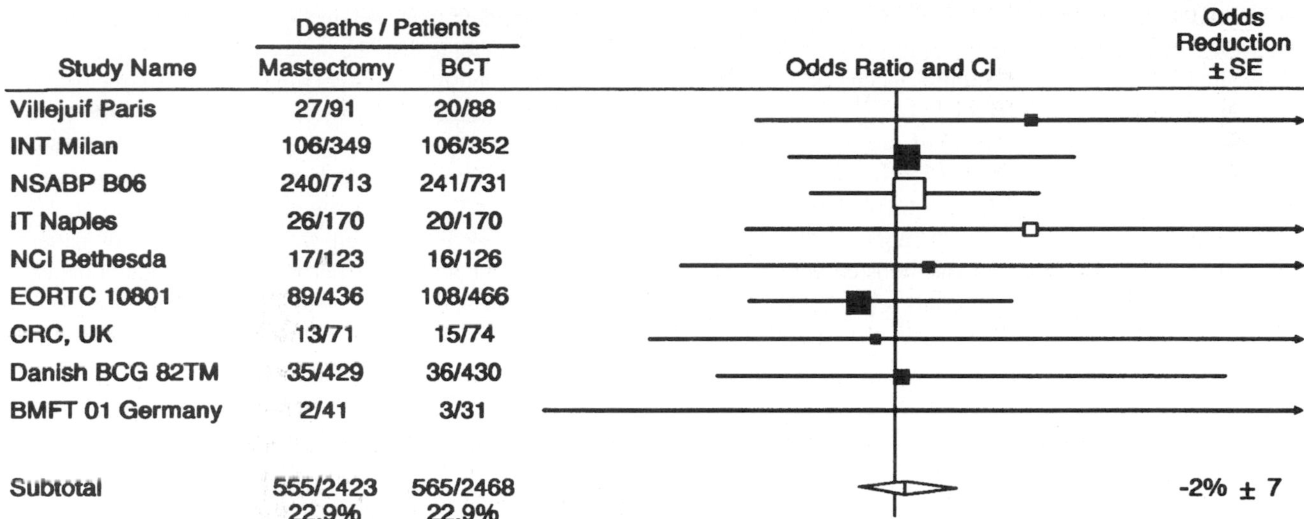

Study Name	Deaths / Patients Mastectomy	BCT	Odds Ratio and CI	Odds Reduction ± SE
Villejuif Paris	27/91	20/88		
INT Milan	106/349	106/352		
NSABP B06	240/713	241/731		
IT Naples	26/170	20/170		
NCI Bethesda	17/123	16/126		
EORTC 10801	89/436	108/466		
CRC, UK	13/71	15/74		
Danish BCG 82TM	35/429	36/430		
BMFT 01 Germany	2/41	3/31		
Subtotal	555/2423 22.9%	565/2468 22.9%		-2% ± 7

FIG. 2. Overview analysis of trials of conservative surgery and radiotherapy versus mastectomy. The squares represent the odds ratio of the annual death rate in the radiotherapy group compared to the control group. The vertical line is an odds ratio of 1, and the 99% confidence interval (CI) is shown by the horizontal line. Squares to the right of the vertical indicate a survival benefit for mastectomy. BCG, Breast Cancer Group; BCT, breast-conserving treatment; BMFT, Bundesminsterium für Forschung und Techologie; CRC, Cancer Research Campaign; EORTC, European Organization for Research and Treatment of Cancer; INT, Instituto Nazionale per lo studio e la Cura dei Tumori; IT, Instituto Tumori; NCI, National Cancer Institute; NSABP, National Surgical Adjuvant Breast and Bowel Project; SE, standard error. (From ref. 40.)

with contraindications to BCT, (b) patient preference for mastectomy, and (c) use of inappropriate selection criteria by physicians. Medical contraindications are not the major factor responsible for underuse of BCT.[51] In a study of 432 patients with stages I and II breast cancer or ductal carcinoma *in situ* (DCIS) who were prospectively evaluated by a multidisciplinary team, only 97 (22%) were found to have contraindications. The incidence and type of contraindications varied with tumor stage and were lowest (10%) for patients with stage I cancer and highest for those with DCIS. Foster et al.[52] report a similar low incidence of contraindications. Contraindications to BCT (discussed in the section Absolute and Relative Contraindications) can be readily identified with a careful history, physical examination, and detailed mammography, including magnification views of the primary site. Morrow et al.[53] evaluated 263 consecutive patients using these parameters. When these parameters suggested a localized tumor, 97% could be treated with BCT.[53] Thus, the available data indicate that a minority of patients have contraindications to BCT and that these are readily identified with standard clinical tools.

National studies indicate that physicians continue to use inappropriate selection criteria for BCT. In a joint study of the American College of Surgeons and the American College of Radiology, 17,931 patients with stages I and II breast cancer were evaluated to determine factors that predicted the use of mastectomy as local therapy.[8] Patients whose tumors had factors associated with a poorer prognosis, such as larger size, the presence of axillary node metastases, and higher histologic grade, were significantly more likely to undergo mastectomy than patients with more favorable features. The presence of an extensive intraductal component (EIC) in association with an invasive cancer was also a predictor of increased use of mastectomy. In addition, patient factors, such as increasing age, insurance status, and geographic location, were found to predict a higher use of mastectomy. These results indicate that inappropriate medical and demographic selection factors continue to be a major cause of high mastectomy rates in the United States.

Local Recurrence

Emphasis has been placed on the problem of recurrence in the breast after BCT. In the randomized studies presented (as shown in Table 2), with widely varying surgical and RT techniques, the rates of recurrence in the breast at 7 to 18 years ranged from 7% to 19%.[32–39] In the corresponding patients treated with mastectomy, local recurrence developed in 4% to 14%, emphasizing that mastectomy does not guarantee freedom from local recurrence, even in women with clinical stages I and II breast carcinoma.

Retrospective studies have helped to establish the incidence of local recurrence and its time course. Ten-year local recurrence rates ranging from 8% to 19% have been reported.[41–48] These rates are similar to the local recurrence rates seen in the randomized trials of CS and RT. However, the nonrandomized studies with the longest follow-up emphasize the prolonged time course to local recurrence in some patients undergoing BCT. Kurtz et al.[47] note that the actuarial incidence of recurrence in the treated breast increased from 7% at 5 years to 14% at 10 years and 20% at 20 years after treatment. These findings were similar to those of other reports describing a persistent risk of recurrence in the breast through 20 years of follow-up.[46,48,54] These results have been contrasted to those seen after mastectomy, in which most local failures occur in the first 3 years after surgery.

Most investigators have classified recurrences in the breast by their location in relation to the original tumor. Recurrences at or near the primary site (presumably representing a recurrence of the original tumor) are classified as either a *true recurrence* (within the boosted region) or a *marginal miss* (adjacent to the boosted region). Other categories of recurrence include those elsewhere in the breast (occurring at a distance from the original tumor and presumably representing a new primary), those primarily involving the skin, and those that are unclassifiable or diffuse in the breast. Gage et al.[48] reported on 1,628 patients with clinical stage I or II invasive carcinoma treated at the JCRT with gross tumor excision and RT, including a dose of at least 60 Gy to the primary site. The median follow-up time in survivors was 116 months. The annual incidence rate for a true recurrence/marginal miss recurrence was between 1.3% and 1.8% for years 2 through 7 after treatment and then decreased to 0.4% by 10 years after treatment. In contrast, the annual incidence rate for recurrence elsewhere in the breast increased slowly to a rate of approximately 0.7% per year at 8 years and remained stable. Recurrences in the skin of the treated breast are a rare event associated with a poor prognosis.[49] Kurtz et al.[47] similarly noticed that 32% of breast recurrences seen after 5 years occurred at a distance from the primary tumor, compared with only 14% of recurrences seen during the first 5 years. The risk of recurrence elsewhere in the breast after the first 5 years after treatment is remarkably similar to the risk of developing a contralateral breast carcinoma.[55] This suggests that although whole breast irradiation is effective at eradicating multicentric breast carcinoma, it does not prevent the subsequent development of new cancers. Thus, patients who elect BCT require lifelong follow-up to screen for the development of new cancers in both the treated and the contralateral breast.

Cosmetic Outcome

A major goal of BCT is the preservation of a cosmetically acceptable breast. To standardize grading of the cosmetic outcome, observer-based scales comparing the degree of deformity of the treated breast with the untreated breast have been developed. In the scoring system recommended by a joint committee of the American College of Surgeons and Radiology along with the College of American Pathologists and the Society of Surgical Oncology[56] and used at the JCRT,[57] the following scores are assigned: *excellent* when the treated and untreated breast are almost identical, *good* when there are minimal differences between the treated and untreated breasts, *fair* when there are obvious differences between the treated and untreated breasts, and *poor* when there are major aesthetic sequelae in the treated breast.

When modern treatment techniques are used, an acceptable cosmetic outcome can be achieved in almost all patients (without compromise of local tumor control). Among a group of patients treated with a whole breast dose of 45 to 46 Gy with a daily dose not greater than 2 Gy, a boost dose of 18 Gy or less, and an accurate matching technique, an excellent cosmetic result at 3 years was seen in 73% of patients, and either an excellent or good result was seen in 96% of patients.[58] Although treatment-related changes in the treated breast stabilize at approximately 3 years, other factors that primarily affect the untreated breast, such as change in size because of weight gain and the normal ptosis seen with aging, continue to affect the symmetry between a patient's breasts.

Although a variety of patient, tumor, and treatment factors have been reported to influence the cosmetic result, the amount of breast tissue resected is the major determinant of appearance when current techniques of RT are used. This is demonstrated in the randomized trial performed at the National Cancer Institute of Milan that compared quadrantectomy combined with RT to gross tumor excision (lumpectomy) combined with RT.[32] One hundred forty-eight consecutive patients participated in a cosmetic evaluation 18 to 24 months after treatment. Twenty-one percent of patients in the quadrantectomy group had a greater than 3-cm difference in height between the nipples, compared with only 7% of patients in the lumpectomy group. Similar discrepancies in the inferior profile of the breast and the distance from the midline to the nipple were observed. In a retrospective analysis from the JCRT, cosmetic outcome was also clearly related to the amount of breast tissue resected (estimated by multiplying the dimensions of the resected breast specimens). When the amount of resected breast tissue was less than 35 cm^3, 85% had excellent scores and 96% had either excellent or good scores. When the resected breast tissue was 36 to 85 cm^3, 78% had excellent scores and 97% had either excellent or good scores. When the resected breast tissue was larger than 85 cm^3, only 51% had excellent scores and 94% had either excellent or good scores. Similar findings have been reported from other studies examining factors that influence cosmetic outcome.[59,60]

In practice, a variety of factors must be considered together (the size of the patient's breast, the size of the tumor, the depth of the tumor within the breast, and the quadrant of the breast in which the tumor is located) to judge the feasibility of a cosmetically acceptable resection. For example, although the removal of a large tumor in the lower portion of the breast often results in distortion of the breast contour, this is only apparent with the arms raised and is acceptable to most women. A similar distortion in the upper inner quadrant of the breast, which is visible in most types of clothing, might not be as acceptable. Techniques such as latissimus dorsi reconstruction of the defect may be appropriate in selected patients to improve the cosmetic appearance after large resections.

Earlier studies suggested that breast size is an important factor influencing the cosmetic results. However, with improved technique, this no longer seems to be true. In particular, the use of higher energies results in improved homogeneity and better cosmetic results. Patients with large breasts can be treated with 8 mV irradiation without bolus and without an increase in local or skin recurrences.[61] With energies higher than 8 mV, a beam spoiler should be considered.

A final factor that has been suggested to influence cosmetic outcome is the use of adjuvant chemotherapy. In studies from the JCRT, patients treated with sequential chemotherapy [typically CMF (cyclophosphamide, methotrexate, and 5-fluorouracil)] and RT had a small decrease in their cosmetic outcome compared to patients not treated with chemotherapy, whereas patients treated with concurrent chemotherapy and RT had a large decrease in their cosmetic outcome.[62] This issue is discussed in greater detail in the section Sequencing of Systemic Therapy and Radiation Therapy.

Risk Factors for Local Recurrence

A large number of studies have been published that attempt to identify prognostic or risk factors. In examining this literature, a number of methodologic considerations are worth mentioning. First, many of the reports examining this issue differ with regard to patient selection, the techniques of surgery and RT, and the use of adjuvant systemic therapy. The risk factors observed to be important may vary because of these differences. Secondly, estimating the risk of local recurrence is complicated by the competing risk of distant recurrence.[63] Actuarial methods (e.g., Kaplan-Meier plots) were developed for analysis of survival data and are not suited for analysis of local recurrence. Actuarial methods require the assumption that the time to local recurrence and the time to distant recurrence are statistically independent, and this is not a reasonable assumption in breast cancer. The effect of a particular factor on local recurrence cannot be assessed separately from its effect on distant recurrence. Because local and systemic recurrence may not be independent, it has been recommended that reports on risk factors for local recurrence provide crude rates of both local and distant recurrence to allow the reader to assess each effect individually.[63] A third consideration is that different types of local recurrence may have different risk factors. It seems likely, for example, that recurrences at sites distant from the original tumor will have risk factors similar to those associated with opposite breast cancer [e.g., young patient age and family history (FH)]. As a result, combining all types of local recurrence may obscure important relationships.

A fourth consideration is that it is important to distinguish between risk factors that are prognostic and those that are predictive. A prognostic factor is used to estimate outcome, whereas a predictive factor is used to estimate the differential effect of a particular treatment. Therefore, if a factor is a risk factor for local recurrence after BCT but is also known to be a risk factor for local recurrence after mastectomy, then this factor is prognostic, not predictive. As a result, such a factor is of no assistance in selecting the best form of local treatment for a patient. Finally, a practical problem in estimating risk factors for local recurrence is projecting estimates too far in time. Estimates beyond the median can seriously underestimate or overestimate the true incidence of local recurrence. In a data set of treated patients, it is typical to first learn about "events," such as local recurrence, compared to learning that a patient is doing well. This "bad news comes first" bias results in an artifactual increase in actuarial rates of local recurrence at times past the median follow-up. To avoid this bias, one should provide crude incidence at the time of minimal follow-up for the entire study population.

Risk factors for recurrence after BCT can be subdivided as follows: patient factors, such as age; tumor factors, such as various histopathologic features; and treatment factors, such as the use of adjuvant systemic therapy. Although many factors for local recurrence have been evaluated, here we review those factors that are currently considered important. (Several factors, such as tumor size and axillary node status, have been shown not to be important risk factors for local recurrence; the data for these were reviewed in the last edition.)

Patient Risk Factors

Young Age

Young age has consistently been observed to be associated with an increased risk of local recurrence after breast-conserving surgery and RT. In the experience of the JCRT, younger age was associated with an increased frequency of various adverse pathologic features, such as lymphatic vessel invasion, grade 3 histology, absence of ERs, and the presence of an EIC. However, even when correction was done for the differing incidence of the pathologic features of the primary tumor between the age groups, younger age still was associated with a decreased survival rate and an increased likelihood of recurrence in the breast.[64] Similar findings were observed in a large series from the Institut Curie.[48,65] On the other hand, in large series from Marseilles[66] and from the European Organization for Research and Treatment of Cancer,[67] pathologic features and less extensive breast resection appeared to explain the higher rate of local recurrence in young patients.

Young age has similarly been associated with a worse outcome after mastectomy. An increase in local failure in younger patients was seen in a study of patients treated with radical mastectomy.[68] In a retrospective analysis from the M. D. Anderson Cancer Center, patients aged 35 years or younger did worse than older patients, but no difference was seen in local recurrence, disease-free survival, or overall survival rates between young patients treated with tumorectomy and irradiation and young patients treated with mastectomy.[69] In a review of 1,703 premenopausal patients treated at the Institut Curie, very young age (younger than 34 years) was associated with a worse outcome independent of type of local treatment.[70] The data from the two randomized trials with longest follow-up do not specifically address the issue of patients younger than 35 years but do not show an advantage for one form of local treatment for younger patients. In the Milan trial,[33] survival was similar after treatment with quadrantectomy and RT or mastectomy among patients younger than 45 years, and in the NSABP trial B-06,[34] survival was similar after treatment with lumpectomy and RT or mastectomy among premenopausal patients. Thus, the available information suggests that young patient age is a prognostic, but not a predictive, factor; it does not seem helpful in selecting the best form of local treatment.

Inherited Susceptibility

An inherited susceptibility to breast cancer and other cancers has recently been linked to germ-line mutations in *BRCA1* and *BRCA2*. Given this, it is important to understand whether patients with such germ-line mutations are at greater risk of local recurrence or other adverse outcomes than patients without such mutations. To begin to evaluate this, the outcome in 201 patients aged 36 years or younger, treated with BCT at the JCRT, was assessed in relation to an FH of a first-degree relative with premenopausal breast cancer or ovarian cancer at any age.[71] Young patients who have a positive FH have a high prior probability of a mutation in *BRCA1* or *BRCA2*. The following was the 5-year crude outcome for patients with a positive FH: no evidence of disease, 69%; local recurrence, 3%; and opposite breast cancer, 14%. This was in comparison to the following outcome for patients with a negative FH: no evidence of disease, 58%; local recurrence, 14%; and opposite breast cancer, 3%. In a multiple variable analysis, a positive FH was associated with a relative risk of 0.2 for local recurrence and a relative risk of 5.7 for opposite breast cancer compared to a negative FH. The increased relative risk for opposite breast cancer was statistically significant. Patients with a positive FH had a similar rate of second nonbreast cancers, complications, and excellent and good cosmetic scores as patients with a negative FH. A higher rate of opposite breast cancer had been noted previously in patients with germ-line mutations in *BRCA1*.[72,73] Also, patients with proven germ-line mutations in *BRCA1* or *BRCA2* have similarly shown a normal reaction to RT to the breast or chest wall.[74] Based on this information, it was concluded that BCT with RT is associated with a higher rate of opposite breast cancer in young women with an FH suggestive of an inherited breast cancer susceptibility compared with young women without such an FH and that this should be taken into account when BCT is considered as a treatment option. The rate of local recurrence in patients with a positive FH was, if anything, lower than in patients with a negative FH. If confirmed, this might be explained by the recent findings linking *BRCA1* and *BRCA2* with radiation repair genes[75,76] or by a greater likelihood of localized (EIC negative) cancers in patients with mutations compared to patients without mutations.[77] Additional studies are currently under way to assess outcome in relation to the findings on genetic testing for mutations. However, until genetic testing can be accomplished rapidly and effectively at the time of diagnosis, the use of young age and FH (and Ashkenazi descent) as surrogates will continue to be of clinical value.

Tumor Risk Factors

Extensive Intraductal Component

An EIC has been shown to be an important risk factor for local recurrence when margins of resection are not evaluated.[78] An EIC applies to infiltrating duct carcinomas in which (a) intraductal carcinoma is prominently present within the tumor and (b) intraductal carcinoma is present in sections of grossly normal adjacent breast tissue. In addition, tumors that are predominantly intraductal but have foci of invasion are considered to have an EIC. EIC-positive cancers are associated with a higher rate of true recurrences or marginal misses but are not associated with an increased rate of recurrence elsewhere in the ipsilateral or the opposite breast or in distant recurrence, compared with EIC-negative cancers. In a study of patients who underwent reexcision of the primary tumor site after an initial gross excision, it was found that those with EIC-positive cancers had a greater incidence of residual tumor in the reexcision specimen than did patients with EIC-negative cancers.[79] For patients with an EIC-positive cancer, the residual tumor often was widespread and was composed predominantly of intraductal carcinoma, whereas residual tumor in patients with an EIC-negative cancer usually consisted of only scattered microscopic foci of infiltrating or intraductal carcinoma. Similar findings were noticed in a study of mastectomy specimens by Holland et al.[22] In this study, approximately 30% of patients with EIC-positive cancers had prominent residual intraductal carcinoma (six or more low-power fields) at least 2 cm beyond the edge of the primary tumor, compared with only 2% of patients with EIC-negative cancers (Fig. 3). These observations indicate that in a substantial minority of patients with an EIC-positive cancer treated with a simple gross excision, there is a large residual tumor burden in the involved quadrant of the breast and that moderate-dose RT is not able to eradicate it. This information also suggests that a larger breast resection in patients with an EIC-positive cancer might result in a smaller residual tumor burden and, therefore, might lower the risk of recurrence in the breast after RT.

The problem of recognizing cancers with such extensive intraductal involvement has been greatly facilitated by the use of mammography.[80] The intraductal component in these lesions frequently shows microcalcifications, and their presence and extent can be detected on high-quality mammograms, particularly with the use of magnification views. The

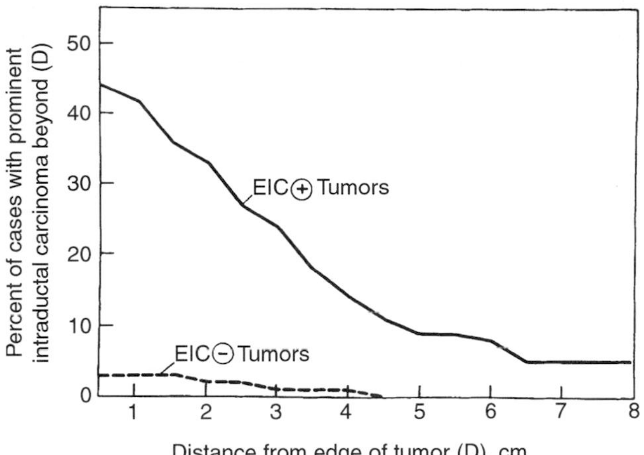

FIG. 3. Frequency of prominent intraductal carcinoma (defined as six or more low-power fields) as a function of the distance from the reference tumor in relation to the presence or absence of an extensive intraductal component (EIC) in the reference tumor. Approximately 30% of EIC-positive tumors have prominent residual intraductal carcinoma 2 cm beyond the reference tumor.

problem of EIC-positive cancers also has to be reconsidered at a time when there is routine evaluation of the microscopic margins of resection; this is discussed in the following section, Margins of Resection. A number of studies (presented below) have demonstrated that patients with an EIC-positive breast cancer but negative margins of resection are reasonable candidates for BCT.

Margins of Resection

Microscopic margins of resection are the major selection factor for BCT in current practice. There are significant technical considerations and limitations in the assessment of margins, and these are discussed in detail in Chapter 30. In addition, there are variations in the definitions of a negative and close margin. Despite these limitations, patients with negative margins of excision (typically defined as the absence of either invasive or ductal *in situ* disease directly at an inked surface) have generally been observed to have low rates of local recurrence after treatment with CS and RT (Table 3).[81–90] In addition, the long-term results of prospective randomized trials of BCT in patients with negative margins of excision have demonstrated low recurrence rates.[34,36] A recent update of the JCRT experience demonstrated an 8-year crude recurrence rate of 7% in 298 patients with negative (including close) inked margins of excision treated with 60 Gy or greater to the tumor bed (Table 4).[84] Of note in this update, all slides were reviewed by study pathologists, and the 8-year end point was chosen because nearly all patients had been followed by that time. Recent studies from the JCRT have also demonstrated that patients with an EIC, but with negative inked margins of excision, are not at an increased risk of local recurrence.[84,91] Other groups have similarly noted no association of EIC and an increased rate of local recurrence when inked margins of excision were routinely evaluated.[85,86,92] Thus, tumors with an EIC that are adequately excised, as judged from inked margin assessment, are not associated with an increased risk of breast recurrence.

TABLE 3. *Recurrence rates (%) by margin status*

Author (institution)	No. of patients (median F/U)	End point	Negative	Close	Positive
Borger et al.[81] (Netherlands)	1,026 (6.5 yr)	5-yr actuarial	2	6	16
Dewar et al.[82] (Gustave-Roussy)	757 (9 yr)	10-yr actuarial	6	—	14
Freedman et al.[83] (Fox Chase)	1,262 (6.3 yr)	5-yr actuarial 10-yr actuarial	4 7	7 14	5 12
Park et al.[84] (JCRT)	340 (10.8 yr)	8-yr crude rate	7	7	14[a]/27[b]
Anscher et al.[85] (Duke)	259 (3.8 yr)	5-yr actuarial	2	—	10
Smitt et al.[86] (Stanford)	289 (6 yr)	10-yr actuarial	2	16	0[a]/9[b]
Peterson et al.[87] (U. Penn.)	1,021 (6.1 yr)	8-yr actuarial	8	17	10
Wazer et al.[88] (Tufts)	498 (6 yr)	10-yr actuarial	2	2	15
Pittinger et al.[89] (U. Rochester)	211 (4.5 yr)	Crude rate (F/U 54 mo)	3	2.9	25
Cowen et al.[90] (Marseilles)	152 (6 yr)	5-yr actuarial	—	—	20

F/U, follow-up; JCRT, Joint Center for Radiation Therapy; U. Penn, University of Pennsylvania; U. Rochester, University of Rochester.
[a]Focally positive.
[b]More than focally positive.

TABLE 4. *Eight-year outcome related to margins of resection (Joint Center for Radiation Therapy)*

Margin status	No. of patients	% Local recurrence	% D/R/O recurrence	% Died with recurrence	% NED
Negative	204	7	25	4	63
Close[a]	94	7	28	6	59
Focally positive[b]	122	14	25	7	54
>Focally positive[b]	66	27	35	3	35

[a]Any *in situ* or invasive disease within 1 mm of inked surface but not present at surface.
[b]*In situ* or invasive disease at inked surface but in three or fewer low-power fields.
D/R/O, distant or regional failure or opposite breast cancer; NED, no evidence of disease.

The outcome of patients with close margins of excision has been less clear (see Table 3). In part, this reflects variability in the definition of "close margins" and, perhaps, the impact of institutional policies that call for escalated radiation doses based on the proximity of cancer cells to the margin of resection. In the JCRT experience, no significant difference was seen in recurrence rates between patients with close margins (1 mm) and those with margins greater than 1 mm using similar doses. Some studies have suggested a high rate of local recurrence at 10 years in patients with close margins; however, the number of patients in these series and the actual follow-up time are limited.[83,86]

Long-term data on the use of BCT in patients with positive margins are more limited. In most analyses, positive margins have been associated with a high risk of breast recurrence.[81–85,88–90] At the JCRT, patients with positive margins had a considerably higher risk of breast recurrence than patients with negative margins. The 8-year crude rate of breast recurrence was 18% for patients with positive margins. However, patients with focally positive margins (any invasive or *in situ* ductal carcinoma at the margin in three or fewer low-power microscopic fields) had a 14% rate of recurrence, compared to a 27% rate in patients with greater than focally positive margins. These data suggest that only patients with focally positive margins should be considered for BCT. As discussed in the section Use of Adjuvant Systemic Therapy, the use of adjuvant systemic therapy results in a large reduction in local recurrence in patients treated with CS and RT. In the JCRT series, among the 45 patients with focally positive margins who received adjuvant systemic therapy, the 8-year local recurrence rate was 8% (95% confidence interval, 1% to 18%).[84] Additional experience is needed to confirm this finding. Patients with more than focally positive margins require more surgery, given that they have a significantly higher rate of breast recurrence, even when the boost dose is escalated.

Treatment Factors

Extent of Resection

The extent of breast resection has a clear association with local recurrence. The rate of local recurrence is much higher after an incisional biopsy than after an excisional biopsy. Beyond gross excision, however, considerable controversy exists regarding the optimal extent of breast resection. In North America, a more limited resection (lumpectomy) is typically performed, whereas in Europe a wider resection (quadrantectomy) is more common. Quadrantectomy was designed to address the segmental nature of involvement of the cancer in the breast; however, the precise limits of these segments are not apparent at the time of surgery. In the Milan II trial, 705 patients with cancers less than 2.5 cm were randomized to either quadrantectomy, axillary dissection, and external beam RT (QUART) or tumorectomy, axillary dissection, external beam RT, and a boost using iridium 192 implantation (TART).[93] Patients treated with TART had positive margins more often than patients treated with QUART (16% versus 5%). With a median follow-up of 113 months, the 10-year rate of local recurrence was higher in the patients treated with TART (19% versus 7%), but no differences were seen in the rate of distant metastases or mortality between patients treated with TART or QUART. Thus, increasing the volume of breast resection is associated with a decrease in the rate of local recurrence but, as previously discussed, also has an adverse effect on the cosmetic result.

Surprisingly little is established concerning the association between radiation treatment factors and recurrence in the breast. As a result, information on the possible importance of radiation factors comes from comparisons within a retrospective review or comparisons between different retrospective reviews, both of which are subject to the potential confounding of treatment factors with other important variables.

Use of a Boost

In particular, the need for a boost to the primary tumor site has been controversial. Many have argued that because the rate of local recurrence in the NSABP B-06 trial (in which a boost was not used) is comparable with that of other series in which a boost is routinely used, a boost is not required in patients with negative margins of resection. On the other side are the arguments that only a very large study could demonstrate the small improvement in local recurrence that might be expected from a policy of routinely using a boost and that the use of a boost does not greatly increase the rate of complications or decrease the cosmetic outcome. In one such trial from Lyons, France, 1,024 patients with cancers measuring 3 cm or less underwent excision and 50-Gy whole-breast RT and then were randomized to a 10-Gy boost or no further treatment. Ninety-eight percent of the patients had negative margins. In a preliminary report with a median follow-up of 3.3 years, the 5-year rate of local recurrence was 3.6% in the patients with a boost and 4.5% in patients without a boost.[94] Another large trial testing the value of a boost has been performed by the European Organization for Research and Treatment of Cancer. In this trial, patients with negative microscopic margins of resection received 50 Gy to the whole breast and then were randomized to receive either no boost or a boost of 15 Gy by interstitial irradiation or 16 Gy by external beam techniques. Patients with positive microscopic margins of resection received 50 Gy to the whole breast and then were randomized either to a low-dose boost of 10 Gy or to a high-dose boost, either 25 Gy by interstitial irradiation or 26 Gy by external beam techniques. Updated results from these trials will be helpful in settling this controversy.

Use of Adjuvant Systemic Therapy

The use of adjuvant systemic therapy is an important factor associated with recurrence in the breast when used in conjunction with CS and RT. The rate of recurrence in the breast has been reported in a number of retrospective series to be lower in patients treated with systemic therapy than in those treated with BCT alone. However, this effect is most clearly demonstrated in three randomized clinical trials. In the NSABP B-13 trial, node-negative estrogen receptor (ER)–negative patients were randomized to chemotherapy or to a no-treatment control group. Among the 235 patients treated with CS and RT, the 8-year rate of recurrence in the ipsilateral breast was 13.4% without chemotherapy and only 2.6% with chemotherapy.[95] Similar results are seen with adjuvant tamoxifen. In NSABP trial B-14, node-negative ER-positive patients were randomized to tamoxifen or to a placebo. Among the 1,062 patients treated with CS and RT, the 10-year rate of recurrence in the ipsilateral breast was 14.7% without tamoxifen and only 4.3% with tamoxifen.[96] A similar result was seen in the Stockholm Breast Cancer Study Group among node-negative patients randomized to tamoxifen or to a placebo. Among the 432 patients treated with CS and RT, the 10-year rate of recurrence in the ipsilateral breast was 12% without tamoxifen and only 3% with tamoxifen.[97]

GUIDELINES FOR PATIENT SELECTION

Based on the extensive information available from prospective and retrospective studies, there is a general consensus on the criteria for patient selection for the use of BCT. It is now established that in most cases, BCT results in a cosmetically satisfactory breast and that it provides survival rates equivalent to those seen after mastectomy. The American College of Surgeons, the American College of Radiology, the College of American Pathologists, and the Society of Surgical Oncology have met to develop standards of care for BCT and published their most recent report in 1998.[56] Key portions of this report are given below, and additional comments are provided in parentheses.

Because of the potential options for treatment of early-stage breast cancer, careful patient selection and a multidisciplinary approach are necessary. The four critical elements in patient selection for BCT are (a) history and physical examination, (b) mammographic evaluation, (c) histologic assessment of the resected breast specimen, and (d) assessment of the patient's needs and expectations. Age, *per se*, whether young or old, is not a contraindication to breast conservation. In the elderly, physiologic age and the presence of comorbid conditions should be the primary determinants of local therapy. Retraction of the skin, nipple, and breast parenchyma are not signs of locally advanced breast cancer and are not contraindications to breast conservation.

Recent (i.e., usually within 3 months) preoperative mammographic evaluation is necessary to determine a patient's eligibility for BCT. It should be done with high-quality, dedicated mammographic equipment. Mammographic evaluation defines the extent of a patient's disease, the presence or absence of multicentricity, and other factors that might influence the treatment decision and evaluates the contralateral breast. The size of the tumor should be included in the mammographic report. If the mass is associated with microcalcifications, an assessment of the extent of the calcifications within and outside the mass should be made. Magnification mammography is important for characterizing microcalcifications.

Histologic subtype other than invasive ductal carcinoma does not appear to be associated with an increased risk of breast cancer recurrence. In particular, patients with invasive lobular cancers are candidates for CS and radiation if the tumor is not diffuse in the breast and can be completely excised with negative margins. Patients with positive axillary nodes do not have an increased risk of breast recurrence when treated with CS and RT. In contrast, in patients undergoing mastectomy, the number of positive axillary nodes correlates with the incidence of chest wall recurrence. The diminished risk of breast recurrence in node-positive patients may be related to the combined effects of chemotherapy or tamoxifen (or both) with RT in these patients. The presence of an EIC is a pathologic indicator that the disease in the breast may be more extensive than is clinically appreciated. Assessment of resection margins in these patients is important in determining treatment options. If negative margins can be achieved, current information suggests that these patients are appropriate candidates for CS and RT. If the reexcision margins remain positive, mastectomy is the preferred treatment.

The influence of the final resection margin on breast cancer recurrence rates varies. In most reported series, positive margins of resection have been associated with an increased risk of breast cancer recurrence, although the magnitude has varied considerably. Ideally, negative margins of resection should be achieved before RT to diminish the risk of a breast cancer recurrence, especially in patients who will not be receiving adjuvant systemic therapy. The ultimate outcome of EIC-negative tumors with focal margin involvement remains to be determined. Presently, reexcision is recommended in patients whose initial margin of resection is unknown or positive. In contrast to DCIS, lobular carcinoma *in situ* is an incidental histologic finding that is considered a marker of increased risk for subsequent breast cancer rather than a malignant lesion requiring surgical excision. The relationship between lobular carcinoma *in situ* and surgical margins is not important.

Perhaps the most difficult aspect of patient evaluation is the assessment of the patient's needs and expectations regarding breast preservation. The patient and her physician must discuss the benefits and risks of mastectomy compared with those of BCT in her individual case. Each woman must evaluate how her choice of treatment is likely to affect her sense of disease control, self-esteem, sexuality, physical functioning, and overall quality of life. The following factors should be considered:

1. Long-term survival
2. The possibility and consequences of local recurrence
3. Psychological adjustment (including the fear of cancer recurrence), cosmetic outcome, sexual adaptation, and functional competence

For most patients, the choice of mastectomy with or without reconstruction or BCT does not influence the likelihood of survival, but it may affect the quality of life.

Psychological research comparing patient adaptation after mastectomy with that after BCT shows no significant differences in global measures of emotional distress. However, women whose breasts are preserved have more positive attitudes about their body image and experience fewer changes in their frequency of breast stimulation and feelings of sexual desirability.

Absolute and Relative Contraindications

Some absolute and relative contraindications and nonmitigating factors exist in the selection of patients for BCT with RT.

Absolute Contraindications

- Women with two or more primary tumors in separate quadrants of the breast or with diffuse malignant-appearing microcalcifications are not considered candidates for BCT.
- A history of previous therapeutic irradiation to the breast region that, combined with the proposed treatment, would result in an excessively high total radiation dose to a significant volume is another absolute contraindication.
- Pregnancy is an absolute contraindication to the use of breast irradiation. However, in many cases, it may be possible to perform breast-conserving surgery in the third trimester and treat the patient with irradiation after delivery.
- Persistent positive margins after reasonable surgical attempts absolutely contraindicate BCT with radiation. The importance of a single, focally positive microscopic margin needs further study and may not be an absolute contraindication. (See updated results from the JCRT, discussed in the section Margins of Resection.)

Relative Contraindications

- A history of collagen vascular disease is a relative contraindication to BCT, because published reports indicate that such patients tolerate irradiation poorly.[98] Most radiation oncologists will not treat patients with scleroderma or active lupus erythematosus, considering either an absolute contraindication. In contrast, rheumatoid arthritis is neither a relative nor an absolute contraindication.[99]
- Patients with multiple gross tumors in the same quadrant and indeterminate calcifications must be carefully assessed for suitability, because studies in this area are not definitive.
- Tumor size is not an absolute contraindication to BCT, although few reports have been published about treating patients with tumors larger than 4 to 5 cm. However, a relative contraindication is the presence of a large tumor in a small breast, in which an adequate resection would result in significant cosmetic alteration.
- Breast size can be a relative contraindication. Women with large or pendulous breasts can be treated by irradiation if reproducibility of patient setup can be ensured and if it is technically possible to obtain adequate dose homogeneity.

Nonmitigating Factors

Certain clinical and pathologic features should not prevent patients from being candidates for BCT. These features include the following:

- The presence of clinical or pathologic involvement in axillary nodes.
- After CS and RT, evaluating the breast for local recurrence is feasible. The changes associated with recurrence can be detected at an early stage by physical examination and mammography.
- The delivery of irradiation in this setting does not result in a meaningful risk of second tumors in either the treated or the untreated area.
- Tumor location is not a factor in the choice of treatment. Tumors in a superficial subareolar location occasionally may require resection of the nipple-areolar complex so that negative margins can be achieved, but this does not affect outcome. The patient and her physician need to assess whether such a resection is preferable to mastectomy.
- An FH of breast cancer is not a contraindication to breast conservation. Little is known about the risk of breast

recurrence in patients with hereditary breast cancer, but currently this is not a contraindication to BCT. (However, such patients should be apprised of their increased risk of opposite breast cancer.)

- A high risk of systemic relapse is not a contraindication for breast conservation but is a determinant of the need for adjuvant therapy.

PREOPERATIVE CHEMOTHERAPY

The use of preoperative chemotherapy in locally advanced breast cancer reduces tumor size by at least 50% in the majority of cases, and complete pathologic responses are seen in approximately 10% of patients (see Chapter 39). This observation has led to a number of studies in patients with stages I and II breast carcinoma to determine if the use of preoperative chemotherapy would allow breast conservation in patients who would otherwise be treated with mastectomy. In an early study, Bonadonna et al.[100] treated 165 patients with tumors 3 cm or larger in size, who would otherwise have been treated with mastectomy at their institution, with three or four cycles of CMF; or fluorouracil, doxorubicin, and cyclophosphamide; or substituted epirubicin for doxorubicin. Complete or partial response was observed in at least 70% of patients in all treatment groups, and progression occurred in only 2%. Response was greatest in smaller tumors and was unrelated to age, menopausal status, ploidy, or thymidine-labeling index. Of the 157 patients who had surgery, 81% had BCT. The authors concluded that this approach allowed the use of BCT in patients who would otherwise have required mastectomy, but the study lacked a control group to definitively support this conclusion. In another nonrandomized study, Smith et al.[101] treated 64 patients with large operable breast cancers (median diameter, 6 cm) with either CMF or mitomycin C/methotrexate/mitoxantrone. Sixty-nine percent of patients achieved an objective response of greater than 50% reduction in tumor size. Complete clinical remission was observed in 17% of patients, and 2% of patients had progression of disease while receiving chemotherapy. Seventy-seven percent of patients had BCT. However, the local recurrence rate was 27%, with a mean follow-up of only 2.5 years.

In addition to increasing the number of patients who can undergo BCT, a second, and more important, rationale for the use of preoperative chemotherapy is to improve survival. However, this can only be assessed in randomized clinical trials. The available randomized trials suggest that the use of preoperative chemotherapy does reduce the need for mastectomy but does not improve survival. Powles et al.[102] randomized 212 patients with palpable, operable breast cancers to surgery followed by eight cycles of chemotherapy, or four cycles of chemotherapy before surgery followed by an additional four cycles postoperatively. An objective response was achieved in 85% of patients who received preoperative therapy, and 10% were found to have a pathologic complete remission. The use of mastectomy was significantly reduced in the preoperative chemotherapy group, with 13% of patients having this procedure compared to 28% of patients who received postoperative chemotherapy ($p < .005$). At a mean follow-up of 28 months, no differences in distant disease-free or overall survival were noted.

The NSABP has reported the results of a large randomized trial in which 1,523 patients with T1-3, N0-1 breast carcinoma were assigned to have surgery followed by four cycles of doxorubicin and cyclophosphamide [Adriamycin-Cytoxan (AC)] or to receive AC before surgery.[103,104] At 5 years of follow-up, no differences in disease-free survival, distant disease-free survival, or overall survival were observed. BCT was used more frequently in the preoperative chemotherapy group, 67.8% versus 59.8% ($p = .003$). Overall, no difference was seen in the incidence of breast recurrence between the preoperative (7.9%) and the postoperative group (5.8%). However, an analysis of breast recurrence rates among patients who were initially eligible for lumpectomy and those who were eligible only after downstaging by chemotherapy demonstrated a local failure rate of 6.9% in those believed to be candidates for lumpectomy before chemotherapy, compared to 14.5% in those who required downstaging ($p = .04$). An increased rate of breast recurrence was noted in downstaged patients, regardless of age or tumor size.

A major practical problem with the use of preoperative chemotherapy to increase rates of BCT is the determination of the extent of residual viable tumor that must be resected. The clinical assessment of response is relatively inaccurate. In one study of 56 patients, the sensitivity of clinical examination was 49%.[105] The sensitivity of mammography was 79%, but the specificity was only 77%. Other studies have confirmed that mammography does not reliably exclude persistent microscopic tumor, and the presence of architectural distortion or calcifications is not always indicative of disease.[106,107] Abraham et al.[108] report that magnetic resonance imaging (MR) accurately predicted the extent of residual disease after induction chemotherapy in 30 of 31 cases, and Gilles et al.[109] demonstrated that MR enhancement accurately predicted the extent of residual disease in 83% of 18 cases. These results are promising, but in many institutions where expertise in breast MR is lacking, decisions about the extent of surgical resection and patient suitability for BCT must be made using clinical, mammographic, and pathologic criteria. We approach these patients by initially resecting any clinically or mammographically abnormal tissue. If viable tumor is present throughout the specimen, even if the initial margins are negative, a reexcision is carried out. If further viable tumor is present in the reexcised specimen, a reevaluation of the patient's suitability for BCT is undertaken. Marking the extent of the tumor before chemotherapy with stereotactically placed clips or skin tattoos is useful for determining the tumor location in patients who have a complete clinical response and may aid in assessing the need for resection of residual abnormalities in patients with a partial response.

The role of neoadjuvant therapy in operable breast cancer remains undefined. There appears to be no rationale, outside

TABLE 5. *Patient characteristics in the trials comparing conservative surgery with and without radiation therapy*

Trial	Years	No. of patients	Tumor size	Nodal status	Type of surgery	Final margins	Adjuvant therapy
NSABP B-06[34]	1976–1984	1,851	≤4 cm	±	Lumpectomy	–	Chemotherapy for node-positive patients
Swedish[110]	1981–1988	381	≤2 cm	–	Sector resection	–	None
Ontario[111]	1984–1989	837	≤4 cm	–	Lumpectomy	–	None
Milan III[33]	1988–1989	567	≤2.5 cm	±	Quadrantectomy	±	Chemotherapy for some node-positive patients
Scottish[112]	1985–1991	585	≤4 cm	±	Lumpectomy	±	CMF for ER-negative patients; tamoxifen for ER-positive patients
English[113]	1981–1990	418	<5 cm	±	Lumpectomy	–	CMF for all patients; tamoxifen given to ER-positive patients

CMF, cyclophosphamide, methotrexate,3-fluorouracil; ER, estrogen receptor; NSABP, National Surgical Adjuvant Breast and Bowel Project.

of a clinical trial, for its routine use in patients who are suitable candidates for BCT. At present, there are no data suggesting that patients with multicentric carcinoma can be converted into appropriate candidates for BCT with the use of preoperative chemotherapy. Initial chemotherapy is appropriate when a large tumor in a small breast would necessitate mastectomy and the patient desires BCT. However, in the study of Morrow et al.,[51] this contraindication to BCT was present in 6% of 336 patients with stages I and II carcinoma. The potential for a higher risk of breast recurrence should be discussed with the patient and the pathology carefully reviewed before it is decided that the patient is a suitable candidate for RT.

CONSERVATIVE SURGERY WITHOUT RADIATION THERAPY

An unresolved question is whether RT is necessary in all patients with invasive breast cancer after CS. Six randomized clinical trials with published results have compared CS alone to CS and RT in patients with early-stage breast cancer.[33,34,110–113] These trials, summarized in Table 5, vary with regard to patient selection, the details of the surgery and RT, the use of adjuvant systemic therapy, and the length of follow-up. The results of these various trials are shown in Tables 5 and 6. These trials all show a large reduction in the rate of local recurrence after RT, with an average crude rate of reduction of approximately 75% (range, 63% to 89%). None of the six trials shows a significant survival benefit for RT; however, in the trials with published data, the survival rate is slightly better for irradiated patients than for nonirradiated patients. In a multivariate analysis of survival in the Ontario trial, for example, the use of RT was associated with a 15% reduction in the relative risk of dying (relative risk, 0.85), but this was not statistically significant (95% confidence interval, 0.59 to 1.23). A very large trial (or perhaps a meta-analysis of multiple smaller trials) is necessary to detect a small but clinically significant difference in survival, if it in fact exists. None of these six has the statistical power to rule out a 10% to 15% proportional reduction in mortality or a 5% to 10% absolute improvement in survival.

Attempts have been made to identify a subgroup of patients (based on various clinical and histologic features) who have a low risk of local recurrence after CS alone. It was not possible to identify such a subgroup within the Ontario and NSABP[34] randomized trials. Local recurrence rates are generally lower in trials that use more extensive surgery than in those using lumpectomy and in older patients than in younger patients. In an analysis of the Milan trials,[33] the 5-year rate of local recurrence after quadrantectomy was approximately 25% in patients aged 55 years or younger but only 10% in patients older than 55 years. However, the use of RT in this age group greatly reduced local recurrence: The

TABLE 6. *Outcome in the trials comparing conservative surgery with and without radiation therapy*

Trial	Median follow-up (mo)	Local recurrences		Survival		Analysis
		CS (%)	CS + RT (%)	CS (%)	CS + RT (%)	
NSABP B-06[34]	144	35	10	58	62	12-yr actuarial
Swedish[110]	64	18	2	90	91	5-yr actuarial
Ontario[111]	91	35	11	76	79	8-yr crude
Milan III[33]	52	18[a]	2[a]	No difference		5-yr actuarial
Scottish[112]	68	25	6	No difference		5-yr actuarial
English[113]	71	35	13	Not available		6-yr crude

CS, conservative surgery; NSABP, National Surgical Adjuvant Breast and Bowel Project; RT, radiation therapy.
[a]Estimated from curves.

annual rate of local recurrence for older patients was 1.53 per 100 patient-years for quadrantectomy alone, compared with only 0.19 per 100 patient-years for quadrantectomy and RT. The JCRT attempted to identify such a subgroup in a prospective single-arm trial in which patients with a very favorable prognosis were offered the option of CS alone. The criteria for entry into this protocol were tumor size of 2 cm or less, histologically negative axillary nodes, absence of both lymphatic vessel invasion and an EIC in the cancer, and no cancer cells visualized within 1 cm of inked margins.[114] All but one patient had a negative reexcision. The median age of patients in this trial was 67 years, and median pathologic size of the cancers was 9 mm. This trial was stopped shortly before it reached its accrual goal of 90 patients because of stopping rules ensuring against an excessively high local recurrence rate. With a median follow-up time of 66 months, the crude rate of local recurrence was 20%. Examination of subsets of patients by age and tumor size did not find any statistically significant differences. Based on the results of this prospective study, it was concluded that even a highly selected group of breast cancer patients have a substantial risk of early local recurrence after treatment with wide excision alone.

The use of adjuvant systemic therapy substantially reduces the rate of local recurrence in patients treated with CS and RT but does not seem to reduce greatly the rate of local recurrence after CS alone. Information on this is available from direct and indirect comparisons within randomized clinical trials for both adjuvant chemotherapy and tamoxifen. In the NSABP trial B-06, an indirect comparison of the effect of adjuvant chemotherapy can be made. Node-positive patients treated with lumpectomy and adjuvant chemotherapy but without RT had a 12-year rate of recurrence in the breast of 41%, compared with only 5% for node-positive patients treated with lumpectomy, RT, and chemotherapy (p <.001).[34] In comparison, node-negative patients treated with lumpectomy without RT had a 12-year rate of recurrence in the breast of 32%, compared with 12% for node-negative patients treated with lumpectomy with RT. A similar observation suggesting that systemic therapy further decreases the rate of local recurrence when combined with RT, but not in its absence, is seen in indirect comparisons within the Milan trials.[33]

In the Scottish trial, patients with ER-negative cancers were treated with adjuvant CMF chemotherapy. With a median follow-up time of approximately 5.7 years, the crude rate of local-regional recurrence was 44% among patients treated with CS but without RT, compared with only 14% among patients treated with RT.[112] A direct comparison of the effect of adjuvant chemotherapy combined with RT is available in NSABP trial B-13, in which node-negative ER-negative patients were randomized to methotrexate and fluorouracil or to a control group. Among the patients treated with CS and RT, the 8-year rate of recurrence in the ipsilateral breast was 13.4% without chemotherapy and only 2.6% with chemotherapy.[95] Similar results are seen with adjuvant tamoxifen. In the Scottish trial, patients with ER-positive cancers were treated with adjuvant tamoxifen. With a median follow-up time of 5.7 years, the crude rate of local-regional recurrence was 25% among patients treated with CS but without RT, compared with only 3% among patients treated with RT.[112] A direct comparison of the effect of tamoxifen given with CS and RT is available in NSABP trial B-14, in which node-negative ER-positive patients were randomized to tamoxifen or to a placebo. Among the 1,062 patients treated with CS and RT, the 10-year rate of recurrence in the ipsilateral breast was 14.7% without tamoxifen and only 4.3% with tamoxifen.[96] A similar result was seen in the Stockholm Breast Cancer Study Group among node-negative patients randomized to tamoxifen or to a placebo. Among the 432 patients treated with CS and RT, the 10-year rate of recurrence in the ipsilateral breast was 12% without tamoxifen and only 3% with tamoxifen.[97] There are no published trials that directly compare CS with and without either chemotherapy or tamoxifen.

There is particular interest in avoiding RT in older patients. It is often less convenient for such patients to receive RT, and their local recurrence rate appears lower after CS alone compared to that of younger patients. The results of retrospective studies of CS alone with or without adjuvant tamoxifen have shown variable results.[115–119] A prospective, randomized clinical trial testing the value of RT in older patients with breast cancer treated by CS and tamoxifen is being conducted in North America by the Cancer and Leukemia Group B (CALGB) and other groups. In addition, the NSABP trial B-21, which opened in 1989 and randomized patients with tumors smaller than 1 cm and with negative margins to either RT, tamoxifen, or both was closed prematurely in 1993 because of slow accrual, but it has been reopened.

It is possible to assess patient preferences (or "utilities") and the cost-effectiveness of routine RT after CS in the assumed absence of a survival benefit. Using the standard gamble technique, patient preferences were assessed among 97 breast cancer patients treated with CS and RT and among 20 medical oncology nurses without a diagnosis of breast cancer.[120] Fear of a local recurrence and an actual local recurrence leading to mastectomy had such a negative impact on quality of life that both groups were willing to accept the risks and inconvenience of RT to avoid them. Using these data in a Markov model, a cost-utility analysis was performed comparing a strategy of RT versus no RT in a hypothetical cohort of 60-year-old women after CS.[121] The addition of RT resulted in an incremental cost-effectiveness ratio of $28,000/quality-adjusted life years (QALY), which is well below $50,000/QALY, a commonly cited threshold for cost-effective care.

In conclusion, the use of breast irradiation after CS is associated with a large reduction in the rate of local recurrence. The available data from the randomized trials do not show a survival benefit; however, none of the available trials has the statistical power to eliminate a small survival difference. A subset at low risk of local recurrence after CS has not been clearly identified, and RT is currently considered standard. The addition of adjuvant systemic therapy to CS alone has not been demonstrated to decrease local recurrence. In frail elderly patients, RT is commonly omitted because of the practical difficulties of delivering such therapy to this group of patients.

TIMING OF BREAST SURGERY

In 1989, Hrushesky et al.[122] reported the results of a retrospective study of 41 premenopausal patients with breast cancer, suggesting that the timing of surgery in relation to the menstrual cycle was an important, independent predictor of survival. In that study, patients who underwent resection during the perimenstrual period (days 0 to 6, 21 to 36) had a 95% survival rate at 10 years, compared with 78% for women who had surgery at other times of the menstrual cycle. Since this report, multiple other studies have been published, and the results are almost evenly divided between studies showing a relationship between menstrual cycle timing and survival and those that do not.[123,124]

The majority of the studies that identified an effect found that surgery during the follicular phase of the cycle (days 0 to 14) was associated with a poorer survival than surgery during the luteal phase.[124–129] However, this effect was only observed in patients with axillary lymph node involvement. Other studies that identified a positive effect divided the menstrual cycle into three groups, with the follicular phase defined as days 3 to 12, and the luteal phase defined as days 0 to 2 and 13 to 32.[125,128–130] These studies also showed a benefit for surgery during the luteal phase, which again was largely confined to patients with positive axillary nodes. However, all of these studies, both positive and negative, suffer from major problems in methodology. Menstrual cycle timing was based on the patient's retrospective recall of the date of her last menstrual period before operation. In some cases, patients were asked to provide this information weeks after surgery, and women with menstrual irregularity and oral contraceptive use were not excluded from the study population in all reports. In addition, although normal menstrual cycle length varies, and between 3% and 20% of women have irregular cycles,[131] these studies assumed a uniform day of ovulation. Other problems that preclude direct comparisons between studies include variations in the number of surgical procedures performed, which surgical procedure was considered the focus of the survival analysis, and lack of standardization of the use of adjuvant systemic therapy.

McGuire et al.[132] hypothesized that the range of positive associations noticed in these reports might simply be due to chance. The impact of testing multiple windows on a single data set was studied by randomly assigning menstrual dates to 675 patients in the San Antonio Database and by dividing the menstrual cycle into two 14-day windows. The experiment was repeated 100 times with different random assignments of menstrual dates, and a significant prognostic period was identified in 28% of the experiments. At present, no definitive conclusions regarding the importance of menstrual cycle timing of surgery can be made. Investigations into possible mechanisms for the positive outcomes observed in some studies have demonstrated that factors potentially involved in invasion and metastases, such as natural killer cell activity,[133] epidermal growth factor receptor levels,[134] and levels of cathepsins and matrix metalloproteinases[135] vary with the menstrual cycle. These observations suggest an underlying biological mechanism and provide further impetus for properly designed prospective trials to address this question. Hagen and Hrushesky[123] report that there are four ongoing or planned prospective studies of the question. Although they believe that the methodology of these studies is imperfect, they will address some of the problems that have been raised.

TECHNIQUE AND COMPLICATIONS OF BREAST-CONSERVING SURGERY

The goal of breast-conserving surgery is to minimize the risk of local recurrence while leaving the patient with a cosmetically acceptable breast. The most common form of breast-conserving surgery used in the United States is referred to as *lumpectomy*. The surgical technique of lumpectomy differs from that used for mastectomy in that lumpectomy is not an *en bloc* cancer operation. *Quadrantectomy* is another type of breast-conserving surgery that is designed to remove an anatomic segment of breast tissue and frequently includes removal of the overlying skin and underlying pectoral fascia. The rationale and results of this procedure are discussed in detail in the section Extent of Research. Because excision of a large amount of breast tissue is the major factor responsible for a poor cosmetic outcome after BCT,[57–60] lumpectomy is considered the appropriate initial surgical approach in the United States. Other surgical factors that influence cosmetic appearance are the size and placement of the incision, the management of the lumpectomy cavity, and the extent of axillary dissection.

A number of technical aspects of lumpectomy are worth emphasizing. In general, the incision should be placed directly over the area of the tumor. This is true even when a biopsy is performed for a mammographically detected lesion. Whereas tunneling for short distances is acceptable to avoid incisions in areas of the breast that may be exposed, extensive tunneling can make it difficult to assess the extent of tumor and to obtain meticulous hemostasis. In the upper part of the breast, incisions should be curvilinear or transverse and follow the natural skin creases (*Langer's lines*) of the breast. In the lower part of the breast, the choice of a curvilinear or radial incision depends on the contour of the patient's breast, the distance from the skin to the tumor, and the amount of breast tissue to be resected. It is not necessary to remove skin (except for very superficial tumors) or to remove needle tracks from core-needle biopsies or fine-needle aspirations. In particular, skin removed with a curvilinear incision in the inferior breast distorts the breast contour and should be avoided.

Preservation of the subcutaneous fat and avoidance of thin skin flaps are also important in maintaining normal breast contour. Raising flaps is necessary only to allow access to the tumor; tumors located deep within the breast parenchyma should be approached by incising the breast tissue superficial to the tumor without raising flaps. Meticulous hemostasis is important, because a large hematoma distorts the appearance of the breast and makes reexcision and follow-up evaluation more difficult. The presence of a postbiopsy hematoma, however, is not a contraindication to BCT. It is best to avoid reapproximation of the breast tissue, because this can result in distortion of the breast contour, which may not be apparent with the patient supine on the operating table. The best cosmetic results usually are obtained by allowing the lumpectomy cavity to fill in with serum and fibrin. For this reason as well, drainage of the lumpectomy cavity should be avoided. Finally, the incision should be closed with a subcuticular suture to avoid cross-hatching of the skin.

A critical step in lumpectomy is the evaluation of the completeness of excision of the tumor. Gross assessment of tumor removal is important, but histologic verification of margin status must also be obtained. To allow adequate histologic evaluation, the specimen should be removed as a single piece of tissue and should not be transected unless the pathologist is present. The use of marking sutures to orient the specimen for the pathologist allows reporting of the status of individual margins. This helps to avoid reexcision of large amounts of normal breast tissue if a single margin is found to be positive. Gross inspection of the specimen in the operating room allows identification of positive or close margins, facilitating immediate reexcision. Frozen section histologic study is sometimes useful to evaluate grossly suspicious areas, but the routine use of frozen sections to evaluate grossly normal margins is of doubtful value, because it represents a minimal sampling that does not preclude the presence of tumor on permanent section. Intraoperative touch preparation cytologic study may be useful for margin assessment, if a cytologist experienced in this technique is available.[136,137] The ideal amount of grossly normal breast tissue around the tumor that should be resected as part of a lumpectomy is uncertain. An attempted resection of 0.5 to 1.0 cm of grossly normal breast tissue resulted in histologically negative margins in 95% of 239 patients in the experience of Kearney and Morrow.[138] Larger resections may be necessary for invasive ductal carcinomas with an EIC[32,79,139] and for infiltrating lobular carcinomas.[140]

When axillary dissection is performed as part of breast-conserving surgery, a separate incision should be used, except in patients with tumors high in the tail of the breast. A curvilinear incision at the edge of the hair-bearing axillary skin provides the best cosmetic result. The incision should not extend anterior to the fold of the pectoralis major or posterior to the latissimus dorsi. Incision across these muscles does not improve access to the apex of the axilla and worsens the cosmetic result. In patients with a narrow axilla, a U-shaped, rather than a transverse, incision should be used. These procedures are described in more detail in Chapter 35.

Indications for Reexcision

The primary indications for a reexcision are positive or unknown histologic margins of resection on the initial excision. Several studies have demonstrated residual carcinoma in approximately one-half of cases when reexcision is performed for positive or unknown margins,[79,138,141] with little difference in the incidence between those patients with positive and those with unknown margins (Table 7). Schmidt Ullrich et al.[142] observed that the likelihood of residual carcinoma in a reexcision specimen done for positive or unknown margins was related to the histologic type of the primary tumor. Sixty-seven percent of invasive tumors with associated DCIS had residual disease, compared with 50% of infiltrating lobular carcinomas and only 35% of cases with infiltrating ductal carcinoma without associated DCIS. Schnitt et al.[79] also found that invasive ductal carcinomas with an EIC predicted a greater likelihood of residual tumor in reexcisions (88% for EIC-positive versus 48% for EIC-negative; $p = .002$).

The question of what is an acceptable margin status for a lumpectomy has not been resolved. It should be remembered when this issue is evaluated that even when margins are determined to be negative, residual cancer is present in a significant number of mastectomy specimens.[21,143,144] As discussed previously, the presence of an EIC *per se* should not be a contraindication to BCT.

Reexcision should be undertaken in patients with unknown margins and in patients with gross tumor or exten-

TABLE 7. *Finding of residual cancer on reexcision in relation to the microscopic margins of resection on the initial specimen*

Authors	No. of cases with positive margins on first excision	Incidence of residual cancer on reexcision (%)	No. of cases with unknown margins on first excision	Incidence of residual cancer on reexcision (%)
Schnitt et al.[79]	29	69	33	64
Gwin et al.[141]	54	65	100	45
Kearney and Morrow[138]	42	45	48	42

sive amounts of microscopic cancer at the margins of resection. The need for reexcision in patients with focal microscopic involvement at the margin of resection is less clear. Whether reexcision, an increased dose of radiation, or the use of adjuvant therapy is the optimal method of maintaining local control in this circumstance requires further evaluation. Cases should be assessed on an individual basis to determine which approach can maximize local control with the least adverse impact on the cosmetic outcome. In addition to margin status, histologic features of the primary tumor should be considered in the decision for reexcision. In patients with an EIC-positive cancer or an infiltrating lobular carcinoma,[36,140] reexcision should be strongly considered in those with focally positive margins of resection.

No consensus exists on the best technique for reexcision. When reexcision is performed within 1 to 2 weeks of the biopsy, it is not usually possible to reexcise an entire biopsy cavity as a single specimen without sacrificing large amounts of breast tissue, and this technique should be attempted only for small biopsy cavities in patients with moderate- to large-sized breasts. The author's (MM) technique of reexcision in most cases is to reexcise each of the walls of the biopsy cavity separately. If the initial specimen was marked with orienting sutures, reexcision can be limited to the involved margins. Otherwise, thin pieces of tissue are shaved off each wall of the biopsy cavity and sent as separate specimens, with the new margin surface marked for the pathologist. When longer intervals have elapsed between the biopsy and the time of reexcision, contraction of the biopsy cavity may allow excision of the entire cavity as a single specimen without sacrifice of excessive amounts of breast tissue. The presence of residual tumor in the reexcision is not a contraindication to BCT. The status of the final margin should be used to determine the patient's suitability for BCT. Kearney and Morrow[138] found that 86 of 90 patients undergoing reexcision for positive or unknown margins were satisfactory candidates for BCT.

Relatively few complications are associated with breast-conserving surgery. Lumpectomy by itself can be performed as an outpatient procedure under local anesthesia with supplemental sedation as needed. Wound infection is infrequent, although rates of infection may be increased when reexcision is performed. Patients with large, pendulous breasts and those who have large lumpectomies may develop dependent erythema of the breast that is mistaken for infection in the postoperative period. This condition is readily distinguished from infection by the absence of fever and pain and the resolution of the erythema over a period of several minutes once the patient is placed in the supine position and the breast is no longer dependent. This condition is due to delayed lymphatic drainage and usually resolves over several months. The late occurrence of breast abscess after BCT has been reported, and the author (MM) has observed four such cases in 420 patients. Keidan et al.[145] noticed a 6% incidence of delayed breast abscess in 112 patients undergoing lumpectomy and RT. The median time to abscess development was 5 months (range, 1.5 to 8.0 months). The use of prophylactic antibiotics, postoperative chemotherapy, the surgeon involved, and whether the excision was primary or secondary did not correlate with abscess formation. The only factor found to correlate with abscess formation was larger size of the lumpectomy specimen. Necrosis of marginally viable fat in the lumpectomy site may be the cause of this problem. Cellulitis of the breast occurring at a median of 4 months after BCT also has been reported in approximately 3% of cases.[146] Altered lymphatic drainage in the breast after axillary dissection and breast irradiation may be an etiologic factor.

TECHNIQUE AND COMPLICATIONS OF MASTECTOMY

The term *modified radical mastectomy* encompasses several different operative procedures, depending on the management of the pectoral nerves, the extent of the axillary dissection, and whether the pectoralis minor muscle is preserved, removed, or divided. All of the operations share the complete removal of the breast tissue, the underlying fascia of the pectoralis major muscle, and the removal of some of the axillary lymph nodes. The modified radical mastectomy initially described by Patey and Dysin[147] is identical to the radical mastectomy, except that the pectoralis major muscle and the lateral pectoral nerve are preserved in the former. In this operation, the pectoralis minor muscle is removed, and the medial pectoral nerve is sacrificed. In contrast, the modified radical mastectomy popularized by Auchincloss[148] preserves the pectoralis minor and the pectoral nerves. Other modifications, involving splitting the pectoralis major[149,150] or dividing the tendon of the pectoralis major[151] to improve access to the apex of the axilla, have also been described.

Modified radical mastectomy is performed through an elliptical transverse incision, which encompasses the nipple-areolar complex and the biopsy scar if an open biopsy has been performed. The abandonment of the Halstedian concepts of *en bloc* surgery also has led to abandonment of the idea that large (4 cm) areas of skin adjacent to the tumor must be excised. The nipple-areolar complex and the biopsy incision must be removed, but the remainder of the skin of the breast can be preserved in early-stage breast cancer if needed for breast reconstruction. With a skin-sparing procedure, additional exposure to allow complete excision of the breast tissue is achieved by incision rather than excision of the skin. Skin flaps are created in the plane between the subcutaneous fat and the underlying breast tissue. Because of the variability in the amount of subcutaneous fat, no single thickness is appropriate for all skin flaps. To encompass all breast tissue, the dissection should extend superiorly to the inferior border of the clavicle, medially to the lateral border of the sternum, inferiorly to the superior extent of the rectus sheath, and laterally to the latissimus dorsi muscle. After skin flaps have been raised, the breast is taken off the chest wall in a superior-to-inferior direction, with the fascia of the pectoralis major muscle as the posterior margin of the specimen. The fascia of the pectoralis major muscle was initially thought to represent an anatomic barrier to the spread of breast cancer. However, the demonstration that lymphatics from the breast penetrate this fascia renders this concept invalid,[4] and the fascia can safely be preserved when needed for breast reconstruction. In general, however, excision posterior to the fascia provides a convenient plane for ensuring removal of most of the breast tissue. At this point, with the breast attached inferiorly and laterally, axillary dissection is carried out. At the conclusion of the procedure, closed suction drains are placed in the apex of the axilla and beneath the inferior skin flap. Skin closure is accomplished with a subcuticular suture. Pressure dressings are not needed with suction drains and may compromise the blood supply to marginally viable skin flaps.

The term *total mastectomy* refers to the removal of the entire breast, with the same limits of dissection as described for the modified radical mastectomy. Care must be taken to remove the axillary tail of Spence, and therefore identification of the latissimus dorsi muscle is important. Both pectoral muscles and the axillary nodes are preserved. Because of the importance of axillary dissection as a staging procedure, total mastectomy has not been considered a standard approach to the management of infiltrating carcinomas. The indications for total mastectomy include patients with DCIS who elect mastectomy, patients undergoing prophylactic surgery to prevent the development of breast cancer, patients in whom a recurrence develops in the breast after BCT that had included an axillary dissection, and, on occasion, patients with metastatic disease who are undergoing toilet mastectomy for local control of the primary tumor.

Mastectomy is an extremely safe operative procedure. A review of the Surveillance, Epidemiology, and End Results (SEER) data for 10,056 patients treated between 1967 and 1973 notes a 30-day operative mortality of 0.35%, and, even for patients older than 75 years, the 30-day operative mortality was 0.87%.[152] For patients with serious comorbid conditions who are at an unacceptably high risk for general anesthesia, mastectomy can be done using a combination of local anesthesia, intercostal blocks, and intravenous sedation.

The reported incidence rate of wound infection with mastectomy ranges from 6% to 14%.[153,154] Infections in the early postoperative period tend to present as cellulitis, whereas those seen later tend to present as abscess formation. The most common organisms are *Streptococcus* or *Staphylococcus aureus*.[154] Factors that predispose to infection include the use of a two-step procedure (i.e, open biopsy preceding mastectomy) and prolonged suction catheter drainage.[154] Beatty et al.[155] observed an 8% incidence rate of wound infection in patients undergoing mastectomy, with a 5% incidence rate for patients undergoing biopsy and mastectomy as a single procedure, compared with a 12% rate of infection for patients undergoing a two-step procedure.

Platt et al.[156,157] analyzed the effect of a single dose of antibiotics (86% cephalosporin) on wound infection rates after breast surgery. Their study consisted of 2,587 breast operations, including 606 that were part of a randomized trial of antibiotic prophylaxis. Forty-six percent of the operations were mastectomies, 41% lumpectomies, 10% reduction mammoplasties, and 4% axillary node dissections. *Wound infection* was defined as a wound with purulent drainage, a wound that was opened, or a wound with erythema and drainage. Because erythema alone was not considered to be infection, the incidence of infections in the mastectomy group might have been underestimated. The overall incidence rate of infection was 3.7%. After adjustment for type and duration of procedure, the relative risk of infection in the group receiving prophylaxis was 0.62, a 38% reduction in the risk of infection ($p = .03$). However, because the overall incidence of infection in these patients was so low, the cost-effectiveness of routine antibiotic prophylaxis for all patients undergoing mastectomy has not been established. A selective policy of antibiotic administration to high-risk patients (e.g., prior biopsy, anticipation of long operating time) seems to be most appropriate.

Necrosis of the skin flaps is a relatively uncommon problem today, but it has been reported in 8% to 60% of cases, particularly in earlier series of patients undergoing radical mastectomy.[158,159] Chilson et al.[160] reported an 18% incidence rate in 351 patients treated between 1983 and 1990. Factors associated with skin flap necrosis include denuding the subcutaneous fat from the flaps, closure under tension, infection, and occlusive pressure dressings.[153,154] Vertical incisions, rarely used today, significantly increase the risk of flap necrosis.[161] Most of these factors are avoidable. Skin incisions should be planned to allow tension-free closure, and if tension is noticed, full-thickness flaps can be raised onto the abdominal wall and above the clavicle. Pressure dressings are not necessary when suction drains are used, and suspected cellulitis should be treated promptly with antibiotics. If skin necrosis develops at the suture line, it can usually be managed with conservative débridement after demarcation and closure by secondary intention.

Seroma formation occurs in 100% of patients after mastectomy and should be considered a side effect, rather than a complication, of the procedure. In a prospective randomized trial, Petrek et al.[162] demonstrated that extensive axillary node involvement was the greatest predictor of prolonged lymphatic drainage after mastectomy, followed by obesity and the performance of a two-step procedure. Prolonged seroma formation, in addition to requiring multiple physician visits, may be associated with delayed wound healing and an increased risk of infection.[153,154,158] Seroma formation can be minimized by leaving drains in place until their combined output is less than 40 mL per 24 hours rather than arbitrarily removing them on a predetermined day. Fluid collections should be managed by aspiration every other day to seal the skin flaps against the chest wall. Chilson and associates[160] have reported on the use of tacking sutures to obliterate the axillary dead space and attach the skin flaps to the pectoral muscle. In a retrospective review of 351 cases, a decrease (39% versus 25%) in seroma formation was noticed in patients who had the tacking procedure. However, a number of other variables that could influence these results were not evaluated in this study, making it difficult to conclude that flap-tacking is of value.

Phantom breast syndrome was first recognized by Ambrose Paré.[163] As many as 50% of patients who undergo mastectomy experience some sensation of a residual breast after mastectomy. The most common complaint is pain, but itching, nipple sensation, erotic sensations, and premenstrual-type breast soreness also are described. Kroner et al.[164] prospectively evaluated a group of patients 3 weeks, 1 year, and 6 years after mastectomy. Phantom pain was reported in 13% of patients at 3 weeks, and nonpainful phantom sensations were present in 15%. At 1 year, these incidences were 13% and 12%, respectively; at 6 years, they were 17% and 12%, respectively. This suggests that symptoms are relatively constant over time. The cause of this syndrome is unknown. However, patient education before mastectomy outlining the possible changes in chest wall sensation and the possibility of phantom breast syndrome may help to relieve patient anxiety if symptoms develop.

ONCOLOGIC CONSIDERATIONS IN IMMEDIATE RECONSTRUCTION

The switch from radical mastectomy to modified radical mastectomy and advances in plastic surgical technique have made immediate breast reconstruction an option for most patients who undergo mastectomy. The technical aspects of immediate reconstruction are discussed in detail in Chapter 34. This discussion considers the impact of immediate reconstruction on breast cancer therapy and its outcome. Concerns about immediate reconstruction have included the potential for the following: (a) an increased incidence of local failure, (b) a delay in the diagnosis of local failure, (c) a delay in the administration of adjuvant chemotherapy because of wound healing problems, (d) an increased incidence of complications when chest wall irradiation is used, and (e) technical problems in the administration of RT, particularly in treatment of the IMNs and the delivery of a boost to the scar.

There have been no prospective randomized trials comparing patients undergoing immediate reconstruction with patients undergoing mastectomy alone. A number of retrospective studies have assessed the incidence of local failure in patients undergoing breast reconstruction in comparison with patients treated by mastectomy alone. Webster et al.[165] compared 85 patients undergoing immediate reconstruction using a variety of techniques with 85 control subjects treated with mastectomy alone who were matched for age, stage, number of involved nodes, and ER status. No differences in the incidence of local or distant recurrence were seen at 30 months. Johnson et al.[166] report a 6% incidence of local failure in 118 patients treated with mastectomy and immediate reconstruction, and 5-year survival rates for reconstructed patients also did not differ from those of historical control subjects treated by mastectomy alone at the same institution. Petit and colleagues[167] compared 146 patients treated with both immediate and delayed silicone gel implant reconstruction with a control group of patients treated with mastectomy alone. The groups were matched for age, year of diagnosis, stage, histologic tumor type and grade, and nodal status. The 10-year rate of local recurrence was 8% for the reconstructed patients and 15% for the patients who had mastectomy alone. Kroll et al.[168] analyzed 87 patients having 100 reconstructions who were followed for a mean of 23 months to determine the impact of skin preservation on the rate of local failure. The nipple-areolar complex and the biopsy scar, if present, were removed, but the remaining skin of the breast was preserved. Two patients developed local recurrences, one of which was associated with widespread metastases. This low rate of local recurrence is consistent with the observation that the extent of skin excision is not a major determinant of the risk of chest wall recurrence after mastectomy alone.[169] Thus, the available data do not indicate a higher risk of local failure in patients undergoing immediate reconstruction, although the data are subject to selection bias.

Concerns that a breast reconstruction may prevent the detection of local recurrence also are not confirmed by the available data. Noone et al.[170] report on 306 patients who had immediate reconstruction and were followed a mean of 6.4 years. Local recurrence as the first site of treatment failure occurred in 5.2% of the group. Fourteen of the 16 isolated local recurrences were in the skin or subcutaneous fat, and four involved the pectoral muscle superficial to the implant. Eberlein et al.[171] also saw no delay in the detection of local recurrence in a study of 216 patients undergoing mastectomy and immediate reconstruction. Thirty-four percent of the patients in this study received chemotherapy, and no delay in the administration of chemotherapy because of complications of reconstruction was observed, a finding also reported by Noone et al.[172]

The expanded role of postmastectomy RT has raised concern about immediate breast reconstruction in patients who may require chest wall irradiation. Barreau-Pouhaer et al.[173] report a 27-fold greater incidence of implant loss in 11 patients who received postoperative RT to the chest wall when compared to 120 patients who received no RT or RT only to the nodal fields. Victor et al.[174] found that the use of bolus technique was significantly associated with a poor cosmetic result. Evans et al.[175] also note a significantly higher rate of complications in patients with implants who received pre- or postoperative radiotherapy. They also examined the effect of radiation exposure when implants were placed beneath latissimus dorsi or rectus abdominis myocutaneous (TRAM) flaps and observed a significant increase in complications compared to patients with the same types of reconstruction who did not receive RT. In contrast, patients reconstructed with TRAM flap reconstructions appear to tolerate postoperative RT well. Hunt et al.[176] report no flap losses and two cases of fat necrosis in 19 patients who received RT after TRAM reconstruction. Eighty-four percent of patients rated their cosmesis as excellent or good.[176] However, Williams et al.[177] compared 19 patients who received postoperative RT after TRAM reconstruction (usually for chest wall recurrence) to 572 who received no radiation. Postradiation changes in the flap were present in 53%, and six required surgical intervention. Fibrosis was the most common complication observed.[177]

In summary, immediate breast reconstruction has not been shown to increase the incidence of local failure or impede the detection of local recurrence. In the hands of an experienced reconstructive surgeon, the incidence of complications associated with the procedure is low (see Chapter 34), and the need for postoperative systemic therapy should not be considered a contraindication to immediate reconstruction. In patients with larger tumors or clinically positive nodes, in which there is a high likelihood that postoperative chest wall RT will be administered, it may be prudent to avoid implant reconstructions.

INDICATIONS FOR POSTOPERATIVE RADIATION THERAPY

Postoperative RT refers to the use of irradiation to the chest wall and draining lymph node regions as an adjuvant treatment after mastectomy. There are three possible reasons for the use of postoperative RT. The first is to reduce the rate of local-regional tumor recurrence (i.e., recurrence on the chest wall or in the axillary, internal mammary, or supraclavicular lymph nodes) by treating residual microscopic disease that has spread beyond the margin of surgical resection. It has been well documented that in the absence of postoperative RT, there is a substantial risk of local recurrence after modified radical (or even radical) mastectomy. This risk is principally related to the presence and extent of axillary nodal involvement; if axillary nodes are involved, local recurrence is seen in approximately 25% of patients, whereas if axillary nodes are uninvolved, local recurrence is seen only in approximately 5% of patients.[178,179] Once a local recurrence is clinically manifest, it can be effectively controlled in only approximately one-half of patients.[180–182] In addition, a local recurrence is often obvious and distressing for afflicted patients. Therefore, postoperative RT can benefit high-risk patients by preventing local recurrence.

The second potential rationale for postoperative RT is, in the absence of effective systemic therapy, to improve survival by eradicating residual local disease that is the only site of persistent cancer after mastectomy and a source of subsequent distant metastases ("seeding"). Patients without residual local disease or patients who already have distant micrometastases do not show any improvement in survival with this form of adjuvant therapy. These groups of patients appear to comprise the large majority of women with breast cancer, and therefore the percentage of patients who could benefit from postoperative RT in the absence of systemic therapy is small.

The third potential rationale for postoperative RT is, in the presence of effective systemic therapy, to improve survival by eradicating residual local disease that is the only site of persistent cancer after mastectomy *and* systemic therapy and a source of subsequent distant metastases ("reseeding"). In this scenario, patients who have both systemic micrometastases and residual local disease after mastectomy might benefit from the use of postoperative RT. Thus, the use of postoperative RT needs to be considered separately in patients treated with and without systemic therapy.

The addition of postoperative RT to mastectomy has been shown to decrease the risk of local recurrence in a number of retrospective series.[183,184] This has been confirmed in a number of randomized clinical trials in which RT consistently resulted in approximately a two-thirds reduction in local-regional recurrence.[40,185] Despite this clear-cut improvement in local control, the effect of adjuvant RT on survival remains controversial. Assessing the survival value of postoperative RT requires evaluation within prospective, randomized clinical trials. However, there are important methodologic considerations in performing such a study properly. A major consideration is that the technical aspects of the RT must be carefully monitored. Postoperative RT can be effective only if the correct volume is treated with the correct dose. Many of the series prior to the 1970s used techniques that either did not ensure adequate coverage of the entire tumor volume, including the draining lymph nodes and chest wall, or did not use a sufficient dose. Some of those trials also used techniques, since considered outmoded, that irradiated large portions of the heart, resulting in excess late cardiac mortality. Another major consideration is the large number of patients required for such a study. The survival benefit from postoperative RT, if it exists, is likely to be small, on the order of 3% to 10%; hence, a very large trial is required to detect this difference. Finally, randomization in these trials must be strict. In some of the first, less controlled studies, it was possible for clinicians to avoid RT for patients who were perceived to have a good prognosis and to select RT for patients with a poor prognosis.

Trials of Postoperative Radiation Therapy without Systemic Therapy

There are six published trials in which patients were randomized after radical or modified radical mastectomy to postoperative RT or no further treatment in the absence of systemic therapy.[186–190] In addition, a number of trials have tested the value of RT after total or "simple" mastectomy.[17,191–193] (These latter trials are not discussed in detail here, as they are no longer relevant to clinical practice.) Table 8 provides the details of treatment and patient accrual

TABLE 8. *Randomized trials testing the value of postoperative radiation therapy without systemic therapy*

Trial	Treatment arms	No. of patients	Years	RT site Type/dose (Gy)/fractions	Follow-up (yr)	Overall survival (%)
Manchester (P and Q trials)[186,a]	RM	752	1949–1955	Quadrate/peripheral techniques	34	11
	RM + RT	709		250 kV/32.5–42.5/15		7
Oslo I[187,a]	RM	264	1964–1967	Chest wall, regional nodes	15	66,[b] 66[c]
	RM + RT	282		200 kV/25–41/20		66,[b] 35[c]
Oslo II[187,a]	RM	277	1968–1972	Regional nodes	15	71,[b] 43[c]
	RM + RT	265		^{60}Co/50/20		60,[b] 41[c]
Heidelberg[188]	RM	58	1969–1972	Regional nodes	5	31
	RM + RT	84		^{60}Co/65/30	Minimum	25
Stockholm[189,190]	RM	321	1971–1976	Chest wall, regional nodes	16	49
	RM + RT	323		7.5–15.0 MeV or ^{60}Co[d]/45/25		57
NSABP[190,b]	RM	317	1961–1968	Regional nodes	5	62
	RM + RT	470		≥200 kV[e]/35–45/—		56
Manchester Regional[191]	TM	359[f]	1970–1975	Chest wall, regional nodes	10	55
	TM + RT	355[f]		300 kV or 4 MeV[g]/37–40/15		62
CRC[192,a]	TM	1,424	1970–1975	Chest wall, regional nodes	16	42
	TM + RT	1,376		Ortho or MeV/28–46/10–24		40
NSABP B-04[17]	TM	365[h]	1971–1974	Chest wall, regional nodes	10	54
	TM + RT	352[h]		MeV/45–50/25		59
Edinburgh[193,a]	TM	175[i]	1974–1979	Chest wall, regional nodes	15	55
	TM + RT	173[i]		6 MeV/42.5–45.0/10		55
Southampton[193,b]	TM	76	1973–?	Chest wall, regional nodes	3	78
	TM + RT	74		MeV/46/20		81

CRC, Cancer Research Campaign; kV, kilovoltage radiation therapy; MeV, megavoltage radiation therapy; NSABP, National Surgical Adjuvant Breast and Bowel Project; ortho, orthovoltage radiation therapy; RM, radical mastectomy; RT, radiation therapy; TM, total mastectomy.
[a]Survival estimated from curves.
[b]Stage I.
[c]Stage II.
[d]Only 9% treated with tangential ^{60}Co fields.
[e]Seventy-five percent received supervoltage, and 25% received orthovoltage.
[f]All patients were clinically stage I.
[g]Nodal.
[h]All patients had clinically negative nodes.
[i]Nodes were either (a) not readily identified by the surgeon or (b) determined to be histologically negative.

for these trials. Some of these are among the earliest clinical trials performed in medicine. In many of these trials, RT was given using orthovoltage equipment, and in most, techniques were used that delivered considerable dose to the heart and are considered outmoded. Despite this, the use of postoperative RT clearly reduced the incidence of local recurrence, but none of these trials demonstrated a clear-cut improvement in the survival rate. In addition, some of these trials showed a late increase in cardiac mortality in patients treated with RT compared with unirradiated patients.[186,187]

The most modern of these trials was conducted at the Radiumhemmet in Stockholm between 1971 and 1976.[189,190] In this trial, 644 patients with operable breast cancer were treated with modified radical mastectomy and randomized to postoperative RT or no further treatment. With a median follow-up time of 16 years, node-negative patients had a decreased rate of local recurrence with postoperative RT, but there was no effect on distant metastases or survival. For node-positive patients, the use of postoperative RT was associated not only with a decrease in local recurrence, but also a decrease in distant metastasis ($p = .02$). The 15-year survival rate was 31% for node-positive patients treated with mastectomy alone, compared with 40% for node-positive patients treated with mastectomy and postoperative RT ($p = .21$). In contrast to the results seen in the Manchester trials, the proportion of patients with persistent local-regional disease at death or last follow-up was decreased in the irradiated group compared to the unirradiated group (6% versus 16%, $p < .01$). When cause-specific mortality was examined in the trial, breast cancer mortality was lower in irradiated than in unirradiated patients (relative risk, 0.8; $p = .07$), but mortality from ischemic heart disease was higher in irradiated patients (relative risk, 1.39; $p = .38$). The dose and volume of heart irradiated were estimated for each of the techniques, and patients were grouped as having either low, intermediate, or high dose-volume. When cause-specific mortality was examined in relation to radiation dose-volume to the heart, increased mortality from ischemic heart disease was higher than for unirradiated patients only in the high group (relative risk = 3.2; $p < .05$). The reduction in breast cancer mortality was similar in all three groups. An overview of randomized trials of postoperative RT after either mastectomy with or without axillary dissection showed no difference was seen in survival when patients treated with RT were compared with those treated without RT over the first 10 years after surgery.[16] After 10 years, however, there was a lower rate of survival associated with the use of RT, but this was not statistically significant. When cause-specific mortality data were examined, there was an excess of cardiac deaths among patients treated with RT that was apparent in the early and more recent trials (p <.001), but this was offset by a reduced number of deaths from breast cancer, especially in the more recent trials. Similar findings were seen in a larger overview, including various types of surgery and with and without adjuvant systemic therapy.[40,188] In the 1999 overview, breast cancer deaths in node-positive patients were reduced from 66.5% to 62.0% at 20 years (p <.01).[188] These studies suggest, but do not establish, that if increased cardiovascular mortality associated with adjuvant irradiation can be avoided by the use of appropriate techniques, a benefit in survival will be seen.

Nevertheless, it remains undetermined whether there is a subset of patients who derive a long-term survival benefit from postoperative RT in the absence of systemic therapy. This issue is less relevant today, given the demonstrated value of adjuvant systemic therapy and hence its widespread use. As a result, the current critical issue is whether it is of value to add RT to adjuvant systemic therapy, and this is discussed in the following section. However, it is first important to consider the effect of systemic therapy combined with mastectomy on local tumor control.

Effect of Systemic Therapy on Local Tumor Control

The effect of adjuvant systemic therapy on local-regional tumor control has been assessed in several clinical trials.[194] In general, they have demonstrated a variable reduction in local-regional recurrence with adjuvant systemic therapy. In the Milan trial, comparing patients treated with CMF with an untreated control group, the 15-year local-regional recurrence rate in the CMF group was 13%, compared with 15% for untreated control patients (p = not significant).[195] In NSABP trial B-05, comparing patients treated with L-phenylalanine mustard with a control group, the cumulative incidence of local recurrence as the site of first failure at 10 years was 14% in the patients who received L-phenylalanine mustard and 24% in the patients who received a placebo.[196] In the NSABP B-13 trial, node-negative ER-negative patients were randomized to methotrexate-fluorouracil chemotherapy or to no treatment. Among the patients treated with mastectomy, the 8-year rate of local-regional recurrence was 13% without chemotherapy and 6% with chemotherapy.[95]

On the other hand, the use of adjuvant tamoxifen seems to be consistently associated with a substantial decrease in local recurrence.[197–199] In NSABP trial B-14, node-negative ER-positive patients were randomized to tamoxifen or to a placebo.[96] Among the patients treated with mastectomy, the 10-year rate of local-regional recurrence was 7.3% without tamoxifen and only 3.3% with tamoxifen. In the Ludwig (International) Group trial IV, 349 postmenopausal patients aged 66 to 80 were randomized to observation or tamoxifen (T) and low-dose prednisone (p).[200] With a median follow-up time of 13 years, isolated local-regional recurrence was 17% for patients randomized to observation and only 7% for prednisone and tamoxifen. In the Ludwig (International) Group trial III, 503 postmenopausal patients aged younger than 66 were randomized to observation, tamoxifen, and low-dose prednisone for 1 year or CMFp for 12 cycles and tamoxifen.[200] With a median follow-up time of 13 years, isolated local-regional recurrence was 17% for patients randomized to observation, 9% for prednisone and tamoxifen, and 8% for CMFpT. The Ludwig trials demonstrate that tamoxifen reduces local-regional recurrence but suggest that the addition of chemotherapy to tamoxifen does not further improve local tumor control.

The effect of chemotherapy dose intensification on local tumor control has been examined in a number of clinical trials. In the CALGB trial 8541, 1,572 women with node-positive breast cancer were randomized to low, moderate, and high dose intensities of Cytoxan, Adriamycin, and 5-fluorouracil.[201] The low dose of chemotherapy was below the doses considered standard. With a median follow-up of 3.4 years, patients treated with moderate or high dose intensity had a significantly improved disease-free and overall survival than those treated with low dose intensity. Patients treated with low dose intensity had a significantly higher number of relapses at all sites than did patients treated with higher dose intensity, but this difference was most apparent in local relapses. No significant differences were seen in outcome for patients treated with high dose intensity compared to moderate dose intensity. In the NSABP trial B-22, 2,305 patients were randomized to either (a) four courses of standard AC, (b) intensified AC with the same total dose of Cytoxan given in two doses, or (c) intensified AC with twice the dose of Cytoxan given in four courses. In a 5-year report, no differences were found in disease-free or overall survival, and local-regional recurrence was 10% in all three groups.[202] Thus, higher intensities of chemotherapy do not appear to further improve local-regional control after mastectomy compared to standard chemotherapy.

A number of other studies have examined the rate of local recurrence in patients treated with mastectomy and adjuvant chemotherapy, but without RT. In a study of patients treated with CMF by Stefanik et al.,[203] the local recurrence rate was 9% in women with one to three positive nodes and 36% in those with four or more positive nodes. Fowble et al.[204] examined the rate of local recurrence in 627 node-positive patients entered into Eastern Cooperative Oncology Group adjuvant systemic therapy trials. The 3-year rate of local recurrence was 7% for patients with one to three positive nodes, 15% with four to seven positive nodes, and 15% with eight or more positive nodes. In a randomized trial from the North Central Cancer Treatment Group, 564 patients were randomized to CFp with or without tamoxifen.[205] The 3-year isolated local-regional recurrence rate was 12% in both arms and was 8% for patients with one to three positive nodes, 14% for women with four to seven positive nodes, and 22% for those with more than seven positive nodes. These studies, as well as the trials discussed in the following section, demonstrate the moderate risk of local-regional recurrence in patients treated with mastectomy and adjuvant systemic therapy, particularly when four or more nodes are involved.

Use of Postoperative Radiation Therapy with Systemic Therapy

A number of studies have examined the issue of adding postoperative RT to adjuvant chemotherapy[206–216] (Table 9). The largest of these are from the Danish Breast Cancer Coop-

TABLE 9. *Randomized trials testing the value of postoperative radiation therapy used in conjunction with adjuvant systemic therapy*

Trial	Treatment arms	No. of patients	Years	Type RT dose (Gy)/fractions	Follow-up (yr)	Survival rate (%)
DFCI/JCRT[209]	CT	100	1974–1984	Supervoltage	5	72
	CT + RT	106		45/20		66
SEG[210]	CMF × 6[a]	133	1976–1981	Supervoltage	10	36[b]
	CMF × 12[a]	61		50/5 wk		22[b]
	RT + CMF × 6[a]	137				43[b]
DBCG[206]	CMF	856	1982–1989	Supervoltage	10	45
	CMF + RT	852		48–50/22–25		
DBCG[207]	Tam	689	1982–1990	Supervoltage	10	36
	Tam + RT	686		48–50/22–25		
Mayo Clinic[211]	L-PAM	85	1973–1980	Supervoltage	5	56
	CFP	112		50/24[c]		66
	RT + CFP	115				68
Piedmont Oncology[212]	L-PAM	43	1977–?	Supervoltage	10	47
	L-PAM + RT	33		45–50/30		60
	CMF	44				58
	CMF + RT	39				46
Glasgow[213]	RT	103	1972–1982	Orthovoltage	5	59[d]
	RT + CMF	111		37.8/15		68[d]
	CMF	108				63[d]
British Columbia[208]	CMF	154	1979–1986	Supervoltage	15	46
	CMF + RT	164		37.5/16		54
Helsinki[214]	CAFt	52	1981–1984	?	8	69
	RT	50		45/15		55
	CAFt + RT	47				65
	CAFt + RT + Tam	50				67
M. D. Anderson[215]	FAC[e]	54	1978–1980	?	3	69[f]
	FAC + RT[e]	43		?		64[f]
South Sweden[216] (premenopausal)	RT	147	1978–1985	Supervoltage	8	62 (both RT groups)[g]
	RT + C	148		38/20		
	C	139				45
South Sweden[216] (postmenopausal)	RT	236	1978–1985	Supervoltage	8	36 (both RT groups)[g]
	RT + Tam	239		38/20		
	Tam	244				54

C, cyclophosphamide; CAFt, cyclophosphamide, doxorubicin, ftorafur; CFP, cyclophosphamide, 5-fluorouracil, prednisone; CMF, cyclophosphamide, methotrexate, and 5-fluorouracil; CT, chemotherapy with L-phenylalanine mustard (PAM) or CMF; DBCG, Danish Breast Cancer Group; DFCI, Dana-Farber Cancer Institute; FAC, fluorouracil, adriamycin, cyclophosphamide; JCRT, Joint Center for Radiation Therapy; RT, radiation therapy; SEG, Southeastern Cancer Study Group; Tam, tamoxifen.
[a]Four positive nodes or more.
[b]Percentage estimated from curves.
[c]Treatment delivered in two 12-day blocks separated by a 4-week interval.
[d]Disease-related mortality.
[e]All patients were randomized to receive FAC with or without bacillus Calmette-Guérin.
[f]Disease-free survival (not survival rate).
[g]Median survival (months).

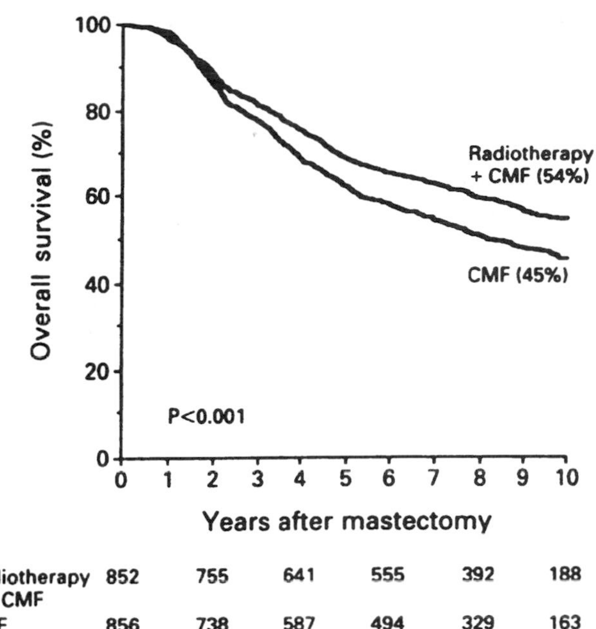

FIG. 4. Survival results in the Danish Breast Cancer Cooperative Group trial 82b comparing CMF (cyclophosphamide, methotrexate, 5-fluorouracil) chemotherapy and radiation therapy to chemotherapy alone in premenopausal patients treated with mastectomy.

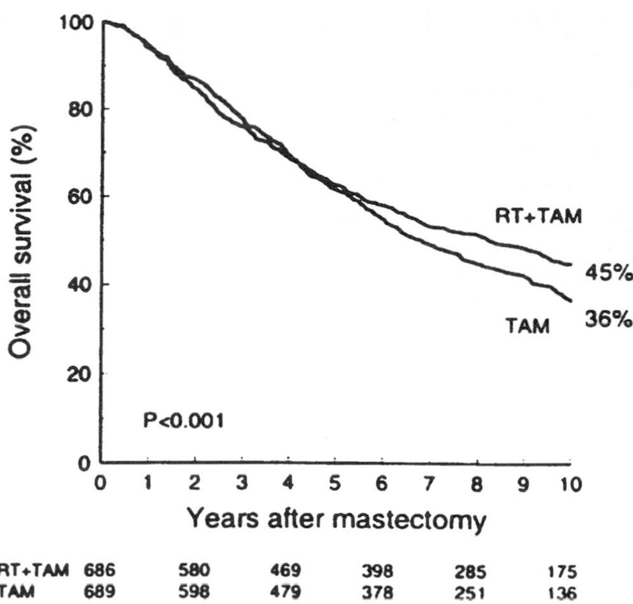

FIG. 5. Survival results in the Danish Breast Cancer Cooperative Group trial 82c comparing tamoxifen (TAM) and radiation therapy (RT) to tamoxifen alone in postmenopausal patients treated with mastectomy.

erative Group (DBCG). In DBCG trial 82b, 1,708 premenopausal patients who had undergone mastectomy for pathologic stage II or III breast cancer were randomly assigned to eight cycles of CMF plus local-regional RT or to nine cycles of CMF alone.[206] With a median follow-up time of 114 months, the 10-year rate of local-regional recurrence was reduced from 32% to 9% with RT, and overall survival improved from 45% to 54% with RT (both p values <.01) (Fig. 4). In DBCG trial 82c, 1,375 postmenopausal patients who had undergone mastectomy for pathologic stage II or III breast cancer were randomly assigned to tamoxifen for 1 year plus local-regional RT or to tamoxifen alone.[207] With a median follow-up time of 123 months, the 10-year rate of local-regional recurrence was reduced from 35% to 8% with RT, and overall survival was improved from 36% to 45% with RT (both p values <.05) (Fig. 5). In a smaller trial from British Columbia, 318 node-positive premenopausal patients treated with modified radical mastectomy were similarly randomized to adjuvant CMF chemotherapy and postoperative RT or chemotherapy alone. The results of this trial were strikingly similar to those of the DBCG trial 82b.[208]

The results of the two Danish trials may be the most relevant to this issue because of their study design, length of follow-up, and large number of patients. The magnitude of the improvement seen in these trials is similar to that seen with adjuvant systemic therapy (chemotherapy, hormonal therapy, or both) and suggests that all node-positive patients should receive postmastectomy RT. However, for a number of reasons, these trials have not resulted in the universal use of postoperative RT in node-positive patients, particularly those with only one to three positive nodes. One reason is that the worldwide overview of all trials of postoperative RT shows only a small, but not statistically significant, survival benefit. However, the overview includes many trials involving a relatively small number of patients treated with heterogeneous treatment volumes and techniques, including many that would now be considered obsolete. In addition, the overview has not subdivided the trials into those with and without adjuvant systemic therapy. Moreover, the results of large, randomized controlled trials are generally regarded as providing a higher source of evidence than meta-analysis.[217] A more substantial reason relates to the issue of generalizing from these results due to differing surgical and systemic treatments. The extent of axillary surgery performed in these trials was less than performed in the United States, and the rates of local-regional recurrence, especially axillary recurrences, observed in the Danish trials were greater than have been observed in U.S. series. In particular, series of patients with one to three positive nodes treated by modified radical mastectomy and adjuvant chemotherapy from the United States show rates of local-regional recurrence in the range of 10%,[203–205] compared to approximately 30% in the two published trials. Also, systemic therapy in the Danish trial may have been suboptimal by current standards. What seems clear is that these trials set forth an important *principle* about the value of establishing local-regional control in the presence of systemic therapy. Without detracting from the importance or validity of the principle, it is legitimate to question the *clinical implica-*

tions of these results for practice in the United States. The final reason for the failure of these trials to translate directly into clinical practice is the concern about long-term complications, especially late cardiac mortality. This is especially relevant in patients receiving chemotherapy with potential cardiac toxicity, such as Adriamycin and paclitaxel (Taxol). However, recent reports from the JCRT and the Danish group have shown no increased cardiac mortality through 12 years of follow-up.[218,219]

To address the issues raised by the available data on postoperative RT, the American Society of Therapeutic Radiology and Oncology (ASTRO) sponsored a symposium on postoperative RT and invited a panel to hear the latest information on this topic and to develop a Consensus Summary Statement. The panel was composed of three radiation oncologists, a medical oncologist, a surgical oncologist, and a consumer activist and included both authors. The panel's recommendations can be found in the following sections.

Patient Selection

Postoperative RT can be given to improve local control or to improve survival. Patients with four or more positive lymph nodes should receive postoperative RT to improve local control. There may also be a survival benefit in these patients. The data regarding patient selection for survival advantage are less clear, but the most recent evidence suggests that the greatest survival benefit is seen in node-positive patients with low tumor burdens (i.e., fewer positive nodes or smaller tumors). RT in these patients for survival benefit is worthy of consideration, pending more definitive data.

To establish the survival benefit of postoperative RT in patients with one to three positive nodes, a large randomized clinical trial should be performed.

Technique

Although both recent trials demonstrating a survival benefit with postoperative RT included treatment to the chest wall, axilla, supraclavicular area, and IMNs, there is controversy about what sites require treatment. In all patients, the chest wall should be treated.

The value of including the IMNs is uncertain and is currently being studied in a large European randomized controlled trial. In patients with positive axillary nodes, the IMNs are known to also be involved in approximately 30% of cases. Treatment of this area is, therefore, worthy of serious consideration, provided that it can be done with acceptable morbidity. After a level I and II axillary dissection, the use of a third field to treat the axillary apex and supraclavicular area is appropriate for selected node-positive patients (particularly those with four or more positive nodes). A posterior axillary radiation field is not routinely indicated after a level I and II axillary dissection. However, if there is concern about the completeness of surgery, the addition of a posterior axillary field may be appropriate. Careful attention must be paid to the morbidity of treatment. In particular, postoperative RT has the potential to cause late cardiac mortality in patients with left-sided cancers. Therefore, the amount of heart (and also lung) in the treatment field must be minimized and documented. Chemotherapy treatment planning is useful in accomplishing this goal.

COMPLICATIONS OF RADIATION THERAPY

Possible complications of RT include arm edema, brachial plexopathy, decreased arm mobility, soft-tissue necrosis, rib fractures, radiation pneumonitis, carcinogenesis (e.g., contralateral breast cancer and sarcoma), and radiation-related heart disease. The data on complications after both postoperative RT and RT as part of BCT are presented here. However, the risks of the various complications may be different after these two uses of RT and are strongly dependent on technique, including dose and fractionation.

Arm edema is the most frequent complication of RT for breast cancer in patients treated to the axilla after axillary surgery. (Arm edema and its management are discussed in greater detail in Chapter 69.) The etiology of the disorder is poorly understood but is probably related to obliteration of lymphatics in the axilla by surgery or RT and enhanced by scarring secondary to thrombophlebitis and infection. Precise volumetric measurements of the arm were made for women in the Stockholm trial that randomized patients to modified radical mastectomy alone, modified radical mastectomy and postoperative RT, and preoperative RT and modified radical mastectomy.[220] RT was delivered to the entire axilla for a total dose of 45 Gy in 5 weeks. In all three groups, some arm edema was observed. Modified radical mastectomy alone resulted in a 2.2% volume increase, compared with a volume increase of 4.5% after preoperative RT and 4.8% after postoperative RT. Severe arm edema was uncommon in all treatment groups: It occurred in 1% of the patients treated with mastectomy alone, 2% of the postoperative RT patients, and 3% of the preoperative RT patients.

The risk of arm edema was reviewed in a group of patients treated with BCT at the JCRT.[221] The entire axilla was irradiated in most patients during this time period. The risk of arm edema was related to the use and extent of axillary surgery. The actuarial risk of arm edema at 6 years was 4% for patients treated without axillary surgery and 13% for patients treated with axillary surgery ($p = .006$). Patients treated with a combination of a full axillary dissection (defined as including a stripping of the axillary vein) and axillary irradiation had a 37% risk of arm edema at 6 years, whereas patients who underwent a lesser axillary dissection and axillary irradiation had only a 7% risk of arm edema ($p < .001$). Arm edema in this series was either mild or moderate, with no patient having severe edema. Similar results were reported from the Institut Gustave-Roussy in Villejuif, France.[82] The available results indicate that both the extent of axillary surgery and the use of axillary irradiation influence the risk of arm edema. In particular, the use of a full axillary dissection and postoperative RT that includes treatment of the axilla significantly increases the risk of arm edema.

One of the possible complications of treatment to the axillary and supraclavicular regions is injury to the brachial plexus. Classic radiation-induced brachial plexopathy is characterized by discomfort in the shoulder and by paresthesias and weakness in the arm and hand and is usually progressive. Typically, there is evidence of soft-tissue fibrosis in the supraclavicular and infraclavicular regions. It is sometimes difficult to distinguish radiation-induced plexopathy from plexopathy caused by involvement by cancer, and this is discussed in greater detail in Chapter 55. The classic radiation-induced injury is dose related and rarely occurs with doses of less than 50 Gy given in 5 weeks.[222,223] In a randomized trial conducted at the Royal Marsden Hospital in London, England, the incidence of brachial plexus neuropathy was related to fraction size.[224] Patients who received 56 Gy in 15 fractions to the axilla had a 5.9% probability of brachial plexus injury at 6 years, compared with only 1% for patients who received 54 Gy in 30 fractions ($p < .01$). Another form of radiation-related brachial plexus injury called *reversible brachial plexopathy* occurs at doses less than 50 Gy, has a short latency period (median, 4.5 months), and is characterized by transient paresthesias and weakness.[225] Neither of these radiation-induced injuries to the brachial plexus has any recognized therapy. At the JCRT, brachial plexopathy developed in 20 of the 1,624 patients (1.2%) treated between 1968 and 1985. The median time to its appearance was 10.5 months (range, 1.5 to 77.0 months). The median age of patients with plexopathy was 44 years old, which was younger than the median age of the entire group. In 16 of the 20 patients (80%), the plexopathy was mild and resolved within 1 year. Plexopathy was restricted to patients who were treated with a third radiation field and was more common with doses above 50 Gy and with the use of adjuvant chemotherapy. Similar findings were observed in a study from Denmark.[226]

The use of postoperative RT can be associated with alterations of soft tissues and bones in the treatment volume. This complication, however, is rare when modern techniques and dose fractionation (1.8 to 2.0 Gy per day) are used. Studies from Sweden[220] and Denmark[227,228] have shown decreased range of movement about the shoulder joint in patients treated with mastectomy, axillary dissection, and postoperative RT compared with patients treated without RT. These changes are more common in patients treated twice a week than in patients treated five times a week and in patients older than 60 years compared with younger patients.[228] At the JCRT, a rib fracture developed in 29 of the 1,624 patients (1.8%) treated between 1968 and 1985.[229] The median time to its occurrence was 12 months (range, 1 to 57 months). Rib fracture was rare in patients treated on a 6- or 8-mV machine but more commonly observed in patients treated on a 4-mV machine. (This is due to increased dose to the lateral rib cage with 4-mV irradiation.) Among patients treated on a 4-mV machine, the likelihood of rib fracture was related to radiation dose given to the entire breast and the use of adjuvant chemotherapy. Of note, it is possible for patients to have persistent but generally mild discomfort in the treated area for years after treatment.[230]

Soft-tissue necrosis is a rare complication after moderate-dose RT, but its incidence can be increased by increasing the radiation dose or by altering the fractionation schedule.[231] At the JCRT, among 1,624 patients treated with CS and RT between 1968 and 1985, 3 (0.4%) developed soft-tissue necrosis that required surgical correction.[229] In two of these patients, the necrosis was located in the region of interstitial implantation. At the University of Pennsylvania, where interstitial implantation was less commonly performed, no cases of necrosis were seen among 697 patients.[45] As previously noted, soft-tissue effects can be more common and more severe in patients with some types of connective tissue disease.[98,99]

Radiation pneumonitis is a recognized but uncommon complication of RT for breast cancer. Patients with radiation pneumonitis typically present 6 to 18 months after treatment with a dry cough, shortness of breath, and low-grade fever. The likelihood and severity of this complication are directly related to the volume of lung irradiated and the use of adjuvant chemotherapy. At the JCRT, radiation pneumonitis developed in 17 of the 1,624 patients (1%) treated between 1968 and 1985.[232] In all cases, the symptoms were transient, and no patient developed permanent respiratory problems. The likelihood of pneumonitis was related to the use of a third radiation field and to the use of adjuvant chemotherapy, particularly when given concurrently with RT. Among these patients in whom the central lung distance[233] (CLD) was limited to 3 cm or less, no apparent correlation was seen between CLD and the appearance of pneumonitis. In one study in which the irradiated lung volume was generally kept to 10% or less of the total lung volume (corresponding to a CLD of approximately 2 cm), there was generally an acute drop in the diffusing capacity of carbon monoxide (DLCO). Two patients developed radiation pneumonitis, and both had baseline deficits in DLCO and had more than 10% of the lung irradiated. However, DLCOs returned to normal levels by 24 months in all patients.[234] At 5 years, there was no discernible decrement in pulmonary function as measured by spirometrics, lung volume, or DLCO in patients treated with either two or three fields. In another study, patients were irradiated with a technique that treated a greater percentage of lung.[235] Symptoms of radiation pneumonitis developed in 26% of patients treated with three-field RT, compared with 13% of patients treated with two-field RT. Patients with radiation pneumonitis showed persistent small changes in pulmonary function tests at 1 year. Thus, the amount of lung irradiated is a key factor predicting the likelihood of radiation pneumonitis. The likelihood of radiation pneumonitis is higher in patients after high-dose chemotherapy, particularly those with pulmonary effects from the chemotherapy.[236] Of note, the use of RT is typically associated with subsequent radiographic changes in the irradiated lung.[237] These changes are characterized by fibrosis and pleural thickening corresponding to the treated area but are not necessarily associated with symptomatic pneumonitis. Such changes are typically better seen on computed tomography scans than on plain radiographs.

One possible complication of RT for breast cancer is the induction of another breast cancer. Breast tissue is known to be sensitive to radiation carcinogenesis (see Chapter 15). The latency period between exposure and the detection of induced cancers is approximately 10 years, and this risk is apparent for many decades after that. The risk of carcinogenesis increases with doses up to 10 Gy, then seems to level off and decline, so for doses in the therapeutic range (greater than 45 Gy), the risk seems to be small.[238,239] It has been hypothesized that radiation results in two competing processes: carcinogenesis and cell inactivation.[240] Carcinogenesis has a linear relationship with radiation dose, whereas cell inactivation occurs as an exponential process with an initial shoulder region. As a result, there is a relatively greater risk of carcinogenesis at lower doses. At higher dose levels, cell inactivation becomes dominant, and the relative risk of carcinogenesis decreases. Because the dose to the opposite breast from a course of RT is in the range of 1 to 3 Gy,[241] tumor induction in the contralateral breast is of greater potential concern than in the ipsilateral breast. Age at exposure to radiation is the other important risk factor for carcinogenesis in human breast tissue.[240,242,243] The highest risk occurs in females exposed at the youngest age. With increasing age, the risk of carcinogenesis declines. The risk for women older than 40 years of age seems to be negligible but is not zero.

A number of studies have addressed the risk of contralateral breast cancer after postoperative RT. Boice et al.[244] conducted a case control study in a cohort of 41,109 patients diagnosed with breast cancer between 1935 and 1982 in Connecticut. Overall, 23% of the women who had a contralateral breast cancer and 20% of the control group had received RT. The average dose of radiation to the contralateral breast, estimated from the original RT records, was 2.82 Gy. Among women who survived for at least 10 years, RT was associated with a small, but marginally significant, elevation in the risk of a contralateral breast cancer (relative risk, 1.33). The increased risk associated with RT was evident among women who were younger than 45 years of age when they were treated (relative risk, 1.59) but not among older women (relative risk, 1.01). In another case control study from Denmark,[245] the incidence of a second primary breast cancer in the contralateral breast was examined among 56,540 women with a first primary breast cancer diagnosed between 1943 and 1978. In that study, RT was not associated with an increased risk of contralateral breast cancer (relative risk, 1.04). These data provide additional evidence that the risk of radiation-induced breast cancer associated with RT is small and is limited to young patients.

It is possible to estimate the increased *absolute* risk of contralateral breast cancer, given the elevated *relative* risk for patients aged 45 or younger seen in the study by Boice et al.[244] (The risk may actually be lower, as suggested by the Danish study.) For patients aged 45 years or younger, the risk of contralateral breast cancer within 15 years is approximately 11% without RT and increases to approximately 12% to 13% with the addition of RT. The risk of contralateral breast cancer within 30 years is approximately 22% without RT and increases to approximately 25% to 26% with RT. Thus, the risk of contralateral breast cancer in young patients, which is already higher than that for older patients, is likely to be further increased to a small extent by the use of RT. Given this, it seems prudent to reduce the dose to the contralateral breast to as low as possible in young patients.

Sarcomas of soft tissue or bone are a rare, but well-documented, complication of RT. In a report from Memorial Sloan-Kettering Cancer Center, a total of 48 patients with a prior history of breast cancer and a subsequent treatment-related sarcoma were seen at the institution over a 43-year period.[246] Lymphangiosarcoma of the extremity accounted for 22, or 46%, of the series. Most of these patients had been treated with radical mastectomy and postoperative RT. The other 26 sarcomas occurred within an RT treatment field and were considered radiation related. Twenty-one of these 26 patients were diagnosed with a soft-tissue sarcoma and 5 with a bone sarcoma. The median latency interval between the diagnosis of breast cancer and the development of sarcoma was 11 years (range, 4 to 44) and was similar for the two types of sarcomas. The survival of these patients was poor. In a registry study from Sweden, 13,490 patients with breast cancer diagnosed between 1960 and 1980 were followed through 1988. Nineteen sarcomas were reported, whereas 8.7 were expected (relative risk, 2.2; absolute risk, $1.7/10^4$ person-years). Twelve of the sarcomas appeared within the radiation fields.[247]

In a series from France, 9 of 7,620 patients treated for breast cancer developed a sarcoma within the irradiated fields.[248] The mean latency period was 9.5 years. The cumulative incidence after initial treatment was 0.2% at 10 years, 0.43% at 20 years, and 0.78% at 30 years. Kurtz et al.[249] report on 2,850 patients with clinical stage I or II breast cancer treated with CS and RT who had survived 5 years without recurrence. Two of these patients (0.1%) developed a chest wall sarcoma, and this represented 9 cases per 100,000 patient-years of observation.

It is of particular interest that a high percentage of sarcomas after treatment with CS and RT are angiosarcomas.[250] The typical initial clinical appearance of this sarcoma is reddish, purplish, or bluish nodules or discolorations of the skin that are often multiple. These initial findings can be subtle, and diagnosis is commonly not made until more advanced signs are present.

Acute nonlymphocytic leukemia is also a well-described, but rare, complication of RT. The median latency period for its appearance is generally 4 to 7 years after exposure.[251] The amount of bone marrow irradiated seems to be a factor influencing risk.[252] The risk of acute nonlymphocytic leukemia is higher after local-regional irradiation than after more localized breast irradiation. An excess of leukemia cases has been seen after low doses of RT (1 to 10 Gy) to the pelvis given for benign conditions[253,254] but is less common after therapeutic levels of RT are given. A small increase in acute nonlymphocytic leukemia has been reported in some cohorts of breast cancer patients treated with postoperative RT; however, in a case control study reported by Curtis et al.[255] using the Connecticut Tumor Registry, an increased risk of leukemia associated with RT could not be detected (relative risk, 1.16; 90% confidence interval, 0.6 to 2.1). Adjuvant chemotherapy (especially with alkylating agents) is also known to be associated with a small increased risk of acute nonlymphocytic leukemia, and the use of local-regional RT in conjunction with chemotherapy seems to increase this risk further.[252]

Lung cancer also appears to be increased in patients irradiated for breast cancer. The latency period from RT to diagnosis is approximately 10 years. In a case-referent study reported by Inskip et al.,[256] using the Connecticut Tumor Registry, a small increased risk of lung cancer was seen among 10-year survivors of breast cancer associated with the use of postoperative RT (relative risk, 1.8; 95% confidence interval, 0.8 to 3.8). The relative risk for the period 15 years or more after RT was 2.8 (95% confidence interval, 1.0 to 8.2); however, it can be difficult to distinguish a late metastasis of breast cancer to lung from a new primary lung cancer, even with a tissue specimen. This increased relative risk suggests that there would be approximately nine cases of RT-induced lung cancer per year among 10,000 breast cancer patients who survived at least 10 years. Similar findings were noted in a study using the SEER database.[257] Another study from this same group suggested that the effects of smoking and RT are multiplicative,[258] although this relationship has not been established with certainty.[259] These studies all examined the risk of lung cancer after local-regional irradiation, and this risk may be higher than that seen after more localized breast irradiation.

Injury to the heart is a possible complication after RT, but its likelihood seems related to the technique of RT used. As discussed in the section on Trials of Postoperative Radiation Therapy without Systemic Therapy, the long-term results from the early trials show an increased risk of cardiac mortality. More recent studies on patients treated with more modern techniques do not show an increased risk[218,219]; however, further long-term experience is needed to be certain of this. It is also possible that RT may increase the risk of cardiomyopathy in patients treated with high-dose doxorubicin.[260]

SEQUENCING OF SYSTEMIC THERAPY AND RADIATION THERAPY

Clinical trials have demonstrated both the effectiveness of adjuvant systemic therapies in prolonging survival and the survival equivalence of BCT and mastectomy. In addition, there is evidence that postmastectomy RT is useful in improving survival in node-positive patients. Consequently, clinicians are commonly faced with the necessity of combining systemic therapy and RT in patients after CS and after mastectomy. In this section, the available information regarding the integration of RT and both chemotherapy and tamoxifen are reviewed. It is worth noting at the onset that the optimal sequencing is still unresolved given (a) the variable agents, duration, and intensity of chemotherapy regimens; (b) variations in RT and surgical techniques; and, chiefly, (c) the limited data from randomized clinical trials addressing this question.

The major goal of the optimal sequencing approach is to obtain the highest rate of survival; however, additional important goals are to maintain a low rate of local recurrence and a low rate of complications. The options for combining RT and chemotherapy are chemotherapy first followed by RT, RT first followed by chemotherapy, RT and chemotherapy simultaneously, or some number of cycles of chemotherapy, then RT, and then more chemotherapy (commonly referred to as *sandwich therapy*). In considering this issue, it would be useful to know whether a delay in either chemotherapy or RT decreases its effect, what the complication rate is for each sequence option, and whether prior RT affects the ability to give maximal doses of chemotherapy.

It seems plausible that delays in the initiation of chemotherapy can decrease its effectiveness; however, firm data demonstrating this are not available. The use of perioperative chemotherapy has not clearly improved survival compared to conventionally timed adjuvant chemotherapy.[261–263] Retrospective reviews of patients treated either with mastectomy or BCT examining the influence of the delay of chemotherapy on outcome have demonstrated conflicting results.[264–266] It is also possible that a delay in the initiation of RT to give chemotherapy first may decrease its effectiveness. The information available on this issue from retrospective reports is also conflicting. Some reports have shown an increased rate of local recurrence with delays in the initiation of RT,[264,267,268] whereas others have not.[269–271] The results from two NSABP adjuvant studies in node-positive breast cancer (B-15 and B-16) did not show any effect with delays of 12 weeks.[272]

Prospective randomized clinical trials are required to test formally the effect of sequencing of chemotherapy and RT on outcome. The JCRT trial is the only published trial specifically designed to address this issue. In this trial, 244 patients at moderate or high risk for relapse (almost all are node positive) were randomly assigned to receive either RT followed by cyclophosphamide, doxorubicin, methotrexate (with leucovorin), fluorouracil, and prednisone given every 21 days for four cycles or this chemotherapy followed by RT.[273] With a median follow-up of 58 months, the 5-year crude incidence of first sites of recurrence suggested that local recurrence was greater with delayed RT and distant recurrence was greater with delayed chemotherapy. The overall actuarial rate of distant failure was higher in the RT–first arm (37% versus 25%, $p = .05$), thus favoring the chemotherapy–first arm. This trial does not specifically address the question of sequencing in node-negative patients or those with longer than 12 weeks of chemotherapy. One can hypothesize that the effect of delay in the initiation of RT is related to the extent of the breast surgery and the final margin status; that is, a delay of 12 to 16 weeks is important only for patients with limited breast surgery and close or positive margins. This hypothesis is suggested by a subset analysis of the JCRT trial; however, this trial was not large enough to allow for such analysis. This hypothesis requires additional support before it should be considered established. At this writing, there are two ongoing unpublished trials in France. In the ARCOSEIN trial, approximately 700 patients treated with breast-conserving surgery are randomized to mitoxantrone, cyclophosphamide, and fluorouracil given every 3 weeks for six cycles followed by RT or to concurrent chemotherapy-RT using the same drugs. In the other trial, patients are randomized to epirubicin, cyclophosphamide, and fluorouracil followed by RT or concurrent mitoxantrone, cyclophosphamide, and fluorouracil and RT.

Another important question regarding sequencing is whether RT and chemotherapy can be given simultaneously without an increase in complications or a decrease in the cosmetic outcome. The use of simultaneous RT and chemotherapy has the advantage of eliminating the necessity for delaying one of the modalities and also might provide an additive or synergistic interaction between the RT and chemotherapy. The interaction between RT and chemotherapy is demonstrated in NSABP trials B-13 and B-19 involving node-negative ER-negative patients. In both trials, RT was initiated within 2 weeks of surgery. In the NSABP B-13 trial, patients were randomized to methotrexate followed by fluorouracil (M > F) chemotherapy or to a no-treatment control group. Among the patients treated with CS and RT, the 8-year rate of recurrence in the ipsilateral breast was 13.4% without chemotherapy and only 2.6% with chemotherapy given *concurrently* with RT.[274] In the NSABP B-19 trial, patients were randomized to M > F or to CMF. Among the patients treated with CS and RT, the 5-year rate of recurrence in the ipsilateral breast was 5.6% with M > F and only 0.6% with CMF again given *concurrently* with RT. Thus, these trials demonstrate a substantial improvement in local control with concurrent CMF and RT compared with RT alone. However, the concurrent use of CMF chemotherapy and full-dose RT can result in more skin reactions compared with patients treated sequentially,[232,274,275] an increased rate of radiation pneumonitis,[232] and a decrease in the long-term cosmetic result.[274]

It may be possible to combine CMF and RT in other, more tolerable, ways. At the University of Pennsylvania, 210 patients were treated with concurrent CF and RT, followed by six cycles of CMF, with excellent results.[276] The JCRT has conducted a prospective pilot study of a modified concurrent CMF-RT regimen using reduced doses of RT designed to lessen treatment side effects by anticipating the known interaction of CMF and RT.[277] One hundred twelve patients with zero to three positive lymph nodes were entered into this prospective study. Patients received six cycles of CMF given every 28 days. On day 14 of cycle 1, patients started tangential field RT, consisting of 39.6 Gy in 22 fractions to the whole breast and a 16-Gy boost to the tumor bed using electrons. The most common acute toxicity observed during or shortly after RT was moist desquamation (seen in 50% of patients). Grade 4 neutropenia was noted in 16 patients during RT, but only 1 patient required hospitalization. Radiation pneumonitis (grade 2) was noted in only one patient. Fifty-one patients were evaluable for cosmetic scoring by JCRT physicians 2 years (± 6 months) after the end of chemotherapy: 47% had excellent, 43% had good, and 10% had fair cosmetic scores. Seventy-nine percent of patients (89 of 112) were evaluable for chemotherapy dosages delivered; overall, 93% of patients received at least 85% of all drug doses. Thus, it seems feasible to consider concurrent treatment with CMF and reduced doses of RT; however, longer-term data are required to substantiate this.

AC given every 3 weeks for four cycles is used more widely than CMF, given its shorter course and at least equivalent outcome. Considering the substantial interaction between doxorubicin and RT, it does not seem feasible to combine these modalities concurrently, even with reduced doses of RT. As noted earlier in this section, it is possible to give mitoxantrone and RT concurrently. The results of the JCRT Upfront-Outback trial provide strong support for the use of AC for four cycles followed by RT in all moderate- and high-risk patients. Preliminary results suggest that AC for four cycles followed by Taxol for four cycles may further improve outcome compared with AC × 4 alone, and the optimal timing of RT in this setting is uncertain. At Dana-Farber/Partners Cancer Care in Boston, Massachusetts, a prospective protocol is under way that is testing the feasibility of AC for four cycles followed by concurrent Taxol and RT.

Another question about sequencing is whether prior RT affects the ability to give full doses of chemotherapy. Nearly full doses of conventional levels of chemotherapy can be given if drug dose reductions are made based on the granulocyte count, rather than total white cell count, and drug doses are reescalated if counts improve.[278,279] Experience has shown that dose reductions should be made based on the granulocyte count, because irradiation can result in a large reduction in the lymphocyte count.

Questions also arise about the sequencing of tamoxifen and RT. There is a hypothetical concern that the concurrent use of tamoxifen and RT might result in a decreased sensitivity to irradiation if cancer cells are made noncycling by tamoxifen. However, the results from laboratory studies do not clearly demonstrate a decrease in radiation sensitivity in the presence of tamoxifen.[280–282] In addition, there is clinical evidence from randomized clinical trials that giving RT and tamoxifen concurrently has a beneficial effect on local control compared to RT alone.[97,283] Tamoxifen does not appear to worsen the cosmetic result after BCT[284] but may increase radiation lung fibrosis when administered concurrently with RT.[285] Given the available information, it is reasonable for clinicians to give tamoxifen with RT or to wait until RT is completed.

THERAPY OF THE REGIONAL NODES

The treatment of the regional nodes is predicated on a knowledge of the lymphatic drainage pathways of the breast, which include drainage to the axillary, internal mammary, and supraclavicular node groups, and on an awareness of the risk of metastatic disease at these sites.

Axillary Node Involvement

The axillary lymph nodes are the major regional drainage site for the breast and receive lymph from all quadrants of the breast. The axillary nodes receive approximately 85% of the lymphatic drainage, with the remainder going to the IMNs.[286] The likelihood of axillary nodal involvement is directly related to the size of the primary tumor, as demonstrated by Haagensen,[286] Nemoto et al.,[287] and studies from the SEER[288] program. Recently, great attention has been focused on the risk of nodal metastases in patients with very small breast cancers, primarily to determine whether a low-risk subset of patients who do not require axillary surgery could be identified. As illustrated in Table 10, reported rates of nodal positivity for tumors of 1 cm or less in size vary considerably, but even for T1a lesions, they may be as high as 12%.[289–295] Part of the reason for the variation among studies may be lack of uniformity in the determination of size. Seidman et al.[296] have demonstrated a significant increase in the incidence of lymph node metastases in small tumors when size is determined based only on the invasive component. The presence of residual tumor in patients undergoing reexcision for positive margins as part of BCT also impacts the incidence of nodal positivity, even though residual microscopic tumor is not factored into size determination by current staging rules. Brenin and Morrow[297] report a 36% incidence of nodal metastases in patients with T1b tumors with residual carcinoma present at reexcision, compared to only 5% in patients with tumors excised to a negative margin with a single procedure or those found to have no tumor at reexcision. This difference was observed, although tumor size, histologic grade, and the presence of lymphatic invasion did not differ significantly between groups.

TABLE 10. *Frequency of axillary node metastases related to tumor size*

Authors	Total no.	% Node positive	
		T1a	T1b
Mustafa et al.[289]	1,641	11	17
Barth et al.[290]	337	4	17
Fein et al.[291]	374	9	13
McGee et al.[292]	359	12	23
Schnabel and Estabrook[293]	604	11	20
Reger et al.[294]	178	3	10
SEER[295]	4,637	12	14

SEER, Surveillance, Epidemiology, and End Results data.

Other factors that influence the risk of nodal positivity are histologic grade and the presence of lymphatic invasion. In the studies of Mustafa et al.,[289] Barth et al.,[290] Fein et al.,[291] and in the SEER data,[295] patients with grade 1 tumors were noted to have a significantly lower rate of nodal positivity, generally approximately one-half that seen with grade 2 or 3 tumors. For example, in the SEER data,[295] patients with grade 1 T1a lesions had a 3.4% incidence of nodal metastases, compared to 21% for those with grade 3 lesions of the same size. The presence of lymphatic invasion was also strongly correlated with the risk of nodal metastases in a number of these studies.[291,292] At present, the only groups of patients reproducibly found to have a risk of axillary metastases of less than 5% are those with a single focus of microinvasion[298–300] and those with grade 1 tumors smaller than 5 mm when lymphatic invasion is not present. A very low risk of nodal metastases in pure tubular carcinomas smaller than 1 cm has also been noted.[301,302]

Evidence supports the theory that the location of the primary tumor in the breast influences the likelihood of axillary node involvement. Several studies have indicated that axillary nodes are more commonly involved when tumors are located in the lateral portion of the breast than when they are in the medial portion. In a 1978 American College of Surgeons survey, 43% of patients with lateral-half tumors had node-positive disease, compared with only 35% of patients with medial-half tumors.[287] Haagensen[286] describes similar results in the frequency of axillary node metastasis from his personal series of 917 patients treated with radical mastectomy. In this series, positive nodes were found in 47% of patients with upper outer quadrant tumors, 38% with lower outer quadrant tumors, 30% with upper inner quadrant tumors, and 23% with lower inner quadrant tumors. Similarly, Fisher et al.[303] found that 52% of patients with lateral-half tumors had positive nodes, compared with 39% of those with medial-half tumors. In the previously noted American College of Surgeons study, the results were examined in relation to tumor size and location. In each category of tumor size, patients with medial tumors were less likely to have positive axillary nodes compared with patients who had lateral tumors. The increased likelihood of axillary involvement for lateral compared with medial tumors is most likely related to preferential drainage of some medial tumors to IMNs. As a result, regional lymph node involvement (either axillary nodes or IMNs) is similar for medial and lateral tumors.

Internal Mammary Node Involvement

The IMNs extend from the fifth intercostal space to the retroclavicular region[286] and receive drainage from all quad-

TABLE 11. *Five-year survival by nodal status*

Authors	Total no. of patients	% 5-yr survival			
		Ax^-IM^-	Ax^+IM^-	Ax^-IM^+	Ax^+IM^+
Bucalossi et al.[308]	610	82	56	79	28
Caceres[309]	425	84	52	56	24
Li and Shen[310]	1,242	90	60	73	38
Urban and Marjani[306]	500	87	68	64	54
Veronesi et al.[311]	995	92	72	88	56

Ax, axillary nodes; IM, internal mammary nodes; $^-$, nodes negative for tumor cells; $^+$, nodes positive for tumor cells.

rants of the breast. Studies by Caceres,[304] Handley et al.,[305] and Urban and Marjani[306] identified the IMNs in the upper three interspaces as those most likely to contain tumor. The extended radical mastectomy was developed to allow the *en bloc* removal of these nodes, but when a prospective randomized trial[21] failed to show a survival benefit for this more extensive procedure, it was abandoned. The lack of survival benefit is not surprising, because isolated metastases to the IMNs are infrequent. Morrow and Foster[307] reviewed 7,070 cases in which the internal mammary and axillary nodes were examined. Although internal mammary metastases were present in 22% of cases, isolated internal mammary nodal metastases were seen in only 4.9%. When the subset of 3,512 patients with negative axillary nodes was considered, internal mammary node metastases were present in 9.9%. Involvement of the IMNs was more frequent for medial than lateral tumors, with isolated internal mammary node metastases seen in 7.6% of medial lesions and 2.9% of lateral lesions. Metastases to the IMNs have historically been considered to be a grave prognostic sign. However, as illustrated in Table 11, the prognosis for patients with metastases to the IMNs alone differs little from that of patients with metastases only to the axillary nodes.[306,308–311] It is only when both nodal groups are involved that a particularly poor prognosis is seen.

The IMNs have been largely ignored since the 1970s due to the widespread use of adjuvant systemic therapy for both node-positive and node-negative breast carcinoma. However, with the advent of sentinel node biopsy and the expanded indications for postmastectomy RT, this node group is assuming new importance. The clinical implications of internal mammary node involvement are discussed later in the section Sentinel Lymph Node Biopsy.

Supraclavicular Lymph Node Involvement

Supraclavicular lymph node involvement is usually associated with extensive axillary node involvement. In one series of patients undergoing routine supraclavicular dissection, involvement of the supraclavicular nodes was found in 23 (18%) of 125 patients who had positive axillary nodes and in 1 of 149 patients whose axillary nodes did not contain tumor cells.[312] The significance of supraclavicular node involvement was first shown by Halsted,[1,2] who performed supraclavicular dissections in 119 patients; of these, 44 patients were found to have involvement of these nodes, with only 2 free of disease at 5 years. Supraclavicular node involvement represents a late stage of axillary node involvement and carries a grave prognosis.

CONVENTIONAL AXILLARY DISSECTION

The appropriate extent of axillary dissection has been defined on either the basis of the number of nodes removed or the anatomic location of the nodes. The axillary nodes are divided into three levels based on their anatomic relationship to the pectoralis minor muscle (Fig. 6). The level I nodes are inferior and lateral to the pectoralis minor muscle, the level II nodes are posterior to the pectoralis minor and below the axillary vein, and the level III nodes are medial to the pectoralis minor and against the chest wall. An accurate determination of which levels of nodes have been removed can only be made if the surgeon marks the specimen for the pathologist.

In order to determine how many levels of the axilla must be removed for accurate staging, a number of authors have looked at the incidence of skip metastases. A *skip metastasis* is defined as the involvement of nodes in the upper axilla

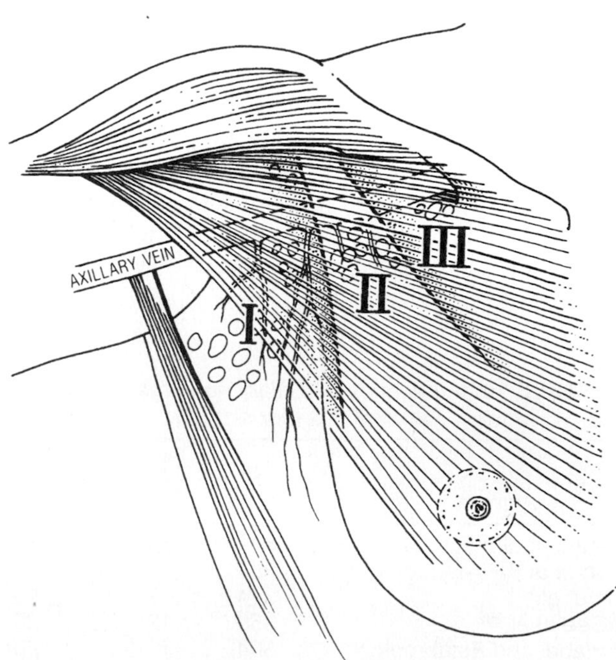

FIG. 6. Axillary lymph nodes by level. Levels I (low axilla), II (midaxilla), and III (apex of the axilla) are defined in relation to the pectoralis minor muscle.

TABLE 12. *Frequency of skip metastases to upper levels in the axilla when lower levels are negative*

Authors	No. of patients with axillary metastases	Negative level I/ positive level II (%)	Negative level I and II/ positive level III (%)
Rosen et al.[313]	429	2	0.2
Veronesi et al.[314]	539	1.5	0.4
Smith et al.[315]	309	16	10
Danforth et al.[316]	65	29	3.1
Chevinsky et al.[317]	93	7	2
Pigott et al.[318]	72	236	1.4
Boova et al.[319]	80	7.5	1.3

TABLE 13. *Role of axillary recurrence after nodal sampling in relation to number of axillary nodes removed*

	Nodes removed (no. of pts)				
Trial	0	<3	<5	>5	>10
Danish Breast Cancer Group[329]	19	10	5	3	—
NSABP[330]	21	—	12	0	—
Fowble et al.[325]	—	21	—	5	2

Risk figures are percentages.
NSABP, National Surgical Adjuvant Breast and Bowel Project.

in the absence of involvement of the level I nodes. In a study of 1,228 specimens with complete axillary dissection, Rosen et al.[313] identified axillary metastases in 429 cases. Isolated disease was present at level III in only 0.2% of the specimens. Similar findings were reported by Veronesi et al.[314] in a study of 539 cases, with skip metastases to level III in only 0.4%. These authors note that level III contained a mean of only 2.2 lymph nodes, which may account for the uniformly low reported incidence of isolated nodal disease in the level III nodes. In contrast, the reported incidence of isolated metastases in level II ranges from 1.5% to 29.0%.[314–319] This variability may be due to differences in the definition of which nodal tissue constitutes level I and level II. The data on skip metastases are summarized in Table 12.[314–319]

Another method of assessing the distribution of axillary node metastases is to examine the incidence of local recurrence in the axilla after the removal of varying levels or numbers of axillary nodes. Haagensen[320] reported an axillary failure rate of 0.25% in 794 patients after complete axillary dissection, and isolated axillary recurrences were seen in 1.5% of patients who had a complete dissection in the NSABP trial B-04.[17] Local recurrence rates after a level I and II axillary dissection as part of BCT are reported to be less than 3%.[321–325]

Other studies have examined the importance of the number of lymph nodes removed, rather than axillary levels, for staging and local control. *Axillary sampling*, an imprecisely defined procedure, refers to the removal of variable amounts of the axillary contents, often without reference to anatomic structures. Its use has been suggested to decrease the morbidity of axillary dissection. Steele et al.[326] report a randomized trial of 401 patients who underwent either axillary sampling or anatomic dissection. The incidence of positive nodes did not differ between groups. A subset of patients underwent sampling followed by dissection, with an increase in the mean number of nodes obtained from 4.1 to 19.7, but no patient's stage was changed by the complete dissection. Another randomized trial reported by Forrest et al.[327] also found no difference in the incidence of nodal positivity between patients undergoing axillary dissection and those who had sampling. In contrast, Kissin et al.[328] report that 24% of patients undergoing axillary sampling would have been erroneously staged, had complete axillary dissection not followed the sampling. The risk of axillary recurrence seems to be inversely related to the number of nodes removed. Several studies have demonstrated axillary failure rates ranging from 5% to 21% in patients with fewer than five lymph nodes removed, whereas the removal of more than five nodes decreased axillary recurrence rates to 3% to 5%.[325,329,330] These findings are illustrated in Table 13.

The preceding information indicates that the removal of the level III nodes is not necessary for staging. Larger sampling procedures resemble level I dissections and result in similar levels of local control and staging accuracy. However, since the numbers of nodes being removed cannot be accurately determined during a nonanatomic sampling, a level I and II anatomic dissection is the preferred operation and was recommended by the National Institutes of Health Consensus Conference in 1991.[331] When grossly positive axillary nodes are identified intraoperatively, a level III dissection usually is carried out to maximize local control.

The increasing use of BCT has eliminated the major morbidity of the loss of the breast. This has focused much greater attention on the sequelae of axillary dissection, and for many women this has become the major cause of long-term morbidity after the local therapy of breast cancer. Major complications of axillary dissection are infrequent occurrences but include injury or thrombosis of the axillary vein and injury to the motor nerves in the axilla. Minor complications are much more common and include seroma formation, shoulder dysfunction, loss of sensation in the distribution of the intercostobrachial nerve, and edema of the arm and breast. Seroma formation is the most frequently occurring complication, and closed-suction drainage is used by most surgeons in an effort to prevent this problem. Siegel et al.[324] describe 259 women who underwent level I and II axillary dissection without drains as part of BCT. They report a 4.2% incidence of seroma formation. However, patients were considered to have seromas only if the fluid accumulation was bothersome, and the average amount of fluid aspirated was 100 mL. Somers et al.[332] performed a randomized study of 227 axillary dissections in which patients were randomized to receive an axillary drain for 24 hours or to be followed expectantly. Any palpable fluid collections were aspirated. The use of a drain was found to decrease the time to seroma resolution, the mean number of aspirations required, and the mean volume of fluid aspirated.

The incidence of many of the other complications of axillary dissection is probably underestimated, because they are not life threatening and do not require hospitalization. Ivens et al.[333] evaluated 106 patients at least 6 months after axillary dissection without RT. The most common complaints were numbness (70%), pain (30%), and weakness (25%), although fewer than 15% of respondents believed that their symptoms were sufficiently severe to interfere with daily living. Numbness and paresthesias in the upper arm are reported in 70% to 80% of patients after division of the intercostobrachial nerve.[333–335] Occasionally, sacrifice of this nerve results in the intercostobrachial nerve syndrome, characterized by severe pain and paresthesias in the upper arm, shoulder, axilla, and anterior chest wall. Because the Halstedian principles of *en bloc* resection that dictated sacrifice of this nerve are no longer believed to be important, the incidence of these symptoms can be minimized by attempting to preserve the superior intercostobrachial nerve.

Hladiuk et al.[335] prospectively assessed subjective feelings of pain and stiffness and objective measures of strength and mobility in 63 patients undergoing axillary dissection using preoperative arm function as a control. Overall, 42% of patients had subjective or objective impairment of arm function 1 year after surgery. Pain and reduced grip strength were the most common problems and were each seen in 16% of patients.

In the study by Lin et al.,[334] 17% of patients had greater than or equal to 15 degrees of restriction of shoulder motion after 1 year, and Keramopoulos et al.[336] found impaired mobility in 17% of 104 patients after axillary dissection. These decreases in mobility may be particularly significant in the patient who already has impaired upper extremity mobility due to degenerative joint disease or neurologic events. Gutman et al.[337] compared range of motion in patients undergoing quadrantectomy, axillary dissection, and RT and in those undergoing modified radical mastectomy. In the early postoperative period, range of motion in the quadrantectomy group was 70% of baseline in 81% of women, compared with 33% of patients in the modified radical mastectomy group. However, range of motion in all patients returned to baseline by 3 months. Lotze et al.[338] compared the effects of early (postoperative day 1) versus late (postoperative day 7) physical therapy on range of motion in 36 patients (21 with breast cancer) undergoing axillary dissection. No significant differences in the percentage of patients achieving functional range of motion were identified at 1, 3, or 6 months after operation. An increase in the number of days in which a drain was required and in wound complications was observed in the early-motion group. Petrek et al.[339] failed to confirm this adverse effect of early arm motion on lymphatic drainage.

In addition to problems with arm function, axillary dissection seems to contribute to the breast edema seen after breast-conserving surgery, but this effect is largely transient.[340] Lymphedema of the arm, the most widely recognized complication of axillary dissection, is discussed in detail in Chapter 69.

Impact of Axillary Node Dissection on Survival

Since the 1970s, the contributions of local control to breast cancer survival have been minimized, in accordance with the prevailing theory that breast cancer is a systemic disease from the time that it is clinically detectable, and variations in local therapy are unlikely to have an impact on survival.[341] However, an increasing body of evidence suggests that the control of local disease does influence survival, raising the possibility that the failure to remove tumor-bearing axillary nodes could be detrimental to the patient with breast cancer.

When considering the systemic disease hypothesis, it is important to remember that a significant number of node-positive patients survive after surgical therapy alone. In the study of Adair et al.,[3] 33% of 30-year survivors had axillary metastases, and Brinkley and Haybittle[342] report that 26% of 20-year survivors had nodal metastases. In a study by Rosen et al.,[343] 40% of patients with T1, N1 breast tumors survived for 20 years.

Evidence that local control has an impact on survival is seen in the second Guy's Hospital trial[344,345] comparing CS and radiation without axillary dissection to radical mastectomy. The dose of axillary irradiation was quite low, and high rates of axillary recurrence were observed. This was associated with an increased rate of distant metastases and a decreased rate of overall survival in the patients treated with breast preservation. More recent support for this concept comes from the Danish and British Columbia studies examining the role of chest wall and nodal irradiation in node-positive women treated by mastectomy.[206,208] Both of these studies (discussed in detail in the section Use of Postoperative Radiation Therapy with Systemic Therapy) demonstrate a reduction in locoregional recurrence and an improvement in overall survival in the patients treated with radiation, suggesting that locoregional therapy may have a survival impact.

In a study at the Institut Curie,[346] 658 patients with clinically negative axillary lymph nodes were randomized to treatment with axillary dissection or nodal irradiation. Patients in the dissection arm with histologically positive nodes received chemotherapy as well. At a mean follow-up of 54 months, a statistically significant improvement in 5-year survival was seen in the axillary dissection group (97% versus 93%; $p = .01$). Although some of this difference was due to the selective use of adjuvant chemotherapy in the axillary dissection group, the magnitude of the difference was too large to be explained by the number of patients receiving chemotherapy. In this regard, it is noteworthy that the combined incidence of axillary and supraclavicular failures in the radiation arm of the study was three times that seen in the dissection arm.

TABLE 14. *Results of lymphatic mapping and sentinel node biopsy*

Study	No. of patients	Technique	Sentinel node identified (%)	Node positive (%)	False-negative rate (%)
Krag et al.[350]	22	R	82	39	0
Giuliano et al.[348]	174	B	66	37	4.4
Albertini et al.[351]	62	B + R	92	32	0
Giuliano et al.[349]	107	R	94	42	0
Veronesi et al.[352]	163	B	98	53	2.5
Shons et al.[353]	243	B + R	92	—	0.5
Galimberti et al.[354]	213	R	99	—	2.9
Guenther et al.[355]	145	B	71	30	3.0
Borgstein et al.[356]	130	R	94	43	1.7
Krag et al.[357]	443	R	91	28	11.0

B, blue dye; R, radioactivity.

The NSABP B-04[17] study, in which clinically node-negative patients were randomized to undergo radical mastectomy or simple mastectomy with observation of the nodes and delayed dissection if clinically evident metastases developed, has been used to argue against a therapeutic role for axillary dissection, because no significant differences in survival have been observed with long-term follow-up. However, it is important to recognize that this study lacks the statistical power to demonstrate a small, but clinically significant, survival difference between groups. Although whether axillary dissection is therapeutic for a subset of patients is still debatable, it is clear that only patients with lymph node involvement have the potential to benefit from the procedure, because normal axillary nodes cannot be expected to act as a source for subsequent tumor dissemination, and their removal should not alter survival.

SENTINEL LYMPH NODE BIOPSY

Sentinel lymph node biopsy offers the possibility of reliably identifying patients with axillary node involvement with a low-morbidity operation, allowing axillary dissection to be limited to patients with nodal metastases who can benefit from the procedure.

The concept of lymphatic mapping and sentinel lymph node biopsy was popularized by Morton et al.[347] in patients with melanoma. The *sentinel node* is defined as the first lymph node that drains a cancer. Morton et al.[347] demonstrated that the intradermal injection of a vital blue dye around the primary melanoma resulted in the identification of a sentinel node in the majority of patients, and the status of this node would predict the status of the remaining nodes in the nodal basin. This technique was subsequently adapted to breast tumors by Giuliano et al.[348,349] In their initial report, they reported 174 patients who underwent sentinel node mapping. Liberal eligibility criteria were used for the study, with all patients with potentially curable breast tumors included. A sentinel node was identified in 65.5% of cases and accurately predicted the status of the remaining axillary nodes in 95.6% of cases.[348] The ability to identify the sentinel node improved as the technique was refined, with a sentinel node found in 58.6% of the first 87 cases and 78% of the last 50 cases.[348] In a subsequent report using a standardized technique in 107 patients, the rate of sentinel node identification was 93.5%, and the sentinel node status accurately predicted the presence or absence of axillary metastases in 100% of patients. In 67% of the node-positive patients (28 of 42), the sentinel node was the only node containing metastases.[349]

After these initial reports, lymphatic mapping with radiolabeled colloids alone, or a combination of a radiolabeled colloid and blue dye, was undertaken by a variety of groups.[348–357] The results of these studies are shown in Table 14. Patient selection criteria and the technique of sentinel node identification varied widely in these studies. For example, only patients with intact primary tumors were eligible for the studies of Albertini et al.[351] and Veronesi et al.[352] The injection of the radiolabeled colloid in the majority of studies was around the tumor site,[350,351] but in the report of Veronesi et al.,[352] subdermal injection was used. The dose of radioactivity, the interval from injection to operation, and the use of lymphoscintigraphy also varied. However, in spite of these variations in patient selection and technique of mapping, it is evident that with experience, a sentinel node can be identified in more than 90% of cases and can predict the status of the remaining axillary nodes with 95% accuracy.

A number of contraindications to sentinel node biopsy have been identified and are listed in Table 15. It should be emphasized that sentinel node biopsy is an appropriate technique only for the patient with a clinically negative axilla. Experience with this technique in tumors larger than 5 cm is extremely limited, and there is a suggestion that the technique is less accurate for larger T2 lesions.[352] Locally advanced

TABLE 15. *Contraindications to sentinel node biopsy*

Suspicious palpable axillary adenopathy
Tumor >5 cm in size or locally advanced
Use of preoperative chemotherapy
Large biopsy cavity
Multicentric carcinoma
Prior axillary surgery
Pregnant or lactating patient

tumors are also problematic, because lymphatics may be blocked with tumor cells. Patients who have received preoperative chemotherapy are unlikely to have nodal metastases reliably identified by lymphatic mapping, because the site of the initial tumor, rather than the residual disease, would need to be mapped. Very large biopsy cavities, particularly if the primary tumor was small, may result in inaccurate mapping, and prior axillary surgery may disrupt lymphatic channels. Finally, neither blue dye nor radioactive colloids is known to be safe in the pregnant or lactating woman.

Another question raised by the sentinel node biopsy technique is the importance of drainage to lymph node basins other than the axilla. As discussed earlier, in the section Internal Mammary Node Involvement, the IMNs contain metastases in 9.9% of axillary node-negative patients.[307] Predictors of internal mammary node metastases include medial location of the primary tumor and tumor size larger than 2 cm.[307] In the study of Albertini et al.,[351] 5 of 62 patients had a technical failure of lymphatic mapping, and all of these patients had inner quadrant tumors. The authors note that no internal mammary node biopsies were performed, due to the inability to adequately localize the sentinel node because of interference from radioactivity at the primary tumor site. An internal mammary node drainage pathway cannot be readily identified with blue dye, and this drainage may account for some of the failures of sentinel node identification with this technique. Although internal mammary node biopsy at the time of mastectomy can be accomplished by splitting the fibers of the pectoralis major, an internal mammary node biopsy in a patient undergoing breast-conserving surgery usually requires a second incision. Since IMNs in the second and third intercostal spaces are the most frequent sites of metastasis, such an incision is likely to be visible in many types of clothing. Until the issue of the management of sentinel nodes in the internal mammary chain is resolved, the use of preoperative lymphoscintigraphy to document axillary drainage of medial tumors seems prudent if a sentinel node biopsy alone is to be performed.

A major issue in the use of sentinel node biopsy is the amount of experience necessary to master the procedure. Cox et al.[358] have found that an individual surgeon must perform approximately 20 procedures to attain competency, whereas Morton[359] recommends 30 to 60. These initial procedures should be done with completion of axillary dissection to ensure that sentinel node identification rates and the predictive status of the sentinel node approximate those in the literature. Although the identification of the sentinel node with radioactivity was initially said to require less of a learning curve than localization with the blue dye technique, Krag et al.[357] found that the success rates of individual surgeons in identifying a sentinel node ranged from 79% to 98% after five training cases. Morrow et al.[360] compared rates of sentinel node identification with blue dye alone or blue dye plus radioactivity in a randomized trial and found no difference between techniques in either the rate of or time to sentinel node identification. Significant variation in learning curves among individual surgeons was noted in this study. At present, no information on the long-term outcome of patients undergoing sentinel node biopsy alone is available. In the absence of any long-term follow-up studies, sentinel node biopsy alone should not be considered the current standard of care. If sentinel node biopsy without completion axillary dissection is undertaken, it has been suggested that it should be done with appropriate informed consent and institutional review board approval.[361]

Sentinel node biopsy also offers the opportunity for the pathologist to perform a much more detailed study of the lymph node that is most likely to contain metastases than is possible when evaluating an entire axillary specimen containing 15 to 25 nodes. It has been known since the 1960s that approximately 20% of lymph nodes in which no tumor is seen after routine processing and light microscopy contain tumor cells that can be identified by serial sectioning or immunohistochemistry (IHC).[362–366] However, these early studies did not find that the presence of these micrometastases was prognostically significant, and the time and expense associated with serial sections or IHC of the entire axillary contents precluded the routine use of these techniques. New interest in the significance of micrometastases has occurred as a result of studies of the sentinel node. Turner et al.[367] report that 64 of 157 sentinel nodes found to be negative by hematoxylin-eosin staining had metastases identified by IHC. In the 60 patients whose sentinel node was negative by hematoxylin-eosin and IHC, examination of 1,087 nonsentinel nodes with IHC revealed only one additional node with metastases. The absence of micrometastases in nonsentinel nodes is reassuring, as it helps to allay concerns that micrometastatic disease that is not surgically removed could result in a high incidence of local recurrence in the axilla or negatively impact survival.

The prognostic implications of micrometastases are more uncertain. Although it may seem intrinsically obvious that such metastases should worsen prognosis, study results are conflicting. As noted, initial studies showed no survival impact,[362–366] but the majority of these studies contained fewer than 100 patients. In 1990, the Ludwig group[368] reported a 9% incidence of immunohistochemically detected metastases in a group of 921 "node-negative" patients, and these were associated with a highly significant decrease in disease-free and overall survival. A significant reduction in disease-free or overall survival, or both, in patients with micrometastases has also been reported by de Mascarel et al.,[369] Hainsworth et al.,[370] McGuckin et al.,[371] and Clare et al.[372] However, the magnitude of this effect is unclear, particularly when patients with gross metastases that were overlooked are excluded. Hartveit and Lilleng[373] have observed that micrometastases in the subcapsular sinus do not alter prognosis, whereas those in nodal tissue are associated with decreased survival. Other authors[374–376] have reported the use of reverse transcriptase polymerase chain reaction to identify RNA from malignant cells in axillary nodes, with positive findings in 30% to 40% of cases. The clinical significance of these findings is completely unknown at this time. Sentinel

TABLE 16. *Technique of sentinel node biopsy with blue dye*

Tumor location	Volume of dye (mL)	Time from injection to incision (min)
Upper outer quadrant	4	4
Upper inner quadrant	4–5	5
Lower outer quadrant	5	7
Lower inner quadrant	5	7
Central	4	6

node biopsy offers the potential for ultrastaging of patients with a refinement of the currently used staging categories of node positive and node negative. However, appropriate prospective studies of the clinical significance of such micrometastases are needed before these findings are incorporated into clinical decision making.

Technique of Sentinel Node Biopsy

Although sentinel biopsy is an apparently simple procedure, meticulous attention to its technical aspects is needed to ensure success rates comparable to those reported in the literature. The technique using lymphazurin blue dye has been well standardized. After the patient is prepped and draped, lymphazurin blue dye is injected around the periphery of the tumor or at the palpable edge of the biopsy cavity. Breast massage is carried out to dilate the breast lymphatics maximally. The recommended amount of blue dye and time from injection to incision are listed in Table 16.[377] The incision is made at the inferior margin of the axillary hair, the subcutaneous fat is divided, and the axillary fascia is entered. At this point, a careful search is made for a blue lymphatic channel leading to a blue stained lymph node. Care must be taken that the node identified as the sentinel node is the most proximal blue node in the axilla, because the transit time of the blue dye is rapid and blue staining of distal, nonsentinel axillary nodes is not uncommon. Failure to identify both a blue lymphatic channel and an associated blue node and failure to remove the most proximal blue node are the two most common technical errors seen with the blue dye technique.

The technique of sentinel node identification using radiocolloid is less well standardized. The majority of studies have used technetium sulfur colloid, but both filtered and unfiltered preparations are used. This has usually been injected in the peritumoral area, although radiolabeled albumin injected intradermally has also been successfully used for mapping.[352] The dose of radioisotope and interval from injection to operation are also variable. The technique used by the M. D. Anderson group is described in Chapter 35. In the absence of a standardized technique, it is important for individuals to document that their results using a radiolabel for localization are equivalent to those reported in the literature.

Although the initial studies clearly seem to indicate that the principle of an anatomic, reproducible, primary route of lymphatic drainage of breast tumors is correct, much work remains to be done to refine our ability to determine which patients are poor candidates for lymphatic mapping and to define the optimal technique of sentinel node identification using radiocolloids. The observation in the initial sentinel node studies that the sentinel node was the only tumor-bearing node in 40% to 60% of cases[348–357] has led to speculation that a completion axillary dissection is not warranted, because the patient has been staged and the need for systemic therapy has been established. Although this is an appropriate research question is being addressed in a prospective, randomized trial by the American College of Surgeons Oncology Group, it is not the current standard of care. Data on the long-term results of sentinel node biopsy in unselected patient populations and information on the ability of surgeons outside of centers of expertise to perform this procedure are needed before it can be determined whether it will replace axillary node dissection as the standard of care for node-negative or node-positive breast cancer.

RADIATION THERAPY FOR TREATMENT OF THE AXILLA

Axillary RT, in the absence of axillary surgery, is also effective in preventing axillary recurrence in patients with clinically negative nodes (N0). *Full axillary RT* is defined here as the use of a third radiation field (in addition to the two tangential radiation fields to the breast or chest wall) encompassing the supraclavicular and upper axillary lymph nodes. Retrospective experience from a number of institutions has demonstrated an axillary recurrence rate of approximately 1% to 2% with RT alone to the axilla. In a series from the JCRT,[323] an 0.8% axillary failure rate was seen in 390 clinically N0 patients at a median follow-up time of 77 months. Clinically, N1 patients had a slightly higher rate of 2.9%. Haffty et al.[378] report a 1.8% axillary failure rate at a median follow-up time of 10.2 years in 327 patients who underwent CS and RT to the breast and regional lymph nodes. Wazer et al.[379] describe a series of 73 older patients managed with conservative breast surgery and RT without dissection. At a median follow-up time of 54 months, an axillary failure rate of 1% was reported. Among 75 patients treated with irradiation to the breast and all regional nodes, Halverson et al.[322] report a 2.7% axillary recurrence rate at a median follow-up time of 55 months.

Three randomized clinical trials with published results have formally assessed the efficacy of axillary dissection compared to axillary RT. In the NSABP B-04 trial, clinically N0 patients were randomized to (a) total mastectomy and axillary dissection, (b) total mastectomy with regional nodal irradiation, or (c) total mastectomy only.[17] Delayed axillary dissection was implemented in the event of an isolated axillary recurrence in the total mastectomy arm. In this arm, the rate of axillary failure treated with delayed dissection was 18%. This is likely an underestimate of the actual axillary recurrence rate, however, because inoperable axillary recurrences and operable axillary recurrences occurring simultaneous with or after distant metastases were excluded. In addition, some patients had lymph node identified within the initial surgical specimen. Among the clinically N0 patients, a 3.1% axillary failure rate was observed in the 183 patients treated with total mastectomy with RT compared with 1.4% in the 197 patients treated with axillary dissection. The Institut Curie randomized patients treated with CS and breast irradiation to either axillary dissection or regional nodal irradiation.[346] Patients treated with dissection and found to have histologic nodal involvement also received RT to the supraclavicular nodes and IMNs; patients with medial or central lesions received radiation to the IMNs. At a mean follow-up time of 54 months, the axillary failure rate was 2.1% (7 of 332) in the radiotherapy arm and 0.9% (3 of 326) in the axillary dissection arm. In the third trial, 381 patients with tumors smaller than 1 cm and a clinically negative axilla treated with BCT were randomized to axillary dissection or irradiation. With a median follow-up time of 26 months, only one axillary recurrence was noted in each treatment arm.[380] Thus, all three trials show low rates of axillary failure after either axillary dissection or irradiation.

Although axillary treatment with either surgery or RT effectively decreases axillary recurrence, such therapy needs to be balanced against the risk of complications. The morbidity of axillary treatment, although infrequent, may not be inconsequential. The risk and severity of arm edema has been correlated with the extent of axillary surgery and the use of full axillary RT. Among patients who received axillary irradiation, Larson et al.[221] report a 36% rate of arm edema in patients who underwent full dissection versus 6% in whom a level I/II dissection was performed. Cabanes et al.[346] found a 2% rate of arm edema for either level I/II dissection or axillary irradiation alone. Impairment of arm function after complete dissection has also been described. Hladiuk et al.[335] report a 42% rate of residual arm dysfunction 1 year after complete dissection. However, this seems much less common in patients who undergo more limited surgery. The risk of arm edema after axillary irradiation alone is low. In the retrospective JCRT series, a 4% actuarial risk of arm edema at 6 years was reported in patients who did not undergo axillary surgery.[323] Other sequelae of full axillary RT have been described, such as brachial plexopathy and radiation pneumonitis. Pierce et al.[229] found a 1.8% incidence of brachial plexopathy among patients who received three-field RT at a median follow-up time of 79 months. Most cases resolved within 1 year. The incidence was significantly higher when the axillary radiation dose was greater than 50 Gy, compared to that seen with doses of 50 Gy or less (5.6% and 1.3%, respectively; $p = .004$). Radiation pneumonitis, also uncommon, has been associated with the use of the third nodal radiation field as well as the addition of chemotherapy.[381,382] In a series from the JCRT, three-field irradiation without chemotherapy yielded a 0.6% incidence of pneumonitis versus 3.3% with the addition of chemotherapy.[382] Even higher rates were reported with concurrent administration versus sequential (8.8% versus 1.3%). Wazer et al.[379] report no significant arm edema (defined as >2 cm increase in circumference) or brachial plexopathy in 73 older patients who received three-field irradiation without axillary dissection. These data suggest that some morbidity is associated with either axillary dissection or axillary irradiation; however, it is uncertain which procedure is less morbid, and this may depend on the precise technique of surgery or irradiation used.

It may be feasible to approach treatment of the axilla in even more limited ways. An alternative to axillary dissection or full axillary RT may be to limit the radiation fields to tangential fields alone. These fields include the lower-echelon axillary nodes (usually most of level I and part of level II). One JCRT retrospective analysis described results in 92 selected patients treated in this manner.[382] Sixty-two percent received adjuvant tamoxifen. Eighty-three percent had T1 tumors; six patients had tumors smaller than 0.5 cm. No isolated regional nodal failures were observed at a median follow-up time of 50 months. One patient was noted to have a microscopically positive axillary node on a salvage mastectomy for a recurrence in the treated breast. Other investigators have reported results of conservative breast surgery and tangential RT. Axillary failure rates in these series were 0% to 5%.[383–385] However, patient numbers and follow-up time were limited in these retrospective analyses, as in the JCRT series. Whether tangential RT is a reasonable option in certain patients remains uncertain. The JCRT has initiated a formal prospective trial of this approach in older patients with clinically node-negative, early-stage disease.

Sentinel node biopsy, described elsewhere in the section Sentinel Lymph Node Biopsy, represents another potentially useful method to determine whether a clinically negative axilla contains metastases. When a sentinel node biopsy is properly performed and is negative, no further treatment is necessary. When it is positive, one could consider treatment with either further axillary surgery or axillary irradiation, or perhaps no further treatment. Studies are currently under way to assess the efficacy and morbidity of each approach.

In conclusion, axillary dissection and full axillary irradiation both yield low, acceptable rates of axillary recurrence and morbidity. Axillary irradiation, however, does not provide the important prognostic information obtained from axillary dissection. This information may be important either for the clinician in formulating the best treatment plan or for the patient to best assess her prognosis.[386] For clinically N0 patients in whom pathologic nodal status is not of interest, axillary RT is a reasonable alternative to dissection. Further studies regarding the feasibility of even more limited approaches, such as tangential radiotherapy or sentinel node biopsy, are currently in progress. The results from the Danish and British Columbia studies,[207,208] however, highlight the importance of obtaining axillary nodal control, particularly when effective systemic therapy is used.

REFERENCES

1. Halsted W. The results of operations for cure of cancer of the breast performed at Johns Hopkins Hospital. *Johns Hopkins Hosp Bull* 1894;4:497.
2. Halsted WS. The results of radical operations for the cure of carcinoma of the breast. *Ann Surg* 1907;66:1.
3. Adair F, Berg J, Joubert L, Robbins GF. Long term follow up of breast cancer patients: the 30 year report. *Cancer* 1974;33:1145.
4. Turner-Warwick R. The lymphatics of the breast. *Br J Surg* 1959;46:574.
5. Urban J. Radical mastectomy with en bloc in continuity resection of the internal mammary lymph node chain. *Surg Clin North Am* 1956;36:1065.
6. Meir P, Ferguson D, Harrison T. A controlled trial of extended radical mastectomy. *Cancer* 1985;55:880.
7. Veronesi U, Valagussa P. Inefficacy of internal mammary node dissection in breast cancer surgery. *Cancer* 1981;47:170.
8. Morrow M, Winchester DP, Chmiel JS, et al. Factors responsible for the under-utilization of breast-conserving therapy. *Proc Am Soc Clin Oncol* 1998;17:98a(abst).
9. Guadagnoli E, Weeks JC, Shapiro CL, Gurwitz JH, Barbas C, Soumerai SB. Use of breast-conserving surgery for treatment of stage I and stage II breast cancer. *J Clin Oncol* 1998;16:101.
10. Nattinger AB, Gottlieb MS, Veum J, Yahuke D, Goodwin JS. Geographic variation in the use of breast-conserving treatment for breast cancer. *N Engl J Med* 1992;326:1102.
11. Robinson D, Van Heerden J, Payne W, et al. The primary surgical treatment of carcinoma of the breast: a changing trend toward modified radical mastectomy. *Mayo Clin Proc* 1976;51:433.
12. Baker R, Montague A, Childs J. A comparison of modified radical mastectomy to radical mastectomy in the treatment of operable breast cancer. *Ann Surg* 1979;189:553.
13. Turner L, Swindell R, Bell W. Radical versus modified radical mastectomy for breast cancer. *Ann R Coll Surg Engl* 1981;63:239.
14. Maddox W, Carpenter J, Laws H, et al. A randomized prospective trial of radical (Halsted) mastectomy versus modified radical mastectomy in 311 breast cancer patients. *Ann Surg* 1983;198:207.
15. Cuzick J, Stewart H, Peto R, et al. Overview of randomized trials of postoperative adjuvant radiotherapy in breast cancer. *Cancer Treat Rep* 1987;71:15.
16. Cuzick J, Stewart H, Rutqvist L, et al. Cause-specific mortality in long-term survivors of breast cancer who participated in trials of radiotherapy. *J Clin Oncol* 1994;12:447.
17. Fisher B, Redmond C, Fisher ER, et al. Ten-year results of a randomized clinical trial comparing radical mastectomy and total mastectomy with or without radiation. *N Engl J Med* 1985;312:674.
18. Lagios MD, Westdahl P, Rose M. The concept and implications of multicentricity in breast carcinoma. In: Sommers SG, ed. *Pathology annual*. New York: Appleton-Century-Crofts, 1981.
19. Qualheim R, Gall E. Breast carcinoma with multiple sites of origin. *Cancer* 1975;35:739.
20. Rosen P, Fracchia A, Urban J, Schottenfeld D, Robbins GF. "Residual" mammary carcinoma following simulated partial mastectomy. *Cancer* 1975;35:739.
21. Holland R, Veling S, Mravunac M, Hendriks JH. Histologic multifocality of Tis, T1-2 breast carcinomas: implications for clinical trials of breast conserving treatment. *Cancer* 1985;56:979.
22. Holland R, Connolly J, Gelman R, et al. Histologic multifocality of Tis, T1-2 breast carcinomas: implications for clinical trials of breast conserving treatment. *J Clin Oncol* 1990;8:113.
23. Lagios M, Richards V, Rose M, Yee E. Segmental mastectomy without radiotherapy: short-term follow-up. *Cancer* 1983,52:2173.
24. Montgomery A, Greening W, Levene A. Clinical study of recurrence rate and survival time of patients with carcinoma of the breast treated by biopsy excision without any other therapy. *J R Soc Med* 1978;71:339.
25. Targart R. Partial mastectomy for breast cancer. *BMJ* 1978;2:1268.
26. Freeman C, Belliveau N, Kim T, Boivin JF. Limited surgery with or without radiotherapy for early breast carcinoma. *J Can Assoc Radiol* 1981;32:125.
27. Fisher B, Redmond C, Poisson R, et al. Eight-year results of a randomized clinical trial comparing total mastectomy and lumpectomy with or without irradiation in the treatment of breast cancer. *N Engl J Med* 1989;320:822.
28. Fletcher G. Local results of irradiation in the primary management of localized breast cancer. *Cancer* 1972;29:545.
29. Kaae S, Johansen H. Does simple mastectomy followed by irradiation offer survival comparable to radical procedures? *Int J Radiat Oncol Biol Phys* 1977;2;1163.
30. Keynes G. Conservative treatment of cancer of the breast. *BMJ* 1937;2:643.
31. Peters MK. Cutting the "Gordian knot" in early breast cancer. *Ann R Coll Phys Surg Can* 1975;8:186.
32. Veronesi U, Luini A, Galimberti V, Zurrida S. Conservation approaches for the management of stage I/II carcinoma of the breast: Milan Cancer Institute trials. *World J Surg* 1994;18:70.
33. Veronesi U, Salvadori B, Luini A, et al. Breast conservation is a safe method in patients with small cancer of the breast. Long-term results of three randomized trials on 1993 patients. *Eur J Cancer* 1995; 31A:1574.
34. Fisher B, Anderson S, Redmond CK, Wolmark N, Wickerham DL, Cronin WM. Reanalysis and results after 12 years of follow-up in a randomized clinical trial comparing total mastectomy with lumpectomy with or without irradiation in the treatment of breast cancer. *N Engl J Med* 1995;333:1456.
35. Jacobson JA, Danforth DN, Cowan KH, et al. Ten-year results of a comparison of conservation with mastectomy in the treatment of stage I and II breast cancer. *N Engl J Med* 1995;332:907.
36. Van Dongen JA, Bartelink H, Fentiman IS, et al. Factors influencing local relapse and survival and results of salvage treatment after breast conserving therapy in operable breast cancer: EORTC trial 1081, breast conservation compared with mastectomy in TNM stage I and II breast cancer. *Eur J Cancer* 1992;28A:801.
37. Arriagada R, Le MG, Rochard F, Contesso G, for the Institute Gustave Roussy Breast Cancer Group. Conservative treatment versus mastectomy in early breast cancer: patterns of failure with 15 years of follow-up data. *J Clin Oncol* 1996;14:1558.
38. van Dongen JA, Bartelink H, Fentiman IS, et al. Randomized clinical trial to assess the value of breast-conserving therapy in stage I and II breast cancer: EORTC 10801 trial. *J Natl Cancer Inst* 1992;11:15.
39. Blichert-Toft M, Rose C, Andersen JA, et al. Danish randomized trial comparing breast conservation therapy with mastectomy: six years of life-table analysis. *J Natl Cancer Inst Monogr* 1992;11:19.
40. Early Breast Cancer Trialists' Collaborative Group. Effects of radiotherapy and surgery in early breast cancer: an overview of the randomized trials. *N Engl J Med* 1995;333:1444.
41. Veronesi U, Salvadori B, Luini A, et al. Conservative treatment of early breast cancer: long-term results of 1232 cases treated with quadrantectomy, axillary dissection, and radiotherapy. *Ann Surg* 1990;211:250.
42. Haffty BG, Goldberg NB, Rose M, et al. Conservative surgery with radiation therapy in clinical stage I and II breast carcinoma: results of a 20-year experience. *Arch Surg* 1989;124:1266.
43. Clark RM, Wilkinson RH, Mahoney LJ, Reid JG, MacDonald WD. Breast cancer: a 21-year experience with conservative surgery and radiation. *Int J Radiat Oncol Biol Phys* 1982;8:967.
44. Clarke D, Le M, Sarrazin D, et al. Analysis of local-regional relapses in patients with early breast cancers treated by excision and radiotherapy: experience of the Institut Gustave-Roussy. *Int J Radiat Oncol Biol Phys* 1985;11:137.
45. Fowble B, Solin L, Schultz D, Goodman RL. Ten-year results of conservative surgery and irradiation for stage I and II breast cancer. *Int J Radiat Oncol Biol Phys* 1991;21:269.
46. Fourquet A, Campana F, Zafrani B, et al. Prognostic factors of breast recurrence in the conservative management of early breast cancer: a 25-year follow-up. *Int J Radiat Oncol Biol Phys* 1989;17:719.
47. Kurtz J, Amalric R, Brandone H, et al. Local recurrence after breast-conserving surgery and radiotherapy: frequency, time course, and prognosis. *Cancer* 1989;63:1912.
48. Gage I, Recht A, Gelman R, et al. Long-term outcome following breast conserving surgery and radiation therapy. *Int J Radiat Oncol Biol Phys* 1995;33:245.
49. Gage I, Schnitt S, Recht A, et al. Skin recurrences after breast conserving therapy for early stage breast cancer. *J Clin Oncol* 1998;16:480.
50. Farrow DC, Hunt WC, Samet JM. Geographic variation in the treatment of localized breast cancer. *N Engl J Med* 1992;326:1097.
51. Morrow M, Bucci C, Rademaker A. Medical contraindications are not a major factor in the underutilization of breast conserving therapy. *J Am Coll Surg* 1998;186:269.

52. Foster RS, Farwell ME, Costanza MC. Breast therapy for breast cancer: patterns of care in a geographic region and estimation of potential applicability. *Ann Surg Oncol* 1995;2:275.
53. Morrow M, Schmidt R, Hassett C. Patient selection for breast conservation therapy with magnification mammography. *Surgery* 1995;118:621.
54. Harris J, Recht A, Amalric R, et al. Time course and prognosis of local recurrence following primary radiation therapy for early breast cancer. *J Clin Oncol* 1984;2:37.
55. Healey E, Cook E, Orav E, Schnitt SJ, Connolly JL, Harris JR. Contralateral breast cancer: clinical characteristics and impact on prognosis. *J Clin Oncol* 1993;11:1545.
56. American College of Radiology, American College of Surgeons, College of American Pathologists, and the Society of Surgical Oncology. Standards for diagnosis and management of invasive breast carcinomas. *CA Cancer J Clin* 1998;48:83.
57. Harris J, Levene M, Svensson G, Hellman S. Analysis of cosmetic results following primary radiation therapy for stages I and II carcinoma of the breast. *Int J Radiat Oncol Biol Phys* 1979;5:257.
58. de la Rochefordiere A, Abner A, Silver B, Vicini F, Recht A, Harris JR. Are cosmetic results following conservative surgery and radiation therapy for early breast cancer dependent on technique? *Int J Radiat Oncol Biol Phys* 1992;23:925.
59. Wazer DE, DiPetrillo T, Schmidt-Ullrich R, et al. Factors influencing cosmetic outcome after conservative surgery and radiotherapy for early stage breast carcinoma. *J Clin Oncol* 1992;10:356.
60. Mills JM, Schultz DJ, Solin LJ. Preservation of cosmesis with low complication risk after conservative surgery and radiotherapy for ductal carcinoma in situ of the breast. *Int J Radiat Oncol Biol Phys* 1997;39:637.
61. Monson MM, Chin L, Nixon A, et al. Is machine energy (4-8 mV) associated with outcome for stage I-II breast cancer patients? *Int J Radiat Oncol Biol Phys* 1997;37:1095.
62. Abner A, Recht A, Vicini F, et al. Cosmetic results after conservative surgery, chemotherapy, and radiation therapy for early breast cancer. *Int J Radiat Oncol Biol Phys* 1991;21:331.
63. Gelman R, Gelber R, Henderson I, Coleman CN, Harris JR. Improved methodology for analyzing local and distant recurrence. *J Clin Oncol* 1990;8:548.
64. Nixon AJ, Neuberg D, Hayes EF, et al. Relationship of patient age to pathologic features of the tumor and prognosis for patients with stage I or II breast cancer. *J Clin Oncol* 1994;12:888.
65. de la Rochefordiere A, Mouret-Fourme E, de Ricke Y, et al. Local and distant relapses in relation to age following breast-conserving surgery and irradiation in premenopausal patients with breast cancer. *Int J Radiat Oncol Biol Phys* 1998;42:180(abst).
66. Kurtz J, Jacquemier J, Amalric R, et al. Why are local recurrences (LR) after breast-conserving surgery more frequent in younger patients? *J Clin Oncol* 1990;8:591.
67. Vrieling C, Collette L, Fourquet A, et al. The higher local recurrence rate after breast conserving therapy in young patients explained by larger tumor size and incomplete excision at first attempt? *Int J Radiat Oncol Biol Phys* 1998;42:125(abst).
68. Donegan W, Perez-Mesa C, Watson F. A biostatistical study of locally recurrent breast carcinoma. *Surg Gynecol Obstet* 1966;122:529.
69. Matthews R, McNeese M, Montague E, Oswald MJ. Prognostic implications of age in breast cancer patients treated with tumorectomy and irradiation or with mastectomy. *Int J Radiat Oncol Biol Phys* 1988;14:659.
70. de la Rochefordiere A, Asselain B, Campana G, et al. Age as a prognostic factor in premenopausal breast carcinoma. *Lancet* 1993;341:1039.
71. Chabner E, Nixon A, Gelman R, et al. Family history and treatment outcome in young women after breast-conserving surgery and radiation therapy for early-stage breast cancer. *J Clin Oncol* 1998;16:2045.
72. Ford D, Easton D, Bishop D, Narod SA, Goldgar DE. Risks of cancer in BRCA1 mutation carriers. *Lancet* 1994;343:692.
73. Verhoog LC, Brekelmans CTM, Seynaeve C, et al. Survival and tumour characteristics of breast cancer patients with germline mutations of BRCA1. *Lancet* 1998;351:316.
74. Gaffney DK, Brohet RM, Lewis CM, et al. Response to radiation therapy and prognosis in breast cancer patients with BRCA1 and BRCA2 mutations. *Radiother Oncol* 1998;47:129.
75. Scully R, Chen J, Plug A, et al. Association of BRCA1 with Rad51 in mitotic and meiotic cells. *Cell* 1997;88:265.
76. Sharan SK, Morimatsu M, Albrecht U, et al. Embryonic lethality and radiation hypersensitivity mediated by Rad51 in mice lacking BRCA. *Nature* 1997;386:804.
77. Marcus JN, Watson P, Page DL, et al. Hereditary breast cancer: pathobiology, prognosis, and BRCA1 and BRCA2 gene linkage. *Cancer* 1996;77:697.
78. Harris JR. Breast-conserving therapy as a model for creating new knowledge in clinical oncology. *Int J Radiat Oncol Phys* 1996; 35:641.
79. Schnitt S, Connolly J, Khettry U, et al. Pathologic findings on reexcision of the primary site in breast cancer patients considered for treatment by primary radiation therapy. *Cancer* 1987;59:675.
80. Healey E, Osteen R, Schnitt S, et al. Can the clinical and mammographic findings at presentation predict the presence of an extensive intraductal component in early stage breast cancer? *Int J Radiat Oncol Biol Phys* 1989;17:1217.
81. Borger J, Kemperman H, Hart A, Peterse H, van Dongen J, Bartelink H. Risk factors in breast-conservation therapy. *J Clin Oncol* 1994;12:653.
82. Dewar JA, Arriagada R, Benhamou S, et al. Local relapse and contralateral tumor rates in patients with breast cancer treated with conservative surgery and radiotherapy (Institute Gustave Roussy 1970-1982). *Cancer* 1995;76:2260.
83. Freedman G, Fowble B, Hanlon A, et al. Patients with close or positive margins treated with conservative surgery and radiation have an increased risk of breast recurrence that is delayed by adjuvant systemic therapy. *Int J Radiat Oncol Biol Phys* 1998;42:126(abst).
84. Park C, Mitsumori M, Recht A, et al. The relationship between pathologic margin status and outcome after breast-conserving therapy. *Int J Radiat Oncol Biol Phys* 1998;42:125(abst).
85. Anscher MS, Jones P, Prosnitz LR, et al. Local failure and margin status in early-stage breast carcinoma treated with conservation surgery and radiation therapy. *Ann Surg* 1993;218:22.
86. Smitt MC, Nowels JW, Zdeblich MJ, et al. The importance of the lumpectomy surgical margin status in long term results of breast conservation. *Cancer* 1995;76:259.
87. Peterson ME, Schultz DJ, Reynolds C, et al. Outcomes in breast cancer patients relative to margin status after treatment with breast-conserving surgery and radiation therapy: the University of Pennsylvania Experience. *Int J Radiat Oncol Biol Phys* 1999;43:1029.
88. Wazer DE, Schmidt-Ullich RK, Ruthazer R, et al. Factors determining outcome for breast-conserving irradiation with margin-directed dose escalation to the tumor bed. *Int J Radiat Oncol Biol Phys* 1998;40:851.
89. Pittinger TP, Maronian NC, Poulter CA, Peacock JL. Importance of margins status in outcome of breast-conserving surgery for carcinoma. *Surgery* 1994;116:605.
90. Cowen D, Largillier R, Bardou V-J, et al. Positive margins after conservative treatments impacts local control and possibly survival in node-negative breast cancer. *Int J Radiat Oncol Biol Phys* 1998;42:126(abst).
91. Gage I, Schnitt SJ, Nixon AJ, et al. Pathologic margin involvement and the risk of recurrence in patients treated with breast-conserving therapy. *Cancer* 1996;78:1921.
92. Fisher ER, Sass R, Fisher B, Gregorio R, Brown R, Wickerham L. Pathologic findings from the National Surgical Adjuvant Breast Project (Protocol 6). II: relation of local breast recurrence to multicentricity. *Cancer* 1986;57:1717.
93. Mariani L, Salvadori B, Marubini E, et al. Ten year results of a randomised trial comparing two conservative treatment strategies for small size breast cancer. *Eur J Cancer* 1998;34:1156.
94. Romestaing P, Lehingue Y, Carrie C, et al. Role of a 10-Gy boost in the conservative treatment of early breast cancer: results of a randomized clinical trial in Lyon, France. *J Clin Oncol* 1997;15:963.
95. Fisher B, Dignam J, Mamounas HP, et al. Sequential methotrexate and fluorouracil for the treatment of node-negative breast cancer patients with estrogen-receptor negative tumors: eight year results from NSAPB B-13 and first report of findings from NSABP B-10 comparing methotrexate and fluorouracil with conventional cyclophosphamide, methotrexate and fluorouracil. *J Clin Oncol* 1996;14:1982.
96. Fisher B, Dignam J, Bryant J, et al. Five versus more than five years of Tamoxifen therapy for breast cancer patients with negative lymph nodes and estrogen receptor-positive tumors. *J Natl Cancer Inst* 1996;88:1529.
97. Dalberg K, Johansson H, Johansson U, Rutqvist L, for the Stockholm Breast Cancer Study Group. A randomized trial of long term adjuvant tamoxifen plus postoperative radiation therapy versus radiation therapy for patients with early stage breast carcinoma treated with breast-conserving surgery. *Cancer* 1998;82:2204.

98. Fleck R, McNeese MD, Ellerbroek NA, Hunter TA, Holmes FA. Consequences of breast irradiation in patients with pre-existing collagen vascular diseases. *Int J Radiat Oncol Biol Phys* 1989;17:829.
99. Morris MM, Powell SN. Irradiation in the setting of collagen vascular disease: acute and late complications. *J Clin Oncol* 1997;15:2728.
100. Bonadonna G, Veronesi U, Brambilla C, et al. Primary chemotherapy to avoid mastectomy in tumors with diameters of three centimeters or more. *J Natl Cancer Inst* 1990;82:1539.
101. Smith IE, Jones AL, O'Brien ME, McKinna JA, Sacks N, Baum M. Primary medical (neoadjuvant) chemotherapy for operable breast cancer. *Eur J Cancer Clin Oncol* 1993;29A:1796.
102. Powles TJ, Hickish TF, Makris A, et al. Randomized trial of chemoendocrine therapy started before or after surgery for treatment of primary breast cancer. *J Clin Oncol* 1995;13:547.
103. Fisher B, Brown A, Mamounas E, et al. Effect of preoperative chemotherapy on local-regional disease in women with operable breast cancer: findings from National Surgical Adjuvant Breast and Bowel Project B-18. *J Clin Oncol* 1997;15:2483.
104. Fisher B, Bryant J, Wolmark N, et al. Effect of preoperative chemotherapy on the outcome of women with operable breast cancer. *J Clin Oncol* 1998;16:2672.
105. Helvie MA, Joynt L, Cody RL, Pierce LJ, Adler DD, Merajver SC. Locally advanced breast carcinoma: accuracy of mammographic versus clinical examination in the prediction of residual disease after chemotherapy. *Radiology* 1996;198:327.
106. Vinnicombe SJ, MacVicar AD, Guy RL. Primary breast cancer: mammographic changes after neoadjuvant chemotherapy with pathologic correlation. *Radiology* 1996;198:333.
107. Cocconi G, Di Blasio B, Alberti G, Bisagni G, Botti E, Peracchia G. Problems in evaluating response of primary breast cancer to systemic therapy. *Breast Cancer Res Treat* 1984;4:309.
108. Abraham DC, Jones RC, Jones SE, et al. Evaluation of neoadjuvant chemotherapeutic response of locally advanced breast cancer by magnetic resonance imaging. *Cancer* 1996;78:91.
109. Gilles R, Guinebretiere JM, Toussaint C, et al. Locally advanced breast cancer: contrast-enhanced subtraction MR imaging of response to reoperative chemotherapy. *Radiology* 1994;191:633.
110. Liljegren G, Holmberg L, Adami HO, Westman G, Graffman S, Bergh J. Sector resection with and without postoperative radiotherapy for stage I breast cancer. Five year results of a randomized trial. *J Natl Cancer Inst* 1994;86:717.
111. Clark RM, Whelan T, Levine M, et al. Randomized clinical trial of breast irradiation following lumpectomy and axillary dissection for node-negative breast cancer: an update. Ontario Clinical Oncology Group. *J Natl Cancer Inst* 1996;88:1659.
112. Forrest AP, Stewart HJ, Everington D, et al. Randomised controlled trial of conservation therapy for breast cancer: 6-year analysis of the Scottish trial. Scottish Cancer Trials Breast Group. *Lancet* 1996;348:708.
113. Renton SC, Gazet JC, Ford HT, Corbishley C, Sutcliffe R. The importance of the resection margin in conservative surgery for breast cancer. *Eur J Surg Oncol* 1996;22:17.
114. Schnitt S, Hayman J, Gelman R, et al. A prospective study of conservative surgery alone in the treatment of selected patients with stage I breast cancer. *Cancer* 1996;77:1094.
115. Nemoto T, Patel J, Rosner D, Dao TL, Schuh M, Penetrante R. Factors affecting recurrence in lumpectomy without irradiation for breast cancer. *Cancer* 1991;67:2079.
116. Kantorowitz DA, Poulter CA, Sischy B, et al. Treatment of breast cancer among elderly women with segmental mastectomy or segmental mastectomy plus postoperative radiotherapy. *Int J Radiat Oncol Biol Phys* 1995;15:263.
117. Reed MWR, Morrison JM. Wide local excision as the sole primary treatment in elderly patients with carcinoma of the breast. *Br J Surg* 1989;76:898.
118. Martelli G, DePalo G, Rossi N, et al. Long-term follow-up of elderly patients with operable breast cancer treated with surgery without axillary dissection plus adjuvant tamoxifen. *Br J Surg* 1995;72:1251.
119. Lee KS, Plowman PN, Gilmore OJA, Gray R. Tamoxifen in breast conservation therapy. *Int J Clin Pharmacol Ther* 1995;33:281.
120. Hayman JA, Fairclough DL, Harris JR, Weeks JC. Patient preferences concerning the trade-off between the risks and benefits of routine radiation therapy after conservative surgery for early stage breast cancer. *J Clin Oncol* 1997;15:1252.
121. Hayman JA, Hillner BE, Harris JR, Weeks JC. Cost-effectiveness of routine radiation following conservative surgery for early-stage breast cancer. *J Clin Oncol* 1998;16:1022.
122. Hrushesky W, Bluning A, Gruber S, et al. Menstrual influence on the surgical care of breast cancer. *Lancet* 1989;2:949.
123. Hagen AA, Hrushesky WJM. Menstrual timing of breast cancer surgery. *Am J Surg* 1998;104:245.
124. Senie RT, Tenser SM. The timing of breast cancer surgery during the menstrual cycle. *Oncology* 1997;11:1509.
125. Senie RT, Rosen PP, Rhodes P, Lesser ML. Timing of breast cancer surgery during the menstrual cycle influences duration of disease-free survival. *Ann Intern Med* 1991;115:337.
126. Veronesi U, Luini A, Mariani L, et al. Effect of menstrual phase on surgical treatment of breast cancer. *Lancet* 1994;343:1545.
127. Saad Z, Bramwell V, Duff J, et al. Timing of surgery in relation to the menstrual cycle in premenopausal women with operable breast cancer. *Br J Surg* 1994;81:217.
128. Badwe RE, Gregory WM, Chaudary MA, et al. Timing of surgery during the menstrual cycle and survival of premenopausal women with operable breast cancer. *Lancet* 1991;337:1261.
129. Gnant MFX, Seifert M, Jakesz R, Adler A, Mittlboeck M, Sevelda P. Breast cancer and timing of surgery during menstrual cycle: a five year analysis of 385 pre-menopausal women. *Int J Cancer* 1992;52:707.
130. Kurebayashi J, Sonoo M, Shimozuma K. Timing of surgery in relation to the menstrual cycle and its influence on the survival of Japanese women with operable breast cancer. *Jpn J Surg* 1995;25:519.
131. Munsterk K, Schmidt L, Helm P. Length and variation in the menstrual cycle: a cross sectional study from a Danish country. *Br J Obstet Gynaecol* 1992;99:422.
132. McGuire W, Hilsenbeck S, Clark G. Optimal mastectomy timing. *J Natl Cancer Inst* 1992;84:346.
133. Sulke AN, Jones DB, Wood PJ. Variation in natural killer activity in peripheral blood during the menstrual cycle. *BMJ* 1985;290:884.
134. Oliver DJ, Ingram DM. Timing of surgery during the menstrual cycle for breast cancer: possible role of growth factors. *Eur J Cancer* 1995;31A:325.
135. Saad Z, Bramwell VH, Wilson SM, O'Malley FP, Jeacock J, Chambers AF. Expression of genes that contribute to proliferative and metastatic ability in breast cancer resected during various menstrual phases. *Lancet* 1998;351:1170.
136. Cox C, Ku N, Reintgen D, Greenberg HM, Nicosia SV, Wangensteen S. Touch preparation cytology of breast lumpectomy margins with histologic correlation. *Arch Surg* 1991;126:490.
137. Ku N, Cox C, Reintgen D, Greenberg HM, Nicosia SV. Cytology of lumpectomy specimens. *Acta Cytol* 1991;35:417.
138. Kearney T, Morrow M. Effect of reexcision on the success of breast conserving surgery. *Ann Surg Oncol* 1995;2:303.
139. Vicini F, Eberlein T, Connolly J, et al. The optimal extent of resection for patients with stages I or II breast cancer treated with conservative surgery and radiotherapy. *Ann Surg* 1992;214:200.
140. Clarke D, Martinez A. Identification of patients who are at high risk for locoregional breast cancer recurrence after conservative surgery and radiotherapy: a review article for surgeons, pathologists, and radiation and medical oncologists. *J Clin Oncol* 1992;10:474.
141. Gwin J, Eisenberg B, Hoffman J, Ottery FD, Boraas M, Solin LJ. Incidence of gross and microscopic carcinoma in specimens from patients with breast cancer after re-excision lumpectomy. *Ann Surg* 1993;218:729.
142. Schmidt-Ullrich R, Wazer D, DiPetrillo T, et al. Breast conservation therapy for early stage breast carcinoma with outstanding local control rates: a case for aggressive therapy to the tumor bearing quadrant. *Int J Radiat Oncol Biol Phys* 1993;27:545.
143. Frazier T, Wong R, Rose D. Implications of accurate pathologic margins in the treatment of primary breast cancer. *Arch Surg* 1989;124:37.
144. Wapnir I, Bancila E, Devereux D, et al. Residual tumor and breast biopsy margins. *Breast Dis* 1989;1:81.
145. Keidan R, Hoffman J, Weese J, et al. Delayed breast abscesses after lumpectomy and radiation therapy. *Am Surg* 1990;56:440.
146. Rescigno J, McCormick B, Brown A, Myskowski PL. Breast cellulitis after conservative surgery and radiotherapy. *Int J Radiat Oncol Biol Phys* 1994;29:163.
147. Patey D, Dysin W. The prognosis of carcinoma of the breast in relation to type of operation performed. *Br J Cancer* 1948;2:71.
148. Auchincloss H. Modified mastectomy. *Am J Surg* 1970;119:506.
149. Kodama H. Modification of muscle preserving radical mastectomy. *Cancer* 1979;44:1517.
150. Croce E. A neoclassical radical mastectomy. *Surg Gynecol Obstet* 1978;1978:147.

151. Roses D, Harris M, Gumport S. Total mastectomy with axillary dissection. *Am J Surg* 1977;134:674.
152. Schneiderman M, Axtell L. Deaths among female patients with carcinoma of the breast treated by a surgical procedure only. *Surg Gynecol Obstet* 1979;148:193.
153. Say C, Donegan W. A biostatistical evaluation of complications from mastectomy. *Surg Gynecol Obstet* 1974;138:370.
154. Aitken D, Minton J. Complications associated with mastectomy. *Surg Clin North Am* 1983;63:1331.
155. Beatty J, Robinson G, Zaia J, et al. A prospective analysis of nosocomial wound infection after mastectomy. *Arch Surg* 1983;118:1421.
156. Platt R, Zucker J, Zaleznik D, et al. Perioperative antibiotic prophylaxis and wound infection following breast surgery. *J Antimicrob Chemother* 1993;31[Suppl B]:43.
157. Platt R, Zucker J, Zaleznik D, et al. Prophylaxis against wound infection following herniorrhaphy or breast surgery. *J Infect Dis* 1992;166:556.
158. Budd D, Cochran R, Sturtz O, Fouty WJ Jr. Surgical morbidity after mastectomy operations. *Am J Surg* 1978;135:218.
159. Myers M, Brock D, Cohn IJ. Prevention of skin slough after radical mastectomy by the use of a vital dye to delineate devascularized skin. *Ann Surg* 1971;173:920.
160. Chilson T, Chan F, Lonser R, Wu TM, Aitken DR. Seroma prevention after modified radical mastectomy. *Am Surg* 1992;58:750.
161. Jolly P, Viar W. Reduction of morbidity after radical mastectomy. *Am Surg* 1981;47:377.
162. Petrek JA, Peters M, Nori S, et al. Axillary lymphadenopathy: a prospective randomized trial of thirteen factors influencing drainage, including early or delayed arm mobilization. *Arch Surg* 1991;125:378.
163. Jamison K, Wellisch DK, Katz RL, Pasnau RO. Phantom breast syndrome. *Arch Surg* 1979;114:93.
164. Kroner K, Knudsen UB, Lundley H, Hvid H. Long-term phantom breast syndrome after mastectomy. *Clin J Pain* 1992;8:346.
165. Webster D, Manse R, Hughes L. Immediate reconstruction of the breast after mastectomy: is it safe? *Cancer* 1984;53:1416.
166. Johnson C, Van Heerden J, Donohue J, et al. Oncological aspects of immediate breast reconstruction following mastectomy for malignancy. *Arch Surg* 1989;124:819.
167. Petit J, Le M, Mouriesse H, et al. Can breast reconstruction with gel-filled silicone implants increase the risk of death and second primary cancer in patients treated by mastectomy for breast cancer? *Plast Reconstr Surg* 1994;94:115.
168. Kroll S, Ames F, Singletary S, et al. The oncologic risks of skin preservation at mastectomy when combined with immediate reconstruction of the breast. *Surg Gynecol Obstet* 1991;172:17.
169. Dao T, Nemoto T. The clinical significance of skin recurrence after radical mastectomy in women with cancer of the breast. *Surg Gynecol Obstet* 1963;117:447.
170. Noone R, Frazier T, Noone G, et al. Recurrence of breast carcinoma following immediate reconstruction: a 13-year review. *Plast Reconstr Surg* 1994;90:96.
171. Eberlein T, Crespo L, Smith B, et al. Prospective evaluation of immediate reconstruction after mastectomy. *Ann Surg* 1993;218:29.
172. Noone R, Murphy J, Spear S, et al. A six-year experience with immediate reconstruction for mastectomy for cancer. *Plast Reconstr Surg* 1985;76:258.
173. Barreau-Pouhaer L, Le M, Rietjens M, et al. Risk factors for failure of immediate breast reconstruction with prostheses after total mastectomy for breast cancer. *Cancer* 1992;70:1145.
174. Victor SJ, Brown DM, Horwitz EM, et al. Treatment outcome with radiation therapy after breast augmentation or reconstruction in patients with primary breast carcinoma. *Cancer* 1998;82:1303.
175. Evans GRD, Schusterman MA, Kroll SS, et al. Reconstruction and the radiated breast: is there a role for implants? *Plast Reconstr Surg* 1995;96:1111.
176. Hunt KA, Baldwin BJ, Strom E, et al. Feasibility of postmastectomy radiation therapy after TRAM flap breast reconstruction. *Ann Surg Oncol* 1997;4:377.
177. Williams JK, Carlson GW, Bostwick J III, Bried JT, Mackay G. The effects of radiation treatment after TRAM flap breast reconstruction. *Plast Reconstr Surg* 1997;100:1153.
178. Valagussa P, Bonadonna G, Veronesi U. Patterns of relapse and survival following radical mastectomy: analysis of 716 consecutive patients. *Cancer* 1978;41:1170.
179. Fisher B, Wolmark N, Bauer M, Redmond C, Gebhardt M. The accuracy of clinical nodal staging and of limited axillary dissection as a determinant of histologic nodal status in carcinoma of the breast. *Surg Gynecol Obstet* 1981;152:765.
180. Bedwinek J, Lee J, Fineberg B, Ocwieza M. Prognostic indicators in patients with isolated local-regional recurrence of breast cancer. *Cancer* 1981;47:2232.
181. Aberizk W, Silver B, Henderson IC, Cady B, Harris JR. The use of radiotherapy for treatment of isolated local-regional recurrence of breast cancer after mastectomy. *Cancer* 1986;58:1214.
182. Chen K, Montague E, Oswald M. Results of irradiation in the treatment of loco-regional breast cancer recurrence. *Cancer* 1985; 56:1269.
183. Fletcher G, McNeese M, Oswald M. Long-range results for breast cancer patients treated by radical mastectomy and postoperative radiation without adjuvant chemotherapy: an update. *Int J Radiat Oncol Biol Phys* 1989;17:11.
184. Uematsu M, Bornstein B, Recht A, et al. Long-term results of postoperative radiation therapy following mastectomy with and without chemotherapy in stage I-III breast cancer. *Int J Radiat Oncol Biol Phys* 1993;25:765.
185. Early Breast Cancer Trialists' Collaborative Group. Favorable and unfavorable effects on long-term survival of radiotherapy for early breast cancer: An overview of the randomized trials (*in press*).
186. Jones JM, Ribeiro GG. Mortality patterns over 34 years of breast cancer patients in a clinical trial of post-operative radiotherapy. *Clin Radiol* 1989;40:204.
187. Host H, Brennhovd IO, Loeb M. Postoperative radiotherapy in breast cancer: long-term results from the Oslo study. *Int J Radiat Oncol Biol Phys* 1986;12:727.
188. Early Breast Cancer Trialists' Group. *Treatment of early breast cancer; world-wide experience, 1985-1990.* Vol. 1. Oxford, UK: Oxford University Press, 1990.
189. Rutqvist L, Pettersson D, Johansson H. Adjuvant radiation therapy versus surgery alone in operable breast cancer: long-term follow-up in a randomized clinical trial. *Radiother Oncol* 1993;26:104.
190. Rutqvist LE, Lax I, Fornander T, Johansson H. Cardiovascular mortality in a randomized trial of adjuvant radiation therapy versus surgery alone in primary breast cancer. *Int J Radiat Oncol Biol Phys* 1992;22:887.
190a. Fisher B, Slack NH, Cavanaugh PJ, Gardner B, Ravdin IG. Postoperative radiotherapy in the treatment of breast cancer: results of the NSABP clinical trial. *Ann Surg* 1970;172:711.
191. Lythgoe JP, Palmer MK. Manchester regional breast study—5 and 10 year results. *Br J Surg* 1982;69:693.
192. Haybittle JL, Brinkley D, A'Hern RP, Baum M. Postoperative radiotherapy and late mortality: evidence from the Cancer Research Campaign trial for early breast cancer. *BMJ* 1989;298:1611.
193. Stewart H, Jack W, Forrest A, et al. South-east Scottish trial of local therapy in node negative breast cancer. *Breast* 1994;3:31.
193a. Turnbull AR, Turner DT, Chant AD, Shepherd JM, Buchanan RB, Fraser JD. Treatment of early breast cancer. *Lancet* 1978;2:7.
194. Fowble B. Postmastectomy radiation: then and now. *Oncology* 1997;11:213.
195. Bonadonna G, Valagussa P, Moliterni A, Zambetti M, Brambilla C. Adjuvant cyclophosphamide, methotrexate and fluorouracil in node-positive breast cancer: the results of 20 years of follow-up. *N Engl J Med* 1995;332:901.
196. Fisher B, Fisher E, Redmond C. Ten year results from the NSABP clinical trial evaluating the use of L-phenylalanine mustard (L-PAM) in the management of primary breast cancer. *J Clin Oncol* 1986;4:929.
197. Rutqvist L, Cedermark B, Fornander T, et al. The relationship between hormone receptor content and the effect of adjuvant tamoxifen in operable breast cancer. *J Clin Oncol* 1989;7:1474.
198. Nolvadex Adjuvant Trial Organization. Controlled trial of tamoxifen as a single adjuvant agent in management of early breast cancer: analysis at six years by the Nolvadex Adjuvant Trial Organization. *Lancet* 1985;1:836.
199. Breast Cancer Trials Committee of the Scottish Cancer Trials Office. Adjuvant tamoxifen in the management of operable breast cancer: the Scottish trial. *Lancet* 1987;2:171.
200. Castiglione-Gertsch M, Johnsen C, Goldhirsch A, et al. The International (Ludwig) Breast Cancer Group trials I-IV: 15-year follow-up. *Ann Oncol* 1994;7:1229.

201. Wood WC, Budman DR, Korzun AH, et al. Dose and dose intensity of adjuvant chemotherapy for stage II, node-positive breast carcinoma. *N Engl J Med* 1994;330:1253.
202. Fisher B, Anderson S, Wickerham DL, et al. Increased intensification and total dose of cyclophosphamide in a doxorubicin-cyclophosphamide regimen for the treatment of primary breast cancer: findings from National Surgical Adjuvant Breast and Bowel Project B-22. *J Clin Oncol* 1997;15:1858.
203. Stefanik D, Goldberg R, Byrne P, et al. Local-regional failure in patients treated with adjuvant chemotherapy for breast cancer. *J Clin Oncol* 1985;3:660.
204. Fowble B, Gray R, Gilchrist K, Goodman RL, Taylor S, Tormey DC. Identification of a subgroup of patients with breast cancer and histologically positive axillary nodes receiving adjuvant chemotherapy who may benefit from postoperative radiotherapy. *J Clin Oncol* 1988;6:1107.
205. Pisansky TM, Ingle JN, Schaid DJ, et al. Patterns of tumor relapse following mastectomy and adjuvant systemic therapy in patients with axillary lymph node-positive breast cancer: impact of clinical, histopathologic and flow cytometric factors. *Cancer* 1993;72:1247.
206. Overgaard M, Hansen PS, Overgaard J, et al. Postoperative radiotherapy in high-risk premenopausal women with breast cancer who receive adjuvant chemotherapy. Danish Breast Cancer Cooperative Group 82b Trial. *N Engl J Med* 1997;337:949.
207. Overgaard M, Jensen M-B, Overgaard J, et al. Randomized controlled trial evaluating postoperative radiotherapy in high-risk postmenopausal breast cancer patients given tamoxifen: report from the Danish Breast Cancer Cooperative Group DBCG 82c Trial. *Lancet* 1999;353:1641.
208. Ragaz J, Jackson SM, Le N, et al. Adjuvant radiotherapy and chemotherapy in node-positive premenopausal women with breast cancer. *N Engl J Med* 1997;337:956.
209. Griem KL, Henderson IC, Gelman R, et al. The 5-year results of a randomized trial of adjuvant radiation therapy after chemotherapy in breast cancer patients treated with mastectomy. *J Clin Oncol* 1987;5:1546.
210. Velez-Garcia E, Carpenter JT Jr, Moore M, et al. Postsurgical adjuvant chemotherapy with or without radiotherapy in women with breast cancer and positive axillary nodes: a South-Eastern Cancer Study Group (SEG) Trial. *Eur J Cancer* 1992;11:1833.
211. Martinez A, Ahmann D, O'Fallon J, et al. An interim analysis of the randomized surgical adjuvant trial for patients with unfavorable breast cancer. *Int J Radiat Oncol Biol Phys* 1984;10[Suppl 2]:106.
212. Muss H, Cooper R, Brockschmidt J, et al. A randomized trial of adjuvant chemotherapy (CT) without radiation therapy (RT) for stage II breast cancer: 11-year follow-up of Piedmont Oncology Association (Protocol no. 74176). *Breast Cancer Res Treat* 1989;14:185.
213. McArdle C, Crawford D, Dykes E, et al. Adjuvant radiotherapy and chemotherapy in breast cancer. *Br J Surg* 1986;73:264.
214. Blomqvist C, Tiusanen K, Elomaa I, et al. The combination of radiotherapy, adjuvant chemotherapy (cyclophosphamide-doxorubicin-ftorafur) and tamoxifen in stage II breast cancer. Long-term follow-up results of a randomised trial. *Br J Cancer* 1992;66:1171.
215. Buzdar AJ, Blumenschein GR, Smith TL, et al. Adjuvant chemotherapy with fluorouracil, doxorubicin, and cyclophosphamide, with or without Bacillus Calmette-Guerin and with or without irradiation in operable breast cancer. A prospective randomized trial. *Cancer* 1984;53:384.
216. Tennvall-Nittby L, Tengrup I, Landberg T. The total incidence of loco-regional recurrence in a randomized trial of breast cancer TNM stage II. The South Sweden Breast Cancer Trial. *Acta Oncol* 1993;32:641.
217. Gelman R. Techniques in the interpretation of clinical trials. *Diseases of the breast.* Harris JR, Lippman ME, Morrow M, Hellman S, eds. Lippincott–Raven, 1996:1002.
218. Nixon AJ, Manola J, Gelman R, et al. No long-term increase in cardiac-related mortality after breast-conserving surgery and radiation therapy using modern techniques. *J Clin Oncol* 1998;16:1374.
219. Hojris I, Overgaard M, Christensen JJ, et al. Morbidity and mortality of ischemic heart disease in 3083 high-risk breast cancer patients given adjuvant systemic treatment with or without postmastectomy irradiation. *Radiother Oncol* 1998;48[Suppl. 1]:S120(abst).
220. Swedborg I, Wallgren A. The effect of pre- and post-mastectomy radiotherapy on the degree of edema, shoulder joint mobility, and gripping force. *Cancer* 1981;47:877.
221. Larson D, Weinstein M, Goldberg I, et al. Edema of the arm as a function of the extent of axillary surgery in patients with stage I and II carcinoma of the breast treated with primary radiotherapy. *Int J Radiat Oncol Biol Phys* 1986;12:877.
222. Match R. Radiation-induced brachial plexus paralysis. *Arch Surg* 1975;110:384.
223. Stoll B, Andrews J. Radiation-induced peripheral neuropathy. *BMJ* 1975;1:834.
224. Powell S, Cooke J, Parsons C. Radiation-induced brachial plexus injury: follow-up of two different fractionation schedules. *Radiother Oncol* 1990;18:213.
225. Salner A, Botnick L, Herzog A, et al. Reversible brachial plexopathy following primary radiation therapy for breast cancer. *Cancer Treat Rep* 1981;65:797.
226. Olsen NK, Pfeiffer P, Johannsen L, Schroder H, Rose C. Radiation-induced brachial plexopathy: neurological follow-up in 161 recurrence-free breast cancer patients. *Int J Radiat Oncol Biol Phys* 1993;26:43.
227. Ryttov N, Holm NV, Qvist N, Blichert-Toft M. Influence of adjuvant irradiation on the development of late arm lymphedema and impaired shoulder mobility after mastectomy for carcinoma of the breast. *Acta Oncol* 1988;27:667.
228. Bentzed S, Overgaard M, Thames H. Fractionation sensitivity of a functional endpoint: impaired shoulder movement after post-mastectomy radiotherapy. *Int J Radiat Oncol Biol Phys* 1989;17:531.
229. Pierce S, Recht A, Lingos T, et al. Long-term radiation complications following conservative surgery (CS) and radiation therapy (RT) in patients with early stage breast cancer. *Int J Radiat Oncol Biol Phys* 1992;23:915.
230. Moore GJ, Mendenhall NP, Kamath SS, et al. Persistent symptomatology after breast-conservation therapy: prevalence and impact on quality of life. *Int J Radiat Oncol Biol Phys* 1998;42:256(abst).
231. Kim J, Chu F, Hilaris B. The influence of dose fractionation on acute and late reactions in patients with postoperative radiotherapy for carcinoma of the breast. *Cancer* 1975;35:1538.
232. Lingos TI, Recht A, Vicini F, et al. Radiation pneumonitis in breast cancer patients treated with conservative surgery and radiation therapy. *Int J Radiat Oncol Biol Phys* 1991;21:335.
233. Bornstein BA, Cheng CW, Rhodes LM, et al. Can simulation measurements be used to predict the irradiated lung volume in the tangential fields in patients treated for breast cancer? *Int J Radiat Oncol Biol Phys* 1990;18:181.
234. Kimsey FC, Mendenhall NP, Ewald LM, Coons TS, Layon AJ. Is radiation treatment volume a predictor for acute or late effect on pulmonary function? A prospective study of patients treated with breast-conserving surgery and postoperative irradiation. *Cancer* 1994;73:2549.
235. Hardman PD, Tweeddale PM, Kerr GR, Anderson ED, Rodger A. The effect of pulmonary function of local and loco-regional irradiation for breast cancer. *Radiother Oncol* 1994;30:33.
236. Marks LB, Halperin EC, Prosnitz LR, et al. Post-mastectomy radiotherapy following adjuvant chemotherapy and autologous bone marrow transplantation for breast cancer patients with greater than or equal to 10 positive axillary lymph nodes. Cancer and Leukemia Group B. *Int J Radiat Oncol Biol Phys* 1992;23:1021.
237. Srinivasan G, Kurtz D, Lichter A. Pleural-based changes on chest x-ray after irradiation for primary breast cancer: correlation with findings on computerized tomography. *Int J Radiat Oncol Biol Phys* 1983;9:1567.
238. Goss PE, Sierra S. Current perspectives on radiation-induced breast cancer. *J Clin Oncol* 1998;16:338.
239. Mattsson A, Ruden B-I, Hall P, Wilking N, Rutqvist LE. Radiation-induced breast cancer: long-term follow-up of radiation for benign breast disease. *J Natl Cancer Inst* 1993;85:1679.
240. Gray L. Radiation biology and cancer. In: *Cellular radiation biology: the M.D. Anderson Hospital and Tumor Institute 18th symposium on fundamental cancer research.* Baltimore: Williams & Wilkins, 1965:7.
241. Fraass B, Roberson P, Lichter A. Dose to the contralateral breast due to primary breast irradiation. *Int J Radiat Oncol Biol Phys* 1985;11:485.
242. Committee on the Biological Effects of Ionizing Radiations, Board on Radiation Effects Research Commission on Life Sciences, National Research Council. *Health effects of exposure to low levels of ionizing radiation: BEIR V.* Washington, DC: National Academy, 1990.
243. Tokunaga M, Land C, Tokuoka S, Nishimori I, Soda M, Skiba S. Incidence of female breast cancer among atomic bomb survivors, 1950–1985. *Radiat Res* 1994;138:209.

244. Boice JD Jr, Harvey EB, Blettner M, Stovall M, Flannery JT. Cancer in the contralateral breast after radiotherapy for breast cancer. *N Engl J Med* 1992;326:781.
245. Storm H, Andersson M, Boice J Jr, et al. Adjuvant radiotherapy and risk of contralateral breast cancer. *J Natl Cancer Inst* 1992;84:1245.
246. Brady MS, Garfein CF, Petrek JA, Brennan MF. Post-treatment sarcoma in breast cancer patients. *Ann Surg Oncol* 1994;1:66.
247. Karlsson P, Holmberg E, Johansson K-A, Kindblom LG, Carstensen J, Wallgren A. Soft tissue sarcoma after treatment for breast cancer. *Radiother Oncol* 1996;38:25.
248. Taghian A, de Vathaire F, Terrier P, et al. Long-term risk of sarcoma following radiation treatment for breast cancer. *Int J Radiat Oncol Biol Phys* 1991;21:361.
249. Kurtz JM, Amalric R, Brandone H, Ayme Y, Spitalier JM. Contralateral breast cancer and other second malignancies in patients treated by breast-conserving therapy with radiation. *Int J Radiat Oncol Biol Phys* 1988;15:277.
250. Wijnmaalen A, van Ooijen B, van Geel B, Henzen-Logmans SC, Treurniet-Donker AD. Angiosarcoma of the breast following lumpectomy, axillary lymph node dissection, and radiotherapy for primary breast cancer: three case reports and a review of the literature. *Int J Radiat Oncol Biol Phys* 1993;26:135.
251. Smith P, Dole R. Age and time-dependent changes in the rates of radiation-induced cancers in patients with ankylosing spondylitis. In: *Late biological effects of ionizing radiation.* Vol. 1. Vienna: International Atomic Energy Agency, 1978:203.
252. Curtis R, Boice J Jr, Stovall M, et al. Risk of leukemia after chemotherapy and radiation treatment for breast cancer. *N Engl J Med* 1992;326:1745.
253. Alderson M, Jackson S. Long-term follow-up of patients with menorrhagia treated with irradiation. *Br J Radiol* 1971;44:295.
254. Doll R, Smith P. The long-term effects of x-irradiation in patients treated for metropathia hemorrhagica. *Br J Radiol* 1968;41:362.
255. Curtis RE, Boice JD Jr, Stovall M, Flannery JT, Moloney WC. Leukemia risk following radiotherapy for breast cancer. *J Clin Oncol* 1989;7:21.
256. Inskip P, Stovall M, Flannery J. Lung cancer risk and radiation dose among women treated for breast cancer. *J Natl Cancer Inst* 1994;86:983.
257. Neugut AI, Robinson E, Lee WC, Murray T, Karwoski K, Kutcher GJ. Lung cancer after radiation therapy for breast cancer. *Cancer* 1993; 71:3054.
258. Neugut A, Murray T, Santos J, et al. Increased risk of lung cancer after breast cancer radiation therapy in cigarette smokers. *Cancer* 1994;73:1615.
259. Inskip P, Boice J Jr. Radiotherapy-induced lung cancer among women who smoke [Editorial]. *Cancer* 1994;73:1541.
260. Shapiro CL, Hardenbergh PH, Gelman R, et al. Cardiac effects of adjuvant doxorubicin and radiation therapy in breast cancer patients. *J Clin Oncol* 1998;16:3493.
261. Ludwig Breast Cancer Study Group. Combination adjuvant chemotherapy for node-positive breast cancer: inadequacy of a single perioperative cycle. *N Engl J Med* 1988;319:677.
262. Kraniner M, Sevelda P, Salzer H, et al. Comparison between the application of intra- versus 3-week postoperative adjuvant chemotherapy in breast cancer. *Eur J Cancer* 1991;27:39(abst).
263. Sertoli M, Pronzato P, Querolo P, et al. Perioperative polychemotherapy for primary breast cancer [Abstract]. In: Gelber R, Goldhirsch A, et al, eds. *Adjuvant therapy breast cancer.* Berlin: Springer-Verlag, 1993:57.
264. Recht A, Come S, Gelman R, et al. Integration of conservative surgery, radiotherapy, and chemotherapy for the treatment of early-stage node-positive breast cancer: sequencing, timing, and outcome. *J Clin Oncol* 1991;9:1662.
265. Glucksberg H, Rivkin S, Rasmussen S, et al. Combination chemotherapy (CMFVP) versus L-phenylalanine mustard (L-PAM) for operable breast cancer with positive axillary nodes: a Southwest Oncology Group study. *Cancer* 1982;50:423.
266. Buzdar A, Smith T, Powell K, Blumenschein GR, Gehan EA. Effect of timing of initiation of adjuvant chemotherapy on disease-free survival in breast cancer. *Breast Cancer Res Treat* 1982;2:163.
267. Buchholz T, Austin-Seymour M, Moe R, et al. Effect of delay in radiation in the combined modality treatment of breast cancer. *Int J Radiat Oncol Biol Phys* 1993;26:23.
268. Hartsell W, Recine D, Griem K, Murthy AK. Delaying the initiation of intact breast irradiation for patients with lymph node positive breast increases the risk of local recurrence. *Cancer* 1995;76:2497.
269. McCormick B, Norton L, Yao TJ, Yahalom J, Petrek JA. The impact of the sequence of radiation and chemotherapy on local control after breast-conserving surgery. *Cancer J Sci Am* 1996;2:39.
270. Wallgren A, Bernier J, Gelber RD, et al. Timing of radiotherapy and chemotherapy following breast conserving surgery for patients with node-positive breast cancer. *Int J Radiat Oncol Biol Phys* 1996;35:649.
271. Leonard CE, Wood ME, Zhen B, et al. Does administration of chemotherapy before radiotherapy in breast patients treated with conservative surgery negatively impact local control? *J Clin Oncol* 1995;13:2906.
272. Mamounas EP, Fisher B, Bryant J, et al. Does delaying breast irradiation in order to administer adjuvant chemotherapy increase the rate of ipsilateral breast tumor recurrence (IBTR)? Results from two NSABP adjuvant studies in node-positive breast cancer (B-15 and B-16). *Breast Cancer Res Treat* 1996;41:219(abst).
273. Recht A, Come SE, Henderson IC, et al. The sequencing of chemotherapy and radiation therapy after conservative surgery for patients with early-stage breast cancer. *N Engl J Med* 1996;334:1356.
274. Botnick L, Come S, Rose C, et al. Primary breast irradiation and concomitant adjuvant chemotherapy. In: Harris J, Hellman S, Silen W, eds. *Conservative management of breast cancer.* Philadelphia: JB Lippincott Co, 1983:321.
275. Meek A, Order S, Abeloff M, Ettinger D, Baker RR, Baral E. Concurrent radiochemotherapy in advanced breast cancer. *Cancer* 1983;51:1001.
276. Markiewicz DA, Fox KR, Schultz DJ, et al. Concurrent chemotherapy and radiation for breast conservation treatment of early-stage breast cancer. *Cancer J Sci Am* 1998;4:185.
277. Dubey AK, Recht A, Shulman L, et al. Outcome following concurrent chemotherapy (CT) and reduced dose radiation therapy (RT) for patients with early stage breast cancer. *Int J Radiat Oncol Biol Phys* 1997;39:267(abst).
278. Lippman M, Lichter A, Edwards B, Gorrell CR, d'Angelo T, DeMoss EV. The impact of primary irradiation treatment of localized breast cancer on the ability to administer systemic adjuvant chemotherapy. *J Clin Oncol* 1984;2:21.
279. Cooper M, Rhyne A, Muss H, et al. A randomized comparative trial of chemotherapy and radiation therapy for stage II breast cancer. *Cancer* 1981;47:2833.
280. Sarkaria J, Miller E, Parker C, Jordan VC, Mulcahy RT. 4-hydroxytamoxifen, an active metabolite of tamoxifen, does not alter the radiation sensitivity of MCF-7 breast carcinoma cells irradiated in vitro. *Breast Cancer Res Treat* 1994;30:159.
281. Wazer D, Joyce M, Chan W, et al. Effects of tamoxifen on the radiosensitivity of hormonally responsive and unresponsive breast carcinoma cells. *Radiat Oncol Investig* 1993;1:20.
282. Kinsella T, Gould M, Mulcahy R, Ritter MA, Fowler JF. Keynote address: integration of cytostatic agents and radiation therapy: a different approach to "proliferating" human tumors. *Int J Radiat Oncol Biol Phys* 1991;20:295.
283. Fisher B, Dignan J, Bryant J, et al. Five versus more than five years of Tamoxifen therapy for breast cancer patients with negative lymph nodes and estrogen receptor-positive tumors. *J Natl Cancer Inst* 1996;88:1529.
284. Wazer DE, Morr J, Erban JK, Schmid CH, Ruthazer R, Schmidt-Ullrich RK. The effects of postradiation treatment with tamoxifen on local control and cosmetic outcome in the conservatively treated breast. *Cancer* 1997;80:732.
285. Bentzen SM, Skoczylas JZ, Overgaard M, Overgaard J. Radiotherapy-related lung fibrosis enhanced by tamoxifen. *J Natl Cancer Inst* 1996;88:918.
286. Haagensen CD. In: Haagensen CD, ed. *Diseases of the breast*, 3rd ed. Philadelphia: WB Saunders, 1986:656.
287. Nemoto T, Vans J, Bedwani RN, Baker HW, McGregor FH, Murphy GP. Management and survival of female breast cancer: results of a national survey by the American College of Surgeons. *Cancer* 1980;45:2917.
288. Carter CL, Allen C, Henson DE. Relation of tumor size, lymph node status and survival in 24,740 breast cancer cases. *Cancer* 1989; 63:181.
289. Mustafa IA, Cole B, Wanebo HJ, Bland KI, Chang HR. The impact of histopathology on nodal metastasis. *Arch Surg* 1997;132:384.
290. Barth A, Craig PM, Silverstein MJ. Predictors of axillary lymph node metastases in patients with T1 breast carcinoma. *Cancer* 1997; 79:1918.

291. Fein DA, Fowble BL, Hanlon AL, et al. Identification of women with T1 and T2 breast cancer at low risk of positive axillary nodes. *J Surg Oncol* 1997;65:34.
292. McGee JM, Youmans R, Clingan F, Malnar K, Bellefeuille C, Berry B. The value of axillary dissection in T1a breast cancer. *Am J Surg* 1996;172:501.
293. Schnabel FR, Estabrook A. Results of axillary node dissection in early breast cancer. *Breast Cancer Res Treat* 1994;32:40(abst).
294. Reger V, Beito G, Jolly PC. Factors affecting the incidence of lymph node metastases in small cancers of the breast. *Am J Surg* 1989;157:501.
295. Ravdin PM. Can patient and tumor characteristics allow prediction of axillary lymph node status? *Semin Breast Dis* 1998;1:141.
296. Seidman JD, Schnaper LA, Aisner SC. Relationship of the size of the invasive component of the primary breast carcinoma to axillary lymph node metastasis. *Cancer* 1995;75:65.
297. Brenin DR, Morrow M. Accuracy of AJCC staging for breast cancer for patients undergoing re-excision for positive margins. *Ann Surg Oncol* 1998;5:719.
298. Wong J, Kopald K, Morton D. The impact of microinvasion on axillary node metastases and survival in patients with intraductal breast cancer. *Arch Surg* 1990;125:1298.
299. Solin L, Fowble B, Yeh IT, et al. Microinvasive ductal carcinoma of the breast treated with breast-conserving surgery and definitive irradiation. *Int J Radiat Oncol Biol Phys* 1992;23:961.
300. Nevin J, Pinzon G, Morton T, Baggerly J. Minimal breast cancer. *Am J Surg* 1980;139:357.
301. McDivitt R, Boyce W, Gersell D. Tubular carcinoma of the breast. Clinical and pathological observations concerning 135 cases. *Am J Surg Pathol* 1982;6:401.
302. Peters G, Wolff M, Haagensen C. Tubular carcinoma of the breast: clinical-pathologic correlations based on 100 cases. *Ann Surg* 1981;193:138.
303. Fisher B, Slack NH, Ausman RK, Bross ID. Location of breast carcinoma and prognosis. *Surg Gynecol Obstet* 1969;129:705.
304. Caceres E. Incidence of metastases in the internal mammary chain in operable cancer of the breast. *Surg Gynecol Obstet* 1959;108:715.
305. Handley R, Patey D, Hand B. Excision of the internal mammary chain in radical mastectomy: results of 57 cases. *Lancet* 1956;1:457.
306. Urban JA, Marjani MA. Significance of internal mammary lymph node metastases in breast cancer. *Am J Roentgenol Radiother Nucl Med* 1971;3:130.
307. Morrow M, Foster RS. Staging of breast cancer. A new rationale for internal mammary node biopsy. *Arch Surg* 1981;116:748.
308. Bucalossi P, Veronesi U, Zingo L, Cantu C. Enlarged mastectomy for breast cancer. Review of 1,213 cases. *Am J Roentgenol Radium Ther Nucl Med* 1971;1:119.
309. Caceres E. An evaluation of radical mastectomy and extended radical mastectomy for cancer of the breast. *Surg Gynecol Obstet* 1967;123:337.
310. Li KYY, Shen ZZ. An analysis of 1242 cases of extended radical mastectomy. *Breast* 1983;10:10.
311. Veronesi U, Cascinelli N, Bufalino R, et al. Risk of internal mammary lymph node metastases and its relevance on prognosis of breast cancer patients. *Ann Surg* 1983;198:681.
312. Dahl Iversen E. Recherches sur les metastases microscopiques des cancers du sein dans las ganglions lymphatiques parasternaux et supraclaviculaires. *Mem Acad Clin* 1952;78:651.
313. Rosen P, Martin M, Kinne D, et al. Discontinuous or "skip" metastases in breast carcinoma: analysis of 1228 axillary dissections. *Ann Surg* 1983;197:276.
314. Veronesi U, Rilke F, Luini A, et al. Distribution of axillary node metastases by level of invasion. An analysis of 539 cases. *Cancer* 1987;59:682.
315. Smith JA III, Gamez-Araujo JJ, Gallager HS, White EC, McBride CM. Carcinoma of the breast: analysis of total lymph node involvement versus level of metastasis. *Cancer* 1977;39:527.
316. Danforth DN Jr, Findlay PA, McDonald HD, et al. Complete axillary lymph node dissection for stage I-II carcinoma of the breast. *J Clin Oncol* 1986;4:655.
317. Chevinsky AH, Ferrara J, James AG, Minton JP, Young D, Farrar WB. Prospective evaluation of clinical and pathologic detection of axillary metastases in patients with carcinoma of the breast. *Surgery* 1990;108:612.
318. Pigott J, Nichols R, Maddox WA, Balch CM. Metastases to the upper levels of the axillary nodes in carcinoma of the breast and its implications for nodal sampling procedures. *Surg Gynecol Obstet* 1984;158:255.
319. Boova R, Bonanni R, Rosato F. Patterns of axillary nodal involvement in breast cancer. Predictability of level one dissection. *Ann Surg* 1982;196:642.
320. Haagensen C. The surgical treatment of mammary carcinoma. In: Haagensen CD, ed. *Diseases of the breast*, 2nd ed. Philadelphia: WB Saunders, 1971;706.
321. Axelsson C, Mouridsen H, Zedeler K, et al. Axillary dissection of level I and II lymph nodes is important in breast cancer classification. *Eur J Cancer* 1992;28A:1415.
322. Halverson KJ, Taylor ME, Perez CA, et al. Regional nodal management and patterns of failure following conservative surgery and radiation therapy for stage I and II breast cancer. *Int J Radiat Oncol Biol Phys* 1993;26:593.
323. Recht A, Pierce SM, Abner A, et al. Regional nodal failure after conservative surgery and radiotherapy for early stage breast carcinoma. *J Clin Oncol* 1991;9:988.
324. Siegel BM, Mayzel KA, Love SM. Level I and II axillary dissection in the treatment of early-stage breast cancer. An analysis of 259 consecutive patients. *Arch Surg* 1990;125:1144.
325. Fowble B, Solin LJ, Schultz DJ, Goodman RL. Frequency, sites of relapse, and outcome of regional node failures following conservative surgery and radiation for early breast cancer. *Int J Radiat Oncol Biol Phys* 1989;17:703.
326. Steele RJ, Forrest AP, Gibson T, Stewart HJ, Chetty U. The efficacy of lower axillary sampling in obtaining lymph node status in breast cancer: a controlled randomized trial. *Br J Surg* 1985;72:368.
327. Forrest AP, Stewart HJ, Roberts MM, Steele RJ. Simple mastectomy and axillary node sampling (pectoral node biopsy) in the management of primary breast cancer. *Ann Surg* 1982;196:371.
328. Kissin MW, Thompson EM, Price AB, Slavin G, Kark AE. The inadequacy of axillary sampling in breast cancer. *Lancet* 1982;1:1210.
329. Graversen HP, Blichert-Toft M, Andersen JA, Zedeler K. Breast cancer: risk of axillary recurrence in node-negative patients following partial dissection of the axilla. *Eur J Surg Oncol* 1988;14:407.
330. Fisher B, Wolmark N, Bauer M, Redmond C, Gebhardt M. The accuracy of clinical nodal staging and of limited axillary dissection as a determinant of histologic nodal status in carcinoma of the breast. *Surg Gynecol Obstet* 1981;152:765.
331. National Institutes of Health Consensus Conference. Treatment of early stage breast cancer. *JAMA* 1991;265:391.
332. Somers RG, Jablon LK, Kaplan MJ, Sandler GL, Rosenblatt NK. The use of closed suction drainage after lumpectomy and axillary node dissection for breast cancer: a prospective randomized trial. *Ann Surg* 1992;215:146.
333. Ivens D, Hoe AL, Podd TJ, Hamilton CR, Taylor I, Royle GT. Assessment of morbidity from complete axillary dissection. *Br J Cancer* 1992;66:136.
334. Lin P, Allison D, Wainstuck J, et al. Impact of axillary lymph node dissection on the therapy of breast cancer patients. *J Clin Oncol* 1993;11:1536.
335. Hladiuk M, Huchcroft S, Temple W, Schnurr BE. Arm function after axillary dissection for breast cancer: a pilot study to provide parameter estimates. *J Surg Oncol* 1992;50:47.
336. Keramopoulos A, Tsionou C, Minaretzis D, Michalas S, Aravantinos D. Arm morbidity following treatment of breast cancer with total axillary dissection: a multivariate approach. *Oncology* 1993;50:445.
337. Gutman H, Kersz T, Barzilai T, Haddad M, Reiss R. Achievements of physical therapy in patients after modified radical mastectomy compared with quadrantectomy, axillary dissection, and radiation for carcinoma of the breast. *Arch Surg* 1990;125:389.
338. Lotze MT, Duncan MA, Gerber LH, Woltering EA, Rosenberg SA. Early versus delayed shoulder motion following axillary dissection: a randomized prospective study. *Ann Surg* 1981;193:288.
339. Petrek JA, Peters MM, Nori S, Knauer C, Kinne DW, Rogatko A. Axillary lymphadenectomy: a prospective, randomized trial of 13 factors influencing drainage, including early or delayed arm mobilization. *Arch Surg* 1990;125:378.
340. Clarke D, Martinez A, Cox RS, Goffinet DR. Breast edema following staging axillary node dissection in patients with breast carcinoma treated by radical radiotherapy. *Cancer* 1982;49:2295.
341. Fisher B. The evolution of paradigms for the management of breast cancer: a personal perspective. *Cancer Res* 1992;52:2371.
342. Brinkley D, Haybittle JL. The curability of breast cancer. *Lancet* 1975;2:95.

343. Rosen PP, Groshen S, Saigo PE, Kinne DW, Hellman S. A long-term follow-up study of survival in stage I (T1N0M0) and stage II (T1N1M0) breast carcinoma. *J Clin Oncol* 1989;7:355.
344. Hayward JL. The Guy's trial of treatment of early breast cancer. *World J Surg* 1977;1:314.
345. Hayward J, Caleffi M. The significance of local control in the primary treatment of breast cancer. *Arch Surg* 1987;122:1244.
346. Cabanes P, Salmon R, Vilcoq J, et al. Value of axillary dissection in addition to lumpectomy and radiotherapy in early breast cancer. *Lancet* 1992;339:1245.
347. Morton DC, Duan-Ren W, Wong JH, et al. Technical details of intraoperative lymphatic mapping and sentinel node biopsy in the management of primary melanoma. *Arch Surg* 1992;127:392.
348. Giuliano AE, Kirgan DM, Guenther JM, Morton DL. Lymphatic mapping and sentinel lymphadenectomy for breast cancer. *Ann Surg* 1994;220:391.
349. Giuliano AE, Jones RC, Brennan M, Statman R. Sentinel lymphadenectomy in breast cancer. *J Clin Oncol* 1997;15:2345.
350. Krag DN, Weaver OJ, Alex JC, Fairbank JT. Surgical resection and radiolocalization of the sentinel node in breast cancer using a gamma probe. *Surg Oncol* 1993;2:335.
351. Albertini JJ, Lyman GH, Cox C, et al. Lymphatic mapping and sentinel node biopsy in the patient with breast cancer. *JAMA* 1996;276:1818.
352. Veronesi U, Paganelli G, Galimberti V, et al. Sentinel-node biopsy to avoid axillary dissection in breast cancer with clinically negative lymph-nodes. *Lancet* 1997;349:1864.
353. Shons A, Joseph E, Cox CE, et al. Predictors of sentinel lymph node metastases in the lymphatic mapping of breast cancer patients. *Breast Cancer Res Treat* 1997;46:24(abst 5).
354. Galimberti V, Zurrida S, Veronesi P, Mazzaol G, Zucali P, Luini A. Can sentinel lymph node biopsy avoid axillary dissection in N0 breast cancer patients? *Breast Cancer Res Treat* 1997;46:24(abst 6).
355. Guenther JM, Krishnamoorthy M, Tan LR. Sentinel lymphadenectomy for breast cancer in a community managed care setting. *Cancer J Sci Am* 1997;3:336.
356. Borgstein PJ, Pijpers R, Cormans EF, van Diest PJ, Boom RP, Meijer S. Sentinel lymph node biopsy in breast cancer: guidelines and pitfalls of lymphoscintigraphy and gamma probe detection. *J Am Coll Surg* 1998;186:275.
357. Krag D, Weaver D, Ashikaga T, et al. The sentinel node in breast cancer. A multicenter validation study. *N Engl J Med* 1998;337:941.
358. Cox CE, Haddad F, Cox JM, et al. Lymphatic mapping in the treatment of breast cancer. *Oncology* 1998;12:1283.
359. Morton DL. Intraoperative lymphatic mapping and sentinel lymphadenectomy: community standard care or clinical investigation? *Cancer* 1997;3:341.
360. Morrow M, Bethke K, Talamonti M, et al. Learning sentinel node biopsy: results of a randomized trial comparing blue dye to blue dye plus radioactivity. *Surgery* (*in press*).
361. Cox CE, Pendas S, Cox JM, et al. Guidelines for sentinel node biopsy and lymphatic mapping of patients with breast cancer. *Ann Surg* 1998;227:645.
362. Pickren JW. Significance of occult metastases. A study of breast cancer. *Cancer* 1961;14:1266.
363. Fisher ER, Swamidoss S, Lee CH, Rockette H, Redmond C, Fisher B. Detection and significance of occult axillary node metastases in patients with invasive breast cancer. *Cancer* 1978;42:2025.
364. Rosen PP, Saigo P, Braun DW Jr, Beattie EJ Jr, Kinne DW. Occult axillary lymph node metastases from breast cancers with intramammary lymphatic tumor emboli. *Am J Surg Pathol* 1982;6:639.
365. Wilkinson EJ, Hause L, Hoffman RG, et al. Occult axillary lymph node metastases in invasive carcinoma: characteristics of the primary tumor and significance of the metastases. *Pathol Annu* 1982;17:67.
366. Saphir O, Amromin GD. Obscure axillary lymph node metastases in carcinoma of the breast. *Cancer* 1948;1:238.
367. Turner RR, Oilila DW, Krasne DL, Guiliano AE. Histopathologic validation of the sentinel node hypothesis for breast carcinoma. *Ann Surg* 1997;226:271.
368. International (Ludwig) Breast Cancer Study Group. Prognostic importance of occult axillary lymph node micrometastases from breast cancer. *Lancet* 1990;335:1565.
369. de Mascarel I, Bonichon F, Coindre JM, Trojani M. Prognostic significance of breast cancer axillary lymph node micrometastases assessed by two special techniques: reevaluation with longer follow up. *Br J Cancer* 1992;66:523.
370. Hainsworth PJ, Tjandra JJ, Stillwell RG, et al. Detection and significance of occult metastases in node-negative breast cancer. *Br J Surg* 1993;80:459.
371. McGuckin MA, Cummings MC, Walsh MD, Hohn BG, Bennett IC, Wright RG. Occult axillary lymph node metastases in breast cancer: their detection and prognostic significance. *Br J Cancer* 1996;73:88.
372. Clare S, Sener SF, Wilkens W, Goldschmidt R, Merkel D, Winchester DJ. Prognostic significance of occult lymph node metastases in node-negative breast cancer. *Ann Surg Oncol* 1997;4:447.
373. Hartveit F, Lilleng PK. Breast cancer: two micrometastatic variants in the axilla that differ in prognoses. *Histopathology* 1996;28:241.
374. Mori M, Mimori K, Inoue M, et al. Detection of cancer micrometastases in lymph nodes by reverse transcriptase-polymerase chain reaction. *Cancer Res* 1995;55:3417.
375. Schoenfeld A, Lugmani Y, Sinnett MD, Shousha S, Coobes RC. Keratin 19mRNA measurement to detect micrometastases in lymph nodes in breast cancer patients. *Br J Cancer* 1996;74:1639.
376. Lockett MA, Baron PL, O'Brien PH, et al. Detection of occult breast cancer micrometastases in axillary lymph nodes using a multimarker reverse transcriptase-polymerase chain reaction panel. *J Am Coll Surg* 1998;187:9.
377. Hansen N. Current status of sentinel node biopsy. *Semin Breast Dis* 1998;1:146.
378. Haffty BG, McKhann C, Beinfield M, Fischer D, Fischer JJ. Breast conservation therapy without axillary dissection. A rational treatment strategy in selected patients. *Arch Surg* 1993;128:1315.
379. Wazer DE, Erban JK, Robert NJ, et al. Breast conservation in elderly women for clinically negative axillary lymph nodes without axillary dissection. *Cancer* 1994;74:878.
380. Greco C, Orecchia R, Valesi G, et al. Randomized clinical trial on the role of axillary radiotherapy in breast conservative management without axillary dissection lesion <1 cm. *Int J Radiat Oncol Biol Phys* 1998;42:250(abst).
381. Lingos T, Recht A, Vicini F, et al. Radiation pneumonitis in breast cancer patients treated with conservative surgery and radiation therapy. *Int J Radiat Oncol Biol Phys* 1991;21:355.
382. Wong JS, Recht A, Beard CJ, et al. Treatment outcome after tangential radiation therapy without axillary dissection in patients with early-stage breast cancer and clinically negative axillary nodes. *Int J Radiat Oncol Biol Phys* 1997;39:915.
383. Hoskin PJ, Rajan B, Ebbs S, Tait D, Milan S, Yarnold JR. Selective avoidance of lymphatic radiotherapy in the conservative management of early breast cancer. *Radiother Oncol* 1992;25:83.
384. Cady B, Stone MD, Wayne J. New therapeutic possibilities in primary invasive breast cancer. *Ann Surg* 1993;218:338.
385. Kuznetsova M, Graybill JC, Zusag TW, Hartsell WF, Griem KL. Omission of axillary lymph node dissection in early-stage breast cancer: effect on treatment outcome. *Radiology* 1995;197:507.
386. Galper SR, Lee S, Tao ML, et al. Assessing patient preferences for axillary dissection: a formal outcomes analysis. *Int J Radiat Oncol Biol Phys* 1998;42:160(abst).

CHAPTER 34

Diseases of the Breast, 2nd ed.,
edited by Jay R. Harris.
Lippincott Williams & Wilkins, Philadelphia © 2000.

Breast Reconstruction

Neil A. Fine, Thomas A. Mustoe, and Geoffery Fenner

Breast reconstruction has undergone tremendous evolution in the last 15 years and continues to evolve from year to year.[1] Currently, advances in flap design, controversy involving implant safety, new implant designs, and changes in the management of the original breast disease are at the forefront of the issues that impact breast reconstruction. The increased use of radiation, in patients in whom breast conservation surgery has failed and postmastectomy, creates added challenges for reconstruction. Additionally, the pursuit of more aggressive breast-conserving surgeries that may require partial reconstruction or reshaping is an example of a change in breast management that is leading to a new subset in breast reconstruction.

Breast reconstruction has a relatively short history, approximately 30 years. Before the availability of myocutaneous flaps, a limited amount of reconstruction was performed with local skin flaps. This required several stages, and results fell short of reasonable symmetry. Silicone gel implants became available in the late 1960s. They were first used alone as a single-stage procedure and were severely limited by deficient tissue. Later, combined with latissimus dorsi myocutaneous flaps in delayed reconstruction, they achieved greater success. With the development of tissue expansion in the 1970s, limitation of skin became less of an issue, and tissue expansion with a second-stage replacement with a permanent implant became a popular technique that has persisted. The transverse rectus abdominis myocutaneous flap (TRAM) was first described by Hartrampf et al. in 1982[2] and rapidly became the autogenous reconstructive method of choice. In 1992, the U.S. Food and Drug Administration (FDA) placed a moratorium on the use of silicone gel implants amidst concerns about health risks and implant leakage. Several months later, the moratorium was lifted for breast cancer patients who agreed to participate in a study protocol. Since that time, saline implants have become the dominant choice for implant reconstruction. Expander/implant reconstruction continues to be the most widely used form of reconstruction.[1,3] However, improved flap techniques, increased numbers of plastic surgeons trained to perform flap reconstruction, and the more natural result obtained by using autologous tissue have led to a steady increase in flap reconstruction in recent years. Methods of nipple reconstruction have also evolved. Simplified methods for forming the nipple with local skin flaps and using tattoo pigment to color the nipple-areolar complex have decreased patient apprehension regarding this step of the reconstruction.

At some time during their reconstructive decision-making process, most women ask, "What is the best reconstruction?" There is, of course, no single "best" operation for all women. Each type of reconstruction, and indeed the decision to proceed with reconstruction at all, is a complex analysis of risk and benefit. Outcome studies are being performed to try and better match women with reconstructive options, but currently a primary goal of a plastic surgical consultation is to fully discuss the pros and cons of each reconstructive technique with the patient and ascertain how the risks and benefits affect them personally.

Immediate reconstruction has gone from a small minority of reconstructions to a majority in most practices. There is considerable evidence that immediate reconstruction is safe, does not delay adjuvant therapies, is cost-effective, and provides the greatest psychological benefit for most women. Historically, women have not undergone immediate reconstruction because of concerns that they would not be accepting of the change in their breast from normal to reconstructed, whereas they would be able to accept the change from nothing to a reconstructed breast.[4] The other main argument against immediate reconstruction was altering the ability to follow for recurrence and delaying adjuvant therapy. Both of these arguments have been refuted by several studies.[5–8] If reconstruction can be performed without delaying or interfering with postoperative adjuvant therapies and surveillance, then virtually all women are potential candidates. With the passage of laws in several states and by the U.S. federal government that require insurance companies to cover breast reconstruction if they cover mastectomy and that mandate coverage for symmetry pro-

N. A. Fine: Division of Plastic Surgery, Northwestern University Medical School, Chicago, Illinois

T. A. Mustoe: Division of Plastic Surgery, Northwestern University Medical School, Chicago, Illinois

G. Fenner: Evanston Northwestern Healthcare, Northwestern University Medical School, Chicago, Illinois

cedures on the opposite breast, discussing reconstructive options with every patient may well become a legal issue.

The development of outcome studies should greatly facilitate our effort to inform patients regarding the "best" reconstruction for their situation. However, the effort is made more difficult by the lack of a true standard for success. In most areas of breast disease, the elimination or control of the disease process or survival is an accepted standard for success. In reconstruction, success can be measured in many ways. The most prevalent in plastic surgery has been how a patient looks in a photograph without clothing.[9] There is room for debate as to whether this represents the most crucial outcome for most women. The use of outcome studies should help to focus success on patient satisfaction issues. An argument against relying too heavily on patient opinion alone is the perception that many patients are satisfied with less than optimal results because they are not aware of "better" alternatives. This is a legitimate concern when satisfaction truly represents an information deficit, but ultimately, patient satisfaction needs to become our gold standard.[10] It remains our goal to fully inform women regarding all available options and then to provide for them the type of reconstruction that best fits their individual needs.

In this chapter, we focus on the three principal methods of breast reconstruction: tissue expansion followed by implant, TRAM flap (free or pedicled), and latissimus dorsi with implant. Alternative choices are also discussed, but in a more limited manner. The issues surrounding silicone gel implants, immediate versus delayed reconstruction, the impact of radiation on choice and timing of reconstruction, and choices of nipple reconstruction are also addressed.

IMMEDIATE VERSUS DELAYED RECONSTRUCTION

In addition to the psychological and historical issues discussed previously, there are technical differences between immediate and delayed reconstruction. A major advantage of immediate reconstruction is that scar formation, with resulting stiffening and contracture, does not distort the breast shape. The skin in immediate reconstruction is more malleable and allows for the reconstruction of a ptotic breast. In delayed reconstruction with a ptotic contralateral breast, mastopexy is virtually always needed to achieve symmetry without a bra.

In the case of implants, the disadvantage of contracted skin is partially offset by the advantage of placing the expander under intact skin in delayed reconstruction. Allowing the skin to heal first eliminates the risk of a mastectomy flap breakdown exposing the expander. This all but eliminates the risk of early implant failure.

In TRAM flap reconstruction, the immediate setting offers technical, aesthetic, and economic advantages and has failed to affect adversely the oncologic outcome.[11] Patients may avoid a lengthy secondary procedure and hospitalization and forgo the emotional, psychosocial, and physical impact of the mastectomy deformity. Concurrent flap harvest during mastectomy, assisted elevation of the mastectomy skin flaps, and at least partial exposure of the recipient thoracodorsal pedicle (for free TRAMs), help expedite the procedure. Preservation of the inframammary fold and the use of skin-sparing mastectomies facilitate flap insetting and lead to a natural and symmetric reconstruction.[12] The mastectomy specimen can be used as a template and expedites accurate volume replacement. Conversely, delayed reconstruction requires elevation of contracted, fibrotic skin flaps and requires inset of a much larger skin paddle from the abdomen. This leads to a less natural result, and the larger TRAM skin paddle increases visible scarring on the reconstructed breast.

Virtually all patients are potential candidates for immediate reconstruction. The most commonly cited reason for delaying reconstruction, the known need for postoperative radiation, is a relative contraindication only. The data from patients with implants who have been radiated show that, although the complications are increased, the majority of patients are able to maintain their reconstructions.[13] Thus, it is our practice to offer high-risk patients reconstruction, including expander/implant reconstruction. One possible approach is to place an expander and allow the postoperative chemotherapy or radiation therapy, or both, to be given and then to address the issue of final reconstruction. In this case, the expander serves as a temporary prosthesis and conserves breast skin. The patient is now in a much more knowledgeable position to determine whether to continue on the expander/implant route and have the implant placed or have the expander removed and proceed with latissimus or TRAM flap reconstruction. Patients who know they have an arduous course of postoperative therapy before them may choose to delay reconstruction, but the option for reconstruction should be discussed.

EXPANDER/IMPLANT

Tissue expansion followed by removal of expander and placement of a permanent implant is the most common form of breast reconstruction in the United States.[3] The reason for its popularity is that it can provide an adequate reconstruction for most women, and it involves the least amount of initial surgery. The procedure is best suited for women with small to moderate-sized breasts and little ptosis who undergo skin-sparing mastectomies (Fig. 1). Skin-sparing surgical techniques minimize the skin deficit. This is particularly important in expander/implant reconstruction, because new skin is not brought in with tissue expansion as it is with latissimus or TRAM reconstruction. Implants do not droop or produce ptosis, a condition that is inherent in larger breasts.

The development of saline expanders and implants that are contoured and textured has improved the aesthetic result

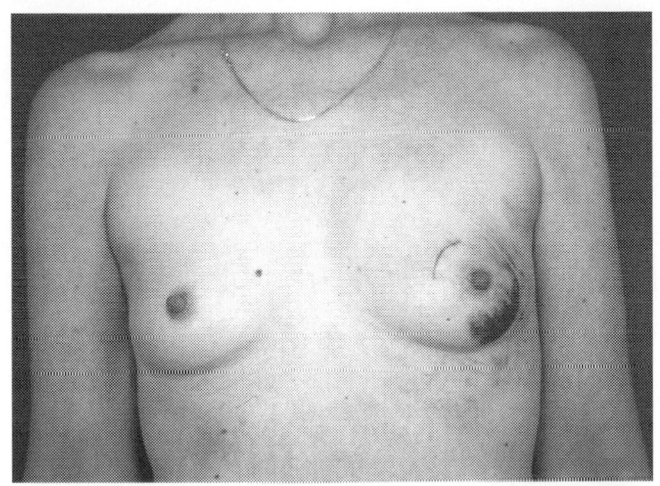

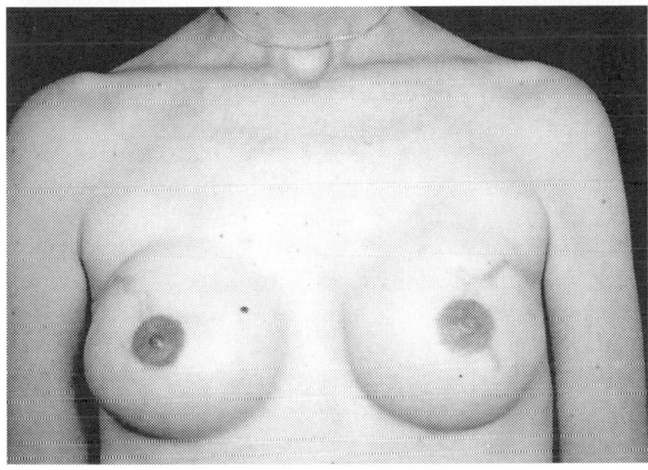

FIG. 1. **A:** Before surgery. **B:** After bilateral tissue expander and saline implant reconstruction.

that can be achieved with implant reconstruction. However, even with the contoured shape, an implant is rarely able to match the subtle curves of a natural breast. As a breast becomes larger and more ptotic, limitations of an implant become more noticeable. The implant appears round, especially in the upper pole. It also lacks normal motion, keeping it upright and forward on the chest even when the woman lies down and the opposite breast flattens and falls to the side.

Most of the visible limitations of implants can be lessened by wearing a bra or by performing surgery on the opposite breast. Surgery on the opposite breast is more frequently an issue with expander/implant reconstruction than with other types, because of the limited ability of an implant to match the appearance of an unoperated breast when the patient wears no clothing. For many, the symmetry obtained by wearing a bra is sufficient, but for others, surgery is an acceptable trade-off in achieving optimal symmetry. The opposite breast can be reduced or lifted to decrease ptosis, improve upper pole fullness, and reduce the size of the implant necessary for reconstruction. This increases symmetry but leaves a scar and requires a brief postoperative recovery, with pain and bruising in the opposite breast. Another possible procedure for the opposite breast is augmentation. This increases the fullness, particularly in the upper pole, providing a better match to the reconstructed breast. Augmentation also requires a scar, postoperative recovery, and the acceptance of another implant. The implant can make screening mammography in the opposite breast more difficult. The increased difficulty with mammography is not believed to be severe enough to limit the use of this procedure, but it needs to be discussed with all patients who undergo breast augmentation. The implant is generally placed in the submuscular position and allows for an increased size range for both breasts.

The rate of significant complications in expander/implant reconstruction should be low in nonradiated patients (i.e., less than 10%).[13] Significant complications include infection; hematoma; extrusion; symptomatic capsular contractures that require reoperation; and deflation, either spontaneous or iatrogenic. Iatrogenic deflation occurs when the expander is punctured in an area other than the resealable expansion port. Spontaneous deflation of saline implants is currently estimated at 1% per year or less.[13] Estimating the true complication rate is difficult, because techniques have changed significantly in the past 5 to 10 years. Older series include many silicone implants that were placed as a single-staged procedure, without tissue expansion.[9,14] This led to an increased complication rate and does not reflect current practice, which is dominated by two-staged tissue expansion and placement of saline implants.

This change in technique and lack of agreement on complication rates are most obvious in women who have had prior radiation or who are likely candidates for postoperative radiation. Many surgeons still believe that radiation is an absolute contraindication for implant reconstruction. However, recent reports have suggested that saline implants can be used in selected cases with a complication rate that is increased (18%) but may be acceptable to women who would strongly prefer this route for their reconstruction.[13,15,16]

The choice of saline versus silicone gel implants for breast reconstruction also requires careful consideration of information that has been highly controversial. Nearly all women have had some exposure to the silicone gel implant controversy and legal maneuvering. There is currently no credible medical evidence that silicone gel causes systemic disease. In general, silicone implants, if they do not develop a significant capsular contracture, are softer and feel more natural than saline implants. If a silicone implant develops a contracture, and the majority do if in place long enough, it is likely to become harder than a saline implant. A saline implant is firmer but holds a shape better if it is contoured and is less likely to develop a contracture and become truly hard.[17] Therefore, a silicone implant may feel softer but often winds up feeling harder. Some patients want to try for the softest implant and choose silicone; others want the more predictable results of saline and do not want to risk the increased contracture rate or the perceived medical risk associated with silicone implants. This topic is covered in more detail in the next section of this chapter.

The surgical technique of expander placement involves placing the expander in a low, medial submuscular (below pectoralis major) position. The low medial placement compensates for a lack of normal motion and the effect of scar contracture, which tends to push the implant superiorly and laterally. In the upright position, a natural breast has more fullness in the lower pole, and the breast physically drops, often placing the nipple at or below the level of the inframammary fold. An implant never drops below the inframammary fold and therefore must generally be placed as low as possible without seeming completely out of place in the upper abdomen. This generally involves lowering the inframammary fold by 2 to 3 cm. This low placement level can cause loss of the inframammary fold. If this occurs and the patient desires correction, a secondary procedure, often at the time of expander/implant exchange, can be performed using internal sutures. Alternatively, an external incision with deepithelialization of adjacent skin and suturing to the thoracic fascia can be performed to reconstruct the fold. This procedure has a higher success rate but adds an additional scar.

Expander/implant reconstruction always requires two operations and often involves three or more. If little change in position is necessary at the second operation to remove the expander and place the permanent implant, then the nipple reconstruction can be performed at the same time. If significant change in position is required, performing the nipple reconstruction at a third procedure leads to more accurate placement. Typically, only the first operation, if it is performed in conjunction with a mastectomy as an immediate reconstruction, requires a general anesthetic and an overnight hospital stay. All secondary surgeries, and even the primary expander placement if performed independently as a delayed reconstruction, can be done as an outpatient procedure, often under monitored local or straight local anesthesia.

The only absolute contraindication to expander/implant reconstruction is infection or a lack of viable skin flaps to close over the expander at the time of placement. Good skin closure is critical to a successful outcome. If the skin flaps do not appear viable, the expander should not be placed. In the postoperative period, if the flaps are found to be necrotic, the necrotic tissue should be excised and closed primarily. If it is not possible to close the skin primarily, a myocutaneous flap can be used. In this situation, a latissimus flap would be used most often.

Relative contraindications include prior history of radiation or planned postoperative radiation, obesity, and smoking. The issues involved with radiation have been covered earlier in this section, and obesity and smoking both decrease vascularity to the skin flaps. This decreased vascularity increases the likelihood of mastectomy skin flap necrosis with exposure of the expander, necessitating removal or salvage with further surgery.

BREAST IMPLANTS

Before silicone gel implants were first marketed in 1962, there were scattered cases of various sponge materials being used for breast reconstruction or breast augmentation, but they were unsatisfactory, both in shape and texture. Silicone gel implants quickly became the standard, and by 1989, an estimated 1 million had been placed in woman, with approximately 20% being used for reconstructive purposes.[18]

Saline implants were also used, but much less frequently, in part because of the viscosity of the filler, which was very different than breast tissue (unlike silicone gel, which was very similar) and also because of litigation secondary to occasional implant deflation. Deflation was believed to be a product liability issue rather than an inevitable occasional outcome of saline implant placement. The most frequent perceived undesirable result of breast implants is capsular contracture leading to an unnatural firmness and, in more severe cases, a distortion in shape of the implant. Some silicone gel implants were coated with polyurethane foam in an effort to prevent capsular contracture, but these were withdrawn from the market around 1990 because of concerns about possible carcinogenic effects of breakdown products from the polyurethane.

In 1992, the FDA reviewed the safety of silicone gel implants. Because they had been used before the 1976 legislation regulating devices, they had been "grandfathered," but several issues regarding their safety had been raised, chiefly questions about the possible associations with connective tissue disorders.[19] The FDA first placed a moratorium on their use and after a few months restricted their use to reconstructive patients, who must enter a clinical trial approved by the FDA. This situation continues. Very quickly, a storm of litigation occurred, including several large class action suits[20,21] with proposed multibillion-dollar settlements. The resulting intense media coverage in 1992 and 1993 had a major impact on patients' perceptions of the risks of silicone gel implants and implants in general.

Currently, most patients choose saline implants for reconstruction. Although the fill of the implant is saline, the shell of a saline implant is made of silicone polymer in solid form. Silicone in this form has yet to be included in legal actions. This solid form of silicone is used in a wide variety of internal devices, including chemotherapy catheters, shunts, porcine heart valves, joint replacements, and pacemaker coatings, without reported disease associations. The FDA currently has saline implants under review, but there is essentially no controversy over their use and no suspected association with disease. Since 1997, their use in breast augmentation has rebounded to the level of 1991 usage for all implants, before the FDA moratorium on silicone gel implants (American Society of Plastic and Reconstructive Surgeons annual statistics, 1998). However, their use in breast reconstruction, in which minimal overlying tissue is present, has significant limitations. In the absence of capsular contracture, the implants can show significant waviness or rippling over the superior pole of the implant, which can be quite apparent and unnatural. With even moderate capsular contracture, which is frequently seen in breast reconstruction, deformation of the implant can occur, leading to an unnatural appearance.

Silicone gel implants are a real option for patients undergoing breast reconstruction, and it is therefore worthwhile to review the potential risks and concerns regarding their use, some of which are applicable to the use of saline implants. The relative risk of breast cancer has been looked at in several studies. The two largest, each involving more than 10,000 women with breast augmentation, failed to show an increased risk of cancer[22,23] and have been confirmed by other studies.[18]

A related and important issue is the potential for breast implants to mask breast cancer and delay its diagnosis. Breast implants filled with either saline or silicone are radiopaque and obscure a significant (30% or more) portion of the breast on routine mammography. This problem is more significant in implants placed in the subglandular position and in patients with capsular contracture, even with special views. However, with both displacement and compression views, a high percentage of the breast can be seen in mammography when the implant is placed in the submuscular position. More significantly, in the large Alberta, Canada, study (more than 10,000 women with breast implants followed for 10 years), in those patients in whom breast cancer developed, the stage of breast cancer at the time of diagnosis[24] was actually earlier than that of the control group. This suggests that breast implants placed in the submuscular position can be used safely, even in the contralateral breast after mastectomy, to achieve symmetry. This is the current practice at Northwestern University Medical School in Chicago, Illinois. One factor that perhaps accounts for this observation is the relative ease of examination of a smaller breast with a smooth underlying breast implant. The issue of radiopaque implants has been the focus of investigation by implant companies, and a radiolucent soybean oil–filled implant was used in a small number of patients on an investigational basis, but it is currently not available in the United States. No other fillers are currently in clinical trials.

The most controversial area regarding silicone gel implants has been the possible association with connective tissue disorders,[19] and this has been the focus of the litigation. Although there have been many well-publicized anecdotal cases, before 1992 there was no epidemiologic evidence of a link. Since that time, two major studies have failed to show any increased risk of connective tissue disease.[25,26] A third, retrospective study of self-reported disease raised the possibility of a slight increase in connective tissue disease.[27] This would still account for only a few cases in the 1 million patients with implants.

The English equivalent of the FDA has concluded that there is no evidence of linkage of silicone breast implants with disease, as has the American Rheumatological Association. In December 1998, a four-member independent panel of court-appointed scientists concluded after a 2-year review that there was no proven link between silicone breast implants and diseases claimed by women suing implant manufacturers.[28] However, the possibility of an association with an as yet undescribed constellation of symptoms constituting a new syndrome has not been completely ruled out. Other conditions, including fibromyalgia and chronic fatigue syndrome, have also been anecdotally linked to silicone gel implants,[18,19] but the epidemiologic evidence is lacking at this time. The largest study to date regarding silicone gel implants, sponsored by the National Cancer Institute, should be published in 1999 or 2000 and offers the promise of further addressing these issues.

Silicone gel implants continue to be available on an investigational basis only for patients undergoing breast reconstruction, but the study is available to any plastic surgeon who wishes to participate. Saline implants are the predominant choice but have some additional limitations in appearance over silicone gel–filled implants. It has been recognized that implant leakage[29,30] and silicone gel bleed[31] are inevitable over time, and the local problems of inflammation and capsular contracture are still unsolved. It is possible that new filler materials will have a viscosity closer to that of breast tissue but will be absorbable, which would combine the best attributes of saline implants and silicone gel. However, none are in clinical trial in the United States.

LATISSIMUS DORSI MYOCUTANEOUS FLAP RECONSTRUCTION

The latissimus dorsi myocutaneous flap popularized by McGraw and Bostwick in the 1970s offered the ability to correct sizable skin deficiencies while using an implant. With the popularity of TRAM flaps and the use of tissue expanders, the latissimus dorsi became less commonly used, decreasing from 62% of all reconstruction from 1979 to 1983 to 12% of all reconstruction from 1988 to 1991 in one series.[32] However, multiple reports detailing high patient satisfaction and low complication rates have led to an increasing enthusiasm for the latissimus flap again.[33–37] For many patients, particularly if a significant amount of skin is removed, the latissimus provides a cosmetic result that is superior to that achieved with expansion and implant alone.[34]

Before 1990, most latissimus flaps were performed in delayed fashion, requiring the use of a large skin paddle, with tissue expansion of the back sometimes being advocated as an additional measure.[38] No additional fatty tissue was harvested with the flap, and therefore the reconstruction tended to keep the globular form of an implant rather than the teardrop shape of the natural breast. The well-known tendency of latissimus flaps to develop troubling seromas was also a drawback. Nevertheless, the flap rate loss was less than 1%, and arm weakness from the donor site was not an issue.[33–36,39]

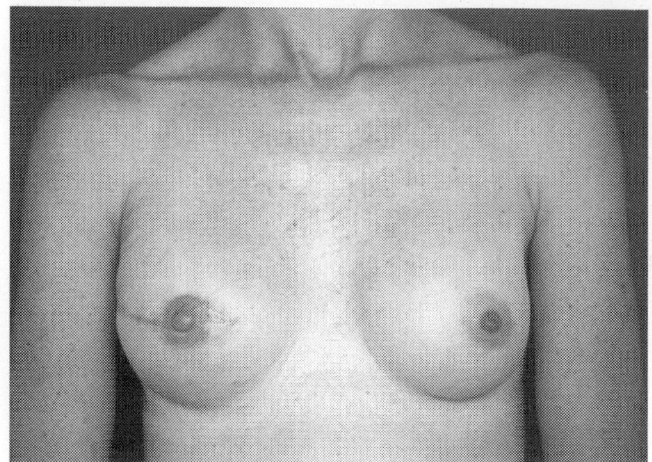
A

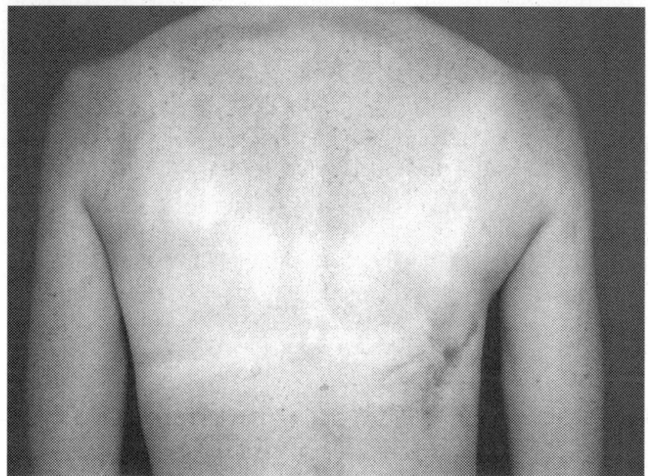
B

FIG. 2. A: Reconstruction with latissimus and implant. **B:** Scar on back after latissimus harvest.

McGraw et al.[40] recognized that if sufficient fatty tissue overlying the latissimus muscle was included in the flap and the skin paddle was made large enough, a completely autogenous tissue reconstruction was possible in selected patients. This autogenous latissimus flap must be distinguished from the more common latissimus with implant reconstruction. Although others[41] have used variations of this method, many patients do not have enough tissue, particularly to match a larger breast, and the donor site scar is much larger.

The use of a modified flap, a latissimus flap with a small skin paddle and preservation of all fatty tissue beneath Scarpa's fascia over most of the latissimus muscle, has enabled significantly smaller breast implants to be used. With this technique, the implant usually forms no more than 50% of the breast volume. When implant volumes are kept low compared to native tissue, a more natural result is obtained. Combining this technique with a skin-sparing mastectomy in immediate breast reconstruction optimizes the aesthetic result[37] (Fig. 2). In addition, by taking more fat with the muscle over the area that will form the inferior pole of the reconstructed breast, a natural teardrop shape can be achieved.

The surgical technique for the latissimus flap has evolved to improve results and decrease complications. For immediate reconstruction, a skin paddle is marked out on the back corresponding to the skin taken at the time of mastectomy. Since 1997, we have been taking an additional section of skin perpendicular to the long axis in a modified fleur-de-lis pattern,[40] which is later deepithelialized and adds volume to the inferior pole of the breast. This also allows a relatively short scar on the back and minimizes the dog-ear. The patient is prepped in the lateral position before the mastectomy and placed on a beanbag, minimizing the time to turn during the operation. Extensive dilute epinephrine solution is injected into the subcutaneous tissue. This allows an entirely sharp dissection, with easy and rapid delineation of the plane of Scarpa's fascia, and essentially eliminates blood loss. With this technique, seromas have been eliminated as a problem. We have had a 10% to 15% incidence of minor fluid reaccumulation, requiring a single-needle aspiration and occasionally two, after removing the drains. We have had no chronic seromas that required other measures. In raising the flap, the nerve is preserved, and the tendon is divided. Dividing the tendon allows greater mobility of the flap and avoids an axillary bulge; preservation of the nerve helps to retain flap volume by maintaining muscle volume. Additionally, endoscopic techniques have been described to raise the latissimus muscle. This is particularly useful when no skin paddle is needed, as a scar on the back is then avoided.[42]

After the patient is turned, the flap is positioned to drape over the entire breast, so the implant adds some additional volume and projection. However, we rely on the latissimus flap and retained breast skin to maintain a natural shape. A permanent implant is then positioned, usually under the pectoralis muscle, to optimize the natural slope of the upper part of the breast.

In delayed reconstruction, because of contraction of the mastectomy skin, there is often a relative deficiency of tissue in both a vertical and horizontal dimension, and a modified *fleur-de-lis* pattern can optimize the shape of the breast. By centering the skin paddle over the future nipple, the scar is not too obtrusive.

Increasingly, patients in whom lumpectomy and radiation have failed, and thus who have received preoperative radiation, are encountered. Capsular contracture rates have remained low in these patients, presumably because the implants are covered by nonradiated tissue. In patients who require postoperative radiation after immediate reconstruction with a latissimus flap, capsular contracture occurs more frequently, but the results are still acceptable to most patients, and it appears to be better tolerated than postoperative radiation after an implant alone.[15]

Long-term studies on latissimus dorsi reconstruction have documented high patient satisfaction, moderate capsular contracture rates, and negligible flap loss. Implant infection has been low (5% or less) and has been reduced further by careful attention to antibiotic irrigation of the wound immediately after the mastectomy and perhaps by placing the implants in a subpectoral position. If an implant does become infected, it is removed and can then be replaced 3 to 6 months later without seriously compromising the quality of the reconstruction.

TRANSVERSE RECTUS ABDOMINIS MYOCUTANEOUS FLAP

The use of autogenous tissue for breast reconstruction has increased significantly in the last decade, and the TRAM flap is the preeminent form of tissue reconstruction.[43] *TRAM* is an acronym that stands for *t*ransverse, *r*ectus *a*bdominis, *m*yocutaneous. Hartrampf[2] first described this flap for breast reconstruction in 1982. This procedure uses skin and fatty tissue from the lower abdomen to replace the skin (nipple-areola and biopsy site) and breast tissue removed by the mastectomy. The flap uses the rectus abdominis muscle as a conduit for blood flow, via perforating vessels, to the overlying subcutaneous fat and skin of the lower abdomen.[44,45] This can be done using one of two available blood supplies to the rectus muscle. The first described was the pedicled TRAM and uses the entire rectus muscle on one side with blood flow provided by the superior epigastric vessels. The second method uses the deep inferior epigastric vessels. This method is referred to as a *free TRAM* and is discussed more fully in the following section, Free Transverse Rectus Abdominis Myocutaneous Breast Reconstruction.

The TRAM flap provides replacement of tissue lost with similar tissue, enabling it to achieve a natural look and feel that are not possible with reconstructions that use implants (Fig. 3). Although the reconstructive result obtained by the TRAM flap can be remarkable, there is a cost. The procedure is complex and technically challenging and leaves a significant scar on the lower abdomen. There is also the added morbidity of a second operative field. Not all women are candidates for TRAM flap reconstruction. There are a few absolute contraindications for this procedure: An upper abdominal incision with previous division of the rectus abdominis muscle precludes a pedicle TRAM flap based on that side. If both muscles have been divided, then a pedicled TRAM cannot be done. Also, if a previous abdominoplasty has been performed, disrupting the continuity of the perforating vessels to the skin and subcutaneous tissue, a TRAM flap is not possible.

Although there are few absolute contraindications, there are many relative contraindications, and balancing and evaluating these is the main job in patient selection for this procedure. The most common factor is age or general medical health as it relates to the length and invasiveness of the procedure. Many women feel they are too old to go through such an involved procedure. Whereas virtually anyone who is medically fit enough to undergo a mastectomy can tolerate an expander placement, the same cannot be said of the extended operative time, blood loss, and stress associated with a TRAM flap procedure. The wide disparity in a willingness to tolerate risk and the ever-changing surgical environment make quantitating or placing artificial limits on this contraindication impossible. However, the importance of proper preoperative medical evaluation for this procedure should be stressed. Other relative contraindications are smoking, obesity, any previous abdominal surgery, diabetes, and hypertension. Being too thin (i.e., not having enough

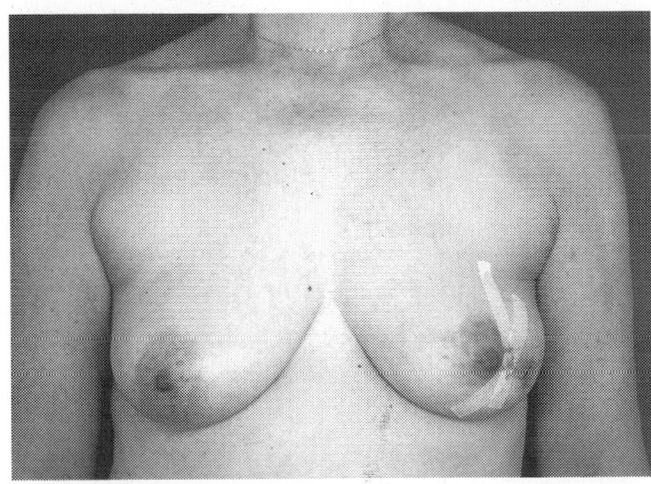
A

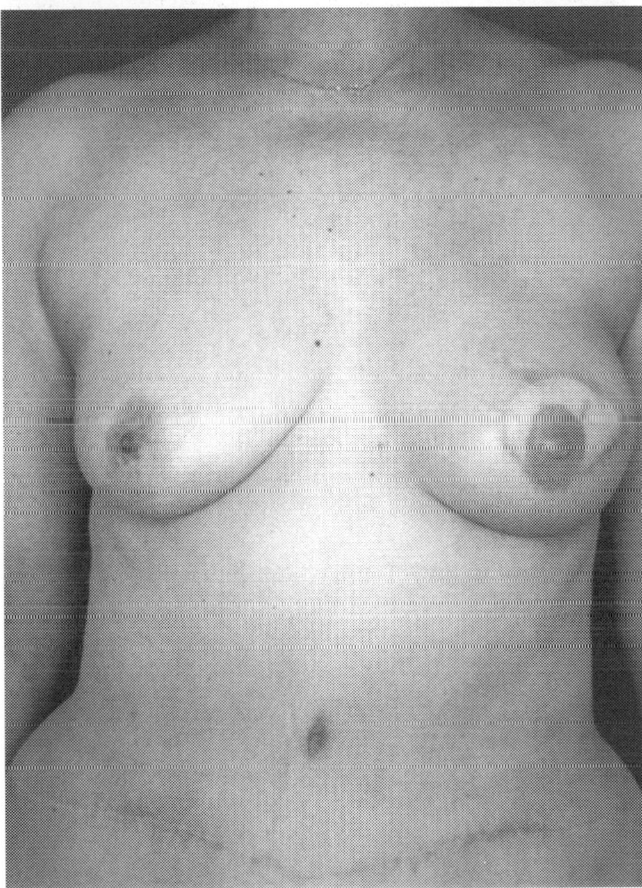
B

FIG. 3. A: Before surgery. **B:** After TRAM flap reconstruction.

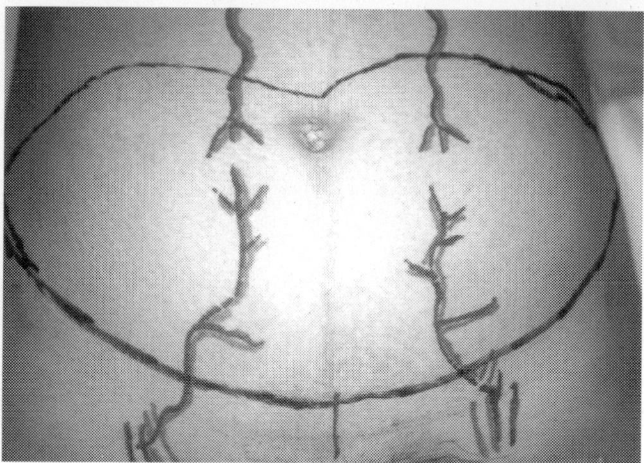

FIG. 4. TRAM flap, illustrating blood supply from the superior and inferior epigastric vessels.

available lower abdominal tissue) is also a relative contraindication. It is surprising how much tissue can be obtained in a thin person, but there are some patients who lack sufficient tissue. Previous term pregnancy nearly always allows for sufficient lower abdominal tissue for breast reconstruction.

Historically, reconstruction was offered to patients with early stage I or II disease. Several studies from 1995 to 1997 have demonstrated the efficacy of immediate autologous reconstruction for stage III patients.[46–48] Immediate TRAM reconstruction may facilitate an aggressive ablation and enable an extensive cutaneous resection without the need for skin grafting. The studies demonstrate no delays in initiation of adjuvant treatment and no tendencies or difficulties toward detecting the presence of local recurrences.

In the future, a greater number of premenopausal patients may be candidates for adjuvant radiation. Radiation fibrosis can affect the ultimate aesthetic result in breast reconstruction and serves as a relative contraindication for preradiation or immediate implant reconstruction. Conversely, autologous flaps can be performed either before or after radiation and provide functional, highly aesthetic results. Compared to nonirradiated TRAM flaps, conventional TRAM flaps that receive either pre- or postreconstruction radiation demonstrated greater, but nonsignificant, percentages of fat necrosis and fibrosis.[12] Immediate free versus conventional TRAM patients who received adjuvant radiotherapy demonstrated less fat necrosis (6% versus 33%) and volume loss, and high patient satisfaction was attained among both groups.[49] Our preference is to perform immediate free TRAM reconstruction, providing 15% to 20% greater volume and ptosis, in anticipation of subsequent volume contraction and radiation fibrosis.

The procedure can be initiated concurrently with the mastectomy to reduce total operative time. The patient can be marked preoperatively or intraoperatively with a tapering transverse ellipse with superior extensions above the umbilicus to capture important superior perforating vessels (Fig. 4). Before incision, the area of dissection surrounding the flap, but not the flap itself, is infiltrated with a dilute solution of epinephrine (1/1,000,000). This significantly decreases blood loss and speeds dissection. The upper abdominal wall is elevated off the rectus fascia, as is the flap to the point where the medial and lateral perforators are seen. At this point, techniques vary; some leave the medial portion of the muscle, some leave the lateral portion of the muscle, and some try to leave a strip of muscle medially and laterally. We believe there is no evidence that leaving a muscle that is denervated increases abdominal wall strength, and there is good evidence that the muscle is denervated by removing the central portion.[50] The denervation occurs because the intercostal motor nerves to the rectus muscle enter the central portion of the muscle on a deep surface and then spread medially and laterally to innovate the entire muscle.[51] Therefore, we believe that it is safer to raise the entire muscle and take both the medial and lateral row of perforators. The deep inferior epigastric vessels are dissected to their origin from the external iliac vessels, ligated, and transferred with the flap. This allows for a microvascular connection to the inferior epigastric vessels in the event that the superior epigastric blood supply proves inadequate.[52] With proper patient selection, this should happen in fewer than 5% of cases.

After the flap is elevated, including the deep inferior epigastric vessels, the flap is passed through a subcutaneous tunnel to the mastectomy defect. The flap is then trimmed and shaped to match the opposite breast. In the case of bilateral reconstructions, we prefer to use the free TRAM technique to preserve muscle. The contralateral muscle is used most often, because the angle of the pedicle requires less twisting when more than 50% of the lower abdominal tissue is to be used. If only 50% of the lower abdominal tissue is to be used, we prefer an ipsilaterally based flap, as this facilitates an inset requiring this volume of tissue.

The abdominal wall fascia is closed meticulously, taking care to include both the internal and external oblique fascia contributions to the anterior rectus fascia. The closure is reinforced with fascial staples. Prolene mesh is used if there is any question concerning the integrity of the fascial closure. Although true hernias are rare, some abdominal wall bulging can be seen in the lower abdomen where the muscle was removed, especially if the relatively loose lower abdominal fascia is not tightened during the abdominal closure.[53]

A bipedicled TRAM flap uses both rectus muscles, providing increased blood flow, but also sacrificing the function of both rectus muscles. Bipedicle TRAM flap reconstruction can be used to either more reliably move more than 60% of lower abdominal tissue in the reconstruction in one breast or to reduce potential healing problems in patients who are at increased risk, primarily smokers and obese patients. The bipedicled TRAM is therefore a nonmicrosurgical alternative to the free TRAM flap for patients who require extra tissue or are at increased risk for a unipedicled TRAM. As a practical matter, this issue is most often decided by the ability of the reconstructive surgeon to perform microsurgery. Those who offer their patients microsurgery generally perform free TRAM flap reconstructions for these patients, and those who do not offer these patients bipedicled TRAM flap surgery. The problem with the bipedicled TRAM is that both rectus muscles are used, and a large number of patients are never able to sit up using abdominal wall strength alone. The proponents of the procedure report that many patients are eventually able to sit up and that those who cannot easily adapt to this loss of abdominal wall strength and are not adversely affected in the majority of day-to-day activities.[54,55]

FREE TRANSVERSE RECTUS ABDOMINIS MYOCUTANEOUS BREAST RECONSTRUCTION

The conventional TRAM flap has revolutionized autologous tissue breast reconstruction. Its primary limitations are due to its secondary blood supply, extensive dissection, and increased morbidity in smokers, the obese, and other high-risk patients. Modifications of the conventional TRAM flap have been developed to try to minimize these limitations.[56] These modifications include "supercharging," performing a microvascular anastomosis to the deep inferior epigastric pedicle in addition to the superior pedicle, the midabdominal harvest, staged delay, and the bipedicle technique. All of these were developed in an attempt to augment vascular reliability and decrease morbidity. The free TRAM flap represents the most advanced modification and offers the advantages of a reliable primary or dominant blood supply, limits the necessary dissection, and provides a more expeditious recovery.

The superior epigastric pedicle, which sustains the conventional TRAM, supplies musculocutaneous perforators only after reconstitution through choke vessels and muscular inscriptions. The superior pedicle represents a secondary blood supply to the lower abdominal tissue. The ipsilateral rectus muscle must be sacrificed during flap elevation and, along with the flap, tunneled subcutaneously into the breast defect. Typically, 40% of the distal flap must be discarded due to insufficient vascularity. Although data confirm objective return of abdominal function at 1 year, during the first 6 weeks patients with pedicled TRAMs show decreased strength when compared to free TRAM patients.[50]

The free TRAM is based on the deep inferior epigastric vessels, the primary blood supply to the lower abdomen[57] (Fig. 5). Using the primary blood supply effectively eliminates the majority of the limitations of the pedicled TRAM. This ensures minimal to no fat necrosis, or partial flap losses, and provides up to 100% of flap volume for reconstruction of women with large or ptotic breasts, or both. This is particularly important in high-risk patients, such as smokers and obese individuals. The use of a free flap does increase the possibility of total flap loss as a result of complications with the microvascular connection. This possibility should be low, 3% or less, and clearly decreases as more experience is gained with the procedure. Schusterman et al.[58] report, in a consecutive series of 211 flaps in 163 patients undergoing free TRAM flap reconstruction, a total flap loss of 1%. Partial flap loss or fat necrosis is harder to quantitate, because the diagnosis is subjective and no standard exists as to how much firmness needs to be present to qualify as fat necrosis. However, even patients at increased risk for fat necrosis who are undergoing free TRAM procedures appear to have less fat necrosis than pedicled TRAM patients. A 1998 study included mammographic evidence of fat necrosis and found 2% of free TRAMs with fat necrosis compared to 13% of pedicled TRAMs.[19]

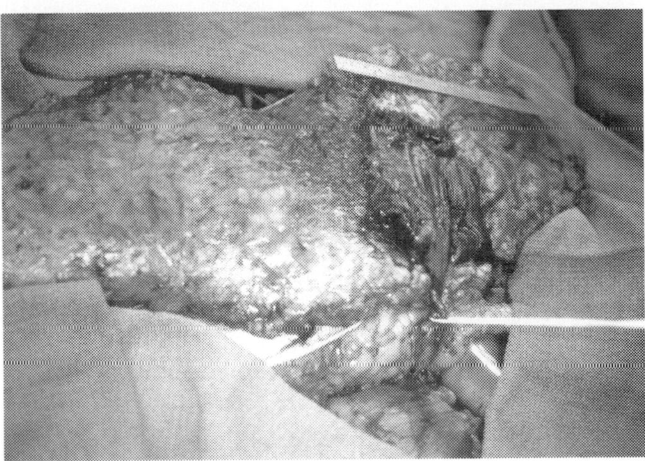

FIG. 5. Free TRAM flap elevated, showing inferior epigastric vessels and the limited removal of rectus muscle.

Recipient vessels for microanastomosis include the thoracodorsal, subscapular, and circumflex scapular as primary choices, and the internal mammary, thoracoacromial, and lateral thoracic pedicles as secondary options. The microanastomosis can be individually sewn, typically with 9.0 suture (Fig. 6) or approximated with the use of a mechanical coupling device. Once perfusion is established, the flap is inset and sculpted to approximate the contralateral breast. The

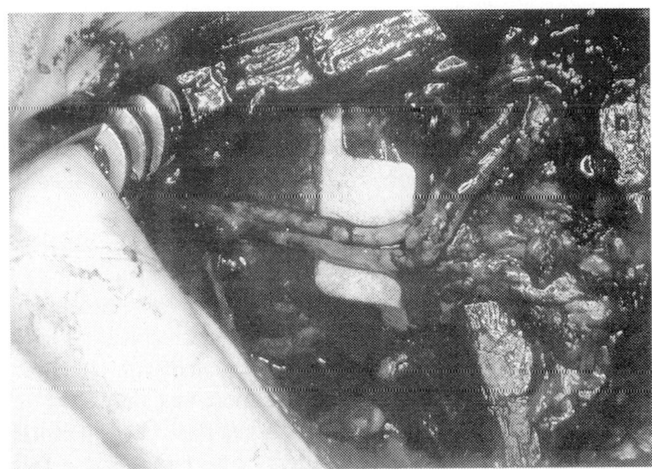

FIG. 6. Sutured microanastomosis of inferior epigastric vessels to thoracodorsal vessels.

lengthy pedicle enables great freedom in positioning of the free TRAM flap, optimizing a symmetric outcome.

Although objective studies do not support the superiority of free TRAM flap reconstruction over pedicled TRAM flaps,[59,60] there are significant advantages for selected patients. The primary indications are in smokers, moderately obese patients, and patients who require more than 60% of their lower abdominal tissue for symmetric reconstruction. We also favor the free TRAM for bilateral reconstruction.[61] Offsetting these advantages is an increased risk of total flap loss, increased operative time, and an increased need for blood transfusion. These negatives are reduced as surgeons gain increased experience with the technique, leading some surgeons to prefer free TRAMs in nearly all patients.

Bilateral Free Transverse Rectus Abdominis Myocutaneous Flap

Contralateral or prophylactic mastectomy may be recommended for women at high risk for breast cancer as an alternative to close surveillance. Public awareness and education, genetic testing, and refinements in reliable natural breast reconstruction have prompted both physician recommendations and patient requests for prophylactic mastectomy. Relative indications for prophylactic mastectomy include a strong family history of premenopausal breast cancer, positive genetic testing, a prior history of breast cancer and mantle irradiation, lobular carcinoma *in situ*, and the presence of risk factors and significant anxiety.

In addition, a growing percentage of women who have undergone early bilateral implant reconstructions are presenting with capsule contractures, migration, asymmetry, rupture, general discontent, or any combination of these, due to the need for repeated secondary procedures. As a result, more patients are presenting for bilateral autologous reconstruction.

The ability to attain an aesthetically pleasing, symmetric result in bilateral reconstructions is facilitated by symmetric simultaneous mastectomies and the harvest and insetting of similar flaps. Timely recognition of high-risk patients and candidacy for prophylactic mastectomy with bilateral immediate reconstruction benefit the patient and produce the ultimate aesthetic result. A patient who undergoes sequential mastectomies cannot use a TRAM flap for the second reconstruction and therefore will lack symmetry in form and scarring, compared to that obtained with a simultaneous bilateral TRAM or latissimus reconstruction.

Bilateral TRAM breast reconstruction requires sufficient lower abdominal tissue. The patient should be expected to tolerate 6 to 8 hours of general anesthesia and a more prolonged recovery. Although bilateral pedicled TRAM reconstruction is faster and technically simpler, it is associated with increased abdominal weakness. Kroll et al.[62] report that only 26% of patients undergoing bilateral conventional flaps could perform sit-ups, compared to 75% of patients who had bilateral free TRAM flaps. Significant abdominal weakness also increases the potential for long-term lower back complications, a leading cause of lost work hours in the United States. For pedicled TRAMs, tunneling both flaps into their respective breast defects necessitates extensive dissection with disruption of the inframammary fold and potential devascularization of the abdominal skin flap and the mastectomy flaps.

The advantages of bilateral free TRAM flap reconstruction benefit both the patient who wishes to retain an active physical status and the high-risk patient with limited reserve. The flaps can be harvested concomitantly with mastectomy to facilitate the procedure. The flap is centrally divided, and both deep inferior epigastric pedicles are exposed. Beveling the superior edge of the flap may attain inclusion of midabdominal, periumbilical soft tissue. Extending the dissection laterally may also attain greater volume. The direct, robust blood supply decreases fat necrosis and allows more aggressive contouring to maximize projection. The vascularity of the upper abdominal skin flap and inferior/medial mastectomy flap is preserved, because extensive tunneling is not required. Maintaining optimal hydration, temperature, and blood pressure, intra- and perioperatively, is critical to an optimal recovery and the avoidance of thrombotic complications.

Bilateral free TRAM reconstruction represents a highly reliable, natural, and aesthetic reconstructive option with the added bonus of a concomitant cosmetic abdominoplasty. The long-term benefits include permanence, acceptable abdominal morbidity for most patients, and little need for secondary surgery. The final result is a highly aesthetic, symmetric outcome with high patient satisfaction.

ALTERNATIVE FLAPS

TRAM flaps are sometimes not available or suitable for patients who need or desire autologous tissue breast reconstruction. Prior surgical incisions, colostomies, previous abdominoplasty, or suction lipectomy may prohibit use of the lower abdomen. Patients may lack the necessary abdominal bulk to reconstruct a large or ptotic breast or may have insufficient tissue for bilateral reconstruction. Alternative flaps are available and are chosen based on the patient's physique, activity status, and understanding of donor morbidity.

The tensor of fascia lata myocutaneous flap encompasses the lateral saddlebag or the upper lateral region of the thigh. This abundant flap may be oriented vertically, obliquely, or horizontally (designated *lateral transverse thigh flap*) along the longitudinal axis and is based on the lateral femoral circumflex artery. Sacrifice of the small tensor muscle does not lead to functional deficits. The pedicle is sufficient (6 to 7 cm), and the arterial caliber averages 1.5 to 2.0 mm. Accurate flap design and conservative resection are critical to avoid lateral contour depressions, "hourglass" deformities, or both, which are difficult to correct. The lateral thigh scars are conspicuous and are the primary objection to this flap. Postoperative morbidity may include prolonged seroma formation. It represents an excellent choice for those who desire bilateral immediate reconstruction, as long as they understand and accept the contour deformity. Flap harvest can be performed concurrently with mastectomy, requires no repositioning, and leads to symmetric donor sites. Achieving an acceptable donor site in a unilateral reconstruction is very difficult.

The Rubens or periiliac flap is a modification of the iliac osteocutaneous flap, without bone, and it includes soft tissue above the posterior ileum, or "love handle" region.[63] This substantial flap is based on the deep circumflex iliac artery. A small cuff of external and internal oblique muscle, as well as transversalis muscle and iliac periosteum, must accompany the flap to ensure the integrity of the blood supply. Reconstruction of this donor wound requires fixation to the iliac crest and may elicit prolonged discomfort and seroma formation. It represents an acceptable choice for lighter patients with an insufficient or unsuitable abdomen. It also represents an option for patients who have had a prior abdominoplasty or TRAM flap. The donor incision is merely an extension of the prior abdominoplasty or TRAM incision.

The superior gluteal myocutaneous flap is technically the most challenging for free flap breast reconstruction and is often relegated to a staged procedure for bilateral reconstructions.[64] Dissection deep within the perisacral region, directly beneath the gluteus maximus, demonstrates the superior gluteal artery, which measures only 1.5 to 2.0 cm in length. This necessitates microanastomosis to a more regional recipient pedicle, such as the internal mammary artery and vein. The gluteal flap is always available, even in the thinnest patients, and provides substantial soft tissue with excellent projection. Two variants, the inferior gluteal flap, based on the inferior gluteal vessels, and the gluteal perforator flap, provide an increase in pedicle length. The inferior gluteal vessels are slightly longer, but the donor site, over the ischial region, is more problematic. The perforator flap extends the pedicle length by dissecting through the muscle and taking only the main perforating blood vessels and no muscle. This extends the pedicle length by the thickness of the muscle, but it prolongs an already lengthy procedure by several hours.

These alternatives provide patients with a spectrum of autologous options. The ultimate reconstructive choice is dependent on each patient's desires and expectations and the expertise of the reconstructive surgeon.

NIPPLE-AREOLAR RECONSTRUCTION

The nipple-areolar complex represents the focal point of breast form and symmetry. The ease of nipple reconstruction belies the magnitude of its visual impact. Nipple reconstruction optimizes the realism of the reconstructed breast. Before the nipple reconstruction, there is a reconstructed breast mound with no visual focal point other than the scars. After nipple reconstruction, there is a "breast," and the scars become less noticeable as the nipple becomes the primary visual focal point. The nipple is typically reconstructed as a second stage, often in conjunction with a mound revision or contralateral symmetry procedure (e.g., reduction, mastopexy, or augmentation). Final nipple position is most accurate if time has been allotted for resolution of postreconstructive edema and induration. It is typical to perform this procedure after the completion of chemotherapy or after the passage of 2 to 3 months, whichever comes first. Symmetric position, height, width, and pigmentation are the ultimate goals in nipple-areolar reconstruction.

The incorporation of skillful areolar tattooing into the reconstructive armamentarium has diminished the need for skin grafting, reducing donor morbidity and patient anxiety. Because of decreased sensation, tattooing can usually be performed with little to no local anesthesia. When necessary, full-thickness skin grafts can be harvested from the groin and concealed within the bikini line. They can also be obtained from excess skin at the lateral portion of a TRAM flap abdominal incision. Grafts are rarely taken from the medial thigh region, because of donor discomfort. Contralateral areola or grafts from the labia have been used in the past but are not used in current practice.

Multiple techniques are available for reconstruction of small to moderate-sized nipple complexes without the need for adjacent skin grafts. Scar contracture, leading to late loss of nipple projection, must be anticipated if a symmetric result is to be attained. The surgeon typically strives for an immediate postoperative projection twice the height of the contralateral nipple. Additionally, in contrast to flap reconstructions, which provide an abundance of local available tissue, nipple reconstructions performed after prosthetic reconstruction may be constrained by thin, expanded mastectomy skin flaps. The skin after expansion is already under tension and lacks projection. Using local tissue for nipple reconstruction may adversely affect shape and projection, but the overall effect is still positive.

Optimal positioning of the anticipated nipple complex is assisted by the use of an adhesive template designed against the contralateral areola. The position is then confirmed with comparative measurements from the sternal notch, midclavicular line, midline, and inframammary fold. Once confirmed, the disc is outlined and serves as a basis for central nipple reconstruction.

The skate flap is used for patients who require substantial nipple height and width and, historically, necessitates skin grafting of the adjacent deepithelialized donor site.[65] A horizontal tangent with a length equal to three times the nipple diameter is drawn at the 12 o'clock or 6 o'clock position of the central nipple complex. The vertical height, measuring two times the contralateral nipple height, is represented by a line extending from the midpoint of this line. The apices are then connected. The bilateral wings are elevated in a deep partial-thickness plane. Centrally, a full-thickness flap, incorporating fat, is elevated while preserving the vertical cutaneous perforators. The wings are then approximated, providing a conical nipple construction, and the donor site is skin grafted.

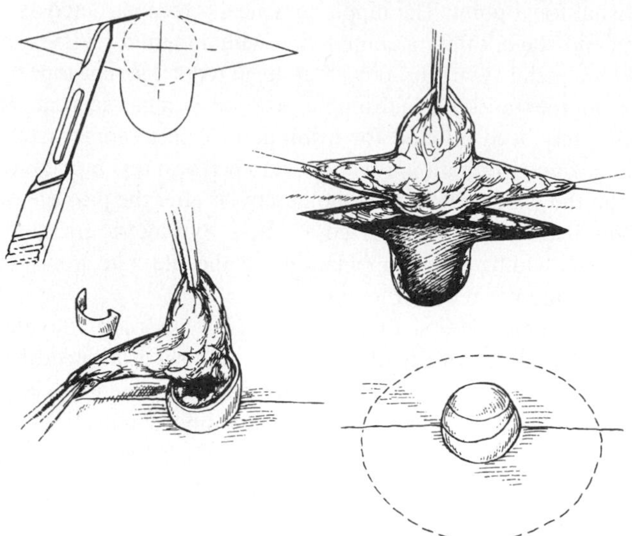

FIG. 7. Nipple reconstruction with three triangular flaps and primary donor site closure. Nipple and surrounding area are tattooed to produce nipple-areolar complex.

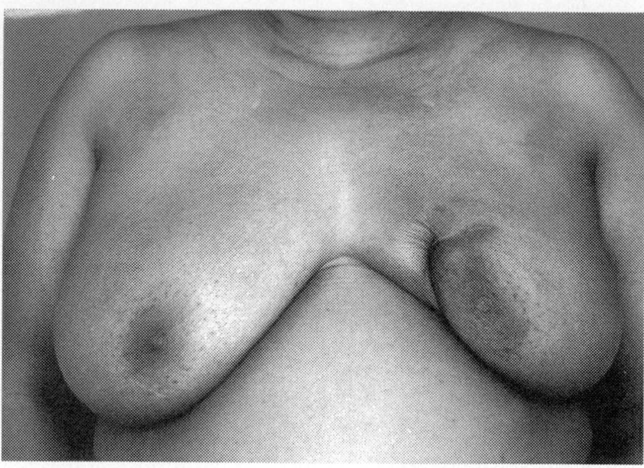

A

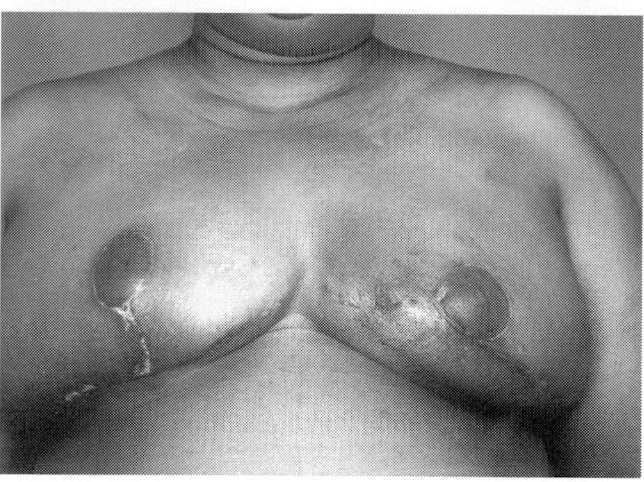

B

FIG. 8. A: Patient with a significant deformity after lumpectomy. **B:** After reduction mammoplasty on the right and a modified "reduction" technique to change the shape of the left breast.

The fishtail, or Star, technique was developed as a modification of the skate flap to ensure primary donor site closure, eliminating the need for a skin graft.[66] This flap can provide moderate nipple projection and is simple to perform. Bilateral triangular flaps, extending to the areolar circumference, are raised in a subdermal plane. These flaps are approximated in a cylindrical manner and topped with a full-thickness "cap" extension, which is incorporated into the center of the design (Fig. 7).

Areolar tattooing provides a realistic, convenient, and expeditious reconstruction that lacks the donor morbidity of skin grafting. It represents an artistic challenge for the reconstructive surgeon and is a final chance to optimize symmetry. It is typically performed 4 to 8 weeks after nipple reconstruction. Templates, again based on the contralateral areolar complex, assist positioning and symmetric realism. Pigments are chosen to match the color of the existing areola, erring to the darker side because substantial lightening will occur with time. Red pigments are added for nipple tattooing to simulate a vascular blush. Subsequent "touch-ups" are common and easily performed.

RECONSTRUCTION OF PARTIAL MASTECTOMY DEFECTS

Patients who undergo partial mastectomy defects are best divided into two groups. One group is comprised of women who are reconstructed with a shifting of remaining breast tissue, generally using a type of breast reduction pattern. The second group is made up of women who require additional tissue, usually a latissimus flap. The flap is used to replace both soft tissue and skin if necessary, thereby correcting or partially correcting the defect.[67–69]

The subject of reconstruction of partial mastectomy defects has received more attention in Europe and Japan than in the United States. This situation will undoubtedly change as information about these techniques becomes more widely known by both patients and general surgeons. The real issue involved is deciding when a lumpectomy defect is sufficiently deforming to warrant corrective surgery. The answer to this is most influenced by three factors: (a) the size of the lumpectomy relative to the size of the breast, (b) the perception and expectation of the patient, and (c) the knowledge that there are alternatives, other than a mastectomy with reconstruction, available to improve the defect that results from breast conservation surgery. It is our goal that the third factor, a lack of knowl-

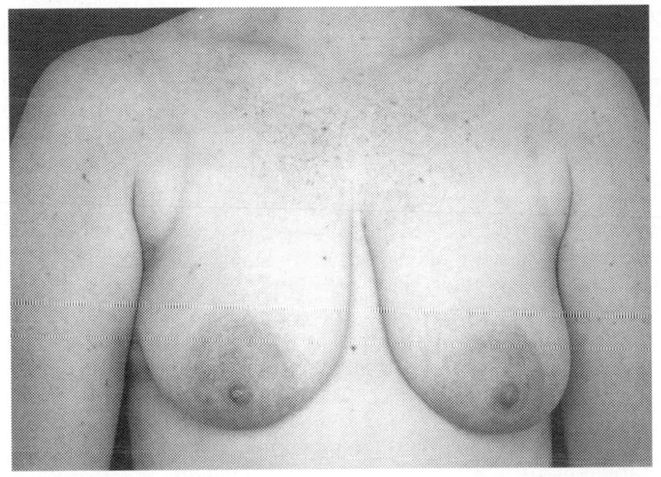

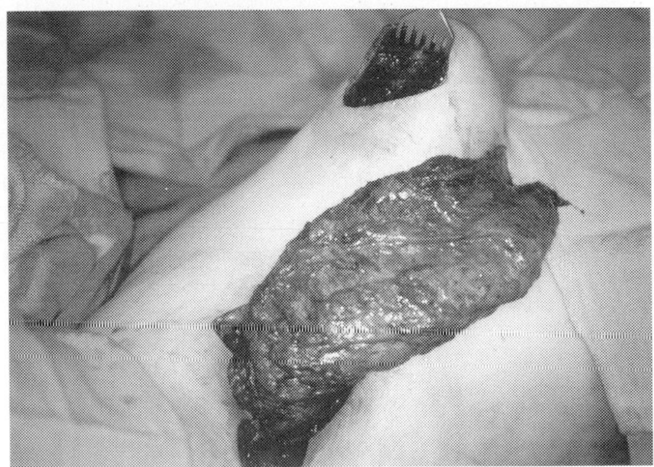

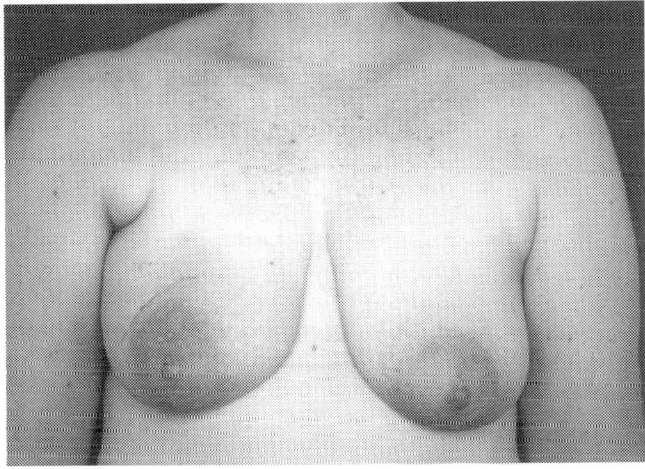

FIG. 9. A: Patient before large central lumpectomy of the right breast. **B:** Latissimus muscle with overlying fat, harvested through the axillary incision, and before placing it in the defect. **C:** Postoperative result of endoscopic latissimus reconstruction of a large central mastectomy defect.

edge that procedures exist to reconstruct partial defects, not be the reason that women do not undergo correction of these defects.

These reconstruction procedures can be performed at the time of lumpectomy or in a delayed manner, after the lumpectomy and radiation therapy. Breast reduction techniques can be altered or modified to accommodate defects in all quadrants (Fig. 8). Latissimus muscle transfer can also be used in all quadrants but is most easily used to reconstruct lateral defects. The latissimus can be used without skin to provide volume or with skin to replace volume and skin deficiency. If the muscle is used without skin, to provide volume replacement, it can be harvested from the axillary dissection access incision using endoscopic techniques (Fig. 9). This procedure, endoscopic harvest of the latissimus muscle, leaves no scar on the back.[42] The ability to improve the contour or shape of the breast without adding any additional scars or visible deformities is appealing to many patients and will become increasingly common as surgeons and patients become more acquainted with this procedure.

SUMMARY

Breast reconstruction is as much an art as it is a science. Determining the optimal type of breast reconstruction for each patient cannot be reduced to an algorithm. It requires careful consideration of the patient's objectives and willingness to take risks or undergo prolonged surgery to maximize the "naturalness" of the result. The experience and training of the reconstructive surgeon are also important factors and may limit or alter the risk-benefit profile of the procedures used in breast reconstruction. The information contained in the comparison of procedures table highlights the most important issues that need to be discussed with each patient (Table 1).

TABLE 1. *Procedure comparison*

	Expander/implant	Latissimus	TRAM
Initial surgery	Minimal	Moderate	Most involved
Secondary surgery in addition to the nipple	Always	Sometimes	Uncommon
Hospitalization	Minimal	Moderate	Longest stay: currently 3–4 days after surgery
Scars	No additional	On back	On lower abdomen
Shape and feel	No ptosis, firm, little motion, no change with weight fluctuation	Moderate to natural ptosis, less firm, more motion, little change with weight fluctuation	Natural ptosis, soft, normal motion, symmetric change with weight fluctuation
Opposite breast	Surgery often required to achieve optimal symmetry	Surgery for symmetry more optional	Surgery for symmetry almost always optional
Impact of radiation	Significant	Moderate	Least impact
Bilateral mastectomy	Advantages magnified, disadvantages minimized	Advantages unchanged, disadvantages somewhat magnifed	Advantages unchanged, disadvantages magnified
Secondary gain	Flexibility with breast size in bilateral cases	None	Flat abdomen similar to an abdominoplasty

TRAM, transverse rectus abdominis flap.

REFERENCES

1. Corral CJ, Mustoe TA. Controversy in breast reconstruction. *Surg Clin North Am* 1996;76:309.
2. Hartrampf CR Jr, Scheflan M, Black PW. Breast reconstruction with a transverse abdominal island flap. *Plast Reconstr Surg* 1982;69:216.
3. ASPRS-Statistics. Arlington Heights, IL: National Clearing House of Plastic Surgery Statistics, 1998.
4. Goldsmith HS, Alday ES. Role of the surgeon and the rehabilitation of the breast cancer patient. *Cancer* 1971;28:1672.
5. Wellisch DK, Schain WS, Noone RB, et al. Psychosocial correlates of immediate vs. delayed reconstruction of the breast. *Plast Reconstr Surg* 1985;76:713.
6. Strax P. Imaging: follow-up of breast cancer reconstruction cases. *Cancer* 1991;68[Suppl]:1157.
7. Wood WC. Nonimaging aspects of follow-up in breast cancer reconstruction. *Cancer* 1991;68[Suppl]:1164.
8. Slavin SA, Love SM, Goldwyn RM. Recurrent breast cancer following immediate reconstruction with myocutaneous flaps. *Plast Reconstr Surg* 1994;93:1191.
9. Kroll SS, Baldwin BA. Comparison of outcomes using three different methods of breast reconstruction. *Plast Reconstr Surg* 1992;90:455.
10. Brown HG. Patient issues in breast reconstruction. *Cancer* 1991; 68:1167.
11. Miller MJ. Immediate breast reconstruction clinics in plastic surgery. *Breast Reconstruction with Autologous Tissue* 1998;25:2.
12. Hidalgo DA. Aesthetic refinement in breast reconstruction: complete skin-sparing mastectomy with autogenous tissue transfer. *Plast Reconstr Surg* 1998;102:63.
13. Spear SL, Majidian A. Immediate breast reconstruction in two stages using textured, integrated-valve tissue expanders and breast implants: a retrospective review of 171 consecutive breast reconstructions from 1989 to 1996. *Plast Reconstr Surg* 1998;101:53.
14. Noone RB, Murphy JB, Spear SL, Little JW. A six year experience with immediate reconstruction after mastectomy for cancer. *Plast Reconstr Surg* 1985;76:258.
15. Evans GR, Schusterman MA, Kroll SS, et al. Reconstruction and the radiated breast: is there a role for implants? *Plast Reconstr Surg* 1995;96:1111.
16. Spear SS, Maxwell GP. Discussion of: reconstruction and the radiated breast: is there a role for implants? *Plast Reconstr Surg* 1995;96:1116.
17. Spear SL, Baker JL. Classification of capsular contracture after prosthetic breast reconstruction. *Plast Reconstr Surg* 1995;96:1119.
18. Brinton LA, Brown SL. Review: breast implants and cancer. *J Natl Cancer Inst* 1997;89:1341.
19. Silverman BG, Brown SL, Bright RA, et al. Reported complications of silicone gel breast implants: an epidemiologic review. *Ann Intern Med* 1996;124:744.
20. Nocera J. Fatal litigation. *Fortune* 1995;Oct 16:60.
21. Angell M. *Science on trial. The clash of medical evidence and the law in the breast implant case*. New York: WW Norton, 1996.
22. Deapen DM, Bernstelin L, Brody GS. Are breast implants anticarcinogenic? A 14-year follow-up of the Los Angeles Study. *Plast Reconstr Surg* 1997;99:1346.
23. Berkel H, Birdsell DC, Jenkins H, Berkel H. Breast augmentation: a risk factor for breast cancer. *N Engl J Med* 1992;326:1649.
24. Birdsell DC, Jenkins H, Berkel H. Breast cancer diagnosis and survival in women with and without breast implants. *Plast Reconstr Surg* 1993;92:795.
25. Gabriel SE, O'Fallon WM, Kurland LT, Beard CM, Woods JE, Melton LJ III. Risk of connective-tissue disease and other disorders after breast implantation. *N Engl J Med* 1994;330:1697.
26. Sanchez-Guerrero J, Coldiztz GA, Karlson EW, Hunter DJ, Speizer FE, Liang MH. Silicone breast implants and the risk of connective-tissue diseases and symptoms. *N Engl J Med* 1995;332:1666.
27. Hennekens CH, Lee IM, Cook NR, et al. Self-reported breast implants and connective-tissue diseases in female health professionals. A retrospective cohort study. *JAMA* 1996;275:616.
28. Silicone breast implants in relation to connective tissue diseases and immunologic dysfunction. A report by an independent National Science Panel appointed by Federal District Judge Sam C. Pointer. Document number 60. Available at http://www.fjc.gov/BRE-IMLIT/mdl9626.htm.
29. De Camara DL, Sheridan JM, Kammer BA. Rupture and aging of silicone gel breast implants. *Plast Reconstr Surg* 1993;91:828.
30. Robinson OG Jr, Bradley EL, Wilson DS. Analysis of explanted silicone implants: a report of 300 patients. *Ann Plast Surg* 1995;34:1.
31. Peters W, Smith D, Lugowksi S, McHugh A, Keresteci A, Baines C. Analysis of silicon levels in capsules of gel and saline breast implants and of penile prostheses. *Ann Plast Surg* 1995;34:575.
32. Trabulsky PP, Anthony JP, Mathes SJ. Changing trends in postmastectomy breast reconstruction: a 13-year experience. *Plast Reconstr Surg* 1994;93:1418.
33. Tschopp H. Evaluation of long-term results in breast reconstruction using the latissimus dorsi flap. *Ann Plast Surg* 1991;26:328.
34. Modena S, Benassuti C, Marchiori L, et al. Mastectomy and immediate breast reconstruction: oncological considerations and evaluation of two different methods relating to 88 cases. *Eur J Surg Oncol* 1995;21:36.

35. Peltoniemi H, Asko-Seljavvaara S, Harma M, Sundell B. Latissimus dorsi breast reconstruction. *Scand J Plast Reconstr Surg Hand Surg* 1993;27:127.
36. Moore T, Farrell L. Latissimus dorsi myocutaneous flap for breast reconstruction: long-term results. *Plast Reconstr Surg* 1992;89:666.
37. Slavin SA, Schnitt SJ, Duda RB, et al. Skin-sparing mastectomy and immediate reconstruction: oncologic risks and aesthetic results in patients with early-stage breast cancer. *Plast Reconstr Surg* 1988;102:49.
38. Slavin SA. Improving the latissimus dorsi myocutaneous flap with tissue expansion. *Plast Reconstr Surg* 1994;93:811.
39. McCraw JB, Maxwell GP. Early and late capsular "deformation" as a cause of unsatisfactory results in the latissimus dorsi breast reconstruction. *Clin Plast Surg* 1988;15:717.
40. McCraw JB, Papp C, Edwards A, McMellin A. The autogenous latissimus breast reconstruction. *Clin Plast Surg* 1994;21:279.
41. Barnett GR, Gianoutsos MP. The latissimus dorsi added flap for natural tissue breast reconstruction: report of 15 cases. *Plast Reconstr Surg* 1996;97:63.
42. Fine NA, Orgill DP, Pribaz JJ. Early clinical experience in endoscopic-assisted muscle flap harvest. *Ann Plast Surg* 1994;33:456.
43. Mustoe TA. Evolving concepts in breast reconstruction. In: Cameron, ed. *Current Surgical Therapy*, St. Louis: Mosby, 1998.
44. Watterson PA, Bostwick J, Hester TR, et al. TRAM flap anatomy correlated with a 10-year clinical experience with 556 patients. *Plast Reconstr Surg* 1995;95:1185.
45. Hendricks DL, Wilkins TH, Witt PD. Blood flow contributions by the superior and inferior epigastric arterial systems in TRAM flaps, based on laser Doppler flowmetry. *J Reconstr Microsurg* 1994;10:249.
46. Godfrey PM, Godfrey NV, Romita MC. Immediate autogenous breast reconstruction in clinically advanced disease. *Plast Reconstr Surg* 1995;95:1039.
47. Styblo TM, Lewis MM, Carlson GW, et al. Immediate breast reconstruction for stage III breast cancer using transverse rectus abdominis musculocutaneous (TRAM) flap. *Ann Surg Oncol* 1996;3:375.
48. Sultan MR, Smith ML, Estabrook A, et al. Immediate breast reconstruction in patients with locally advanced disease. *Ann Plast Surg* 1997;38:345.
49. Kroll SS, Gherardini G, Martin JE, et al. Fat necrosis in free and pedicled TRAM flaps. *Plast Reconstr Surg* 1998;102:1502.
50. Kind GM, Radamaker AW, Mustoe TA. Abdominal wall recovery following TRAM flap: a functional outcome study. *Plast Reconstr Surg* 1997;99:41.
51. Lejour M, Dome M. Abdominal wall function after rectus abdominis transfer. *Plast Reconstr Surg* 1991;87:1054.
52. Harashina T, Stone K, Inoue T, et al. Augmentation of circulation of pedicled transverse rectus abdominis musculocutaneous flaps by microvascular surgery. *Br J Plast Surg* 1987;40:367.
53. Kroll SS, Marchi M. Comparison of strategies for preventing abdominal-wall weakness after TRAM flap breast reconstruction. *Plast Reconstr Surg* 1992;89:1045.
54. Mizgala CL, Hartrampf CR, Bennett GK. Assessment of the abdominal wall after pedicled TRAM flap surgery: 5 to 7-year follow-up of 150 consecutive patients. *Plast Reconstr Surg* 1994;93:988.
55. Paige KT, Bostwick J, Bried JT, Jones G. A comparison of morbidity from bilateral, unipedicled and unilateral, unipedicled TRAM flap breast reconstructions. *Plast Reconstr Surg* 1998;101:1819.
56. Codner MA, Bostwick J III, Nahai F, Bried JT, Eaves FF. TRAM flap vascular delay for high-risk breast reconstruction. *Plast Reconst Surg* 1995;96:1615.
57. Boyd JB, Taylor GI, Corlett R. The vascular territories of the superior epigastric and the deep inferior epigastric systems. *Plast Reconstr Surg* 1984;73:1.
58. Schusterman MA, Kroll SS, Miller MJ, et al. The free transverse rectus abdominis musculocutaneous flap for breast reconstruction: one center's experience with 211 consecutive cases. *Ann Plast Surg* 1994;32:234.
59. Serletti JM, Moran SL. Free versus the pedicled TRAM flap: a cost comparison and outcome analysis. *Plast Reconstr Surg* 1997;100:1418.
60. Mustoe TA, Fine NA. Discussion of: free versus the pedicled TRAM flap: a cost comparison and outcome analysis. *Plast Reconstr Surg* 1997;100:1425.
61. Baldwin BJ, Schusterman MA, Miller MJ, et al. bilateral breast reconstruction: conventional versus free TRAM. *Plast Reconstr Surg* 1994;93:1410.
62. Kroll SS, Schusterman MA, Reece GP, Miller MJ, Robb GL, Evans G. Abdominal wall strength, bulging, and hernia after TRAM flap breast reconstruction. *Plast Reconstr Surg* 1995;96:616.
63. Hartrampf CR, Noel RT, Drazan L, et al. Ruben's fat pad for breast reconstruction: a peri-iliac soft tissue free flap. *Plast Reconstr Surg* 1994;93:402.
64. Shaw WW. Bilateral free flap breast reconstruction. *Clin Plast Surg* 1994;21:297.
65. Little JW, Spear SL. The finishing touches in nipple areolar reconstruction. *Perspect Plast Surg* 1998;2:1
66. Little JW. Nipple-areolar reconstruction. In: Spear SL, ed. *The breast: principles and art*. Philadelphia: Lippincott–Raven, 1998;661.
67. Papp C, Wechselberger G, Schueller T. Autologous breast reconstruction after breast-conserving cancer surgery. *Plast Reconstr Surg* 1998;102:1932.
68. Clough KB, Nos C, Salmon, RJ, et al. Conservative treatment of breast cancers by mammaplasty and irradiation: a new approach to lower quadrant tumors. *Plast Reconstr Surg* 1995;96:363.
69. Bold RJ, Kroll SS, Baldwin BJ, et al. Local rotational flaps for breast conservation therapy as an alternative to mastectomy. *Ann Surg Oncol* 1997;4:540.

Diseases of the Breast, 2nd ed.,
edited by Jay R. Harris.
Lippincott Williams & Wilkins, Philadelphia © 2000.

CHAPTER 35

Techniques of Surgery

S. Eva Singletary

Determining the most appropriate treatment plan for a patient with breast cancer requires knowledge of the cancer's anticipated biological behavior and of the patient's physical, emotional, and rehabilitation needs. Therapeutic options are diverse and often require the interaction of a multidisciplinary team of specialists. To communicate effectively, the members of this team must understand the concepts and current practice of the surgical management of breast cancer. This chapter addresses the basic principles and surgical techniques of segmental mastectomy (wide local excision), axillary node dissection, lymphatic mapping and sentinel lymph node biopsy, and skin-sparing mastectomy with immediate breast reconstruction.

SEGMENTAL MASTECTOMY (WIDE LOCAL EXCISION)

Patients who are candidates for breast-conservation surgery should be seen by a radiotherapist before surgery. This referral ensures that the patient is adequately informed concerning the plan for delivering radiation therapy (location of the radiation center and duration of treatment) and the potential short-term and long-term effects and complications of irradiation. The surgeon and patient should discuss whether the patient desires to proceed with a total mastectomy if negative margins cannot be obtained at the time of surgery. For patients who have received preoperative chemotherapy, the surgeon must carefully examine both the initial diagnostic mammogram and a mammogram obtained after chemotherapy before surgery. Evidence of multicentricity on the initial mammogram or extensive microcalcifications remaining or developing after chemotherapy would contraindicate breast-conservation surgery.[1] If total mastectomy is required, and the patient desires immediate reconstruction, deferring the total mastectomy with or without an axillary lymph node dissection and performing it as a second-stage procedure is usually more practical, especially when an autogenous flap reconstruction is likely.

The skin incision should be placed directly over the breast mass. An ellipse of skin is included if the lesion is superficial or has previously been biopsied. Usually, a curvilinear transverse incision that conforms to the contour of the breast achieves the best cosmetic result. If the patient is a borderline candidate for breast conservation, however, the skin incision should be oriented so that it can be easily included in a mastectomy specimen, especially if the probability is high of performing a skin-sparing mastectomy with immediate reconstruction. When the lesion is large, or considerable skin sacrifice is required, particularly for tumors in the lower aspect of the breast, consultation with a plastic surgeon is helpful before attempting segmental mastectomy. Potential strategies for avoiding a poor cosmetic result—for example, Z-plasty closure or a local rotational flap (Fig. 1)—can be discussed preoperatively.[2,3] The incision for the segmental mastectomy should be separate from the incision for the axillary lymph node dissection, unless the lesion is in the tail of the breast (Fig. 2). Separate incisions diminish subsequent retraction of the breast toward the axilla after irradiation and allow the radiotherapist the option of delivering a boost to the tumor bed if needed.

In general, the tumor or biopsy cavity is excised *en bloc*, along with a 1-cm or larger margin of normal breast tissue in all three dimensions.[4] The skin flaps should be relatively thick, unless the tumor is superficial. For lesions deep in the breast, the pectoralis fascia may be included. If the tumor invades the pectoralis major muscle, a wide local excision of the involved muscle should be performed. If the surgeon who performed the prior excisional biopsy is certain of the location of the close or positive margins, then reexcision of the involved biopsy cavity wall through the original surgical incision is also an acceptable technique.[5] The surgeon should use radiopaque hemoclips to mark the base of the biopsy site in the breast to assist the radiotherapist in planning the treatment field (Fig. 3).

The surgeon should personally orient the specimen for the pathologist and request that any close margins be checked with frozen section analysis (Fig. 4). At least two of the mar-

S. E. Singletary: Department of Surgical Oncology, Surgical Breast Service, University of Texas M. D. Anderson Cancer Center, Houston, Texas

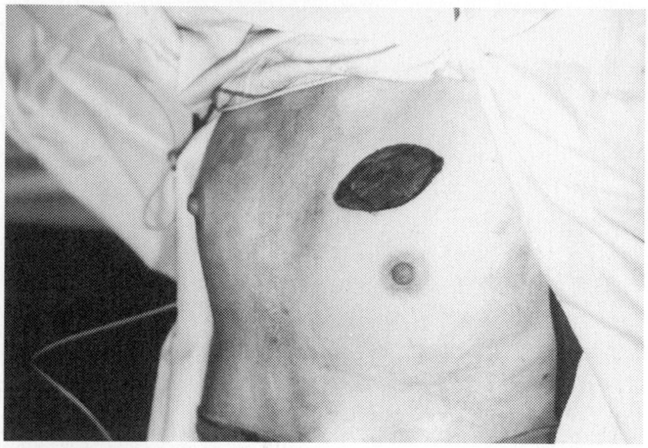

A

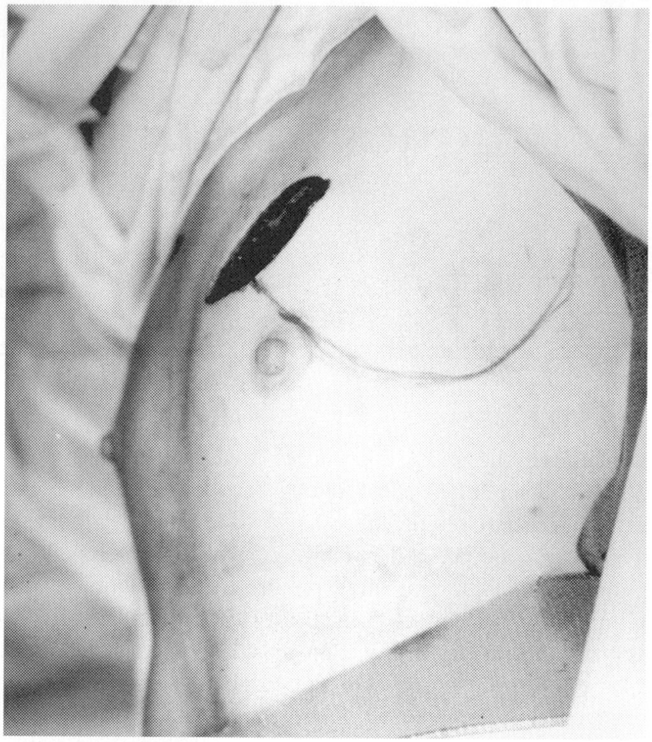

B

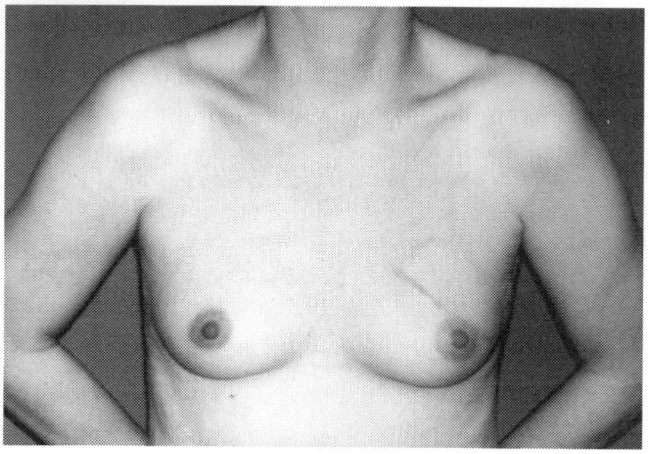

C

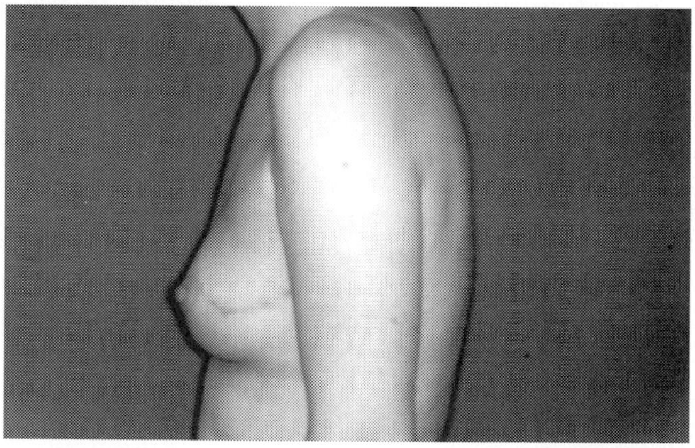

D

FIG. 1. A: Operative defect in the upper inner quadrant of the breast following excision of a T2 breast carcinoma. **B:** Plan for a superiorly based flap. **C–D:** Results 1 year later. (From ref. 2, with permission.)

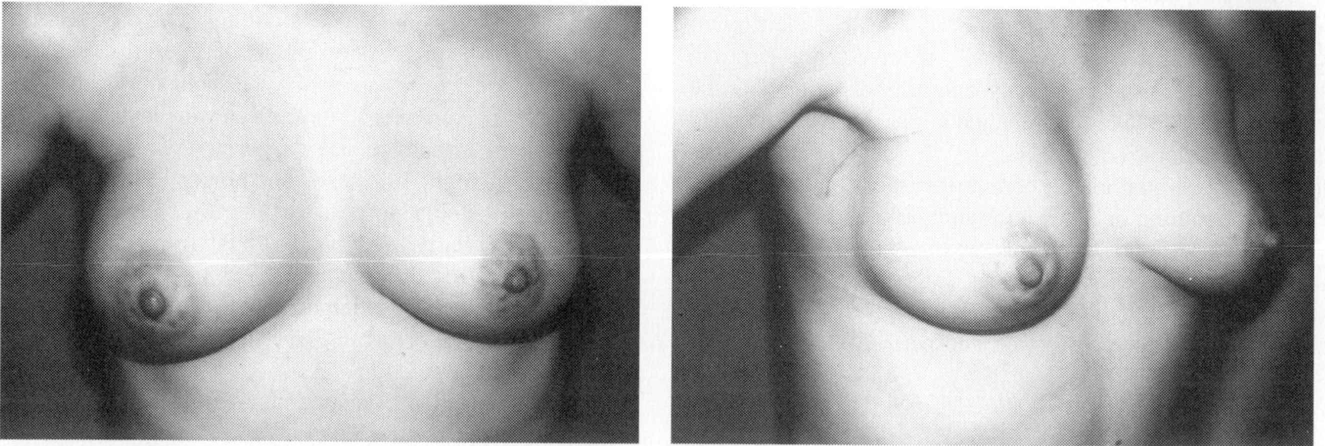

FIG. 2. Postoperative results of a segmental mastectomy and axillary node dissection for a 1-cm invasive ductal carcinoma arising in the tail of the breast adjacent to the axilla.

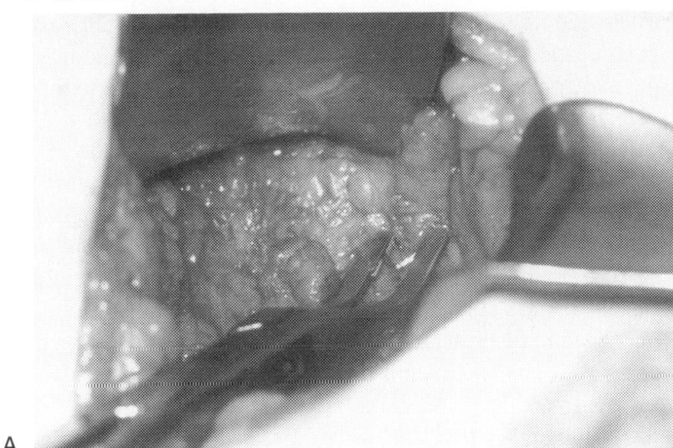

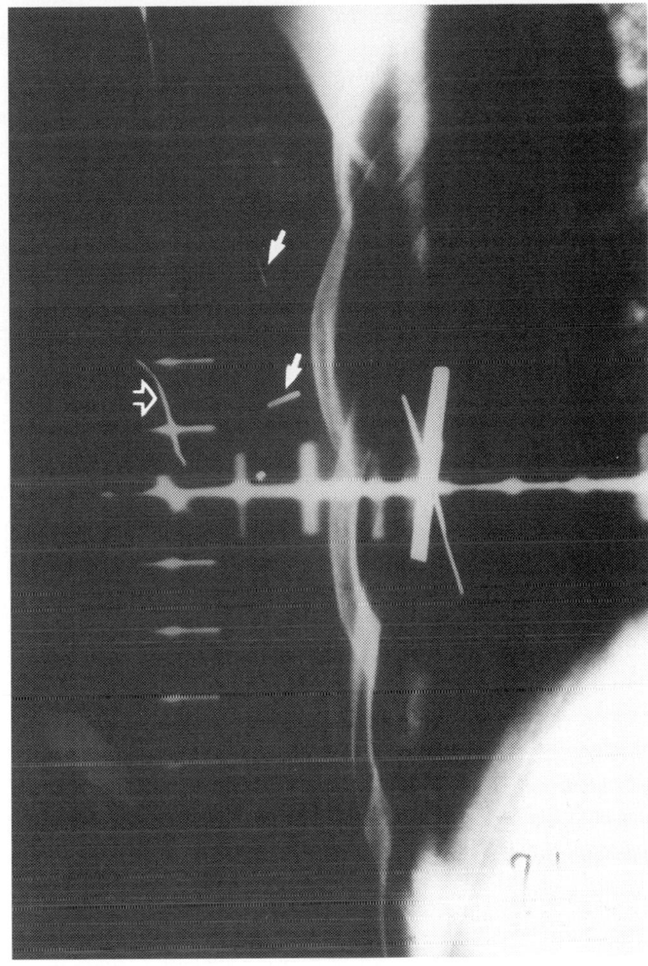

FIG. 3. **A:** Hemoclips are inserted at the base of the biopsy site after frozen section evaluation documented the lesion was malignant. **B:** Radiotherapy tangential field simulation of a patient following segmental mastectomy. The solid arrows denote radiopaque hemoclips placed at the time of surgery to demarcate the margins of resection. The open arrow denotes a wire placed over the skin incision by the radiotherapist.

gins should be identified by either hemoclips or sutures. Careful hemostasis should be obtained before closure. The defect inside the breast is not closed with sutures, and drains are not necessary. The skin is closed with absorbable interrupted inverted sutures of the deep dermis, followed by a running subcuticular 4-0 or 5-0 absorbable suture. Steri-strips are used to approximate the skin edges. Bulky pressure dressings and heavy tape are not necessary and are uncomfortable to the patient. A lightweight stretch bra supports the breast and may decrease tension on the incision from the weight of the breast itself.

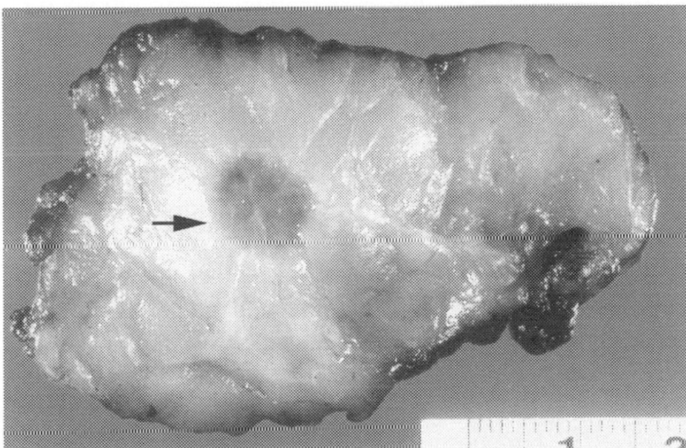

FIG. 4. After the specimen is inked circumferentially and then transected by the pathologist, a frozen section is obtained of any margin within 10 mm of the grossly evident tumor.

AXILLARY NODE DISSECTION

The standard of care for operable invasive breast cancer is to perform a level 1–2 axillary lymph node dissection (removal of axillary lymph nodes lateral and posterior to the pectoralis minor muscle). An axillary lymph node dissection can be omitted in patients with localized ductal carcinoma *in situ*, lobular carcinoma *in situ*, and limited microinvasive disease.[6] In patients with a limited life expectancy or severe comorbid conditions, the value of the surgical procedure must be weighed against the possible complications or side effects.

In preparation for the procedure, the patient is placed in the supine position with the ipsilateral arm extended. A small roll is placed beneath the patient's back longitudinally to elevate the axilla from the operating table. To avoid possible brachial plexus injury from excessive traction, folded sheets should be used to raise the extended arm to the same height as the axilla. The arm must not be hyperextended. The entire breast and ipsilateral arm are then prepared. If immediate reconstruction is planned, the opposite breast should be included in the surgical field to allow the plastic surgeon to compare symmetry between the breasts. The ipsilateral arm is draped separately from the field so that, if necessary, the surgeon can lift the arm to gain access to the high axilla either for removal of nodal disease or for control of any unexpected hemorrhage.

In patients who undergo axillary lymph node dissection with breast-conservation surgery, a separate transverse S-shaped incision is made 2 to 3 cm beneath the axillary skin fold. If possible, the incision should be placed below the hair follicles to facilitate shaving in the future. The anterior cephalad extension of the S-shaped incision is the lateral border of the pectoralis major muscle. The posterior caudad extension of the S-shaped incision is the anterior border of the latissimus dorsi muscle.

The extent of the axillary lymph node dissection is the same regardless of whether the patient is undergoing breast-conservation surgery or total mastectomy. First, the superior skin flap is raised with the electrocautery unit; fine-tipped skin hooks are used for skin retraction. The plane of dissection is usually approximately 5 mm beneath the skin to ensure adequate cutaneous blood supply. The cephalad portion of the pectoralis major muscle is identified and used as an anatomic landmark for the anticipated location of the axillary vein. Then the inferior skin flap is elevated to at least the level of the fifth intercostal space to ensure that the lowest axillary lymph nodes are included with the specimen.

The lateral border of the pectoralis major muscle is exposed, and the anterior border of the latissimus dorsi muscle is identified. The dissection follows the tendinous insertion of the latissimus dorsi muscle, until the axillary vein is visualized. The axillary fascia, immediately medial to the anterior border of the latissimus muscle, is incised to expose the thoracodorsal vessels. The fascia on the lateral surface of the thoracodorsal trunk is dissected free, allowing the vessels and thoracodorsal nerve to fall laterally as the specimen is retracted medially. A perpendicular branch from the medial side of the thoracodorsal vessels often points to the location of the long thoracic nerve. The fascia anterior to the long thoracic nerve is incised to allow the specimen to be moved more medially. The thoracodorsal trunk and the long thoracic nerve are identified early in the procedure so that, if unexpected hemorrhage occurs, the specimen can be removed without damaging these important structures.

The specimen is then dissected off the lateral aspect of the pectoralis major muscle, exposing the underlying pectoralis minor muscle. The fascia covering the pectoralis major muscle is incised, with care taken to preserve the pectoralis minor neurovascular bundle. Preservation of the nerve branch coursing through this bundle to the pectoralis major muscle may avoid atrophy of the lateral one-third of the pectoralis major muscle. The nodal tissue is dissected free from the axillary vein either from a lateral-to-medial direction or *vice versa*, depending on the surgeon's preference. Larger tributaries from the axillary vein into the specimen are divided and ligated with a 3-0 suture. At the medial aspect of the dissection, a retractor is used to elevate the pectoralis minor muscle to gain exposure to the level 2 lymph nodes. Division of the pectoralis minor muscle is seldom required in a lymph node dissection done for staging of breast cancer. When preservation of any of the intercostal brachial cutaneous nerves is attempted, the specimen may need to be bivalved where the cutaneous nerves enter the chest wall. The specimen is then dissected from the chest wall, leaving intact the fascia over the serratus anterior muscle.

The wound is irrigated with saline solution, and meticulous hemostasis is achieved. A single quarter-inch, closed-suction Silastic drainage catheter is inserted through the inferior skin flap into the axilla. The catheter should not be in direct contact with the axillary vein. To prevent an air leak, the surgeon should make sure that the most distal perforations of the catheter are not too close to the exit wound. The catheter is secured to the skin with a single 3-0 nylon suture. To allow easy removal, the suture should not loop the skin too tightly; however, the skin loop should not be too large, as this could allow the catheter to slide in and out of the axilla and become contaminated. The skin flaps are reapproximated with 3-0 or 4-0 synthetic absorbable sutures on the deep dermis and a running subcuticular 4-0 or 5-0 synthetic absorbable suture on the skin. Steri-Strips are applied along the length of the wound for coverage, and a small 4×4-inch gauze dressing is placed over the drain site and covered with a small amount of antibacterial ointment. No other dressings are necessary.

LYMPHATIC MAPPING AND SENTINEL LYMPH NODE BIOPSY

Lymphatic mapping and sentinel lymph node (SLN) biopsy have received much attention as a possible alternative to axillary node dissection. This technique was initially used as a method for detecting occult lymph node metastases in patients with melanoma. Morton et al.[7] observed that specific areas drained by way of afferent lymphatics to a sentinel node before draining to other lymph nodes in the basin. If the SLN is negative, the other nodes are presumed also to be negative. Thus, the morbidity of axillary node dissection can be avoided in patients who are unlikely to benefit from it.

The SLN is identified by injecting either a vital dye or a colloidal suspension of radioactively tagged substance into the periphery of the primary tumor site. When vital dye is used, the SLN is detected visually during the surgery (Fig. 5). When the radioactive tag method is used, the SLN can be localized by lymphoscintigraphy before surgery or by use of a handheld gamma-ray detector during surgery.

Although SLN biopsy is being actively studied at only a few sites, the results are impressive.[8–18] Five of the six sites

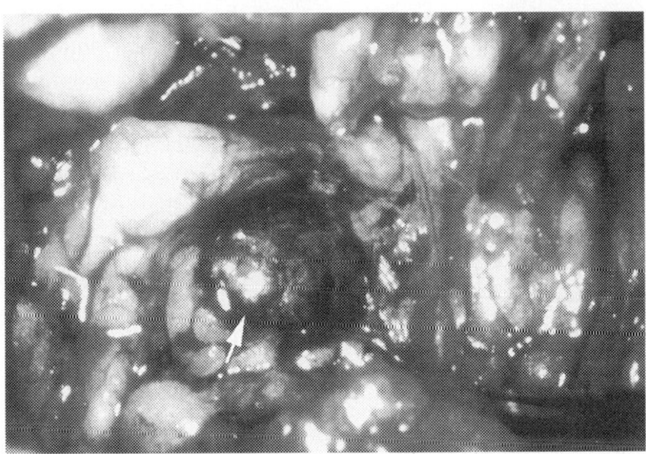

FIG. 5. The sentinel lymph node is carefully dissected from the surrounding fat with ligation of the lymphatic channels to avoid extravasation of the blue dye during the procedure. (Photograph courtesy of Dr. Henry Kuerer.)

are using the radioactive tag method with technetium (Tc) 99m, either alone or in combination with vital dye; the sixth site uses vital dye alone. No significant differences in outcome are seen as a function of protocol. At all sites, the SLN can now be successfully identified in approximately 95% of cases, and in these cases, the status of the SLN accurately predicts the status of the remaining lymph nodes in essentially 100% of cases.

The limited success of SLN biopsy shown in reports from the John Wayne Cancer Center indicate that this technique is associated with a learning curve. At the John Wayne Cancer Center, within a 2-year period, the percentage of cases in which the SLN was identified rose from 65% to 93%, whereas the number of those cases in which SLN status predicted overall nodal status increased from 95% to 100%. Whether this learning curve is associated with the use of the dye marker alone and can be avoided by using radioactive detection or both methods in combination remains to be demonstrated.

An important potential development in SNL biopsy will be the use of molecular and immunohistochemical markers to detect occult micrometastases in the SLN. Although not a practical approach for standard assessment of all lymph nodes from an axillary node dissection, use of these techniques is certainly possible in a single specified lymph node. Nodal micrometastases detected by this method may be associated with a reduction of survival rates by 10% to 15% compared with the survival rate predicted by a negative histologic nodal status based on routine processing of the axillary lymph node dissection specimen. Thus, intensive study of the SLN may actually result in a more accurate prediction of survival than processing of the standard axillary node dissection specimen.

The technical aspects of SNL biopsy are evolving. The vital dye method is the simplest technique, but it requires more experience. When the breast lesion is palpable, 4 to 5 mL of 1% isosulfan blue is injected circumferentially directly around the primary tumor or in the periphery of the excisional biopsy site. Our current practice is to inject 1 mL of dye at the nine o'clock, twelve o'clock, three o'clock, and six o'clock positions with a 1-mL tuberculin syringe. Care must be taken to avoid staining of the overlying skin. However, most staining of the skin resolves within 2 weeks. The patient should be informed that the urine will be green for 24 hours.

The injection is performed before skin preparation, so that 8 to 10 minutes have elapsed between the time of injection and the initiation of the SNL biopsy. For nonpalpable tumors, dye can be injected under ultrasonic guidance in the operating room. The axillary incision is marked using the standard anatomic landmarks. Within 10 minutes of dye injection, a small incision is made in the axilla in such a way that it could be incorporated into the standard incision should a formal dissection be required. Electrocautery is used to incise the subcutaneous tissue and open the axillary fascia. Careful dissection is then performed to identify the lymphatic channel and sentinel node. The sentinel node is excised, and the vascular pedicle is clamped and ligated. The dermis is closed with interrupted 3-0 or 4-0 absorbable sutures, and the skin is closed with a running 4-0 absorbable suture in a subcuticular fashion.

The use of a radioactively tagged marker provides added insurance that the SLN has been correctly identified. Which type of colloidal suspension to use and whether the suspension should be filtered or unfiltered remains controversial, however.[19] Our current practice is to used filtered Tc 99m–sulfur colloid (450 μCi) injected 2 to 6 hours before the operative procedure. This dose is diluted in 6 mL of saline that is divided into six 1-mL aliquots injected around the periphery of the tumor or previous biopsy site (using ultrasonic guidance if necessary). Lymphoscintigraphy is performed using a large-field-of-view gamma camera set at a 20% window and fitted with a low-energy, high-resolution parallel hole collimator. The patient's arm is abducted above the head to increase the distance between the primary tumor injection site and the regional nodal basins and to permit visualization of the axilla in two planes. Scans of the site of the primary tumor and adjacent nodal basins are made immediately on injection, and a dynamic flow study is obtained to identify the SLN(s). Delayed images are also obtained at 2 hours, or until tracer is detected in the liver, to document the drainage pathway.

Intraoperatively, a handheld gamma ray–detecting probe is used to detect the SLN. The axillary incision is placed in the area of greatest radioactivity. An SLN is defined as any blue or radioactive ("hot") node with a 10:1 *ex vivo* gamma-probe radioactivity ratio of SLN to non-SLN. After all SLNs have been removed, the axilla is scanned with the probe to document that activity levels have returned to background levels.

Each SLN is submitted separately to the pathology suite for serial sectioning at 2- to 3-mm intervals for routine histologic examination. If the SLN is negative by hematoxylin-eosin staining, then the SLN is submitted for immunohistochemical staining using a cytokeratin monoclonal antibody for detection of occult metastases.[20] Frozen section analysis is avoided, unless gross metastasis is evident and a complete axillary node dissection is planned in the same operative setting.

SKIN-SPARING MASTECTOMY WITH IMMEDIATE RECONSTRUCTION

Skin-sparing mastectomy refers to a standard mastectomy with minimal unnecessary skin sacrifice.[21] The procedure is performed when immediate reconstruction is planned. Aside from the sparing of skin, the mastectomy is the same as a standard modified radical mastectomy, with removal of all breast tissue and a level 1–2 axillary lymph node dissection. Preservation of uninvolved breast skin provides an ideal color and texture match between the reconstructed breast and the opposite breast. It also aids the plastic surgeon in creating a normal breast shape by providing a properly shaped breast skin envelope that the surgeon simply needs to fill.

Creativity should be used in outlining the breast skin to be removed (Fig. 6). Removal of the commonly used standard wide ellipse of skin is not necessary, nor is removal of a predetermined skin margin around the nipple-areolar complex. Skin can often be preserved between the biopsy site and the areola by altering the direction of the incision line to encompass the biopsy scar or by excising the biopsy scar separately. If the cancer diagnosis was obtained with fine-needle aspiration biopsy and the lesion is deep within the breast, no skin overlying the area of the tumor needs to be excised. Input from the plastic surgeon is useful during the planning stages, but the final decision on the design of the skin flaps must always rest with the oncologic surgeon. The surgeon should not hesitate to remove any breast skin required to obtain a negative margin.

A scalpel with a size 15 blade is used for the skin incision, because a small blade facilitates following unusual or short skin markings. An electrocautery unit is used for flap elevation, and fine-tipped skin hooks are held perpendicular for skin retraction. The thickness of the mastectomy flaps should be the same as in a standard modified radical mastectomy. The keys to success are to ensure that the flap thickness is uniform and to avoid thin spots. The biopsy cavity site, along with its scar, should be included intact with the mastectomy specimen when the flaps are elevated. The inframammary fold should be left undisturbed without extending the dissection inferiorly on the rectus muscle. This allows a more normal contour of the reconstructed breast mound than when a plastic surgeon attempts to recreate an inframammary fold. The remainder of the skin-sparing mastectomy is performed as in a standard mastectomy. It is very helpful for the oncologic surgeon to assist the pathologist in orienting the mastectomy specimen and inking both the anterior and posterior breast surfaces of the specimen. Any margin close to the tumor or biopsy site should be submitted for frozen section evaluation. If additional skin must be resected because of an inadequate margin, it should be removed without hesitation.

The two basic methods of breast reconstruction are reconstruction with saline-filled implants and reconstruction with autogenous tissue. In implant procedures, the prosthesis is used to replace missing breast volume, and skin is replaced either through tissue expansion or with a regional tissue flap, such as the latissimus dorsi flap. In autogenous tissue-based reconstruction, a large myocutaneous flap is used to replace both breast skin and breast volume.

The primary advantage of using implants for immediate breast reconstruction is that they can be easily and quickly inserted, usually in less than 1 hour. The patient should be made aware that tissue expansion requires gradual inflation over 4 to 6 months, with eventual overinflation to stretch the mastectomy skin envelope to twice the size of the opposite breast. This period involves numerous office visits, and the inflation is generally associated with some discomfort. Once inflation is complete, a second surgical procedure is needed to replace the tissue expander with an implant, unless a combination expander/implant is used (Fig. 7). The disadvantage of implants is the continual risk of implant failure in the form of infection, rupture, extrusion, or capsular contracture. A thorough discussion with the patient regarding the controversy surrounding implants is mandatory, as even the saline-filled implants have a silicone envelope. Although no conclusive determination has been made as to whether implants contribute to or induce secondary diseases such as autoimmune disorders, preliminary data suggest that no link exists between silicone implants and autoimmune diseases.[22–24]

Although initially more complex and expensive, autogenous tissue-based breast reconstruction avoids all of the potential complications of breast reconstruction with implants and provides a reconstructed breast mound that better simulates the normal breast. When all costs associated with implant revisions over 5 years of follow-up are evaluated, autogenous-tissue reconstructions actually cost less than implant-based reconstructions.[25]

The most common method of autogenous tissue breast reconstruction is use of a transverse rectus abdominis myocutaneous (TRAM) flap, which is taken from the lower abdomen (Fig. 8). In the conventional TRAM flap technique, the flap is transferred with the muscle pedicle based superiorly, and the blood supply is from the superior epigastric vessels. This method requires sacrifice of most of the rectus muscle, which can lead to subsequent weakening of the abdominal wall. Because the major blood supply to the lower abdominal skin comes from the inferior epigastric system, ischemia and partial flap loss may occur with the superiorly based TRAM flap.

With the free TRAM flap technique, the flap receives its blood supply from the deep inferior epigastric vessels, which are divided and then joined to the thoracodorsal vessels using

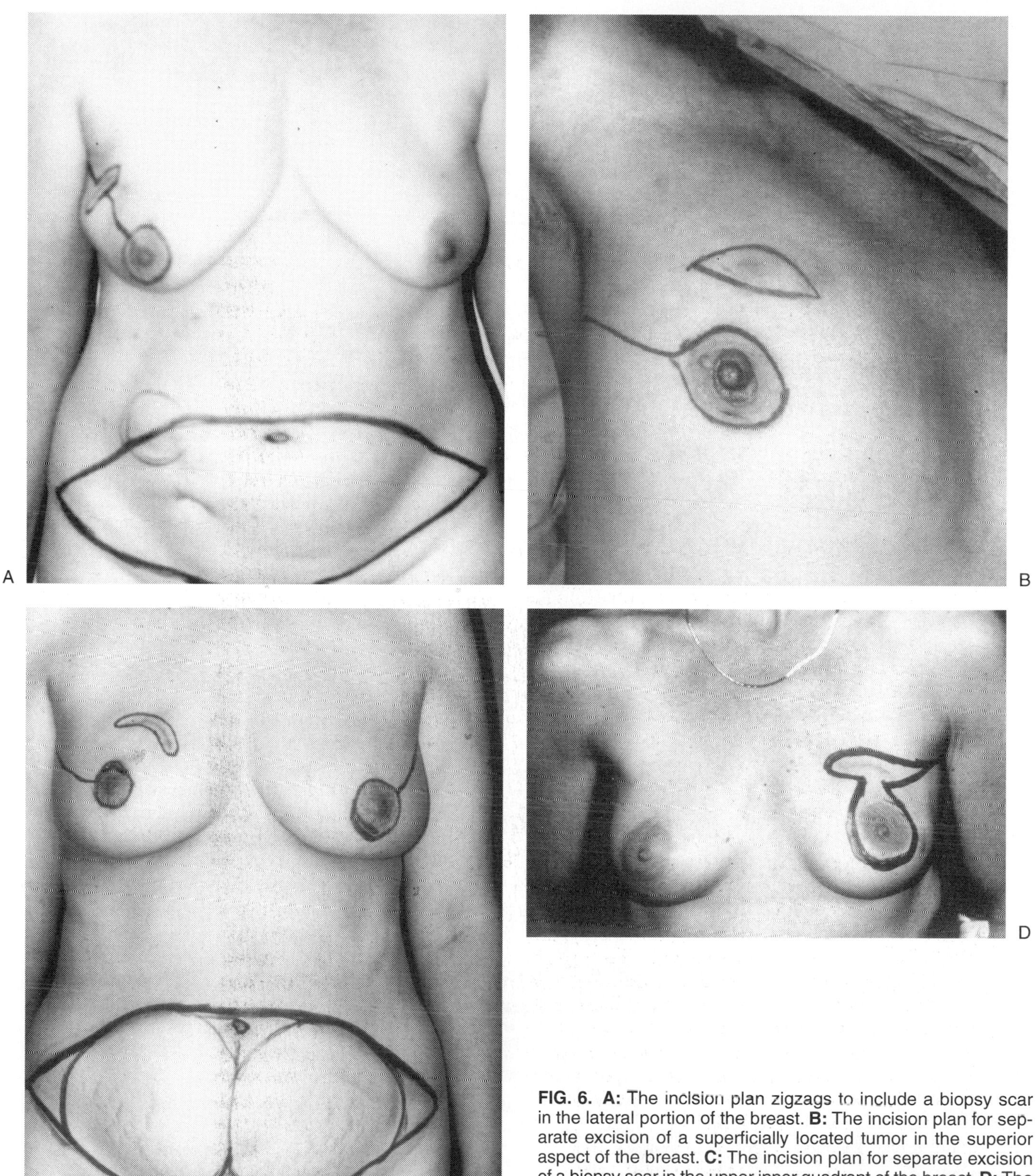

FIG. 6. A: The incision plan zigzags to include a biopsy scar in the lateral portion of the breast. **B:** The incision plan for separate excision of a superficially located tumor in the superior aspect of the breast. **C:** The incision plan for separate excision of a biopsy scar in the upper inner quadrant of the breast. **D:** The incision plan to include the skin bridge between the biopsy scar and the nipple-areolar complex.

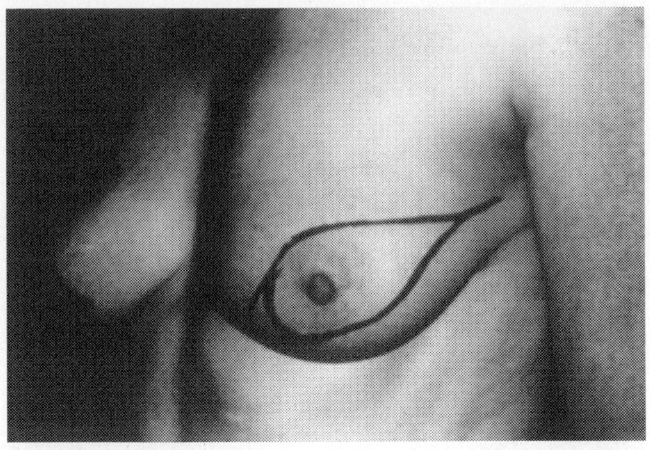
A

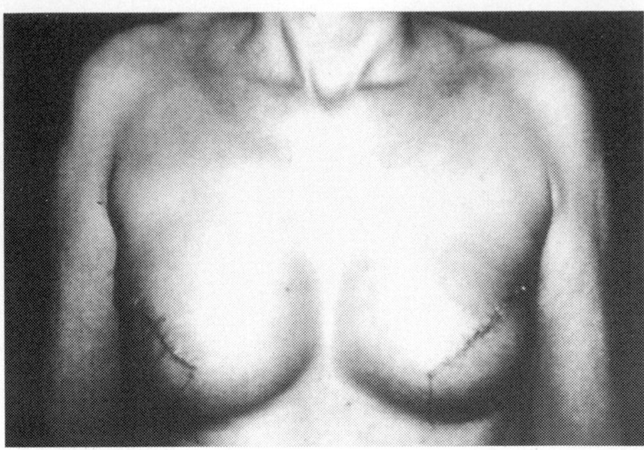
B

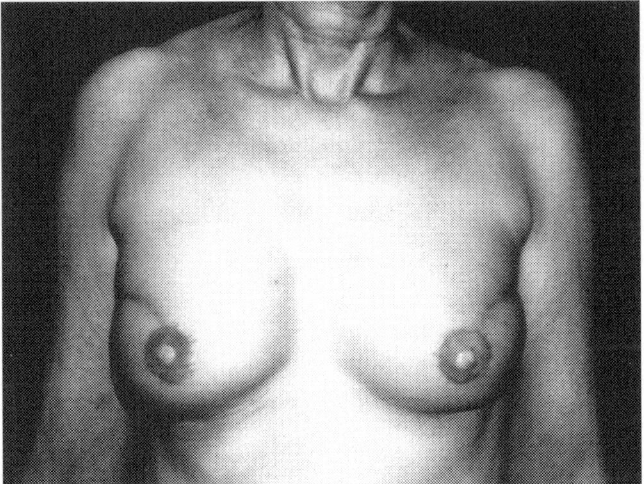
C

FIG. 7. A: Incision plan for left modified radical mastectomy and a right prophylactic mastectomy with maximum preservation of the patient's own breast skin. As reconstruction with tissue expanders is planned, the incision extends medially to allow primary closure in a linear fashion. **B:** Silicone tissue expanders inserted at the time of mastectomy beneath the pectoralis major muscles are gradually inflated with saline through a subcutaneous sideport. **C:** Expanders are replaced several weeks later with permanent prostheses and nipples are reconstructed from double-opposing-tab skin flaps from the adjacent chest wall. The areola was simulated by tattooing. (Reprinted with permission from Singletary SE. Selection of alternatives in the treatment of early breast cancer. *Clin Consult Obstet Gynecol* 1991;3:106.)

microvascular anastomoses.[26] This technique allows less sacrifice of the rectus muscle and thus a stronger abdominal wall after surgery. As tunneling of the pedicle is eliminated, an improved cosmetic result is achieved, with no bulging evident in the medial contour of the reconstructed breast mound.

For patients with extensive abdominal wall scars and patients who developed a new contralateral breast cancer after a previous unilateral TRAM flap reconstruction, alternative sources of autogenous tissue are available.[27] The extended latissimus dorsi flap is similar to the standard latissimus dorsi flap, except that additional subcutaneous

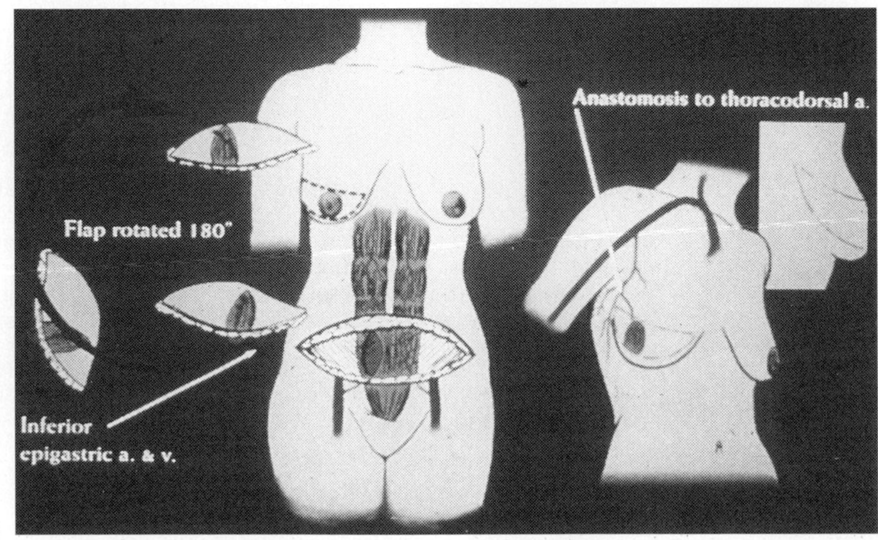

A

FIG. 8. Transverse rectus abdominis myocutaneous (TRAM) flap, the so-called tummy-tuck flap. **A:** With this technique, a large area of abdominal skin and fat is outlined and raised with a portion of the rectus muscle and its blood supply, the inferior epigastric vessels. The flap is directly transferred by free microvascular anastomoses of the inferior epigastric vessels to the axillary thoracodorsal vascular pedicle. (*Continued*)

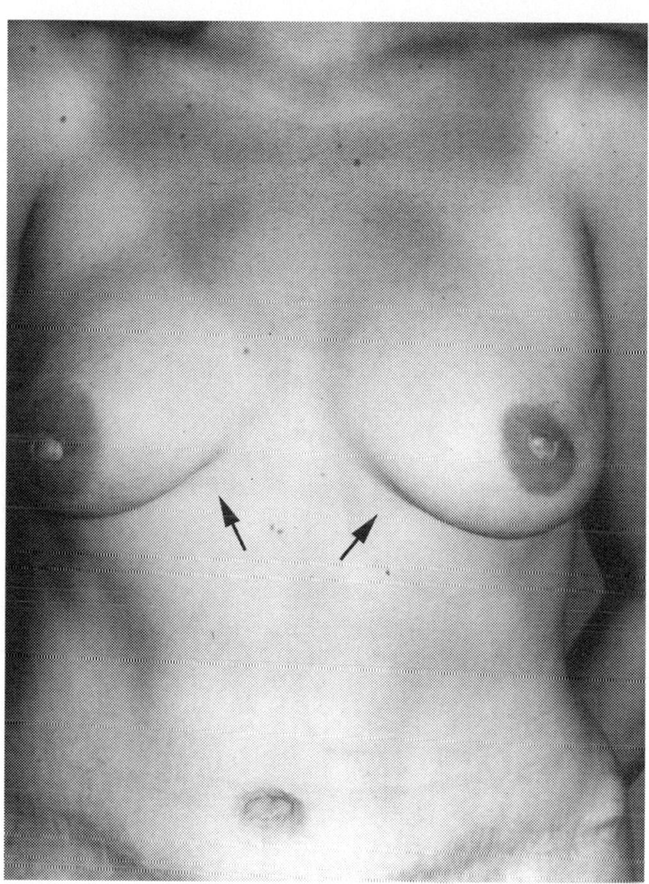

B

FIG. 8. *Continued.* **B:** Postoperative results after bilateral skin-sparing mastectomies and TRAM flap reconstruction using microvascular anastomoses. Note that there is no bulging of the medial inframammary contour of the reconstructed breast, which often occurs with a pedicled TRAM flap that is tunneled under the abdominal skin.

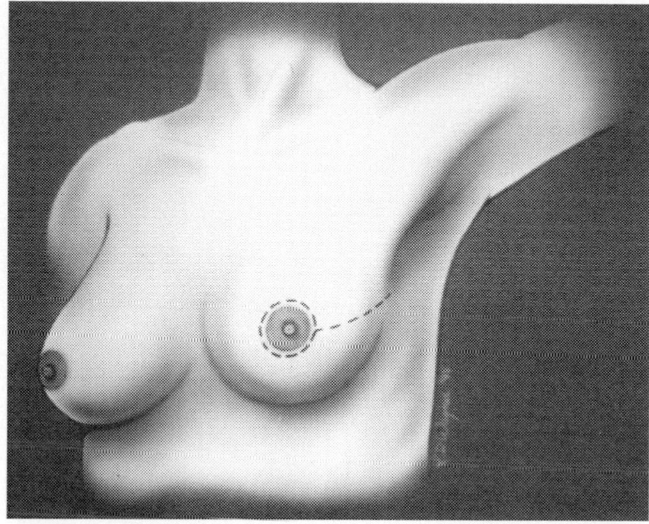

A

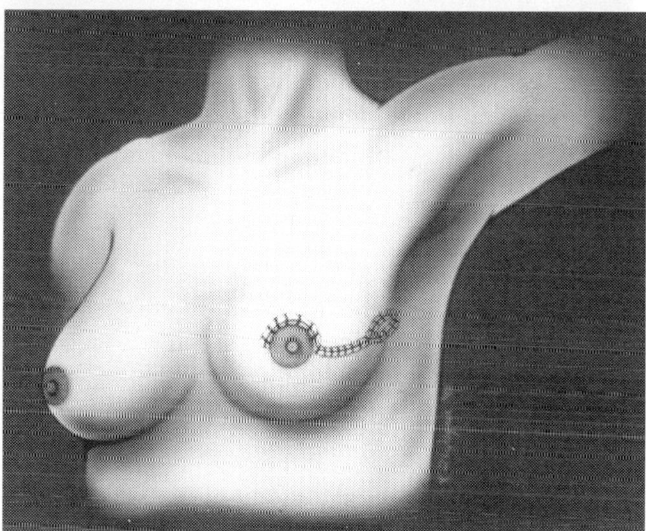

B

FIG. 9. A: Preoperative markings for standard skin-sparing mastectomy. **B:** Incision plan for a nipple-areolar complex-sparing mastectomy. The incision is made along the superior border of the nipple-areolar complex from medial to lateral and then continues transversely from the lateral border of the complex toward the axilla. A small window is created in the lateral aspect of the incision to monitor the viability of the autogenous tissue flap. (*Continued*)

fat and skin are transferred so that an implant is usually unnecessary. However, shaping of the reconstructed breast mound may be more difficult with the latissimus dorsi flap than with a free TRAM flap, and donor site deformity is more apparent when the patient wears a bathing suit. The gluteal free flap is used only rarely, because reconstruction with this flap is technically more difficult than reconstruction with the other flaps and often requires a vein graft.[28] Another disadvantage of the gluteal free flap is flattening of the hip contour, which is noticeable even when the patient is clothed. Reconstruction with a "Ruben's fat pad" flap, which uses fatty tissue in the flank overlying the iliac crest, is technically easier than reconstruction with the gluteal free flap but also may cause a contour change when performed unilaterally.[29]

Nipple reconstruction is deferred until postoperative edema has resolved, usually approximately 8 to 12 weeks after surgery. The current method of creating the nipple projection is to use small, local double-opposing-tab flaps elevated from the breast mound.[30] The areola is simulated using micropigmentation with a medical-grade tattoo performed under local anesthesia without sedation.

Another alternative is to preserve the nipple-areolar complex as part of the skin-sparing mastectomy. The dogma that the nipple-areolar complex must be removed with the mastectomy specimen was based on several studies in the 1970s and 1980s that demonstrated occult tumor in the vicinity of the nipple-areolar complex.[31–38] The nipple sampling technique varied among these studies, however. Most often, the technique was to serially section the nipple vertically and the areola horizontally at 5-mm intervals with a depth that ranged from 5 to 20 mm. The risk of tumor involvement was higher if the primary tumor was subareolar, larger than 2 cm

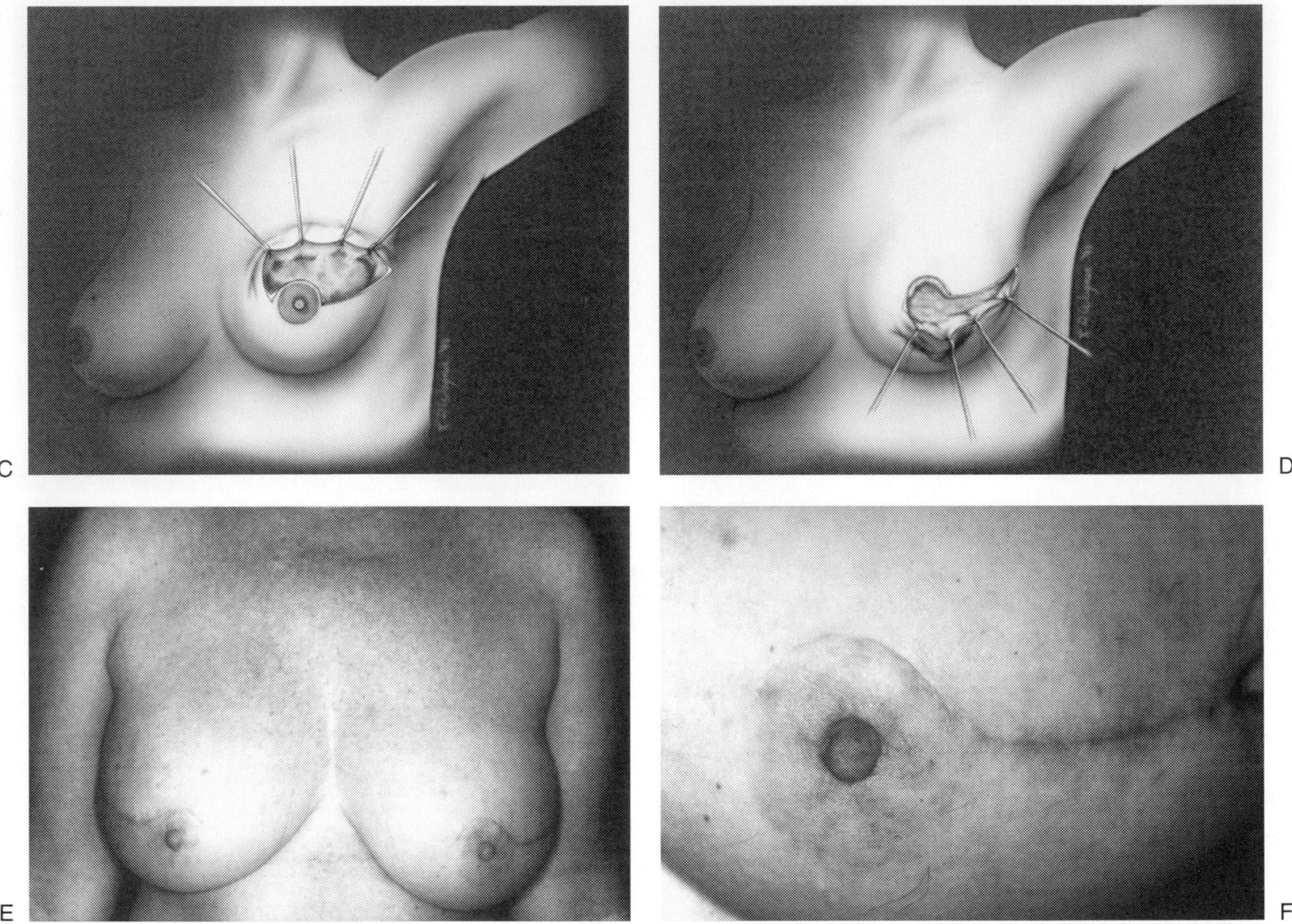

FIG. 9. *Continued.* **C:** The superior mastectomy flap is raised in the superficial plane (approximately 3 mm in thickness) as done for a standard modified radical mastectomy. **D:** The inferior mastectomy flap is similarly raised but includes the nipple-areolar complex. **E:** Six-week postoperative result of bilateral nipple-areolar complex-sparing mastectomies. **F:** Postoperative close-up view of the preserved nipple-areolar complex. The subareolar margins were negative on intraoperative frozen section evaluation. (Reprinted with permission from Laronga C, Robb GL, Singletary SE. Feasibility of skin-sparing mastectomy with preservation of the nipple-areola complex. *Breast Dis: A Yearbook Quarterly* 1998;9:125.)

in size, or associated with positive axillary lymph nodes. In the technique to spare the nipple-areolar complex, the nipple-areolar flap is usually less than 3 mm thick (Fig. 9). This shallow depth eliminates most of the tumors that were detected in previous studies of the nipple-areolar complex, especially if the primary tumor is small and located peripherally in the breast. Intraoperative examination of frozen sections at the subareolar margin also determines whether the nipple-areolar complex can be preserved. The patient should be informed preoperatively that the nipple-areolar complex will be sacrificed if occult tumor is discovered or if the vascularity of the flap is questionable. If the reconstruction is performed using an autogenous flap, a small island of skin from the autogenous flap can be left visible from the lateral extension of the mastectomy incision to monitor flap viability (see Fig. 9B).

POSTOPERATIVE CARE

Postoperative care after a segmental or total mastectomy with axillary lymph node dissection involves only daily inspection of the wound and daily dressing changes over the suction-drain exit site. With thorough instruction in wound care for the patient and her primary caregiver, most patients can be discharged from the hospital as soon as they recover from the general anesthesia, usually within 24 hours.[39] Patients are instructed to call if their temperature exceeds 101°F, if they have excessive bloody drainage (200 mL or more over an 8-hour period), or if any signs of infection or difficulty with the drainage system are present. Suction catheters are removed when the drainage is less than 30 mL over a 24-hour period. Range of motion of the ipsilateral arm is not restricted postoperatively. However, range-of-motion exercises are deferred until the day after catheter removal. If feasible, patients are seen the week after drain removal to check for seroma formation in the axilla. Most seromas can be managed by needle aspiration. If a seroma reaccumulates despite multiple aspirations, a catheter may have to be reinserted.

For patients who undergo mastectomy and immediate reconstruction with autogenous tissue, the hospital stay is usually 5 days. The blood supply of the flap is carefully monitored with a Doppler ultrasonic probe. Occasionally, a low-dose intravenous drip of heparin sodium is used, depending on the plastic surgeon's preference. Range-of-motion exercises are delayed for 2 weeks if a microvascular procedure is done.

Routine postoperative follow-up for invasive cancers requires a thorough history and physical examination every 3 to 4 months for the first 2 years, every 6 months during years 3 through 5, and yearly thereafter for the patient's lifetime. Only annual diagnostic mammograms of the contralateral breast and, if intact, the treated breast, are required. However, an initial baseline mammogram 6 months after completion of radiation therapy for patients who have undergone breast-conservation surgery is often helpful for future comparisons. Mammograms of the reconstructed breast mound are not useful and may even create confusion if fat necrosis is present. Extensive laboratory or radiologic studies obtained on routine patient follow-up have not been shown to affect survival or quality of life in the absence of symptoms and are not cost-effective.[40–42] In cases of carcinoma *in situ* or limited microinvasive disease, only yearly follow-up with diagnostic mammograms is needed.

SUMMARY AND FUTURE DIRECTIONS

Patient rehabilitation should begin at the time of diagnosis, because the outcome of treatment depends in part on the patient's perception of how her goals have been achieved. For some patients, an irradiated but intact breast may offer the best quality of life; others experience greater peace of mind with a total mastectomy and possibly breast reconstruction.

The strength of progress in the management of breast cancer lies in the team approach of multimodal care, which offers treatment based on the latest advances in research within each discipline—pathology, surgery, radiation therapy, and medical oncology. Treatment strategies based on the genetic or biological features of breast cancer in the individual patient propel the surgeon into a new surgical era of minimally invasive approaches to the primary tumor. The traditional approach to surgical margins may be replaced in the future with a theory of control of the abnormal molecular or genetic field defect of the primary tumor. The surgeon should not fear these advances but should accept the challenge to explore new therapies for control of tumor growth.

REFERENCES

1. Singletary SE, McNeese MD, Hortobagyi GN. Feasibility of breast conservation surgery after induction chemotherapy for locally advanced breast carcinoma. *Cancer* 1992;69:2849.
2. Bold RJ, Kroll SS, Baldwin B, Ross MI, Singletary SE. Local rotational flaps for breast conservation treatment (BCT) as an alternative to mastectomy. *Ann Surg Oncol* 1997;4:540.
3. Kroll S, Singletary SE. Repair of partial mastectomy defects. *Clin Plast Surg* 1998;25(2):303.
4. Singletary SE. Breast surgery. In: Roh MS, Ames FC, eds. *Atlas of advanced oncologic surgery*. New York: Gower Medical, 1993:14.1.
5. Winchester DP, Cox JD. Standards for diagnosis and management of invasive breast carcinoma. *CA Cancer J Clin* 1998;48:83.
6. Winchester DP, Strom EA. Standards for diagnosis and management of ductal carcinoma in situ (DCIS) of the breast. *CA Cancer J Clin* 1998;48:108.
7. Morton DL, Wen D-R, Wong JH, et al. Technical details of intraoperative lymphatic mapping for early stage melanoma. *Arch Surg* 1992;127:392.
8. Veronesi U, Paganelli G, Galimberti V, et al. Sentinel-node biopsy to avoid axillary dissection in breast cancer with clinically negative lymph nodes. *Lancet* 1997;349:1864.
9. Meijer S, Collet GH, Pijpers HJ, et al. Less axillary dissection necessary due to sentinel node biopsy in patients with breast carcinoma. *Ned Tijdschr Geneeskd* 1996;140:2239.
10. Cox CE, Pendas S, Cox JM, et al. Guidelines for sentinel node biopsy and lymphatic mapping of patients with breast cancer. *Ann Surg* 1998;227:645.
11. Albertini JJ, Lyman GH, Cox C, et al. Lymphatic mapping and sentinel node biopsy in the patient with breast cancer. *JAMA* 1996;276:1818.
12. Albertini J, Cox C, Yeatman T, et al. Lymphatic mapping and sentinel node biopsy in the breast cancer patient. *Proc Am Soc Clin Oncol* 1995;14:A99(abst).
13. O'Hea BJ, Hill AD, El-Shirbiny AM, et al. Sentinel lymph node biopsy in breast cancer: initial experience at Memorial Sloan-Kettering Cancer Center. *J Am Coll Surg* 1998;186:423.
14. Barnwell JM, Arredondo MA, Kollmorgen D, et al. Sentinel node biopsy in breast cancer. *Ann Surg Oncol* 1998;5(2):126.
15. Giuliano AE, Jones RC, Brennan M, et al. Sentinel lymphadenectomy in breast cancer. *J Clin Oncol* 1997;15:2345.
16. Statman RD, Jones RC, Cabot MC, et al. Sentinel lymphadenectomy. A technique to eliminate axillary dissection in node-negative breast cancer. *Proc Am Soc Clin Oncol* 1996;15:A167(abst).
17. Giuliano AE, Kirgan DM, Guenther JM, et al. Lymphatic mapping and sentinel lymphadenectomy for breast cancer. *Ann Surg* 1994;220:391.
18. Beitsch PD, Kirgan DM, Guenther JM, et al. Improved microstaging of axillary lymph nodes in breast cancer. *Breast Cancer Res Treat* 1994;32:94(abst).
19. Krag DN, Ashikaga T, Harlow SP, Weaver DL. Development of sentinel node targeting technique in breast cancer patients. *Breast J* 1998;4:67.
20. Jannick I, Fan M, Nagy S, Rayudu G, Dowlatshahi K. Serial sectioning of sentinel nodes in patients with breast cancer: a pilot study. *Ann Surg Oncol* 1998;5(4):310.
21. Singletary SE. Skin-sparing mastectomy with immediate breast reconstruction: the M.D. Anderson Cancer Center experience. *Ann Surg Oncol* 1996;3:411.
22. Hennekens CH, Lee I M, Cook NR, et al. Self-reported breast implants and connective-tissue diseases in female health professionals: a retrospective cohort study. *JAMA* 1996;275:616.
23. Deapen DM, Bernstein L, Brody GS. Are breast implants anticarcinogenic? A 14-year follow-up of the Los Angeles Study. *Plast Reconstr Surg* 1997;99:1346.
24. Brody GS, Conway DP, Deapen DM, et al. Consensus statement on the relationship of breast implants to connective-tissue disorders. *Plast Reconstr Surg* 1992;90:1102.
25. Kroll SS, Evans GRD, Reece GP, et al. Comparison of resource costs between implant-based and TRAM flap breast reconstruction. *Plast Reconstr Surg* 1996;97:364.
26. Schusterman MA, Kroll SS, Miller MJ, et al. The free TRAM flap for breast reconstruction: a single center's experience with 211 consecutive cases. *Ann Plast Surg* 1994;32:234.
27. Kroll SS, Asko-Seljavaara S. Overview of breast reconstruction. In: Kavanagh JJ, Singletary SE, Einhorn N, DePetrillo AD, eds. *Cancer in women*. Boston: Blackwell Science, 1998:124.

28. Codner MA, Nahai F. The gluteal free flap breast reconstruction: making it work. *Clin Plast Surg* 1994;21:289.
29. Hartrampf CR Jr, Noel RT, Drazan L, et al. Ruben's fat pad for breast reconstruction: a peri-iliac soft-tissue free flap. *Plast Reconstr Surg* 1994;93:402.
30. Kroll SS. Nipple and areolar reconstruction. In: Kroll SS, ed. *Oncologic plastic surgery: reconstructive surgery for cancer patients*. Philadelphia: Mosby, 1996:414.
31. Lagios MD, Gates EA, Westdahl PR, et al. A guide to the frequency of nipple involvement in breast cancer. A study of 149 consecutive mastectomies using a serial subgross and correlated radiographic technique. *Am J Surg* 1979;138:135.
32. Fisher ER, Gregorio RM, Fisher B, et al. The pathology of invasive breast cancer. *Cancer* 1975;36:1.
33. Wertheim U, Ozello L. Neoplastic involvement of nipple and skin flap in carcinoma of the breast. *Am J Surg Pathol* 1980;4:543.
34. Smith J, Payne WS, Carney JA. Involvement of the nipple and areola in carcinoma of the breast. *Surg Gynecol Obstet* 1976;143:546.
35. Parry RG, Cochran TC, Wolfort FG. When is there nipple involvement in carcinoma of the breast? *Plast Reconstr Surg* 1977; 59:535.
36. Santini D, Taffurelli M, Gelli MC, et al. Neoplastic involvement of nipple-areolar complex in invasive breast cancer. *Am J Surg* 1989;158:399.
37. Suehiro S, Inai K, Tukuoka S, et al. Involvement of the nipple in early carcinoma of the breast. *Surg Gynecol Obstet* 1989;168:244.
38. Mormoto T, Komaki K, Inui K, et al. Involvement of nipple and areola in early breast cancer. *Cancer* 1985;55:2459.
39. Feig BW. Outpatient mastectomy. In: Singletary SE, ed. *Breast cancer*. New York: Springer-Verlag, 1999:224.
40. Judkins AF, Singletary SE. Surveillance studies and long term follow-up care. In: Singletary SE, ed. *Breast cancer*. New York: Springer-Verlag, 1999:233.
41. GIVIO Investigators. Impact of follow-up testing on survival and health-related quality of life in breast cancer patients: a multicenter randomized controlled trial. *JAMA* 1994;271:1587.
42. Del Turco MR, Palli D, Cariddi A, et al. Intensive diagnostic follow-up after treatment of primary breast cancer: a randomized trial. *JAMA* 1994;271:1593.

CHAPTER 36

Diseases of the Breast, 2nd ed.,
edited by Jay R. Harris.
Lippincott Williams & Wilkins, Philadelphia © 2000.

Techniques of Radiation Therapy

Allen S. Lichter and Lori J. Pierce

Radiation therapy has been used in the treatment of breast cancer since the early 1900s. The earliest uses involved treatment of chest wall recurrences and primary therapy for advanced inoperable cases. Over the decades, the major uses of radiotherapy have shifted. Today, radiation oncologists are called on to treat many patients who have an intact breast after lumpectomy, as well as many patients who are postmastectomy but at high risk for local chest wall or regional lymph node failure. The importance of technical excellence in irradiating the intact breast or chest wall cannot be overemphasized. Many patients live for decades after treatment. Thus, efforts must be made to minimize the technical factors associated with long-term complications, especially in the lung and heart. Furthermore, a local recurrence, either in the breast or on the chest wall, can have devastating consequences for patients. Therefore, one must ensure that an adequate dose has been delivered to appropriate targets to minimize recurrence risk. This chapter presents an overview of the technical aspects of radiation therapy to the breast, chest wall, and regional lymph nodes.

TARGET VOLUME PLANNING

Three important anatomic regions must be considered in target volume definition: (a) the breast or chest wall itself, (b) the internal mammary lymph node region, and (c) the supraclavicular fossa and axilla. Depending on the clinical situation, one, two, or all three volumes need to be treated in a single patient. For purposes of this discussion, however, these volumes are discussed separately.

Intact Breast or Chest Wall

The breast or chest wall is typically defined clinically. Medially, the target volume is extended to the midline, although in some cases it can certainly fall short of the midline by 1 cm or more, depending on the shape of the patient and the amount of underlying lung included in the radiation field (the farther away from midline, the less lung subtended by the deep field edge). Laterally, the field is typically carried to the midaxillary line. In a patient with an intact breast, the end of breast tissue can usually be palpated, and the field can be extended 1 cm beyond this palpable border. In chest wall irradiation, the lateral field edge often must extend beyond the mastectomy scar. Inferiorly, the field comes below the inframammary fold in the intact breast or the contralateral inframammary fold when the chest wall is treated. Superiorly, the field typically extends to the base of the clavicular head. In the case of an intact breast, the superior extent of breast tissue can be palpated, and the field can be extended 1 cm beyond this palpably defined boundary.

Internal Mammary Nodes

The internal mammary lymph nodes are located, along with the internal mammary artery and vein, superior to the pleura and lateral to the sternum. On a computed tomographic (CT) scan (Fig. 1), these vessels can easily be seen to contain contrast material. When treating the internal mammary lymph node chain, one must recognize that lymph nodes in the first three interspaces are more likely to be pathologically involved with tumor than those in the lower interspaces.[1] Thus, these three interspaces typically are marked with a catheter in patients in whom these nodes are to be treated, so that the location of these interspaces is clearly indicated on the CT scan. One can then draw the target volume of the internal mammary nodes quite easily.

Axilla and Supraclavicular Fossa

The supraclavicular target volume lies superior to the upper border of the breast or chest wall field, and the junction of these two target areas is carefully matched, as is discussed in the section Supraclavicular and Axillary Field and Field Matching. Superiorly, the field extends to cover the top of the first rib and may or may not extend beyond the skin of the

A. S. Lichter: Department of Radiation Oncology, University of Michigan Medical School, Ann Arbor, Michigan
L. J. Pierce: Department of Radiation Oncology, University of Michigan Medical School, Ann Arbor, Michigan

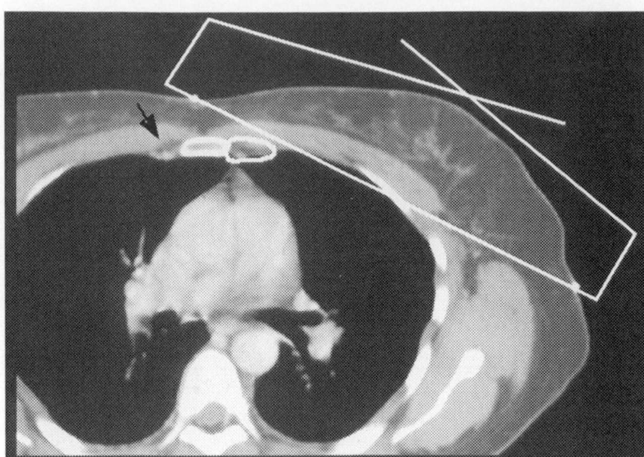

FIG. 1. Cross-sectional computed tomographic (CT) scan illustrating the typical tangent fields and location of the internal mammary nodes. In a contrast-enhanced CT, the internal mammary, artery, and vein can be seen as small white dots lateral to the sternum (see arrow on contralateral side). The internal mammary lymph node volume is outlined next to the sternum on the ipsilateral side. Two catheter dots mark the medial and lateral entrance points for the standard tangent fields designed to treat the breast only in this patient.

supraclavicular fossa, depending on physician preference. Medially, the field extends to the pedicles of the cervical spine. Laterally, the field is relatively narrow if only the supraclavicular nodes and apex of the axilla are treated; its width is extended if the full axilla is to be included. The apex of the axilla corresponds anatomically to the coracoid process, which can easily be seen on a simulator film. When surgical clips mark the boundaries of a full axillary dissection, the superior clip is frequently seen to lie at the point where the first rib crosses the clavicle, and this can be another anatomic marker for the axillary apex. Extending 1 to 2 cm laterally beyond the crossing of the first rib and clavicle or to the coracoid process treats the apex of the axilla, and this area is always included in the supraclavicular field. Typically, this port is 7 to 8 cm wide. If the full axilla is to be treated, the field extends further laterally to split the humeral head.[2]

TECHNIQUES OF TREATMENT

Intact Breast

The breast is treated with a pair of tangential fields that enter and exit through the previously determined medial and lateral borders of breast target volume as defined previously (see Fig. 1). The exact technique of setting up these fields is discussed in the section Simulation Techniques. Several important factors should be noted concerning this tangential pair. First, the deep edges of the field are coplanar. This allows all divergence to be directed into the air above the breast of the patient and not deeper into the lung. This coplanar edge can be achieved by angling the fields a few degrees beyond 180 degrees opposed. Another technique used with modern linear accelerators and asymmetric collimator jaws is to set the isocenter at the deep edge and to half-beam block the field using the asymmetric collimator. Half-beam blocking with a beam splitter is strongly discouraged. These external blocks still transmit 3% to 5% of the incident radiation and contribute an unnecessary dose to the contralateral uninvolved breast.[3,4]

The radiation oncologist should be aware of two important normal tissues within the breast radiation fields—namely, the lung and heart. The amount of lung projected on the tangential field at the central axis correlates reasonably well with the volume of ipsilateral lung irradiated.[5,6] In the authors' experience, if the amount of lung projected at central axis is 2 cm or less, the risk of subsequent radiation pneumonitis is extremely small, less than 1%. For only the rare patient can the medial and lateral field edges not be adjusted so that the amount of lung treated is within this 2-cm desired limit. The amount of heart included in modern radiotherapy treatment fields is quite small. In a study from Scandinavia, fewer than 5% of patients treated with tangential breast fields had heart volumes that would place them at risk for subsequent cardiac damage.[7] A study from Boston showed that left-sided patients followed out to 12 years did not have an incidence of cardiac events greater than that of right-sided patients or greater than expected from an age-matched population.[8] When an undesirable amount of heart is in the field, one can attempt to shape the fields using custom blocks to eliminate some of this heart volume.[9] Such shielding must be done with great care, however, to make sure that meaningful amounts of breast tissue are not also shielded.

Chest Wall

The chest wall can also be treated with tangential fields set up much as for the intact breast. The field borders are the same, and the considerations regarding underlying volume of heart and lung included in the tangential fields are identical. Photon fields exhibit skin sparing, and because the skin is at risk for harboring cancer cells, bolus material must be used to help ensure that the skin receives full dose. The authors typically begin this bolus every other day to produce a brisk erythema over the chest wall by the end of treatment. Because room must exist for this bolus, sufficient flash must be left over the chest wall when tangential photon fields are used to allow the bolus to fit comfortably within the field.

The chest wall is also treated quite satisfactorily using an electron beam. Such treatment can take several different forms. Some radiation oncologists use a single electron field either directly anterior or angled laterally 20 to 30 degrees, thus avoiding the need for field matching. Dosimetry must be performed carefully, however, to make sure that falloff at the edges of the field is not too great. Others use a combination of fields: a direct anterior field with higher energy over the medial portion of the chest wall, especially if the internal mammary nodes are to be treated, matched to a second field over the thinner part of the chest wall as it moves laterally. Care must be taken in abutting these fields so that undue hot or cold spots do not occur.

Internal Mammary Nodes

Although a variety of techniques are available to treat the internal mammary lymph node chain, two techniques have been used that should be discouraged. The first is the use of full tangent fields that are brought across the midline of the patient to try to include the internal mammary lymph node inside the high-dose volume ("deep tangents").[2] When this technique is used, the amount of lung that needs to be included inside the tangential fields to obtain reliable coverage of the internal mammary region is, in general, prohibitive. This technique has largely been abandoned. The second technique is the use of an *en face* internal mammary photon field matched to shallow tangents whose medial entrance point is the lateral border of the internal mammary field.[2] A "cold triangle" of tissue cannot be avoided at the junction of the medial tangent and the anterior internal mammary field, and this is especially significant in the setting of the intact breast. These photon fields also deliver a substantial amount of radiation to the heart, which can later produce an increase in cardiac events, such as myocardial infarction.[10]

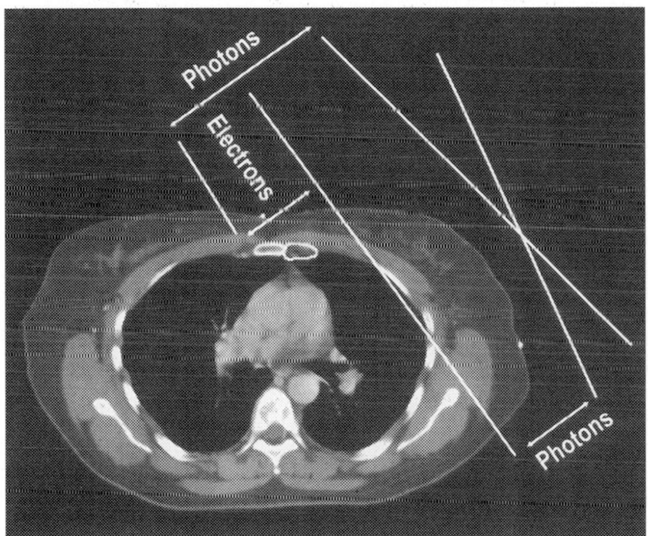

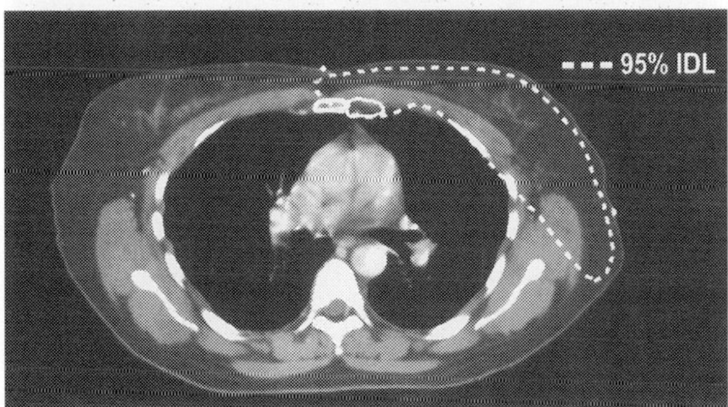

FIG. 2. Technique designed to treat the internal mammary lymph node volume without using deep tangents. A pair of shallow tangents treats the majority of the breast or chest wall. An electron field is angled to match the angle of the medial tangent field. The 95% isodose line (IDL) covers the treatment volume quite adequately.

Because of the deficiencies of deep tangents or of a direct anterior internal mammary field matched to shallow tangents, numerous other techniques have emerged to allow inclusion of the internal mammary nodal volume while treating the chest wall or the intact breast. One technique that is particularly useful is to include the internal mammary region in the medial tangent but not in the lateral tangent, and then to supplement for the missing dose with angled electron fields (Fig. 2).[1,11] In the authors' experience, these treatment techniques can produce satisfactory dose distribution in the majority of patients. One must carefully calculate the amount of lung dose given in these cases so as not to increase the risk

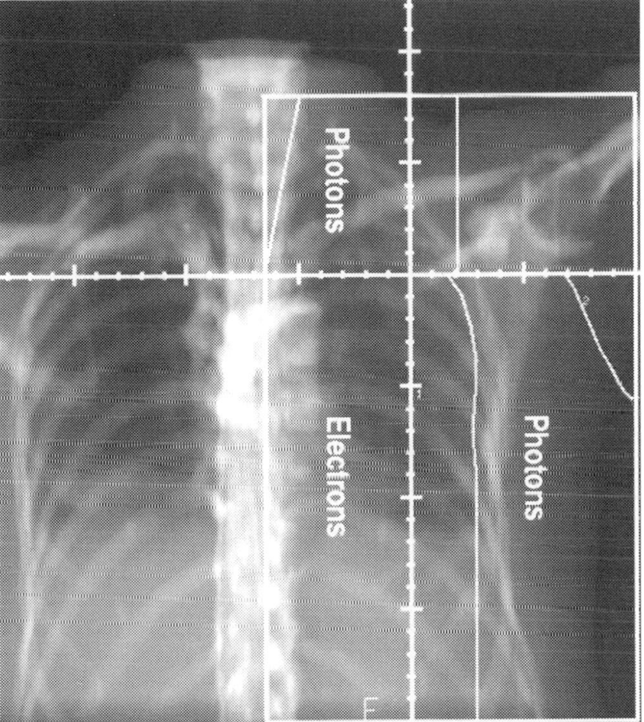

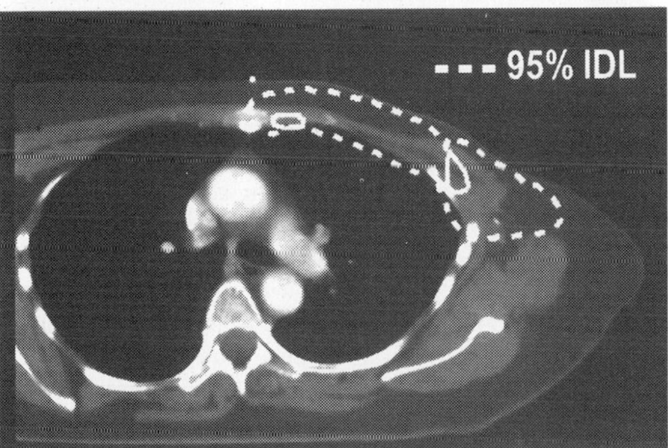

FIG. 3. "Reverse hockey stick" technique to treat the chest wall and internal mammary lymph nodes. A photon beam is used to treat the supraclavicular fossa (with or without the axilla) and the lateral chest wall. The medial chest and internal mammary nodes are treated with an electron beam. The 95% isodose line (IDL) covers the target volume.

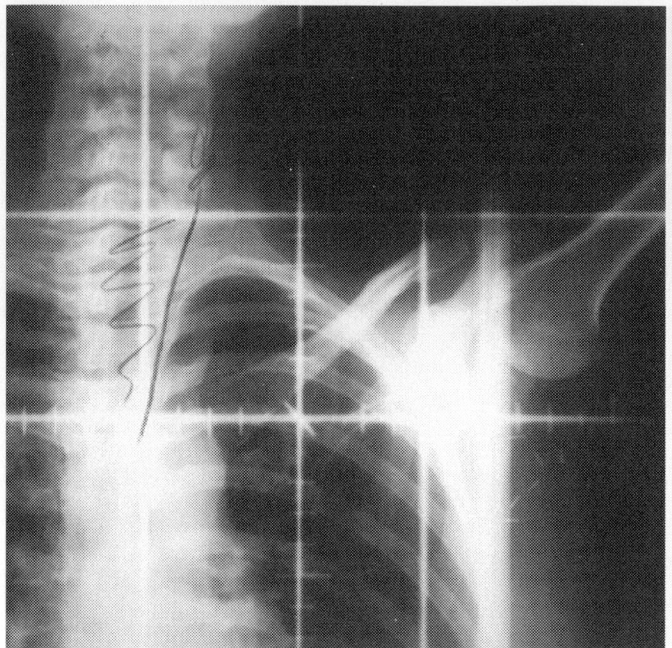

A

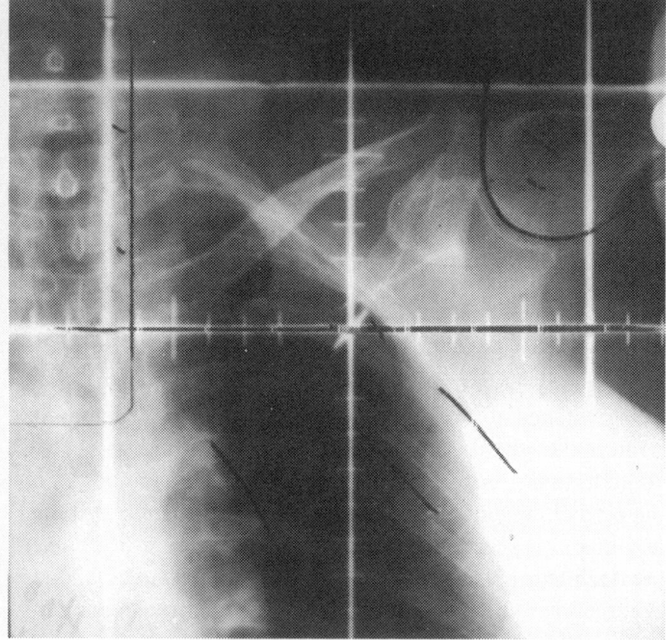

B

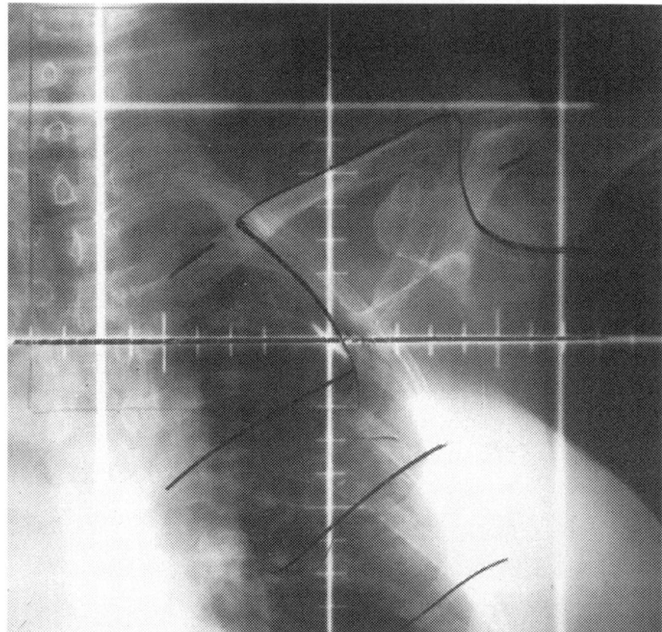

C

FIG. 4. Fields for the treatment of the supraclavicular fossa and axilla. **A:** Anterior field to treat the supraclavicular lymph nodes only. The inferior border of the field matches with the tangent chest wall or breast fields and is half-beam–blocked. Superiorly, the entire first rib is covered. Medially, the field abuts the bony spine. Laterally, the field extends to the coracoid process, beyond the point at which the first rib crosses the clavicle. **B:** Full supraclavicular and axillary field. The field is brought out laterally to include the entire axilla. The humoral head is blocked. **C:** Posterior axillary boost. This field is isocentric with the field in **B**. A block is used to shield the lung, the tissues above the clavicle, and the humoral head.

of radiation pneumonitis. Also, the angled electron field may have to travel a significant distance through tissue to reach the deep aspect of the internal mammary volume, and in some patients, especially those with an intact breast, this depth may require a very high energy electron beam. These cases all require individualized dosimetry plans, preferably using CT-based technology (see the section Dosimetry).

Another technique that is useful for treating the internal mammary nodes in the setting of postmastectomy radiation is what some have referred to as a "reverse hockey stick" technique (Fig. 3). In this technique, anterior or anterior-posterior opposed photon beams are used to treat the lateral chest wall, axilla, and supraclavicular lymph nodes, and the majority of the chest wall is left untreated. Then, an anterior electron beam fills in this area with an electron depth chosen to match the depth of the internal mammary nodes. The electron field includes chest wall laterally that is not as thick, so a bolus is used as a tissue substitute to minimize dose to underlying lung.[12] A technique very similar to this was used by the Danish Breast Cancer Cooperative Group in their large randomized trial showing a survival advantage for postmastectomy chest wall radiation.[13]

Finally, another technique is to treat the chest wall entirely with an electron beam.[14] Although this technique can be quite successful, it must be used with great care. If a single oblique angle is used, then the electron beam approaches the internal mammary nodal volume through an oblique path in tissue, which increases the path length and thus increases the electron energy required. This energy probably is too high for the majority of the chest wall, and thus a bolus must be used to attenuate the beam, or multiple fields with multiple energies must be used. If an anterior direct electron field is used to treat the internal mammary region, then to approach it with the shortest path length, a second electron field of lower energy must be matched to the lateral chest wall; although this can be done, it represents a dosimetric challenge. Finally, the electron beam deposits a very high dose to the superficial skin on a daily basis, and no means are available to modify this dose from day to day. Patients with sensitive skin can develop a brisk skin reaction before the treatment is concluded, making the last few days of treatment extremely uncomfortable. An advantage to using a photon beam is the ability to titrate the application of bolus in response to the patient's individual skin reaction. We thus prefer photon techniques for the chest wall, but we have used electron techniques successfully on selected patients.

Axilla and Supraclavicular Fossa

In virtually every treatment technique, this volume is treated with an anterior photon field. The fields used to treat this volume are illustrated in Fig. 4. When treating the supraclavicular fossa and the apex of the axilla only, the field is typically 7 to 8 cm wide. The recommendation is that the field be angled 10 degrees laterally so the cervical spine is not treated, in case this region needs palliative treatment later in the patient's disease course. When the full axilla needs treatment, the field is extended laterally to include a part of the humeral head. A posterior axillary boost is commonly added, because the supraclavicular nodes are typically dosed to a depth of 3 cm, whereas the average midaxillary depth is in the range of 7 cm. This dose deficiency is made up through the use of a posterior axillary boost, which provides a small amount of treatment daily or two to three times per week.

SIMULATION TECHNIQUES

Starting in the early 1980s, many authors have published reports on a variety of simulation and setup techniques for treating the intact breast.[15–25] All of these techniques are variations that generally incorporate the following four basic principles:

1. Almost all of the techniques are isocentric.
2. All keep the deep edges of the treatment field coplanar, so divergence is directed into air rather than into lung.
3. Most define the deep edge of the field using the primary collimator jaw rather than an external block.
4. All attempt to provide acceptable dosimetry (avoidance of extreme hot or cold spots) at the junction of fields.

Today, breast simulation can be performed in one of two ways: either *actual*, in the simulator, or *virtual*, on a CT-based

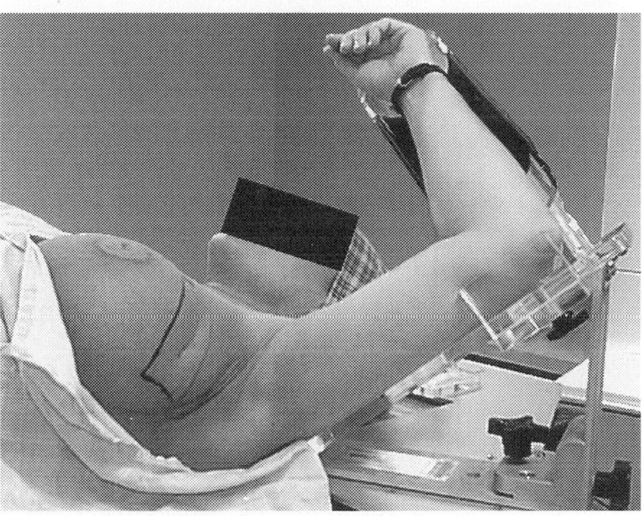

FIG. 5. Patient in an arm board support ready for treatment. The arm is held comfortably in place and is well supported. Many adjustments on the arm board accommodate different flexibilities and range of motion from one patient to the next.

data set. For either technique, providing good immobilization for the patient is critically important. For many years, the authors have used a universal arm board, illustrated in Fig. 5. Although the device is custom made, such devices are now commercially available. The device supports the patient's arm in a reproducible position each day and provides enough flexibility that the board can be customized from patient to patient. The device flips to accommodate right- or left-sided treatments. A major disadvantage of this board, however, is that it does not fit through a standard CT aperture. Thus, when a virtual simulation is performed, the patient is positioned in a customized foam immobilization device with the arm much more elevated, so that the entire torso fits through the scanner, from the top of the supraclavicular fossa all the way through the bottom of the treatment field. We have not changed our standard simulation techniques since the early 1980s, and the technique has been described in some detail in previous publications.[2,17] Briefly, a breast bridge is used to measure the angle relative to vertical of a line that connects the medial and lateral entrance points. At the same time, the spatial separation between these two points is measured. With the aid of a simple computer program, the location of the isocenter within the breast, relative to the entrance point of the medial tangent field, is calculated. This isocenter is then set up using table shifts, starting with the field centered at the appropriate depth over the medial tangent entrance point. The computer program also calculates the medial and lateral gantry angles. Typically, a simulation of a two-field breast treatment (medial and lateral tangent) takes 15 to 20 minutes. The deep edges of the field are made coplanar; a BB-sized dot is placed at the medial entrance point, and short wire at the lateral entrance point. If the setup is done correctly, these two markers should line up with one another, confirming that divergence has been eliminated from the setup. A typical simulator film for our

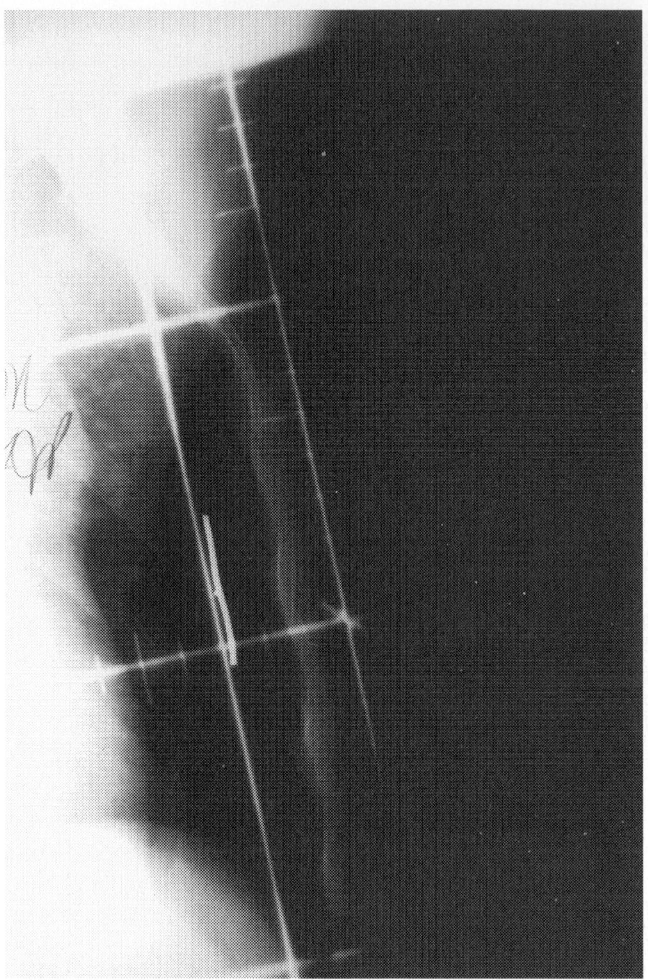

FIG. 6. Typical simulator film for a tangent breast field. The BB dot is on the medial border and the wire is on the lateral border of the field. Note that the deep edge of the tangents includes both of these points, confirming the nondivergent nature of these fields. The collimator is angled to parallel the chest wall.

tangential breast technique is shown in Fig. 6. In the treatment room, daily setup is fast and accurate. After the patient is positioned in the immobilization device, the field center is placed over the medial entrance point on the patient's skin, which is identified by the sole tattoo mark. The appropriate source-skin distance is set. Then the table is shifted laterally by the precalculated amount, and the gantry can be rotated to the medial and lateral gantry angles to deliver the appropriate therapy. Collimator rotation typically is used to make the tangent field parallel to the chest wall. An acceptable alternative is to elevate the patient on a tilt board until the sternum is level and no collimator rotation is required.

Using modern CT technology, many institutions are beginning to use virtual simulation for their breast setup.[26] For this technique, the patient is brought into the department, and an immobilization device is created. The use of radiopaque catheters to clinically mark the borders of the field, scars, and any match line junction, such as the plane in which the tangential fields abut the supraclavicular/axillary field, is extremely helpful. The patient then is taken to the CT scanner, and slices are taken from the top through the bottom of the volume. Three-millimeter slice spacing produces high-resolution digitally reconstructed radiographs; with a modern helical scanner, this entire procedure takes less than 15 minutes. The scan information is then brought up on the treatment-planning console, and one can treat the data set much as one would treat the actual patient in the simulator room. For us, this means calculating the location of the isocenter using the medial and lateral tangent entrance points, calculating the appropriate gantry angles, and then performing the setup on the virtual patient, looking at digitally reconstructed radiographs to confirm that we have the entire target volume inside the field without excessive amounts of lung and heart. Just as in an actual simulation, if the virtual simulation shows that the constraints have not been met, the entrance points of the tangential fields can be varied until one is satisfied with the simulation. A display from our computer screen during a virtual simulation is shown in Fig. 7. Note that the heart is well visualized and that the heart volume can be calculated using CT techniques, a marked advantage over standard simulation. After the patient has been simulated, daily treatment progresses just as with those cases that have had an actual simulation.

Patients with large breast size represent an important challenge. The dosimetry of tangential breast treatment can be quite inhomogeneous as breast size increases (see below), and elevating the breast off the anterior abdominal wall is critically important to avoid an undesirable skin reaction and late long-term telangiectasia and fibrosis. The authors have often used the barrel of a 50-mL syringe placed in the inframammary fold to keep the breast elevated. Others have described a ring device that helps elevate the breast.[27] Still others have advised treating patients with large breast volumes in a prone position.[28] Not only can homogeneity be improved using this technique, but some have also suggested that scatter dose to other tissues is actually reduced by using a prone position.[29] If this technique is used, however, great care must be taken to define target volumes so as not to miss critical tissue, especially if the tumor bed is close to the chest wall.[30]

Simulation techniques for the chest wall are very similar to those for the intact breast. The patient can undergo an actual or a virtual simulation. If tangential photon fields are used, the simulation techniques do not vary from those of the intact breast. Electron fields are typically simulated clinically and can be verified with CT dosimetry (see the section Dosimetry).

When the internal mammary lymph nodes are to be added to the volume, CT-based simulation techniques are extremely valuable. Although the authors have experimented with templated plans that can be used without three-dimensional treatment planning, the variation in body size and shape and the thickness of the chest wall make finding a templated solution to internal mammary lymph node coverage quite challenging. Thus, the authors currently use CT simulation in every

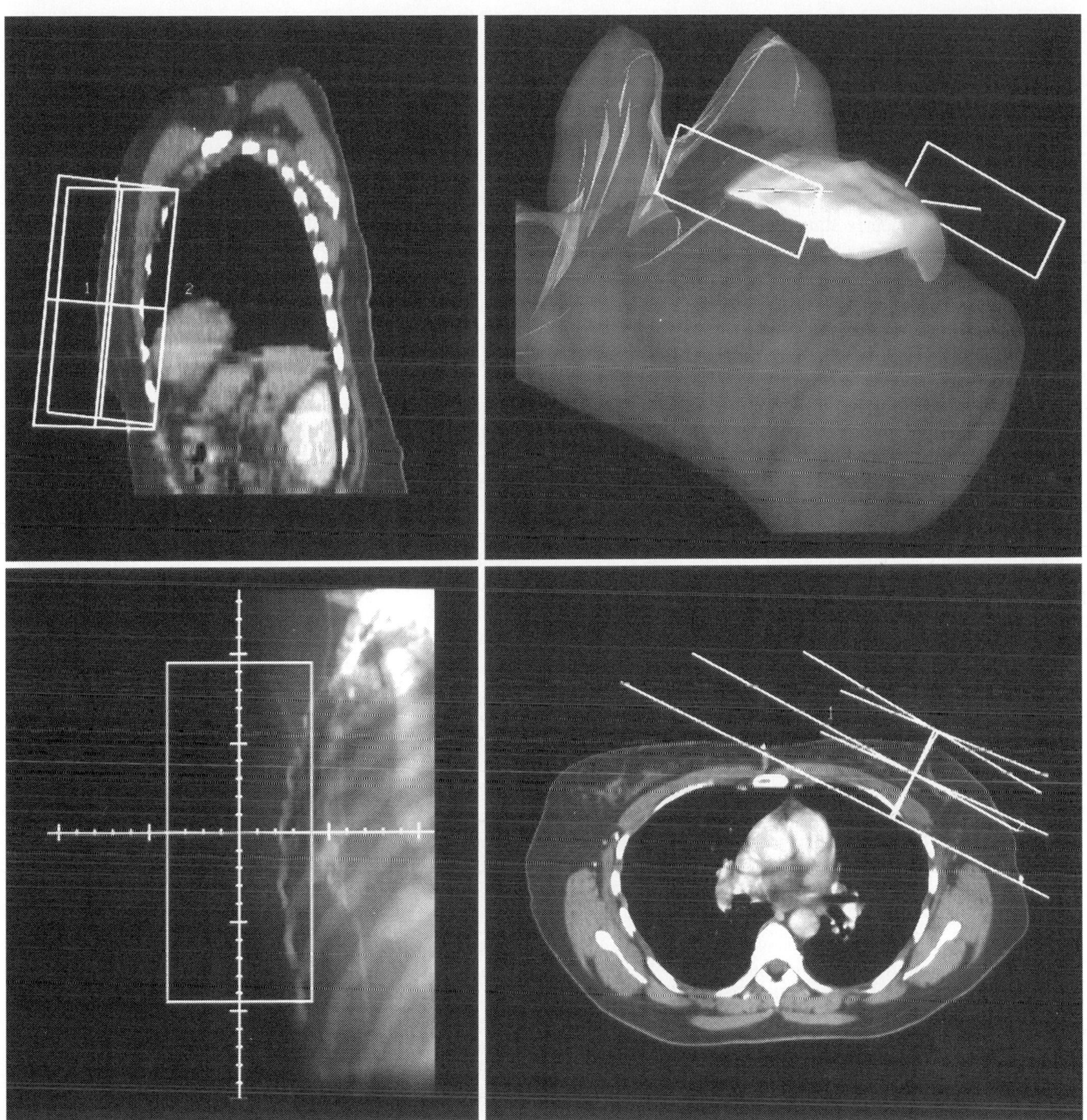

FIG. 7. Typical display for a virtual simulation. At upper left is a sagittal computed tomographic (CT) reconstruction with the projection of the treatment fields. At lower left is a digitally reconstructed radiograph that would mimic a simulator film. At upper right is a three-dimensional view of the target volume with the two tangent fields. At lower right is a standard CT view. Catheters mark the medial and lateral field borders, which have been palpated clinically.

case in which internal mammary lymph node coverage is desired. Our favored setup technique is to treat the internal mammary lymph nodes with a combination of photon and electron beams, with these fields angled to parallel the angle of the tangential breast or chest wall fields. As mentioned previously, however, other techniques, including electron techniques, have been described and can be used quite satisfactorily. We typically attempt to treat only the internal mammary lymph node chain in intercostal spaces 1–3. This allows the internal mammary field to end at or above the level of the heart and can spare cardiac dose, which may reduce long-term complications of treatment.

SUPRACLAVICULAR AND AXILLARY FIELD AND FIELD MATCHING

The location and shape of the supraclavicular and axillary apex field were previously illustrated in Fig. 4. Typically, these fields are set to a depth of 3 cm from the anterior and dosed at that level. They are half-beam–blocked so they do not overlap into the tangential fields, and they are angled 10 degrees away from the spine to avoid unintentional cervical spine irradiation. If the full axilla is to be treated, the dose falloff at the midplane of the axilla often needs to be compensated by use of a posterior axillary boost. Because the prescription depth for the anterior field is at 3 cm and the typical axillary middepth is 7 cm, a 10% to 15% underdose (using 6-mV photons) at this level is easily compensated using the posterior axillary boost field. We typically set up our posterior axillary boost isocentrically with the anterior field, and treating the area on a daily basis is straightforward.

Overlap of the tangential fields into the half-beam–blocked supraclavicular and axillary field must be eliminated to avoid an area of overdosage that can lead to fibrosis at the match line. A number of techniques have been advocated and are successful at avoiding this overlap and matching these fields appropriately.[2] If asymmetric jaws are used to set up not only the supraclavicular field but also the tangential field,[25] then any match line problems are automatically resolved. If a divergent tangential field is used, then some maneuver must be made to eliminate the divergence. If collimator rotation has been used, then a block must be placed at the top of the tangential fields, and the couch angle must be rotated to define an appropriate match. If the patient is treated on a tilt board without collimator rotation, then only rotation of the couch angle is required. Which of the many techniques is used to create an appropriate match line is unimportant. The critical point is that attention be paid to this important aspect of the setup for the intact breast or the postmastectomy chest wall.

DOSIMETRY

Whether the intact breast or the postmastectomy chest wall is being treated, treatment must be individualized to minimize the dosimetric variation that can occur from case to case when standard templated treatment plans are used.[31] Dosimetry can be accomplished using manually derived single-slice contours or in a full three-dimensional mode using multislice CT scans. The authors have used single-slice hand-derived contours for many years. On these contours, we draw the location of the underlying lung, using the tangential breast simulator films along with an anterior and lateral film taken isocentrically.[2] More sophisticated models have been developed to ascertain the shape of the lung from simulator films,[32] but rather straightforward techniques seem to do as well. The reason to take lung density into account in the treatment planning of breast fields has been detailed by Fraass[33] and others.[34] Plans that correct for lung density have fewer hot spots than plans that do not take lung density into account. Furthermore, correction of plans for lung density allows reduction of the amount of tissue compensation performed with wedge filters. Such wedges are responsible for a substantial amount of the dose scattered to the contralateral breast; thus, reducing the amount of wedging has the beneficial side effect of reducing contralateral breast scatter. Many of our patients require only a single 15-degree wedge placed in the lateral beam. Eliminating the use of wedge filters in the medial beam greatly reduces dose to the contralateral breast, and this should be encouraged.[33,35] Just how many institutions use density-corrected plans today is not clear, although the number appears to be growing due to the availability of CT simulation with ready access to density information.

The breast is a complex three-dimensional structure, and central-axis dosimetry does not easily reflect the dose that occurs in other planes that are off the central axis.[35] Areas receiving 10% to 15% more than the isocentric dose are commonly seen, and the situation is even worse as breast size increases.[35,36] Although some have advocated making individual treatment compensators to correct for these areas of excess dose,[37] the authors have not seen major short-term or long-term consequences of treating without a compensator as long as these areas of inhomogeneity are small and lung density correction is used in treatment planning. Of course, if CT simulation is done and one has a full three-dimensional data set to use, one can calculate these off-axis doses with considerable accuracy and determine whether to compensate.

Once we have calculated a treatment plan, we normalize the plan to isocenter and then prescribe to the isodose line that entirely covers the breast tissue. We use wedging and varied beam weighting to try to maximize homogeneity and minimize hot spots.

A variety of single-point methods exist to prescribe breast dose, including 1.5 cm from the deep tangent field, at the chest wall interface, at one-third the height of the breast, and at the midheight of the breast.[38] This creates wide variation in actual doses delivered, although different institutions may quote the same dose prescription in their papers. One must become familiar with a single method of dose prescription and then evaluate the outcome accordingly. Standardization of dose prescription to the breast would be ideal, but such standardization is unlikely to occur in the near future.

After delivering doses of 45 to 50 Gy over 5.0 to 5.5 weeks, most treatment centers deliver a boost to the tumor bed in the intact breast. Whether this treatment is necessary is the subject of vigorous debate and considerable research within the radiation oncology community.

Historically, interstitial implants were used to boost the breast, and such implantation with iridium can be performed either after the completion of all external beam therapy or at the time of the lumpectomy to allow for direct visualization of the tumor bed. In general, relatively few institutions continue to use interstitial implants; the use of an electron beam boost has generally become the method of choice. However, renewed interest has been seen in the use of interstitial radiation as the sole treatment for selected patients with breast cancer, and early results with this therapy are encouraging.[39,40]

For delivery of the electron boost to be most effective, identification of the tumor bed with surgical clips at the time of lumpectomy is recommended.[41,42] This is the best way to minimize error in placement of the boost, because the surgical scar does not always correspond to the area of tumor removal. The use of surgical clips also minimizes errors when choosing the depth of the electron beam to be used. Others have used ultrasonography to help define the tumor bed.[43] Another method is the use of CT scans,[44] the technique the authors now favor. If the patient's treatment has not been planned using CT, the authors usually get a limited number of CT slices through the potential tumor bed. Use of CT helps to determine the shape of the field and the depth of the tumor bed for proper electron dosimetry. The typical electron boost dose used by the authors is 14 Gy, which, when added to the 46 Gy delivered to the whole breast, results in a final tumor bed dose of 60 Gy. In patients with focally positive margins (in the absence of an extensive intraductal component) or with an extensive intraductal component and negative margins, a 20-Gy boost is typically given, for a total dose of 66 Gy to the tumor bed.

When the chest wall is treated after mastectomy, a boost is not necessary in routine cases. A dose of 50 Gy in 25 treatments over 5 weeks eliminates the overwhelming majority of recurrences. In patients with positive margins after mastectomy, stage III disease, or a resected chest wall recurrence with negative margins, a 10-Gy boost is generally delivered to the recurrence area or to the mastectomy scar. In patients who have gross residual disease on the chest wall, doses of 70 Gy or more are often required for optimum tumor control.

REFERENCES

1. Marks LB, Hebert ME, Bentel G, Spencer DP, Sherouse GW, Prosnitz LR. To treat or not to treat the internal mammary nodes: a possible compromise. *Int J Radiat Oncol Biol Phys* 1994;29:903.
2. Lichter AS, Fraass BA, Yanke B. Treatment techniques in the conservative management of breast cancer. *Semin Radiat Oncol* 1992;2:94.
3. Fraass BA, Roberson PL, Lichter AS. Dose to the contralateral breast due to primary breast irradiation. *Int J Radiat Oncol Biol Phys* 1985;11:485.
4. Kelly CA, Wang XY, Chu JC, Hartsell WF. Dose to contralateral breast: a comparison of four primary breast irradiation techniques. *Int J Radiat Oncol Biol Phys* 1996;34:727.
5. Bornstein BA, Cheng CW, Rhodes LM, et al. Can simulation measurements be used to predict the irradiated lung volume in the tangential fields in patients treated for breast cancer? *Int J Radiat Oncol Biol Phys* 1990;18:181.
6. Neal AJ, Yarnold JR. Estimating the volume of lung irradiated during tangential breast irradiation using the central lung distance. *Br J Radiol* 1995;68:1004.
7. Rutqvist LE, Liedberg A, Hammar N, Dalberg K. Myocardial infarction among women with early-stage breast cancer treated with conservative surgery and breast irradiation. *Int J Radiat Oncol Biol Phys* 1998;40:359.
8. Nixon AJ, Manola J, Gelman R, et al. No long-term increase in cardiac-related mortality after breast-conserving surgery and radiation therapy using modern techniques. *J Clin Oncol* 1998;16:1374.
9. Hartsell WF, Murthy AK, Kiel KD, Kao M, Hendrickson FR. Technique for breast irradiation using custom blocks conforming to the chest wall contour. *Int J Radiat Oncol Biol Phys* 1990;19:189.
10. Cuzick J, Stewart H, Rutqvist L, et al. Cause-specific mortality in long-term survivors of breast cancer who participated in trials of radiotherapy. *J Clin Oncol* 1994;12:447.
11. Kuske RR. Adjuvant chest wall and nodal irradiation: maximize cure, minimize late cardiac toxicity. *J Clin Oncol* 1998;16:2579.
12. Steeves RA, Thomadsen BR, Hansen H, Phromratanapongse P, Paliwal BR. A practical alternative to conventional five-field irradiation postmastectomy for locally advanced breast cancer. *Med Dosim* 1994;19:135.
13. Overgaard M, Christensen JJ, Johansen H, et al. Postmastectomy irradiation in high-risk breast cancer patients: present status of the Danish Breast Cancer Cooperative Group trials. *Acta Oncologica* 1998;27:707.
14. Gaffney DK, Prows J, Leavitt DD, Egger MJ, Morgan JG, Stewart JR. Electron arc irradiation of the postmastectomy chest wall: clinical results. *Radiother Oncol* 1997;42:17.
15. Siddon RL, Buck BA, Harris JR, Svensson GK. Three-field technique for breast irradiation using tangential field corner blocks. *Int J Radiat Oncol Biol Phys* 1983;9:583.
16. Svensson GK, Bjarngard BE, Larsen RD, Levene MB. A modified three-field technique for breast treatment. *Int J Radiat Oncol Biol Phys* 1980;6:689.
17. Lichter AS, Fraass BA, van de Geijn J, Padikal TN. A technique for field matching in primary breast irradiation. *Int J Radiat Oncol Biol Phys* 1983;9:263.
18. Podgorsak EB, Gosselin M, Kim TH, Freeman CR. A simple isocentric technique for irradiation of the breast, chest wall and peripheral lymphatics. *Br J Radiol* 1984;57:57.
19. Chu JC, Solin LJ, Hwang CC, Fowble B, Hanks GE, Goodman RL. A nondivergent three field matching technique for breast irradiation. *Int J Radiat Oncol Biol Phys* 1990;19:1037.
20. Conte G, Nascimben O, Turcato G, et al. Three field isocentric technique for breast irradiation using individualized shielding blocks. *Int J Radiat Oncol Biol Phys* 1988;14:1299.
21. Lebesque JV. Field matching in breast irradiation: an exact solution to a geometrical problem. *Radiother Oncol* 1986;5:47.
22. Galvin JM, Powlis W, Fowble B, Goodman RL. A new technique for positioning tangential fields. *Int J Radiat Oncol Biol Phys* 1993;26:877.
23. Rosenow UF, Valentine ES, Davis LW. A technique for treating local breast cancer using a single set-up point and asymmetric collimation. *Int J Radiat Oncol Biol Phys* 1990;19:183.
24. Marshall MG. Three-field isocentric breast irradiation using asymmetric jaws and a tilt board. *Radiother Oncol* 1993;28:228.
25. Klein EE, Taylor M, Michaletz-Lorenz M, Zoeller D, Zoeller D, Umfleet W. A mono isocentric technique for breast and regional nodal therapy using dual asymmetric jaws. *Int J Radiat Oncol Biol Phys* 1994:28:753.
26. Butker EK, Helton DJ, Keller JW, Hughes LL, Crenshaw T, Davis LW. A totally integrated simulation technique for three-field breast treatment using a CT simulator. *Med Phys* 1996;23:1809.
27. Bentel GC, Marks LB. A simple device to position large/flaccid breasts during tangential breast irradiation. *Int J Radiat Oncol Biol Phys* 1994;29:879.
28. Merchant TE, McCormick B. Prone position breast irradiation. *Int J Radiat Oncol Biol Phys* 1994;30:197.
29. Bieri S, Russo M, Rouzaud M, Kurtz JM. Influence of modifications in breast irradiation technique on dose outside the treatment volume. *Int J Radiat Oncol Biol Phys* 1997;38:117.
30. Algan O, Fowble B, McNeeley S, Fein D. Use of the prone position in radiation treatment for women with early stage breast cancer. *Int J Radiat Oncol Biol Phys* 1998;40:1137.
31. Dunlap B, Olch A, Wollin M, Kagan AR. The need for individualized dosimetry for tangential breast treatment. *Med Dosim* 1997;22:315.
32. Chen W, Chu JC, Griem K, Hartsell WF, Saxena VS. Using simulation data to predict lung geometry for inhomogeneity corrections in breast cancer treatments. *Int J Radiat Oncol Biol Phys* 1995;33:683.
33. Fraass BA, Lichter AS, McShan DL, et al. The influence of lung density corrections on treatment planning for primary breast cancer. *Int J Radiat Oncol Biol Phys* 1988;14:179.
34. Mijnheer BJ, Heukelom S, Lanson JH, van Battum LJ, van Bree NA, van Tienhoven G. Should inhomogeneity corrections be applied during

treatment planning of tangential breast irradiation? *Radiother Oncol* 1991;22:239.
35. Buchholz TA, Gurgoze E, Bice WS, Prestidge BR. Dosimetric analysis of intact breast irradiation in off-axis planes. *Int J Radiat Oncol Biol Phys* 1997;39:261.
36. Neal AJ, Torr M, Helyer S, Yarnold JR. Correlation of breast dose heterogeneity with breast size using 3D CT planning and dose-volume histograms. *Radiother Oncol* 1995;34:210.
37. Neal AJ, Mayles WP, Yarnold JR. Invited review: tangential breast irradiation—rationale and methods for improving dosimetry. *Br J Radiol* 1994;67:1149.
38. Das IJ, Cheng CW, Fein DA, Fowble B. Patterns of dose variability in radiation prescription of breast cancer. *Radiother Oncol* 1997;44:83.
39. Vicini FA, Chen PY, Fraile M, et al. Low-dose-rate brachytherapy as the sole radiation modality in the management of patients with early-stage breast cancer treated with breast-conserving therapy: preliminary results of a pilot trial. *Int J Radiat Oncol Biol Phys* 1997;38:301.
40. Kuske RR, Bolton JS, McKinnon WMP, Scroggins TG, Zakris EL, Wilenzick RW. 5-year results of a prospective phase II trial of wide-volume brachytherapy as the sole method of breast irradiation in Tis, T_1, T_2, N_{o-1} breast cancer. *Int J Radiat Oncol Biol Phys* 1998;181: 113(abst).
41. Hunter MA, McFall TA, Hehr KA. Breast-conserving surgery for primary breast cancer: necessity for surgical clips to define the tumor bed for radiation planning. *Radiology* 1996;200:281.
42. Harrington KJ, Harrison M, Bayle P, et al. Surgical clips in planning the electron boost in breast cancer: a qualitative and quantitative evaluation. *Int J Radiat Oncol Biol Phys* 1996;34:579.
43. DeBiose DA, Horwitz EM, Martinez AA, et al. The use of ultrasonography in the localization of the lumpectomy cavity for the interstitial brachytherapy of the breast. *Int J Radiat Oncol Biol Phys* 1997;38:755.
44. Messer PM, Kirikuta IC, Bratengeier K, Flentje M. CT planning of boost irradiation in radiotherapy of breast cancer after conservative surgery. *Radiother Oncol* 1997;42:239.

Diseases of the Breast, 2nd ed.,
edited by Jay R. Harris.
Lippincott Williams & Wilkins, Philadelphia © 2000.

CHAPTER 37

Adjuvant Systemic Therapy of Primary Breast Cancer

C. Kent Osborne and Peter M. Ravdin

Adjuvant systemic therapy is defined as the administration of cytotoxic chemotherapy or the use of ablative or additive endocrine therapy after primary surgery of breast cancer to kill or inhibit clinically occult micrometastases. Death from breast cancer results from growth of micrometastases that are present at distant sites beyond the confines of the surgically resected breast and regional lymphatics. These metastases, which are rarely clinically evident at the time of diagnosis, account for the high treatment failure rate in breast cancer patients treated only with local modalities, such as surgery and irradiation.

HISTORICAL PERSPECTIVE AND RATIONALE FOR ADJUVANT THERAPY

In the late 1800s, Halsted devised the radical mastectomy for breast cancer treatment based on his belief that the disease usually spreads slowly, metastasizing under the skin, along fascial planes, and by lymphatics, but not hematogenously. He thought that the cancer remained localized and confined for a time in the breast and in regional lymph nodes, which served as barriers to distant migration. *En bloc* removal of all these tissues (radical mastectomy) should thus increase curability of the disease. Only 12% of patients treated by Halsted and his students survived 10 years, however, and later attempts to perform even more radical surgery failed to improve survival, leading to the conclusion that distant metastases were already present in many patients by the time of the initial diagnosis.[1,2]

More recent surgical studies, completed in an era when patients were diagnosed earlier with smaller tumors, provided more encouraging results from radical mastectomy, with 50% of all patients remaining disease free at 10 years. Still, 30% of node-negative patients and 75% of node-positive patients eventually have recurrences and die of their disease when it is treated by surgery alone.[2] The recognition that patients with breast cancer have a relatively poor prognosis despite radical surgery had two major clinical implications. First, it was hypothesized that less disfiguring breast surgical procedures would improve cosmesis and quality of life (QOL) without jeopardizing survival, which is predetermined by the presence or absence of micrometastases. Second, improvements in breast cancer survival would require better methods to diagnose the disease in its premetastatic phase or methods of effective systemic therapy to eradicate micrometastases at the time of diagnosis of the primary tumor, when the number of metastatic foci is smallest. In the 1950s, the paradigm for adjuvant systemic therapy was established by studies in preclinical animal models demonstrating curability of cancer with a combined treatment approach of surgical resection and chemotherapy.[3,4] Later, investigators recognized that early administration of chemotherapy in animal models, when the tumor burden was low and when growth kinetics were most favorable, could eradicate cancers that became incurable when treatment was delayed.[5]

Historically, the first randomized trial of breast cancer adjuvant therapy, initiated in 1948 (in fact, one of the first randomized trials of any sort), involved ovarian ablation by irradiation.[6] This study was based on earlier observations that ovarian ablation could induce regressions of advanced breast cancer in premenopausal patients. Accrual to the first chemotherapy adjuvant study was begun in 1958. This study and other early adjuvant trials were designed on the premise that breast cancer metastases were caused by surgical manipulation of the tumor, which "seeded" the bloodstream, a hypothesis supported by experimental observations.[7–10]

Contemporary adjuvant chemotherapy trials, in which prolonged postoperative treatment was used to inhibit established micrometastases, were begun in the late 1960s and early 1970s. Initial studies focused on patients with axillary

C. K. Osborne: Breast Center, Baylor College of Medicine, Houston, Texas
P. M. Ravdin: Department of Medical Oncology, University of Texas Health Science Center at San Antonio, San Antonio, Texas

lymph node metastases in the mastectomy specimen; such patients have a high risk of disease recurrence, justifying the use of potentially toxic therapy. Trials using a new endocrine therapy, the antiestrogen tamoxifen, were initiated in the mid-1970s. The 1980s brought studies of doxorubicin-based chemotherapy regimens, clinical trials of adjuvant therapy in patients without axillary nodal involvement, studies of combined chemoendocrine therapy, and a renewed interest in ovarian ablation using the new luteinizing hormone–releasing hormone antagonists. The 1990s has been the decade for studies of chemotherapy dose intensity, including trials of extremely high-dose chemotherapy with autologous bone marrow transplantation, studies of preoperative (neoadjuvant) chemotherapy, and trials evaluating the introduction of taxanes into adjuvant programs.

More than 100 randomized clinical trials of breast cancer adjuvant therapy have now been completed. Many of these studies have more than 15 to 20 years of patient follow-up, and definitive conclusions about the value of treatment in different patient subsets can be drawn. Although many questions remain, it is clear that appropriately administered adjuvant treatment improves disease-free and overall survival (OS) of patients with early-stage disease.

INTERPRETATION OF ADJUVANT CLINICAL TRIAL RESULTS

An understanding by the clinician of the various methods of analysis of clinical trials of adjuvant therapy is crucial for proper data interpretation and for accurate estimation of treatment benefit. Such estimates provide critical information for the patient and physician in making clinical treatment decisions. (See Chapter 74 for a more detailed discussion.)

Randomized Adjuvant Therapy Trials

Progress in the adjuvant therapy of breast cancer comes from randomized, controlled clinical studies. Uncontrolled or historically controlled trials are acceptable only for testing the safety of new regimens and for generating hypotheses, but large randomized studies are mandatory for definitive information on safety and efficacy of a new treatment approach, especially when the difference in treatment outcome is small. As an example, three-drug chemotherapy combined with bacillus Calmette-Guérin (BCG) immunotherapy was promoted as effective adjuvant therapy for breast cancer in the late 1970s, based on a retrospective comparison of treated patients to a historical control population that did not receive adjuvant therapy.[11] These data generated a series of randomized trials that eventually concluded that not only was BCG immunotherapy ineffective, but its addition to chemotherapy resulted in increased mortality.[12]

Thus, the major contribution of randomized trials is to correct false-positive results produced by nonrandomized trials. Many randomized trials of adjuvant therapy for breast cancer are inadequate and inconclusive, however, because of their small size. Such trials may produce false-negative results (a study shows "no difference" between the two treatments tested when a true difference exists) if the study population is not large enough. Several individual randomized trials failed to show a statistically significant survival benefit for chemotherapy in postmenopausal patients or for tamoxifen in lymph node–negative patients. In contrast, later meta-analyses of these studies clearly demonstrated a small but worthwhile mortality reduction with these therapies. The potential problems inherent in small randomized trials are magnified by the need to examine major patient subsets (e.g., menopausal status, nodal status), a need that further reduces the statistical power to detect treatment differences.

Trial End Points

Disease-free survival (*DFS*), defined as the time from randomization to first evidence of treatment failure or death, and *OS*, defined as the time from randomization to death from any cause, are the major end points of interest in most randomized adjuvant treatment trials. Distant DFS is the time from randomization to first evidence of treatment failure outside the primary disease site or death from any cause. Breast cancer–specific DFS or OS is used less commonly, because deaths from other causes are potentially related in some way to the disease itself or its treatment. OS is probably the most important efficacy end point in adjuvant therapy trials; however, it is influenced not only by the impact of the adjuvant therapy but also by treatment given after relapse, which is usually not standardized in clinical trials. OS is also influenced by deaths from other causes, which can be a major factor in an elderly population. DFS focuses on the efficacy of the primary disease treatment, but it ignores what happens to the patient after disease recurrence, which might be influenced by the adjuvant treatment received. Thus, although adjuvant treatments that prolong DFS might also be expected to prolong OS, this might not occur if the adjuvant treatment decreases response to treatments given after relapse, resulting in shorter postrelapse survival. Similarly, prolongation of DFS or OS by adjuvant treatment does not necessarily indicate that any patients are cured or that they will not relapse or die from breast cancer during their expected lifetime. Disease recurrence or mortality may simply be delayed by some period of time that, if long enough, may still justify the toxicity and cost of treatment. Although substantial prolongations in DFS and OS have been observed with adjuvant therapy of breast cancer, whether these treatments are curative in any patients is still uncertain. This point becomes less important if patients survive long enough to die of other causes before relapse of breast cancer.

The results from randomized clinical trials are frequently depicted by Kaplan-Meier life-table plots, in which the proportion of patients who remain disease free or alive is shown

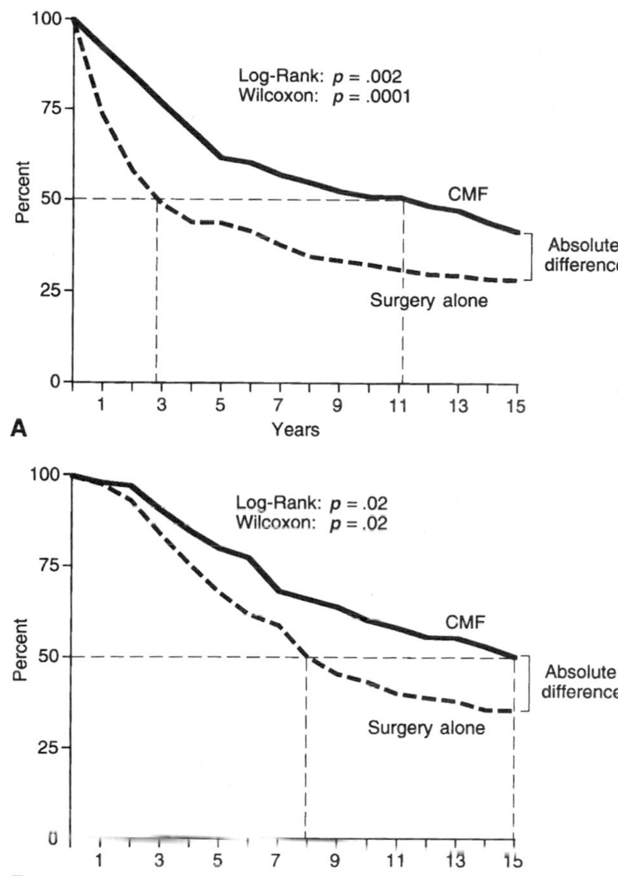

FIG. 1. Kaplan-Meier plot of relapse-free survival **(A)** and overall survival **(B)** in premenopausal patients in the first Milan study of adjuvant CMF (cyclophosphamide, methotrexate, 5-fluorouracil). (From ref. 13, with permission.)

TABLE 1. *Absolute reduction in mortality at 10 years per 100 patients treated*

Estimated 10-yr death rate with no therapy	Hypothetical proportional reduction in mortality due to treatment				
	50%	40%	30%	20%	10%
70% (several positive nodes)	25	19	13	8	4
50% (5-cm tumor, negative nodes)	21	16	12	7	4
30% (average tumor diameter, negative nodes)	14	11	8	5	3
10% (≤1-cm tumor, negative nodes)	5	4	3	2	1

as a function of the time after randomization (Fig. 1). Results are sometimes also presented as a *hazard function*, defined as the risk of failure per unit time. In comparing two treatment groups, the hazard ratio is the ratio of the hazard function of the control group to that of the experimental treatment group; therefore, when the ratio is close to one, no difference in efficacy exists between the two groups. A hazard ratio greater than one indicates a higher relapse or death rate in the control group, whereas a ratio less than one indicates more untoward events in the experimental group. Although these numbers are useful in interpreting quantitative differences between two treatment groups, they provide little useful information to the physician or patient trying to make a treatment decision.

Closer examination of life-table plots can produce clinically useful information (see Fig. 1). A common method of analyzing such plots is to calculate the absolute difference between the two treatment groups at a defined point in time. To be most accurate, the chosen point in time should be equal to or shorter than the median follow-up time of all patients in the study. Figure 1 shows the long-term relapse-free survival and OS of premenopausal women enrolled in one of the first randomized trials of adjuvant combination chemotherapy in axillary lymph node–positive women.[13] At 15 years of follow-up (an appropriate time, given that all the patients in the study had been followed for more than 15 years), approximately 42% of patients receiving cyclophosphamide, methotrexate, 5-fluorouracil (CMF) therapy after surgery remained relapse free, and 50% remained alive, compared with 28% and 35%, respectively, of control patients. Thus, the difference in relapse-free survival is 14%, and the difference in OS is 15%. This difference is defined as the absolute benefit or the number of recurrences or deaths avoided (in this case, at 15 years) per 100 women treated. Some investigators report results in terms of the proportional benefit or the average annual percentage reduction in the odds of recurrence or death. In the study shown in Fig. 1, 65% of the group of patients treated by surgery alone had died by 15 years, whereas only 50% of CMF-treated patients had died. These results correspond roughly to a 30% to 35% proportional reduction in the annual odds of death with adjuvant CMF therapy.

Physicians must understand the difference between absolute benefit (15% in the example above) and proportional benefit (30% to 35%) in discussing treatment options with patients. This is especially important in patients with a lower risk of recurrence. Table 1 shows the number of deaths avoided per 100 patients treated in several hypothetical subsets of patients with markedly different estimated 10-year death rates (range, 10% to 70%) without adjuvant treatment as a function of different estimates of treatment benefit shown as proportional reductions in mortality if they did receive treatment. The calculations assume exponential death with a constant hazard ratio and do not consider deaths from other causes, which can be significant in older patients. Approximately 13 of every 100 patients treated in the poorest risk group benefited at 10 years because of the treatment, given a 30% proportional reduction in mortality by the adjuvant therapy. These data are similar to the results obtained in the Milan CMF trial in premenopausal patients described earlier (see Fig. 1). In contrast, only 3 of every 100 patients treated in the best prognostic group benefited at 10 years from the same treatment; most of the patients in this group failed to benefit because they were already cured by surgery and could not possibly benefit from adjuvant treatment. The absolute benefit would be greater if treatment provided a greater proportional reduction in mortality, but reductions in the 40% to 50% range have not been observed consistently with current chemotherapy regimens. In patients with high tumor estrogen-receptor (ER) levels, 5 years of adjuvant tamoxifen provided annual reductions in recurrence of 50% to 60%, although deaths were reduced by only one-third (see the section Adjuvant Therapy with Tamoxifen). Proportional reductions in mortality in the 10% to 15% range, typical of the effects of adjuvant chemotherapy in older women, lead to still lower absolute benefits.

Although the absolute benefit is perhaps the most important and simplest parameter in helping patients make treatment decisions, it underestimates the true value of adjuvant therapy. In Fig. 1, one might incorrectly assume that only 15 patients benefited out of every 100 patients treated with CMF. However, other patients who had already died by year 15 might have had a substantial delay in their death by treatment. An alternative method of evaluating the benefits of therapy is to calculate the difference in median DFS or OS. In the CMF study, the median times to recurrence and median survival were approximately 3 and 8 years, respectively, in the control group, compared with 11 and 15 years in the group treated with chemotherapy (see Fig. 1). Thus, although many patients eventually had recurrences and died despite receiving 1 year of CMF chemotherapy, they still benefited substantially in terms of a prolonged time to recurrence and death.

Two other cautions need to be considered in the interpretation of randomized trials. Small trials can produce not only false-negative results because of insufficient statistical power but also false-positive results simply by the play of chance. Trials that produce positive results are more likely to be published in widely read journals, whereas negative studies may be relegated to more obscure journals or are not published at all. This publication bias may influence medical practice for years, until subsequent trials fail to confirm results. As an example, the initial report of the first Milan CMF trial showed equally promising results in premenopausal and postmenopausal patients, and these results led to widespread use of this regimen in both subsets.[14] Later analyses of this study failed to show a benefit in postmenopausal patients, and subsequent analyses of multiple studies have established that the benefit of chemotherapy in these women is much less than in younger patients.

Another hazard in the reporting of randomized trials is multiple-subset analysis. Most trials report treatment differences in numerous subsets of patients categorized by nodal status, menopausal status, receptor status, and so forth. Analysis of multiple subsets is bound to yield a misleadingly positive result simply by statistical chance, even if a true treatment difference does not exist. Subset analyses, unless taken into consideration in the original statistical design of a study, can only be used to generate new hypotheses, and they do not usually provide conclusive information.

Treatment Toxicity and Quality of Life

Treatment side effects, long-term toxicities, and their impact on patient QOL are additional important gauges of the efficacy of adjuvant treatment. Patients' side effects recorded by a nurse or physician, although providing important information, frequently underestimate the incidence or severity of various toxicities, because these parameters are not sought in a formal, prospective fashion in some trials, especially those performed many years ago. Furthermore, these estimates represent physicians' estimates of severity rather than the patient's, and they tend to focus on laboratory values or purely physical parameters rather than on more subjective evidence of morbidity affecting the patient's lifestyle. An accurate portrayal of the adverse effects of treatment is necessary when comparing the overall efficacy of two treatments that happen to provide similar mortality reductions. An accurate toxicity profile is also mandatory for women to make an informed decision about adjuvant therapy, especially patients with a low risk of disease recurrence when the toxicity-benefit ratio may be close to one.

QOL studies using questionnaires administered to patients during and after adjuvant therapy have confirmed the feasibility of such studies, and some randomized trials now include QOL end points.[15–18] Although DFS and OS are commonly considered the most important end points, for adjuvant regimens with nearly equal efficacy, QOL during and particularly after adjuvant therapy can help to determine treatment selection.

An interesting QOL assessment tool developed by the International Breast Cancer Study Group is known as *Q-TWiST* (QOL-adjusted analysis of time without symptoms and toxicity).[19] This modified survival analysis calculates adjusted survival time, after subtracting from OS the time during which the patient was experiencing treatment-related toxicity, the time needed to recover from treatment given for local recurrence, and the survival period after a systemic relapse of disease. Thus, Q-TWiST incorporates treatment effectiveness and morbidity into a single parameter. An analysis using the Q-TWiST method of the possible advantage for chemoendocrine therapy compared with endocrine therapy alone in postmenopausal patients concluded that there was no net benefit for tamoxifen plus chemotherapy over tamoxifen alone in quality-adjusted years for the average patient participating in these trials.[20] Although this conclusion is somewhat controversial in that it is highly dependent on the QOL estimates for different disease and toxicity states, it highlights areas in which additional research may have particular value.

Meta-Analyses

Given the more than 100 randomized, prospective, adjuvant therapy breast cancer trials that have been reported, solely on the basis of chance some of these trials are likely to be misleadingly promising, whereas others may be misleadingly negative. Furthermore, many individual studies are far too small to detect modest but worthwhile treatment benefits that would have major public health implications given the high incidence of breast cancer.

One method of overcoming these pitfalls is the overview, or meta-analysis, technique. In general, this approach uses information from all trials addressing the same question (i.e., adjuvant tamoxifen versus no adjuvant tamoxifen) by calculating the annual difference between the number of observed recurrences or deaths in the treatment group and the number expected if the events in the treatment group and control group were the same.[12] The values of observed events minus expected events from each trial can be added together to give an overall effect. Large trials with longer follow-up and more events have more weight than small trials. The large numbers of patients contributed by all individual trials provide great statistical power and enable meta-analyses to detect reliably modest advantages for one treatment over another and, thus, to correct false-negative results produced by small randomized trials.

Even meta-analyses, however, have potential problems. For instance, the meta-analysis for adjuvant chemotherapy of breast cancer is likely to be an underestimate of the actual benefit achievable in a compliant patient population given the best drug regimen, because the analysis combines the results of studies using a variety of different chemotherapy regimens with various drug doses and schedules, some of which must be more or less effective than others. Overview results of the tamoxifen or ovarian ablation trials are likely to be more accurate, because compliance and differences in the treatment administered are not an issue. Nevertheless, the meta-analysis of breast cancer adjuvant therapy has contributed substantially to our current medical practice patterns by providing more certain evidence of the efficacy of adjuvant therapy, by resolving controversies originating in previously conflicting results, and by generating testable hypotheses for future studies. Data from the breast cancer meta-analyses are used extensively in this chapter to emphasize certain points.

EVIDENCE FOR THE EFFECTIVENESS OF ADJUVANT CHEMOTHERAPY

Overall Results

Randomized trials of prolonged, postoperative adjuvant chemotherapy were first initiated in the 1970s. The early trials focused on patients with positive axillary lymph nodes, because the high risk of recurrence and death (75% overall at 10 years) of these patients was thought to justify the use of potentially toxic chemotherapy. Based on estimates derived from animal studies and mathematical models, as well as a certain degree of empiricism, most early studies used 1 to 2 years of adjuvant treatment. Most trials were small, accruing fewer than 500 patients.

Studies of adjuvant chemotherapy proceeded in a logical series of experiments. First, patients who received one-drug or multiple-drug regimens were compared with those given placebo or with a no-treatment control group. Multiple-drug regimens were then compared with single-drug regimens, and shorter durations of treatment were compared with longer durations. Later trials evaluated doxorubicin-based regimens or compared combination chemoendocrine therapy with each modality used alone. Very recent trials compare dose-intensive chemotherapy with conventional regimens.

Two adjuvant chemotherapy studies, begun in 1972 and 1973, had the most impact on changing the patterns of care for patients with breast cancer.[14,21] A study of 349 node-positive patients performed by the National Surgical Adjuvant Breast and Bowel Project (NSABP) compared 2 years of single-agent melphalan with placebo, and a similar study of 386 patients carried out at the Instituto Nazionale Tumori in Milan, Italy, compared a group of patients given a regimen of CMF for 1 year with a group of patients treated with surgery alone. Both studies showed an overall statistically significant DFS advantage for chemotherapy; a trend for improved OS was also evident in both studies, but the differences failed to reach statistical significance. Subset analyses suggested that the chemotherapy advantage was confined to premenopausal patients or patients younger than 50 years of age. Acute toxicity was deemed acceptable, especially with melphalan, although life-threatening or fatal reactions did occur with these treatments. Although outcomes were similar, CMF soon became the standard chemotherapy regimen for adjuvant breast cancer therapy. The shorter duration of treatment (1 year versus 2 years), the documented superiority of CMF in advanced breast cancer, and the fear of the leukemogenic potential of melphalan all contributed to the popularity of CMF.

Numerous other controlled, randomized studies of a variety of chemotherapy regimens have now been completed. Many of these studies suggested trends for benefit in postmenopausal patients and in node-negative patients, but most of them individually lacked the statistical power to address the efficacy of chemotherapy in these clinically important subsets. Realizing this weakness of the individual studies, an international collaboration, the Early Breast Cancer Trialists' Collaborative Group, conducted meta-analyses on all major randomized trials, publishing the results in 1988,[12] 1992,[22] and 1998.[23]

The 1988 analysis came to three major conclusions about adjuvant chemotherapy trials.[12] (a) Adjuvant chemotherapy imparted a statistically significant reduction in the risk of relapse and death at 5 years of follow-up (with a hazard reduction of approximately one-fourth). Trends for benefit among women older than 50 and for women who were node negative did not reach statistical significance. (b) Indirect comparisons showed that combination chemotherapy was significantly more effective than single-agent therapy. (c) The

TABLE 2. *Meta-analysis of the effects of polychemotherapy*

		Reduction in annual odds	
Regimen	No.[a]	Recurrence (%)	Death (%)
All polychemotherapy	9,426/9,362	24 ± 2	15 ± 2
CMF	4,103/4,047	24 ± 3	14 ± 4
CMF + extracytotoxics	1,622/1,596	20 ± 2	15 ± 5
Other polychemotherapy	3,701/3,719	25 ± 4	17 ± 4

CMF, cyclophosphamide, methotrexate, 5-fluorouracil.
[a]Number of patients in the trials who received polychemotherapy versus the number who did not. [The % of reduction ± the standard error (SE). Two times the SE defines the limits of the 95% confidence interval.]
Adapted from ref. 23.

TABLE 3. *Meta-analysis of the effects of polychemotherapy: relationship with age*

		Reduction in annual odds	
Age (yr)	No.	Recurrence (%)	Death (%)
<40	694/675	37 ± 7	27 ± 5
40–49	1,629–1,531	34 ± 5	27 ± 5
50–59	3,362/3,411	22 ± 4	14 ± 4
60–69	3,394/3,413	18 ± 4	8 ± 4
≥70	307/302	NS	NS
Overall	**9,386/9,332**	**24 ± 2**	**15 ± 2**

NS, not significant.
Adapted from ref. 23.

data suggested that administration of chemotherapy for 8 to 24 months may offer no survival advantage over administration of the same chemotherapy for 4 to 6 months.

The 1992 results with 10 years of follow-up confirmed and extended the 1988 analysis.[22] (a) Adjuvant chemotherapy conferred benefit to both premenopausal and postmenopausal patients (although to a lesser degree) and to node-positive and node-negative patients (to the same proportional degree). (b) Polychemotherapy was superior to single-agent regimens. (c) Both direct and indirect comparisons showed that long-term polychemotherapy (e.g., 12 months) was no better than shorter (e.g., 6 months) regimens. (d) Finally, between ages 50 and 69, direct comparisons showed that combined chemotherapy plus tamoxifen was more effective than either chemotherapy or tamoxifen alone.

These results have been extended further by the most recent 1998 analysis.[23] Many trials have now had more than 15 years of follow-up, giving the analyses more statistical power. The analysis of chemotherapy versus no chemotherapy is based on 47 trials that contained 17,723 patients. Analysis of longer versus shorter chemotherapy is based on 11 trials with 6,104 patients, and analysis of anthracycline-containing regimens versus nonanthracycline CMF-based regimens is based on 11 trials with 5,942 patients.

The results of the 1998 overview show a highly statistically significant benefit from several months of polychemotherapy for the average patient participating in these trials[23] (Table 2). Considering all patients, approximately one of every four recurrences and one of every seven deaths is avoided each year with chemotherapy. Quantitative differences in the benefit from chemotherapy are evident in several clinically relevant subsets.

Age and Menopausal Status

Age had an important effect on the benefits from adjuvant chemotherapy.[23] The youngest patients had the greatest benefit (Table 3). More than one-third of recurrences and one-fourth of deaths each year were avoided with treatment. There was a general trend for less benefit in older patients, although differences between chemotherapy and no chemotherapy were still statistically significant. Relatively few patients older than age 70 participated in these studies (n = 609), making the results less reliable and inconclusive, but these elderly patients had no statistically significant benefit. The results, however, cannot rule out the possibility that these individuals benefited as much as other patients older than 50, nor can they rule out the possibility that there is no benefit at all. Still, the annual reductions in the odds of recurrence and death are very modest for the average woman 50 years of age or older, with only approximately one of every ten deaths avoided each year with chemotherapy.

The quantitatively greater benefit of adjuvant chemotherapy in younger women suggests the possibility of a dual mechanism: cytotoxic effects of chemotherapy on the tumor cells plus an endocrine effect derived from the ovarian ablative effects of chemotherapy. This possibility is supported by studies correlating chemotherapy-induced amenorrhea with improved outcome in younger patients.[24,25] Interestingly, however, for women who were younger than age 50 at the time of randomization, the effect of polychemotherapy on the risk of recurrence or death was approximately the same in postmenopausal as in premenopausal women in this age group, although the relatively small number of young postmenopausal patients makes this comparison less reliable (Table 4). The results suggest that age may be more important than menopausal status in defining the benefit achieved from polychemotherapy.

The meta-analysis confirms the conclusions of the earliest chemotherapy trials, that adjuvant chemotherapy is more effective in younger women. The results show, however, that older women do benefit from adjuvant chemotherapy, although only approximately one in nine or ten deaths annually is avoided by treatment. Why older women benefit less than younger women is not totally clear. In addition to the endocrine ablative effects of chemotherapy in younger women, other possible contributing factors include age-related

TABLE 4. *Meta-analysis of the effects of polychemotherapy: menopausal status*

	Reduction in annual odds		
	No.	Recurrence (%)	Death (%)
Age <50 yr			
Pre/perimenopausal	2,105/1,959	34 ± 4	27 ± 5
Postmenopausal	227/249	44 ± 13	28 ± 15
Age 50–69 yr			
Pre/perimenopausal	710/759	24 ± 7	19 ± 8
Postmenopausal	6,077/6,094	20 ± 3	10 ± 3

Adapted from ref. 23.

TABLE 5. *Meta-analysis of the effects of chemotherapy: influence of estrogen receptor (ER)*

	Reduction in annual odds		
ER	No.	Recurrence (%)	Death (%)
Age <50 yr			
ER poor	710/688	40 ± 7	35 ± 9
ER positive	565/550	33 ± 8	20 ± 10
Age 50–69 yr			
ER poor	1,647/1,593	30 ± 5	17 ± 6
ER positive	3,359/3,434	18 ± 4	9 ± 5

Adapted from ref. 23.

differences in tumor biology (for instance, ER level is related to age) or the reduced doses arbitrarily given to older women in some trials because of the fear of excessive toxicity.[26]

More recent trials raise questions about the relative ineffectiveness of adjuvant chemotherapy in older patients. Trials of CMF and MF in node-negative patients, trials of other multiple-drug regimens, and trials of doxorubicin-based therapy reveal similar benefits in younger and older patients.[27–31]

Axillary Lymph Node Status

Some of the early randomized trials of adjuvant chemotherapy included node-negative patients, but these trials were not designed prospectively to assess the benefit in this subgroup, and most trials contained too few patients to draw definitive conclusions. Many physicians were reluctant to treat node-negative patients with chemotherapy because of the potential toxicity and because of the relatively favorable prognosis of this group of women.

Although 75% of node-positive patients treated by surgery alone die within 10 years, only 25% to 30% of node-negative patients have recurrences and die of breast cancer during this time. Studies with very long-term follow-up suggest that additional recurrences and deaths, perhaps one-fourth of the total, can occur after more than 10 years in patients with initially negative lymph nodes, but the majority of patients with breast cancer who do not have nodal metastases do not succumb to breast cancer and are cured by surgery alone.[32] Obviously, these patients could not benefit from adjuvant treatment designed to eliminate viable micrometastases that they do not have.

The node-negative breast cancer population is a heterogeneous group of patients with widely disparate prognoses. Other prognostic factors, reviewed in Chapter 32, can be used to distinguish node-negative patients with an extremely low risk of breast cancer recurrence and death from other groups with a 10-year survival just as poor as some patients with positive lymph nodes. Patients with tumors 1 cm in diameter or smaller have only a 10% to 15% chance of ever having a recurrence, whereas those with tumors 3 cm or larger have a 50% or greater chance of disease recurrence.[27] Patients with ER-positive tumors have a somewhat lower risk of recurrence over the first 5 years of follow-up compared to those with ER-negative tumors, but this difference tends to disappear with longer follow-up.[33] Some of these prognostic factors were used to identify higher-risk node-negative patients for adjuvant chemotherapy studies focusing on this subgroup that were initiated in the early 1980s.

One of the first studies of adjuvant chemotherapy in node-negative patients was initiated in the mid-1970s, and it showed no significant DFS or OS benefit; however, the chemotherapy regimen used would be considered inappropriate by today's standards.[34] Interest in adjuvant treatment of patients with node-negative breast cancer rose with the publication of the results of several other trials completed in the 1980s.[13,27,28,35–39] Three of these trials examined CMF-like regimens given in appropriate doses, and all of them showed highly significant DFS benefits in node-negative patients.[13,38,39]

A greater degree of certainty of the DFS and OS benefits of adjuvant chemotherapy in node-negative patients comes from the recent meta-analysis.[23] Quantitatively, the proportional improvements in DFS and in OS were similar in node-negative and node-positive patients. Given the better prognosis of node-negative patients when they are treated with surgery alone, however, the absolute number of patients with negative nodes who benefit from adjuvant chemotherapy is less than the subset with positive lymph nodes.

Estrogen-Receptor Status

Inconsistent results were reported in numerous prior studies examining the relationship between chemotherapy benefit and ER status of the tumor. The question of whether ER expression influences the results of adjuvant polychemotherapy was addressed by the 1998 overview (Table 5).[23] ER-negative tumors have a slightly higher proliferative rate and on a cell kinetic basis might be expected to respond better to cytotoxic drugs; in the meta-analysis, in both younger and older patients, there was a trend for ER-poor tumors to benefit more from adjuvant chemotherapy. Most notably, among women 50 to 69 years of age, polychemotherapy reduced the risk of recurrence and mortality in patients with both ER-positive and ER-poor tumors. However, patients with ER-poor tumors were almost twice as likely to benefit. These data suggest that patients with ER-poor tumors may respond somewhat better to chemotherapy than those with ER-positive tumors, who benefit more from tamoxifen. It is possible that this modest relationship is partly dependent on the particular drugs used in a given regimen, but an analysis of this type has not been done.

Optimal Adjuvant Chemotherapy Regimen

After the initial studies of adjuvant chemotherapy produced encouraging results, subsequent studies were done to define the optimal chemotherapy regimen. Although these studies have not identified a "standard" regimen used by all oncologists, they do provide important general conclusions and a menu of possible regimens to be considered by the practicing physician.

Single Agents Compared with Combination Chemotherapy

In 1975, the results of the NSABP trial comparing melphalan with placebo demonstrated the superiority of adjuvant chemotherapy.[21] At the time, combination chemotherapy was proving superior to single agents in advanced breast cancer, and therefore the next logical step was to compare a multiple-drug regimen with melphalan in the adjuvant setting.

In 1975, the Southwest Oncology Group (SWOG) compared 2 years of melphalan with 1 year of continuous CMFVP, a regimen in which cyclophosphamide is given daily by mouth, methotrexate and 5-fluorouracil weekly intravenously, and vincristine and prednisone intravenously and orally, respectively, only for the first 10 weeks.[40] The results, now at 20 years, conclude that the combination is superior to the single agent in both DFS and OS.[41] Median survival with CMFVP is 12.1 years, compared to 7.2 years with melphalan. Similar results were observed in a second-generation NSABP study that compared melphalan with melphalan combined with 5-fluorouracil.[42]

The 1992 meta-analysis included 13 studies of combination chemotherapy compared with single-agent therapy.[22] A trend for an advantage for combination therapy was apparent in 10 of these studies. Overall, polychemotherapy produced a 13% ± 5% and 17% ± 5% reduction in the annual odds of recurrence and death, respectively. The cumulative data thus suggest that combination drug therapy provides a modest advantage over single-agent therapy. It should be noted that none of the single-agent versus combination studies used the single agent optimally in terms of dose. Thus, the greater effectiveness of polychemotherapy over single-agent regimens might conceivably be due in part to simple differences in dose intensity. It is theoretically possible that a single agent given at its optimal dose and schedule would be equivalent, or even superior, to combination therapy given in a traditional schedule. This strategy is being investigated in randomized clinical trials.

Duration of Therapy

Most early trials of adjuvant chemotherapy in breast cancer empirically chose a treatment duration of 1 or 2 years. Second- and third-generation trials compared treatment given for shorter durations. Most of these studies evaluated CMF or CMF-based regimens.

In the mid-1970s, two studies compared the standard 12-month CMF regimen with a similar regimen given for either 4 or 6 months.[13,43,44] These studies found that the shorter durations of treatment were as effective as the longer durations.

Another study asked whether prolonging chemotherapy from 1 year to 2 years would improve DFS or OS in a poor-prognosis subset of ER-negative node-positive patients.[45] The prolonged treatment regimen was poorly tolerated, with only 37% of patients completing the assigned full 2 years; overall, no advantage to the more prolonged schedule was seen.

Durations of CMF regimens shorter than 4 months may be suboptimal. One month (one cycle) of treatment after surgery was significantly inferior to a 6-month course.[46] In another study, 12 weeks of adjuvant chemotherapy was significantly inferior to 36 weeks of treatment.[47]

Eleven trials are included in the meta-analysis investigating the duration of adjuvant chemotherapy (Table 6).[23] Overall, no clinically important differences between a few months of adjuvant chemotherapy compared to longer durations were observed. The cumulative data suggest that durations of chemotherapy in the range of 3 to 6 months are better tolerated and as effective as longer-duration regimens in treating patients with breast cancer. However, the treatment duration question has not been rigorously evaluated for all drug regimens, including the popular regimen combining doxorubicin and cyclophosphamide (AC) every 3 weeks for four cycles. One interpretation for the recently reported study showing an advantage for the addition of four cycles of paclitaxel (Taxol) to four cycles of AC compared to four cycles of AC alone is that the observed advantage is not due to the Taxol but simply to more prolonged chemotherapy.[48] A third arm giving eight cycles of AC would have been desirable to fully interpret these results.

TABLE 6. *Meta-analysis of adjuvant chemotherapy: duration of treatment*

	Reduction in annual odds		
Regimen	No.	Recurrence (%)	Death (%)
Longer vs shorter	3,049/3,055	7 ± 4	−1 ± 5

Adapted from ref. 23.

Anthracycline-Based Chemotherapy

Modifications of the basic CMF treatment program, including the deletion, substitution, or addition of certain drugs, have been tested in randomized clinical trials. The combination of MF was superior to no adjuvant therapy in a group of node-negative patients, and the addition of cyclophosphamide to MF resulted in a statistically significant DFS and OS advantage.[49] These data suggest that, although CMF is superior to MF, MF might offer an alternative for some women in whom drug toxicity is a major issue.

Anthracycline-based regimens, usually using doxorubicin or epirubicin, have also been compared to CMF-based regimens. The addition of doxorubicin to melphalan and 5-fluorouracil improved DFS and OS.[50] Ten-year results of the Oncofrance trial in node-positive patients demonstrated a significant DFS and OS advantage for doxorubicin/vincristine/cyclophosphamide/5-fluorouracil compared with CMF.[51] Another SWOG study compared a 20-week regimen combining 5-fluorouracil/doxorubicin/cyclophosphamide/methotrexate with CMFVP for 1 year in receptor-negative node-positive patients.[52] At 5 years of follow-up, a nonsignificant trend in favor of CMFVP was evident. An NSABP trial compared four cycles of AC with six cycles of CMF, with a third arm of AC followed in 6 months by CMF to test the idea of interval reinduction.[53] AC was similar in efficacy to CMF in this study. Because the AC regimen was completed in less than one-half the time of CMF, and because it was associated with fewer physician visits, fewer treatment days, and fewer days of nausea, many investigators conclude that AC is the preferred regimen.

Other trials have evaluated the use of sequential or alternating regimens, one of which contains doxorubicin. In one trial, 12 courses of intravenous CMF were compared to 8 cycles of CMF followed by 4 courses of doxorubicin.[54] There was no advantage for the sequential doxorubicin regimen. In another study, doxorubicin for 4 cycles followed by intravenous CMF for 8 courses was compared to the sequential use of CMF for 2 cycles followed by doxorubicin for 1 cycle, for a total of 12 courses.[55] This study showed highly significant DFS and OS advantages for the sequential regimen compared to the alternating regimen. No CMF-alone arm was included in this trial, but historical comparisons with the original CMF study and with results of other drug regimens suggest that the sequential regimen of doxorubicin followed by CMF may be superior.

The meta-analysis evaluated a total of 11 trials in which patients were randomized between anthracycline- and nonanthracycline-containing adjuvant polychemotherapy.[23] Anthracycline-containing regimens were modestly superior in reducing recurrence and death to those regimens without anthracyclines (Table 7). The absolute difference in overall mortality at 5 years for the average patient in these trials was 3%. Long-term benefits from anthracyclines are still uncertain, given the relatively short follow-up in many of these trials. Furthermore, approximately 70% of the women in these trials were premenopausal, making it difficult to assess with certainty the relative effectiveness in older patients. A recently reported large trial randomized 2,691 node-negative patients to six cycles of CAF (cyclophosphamide, anthracycline, 5-fluorouracil) versus six cycles of CMF both with or without tamoxifen.[56] The doxorubicin-containing regimen was superior in both pre- and postmenopausal patients. The cumulative data thus suggest that doxorubicin-containing regimens are modestly superior to regimens without an anthracycline. Doxorubicin-containing regimens have grown in popularity not only because they are somewhat more effective, but also because regimens such as AC for four cycles can be given over a short period of time and are well tolerated.

TABLE 7. *Meta-analysis of adjuvant anthracycline versus nonanthracycline regimen*

	Reduction in annual odds		
Regimen	No.	Recurrence (%)	Death (%)
With anthracyclines vs without	3,477/3,473	12 ± 4	11 ± 5

Adapted from ref. 23.

New Agents

In the past few years, several new agents have been shown to be as effective, or more effective, than older drugs in the treatment of advanced breast cancer. Their incorporation into studies of adjuvant therapy, however, is just now being studied. These agents include the taxanes, paclitaxel and docetaxel, vinorelbine, and herceptin (a humanized antibody against the c-*erb*-b2 oncogene product). The taxanes are of great interest because of their high activity in metastatic breast cancer and because they demonstrate non–cross-resistance with anthracyclines. Trials using docetaxel in combination with cyclophosphamide or given sequentially after AC are in progress. A recently reported large randomized trial suggests that the sequential use of paclitaxel after AC may offer an advantage.[48] In this trial, lymph node–positive pre- and postmenopausal patients were randomized to four cycles of one of three dose levels of AC and then either no additional therapy or four additional cycles of paclitaxel. Women who received paclitaxel had a statistically significant improvement in DFS (90% versus 86%) and OS (97% versus 95%) at a median follow-up time of only 2 years. This represents a 22% reduction in the odds of relapse and a 26% reduction in the odds of death—a significant improvement if the differences observed persist with longer follow-up. As described earlier in this section, under Duration of Therapy, we do not yet know whether this difference is due to the incorporation of paclitaxel or simply to more prolonged therapy. At this time, no data are available from adjuvant studies on the use of the other new agents, and they should not be used outside of the research setting until their efficacy and safety have been demonstrated in randomized clinical trials. Although herceptin has activity in metastatic breast cancer and appears to have an additive effect when combined with doxorubicin or paclitaxel, it should not yet be used for routine adjuvant therapy until its safety profile has been established.[57,58] Approximately 5% of patients with advanced breast cancer experience cardiac toxicity when herceptin is used as a single agent, and significantly more patients suffer cardiac toxicity when it is combined with doxorubicin. Trials evaluating herceptin in adjuvant therapy regimens are currently being planned.

Adjuvant Therapy Using Bisphosphonates

Other drugs that are not strictly cytotoxic are also being investigated in combination with standard adjuvant therapy strategies. The most interesting of these agents are the bisphosphonates. As described in Chapter 60 in more detail, bisphosphonates inhibit the osteoclast overactivity in bone that results from metastatic tumor cells. They inhibit bone resorption and, secondarily, the release of growth factors from bone that may be important for tumor cell viability and growth. They reduce the incidence of bone metastases in experimental animal models and in patients with metastatic disease.[59–61] Conceivably, they could also improve DFS or OS when used as adjuvant therapy by indirectly inducing tumor cell apoptosis and by retarding the growth and secondary metastases arising from subclinical microscopic bone marrow involvement that is commonly detected in patients with primary breast cancer. The results of a European adjuvant trial with clodronate, an oral bisphosphonate, are provocative.[62] Patients with primary breast cancer who had microscopic bone marrow involvement detected by sensitive assays received standard adjuvant therapy and were then randomized either to receive, or not to receive, clodronate for 2 years. At 3 years of follow-up, patients who received clodronate not only had a reduction in the incidence of bone metastasis but also a reduced incidence of soft-tissue and visceral metastases.[62] Preliminary results of a second trial also showed a significant reduction in the development of bone metastases when the drug was used as an adjuvant to other treatment modalities.[63] These exciting data prompted the autumn 1999 activation of a large confirmatory intergroup trial.

DOSE-INTENSIVE ADJUVANT CHEMOTHERAPY

One strategy that has been the subject of several recent clinical trials is to increase the doses of chemotherapy or to increase the frequency of administering a standard dose. The surge in popularity of dose-intensive chemotherapy is related to the availability of hematopoietic growth factors to reduce toxicity from myelosuppression, to improvements in other methods of supportive care, and to the results of pilot studies and retrospective calculations of dose intensity suggesting possible advantages to this approach. Steep dose-response curves for certain drugs in preclinical models and high response rates in patients with metastatic breast cancer indicate that drug resistance can be overcome partially by raising drug dose.

Two different strategies for dose intensification are under investigation (see Chapter 38 for a more detailed discussion). One method is to use extremely high myeloablative doses of chemotherapy that require hematopoietic reconstitution with autologous bone marrow transplantation, peripheral progenitor cell support, or both. The high blood levels of drugs achieved, even for a brief time, may be sufficient to kill cells that are resistant to the same classes of drugs used at conventional doses. The need for supportive care and prolonged hospitalization, high cost, and relatively high morbidity and occasional mortality are issues that complicate the widespread application of this approach.

A second method of dose intensification is to increase the amount of drug delivered per unit time (dose density). High dose density can be achieved by raising drug doses in standard regimens, such as CMF or AC, or by shortening the interval between drug treatments. The measure of dose density is frequently expressed as milligrams of drug received per square meter of body surface area per week. Thus, a 50% increase in dose intensity can be achieved by administering the same doses of AC every 2 weeks instead of every 3 weeks or by increasing the dose given every 3 weeks. Dose-intensive regimens designed in this way can be given on an outpatient basis and can be administered repeatedly for prolonged periods, an attractive feature for a slow growing, low-growth growth fraction tumor such as breast cancer.

Dose Intensification of Standard Regimens

The issue of dose intensity first received wide attention in 1981, when the Milan group reported a retrospective analysis of their original CMF adjuvant study suggesting that only those patients who received at least 85% of their planned CMF dose benefited significantly from adjuvant therapy, whereas those receiving less than 65% of the planned dose had the same DFS and OS as the group of control patients treated by surgery alone.[26] Unfortunately, this type of analysis has been questioned for a variety of reasons, most notably that distinguishing among several plausible explanations for a relationship between DFS and chemotherapy dose received is impossible.[64] Patients may have a recurrence because they received a lower drug dose. Alternatively, patients who received a lower drug dose may have done so because they did not tolerate chemotherapy as a result of factors also associated with a greater likelihood of disease recurrence. For example, patients with subclinical bone marrow metastases who are destined to have a recurrence may tolerate chemotherapy less well than other patients and may require dose reductions.

Another technique to analyze dose intensity retrospectively was reported by Hryniuk and Levine.[65] An analysis of the planned dose intensity of a variety of CMF-based adjuvant regimens showed that it significantly correlated with DFS independent of other factors. These data provided additional support for the hypothesis that dose intensity might be important in the adjuvant therapy of breast cancer, but more definitive prospective studies were needed.

The major question addressed in dose intensification studies is whether the efficacy of a given therapy increases linearly with dose or dose density or whether it plateaus at a level close to that now considered conventional. Three recently reported studies suggest that modest dose escalation beyond currently accepted standard doses does not improve the efficacy of adjuvant therapy.[66–68] The Cancer and Leukemia Group B trial randomly assigned 1,572 women to three treatment groups given different doses and schedules of CAF.[66] The high-dose arm had twice the dose intensity and twice the drug dose as the low-dose arm. The moderate-dose arm had two-thirds the dose intensity as the high-dose arm but the same total drug dose. None of these schedules is really dose intensive by today's standards. At a median follow-up of 9 years, DFS and OS for patients on the moderate- and high-dose arms are superior to those for patients on the low-dose arm. There was no difference in DFS or OS between the moderate- and the high-dose arms. The authors concluded that within the conventional dose range for this chemotherapy regimen, a higher dose is associated with better outcome, but it is just as reasonable to argue that reducing the doses of standard treatment regimens should be avoided unless necessitated by severe toxicity.

Other randomized trials have explored an alternative approach of significantly increasing the doses of either cyclophosphamide or doxorubicin in the standard AC regimen. One study randomized patients between the standard four cycles of AC with the dose of doxorubicin at 60 mg per m^2 and cyclophosphamide at 600 mg per m^2 and two other arms in which the dose of cyclophosphamide was intensified. The second arm in this study kept the doxorubicin dose stable but increased cyclophosphamide to 1,200 mg per m^2 for two courses. A third arm gave cyclophosphamide for four courses at 1,200 mg per m^2.[67] Thus, this study examined both dose intensification and increasing the total dose of drug given. Neither strategy resulted in significant improvement in either DFS or OS. A large follow-up study of 1,548 node-positive patients randomized patients to three different arms in which the doxorubicin dose was fixed at 60 mg per m^2 and the dose of cyclophosphamide was escalated. One group received cyclophosphamide at 1,200 mg per m^2 for four cycles, the second group received 2,400 mg per m^2 for two cycles, and the third received 2,400 mg per m^2 for four cycles; all patients received granulocyte colony stimulating factor (G-CSF) prophylaxis.[68] Preliminary results of this study also failed to show any advantage for escalating cyclophosphamide to a dose four times that which is now considered standard.

Escalating the dose of doxorubicin has also been explored in an intergroup trial in which the cyclosphosphamide dose was fixed at 600 mg per m^2.[48] In this trial, 3,120 women with node-positive breast cancer were randomized to standard AC or to AC in which the doxorubicin dose was escalated either to 75 mg per m^2 in one group or to 90 mg per m^2 in another. G-CSF prophylaxis was permitted for the intermediate and high-dose arms. All patients had a second randomization to four cycles of Taxol or no additional therapy, as described previously. At 2 years of follow-up, no advantage has emerged for dose escalation of doxorubicin. Thus, escalation of cyclophosphamide or doxorubicin in the standard AC regimen offers no therapeutic advantage and is associated with greater toxicity.

Myeloablative Chemotherapy with Stem Cell Support

Studies of extremely high-dose chemotherapy and autologous bone marrow transplantation or stem cell support are being performed in patients at high risk of disease recurrence, such as those with ten or more positive axillary nodes. More than 90% of these patients relapse within 10 years when treated with surgery alone; more than 50% relapse within 5 years and more than 70% within 10 years even when they are treated with adjuvant chemotherapy.

Two very small randomized trials have been reported.[69,70] A Dutch study randomized 81 patients with infraclavicular-involved nodes to a CEF (cyclophosphamide, epirubicin, 5-fluorouracil) regimen or a CEF regimen plus a high-dose regimen with stem cell support.[69] The 4-year OS was 79% compared to 72%, and DFS was 45% compared to 56% for the high-dose and conventional chemotherapy arms, respectively. These differences were not statistically significant, but the trend for worse DFS in the high-dose arm suggests that this therapy could not offer a major advantage. In addition to the documented acute morbidity and occasional mortality from this approach, this study also reports impaired cognitive function in patients who receive high-dose chemotherapy.[71] A small American trial randomized 78 patients with ten or more involved axillary nodes at primary surgery or four or more nodes after neoadjuvant therapy to either standard FAC (5-fluorouracil, doxorubicin, cyclophosphamide) or FAC plus high-dose therapy and stem cell support.[70] The trend for worse outcome in patients on the high-dose arm was not statistically significant, but, as with the Dutch trial, a major advantage for high-dose therapy seems very unlikely.

Two large, North American, intergroup randomized trials of high-dose chemotherapy with autologous bone marrow support that have the statistical power to detect small differences in outcome have recently completed accrual. The Cancer and Leukemia Group B study randomized patients with ten or more positive axillary nodes to standard CAF followed by low-dose cyclophosphamide, cisplatin, and carmustine or to CAF followed by high doses of the same drugs combined with autologous bone marrow support. Both groups receive tamoxifen, and chest wall radiation is given because of the high risk of local recurrence in these patients. Preliminary results of this trial show no overall advantage for the high-dose arm.[72] A slight reduction in breast cancer–specific recurrence is offset by higher mortality in the transplant group. The Eastern Cooperation Oncology Group (ECOG) intergroup study randomizes the same subset of patients to CAF followed by radiation and tamoxifen or to CAF followed by high-dose cyclophosphamide plus thiotepa along with bone marrow support, tamoxifen, and radiation. Results from this trial are not yet available. Taken together, the data do not support the routine use of either moderate dose escalations of cyclophosphamide or doxorubicin in the standard AC regimen or the use of very high-dose chemotherapy with marrow or stem cell support. The latter approach should be confined to experienced research centers.

PERIOPERATIVE AND PREOPERATIVE (NEOADJUVANT) CHEMOTHERAPY

Perioperative Adjuvant Chemotherapy

Chemotherapy given at the time of or just after surgery offers several theoretical advantages. The drugs may kill circulating tumor cells that conceivably are dislodged at the time of surgery. Furthermore, after removal of the primary tumor, DNA synthesis and proliferation of distant micrometastases increase almost immediately, perhaps increasing their vulnerability to cytotoxic drugs.[73] Finally, immediate treatment might kill metastatic cells before the spontaneous emergence of drug resistance.[74] Although some early trials suggested that perioperative chemotherapy might be beneficial, two large randomized studies demonstrated that the benefit is substantially less than that observed with several cycles of postoperative conventional polychemotherapy. In one study, node-negative breast cancer patients were randomized to receive either one cycle of perioperative CMF starting within 36 hours of surgery or no adjuvant treatment.[75] Interestingly, a statistically significant 20% reduction in the odds of recurrence was achieved with the single cycle of perioperative therapy, approximately one-half of what might be expected from a conventional six-cycle program. This trial suggests that the first cycles of a prolonged regimen might be the most important, and it is consistent with lack of additional benefit achieved by prolonging chemotherapy beyond 3 to 6 months. Another trial in node-positive patients compared one cycle of perioperative CMF, one cycle of perioperative therapy combined with six subsequent cycles of CMF, or a conventional six-cycle CMF program.[46] The single cycle of perioperative CMF was significantly inferior to the longer regimens, and the addition of a single cycle of perioperative therapy added nothing to six cycles of standard CMF. A 1997 meta-analysis of perioperative trials showed a modest improvement in DFS but no OS benefit.[76] Data do not support the use of chemotherapy given around the time of primary breast cancer surgery.

Neoadjuvant Chemotherapy

Several potential advantages and disadvantages also exist for the administration of chemotherapy before definitive surgery. The presence of a measurable mass permits assessment of response as a direct *in vivo* measure of the sensitivity of the tumor cells to the particular drugs used. Early detection of a resistant tumor would enable the oncologist to both discontinue a worthless therapy, thus avoiding unnecessary toxicity, and change to a potentially more effective regimen. In addition, the earlier the disease is treated, the less likely that resistant tumor clones will have emerged spontaneously. Theoretically, even a short delay in administering systemic therapy could adversely affect outcome.[77] Finally, preoperative chemotherapy may shrink large primary tumors sufficiently to allow breast-preserving surgery rather than mastectomy.

Disadvantages of preoperative chemotherapy include the reliance on a fine-needle aspirate or core biopsy for histologic diagnosis. Although in experienced hands mistakes in diagnosis using these techniques are uncommon, it is possible that palpable *in situ* cancers may be mislabeled as invasive cancers (especially with fine-needle aspiration) and that patients will then be treated inappropriately with chemotherapy. Prognostic factor analyses, such as receptor status, DNA flow cytometry, and other markers that may be useful in some clinical situations, are more difficult to perform (although not impossible) on these small specimens. Most important, however, axillary nodal status is not known before the selection of adjuvant chemotherapy, and an accurate estimate may never be possible in some responding patients. Axillary nodal status provides important prognostic information to the physician and patient, information that may be crucial in planning both for the intensity of adjuvant chemotherapy and for chest wall and regional lymphatic irradiation.

Preoperative chemotherapy has been used extensively in inoperable, locally advanced breast cancer to achieve tumor reduction and, thus, to facilitate mastectomy or irradiation. More recently, this strategy has been studied in operable primary breast cancer, most commonly in patients with tumors 3 cm or larger in diameter. A comprehensive phase II study from Milan investigating five different chemotherapy regimens [CMF, FAC, FEC, FNC (mitoxantrone substituting for doxorubicin), and doxorubicin alone] demonstrated partial response rates ranging from 62% (tumors larger than 5 cm) to 93% (3- to 4-cm tumors).[78] Overall response rates approached 80%, and no differences were observed among the various regimens employed. Response to single-agent doxorubicin was equivalent to that of the combinations. Breast-preserving surgery (quadrantectomy) was possible in 91% of the patients. More than 73% of patients with tumors larger than 5 cm became candidates for breast preservation based on tumor size. At a median follow-up of 18 months, only 1 of 201 patients treated by quadrantectomy and radiation suffered a local recurrence, but it is far too early to draw conclusions about local control.

Although partial responses are common, pathologic complete response (CR) is uncommon with preoperative chemotherapy, occurring in only 10% to 20% of patients.[79–81] Importantly, patients who enjoy a CR have a better prognosis than patients who do not achieve pathologic CR. One of the possible advantages of neoadjuvant therapy is to assess chemosensitivity of tumors *in vivo* and to obtain information on tumor biology. Nonrandomized studies with pre- and postchemotherapy tumor sampling show that residual cell populations after treatment may have different characteristics, such as a lower mitotic rate, than those of pretreatment populations.[82,83]

The largest trial evaluating neoadjuvant therapy randomized 1,523 patients to surgery followed by four cycles of AC or to four cycles of AC followed by surgery.[84] Tumor size was reduced in 80% of patients after preoperative therapy, and 36% had a clinical CR. Only 26% of women with a clinical CR had a pathologic CR. Preoperative therapy resulted in a 37% increase in the incidence of pathologically negative axillary nodes. Although patients were downstaged by preoperative chemotherapy, it did not improve DFS, distant DFS, or OS. More patients treated preoperatively than postoperatively underwent lumpectomy and radiation therapy (68% versus 60%, respectively), presumably because of smaller tumors after chemotherapy. Because some patients are likely to have residual disease near the margins of the original (before chemotherapy) extent of the tumor, local recurrence is a potential problem. Considerable microscopic residual disease may be left behind. So far, the rate of local recurrence is acceptable in these patients, but longer follow-up is necessary to assess local control. Outcome was better in women whose tumors showed a pathologic CR than in those whose did not, even when baseline prognostic variables were considered.

Another randomized neoadjuvant study included 212 patients and reported an overall clinical response rate of 85%, with a complete histologic response rate of 10%.[85] There was a modest but statistically significant reduction in the requirement for mastectomy in patients who received neoadjuvant treatment (13% versus 28%), but DFS and OS have not yet been reported.

A French study of 272 women with tumors larger than 3 cm randomized patients to primary chemotherapy with three cycles of epirubicin, vincristine, and methotrexate followed by three cycles of mitomycin, thiotepa, and vindesine followed by local treatment, versus mastectomy and the same chemotherapy if the patients were found to be node positive or ER negative.[86] The breast was conserved in 63% of patients in the preoperative chemotherapy arm. At a median follow-up of approximately 3 years, local control was acceptable, and survival was longer in the early chemotherapy group.

Taken together, preoperative chemotherapy may allow breast preservation in some patients with large tumors who would not otherwise be candidates. On the other hand, control of distant micrometastases is not improved, staging of the axilla is problematic, and pretreatment assessment of molecular markers is more difficult. Preoperative therapy may be appropriate for those women with larger tumors who strongly desire breast preservation.

ESTIMATING ABSOLUTE BENEFITS OF ADJUVANT CHEMOTHERAPY

Using data from the meta-analysis, major subsets of patients (generated on the basis of nodal status: negative versus positive, and age: younger than 50 years versus 50 to 69 years) enjoy a statistically significant reduction in relapse and death at 10 years (Table 8).[23] For certain subsets, such as younger patients with positive nodes, the benefits are substantial. The absolute benefits are more modest for the average postmenopausal or node-negative patient. Some node-negative patients (tumors ≤1 cm) have a much lower than average risk of recurrence (10% or less), and the absolute benefit is even less (two or three out of 100 patients treated), making it difficult to justify the risks and expense of chemotherapy. Other factors may also modify these estimates. Older women with

TABLE 8. *Absolute benefits of adjuvant chemotherapy by age and nodal status*

	With polychemotherapy (%)	With no polychemotherapy (%)	Absolute benefit (%)
Disease-free survival			
Age <50 yr			
Node negative	68.3	58.0	10.3
Node positive	47.6	32.2	15.4
Age 50–69 yr			
Node negative	65.6	59.9	5.7
Node positive	43.4	39.0	5.4
Overall survival			
Age <50 yr			
Node negative	77.6	71.9	5.7
Node positive	53.8	41.4	12.4
Age 50–69 yr			
Node negative	71.2	64.8	6.4
Node positive	48.6	46.3	2.3

Adapted from ref. 23.

TABLE 9. *Popular chemotherapy regimens useful in the adjuvant therapy of breast cancer*

Regimen[a]	Dose and schedule	Cycle interval (d)	Cycles
CMF (standard)			
Cyclophosphamide	100 mg/m^2/d p.o. x 14 d	28	6
Methotrexate	40 mg/m^2 i.v. d 1 & 8	28	6
5-Fluorouracil	600 mg/m^2 i.v. d 1 & 8	28	6
CMF (i.v.; tested in node-negative patients only)			
Cyclophosphamide	600 mg/m^2 i.v.	21	12
Methotrexate	40 mg/m^2 i.v.	21	12
5-Fluorouracil	600 mg/m^2 i.v.	21	12
CAF			
Cyclophosphamide	100 mg/m^2 p.o. x 14 d	28	6
Doxorubicin	30 mg/m^2 i.v. d 1 & 8	28	6
5-Fluorouracil	500 mg/m^2 i.v. d 1 & 8	28	6
CAF			
Cyclophosphamide	600 mg/m^2 i.v. d 1	21–28	4–6
Doxorubicin	60 mg/m^2 i.v. d 1	21–28	4–6
5-Fluorouracil	600 mg/m^2 i.v. d 1 & 8	21–28	4–6
AC			
Doxorubicin	60 mg/m^2 i.v. d 1	21	4
Cyclophosphamide	600 mg/m^2 d 1	21	4
AC → Taxol			
Doxorubicin	60 mg/m^2 i.v. d 1	21	4
Cyclophosphamide	600 mg/m^2 i.v. d 1	21	4
Taxol	175 mg/m^2 i.v. d 1	21	4 (after AC)
AC → CMF (tested in node-positive patients only)			
Doxorubicin	75 mg/m^2 i.v. d 1	21	4
Cyclophosphamide	600 mg/m^2 i.v.	21	8 (cycles 5–12)
Methotrexate	40 mg/m^2 i.v.	21	8 (cycles 5–12)
5-Fluorouracil	600 mg/m^2 i.v.	21	8 (cycles 5–12)

[a]Some institutions use a 48- to 96-hour continuous infusion of doxorubicin to reduce the potential for cardiac toxicity.

ER-negative tumors may benefit more from adjuvant chemotherapy than the average woman older than 50 years (see Table 5). Furthermore, overexpression of the c-*erb*-b2 oncogene may also modify the magnitude of the benefit observed with chemotherapy (reviewed in detail in Chapter 32). Although this is still controversial, tumors that express c-*erb*-b2 may be less responsive to CMF-based chemotherapy and to tamoxifen, whereas they may respond well to adequate doses of doxorubicin-based chemotherapy.[87–89]

The absolute risk reduction (the number of patients benefiting per 100 treated) cannot be accurately calculated simply by multiplying the risk of recurrence or death in the absence of therapy by the proportional risk reduction. This is because the proportional risk reduction presented in the meta-analysis is calculated as an *annual* risk. However, understanding the absolute benefits of treatment in patient subsets with a variety of risks of recurrence (or death) can help physicians and patients to make more informed treatment decisions. Tables 1 and 8 may be helpful in this regard. Commonly used adjuvant chemotherapy regimens are shown in Table 9.

ADJUVANT THERAPY WITH TAMOXIFEN

Tamoxifen is the most commonly prescribed drug for the treatment of breast cancer. The drug is a nonsteroidal compound that binds to ER and displays both estrogen antagonist and estrogen agonist properties.[90] Drugs that exhibit such dual activities are now referred to as *SERMs* (selective ER modulators). Tamoxifen, much like estrogen, preserves bone mineral density in postmenopausal women,[91] and it exerts a favorable effect on blood lipid profiles,[92] both attractive features in women for whom estrogen-replacement therapy may be hazardous. Tamoxifen's antiestrogenic effects are mediated by competitive blockade of ER, resulting in reduced transcription of estrogen-regulated genes.[90] The net result is a blockade of cell cycle transit in G_1 phase and inhibition of tumor growth. Some evidence suggests that programmed cell death may also be induced by tamoxifen.[93] A reduction in serum insulinlike growth factor I (IGF-I) concentration and an increase in IGF-binding protein levels provide another mechanism for tumor growth inhibition, although the lack of effectiveness of tamoxifen in tumors that do not express ER suggests that inhibition of ER-mediated activity is the dominant mechanism.[94]

Because of its favorable toxicity profile and its activity in advanced breast cancer, tamoxifen entered clinical trials of adjuvant therapy in the middle to late 1970s. More than 37,000 patients in 55 tamoxifen trials were included in a 1998 meta-analysis, and definitive conclusions are available.[95]

Tamoxifen in Premenopausal and Postmenopausal Patients

More than 20 trials have compared at least 1 year of tamoxifen therapy with a no-treatment control arm.[12,22,95] Many of these trials focused on postmenopausal patients, although a few included some premenopausal patients. Most of these studies included both node-positive and node-negative patients, although a large trial from the NSABP studied node-negative patients exclusively.[35] ER-positive and ER-negative patients were included in many of these studies, and the duration of tamoxifen varied from 1 to more than 5 years. Nearly all of these studies found a statistically significant DFS advantage for tamoxifen, but only two large studies, the North American Treaty Organization trial and the Scottish trial,[96,97] showed a significant OS advantage. A survival trend in favor of tamoxifen was found in most of the other trials.

Earlier meta-analyses suggested that tamoxifen had no benefit in women younger than age 50.[12,22] However, because of the inclusion of women with ER-negative tumors, and because the duration of tamoxifen treatment was usually only 1 or 2 years in these early trials, definitive conclusions could not be drawn. There is now convincing evidence showing that more prolonged treatment (approximately 5 years) results in a significant benefit in women younger than 50 years old, as well as in older women, as long as their tumors are ER positive. In the previously mentioned NSABP node-negative adjuvant trial of tamoxifen versus placebo in ER-positive patients, tamoxifen was more effective than placebo both in women who had reached menopause and in those who had not.[35] The recent meta-analysis confirms these results (Table 10).[95] In the entire group of patients with ER-positive tumors, there is nearly a 50% reduction in the annual odds of recurrence and a 26% reduction in the annual odds of death. Women younger than age 50 years, most of whom would be expected to be premenopausal, benefit from tamoxifen as much as older women, and even women younger than age 40 benefit, with reduced recurrence and mortality. The benefits found with 5 years of tamoxifen in younger women, along with the lack of benefit with the shorter durations used in earlier studies, strongly suggest that longer treatment is very important in this age group. These data also indicate that tamoxifen can inhibit the proliferation of breast cancer cells even in the presence of high serum levels of estrogen, which are common in premenopausal patients who take the drug, and they demand that oncologists reexamine the traditional approach of reserving tamoxifen for postmenopausal women and treating premenopausal women with chemotherapy only. Whether tamoxifen is equivalent or even superior to chemotherapy in premenopausal women, as it appears to be in older women who have ER-positive tumors, remains a question. Although the data from the meta-analysis suggest that tamoxifen is at least as effective as adjuvant chemotherapy in women younger than age 50 with ER-positive tumors, few studies have directly addressed this question. In a single small trial of premenopausal women with ER-positive tumors, chemotherapy was superior to tamoxifen, but the duration of tamoxifen treatment was only 2 years.[98] In a 1997 large randomized trial that compared chemotherapy plus tamoxifen with tamoxifen alone, the combination was more effective.[99] However, this study did not have a chemotherapy-alone arm to assess the relative effectiveness of each single modality.

TABLE 10. *Effects of tamoxifen given for 5 years in women with estrogen receptor–positive tumors by age*

Age (yr)	Reduction in annual odds	
	Recurrence (%)	Death (%)
All patients	47 ± 3	26 ± 4
<40	54 ± 13	52 ± 17
40–49	41 ± 10	22 ± 13
<50	45 ± 8	32 ± 10
50–59	37 ± 6	11 ± 8
60–69	54 ± 5	33 ± 6
70+	54 ± 13	34 ± 13

Adapted from ref. 95.

In any event, with more than 15 years of follow-up from many studies, it is now clear that if tamoxifen is given for 5 years to patients selected on the basis of ER status, it is effective in both younger and older patients. It is also important to note that the differences in outcome between tamoxifen and no tamoxifen observed after 5 years of follow-up grew even larger during the next 5 years, indicating that the benefits of tamoxifen are very durable over time.[95]

Tamoxifen in Node-Negative and Node-Positive Patients

No biological reason suggests that women with node-negative breast cancer would respond differently to adjuvant tamoxifen (or chemotherapy) than those with positive nodes, and many trials of adjuvant tamoxifen included both node-negative and node-positive patients. Fewer recurrences and deaths in the node-negative subset make it more difficult to show significant differences between tamoxifen and no treatment, but strong trends were evident in the larger studies.[96,97] NSABP trial B-14 is by far the largest trial of adjuvant tamoxifen (2,644 patients), and it focused on patients with histologically negative axillary nodes.[35,100] Both patients younger than 50 years of age (820 patients) and older patients (1,824 patients) were eligible, and all patients had ER-positive disease. Patients were randomly assigned to receive placebo or tamoxifen for 5 years, and those who received tamoxifen were reassigned at 5 years to stop therapy or to continue for 5 additional years. Significantly fewer recurrences and deaths occurred in both premenopausal and postmenopausal patients given tamoxifen for at least 5 years than in those given placebo. Tamoxifen-treated patients also had fewer ipsilateral breast, local-regional, and distant recurrences than placebo-treated patients, and they had a substantial reduction (approximately 50%) in contralateral breast cancer.

The meta-analysis also suggests that the benefit with adjuvant tamoxifen is similar for node-negative and node-positive patients.[12,22,95] The reduction in the annual odds of recurrence was 49% ± 4% for node-negative patients and 43% ± 5% for node-positive women given tamoxifen for 5 years (see Table 10). Tamoxifen also reduced the annual odds of death from any cause in both groups (25% ± 5% and 28% ± 6%, respectively). Thus, the cumulative data suggest that tamoxifen improves survival in both node-negative patients, who already have a lower risk of recurrence and death, and in node-positive patients. Because of its favorable toxicity profile, tamoxifen is especially attractive for treating women who have a lower risk of disease recurrence. Although the absolute benefit of tamoxifen is modest in this group of patients because most are cured by surgery alone, they experience less morbidity than with chemotherapy, and they may also enjoy the ancillary benefits of tamoxifen described in the following section.

TABLE 11. *Duration of tamoxifen therapy by age and nodal status*

G roup	Reduction (SD) in annual odds	
	Recurrence	Death
Tamoxifen ~ 1 yr		
Node negative	17 (8%)	13 (8%)
Node positive	21 (3%)	12 (4%)
Age <50 yr	2 (7%)	−2 (8%)
Age 50–59 yr	28 (6%)	21 (6%)
Age 60–69 yr	26 (6%)	12 (6%)
Age 70+ yr	22 (9%)	8 (8%)
Total	**20 (3%)**	**11 (3%)**
Tamoxifen ~ 2 yr		
Node negative	28 (5%)	11 (6%)
Node positive	30 (3%)	19 (3%)
Age <50 yr	14 (5%)	10 (6%)
Age 50–59 yr	32 (4%)	19 (5%)
Age 60–69 yr	33 (4%)	12 (5%)
Age 70+ yr	42 (8%)	36 (7%)
Total	**29 (3%)**	**17 (3%)**
Tamoxifen ~ 5 yr		
Node negative	49 (4%)	25 (5%)
Node positive	43 (5%)	28 (6%)
Age <50 yr	45 (8%)	32 (10%)
Age 50–59 yr	37 (6%)	11 (8%)
Age 60–69 yr	54 (5%)	33 (6%)
Age 70+ yr	54 (13%)	34 (13%)
Total	**47 (3%)**	**26 (4%)**

Estrogen receptor–poor tumors are excluded.
Adapted from ref. 95.

Optimal Duration of Tamoxifen Therapy

Theoretical reasons exist for prolonged or even indefinite tamoxifen therapy, but published studies suggest that extending treatment to 5 years, but not longer, may be optimal. Several trials compared shorter versus longer tamoxifen adjuvant treatment directly. In two large European trials from Britain and Sweden, respectively, women treated with tamoxifen for 5 years had fewer recurrences and deaths than those treated for only 2 years.[101,102] Two North American trials, the large trial from the NSABP and a much smaller trial, compared tamoxifen treatment for 5 years with treatment that lasted for approximately 10 years,[100,103] and a trial from Scotland compared 5 years with indefinite tamoxifen treatment.[104] Although the numbers of recurrences and deaths are small given the short follow-up time in some of these trials, there is no convincing evidence that treatment lasting longer than 5 years is beneficial. In fact, in two of these trials there was a trend, highly statistically significant in one, toward a detrimental effect after treatment for more than 5 years.[100,104] Furthermore, more prolonged administration of tamoxifen did not further reduce the incidence of contralateral breast cancer compared to just 5 years of treatment.

A 1998 meta-analysis compared trials of tamoxifen adjuvant therapy for approximately 1 year, 2 years, or 5 years (Table 11).[95] After excluding patients with known ER-poor tumors, treatment for 5 years produced significantly superior recurrence and mortality benefits. Women younger than 50 years of age especially benefited from the longer-term treatment. Other trials are currently readdressing the issue of very long-term tamoxifen, but until the results of these trials are available, it seems reasonable to recommend that tamoxifen be given for 5 years, regardless of age or nodal status.

Given the trends for poorer outcome with tamoxifen treatment for longer than 5 years in two large trials and the failure of more prolonged treatment to reduce further contralateral breast cancer risk, the practice of extending tamoxifen beyond 5 years for its favorable effects on bone density and cholesterol is not justified. Furthermore, switching from tamoxifen to other similar drugs, such as toremifene or raloxifene, after 5 years seems hazardous until this strategy has been adequately tested in randomized trials. The possibly inferior results in studies of very long-term tamoxifen could be due to tamoxifen-stimulated growth, which may be one mechanism for acquired tamoxifen resistance.[105] Toremifene, like tamoxifen, stimulated tumor growth after months of treatment in an *in vivo* experimental model, and the effects of raloxifene are not yet known.[106]

Tamoxifen in Patients with Estrogen Receptor–Rich or Estrogen Receptor–Poor Tumors

Many of the early tamoxifen adjuvant trials included patients with ER-negative or ER-poor as well as ER-positive and ER-unknown tumors. These studies helped to assess the potential benefits of tamoxifen in both subsets. The results are difficult to interpret, however, because of varying definitions of *ER-positive* and *ER-negative* and because only a fraction of the patients included in some of these studies had ER assays performed. Most studies of breast cancer cells grown in tissue culture or studies using animal models show little or no effects of tamoxifen in ER-negative cells at drug concentrations achieved in patients.[107,108] However, tamoxifen has numerous effects on cells that are not mediated through the ER that would affect receptor-negative tumors. Alternatively, the effects of the drug on the few ER-positive cells present in an "ER-negative" tumor could conceivably indirectly also inhibit cell populations that lack receptors. Finally, the drug has systemic effects, such as lowering serum IGF-I levels, that could inhibit growth of tumors regardless of ER content.[94,109] Antitumor activity, even in ER-negative tumors, is therefore plausible. However, the low response rates observed with tamoxifen in ER-negative metastatic disease (5% to 10%) argue that these ancillary cellular effects of tamoxifen are clinically unimportant and suggest that the benefit is likely to be modest in the adjuvant setting. The few responses observed in such patients are more consistent with false-negative ER assays.

Nevertheless, several trials have reported some advantage for tamoxifen in "ER-poor" patients. The North Atlantic Treaty Organization trial measured ER on a proportion of their patients.[96] When 5 fmol per mg protein was used to distinguish ER-positive from ER-negative, ER-negative patients in the untreated group did not have the expected more rapid rate of recurrence than those with ER-positive tumors, raising questions about the validity of the assay. Using this cutoff, the beneficial effects of tamoxifen were just as great in the ER-negative as in the ER-positive group. This study did find a correlation between tamoxifen response and histologic grade, which can be thought of as a surrogate marker for ER status.[110] Patients with grade 1 and 2 tumors, which are more likely to be ER positive, benefited from tamoxifen, whereas those with grade 3 tumors did not.

The Scottish tamoxifen trial did report a relationship between ER status and tamoxifen benefit.[97] The higher the ER, the greater the difference between tamoxifen and control patients in DFS at 3 years. However, even patients with low tumor ER had a statistically significant benefit. NSABP study B-09 randomized patients to chemotherapy alone or to chemotherapy and tamoxifen.[111] Overall, no significant benefit was observed for tamoxifen in patients with tumor ER less than 10 fmol per mg protein, whereas a significant improvement in DFS was observed in the ER-positive group. However, multiple-subset analysis by age and ER status showed that women aged 60 to 70 years received some benefit from tamoxifen even if their tumor had an ER content of 0 to 9 fmol per mg protein. The authors concluded that this result was probably related to analytical errors in receptor measurement. It might also have been related to chance, given the multiple subsets analyzed.

TABLE 12. *Effects of tamoxifen for 5 years according to estrogen-receptor level*

Estrogen-receptor level	Reduction (SD) in annual odds: Recurrence	Reduction (SD) in annual odds: Death
Poor (<10 fmol/mg)	6 (11%)	−3 (11%)
Unknown	37 (8%)	21 (9%)
Positive (≥10 fmol/mg)	50 (4%)	28 (5%)
10–99 fmol/mg	43 (5%)	23 (6%)
≥100 fmol/mg	60 (6%)	36 (7%)

Adapted from ref. 95.

Earlier meta-analyses suggested a small but statistically significant survival benefit in women with ER-poor tumors treated with adjuvant tamoxifen, but the most recent meta-analysis with longer follow-up and a larger sample size did not[22,95] (Table 12). Patients with ER-poor tumors, a subset that includes tumors in which ER is undetectable or borderline positive (3 to 10 fmol per mg protein by ligand-binding assay), showed no reduction in the annual odds of recurrence or death. The ER-unknown group (approximately 70% would be expected to be positive) had a 37% reduction in the annual odds of recurrence and a 21% reduction in the annual odds of death. Women with tumors known to be definitely positive for ER had a 50% reduction in the annual odds of recurrence and a 28% reduction in the annual odds of death with 5 years of tamoxifen, and those with high levels of ER (≥100 fmol per mg protein) enjoyed even greater reductions in recurrence and mortality.

The only prospective randomized trial addressing the value of 5 years of tamoxifen in ER-positive and ER-negative patients was presented in preliminary form, although the results have not yet been published.[56] This trial randomized both ER-positive and ER-negative node-negative patients to either chemotherapy alone or chemotherapy plus tamoxifen, and ER was measured in quality-controlled laboratories. This trial now shows a strong trend, which reaches statistical significance in premenopausal patients, for a detrimental effect on DFS and OS when tamoxifen is used in patients whose tumors have very low or undetectable ER.

Relatively few studies have included measurements of progesterone receptors (PgR) in tumor tissue. However, in the meta-analysis, among women with ER-positive tumors, the efficacy of tamoxifen was independent of the concentration of PgR in the tumor tissue.[95] Among women with ER-negative tumors, those few whose tumors contained PgR did benefit from tamoxifen, data similar to those in studies of patients with metastatic disease.

Until more data are available, it seems prudent to restrict the use of tamoxifen to women with ER- or PgR-positive tumors, or both. Additional study is required to determine whether the risk of recurrence is indeed somewhat higher when tamoxifen is used in ER-negative patients, a detrimental effect that would outweigh any ancillary benefits of tamoxifen on osteoporosis, lipid profiles, and reduction in contralateral breast cancer.

Tamoxifen in Elderly Patients

Because it is generally well tolerated, tamoxifen has been used to treat elderly patients with breast cancer. The meta-analysis demonstrates a significant mortality reduction in patients older than 70 years treated with adjuvant tamoxifen (see Table 10).[95] Furthermore, some individual trials have specifically targeted this population. The ECOG randomized 181 patients 65 years of age or older to tamoxifen or placebo for 2 years.[112] The drug was well tolerated, and significant reductions in recurrence and borderline significant reductions in mortality were observed. Tamoxifen also reduced the incidence of contralateral breast cancers. The majority of the patients who died in this study (61%) succumbed to breast cancer, although, as anticipated, a significant number of these older women (22%) died of illness not related to cancer, a factor that must be considered when making adjuvant therapy decisions.

ANCILLARY BENEFITS OF TAMOXIFEN

Although we think of tamoxifen as an estrogen antagonist because of its antiproliferative properties in the breast, it is more appropriately classified as a SERM, because it has estrogen agonist properties in certain tissues and cells and on certain genes, whereas it has estrogen antagonist properties on others. These unique dual activities of tamoxifen provide additional potential benefits for women taking the drug.[113]

Serum Lipoproteins and Mortality from Cardiovascular Causes

In contrast to earlier meta-analyses, a 1998 meta-analysis does not demonstrate a reduction in the incidence of non–cancer-related deaths.[12,95] However, it includes data from many different areas of the world, and accurate causes of death are difficult to obtain in some countries. Furthermore, the meta-analysis includes data from patients who took tamoxifen for variable periods of time, ranging from less than a year to more than 5 years. Most of the ancillary benefits of tamoxifen might be expected to require at least several years of therapy. Individual trials of tamoxifen adjuvant therapy do suggest that the rate of non–breast cancer–related deaths (deaths before relapse), may be reduced.[97,113–116] This mortality reduction is largely due to a decrease in deaths from cardiovascular causes. In addition, fewer hospitalizations for cardiac events have been reported for patients taking tamoxifen.[115] The estrogen agonist properties of tamoxifen may account for these reductions. Serum concentrations of total cholesterol and low-density lipoprotein cholesterol are reduced by tamoxifen, and it may also inhibit atherogenesis by directly affecting the metabolism of low-density lipoproteins in the arteries.[115,117–119]

Bone Mineral Density

Tamoxifen also has estrogen agonist properties in bone. In postmenopausal women, long-term tamoxifen treatment increases the bone density of the axial skeleton and stabilizes the bone density of the appendicular skeleton.[91,120] In premenopausal women, however, tamoxifen may decrease bone mineral density by antagonizing the more potent activity of endogenous estrogen.[121] Although evaluating osteoporotic fracture rates in patients with a diagnosis of metastatic breast cancer is difficult, a 1998 prevention trial of tamoxifen does show a significant reduction in fractures with 5 years of treatment.[122]

Contralateral Breast Cancer and Prevention of Breast Cancer in Women at High Risk

Individual clinical trials in patients with invasive breast cancer as well as the updated meta-analysis indicate that there is nearly a 50% reduction in the risk of contralateral breast cancer after approximately 5 years of tamoxifen treatment.[95,100,123,124] This reduction in the incidence of contralateral breast cancer, as well as the potentially beneficial effects of tamoxifen on cardiovascular disease and osteoporosis, provided the rationale for trials assessing the use of tamoxifen and raloxifene for the prevention of breast cancer.[122,125–127] Two of these trials, one using tamoxifen (NSABP P-1) and the other employing a similar SERM, raloxifene, and both with a short follow-up of 3 to 4 years, show a 50% to 70% reduction in the risk of breast cancer.[122,125] Two smaller studies using tamoxifen failed to confirm these results.[126,127] The explanation for these disparate results is not clear, but it could be related to differences in the population of women studied, differences in compliance rates, or the use of estrogen replacement therapy along with tamoxifen in the two negative studies. The incidence of fractures is also lower in the raloxifene and NSABP tamoxifen trials, whereas the incidence of endometrial cancer is higher with tamoxifen.[122,125] No difference has arisen between placebo and tamoxifen in the incidence of ischemic heart disease. Whether tamoxifen is just preventing the clinical appearance of occult cancers that must have been present in some women at entry into the trial or whether it will have a true prevention effect by blocking or reversing premalignant progression requires longer follow-up of women in these trials.

TAMOXIFEN SUMMARY

Taking tamoxifen for 5 years prolongs DFS and OS in patients with ER-positive tumors regardless of axillary lymph node status. Equally beneficial effects are seen in premenopausal and postmenopausal women. Tamoxifen adjuvant therapy should be considered for nearly all such patients, except perhaps those with a very low risk of disease recurrence, in whom the absolute benefit of tamoxifen is small. These patients might also benefit, however, from the ancillary effects of tamoxifen on bone, lipids, and contralateral breast cancer, although the potential for occasional serious toxicity exists (see the section Toxicity of Adjuvant Therapy).

OTHER FORMS OF ADJUVANT ENDOCRINE THERAPY

Adjuvant Ovarian Ablation

Among the first randomized trials of adjuvant therapy in breast cancer were studies of adjuvant ovarian ablation either by surgical oophorectomy or by irradiation.[12,128] Some of these trials were not properly randomized by modern standards.[6] Many were small, a few included both premenopausal and postmenopausal women, and none included ER analyses, which were not yet available. Most of these trials found a significant DFS advantage for ovarian ablation, and two reported a significant OS advantage.[129,130]

The meta-analysis included data from 12 properly randomized trials of ovarian ablation involving 2,102 patients younger than 50 years of age; 7 of these trials compared ovarian ablation with no adjuvant therapy, and 5 compared ovarian ablation and chemotherapy with the same chemotherapy alone.[128] As expected, no significant benefit was observed for oopharectomy among 1,354 women older than 50 years of age, most of whom were postmenopausal, when randomized. Younger women had a significant DFS and OS advantage with ovarian ablation compared to no adjuvant therapy (25% ± 7% reduction in the odds of recurrence and 24% ± 7% reduction in the odds of death) (Table 13). Data are insufficient, even in the meta-analysis, to determine whether ovarian ablation reduces the incidence of contralateral breast cancer. These results are comparable to those achieved with chemotherapy in women younger than 50 years of age. Different quantitative results were noted in the studies of ovarian ablation alone compared with those studies in which the procedure was combined with chemotherapy (see Table 13).[128] In the presence of chemotherapy, which itself results in a chemical ablation in many patients, the benefit of ovarian ablation was much smaller and not statistically significant. However, the relatively small number of patients precludes definitive statements about the benefits of ovarian ablation when combined with chemotherapy. Preliminary results of a large intergroup trial randomizing ER-positive node-positive premenopausal women to chemotherapy alone, chemotherapy combined with chemical ablation with goserelin, or chemotherapy plus goserelin plus tamoxifen suggest that ovarian ablation adds little to chemotherapy.[131] Outcome was similar for patients randomized to chemotherapy alone or combined with goserelin. The addition of tamoxifen, however, improved DFS.

TABLE 13. *Meta-analysis of the effects of ovarian ablation*

Group	Reduction in annual odds: Recurrence (%)	Reduction in annual odds: Death (%)
Ovarian ablation vs no adjuvant therapy	25 ± 7	24 ± 7
Ovarian ablation + chemotherapy vs chemotherapy	10 ± 9	8 ± 10

Modified from ref. 128.

Because chemotherapy plus goserelin produced no better results than chemotherapy alone, one might argue that ovarian ablation alone would not likely be superior to chemotherapy alone in premenopausal ER-positive patients. However, another smaller trial suggests that it might be.[132] More than 300 node-positive premenopausal patients were randomized to intravenous CMF given every 3 weeks for six or eight cycles or to ovarian ablation, each with or without prednisolone, 7.5 mg per day, for 5 years. Prednisolone offered no advantage. At a median follow-up of approximately 6 years, no overall difference was noted between CMF and ovarian ablation. ER status was known for 81% of the patients in this trial, however, and analysis by ER status yielded interesting results. Patients with low ER (less than 20 fmol per mg protein) benefited more from chemotherapy, and those with high ER (20 fmol per mg protein or higher) benefited more from ovarian ablation. These results suggest that chemotherapy works through a cytotoxic mechanism in addition to the endocrine effects achieved in patients who had chemical castration. Otherwise, the benefits of chemotherapy in the ER-negative subset would be more modest. Thus, the relative benefits of chemotherapy and ovarian ablation in young patients remain inconclusive, and they may depend on the type of chemotherapy administered and the incidence of chemotherapy-induced ovarian ablation.

The database from which to draw definitive conclusions on the value of ovarian ablation is much less substantial than that for adjuvant tamoxifen and chemotherapy. Other studies are comparing ovarian ablation with or without chemotherapy. More information on the long-term consequences of inducing ovarian failure in young women is also needed. Premature coronary artery disease and osteoporosis might be expected in some patients. Even short-term treatment with goserelin in premenopausal women with endometriosis was associated with bone loss.[133] The meta-analysis does not yet show increased vascular deaths in women with breast cancer treated by ovarian ablation, but the database is small.[12,128] Considering the relatively limited database, it is difficult to know where ovarian ablation fits in our current armamentarium of adjuvant therapies for premenopausal patients. It might be considered in those who refuse other therapies or in patients with hereditary breast cancer syndrome who have a high risk of developing ovarian cancer.

Other Trials of Adjuvant Endocrine Therapy

Individual small trials of other forms of endocrine therapy have been reported, but data are insufficient to draw conclusions or to make recommendations. High-dose diethylstilbestrol, which is too toxic for routine use in the adjuvant setting, was similar to tamoxifen in improving DFS in postmenopausal patients in a Danish study.[134] Eight-year follow-up of an English trial in which 354 postmenopausal node-positive patients were randomized to aminoglutethimide (an aromatase inhibitor that lowers estrogen levels) and hydrocortisone or to placebo for 2 years indicated no overall DFS or OS benefit.[135] Strong favorable trends were evident, however, in ER-positive patients treated with aminoglutethimide, and trials of new aromatase inhibitors are in progress. Preliminary results of a trial using high-dose medroxyprogesterone acetate or no adjuvant therapy in 240 node-negative patients showed significant improvements in both DFS and OS.[136] All of these therapies, however, are more toxic than tamoxifen, and in the absence of additional data, they cannot be recommended for adjuvant therapy, except perhaps in the rare situation in which tamoxifen is not tolerated.

ADJUVANT CHEMOENDOCRINE THERAPY

The benefits of adjuvant chemotherapy and endocrine therapy used as single modalities prompted investigators to consider a combined approach based on the basic oncology principle of using multiple therapies or drugs that have different mechanisms of action and nonoverlapping toxicities. Conceptually, cells in a heterogeneous tumor could be sensitive only to endocrine therapy, sensitive only to chemotherapy, sensitive to both therapies, or resistant to both. A combined approach might then provide an additive beneficial antitumor effect. The panoply of cellular effects of endocrine therapy could also, on the other hand, interact with cytotoxic agents to alter chemosensitivity. Tamoxifen and estrogen deprivation are predominantly cytostatic and slow cell proliferation by blocking cell cycle transit.[137–139] These cell cycle alterations could conceivably render cells less sensitive to cell cycle–active chemotherapeutic agents. Tamoxifen has a variety of other effects on the cell that could also alter sensitivity to cytotoxic agents. It antagonizes calmodulin and is an effective Ca^{2+} channel antagonist—effects that could alter drug uptake.[140,141] Membrane lipids are altered by tamoxifen, an effect that could change the diffusion rates of certain drugs.[142] Tamoxifen and progestins inhibit p-glycoprotein, an effect that could enhance sensitivity to drugs such as doxorubicin.[143,144] Finally, the apoptosis inhibitor Bcl-2 is down-regulated by tamoxifen, possibly enhancing sensitivity to drugs using this cell death pathway.[145]

Preclinical studies investigating interactions between tamoxifen and various chemotherapeutic drugs have not always produced consistent results, but they do provide some evidence for both antagonistic and additive interactions, depending on the drug.[146] Tamoxifen antagonized the cytotoxicity of melphalan and 5-fluorouracil in human breast cancer cells, a finding that perhaps explains the poorer results obtained by adding tamoxifen to these agents in premenopausal receptor-negative patients in an NSABP study.[111,146,147] On the other hand, tamoxifen demonstrated an additive effect when it was combined with doxorubicin and cyclophosphamide *in vitro*,[146] and one of the few trials showing a significant survival advantage for chemotherapy plus tamoxifen compared with tamoxifen alone used cyclophosphamide and doxorubicin.[148] These *in vitro* drug interactions were independent of ER status and were not related to the cell cycle effects of tamoxifen.[146]

Clinical trials of chemoendocrine therapy have been designed in several ways. A few early trials compared a CMF-based chemotherapy regimen including tamoxifen with a no-treatment control arm in postmenopausal, node-positive patients.[149–151] These trials were small, and although all showed prolonged DFS with the adjuvant treatment, only the largest study demonstrated a significant OS advantage. Given the proven benefit for chemotherapy in women younger than 50 years of age and the proven benefits of tamoxifen in older patients, especially those with ER-positive tumors, the two questions of greatest interest to the clinician are the following: (a) Is it advantageous to add endocrine therapy (tamoxifen or ovarian ablation) to chemotherapy in younger women? (b) Should chemotherapy be added to tamoxifen therapy in older women? Many studies have now been completed comparing chemotherapy alone and combined with endocrine therapy in premenopausal patients and comparing tamoxifen with or without chemotherapy in postmenopausal patients.[23,95]

Chemoendocrine Therapy in Premenopausal Patients

Because chemotherapy has been considered standard therapy in premenopausal patients for many years, trials comparing endocrine therapy, such as tamoxifen, in one group with chemotherapy plus tamoxifen in another are few. The largest was reported by the NSABP in 1997 and shows an advantage for the combination in ER-positive patients.[99] Abundant data, however, are available from trials comparing chemotherapy with or without endocrine therapy.

Chemotherapy and Ovarian Ablation

As described in the section Adjuvant Ovarian Ablation, trials of chemotherapy alone versus chemotherapy and ovarian ablation are complicated by the fact that chemotherapy itself induces chemical ovarian ablation, the frequency of which depends on the age of the patient and the chemotherapy regimen used. (See Chapter 71 for more details.) Furthermore, few trials have measured blood estrogen levels, and amenorrhea, although a valuable surrogate marker, may not always indicate complete loss of ovarian function. Two small studies provide somewhat conflicting results.[152,153] One study suggests a slight advantage for the combination of CMF plus prednisone (CMFP) plus oophorectomy compared with CMFP alone.[152] The other study compared one year of CMFVP versus the same chemotherapy combined with oophorectomy in premenopausal patients with ER-positive tumors.[153] No advantage for adding ovarian ablation was evident at 5 years, although a trend existed in patients with four or more positive axillary lymph nodes. A large intergroup study of more than 1,500 premenopausal patients with ER-positive tumors and positive axillary lymph nodes suggests that drug-induced ovarian ablation using goserelin for 5 years after CAF chemotherapy is no better than CAF chemotherapy alone.[131] Presently, therefore, there are no data to support the use of ovarian ablation and chemotherapy in young women.

Chemotherapy and Tamoxifen in Premenopausal Patients

Whether tamoxifen adds to the benefits achieved with chemotherapy in younger patients has been addressed by numerous randomized trials.[12,22,95]

As described in the introduction to the section Adjuvant Chemoendocrine Therapy, the NSABP B-09 randomly assigned 1,858 patients (779 premenopausal) to receive melphalan and 5-fluorouracil therapy or chemotherapy and tamoxifen.[111] An advantage for tamoxifen was observed in postmenopausal patients but not in premenopausal women, who actually had worse DFS and OS. This trial raised the question of an antagonistic drug interaction, and we now know that tamoxifen inhibits cellular uptake of melphalan.[146,147] These results also convinced some oncologists to begin tamoxifen after chemotherapy is completed to avoid possible antagonism. However, it is also possible that with certain drugs, tamoxifen may be additive or even synergistic because of the many different pathways that it affects in cells. Results of a completed intergroup trial evaluating combined versus sequential tamoxifen with CAF chemotherapy in postmenopausal ER-positive patients should be available in 2000.[31]

Several other older studies found either no advantage to the addition of tamoxifen to CMF-based chemotherapy or, in one study, even a trend for a survival detriment.[154–156] However, in all of these studies, tamoxifen was only given for 1 year—a duration that is now considered suboptimal. An Italian study used CMF followed by epirubicin chemotherapy with or without tamoxifen for 5 years in ER-positive premenopausal patients.[157] A trend in favor of the addition of tamoxifen did not reach statistical significance in this small study.

Two large intergroup trials and the most recent meta-analysis clearly demonstrate that there is an additional benefit for adding tamoxifen for 5 years in premenopausal patients treated with chemotherapy whose tumors are ER positive. In one study directed by SWOG, more than 2,000 pre- and postmenopausal patients who had high-risk node-negative disease based on tumor size, ER status, and proliferation rates measured by DNA flow cytometry were randomized initially to CMF or CAF chemotherapy and then to tamoxifen or not for 5 years.[56] The study intentionally included both ER-positive and ER-negative patients to directly test the value of the addition of tamoxifen in each subset. Initial results of the trial demonstrate that CAF is somewhat superior to CMF and that tamoxifen is significantly better than no tamoxifen but only in ER-positive patients. In fact, DFS and OS are slightly worse (statistically significantly so in the premenopausal group) in patients whose tumors are ER negative. The trial suggests that tamoxifen should not be routinely given to all patients, especially if their tumors are receptor negative.

TABLE 14. *Meta-analysis of chemotherapy plus 5 years of tamoxifen*

Group	Reduction in annual odds: Recurrence (%)	Reduction in annual odds: Death (%)
All ages		
C + T vs T	Not reported	Not reported
C+T vs C	52 ± 8	47 ± 9
Age <50 yr		
C + T vs T	21 ± 13	25 ± 14
C + T vs C	40 ± 19	39 ± 22
Age ≥50 yr		
C + T vs T	19 ± 3	11 ± 4
C + T vs C	54 ± 8	49 ± 10

C, chemotherapy; T, tamoxifen.
Adapted from refs. 23 and 95.

A trial reported in 1999, directed by the ECOG compared CAF chemotherapy alone, CAF chemotherapy followed by 5 years of goserelin (Zoladex), or 5 years of Zoladex and tamoxifen in premenopausal, node-positive ER-positive patients.[131] As described in the section Chemotherapy and Ovarian Ablation, this trial showed no advantage for the addition of Zoladex alone to CAF chemotherapy but did demonstrate an advantage for the addition of Zoladex and tamoxifen. Given the wealth of data reviewed earlier, it is doubtful that Zoladex contributed much, if anything, to the favorable outcome for patients on the third arm.

The 1998 meta-analysis also reports the effects of chemoendocrine therapy in women younger than 50 years of age[23,95] (Table 14). Relatively few studies compare chemotherapy plus tamoxifen versus tamoxifen alone, and, furthermore, the meta-analysis included studies of all durations of tamoxifen and studies that contained ER-negative patients. The results suggest that the addition of chemotherapy to tamoxifen provides a modest advantage compared to tamoxifen alone. However, the large NSABP trial in ER-positive patients comparing tamoxifen alone for 5 years versus chemotherapy plus tamoxifen for 5 years did show a significant advantage for the addition of chemotherapy, especially in women younger than 50 years of age.[99]

It is perhaps a more relevant clinical question to ask whether 5 years of tamoxifen adds to the benefits of chemotherapy in women younger than 50 years of age. Although the meta-analysis data are less reliable because of relatively small numbers, they do suggest that the addition of tamoxifen to chemotherapy in ER-positive patients provides significant additional benefit (see Table 14).[95] These data are supported by those from the intergroup trial described two paragraphs earlier show an advantage for chemotherapy plus tamoxifen only in patients with ER-positive tumors.[56] Thus, in women younger than 50 years of age with breast cancer of sufficient risk to warrant adjuvant systemic therapy, it would seem reasonable to add 5 years of tamoxifen to adjuvant chemotherapy, but only if the tumor is ER positive. Because of its favorable toxicity profile, it might even be reasonable to use tamoxifen alone in some premenopausal patients with relatively lower-risk, ER-positive tumors.

Chemoendocrine Therapy in Postmenopausal Patients

Many randomized trials have investigated chemoendocrine therapy in postmenopausal women 50 years of age and older, most of whom are postmenopausal. Some trials directly compared chemotherapy alone with chemotherapy plus tamoxifen, whereas others compared chemotherapy plus tamoxifen versus tamoxifen alone. In early studies, a CMF-based regimen was used most frequently. Most of the trials assessing the addition of tamoxifen to chemotherapy found a highly significant benefit, which is not surprising, considering the meager benefits of chemotherapy and the more substantial benefits of tamoxifen in this age group. A more pressing clinical question, however, is whether the addition of chemotherapy with its associated toxicities is better than tamoxifen alone.

Several mature trials have addressed this question.[151,158,159] These studies are difficult to interpret, however, because either they did not focus on ER-positive patients or because tamoxifen was given for only 1 year, or both. The studies also used a CMF-based regimen and usually gave chemotherapy concomitantly with tamoxifen. These studies typically showed either no benefit for the addition of chemotherapy or a modest benefit in DFS but not OS.

A more recent trial reported in 1997 from Canada compared the all-intravenous, every-3-week CMF regimen for eight cycles combined with tamoxifen for 2 years versus tamoxifen alone in receptor-positive postmenopausal women.[160] No significant differences were found in DFS or OS between the two arms, but chemotherapy added substantial toxicity.

In a 1997 trial from the International Group comparing tamoxifen alone for 5 years versus tamoxifen combined with CMF-based chemotherapy, a significant advantage was observed for the combination approach if the tumor was ER positive.[161] In contrast, in patients with ER-negative tumors, tamoxifen plus CMF was associated with a nonsignificant increased risk of relapse, similar to the trial discussed earlier.[56]

Two studies that used doxorubicin-based chemotherapy regimens in ER-positive postmenopausal patients have reported significant advantages for the addition of chemotherapy to 5 years of tamoxifen.[31,148] NSABP B-16 compared tamoxifen alone in one arm, AC for 4 cycles plus tamoxifen in a second, and PAF (melphalan, doxorubicin, 5-fluorouracil) for 17 cycles plus tamoxifen in a third. AC plus tamoxifen significantly improved both DFS and OS compared with tamoxifen alone. The SWOG Intergroup trial compared tamoxifen alone for 5 years, CAF for six cycles plus tamoxifen starting at the same time as the chemotherapy, and CAF for six cycles followed by 5 years of tamoxifen.[31] No data are yet available on the optimal sequence of CAF plus tamoxifen, but chemotherapy provided a significant DFS advantage compared to tamoxifen alone. The HER-2/neu oncogene was measured in a subset of patients in this trial.[162] In HER-2/neu–negative patients, CAF chemotherapy provided no significant DFS advantage, but the outcome in HER-2/neu–positive patients treated with tamoxifen alone was relatively poor, and the addition of chemotherapy provided a sizable benefit. The relationship between HER-2/neu status and tumor responsiveness to chemoendocrine therapy requires more study, but if other trials can confirm these results, then postmenopausal patients with ER-positive, HER-2/neu–negative tumors might be spared the additional toxicity and cost of adjuvant chemotherapy because it would offer few additional clinical benefits. The addition of chemotherapy would then be reserved for those few patients who have HER-2/neu–positive tumors.

The meta-analysis confirms that the addition of chemotherapy to tamoxifen provides moderate benefits in women 50 years of age and older (see Table 14).[23,95] Thus, the cumulative data would suggest that the addition of chemotherapy to tamoxifen should be considered in postmenopausal women with ER-positive tumors. However, this modest benefit together with the additional toxicity associated with chemotherapy need to be considered. In one trial discussed earlier, chemoendocrine therapy did not provide more quality-adjusted survival time than tamoxifen alone in this group of patients.[20] Individualization of treatment, after careful discussion of the risks and benefits with the patient, is necessary for an informed decision.

ADJUVANT IMMUNOTHERAPY

More than 20 randomized trials of adjuvant immunotherapy have been completed.[12,22] Most of these trials included other therapies in addition to treatment with BCG, levamisole, or a variety of other nonspecific immune stimulants. None of these individual trials demonstrated a significant DFS or OS benefit for immunotherapy. Even the meta-analyses of all trials, which included more than 6,000 patients, could not find a hint of benefit. In fact, the analysis of the BCG trials showed a sizable and statistically significant adverse impact on both DFS and OS (odds reduction for DFS, –17% ± 8%;

odds reduction for OS, –20% ± 8%). Currently, no evidence supports the use of immunotherapy in the adjuvant treatment of breast cancer.

TOXICITY OF ADJUVANT THERAPY

Toxicity of Adjuvant Chemotherapy

Acute Toxicity

In general, women with early breast cancer tolerate adjuvant chemotherapy well, better than those with metastatic disease, whose health may be compromised by a larger tumor burden and visceral dysfunction. Modifications of normal lifestyle are required during the treatment period of usually 4 to 6 months, but most patients are able to continue working and performing their daily routines. Death caused by the complications of adjuvant therapy is uncommon, but it can be devastating when an apparently healthy woman with a curable cancer dies of neutropenic infection. No deaths were reported in a large trial of more than 2,000 node-positive patients (75% younger than 50 years old) treated with AC or CMF chemotherapy.[53] Another trial of 966 postmenopausal patients with positive lymph nodes treated with 4 or 12 cycles of CMF reported nine treatment-related deaths (0.9%), most from neutropenic sepsis or thromboembolism. Thromboembolic events are more common in patients treated with chemotherapy, especially when it is combined with tamoxifen.[44,158,160,163] In another study of chemotherapy in postmenopausal patients, four deaths were reported in 600 patients (0.6%) who received 1 year of CMFVP chemotherapy alone (one death) or combined with tamoxifen (three deaths).[158] The cumulative data suggest that lethal toxicities occur in approximately 1 of every 200 to 500 patients who receive adjuvant chemotherapy, that toxic deaths may occur more frequently in postmenopausal patients, and that the addition of tamoxifen to chemotherapy increases toxicity because of an increased risk for thromboembolism.

Although lethal toxicities are uncommon, other acute side effects are bothersome to patients. NSABP B-15 compared the toxicities of AC for four cycles and standard CMF for six cycles, both commonly used treatment regimens.[53] Cardiac toxicity was not problematic in this study with either treatment. The most common side effects were alopecia, nausea and vomiting, weight gain, and grade 3 or 4 neutropenia. Infection was uncommon. CMF was associated with slightly more neutropenia, nausea without vomiting, and weight gain. Alopecia and vomiting were more frequent with AC. Another way to evaluate toxicity is by the duration of symptoms and the total number of patient visits to the physician. The AC regimen consists of only four intravenous drug treatments 3 weeks apart; CMF includes oral cyclophosphamide for 2 weeks and intravenous MF on days 1 and 8 of each 4-week cycle repeated six times, for a total of 84 treatment days and 12 intravenous treatments. Thus, on average, AC was completed in 63 days, compared with 154 days for CMF. Patients given CMF required three times the number of physician visits. Finally, antiemetic medication was prescribed for a total of 84 days with CMF and only 12 days with AC. Fatigue is another common side effect of chemotherapy that is difficult to quantify, and its incidence was not reported in this study.

Anxiety and psychological distress have not been studied in detail, and separating the impact of the recent diagnosis of a life-threatening disease from the impact of treatment is also difficult. Mild symptoms of distress have been reported in patients who received chemotherapy, especially with prolonged treatment.[164,165] A small sample from a randomized, controlled treatment trial suggested more anxiety for patients assigned to no treatment than for those assigned to chemotherapy, perhaps because of a placebo effect associated with active treatment and the hope that the intervention can improve the chance for cure.[166]

Long-Term Adverse Effects of Adjuvant Chemotherapy

Complications of adjuvant chemotherapy that may occur months to years after completion of treatment are more difficult to identify, but they can be extremely important considerations when treating patients who have a low risk of death from breast cancer. Even uncommon but serious adverse events can cancel out the small absolute benefits of chemotherapy in node-negative patients with small or moderate-sized tumors or in postmenopausal patients. The major potential long-term toxicities to consider are cardiac dysfunction, premature menopause, and the development of second cancers.

The cardiomyopathy due to doxorubicin may occur during treatment, shortly after its completion, or many months later. The incidence of congestive heart failure in patients treated with doxorubicin-based adjuvant therapy varies according to the total cumulative dose received and, perhaps, according to the peak blood levels. In the NSABP trial of AC for four cycles, heart failure was not observed (maximum total dose of doxorubicin, 240 mg per m^2).[53] In two studies from Milan using sequenced CMF and doxorubicin (maximum total dose, 300 mg per m^2), congestive heart failure was observed in one patient who received CMF and in one patient treated with doxorubicin, both of whom also were treated with irradiation to the left breast.[54,55] The incidence of cardiomyopathy was higher in two other studies (4% to 7%), but it was less than 1% when the total cumulative doxorubicin dose was less than 300 mg per m^2.[167,168] Cardiomyopathy may be less common when doxorubicin is administered by a 2- to 4-day continuous infusion, but this technique requires an indwelling venous catheter that itself has a high complication rate. Whether continuous infusion of doxorubicin has equivalent antitumor activity in the adjuvant therapy of breast cancer has not been studied definitively.

The low incidence of acute doxorubicin-induced cardiomyopathy when the cumulative dose is kept at or below

300 mg per m^2 seems acceptable for higher-risk breast cancer patients, but it may be less so for patients with a low risk of disease recurrence, the majority of whom are already cured by surgery alone. Although doxorubicin-based chemotherapy may be slightly superior to CMF, the latter, or even no chemotherapy, may be preferred by some low-risk patients and their physicians.[23,56] Another concern that is difficult to study is the possibility that patients given doxorubicin early in life could have premature heart disease when they get older. Although no data support this worry at the present time, this concern emphasizes the need for long-term follow-up studies of cardiac events in randomized trials and the need for caution in prescribing doxorubicin to patients in whom the potential benefit is small.

Another concern is chemotherapy-induced ovarian failure. The overall incidence of treatment-induced amenorrhea is approximately 70%, although it varies according to patient age and the dose and type of alkylating agent.[169–171] Permanent ovarian dysfunction with standard chemotherapy is less common in patients younger than 35 years old, whereas it is nearly universal in women older than 45 years of age. Chemical ovarian ablation may be a "desirable" side effect in higher-risk patients because it may provide an advantage in reducing the odds of breast cancer recurrence and death. In low-risk patients, however, the minimal absolute benefits of ovarian ablation may be exceeded by the discomforts related to menopausal symptoms and by the theoretical increased risk of premature osteoporosis and cardiovascular disease. Premenopausal patients treated in the first-generation adjuvant trials are just now reaching the age at which these problems may emerge, and careful study of these and other long-term effects is needed. Rapid bone loss after chemotherapy-induced ovarian failure that was significantly reduced by bisphosphonate treatment was reported in a 1997 study.[172]

Many cytotoxic drugs are carcinogens, and a possible increased risk of second malignant disease is another concern. An increased risk of treatment-induced myeloproliferative disease and acute leukemia in breast cancer patients treated with adjuvant chemotherapy has been established. Data from the Surveillance Epidemiology and End Results program indicate an increased risk of leukemia (cumulative incidence, 0.7% at 10 years) related to the cumulative dose and to the type of alkylating agent used.[173] Overall, a five-fold increased risk of developing leukemia and an 11.5-fold increased risk of acute nonlymphocytic leukemia were observed. No increased risk was observed in patients treated by surgery alone. Leukemia risk was higher with more prolonged treatment regimens, and it was strongly related to the use of melphalan [relative risk (RR), 45]. Similar data were reported by the NSABP.[174]

A larger 1992 study of 82,700 patients from five regions of the United States provides more information on the leukemia risk associated with breast cancer treatment.[175] The risk of acute nonlymphocytic leukemia was increased after regional radiotherapy (RR, 2.4), alkylating agents alone (RR, 10), and combined chemotherapy and radiation (RR, 17.4). The risk associated with melphalan was ten times that related to cyclophosphamide (RR, 31.4 versus 3.1). Patients who received cyclophosphamide for less than 12 months or who received less than 20 g total dose had almost no detectable increase in leukemia risk. A review of the leukemia and myelodysplastic syndrome risk associated with standard-dose cyclosphosphamide in a series of cooperative group studies suggests that this risk is not much higher than that of the general population.[176] Thus, the cumulative data suggest that the leukemia risk associated with the cyclophosphamide-containing regimens used most frequently today is extremely low. Regional radiation increases this risk. The leukemia risk is somewhat higher in women treated with higher than standard doses of cyclophosphamide combined with an anthracycline. Fourteen cases of leukemia from a total of 1,474 patients treated with FAC were reported from M. D. Anderson Hospital in Houston.[177] Twelve of the 14 had also received radiotherapy. The 10-year estimated leukemia rate was 1.5% overall, 2.5% in the group also receiving radiation, and 0.5% in patients who received only chemotherapy. Relatively short follow-up of NSABP B-25, in which patients were treated with an AC regimen that included higher doses of cyclophosphamide, found 17 cases of leukemia or myelodysplastic syndrome in 2,548 patients (0.7%).[178] Finally, acute leukemia developed in 5 of 351 (1.4%) patients treated at 5 years with an epirubicin-cyclophosphamide–containing regimen.[179] This worrisome, although uncommon, toxicity needs to be considered when treating relatively low-risk patients with these more aggressive regimens.

Most treatment-induced leukemias occur within the first few years after exposure to the cytotoxic agent, but solid tumors have a much longer latency period. Thus, to draw conclusions about the risk of solid tumors in patients treated with adjuvant chemotherapy for breast cancer is premature, because relatively few patients in prospective trials have been followed for more than 15 years.[180] The already increased risk of other tumors, such as ovarian, endometrial, and colorectal cancer, in patients with a history of breast cancer complicates estimates of risk from chemotherapy. No evidence suggesting an increased risk of second malignancy has been found in long-term follow-up studies from Milan of patients treated with CMF.[181] Additional reassurance, comes from the meta-analysis.[23] The rate of non–breast cancer–related deaths was slightly lower, not higher, in patients randomized to adjuvant chemotherapy (Table 15). In any event, the slight risk of leukemia and the absence of an indication of an increased risk of solid tumors with adjuvant chemotherapy are of little concern for patients with breast cancer in whom the risk of breast cancer recurrence is substantial. These small risks for second malignant disease, however, are potentially more important in treating patients at low risk of breast cancer recurrence, and they should be considered in making treatment decisions in such patients.

TABLE 15. *Effects of adjuvant polychemotherapy on non–breast cancer–related breast cancer and incidence of second breast cancers*

	10-yr risk per 1,000 patients		
	Chemotherapy	Control	Significant difference?
Non–breast cancer mortality	66	75	No
Contralateral breast cancer incidence	44	55	Yes

Adapted from ref. 23.

Toxicity of Tamoxifen Adjuvant Therapy

In general, tamoxifen is well tolerated by most patients with breast cancer. In early trials of adjuvant therapy, fewer than 5% of patients discontinued therapy early because of toxicity.[182,183] In one of the largest randomized placebo-controlled trials, 7% of tamoxifen-treated patients and 5% of placebo-treated patients withdrew from the study early for reasons that were possibly related to toxicity.[35,100]

Menopausal Symptoms

The most frequently reported side effects in patients taking tamoxifen are menopausal symptoms.[35,100,184] At least 50% to 60% of these women report some hot flashes, but 40% to 50% of placebo-treated patients report similar episodes. Tamoxifen may cause hot flashes more commonly in premenopausal women than in older women. Many postmenopausal patients have hot flashes before starting tamoxifen because of natural causes or because of the withdrawal of estrogen replacement therapy when breast cancer is diagnosed. Approximately 20% of patients report severe hot flashes while taking tamoxifen, compared with 3% of placebo patients. Vaginal discharge and irregular menses are also slightly more common in patients taking tamoxifen than in those receiving placebo. In one study, general quality of life scores were similar for tamoxifen and placebo.[184] Headaches were reported less frequently with tamoxifen. The incidence of nausea, arthralgias, insomnia, restlessness, depression, and fatigue was similar with tamoxifen and placebo.

Depression has not been reported to be increased in randomized, placebo-controlled trials, but this may reflect underreporting of symptoms that may be brought out by more careful and detailed questioning. Many oncologists would contend, based on their own experience, that depression is an uncommon but real side effect of tamoxifen treatment. A nonrandomized single-institution study suggests that symptoms of depression can be identified in up to 10% of patients taking tamoxifen.[185] Symptoms are occasionally severe and may require dose reduction, antidepressant medication, or even discontinuation of the drug. However, the failure to identify depression as a side effect in placebo-controlled trials suggests that discontinuation of estrogen replacement therapy may be causally more important than tamoxifen itself.

Ocular Toxicity

Ocular toxicity has been reported with high tamoxifen doses.[186] An uncontrolled study concluded that ocular toxicity in the form of retinopathy or keratopathy was a side effect of conventional doses of tamoxifen, a result not confirmed in a controlled study in which complete ophthalmologic examinations were performed in a blinded fashion.[187,188] Other reports of ocular toxicity have been inconsistent.[189–191] In one large study and in preliminary results from the NSABP tamoxifen prevention trial, women with preexisting cataracts who were taking tamoxifen had a slightly increased risk of posterior subcapsular opacities and need for cataract surgery, but no vision-threatening ocular toxicity was found.[191] Occasional ophthalmologic examination should be sufficient monitoring for patients with breast cancer who are receiving long-term tamoxifen therapy.

Thromboembolic and Hematologic Toxicities

An increased incidence of thromboembolic events has also been reported from studies of tamoxifen adjuvant therapy in patients with breast cancer as well as from tamoxifen prevention studies in high-risk women.[35,122,182,192–195] This complication occurs more frequently when tamoxifen is combined with chemotherapy. Most patients reported with this complication have superficial phlebitis and do not require hospitalization. Severe thromboembolic phenomena occur in fewer than 1% of patients given the drug. However, deaths due to thromboembolism have been reported in patients with cancer and in normal women in the prevention trials. Thrombocytopenia and leukopenia have also been reported with tamoxifen, but they are unusual and rarely require cessation of therapy.

Endometrial and Other Cancers

The most troublesome side effect of long-term tamoxifen is related to its possible carcinogenic activity. Although the drug is not a mutagen in the Ames assay, it is genotoxic. Electrophilic metabolites produced by rat and human liver P450 enzymes can form covalent DNA adducts, at least in the rat.[196,197] Tamoxifen is a potent hepatocarcinogen in the rat, but not in the mouse.[198,199] The presence of adducts has not yet been confirmed in human liver, but the microsomal enzymes in human liver are capable of producing reactive metabolites *in vitro*. Although abnormal liver function tests are occasionally observed in patients receiving tamoxifen, only a few anecdotal cases of hepatoma have, thus far, been reported, and the incidence of hepatoma since the introduction of tamoxifen has not increased.[200,201] Careful long-term follow-up studies of tamoxifen users are needed in view of the preclinical data and given the long latency period usually associated with carcinogen-induced solid tumors.

Tamoxifen use, much like estrogen therapy, is clearly related to an increased incidence of endometrial cancer.[125,202,203] Even just 1 year of adjuvant tamoxifen is associated with a slightly increased incidence, but the risk rises with more prolonged treatment. Interpretation of these results is a problem, because many women taking tamoxifen were treated with estrogen replacement therapy before the diagnosis of breast cancer. Nevertheless, 8-year follow-up of NSABP B-14, in which 2,843 patients were randomly assigned to receive at least 5 years of tamoxifen or placebo, indicate that tamoxifen was associated with an annual hazard rate of 1.7 per 1,000, an RR of 2.2 compared with population-based rates of endometrial cancer from Surveillance Epidemiology and End Results program data.[204] The type of endometrial cancer in patients taking tamoxifen is similar to that in patients not exposed to tamoxifen. Eighteen of the 23 cancers in NSABP B-14 were of low histologic grade, and most were stage I. Four patients died of uterine cancer, however, indicating the lethal potential of this complication and the need for regular gynecologic examinations. The role of endometrial cancer screening by vaginal ultrasound or endometrial biopsy and the role of progestins in reducing the risk of endometrial cancer are now being evaluated. The high incidence of uterine cancers with an unfavorable prognosis reported in tamoxifen-treated patients in a small retrospective study is most likely due to referral bias.[205]

An increased incidence of endometrial cancer has also been observed in a large prevention trial in women without breast cancer, but all of the cases reported have a very favorable histology.[206] Increased endometrial thickness and the incidence of hyperplasia, polyps, and ovarian cysts can be increased by tamoxifen.[125,207,208] Data from the NSABP and the large Swedish randomized trials indicate that tamoxifen adjuvant therapy has not yet resulted in an increased incidence of other solid tumors.[125,196,198,200,204,209] Although these adverse effects of tamoxifen do not detract from the proven substantial survival benefits in patients with invasive breast cancer, they do raise caution for the use of tamoxifen in benign conditions or for breast cancer prevention.

COST-EFFECTIVENESS OF ADJUVANT THERAPY

Given the high incidence of breast cancer and the moderate survival benefits of adjuvant therapy, one must evaluate both efficacy and cost-effectiveness from a public health perspective. Several such studies have been reported.[210–212] Using a decision-analysis model and reasonable assumptions of risk and benefit, adjuvant therapy increases the quality-adjusted life expectancy of an average woman at a cost similar to that of other widely accepted therapies. Treatment is more cost-effective in higher-risk patients, but even node-negative patients benefit.[210] Cost-effectiveness is greater for premenopausal than for postmenopausal patients, but still some elderly patients benefit.[212] The cost of the benefit in elderly patients is comparable to that of other reimbursed procedures until a point between ages 75 and 80 years. Cost-benefit ratios can be significantly improved by selection of patients at high risk of disease recurrence or those who are most likely to benefit from treatment. A discussion of prognostic and predictive biomarkers is found in Chapter 32.

MAKING ADJUVANT TREATMENT DECISIONS

Breast cancer is a heterogeneous disease. Some patients have aggressive disease that is refractory to treatment; survival duration may be only a few months. Many patients have more indolent disease that is responsive to hormone therapy or chemotherapy. Today, with the increasing use of mammography, the majority of patients (approximately 60%) are cured by surgery alone and do not need adjuvant treatment. Given the modest benefits of adjuvant treatment, it makes little sense to recommend therapy to all patients when many do not need it and only a few benefit. A more rational approach is to consider each patient individually and to estimate risk-benefit profiles for each patient.

Clinical decision making requires an assessment of the risk of recurrence and death, the benefits of treatment, and the costs and toxicity of treatment. Many patients overestimate or underestimate their chance of being cured by breast cancer surgery, and physicians and patients tend to overestimate the benefits of adjuvant therapy.[213,214] An accurate estimate of both is crucial for meaningful discussions about the value of adjuvant therapy.

Estimates of the impact of the disease and the benefits of adjuvant therapy on 10-year survival can be made using patient age, natural mortality from other causes, breast cancer mortality, and mortality reductions derived from the meta-analysis data on chemotherapy and tamoxifen (Table 16). The low-risk subset in each age group might represent patients with tumors of 1 cm or smaller and negative lymph nodes; the intermediate-risk group represents the typical node-negative patient; and the high-risk group typifies patients with one or two positive lymph nodes. The natural mortality in patients of similar age without a diagnosis of breast cancer is nearly 10 times higher in a 65-year-old than in a 40-year-old. Competing causes of mortality are significant in older women and must be considered. This natural mortality would be even higher in women with preexisting medical illness, such as diabetes or heart disease. Assuming

TABLE 16. *Survival estimates at 10 years by age and risk of breast cancer death, with and without adjuvant therapy*

Hypothetical risk[a] of breast cancer death	Natural mortality without breast cancer, next 10 yr (%)	Alive at 10 yr		
		No adjuvant therapy	Adjuvant therapy[b]	Absolute benefit
40 yr old				
10% (low risk)	2	88	90	2
28% (intermediate risk)	2	71	77	6
57% (high risk)	2	41	51	10
65 yr old				
9% (low risk)	19	73	75	2
26% (intermediate risk)	19	58	63	5
54% (high risk)	19	34	43	9

[a]Values shown are derived from three different risk estimates and assume exponential death with a constant hazard ratio. The differences between 40 and 65 years of age reflect deaths from other causes.
[b]Based on a 25% annual reduction in the odds of death, a reasonable estimate of the benefits of chemotherapy in premenopausal patients and tamoxifen in an estrogen receptor–positive postmenopausal patient.

a 25% annual reduction in the odds of death by treatment, the absolute benefit (the number of patients alive per 100 patients treated) increases as the risk of death from breast cancer increases. The total number of patients who receive some benefit from adjuvant treatment is likely to be greater than the absolute benefit, however, because some patients whose cancer recurred and who died by 10 years may have had their death delayed several years by therapy. Nevertheless, the benefits are modest, particularly in the subsets with a low risk of death. Given the morbidity, possible mortality, and cost of adjuvant treatment, many patients and physicians would argue that adjuvant chemotherapy is not indicated routinely in such low-risk patients. The mortality reductions (and, thus, the absolute benefit) from treatment would be even smaller than the 25% shown in the example in Table 16 for adjuvant chemotherapy in postmenopausal patients with ER-positive tumors, in whom proportional benefits approach 10%. Patients must also be aware that the differences in 10-year survival (absolute benefit) do not necessarily indicate that any patients are cured by treatment. Without longer follow-up, one cannot differentiate between a substantial prolongation of life with persistent subclinical cancer and a cure with complete tumor eradication in some treated patients.

Thus, the real question is at what level of benefit adjuvant therapy is indicated. This question is difficult to answer. Clinical experience suggests that some patients or physicians are willing to accept the toxicity and costs of treatment for a relatively meager potential benefit, whereas others require more substantial gains.[215] Some patients may select a less toxic therapy, such as tamoxifen alone, even though it may be slightly less effective than chemotherapy plus tamoxifen. The 1990 National Institutes of Health Consensus Panel concluded that patients with node-negative tumors 1 cm or smaller in diameter "have an excellent prognosis and do not require adjuvant systemic therapy outside of clinical trials."[216] Such patients have a 10-year recurrence risk of approximately 10%.[217] As discussed in Chapter 32, other prognostic factors can be used to identify a group of node-negative patients with a similarly excellent prognosis. Patients with histologic or nuclear grade 1 tumors; those with a special tumor type, such as tubular, mucinous, or papillary carcinoma; patients with ductal carcinoma *in situ* with or without microinvasion; and even patients with tumors between 1 and 2 cm in diameter with other good prognostic factors, such as positive ER and a low proliferative index, have 10-year recurrence rates that range from 2% to 15%. No adjuvant chemotherapy is an appropriate consideration in such patients. Rather than setting some arbitrary cutoff to discriminate patients who should not receive adjuvant therapy from those who should, a better strategy is to present an accurate risk-benefit profile to each patient and make recommendations based on a global assessment of the patient's tumor characteristics, age, and coincidental medical illness, as well as the patient's own response to the disease and the potential treatment benefits. Finally, these analyses illustrate the need for the development of additional prognostic factors to predict the risk of disease recurrence accurately and for the identification of accurate predictive factors to determine the responsiveness of a tumor to chemotherapy. A biomarker for chemotherapy sensitivity equivalent to ER in predicting response to endocrine therapy would greatly facilitate treatment decisions.

Timing of Adjuvant Chemotherapy and Tamoxifen

Most randomized trials of adjuvant chemotherapy dictated that treatment commence from 2 to at most 12 weeks after definitive surgery. Whether delays within this range or longer adversely affect outcome has not been studied well, but it seems prudent to start chemotherapy as early as medically justified, avoiding all but necessary delays for such things as wound infections or other concomitant illness. One randomized trial investigating the timing of breast irradiation and initiation of chemotherapy after lumpectomy reports that delaying chemotherapy until the completion of radiation resulted in an increased distant recurrence rate, whereas a delay of 12 weeks in starting radiation caused slightly more breast recurrences.[218] Because distant recurrences more directly impact survival, it is rational to give chemotherapy early, before radiation, except perhaps in those patients with a relatively low risk for distant recurrence. Of course, no chemotherapy at all is also an attractive option for these patients. Based on the available data, there is no rationale for starting chemotherapy in patients who have had surgery more than 3 to 6 months earlier. For a more detailed discussion of the timing of radiation and chemotherapy, see Chapter 33.

Most studies of adjuvant tamoxifen alone started the drug 2 to 6 weeks after mastectomy. Trials of chemotherapy plus tamoxifen either initiated both treatments simultaneously or began tamoxifen 3 to 6 months later when chemotherapy was complete to avoid possible antagonism. Results of one study that addresses this question are pending.[31] Until they are available, physician judgment should be used to decide on the timing of these agents. In patients who receive only tamoxifen, it can be started soon after definitive surgery. There is no good clinical evidence to suggest that tamoxifen should not be used during breast irradiation.

FUTURE DIRECTIONS

Adjuvant systemic therapy reduces recurrence rates by 30% to 50%, depending on the patient and the characteristics of the tumor. Ongoing and planned clinical trials are necessary to refine current treatment approaches and to test new strategies.

A host of trials addressed the role of increasing chemotherapy dose intensity, including high-dose chemotherapy and stem cell support. The results of these studies are not very promising, and future trials using this approach are likely to be smaller phase II trials testing new agents, combinations, or repeated cycles of therapy. Given the relatively exciting results obtained with studies of bisphosphonates as adjuvant agents, a large confirmatory intergroup randomized trial will be activated in 1999 evaluating the role of zoledronate after standard adjuvant therapy. This drug is 20 times more potent than older drugs that have been studied in breast cancer, and it has the advantage of requiring only a short intravenous infusion time. Other chemotherapy trials are evaluating the role of sequential single-agent chemotherapy, giving each agent at its full dose intensity in sequence, compared to standard combination therapy. Mathematical modeling suggests that this approach may offer an advantage. One such trial comparing the combination of doxorubicin and cyclophosphamide with the same drugs in sequence has been completed, and the results should be available in a year or two. Finally, docetaxel, an agent that has high activity in metastatic breast cancer, is being incorporated into adjuvant regimens either in combination with cyclophosphamide or after the completion of the standard AC regimen. These studies should help to confirm and extend the promising study using paclitaxel.[48]

Herceptin, the humanized monoclonal antibody recognizing the external domain of the HER-2/neu oncogene growth factor receptor, has shown additive activity when combined with doxorubicin or taxane-containing regimens and has modest single-agent activity itself in patients who overexpress this protein. The high rate of cardiac toxicity when this drug is combined with doxorubicin makes adjuvant trials more difficult, but studies are now being planned to incorporate herceptin into adjuvant therapy regimens avoiding concomitant administration with doxorubicin.

Several new endocrine approaches are currently in clinical trial, or studies will soon be activated. A large intergroup adjuvant trial will address the role of adding an aromatase inhibitor in patients who have completed 5 years of tamoxifen compared to 5 years of tamoxifen alone. Raloxifene, a selective ER modulator similar to tamoxifen, but without agonist activity in the endometrium, also should be studied in patients with primary and metastatic breast cancer. Raloxifene is now being given by many gynecologists to patients with breast cancer who have completed tamoxifen therapy to reduce bone resorption. A study is needed to confirm the safety of this approach, because the studies reviewed earlier of prolonged tamoxifen suggest the possibility that therapy beyond 5 years may actually be detrimental. Because tamoxifen and raloxifene have a similar spectrum of activity, it is possible that the results seen with prolonged raloxifene may be no different than those reported with prolonged tamoxifen. Pure antiestrogens, which are more potent in preclinical models and which have activity in patients with tamoxifen resistance, are now in phase III clinical trials in patients with metastatic disease. If these agents prove more effective, then their rapid introduction into the adjuvant setting will be of interest.

MANAGEMENT SUMMARY

Recommendations for the use of adjuvant therapy in clinical practice are shown in Table 17. No recipe exists with which everyone agrees, because uncertainty about the role of certain treatment approaches is still considerable. Experience and clinical judgment are required to make appropriate decisions in individual patients. Participation in clinical trials is encouraged to expedite answers to important questions. Progress would be faster if more than 4% (current rate) of patients with breast cancer were enrolled in randomized clinical trials. In the meantime, most oncologists agree that very low-risk patients (<10% risk of distant recurrence) should not receive chemotherapy because relatively few patients stand to benefit, and the cost-benefit ratio does not justify it. Tamoxifen, because of its lower toxicity profile and greater reduction in recurrence, might be considered in some of these patients depending on the circumstances. The risk-benefit ratio in other node-negative patients favors the use of adjuvant therapy. Chemotherapy for at least several months is optimal in the premenopausal ER-negative subset, whereas

TABLE 17. *Recommendations for the use of adjuvant therapy in clinical practice*

Patient subset	Recommended treatment
Node negative, low risk[a]	Physician judgment; no treatment or tamoxifen if ER positive
Node negative, higher risk	
ER+	Tamoxifen or chemotherapy + tamoxifen
ER−	Chemotherapy
Node positive	
ER+	Chemotherapy + tamoxifen or tamoxifen alone
ER−	Chemotherapy

ER, estrogen receptor.
[a]*Low risk* defined as negative axillary nodes and tumor ≤1 cm, nuclear grade 1, special histologic type, or 1- to 2-cm tumor along with ER+ tumor with low proliferation index.

tamoxifen alone or combined with chemotherapy is considered standard treatment for premenopausal and postmenopausal ER-positive patients. Depending on the patient, no treatment at all might be considered for older women whose tumors are ER negative. Chemotherapy might be considered in other postmenopausal, ER-negative patients. Substantial data justify the use of chemotherapy in premenopausal node-positive patients, and new data suggest that the addition of 5 years of tamoxifen further improves outcome if the tumor is ER positive. Although data suggest that ovarian ablation may be beneficial in premenopausal patients, additional study of the efficacy and long-term consequences of ovarian ablation are needed. It should not be used in conjunction with chemotherapy. Adjuvant tamoxifen alone or combined with chemotherapy should be considered in all postmenopausal, node-positive ER-positive patients.

Adjuvant therapy improves long-term survival of patients with primary breast cancer. The benefits are modest but real, and given the high incidence of breast cancer, the mortality reductions achieved today with standard approaches should prevent or substantially delay hundreds of thousands of deaths worldwide in this decade.

REFERENCES

1. Lewis D, Rienhoff WF Jr. A study of the results of operations for the cure of cancer of the breast. *Ann Surg* 1932;95:336.
2. Fisher B, Gebhardt MC. The evolution of breast cancer surgery: past, present, and future. *Semin Oncol* 1978;5:385.
3. Cruz EP, McDonald GO, Cole WH. Prophylactic treatment of cancer: the use of chemotherapeutic agents to prevent tumor metastasis. *Surgery* 1956;40:291.
4. Shapiro DM, Fugmann RA. A role of chemotherapy as an adjunct to surgery. *Cancer Res* 1957;17:1098.
5. Skipper HE. Kinetics of mammary tumor cell growth and implications for therapy. *Cancer* 1971;28:1479.
6. Cole MP. A clinical trial of an artificial menopause in carcinoma of the breast. *INSERM* 1975;55:143.
7. Fisher B, Ravdin RG, Ausman RK, et al. Surgical adjuvant chemotherapy in cancer of the breast: results of a decade of cooperative investigation. *Ann Surg* 1968;168:337.
8. Nissen-Meyer R. One short chemotherapy course in primary breast cancer: 12-year follow-up in series 1 of the Scandinavia adjuvant chemotherapy study group. In: Jones SE, Salmon SE, eds. *Adjuvant therapy of cancer*, vol 2. New York: Grune & Stratton, 1979:207.
9. Roberts S, Watne A, McGrath R, et al. Technique and results of isolation of cancer cells from the circulating blood. *Arch Surg* 1958;76:334.
10. Jonasson O, Long L, Roberts S, et al. Cancer cells in the circulating blood during operative management of genitourinary tumors. *J Urol* 1961;85:1.
11. Buzdar A, Blumenschein G, Gutterman J, et al. Adjuvant therapy with 5-fluorouracil, Adriamycin, cyclophosphamide and BCG (FAC-BCG) for stage II or III breast cancer. In: Jones SE, Salmon SE, eds. *Adjuvant therapy of cancer*, vol 2. New York: Grune & Stratton, 1979:277.
12. Early Breast Cancer Trialists' Collaborative Group. Effects of adjuvant tamoxifen and of cytotoxic therapy on mortality in early breast cancer: an overview of 61 randomised trials among 28,896 women. *N Engl J Med* 1988;319:1681.
13. Bonadonna G. Evolving concepts in the systemic adjuvant treatment of breast cancer. *Cancer Res* 1992;52:2127.
14. Bonadonna G, Brusamolino E, Valagussa P, et al. Combination chemotherapy as an adjuvant treatment in operable breast cancer. *N Engl J Med* 1976;294:405.
15. Bernhard J, Hurny C, Coates AS, et al. Quality of life assessment in patients receiving adjuvant therapy for breast cancer: the IBCSG approach. The International Breast Cancer Study Group [Published erratum appears in *Ann Oncol* 1998;9:231]. *Ann Oncol* 1997;8:825.
16. Ganz PA, Day R, Costantino J. Compliance with quality of life data collection in the National Surgical Adjuvant Breast and Bowel Project (NSABP) breast cancer prevention trial. *Stat Med* 1998;17:613.
17. Fetting JH, Gray R, Fairclough DL, et al. Sixteen-week multidrug regimen versus cyclophosphamide, doxorubicin, and fluorouracil as adjuvant therapy for node-positive, receptor-negative breast cancer: an Intergroup study. *J Clin Oncol* 1998;16:2382.
18. Bernhard J, Hurny C, Coates AS, et al. Factors affecting baseline quality of life in two international adjuvant breast cancer trials. International Breast Cancer Study Group (IBCSG). *Br J Cancer* 1998;78:686.
19. Gelber RD, Goldhirsch A, Cavalli F, et al. Quality-of-life-adjusted evaluation of adjuvant therapies for operable breast cancer. *Ann Intern Med* 1991;114:621.
20. Gelber RD, Cole BF, Goldhirsch A, et al. Adjuvant chemotherapy plus tamoxifen compared with tamoxifen alone for postmenopausal breast cancer: meta-analysis of quality-adjusted survival [See comments]. *Lancet* 1996;347:1066.
21. Fisher B, Carbone P, Economou SG, et al. L-Phenylalanine mustard (L-PAM) in the management of primary breast cancer: a report of early findings. *N Engl J Med* 1975;292:117.
22. Early Breast Cancer Trialists' Collaborative Group. Systematic treatment of early breast cancer by hormonal, cytotoxic, or immune therapy: 133 randomised trials involving 31,000 recurrences and 24,000 deaths among 75,000 women. *Lancet* 1992;339:1,71.
23. Early Breast Cancer Trialists' Collaborative Group. Polychemotherapy for early breast cancer: an overview of the randomised trials. *Lancet* 1998;352:930.
24. Padmanabhan N, Howell A, Rubens RD. Mechanism of action of adjuvant chemotherapy in early breast cancer. *Lancet* 1986;2:411.
25. Henderson IC. Adjuvant chemotherapy: a chemical oohorectomy? *Breast Dis Year Book Q* 1994;5:16.
26. Bonadonna G, Valagussa P. Dose-response effect of adjuvant chemotherapy in breast cancer. *N Engl J Med* 1981;304:10.
27. Mansour EG, Gray R, Shatila AH, et al. Survival advantage of adjuvant chemotherapy in high-risk node-negative breast cancer: ten-year analysis—an intergroup study. *J Clin Oncol* 1998;16:3486.
28. Fisher B, Redmond C, Dimitrov NV, et al. A randomized clinical trial evaluating sequential methotrexate and fluorouracil in the treatment of patients with node-negative breast cancer who have estrogen-receptor-negative tumors. *N Engl J Med* 1989;320:473.
29. Tormey DC, Weinberg VE, Holland JF, et al. A randomized trial of five and three drug chemotherapy and chemoimmunotherapy in women with operable node positive breast cancer. *J Clin Oncol* 1983;1:138.
30. Wood WC, Budman DR, Korzun AH, et al. Dose and dose intensity of adjuvant chemotherapy for stage II, node-positive breast carcinoma. *N Engl J Med* 1994;330:1253.
31. Albain K, Green S, Osborne K, et al. Tamoxifen vs cyclophosphamide, Adriamycin, and 5-FU plus either concurrent or sequential tamoxifen in postmenopausal receptor+ node+ breast cancer: a South-

west Oncology Group Phase III Intergroup Trial (SWOG-8814, Int-0100). *Proc Am Soc Clin Oncol* 1997;16:1a(abst 450).
32. Rosen PP, Groshen S, Saigo PE, et al. A long-term follow-up study of survival in stage 1 (T1N0M0) and stage II (T1N1M0) breast carcinoma. *J Clin Oncol* 1989;7:355.
33. Hilsenbeck SG, Ravdin PM, de Moor CA, Chamness GC, Osborne CK, Clark GM. Time dependence of hazard ratios for prognostic factors in primary breast cancer. *Breast Cancer Res Treat* 1998:52.
34. Morrison JM, Howell A, Kelly KA, et al. West Midlands Oncology Association trials of adjuvant chemotherapy in operable breast cancer: results are a median follow-up of 7 years. II. Patients without involved axillary lymph nodes. *Br J Cancer* 1989;60:919.
35. Fisher B, Costantino J, Redmond C, et al. A randomized clinical trial evaluating tamoxifen in the treatment of patients with node-negative breast cancer who have estrogen-receptor-positive tumors. *N Engl J Med* 1989;320:479.
36. Ludwig Breast Cancer Study Group. Prolonged disease-free survival after one course of perioperative adjuvant chemotherapy for node-negative breast cancer. *N Engl J Med* 1989;320:491.
37. Bonadonna G. Conceptual and practical advances in the management of breast cancer. Karnofsky Memorial Lecture. *J Clin Oncol* 1989;7:1380.
38. Fisher B, Wickerham DL, Redmond C. Recent developments in the use of systemic adjuvant therapy for the treatment of breast cancer. *Semin Oncol* 1992;19:263.
39. Mansour EG, Eudey L, Tormey DC, et al. Chemotherapy versus observation in high-risk node-negative breast cancer patients. *J Natl Cancer Inst Monogr* 1992;11:97.
40. Rivkin SE, Green S, Metch B, et al. Adjuvant CMFVP versus melphalan for operable breast cancer with positive axillary nodes: 10-year results of a Southwest Oncology Group Study. *J Clin Oncol* 1989;7:1229.
41. Rivkin SE, Green S, O'Sullivan J, et al. Adjuvant CMFVP versus melphalan for operable breast cancer with positive axillary nodes: 20-year results of a Southwest Oncology Group study. *Proc Am Soc Clin Oncol* 1997;16a(abst 457).
42. Wolmark N, Fisher B, and contributing NSABP investigators. Adjuvant chemotherapy in stage-II breast cancer: an overview of the NSABP clinical trials. *Breast Cancer Res Treat* 1983;3[Suppl 1]:19.
43. Tancini G, Bonadonna G, Valagussa P, et al. Adjuvant CMF in breast cancer: comparative 5-year results of 12 versus 6 cycles. *J Clin Oncol* 1983;1:2.
44. Falkson HC, Gray R, Wolberg WH, et al. Adjuvant trial of 12 cycles of CMFPT followed by observation or continuous tamoxifen versus four cycles of CMFPT in postmenopausal women with breast cancer: an Eastern Cooperative Oncology Group Phase III study. *J Clin Oncol* 1990;8:599.
45. Rivkin SE, Green S, Metch B, et al. One versus 2 years of CMFVP adjuvant chemotherapy in axillary node-positive and estrogen receptor-negative patients: a Southwest Oncology Group study. *J Clin Oncol* 1993;11:1710.
46. Ludwig Breast Cancer Study Group. Combination adjuvant chemotherapy for node-positive breast cancer: inadequacy of a single perioperative cycle. *N Engl J Med* 1988;319:677.
47. Levine MN, Gent M, Hryniuk WM, et al. A randomized trial comparing 12 weeks with 36 weeks of adjuvant chemotherapy in stage II breast cancer. *J Clin Oncol* 1990;8:1217.
48. Henderson IC, Berry D, Demetri G, et al. Improved disease-free and overall survival from the addition of sequential paclitaxel but not from the escalation of doxorubicin dose level in the adjuvant chemotherapy of patients with node-positive primary breast cancer. *Proc Am Soc Clin Oncol* 1998;17:101a(abst 390A).
49. Fisher B, Dignam J, Mamounas EP, et al. Sequential methotrexate and fluorouracil for the treatment of node-negative breast cancer patients with estrogen receptor-negative tumors: eight-year results from National Surgical Adjuvant Breast and Bowel Project (NSABP) B-19 comparing methotrexate and fluorouracil with conventional cyclophosphamide, methotrexate, and fluorouracil. *J Clin Oncol* 1996;14:1982.
50. Fisher B, Redmond C, Wickerham DL, et al. Doxorubicin-containing regimens for the treatment of stage II breast cancer: the National Surgical Adjuvant Breast and Bowel Project experience. *J Clin Oncol* 1989;7:572.
51. Misset JL, Gil-Dalgado M, Chollet Ph, et al. Ten-year results of the French trial comparing adriamycin, vincristine, 5-fluorouracil and cyclophosphamide to standard CMF as adjuvant therapy for node positive breast cancer. *Proc Am Soc Clin Oncol* 1992;11:54(abst).
52. Budd GT, Green S, O'Bryan RM, et al. Short-course FAC-M versus 1-year of CMFVP in node-positive, hormone receptor-negative breast cancer: an intergroup study. *J Clin Oncol* 1995;13:831.
53. Fisher B, Brown AM, Dimitrov NV, et al. Two months of doxorubicin-cyclophosphamide with and without interval reinduction therapy compared with 6 months of cyclophosphamide, methotrexate, and fluorouracil in positive-node breast cancer patients with tamoxifen-nonresponsive tumors: results from the National Surgical Adjuvant Breast and Bowel Project B-15. *J Clin Oncol* 1990;8:1483.
54. Moliterni A, Bonadonna G, Valagussa P, et al. Cyclophosphamide, methotrexate, and fluorouracil with and without doxorubicin in the adjuvant treatment of resectable breast cancer with one to three positive axillary nodes. *J Clin Oncol* 1991;9:1124.
55. Bonadonna G, Zambetti M, Valagussa P. Sequential or alternating doxorubicin and CMF regimens in breast cancer with more than three positive nodes. Ten-year results. *JAMA* 1995;273:542.
56. Hutchins L, Green S, Ravdin P, et al. CMF versus CAF with and without tamoxifen in high-risk node-negative breast cancer patients and a natural history follow-up study in low-risk node-negative patients: first results of intergroup trial INT 0102. *Proc ASCO* 1998;17:1a(abst 2).
57. Cobleigh MA, Vogel CL, Tripathy NJ, et al. Efficacy and safety of herceptin (humanized anti-HER2 antibody) as a single agent in 222 women with HER2 overexpression who relapsed following chemotherapy for metastatic breast cancer. *Proc Am Soc Clin Oncol* 1998;17:97a(abst 376).
58. Slamon D, Leyland-Jones B, Shak S, et al. Addition of herceptin (humanized anti-HER2 antibody) to first line chemotherapy for HER2 overexpressing metastatic breast cancer (HER2+/MBC) markedly increases anticancer activity: a randomized multinational controlled phase III trial. *Proc Am Soc Clin Oncol* 1998;17:98a(abst 377).
59. Mundy GR, Yoneda T. Bisphosphonates as anticancer drugs [Editorial]. *N Engl J Med* 1998;339:398.
60. Kanis JA, McCloskey EV. Clodronate. Skeletal complications of malignancy. *Cancer Suppl* 1997;80:1691.
61. Hortobagyi GN, Theriault RL, Porter L, et al. Efficacy of pamidronate in reducing skeletal complications in patients with breast cancer and lytic bone metastases. *N Engl J Med* 1996;335:1785.
62. Diel IJ, Solomayer EF, Costa SD, et al. Reduction in new metastases in breast cancer with adjuvant clodronate treatment. *N Engl J Med* 1998;339:357.
63. Powles TJ, Paterson AHG, Nevantaus A, et al. Adjuvant clodronate reduces the incidence of bone metastases in patients with primary operable breast cancer. *Proc Am Soc Clin Oncol* 1998;17:123a(abst 468).
64. Redmond C, Fisher B, Wieand HS. The methodologic dilemma in retrospectively correlating the amount of chemotherapy received in adjuvant therapy protocols with disease-free survival. *Cancer Treat Rep* 1983;67:519.
65. Hryniuk W, Levine MN. Analysis of dose intensity for adjuvant chemotherapy trials in stage II breast cancer. *J Clin Oncol* 1986;4:1162.
66. Budman DR, Berry DA, Cirrincione CT, et al. Dose and dose intensity as determinants of outcome in the adjuvant treatment of breast cancer. The Cancer and Leukemia Group B. *J Natl Cancer Inst* 1998;90:1205.
67. Fisher B, Anderson S, Wickerham DL, et al. Increased intensification and total dose of cyclophosphamide in a doxorubicin-cyclophosphamide regimen for the treatment of primary breast cancer: findings from National Surgical Adjuvant Breast and Bowel Project B-22. *J Clin Oncol* 1997;15:1858.
68. Fisher B, Anderson S, DeCillis A, et al. Further evaluation of intensified and increased total dose of cyclophosphamide for the treatment of primary breast cancer: findings from National Surgical Adjuvant Breast and Bowel Project B-25. *J Clin Oncol* 1999 (*in press*).
69. Rodenhuis S, Richel DJ, Van der Wall E, et al. A randomized trial of high dose chemotherapy and hematopoietic progenitor cell support in operable breast cancer with extensive axillary lymph node involvement. *Proc Am Soc Clin Oncol* 1998;17:470(abst).
70. Hortobagyi GN, Buzdar AU, Champlin R, et al. Lack of efficacy of adjuvant high-dose tandem combination chemotherapy for high risk primary breast cancer—a randomized trial. *Proc Am Soc Clin Oncol* 1998;17:123a(abst 471).
71. van Dam FSAM, Schagen SB, Muller MJ, et al. Impairment of cognitive function in women receiving adjuvant treatment for high-risk breast cancer: high-dose standard-dose chemotherapy. *J Natl Cancer Inst* 1998;90:210.

72. Peters WP, Rosner G, Vredenburgh J, et al. A prospective randomized comparison of two doses of combination alkylating agents as consolidation after CAF in high-risk primary breast cancer involving ten or more axillary lymph nodes: preliminary results of CALGB 90B2/SWOG 9114/NCIC MA-13. *Proc Am Soc Clin Oncol* 1999 (*in press*).
73. Fisher B, Gunduz N, Saffer EA. Influence of the interval between primary tumor removal and chemotherapy on kinetics and growth of metastases. *Cancer Res* 1983;43:1488.
74. Goldie JH. Scientific basis for adjuvant and primary (neoadjuvant) chemotherapy. *Semin Oncol* 1987;14:1.
75. Ludwig Breast Cancer Study Group. Prolonged disease-free survival after one course of perioperative adjuvant chemotherapy for node-negative breast cancer. *N Engl J Med* 1989;320:491.
76. Clahsen PC, van de Velde CJH, Goldhirsch A, et al. Overview of randomized perioperative polychemotherapy trials in women with early-stage breast cancer. *J Clin Oncol* 1997;15:2526.
77. Goldie JH. Scientific basis for adjuvant and primary (neoadjuvant) chemotherapy. *Semin Oncol* 1987;14:1.
78. Bonadonna G, Valagussa P, Brambilla C, et al. Adjuvant and neoadjuvant treatment of breast cancer with chemotherapy and/or endocrine therapy. *Semin Oncol* 1991;15:515.
79. Kuerer HM, Newman LA, Buzdar AU, et al. Pathologic tumor response in the breast following neoadjuvant chemotherapy predicts axillary lymph node status [See comments]. *Cancer J Sci Am* 1998;4:230.
80. Machiavelli MR, Romero AO, Perez JE, et al. Prognostic significance of pathological response of primary tumor and metastatic axillary lymph nodes after neoadjuvant chemotherapy for locally advanced breast carcinoma. *Cancer J Sci Am* 1998;4:125.
81. Brain E, Garrino C, Misset JL, et al. Long-term prognostic and predictive factors in 107 stage II/III breast cancer patients treated with anthracycline-based neoadjuvant chemotherapy. *Br J Cancer* 1997;75:1360.
82. Ellis PA, Smith IE, Detre S, et al. Reduced apoptosis and proliferation and increased Bcl-2 in residual breast cancer following preoperative chemotherapy. *Breast Cancer Res Treat* 1998;48:107.
83. Bottini A, Berruti A, Bersiga A, et al. Effect of neoadjuvant chemotherapy on Ki67 labelling index, c-erbB-2 expression and steroid hormone receptor status in human breast tumours. *Anticancer Res* 1996;16:3105.
84. Fisher B, Bryant J, Wolmark N, et al. Effect of preoperative chemotherapy on the outcome of women with operable breast cancer. *J Clin Oncol* 1998;16:2672.
85. Powles TJ, Hickish TG, Makris A, et al. Randomized trial of chemoendocrine therapy started before or after surgery for treatment of primary breast cancer. *J Clin Oncol* 1995;13:547.
86. Mauriac L, Durand M, Avril A, et al. Effects of primary chemotherapy in conservative treatment of breast cancer patients with operable tumors larger than 3 cm: results of a randomized trial in a single center. *Ann Oncol* 1991;2:347.
87. Allred DC, Clark GM, Tandon AK, et al. HER-2/neu in node-negative breast cancer: prognostic significance of overexpression influenced by presence of in-situ carcinoma. *J Clin Oncol* 1992;10:599.
88. Carlomagno C, Perrone F, Gallo C, et al. c-erbB2 overexpression decreases the benefit of adjuvant tamoxifen in early breast cancer without axillary lymph node metastases. *J Clin Oncol* 1996;14:2702.
89. Muss HB, Thor AD, Berry DA, et al. c-erbB-2 expression and response to adjuvant therapy in women with node-positive early breast cancer. *N Engl J Med* 1994;330:1260.
90. Osborne CK. Steroid hormone receptors in breast cancer management. *Breast Cancer Res Treat* 1998;51:227.
91. Love RR, Mazess RB, Barden HW, et al. Effects of tamoxifen on bone mineral density in postmenopausal women with breast cancer. *N Engl J Med* 1992;326:852.
92. Love RR, Newcombe PA, Wiebe DA, et al. Effects of tamoxifen therapy on lipid and lipoprotein levels in postmenopausal patients with node-negative breast cancer. *J Natl Cancer Inst* 1990;82:1327.
93. Ellis PA, Saccani-Jotti G, Clarke R, et al. Induction of apoptosis by tamoxifen and ICI 182780 in primary breast cancer. *Int J Cancer* 1997;72:608.
94. Lahti EI, Knip M, Laatikainen TJ. Plasma insulin-like growth factor I and its binding proteins 1 and 3 in postmenopausal patients with breast cancer receiving long-term tamoxifen. *Cancer* 1994;74:618.
95. Early Breast Cancer Trialists' Collaborative Group. Tamoxifen for early breast cancer: an overview of the randomised trials. *Lancet* 1998;351:1451.
96. NATO Steering Committee. Controlled trial of tamoxifen as a single adjuvant agent in the management of early breast cancer. *Br J Cancer* 1988;57:608.
97. Report from the Breast Cancer Trials Committee, Scottish Cancer Trials Office, Edinburgh. Adjuvant tamoxifen in the management of operable breast cancer: the Scottish trial. *Lancet* 1987;8552.
98. Kaufman M, Jonat W, Abel U, et al. Adjuvant randomized trials of doxorubicin/cyclophosphamide/tamoxifen and CMF chemotherapy versus tamoxifen in women with node-positive breast cancer. *J Clin Oncol* 1993;11:454.
99. Fisher B, Dignam J, Wolmark N, et al. Tamoxifen and chemotherapy for lymph node-negative, estrogen receptor-positive breast cancer. *J Natl Cancer Inst* 1997;89:1673.
100. Fisher B, Dignam J, Bryant J, et al. Five versus more than five years of tamoxifen therapy for breast cancer patients with negative lymph nodes and estrogen receptor-positive tumors. *J Natl Cancer Inst* 1996;1529.
101. Swedish Breast Cancer Cooperative Group. Randomized trial of two versus five years of adjuvant tamoxifen for postmenopausal early stage breast cancer. *J Natl Cancer Inst* 1996;88:1543.
102. Current Trials Working Party of the Cancer Research Campaign Breast Cancer Trials Group. Preliminary results from the Cancer Research Campaign trial evaluating tamoxifen duration in women aged fifty years or older with breast cancer. *J Natl Cancer Inst* 1996;88:1834.
103. Tormey DC, Gray R, Falkson HC. Postchemotherapy adjuvant tamoxifen therapy beyond five years in patients with lymph node–positive breast cancer. *J Natl Cancer Inst* 1996;88:1828.
104. Stewart HJ, Forrest AP, Everington D, et al. Randomised comparison of 5 years of adjuvant tamoxifen with continuous therapy for operable breast cancer. The Scottish Cancer Trials Breast Group. *Br J Cancer* 1996;74:297.
105. Wiebe VJ, Osborne CK, Fuqua SAW, et al. Tamoxifen resistance in breast cancer. *Crit Rev Oncol Hematol* 1993;14:173.
106. Osborne CK, Jarman M, McCague R, Coronado EB, Hilsenbeck SG, Wakeling AE. The importance of tamoxifen metabolism in tamoxifen-stimulated breast tumor growth. *Cancer Chemother Pharmacol* 1994;34:89.
107. Lippman ME, Osborne CK, Knazek R, Young N. *In vitro* model systems for the study of hormone dependent human breast cancer. Beth Israel seminars in medicine. *N Engl J Med* 1977;296:154.
108. Osborne CK, Hobbs K, Clark GM. Effect of estrogens and antiestrogens on growth of human breast cancer cells in athymic nude mice. *Cancer Res* 1985;45:584.
109. Pollak M, Costantino J, Polychronakos C, et al. Effect of tamoxifen on serum insulin-like growth factor 1 levels in stage 1 breast cancer. *J Natl Cancer Inst* 1990;82:1693.
110. Fisher ER, Osborne CK, McGuire WL, et al. Correlation of primary breast cancer histopathology and estrogen receptor content. *Breast Cancer Res Treat* 1981;1:37.
111. Fisher B, Redmond C, Brown A, et al. Adjuvant chemotherapy with and without tamoxifen in the treatment of primary breast cancer: 5-year results from the National Surgical Adjuvant Breast and Bowel Project trial. *J Clin Oncol* 1986;4:459.
112. Cummings FJ, Gray R, Tormey DC, et al. Adjuvant tamoxifen versus placebo in elderly women with node-positive breast cancer: long-term follow-up and causes of death. *J Clin Oncol* 1993;11:29.
113. Osborne CK. Drug therapy: tamoxifen in the treatment of breast cancer. *N Engl J Med* 1998;339:1609.
114. McDonald CC, Stewart HJ. Fatal myocardial infarction in the Scottish Adjuvant Tamoxifen trial: the Scottish Breast Cancer Committee. *BMJ* 1991;303:435.
115. Rutqvist LE, Mattsson A for the Stockholm Breast Cancer Study Group. Cardiac and thromboembolic morbidity among postmenopausal women with early-stage breast cancer in a randomized trial of adjuvant tamoxifen. *J Natl Cancer Inst* 1993;85:1398.
116. Costantino JP, Kuller LH, Ives DG, Fisher B, Dignam J. Coronary heart disease mortality and adjuvant tamoxifen therapy. *J Natl Cancer Inst* 1997;89:776.
117. Rossner S, Wallgren A. Serum lipoproteins and proteins after breast cancer surgery and effects of tamoxifen. *Atherosclerosis* 1984;52:339.
118. Love RR, Newcombe PA, Wiebe DA, et al. Effects of tamoxifen therapy on lipid and lipoprotein levels in postmenopausal patients with node-negative breast cancer. *J Natl Cancer Inst* 1990;82:1327.
119. Williams JK, Wagner JD, Li Z, Golden DL, Adams MR. Tamoxifen inhibits arterial accumulation of LDL degradation products and pro-

gression of coronary artery atherosclerosis in monkeys. *Anterioscler Thromb Vasc Biol* 1997;17:403.
120. Kristensen B, Ejlertsen B, Dalgaard P, et al. Tamoxifen and bone metabolism in postmenopausal low-risk breast cancer patients: a randomized study. *J Clin Oncol* 1994;12:992.
121. Powles TJ, Hickish T, Kanis JA, Tidy A, Ashley S. Effect of tamoxifen on bone mineral density measured by dual-energy x-ray absorptiometry in healthy premenopausal and postmenopausal women. *J Clin Oncol* 1996;14:78.
122. Fisher B, Constantino JP, Wickerham DL, et al. Tamoxifen for prevention of breast cancer: report of the National Surgical Adjuvant Breast and Bowel Project P-1 Study. *J Natl Cancer Inst* 1998;90:1371.
123. Rutqvist LE, Cedermark B, Glas U, et al. Contralateral primary tumors in breast cancer patients in a randomized trial of adjuvant tamoxifen therapy. *J Natl Cancer Inst* 1991;83:1299.
124. Wilking N, Isaksson E, von Schoultz E. Tamoxifen and secondary tumours: an update. *Drug Saf* 1997;16:104.
125. Cummings SR, Norton L, Eckert S, et al. Raloxifene reduces the risk of breast cancer and may decrease the risk of endometrial cancer in post-menopausal women. Two-year findings from the Multiple Outcomes of Raloxifene Evaluation (MORE) trial. *Proc Am Soc Clin Oncol* 1998;17:2a(abst).
126. Powles T, Eeles R, Ashley S, et al. Interim analysis of the incidence of breast cancer in the Royal Marsden Hospital tamoxifen randomised chemoprevention trial. *Lancet* 1998;352:98.
127. Veronesi U, Maisonneuve P, Costa A, et al. Prevention of breast cancer with tamoxifen: preliminary findings from the Italian randomised trial among hysterectomised women. Italian Tamoxifen Prevention Study. *Lancet* 1998;352:93.
128. Early Breast Cancer Trialists' Collaborative Group. Ovarian ablation in early breast cancer: overview of the randomised trials. *Lancet* 1996;348:1189.
129. Bryant AJ, Weir JA. Prophylactic oophorectomy in operable instances of carcinoma of the breast. *Surg Gynecol Obstet* 1981;153:660.
130. Meakin JW, Allt WEC, Beale FA, et al. Ovarian irradiation and prednisone therapy following surgery and radiotherapy for carcinoma of the breast. *Can Med Assoc J* 1979;120:1221.
131. Davidson N, O'Neill A, Habermann T, Osborne CK, Martino S, White D, Abeloff MD for ECOG, SWOG, and CALGB. Effect of chemohormonal therapy in premenopausal, node(+), receptor(+) breast cancer: an Eastern Cooperation Oncology Group Phase III Intergroup Trial (E5188, INT-0101). Submitted to the American Society Clinical Oncology Annual Meeting, May 1999.
132. Scottish Cancer Trials Breast Group and ICFR Breast Unit, Guy's Hospital. Adjuvant ovarian ablation versus CMF chemotherapy in premenopausal women with pathological stage II breast carcinoma: the Scottish Trial. *Lancet* 1993;341:1293.
133. Stevenson JC, Lees B, Gardner R, Shaw RW. A comparison of the skeletal effects of goserelin and danazol in premenopausal women with endometriosis. *Horm Res* 1989;32:161.
134. Palshof T, Carstensen B, Mouridsen HT, et al. Adjuvant endocrine therapy in pre- and postmenopausal women with operable breast cancer. *Rev Endocr Rel Cancer* 1985;s17:43.
135. Jones AL, Powles TJ, Law M, et al. Adjuvant aminoglutethimide for postmenopausal patients with primary cancer. analysis at 8 years. *J Clin Oncol* 1992;10:1547.
136. Focan C, Baudoux A, Beauduin M, et al. Adjuvant treatment with high dose medroxyprogesterone acetate in node-negative early breast cancer. *Acta Oncol* 1989;28:237.
137. Osborne CK, Boldt DH, Clark GM, et al. Effects of tamoxifen on human breast cancer cell cycle kinetics: accumulation of cells in early G1. *Cancer Res* 1983;43:3583.
138. Osborne CK, Boldt DH, Estrada P. Human breast cancer cell cycle synchronization by estrogens and antiestrogens in culture. *Cancer Res* 1984;44:1433.
139. Osborne CK, Coronado EB, Robinson JP. Human breast cancer in the athymic nude mouse: cytostatic effects of long-term antiestrogen therapy. *Eur J Cancer Clin Oncol* 1987;23:1189.
140. Greenberg DA, Carpenter CL, Messing RO. Calcium channel antagonist properties of the antineoplastic antiestrogen tamoxifen in the PC12 neurosecretory cell line. *Cancer Res* 1987;47:70.
141. Lam H-YP. Tamoxifen is a calmodulin antagonist in the activation of cAMP phosphodiesterase. *Biochem Biophys Res Commun* 1984; 118:27.
142. Se H-D, Mazzei GJ, Vogler WR, et al. Effect of tamoxifen, a nonsteroidal antiestrogen, on phospholipid/calcium-dependent protein kinase and phosphorylation of its endogenous substrate proteins from the rat brain and ovary. *Biochem Pharmacol* 1985;34:3649.
143. Berman E, Adams M, Duigou-Osterndorf R, et al. Effect of tamoxifen on cell lines displaying the multidrug-resistant phenotype. *Blood* 1991;77:818.
144. Naito M, Yusa K, Tsuruo T. Steroid hormones inhibit binding of Vinca alkaloid to multidrug resistance related p-glycoproteins. *Biochem Biophys Res Commun* 1989;158:1066.
145. Elledge RM, Green S, Howes L, et al. bcl-2, p53, and response to tamoxifen in ER-positive metastatic breast cancer: a Southwest Oncology Group study. *J Clin Oncol* 1997;15:1916.
146. Osborne CK, Kitten L, Arteaga CL. Antagonism of chemotherapy-induced cytotoxicity for human breast cancer by antiestrogens. *J Clin Oncol* 1989;7:710.
147. Goldenberg GJ, Froese EK. Antagonism of the cytocidal activity and uptake of melphalan by tamoxifen in human breast cancer cells in vitro. *Biochem Pharmacol* 1985;34:763.
148. Fisher B, Redmond C, Legault-Poisson S, et al. Postoperative chemotherapy and tamoxifen compared with tamoxifen alone in the treatment of positive-node breast cancer patients aged 50 years and older with tumors responsive to tamoxifen: results from the National Surgical Adjuvant Breast and Bowel Project B-16. *J Clin Oncol* 1990;8:1005.
149. Ingle JN, Everson LK, Wieand HS, et al. Randomized trial of observation versus adjuvant therapy with cyclophosphamide, fluorouracil, prednisone with or without tamoxifen following mastectomy in postmenopausal women with node-positive breast cancer. *J Clin Oncol* 1988;6:1388.
150. Taylor SG, Knuiman KW, Sleeper LA, et al. Six-year results of the Eastern Cooperative Oncology Group trial of observation versus CMFP versus CMFPT in postmenopausal patients with node-positive breast cancer. *J Clin Oncol* 1989;7:879.
151. Goldhirsch A, Gelber RD. Adjuvant chemo-endocrine therapy or endocrine therapy alone for postmenopausal patients: Ludwig studies III and IV. In: Senn H, Goldhirsch A, Gelber RD, et al, eds. *Recent results in cancer research: adjuvant therapy of primary breast cancer*. Berlin: Springer-Verlag, 1989:153.
152. The International Breast Cancer Study Group. Late effects of adjuvant oophorectomy and chemotherapy upon premenopausal breast cancer patients. *Ann Oncol* 1990;1:30.
153. Rivkin S, Green S, Metch B, et al. Adjuvant combination chemotherapy (CMFVP) vs oophorectomy followed by CMFVP (OCMFVP) for premenopausal women with ER+ operable breast cancer with positive axillary lymph nodes: an intergroup study. *Proc Am Soc Clin Oncol* 1991;10:47.
154. Dombernowsky P, Brincker H, Hansen M, et al. Adjuvant therapy of premenopausal and menopausal high-risk breast cancer patients. *Acta Oncol* 1988;27:691.
155. Tormey DC, Gray R, Gilchrist K, et al. Adjuvant chemohormonal therapy with cyclophosphamide, methotrexate, 5-fluorouracil, and prednisone (CMFP) or CMFP plus tamoxifen compared with CMF for premenopausal breast cancer patients. *Cancer* 1990;65:200.
156. Ingle JN, Everson LK, Wieand HS, et al. Randomized trial to evaluate the addition of tamoxifen to cyclophosphamide, 5-fluorouracil, prednisone adjuvant therapy in premenopausal women with node-positive breast cancer. *Cancer* 1989;63:1257.
157. Boccardo F, Rubagotti A, Bruzzi P, et al. Chemotherapy versus tamoxifen versus chemotherapy plus tamoxifen in node-positive, estrogen receptor-positive breast cancer patients: results of a multicentric Italian study. *J Clin Oncol* 1990;8:1310.
158. Mouridsen HT, Rose C, Overgaard M, et al. Adjuvant treatment of postmenopausal patients with high risk primary breast cancer. *Acta Oncol* 1988;27:699.
159. Rivkin SE, Green S, Metch B, et al. Adjuvant CMFVP versus tamoxifen versus concurrent CMFVP and tamoxifen for postmenopausal, node-positive and estrogen receptor-positive breast cancer patients: a Southwest Oncology Group study. *J Clin Oncol* 1994;12:2078.
160. Pritchard KI, Paterson AHG, Fine S, et al. Randomized trial of cyclophosphamide, methotrexate, and fluorouracil chemotherapy added to tamoxifen as adjuvant therapy in postmenopausal women with node-positive estrogen and/or progesterone receptor-positive breast cancer: a report of the National Cancer Institute of Canada Clinical Trials Group. *J Clin Oncol* 1997;15:2302.

161. The International Breast Cancer Study Group. Effectiveness of adjuvant chemotherapy in combination with tamoxifen for node-positive postmenopausal breast cancer patients. *J Clin Oncol* 1997;15:1385.
162. Ravdin PM, Green S, Albain KS, et al. Initial report of the SWOG biological correlative study of c-erbB-2 expression as a predictor of outcome in a trial comparing adjuvant CAF T with tamoxifen alone. *Proc Am Soc Clin Oncol* 1998;17:97a(abst).
163. Levine MN, Gent M, Hirsh J, et al. The thrombogenic effect of anticancer drug therapy in women with stage II breast cancer. *N Engl J Med* 1988;318:404.
164. Knobf MT. Physical and psychologic distress associated with adjuvant chemotherapy in women with breast cancer. *J Clin Oncol* 1986;4:678.
165. Hughson AVM, Cooper AF, McArdle CS, et al. Psychological impact of adjuvant chemotherapy in the first two years after mastectomy. *BMJ* 1986;293:1268.
166. Cassileth BR, Knuiman MW, Abeloff MD, et al. Anxiety levels in patients randomized to adjuvant therapy versus observation for early breast cancer. *J Clin Oncol* 1986;4:972.
167. Buzdar AU, Marcus C, Smith TL, et al. Early and delayed clinical cardiotoxicity of doxorubicin. *Cancer* 1985;55:2761.
168. Griem KL, Henderson IC, Gelman R, et al. The 5-year results of a randomized trial of adjuvant radiation therapy after chemotherapy in breast cancer treated with mastectomy. *J Clin Oncol 1*987;5:1546.
169. Padmanabhan N, Wang DY, Moore JW, et al. Ovarian function and adjuvant chemotherapy for early breast cancer. *Eur J Cancer Clin Oncol* 1987;23:745.
170. Gradishar WJ, Schilsky RL. Ovarian function following radiation and chemotherapy for cancer. *Semin Oncol* 1989;16:425.
171. Bines J, Oleske DM, Cobleigh MA. Ovarian function in premenopausal women treated with adjuvant chemotherapy for breast cancer. *J Clin Oncol* 1996;14:1718.
172. Saarto T, Blomqvist C, Välimäki M, Mäkelä P, Sarna S, Elomaa I. Chemical castration induced by adjuvant cyclophosphamide, methotrexate, and fluorouracil chemotherapy causes rapid bone loss that is reduced by clodronate: a randomized study in premenopausal breast cancer patients. *J Clin Oncol* 1997;15:1341.
173. Curtis RE, Boice JD Jr, Moloney WC, et al. Leukemia following chemotherapy for breast cancer. *Cancer Res* 1990;50:2741.
174. Fisher B, Rockette H, Fisher ER, et al. Leukemia in breast cancer patients following adjuvant chemotherapy or postoperative radiation: the NSABP experience. *J Clin Oncol* 1985;3:1640.
175. Curtis RE, Boice JD, Stovall M, et al. Risk of leukemia after chemotherapy and radiation treatment for breast cancer. *N Engl J Med* 1992;326:1745.
176. Tallman MS, Gray R, Bennett JM, et al. Leukemogenic potential of adjuvant chemotherapy for early-stage breast cancer: the Eastern Cooperative Oncology Group experience. *J Clin Oncol* 1995;13:1557.
177. Diamandidou E, Buzdar AU, Smith TL, Frye D, Witjaksono M, Hortobagyi GN. Treatment-related leukemia in breast cancer patients treated with fluorouracil-doxorubicin-cyclophosphamide combination adjuvant chemotherapy. *J Clin Oncol* 1996;14:2722.
178. DeCillis A, Anderson S, Bryant J, et al. Acute myeloid leukemia and myelodysplastic syndrome in NSABP B25. *Proc Am Soc Clin Oncol* 1997;16:459(abst).
179. Levine MN, Bramwell VH, Pritchard KI, et al. Randomized trial of intensive cyclophosphamide, epirubicin, and fluorouracil chemotherapy compared with cyclophosphamide, methotrexate, and fluorouracil in premenopausal women with node-positive breast cancer. *J Clin Oncol* 1998;16:2651.
180. Henderson IC, Gelman R. Second malignancies from adjuvant chemotherapy? Too soon to tell [Editorial]. *J Clin Oncol* 1987;5:1135.
181. Valagussa P, Tancini G, Bonadonna G. Second malignancies after CMF for resectable breast cancer. *J Clin Oncol* 1987;5:1138.
182. Adjuvant tamoxifen in the management of operable breast cancer: the Scottish trial. Report from the Breast Cancer Trials Committee, Scottish Cancer Trials Office (MCR), Edinburgh. *Lancet* (8552) 1987;171.
183. Ribeiro G, Swindell R. The Christie Hospital adjuvant tamoxifen trial—status at 10 years. *Br J Cancer* 1988;57:601.
184. Love RR, Cameron L, Connell BL, et al. Symptoms associated with tamoxifen treatment in postmenopausal women. *Arch Intern Med* 1991;151:1842.
185. Cathcart CK, Jones SE, Pumroy CS, et al. Clinical recognition and management of depression in node negative breast cancer patients treated with tamoxifen. *Breast Cancer Res Treat* 1993;27:277.
186. Kaiser-Kupfer MI, Lippman ME. Tamoxifen retinopathy. *Cancer Treat Rep* 1978;62:315.
187. Pavlidis NA, Petris C, Briassoulis E, et al. Clear evidence that long-term, low-dose tamoxifen treatment can induce ocular toxicity. *Cancer* 1992;69:2961.
188. Longstaff S, Sigurdsson H, O'Keeffe M, Ogston S, Preece P. A controlled study of the ocular effects of tamoxifen in conventional dosage in the treatment of breast carcinoma. *Eur J Cancer Clin Oncol* 1989; 25:1805.
189. Nayfield SG, Gorin MB. Tamoxifen-associated eye disease: a review. *J Clin Oncol* 1996;14:1018
190. Gorin MB, Day R, Costantino JP, et al. Long-term tamoxifen citrate use and potential ocular toxicity. *Am J Ophthalmol* 1998;125:493
191. Communication from the Department of Health and Human Services, National Institutes of Health, National Cancer Institute, January 27, 1997. Tamoxifen-associated eye toxicity.
192. "Nolvadex" Adjuvant Trial Organisation. Controlled trial of tamoxifen as a single agent in the management of early breast cancer. *Br J Cancer* 1988;57:608.
193. Rutqvist LE, Mattsson A for the Stockholm Breast Cancer Study Group. Cardiac and thromboembolic morbidity among postmenopausal women with early-stage breast cancer in a randomized trial of adjuvant tamoxifen. *J Natl Cancer Inst* 1993;85:1398.
194. Pritchard KI, Paterson AHG, Paul NA, Zee B, Fine S, Pater J. Increased thromboembolic complications with concurrent tamoxifen and chemotherapy in a randomized trial of adjuvant therapy for women with breast cancer. *J Clin Oncol* 1996;14:2731.
195. Levine MN. Prevention of thrombotic disorders in cancer patients undergoing chemotherapy. *Thromb Haemost* 1997;78:133.
196. Potter GA, McCague R, Jarman M. A mechanistic hypothesis for DNA adduct formation by tamoxifen following hepatic oxidative metabolism. *Carcinogenesis* 1994;15:439.
197. Styles LA, Davies A, Lim CK, et al. Genotoxicity of tamoxifen, tamoxifen epoxide and toremifene in human lymphoblastoid cells containing human cytochrome P450s. *Carcinogenesis* 1994;15:5.
198. Hard GC, Iatropoulos MJ, Jordan K, et al. Major difference in the hepatocarcinogenicity and DNA adduct forming between toremifene and tamoxifen in female Crl:CD(BR) rats. *Cancer Res* 1993;53:4534.
199. Ahotupa M, Hirsimaki P, Rarssinen R, et al. Alterations of drug metabolizing and antioxidant enzyme activities during tamoxifen-induced hepatocarcinogenesis in the rat. *Carcinogenesis* 1994;15:863.
200. Fornander T, Cedermark B, Mattsson A, et al. Adjuvant tamoxifen in early breast cancer: occurrence of new primary cancers. *Lancet* 1989; 1:117.
201. Muhlemann K, Cook LS, Weiss NS. The incidence of hepatocellular carcinoma in US white women with breast cancer after the introduction of tamoxifen in 1977. *Breast Cancer Res Treat* 1994;30:201.
202. Jordan VC, Morrow MM. Should clinicians be concerned about the carcinogenic potential of tamoxifen? *Eur J Cancer* 1994;30A:1714.
203. Assikis VJ, Jordan VC. Gynecological effects of tamoxifen and the association with endometrial cancer. *Int J Gynecol Obstet* 1995; 9:241.
204. Fisher B, Costantino JP, Redmond CK, et al. Endometrial cancer in tamoxifen-treated breast cancer patients: findings from the National Surgical Adjuvant Breast and Bowel Project (NSABP) B-14. *J Natl Cancer Inst* 1994;86:527.
205. Magriples U, Naftolin F, Schwartz PE, et al. High-grade endometrial carcinoma in tamoxifen-treated breast cancer patients. *J Clin Oncol* 1993;11:485.
206. Fisher B, Costantino JP, Wickerham DL, et al. Tamoxifen for prevention of breast cancer: report of the National Surgical Adjuvant Breast and Bowel Project P-1 Study. *J Natl Cancer Inst* 1998;90:1371.
207. Hann LE, Giess CS, Bach AM, Tao Y, Baum HJ, Barakat RR. Endometrial thickness in tamoxifen-treated patients: correlation with clinical and pathologic findings. *AJR Am J Roentgenol* 1997;168:657.
208. Shushan A, Peretz T, Uziely B, Lewin A, Mor-Yosef S. Ovarian cysts in premenopausal and postmenopausal tamoxifen-treated women with breast cancer. *Am J Obstet Gynecol* 1996;174:141.
209. Andersson M, Storm HH, Mouridsen HT. Incidence of new primary cancers after adjuvant tamoxifen therapy and radiotherapy for early breast cancer. *J Natl Cancer Inst* 1991;83:1013.
210. Hillner BE, Smith TJ. Efficacy and cost effectiveness of adjuvant chemotherapy in women with node-negative breast cancer. *N Engl J Med* 1991;324:160.

211. Smith TJ, Hillner BE. The efficacy and cost-effectiveness of adjuvant therapy of early breast cancer in premenopausal women. *J Clin Oncol* 1993;11:771.
212. Desch CE, Hillner BE, Smith TJ, et al. Should the elderly receive chemotherapy for node-negative breast cancer? A cost-effectiveness analysis examining total and active life-expectancy outcomes. *J Clin Oncol* 1993;11:777.
213. Siminoff LA, Fetting JH, Abeloff MD. Doctor-patient communication about breast cancer therapy. *J Clin Oncol* 1989;7:1192.
214. Rajagopal S, Goodman PF, Tannock IF. Adjuvant chemotherapy for breast cancer: discordance between physicians' perception of benefit and the results of clinical trials. *J Clin Oncol* 1994;12:1296.
215. Coates AS, Simes RJ. Patient assessment of adjuvant treatment in operable breast cancer. In: Williams CJ, ed. *Introducing new treatments for cancer: practical, ethical, and legal problems.* New York: John Wiley & Sons, 1992:447.
216. NIH Consensus Development Panel. Consensus statement: treatment of early-stage breast cancer. *J Natl Cancer Inst Mongr* 1992;11:1.
217. Rosen PP, Groshen S, Saigo PE, et al. Pathological prognostic factors in stage I (T1N1M0) breast carcinoma: a study of 644 patients with median followup of 18 years. *J Clin Oncol* 1989;7:1239.
218. Recht A, Come SE, Henderson IC, et al. The sequencing of chemotherapy and radiation after conservative surgery for early-stage breast cancer. *N Engl J Med* 1996;334:1356.

Diseases of the Breast, 2nd ed.,
edited by Jay R. Harris.
Lippincott Williams & Wilkins, Philadelphia © 2000.

CHAPTER 38

Dose-Intensive Chemotherapy

Nancy E. Davidson, M. John Kennedy, and Deborah K. Armstrong

Despite nearly 20 years of research, the importance of chemotherapy drug dose in the treatment of breast cancer remains an unanswered question. That dose might be correlated with outcome was first suggested by the retrospective analysis of adjuvant chemotherapy with cyclophosphamide, methotrexate, and 5-fluorouracil (CMF) performed by Bonadonna et al. in 1981.[1] The authors reported that women with node-positive breast cancer who received more than 85% of the planned dose of CMF had a better clinical outcome than those who received less. Indeed, those who received less than 65% of the intended dose fared no better than women in the untreated control group. Of course, it was not clear whether the better outcome was a result of the increased therapy *per se*, or whether individuals who were able to tolerate the highest doses of chemotherapy were destined to do better for other reasons. Subsequently, a number of such retrospective analyses of the relationship between dose and outcome in individual trials appeared, some supporting and others refuting this hypothesis.

A second type of support from the clinical literature for the dose hypothesis in breast cancer emanated from the work of Hryniuk et al.[2,3] They devised the concept of dose intensity—that is, a measure of the amount of drug given per unit of time, to serve as a common denominator for comparison between trials. Their initial retrospective analysis of the importance of dose intensity for chemotherapy examined the dose intensity of Cooper-like regimens in patients with stage IV breast cancer.[2] A higher likelihood of response was noted with increasing delivered drug dose of these CMF-based regimens. A second analysis of cyclophosphamide, doxorubicin (A), and 5-fluorouracil (CAF)-type regimens gave similar results. This technique of analysis was also applied to CMF-based regimens administered in the adjuvant setting.[3] Again, dose intensity was significantly correlated with 3-year disease-free survival (DFS). Thus, these studies of dose intensity versus outcome in both adjuvant[3] and metastatic[2] trials added support to the provocative hypothesis that higher doses of chemotherapy do impart better outcome in breast cancer.

However, both of these types of studies, which are retrospective in nature, are best regarded as hypothesis generating. For this reason, the concepts of dose and dose intensity have been the major focus of a number of prospective randomized trials. These have been made possible in large part by advances in supportive care measures, such as improved antiemetics and antibiotics, use of colony-stimulating factors, and widespread availability of technologies to harvest, store, and reinfuse autologous bone marrow or peripheral blood stem cells. It is the goal of this chapter to provide information about clinical trials that have prospectively addressed the dose issue in both the subtransplant and transplant settings.

DOSE ESCALATION IN THE SUBTRANSPLANT RANGE

In a recent editorial, Biganzoli and Piccart[4] provided a conceptual framework for the analysis of clinical trial–based evidence of the dose issue. They postulated the existence of at least five models that could permit the delivery of higher overall chemotherapy dose in both early and advanced stages of breast cancer. These hypothetical models are listed in Table 1. Most, but not all, have actually been tested in randomized clinical trials, the results of which are summarized here. In general, these trials have sought to evaluate the dose or dose intensity, or both, of anthracyclines (doxorubicin or epirubicin) or cyclophosphamide.

Chemotherapy for Advanced Breast Cancer

One of the first randomized trials to test the dose hypothesis prospectively compared two dose levels of CMF in 133 patients with previously untreated advanced breast cancer.[5] Low-dose CMF (cyclophosphamide, 300 mg/m^2; methotrexate, 20 mg/m^2; and 5-fluorouracil, 300 mg/m^2 intravenously on day 1 of 21-day cycles) was compared with standard-dose CMF, which was administered at twice the doses (600, 40, and 600 mg/m^2, respectively). Response rates were 26% for

N. E. Davidson: Johns Hopkins Oncology Center, Johns Hopkins University School of Medicine, Baltimore, Maryland

M. J. Kennedy: Department of Hematology/Oncology, St. James Hospital Dublin, Dublin, Ireland

D. K. Armstrong: Department of Oncology, Johns Hopkins University School of Medicine, Baltimore, Maryland

TABLE 1. *Some potential models to allow enhanced dose intensity in breast cancer*

Model	Dose/course	Cycle interval	Cumulative dose
I	Increased	Unchanged	Unchanged
II	Increased	Unchanged	Increased
III	Increased	Unchanged	Reduced
IV	Reduced	Reduced	Unchanged
V	Unchanged	Reduced	Unchanged

Adapted from ref. 4.

the standard-dose arm and 11% for the low-dose arm. Median survival was 15.6 and 12.8 months on the standard- and low-dose arms, a nonsignificant difference after adjustment for an imbalance in pretreatment characteristics.

The impact of dose intensity on the efficacy of single-agent doxorubicin has also been assessed in 48 women with metastatic breast cancer.[6] Patients received doxorubicin, 70 mg/m^2 intravenously, every 3 weeks for 8 cycles or 35 mg/m^2 intravenously every 3 weeks for 16 cycles. Thus, the total intended dose was identical (560 mg/m^2), but the first treatment was more dose intense according to the definition of Hryniuk and Bush.[2] Patients on the 70-mg per m^2 arm had improved response rate, response duration, and survival. These two small trials suggest that dose reduction below standard dose is associated with inferior outcome.

Results of six larger randomized trials reported in the 1990s that examined the impact of epirubicin dose on outcome for women with advanced breast cancer are summarized in Table 2.[7–12] These trials include studies of epirubicin (E) alone or in combination with cyclophosphamide with or without 5-fluorouracil (EC or FEC). The increased dose intensity of epirubicin across all of these trials ranged from approximately 1.5- to 3.5-fold; most examined a dose intensity that was approximately twice that of the control arm. In these trials, the intended dose intensity and the dose intensity actually delivered are generally similar. The clinical results are strikingly uniform. Increased dose intensity was associated with improved response rate up to a point. Median time to progression was prolonged in some, but not all, trials. However, in no case was an impact on survival appreciated. These trials were relatively small (fewer than 400 women) and thus not of sufficient statistical power to detect small differences in survival. Nonetheless, in aggregate, they appear to support the concept of a dose threshold; that is, clinical outcome as judged by response rate is compromised by low epirubicin dose intensity. However, within the confines of these trials, there is little evidence for substantial benefit of epirubicin dose escalation beyond standard dose.

A randomized study of the impact of paclitaxel dose in advanced breast cancer has also been reported.[13] Cancer and Acute Leukemia Group B (CALGB) 9342 randomized 475 women with stage IV breast cancer to paclitaxel doses of 175, 210, or 250 mg per m^2, all infused over 3 hours. Response rates were similar for the 375 women assessed thus far (21%, 28%, and 22%, respectively), as was median survival (9.8, 11.8, and 11.9 months, respectively). There was a correlation of borderline significance ($p = .03$) between paclitaxel dose and time to treatment failure: 3.8, 4.1, and 4.8 months for 175, 210, and 250 mg per m^2, respectively. Neurosensory and hematologic toxicity was also directly related

TABLE 2. *Trials of epirubicin dose in advanced breast cancer*

	Schedule	No. of evaluable patients	Median delivered dose intensity of epirubicin (mg/m^2/wk)	RR (%)	Median TTP (mo)	Median survival (mo)	Reference
Model 1							
E	50 mg/m^2 × 16	209	5.2	23	—	10	7
	100 mg/m^2 × 8	—	25	41[a]	NS	10	—
E	40 mg/m^2	263	12.7	20	4.4	13.6	8
	60 mg/m^2	—	18.4	19.7	4.7	14.0	—
	90 mg/m^2	—	26.4	37.5[a]	8.4[a]	14.6	—
	135 mg/m^2	—	37.8	36.2[a]	8.4[a]	11.3	—
Model 2							
FEC	50 mg/m^2	390	15.5	41	7	17	9
	100 mg/m^2	—	29.5	57[a]	7.6	18	—
FEC	50 mg/m^2 day 1	141	14.9	41	8	23.6	10
	50 mg/m^2 days 1 and 8	—	25.4	69[a]	19[a]	27.1	—
EC	60 mg/m^2	197	NS	47	NS	9.6	11
	120 mg/m^2	—	—	63[a]	—	9.9	—
Model 5							
E	110 mg/m^2 q4wk	167	27.2	49	7.2	14.6	12
	110 mg/m^2 q2wk	—	52.9	53	7.4	14.9	—

C, cyclophosphamide; E, epirubicin; F, 5-fluorouracil; NS, not stated; RR, response rate; TTP, time to progression.
[a]Significant difference from lowest dose.

to dose of paclitaxel. Thus, based on this trial, there is no clear rationale for routine dose escalation of paclitaxel beyond the dose of 175 mg per m^2 over 3 hours. It is not certain whether this dose is more effective than 135 mg per m^2, as this lower dose was not explicitly tested in the trial.

Neoadjuvant Therapy for Locally Advanced Breast Cancer

A large trial has provided information on the role of dose intensity of primary chemotherapy for locally advanced breast cancer.[14] The EORTC-NCIC-SAKK trial randomized 448 patients with locally advanced breast cancer (241 women with noninflammatory and 267 women with inflammatory cancer) to a standard therapy of six cycles of 5-fluorouracil, 500 mg per m^2 on days 1 and 8; epirubicin, 60 mg per m^2 on days 1 and 8; and cyclophosphamide, 75 mg per m^2 by mouth on days 1 to 14 of a 28-day cycle or six cycles of epirubicin, 120 mg per m^2 on day 1 and cyclophosphamide, 830 mg per m^2 on day 1 given every 2 weeks with granulocyte-colony stimulating factor support. The type of local therapy to be used after induction chemotherapy was not mandated, but individualized, according to physician and patient preference. With a median follow-up of 27 months, no clear advantage for the more intense approach has emerged, although longer follow-up is clearly needed.

Adjuvant Therapy for Early-Stage Breast Cancer

It is arguable that the results summarized in the previous section, which were generally obtained through dose escalation of one drug in the metastatic setting, cannot be broadly applied to all scenarios of breast cancer. For example, it is possible that escalating dose intensity of other drugs (e.g., cyclophosphamide) or combinations of drugs might improve outcome. It is also conceivable that modest escalations of dose intensity that have little value in a state of high tumor burden could nonetheless have impact in the setting of micrometastatic disease. Several trials have therefore assessed the importance of dose and dose intensity in the adjuvant setting, and they are reviewed here.

A pivotal trial, CALGB 8541, tested the value of dose intensity in the standard-dose range in 1,572 women with node-positive breast cancers.[15] These patients were allocated to receive (a) cyclophosphamide, 300 mg per m^2 on day 1; doxorubicin, 30 mg per m^2 on day 1; and 5-fluorouracil, 300 mg per m^2 on days 1 and 8 of every 28 days for four cycles (low); (b) C, 400 mg per m^2 on day 1; A, 40 mg per m^2 on day 1; and F, 400 mg per m^2 on days 1 and 8 for six cycles (moderate); or (c) C, 600 mg per m^2 on day 1; A, 60 mg per m^2 on day 1; and F, 600 mg per m^2 on days 1 and 8 for four cycles (high). Thus, the high- and moderate-dose arms had different dose intensity but identical cumulative dose, whereas the low-dose arm had reduced dose intensity and cumulative dose. In the initial report of this study, the low-dose arm gave inferior results in all clinical outcomes at 3 years when compared with the moderate- or high-dose arms. However, no major difference could be perceived in results between patients assigned to the moderate- and high-dose arms. DFS at 3 years was 63%, 70%, and 74%, and overall survival was 84%, 90%, and 92% for the low-, moderate-, and high-dose arms, respectively. Results of the study were updated in 1998, and, after 9 years' median follow-up, continued to show benefit for the moderate- and high-dose arms compared to the low-dose group, without any substantial difference in outcome between the first two arms.[16] At 5 years, overall survival was 79% for patients on the high-dose arm, 77% for those on the moderate-dose arm, and 72% for patients on the low-dose arm. DFSs were 66%, 61%, and 56%, respectively.

A provocative finding from this trial was the observation that high expression of the HER-2/neu gene was associated with patient response to the high-dose arm.[17] An initial analysis of tumors derived from 397 patients enrolled in CALGB 8541 demonstrated that those assigned to the high-dose but not the low- or moderate-dose arms had significantly longer DFS and overall survival if their tumors were high expressors of the HER-2/neu protein.[17] However, a second analysis that included a further 595 patients was not as compelling.[18] Nonetheless, this study points to the need to identify predictive markers for dose-intensive therapy.

A similarly designed trial was reported by the French Adjuvant Study Group.[19] In it, 534 evaluable women with poor-prognosis node-positive breast cancer (one to three nodes with poor-grade and negative steroid receptors or more than three nodes) were randomized to receive six cycles of F, 500 mg per m^2; E, 50 mg per m^2; and C, 500 mg per m^2 on day 1 every 3 weeks (FEC 50) or the same regimen but with E, 100 mg per m^2 (FEC 100). Although toxicity was less in the FEC 50 group, clinical outcome was also inferior. After 5 years of follow-up, DFS was 59% and 70%, and survival was 70% and 80% for FEC 50 and FEC 100, respectively. Taken together, the results of these two trials are consistent with a dose-threshold hypothesis, arguing that an adequate dose of chemotherapy is necessary. However, neither trial provides compelling support for dose escalation of these agents beyond standard doses.

Further dose escalation of cyclophosphamide has been tested in two sequential trials of cyclophosphamide and doxorubicin as adjuvant treatment for women with node-positive breast cancer.[20,21] Both trials used a fixed dose of doxorubicin at 60 mg per m^2 given every 3 weeks for a total of four cycles and varied the cyclophosphamide dose. In the National Surgical Adjuvant Breast and Bowel Project (NSABP) B-22, the standard-dose arm administered 600 mg per m^2 cyclophosphamide in each cycle, whereas the high-dose arm provided 1,200 mg per m^2 in each of the four cycles.[20] An intermediate arm gave 1,200 mg per m^2 cyclophosphamide during the first two cycles only, thus providing the same total cyclophosphamide dose as in the standard-dose arm, but at higher dose intensity, because it was administered only during the first two cycles. No colony-stim-

TABLE 3. *Dose escalation trials in the adjuvant setting*

Trial (reference)	Dose (mg/m²) C	A	F	No. of cycles	Benefit in Disease-free survival	Survival
CALGB 8541 (15,16)	300	30	300	4	—	—
	400	40	400	6	Yes	Yes
	600	60	600	4	Yes	Yes
FASG (19)	500	50[a]	500	6	—	—
	500	100[a]	500	6	Yes	Yes
NSABP B-22 (20)	600	60	—	4	—	—
	1,200	60	—	2[b]	No	No
	1,200	60	—	4	No	No
NSABP B-25 (21)	1,200	60	—	4	—	—
	2,400	60	—	2[b]	No	No
	2,400	60	—	4	No	No
CALGB 9344 (22)	600	60	—	4	—	—
	600	75	—	4	No	No
	600	90	—	4	No	No

A, doxorubicin; C, cyclophosphamide; CALGB, Cancer and Acute Leukemia Group B; F, 5-fluorouracil; FASG, French Adjuvant Study Group; NSABP, National Surgical Adjuvant Breast and Bowel Project.
[a]Epirubicin used in place of doxorubicin.
[b]Cyclophosphamide given for two cycles and doxorubicin for four cycles.

ulating factors were used. More than 2,300 patients were randomized on this trial. Three-year results were identical to those obtained at 3 years with the high-dose arm of CALGB 8541, discussed earlier. Also, no significant differences were seen in DFS or overall survival through 5 years. Five-year DFS was 62%, 60%, and 64% for the standard-, intermediate-, and high-dose arms, respectively, and overall survival was 78%, 77%, and 77%. A careful analysis failed to show any differences in outcome among the groups when differences in actual amount or intensity of therapy or dose delays were considered. Not surprisingly, toxicities worsened with treatment intensity. The frequency of grade 4 toxicity of any type was 6.5% in the standard-dose group, 16.4% in the intermediate group, and 20.6% in the high-dose group. Of particular concern, acute myelogenous leukemia or myelodysplastic syndrome was reported in two patients in the standard group, in one patient in the intermediate arm, and in three patients in the high-dose cohort. Thus, in this trial, administration of cyclophosphamide at a twofold higher dose intensity had no benefit and was associated with excess toxicity.

Begun before the results of NSABP B-22 were reported, NSABP B-25 explored the value of even greater cyclophosphamide dose escalation.[21] This trial again randomized 2,548 node-positive patients to four cycles of variable doses of cyclophosphamide with fixed doxorubicin dose at 60 mg per m^2 per cycle. The three cyclophosphamide levels were 1,200 mg per m^2 per cycle for four cycles; 2,400 mg per m^2 per cycle for two cycles; and 2,400 mg per m^2 per cycle for four cycles. All patients received G-CSF prophylaxis at 5 μg per kg per day beginning on day 2. Preliminary results from this trial again failed to show any statistically significant benefit for the use of cyclophosphamide intensified fourfold over standard dose, although follow-up continues. At 5 years, the DFS of women in the three groups was 60%, 61%, and 66%, respectively, a nonsignificant difference. Survival was identical across the three groups at 77%, 76%, and 78%, respectively. Attempts to identify a patient subset that benefited from the higher doses were not successful. Of note, 14 patients enrolled on this trial have developed acute myelogenous leukemia, and a further 7 patients have been found to have myelodysplastic syndrome, resulting in a 0.8% incidence of these disorders, higher than that observed in the cumulative NSABP experience using cyclophosphamide at 600 mg per m^2. These cases appear to be clinically and cytogenetically similar to those previously associated with topoisomerase II inhibitors. Based on the combined results of NSABP B-22 and B-25, it would appear that dose escalation of cyclophosphamide beyond standard dose in this type of outpatient regimen is not a useful clinical strategy and is clearly associated with greater toxicity. The results from this series of trials are summarized in Table 3.

Doxorubicin is also an active agent in breast cancer, and studies of its use as a single agent in metastatic breast cancer provided evidence of a dose-response relationship. Therefore, a trial investigating the use of escalation of doxorubicin dose in the adjuvant setting has also been completed.[22] An intergroup trial, CALGB 9344, randomized 3,120 women with node-positive breast cancer in a 3-×-2 factorial trial design to a fixed dose of cyclophosphamide at 600 mg per m^2 plus doxorubicin at 60, 75, or 90 mg per m^2 given every 3 weeks, for a total of four cycles followed by paclitaxel, 175 mg per m^2, every 3 weeks for four cycles or not. Use of G-CSF prophylaxis was permitted for the intermediate dose of doxorubicin and required for the highest dose. Kaplan-Meier estimates of DFS and overall survival at 18 months were 86% and 90%, respectively, for the combined doxorubicin-cyclophosphamide arms and did not vary by doxorubicin dose. No evidence has been found of excess cardiac toxicity with higher doses of doxorubicin. Although it is possible that differences could emerge with time, as the follow-up on this trial is extremely short, the initial results would argue that a 50% increase in doxorubicin dose is not beneficial in the adjuvant treatment of node-positive breast cancer.

Another means of intensifying dose has been proposed by Hudis et al.[23] Termed *dose density*, this approach seeks to administer single agents in an intensive fashion, but in sequence rather than in combination. Support for this type of strategy was derived indirectly from a trial of the Milan Cancer Institute that showed superior outcomes in women with more than three positive axillary nodes who were treated with four cycles of doxorubicin followed by eight cycles of CMF, as opposed to alternating doxorubicin and CMF.[24] The concept of dose density is currently undergoing prospective evaluation through two U.S. intergroup studies. One trial, S9313, has already enrolled more than 3,000 women with high-risk node-negative or one to three node-positive breast cancer to six cycles of doxorubicin and cyclophosphamide in combination versus a sequence of doxorubicin followed by cyclophosphamide. The two arms of the trial were designed so the cumulative dose of each drug and the duration of all therapies are identical in both arms. Thus, the question of sequence and dose density can be specifically addressed. A second trial, CALGB 9741, will further dissect the value of this approach through a four-arm trial of AC followed by paclitaxel versus doxorubicin followed by paclitaxel followed by cyclophosphamide administered to node-positive women at 2- or 3-week intervals.

Finally, a third intergroup trial is testing the relative value of a dose-dense approach (A→T→C) similiar to that just described, with a strategy that includes high-dose chemotherapy with autologous stem cell support. This trial, which targets women with involvement of four to nine axillary nodes, will provide a link between trials testing these various methods of increasing dose.

DOSE ESCALATION IN THE TRANSPLANT SETTING

High-dose chemotherapy with stem cell transplantation represents the ultimate expression of dose intensification with single courses of treatment. Initial studies of this modality investigated single and combination therapy with alkylating agents in patients with resistant metastatic breast cancer.[25] These studies were characterized by substantial toxicity but also by responses, including occasional complete responses, in some heavily pretreated patients. This activity prompted evaluation of high-dose therapy with stem cell support in patients with earlier stages of disease. As a consequence of the high incidence of breast cancer and great enthusiasm for this approach, breast cancer has become the most common indication for autologous transplantation. Statistics maintained by the Autologous Blood and Marrow Transplantation Registry of North America (ABMTR) suggest that approximately 40% of autologous transplants done in the United States in 1995 were performed in patients with breast cancer.[26]

Transplantation in Advanced Breast Cancer

Phase II studies evaluating outcomes for transplantation in patients with chemotherapy-sensitive metastatic breast cancer provoked considerable initial interest in this modality. A series of trials with small numbers of patients indicated that a small proportion, between 10% and 20%, remained free of progression after time periods that ranged from 2 to 5 years after transplant.[27–30] Whether these data suggest superior outcome, thereby supporting the use of high-dose chemotherapy in the treatment of patients with metastatic breast cancer, is a topic of intense debate. This is because new data indicate that some patients with metastatic disease who undergo standard-dose, doxorubicin-based combination chemotherapy also achieve long-term remissions. Greenberg et al.,[31] from the M. D. Anderson Cancer Center in Houston, reported the results of an analysis of 1,581 women with stage IV breast cancer who received FAC-based chemotherapy. In this review, 16.6% of patients with metastatic breast cancer achieved a complete response to such treatment. Of this group, 18% remained disease free for more than 5 years after treatment.

In addition, it has been shown by several authors that patient selection can have a significant impact on outcome for women with metastatic breast cancer independent of therapy. Rahman et al.[32] reviewed outcomes for 1,581 women with metastatic breast cancer who were treated with standard-dose, doxorubicin-based combination chemotherapy at the M. D. Anderson Cancer Center and categorized patients according to whether they would have been eligible for high-dose therapy trials based on age, performance status, laboratory values, and response to chemotherapy. Of these women, 645 were candidates for high-dose chemotherapy by these criteria, whereas 936 were not. The complete response rate was 27% for high-dose candidates and 7% for noncandidates. Median progression-free survival was 16 and 8 months, and median survival was 30 and 17 months, respectively. Five-year survival was 21% and 6% for high-dose candidates and noncandidates, respectively. These results speak to the potent impact of patient demographics on outcome, independent of therapy administered. Thus, it is not possible to use results of phase II trials of high-dose chemotherapy to discern whether the proportion of patients who achieve prolonged remissions with this modality has increased. Resolution of this question awaits the results of randomized phase III clinical trials. A summary of randomized trials whose results have been released is shown in Table 4.

The first randomized clinical trial evaluating the potential role of high-dose therapy in the treatment of patients with metastatic breast cancer was reported in 1995 by Bezwoda

TABLE 4. *Randomized trials of autologous transplant for stage IV breast cancer*

Design	Patient no.	Significant benefit with ABMT for		Reference
		Disease-free survival	Survival	
Immediate ABMT vs standard chemotherapy in new stage IV	90	Yes	Yes	33, 34
ABMT vs continuing chemotherapy in chemotherapy responders	61	Yes	No	37
ABMT vs continuing chemotherapy in chemotherapy responders	180	No	No	38
Immediate ABMT vs ABMT at progression for complete responders after chemotherapy	98	Yes	No—worse	39, 40

ABMT, autologous bone marrow transplant.

et al. from the University of Witwatersrand in South Africa.[33] The trial included 90 women with metastatic breast cancer who had not received chemotherapy for metastatic disease. They were randomly assigned to high-dose chemotherapy with cyclophosphamide, mitoxantrone, and etoposide for two courses with stem cell transplantation or to lower doses of similar chemotherapy (cyclophosphamide, mitoxantrone, and vincristine) administered without stem cell support for six to eight courses.

This small study produced striking results. Complete responses were observed in 51% of patients treated with high-dose therapy, and the overall response rate was 95%. In contrast, in the standard-dose arm, the overall response rate was 53%, and complete responses were seen in 4% of patients. In this trial, median response duration was 36 weeks for standard-dose therapy and 80 weeks for high-dose therapy. Median survival was doubled from 52 weeks for standard-dose therapy to 108 weeks for high-dose therapy. All these differences were highly significant. Interestingly, in 1998, Bezwoda[34] reported updated information from this study indicating that all nine women who remained in remission in the high-dose arm at the time of the 1995 report were still in remission after 5 years of follow-up. No patient in the standard-dose arm remained in remission. Despite these encouraging results, the findings from this randomized trial must be viewed with caution for several reasons.

It has been suggested that the response rate in the standard-dose arm in this trial is unusually low, thereby causing the high-dose arm to appear more active than it would if it were compared with a more active "standard" regimen. However, this regimen had been evaluated in the past in a phase II study by the same group of investigators, and substantial numbers of complete and overall responses were observed, suggesting that it is an active regimen.[35] In addition, several reports have suggested that response rates for standard-dose regimens may currently be less than previously supposed. For example, the Eastern Cooperative Oncology Group has shown that the combination of doxorubicin and paclitaxel produces a 46% response rate in a large cohort of women who had not received previous chemotherapy for metastatic disease.[36] This generalized reduction in response rates seen in large stage IV trials may reflect the increasing numbers of patients in such studies who have previously been exposed to adjuvant chemotherapy. Taken together, these data suggest that the response rates in the standard-dose arm in this trial may not be unrealistically low. In addition, the high complete response rate observed in the high-dose arm is entirely consistent with results reported from numerous phase II studies of high-dose chemotherapy.

A potential confounding factor in this study, however, relates to the use of hormonal therapy. By trial design, only patients who responded to chemotherapy in either arm of the trial were subsequently treated with tamoxifen. As there were greater numbers of responders in the high-dose arm, more patients in this group received tamoxifen. This represents a confounding variable in the study that might have had an impact on the DFS as it was subsequently evaluated.

Another factor is that the median survival reported for standard-dose chemotherapy—1 year—is unusually short in this trial. In the Eastern Cooperative Oncology Group trial of taxane and anthracycline mentioned in the previous paragraph, median survival was approximately 2 years in all arms, identical to that seen with the high-dose therapy in the Bezwoda trial.[33] For these reasons, this trial should be viewed as promising but not definitive.

Initial results from another small randomized trial have also been reported.[37] The PEGASE 4 trial from France randomized 61 patients with stage IV breast cancer who responded to four to six cycles of conventional chemotherapy to continuation of the same therapy (29 patients) or treatment with a high-dose regimen of mitoxantrone, cyclophosphamide, and melphalan with stem cell support (32 patients). Median progression-free survivals were 15.7 and 26.9 months in the standard- and high-dose groups (p = .04), and median overall survivals were 15.7 and 36.1 months, respectively (p = .08). Thus, this small trial also provides promising results.

Initial results from a third large, randomized clinical trial designed to determine whether high-dose chemotherapy results in superior DFS or overall survival for women with metastatic breast cancer have also been presented.[38] This trial enrolled women with newly diagnosed stage IV breast cancer who received induction chemotherapy with CAF or CMF. Those who achieved a complete or partial response (PR) were then randomly assigned to continuation of CMF for up to 2 years or high-dose chemotherapy with cyclophosphamide, carboplatin, and thiotepa (STAMP V) and autologous bone marrow or stem cell support, or both. Preliminary results from this trial show that 553 women received induction therapy with four to six cycles of CAF (507 patients) or CMF (46 patients), and 303 achieved a response [PR in 247 and complete remission (CR) in 56]. Of these responders, 199 were randomized and 180 were eligible for response analysis at the time of this first analysis, 101 in the high-dose arm and 79 in the maintenance CMF arm. Fifteen patients did not adhere to their randomization assignment; four declined high-dose chemotherapy, and 11 refused to take maintenance CMF.

No significant differences were seen between the two treatment groups with regard to age, dominant site of disease, response to induction therapy, or estrogen receptor status. An intention to treat analysis was performed and showed no difference in overall survival between the two groups. Two-year overall survival was 46% for patients on the high-dose arm and 52% for patients assigned to the CMF arm. There was also no difference in survival between the two treatment groups for women who achieved a CR with induction therapy; 2-year survival was 58% in both groups. Similarly, there was no survival benefit for high-dose chemotherapy for women who achieved a PR to induction chemotherapy. Two-year overall survival was 39% for partial responders assigned to high-dose chemotherapy and 51% for those assigned to continuing CMF. Therapy-related mortality was rare on this trial. Five patients died during induction chemotherapy, one patient died from venoocclusive disease of the liver during high chemotherapy, and no patient succumbed to a chemotherapy-related toxicity during maintenance CMF. Progression-free survival was identical in these two arms. The number of individuals who were converted from partial to complete responders was also identical in the two arms. Crucial information about quality of life and economic costs is not yet available. However, initial results do not demonstrate a major difference in 2-year progression-free or overall survival or treatment-related mortality between these two approaches. This trial has been criticized because of the small fraction of enrolled patients who were actually randomized. Nonetheless, it represents the largest randomized trial of a transplant approach versus a conventional approach in metastatic breast cancer.

Preliminary results of a fourth randomized trial of unusual design have also been made public. Peters et al.,[39] from Duke University in Durham, North Carolina, presented data from a randomized comparison in patients who achieved an initial complete response to standard-dose chemotherapy of (a) high-dose chemotherapy at the time of initial complete response or (b) high-dose chemotherapy administered at the time of second relapse. In this trial, ninety-eight patients with metastatic breast cancer achieved a complete response with initial induction chemotherapy with doxorubicin, 5-fluorouracil, and methotrexate (AFM) and were randomly assigned to observation, with subsequent transplant at the time of relapse or to immediate transplant after achieving first CR. The STAMP I alkylator regimen of cyclophosphamide, BCNU, and cis-platinum was used in both arms of the trial. Median follow-up for patients on this study is approximately 5 years. Median DFS for patients who underwent high-dose therapy at first remission was 14 months. Not surprisingly, it was only 4 months for patients who were observed after the first CR. Thus, high-dose therapy apparently results in improved DFS compared with observation. However, it is not clear that transplant is superior to other potential forms of "consolidation" therapy, such as radiation, hormonal therapy, or continuation of standard-dose outpatient chemotherapy. Therefore, it is not necessarily true that high-dose therapy produces superior DFS when compared to continuation of a "standard" treatment, but rather that it results in superior DFS when compared to observation.

Paradoxically, overall survival in this trial was better for women who underwent high-dose therapy at second relapse—that is, after a period of observation in first CR. Median survival was 2.3 years for patients who underwent high-dose therapy at the time of first CR and 3.2 years for the patients who received transplant after observation at the time of second recurrence. This is a provocative finding, but one of uncertain significance, and, as the trial is a small one, this result may be a statistical artifact. However, a variety of explanations can be invoked for the observed results. One possibility is that the improved survival associated with a delay in high-dose therapy until the time of second relapse might be caused by a lead-time bias associated with high tumor cell kill that can be achieved with high-dose chemotherapy no matter when it is administered. Alternatively, the superior survival associated with the delayed transplant might be due to resolution of immunosuppression because of prior outpatient chemotherapy or to improved kinetic parameters within the tumor after chemotherapy has been discontinued. Whatever the reason for this result, the issue of optimal timing of high-dose therapy is being evaluated in ongoing randomized phase III trials.

The Peters trial of immediate versus delayed transplant was part of a larger trial that included at the outset 425 patients with new stage IV breast cancer. A report of this trial showed that 113 patients enrolled achieved a CR, whereas 202 had a PR with AFM, giving an overall response rate of 74%.[40] Of these women, 299 proceeded to high-dose therapy, either via randomization if they had achieved a CR or direct assignment if they had a PR. Median follow-up is 5.6 years. The 5-year DFS is 16%, and the 5-year overall survival is 20% for all women who received high-dose chemotherapy. Results are somewhat better for those who achieved a CR with AFM with 5-year DFS and survival of 20% and 38%, respectively.

Finally, a survey of results of autotransplants for stage IV breast cancer has been made available through the ABMTR.[26]

TABLE 5. *Three-year Kaplan-Meier estimates of progression-free and overall survival after autologous transplantation for breast cancer*

Disease stage	PFS (%)	Survival (%)
II	65	74
III	60	70
III B (inflammatory)	42	52
IV	18	30
CR after chemotherapy	32	46
PR after chemotherapy	13	29
NR after chemotherapy	7	16

CR, complete response; NR, no response; PFS, progression-free survival; PR, partial response.
Adapted from ref. 26.

This review includes results from 3,451 patients who underwent autologous transplantation for stage IV breast cancer between 1989 and 1995. The 100-day mortality was 10%. The major findings are summarized in Table 5. The critical finding is that the likelihood of progression-free and overall survival at 3 years is directly correlated with the extent of disease and response to induction chemotherapy. Thus, individuals who achieved a complete response to induction chemotherapy had 3-year progression-free and overall survivals of 32% and 46%, respectively, whereas those who did not respond to initial chemotherapy demonstrated 3-year progression-free and overall survivals of 7% and 16%. These composite data are supportive of current practice, in which high-dose chemotherapy options are generally limited to those who manifest a response to induction chemotherapy.

This database was also used to carry out a nonrandomized comparison of survival after conventional versus high-dose therapy for stage IV breast cancer.[41] In this analysis, 657 women who had received standard chemotherapy with a doxorubicin-containing regimen in four different CALGB trials and would have met conventional criteria for autologous transplant were compared to 560 women who had received high-dose therapy identified from the ABMTR. A univariant analysis showed a significant 14% reduction in risk of death with high-dose therapy. However, a multivariant analysis that took into account standard breast cancer prognostic factors, such as disease-free interval and performance status, showed no significant difference between the two modes of therapy.

Transplantation for Early-Stage Breast Cancer

In the high-risk adjuvant setting, preliminary results from a number of phase II single-arm studies of high-dose therapy suggested that DFS might be improved by transplantation. Peters et al.[42] treated 85 women with tumor that involved more than nine axillary lymph nodes with high-dose cyclophosphamide, cis-platinum, and BCNU (STAMP I) after four courses of standard-dose FAC chemotherapy. Data from this study indicate that the 5-year DFS for patients so treated is 71%. By comparison, data from historical age- and stage-matched control populations derived from cooperative group trials suggest a DFS of approximately 30% with the standard chemotherapy. Overall survival is reported as 78% versus an overall survival of less than 50% for the nonrandomized historical controls treated with standard-dose chemotherapy. Similar results were obtained by Gianni et al.[43] from the National Cancer Institute of Milan, who administered a high-dose regimen to 67 patients with ten or more positive lymph nodes. These women were treated with a regimen of high-dose cyclophosphamide initially followed by vincristine, methotrexate, and cis-platinum and subsequent high-dose consolidation with melphalan with stem cell support. Four-year disease-free survival was 57%, compared with a 41% 4-year DFS in women in a historical standard-dose chemotherapy population. Also, Basser et al.[44] observed parallel results in 99 women with breast cancer that involved ten or more axillary nodes who received three cycles of high-dose epirubicin and cyclophosphamide with peripheral blood stem cell support after each cycle. The actuarial distant DFS and overall survival rates at 5 years of follow-up were 64% and 67%, respectively.

Results from these small trials could suggest that high-dose adjuvant therapy might improve outcomes for women at high risk of recurrence because of extensive lymph node involvement. Such an interpretation, however, has provoked intense controversy. It has been pointed out that the outcome difference that apparently exists between patients who receive high-dose chemotherapy and those who receive standard-dose chemotherapy might simply be the result of patient selection. That possibility might be enhanced by the more rigorous eligibility criteria and screening procedures that have been implemented in the transplant studies. Crump et al.[45] report the results of intensive screening for women with high-risk breast cancer who underwent protocol-mandated evaluation for possible participation in a randomized cooperative group trial of transplant. Thirty potentially eligible women underwent staging with bilateral bone marrow biopsies and computed tomography of the head, chest, abdomen, and pelvis. Seven (23%) of these women had occult metastatic disease identified solely by these screening procedures. The exclusion of such patients from single-arm studies of high-dose therapy may well have contributed to the apparently favorable results of such trials, in contrast to standard-dose studies that did not require similar extensive staging. Thus, it is possible that the seemingly improved results are due to stage migration as much as to the therapeutic benefits of high-dose chemotherapy. Until large randomized trials evaluating this therapy in this patient population have been completed, it is impossible to say whether this apparent benefit in outcome is due to patient selection, treatment effects, or both. Results from randomized trials of high-dose chemotherapy for women with high-risk breast cancer are summarized in Table 6.

Three small randomized trials of high-dose therapy have been reported. Rodenhuis et al.[46] treated 97 patients who were believed to have extensive axillary node metastases because of a positive infraclavicular lymph node biopsy at the time of diagnosis of breast cancer with three courses of

TABLE 6. *Randomized trials of autologous transplant for high-risk stage II to III breast cancer*

Design	No. of patients	Median follow-up	Significant benefit with ABMT for DFS	Significant benefit with ABMT for Survival	Reference
FEC vs FEC + ABMT	97	4 yr	No	No	46
FAC vs FAC + ABMT	78	4 yr	No	No	47
Immediate ABMT vs CAF	150	5 yr	Yes	Yes	48
FEC × 9 vs FEC × 3 + ABMT	525	2 yr	No	No	49
CAF + intermediate or high-dose chemotherapy	874	3 yr	No	No	50

ABMT, autologous bone marrow transplant; CAF, cyclophosphamide + doxorubicin + 5-fluorouracil; DFS, disease-free survival; FAC, 5-fluorouracil + doxorubicin + cyclophosphamide; FEC, 5-fluorouracil + epirubicin + cyclophosphamide.

preoperative FEC. Responding patients were subsequently randomized and underwent definitive surgical therapy, a fourth course of FEC chemotherapy, radiation, and tamoxifen. In addition, one-half of the patients received high-dose chemotherapy with cyclophosphamide, thiotepa, and carboplatin with stem cell support after the final course of FEC. Eighty-one patients were randomized. Of the remainder, 11 refused to continue because of unwillingness to receive high chemotherapy, and five were believed to have chemotherapy-unresponsive disease. After randomization, five more patients assigned to high-dose chemotherapy refused to take that therapy, and one patient could not undergo high-dose therapy because of inadequate stem cell collection. Thus, only 35 of the 41 patients assigned to high-dose chemotherapy actually received the intended treatment. With a median follow-up of approximately 4 years, the 4-year overall and relapse-free survivals for all 97 patients entered on trial were 75% and 54%, respectively. No difference has been observed in progression-free or overall survival between the two arms. This trial was carried out as a pilot trial to assess feasibility in preparation for an ongoing multicenter Dutch trial of transplant for women with four or more axillary lymph node breast cancer. Thus, its statistical power is limited; indeed, this study was not large enough to exclude a reduction of odds of relapse of up to 40%.

Hortobagyi et al.[47] report 4-year results of a randomized trial in which 78 patients with more than nine axillary nodes at initial surgery or more than three nodes after primary chemotherapy underwent chemotherapy with FAC before randomization to a control arm of radiation and tamoxifen or an intensive treatment arm of two courses of high-dose therapy with cisplatin, etoposide, and cyclophosphamide with stem cell support before radiation therapy and tamoxifen. This trial, like the Rodenhuis trial, has thus far shown no evidence of an improved outcome for patients treated on the high-dose arm. Both of these trials are very small, however. Even when evaluated together, they cannot exclude a 30% improvement (or worsening) in survival associated with the use of high-dose therapy.

In contrast, a third small study with a different design gave very positive results. Bezwoda[48] enrolled 154 women on a trial of two cycles of immediate high-dose chemotherapy with cyclophosphamide, mitoxantrone, and etoposide with stem cell support versus six cycles of CAF. Participants were at high risk for recurrence because of involvement of ten or more axillary lymph nodes or a combination of tumor size of at least 5 cm and involvement of seven to nine nodes. With a median follow-up of 278 weeks, the median relapse-free and overall survivals were more than 400 weeks for the high-dose group and 190 and 320 weeks, respectively, for the CAF group. This difference was statistically significant, favoring the approach of two cycles of high-dose therapy.

These data emphasize the need for results from the several large randomized trials that have or are currently finishing accrual before one can state definitively whether high-dose chemotherapy is appropriate treatment for patients at high risk of recurrence because of extensive lymph node burden. Two such trials have been reported; results from several other trials are eagerly awaited.

The Scandinavian Breast Cancer Study Group 9401 trial was a population-based study of nine cycles of FEC at doses tailored to individual hematologic tolerance versus three cycles of FEC followed by STAMP V with autologous hematopoietic support.[49] Participants were selected because their 5-year risk of relapse was at least 70% based on Scandinavian databases, and more than one-half of the eligible patients participated, making this the most representative of the high-dose trials to date. With a median follow-up of less than 2 years, no difference was found in relapse-free or overall survival. A higher incidence of acute myelogenous leukemia and myelodysplastic syndrome was seen in the women who received tailored FEC.

The largest of the adjuvant transplant trials reported to date, CALGB 9082, included women with high-risk primary breast cancer that involved at least ten axillary lymph nodes.[50] All received four cycles of CAF and were then randomized to either high-dose STAMP I or intermediate-dose STAMP I, a dose that required G-CSF but not stem cell support. With a median follow-up of 37 months, event-free survivals were 68% and 64% for 783 randomized women who were given high-dose and intermediate-dose chemotherapy, respectively. Survival was identical at 78% and 80%. Although fewer relapses were noted in the high-dose arm, 29 treatment-related deaths occurred in the high-dose arm and none in the intermediate-dose arm. A key feature of this multiinstitutional trial is that treatment-related mortality was twice as high in centers that performed fewer than 50 transplants: 6% for higher-volume centers versus 11% for lower-volume centers.

The ABMTR also includes composite results for 1,747 women who have undergone autotransplantation for stage II or III breast cancer.[26] The results are shown in Table 5. Of note, the 100-day mortality for women with these early stages of breast cancer was 3%. It is otherwise difficult to interpret the clinical outcomes for these results from non-randomized trials.

Allogeneic Bone Marrow Transplantation for Breast Cancer

Initial enthusiasm concerning the potential value of high-dose therapy with autologous stem cell support in the treatment of advanced and high-risk breast cancer has been tempered with skepticism as more mature data have emerged. Thus, some investigators have begun to evaluate the possible role of allogeneic transplantation in women with advanced metastatic disease. This approach has the theoretical advantages of using a stem cell source uncontaminated with tumor cells and engineering a graft-versus-tumor effect against residual tumor cells. Eibl et al.[51] treated a woman with metastatic breast cancer with high-dose chemotherapy and allogeneic transplantation and observed the resolution of hepatic metastases during the evolution of graft-versus-host disease (GVHD). Although this patient subsequently died from progressive hepatic metastases, this case report has been extended through a series from Ueno et al.,[52] in which ten women with poor-risk metastatic disease underwent similar therapy. Six patients responded, one with a complete response, and two showed evidence of disease regression during the time of development of GVHD. Although of great interest, these reports suggest only that further study of this approach is warranted. Proof of the existence of an antitumor effect associated with the development of GVHD that can be directed against human breast cancer requires much intensive clinical investigation, either through trials of allogeneic transplantation or trials designed to induce a transient GVHD-like state by pharmacologic means.[53]

MANAGEMENT SUMMARY

The hypothesis that dose of chemotherapy might influence outcome with breast cancer has been an area of active investigation for more than 15 years. It was initially predicated on preclinical data suggesting a clear dose-response relationship for a number of cytotoxic agents, as well as clinical experience that supported the dose hypothesis in treatment of other types of malignancy. However, the evidence derived from prospectively designed clinical trials testing this hypothesis in breast cancer is most consistent with a dose-threshold effect. Aggregate results from these trials suggest that underdosing is associated with poorer clinical outcome, but trials using colony-stimulating factors to enhance chemotherapy dose beyond the "standard" range have not yet shown an advantage for dose escalation. Furthermore, this type of dose escalation may be associated with serious toxicities, such as infections and second malignancies. Thus, based on current evidence, dose escalation in the subtransplant range should not be used in routine practice.

Likewise, although provocative pilot data exist, approaches using high-dose chemotherapy with autologous or allogeneic hematopoietic support for breast cancer should be viewed as appropriate only in the setting of a clinical trial. Randomized trials of autologous transplantation have given ambiguous results in both adjuvant and metastatic settings. We hope that longer follow-up of these trials, as well as emergence of results from other ongoing or completed trials, will provide more definitive information. In the interim, physician and patient enthusiasm for this technology should be tempered by the absence of clear information from clinical trials to establish any superiority for this approach.

REFERENCES

1. Bonadonna G, Valagussa P. Dose-response effect of adjuvant chemotherapy in breast cancer. *N Engl J Med* 1981;304:10–15.
2. Hryniuk W, Bush H. The importance of dose-intensity in chemotherapy of metastatic breast cancer. *J Clin Oncol* 1984;2:1281–1288.
3. Hryniuk W, Levine MN. Analysis of dose-intensity for adjuvant chemotherapy trials in stage II breast cancer. *J Clin Oncol* 1986; 4:1162–1170.
4. Biganzoli L, Piccart MJ. The bigger the better? . . . Or what we know and what we still need to learn about anthracycline dose, dose per course, dose density and cumulative dose in the treatment of breast cancer. *Ann Oncol* 1997;8:1177–1182.
5. Tannock IF, Boyd NF, DeBoer G, et al. A randomized trial of two dose levels of cyclophosphamide, methotrexate, and fluorouracil chemotherapy for patients with metastatic breast cancer. *J Clin Oncol* 1988;6: 1377–1387.
6. Carmo-Pereira J, Oliveira Costa F, Henriques E, et al. A comparison of two doses of adriamycin in the primary chemotherapy of disseminated breast carcinoma. *Br J Cancer* 1987;56:471–473.
7. Habeshaw T, Paul R, Jones R, et al. Epirubicin at two dose levels with prednisolone as treatment for advanced breast cancer: the results of a randomized trial. *J Clin Oncol* 1991;9:295–304.
8. Bastholt L, Dalmark M, Gjedde SB, et al. Dose-response relationship of epirubicin in the treatment of postmenopausal patients with metastatic breast cancer: a randomized study of epirubicin at four different dose levels performed by the Danish Breast Cancer Cooperative Group. *J Clin Oncol* 1996;14:1146–1155.
9. Brufman G, Corajort E, Ghilezan N, et al. Doubling epirubicin dose intensity (100 mg/m^2 versus 50 mg/m^2) in the FEC regimen significantly increases response rate: an international randomized phase III study in metastatic breast cancer. *Ann Oncol* 1997;8:155–162.
10. Focan C, Andrien JM, Closon M, et al. Dose-response relationship of epirubicin-based first-line chemotherapy for advanced breast cancer: a prospective randomized trial. *J Clin Oncol* 1993;11:1253–1263.
11. Marschner N, Kreienberg R, Souchon R, et al. Evaluation of the importance and relevance of dose intensity using epirubicin and cyclophosphamide in metastatic breast cancer: interim analysis of a prospective randomized trial. *Semin Oncol* 1994;21[Suppl 1]:10–16.
12. Fountzilas G, Athanassiades A, Giannakkais T, et al. A randomized

study of epirubicin monotherapy every four or every two weeks in advanced breast cancer: a Hellenic Cooperative Oncology Group study. *Ann Oncol* 1997;8:1213–1220.

13. Winer E, Berry D, Duggan D, et al. Failure of higher dose paclitaxel to improve outcome in patients with metastatic breast cancer—results from CALGB 9342. *Proc Am Soc Clin Oncol* 1998;17:101a.
14. Therasse P, Mauriac L, Welnicka M, et al. Neo-adjuvant dose intensity chemotherapy in locally advanced breast cancer (LABC): an EORTC-NCIC-SAKK randomized phase III study comparing FEC (5FU, epirubicin, cyclophosphamide) vs high dose intensity EC + G-CSF (Filgrastim). *Proc Am Soc Clin Oncol* 1998;17:124a.
15. Wood WC, Budman DR, Korzun AH, et al. Dose and dose intensity of adjuvant chemotherapy for stage II, node-positive breast carcinoma. *N Engl J Med* 1994;330:1253–1259.
16. Budman DR, Berry DA, Cirrincone CT, et al. Dose and dose intensity as determinants of outcome in the adjuvant treatment of breast cancer. *J Natl Cancer Inst* 1998;90:1205–1211.
17. Muss HB, Thor AD, Berry DA, et al. C-erbB-2 expression and response to adjuvant therapy in women with node-positive early breast cancer. *N Engl J Med* 1994;330:1260–1266.
18. Thor AD, Berry DA, Budman DR, et al. C-erb-2, p53, and efficacy of adjvuant therapy in lymph node-positive breast cancer. *J Natl Cancer Inst* 1998;90:1346–1360.
19. Bonneterre J, Roché H, Bremond A, et al. Results of a randomized trial of adjuvant chemo-therapy with FEC50 vs FEC100 in high node-positive breast cancer patients. *Proc Am Soc Clin Oncol* 1998; 17:124a.
20. Fisher B, Anderson S, Wickerham DL, et al. Increased intensification and total dose of cyclophosphamide in a doxorubicin-cyclophosphamide regimen for the treatment of primary breast cancer: findings from the National Surgical Adjuvant Breast and Bowel Project B-22. *J Clin Oncol* 1997;15:1858–1869.
21. Fisher B, Anderson S, DeCillis A, et al. Further evaluation of intensified and increased total dose of cyclophosphamide for the treatment of primary breast cancer: findings from National Surgical Adjuvant Breast and Bowel Project B-25. *J Clin Oncol (in press)*.
22. Henderson IC, Berry D, Demetri G, et al. Improved disease-free (DFS) and overall survival (OS) from the addition of sequential paclitaxel (T) but not from escalation of doxorubicin (A) dose level in the adjuvant chemotherapy of patients (pts) with node-positive breast cancer (BC). *Proc Am Soc Clin Oncol* 1998;17:101a.
23. Hudis C, Seidman A, Baselga JG, et al. Sequential dose-dense doxorubicin, paclitaxel, and cyclophosphamide for resectable high-risk breast cancer: feasibility and efficacy. *J Clin Oncol* 1999;17: 93–100.
24. Bonadonna G, Zambetti M, Valagussa P. Sequential or alternating doxorubicin and CMF regimens in breast cancer with more than three positive nodes: ten-year results. *JAMA* 1995;273:542–547.
25. Eder JP, Antman K, Peters W, et al. High-dose combination alkylating agent chemotherapy with autologous bone marrow support for metastatic breast cancer. *J Clin Oncol* 1986;4:1592–1597.
26. Antman KH, Rowlings PA, Vaughan WP, et al. High-dose chemotherapy with autologous hematopoietic stem-cell support for breast cancer in North America. *J Clin Oncol* 1997;15: 1870–1879.
27. Williams SF, Mick R, Desser R, et al: High-dose consolidation therapy with autologous stem cell rescue in stage IV breast cancer. *J Clin Oncol* 1989;7:1824–1830.
28. Kennedy MJ, Beveridge RA, Rowley SD, et al. High dose chemotherapy with reinfusion of purged autologous bone marrow following dose-intense induction as initial therapy for metastatic breast cancer. *J Natl Cancer Inst* 1991;83:920–926.
29. Antman K, Ayash L, Elias A, et al. A phase II study of high-dose cyclophosphamide, thiotepa and carboplatin with autologous marrow support in women with measurable advanced breast cancer responding to standard-dose chemotherapy. *J Clin Oncol* 1992;10: 102–110.
30. Peters WP, Shpall EJ, Jones RB, et al. High-dose combination alkylating agents with bone marrow support as initial treatment for metastatic breast cancer. *J Clin Oncol* 1988;6:1368–1376.
31. Greenberg PAC, Hortobagyi GN, Smith T, et al. Long-term follow-up of patients with complete remission following combination chemotherapy for metastatic breast cancer. *J Clin Oncol* 1997;14: 2197–2205.
32. Rahman ZU, Frye DK, Buzdar AU, et al. Impact of selection process on response rate and long-term survival of potential high-dose chemotherapy candidates treated with standard dose doxorubicin containing chemotherapy in patients with metastatic breast cancer. *J Clin Oncol* 1997;15:3171–3177.
33. Bezwoda WR, Seymour L, Dansey RD. High-dose chemotherapy with hematopoietic rescue as primary treatment for metastatic breast cancer: a randomized trial. *J Clin Oncol* 1995;13:2483–2489.
34. Bezwoda WR. Primary high-dose chemotherapy for metastatic breast cancer: update and analysis of prognostic factors. *Proc Am Soc Clin Oncol* 1998;17:445a.
35. Bezwoda WR, Dansey R, Seymour L. First line chemotherapy of advanced breast cancer with mitoxantrone, cyclophosphamide and vincristine. *Oncology* 1989;46:208–211.
36. Sledge GW, Neuberg D, Ingle J, et al. Phase III trial of doxorubicin (A) vs paclitaxel (T) vs doxorubicin + paclitaxel (A+T) as first-line therapy for metastatic breast cancer (MBC): an intergroup trial. *Proc Am Soc Clin Oncol* 1997;16:1a.
37. Lotz J-P, Curé H, Janvier M, et al. High-dose chemotherapy (HD-CT) with hematopoietic stem cells transplantation (HSCT) for metastatic breast cancer (MBC): results of the French protocol PEGASE 04. *Proc Am Soc Clin Oncol* 1999;18:43a.
38. Stadtmauer EA, O'Neill A, Goldstein LJ, et al. Phase III randomized trial of high-dose chemotherapy (HDC) and stem cell support (SCT) shows no difference in overall survival or severe toxicity compared to maintenance chemotherapy with cyclophosphamide, methotrexate, and 5-fluorouracil (CMF) for women with metastatic breast cancer who are responding to conventional induction chemotherapy: the Philadelphia intergroup study (PBT-1). *Proc Am Soc Clin Oncol* 1999;18:1a.
39. Peters WP, Jones RB, Vredenburgh J, et al. A large prospective randomized trial of high-dose combination alkylating agents (CPB) with autologous cellular support (ABMS) as consolidation for patients with metastatic breast cancer achieving complete remission after intensive doxorubicin-based induction therapy (AFM). *Proc Am Soc Clin Oncol* 1996;15:149.
40. Rizzieri DA, Vredenburgh JJ, Chao NJ, Broadwater G, Berry D, Peters WP. Long term disease free survival for patients undergoing aggressive induction therapy followed by high dose therapy with hematopoietic support. *Blood* 1998; 92[Suppl 1]:323a.
41. Berry DA, Broadwater G, Perry MC, et al. Conventional vs high-dose therapy for metastatic breast cancer: comparison of Cancer and Leukemia Group B (CALGB) and Blood and Marrow Transplant Registry (ABMTR) patients. *Proc Am Soc Clin Oncol* 1999; 18:128a.
42. Peters WP, Ross M, Vredenburgh J, et al. High-dose chemotherapy and autologous bone marrow support after standard-dose adjuvant therapy for high-risk primary breast cancer. *J Clin Oncol* 1993;11: 1132–1143.
43. Gianni AM, Siena S, Bregni M, et al. Efficacy, toxicity and applicability of high-dose sequential chemotherapy as adjuvant treatment in operable breast cancer with 10 or more involved axillary nodes: five-year results. *J Clin Oncol* 1997;15:2312–2321.
44. Basser RL, To LB, Collins JP, et al. Multicycle high-dose chemotherapy and filgrastim-mobilized peripheral-blood progenitor cells in women with high-risk stage II or III breast cancer: five-year follow-up. *J Clin Oncol* 1999;17:82–92.
45. Crump M, Goss PE, Prince M, et al. Outcome of extensive evaluation before adjuvant therapy in women with breast cancer and 10 or more positive axillary nodes. *J Clin Oncol* 1996;14:66–69.
46. Rodenhuis S, Richel DJ, van der Waal E, et al. Randomised trial of high-dose chemotherapy and haematopoietic progenitor-cell support in operable breast cancer with extensive axillary lymph-node involvement. *Lancet* 1998;352:515–521.
47. Hortobagyi GN, Buzdar AU, Champlin R, et al. Lack of efficacy of adjuvant high-dose (hd) tandem combination chemotherapy (ct) for high risk primary breast cancer. *Proc Am Soc Clin Oncol* 1998; 17:417a.
48. Bezwoda WR. Randomized, controlled trial of high dose chemotherapy (HD-CNVp) versus standard dose (CAF) chemotherapy for high risk, surgically treated, primary breast cancer. *Proc Am Soc Clin Oncol* 1999;18:2a.
49. The Scandinavian Breast Cancer Study Group 9401. Results from a randomized adjuvant breast cancer study with high dose chemother-

apy with CTC_b supported by autologous bone marrow stem cells versus dose escalated and tailored FEC. *Proc Am Soc Clin Oncol* 1999; 18:2a.
50. Peters W, Rosner G, Vredenburgh J, et al. A prospective, randomized comparison of two doses of combination alkylating agents (AA) as consolidation after CAF in high-risk primary breast cancer involving ten or more axillary lymph nodes (LN): preliminary results of CALGB 9082/SWOG 9114/NCIC MA-13. *Proc Am Soc Clin Oncol* 1999; 18:1a.
51. Eibl B, Schwaighofer H, Nachbaur D, et al. Evidence for a graft versus tumor effect in a patient treated with marrow ablative chemotherapy and allogeneic bone marrow transplantation for breast cancer. *Blood* 1996;88:1501–1508.
52. Ueno NT, Rondon G, Mirza NQ, et al. Allogeneic peripheral blood progenitor cell transplantation for poor risk patients with metastatic breast cancer. *J Clin Oncol* 1998;16:986–993.
53. Kennedy MJ, Vogelsang GB, Jones RJ, et al. Phase I trial of interferon gamma to potentiate cyclosporine-induced graft-versus-host disease in women undergoing autologous bone marrow transplantation for breast cancer. *J Clin Oncol* 1994;12:249–257.

CHAPTER 39

Diseases of the Breast, 2nd ed.,
edited by Jay R. Harris.
Lippincott Williams & Wilkins, Philadelphia © 2000.

Treatment of Locally Advanced and Inflammatory Breast Cancer

Gabriel N. Hortobagyi, S. Eva Singletary, and Eric A. Strom

Locally advanced breast cancer (LABC), despite its decreasing frequency, remains an important and challenging problem in practice. In mammographically screened populations, stage III breast cancer seldom amounts to 5% of those diagnosed; however, in medically underserved areas of the United States and in many other countries, LABC represents 30% to 50% of newly found malignant breast neoplasms.[1–3]

LABC generally refers to large primary tumors (greater than 5 cm) associated with skin or chest wall involvement or with fixed (matted) axillary lymph nodes (T3 and T4; N2).[4] Inflammatory breast cancer is usually included in this group, although some studies suggest that it differs in histologic characteristics, growth pattern, and prognosis from noninflammatory LABC.[5] In this chapter, inflammatory breast cancer is considered a form of LABC, as are tumors associated with disease in the ipsilateral supraclavicular nodal region. Tumors associated with supraclavicular disease have been reclassified as stage IV disease; however, patients with metastases confined to supraclavicular nodes have a better prognosis than patients with metastases at other distant sites and can be rendered disease free with locoregional therapy.[6] Large primary tumors (larger than 5 cm) with no evidence of nodal involvement (T3 N0, stage IIB disease) have a more favorable prognosis than LABC, with a 5-year survival rate of 70% to 80%. However, for the purposes of treatment, T3 N0 tumors are also addressed in this chapter. The management of patients with LABC has evolved substantially over the last three decades, and this chapter summarizes the various therapeutic options in use.[7]

HISTORICAL PERSPECTIVE

Adjuvant systemic treatments have become integral components of the curative management of primary breast cancer.[8,9] Information derived from multiple randomized clinical trials, and from the Oxford meta-analysis, indicates that postoperative adjuvant chemotherapy and hormone therapy decreases the odds of recurrence and death from breast cancer for patients with both node-negative and node-positive tumors. Only limited information exists regarding the efficacy of postoperative adjuvant systemic therapy specifically for stage III breast cancer; however, a few randomized trials have suggested that adjuvant systemic therapies also decrease the probability of recurrence and death in this group of patients.[9–12] Furthermore, most of the randomized clinical trials considered in a world overview included patients with operable stage III breast cancer, and the analysis did not identify any subgroup that did not benefit from adjuvant systemic therapy.[9]

Historically, patients with LABC were treated with a radical mastectomy, when technically possible. On the basis of this experience, Haagensen and Stout defined the concepts of operable and inoperable breast cancer.[13] Skin ulceration, edema, and fixation, as well as fixation of the tumor to the chest wall, were all correlated with almost universal treatment failure, and therefore were considered markers of inoperability. After publication of this landmark work, patients with inoperable tumors were treated with radiation therapy alone or radiation therapy combined with surgical resection.[7,14,15] Large dosages of radiation were necessary to optimize local control, however, and at these dosages, radiotherapy was often associated with long-term complications, including skin and chest wall fibrosis, skin ulceration, rib necrosis or resorption, brachial plexopathy, and lymphedema of the arm.[16–18] The combination of surgery and radiation therapy improved local control rates but did not affect overall survival duration.[7]

Virtually all the historical data regarding locally advanced and inflammatory breast cancer derive from open phase II studies or from retrospective reviews of single-institution experiences with a given treatment strategy. Combinations of systemic therapies and locoregional therapies are preferred. The emphasis on the combined-modality approach is

G. N. Hortobagyi: Department of Breast Medical Oncology, University of Texas M. D. Anderson Cancer Center, Houston, Texas

S. E. Singletary: Department of Surgical Oncology, Surgical Breast Service, University of Texas M. D. Anderson Cancer Center, Houston, Texas

E. A. Strom: Department of Radiation Oncology, University of Texas M.D. Anderson Cancer Center, Houston, Texas

based on the view that successful treatment of breast cancer depends, for most patients, on the eradication of occult micrometastases.[19] With the increasing use of combinations of systemic and local therapies, continual developments have been made in the extent and timing of each treatment modality in the overall treatment strategy.

DIAGNOSIS AND STAGING

Most LABCs and inflammatory breast cancers are easily palpable and even visible. However, some present with diffuse infiltration of the breast and without a dominant mass. These require mammographic assessment and often present as large areas of calcification or parenchymal distortion; sometimes skin thickening is also present.

A core-needle biopsy usually establishes the histologic diagnosis; incisional biopsies are seldom required, although a full-thickness skin biopsy is often obtained when inflammatory breast cancer is suspected. If an experienced cytopathologist is available, diagnosis can be confirmed by fine-needle aspiration cytology. Nuclear grade, flow cytometry, estrogen-receptor and progesterone-receptor status can all be assayed on samples from fine-needle aspiration cytology; so can most other proposed prognostic indicators (e.g., presence of PCNA, Ki67, HER-2/neu, p53). However, fine-needle aspiration cytology cannot differentiate invasive and noninvasive tumors.

Once the diagnosis is established, the extent of tumor involvement is ascertained. A biochemical survey, tumor marker assays, and chest radiographs and bone scan complement a complete physical examination, with quantitative documentation of all palpable abnormalities. If liver function tests or tumor marker assays are abnormal, abdominal imaging (computerized tomography or ultrasonography) is recommended; areas of increased radionuclide uptake on bone scan are assessed by radiography. A contralateral mammogram serves to rule out the presence of synchronous bilateral cancer or contralateral metastases, and ultrasonography serves to further define tumor dimensions and regional lymph node involvement. Other tests are indicated only in the presence of specific symptoms or for investigational purposes.

DEVELOPMENT OF COMBINED-MODALITY STRATEGIES

Systemic therapy was introduced in the management of inoperable breast cancers in the 1950s.[20] Systemic therapy was followed in these trials by surgery or radiation therapy, or both. Perhaps the most important aspect of combined-modality therapies is the conceptual framework. For optimal use of all treatment modalities, all interested specialists (radiologist, pathologist, and surgical, radiation, and medical oncologists) review the data, examine the patient jointly, and determine the optimal type and sequence of therapies. Thus, teamwork has replaced the single-specialty orientation. Treatment strategies that include induction chemotherapy (or hormone therapy) have several potential advantages (Table 1): early initiation of systemic therapy, *in vivo* assessment of response, and downstaging of primary tumor and regional lymphatic metastases, which makes breast-conserving surgery an option for many. The potential (theoretical) shortcomings include delay in local treatment, induction of drug resistance, and unreliability of clinical staging. In practice, the advantages have exceeded the disadvantages. The ability to monitor response to therapy by serial measurements of the primary tumor, and the achievement of downstaging that often permits breast conservation, are the two major clinical advantages of these treatment strategies.

TABLE 1. *Characteristics of combined-modality therapeutic strategies that include induction chemotherapy*

Advantages
Early initiation of systemic treatment
Inhibition of postsurgical growth spurt
Delivery of chemotherapy through intact tumor vasculature
In vivo assessment of response
Downstaging of primary tumor and lymph node metastases
Less radical locoregional therapy needed
Breast conservation possible
Good biological model to evaluate effects of chemotherapy on the tumor
Disadvantages
Local treatment delayed for nonresponders
Induction of drug resistance
Large tumor burden
Only clinical staging available; imprecise
Possible increased risk in surgical and radiotherapy-related complications

INDUCTION CHEMOTHERAPY

The first clinical trials with induction (neoadjuvant) chemotherapy started in the late 1960s, but the earliest reports were published in the 1970s.[21] Since then, reports of the results of this strategy have multiplied, documenting the effectiveness of primary chemotherapy in this group of patients.[7,22–28] In most reports, the majority (60% to 80%) of patients achieved a major objective regression in primary tumor volume and enlarged regional lymph nodes.[21,22,24–26,29–38] Although a few patients experienced mixed responses (response in the primary tumor and no response in the regional lymph nodes, or vice versa), for most patients, response was similar in all sites of tumor involvement.[38–41] Clinical complete remissions were reported in 10% to 20% of patients treated in this manner in most clinical trials.[24,29,33,38,42] In one trial, induction chemotherapy was continued until maximum response was reached (by force, a retrospective definition).[41] Great het-

TABLE 2. *Locally advanced breast cancer: correlation of clinical and pathologic complete remissions after induction chemotherapy*

Study	Treatment program	No. of patients	Patients with complete remission (%)	
			Clinical	Pathologic
Hobar et al.[32]	CT + S ± RT + CT	36	8	11
Conte et al.[24]	CT + S + CT	39	15	8
Lippman et al.[41]	CT ± S + RT + CT	51	52	33
Cocconi et al.[43]	CT + S + CT + RT	49	8	14
Hortobagyi et al.[38]	CT ± S + RT – CT	174	17	8

CT, chemotherapy; RT, radiation therapy; S, surgery.

erogeneity was seen in patient responses; some patients achieved maximum tumor reduction after only one cycle of therapy, whereas others required up to 8 months of treatment to reach that point. Thus, individualizing the duration of induction chemotherapy appears to improve the rate of complete remission; such individualization might be desirable if breast conservation is a major objective of therapy.

Clinical measurements of breast masses are often inaccurate, and substantial interindividual variation exists among examiners.[43] Therefore, imaging methods are often used to document the extent of disease more reliably.[43–45] Combining physical examination with either mammography or ultrasonography yields measurements that closely approach those achieved by histopathology and reduces error rates in serial monitoring of response to systemic therapy.[45] A determination of clinical complete remission requires that no residual disease be present by physical examination or by imaging (mammography or ultrasound) in the breast or regional lymph nodes.[38] Even when these criteria are followed, only two-thirds of patients thought to have a clinical complete remission are found to have a pathologic complete remission (i.e., no residual disease) (Table 2).[10,24,29,38,41,42] Conversely, one-third of patients with no residual disease on histologic examination have residual clinical or imaging abnormalities that preclude the diagnosis of clinical complete remission. The careful determination of complete remission after induction chemotherapy is important, because patients classified in this group have a markedly better long-term prognosis than patients who achieve less marked or no response.[25,46] Furthermore, these patients are excellent candidates for breast-conserving procedures, with or without surgical intervention.

APPROACHES TO LOCAL THERAPY

For patients with operable (stage IIIA) LABC, a modified radical mastectomy followed by systemic adjuvant therapy, represents an effective treatment option.[47] Selected patients with small T4 tumors may also be given surgery as their initial treatment modality.[48] In recent years, an increasing number of patients with stage IIIA breast cancer have been treated with induction chemotherapy followed by various locoregional approaches, a strategy favored by the authors and others.[47,49] Major objective responses after induction chemotherapy have resulted in downstaging for approximately 70% of patients.[38,42,49] After induction chemotherapy, surgery alone,[21,31,34,49] radiotherapy alone,[21,22,25,50–53] or a combination of both[21,26,53,54] has been used in the context of multidisciplinary management. Surgical therapy may require a total mastectomy or only a wide excision (lumpectomy or quadrantectomy), both accompanied by an axillary dissection, especially in the presence of palpable axillary lymph nodes. In randomized trials, total mastectomy alone has been compared with radiation therapy alone, both after primary chemotherapy (Table 3).[21,34,53,55] Early reports of these trials

TABLE 3. *Randomized clinical trials to define optimal local therapy for locally advanced breast cancer treated with combined-modality approach*

Study	Treatments compared	No. of patients	CR (%)	CR + PR (%)	Failure	
					Local	Distant
DeLena et al.[21]	CT, S	65	78	78	30	43
	CT, RT	67	51	85	31	26
Perloff et al.[34]	CT, S	43	100	100	19	26
	CT, RT	44	52	77	27	23
Papaioannou et al.[54]	CT, S, CT	57	57	57	11	11
	CT, S + RT, CT	48	48	48	8	19

CR, complete remission; CT, chemotherapy; PR, partial remission; RT, radiation therapy; S, surgery.

suggested that the two strategies were equivalent; indeed, to date, no significant differences in survival have been demonstrated in these studies. Based mostly on indirect comparisons, local control rates seem to be higher when both surgical excision and radiation therapy (after primary chemotherapy) are included in the treatment strategy[21,24,26,29,32,33,36,37,56–58] than when only one local treatment is given. However, the need to use chemotherapy followed by both surgery and radiation therapy for all patients with LABC has not been confirmed in randomized trials. Therefore, additional controlled trials are needed to establish the optimal sequence and composition of multimodality treatments.

ROLE OF RADIATION THERAPY IN LOCALLY ADVANCED BREAST CANCER

Comprehensive irradiation is an effective therapy for eliminating occult deposits of tumor in locoregional tissues after surgical removal of macroscopic tumor. Patients with stage III breast cancer have a 30% to 50% risk of locoregional recurrence when surgery or radiation is used as the sole local treatment.[21,23,31,34,56] For operable stage III breast cancer, the postoperative administration of chemotherapy and radiotherapy resulted in better local control and higher overall survival rates than the use of either adjuvant treatment alone.[10] For locoregional treatment to be effective, it must encompass all the volumes at risk, and it must eliminate any tumor cells therein. For LABC, this means treating the entire soft tissue of the chest wall, including any residual breast tissue, surrounding skin, connective tissue, and regional lymphatics. Most local recurrences occur on the chest wall; these are followed in order of frequency by recurrences in the axillary and supraclavicular chain and, infrequently, in the internal mammary chain. Failure in the dissected axilla is unusual, provided no gross disease remains. In the presence of known residual disease, higher dosages of radiation therapy are required, with a consequent increase in acute and long-term complications. For this reason, if residual disease remains after induction chemotherapy, the authors prefer a surgical excision, followed by adjuvant chemotherapy and radiotherapy. Usually, the chest wall is treated at our institution with tangential 6-mV photon beam fields, although electron beam fields may be used for treatment of patients with favorable anatomic configurations. An adjacent, matching electron beam field is used to treat the lymph nodes of the internal mammary chain. With this technique, the left ventricle can be completely excluded from the irradiated volume, and a maximum of 2 to 3 cm of lung is treated. Alternatively, a series of electron beam fields can be used to treat the chest wall and internal mammary nodes. The undissected lymphatics of the axillary apex and supraclavicular fossa are treated with low-energy photon or electron beams. Fifty Gy is delivered in 25 fractions followed by a boost to the chest wall, for a total dose of at least 60 Gy. Areas of initial nodal involvement not removed at surgery are also boosted to achieve a total dose of 60 to 66 Gy. In patients with an N2 presentation, or those with gross (macroscopic) extranodal extension or free tumor in the axillary fat, the midplane axilla is supplemented through a posterior field to achieve a midplane dose of 40 to 50 Gy. Combined-modality therapy offers excellent local control for 80% or more of those with stage IIIB or stage IV breast cancer, and an even higher proportion of those with stage IIIA disease.[38] If any part of the multidisciplinary treatment strategy is suboptimal, however, it compromises the efficacy of the entire program.

The therapeutic modalities used to treat for breast cancer may be combined or sequenced in many possible ways. The high incidence of distant metastases in patients with LABC makes the early introduction of systemic therapy reasonable. Whether simultaneous chemotherapy and radiotherapy result in improved local and distant control remains to be established.[58,59] Therefore, most combined-modality strategies for inoperable LABC start with induction chemotherapy, usually with an anthracycline-containing multidrug regimen. The subsequent sequence of local, regional, and additional systemic treatments is poorly defined. The authors find that induction chemotherapy followed by surgical resection, adjuvant chemotherapy, and consolidation radiotherapy is a well-tolerated, safe, and effective sequence of therapies for patients with LABC.[38]

BREAST PRESERVATION AFTER INDUCTION CHEMOTHERAPY

Clinical trials of primary chemotherapy provide increasing evidence that many patients with stage III breast cancer, including some with LABC, can be treated appropriately with breast-conserving techniques.[21,22,25,26,29,31,34,49,50,52] Clinical trials with induction chemotherapy and radiation therapy performed at the M. D. Anderson Cancer Center in Houston,[29] the Milan Cancer Institute,[21] the U.S. National Cancer Institute in Bethesda, Maryland,[26] and several European centers[25,37,50,60] have demonstrated that patients with LABC were downstaged to the extent that 15% to 95% of them could be treated with radiation therapy without surgical resection. These reports revealed that breast conservation was clearly possible after induction chemotherapy; however, the fraction of patients offered breast-conserving treatment varied markedly among institutions, because the size of the tumor was only one of several criteria used to select patients for breast-conservation therapy. Many characteristics of the patient and the tumor must be considered in selecting candidates for breast-conserving therapy. Age, tumor histologic type, tumor differentiation, and availability of family and social support systems are among the factors considered in making this decision. Very few absolute contraindications to breast-conserving therapy exist, although each of the factors cited may moderately influence the risk of recurrence within the breast. Although these criteria are used for patients treated with induction chemotherapy, they were originally derived from patients with early (stages I and II) breast cancer. Therefore, selection of patients with LABC for breast-conserving therapy should be performed with caution and implemented only by groups with experience in combined-modality therapy.

To assess the feasibility of breast-conservation surgery after tumor downstaging at our institution, we performed a retrospective review that correlated the clinical and mammographic responses with the histologic findings in the mastectomy specimen after induction chemotherapy and with the risk of locoregional relapse.[61] The study population (1985 through 1989) consisted of 143 patients with LABC who had either a complete response (16%) or a partial response (84%) to doxorubicin hydrochloride–based combination chemotherapy.[62] We applied strict eligibility criteria for breast conservation: complete resolution of skin edema, residual tumor size of less than 5 cm, no evidence of multicentric lesions, and the absence of extensive intramammary lymphatic invasion or extensive microcalcifications (in addition to the usual absolute contraindications). According to these criteria, 33 (23%) of the 143 patients who responded to induction chemotherapy would have been considered eligible for a segmental mastectomy and axillary node dissection rather than a modified radical mastectomy. None of these 33 patients was found to have tumor in other quadrants of the breast in the total mastectomy specimens, and at a median follow-up of 34 months, none had experienced a chest wall recurrence. In contrast, of the 110 patients who were not considered to be good candidates for breast-conservation surgery, 55 (50%) had tumor in other quadrants.

The factors most commonly associated with multiple-quadrant involvement were persistent skin edema (65%), residual tumor size larger than 4 cm (56%), extensive intramammary lymphatic invasion (20%), and mammographic evidence of multicentric disease (16%). Of the 110 patients who were not candidates for breast conservation, 17 (15%) had recurrence on the chest wall after radiotherapy. Of these 17, 13 (76%) had persistent skin edema before mastectomy, two (12%) had extensive intramammary lymphatic invasion, and two (12%) had extensive multicentric disease.

Ninety-three patients with large or locally advanced breast cancer were treated with induction FAC (5-fluorouracil, doxorubicin, cylcophosphamide) chemotherapy and breast-conservation surgery at our institution between 1982 and 1994.[63] The initial distribution of cancer stages was the following: stage IIA, 22.6%; stage IIB, 24.7%; stage IIIA, 32.3%; stage IIIB, 16.1%; and stage IV (supraclavicular metastases only), 4.3%. After segmental mastectomy and axillary node dissection, patients received four to eight cycles of adjuvant chemotherapy followed by radiation therapy. Of the 93 patients, 86 completed postoperative therapy. Overall, nine patients had a local recurrence, for a local failure rate of 9.7%. The median time to local recurrence in these patients was 55 months. Therefore, the local recurrence rate was similar to the local failure rate observed for breast-conservation therapy in patients with early-stage breast cancer.

The six patients with local recurrence only or local recurrence before distant metastases had an overall survival rate of 83% at a median follow-up of 88 months. This survival rate was similar to the overall survival rate of 89% for the entire group of 93 patients (median follow-up, 73 months).

The radiotherapeutic technique for breast conservation in patients with LABC is particularly challenging, because the target volume extends beyond the intact breast to include the regional lymphatics. The use of multiple adjacent fields is thus involved. Ideally, noncoplanar beams are used with precise matching techniques when photon fields abut one another. Typically, the breast and undissected lymphatics are treated to a dose of 50 Gy in 25 fractions over 5 weeks, followed by a 10-Gy boost to the tumor bed, which is marked intraoperatively with clips. In patients with LABC downstaged with systemic therapy, our current practice is to design treatment fields based on the original extent of disease.

The use of induction chemotherapy has been extended to stage I and stage II breast cancer.[40,49,64–67] To date, clinical trials in early breast cancer have confirmed the efficacy of these regimens and suggest that downstaging is even more likely in early stages.[40,49,67,68] Furthermore, the preliminary report of a large multicenter trial confirmed that substantial downstaging after induction chemotherapy also occurred at the level of regional lymph nodes, suggesting that a similar effect might extend to distant micrometastases.[40]

The role of axillary node dissection after induction chemotherapy in patients with LABC is being reassessed. Four main arguments are voiced against the routine use of axillary node dissection in this setting. First, induction chemotherapy in patients with LABC and operable breast cancer has been shown to downstage positive axillary lymph nodes to negative lymph nodes in 25% to 44% of patients.[40,68–72] Second, in most treatment protocols, patients with LABC routinely receive additional postoperative chemotherapy and radiotherapy, regardless of the findings at axillary node dissection. Third, some LABC series have reported equivalent axillary control rates after induction chemotherapy followed by axillary node dissection alone, axillary irradiation alone, and a combination of surgery and irradiation.[28,31,62] Fourth, high-dose chemotherapy off protocol cannot be recommended in the absence of prospective randomized data demonstrating a survival advantage for high-dose chemotherapy over standard anthracycline-based chemotherapy in patients with multiple positive axillary nodes after induction chemotherapy.[73] Proponents of axillary node dissection in patients receiving induction chemotherapy assert that the number of positive nodes detected after tumor downstaging may affect whether patients are crossed over to a different chemotherapeutic agent. For example, phase II trials have demonstrated high activity of taxane-based chemotherapy (paclitaxel and docetaxel) in anthracycline-resistant breast cancer.[74,75] However, if the trend in therapy is toward a sequential approach using anthracycline and taxane-based regimens before (or after) local therapy, with no further systemic intervention planned, then the histologic assessment of the axilla becomes only a prognostic tool with no influence on the treatment plan.

To determine whether there may be an alternative to axillary node dissection after tumor downstaging, we analyzed 147 consecutive patients with LABC treated at our institution between 1992 and 1996 in a prospective trial of neoadjuvant chemotherapy using FAC.[72,76] Downstaging to a negative axilla, as assessed by physical and ultrasonographic evaluation, occurred after induction chemotherapy in 43 patients with palpable axillary disease on initial examination. A pathologic complete axillary lymph node response was found in 30 patients. Of the 72 patients with axillary metastases that were cytologically proven by fine-needle aspiration on initial evaluation, 15 patients (21%) were confirmed to have histologically negative axillary lymph nodes after induction chemotherapy.

Whether the excellent results obtained in patients with early-stage breast cancer treated with axillary irradiation without surgery can be achieved in patients with LABC downstaged to a clinically negative axilla is unknown.[77–80] Sentinel lymph node mapping and biopsy in patients with LABC has not been studied and will prove accurate only if metastatic deposits within each axillary lymph node respond identically to the effect of chemotherapy.

INFLAMMATORY BREAST CANCER

Inflammatory breast cancer, perhaps the most aggressive form of breast neoplasia, represents 1% to 3% of newly diagnosed breast malignancies and is often considered together with LABC, despite specific differential features.[81] This entity is diagnosed on clinical grounds, based on the presence of erythema and edema (*peau d'orange*) of the skin of the breast, as well as ridging. Although a dominant mass is present in many cases, most inflammatory cancers present as diffuse infiltration of the breast without a well-defined tumor. The absence of a well-defined tumor often suggests an inflammatory etiology. Very often, these patients are treated with antibiotics for several weeks before the appropriate diagnosis is made because of the extensive inflammatory signs without the signs of a malignant neoplasm. Dermal lymphatic invasion is present in most patients, but this feature is not a necessary component of the diagnostic complex. Most inflammatory breast cancers are poorly differentiated ductal carcinomas and are estrogen receptor– and progesterone receptor–negative. Compared to noninflammatory LABC, the median thymidine-labeling index is significantly higher for inflammatory breast cancer than for LABC. HER-2/neu-overexpression and p53 gene mutations are also abnormalities frequently found in inflammatory breast cancer. A history of rapid onset (less than 3 months) is often used to differentiate inflammatory breast cancer from locally advanced breast cancer with secondary inflammatory features.[82] This differentiation is important, because some of the secondary inflammatory breast cancers follow an indolent course and are often hormone responsive.

Before the introduction of systemic therapy in combined-modality treatment programs, inflammatory breast cancer was a uniformly fatal disease.[7] Patients with inflammatory breast cancer treated with surgery or radiation therapy, or a combination of both, had an extremely poor prognosis: The local recurrence rate was very high (50% to 80%), metastases developed in more than 90% of patients in less than 2 years, and 5-year survival rates were consistently less than 5%.[7,83]

With the development of strategies that contained induction chemotherapy, a most dramatic change occurred in the natural history of inflammatory breast cancer (Table 4).[7,21,25,26,84–95] Now, objective response rates after induction chemotherapy consistently reach 80% in patients with inflammatory breast cancer, and most patients (more than 95%) can be rendered disease free after combined-modality therapy. Three-year survival rates after these treatments now range from 40% to 70%, and at five years, up to 50% of patients remain alive. In reports with longer follow-up, 35% remain disease free at 10 years, and even longer.[94] In fact, late relapses of inflammatory breast cancer are uncommon.

Locoregional therapy for inflammatory breast cancer presents special challenges. Because of the diffuse nature of this type of breast cancer, determining the extent of disease preoperatively or even intraoperatively might be difficult. In addition, even after induction chemotherapy, complete normalization of cutaneous abnormalities is distinctly uncommon. Before the introduction of combined systemic and regional treatment strategies, the locoregional failure rate was 50% to 75% for this group of patients after surgery alone, radiation therapy alone, or a combination of both.[7,83] These results led to the conclusion that surgical removal of the breast served no useful purpose, and surgery was considered contraindicated for inflammatory breast cancer. The relative success of combination chemotherapy regimens, however, prompted a reevaluation of surgical resection in the management of inflammatory breast cancer. Most series that attempt to define the benefit of mastectomy in inflammatory breast cancer are limited by an inherent patient bias: Patients with the best response to induction chemotherapy have their disease rendered technically resectable and are the only ones offered surgical treatment.[94–100] A retrospective review of the experience with 178 women treated for inflammatory breast cancer with doxorubicin-hydrochloride-based multimodality therapy protocols between 1974 and 1993 suggested that the addition of mastectomy might lead to a modest improvement in locoregional disease control for patients who achieved a partial remission after chemotherapy.[101] Locoregional relapse rates were 16.3% (16 of 98 patients) for patients who underwent chemotherapy, mastectomy, and radiation therapy, and 35.7% (15 of 42 patients) for patients who underwent only chemotherapy and radiation therapy ($p = .016$). In addition, patients who had a complete or partial clinical response to induction

TABLE 4. *Results of combined-modality treatment programs for inflammatory breast carcinoma*

Study	Treatment program	No. of patients	Patients rendered disease free (%)	Median survival time (mo)	5-year survival rate (%)
DeLena et al.[21]	CT + RT ± CT	36	73	25	NA
Chu et al.[84]	RT + H	14	NA	15	NA
	RT + CT	16	NA	>26	NA
Pouillart et al.[85]	CT + RT + CT	77	51	34	NA
Zylberberg et al.[86]	CT + S + CT ± RT	15	100	>50	70
Pawlicki et al.[27]	CT ± S + RT	72	NA	NA	NA
Loprinzi et al.[87]	S + CT + RT + CT	9	100	>25	55
Keiling t al.[88]	CT + S + CT	41	100	NR	63
Jacquillat et al.[115]	CT + RT + CT + H	66	100	NR	66
Alberto et al.[135]	CT + S + CT + RT	22	95	26	10
Ferriere et al.[136]	CT + RT ± S + CT	75	93	NR	54
Pourny et al.[137]	CT + S ± RT + CT	33	82	70	60
Chevallier et al.[138]	CT + RT ± CT ± S	178	83	37	32
Rouesse et al.[89]	CT + RT + CT + H	91	41	36	40
Israel et al.[90]	CT + S + CT	25	96	NR	62
Krutchik et al.[91]	CT + RT + CT	32	NA	24	NA
Brun et al.[100]	CT + RT + S + CT	26	NA	31	NA
Thoms et al.[92]	CT + S + CT + RT	61	NA	61	35
Swain et al.[26]	CT + RT + S + CT + H	45	NA	36	NR
Fields et al.[93]	CT + S + RT + CT	37	NA	49	44
Maloisel et al.[139]	CT + S + CT + RT + H	43	NA	46	75
Koh et al.[94]	CT + RT + CT	40	NA	39	37
	CT + S + CT + RT	23	NA	38	30
	CT + S + CT + RT	43	NA	31	40

CT, chemotherapy; H, hormone therapy; NA, not available; NR, not reached; RT, radiation therapy; S, surgery.

chemotherapy and were treated with mastectomy in addition to chemotherapy and irradiation had significantly improved 5-year disease-specific survival compared with patients who had a similar response to induction chemotherapy but did not undergo mastectomy (survival rate of 62.0% versus 43.0%, respectively; $p = .018$). No improvement in outcome was detected with the addition of mastectomy in patients who had no significant response to induction chemotherapy, nor did overall survival improve in these patients. The results of this retrospective analysis need confirmation from prospective trials. Other benefits of mastectomy include a more accurate assessment of the amount of residual disease after induction chemotherapy and the ability to use lower dosages of radiation therapy, because gross disease has been removed.[100,101]

Accelerated fractionation schedules of radiotherapy have been proposed to exploit the biological characteristics of inflammatory breast cancer. Since 1986, in cases of inflammatory breast cancer, the chest wall and peripheral lymphatics have been treated at our institution with irradiation of 51 Gy at 1.5 Gy per fraction, twice daily, with a minimum 6-hour interfraction interval. The dissected axilla is supplemented in selected patients, just as in patients with noninflammatory breast cancer, as indicated previously. Vigorous bolus schedules are used to achieve brisk erythema in most patients, but excessive moist desquamation that would result in treatment breaks is avoided. Subsequently, the mastectomy flaps are boosted and an additional 15 Gy is given, at 1.5 Gy per fraction, twice daily, to achieve a total dose in the boosted volume of 66 Gy in 4.5 weeks. A retrospective analysis of the results of this strategy suggests improved locoregional control rates compared with those of historical controls at M. D. Anderson Cancer Center. The locoregional control rates for the new series were 91.2% at 5 years and 84.6% at 10 years. The disease-free survival rates for the series were 39.3% at 5 years and 35.6% at 10 years, respectively. Long-term complications, such as arm edema, rib fracture, severe chest wall fibrosis, and symptomatic pneumonitis were comparable to those of prior series, indicating that the radiation dosage escalation did not result in increased morbidity.[102] These results should be confirmed in a prospective study before they are universally adopted, however.[92,103] Some investigators have attempted to conserve the breast by substituting interstitial irradiation for mastectomy in patients who experience significant tumor reduction with chemotherapy; however, the experience with this approach is limited. Brun et al. found local recurrences in 7 of 13 patients treated with breast conservation therapy and interstitial irradiation.[100]

TOLERANCE AND TOXICITY

Combined-modality regimens have been well tolerated, and no increase in surgical complications has been reported.[104] Surgery is usually sandwiched between cycles

TABLE 5. *Survival of patients with stage III breast cancer after combined-modality treatment based on induction chemotherapy followed by local treatment (nonrandomized trials)*

Study	Treatment program	No. of patients	Patients rendered disease free (%)	Median survival time (mo)	Survival rate (%)	
					3 yr	5 yr
DeLena et al.[21]	CT + RT ± CT	110	83	36	50	NR
Hortobagyi et al.[31]	CT + RT ± S + CT	52	94	65	65	55
Bedwinek et al.[105]	CT + RT + CT	22	78	28	40	NR
Pawlicki et al.[27]	CT	40	NA	NA	13	NR
	CT + RT + CT	34	NA	NA	32	NR
	CT + S + RT + CT	13	NA	NA	62	NR
Valagussa et al.[23]	CT + RT	72	64	30	43	20
	CT + RT + CT	126	75	42	60	36
	CT + S + CT	79	82	58	64	49
Balawajder et al.[28]	CT + RT	23	NA	NA	NA	46
	CT + RT + S	30	NA	NA	NA	38
Conte et al.[24]	H + CT + S + H + CT ± RT	39	92	NR	60	NR
Pouillart et al.[51]	CT + S + RT	82	100	NR	85	NR
Jacquillat et al.[25]	CT + RT + CT	98	100	NR	77	NR
Hortobagyi et al.[38]	CT + RT + S + CT	174	96	66	65	55
Swain et al.[26]	CT + RT + S + CT	75	100	39	42	NR

CT, chemotherapy; H, hormone therapy; NA, not available; NR, not reached; RT, radiation therapy; S, surgery.

of chemotherapy, and systemic treatment seldom needs to be interrupted. The expected acute toxic effects of combination chemotherapy are observed without apparent increase in frequency or intensity. In studies of simultaneous radiation therapy and chemotherapy, a slight increase in hematologic toxicity and enhancement of acute radiation effects (erythema, moist desquamation) have been reported.[105–108] Simultaneous administration of chemotherapy and radiation therapy impairs the cosmetic results of breast-conserving therapy to some extent. Although some impairment of cosmesis is also observed with the sequential use of chemotherapy and radiotherapy, this effect is not clinically important for most patients. For patients with left-breast cancer, synergistic cardiac toxicity is a danger with simultaneous therapy.[107,108] However, a modification in radiotherapy techniques and careful attention to the total dosage of anthracyclines minimizes this risk. The administration of doxorubicin hydrochloride by 48-hour or 96-hour continuous infusion schedules also reduces the risk of cardiac toxicity substantially.[109]

SURVIVAL EFFECTS OF COMBINED-MODALITY STRATEGIES

The bulk of the information regarding the multidisciplinary treatment of stage III and locally advanced breast cancer was obtained from open (uncontrolled) phase II trials; therefore, assessments of the effects of these treatments on survival are tentative at best, and definitive conclusions must await the completion of prospective randomized trials. Such trials are possible for patients with operable stage III breast cancer; however, for patients with inoperable stage III or inflammatory breast cancer, the window of opportunity to perform such trials may have been closed many years ago. The results of phase II trials compare favorably with the outcomes of historical control series or literature controls and suggest higher 5- and 10-year survival rates, especially for subgroups with the worst prognosis, such as those with inflammatory breast cancer (Tables 4 and 5),[7,81] patients with supraclavicular lymph node involvement,[38] and patients with T4 primary lesions. Fig. 1 shows the disease-free survival rates for patients with stage IIIA and stage IIIB cancer treated at this institution with induction chemotherapy followed by surgery, radiation therapy, and adjuvant chemotherapy; the maximum follow-up now exceeds 20 years. The two curves are compared with those for patients with similar-stage disease (IIIA and IIIB) treated at this same institution with surgery and radiation therapy but without systemic treatment. Fig. 2 shows the overall survival curves from the same four groups of patients. Disease-free and overall survival appear to improve substantially for patients who received the combined-modality treatment, including induction chemotherapy. The median relapse-free and overall survival times for patients with stage IIIA breast cancer treated with surgery and radiotherapy were 102 and 140 months, respectively, whereas they have not been reached at 200 months by patients treated also with induction chemotherapy. The differences in both disease-free and overall survival for patients with stage IIIB breast cancer treated with these two strategies were 10 and 13 months, respectively. The 5- and 10-year disease-free and overall survival rates were approxi-

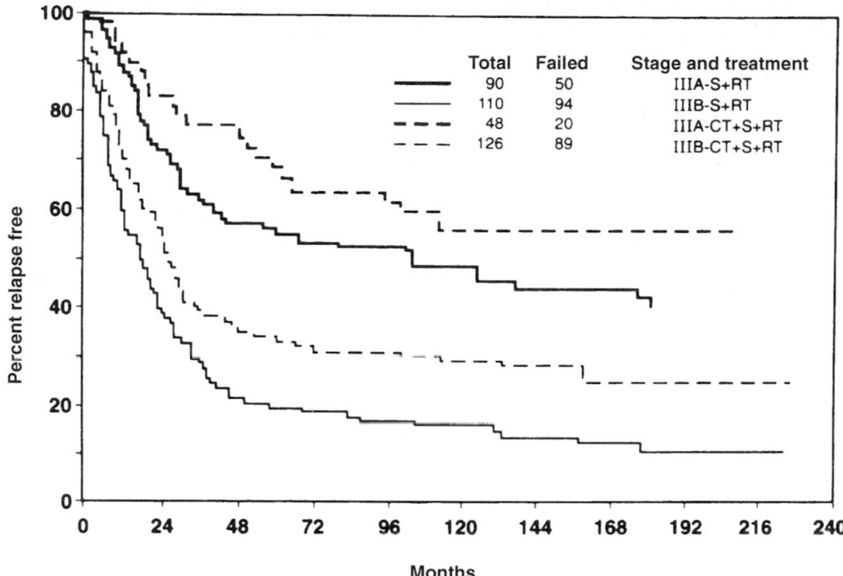

FIG. 1. Relapse-free survival rates of patients with stage IIIA and stage IIIB breast cancer treated with induction chemotherapy (FAC) followed by surgical resection, radiation therapy, and adjuvant chemotherapy between 1973 and 1984. The control groups consist of patients with stage IIIA and stage IIIB breast cancer treated at the same institution with surgery and radiation therapy before 1974. (CT, chemotherapy; RT, radiation therapy; S, surgery.)

mately ten points higher for patients treated with all three modalities in sequence than for the historical controls. These differences have persisted beyond 10 years of follow-up and are projected to continue beyond 20 years after diagnosis and treatment. Patients with stage III breast cancer treated with local therapy followed by postoperative adjuvant chemotherapy are generally considered to remain relapse free for significantly longer[9–11,50,110,111] and sometimes to achieve significantly greater overall survival rates[9–11,111] than those treated with only local therapy, although not all studies have confirmed this observation.[52] The results of randomized trials comparing induction (or preoperative) chemotherapy with postoperative chemotherapy in the context of combined-modality treatment suggest that the results obtained with induction chemotherapy are at least equivalent to those observed after postoperative chemotherapy (Table 6).[40,64,65,67,112] In two of these studies,[22,52] however, the dosage of radiation therapy administered was too low to provide appropriate local control, and by today's standards, the dose-intensity of chemotherapy was also low. In addition, three of the six studies shown in Table 6 have sample sizes insufficient to detect even large differences in outcome. Additional well-designed trials, with adequate statistical power and sufficient follow-up, are needed to define the survival benefit obtained and the relative benefits of induction versus postoperative adjuvant systemic therapy.

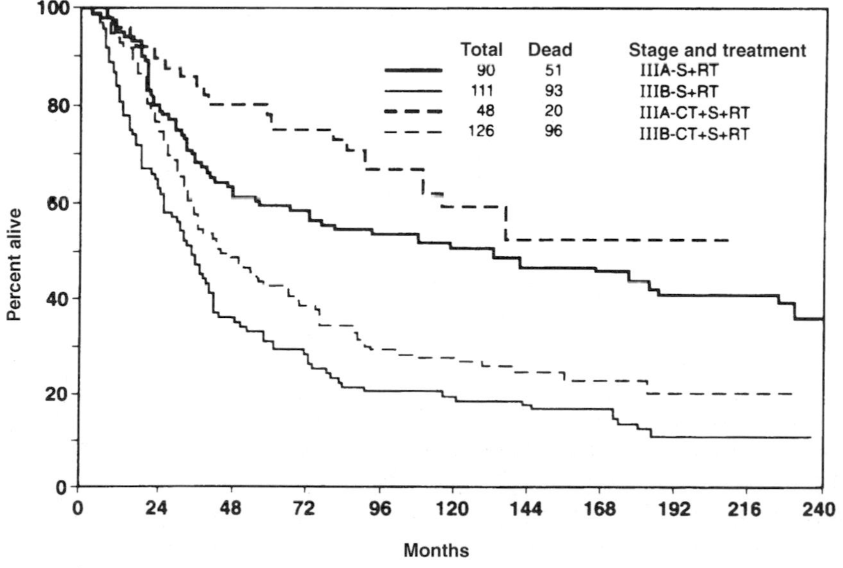

FIG. 2. Overall survival rates of patients with stage IIIA and stage IIIB breast cancer treated with induction chemotherapy (FAC) followed by surgical resection, radiation therapy, and adjuvant chemotherapy between 1973 and 1984. The control groups consist of patients with stage IIIA and stage IIIB breast cancer treated at the same institution with surgery and radiation therapy between 1965 and 1974. (CT, chemotherapy; RT, radiation therapy; S, surgery.)

TABLE 6. *Survival of patients with stage II–III breast cancer after combined-modality treatment based on induction chemotherapy followed by local treatment (randomized trials)*

Study	Treatment program	No. of patients	Patients rendered disease free (%)	Median survival time (mo)	Survival rate (%)	
					3 yr	5 yr
Rubens et al.[22]	CT + RT[a] + CT	12	67	36	50	NR
	RT[a] + CT	12	75	36	50	NR
Mauriac et al.[65]	S + CT	138	99	NR	87	NR
	CT + S	134	99	NR	94	NR
Scholl et al.[64]	RT + S + CT	190	NA	NR	87	78
	CT + RT + S	200	NA	NR	92	86
Schaake-Koning et al.[52]	RT[a]	45	75	42	59	37
	RT[a] + CT	71	50	45	59	37
	CT + RT[a] + CT	39	71	50	61	37
Valagussa et al.[23]	CT + RT[a] + CT	59	51	34	NA	33
	RT[a] + CT	60	42	24	NA	32
Fisher et al.[112]	CT → S[b]	760	100	NR	90	80
	S → CT[b]	763	100	NR	90	80

[a]Low-dose radiation therapy, probably inadequate for optimal local control.
[b]Most patients in this study had stage II breast cancer.
CT, chemotherapy; NA, not available; NR, not reached; RT, radiation therapy; S, surgery.

PROGNOSTIC FACTORS

The ability to predict outcome changes with the efficacy of the treatments used. For LABC treated with regional therapies only, large tumor size, involvement of axillary lymph nodes, involvement of supraclavicular lymph nodes, skin edema, inflammatory breast cancer, diffuse primary tumor, and short duration of symptoms were predictive of decreased relapse-free and overall survival rates.[13,113,114] Evaluation of the prognostic value of axillary lymph node involvement after induction chemotherapy showed that the number of involved nodes was the best predictor for both relapse and death in a multivariate analysis.[69] Division into the pathologic nodal subgroups of 0, 1–3, 4–10, and more than ten positive lymph nodes after induction chemotherapy predicted a prognostic distribution similar to that found in previously untreated patients. Other important and independent factors found in this study by multivariate analysis were clinical tumor stage at presentation, clinical response to induction chemotherapy, and menopausal status. Clinical response to induction chemotherapy—or its surrogate, histologically detected extent of residual disease—has also been reported by other investigators to be an important prognostic indicator.[66,115]

Response (and especially complete response) to induction chemotherapy occurs significantly more often in patients with poorly differentiated tumors than in patients with well-differentiated tumors in some[39,66,116] but not all[37,117] reported series. Provocative data from pilot studies suggested that responses were more common in patients with aneuploid tumors and in those with high proliferative fraction.[118,119] Although biologically plausible, these data need additional prospective confirmation. The results of retrospective analyses of randomized clinical trials have suggested that tumors that overexpress the HER-2 oncoprotein might be relatively resistant to the CMF (cyclophosphamide, methotrexate, and 5-fluorouracil) combination and to hormonal therapy with tamoxifen citrate. Other analysis has suggested that higher dosages of doxorubicin hydrochloride might be more effective in this same group. Preliminary reports suggest that p53 overexpression is associated with poorer prognosis and relative resistance to chemotherapy, whereas Bcl-2 overexpression is a predictor of good prognosis but resistance to chemotherapy. The results of all this research need to be confirmed in prospective studies before these molecular markers can be adopted to select optimal systemic therapy.

Other studies have assessed the prognostic importance of various factors in terms of relapse-free and overall survival. Initial TNM stage, clinical tumor size, clinical nodal stage, and histologic grade have been shown to correlate with both these end points in univariate analyses.[25,29,37,38,65] In multivariate analyses, histologic and nuclear grade, both clinical and surgical nodal stage, initial tumor size, and response to induction chemotherapy were significant predictors of disease-free survival,[38,66,69] whereas tumor size, nodal status, grade, and response to induction chemotherapy correlated with overall survival.[38,66,69]

The value of prognostic factors for inflammatory breast cancer is harder to determine because of the small numbers of patients included in individual studies. However, large tumor size,[93] presence of diffuse tumor,[93] extent of initial erythema,[120] extent of erythema after chemotherapy,[120] extent of skin edema,[120] no systemic therapy,[93] no surgical therapy,[93,120] negative estrogen-receptor status,[121] no response to chemotherapy,[120] and extent of residual disease after treatment[120] have been reported to be correlated with lower relapse-free survival rates in univariate analyses. When overall survival was the end point, large tumor size,[95] diffuse type,[95] extent of erythema and edema,[120] N2 or N3 stage,[93,120] no systemic therapy or mastectomy,[93,120] extent of residual tumor,[120] negative estrogen-receptor status,[121] negative progesterone-receptor status,[122] and high labeling index[122] were reported as adverse factors. In multivariate analyses, race,[93] presence of diffuse mass,[93] extent of erythema,[120] lymph node involvement,[120] and no chemotherapy or mastectomy[93] were the only important adverse factors.

DOSE-INTENSIVE THERAPY FOR LOCALLY ADVANCED AND INFLAMMATORY BREAST CANCER

The major obstacle to long-term survival for patients with LABC is the development of distant metastases. Therefore, to improve the effectiveness of treatment, more effective systemic therapies are required. One research approach to improving the efficacy of chemotherapy and the survival of patients with stage III and locally advanced breast cancer is dose intensification of induction chemotherapy or postoperative (postradiotherapy) consolidation treatment. The results of a few small phase II trials that included patients with stage III or inflammatory breast cancer treated with dose-intensive chemotherapy have been encouraging but inconclusive.[123] The maximum follow-up reported in any of these studies was 53 months, and sample sizes were small.[124] The results of two randomized phase II trials comparing standard-dose and high-dose chemotherapy in the context of multidisciplinary management of LABC were reported.[125,126] The risk of recurrence for appropriately treated patients with LABC or inflammatory breast cancer is still very high, and more effective treatments are needed. However, high-dose chemotherapy remains an investigational tool, because its use has not been demonstrated to affect survival in any subgroup of patients with breast cancer.

FUTURE PROSPECTS

New cytotoxic agents with demonstrated antitumor efficacy against metastatic breast cancer have been developed.[127] The taxanes (paclitaxel and docetaxel), the anthrapyrazoles, and vinorelbine tartrate have been reported to be highly effective, with objective responses reported in 50% to 70% of patients, including some with tumors with clear-cut resistance to anthracyclines.[127–129] Gemcitabine hydrochloride, miltefosin, capecitabine, liposomal doxorubicin derivatives, and several antifols have also shown modest activity, in the 20% to 45% range.[127] As they are gradually integrated into multidrug regimens, these new cytotoxic agents are likely to improve the efficacy of breast cancer chemotherapy. A tendency is already seen, although as yet unsupported by clinical trials, to introduce a non–cross-resistant regimen (most often a taxane) into the preoperative or postoperative treatment of patients who have an unsatisfactory response to an induction anthracycline-containing regimen.

Developments are occurring in biological therapy as well. Monoclonal antibodies against breast cancer–related antigens,[130] autocrine or paracrine growth factors, or their receptors[131] are entering clinical trials. Although antibodies alone have not shown major antitumor efficacy, they may function as vehicles to deliver cytotoxic therapy,[132] radioisotopes, or natural toxins (immunoconjugates or immunotoxins). A monoclonal antibody against the extracellular domain of the HER-2 oncoprotein has now been approved by the Food and Drug Administration on the basis of clear-cut antitumor activity in patients with metastatic breast cancer[133] and the potentiation of the efficacy of chemotherapy in a randomized clinical trial.[134]

Recognition of the many remaining questions regarding the optimal sequence of local and systemic treatments in combined-modality therapy prompted the development of clinical trials to assess the relative efficacy of various sequences of administration and to evaluate the efficacy of limited surgery and several modifications of radiotherapy technique to minimize toxicity without compromising outcome.

Combined-modality therapy that includes induction chemotherapy permits optimal local control with less radical surgical and radiotherapeutic intervention. By downstaging primary and regional tumors, such therapy allows breast-conservation treatment to become an option for some patients. In addition, the multidisciplinary management of stage III and locally advanced breast cancer provides an excellent biological model to assess the effects of systemic therapy on the primary tumor. On the clinical side, this provides *in vivo* assessment of response and the possibility of modifying subsequent therapy based on this evaluation of response.

Thus, this subgroup of patients, although receiving what is considered optimal therapy today, provides clear scientific opportunities for optimizing therapies for primary breast cancer.

MANAGEMENT SUMMARY

Combined-modality strategies represent the treatment of choice for patients with locally advanced and inflammatory breast cancer. Effective and well-tolerated strategies are shown in Figures 3 and 4.

Although initial prognostic evaluation is important for the determination of optimal therapy, treatment must be individualized during the course of treatment, depending on response to and tolerance of therapy.

Aggressive induction chemotherapy, careful multimodal evaluation and monitoring, and effective strategies for locoregional control are the key to the success of the overall treatment strategy.

Close and continued interaction between all therapeutic and diagnostic specialists is needed to deliver optimal therapy.

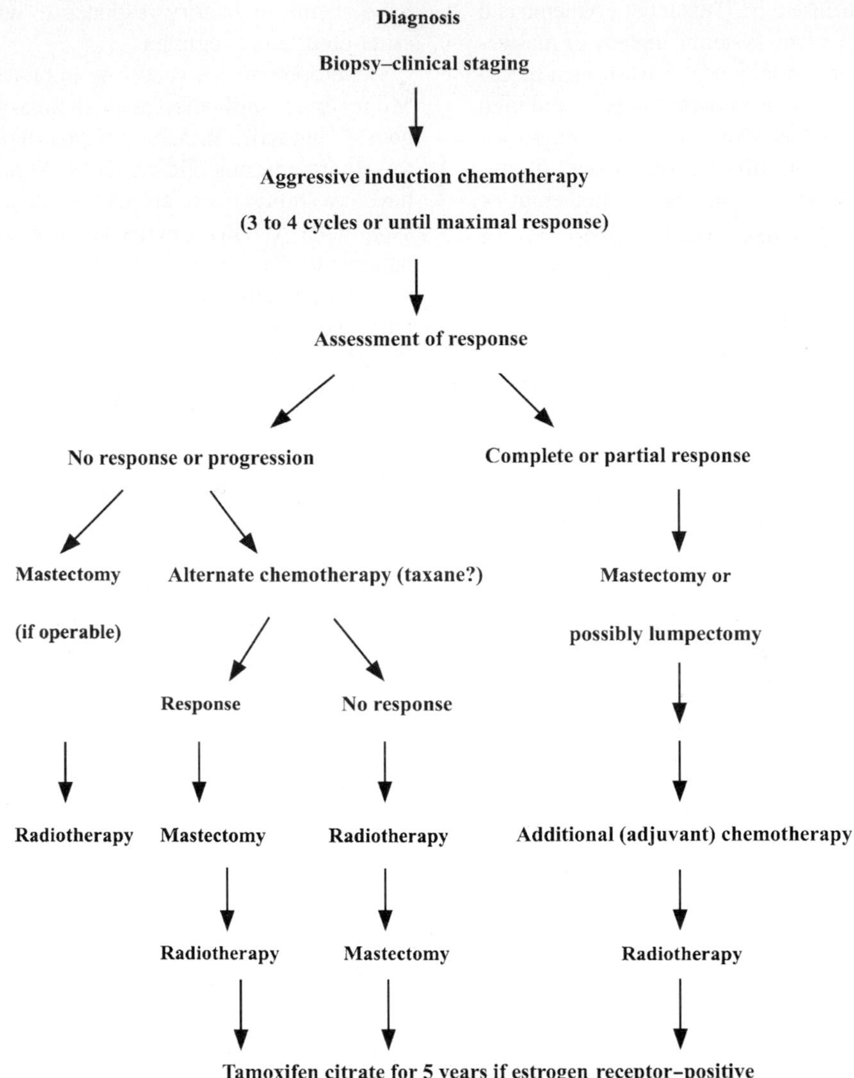

FIG. 3. Flow diagram for the treatment of patients with locally advanced breast cancer.

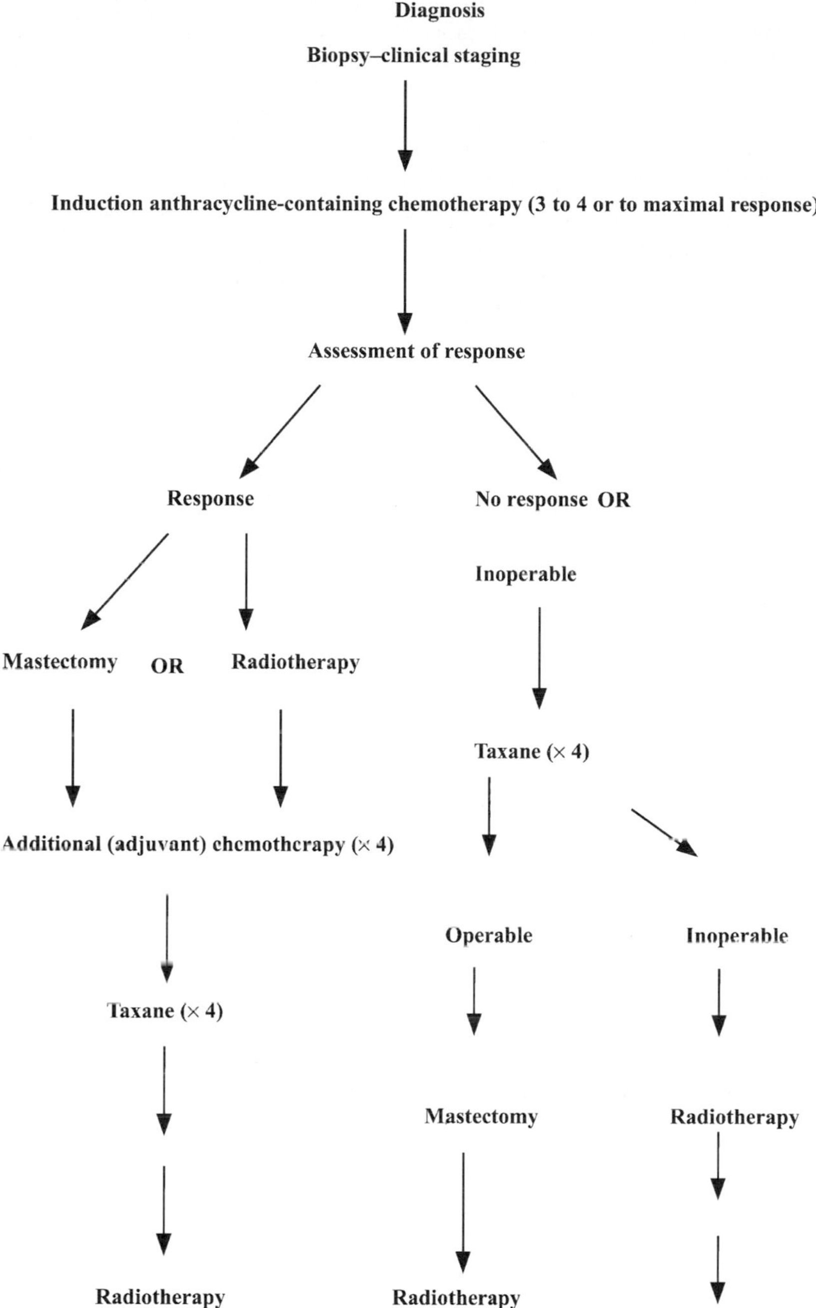

FIG. 4. Flow diagram for the treatment of patients with inflammatory breast cancer.

REFERENCES

1. Seidman H, Gelb SK, Silverberg E, LaVerda N, Lubera JA. Survival experience in the Breast Cancer Detection Demonstration Project. *Cancer J Clinicians* 1987;37:258.
2. Zeichner GI, Mohar BA, Ramirez UMT. Epidemiologia del cancer de mama en el Instituto Nacional de Cancerologia (1989–1990). *Cancerologia* 1993;39:1825.
3. Moisa FC, Lopez J, Raymundo C. Epidemiologia del carcinoma del seno mamario en Latino America. *Cancerologia* 1989;35:810.
4. Anonymous. Breast. In: Fleming ID, Cooper JS, Henson DE, et al, eds. *AJCC cancer staging manual*, 5th ed. Philadelphia: Lippincott–Raven 1997:171.
5. Levine PH, Steinhorn SC, Ries LG, Aron JL. Inflammatory breast cancer: the experience of the Surveillance, Epidemiology, and End Results (SEER) program. *J Natl Cancer Inst* 1985;74:291.
6. Strom EA, McNeese MD, Fletcher GH, Romsdahl MA, Montague ED, Oswald MJ. Results of mastectomy and postoperative irradiation in the management of locoregionally advanced carcinoma of the breast. *Int J Radiat Oncology Biol Phys* 1991;21:319.
7. Hortobagyi GN, Buzdar AU. Locally advanced breast cancer: a review including the M.D. Anderson experience. In: Ragaz J, Ariel IM, eds. *High-risk breast cancer*. Berlin: Springer-Verlag, 1991:382.
8. Early Breast Cancer Trialists' Collaborative Group. Effects of adjuvant tamoxifen and of cytotoxic therapy on mortality in early breast cancer. An overview of 61 randomized trials among 28,896 women. *N Engl J Med* 1988;319:1681.
9. Early Breast Cancer Trialists' Collaborative Group. Polychemotherapy for early breast cancer: an overview of the randomised trials. *Lancet* 1998;352:930.
10. Grohn P, Heinonen E, Klefstrom P, Tarkkanen J. Adjuvant postoperative radiotherapy, chemotherapy, and immunotherapy in stage III breast cancer. *Cancer* 1984;54:670.
11. Bartelink H, Rubens RD, van der Schueren E, Sylvester R. Hormonal therapy prolongs survival in irradiated locally advanced breast cancer: a European Organization for Research and Treatment of Cancer phase III trial. *J Clin Oncol* 1997;15:207.
12. Rivkin SE, Green S, Metch B, et al. Adjuvant CMFVP versus melphalan for operable breast cancer with positive axillary nodes: 10-year results of a Southwest Oncology Group study. *J Clin Oncol* 1989;7:1229.
13. Haagensen CD, Stout AP. Carcinoma of the breast. Criteria of inoperability. *Am Surg* 1943;118:859.
14. Zucali R, Uslenghi C, Kenda R, Bonadonna G. Natural history and survival of inoperable breast cancer treated with radiotherapy and radiotherapy followed by radical mastectomy. *Cancer* 1976;37:1422.
15. Harris JR, Sawicka J, Gelman R, Hellman S. Management of locally advanced carcinoma of the breast by primary radiation therapy. *Int J Radiat Oncol Biol Phys* 1983;9:345.
16. Baclesse F. Roentgen therapy as the sole method of treatment of cancer of the breast. *AJR Am J Roentgenol* 1949;62:311.
17. Fletcher GH, Montague ED. Radical irradiation of advanced breast cancer. *AJR Am J Roentgenol* 1965;93:573.
18. Spanos WJ, Montague ED, Fletcher FH. Late complications of radiation only for advanced breast cancer. *Int J Radiat Oncol Biol Phys* 1980;6:1473.
19. Fisher B, Ravdin RD, Ausman RK, Slack NH, Moore GE, Noer RJ. Surgical adjuvant chemotherapy in cancer of the breast: results of a decade of cooperative investigation. *Ann Surg* 1968;168:337.
20. Kennedy BJ, Kelley RM, White G, Nathanson IT. Surgery as an adjunct to hormone therapy of breast cancer. *Cancer* 1957;10:1055.
21. DeLena M, Zucali R, Viganotti G, Valagussa P, Bonadonna G. Combined chemotherapy-radiotherapy approach in locally advanced (T_{3b}-T_4) breast cancer. *Cancer Chemother Pharmacol* 1978;1:53.
22. Rubens RD, Sexton S, Tong D, Winter PJ, Knight RK, Hayward JL. Combined chemotherapy and radiotherapy for locally advanced breast cancer. *Eur J Cancer* 1980;16:351.
23. Valagussa P, Zambetti M, Bignami PD, et al. T3b-T4 breast cancer: factors affecting results in combined modality treatment. *Clin Exp Metastasis* 1983;1:191.
24. Conte PF, Alama A, Bertelli G, et al. Chemotherapy with estrogenic recruitment and surgery in locally advanced breast cancer: clinical and cytokinetic results. *Int J Cancer* 1987;40:490.
25. Jacquillat C, Baillet F, Weil M, et al. Results of a conservative treatment combining induction (neoadjuvant) and consolidation chemotherapy, hormonotherapy, and external and interstitial irradiation in 98 patients with locally advanced breast cancer (IIIA-IIIB). *Cancer* 1988;61:1977.
26. Swain SM, Sorace RA, Bagley CS, et al. Neoadjuvant chemotherapy in the combined modality approach of locally advanced nonmetastatic breast cancer. *Cancer Res* 1987;47:3889.
27. Pawlicki M, Skolyszewki J, Brandys A. Results of combined treatment of patients with locally advanced breast cancer. *Tumori* 1983;69:249.
28. Balawajder I, Antich PP, Boland J. An analysis of the role of radiotherapy alone and in combination with chemotherapy and surgery in the management of advanced breast cancer. *Cancer* 1983;51:574.
29. Burn I. Primary endocrine therapy of advanced local breast cancer. *Rev Endocrine-related Cancer* 1985;[Suppl]16:5.
30. DeLena M, Varini M, Zucali R, et al. Multimodal treatment for locally advanced breast cancer. Results of chemotherapy-radiotherapy versus chemotherapy-surgery. *Cancer Clin Trials* 1981;4:229.
31. Hortobagyi GN, Blumenschein GR, Spanos W, et al. Multimodal treatment of locoregionally advanced breast cancer. *Cancer* 1983;51:763.
32. Hobar PC, Jones RC, Schouten J, Leitch AM, Hendler F. Multimodality treatment of locally advanced breast carcinoma. *Arch Surg* 1988;123:951.
33. Cocconi G, di Blasio B, Bisagni G, Alberti G, Botti E, Anghinoni E. Neoadjuvant chemotherapy or chemotherapy and endocrine therapy in locally advanced breast carcinoma. *Am J Clin Oncol* 1990;13:226.
34. Perloff M, Lesnick GJ, Korzun A, et al. Combination chemotherapy with mastectomy or radiotherapy for stage III breast carcinoma: a cancer and leukemia group B study. *J Clin Oncol* 1988;6:261.
35. Rosso R, Gardin G, Conte PF, et al. Combined modality approach in locally advanced breast cancer. *Ann Oncol* 1990;1[Suppl]:22a(abst P3:21).
36. Poddubnaya I, Letjagin V, Ognerubov N, Cancer Research Center of RAMS R. Neoadjuvant chemotherapy in the complex treatment of local advanced mammae cancer. Proceedings of the Biennial Meeting of the International Association of Breast Cancer Research, Banff, Canada, April 25–28, 1993;76(abst).
37. Touboul E, Lefranc JP, Blondon J, et al. Multidisciplinary treatment approach to locally advanced noninflammatory breast cancer using chemotherapy and radiotherapy with or without surgery. *Radiother Oncol* 1992;25:167.
38. Hortobagyi GN, Ames FC, Buzdar AU, et al. Management of stage III primary breast cancer with primary chemotherapy, surgery, and radiation therapy. *Cancer* 1988;62:2507.
39. Kemeny F, Vadrot J, d'Hubert E, de Maublanc MA, Collet JF, Misset JL. Evaluation histologique e radioclinique de l'effet de la chimiotherapie premiere sur les cancers non inflammatoires du sein. *Cahiers Cancer* 1991;3:705.
40. Fisher B, Brown A, Mamounas E, et al. Effect of preoperative chemotherapy on local-regional disease in women with operable breast cancer: findings from National Surgical Adjuvant Breast and Bowel Project B-18. *J Clin Oncol* 1997;15:2483.
41. Lippman ME, Sorace RA, Bagley CS, Danforth DW, Lichter A, Wesley MN. Treatment of locally advanced breast cancer using primary induction chemotherapy with hormonal synchronization followed by radiation therapy with or without debulking surgery. *NCI Monogr* 1986;1:153.
42. Schwartz GF, Cantor RI, Biermann WA. Neoadjuvant chemotherapy before definitive treatment for stage III carcinoma of the breast. *Arch Surg* 1987;122:1430.
43. Cocconi G, di Blasio B, Alberti G, Bisagni G, Botti E, Peracchia G. Problems in evaluating response of primary breast cancer to systemic therapy. *Breast Cancer Res Treat* 1984;4:309.
44. Fornage BD, Toubas O, Morel M. Clinical, mammographic, and sonographic determination of preoperative breast cancer size. *Cancer* 1987;60:765.
45. Herrada J, Iyer RB, Atkinson EN, Sneige N, Buzdar AU, Hortobagyi GN. Relative value of physical examination, mammography, and breast sonography in evaluating the size of the primary tumor and regional lymph node metastases in women receiving neoadjuvant chemotherapy for locally advanced breast carcinoma. *Clin Cancer Res* 1997;3:1565.
46. Feldman LD, Hortobagyi GN, Buzdar AU, Ames FC, Blumenschein GR. Pathological assessment of response to induction chemotherapy in breast cancer. *Cancer Res* 1986;46:2578.
47. Rubens RD, Bartelink H, Engelsman E, et al. Locally advanced breast cancer: the contribution of cytotoxic and endocrine treatment to radiotherapy. *Eur J Cancer* 1989;25:667.
48. Hortobagyi GN. Drug therapy: treatment of breast cancer. *N Engl J Med* 1998;339:974.

49. Zucali R, Kenda R. Small size T4 breast cancer: natural history and prognosis. *Tumori* 1981;67:225.
50. Bonadonna G, Veronesi U, Brambilla C, et al. Primary chemotherapy to avoid mastectomy in tumors with diameters of three centimeters or more. *J Natl Cancer Inst* 1990;82:1539.
51. Pouillart P, Palangie T, Jouve M, et al. Essai pilote de chimiotherapie neoadjuvante dans le cancer du sein. In: Jacquillat C, Weil M, Khayat D, eds. *Neo-adjuvant chemotherapy*. Paris: John Libbey, 1986:257.
52. Schaake-Koning C, van der Linden EH, Hart G, Engelsman E. Adjuvant chemo- and hormonal therapy in locally advanced breast cancer: a randomized clinical study. *J Radiat Oncol Biol Phys* 1985;11:1759.
53. Olson JE, Gray R, Sponzo R, Damsker J, Tormey D, Cummings F. Primary chemotherapy for nonresectable locally advanced breast cancer: 8 yr results of an ECOG trial. *Breast Cancer Res Treat* 1990;16:148a(abst 15).
54. Papaioannou A, Lissaios B, Vasilaros S, et al. Pre- and postoperative chemoendocrine treatment with or without postoperative radiotherapy for locally advanced breast cancer. *Cancer* 1983;51:1284.
55. Valagussa P, Zambetti M, Bonadonna G, Zucali R, Mezzanotte G, Veronesi U. Prognostic factors in locally advanced noninflammatory breast cancer. Long-term results following primary chemotherapy. *Breast Cancer Res Treat* 1990;15:137.
56. Aisner J, Morris D, Elias G, Wiernik PH. Mastectomy as an adjuvant to chemotherapy for locally advanced or metastatic breast cancer. *Arch Surg* 1982;117:882.
57. Boyages J, Langlands AO. The efficacy of combined chemotherapy and radiotherapy in advanced non-metastatic breast cancer. *Int J Radiat Oncol Biol Phys* 1987;14:71.
58. Piccart MJ, de Valeriola D, Paridaens R, et al. Six-year results of a multimodality treatment strategy for locally advanced breast cancer. *Cancer* 1988;62:2501.
59. Bedwinek JM, Ratkin GA, Philpott GW, Wallack M, Perez CA. Concurrent chemotherapy and radiotherapy for nonmetastatic, stage IV breast cancer. *Am J Clin Oncol* 1983;6:159.
60. Hery M, Namer M, Moro M, Boublil JL, LaLanne CM. Conservative treatment (chemotherapy/radiotherapy) of locally advanced breast cancer. *Cancer* 1986;57:1744.
61. Singletary SE, McNeese MD, Hortobagyi GN. Feasibility of breast conservation surgery after induction chemotherapy for locally advanced breast carcinoma. *Cancer* 1992;69:2849.
62. Peoples G, Quan R, Heaton K, et al. Breast conservation therapy for large primary and locally advanced breast cancer after induction chemotherapy. *Ann Surg Oncol* 1999 (*in press*).
63. Hunt KK, Singletary SE, Smith TL, et al. Conservation surgery and radiation: the M.D. Anderson Cancer Center experience. In: Bland KI, Copeland EM III, eds. *The breast*, 2nd ed. Philadelphia: WB Saunders, 1998:1179.
64. Scholl SM, Fourquet A, Asselain B, et al. Neoadjuvant versus adjuvant chemotherapy in premenopausal patients with tumors considered too large for breast conserving surgery: preliminary results of a randomised trial: S6. *Eur J Cancer* 1994;30A:645.
65. Mauriac L, Durand M, Avril A, Dilhuydy JM. Effects of primary chemotherapy in conservative treatment of breast cancer patients with operative tumors larger than 3 centimeters: results of a randomized trial in a single center. *Ann Oncol* 1991;2:347.
66. Jacquillat C, Weil M, Baillet F, et al. Results of neoadjuvant chemotherapy and radiation therapy in the breast-conserving treatment of 250 patients with all stages of infiltrative breast cancer. *Cancer* 1990; 66:119.
67. Mauriac L, Durand M, Dilhuydy JM, Avril A, FBBGS. Randomized trial comparing induction chemotherapy to mastectomy for operable breast cancer larger than 3 cm. *Breast Cancer Res Treat* 1992;23:181a(abst 202).
68. Scholl SM, Asselain B, Beuzeboc P, et al. Improved survival rates following first line chemotherapy in operable breast cancer. 4-year results of a randomized trial. *Proc Fourth Int Congress Anticancer Chemother* 1993;64a(abst 27).
69. McCready DR, Hortobagyi GN, Kau SW, Smith TL, Balch CM. The prognostic significance of lymph node metastases after preoperative chemotherapy for locally advanced breast cancer. *Arch Surg* 1989;124:21.
70. Bonnadonna G, Veronesi U, Brambilla C, et al. Primary chemotherapy to avoid mastectomy in tumors with diameters of three centimeters or more. *J Natl Cancer Inst* 1990;82:1539.
71. Schwartz GF, Birchansky CA, Komarnicky LT, et al. Induction chemotherapy followed by breast conservation for locally advanced carcinoma of the breast. *Cancer* 1994;73:362.
72. Kuerer HM, Newman LA, Fornage BD, et al. Role of axillary lymph node dissection after tumor downstaging with induction chemotherapy for locally advanced breast cancer. *Ann Surg Oncol* 1998;5:673.
73. Rahman ZU, Frye DK, Buzdar AU, et al. Impact of selection process on response rate and long-term survival of potential high-dose chemotherapy candidates treated with standard-dose doxorubicin-containing chemotherapy in patients with metastatic breast cancer. *J Clin Oncol* 1997;15:3171.
74. Valero V, Holmes FA, Walters RS, et al. Phase II trial of docetaxel, a new highly effective antineoplastic agent in the management of patients with anthracycline-resistant breast cancer. *J Clin Oncol* 1995; 13:2886.
75. Vermorken JB, ten Bokkel Huinink WW, Mandjes IA, et al. High dose paclitaxel with granulocyte colony-stimulating factor in patients with advanced breast cancer refractory to anthracycline therapy: European cancer center trial. *Semin Oncol* 1995;22[Suppl 8]:16.
76. Dhingra K, Singletary E, Strom E, et al. Randomized trial of G-CSF (Filgrastim)-supported dose-intensive neoadjuvant chemotherapy in locally advanced breast cancer. *Proc Am Soc Clin Oncol* 1995;14:94.
77. Osborne MP, Ormiston N, Harmer OL, McKinna JA, Baker J, Greening WP. Breast conservation in the treatment of early breast cancer: a 20-year follow-up. *Cancer* 1984;53:349.
78. Delouche G, Bachelot F, Premont M, Kurts JM. Conservation treatment of early breast cancer: long term results and complications. *Int J Radiat Oncol Biol Phys* 1987;13:29.
79. Wazer DE, Erban JK, Robert NJ, et al. Breast conservation in elderly women for clinically negative axillary lymph nodes without axillary dissection. *Cancer* 1994;74:878.
80. Early Breast Cancer Trialists' Collaborative Group. Effects of radiotherapy and surgery in early breast cancer. *N Engl J Med* 1995;333:1444.
81. Jaiyesimi IA, Buzdar AU, Hortobagyi G. Inflammatory breast cancer: a review. *J Clin Oncol* 1992;10:1014.
82. Taylor GW, Metzer A. Inflammatory carcinoma of the breast. *Am J Cancer* 1938;33:33.
83. Singletary SE, Ames FC, Buzdar AU. Management of inflammatory breast cancer. *World J Surg* 1994;18:87.
84. Chu AM, Wood WC, Doucette JA. Inflammatory breast carcinoma treated by radical radiotherapy. *Cancer* 1980;45:2730.
85. Pouillart P, Palangie T, Jouve M, et al. Cancer inflammatoire du sein traite par une association de chimiotherapie et d'irradiation: resultats d'un essai randomise etudiant le role d'une immunotherapie par le BCG. *Bull Cancer (Paris)* 1981;68:171.
86. Zylberberg B, SalatBaroux J, Ravina JH, et al. Initial chemoimmunotherapy in inflammatory carcinoma of the breast. *Cancer* 1982;49:1537.
87. Loprinzi CL, Carbone PP, Tormey DC, et al. Aggressive combined modality therapy for advanced local-regional breast carcinoma. *J Clin Oncol* 1984;2:157.
88. Keiling R, Guiochet N, Calderoli H, Hurteloup P, Krzisch C. Preoperative chemotherapy in the treatment of inflammatory breast cancer. In: Wagener DJT, Blijham GH, Smeets JBE, Wils JA, eds. *Primary chemotherapy in cancer medicine*. New York: Alan R. Liss, 1985:95.
89. Rouesse J, Friedman S, Sarrazin D, et al. Primary chemotherapy in the treatment of inflammatory breast carcinoma: a study of 230 cases from the Institut Gustave-Roussy. *J Clin Oncol* 1986;4:1765.
90. Israel L, Breau JL, Morere JF. Neo-adjuvant chemotherapy without radiation therapy in inflammatory breast carcinoma. In: Jacquillat C, Weil M, Khayat D, eds. *Neo-adjuvant chemotherapy*, 169th ed. Paris: John Libbey, 1988:207.
91. Krutchik AN, Buzdar AU, Blumenschein GR, et al. Combined chemoimmunotherapy and radiation therapy of inflammatory breast carcinoma. *J Surg Oncol* 1979;11:325.
92. Thoms WW, McNeese MD, Fletcher GH, Buzdar AU, Singletary SE, Oswald MJ. Multimodal treatment for inflammatory breast cancer. *Int J Radiat Oncol Biol Phys* 1989;17:739.
93. Fields JN, Kuske RR, Perez CA, Fineberg BB, Bartlett N. Prognostic factors in inflammatory breast cancer. *Cancer* 1989;63:1225.
94. Koh EH, Buzdar AU, Ames FC, et al. Inflammatory carcinoma of the breast: results of a combined-modality approach—MD Anderson Cancer Center experience. *Cancer Chemother Pharmacol* 1990;27:94.
95. Fields JN, Perez CA, Kuske RR, et al. Inflammatory carcinoma of the breast: treatment results on 107 patients. *Int J Radiat Oncol Biol Phys* 1989;17:249.
96. Knight CD, Martin JK, Welch JS, et al. Surgical considerations after chemotherapy and radiation therapy for inflammatory breast cancer. *Surgery* 1986;99:385.

97. Hagelberg RS, Jolly PC, Anderson RP. Role of surgery in the treatment of inflammatory breast carcinoma. *Am J Surg* 1984;148:124.
98. Moore MP, Ihde JK, Crowe JP Jr, et al. Inflammatory breast cancer. *Arch Surg* 1991;126:3304.
99. Schafer P, Alberto P, Forni M, Obradovic D, Pipard G, Krauer F. Surgery as part of a combined modality approach for inflammatory breast carcinoma. *Cancer* 1987;59:1063.
100. Brun B, Ottmezguine Y, Feuilhade F, et al. Treatment of inflammatory breast cancer with combination chemotherapy and mastectomy versus breast conservation. *Cancer* 1988;61:1096.
101. Liao Z, Strom EA, Buzdar AU, et al. Locoregional irradiation for inflammatory breast cancer: effectiveness of dose escalation in decreasing recurrences. *Int J Radiat Oncol Biol Phys* 1997;39:262.
102. Fleming RY, Asmar L, Buzdar AU, et al. Effectiveness of mastectomy by response to induction chemotherapy for control in inflammatory breast carcinoma. *Ann Surg Oncol* 1997;4:452.
103. Barker JL, Montague ED, Peters LJ. Clinical experience with irradiation of inflammatory carcinoma of the breast with and without elective chemotherapy. *Cancer* 1981;45:625.
104. Broadwater JR, Edwards MJ, Kuglen C, Hortobagyi GN, Ames FC, Balch CM. Mastectomy following preoperative chemotherapy. *Ann Surg* 1991;213:126.
105. Bedwinek JM, Ratkin GA, Philpott GW, Wallack M, Perez CA. Concurrent chemotherapy and radiotherapy for nonmetastatic, stage IV breast cancer. A pilot study by the Southeastern Cancer Study Group. *Am J Clin Oncol* 1983;6:159.
106. Recht A, Come SE. Sequencing of irradiation and chemotherapy for early-stage breast cancer. *Oncology* 1994;8:19.
107. Buzzoni R, Bonadonna G, Valagussa P, Zambetti M. Adjuvant chemotherapy with doxorubicin plus cyclophosphamide, methotrexate, and fluorouracil in the treatment of resectable breast cancer with more than three positive nodes. *J Clin Oncol* 1991;9:2134.
108. Valagussa P, Moliterni A, Zambetti M, Bonadonna G. Long-term sequelae from adjuvant chemotherapy. In: Senn HJ, Goldhirsch A, Gelber RD, Thurlimann B, eds. *Adjuvant therapy of breast cancer IV. Papers stemming from the 4th International Conference on Adjuvant Therapy of Primary Breast Cancer held in St. Gallen, Switzerland in 1992*, 127th ed. Berlin: Springer-Verlag, 1993:248.
109. Hortobagyi GN, Frye D, Buzdar AU, et al. Decreased cardiac toxicity of doxorubicin administered by continuous intravenous infusion in combination chemotherapy for metastatic breast cancer. *Cancer* 1989;63:37.
110. Arbeitskreis RH for Perioperative Chemotherapie. Prospective randomized clinical trial of primary therapy in breast cancer stages T3/4, N+/–, M0 chemo versus radiotherapy. In: Salmon SE, ed. *Adjuvant therapy of cancer VI*. Philadelphia: WB Saunders, 1990:232.
111. Caceres E, Zaharia M, Lingan M, Valdivia S, Moran M, Tejada F. Combined therapy of stage III adenocarcinoma of the breast. *Proc Am Assoc Cancer Res* 1980;21:199a(abst 798).
112. Fisher B, Bryant J, Wolmark N, et al. Effect of preoperative chemotherapy on the outcome of women with operable breast cancer. *J Clin Oncol* 1998;16:2672.
113. Stewart JH, King RJB, Winter PJ, Tong D, Hayward JL, Rubens RD. Oestrogen receptors, clinical features and prognosis in stage III breast cancer. *Eur J Cancer Clin Oncol* 1982;18:1315.
114. Fourquet A, Vilcoq JR, Julien D, Calle R, Ghossein NA. The Prognostic significance of initial nodal involvement in patients with locally advanced breast cancer treated by radical radiotherapy. *Am J Clin Oncol* 1984;7:118a(abst).
115. Jacquillat C, Weil M, Auclerc G, et al. Neo-adjuvant chemotherapy in the conservative management of breast cancers—study on 205 patients. In: Jacquillat C, Weil M, Khayat D, eds. *Neo-adjuvant chemotherapy*. London: John Libbey, 1986:197.
116. AbuFarsakh H, Sneige N, Atkinson N, Hortobagyi G. Pathologic predictors of tumor response to preoperative chemotherapy in patients with locally advanced breast carcinoma. *Breast J* 1995;1:96.
117. Belembaogo E, Feillel V, Chollet P, et al. Neoadjuvant chemotherapy in 126 operable breast cancers. *Eur J Cancer* 1992;28A:896.
118. Spyratos F, Brifford M, Tubiana-Hulin M, et al. Sequential cytopunctures during preoperative chemotherapy for primary breast carcinoma. *Cancer* 1992;69:470.
119. Remvikos Y, Jouve M, Beuzeboc P, Viehl P, Magdalenat H, Pouillart P. Cell cycle modifications of breast cancers during neoadjuvant chemotherapy: a flow cytometry study on fine needle aspirates. *Eur J Cancer* 1995;29A:1843.
120. Chevallier B, Asselain B, Kunlin A, Veyret C, Bastit P, Graic Y. Inflammatory breast cancer—determination of prognostic factors by univariate and multivariate analysis. *Cancer* 1987;60:897.
121. Delarue JC, May-Levin F, Mouriesse H, Contesso G, Sancho-Garnier H. Oestrogen and progesterone cytosolic receptors in clinically inflammatory tumours of the human breast. *Br J Cancer* 1981;44:911.
122. Paradiso A, Tommasi S, Brandi M, et al. Cell kinetics and hormonal receptor status in inflammatory breast carcinoma. *Cancer* 1989; 64:1922.
123. Antman KH. Dose-intensive therapy in breast cancer. In: Armitage JO, Antman KH, eds. *High-dose cancer therapy*. Baltimore: Williams & Wilkins, 1992:701.
124. Ayash LJ, Elias A, Ibrahim J, et al. High-dose multimodality therapy with autologous stem-cell support for stage IIIB breast carcinoma. *J Clin Oncol* 1998;16:1000.
125. Rodenhuis S, Richel DJ, van der Wall E, et al. Randomised trial of high-dose chemotherapy and haemopoietic progenitor-stem cell support in operable breast cancer with extensive axillary lymph node involvement. *Lancet* 1998;352:515.
126. Hortobagyi GN, Buzdar AU, Champlin R, et al. Lack of efficacy of adjuvant high-dose tandem combination chemotherapy for high-risk primary breast cancer—a randomized trial. *Proc Am Soc Clin Oncol* 1998;17:123a(abst 471).
127. Hortobagyi GN. Overview of new treatments for breast cancer. *Breast Cancer Res Treat* 1992;21:3.
128. Holmes FA, Walters RS, Theriault RL, et al. Phase II trial of Taxol, an active drug in the treatment of metastatic breast cancer. *J Natl Cancer Inst* 1991;83:1797.
129. Pazdur R, Kudelka AP, Kavanagh JJ, Cohen PR, Raber MN. The taxoids: paclitaxel (TAXOL) and docetaxel (Taxotere). *Cancer Treat Rev* 1993;19:351.
130. Goodman GE, Hellstrom I, Brodzinsky L, et al. Phase I trial of murine monoclonal antibody L6 in breast, colon, ovarian, and lung cancer. *J Clin Oncol* 1990;8:1083.
131. Baselga J, Norton L, Masui H, et al. Antitumor effects of doxorubicin in combination with antiepidermal growth factor receptor monoclonal antibodies. *J Natl Cancer Inst* 1993;85:1327.
132. Trail PA, Willner SJ, Lasch AJ, et al. Cure of xenografted human carcinomas by BR96-doxorubicin immunoconjugates. *Science* 1993;261:212.
133. Baselga J, Tripathy D, Mendelsohn J, et al. Phase II study of weekly intravenous recombinant humanized anti-p185HER2 monoclonal antibody in patients with HER2/neu-overexpressing metastatic breast cancer [See comments]. *J Clin Oncol* 1996;14:737.
134. Slamon D, Leyland-Jones B, Shak S, et al. Addition of Herceptin (humanized anti-HER2 antibody) to first line chemotherapy for HER2 overexpressing metastatic breast cancer markedly increases anticancer activity: a randomized, multinational controlled phase III trial. *Proc Am Soc Clin Oncol* 1998;17:98a(abst 377).
135. Alberto P, Schafer P, Mermillod B, et al. Traitement combine des cancers inflammatoires du sein par chimiotherapie suivie de chirurgie et de radiotherapie. In: Jacquillat C, Weil M, Khayat D, eds. *Neo-adjuvant chemotherapy*. London: John Libbey, 1986:237.
136. Ferriere JP, Bignon YJ, Legros M, et al. Resultats du traitement des cancers inflammatoires du sein par une association therapeutique comportant une chimiotherapie initiale. In: Jacquillat C, Weil M, Khayat D, eds. *Neo-adjuvant chemotherapy*. London: John Libbey, 1986:271.
137. Pourny C, Nguyen TD, Nzengu B, Cattan A. Traitements par chimiotherapie premiere de cancers du sein MO, localement avances (T3T4) ou s'accompagnant de signes inflammatoires locaux. In: Jacquillat C, Weil M, Khayat D, eds. *Neo-adjuvant chemotherapy*. London: John Libbey, 1986:293.
138. Chevallier B, Bastit P, Graic Y, et al. The centre H. Becquerel studies in inflammatory non-metastatic breast cancer. Combined modality approach in 178 patients. *Br J Cancer* 1993;67:594.
139. Maloisel F, Dufour P, Bergerat JP, et al. Results of initial doxorubicin, 5-fluorouracil, and cyclophosphamide combination chemotherapy for inflammatory carcinoma of the breast. *Cancer* 1990;65:851.

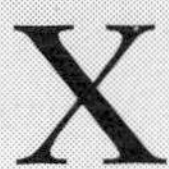

X

Diseases of the Breast, 2nd ed.,
edited by Jay R. Harris.
Lippincott Williams & Wilkins, Philadelphia © 2000.

Special Therapeutic Problems

CHAPTER 40

Male Breast Cancer

William J. Gradishar

EPIDEMIOLOGY

Male breast cancer (MBC) is a rare disease in all parts of the world. In the United States, in 1998, approximately 1,600 new cases of MBC were diagnosed and 400 deaths occurred as a result of MBC.[1]

MBC accounts for approximately 1% of all breast cancers and fewer than 1% of all annual cancer deaths in males. The overall ratio of female breast cancer to MBC in most white Western populations is 100 to 1; however, in the U.S. African-American population, the female-male ratio of breast cancer is 100 to 1.4.[2] Limited registry data from black African populations suggest a lower female-male ratio of 100 to 6 in a narrow geographic band stretching across Africa from Angola to Tanzania.[3] The incidence rate of MBC in nearly all populations for which data are available is on the order of 1 case per 100,000 human-years or less.[4] Muir et al.[4] report that the highest incidence rate for MBC was 3.4 cases per 100,000 human-years in Recife, Brazil, whereas incidence rates of 0.1 cases per 100,000 have been reported in parts of Colombia, Singapore, Hungary, and Japan. An analysis of death certification rates for MBC in the United States and Europe suggests no evidence for an increase in the disease since the 1960s.[5,6] In contrast, an increase in incidence rates of female breast cancer in both the United States and European countries has been observed over the same time period and may reflect the effect of widespread mammography screening in women or a change in risk factors that are specific to women, or both.[7]

Although MBC has been described in children as young as 5 years old,[8] most large series report a median age of onset between 65 and 67 years, which is approximately 10 years later than for female breast cancer.[7] Sasco et al.,[2] in a meta-analysis of case control studies, found that the risk of developing MBC was elevated in men with the following characteristics: never married, Jewish descent, previous benign breast disease, gynecomastia, history of testicular pathology or liver disease, a family history of breast cancer, and prior chest wall irradiation.

Several of the risk factors detected by epidemiology studies suggest that some cases of MBC may be caused by conditions that result in relative estrogen excess or lack of androgen.[2,7] Cases of MBC have been described in patients

W. J. Gradishar: Breast Medical Oncology, Robert H. Lurie Comprehensive Cancer Center, Northwestern University Medical School, Chicago, Illinois

with a prior history of orchitis, undescended testes, and testicular injury.[7,9–11] Although the association between these conditions and the development of MBC suggests that hormonal abnormalities may play a causative role, it remains uncertain whether testosterone levels are actually abnormal at the time of diagnosis.[12]

The strongest risk factor for developing MBC is Klinefelter's syndrome, a rare condition that results from the inheritance of an additional X chromosome.[7,13–15] Men with this condition have atrophic testes, gynecomastia, high levels of gonadotropins (follicle-stimulating hormone, luteinizing hormone), and low plasma levels of testosterone. The effect is a high estrogen-testosterone ratio. Men with this condition are usually exposed to this aberrant hormonal milieu for decades before breast cancer arises. The risk of MBC in these individuals is up to 50 times higher than for men with a normal genotype.[7]

In men with chronic liver disorders, such as cirrhosis,[16–18] chronic alcoholism,[11] and schistosomiasis,[19,20] the risk of MBC may be increased. Individuals with cirrhosis have an impaired ability to metabolize endogenously produced estrogen, resulting in a relative hyperestrogenic state (e.g., increased estrogen-testosterone ratio). In addition, several studies suggest that women who consume more than moderate amounts of ethanol may be at increased risk of developing breast cancer. Ethanol is a metabolic modifier for mammary epithelium and may promote the most carcinogenic pathway of estradiol metabolism to catechol estrogen. However, most patients with cirrhosis have a relatively short life span compared to individuals with Klinefelter's syndrome, perhaps accounting for the relatively few cases of MBC described in patients with cirrhosis and chronic alcoholism.

Gynecomastia and drugs that cause it (i.e., digoxin, thioridazine, etc.) have been associated with an increased risk of MBC.[7,10] MBC has been described in three men who were prescribed finasteride (Proscar), a drug approved for the treatment of prostatic hyperplasia.[21] Gynecomastia, which has been the most common side effect associated with the use of finasteride, is caused by an increased estrogen-testosterone ratio. Other conditions, such as obesity, thyroid disease, use of marijuana, and exogenous estrogen ingestion (i.e., transsexuals, treatment of prostate cancer) in which either an increased estrogen-testosterone ratio or an association with gynecomastia, or both, is present, have a more tenuous relationship to MBC.[7,10]

Prolactin can act as an initiator and promoter of cancer in animal experiments; however, physiologic states of prolactin excess, such as multiple pregnancies, do not increase the risk of breast cancer in women but may actually be protective. Several case reports[22–24] have described the development of MBC in association with a prolactinoma, a setting in which low plasma testosterone levels are frequently observed. Whether prolactin excess is actually a risk factor for the development of MBC remains unclear.

Androgens may convey a protective effect on breast tissue by inhibiting cell proliferation. Mutations in the androgen receptor (AR) gene have been implicated as playing a role in the development of MBC in two reports.[25,26] These mutations occurred in the DNA-binding domain, in two adjacent amino acid positions in the second zinc-finger, believed to be an area responsible for transcriptional control. More recently, in 1996, tumor material from 11 MBC patients without clinical evidence for androgen insensitivity was carefully analyzed and found to have no evidence for AR gene mutations.[27]

Approximately 5% to 10% of all breast cancer is thought to have a genetic predisposition. The recently identified breast/ovarian cancer genes BRCA1 and BRCA2 are estimated to account for 80% of multiple-case breast cancer families with an autosomal dominant pattern of inheritance.[28–31] Limited evidence exists supporting a link between BRCA1 germ-line mutations and the risk of developing MBC. One Dutch and one American BRCA1 family, each with multiple associated female breast cancer cases, had one associated case of MBC.[32,33]

In women who carry a BRCA1 or BRCA2 mutation, the lifetime risk of developing breast cancer approaches 85%, and men who carry a BRCA2 mutation are believed to have an increased risk of developing breast cancer.[28,29] In a report by Couch et al.,[34] 50 MBC cases were analyzed for BRCA2 germ-line mutations, but the mutation was detected in only 14% of patients, 85% of whom (6/7) had a family history of male or female breast cancer. Similarly, Friedman et al.[35] report on a population-based series of 54 MBC cases that were analyzed for germ-line mutations in BRCA1 and BRCA2. Nine of the patients (17%) had a family history of breast or ovarian cancer, or both, in at least one first-degree relative. No BRCA1 germ-line mutations were detected, and only two patients (4%) were found to have BRCA2 germ-line mutations. Only one of the two patients with a BRCA2 mutation had a family history of cancer, with one case of ovarian cancer in a first-degree relative. The possibility that BRCA2 mutation carriers may not manifest the cancer phenotype (e.g., variable penetrance) is also suggested from the report on Icelandic populations, in which 3 of 12 patients with MBC who carry the same BRCA2 mutations have no family history of breast cancer.[36] Alternatively, the MBC cases with an associated family history of breast or ovarian cancer, or both, that do not carry a BRCA2 mutation may be explained by insensitive mutation screening techniques, chance clustering due to the high frequency of sporadic female breast cancer in the general population, or other inherited breast cancer susceptibility genes that have yet to be characterized.

CLINICAL FEATURES

The majority of rudimentary breast tissue in males is located in the subareolar area. As a result, MBC typically presents as a painless, firm subareolar mass. A mass in the upper outer quadrant is the second most common presentation. There is a slight predilection for the left breast in multiple series, and bilateral breast cancer is distinctly unusual

(<1%).[37] Nipple discharge is an unusual presentation of the disease; however, serosanguineous or bloody discharge is frequently associated with an underlying cancer. Other findings at presentation include nipple retraction, ulceration of the nipple or skin, fixation to skin or muscle, tumor tenderness, and enlarged axillary adenopathy.[37]

The differential diagnosis of a breast mass in men should include gynecomastia, breast abscess, metastases to the breast, and malignancies such as sarcomas that are not related to breast cancer. Gynecomastia is common, occurring in up to 40% of men without MBC and an equal fraction of MBC tumor specimens.[38,39] Gynecomastia presents as either unilateral or bilateral symmetric enlargement of the breast with poorly defined borders. Mammography criteria can usually distinguish between malignancy and gynecomastia.[40] Radiologic features of malignancy include a well-defined mass eccentric to the nipple, spiculated margins, and, occasionally, microcalcifications. Gynecomastia typically appears as a round or triangular area of increased density positioned symmetrically in the retroareolar region. Although small series have shown that mammography can detect abnormalities in 80% to 90% of patients with MBC,[39,41] tumors may not appear on mammograms or may be obscured by associated gynecomastia.[42] Due to the low incidence of MBC in all populations, there is no role for screening mammography.

DIAGNOSIS

Once a suspicious breast mass has been identified, tissue confirmation of the diagnosis is mandatory. In centers with an experienced cytopathologist, fine-needle aspiration (FNA) can be performed. A 1998 report suggested that mammography added no additional diagnostic information to the combination of physical examination and FNA.[43] Compared with routine open biopsy, the combination of physical examination and FNA avoided surgical biopsy in 59% of cases. The efficacy of FNA in diagnosing MBC is difficult to establish due to the small number of cases described in each report. However, if inadequate tissue is obtained or if it is not feasible to perform FNA, a core biopsy or an open biopsy should be performed. An adequate tissue sample is important for establishing the diagnosis and for performing estrogen and progesterone receptor assays.

PATHOLOGY

The most common histopathologic type of MBC is invasive ductal carcinoma, which accounts for up to 85% of cases.[44–48] In most series, lobular carcinoma is rare or has not been reported, in contrast to female breast cancer, in which lobular carcinoma accounts for up to 15% of cases.[49,50] The rarity of lobular carcinoma in males is thought to be due to the lack of acini and lobules in normal male breast tissue. The male breast can be induced to resemble the female breast, with the development of true acini and lobules, after exposure to estrogenic stimulation (i.e., treatment for prostate cancer and Klinefelter's syndrome). Ductal carcinoma *in situ* accounts for 20% to 25% of all cases of female breast cancer. In contrast, the frequency of ductal carcinoma *in situ* in men ranges from 0 to 17%, with an average of 7%.[51] Lobular carcinoma *in situ* has been reported in a phenotypically and genotypically normal male.[52] Paget's disease of the breast accounts for 1% to 5% of all female breast tumors, but only 32 cases of Paget's disease of the male breast have been described. All other subtypes of breast cancer have been reported in men.[53]

In females with breast cancer, tumors are estrogen receptor (ER) positive or progesterone positive, or both, in 60% to 70% of cases. In contrast, series of MBC in which steroid hormone receptors have been evaluated report that up to 91% of tumors are ER positive, and 96% are progesterone positive.[37,54]

Limited information is available regarding other molecular markers in MBC. In a series of 111 MBC patients from the Mayo Clinic, tumor samples were analyzed for AR, the protooncogenes p53 and HER-2, cell cycle regulatory proteins cyclin D_1 and MIB1, and the marker of apoptosis bcl-2.[54] AR was positive in 95% of cases, a finding consistent with other reports. Bcl-2 expression in female breast cancer has been associated with expression of ER. Bcl-2 was expressed in 95% of MBC cases. HER-2 is overexpressed in approximately 30% of female breast cancer cases, and in the Mayo series it was positive in 29% of MBC cases. Cyclin D_1 complexes with cyclin-dependent kinases that bind and phosphorylate the retinoblastoma gene protein and are the rate-limiting step for cell entry into S phase. In female breast cancer approximately 50% of tumors overexpress cyclin D_1, similar to 58% of MBC samples. MIB1 is an antibody directed against Ki67, a proliferation-associated antigen. Thirty-eight percent of MBC samples were found to be MIB1 positive. p53 was positive in 21% of MBC cases, somewhat lower than other reports in which up to 54% of samples are p53 positive.[54]

TREATMENT: SURGICAL MANAGEMENT

The traditional surgical approach for localized disease had been radical mastectomy, but with clinical trials in female breast cancer showing no improvement in outcome for patients treated with radical mastectomy compared to modified radical mastectomy, the latter has become the standard treatment in men. Rarely, patients with extensive chest wall muscle involvement or involvement of Rotter's nodes may benefit from radical mastectomy.[39] Although breast conservation (lumpectomy and breast irradiation) should be strongly considered in women with early-stage breast cancer, breast-conserving therapy is not an option in men because of the lack of breast tissue and the central location of most tumors.

PROGNOSTIC FACTORS

MBC and female breast cancer are staged according to the American Joint Committee Clinical Staging System. Similar to women with breast cancer, stage, tumor size, and axillary lymph node status appear to be the most important factors influencing outcome. Guinee et al.[55] report on 335 MBC cases registered over a 20-year period. The survival rate at 10 years was 84% for patients with histologically negative nodes, 44% for those with one to three positive nodes, and 14% for the group with four or more histologically positive nodes. Joshi and Pande[45] report on 42 well-characterized patients with invasive MBC. Analysis of adjusted survival by stage revealed a 5-year survival of 100% for stage I patients, 83% for stage II patients, 60% for stage III patients, and 25% for stage IV patients. Patients with axillary nodal involvement had a decreased 10-year adjusted and disease-free survival compared to patients without axillary nodal involvement (36% versus 58%, 18% versus 44%, respectively). Donegan et al. reported on 217 MBC cases accessioned from tumor registries at 18 institutions in Wisconsin between 1953 and 1995. Consistent with other reports, 5-year survival declined with increasing stage of disease and increasing number of involved axillary lymph nodes. Donegan et al.[46] also found that since 1986, patients have presented with earlier-stage disease and have been more likely to be treated with modified radical mastectomy and adjuvant systemic therapy. These changes compared to earlier times coincided with an improved 5-year survival. Other series have reported similar findings.[41,47,48,56–60]

The usefulness of other prognostic factors in MBC is questionable, because the disease is rare and none of the clinical series were large enough or designed prospectively to evaluate a specific molecular or pathologic marker. Although many reports describe various molecular markers in MBC (i.e., DNA ploidy, nuclear differentiation, MIB1 positivity, cathepsin D, HER-2, etc.), their correlation with prognosis has not been confirmed.[54,61,62]

Although some reports have suggested that MBC has a poorer prognosis than breast cancer occurring in women, most recent reports carefully matched for stage do not substantiate a difference in outcome between genders.[63,64]

TREATMENT OF METASTATIC DISEASE

Hormonal manipulation has played an important role in the management of metastatic MBC because bilateral orchiectomy was reported to impact on disease progression in 1942.[65] Multiple reports of orchiectomy as treatment of metastatic MBC indicate response rates between 32% and 67%, with a median survival of 56 months in responding patients versus 38 months in nonresponding patients.[37] Other ablative surgical procedures have been evaluated in metastatic MBC either as primary treatment or at the time of disease progression after orchiectomy. Adrenalectomy and hypophysectomy are associated with response rates of 76% and 58%, respectively.[37] Due to the unwillingness of many men to accept orchiectomy for psychological reasons, the morbidity associated with ablative surgical procedures, and the introduction of medical management of metastatic disease, these surgical procedures are rarely used today.

Because the majority of breast cancers in men express ER, tamoxifen is the endocrine treatment of choice for metastatic disease. Objective response rates as high as 81% have been reported in ER-positive MBC treated with tamoxifen.[66] Other endocrine therapies have also been evaluated in metastatic MBC, including aminoglutethimide, estrogen, megestrol acetate, androgens, steroids, and luteinizing hormone–releasing hormone analogues. In most reports clinical information is limited, but response rates in excess of 40% are observed in ER-positive tumors.[66] Alternative endocrine therapy can be considered in men with ER-positive tumors who develop disease progression after treatment with tamoxifen and who do not have life-threatening visceral disease.

Chemotherapy should be considered for patients with ER-negative tumors or for those with rapidly progressing disease. Numerous anecdotal reports have appeared in the medical literature describing the activity of single-agent chemotherapy or combination chemotherapy regimens in MBC.[66] Although the optimal chemotherapy regimen has not been defined for MBC, treatment guidelines used for women are reasonable considerations in men.

ADJUVANT SYSTEMIC THERAPY

A recommendation for adjuvant endocrine or chemotherapy, or both, is based largely on the benefits of this therapy that have been observed in clinical trials in women with early-stage breast cancer. The low incidence of MBC precludes the development and timely completion of clinical trials to assess the efficacy of adjuvant therapy.

Because the majority of MBC patients have ER-positive tumors, adjuvant tamoxifen therapy for 5 years is frequently recommended. Ribeiro and Swindell[67] report improved 5-year actuarial survival and disease-free survival in 39 patients who received tamoxifen compared to a historical control group (61% versus 44% and 56% versus 28%, respectively). Tamoxifen is generally well tolerated, but a 1994 report described the side effects experienced by 24 patients who received adjuvant tamoxifen.[68] The most common side effects were decreased libido (29%), weight gain (25%), hot flashes (21%), mood alteration (21%), and depression (17%). In addition, 21% of patients discontinued tamoxifen because of side effects; the attrition was 4% in women who received adjuvant tamoxifen.

There are a similar lack of data for the benefit of adjuvant chemotherapy in MBC. Patel et al.[69] report on 11 stage II/III patients who were treated with adjuvant CMF (cyclophosphamide, methotrexate, and 5-fluorouracil) after local therapy. Compared to the untreated historical control group, adjuvant CMF appeared to favorably influence the risk of

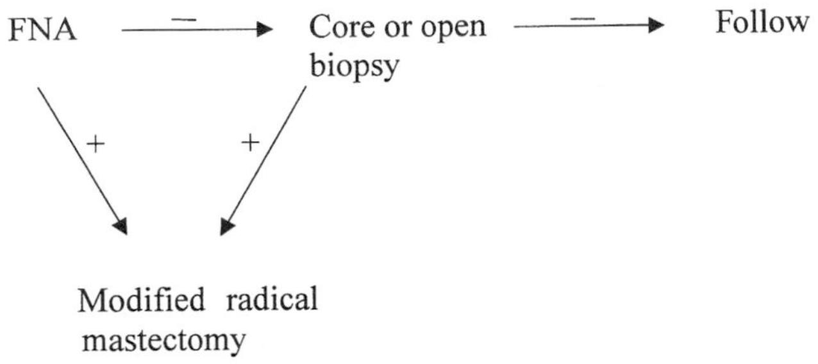

FIG. 1. Management summary. FNA, fine-needle aspiration; –, no cancer cells; +, positive cancer cells.

recurrence and survival. At the National Cancer Institute, 24 patients with axillary node–positive, stage II MBC were treated with adjuvant CMF chemotherapy for up to 12 cycles.[70] Only 17 of 24 patients were able to complete all 12 cycles of therapy, but the 5-year survival of more than 80% and median overall survival of 98 months for treated patients suggested a benefit from adjuvant chemotherapy compared to the historical control group. Recommendations for adjuvant therapy that have been adopted for women with early-stage breast cancer would generally be a rational consideration for patients with early-stage MBC.

ADJUVANT RADIATION THERAPY

No prospective, randomized clinical trials are available that evaluate the clinical impact of postoperative, adjuvant radiation therapy. In several series, postoperative radiation therapy was administered to some patients, but the technical aspects of radiotherapy varied between series and over time, making any assessment of clinical impact difficult. Postmastectomy radiation therapy for MBC appears to reduce local-regional recurrence but has had no apparent impact on overall survival.[46,71,72] However, the publications of two clinical trials showing a survival advantage for women with stage II breast cancer who received postmastectomy radiation therapy may be applicable to similar patients with MBC.[73,74]

MANAGEMENT SUMMARY

A suspicious breast mass in a man must be evaluated by obtaining an adequate tissue sample with FNA or biopsy (Fig. 1). If invasive cancer is detected, definitive local therapy is a modified radical mastectomy. As in women, chest wall and regional lymph node irradiation can be considered after mastectomy for men determined to be at high risk of relapse due to axillary lymph node involvement or the presence of features of locally advanced disease, or both.

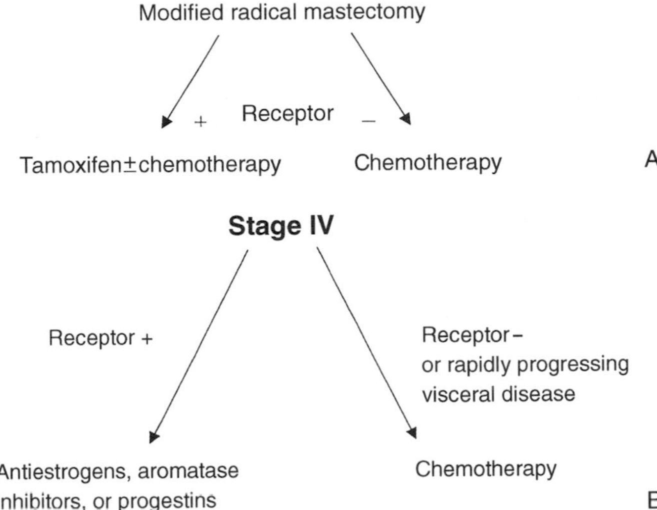

FIG. 2. A: Stage I, II, and III. Radiation therapy to the chest wall and regional nodes should be considered for stages II and III. **B:** Stage IV.

Adjuvant therapy recommendations are similar to those in women with the same stage of disease (Fig. 2A). For patients with tumors that express steroid hormone receptors, adjuvant tamoxifen with or without chemotherapy should be recommended. For patients with hormone receptor–negative disease, chemotherapy should be recommended. For metastatic disease (Fig. 2B), chemotherapy should be recommended to patients with rapidly progressing disease or hormone receptor–negative disease, or both. Antiestrogens, aromatase inhibitors, and progestins can be considered for patients with hormone receptor–positive disease.

REFERENCES

1. Landis SH, Murray T, Bolden S, Wingo PA. Cancer statistics, 1998. *CA Cancer J Clin* 1998;48:6.
2. Sasco AJ, Lowenfels AB, Pasker-de Jong P. Review article: epidemiology of male breast cancer. A meta-analysis of published case-control studies and discussion of selected etiological factors. *Int J Cancer* 1993;53:538.
3. Parkin DM, Cancer occurrence in developing countries. *IARC scientific publications 75.* Lyon: International Agency for Research on Cancer, 1986.
4. Muir C, Waterhouse J, Mack T, Powell J, Whelan S. *Cancer incidence in five continents*, vol 5. IARC Scientific Publications. Lyon: International Agency for Research on Cancer, 1987:882.
5. La Vecchia C, Levi F, Lucchini F. Descriptive epidemiology of male breast cancer in Europe. *Int J Cancer* 1992;51:62.
6. La Vecchia C, Lucchini F, Negri E, Boyle P, Maisonneuve P, Levi F. Trends of cancer mortality in Europe, 1955–1989: III, Breast and genital sites. *Eur J Cancer* 1992:927.
7. Thomas DB. Breast cancer in men. *Epidemiol Rev* 1993;15:220.
8. Simpson JS, Barson AJ. Breast tumours in infants and children: a 40-year review of cases at a children's hospital. *Can Med Assoc J* 1969; 101:100.
9. Mabuchi K, Bross DS, Kessler, II. Risk factors for male breast cancer. *J Natl Cancer Inst* 1985;74:371.

10. Thomas DB, Jimenez LM, McTiernan A, et al. Breast cancer in men: risk factors with hormonal implications. *Am J Epidemiol* 1992; 135:734.
11. Olsson H, Ranstam J. Head trauma and exposure to prolactin-elevating drugs as risk factors for male breast cancer. *J Natl Cancer Inst* 1988;80:679.
12. Ballerini P, Recchione C, Cavalleri A, Moneta R, Saccozzi R, Secreto G. Hormones in male breast cancer. *Tumori* 1990;76:26.
13. Harnden DG, Maclean N, Langlands AO. Carcinoma of the breast and Klinefelter's syndrome. *J Med Genet* 1971;8:460.
14. Scheike O, Visfeldt J, Petersen B. Male breast cancer. 3. Breast carcinoma in association with the Klinefelter syndrome. *Acta Pathol Microbiol Scand* [A] 1973;81:352.
15. Hultborn R, Hanson C, Kopf I, Verbiene I, Warnhammar E, Weimarck A. Prevalence of Klinefelter's syndrome in male breast cancer patients. *Anticancer Res* 1997;17:4293.
16. Lenfant-Pejovic MH, Mlika-Cabanne N, Bouchardy C, Auquier A. Risk factors for male breast cancer: a Franco-Swiss case-control study. *Int J Cancer* 1990;45:661.
17. Misra SP, Misra V, Dwivedi M. Cancer of the breast in a male cirrhotic: Is there an association between the two? *Am J Gastroenterol* 1996;91:380.
18. Sorensen HT, Friis S, Olsen JH, et al. Risk of breast cancer in men with liver cirrhosis. *Am J Gastroenterol* 1998;93:231.
19. El-Gazayerli MM, Abdel-Aziz AS. On bilharziasis and male breast cancer in Egypt: a preliminary report and review of the literature. *Br J Cancer* 1964;17:566.
20. Bhagwandeen SB. Carcinoma of the male breast in Zambia. *East Afr Med J* 1972;49:89.
21. Green L, Wysowski DK, Fourcroy JL. Gynecomastia and breast cancer during finasteride therapy [letter]. *N Engl J Med* 1996;335:823.
22. Olsson H, Alm P, Aspegren K, Gullberg B, Jonsson PE, Ranstam J. Increased plasma prolactin levels in a group of men with breast cancer— a preliminary study. *Anticancer Res* 1990;10:59.
23. Haga S, Watanabe O, Shimizu T, et al. Breast cancer in a male patient with prolactinoma. *Surg Today* 1993;23:251.
24. Volm MD, Talamonti MS, Thangavelu M, Gradishar WK. Pituitary adenoma and bilateral male breast cancer: an unusual association. *J Surg Oncol* 1997;64:74.
25. Wooster R, Mangion J, Eeles R, et al. A germline mutation in the androgen receptor gene in two brothers with breast cancer and Reifenstein syndrome. *Nat Genet* 1992;2:132.
26. Lobaccaro JM, Lumbroso S, Belon C, et al. Androgen receptor gene mutation in male breast cancer. *Hum Mol Genet* 1993;2:1799.
27. Hiort O, Naber SP, Lehners A, et al. The role of androgen receptor gene mutations in male breast carcinoma. *J Clin Endocrinol Metab* 1996;81:3404.
28. Wooster R, Bignell G, Lancaster J, et al. Identification of the breast cancer susceptibility gene BRCA2. *Nature* 1995;378:789.
29. Easton DF, Bishop DT, Ford D, Crockford GP. Genetic linkage analysis in familial breast and ovarian cancer: results from 214 families. The Breast Cancer Linkage Consortium. *Am J Hum Genet* 1993; 52:678.
30. Hall JM, Lee MK, Newman B, et al. Linkage of early-onset familial breast cancer to chromosome 17q21. *Science* 1990;250:1684.
31. Miki Y, Swensen J, Shattuck-Eidens D, et al. A strong candidate for the breast and ovarian cancer susceptibility gene BRCA1. *Science* 1994;266:66.
32. Hogervorst FB, Cornelis RS, Bout M, et al. Rapid detection of BRCA1 mutations by the protein truncation test. *Nat Genet* 1995;10:208.
33. Struewing JP, Brody LC, Erdos MR, et al. Detection of eight BRCA1 mutations in 10 breast/ovarian cancer families, including 1 family with male breast cancer. *Am J Hum Genet* 1995;57:1.
34. Couch FJ, Farid LM, DeShano ML, et al. BRCA2 germline mutations in male breast cancer cases and breast cancer families. *Nat Genet* 1996;13:123.
35. Friedman LS, Gayther SA, Kurosaki T, et al. Mutation analysis of BRCA1 and BRCA2 in a male breast cancer population. *Am J Hum Genet* 1997;60:313.
36. Thorlacius S, Sigurdsson S, Bjarnadottir H, et al. Study of a single BRCA2 mutation with high carrier frequency in a small population. *Am J Hum Genet* 997;60:1079.
37. Donegan WL, Redlich PN. Breast cancer in men. *Surg Clin North Am* 1996;76:343.
38. Heller KS, Rosen PP, Schottenfeld D, Ashikari R, Kinne DW. Male breast cancer: a clinicopathologic study of 97 cases. *Ann Surg* 1978;188:60.
39. Borgen PI, Wong GY, Vlamis V, et al. Current management of male breast cancer. A review of 104 cases. *Ann Surg* 1992;215:451.
40. Cooper RA, Gunter BA, Ramamurthy L. *Mammography in radiology.* 1994;191:651.
41. Salvadori B, Saccozzi R, Manzari A, et al. Prognosis of breast cancer in males: an analysis of 170 cases. *Eur J Cancer* 1994;7:930.
42. Dershaw DD, Borgen PI, Deutch BM, Liberman L. Mammographic findings in men with breast cancer. *Am J Roentgenol* 1993;160:267.
43. Vetto J, Schmidt W, Pommier R, et al. Accurate and cost-effective evaluation of breast masses in males. *Am J Surg* 1998;175:383.
44. Willsher PC, Leach IH, Ellis IO, et al. Male breast cancer: pathological and immunohistochemical features. *Anticancer Res* 1997; 17:2335.
45. Joshi N, Pande C. Papillary carcinoma of the male breast diagnosed by fine needle aspiration cytology. *Indian J Pathol Microbiol* 1998; 41:103.
46. Donegan WL, Redlich PN, Lang PJ, Gall MT. Carcinoma of the breast in males: a multiinstitutional survey. *Cancer* 1998;83:498.
47. Cutuli B, Lacroze M, Dilhuydy JM, et al. Male breast cancer: results of the treatments and prognostic factors in 397 cases. *Eur J Cancer* 1995;31A:1960.
48. Ciatto S, Iossa A, Bonardi R, Pacini P. Male breast carcinoma: review of a multicenter series of 150 cases. Coordinating center and writing committee of FONCAM (National Task Force for Breast Cancer), Italy. *Tumori* 1990;76:555.
49. San Miguel P, Sancho M, Enriquez JL, Fernandez J, Gonzalez-Palacios F. Lobular carcinoma of the male breast associated with the use of cimetidine. *Virchows Arch* 1997;430:261.
50. Michaels BM, Nunn CR, Roses DF. Lobular carcinoma of the male breast. *Surgery* 1994;115:402.
51. Camus MG, Joshi MG, Mackarem G, et al. Ductal carcinoma in situ of the male breast. *Cancer* 1994;74:1289.
52. Nance KV, Reddick RL. In situ and infiltrating lobular carcinoma of the male breast. *Hum Pathol* 1989;20:1220.
53. Desai DC, Brennan EJ Jr, Carp NZ. Paget's disease of the male breast. *Am Surg* 1996;62:1068.
54. Rayson D, Erlichman C, Suman VJ, et al. Molecular markers in male breast carcinoma. *Cancer* 1998;83:1947.
55. Guinee VF, Olsson H, Moller T, et al. The prognosis of breast cancer in males. A report of 335 cases. *Cancer* 1993;71:154.
56. Kinne DW. Management of male breast cancer. *Oncology* 1991;5:45.
57. Williams WL Jr, Powers M, Wagman LD. Cancer of the male breast: a review. *J Natl Med Assoc* 1996;88:439.
58. Stierer M, Rosen H, Weitensfelder W, et al. Male breast cancer: Austrian experience. *World J Surg* 1995;19:687.
59. Crocetti E, Buiatti E. Male breast cancer: incidence, mortality and survival rates from an Italian population-based series [letter]. *Eur J Cancer* 1994;11:1732.
60. Izquierdo MA, Alonso C, De Andres L, Ojeda B. Male breast cancer. Report of a series of 50 cases. *Acta Oncol* 1994;33:767.
61. Hecht JR, Winchester DJ. Male breast cancer. *Am J Clin Pathol* 1994;102:S25.
62. Weber-Chappuis K, Bieri-Burger S, Hurlimann J. Comparison of prognostic markers detected by immunohistochemistry in male and female breast carcinomas. *Eur J Cancer* 1996;32A:1686.
63. Borgen PI, Senie RT, McKinnon WM, Rosen PP. Carcinoma of the male breast: analysis of prognosis compared with matched female patients. *Ann Surg Oncol* 1997;4:385.
64. Willsher PC, Leach IH, Ellis IO, Bourke JB, Blamey RW, Robertson JF. A comparison outcome of male breast cancer with female breast cancer. *Am J Surg* 1997;173:185.
65. Farrow JH, Adair FE. Effect of orchiectomy on skeletal metastases from cancer of the male breast. *Science* 1942;95:654.
66. Jaiyesimi IA, Buzdar AU, Sahin AA, Ross MA. Carcinoma of the male breast. *Ann Intern Med* 1992;117:771.
67. Ribeiro G, Swindell R. Adjuvant tamoxifen for male breast cancer (MBC). *Br J Cancer* 1992;65:252.

68. Anelli TF, Anelli A, Tran KN, Lebwohl DE, Borgen PI. Tamoxifen administration is associated with a high rate of treatment-limiting symptoms in male breast cancer patients. *Cancer* 1994;74:74.
69. Patel HZ Jr., Buzdar AU, Hortobagyi GN. Role of adjuvant chemotherapy in male breast cancer. *Cancer* 1989;64:1583.
70. Bagley CS, Wesley MN, Young RC, Lippman ME. Adjuvant chemotherapy in males with cancer of the breast. *Am J Clin Oncol* 1987;10:55.
71. Erlichman C, Murphy KC, Elhakim T. Male breast cancer: a 13-year review of 89 patients. *J Clin Oncol* 1984;2:903.
72. Schuchardt U, Seegenschmiedt MH, Kirschner MJ, Renner H, Sauer R. Adjuvant radiotherapy for breast carcinoma in men: a 20-year clinical experience. *Am J Clin Oncol* 1996;19:330.
73. Overgaard M, Hansen PS, Overgaard J, et al. Postoperative radiotherapy in high-risk premenopausal women with breast cancer who receive adjuvant chemotherapy. Danish Breast Cancer Cooperative Group 82b trial. *N Engl J Med* 1997;337:949.
74. Ragaz J, Jackson SM, Le N, et al. Adjuvant radiotherapy and chemotherapy in node-positive premenopausal women with breast cancer. *N Engl J Med* 1997;337:956.

Diseases of the Breast, 2nd ed.,
edited by Jay R. Harris.
Lippincott Williams & Wilkins, Philadelphia © 2000.

CHAPTER 41

Phyllodes Tumors

Jeanne A. Petrek

Since 1838, when its physical appearance was described by Johannes Muller,[1] cystosarcoma phyllodes has had dozens of names and synonymous designations.[2] It is a rare distinctive tumor of the breast without counterpart in other organs. Believing that the tumor was entirely benign, Muller stressed its difference from breast cancer and apparently chose the term *sarcoma*, not to indicate the rare malignant subgroup, but to describe the fleshy appearance.

It was only in 1931,[3] at Memorial Hospital in New York City, that the first case of metastatic phyllodes tumor was described. Nevertheless, the name *cystosarcoma phyllodes* overstates the malignant potential of the vast majority of such tumors; thus, it is unduly alarming to patients and physicians alike. The term *sarcoma* is not objectionable when it refers to the malignant and borderline varieties, both of which occur infrequently. *Cysto-* implies that the lesion contains macroscopic cysts, although this is not always the case.

In modern times, the internationally accepted term[4] is *phyllodes tumor*, with the extra qualification according to the pathologist's assessment of its microscopic appearance and therefore its likely biologic behavior. The entity produces a spectrum of diseases that range from benign, with significant risk of local recurrence, to malignant, sometimes with rapidly growing metastases.

MACROSCOPIC APPEARANCE

The size of phyllodes tumors is variable, ranging from 1 cm[5] to larger than 40 cm.[6] In modern series and with greater incidence of presentation on screening mammography, it is common to diagnose the majority in the smaller sizes.[7] Most phyllodes tumors, benign or malignant, appear well circumscribed grossly, although they lack a true capsule. This may occur because, being so hypercellular, they present a hard barrier that compresses and pushes the softer surrounding breast tissue.

J. A. Petrek: Evelyn Lauder Breast Center, Memorial Sloan-Kettering Cancer Center, New York, New York

Muller[1] described the lesion as greyish-white and resembling a head of cauliflower. The barely visible surface projections make complete surgical excision with narrow margins difficult, and inadvertent amputation predisposes to tumor recurrence. The cut surface is slimy or mucoid and tends to bulge outward. Firm fibrous areas alternate with soft fleshy areas and, occasionally, with cysts filled with clear or semisolid bloody fluid. Yellow fatty areas and areas of hemorrhage and necrosis can occur. Leaflike ("phyllodes") papillary protrusions of stromal connective tissue lined with epithelium often extend into the cystic areas.

MICROSCOPIC APPEARANCE

Histologically, phyllodes tumor, like fibroadenoma, is composed of epithelial elements and a connective tissue stroma. Cuboidal epithelium, resembling ductal epithelium of the surrounding breast tissue, lines the canaliculi, which appear as ductal spaces. These epithelial areas can become irregularly flattened in rapidly growing lesions, presumably by the pressure of the enlarging stroma. The epithelium may be hyperplastic and may have varying degrees of atypia in benign or malignant phyllodes tumors. Apocrine and squamous metaplasia of the epithelial elements, although rare, have also occurred.[5] There have been rare case reports in which the epithelium had changes of carcinoma.[8]

Characteristics of the stroma alone determine whether a phyllodes tumor should be classified as benign or malignant, just as the appearance of the connective tissue distinguishes a benign phyllodes tumor from fibroadenoma (Fig. 1). In general, stroma from malignant phyllodes tumor contain marked cellularity with pleomorphism and nuclear atypia, increased mitotic activity, and overgrowth of the stromal element[9,10] (Fig. 2). Often, the malignant areas are focal and can be overlooked if multiple areas are not sampled.[11,12]

There are two common stromal patterns. In the first type, cells are spindle shaped, resembling a fibrosarcoma. In the second, the cells are looser and myxoid in appearance, resembling a myxoliposarcoma.[5,13] Both patterns are usually found intermixed in the same tumor. The stroma can also show mul-

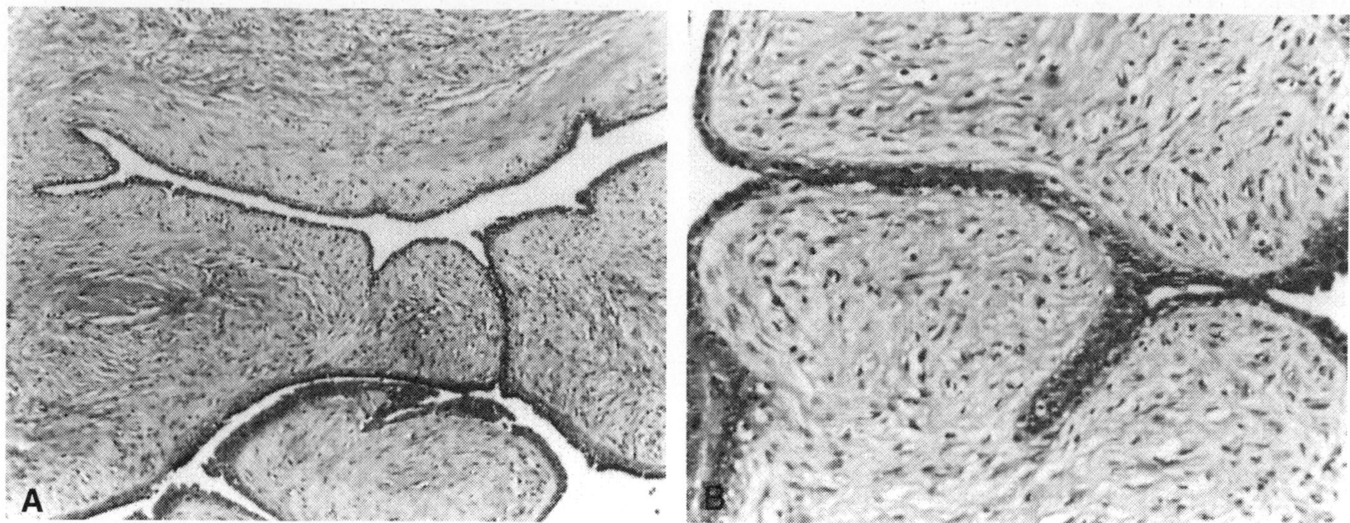

FIG. 1. Benign cystosarcoma phyllodes. **A:** Low-power view showing characteristic epithelium-lined clefts, which outline islands of stroma composed of spindle cells and collagen. **B:** High-magnification view showing thin layers of benign epithelial cells and benign stroma. Mitoses and nuclear pleomorphism are absent from the stroma.

tidirectional differentiation into mesenchymal elements, which are, in order of frequency, fibrosarcoma, liposarcoma, chondrosarcoma, osteosarcoma, and leiomyosarcoma.[5,10]

HISTOLOGIC CLASSIFICATION AND CLINICAL BEHAVIOR

The association of histologic appearance with the clinical course has been studied in various retrospective surveys, including several reviews (Table 1). In the 1950s, the large series of Lester and Stout[12] (58 patients) and that of Treves and Sunderland[9] (77 patients) tried to relate the clinical behavior of phyllodes tumors to two characteristics of the stroma: cellular atypia and increased mitotic activity. Both groups found this classification unreliable, because some patients with characteristics of malignancy had a benign course, and patients with metastases had tumors with only benign or borderline characteristics.

In 1967, Norris and Taylor[14] used the same two characteristics—cellular atypia and mitotic activity—and added a third, tumor margin (pushing versus infiltrating), as determinants of malignant potential. These three criteria, when considered together, improve reliability.

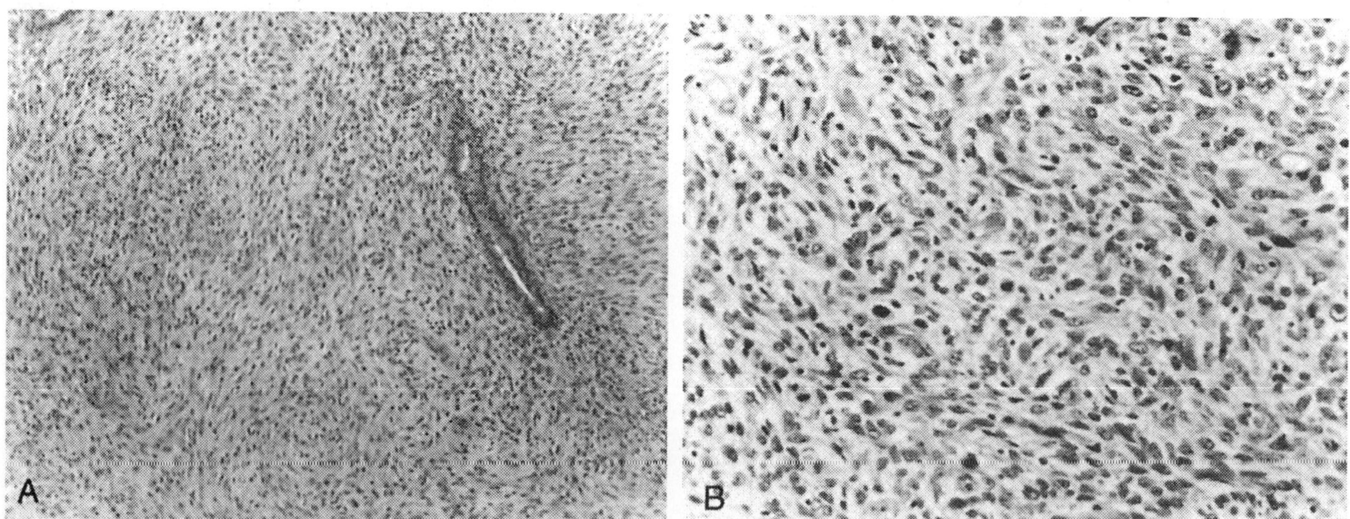

FIG. 2. Malignant cystosarcoma phyllodes. **A:** Low-magnification view showing highly cellular stroma and relatively inconspicuous epithelium. **B:** At higher magnification, the cellular stoma reveal considerable nuclear pleomorphism and several mitotic figures.

TABLE 1. *Histologic considerations in the classification of phyllodes tumors as benign, borderline, and malignant*

Accepted and standard characteristics
Cellular atypia[9,12,14–17]
Miotic activity[9,12,14–17]
Tumor margins[14,15]
Stromal overgrowth[13,16,17,25–29]
Nonstandard or unproven characteristics
Vascularity[16,17]
Flow cytometric analyses[16–22]
Pleomorphism[16,17]
Electron microscopic characteristics[24]

Pietruszka and Barnes,[15] refining the criteria of Norris and Taylor, attempted to correlate clinical behavior with classification as benign [zero to four mitoses in ten high-power fields (HPF)], borderline (five to nine mitoses in ten HPF, pushing or infiltrating margins, minimal stromal cellular atypia), or malignant (ten or more mitoses in ten HPF, infiltrating margins, moderate to marked stromal cellular atypia). Although mitotic rate was the most important determinant, the authors found increased predictability with the combination criteria. Metastases occurred only in the malignant category. Nevertheless, metastatic disease developed in only 23.5% of patients diagnosed with a malignant phyllodes tumor.

Studies[16,17] from the Northwestern University Hospitals have used a grading system (based on cellularity, pleomorphism, differentiation, mitoses, and also adding vascularity) to be an indicator of aggressive behavior. Their studies with flow cytometric analysis of DNA ploidy and proliferative index also correlated with the grading system.[17]

Although the role of flow cytometric analysis is still being evaluated, several reports have not shown this tool to be particularly useful. Five series[18–22] published in the 1990s with small numbers, ranging from 8 to 30 patients, have evaluated the correlation of flow cytometry with standard pathologic variables and clinical behavior. Three studies[18,19,21] show poor correlation, and one shows that DNA content is a significant predictor on multivariate analysis.[22] In a very small series of nine women with phyllodes tumors, p53 was demonstrated immunohistochemically in the borderline and malignant tumors but not in the benign phyllodes tumors.[23] Finally, electron microscopy has not contributed to the differentiation of benign from malignant tumors.[24]

Stromal overgrowth (at the expense of epithelial elements) has been found to be a reliable and perhaps the most important predictor of aggressive behavior in many recent studies.[13,16,17,25–29] The only large series (77 patients) in which this factor was not predictive is that of the Swedish Cancer Registry.[25] *Stromal overgrowth* has been most commonly defined as disproportionate proliferation of the stromal components so that at least one 40-power field (other than in the large papillary regions) contains no ductal epithelium.[29]

Probably because of the diverse criteria, the percentage of all phyllodes tumors classified as malignant ranges between 23%[11] and 50%.[30] One review article concluded that the accepted incidence of histologically malignant tumors is approximately 25%.[31] Metastases occur in 6.2%[32] to 22%[33] of all cases.

Precise classification by individual pathologists of this uncommon tumor into benign, borderline, and malignant is partly responsible for this wide range. Referral patterns favor malignancy in series from specialized institutions, such as Memorial Sloan-Kettering Cancer Center[5,11] or the Armed Forces Institute of Pathology.[14] Haagensen[32] asserted that a realistic figure of metastatic disease from all phyllodes tumors is that from his series (6.2%), which originated in a general surgical center.

HISTOGENESIS

The origin of phyllodes tumors has been difficult to investigate, presumably because of their relative rarity and because incipient tumors and microscopic disease are rarely encountered. One group believes that most phyllodes tumors arise in preexisting fibroadenoma.[34] Occasionally, patients have noted small lumps in their breast for as long as 45 years before growth of the nodule, biopsy, and diagnosis of phyllodes tumors.[35] In some tumors, the more dense fibrous parts appear localized into a distinctly ovoid outline, an appearance that has been interpreted as the residual benign fibroadenoma that gave rise to phyllodes tumors.[32]

STEROID RECEPTORS

Estrogen and progesterone receptor analysis has recently been performed on tumor tissue from patients with phyllodes tumors. Variability of results has been noted[36–38] and may reflect, in part, the relative amounts of epithelium (which contains the receptors) versus stroma in the tumors. There is no known value to hormonal treatment, because only the stromal component metastasizes.

CLINICAL AND IMAGING FEATURES

In almost all cases, a phyllodes tumor (whether benign or malignant) is discovered as a painless breast mass that is smooth, rounded, and multinodular. Most patients have continuous growth, although some individuals have had rapid growth in a previously stable, long-standing nodule. When the tumor grows large, it often does so rapidly, but this does not necessarily indicate malignancy. Shiny, stretched, and attenuated skin with varicose veins overlying a phyllodes tumor can occur. In these circumstances, skin ulceration is due to ischemia secondary to stretching and pressure. With ulceration due to carcinoma, the ulcerated skin also has dimpling or *peau d'orange*. The nipple may be effaced, but it is not invaded or retracted.

A notable feature of phyllodes tumor is the usual absence of suspicious axillary lymph nodes despite a large-sized mass, a situation that occurs infrequently with breast cancer. Axillary lymph node enlargement can occur (in as many as 20% of cases in one series).[14] This is virtually never the result of metastatic disease but is usually caused by necrotic, and sometimes infected, tumor.

On mammography, the appearance of phyllodes tumors is very much like that of fibroadenoma, with smooth, polylobulated margins, although some margins may be irregular, suggesting local invasion.[39–41] Similarly, on ultrasonography, these tumors cannot be differentiated from fibroadenomas and well-circumscribed malignant tumors.[39,40] On ultrasonography, fluid-filled elongated clefts may be found within an otherwise solid mass with no significant posterior shadowing. Phyllodes tumor, therefore, should be considered if cysts are demonstrated with a solid circumscribed lesion. In 1996, Memorial Sloan-Kettering Cancer Center published a large review of mammographic and ultrasonographic features of 51 phyllodes tumors.[42]

Magnetic resonance imaging is probably not useful in phyllodes tumors except possibly in demonstrating the full extent before wide surgical excision, although ultrasonography should suffice.[43] There is significant overlap in the rate of contrast enhancement between fibroadenoma and benign cystosarcoma and between benign and malignant cystosarcoma.

PATIENT CHARACTERISTICS

Phyllodes is rare, reported to be from 2%[9,12,32] to 4.4%[44] as numerous as fibroadenomas diagnosed in the same institution. A population-based study from California noted a higher risk in Latino women than in white or Asian women. The overall risk of malignant phyllodes tumors in this study was 2.1 per million women.[45]

The mean age of patients in large series is in the fourth decade,[5,11,15,32] which is 10 to 20 years older than the mean age for fibroadenoma. A wide range is recorded in most series, and phyllodes tumor has been recorded in prepubertal and adolescent ages.[46,47] The mean age of patients with benign phyllodes is younger than that of patients with malignant phyllodes.[5,34] Bilaterality is rare with either benign[14,32] or malignant tumors. A 30% incidence of bilaterality was found in only one report[48] and is a notable exception.

Phyllodes tumor is rarely, if ever, found in men. A large series is from the Armed Forces Institute of Pathology.[49] All reported cases in men seem to occur in the background of gynecomastia and lobular development.[49]

Histologically malignant epithelium is quite rare, as witnessed by the few cases reported. Intraductal cancer,[8,14,32,50] infiltrating duct cancer,[50,51] lobular carcinoma *in situ* (lobular neoplasia), and squamous carcinoma[8,9,32,52] all have been described. A study from Denmark[53] presented similar conclusions about the rare occurrence. Nevertheless, as any associated carcinoma is quite rare, principles of management for phyllodes tumors should generally not take this possibility into account.

NATURAL HISTORY

Local and Regional Recurrence

Numerous investigators have concluded that, overall, phyllodes tumors recur locally in approximately 20% of the cases.[10,32,34,54] The recurrence may be easily excised or, as evidenced from the rare case report, may be quite aggressive, invading the chest wall and thoracic cavity.[11,55,56]

In general, there is little difference in the tendency for benign versus malignant tumors to recur locally. A series of malignant phyllodes tumors (not necessarily metastatic)[57] at Memorial Hospital found a low 8% local recurrence rate. This probably occurred because more extensive margin was obtained, compared with benign phyllodes tumors, which have a higher local recurrence rate. In another series, a local recurrence developed in one-half of patients in the course of their metastatic disease.[31]

Most locally recurrent tumors are histologically similar to the original. In the Memorial Hospital series, only 2 of the 28 locally recurrent benign lesions had histologic "malignant transformation" at reexcision.[57] A small series noted such transformation in one of seven local recurrences.[56] Other authors note malignant transformation of the recurrence less commonly than the Memorial Hospital series.[32,58,59]

The Memorial Hospital series[57] reported earlier recurrences when the original lesion was classified as malignant (6 to 24 months) rather than benign (18 to 24 months). In a large series of 216 consecutive patients, the Milan authors had similar findings: They found an "average" interval to local recurrence of 32 months for benign, 22 months for malignant, and 18 months for borderline phyllodes tumors.[60]

Regional lymph node metastases very rarely develop from malignant phyllodes tumors. Clinical enlargement of the lymph nodes is present in approximately 20%,[14,61] although this must be due to necrotic tumor or other factors because the incidence of lymph node metastases in various series of malignant phyllodes tumor is less than 5%.[61–63] One patient with axillary lymph node metastases was reported as being cured.[64]

Systemic Recurrence

All metastatic lesions except one possible case[65] have resembled sarcomas, being devoid of all the epithelial elements. Fewer than 5% of all phyllodes tumors (benign, borderline, and malignant) metastasize. Approximately one-fourth of those classified as histologically malignant metastasize, depending, as always, on the histologic criteria used for classification.

In a review of all reported cases of metastatic phyllodes tumors (67 cases), Kessinger and colleagues[31] reported in

1972 that the average survival time after diagnosis of metastasis was 30 months. Metastatic lesions have been reported as early as at the initial diagnosis of the primary tumor and as late as 12 years after diagnosis. The longest survival time after diagnosis with metastatic disease was 14.5 years. The most common site of the initially diagnosed distant metastasis was the lungs. After lungs, the bones, liver, heart, and distant lymph nodes were the other metastatic sites (in a roughly descending order of frequency).[31,61]

MANAGEMENT CONSIDERATIONS

Initial Diagnosis

Because of its similarity to fibroadenoma on physical examination and mammography and during operation, phyllodes tumors are often enucleated (excised with no margin), which is the standard for fibroadenoma. Approximately 20% of phyllodes tumors recur locally if excised with no margin or with a margin of only a few millimeters. The proportion may be somewhat higher with borderline or malignant varieties and lower with benign phyllodes tumors. Local recurrence rates as high as 20%,[57] 28%,[32] and 33%[14] have been reported.

Even when agreeing with the general number of 20% local recurrence, authors differ as to whether immediate reexcision should be undertaken to obtain the recommended margin of 2 cm when an unsuspected phyllodes is diagnosed on permanent section. At Memorial Hospital, with patients informed of these statistics and of the alternatives, risks, and benefits, most undergo reexcision approximately 4 weeks later.

In a review of 106 benign phyllodes tumor patients from Singapore, Chua and associates[66] concluded that because only 16% of patients presumptively operated on for fibroadenoma develop a local recurrence, a policy of close follow-up is usually acceptable. If, however, microscopic assessment shows definite transection of the tumor, they recommend immediate reoperation. A pitfall in the "watch and wait" policy is demonstrated by the fact that 7 of 106 patients who received long-term follow-up had "pseudorecurrences," with only scar tissue and benign fibrocystic changes found on second operation.[67] In another series, in six benign tumors that recurred, the authors experienced initial incomplete excision, which confirms the recommendation of immediate reoperation if that is demonstrated.[56]

The largest series reported thus far, with 216 consecutive patients from Milan, also addressed the issue of phyllodes tumor found unexpectedly on permanent section analysis.[60] With a variety of breast resection procedures, 7.9% of the benign phyllodes tumors recurred. The authors found no difference in local recurrence rates with narrow margins versus no margin. Five of 55 patients were treated with enucleation, and 5 of 52 were treated with narrow (otherwise undefined) resections. In the small group of malignant phyllodes, 23.3% recurred, and in the borderline group, 19.6% recurred. This is logical, because the borderline and malignant varieties recur earlier, probably due to faster growth, although benign phyllodes eventually have a similar local recurrence.

Methods that have been evaluated but do not have an important place in the management of phyllodes tumors include preoperative fine-needle aspiration of all apparent fibroadenomas, intraoperative frozen section, or both. Theoretically, this could lead to identification of phyllodes tumor and would lead the surgeon to perform a wide rather than a close excision as the initial surgical procedure.

To diagnose a phyllodes tumor on fine-needle aspiration, the smear must yield a dimorphic pattern of stromal elements (tissue fragments or single spindle cells) and benign epithelial tissue. Fine-needle aspiration failed in 22%[68] and 86%[30] of cases in two reports; in another report[69] containing four benign phyllodes tumors, two were mistakenly diagnosed as carcinoma, one was suspicious for carcinoma, and one was summarized descriptively as "benign duct epithelium." The largest report catalogs the cytologic findings of 22 cases of histologically confirmed phyllodes and concludes that cytopathologists "should be careful."[23]

Performing an intraoperative frozen section on all apparent fibroadenomas would not be judicious. Apart from the great expense and intraoperative time involved for the rare occurrence, the differentiation of benign phyllodes from cellular fibroadenoma can be quite difficult on frozen section. Furthermore, the sarcomatous element in phyllodes tumors can be mistakenly diagnosed as an undifferentiated carcinoma, thereby leading to unnecessary radical procedures.

Special Considerations for Malignant Phyllodes Tumors

Most authors agree on the initial wide excision for benign phyllodes tumors. However, for histologically malignant phyllodes tumors, some authors,[14,31,34,35,53,59,65,69] have recommended total mastectomy as routine initial treatment.

Haagensen[32] was one of the first to advocate a wide excision instead of a mastectomy if the tumor-to-breast size would permit, because the objective is local control. With multicentricity not an issue as in breast cancer, breast preservation without radiation therapy has been accomplished successfully with malignant phyllodes tumors in more recent series.[61,62,70]

Because regional lymph node metastases rarely occur with phyllodes tumors, it is virtually never necessary to perform a formal axillary dissection.[14,61,62] If clinically enlarged and suspicious lymph nodes exist, excisional biopsy invariably proves these lymph nodes to be hyperplastic.

Local Recurrence

For the local recurrence of a benign phyllodes tumor, reexcision with at least a 2- to 3-cm margin is advised. Almost all recurrences retain the histologic pattern of the primary tumor, and more aggressive treatment for the small possibility of malignant transformation is not advised. Rarely, with a large tumor relative to a small breast size, the recommended margin necessitates a mastectomy. Sometimes, the wide excision or mastectomy may include a portion of the pectoralis fascia or even a portion of full-thickness pectoralis muscle, if necessary, for 2 to 3 cm of posterior margin.

With local recurrence after a malignant phyllodes, a total mastectomy is most often recommended. Although acknowledging that no patient with a malignant phyllodes treated by simple mastectomy in his practice had a recurrence, Haagensen[32] pointed out that with local recurrence after wide excision, mastectomy was successful at that time.

Systemic Disease

Therapy for metastatic disease has been discouraging, with no sustained remissions from radiation,[11,12,65,71,72] additive hormones,[11] castration,[34,73] or chemotherapy.[31,65,71] A recent report attempted to evaluate the role of radiation in this disease. It concluded that little had been published, probably because early experience found no effect of radiation, and these results deterred further attempts.[74] There are no reported cases of response to hormonal manipulation,[11,14,31,71,72] even if hormone receptors were present. Ifosfamide, and secondly doxorubicin, may be the most active on metastatic disease.[71,75,76]

At the opposite end of the spectrum are the rare cases that prove fatal by direct extension without distant metastases.[15,77] As with sarcomas in general, distant pulmonary metastases may be resectable for possible cure.[10,64]

MANAGEMENT SUMMARY

Because of its similarity to fibroadenoma on physical examination/mammography and during operation, phyllodes tumors are often enucleated or excised with narrow margins, which is standard treatment for fibroadenoma. In this situation, a local recurrence rate of 20% can be expected.

If permanent histology shows phyllodes tumor at the margin, reoperation to obtain a 2-cm negative margin is recommended. For negative margins that are less, reoperation for wider excision or close follow-up has been recommended.

The use of systemic therapy for metastatic disease of phyllodes tumor is based on the guidelines for treating sarcomas, not breast carcinoma.

REFERENCES

1. Muller J. *Uber den feineran Bau and die Forman der krankhaften Geschwilste.* Berlin: G Reimer, 1838.
2. Fiks A. Cystosarcoma phyllodes of the mammary gland: Muller's tumor. *Virchows Arch* 1981;392:1.
3. Lee B, Pack G. Giant intracanalicular fibroadenomyxoma of the breast. *Am J Cancer* 1931;15:2583.
4. Anonymous. Histological typing of breast tumors. *Tumori* 1982;68:181.
5. McDivitt RW, Stewart FW, Berg JW. Tumors of the breast. In: *Atlas of tumor pathology.* Series 2, fascicle 2. Washington: Armed Forces Institute of Pathology, 1968.
6. Lee B, Pack G. Giant intracanalicular fibroadenomyxoma. The so-called cystosarcoma phyllodes mammae of Johannes Muller. *Ann Surg* 1931;93:250.
7. Bartoli C, Zurrida S, Veronesi P, et al. Small sized phyllodes tumor of the breast. *Eur J Surg Oncol* 1990;16:215.
8. Rosen PP, Urban JA. Coexistent mammary carcinoma and cystosarcoma phyllodes. *Breast* 1975;1:9.
9. Treves N, Sunderland D. Cystosarcoma phyllodes of the breast: a malignant and a benign tumor. *Cancer* 1951;4:1286.
10. Hart WR, Bauer RC, Oberman HA. A clinicopathologic study of twenty-six hypercellular periductal stromal tumors of the breast. *Am J Clin Pathol* 1978;70:211.
11. Treves N. A study of cystosarcoma phyllodes. *Ann N Y Acad Sci* 1964; 114:922.
12. Lester J, Stout A. Cystosarcoma phyllodes. *Cancer* 1954;7:335.
13. Azzopardi JG. Sarcomas of the breast. In: Bennington JL, ed. *Problems in breast pathology.* Vol 2. Philadelphia: WB Saunders, 1979.
14. Norris HJ, Taylor HB. Relationship of histologic features to behavior of cystosarcoma phyllodes. Analysis of ninety-four cases. *Cancer* 1967;20:2090.
15. Pietruszka M, Barnes I. Cystosarcoma phyllodes: a clinicopathologic analysis of 42 cases. *Cancer* 1978;41:1974.
16. Hines JR, Murad TM, Beal JM. Prognostic indicators in cystosarcoma phyllodes. *Am J Surg* 1987;153:276.
17. Murad TM, Hines JR, Beal J, et al. Histological and clinical correlations of cystosarcoma phyllodes. *Arch Pathol Lab Med* 1988;112:752.
18. Rowell MD, Perry RR, Hsiu JG, Barranco SC. Phyllodes tumors. *Am J Surg* 1993;165:376.
19. Keelan PA, Myers JL, Wold LE, Katzmann JA, Gibney DJ. Phyllodes tumor: clinicopathologic review of 60 patients and flow cytometric analysis in 30 patients. *Hum Pathol* 1992;23:1048.
20. Grimes MM. Cystosarcoma phyllodes of the breast: histologic features, flow cytometric analysis, and clinical correlations. *Mod Pathol* 1992;5:232.
21. Palko MJ, Wang SE, Shackney SE, Cottington EM, Levitt SB, Hartsock RJ. Flow cytometric S fraction as a predictor of clinical outcome in cystosarcoma phyllodes. *Arch Pathol Lab Med* 1990;114:949.
22. El-Naggar AK, Ro JY, McLemore D, Garnsy L. DNA content and proliferative activity of cystosarcoma phyllodes of the breast. *Am J Clin Pathol* 1990;93:480.
23. Shabalova IP, Chemeris GJ, Ermilova VD, Rodionova LM, Pavlikova NA, Syrjanen KJ. Phyllodes tumour: cytologic and histologic presentation of 22 cases, and immunohistochemical presentation of p53. *Cytopathology* 1997;8:177.
24. Kesterson GHD, Georgiade N, Seigler HF, et al. Cystosarcoma phyllodes: a steroid receptor and ultrastructure analysis. *Ann Surg* 1988; 190:640.
25. Cohn-Cedermark G, Rutqvist LE, Rosendahl I, Silfversward C. Prognostic factors in cystosarcoma phyllodes: a clinicopathologic study of 77 patients. *Cancer* 1991;68:2017.
26. Kario K, Maeda S, Mizuno Y, Makino Y, Tankawa H, Kitazawa S. Phyllodes tumor of the breast: a clinicopathologic study of 34 cases. *J Surg Oncol* 1990;45:46.
27. Hawkins RE, Schofield JB, Fisher C, Wiltshaw E, McKinna JA. The clinical and histologic criteria that predict metastases from cystosarcoma phyllodes. *Cancer* 1992;69:141.
28. Inoshita SI. Phyllodes tumor (cystosarcoma phyllodes) of the breast. *Acta Pathol Jpn* 1988;28:21.
29. Ward RM, Evans HL. Cystosarcoma phyllodes. A clinicopathology study of 26 cases. *Cancer* 1986;58:2282.
30. Salvadori B, Cusumano F, Del Bo R, et al. Surgical treatment of phyllodes tumors of the breast. *Cancer* 1989;63:2532.
31. Kessinger A, Foley JF, Lemon HM, et al. Metastatic cystosarcoma phyllodes: a case report and review of the literature. *J Surg Oncol* 1972;4:131.
32. Haagensen CD. *Diseases of the breast,* 2nd ed. Philadelphia: WB Saunders, 1975:227.
33. Oberman HA. Cystosarcoma phyllodes: a clinicopathologic study of hypercellular periductal stromal neoplasms of the breast. *Cancer* 1965;18:697.

34. McDivitt RW, Urban JA, Farrow JH. Cystosarcoma phyllodes. *Johns Hopkins Med J* 1966;120:33.
35. Maier WP, Rosemond GP, Wittenberg R, et al. Cystosarcoma phyllodes mammae. *Oncology* 1968;22:145.
36. Pashof T. Estradiol binding protein in cystosarcoma phyllodes of the breast. *Eur J Cancer Clin Oncol* 1980;16:591.
37. Porton WM, Poortman J. Estrogen receptors in cystosarcoma phyllodes of the breast. *Eur J Cancer Clin Oncol* 1981;17:1147.
38. Brentani MM, Nagai MA, Oshimi CTF, et al. Steroid receptors in cystosarcoma phyllodes. *Cancer Detect Prev* 1982;5:211.
39. Buchberger W, Strasser K, Heim K, Muller E, Schrocksnadel H. Phyllodes tumor: findings on mammography, sonograph, and aspiration cytology in 10 cases. *AJR Am J Roentgenol* 1991;157:715.
40. Dorsi CJ, Feldhaus L, Sonnenfeld M. Unusual lesions of the breast. *Radiol Clin North Am* 1983;21:67.
41. Cosmacini P, Zurrida S, Veronesi P, Bartoli C, Coopmans de Yoldi GF. Phyllodes tumor of the breast: mammographic experience in 99 cases. *Eur J Radiol* 1992;15:11.
42. Liberman L, Bonaccio E, Hamele-Bena D, Abramson AF, Cohen MA, Dershaw DD. Benign and malignant phyllodes tumors: mammographic and sonographic findings. *Radiology* 1996;198:121.
43. Farria DM, Gorczyca DP, Barsky SH, Sinha S, Bassett LW. Benign phyllodes tumor of the breast: MR imaging features. *AJR Am J Roentgenol* 1996;167:187.
44. Dyer NH, Bridger JE, Taylor RS. Cystosarcoma phyllodes. *Br J Surg* 1966;53:450.
45. Bernstein L, Deapen D, Ross RK. The descriptive epidemiology of malignant cystosarcoma phyllodes tumors of the breast. *Cancer* 1993; 71:3020.
46. Rajan PB, Cranor ML, Rosen PP. Cystosarcoma phyllodes in adolescent girls and young women. A study of 45 patients. *Am J Surg Pathol* 1998;22:64.
47. Gibbs BR Jr, Roe RD, Thomas DF. Malignant cystosarcoma phyllodes in a pre-pubertal female. *Ann Surg* 1968;167:229.
48. McDonald JR, Harrington SW. Giant fibro-adenoma of the breast: cystosarcomas phyllodes. *Ann Surg* 1950;131:243.
49. Ansah-Boateng Y, Tavassoli F. Fibroadenoma and cystosarcoma phyllodes of the male breast. *Mod Pathol* 1992;5:114.
50. Klausner JM, Lelcuk S, Ilia B, et al. Breast carcinoma originating in cystosarcoma phyllodes. *Clin Oncol* 1983;9:71.
51. Philip PJ. Carcinosarcoma of the breast. *J R Coll Surg Edinb* 1976; 21:229.
52. Cornog JL, Mobini SE, Enterline HT. Squamous carcinoma of the breast. *Am J Clin Pathol* 1971;55:410.
53. Christensen L, Nielsen M, Madsen PM. Cystosarcoma phyllodes: a review of 19 cases with emphasis on the occurrence of associated breast carcinoma. *Acta Pathol Microbiol Immunol Scand* 1986;94:35.
54. Contarini O, Urdaneta LF, Hagan W, et al. Cystosarcoma phyllodes of the breast: a new therapeutic proposal. *Am Surg* 1982;48:157.
55. Ross DE. Malignancy occurring in cystosarcoma phyllodes. *Am J Surg* 1954;88:243.
56. Moffat CJC, Pinder SE, Dixon AR, Elston CW, Blamey RW, Ellis IO. Phyllodes tumors of the breast: a clinicopathological review of thirty-two cases. *Histopathology* 1995;27:205.
57. Hajdu S, Espinosa MH, Robbins GF. Recurrent cystosarcoma phyllodes: a clinicopathologic study of 32 cases. *Cancer* 1975;38:1402.
58. Al-jurf A, Hawks WA, Crile G Jr. Cystosarcoma phyllodes. *Surg Gynecol Obstet* 1978;146:358.
59. Rix DB, Tredwell SJ, Forward AD. Cystosarcoma phyllodes (cellular intracanalicular fibroadenoma): clinicopathologic relationships. *Can J Surg* 1971;14:31.
60. Zurrida S, Bartoli C, Galimberti V, et al. Which therapy for unexpected phyllode tumour of the breast? *Eur J Cancer* 1992;28:654.
61. Reinfuss M, Mitus J, Smolak K, et al. Malignant phyllodes tumors of the breast: a clinical and pathological analysis of 55 cases. *Eur J Cancer* 1993;29A:1252.
62. Palmer ML, De Risi DC, Pelikan A, et al. Treatment options and recurrence potential for cystosarcoma phyllodes. *Surg Gynecol Obstet* 1990;170:193.
63. Reinfuss M, Mitus J, Duda K, Stelmach A, Rys J, Smolak K. The treatment and prognosis of patients with phyllodes tumor of the breast: an analysis of 170 cases. *Cancer* 1996;77:910.
64. Fernandez BB, Hernandez FJ, Spindler W. Metastatic cystosarcoma phyllodes: a light and electron microscopic study. *Cancer* 1976; 37:1737.
65. West L, Weiland LH, Clagett OT. Cystosarcoma phyllodes. *Ann Surg* 1971;173:520.
66. Chua CL, Thomas A, Ng BK. Cystosarcoma phyllodes: a review of surgical options. *Surgery* 1989;105:141.
67. Chua CL, Thomas A. Cystosarcoma phyllodes tumors. *Surg Gynecol Obstet* 1988;166:302.
68. Stanley MW, Tani EM, Rutqvist LE, et al. Cystosarcoma phyllodes of the breast: a cytologic and clinicopathologic study of 23 cases. *Diagn Cytopathol* 1989;5:29.
69. Dusenbery D, Frable WJ. Fine needle aspiration cytology of phyllodes tumor: potential diagnostic pitfalls. *Acta Cytologica* 1992; 36:215.
70. Zissis C, Apostolikas N, Konstantinidou A, Griniatsos J, Vassilopoulos PP. The extent of surgery and prognosis of patients with phyllodes tumor of the breast. *Breast Cancer Res Treat* 1998;48:205.
71. Burton GV, Hart LL, Leight GS Jr, et al. Cystosarcoma phyllodes: effective therapy with cisplatin and etoposide chemotherapy. *Cancer* 1989;63:2088.
72. Vorherr H, Vorherr VF, Kutvirt DM, et al. Cystosarcoma phyllodes: epidemiology, pathohistology, pathobiology, diagnosis, therapy, and survival. *Arch Gynecol* 1985;236:173.
73. Geist D. Cystosarcoma phyllodes of the female breast. *Am Surg* 1964;30:105.
74. Hopkins ML, McGowan TS, Rawlings G, et al. Phyllodes tumor of the breast: a report of 14 cases. *J Surg Oncol* 1994;56:108.
75. Hawkins RE, Schofield JB, Wiltshaw E, Fisher C, McKinna JA. Ifosfamide is an active drug for chemotherapy of metastatic cystosarcoma phyllodes. *Cancer* 1992;69:2271.
76. Turalba CIC, El-Mahdi AM, Ladaga L. Fatal metastatic cystosarcoma phyllodes in an adolescent female: case report and review of treatment approaches. *J Surg Oncol* 1986;33:176.
77. Aronson W. Malignant cystosarcoma phyllodes with liposarcoma. *Wis Med J* 1966;65:184.

CHAPTER 42

Diseases of the Breast, 2nd ed.,
edited by Jay R. Harris.
Lippincott Williams & Wilkins, Philadelphia © 2000.

Paget's Disease

Carolyn M. Kaelin

In 1307, John of Arderne recorded the several-year evolution of nipple ulceration in a male priest, with the subsequent development of a breast cancer.[1] In 1840, Velpeau[2] described the visual surface lesion of Paget's disease in two patients and is typically credited with the first clinical description of the condition. In 1874, Sir James Paget[3] recorded the association of the clinical findings with an underlying breast cancer in 15 patients, although he speculated that the chronic skin condition was benign. It was Thin,[4] in 1881, who concluded that the clinical Paget's nipple was not a benign entity, but rather a malignancy. Darier[5] described the microscopic appearance of the Paget's cell in 1889, although he mistook it for a "psorosperm" or coccidia. In 1928, Pautrier[6] advanced the theory that the Paget's cell is malignant.

PATHOGENESIS

There are two main theories for the origin of Paget's disease. The epidermotropic theory, first described by Jacobeus,[7] suggests that the Paget's cells arise in breast ducts and spread by way of the lactiferous sinuses to the nipple epidermis. This view is supported by the fact that more than 97% of patients with Paget's disease have an underlying breast carcinoma[8] and that in the majority of cases, the immunophenotype of the Paget's cell is the same as the breast cancer.[9–11]

The intraepidermal transformation theory proposes that the Paget's cells arise in the terminal portion of the lactiferous duct at its junction with the epidermis; they are altered epidermal cells that have been transformed *in situ.* Support for this theory is found in the rare cases of Paget's disease without an underlying breast carcinoma[12–16] or cases in which the Paget's disease and the underlying carcinoma appear to be separate tumors.[17]

Histologically, the Paget's cell is a large, pale-staining cell with round or oval nuclei and large nucleoli. The cells are between the normal keratinocytes of the nipple epidermis, occurring singly in the superficial layers, and in clusters toward the basement membrane. Serous fluid can seep through the disrupted keratinocyte layer, resulting in the crusting and scaling of the nipple skin. Paget's cells can traverse the epithelium and thus sometimes are found in the superficial layers (Fig. 1). The basement membrane of the lactiferous sinuses is in continuity with the basement membrane of the skin. Paget's cells do not invade through the dermal basement membrane and therefore are a form of carcinoma *in situ.* Paget's disease is frequently associated with a chronic inflammatory infiltrate in the dermis.

C. M. Kaelin: Department of Surgery, Harvard Medical School; Comprehensive Breast Health Center, Brigham and Women's Hospital, Dana-Farber Cancer Institute, Boston, Massachusetts

CLINICAL PRESENTATION AND DIAGNOSIS

Paget's disease initially presents with erythema and mild eczematous scaling and flaking of the nipple skin. Without treatment, the condition advances to crusting, skin erosion, and ulceration, with exudation or frank discharge. At times, it is associated with tingling, pruritus, hypersensitivity, burning, or pain. Kister[18] has observed in 117 patients with Paget's disease that the skin changes always begin on the nipple and secondarily extend to the areola (Fig. 2). Given that the ductal system may connect directly with the areola, Paget's disease may be confined to the areola,[19] thus mimicking eczema.

The clinical differential diagnosis of scaling skin and erythema of the nipple-areolar complex includes eczema, contact dermatitis, postradiation dermatitis, and Paget's disease. Bilateral symptoms are most consistent with eczema or contact dermatitis, although bilateral Paget's disease has been reported.[20,21] Skin changes that are confined to the areola and spare the nipple are typically attributed to eczema,[22] although they can occur rarely in Paget's disease as well.[19] The clinical differential diagnosis has prompted initial topical steroid treatment, often with transient improvement of symptoms.[23] Other patients have been treated with antibiotics.[24] Paget's disease may mimic postradiation scaling in patients who have undergone breast conservation treatment for primary breast cancer. Given the infrequency of Paget's

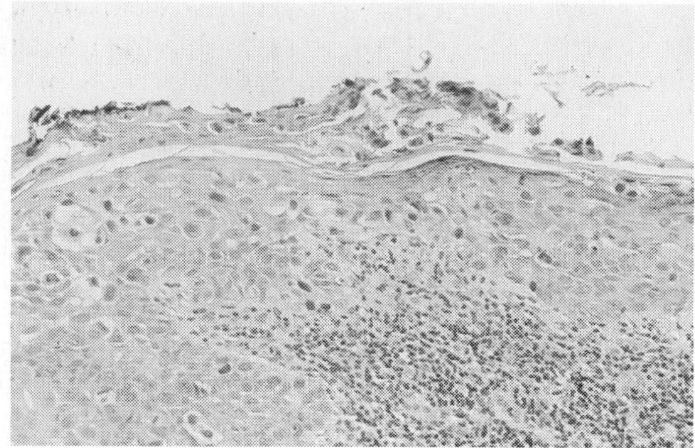

FIG. 1. A perpendicular section through the nipple epidermis demonstrating Paget's cells in the nipple crust. Large, pale-staining Paget's cells are more densely concentrated toward the basement membrane. (Hematoxylin-eosin stain; original magnification, ×300.) (Courtesy of Susan Lester, M.D., Ph.D., Department of Pathology, Brigham and Women's Hospital, Boston, Massachusetts.)

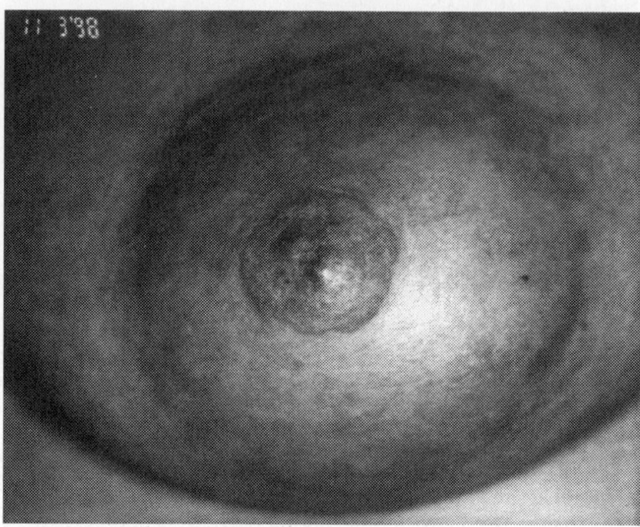

FIG. 2. Photograph of a Paget's nipple. The nipple skin is eczematous and has flattened and splayed, blending into the surrounding areola.

disease in this setting, the diagnosis of Paget's disease may be delayed.[25–27] Symptom duration preceding the diagnosis of Paget's disease averages 6.5 to 27.0 months, with a range of 1 week to 20 years.[24,28–32]

Less common diagnoses in the clinical differential of mammary Paget's disease include nipple adenoma,[33] papillomatosis,[34,35] melanoma,[36] and Bowen's disease,[37] and rarely basal cell carcinoma,[38] squamous carcinoma, sebaceous carcinoma, Merkel's cell carcinoma, infiltrating lobular carcinoma, cutaneous T-cell lymphoma, Spitz nevus, epidermatropic metastases,[39] syringomatous adenoma,[40] pseudoxanthoma elasticum,[41] and pemphigus vulgaris.[42]

The diagnosis can be obtained by scrape cytology,[36] a superficial epidermal shave biopsy, a 2-mm punch biopsy, a wedge incisional biopsy, or nipple excision.[43] The ideal specimen contains adequate epidermis to provide Paget's cells and a lactiferous duct. Paget's cells may be distributed in a patchy fashion throughout the nipple, and thus additional specimen sampling may be required to secure the diagnosis.[43]

The histologic differential diagnosis of Paget's disease includes superficial spreading melanoma, squamous cell carcincoma *in situ* (Bowen's disease), and clear cell changes of squamous cells of the epidermis (Toker cells). The cell type can be determined by immunohistochemical studies including low-molecular-weight keratins (CK7, CAM-5.2), broad-spectum keratins, melanoma antibodies, and mucin stains.

Paget's cells are immunoreactive for keratins (CK7,[44] CAM-5.2,[45,46] AE1/AE3[39]), occasionally are immunoreactive for S100 (26%),[47] and are not immunoreactive for HMB45[46] or high-molecular-weight keratins.[48] In one study, mucin was present in 55% of 20 cases and, thus, was not informative in 45% of cases.[46] Paget's cells can phagocytose melanin from adjacent epidermal melanocytes[46,49] and may be mistaken for melanoma if immunohistochemistry is not performed. Melanomas are immunoreactive for S100,[46,47,50] are frequently immunoreactive for HMB45,[46,50–53] and are only very rarely immunoreactive for low-molecular-weight (CAM-5.2)[45,52] broad-spectrum keratins (AE1/AE3)[39,48] or mucin stains.[45] Squamous cells are immunoreactive for low-molecular-weight keratins[48] and broad-spectrum keratins (AE1/AE3),[39] are infrequently immunoreactive for S100,[47] and are not immunoreactive for CAM-5.2,[45] HMB45,[39] or mucin stains.[45] Toker cells,[54] or clear-cell changes of the epidermal squamous cells, are a nonneoplastic alteration of keratinocytes present in 10% of normal nipples.[39] Toker cells can be distinguished from Paget's cells by their lack of nuclear pleomorphism or cytologic atypia and their absence of mucin.[39]

In 807 patients with clinical Paget's disease from 12 series, 371 (46%) presented with a breast mass, and 436 (54%) presented without a mass.[8,14,22,24,28–32,55–57] In patients with a mass, 93% had an invasive breast cancer, and 7% had ductal carcinoma *in situ* (DCIS). In patients without a mass, 38% had an invasive breast cancer, and 62% had DCIS.[8,14,22,28,31,32,55] In Kister and Haagensen's[29] series of 159 patients with histologically confirmed Paget's disease, the mean age of patients with an associated breast mass was 49 and without a mass 58 ($p = .01$).

In patients with clinical Paget's disease without a palpable breast mass, mammography has been reported as normal in 2.5% to 100% of patients.[24,55,58–63] Of the 212 total patients in these combined series, 91 (43%) had normal mammograms. In seven series, breast histology was evaluated in those patients with clinical Paget's disease and normal mammograms. All patients had an underlying malignancy in four of these series (combined n = 44),[23,59–61] 12 of 14 (85%) patients had an associated malignancy in the fifth series,[55] 9 of 17 (53%) patients had an associated malignancy in the sixth series,[63] and four of ten (40%) had an associated malignancy in the seventh.[58] These retrospective studies included patients accrued in the late 1970s, when xeromammography was still in use[60] and retroareolar spot compression views were not routine.[61]

INCIDENCE

Paget's disease is a more common pathologic than clinical entity.[24,28,30,64] Its clinical incidence ranges from 0.5% to 2.6%, with a mean of 1.1% in more than 44,000 patients combined from eight studies.[24,28–32,64,65] Histologic evidence of Paget's cells is present in 0.5% to 4.7% of nipples from breast cancer specimens[8,24,28–30,64,66,67] In a series by Lagios et al.[66] of 3,000 consecutive breast cancer mastectomy specimens, 21 (0.7%) had clinical evidence of Paget's disease and 147 (4.9%) had Paget's cells histologically, thus yielding a sevenfold difference.

Of the 158,621 microscopically confirmed female and male breast cancer registrants from the Surveillance Epidemiology and End Results registry of the National Cancer Institute,[67] 1,775 (1.1%) had histologic Paget's disease. Of breast cancer patients from this database, Paget's disease was histologically identified in 1.1% of white female patients, 1.3% of African-American female patients, 1.1% of white male patients, and no African-American male patients. Clinical Paget's disease has been reported in patients ranging in age from 26 to 88, with means ranging from 53 to 58 years.[24,29–32,57] In a further analysis of the Surveillance Epidemiology and End Results data,[68] the mean age of women with Paget's disease was 62 years and of men, 69 years. This was not significantly different from female (61 years) and male (67 years) patients with ductal breast cancer.

TREATMENT

Treatment for Paget's disease has followed the evolution of surgical options for patients with an invasive breast cancer,[69–72] with patients with Paget's disease confined to the nipple-areolar complex now being considered potential candidates for breast preservation. Physical examination and mammography are used in efforts to identify multicentric disease and thus the requirement for mastectomy. Identification of a coexistent invasive breast cancer dictates the role of axillary nodal evaluation.

Breast magnetic resonance imaging (MRI) has shown promise in identifying clinically and mammographically occult breast cancers.[73] In patients with clinical Paget's disease of the nipple and physical examination and mammography findings confined to the nipple-areolar complex, MRI may identify multicentric sites of disease.[74] In this role, it may facilitate selection of patients in whom breast conservation surgery is not appropriate.

Peripheral breast cancers may not be identified when surgery is limited to excision of the nipple-areolar complex. In a study of 50 patients with Paget's disease by Paone and Baker,[56] an underlying cancer was 2 cm or greater from the nipple in 6 (12%) patients, and, despite multiple microscopic sections, no anatomic connection between the Paget's lesion and the underlying breast carcinoma could be identified. Ikeda et al.[59] described 11 patients with clinical Paget's disease without breast masses and with normal mammograms treated with mastectomy in which DCIS was identified far from the nipple in 6 patients and in two or more quadrants in 5. Kollmorgen et al.[63] identified 28 patients with Paget's disease and no breast mass who were found to have an occult tumor on histologic review. One-half of these were located centrally (within 2 cm of the areolar margin) and one-half peripherally. Within this group, 17 patients had normal mammograms. Yim et al.[55] described 11 patients with clinical Paget's disease, no palpable mass, and pathologically confirmed multifocal disease. In these 11 patients, mammography identified multifocal disease in 4 (36%) patients and failed to identify multifocal DCIS in 7 (64%) patients, 2 of whom also had mammographically occult invasive ductal carcinoma in noncentral breast quadrants. In an analysis of 100 consecutive mastectomy specimens, Wertheim and Ozzello[64] identified 18 cases of Paget's disease, 4 (22%) of which had invasive cancers in peripheral quadrants of the breast.

Breast Conservation without Radiation

Failure to identify peripheral cancers when patients are treated with breast conservation surgery without irradiation may yield increased local failure rates. In a series reported by Dixon et al.,[23] ten patients with Paget's disease without an associated mass and with negative mammographic findings or findings suggestive of *in situ* changes confined to the immediate nipple area underwent excision of the nipple-areolar complex with underlying cone biopsy. All ten specimens had underlying DCIS, one had an associated invasive breast cancer, and all had negative surgical margins. With a median follow-up of 40 months, there were four local recurrences, one as Paget's in the surgical scar and the other three as invasive cancers. Metastatic disease subsequently developed in two patients. Dixon et al. conclude by advocating simple mastectomy for treatment of patients with clinical Paget's disease even in the absence of an associated breast mass. In contrast, Paone and Baker[56] described five patients with Paget's disease without an associated breast mass treated with nipple excision and underlying breast wedge resection. Although there were no recurrences, the length of follow-up is not specified. Lagios et al.[16] reported on five patients with clinical Paget's disease without an associated palpable mass or mammographic abnormality. Treatment involved breast conservation surgery alone. Of the four patients undergoing total excision of the nipple-areolar complex, no recurrences were seen at 16 to 55 months (median, 36 months) after treatment. In the patient who underwent partial resection, the remainder of the nipple-areolar complex was resected at the time of recurrence

TABLE 1. *Paget's disease treated with radiotherapy alone*

Author	No.	Median follow-up (mo)	Recurrence	Form of recurrence			
				Paget's	Microinvasive DCIS	Invasive	Death
Bulens et al.[79]							
Christiaens et al.[80]	27	79	4	3	0	1	1
Stockdale et al.[81]	19	63	3	0	2	1	0
Forquet et al.[82]	17	90	3	3	0	0	0

DCIS, ductal cardinoma *in situ.*

12 months after the initial resection. The patient has no evidence of further recurrence at 43 months. Detailed pathologic review of these five specimens demonstrated *in situ* disease confined to the protuberant nipple in two patients and DCIS to a depth not exceeding 8 mm in three patients. A sixth patient had undergone mastectomy, and a single involved lactiferous duct was identified to a depth of 15 mm.

Breast Conservation with Radiation

The addition of radiotherapy (XRT) may add to the efficacy of breast-conserving surgery for patients with Paget's disease. In an abstract from Memorial Sloan-Kettering Cancer Center,[75] 14 patients with clinical Paget's disease without evidence of invasion underwent central quadrantectomy achieving negative surgical margins. Of the nine patients who received XRT (6,120 cGy), one had a recurrence. Of the five patients not receiving XRT, three had recurrences. Time to recurrence was not specified.

Pierce et al.[76] present 30 patients with Paget's disease without a palpable mass or mammographic density from seven institutions. All patients were treated with breast irradiation with varying extents of surgical excision. Mammography review was available for 29 patients; in 24, it was negative; in 3, it demonstrated nipple thickening; in 2, retroareolar calcifications; and in 1, calcifications elsewhere in the breast. Twenty-two patients underwent complete excision of the nipple (3) or nipple-areolar (19) complex, 6 underwent partial excision of the nipple (4) or nipple-areolar (2) complex, and 2 patients underwent incisional biopsy only for histologic confirmation of Paget's disease. All patients received whole breast irradiation to a median dose of 50 Gy, with 97% receiving a boost to the tumor bed for a median total dose of 61.5 Gy. With median follow-up of 62 months, five inbreast recurrences were detected, three (14%) in the group treated with complete excision of the nipple or nipple-areolar complex and two (33%)[84-88] in the group treated with partial excision. Additionally, one patient had an ipsilateral axillary recurrence in 6 of 19 involved lymph nodes, and another patient had a contralateral axillary occurrence. Two patients are alive with distant disease, one patient having a local failure first and the other having the contralateral axillary occurrence (L. J. Pierce, *personal communication*, 14 January 1999). Pierce concludes that breast-conserving therapy involving complete nipple-areolar excision followed by XRT should be considered in patients with localized Paget's disease, given the adequate local control and high rates of disease-free survival. The efficacy of central quadrantectomy and XRT (50 Gy) in patients with Paget's disease and DCIS limited to the retroareolar ducts will be further defined in the ongoing nonrandomized study of 100 patients by the European Organization for Research and Treatment of Cancer.[77]

Radiation without Surgery

The possibility of radiation treatment alone for patients with Paget's disease without a palpable mass or abnormal mammogram has been reported. In a photographic case report by Hareyama et al.,[78] a patient with advanced Paget's disease involving the entire nipple-areolar complex was treated with whole-breast irradiation to 5,400 cGy. At 6 years posttreatment, she is without evidence of recurrence and has an excellent cosmetic result. El Sharkawi and Waters[79] provide a similar photographic essay in three patients 3 to 5 years after treatment with XRT of 3,500 to 4,500 cGy focused to the nipple-areolar region alone. Table 1 presents four reports of patients with histologically confirmed Paget's disease without evidence of invasion and treated with irradiation alone.[80–83] At a median follow-up of 63 to 90 months after treatment, 10 of the 63 patients (16%) developed inbreast recurrences, 6 as Paget's disease, 2 as microinvasive DCIS, and 2 as invasive breast cancer. The patient with an invasive recurrence died of metastatic disease 9.5 years after initial treatment.

Axillary Dissection

The indication for axillary dissection in the patient with clinical Paget's disease without other physical examination or radiologic findings is not well defined. In 15 combined series[8,14,24,28,29,31,32,36,56,57,84–88] of patients with clinical Paget's disease without a palpable mass, axillary metastases were identified in 50 of 417 (12%) patients (range, 0 to 25%). These studies were predominantly from the premammography era. Kollmorgen[63] recommends axillary dissection in all patients with Paget's disease. In his series of 68 patients with clinical Paget's disease, a subset of 32 without a palpable mass underwent axillary dissection, with nodal positivity identified in 6 patients (19%). Neither the mammography findings of this patient subset nor whether these six patients had a concurrent invasive breast cancer is specified.

MANAGEMENT SUMMARY

The diagnosis of Paget's disease is confirmed by nipple scrape cytology or biopsy.

Retroareolar spot compression views of the ipsilateral breast should be added to standard bilateral mammography. If available, preoperative breast MRI can be obtained to evaluate for possible occult disease in patients who are considering breast preservation. Patients with disease identified beyond the central portion of the breast by physical examination or breast imaging studies should undergo mastectomy. For patients choosing breast conservation therapy, strong consideration should be given to combining surgery and radiation in efforts to minimize future local recurrence. For patients undergoing either mastectomy or breast conservation, the decision for axillary node dissection should be based on the presence of an invasive breast cancer. Adjuvant therapy decisions are based on the final pathology.

Patients with clinical and mammographic disease limited to the retroareolar area can be considered candidates for breast conservation. Surgery should include excision of the full nipple-areolar complex with at least a 2-cm cone of retroareolar tissue and complete excision of abnormal retroareolar radiologic findings. For patients with positive margins after central quadrantectomy, consideration for mastectomy should be given. Patients with negative surgical margins should undergo irradiation.

ACKNOWLEDGMENTS

The author gratefully acknowledges Susan Lester, M.D., Ph.D., for her editorial comments and Kathy Bear for her invaluable assistance in the preparation of this chapter.

REFERENCES

1. Graham H. *The story of surgery*, 1st ed. New York: Doubleday, Doran & Company, Inc., 1939.
2. Velpeau A. *Lecons orales de clinique chirurgicale faites a l'hospital de la charite*. Vol 2. Paris: G. Bailliere, 1840.
3. Paget J. On disease of the mammary areola preceding cancer of the mammary gland. *St. Barts Hospital Rep* 1874;10:87.
4. Thin G. On the connection between diseases of the nipple and areola and tumors of the breast. *Trans Path Soc London* 1881;32:218.
5. Darier J. Surune nouvelle forme de psorospermose cutanu:la maladie de Paget du mamelon. *Compt Rend Soc Biol* (ser. 9) 1889;1:294.
6. Pautrier LM. Paget's disease of the nipple. *Arch Dermatol Syph* 1928;17:767.
7. Jacobeus HC. Paget's disease und sein verhaltnis zum milch-drusenkarzinom. *Virchows Arch Path Anat* 1904;178:124.
8. Ashikari R, Park K, Huvos AG, et al. Paget's disease of the breast. *Cancer* 1970;26:680.
9. Jahn H, Osther P, Nielsen E, Rasmussen G, Anderson J. An electron microscopic study of clinical Paget's disease of the nipple. *APMIS* 1995;103:628.
10. Cohen C, Guarner J, DeRose PB. Mammary Paget's disease and associated carcinoma: an immunohistochemical study. *Arch Pathol Lab Med* 1993;117:291.
11. Wood W, Hegodus C. Mammary Paget's disease and intraductal carcinoma: histologic histochemical and immunocytochemical comparison. *Am J Dermatopathol* 1988;10:183.
12. Sagebiel RW. Ultrastructural observations on epidermal cells in Paget's disease of the breast. *Am J Pathol* 1969;57:49.
13. Rosen PP, Oberman HA. *Atlas of tumor pathology: tumors of the mammary gland. Third series*. Vol. 7. Armed Forces Institute of Pathology. Washington: Fasciclez, 1993:266.
14. Nance FC, De Loach DH, Welsh RA, et al. Paget's disease of the breast. *Ann Surg* 1970;171:864.
15. Jones RE Jr. Mammary Paget's disease without underlying carcinoma. *Am J Dermatopathol* 1985;7:361.
16. Lagios MD, Westdahl PR, Rose MR, et al. Paget's disease of the nipple: alternative management in cases without or with minimal extent of underlying breast carcinoma. *Cancer* 1984;54:545.
17. Muir R. Further Observations on Paget's disease of the nipple. *J Pathol Bacteriol* 1939;49:299.
18. Kister SJ, Haagensen CD. Paget's disease of the breast. *Am J Surg* 1970;119:606.
19. van der Putte S, Toonstra J, Hennipman A. Mammary Paget's disease confined to the areola and associated with multifocal Toker cell hyperplasia. *Am J Dermatopathol* 1995;17:487.
20. Anderson WR. Bilateral Paget's disease of the nipple: a case report. *Am J Obstet Gynecol* 1979;134:877.
21. Fernandes FJ, Costa MM, Bernardo M. Rarities in breast pathology. Bilateral disease of the breast—a case report. *Eur J Surg Oncol* 1990; 16:172.
22. Colcock BP, Sommers SC. Prognosis in Paget's disease of the breast. *Surg Clin North Am* 1954;35:773.
23. Dixon R, Galea MH, Ellis IO, Elston CW, Blamey RW. Paget's disease of the nipple. *Br J Surg* 1991;78:722.
24. Freund H, Maydovnik M, Laufer N, Durst AL. Paget's disease of the nipple. *J Surg Oncol* 1977;9:93.
25. Menzies D, Barr L, Ellis H. Paget's disease of the nipple occurring after wide excision and radiotherapy for carcinoma of the breast. *Surg Oncol* 1989;115:271.
26. Markopoulous CH, Gazet JC. Paget's disease of the nipple occurring after conservative management of early breast cancer. *Eur J Surg Oncol* 1988;14:77.
27. Plowman PN, Gilmore OJA, Curling M, et al. Paget's disease of the nipple occurring after conservative management of early infiltrating breast cancer. *Br J Surg* 1986;73:45.
28. Kay S. Paget's disease of the nipple. *Surg Gynecol Obstet* 1966; 123:1010.
29. Kister SJ, Haagensen CD. Paget's disease of the breast. *Am J Surg* 1970;119:606.
30. Rissanen PM, Holsti P. Paget's disease of the breast. The influence of the presence or absence of an underlying palpable tumor on the prognosis and of the choice of treatment. *Oncology* 1969;23:209.
31. Ascensao AC, Marques MSJ, Capitao-Mor M. Paget's disease of the nipple: clinical and pathological review of 109 female patients. *Dermatologica* 1985;170:170.
32. Chaudary MA, Millis RR, Lane B, et al. Paget's disease of the nipple: a ten-year review including clinical pathological and immunohistochemical findings. *Breast Cancer Res Treat* 1986;8:139.
33. Perzin KH, Lattes R. Papillary adenoma of the nipple: a clinicopathologic study. *Cancer* 1972;9:996.
34. Rosen PP, Caicco J. Florid papillomatosis of the nipple: a study of 51 patients including nine having mammary carcinoma. *Am J Surg Pathol* 1986;10:87.
35. Scott P, Kissin MW, Collins C, Webb AJ. Florid papillomatosis of the nipple: a clinico-pathological surgical problem. *Eur J Surg Oncol* 1991;17:211.
36. Culberson JD, Horn RC Jr. Paget's disease of the nipple: a review of 25 cases with special reference to melanin pigmentation of Paget cells. *Arch Surg* 1956;72:224.
37. Venkataseshan VS, Budd DC, Un KD, Hutter RV. Intraepidermal squamous carcinoma (Bowen's disease) of the nipple. *Hum Pathol* 1994;25:1371.
38. Sauven P, Roberts A. Basal cell carcinoma of the nipple. *J R Soc Med* 1983;76:699.
39. Kohler S, Rouse RV, Smoller RR. The differential diagnosis of Pagetoid cells in the epidermis. *Mod Pathol* 1998;11:79.
40. Rosen PP. Syringomatous adenoma of the nipple. *Am J Surg Pathol* 1983;7:739.
41. Von Dach B, Neuweiler J, Haller U. Zur differentialdiagnose von mammatumoren mit ekzematosen mamillenveranderungen:zwe;seltene falle. *Helv Chir Acta* 1992;59:217.

42. Rae V, Gould E, Ibe MJ, Penneye NS. Coexistent pemphigus vulgaris and Paget's disease of the nipple. *J Am Acad Dermatol* 1987;16:235.
43. Rosen PP. Paget's disease of the nipple. In: Rosen PP. *Rosen's breast pathology*. Philadelphia: Lippincott–Raven, 1996:493.
44. Smith K, Tuur S, Corvette D, Lupton G, Skelton H. Cytokeratin-7 staining in mammary and extramammary Paget's disease. *Mod Pathol* 1997;10:1069.
45. Hitchcock A, Tophams S, Bell J, et al. Routine diagnosis of mammary Paget's disease: a modern approach. *Am J Surg Pathol* 1992;16:58.
46. Ramachandra S, Gillett C, Millis R. A comparative immunohistochemical study of mammary and extramammary Paget's disease and superficial spreading melanoma with particular emphasis on melanocytic markers. *Virchows Arch* 1996;429:371.
47. Gillet CE, Bobrow LG, Millis RR. S100 protein in human mammary tissue—immunoreactivity in breast carcinoma including Paget's disease of the nipple and value as a marker of myoepithelial cells. *J Pathol* 1990;160:19.
48. Shah KD, Tabibzadeh SS, Gerber MA. Immunohistochemical distinction of Paget's disease from Bowen's disease and superficial speading melanoma with the use of monoclonal cytokeratin antibodies. *Am J Clin Pathol* 1987;88:689.
49. Requena L, Sanchez Y, Nunez C, White C, Sangueza O. Epidermotropically metastatic breast carcinomas. Rare histopathologic variants mimicking melanoma and Paget's disease. *Am J Dermatopathol* 1996;18:385.
50. Ben-Izhak O, Stark P, Levy R, Bergman R, Lichtig C. Epithelial markers in malignant melanoma: a study of primary lesions and their metastases. *Am J Dermatopathol* 1994;16:241.
51. Gown AM, Vogel AM, Hoak D, Gough F, McNutt MA. Monoclonal antibodies specific for melanocytic tumors distinguish subpopulations of melanocytes. *Am J Pathol* 1986;123:195.
52. Bishop PW, Menasce LP, Yates AJ, Win NA, Bunerjee SS. An immunophenotypic survey of malignant melanomas. *Histopathology* 1993;23:159.
53. Wick M, Swanson P, Rocamora A. Recognition of malignant melanoma by monoclonal antibody HMB-45: an immunohistochemical study of 200 paraffin-embedded cutaneous tumors. *J Cutan Pathol* 1988;15:201.
54. Toker C. Clear cells of the nipple epidermis. *Cancer* 1970;25:601.
55. Yim J, Wick M, Philpott G, Norton J, Doherty G. Underlying pathology in mammary Paget's disease. *Ann Surg Oncol* 1997;4:287.
56. Paone JF, Baker PR. Pathogenesis and treatment of Paget's disease of the breast. *Cancer* 1981;48:825.
57. Maier WP, Rosemond GP, Harasym EL, et al. Paget's disease of the female breast. *Surg Gynecol Obstet* 1969;128:1253.
58. Stomper P, Penetrante R, Carson W. Sensitivity of mammography on patients with Paget's disease of the nipple. *Breast Dis* 1995;8:173.
59. Ikeda DM, Helvie MA, Frank TS, et al. Paget's disease of the nipple: radiologic-pathologic correlation. *Radiology* 1993;189:89.
60. Edeiken S. Mammography in the symptomatic woman. *Cancer* 1989;63:1412.
61. Sawyer RH, Asbury DL. Mammographic appearances in Paget's disease of the breast. *Clin Radiol* 1994;49:185.
62. Egan RE. *Breast imaging*. London: WB Saunders, 1988:426.
63. Kollmorgen DR, Varanasi JS, Edge SB, Carson WE. 3rd Paget's disease of the breast: a 33-year experience. *J Am Coll Surg* 1998;187:171.
64. Wertheim U, Ozzello L. Neoplastic involvement of nipple and skin flap in carcinoma of the breast. *Am J Surg Pathol* 1980;4:543.
65. Ceccherini AF, Evans AJ, Pinder SE, et al. Is ipsilateral mammography worthwhile in Paget's disease of the breast? *Clin Radiol* 1996;51:35.
66. Lagios MD, Gates EA, Westdahl PR, et al. A guide to the frequency of nipple involvement in breast cancer. *Am J Surg* 1979;138:135.
67. Berg JW, Hutter RV. Breast cancer. *Cancer* 1995;75[Suppl 1]:257.
68. Stalsberg H, Thomas DB. Age distribution of histologic types of breast carcinoma. *Int J Cancer* 1993;54:1.
69. Turner L, Swindell R, Bell WG, et al. Radical versus modified radical mastectomy for breast cancer. *Ann R Coll Surg Engl* 1981;63:239.
70. Maddox WA, Carpenter JT Jr, Laws HL, et al. A randomized prospective trial of radical (Halsted) mastectomy versus modified radical mastectomy in 311 breast cancer patients. *Ann Surg* 1983;198:207.
71. Veronesi U, Salvadori B, Luini A, et al. Breast conservation is a safe method in patients with small cancers of the breast. Long-term results of three randomized trials on 1973 patients. *Eur J Cancer* 1995;31A:1574.
72. Fisher B, Anderson S, Redmond CK, et al. Reanalysis and results after 12 years of follow-up in a randomized clinical trial comparing total mastectomy with lumpectomy with or without irradiation in the treatment of breast cancer. *N Engl J Med* 1995;333:1456.
73. Brenner R, Rothman B. Detection of primary breast cancer in women with known adenocarcinoma metastatic to the axilla: use of MRI after negative clinical and mammographic examination. *J Magn Reson Imaging* 1997;7:1153.
74. Friedman E, Hall-Craggs M, Mumtaz H, Schneidau A. Breast MR and the appearance of the normal and abnormal nipple. *Clin Radiol* 1997;52:854.
75. Anelli A, Anelli TF, McCormick B, Senie R, Borgen PL. Conservative management of Paget's disease of the nipple (meeting abstract). Proc Annual Meeting First European Breast Cancer Conference. *Am Soc Clin Oncol* 1995;A100(abst).
76. Pierce L, Haffty BG, Solin LJ, et al. The conservative management of Paget's disease of the breast with radiotherapy. *Cancer* 1997;80:1065.
77. EORTC 10873 Phase II Study Breast conserving therapy in Paget's disease of the nipple.
78. Hareyama M, Saito A, Oocubo T, et al. A case report of Paget's disease of the breast treated with radiotherapy alone. *Radiat Med* 1990;8:152.
79. El-Sharkawi A, Waters JS. The place for conservative treatment in the management of Paget's disease of the nipple. *Eur J Surg Oncol* 1992;18:301.
80. Bulens P, Vanuytsel L, Rijnders A. Breast conserving treatment of Paget's disease. *Radiother Oncol* 1990;17:305.
81. Christiaens MR, Knol J, Van den Bogaert W, VanLimbergen E. Treatment of Paget's disease of the breast with radiotherapy only. *Proc Annu Meet Am Soc Clin Oncol* 1998:258.
82. Stockdale AD, Brierley JD, White WF, Folkes A, Rostom AY. Radiotherapy for Paget's disease of the nipple: a conservative alternative. *Lancet* 1989;2:664.
83. Forquet A, Campana F, Viech P, et al. Paget's disease of the nipple without detectable breast tumor: conservative management with radiation therapy. *Int J Radiat Oncol Biol Phys* 1987;13:1463.
84. McGregor JK, McGregor DD. Paget's disease of the breast. A twenty-two year survey of cases presenting at a large general hospital. *Surgery* 1959;45:562.
85. Ridenhour CE, Perez-Mesa C, Husi JM. Paget's disease of the nipple. *Cancer Bull* 1969;21:15.
86. West JP, Nickel WF Jr. Paget's disease of the nipple. *Ann Surg* 1942;116:19.
87. Helman P, Kliman M. Paget's disease of the nipple. A clinical review of 27 cases. *Br J Surg* 1956;43:481.
88. Lattes R, Haagensen CD. Proceedings of II International Symposiums on Mammary Cancer at University of Perugia, Italy. 1957:189.

CHAPTER 43

Diseases of the Breast, 2nd ed.,
edited by Jay R. Harris.
Lippincott Williams & Wilkins, Philadelphia © 2000.

Other Cancers of the Breast

Carl Freter

The most frequently encountered non-epithelial malignancies of the breast presenting as primary breast masses are lymphomas, sarcomas, and malignant melanomas. Metastatic cancer to the breast is occasionally the first presenting sign of a distant malignancy, and a wide variety of malignancies may at some time during their clinical courses involve at least one anatomic component of the breast. Although each of these malignancies involving the breast is uncommon to rare compared to epithelial breast malignant disease, knowledge of their unique features in terms of clinical characteristics, pathology, molecular biology, appropriate diagnosis, staging, and treatment is necessary to preserve optimal care and outcomes. In contrast to epithelial breast cancer, the role of surgery in breast lymphomas is largely limited to obtaining diagnostic tissue. Diagnostic and staging procedures are frequently very different and treatment is based on chemotherapy, with radiation therapy sometimes playing a role. Breast sarcomas are a heterogeneous group of diseases spanning a wide spectrum from relatively benign to aggressively malignant with high metastatic potential. As in epithelial breast cancer, surgery plays a dominant therapeutic role within a multi modality approach, which also frequently involves radiation therapy and chemotherapy, with the latter therapy specific for sarcoma treatment. Malignant melanoma is an initially cutaneous disease whose prognosis heavily rests on a unique staging system focused on vertical and anatomic extent of skin involvement. Surgery is the primary initial therapeutic modality, with additional less clearly defined roles for chemotherapy, radiation therapy, and other biological agents that are sometimes used for more extensive disease. Metastatic disease to the breast from an occult primary site often involves a pathologic tour de force of analysis of a primary breast metastatic cancer tissue sample involving conventional histologic sections, special stains, examination of cell surface and other markers with immunohistochemistry and flow cytometry, cytogenetics, electron microscopy, and molecular identification of any of an increasingly wide variety of aberrant or aberrantly expressed genes. Such an approach in the primary tumor tissue may be complemented at times by an almost equally complex effort to identify the primary source of the malignancy within the patient.

PRIMARY BREAST LYMPHOMA

Primary breast lymphomas are thought to arise from the malignant transformation of lymphocytes either in residence or in transit in intramammary lymph nodes or from lymphatics representing less than 1 per 1,000 malignant breast tumors.[1,2] Occasional observations of bilateral primary breast lymphoma[3,4] associated with pregnancy or lactation, or both,[5–7] and the presence of estrogen or progesterone receptors[5,8] suggest complex biological-hormonal-trophic relationships between organs of origin and breast lymphomas, whose precise natures and etiologic roles remain uncertain. The clinical presentation of lymphoma in the breast is similar to presentation at other sites, with a typically single, painless, round, "rubbery" (as opposed to hard), immobile (as opposed to mobile enlarged peripheral) mass within the breast parenchyma. Typically, primary breast lymphomas do not involve fixation to underlying chest wall or overlying cutaneous changes (which, if present, are nearly uniformly associated with intermediate or high-grade lymphomas within the Working Formulation classification).[2,6,8] Skin thickening, redness, hypervascularity, or ulceration all suggest direct extension into the skin, often with a T-lymphocyte phenotype in contrast to the 90% B-lymphocyte predominance of non-Hodgkin's lymphomas (NHLs) in general. Primary lymphomas of the skin overlying the breast include true epidermotropic mycosis fungoides, "peripheral" T-cell lymphomas, or cutaneous B-cell lymphomas. Radiographic imaging characteristics of breast lymphomas are relatively nonspecific, with the exception that microcalcifications are rare.[9,10] Imaging modalities depending on a differentially nonincreased metabolic or growth rate (e.g., gallium or positron emission tomography scans) may be of some use in distinguishing breast lymphomas from other breast neoplasms after response to therapy and in determining remission status in the presence of

C. Freter: Lombardi Cancer Center, Georgetown University Medical Center, Washington, D.C.

TABLE 1. *Ann Arbor Staging System*

Stage	Description
I	Involvement of a single lymph node region (I) or a single extralymphatic organ or site (IE).
II	Involvement of two or more lymph node regions on the same side of the diaphragm (II) or localized involvement of an extralymphatic organ or site (IIE).
III	Involvement of lymph node regions on both sides of the diaphragm (III) or localized involvement of an extralymphatic organ or site (IIIE) or spleen (IIIS) or both (IIISE).
IV	Diffuse or disseminated involvement for one or more extralymphatic organs with or without associated lymph node involvement.

Identification of the presence or absence of symptoms should be noted with each stage designation. *A* added to stage number represents asymptomatic; *B* added to stage number represents fever, sweats, and weight loss of more than 10% of body weight.

minimal residual masses determined by physical examination or other imaging techniques.[11–13]

The most commonly used pathologic classification systems for NHL are the Working Formulation classification system[14] and the Revised European American Lymphoma classification system,[15] which both roughly divide NHL into three distinct groups characterized as low grade, intermediate grade, and high grade. With more sophisticated molecular subclassifications of NHL, however, less clear distinctions exist between some members of these groups, although for therapeutic purposes these distinctions remain useful. Pathologic diagnostic analysis of NHL typically includes, in addition to standard hematoxylin and eosin stain, light microscopy cell surface markers for T- versus B-cell lineage, monoclonality, and other characteristics by immunohistochemistry and flow cytometry, cytogenetics, and molecular studies for immunoglobulin and T-cell receptor gene rearrangements. Cytogenetics and gene rearrangement studies in particular may be useful in defining tumor or patient-specific disease markers detectable by sensitive polymerase chain reaction-based tests or other methods to evaluate the presence of submicroscopic disease for both staging and assessing completeness of treatment response. Histologic features suggestive of lymphoma in limited needle biopsy specimens obtained from breast masses are absence of *in situ* carcinoma, frequent individual karyorrhectic cells, lymphoepithelial lesions, and cellular discohesiveness.[16]

The Ann Arbor Staging System (Table 1) developed originally for Hodgkin's disease is also used for NHL. The International Prognostic Index has defined clear prognostic groups within the Ann Arbor stages,[17] but neither primary breast lymphoma nor breast involvement are explicitly recognized prognostic factors. Typically, staging procedures include contrast computed tomography scans of the chest, abdomen, and pelvis, and bilateral bone marrow biopsies and aspirates. Other staging studies may include head computed tomography scans, magnetic resonance imaging scans, gallium scans, positron emission tomography scans, lymphangiography, and lumbar puncture with evaluation of cerebrospinal fluid chemistry and cytology depending on the clinical presentation and histologic subtype of lymphoma. A variety of biopsy techniques, including gastrointestinal endoscopy, bronchoscopy, mediastinoscopy, thoracoscopy, laparoscopy, thoracotomy, or laparotomy, may be indicated in the process of diagnosis and staging.[18]

The published clinical series of primary breast lymphomas reflect the heterogeneity of NHL[8]; however, the overall experience with primary breast lymphomas is that they behave similarly to primary lymphomas in other sites, including distribution of histologic subtypes, clinical course, response to therapy, and prognosis. A retrospective review of 23 previously untreated patients with localized primary lymphoma of the breast contained two patients with low-grade lymphomas, 18 with intermediate, and two with high-grade lymphomas (one patient was unclassifiable). The overall 5-year relapse-free survival rate for the various treatment approaches for the entire group was 73%, and was 70% for the 17 patients with diffuse large cell lymphoma, results comparable to those for similar series of Stage I or II lymphomas of other sites.[19] A small, distinct, and notable group of patients present during pregnancy or lactation with bilateral, diffuse, extremely aggressive disease with a high-grade Burkitt's histology, which is usually rapidly fatal despite aggressive combination chemotherapy.[5] These lymphomas are often reported to have estrogen receptors or progesterone receptors, as has been the case in four such patients treated by the author. Another distinctive monocytoid B-cell primary breast lymphoma suggested to be related to the mucosa-associated lymphoid tissue lymphomas has been described, but has not been generally recognized.[5]

Treatment recommendations for primary breast lymphomas are the same for primary lymphomas presenting in other nodal or extranodal sites. Pathologic stage I disease (low grade) requires involved field radiation therapy; intermediate or high grade requires "short-course" combination chemotherapy followed by involved field radiation therapy.[18] High-grade presentations with bilateral or systemic disease in pregnant or lactating women should be treated with high-grade lymphoma regimens and considered for high-dose therapy in the context of autologous or allogeneic bone marrow or stem cell transplantation.

The acquired immunodeficiency syndrome (AIDS)–associated NHLs represent a particular challenge for treatment because they are aggressive, often high-grade, stage IV lesions occurring in multiple nodal and extranodal sites whose treatment is complicated by poor performance status, bone marrow function, opportunistic infections, and severe immunosuppression. Primary, isolated breast disease in this setting is extremely uncommon, although breast involvement during the course of AIDS-associated lymphoma is not rare. A number of chemotherapy regimens and treatment plans have been developed for treatment of AIDS-related lymphomas.[20–22] The interested reader is referred to more detailed discussion and description of treatment regimens for NHL.[18] Other hematologic malignancies that rarely present in the breast include Hodgkin's disease, multiple myeloma, and granulocytic sarcoma.[16]

PRIMARY BREAST SARCOMAS

Primary malignancies of the breast stromal elements and sarcomas of mesenchymal origin comprise less than 1% of all breast neoplasms, and are a highly heterogeneous group of tumors.[23–45] Although the extensive histologic array of breast sarcomas does not differ greatly from those of other sites in the body, the majority are made up of malignant fibrous histiocytomas, fibrosarcomas, liposarcomas, and the less common angiosarcomas; true "stromal sarcomas" of the breast are distinctly rare.[46] Although malignant fibrous histiocytomas and fibrosarcomas tend to predominate in reported surgical and pathologic series of "spontaneous" primary breast sarcomas, some series of sarcomas arising in previously therapeutically irradiated breasts have reported angiosarcomas with increasing frequency following the initial description by Body et al. in 1987.[47–52] However, the etiology of the increasing use of radiation therapy in the treatment of epithelial breast cancer in breast preservation therapeutic strategies is uncertain, as discussed in Primary Angiosarcomas of the Breast. Cystosarcoma phyllodes, or phyllodes tumors, are not formally true sarcomas because they are composed of epithelial elements within a cellular connective tissue stroma and are considered in Chapter 41.

Primary breast sarcomas typically clinically present with a unilateral mass of variable growth rate, a rate that is often rapid compared to that of epithelial breast cancer. In contrast to epithelial breast cancer, the dominant mode of metastatic spread in primary breast sarcoma is hematogenous, with axillary or other local lymph node involvement being comparatively rare.[26–37] The most common sites of initial metastatic spread are the lungs, bone marrow, and liver, although hematogenous metastases can appear in virtually any anatomic site.[23–45] Radiographic imaging characteristics are nonspecific, except that tumor inhomogeneity is commonly consistent with areas of necrosis, and mirocalcifications are rare and suggest a malignancy of epithelial origin.[31,32,37,39]

Diagnostic tissue is infrequently obtained from fine-needle or small core biopsies, and sufficient tissue for diagnosis and histologic grading usually requires large-needle core, incisional, or excisional biopsy. Excisional biopsy is clearly preferred in limiting hematogenous dissemination if a suspicion of a sarcoma is entertained on the basis of clinical, radiographic, or previous cytologic or histologic evidence. Aside from histologic classification, the most critical pathologic judgment is histologic grade,[26] which is central to the staging system and also includes determination of primary tumor size, presence or absence of local nodal or distant metastasis (Table 2), and, although not formally part of the staging system, anatomic location. Other studies in pathologic analysis and differentiation from other malignancies can include cell surface markers, immunohistochemical studies, cytogenctics, molecular determination of altered expression of tumor suppressor or oncogenes, and, in some cases, ultrastructural electron microscopic studies.

TABLE 2. *American Joint Committee on Cancer staging system for soft-tissue sarcomas: International Union against Cancer*

Tumor, node, metastasis definitions	
Histologic grade	
G1	Low grade
G2	Moderate grade
G3	High grade
Primary tumor	
T1	Tumor smaller than 5 cm
T2	Tumor 5 cm or larger
Regional nodes	
N0	No histologically verified metastases to regional nodes
N1	Histologically verified regional lymph node metastases
Distant metastasis	
M0	No distant metastasis
M1	Distant metastasis present
Stage grouping	
Stage IA	G1, T1, N0, M0
Stage IB	G1, T2, N0, M0
Stage IIA	G2, T1, N0, M0
Stage IIB	G2, T2, N0, M0
Stage IIIA	G3, T1, N0, M0
Stage IIIB	G3, T2, N0, M0
Stage IVA	Any G, any T, N1, M0
Stage IVB	Any G, any T, N1, M1

From Beahrs OH, Henson DE, Hutter RVP, Kennedy BJ, eds. *Manual for staging of cancer*, 4th ed. Philadelphia: JB Lippincott, 1992. With permission.

In general, the treatment for primary breast sarcomas is excision with or without mastectomy depending on tumor size, histology, grade, and margins.[53–57] The additional roles of radiation therapy and chemotherapy, although not clearly established, also depend on the preceding variables.[53–58] Optimum treatment is best individualized in a multi modality approach involving a collaborative effort in planning therapy between surgeon, radiation oncologist, and medical oncologist.[59] For metastatic disease, the approach to breast sarcomas is the same as for other sarcomas of the same histology and grade, and should likewise involve a multi modality approach. The interested reader is referred to a more extensive review of specific therapeutic approaches to individual sarcomas.[60]

Several sarcomas of note with respect to primary breast presentations are individually discussed in the following sections.

Primary Angiosarcoma of the Breast

Angiosarcomas have a predilection for involvement of the breast as opposed to other anatomic sites.[61] Typical presentation is a rapidly expanding breast mass, frequently with an observed violaceous or bluish color of the overlying skin and a significant incidence of bilaterality.[61–63] Specific histopathologic findings include hyperchromatic nuclei and the presence of interanastomosing vascular channels within the breast parenchyma, and prognostically significant subgroups based on degree of differentiation or other histologic features, or both, have been proposed.[61,64] As with other sarcomas, prognosis is most closely linked to histologic grade, with tumor size and the ability to obtain adequate resection with clear margins determining whether an excisional approach versus mastectomy is used. Traditionally, axillary dissection has not been recommended, and the roles of adjuvant chemotherapy or radiation therapy are unclear. Although angiosarcomas in the context of breast-conserving surgery and radiation therapy for epithelial breast cancer have been increasingly described since 1987, a study of 122,991 women treated for breast cancer in the Swedish Cancer Register identified 116 sarcomas, 40 of which were angiosarcomas.[65] In this case-control study, angiosarcoma correlated significantly with lymphedema of the arm with an odds ratio of 9.5 (95% confidence interval, 3.2–28.0). No correlation with radiation therapy was observed, although a correlation with integral radiation dose did appear to exist with other sarcomas. Similarly, in a published series of 20,000 women treated with breast-conserving surgery and radiation therapy from French comprehensive cancer centers, nine angiosarcomas were identified, representing a prevalence of 5 per 10,000, which is the same prevalence observed in France in healthy breasts.[66] The median latency between treatment and angiosarcoma was 74 months, with all recurrences of angiosarcoma after mastectomy for angiosarcoma occurring within 16 months. In this setting, patients with angiosarcoma had a poor prognosis, with a median survival of 15.5 months.

Extraskeletal Primary Osteogenic Sarcoma of the Breast

Extraskeletal osteogenic sarcomas are associated with the diagnostic mammographic finding of osseous trabeculae within a breast mass.[38,67,68] A retrospective series of 50 cases of primary pure osteosarcoma of the breast diagnosed between 1957 and 1995 at the Armed Forces Institute of Pathology presented with a median age of 64.5 years; only one patient had received ipsilateral radiation therapy for breast carcinoma 9 years previously.[67] All 20 cases in which axillary node dissection was carried out were free of tumor. Of 39 patients with follow-up, locally recurrent (n = 11) or metastatic disease (n = 15) was observed in 59% at means of 10.5 and 14.5 months from diagnosis, respectively.[67]

Primary Embryonal Rhabdomyosarcoma of the Breast

Primary breast embryonal rhabdomyosarcomas (RMS) are malignancies of adolescent and young women, although they have been occasionally described in older women as well.[69–71] Of 26 patients with either primary or secondary RMS identified from 1972–1992 by the Intergroup Rhabdomyosarcoma Study, all were female with a median age of 15.2 years (11.5–20.2). Twenty-four were of alveolar histologic subtype with seven tumors primary in the breast and 19 tumors metastatic to the breast. Fifty percent of patients with primary breast disease and 15% of those with metastatic breast disease were long-term survivors after risk-based treatment, according to extent and site of disease.[71]

Stewart-Treves Syndrome (Lymphedema-Associated Lymphangiosarcoma)

In 1948, Stewart and Treves described six cases of lymphangiosarcoma in edematous upper extremities of women treated with radical mastectomy and radiation therapy for breast carcinoma.[72] The recognized incidence of this eponymous syndrome is approximately 0.5% in such patients with an aggressive fatal clinical course, with 5-year survival of less than 5% with multimodality treatment.[73,74]

CUTANEOUS MALIGNANT MELANOMA OF THE BREAST

Melanoma is one of the common tumors metastasizing to either the breast parenchyma or overlying skin although primary cutaneous melanomas of the skin overlying the breast only account for a small percentage of cutaneous melanomas.[75–77] Cutaneous melanoma of the skin of the breast is diagnosed at an average age of 40 years, more frequently in men but at a younger age in women; therefore, the role of differential sun exposure is uncertain.[75–78] Melanomas may also occur (although uncommonly) in the nipple-areolar complex, and must be pathologically distinguished from Paget's disease with phagocytosis of melanin by Paget's cells.[79–81] Symptoms and signs suggestive of melanoma in pigmented cutaneous lesions of the breast are the same as elsewhere and include changes in size, pigmentation, ulceration, and bleeding.[75–78] Similarly, risk factors for metastatic spread include a vertical growth phase pattern, ulceration, Clark level III or higher,[82] or thickness greater than 1.5 mm as described by Breslow[83] (Table 3).

Current treatment recommendations are for excisional biopsy of suspicious skin lesions followed by wide local excision of primary diagnostic skin lesions.[75,77] The extent of resection is traditionally based on the thickness of the primary lesion with 1-cm margins for lesions smaller than 1-mm and 2- to 3-cm margins for thicker lesions.[84,85] Although axillary node involvement increases with tumor thickness, the appropriate setting and role of lymphadenectomy remains controversial, although resection of clinically positive nodes appears to achieve improved local control and improve survival.[77,85,86] Lesion thickness has generally been used as a criterion for elective dissection of a clinically negative axillary basin, although the sentinel lymph node tech-

TABLE 3. *New staging system for melanoma adopted by the American Joint Committee on Cancer*

Stage	Description
IA	Localized melanoma ≤0.75 mm or level II[a] (T1, N0, M0)
IB	Localized melanoma 0.76–1.50 mm or level III[a] (T2, N0, M0)
IIA	Localized melanoma 1.5–4.0 mm or level IV[a] (T3, N0, M0)
IIB	Localized melanoma >4 mm or level V[a] (T4, N0, M0)
III	Limited nodal metastases involving only one regional lymph node basin or fewer than five in-transit metastases without nodal metastases (any T, N1, M0)
IV	Advanced regional metastases (any T, N2M0) or any patient with distant metastases (any T, any N, M1 or M2)

[a]When the thickness and level of invasion criteria do not coincide within a T classification, thickness should take precedence.
From Ketcham AS, Balch CM. Classification and staging systems. In: Balch CM, Milton GW, eds. *Cutaneous melanoma: clinical management and treatment results worldwide.* Philadelphia: JB Lippincott, 1985:55. With permission.

nique has been reported to be an acceptable, less invasive method for assessment of axillary node status.[86–90] The prognoses for cutaneous melanomas of the breast are similar to those for melanomas in other anatomic sites, with one series reporting a 72% overall survival rate with a median follow-up of 58 months.[77]

METASTASES TO THE BREAST

The most common malignancy to metastasize to the breast in women is contralateral breast cancer by a "cross-lymphatic" route.[91,92] (In men, it is prostate cancer by hematogenous metastases.[93,94]) In children and adolescent females, RMS is the most common metastatic lesion to the breast, as previously discussed (see Primary Breast Sarcomas).[69–71] Overall, metastatic cancer to the breast is seen in premenopausal women older than 30 years.[95,96] The most common non-breast primary malignancies with hematogenous metastases to the breast are NHL leukemias, melanoma, and lung cancer, particularly small cell carcinoma.[92,93,96–98] Gynecologic cancers metastasizing to the female breast are commonly reported, suggesting incompletely defined hormonal or trophic effects and biology; the most common are ovarian and cervical carcinomas, followed by carcinomas of the vagina, endometrium, and peritoneum.[99] Soft-tissue sarcomas, gastrointestinal adenocarcinomas, and other genitourinary tumors are also metastatic to the breast, although uncommon.[92,97,98,100–105] Rare metastases to the breast have been reported in fallopian tube cancer,[106] ovarian dysgerminoma,[107] medullary thyroid cancer,[108,109] carcinoid,[110] medulloblastoma,[111] malignant schwannoma,[112] and pharyngeal carcinoma.[113]

Mammographic findings in women with breast metastases are nonspecific with single or multiple masses, often with skin thickening or axillary adenopathy, although metastatic lymphomas or chloromas may be associated with a diffuse increase in stromal density of surrounding breast tissue and absent microcalcifications.[92,98] Fine-needle aspiration cytology specimens may sometimes be useful in distinguishing metastatic from primary breast tumors, but open biopsy is frequently necessary to obtain adequate tissue for pathologic analysis. Pathologic analysis can include cytochemistry, immunohistochemistry, cytogenetics, flow cytometric analysis, electron microscopy and other molecular studies and can confirm a primary metastatic site or aid in its identification in the case of an occult primary malignancy.[96–98,104] The possibility of synchronous or metachronous metastatic disease coexisting with primary breast epithelial carcinoma must prompt careful evaluation of bilateral breast masses or disease to clarify overall diagnosis, management approach, and treatment.[114–116] Factors suggesting contralateral metastatic breast cancer include short disease-free interval, medial location, multiple breast lesion, and known metastatic breast cancer at other distant sites.[115–118] Factors suggesting non-breast metastatic disease include location in fat or subcutaneous tissue as opposed to breast parenchyma, lack of *in situ* disease, and lack of microcalcifications.[114–121]

Metastatic disease to the breast is associated with an overall poor prognosis with a median survival of less than 1 year, except in the case of lymphoma or other hematologic malignancies.[96,98] Oncologic management of cancer metastatic to the breast should focus on diagnosis and appropriate treatment for the primary lesion with palliation and local control of disease at metastatic sites as necessary. If the primary versus metastatic nature of a new epithelial breast cancer is uncertain, treatment should be undertaken for a presumed new primary lesion. Similarly, in cases of histologic or anatomic uncertainty regarding metastatic disease, treatment efforts should be focused on a balance between the probable histologic identity and primary site of the lesion and the known therapeutic efficacy of treatment for the presumed primary cancer.

REFERENCES

1. Tavassoli FA. *Pathology of the breast.* New York: Elsevier, 1992:625.
2. Giardini R, Piccolo C, Rilke F. Primary non-Hodgkin's lymphomas of the female breast. *Cancer* 1992;69:725.
3. Wiseman C, Liao K. Primary lymphoma of the breast. *Cancer* 1972;29:1705.
4. Arber D, Simpson J, Weiss L, et al. Non-Hodgkin's lymphoma involving the breast. *Am J Surg Pathol* 1994;18:288.
5. Hugh JC, Jackson FI, Hanson JP, et al. Primary breast lymphoma: an immunohistologic study of 20 new cases. *Cancer* 1990: 66:2602.
6. Abbondanzo SL, Seidman JD, Lefkowitz M, Tavassoli FA, Krishnan J. Primary diffuse large B-cell lymphoma of the breast: a clinicopathologic study of 31 cases. *Pathol Res Pract* 1996;192:37.
7. Kirkpatrick AW, Bailey DJ, Weizel HA. Bilateral primary lymphoma in pregnancy: a case report and literature review. *Can J Surg* 1996; 39(4):333.

8. Bobrow LG, Richards MA, Haperfield LC, et al. Breast lymphomas: a clinicopathologic review. *Hum Pathol* 1992;24:274.
9. Mussurakis S, Carleton PJ, Turnbull LW. Imaging of primary non-Hodgkin's breast lymphoma: a case report. *Acta Radiol* 1997;38:104.
10. Liberman L, Giess CS, Dershaw DD. Non-Hodgkin's lymphoma of the breast: imaging characteristics and correlation with histopathologic findings. *Radiology* 1994;192:157.
11. Gasparini M, Bombardieri E, Castellani M, et al. Gallium-67 scintigraphy evaluation of therapy in non-Hodgkin's lymphoma. *J Nucl Med* 1998;39:1586.
12. Hussain R, Christie DR, Gebski V, Barton MB, Gruenewald SM. The role of the gallium scan in primary extranodal lymphoma. *J Nucl Med* 1998;39:95.
13. Delbeke D. Oncological applications of FDG PET imaging: brain tumors, colorectal cancer, lymphoma and melanoma. *J Nucl Med* 1999;40:591.
14. National Cancer Institute-sponsored study of classification of non-Hodgkin's lymphomas: the Non-Hodgkin's Lymphoma Pathologic Classification Project. *Cancer* 1982;49:2112.
15. Jaffe ES, Harris NL, Diebold J, Muller-Hermelink HK. World Health Organization classification of lymphomas: a work in progress. *Ann Oncol* 1998;9[Suppl 5]:S25.
16. Lin Y, Govindan R, Hess JL. Malignant hematopoietic breast tumors. *Am J Clin Pathol* 1997;107:177.
17. Coiffier B, Shipp MA, Cabanillas F, Crowther D, Armitage JO, Canellos GP. Report of the first workshop on prognostic factors in large-cell lymphomas. *Ann Oncol* 1991;2[Suppl 2]:213.
18. Shipp MA, Mauch PM, Harris NL. Non-Hodgkin's lymphomas. In: DeVita VT, Hellman S, Rosenberg SA, eds. *Cancer principles and practice of oncology*, 5th ed. Lippincott–Raven, 1997:2165.
19. Ha CS, Dubey P, Goyal LK, et al. Localized primary non-Hodgkin lymphoma of the breast. *Am J Clin Oncol* 1998:21:376.
20. Brockmeyer N, Barthel B. Clinical manifestations and therapies of AIDS associated tumors. *Eur J Med Res* 1998;3(3):127.
21. Straus DJ. Human immunodeficiency virus-associated lymphomas. *Med Clin North Am* 1997;81(20):495.
22. Freter CE. Acquired immunodeficiency syndrome-associated lymphomas. *J Monogr Natl Cancer Inst* 1990;10:45.
23. Barnes L, Pietruszka M. Sarcomas of the breast. *Cancer* 1977;40:1577.
24. Callery CD, Rosen PP, Kinne DW. Sarcoma of the breast. *Ann Surg* 1985;201:527.
25. Khana S, Gupta S, Khana NN. Sarcomas of the breast: homogeneous or heterogenous. *J Surg Oncol* 1981;18:119.
26. Costa J, Wesley RA, Glastein E, et al. The grading of soft tissue sarcomas: results of a clinicopathologic correlation in a series of 163 cases. *Cancer* 1984;53:530.
27. Pollard SG, Marks PV, et al. Breast sarcoma: a clinicopathologic review of 25 cases. *Cancer* 1991;66:941.
28. McGregor GI, Knowling MA, Este FA. Sarcoma and cystosarcoma phyllodes tumors of the breast: a retrospective review of 58 cases. *Am J Surg* 1994;167:477.
29. Terrier PH, Terrier-Lacombe MJ, Mourisse H, et al. Primary breast sarcoma: a review of 33 cases with immunohistochemistry and prognostic factors. *Breast Cancer Res Treat* 1989;13:39.
30. Norris HJ, Taylor HB. Sarcomas and related mesenchymal tumors of the breast. *Cancer* 1968;22:22.
31. D'Orsi, CJ, Feldhaus L, Sonnenfeld M. Unusual lesions of the breast. *Radiol Clin North Am* 1983;21:67.
32. Langham MR Jr, Mills AS, DeMay RM, et al. Malignant fibrous histiocytoma of the breast. *Cancer* 1984;54:558.
33. Austin RM, Dupree WB. Liposarcoma of the breast: a clinicopathologic study of 20 cases. *Hum Pathol* 1986;17:906.
34. Chen KTK, Kuo TT, Hoffmann KD. Leiomyosarcoma of the breast. *Cancer* 1981;47:1883.
35. Pardo-Mindan J, Garcia-Julian G, Altuna ME. Leiomyosarcoma of the breast. *Am J Clin Pathol* 1974;62:477.
36. Pitts WC, Rojas VA, Gaffey MJ, et al. Carcinomas with metaplasia and sarcomas of the breast. *Am J Clin Oncol* 1991;95:623.
37. Roditi G, Prasad S. Case report radiology of stromal sarcoma of the breast with ossifying pleural metastases. *Br J Radiol* 1994;67:212.
38. Jernstrom P, Lindberg AL, Meland ON. Osteogenic sarcoma of the mammary gland. *Am J Clin Pathol* 1963;40:521.
39. Elson BC, Ikeda DM, Anderson I, et al. Fibrosarcoma of the breast: mammographic findings in five cases. *AJR Am J Roentgenol* 1992; 158:993.
40. Myerowitz RL, Pietruszka M, Barnes EL. Primary angiosarcoma of the breast. *JAMA* 1978;30:239.
41. Rainewater LM, Martin JK, Gaffey TA, et al. Angiosarcoma of the breast. *Arch Surg* 1986;121:669.
42. Chen KT, Kirkegaard DD, Bocian JJ. Angiosarcoma of the breast. *Cancer* 1980;46:368.
43. Antman KH, Corson J, Greenberg J, et al. Multimodality therapy in the management of angiosarcoma of the breast. *Cancer* 1982;50:2000.
44. Merino MJ, Berman M, Carter D. Angiosarcoma of the breast. *Am J Surg Pathol* 1983;7:53.
45. Roger PP, Kimmel M, Ernsberger D. Mammary angiosarcoma: the prognostic significance of tumor differentiation. *Cancer* 1988;62:2145.
46. Berg JW, DeCrosse JJ, Fracchia AA, et al. Stromal sarcomas of the breast. *Cancer* 1962;15:418.
47. Body G, Sauvanet E, Calais G, et al. Angiosarcoma of the breast following adenocarcinome mammaire opere et irradie. *J Gynecol Obstet Biol Reprod* 1987;16:479.
48. Timmer SJ, Osuch JR, Colony LH, et al. Angiosarcoma of the breast following lumpectomy and radiation therapy for breast carcinoma: case report and review of the literature. *Breast J* 1997;3:40.
49. Buatti JM, Harari PM, Leigh BR, et al. Radiation-included angiosarcoma of the breast. *Am J Clin Oncol* 1994;17:444.
50. Provencio M, Bonilla F, Espana, P. Breast angiosarcoma after radiation therapy. *Acta Oncol* 1995;34:969.
51. Turner WH, Greenall MJ. Sarcoma induced by radiotherapy after breast conservation surgery. *Br J Surg* 1991;78:1317.
52. Zucali R, Merson M, Placucci M, et al. Soft tissue sarcoma of the breast after conservative surgery and irradiation for early mammary cancer. *Radiother Oncol* 1994;30:271.
53. Gutman H, Polloch RE, Ross MI, et al. Sarcoma of the breast: implications for extent of therapy: the M. D. Anderson Experience. *Surgery* 1994;116:505.
54. Devereux DF, Wilson RE, et al. Surgical treatment of low-grade tissue sarcomas. *Am J Surg* 1982;143:490.
55. Savage R. The treatment of angiosarcoma of the breast. *J Surg Oncol* 1981;18:129.
56. Rosner D. Angiosarcoma of the breast: long-term survival following adjuvant chemotherapy. *J Surg Oncol* 1988;39:90.
57. Hunter TB, Martin PC, Dietzen CD, et al. Angiosarcoma of the breast. *Cancer* 1985;56:2099.
58. Johnstone PA, Pierce LJ, Merino MJ, et al. Primary soft tissue sarcomas of the breast: local-regional control with post-operative radiotherapy. *Int Radio Oncol Bio Phys* 1993;27:671.
59. Brennan MF, Casper ES, et al. The role of multimodality therapy in soft-tissue sarcoma. *Ann Surg* 1991;214:328.
60. Shipp MA, Mauch PM, Harris NL. Non-Hodgkin's lymphomas. In: DeVita VT, Hellman S, Rosenberg SA, eds. *Cancer principles and practice of oncology*, 5th ed. Lippincott–Raven Publishers, 1997:1738.
61. Donnell RM, Rosen PP, Lieberman PH, et al. Angiosarcoma and other vascular tumors of the breast. *Am J Surg Pathol* 1981;5:629.
62. Chen KTK, Kirkgaard DD, Bocian JJ. Angiosarcoma of the breast. *Cancer* 1980;46:368.
63. Rosen PP, Kimel M, Ernsberg D. Mammary angiosarcoma. *Cancer* 1988;62:2145.
64. Merino MJ, Berman M, Carter D. Angiosarcoma of the breast. *Am J Surg Pathol* 1983;7:53.
65. Karlsson P, Holmberg E, Samuelsson A, Johansson KA, Wallgren A. Soft tissue sarcoma after treatment for breast cancer—a Swedish population-based study. *Eur J Cancer* 1998;4130:2068.
66. Marchal C, Weber B, de Lafontan B, et al. Nine angiosarcomas after conservative treatment for breast carcinoma: survey from French comprehensive cancer centers. *Int J Radiat Oncol Biol Phys* 1999;44(1):113.
67. Silver SA, Tavassoli FA. Primary osteogenic sarcoma of the breast: a clinicopathologic analysis of 50 cases. *Am J Surg Pathol* 1998;22:925.
68. Brown AL, Holwill SD, Thomas VA, Sacks NP, Given-Wilson R. Case report. Primary osteosarcoma of the breast: imaging and histological features. *Clin Radiol* 1998;53(12):920.
69. Kyriazis AP, Kyriazis AA. Primary rhabdomyosarcoma of the female breast: report of a case and review of the literature. *Arch Pathol Lab Med* 1998;122:747.
70. Chateil JF, Arboucalot F, Perel Y, Brun M, Boisseric-Lacroix M, Diard F. Breast metastases in adolescent girls: US findings. *Pediatr Radiol* 1998;110:832.

71. Hays DM, Donaldson SS, Shimada H, et al. Primary metastatic rhabdomyosarcoma in the breast: neoplasms of adolescent females. A report from the Intergroup Rhabdomyosarcoma Study. *Med Pediatr Oncol* 1997;293:181.
72. Stewart FW, Treves N. Lymphoma in post-mastectomy lymphoedema. *Cancer* 1948;1:64.
73. Clements WD, Kirk SJ, Spence RA. A rare late complication of breast cancer treatment. *Br J Clin Pract* 1993;47(4):219.
74. Aygit AC, Yildirim AM, Dervisoglu S. Lymphangiosarcoma in chronic lymphoedema: Stewart-Treves syndrome. *J Hand Surg [Br]* 1999;24(1):135.
75. Roses DF, Harris MN, Stern JS, et al. Cutaneous melanoma of the breast. *Ann Surg* 1978;189:112.
76. Ariel IM, Caron AS. Diagnosis and treatment of malignant melanoma arising from the skin of the female breast. *Am J Surg* 1972;124:384.
77. Greenberg BM, Hamilton R, Rothkopf DM, et al. Management of cutaneous melanoma of the female breast. *Plast Reconstr Surg* 1987;80:409.
78. Papachristou DN, Kinne DW, Rosen PP, et al. Cutaneous melanoma of the breast. *Surgery* 1979;85:322.
79. Cuberson JD, Horn RC. Paget's disease of the nipple: review of 25 cases with special reference to melanin pigmentation of Paget's cells. *Arch Surg* 1956;72:224.
80. Peison B, Benisch B. Paget's disease of the nipple simulating malignant melanoma in a black woman. *Am J Dermatopathol* 1985;7:165.
81. Sau P, Solis J, Lupten GP, et al. Pigmented breast carcinoma: a clinical and histopathologic simulator of malignant melanoma. *Arch Dermatol* 1989;125:536.
82. Clark WH, From L, Bernardino EH, et al. Histogenesis and biologic behavior of primary human malignant melanoma of the skin. *Cancer Res* 1969;29:705.
83. Breslow A. Thickness, cross-sectional area and depth of invasion in prognosis of cutaneous melanoma. *Ann Surg* 1970;172:902.
84. Balch CM, Cascinelli N, Drzewiecki KT, et al. A comparison of prognostic factors worldwide: epidemiologic features of melanoma prognostic factors. In: Balch CM, Houghton AN, Milton GW, et al, eds. *Cutaneous melanoma*, 2nd ed. Philadelphia: JB Lippincott, 1992:188.
85. Singletary SE, Balch CM, Urist MM, et al. Surgical treatment of primary melanoma: epidemiologic features of melanoma prognostic factors. In: Balch CM, Houghton AN, Milton GW, et al, eds. *Cutaneous melanoma*, 2nd ed. Philadelphia: JB Lippincott, 1992:269.
86. Krag DN, Meijer SJ, Weaver DL, et al. Minimal access surgery for staging of malignant melanoma. *Arch Surg* 1995;130:654.
87. Alex JC, Krag DN. Gamma-probe guided localization of lymph nodes. *Surg Oncol* 1993;2:137.
88. Alex JC, Weaver DL, Fairbank JT, et al. Gamma-probe guided lymph node localization in malignant melanoma. *Surg Oncol* 1993;2:303.
89. Albertini JJ, Cruse CW, Rappaport D, et al. Intra-operative radio lymphoscintigraphy improves sentinel lymph node identification for patients with melanoma. *Ann Surg* 1996;223:217.
90. Dale PS, Foshag LJ, Wanek LA, et al. Metastasis of primary melanoma to two separate lymph node basins: prognostic significance. *Ann Surg Oncol* 1997;4:13.
91. Sandison AT. Metastatic tumors in the breast. *Br J Surg* 1959;47:54.
92. Paulus DD, Libshitz HI. Metastasis to the breast. *Radiol Clin North Am* 1982;20:561.
93. Allen FJ, Van Velden JJ. Prostate carcinoma metastasis to the male breast. *Br J Urol* 1991;67:434.
94. Lo MC, Chomat B, Rubenstone AI. Metastatic prostatic adenocarcinoma of the male breast. *Urology* 1978;11:641.
95. Arora R, Robinson WA. Breast metastases from malignant melanoma. *J Surg Oncol* 1992;50:27.
96. Hajdu SI, Urban JA. Cancers metastasis to the breast. *Cancer* 1972;29:1691.
97. Gorczyca W, Osszewski W, Tuziak T, et al. Fine needle aspiration cytology of rare malignant tumors of the breast. *Acta Cytol* 1992;36:918.
98. Sneige N, Zachariah S, Fanning TV, et al. Fine needle aspiration cytology of metastatic neoplasms in the breast. *Am J Clin Pathol* 1989;92:27.
99. Moore DH, Wilson DK, Hurteau JA, et al. Gynecologic cancers metastatic to the breast. *J Am Coll Surg* 1998;187:178.
100. Hamby LS, McGarth PC, Cibull ML, et al. Gastric carcinoma metastatic to the breast. *J Surg Oncol* 1991;48:117.
101. Alvarez RD, Gleason BP, Gore H, et al. Coexisting intraductal breast carcinoma and metastatic choriocarcinoma presenting as a breast mass. *Gynecol Oncol* 1991;43:295.
102. Kumar PV, Esfahani FN, Salimi A. Choriocarcinoma metastatic to the breast diagnosed by fine needle aspiration. *Acta Cytol* 1991;35.
103. Lesho EP. Metastatic renal cell carcinoma presenting as a breast mass. *Postgrad Med J* 1992;91:145.
104. Silverman JF, Feldman PS, Covell JL, et al. Fine needle aspiration cytology of neoplasm metastatic to the breast. *Acta Cytol* 1987;31: 291.
105. Di Bonito L, Luchi M, Giarelli L, et al. Metastatic tumors to the female breast: an autopsy study of 12 cases. *Pathol Res Pract* 1991;187:432.
106. Fishman A, Steel BL, Girtanner RE, et al. Fallopian tube cancer metastatic to the breast. *Eur J Gynaecol Oncol* 1994;15:101.
107. Kattan J, Droz JP, Charpentier P, et al. Ovarian dysgerminoma metastatic to the breast. *Gynecol Oncol* 1992;46:104.
108. Soo MS, Williford ME, Elenberger CD. Medullary thyroid carcinoma metastatic to the breast: mammographic appearance. *AJR Am J Roentgenol* 1995;165:65.
109. Ali SZ, Teichberg S, Attie JN, et al. Medullary thyroid carcinoma metastatic to breast masquerading as infiltrating lobular carcinoma. *Ann Clin Lab Sci* 1994;24:441.
110. Fishman A, Kim HS, Girtanner RE, et al. Solitary breast metastasis as first manifestation of ovarian carcinoid tumor. *Gynecol Oncol* 1994;54:222.
111. Baliga M, Holmquist ND, Espinoza CG. Medulloblastoma metastatic to breast diagnosed by fine-needle aspiration biopsy. *Diagn Cytopathol* 1994;10:33.
112. Matusda M, Sone H, Ishiguro S, et al. Fine needle-aspiration cytology of malignant schwannoma metastatic to the breast. *Acta Cytol* 1989;33:372.
113. Nunez DA, Sutherland CG, Sood RK. Breast metastasis from a pharyngeal carcinoma. *J Laryngol Otol* 1989;103:227.
114. Harvey EB, Britton LA. Second cancer following cancer of the breast in Connecticut, 1935–82. *J Natl Cancer Inst Monogr* 1985;68:99.
115. Leis HP. Managing the remaining breast. *Cancer* 1980;46:1026.
116. Lewision EF. The follow-up examination of the contralateral breast from the viewpoint of the surgeon. *Cancer* 1969;23-809.
117. Finney GG, Finney GG, Montague ACW, et al. Bilateral breast cancer: clinical and pathological review. *Ann Surg* 1972;175;635.
118. Fisher ER, Fisher B, Sass R, et al. Pathologic findings from the National Surgical Adjuvant Breast and Bowel Project (protocol no 4). XI. Bilateral breast cancer. *Cancer* 1984;54:3002.
119. Lewison EF, Neto AS. Bilateral breast cancer at the Johns Hopkins Hospital: a discussion of the dilemma of the contralateral breast. *Cancer* 1971;28;1297.
120. Chaudrary MA, Millis RR, Hoskins EOL, et al. Bilateral primary breast cancer: a prospective study of disease incidence. *Br J Surg* 1984;71:711.
121. Egan RI. Bilateral breast carcinomas: role of mammography. *Cancer* 1976;38:931.

Diseases of the Breast, 2nd ed.,
edited by Jay R. Harris.
Lippincott Williams & Wilkins, Philadelphia © 2000.

CHAPTER 44

Breast Cancer Treatment in Pregnant or Postpartum Women and Subsequent Pregnancy in Breast Cancer Survivors

Jeanne A. Petrek and Anne Moore

BREAST CANCER TREATMENT IN PREGNANT OR POSTPARTUM PATIENTS

Studying the coexistence of breast cancer and pregnancy is difficult. Although pregnancy and the diagnosis of breast cancer are occasionally concurrent, a greater number of patients have had an unknown subclinical breast cancer while pregnant, given that the occult preclinical breast cancer growth is several years.[1] This issue has only recently been addressed.

A 1994 study of young patients with breast cancer at nine American and European cancer centers demonstrated that a recent previous pregnancy (up to 4 years before diagnosis) was associated with a worse prognosis.[2] To put it the opposite way, for each additional year in the time between pregnancy and breast cancer diagnosis, the risk of dying decreased by 15%. The effect of recent pregnancy could substantially contribute to the observation of the poorer prognosis in the young,[3,4] considering that the reproductive rate is high in this group and that the documented effect lingers for 4 years.[2] Since 1994, two studies have found significantly decreased survival with shorter interval of breast cancer diagnosis to previous pregnancy: a population-based tumor registry and birth record linkage from Denmark[5] and a case control series of 540 women from the Memorial Sloan-Kettering Cancer Center.[6] Two other studies have not noted this,[7,8] possibly because of combining completed pregnancies and abortions or other factors.

Nevertheless, although pregnancy and microscopic incipient breast cancer have coexisted in unknown large numbers of young women, it is necessary to define and limit the definition of pregnancy-associated breast cancer. The traditional definition is that the diagnosis of breast cancer is made during pregnancy or within 1 year afterward, and that is the definition used here. With that definition, one review noted an incidence reported between 0.2% to 3.8% in 32 series over the past several decades.[9]

Diagnosed breast cancers occur in 1:10,000 to 1:3,000 pregnancies,[10,11] making the malignancy approximately as common as that of the uterine cervix.[12] The incidence among breast cancer patients younger than 40 years old using the traditional definition is approximately 15%.[9] As more modern women are bearing children in their 30s and even 40s, an age when breast cancer is more common, the incidence of pregnancy-associated breast cancer is expected to rise.

Prognosis of Pregnancy-Associated Breast Cancer

The earliest reports, several decades ago, noted a dismal prognosis. Kilgore and Bloodgood[13] reported no survivors, and White's collective series[14] in 1954 reported a 17% 5-year survival rate. Haagensen and Stout[15] reported only an 8.6% overall 5-year rate.

Harrington[16] at the Mayo Clinic (1937) is credited with reviving optimism on finding a 61% 5-year survival rate among those with negative lymph nodes. Unfortunately, presentation with lymph node metastases was, and remains, common in the pregnant woman. Eight papers published during the 1960s,[17–24] reporting numbers of patients ranging from 29 to 117, found a rate of positive lymph nodes ranging from 53% to 74% (median, 65%). Four similar papers[11,25–27] published during the 1970s found a rate of positive lymph nodes from 56% to 81%. Few studies have attempted to put these percentages into the context of the age, decade of diagnosis, and similar demographics by designating a nonpregnant comparison group.

At Memorial Hospital in New York, the author compared 56 patients with pregnancy-associated breast cancer [American

J. A. Petrek: Evelyn Lauder Breast Center, Memorial Sloan-Kettering Cancer Center, New York, New York

A. Moore: Department of Hematology and Oncology, Joan and Sanford I. Weill Medical College, New York Presbyterian Hospital - Cornell University, New York, New York

Joint Committee (AJC) stages I/II/III] diagnosed between 1960 and 1980 with nonpregnant control patients from a consecutive mastectomy series of the same age, diagnosed and treated at the same hospital, during the same time period, and by the same physicians.[28] Sixty-two percent of the pregnancy-associated patients had positive lymph nodes versus 39% of their nonpregnant counterparts. Only 31% of the pregnant patients had pathologic tumors smaller than 2 cm versus 50% of their counterparts. A more recent publication[29] on a smaller series of women from Memorial Hospital had the same findings. In a series published in 1985 composed of twice as many women, 74% of pregnant patients, compared with only 37% of similarly aged nonpregnant patients, had cancer in their axillary lymph nodes.[30] The findings are similar to those of other studies,[21,31–33] which also include a comparison group.

The patients with pregnancy-associated breast cancer who had negative lymph nodes had an 82% 5-year survival rate compared with 82% in their nonpregnant counterparts. The pregnancy-associated patients with positive lymph nodes had a 47% 5-year survival rate compared with 59% in their counterparts. Among pregnancy-associated patients who were eligible, the 10-year survival rate was 77% for those with negative lymph nodes and 25% for those with positive lymph nodes. In comparison, the 10-year survival rate was 75% for the nonpregnant patients with negative nodes and 41% for the nonpregnant patients with positive nodes. The differences in 5- and 10-year survival times in patients grouped by stage are not statistically significant.

There are only two modern case control series indicating that pregnancy is a risk factor independent of stage at diagnosis. A small series from Norway contained 20 patients.[34] More important is the 1997 study of 154 women, each matched with two control subjects.[35] In this group of countrywide French patients, multivariate analysis demonstrated that pregnancy was an independent and significant prognostic factor.

Other recent reports indicate that pregnancy is associated with a more advanced stage at diagnosis but not a worse survival within that stage. In Toronto, 118 women with pregnancy-associated breast cancer from 1958 to 1987 were reported. No statistically significant difference was found in survival between pregnant and nonpregnant patients when matched by age, stage, and year of diagnosis.[36] Showing the tendency to present with advanced disease, the pregnant women had a 2.5-fold higher risk of diagnosis with metastatic breast cancer and a significantly decreased chance of a stage I diagnosis. A 1992 study published in a Japanese cancer journal, also with a large number of patients, shows similar findings.[37] A New Zealand report[38] of 20 women and a Saudi Arabian report[39] of 28 women showed the same findings.

In summary, almost all reports note a worse survival rate for pregnancy-associated breast cancer overall. However, when the patients with pregnancy-associated breast cancer are evaluated with nonpregnant control subjects, the pregnancy-associated group has an equivalent survival rate, at least in the early stages. Overall, pregnancy-associated breast cancer bears a worse prognosis, because it is regularly associated with more advanced disease at presentation. It is unknown whether this is due to (a) a more aggressive growth pattern secondary to the biological effects of pregnancy, (b) delayed diagnosis secondary to the breast changes of pregnancy, or (c) a combination of the two.

Considerations of the Fetus in Staging and Treatment

The aspects of breast biopsy and diagnosis of the primary tumor are discussed in Chapter 7 and not within this chapter. In cancer diagnosis and treatment, dangers to the fetus include those of development, such as the teratogenicity possibly caused by radiation, chemotherapy, and general anesthesia. In addition to congenital abnormalities, various other risks, such as intrauterine growth retardation, prematurity, or both, and possible postnatal neoplasia must also be considered. The effects overall on the fetus for chemotherapy and radiation without considering specific diseases have been reviewed.[40]

Radiation Risk to the Fetus

In rodents and humans, the principal effect of radiation during the preimplantation period (from conception to days 10 to 14) is embryo death. The second period, that of organogenesis (lasting from days 10 to 14 through the eighth week), is undoubtedly the most sensitive to ionizing radiation. Radiation exposure beyond 8 weeks is less likely to produce congenital abnormalities in any site, although there has been concern about radiation-induced neurologic abnormalities. In the pregnant women of Hiroshima and Nagasaki, an air dose of 1 to 9 cGy during weeks 6 through 11 of pregnancy resulted in an 11% incidence of microcephaly and mental retardation in children, compared with 4% in a Japanese nonirradiated control population.[41]

In humans, microcephaly has been observed with radiation exposure after 8 weeks of getstation, but, dose for dose, the incidence is four to five times less than after exposure during the earlier organogenesis period.[41] A 1998 review summarizes the concern about prenatal irradiation for the developing brain.[42]

The atomic bomb experience and animal experimentation data lead to the conclusion that 5 cGy is the dose level for early pregnancy at which radiation-induced anomalies become meaningful. The American Academy of Pediatrics and other organizations support the conclusion of the American College of Radiology that interruption of pregnancy is not routinely recommended if the fetus was exposed to less than 5 cGy.[9] (In this discussion, we do not consider that even low doses could have genetic effects that will be manifested only in subsequent generations derived from this offspring.)

Another theoretical risk of radiation is carcinogenesis in the offspring. Retrospective studies indicate an association between prenatal x-ray exposure (usually via maternal pelvimetry) and future childhood cancers. The reported risk of leukemia at 10 years after a 2-cGy exposure may be 1:2,000 versus 1:3,000 in unexposed controls.[43] A 1997 review[44] evaluates the data and concludes that small radiation doses, on the order of 1 cGy, produce a detectable increase in the risk of childhood cancer. Blood-borne carcinogenesis (transplacental) was reviewed in 1986.[45]

Staging Procedures during Pregnancy and Fetal Risk

Accurate staging and appropriate treatment depend on comprehensive evaluation for metastatic disease, and most tests use ionizing radiation. Published estimates of the approximate fetal and maternal exposures are available.[46] The radiation dose to the embryo, fetus, or even a particular fetal organ can also be specifically calculated by a medical physicist when the relevant parameters are known: for x-ray examinations, these include beam quality, kilovoltage, exposure time, distance, film size, and view; for nuclear medicine procedures, they include type of agent, total activity, target organ, and effective half-life.[47]

Some guidelines can be made for recommended staging tests. There is no contraindication to a chest x-ray, which is sometimes performed with abdominal and pelvic shielding. Late in pregnancy, with the gravid uterus directly under the diaphragm, fetal shielding would obscure the lower lung parenchyma. Nevertheless, exposing the third-trimester fetus to a chest x-ray presents no great concern.

As regards evaluation for bone metastases, serum alkaline phosphatase is elevated due to pregnancy itself. Conventional radiography, excluding the pelvis and abdomen, can be performed (e.g., skull, long bones). There is no adequate substitute for a bone scan. A recent article notes modification of the bone-scanning technique for pregnant patients.[48] If the bone scan result will not change the immediate treatment, it should be delayed until after delivery. Thus, in a patient with clinical stage I or II disease, bone scan can usually be avoided, because the incidence of diagnosable bone metastases is so low.[49] On the other hand, in clinical stage III pregnant patients with increased rate of bone metastases found on bone scan, it is possible that the results of this test may change treatment.

Magnetic resonance imaging is accurate and seems safe for the fetus, although the Safety Committee of the Society for the Magnetic Resonance Imaging states, "The safety of MR imaging during pregnancy has not been proven."[50] Reports on its use for fetal imaging in prenatal diagnosis contain limited follow-up of the infants, with no untoward effects reported.[51,52] It may be particularly useful for the diagnosis or confirmation of bone metastases, liver metastases, or even brain metastases (although a head computed tomogram with abdominal shielding should yield only small amounts of fetal exposure).

Breast or Chest Wall Radiotherapy during Pregnancy

The fetal dose can be estimated by thermoluminescent dosimeters placed in an anatomic phantom shielding. However, as explained in the next paragraph, the standard breast radiotherapy course of approximately 5,000 cGy exposes the fetus to between 10 cGy early in pregnancy to 200 or more cGy late in pregnancy and therefore should be rejected as a treatment option.

The developing fetus receives from several tenths of a percent to several percent of the total breast dose. The radiation leakage from the radiotherapy unit should not exceed 0.1% of the direct beam exposure rate, as measured at a distance of 1 m from the radiation source.[53] A larger amount of radiation, however, reaches the fetus from internal scatter by the mother's tissues (which cannot be reduced by external shielding). The quantity of such radiation depends on (a) the distance of the fetus from the field center, (b) the field size, and (c) the energy source of the radiation. A 6-megavolt linear accelerator produces less fetal dose by internal scatter than a 1.25-megavolt cobalt 60 unit.

For example, when the fetus is less than 12 weeks old (i.e., is still in the true pelvis and perhaps 40 cm from field center), the dose from a field that is 10 cm × 10 cm and is produced by a 4-megavolt unit would be in the range of 0.2% to 0.3% of the tumor dose. This could result in 10 to 15 cGy early in pregnancy, for a breast treatment course of 5,000 cGy. Toward the end of pregnancy, if a fetal part is 10 cm distant, it will receive 200 cGy for the same treatment course.

Much of the information concerning radiation (and also chemotherapy) must be obtained in reports concerning treatment of pregnant women with lymphoma and leukemia. A recent report from the M.D. Anderson Cancer Center[54] in Houston, Texas evaluated 14 patients with Hodgkin's disease who had various fields of radiation to 3,500 to 4,000 cGy while in the second and third trimester. This is approximately three-fourths of the dose necessary to treat breast cancer. With specialized techniques, they were able to decrease the total estimated midfetus dose to 1.4 to 13.6 cGy. The dose to the closest fetal part was not estimated.

Likewise, radiation after mastectomy involves similar doses to the chest wall and poses the same hazard to the fetus. Even with medial breast cancers, postmastectomy irradiation is of arguable benefit in the routine case; it therefore should be postponed in similar-staged pregnant women. Postmastectomy irradiation in late stage is often indicated because of the high risk of local recurrence. Nevertheless, it is probably wisest to delay the radiotherapy until the patient is no longer pregnant. If local recurrence occurs before delivery, it can be excised to the extent possible to enable further postponement of irradiation at least until late in pregnancy, when fetal risk is greatly lessened.

To accomplish breast preservation in the pregnant woman, the plan of lumpectomy during pregnancy followed by radiation therapy after delivery has been suggested. To advocate this approach, one must extrapolate from the data obtained in the nonpregnant woman. However, the pregnant woman's breast, with the large interanastomosing network of ducts and sizable lymph/blood vessels, is not anatomically and physiologically similar to the less active breast of the premenopausal young woman. The duct structure itself might predispose to lengthy intraductal spread. It is not certain that the same results after lumpectomy and irradiation will occur with lumpectomy during pregnancy and delayed postpartum radiation.

A situation due to endogenous hormones changing anatomic structure of the breast and resulting in increased local recurrence rates (with quadrantectomy and no radiation) is hypothesized in the 1993 Milan study.[55] Authors of this study found 3.8% local recurrences in women older than 55 years, 8.7% in women aged 46 to 55 years, and 17.5% in women aged 45 years or younger. They surmise that treatment response differed by age as a result of the duct structure. After menopause, the complex structures of the breast disappear, and the breast becomes "a fatty organ with scattered islands of fibroepithelial tissue without connection between them." The anatomic difference between the pregnant and nonpregnant breast of the same individual seems greater than that between the pre- and postmenopausal breast.

There has been a limited experience[56] with a median follow-up of 24 months of nine women with pregnancy-associated breast cancer who were treated conservatively. Six were pregnant, and three were within 1 year postpartum. Two of the six pregnant women were in the first trimester and underwent abortion. Median tumor size was 1.5 cm. No local recurrences and three distant recurrences occurred in this short follow-up study.

Chemotherapy during Pregnancy

The decision to recommend chemotherapy to a pregnant woman is one of the most difficult decisions in the management of women with breast cancer. The treatment involves not only the patient and the medical oncologist, but also the family, the obstetrician, the neonatologist, and, of course, the unborn fetus.

Chemotherapeutic drugs exert their effort by inhibiting cells from dividing. Pregnant women are concerned about the side effects of chemotherapy, both for themselves and for the fetus. The physiologic changes of pregnancy on blood volume, glomerular filtration rate, and other parameters may affect maternal chemotherapy drug metabolism, but there are few pharmacokinetic studies of chemotherapy in pregnant patients. Detailed studies of transplacental passage of chemotherapeutic agents to human fetuses are also not available. The potential adverse effects of antineoplastic agents on the fetus and neonate involve immediate effects, such as spontaneous abortion, teratogenesis, or organ damage, and delayed effects, such as growth retardation or gonadal dysfunction. Organogenesis primarily occurs within the first 10 weeks of pregnancy. The delivery of chemotherapy in the first trimester is associated with an increased incidence of stillbirths and congenital malformations.[57] In one series of 13 women exposed to chemotherapy during the first trimester, four spontaneous abortions, four therapeutic abortions, and two major fetal malformations occurred among the five term infants.[58] Because central nervous system development continues during the second trimester, there is a theoretical concern that chemotherapy may interfere with this process and result in delayed cognitive damage. The long-term follow-up of children exposed to *in utero* chemotherapy during maternal treatment for breast cancer is important.

Chemotherapy agents most commonly used in the initial management of a woman with breast cancer are relatively safe to administer during the second and third trimesters. Drugs that have been given after the first trimester without a reported increased risk of birth defects include cyclophosphamide,[59] doxorubicin,[60] and 5-fluorouracil.[61] Methotrexate, a folic acid antagonist, has also been given without serious sequelae in the second and third trimesters; however, because the folic acid antagonists have been the most frequently reported drugs to cause first-trimester fetal abnormalities, and because there is a concern about the metabolism of methotrexate in the presence of the third space provided by the amniotic fluid, most oncologists prefer to avoid prescribing methotrexate during pregnancy. Taxanes have not been studied and for that reason should be avoided during pregnancy. For the same reason, growth factors (e.g., granulocyte colony stimulating factor) should not be used routinely in a pregnant woman. Because laboratory studies have suggested that tamoxifen is teratogenic, it is not indicated during pregnancy.

One prospective study of 24 women with breast cancer treated with a uniform chemotherapy program during the second and third trimesters of pregnancy is particularly informative.[61] Twenty-two women were treated for primary breast cancer, mainly stage II or III, including two women with inflammatory breast cancer. Two women had metastatic disease. Cyclophosphamide, doxorubicin, and 5-fluorouracil were given every 21 to 28 days for a maximum of four treatments, with no evidence of fetal compromise or adverse effects on early development. The disease-free survival of the mothers was similar to that of nonpregnant patients and was dependent on the stage of the breast cancer at diagnosis. Table 1 offers a guide for management of chemotherapy in the pregnant patient with operable breast cancer.

In planning chemotherapy for pregnant women, it is preferable to allow at least 2 weeks between the last dose

TABLE 1. *Suggestions for adjuvant chemotherapy during pregnancy*

1. Avoid chemotherapy during the first trimester.
2. For women with positive lymph nodes,
   - Begin chemotherapy within 6 weeks of surgery if possible; however, a delay for several weeks to allow delivery before initiating chemotherapy is reasonable.
   - Drugs of choice: cyclophosphamide and doxorubicin with or without 5-fluorouracil.
3. For women with negative nodes,
   - If high risk (tumor >2 cm, tumor <2 cm but >1 cm with unfavorable factors), begin chemotherapy as in 2. Within 12 weeks of surgery if possible.
   - If low risk (tumor <1 cm), no chemotherapy.
   - If intermediate risk, assess benefits and schedule of chemotherapy with each patient individually.

and delivery. This minimizes the risk of delivering a neutropenic infant from a neutropenic mother. In addition, fetal drug metabolism switches from the placenta to the kidney and liver at delivery. If the fetus is delivered soon after chemotherapy, the drugs may persist for a prolonged period in the newborn.[62] Women who have recently received chemotherapy should be advised against breast-feeding.

The management of the pregnant woman with breast cancer involves close communication with the patient, her family, and the medical team involved in her care. Full disclosure about what is known and not known about the real benefits of chemotherapy to the mother and the long-term effects of chemotherapy on the fetus are of crucial importance.

Metastatic Disease in the Fetus and Placenta

Melanoma, hematopoietic malignancies, hepatoma, and choriocarcinoma have been reported to cause actual fetal metastases, but breast cancer has not been reported.[63,64] Placental metastases have been reported in 30 patients with solid tumor, including several breast cancers.[65] Microscopic examination of the placenta, especially of the intervillous space, is important, as only one-half the patients had visible metastases.[66]

Anesthetic Considerations

General anesthesia is necessary for a mastectomy or axillary dissection and rarely for an adequate wide excision. General anesthesia during pregnancy is difficult because of factors including increased blood volume, increased heart rate and cardiac output, increased platelet count and fibrinogen level, supine positional hypotension, decreased pulmonary functional residual capacity, elevated diaphragms, prolonged gastric emptying, and hypervascularity of the respiratory tract mucosa. As compared with the risks of teratogenesis from radiation and chemotherapy, those associated with the general anesthetic drugs are almost nonexistent. A recent review[67] details anesthetic and other precautions to be taken in the pregnant woman.

Despite the fact that nitrous oxide and halothane interfere *in vitro* with nucleic acid synthesis, no deleterious effects can be detected in humans.[68] These potent inhalational agents have the theoretical advantage of relaxing uterine musculature and forestalling premature labor. In fact, premature labor seems to depend more on the surgical site—being more common with lower abdominal or pelvic operations—than on anesthetic technique and is not likely with breast operations. In any event, obstetricians have several drugs for reversal of premature labor. Fetal monitoring should be used whenever possible, so patterns of fetal distress can be followed immediately by fine adjustments of anesthetic technique.

A large population-based study from Sweden studied 5,405 nonobstetric operations during pregnancy and compared them to 720,000 pregnancies in which the women did not have general anesthesia.[69] The major problems are increased incidence of low birth weight, which is due to prematurity and to intrauterine growth retardation, and an increased incidence of infants born alive who die within 7 days. These adverse effects are not necessarily attributable to the surgical operation, because the illness or injury that necessitated the surgery must have a significant role.[69] On the positive side, the incidence of congenital anomalies was not increased in women who had first-trimester operations, and general anesthesia with nitrous oxide was not associated with an increased incidence of adverse outcomes.

The Question of Therapeutic Abortion

The traditional view of concurrent breast cancer and pregnancy as an especially dreaded situation may have contributed to zealous enthusiasm for abortion in the past, usually combined with oophorectomy. For example, Haagensen and Stout[15] recommended refusing mastectomy to any patient whose breast cancer was diagnosed during pregnancy or lactation as being categorically incurable (although they later changed their opinion).[70] In 1953, Adair[71] of Memorial Hospital noted longer crude survival rates after therapeutic abortion, especially for patients with positive axillary lymph nodes (these differences were not statistically significant).

Gradually thereafter, the opinion on the uniformly lethal nature of concurrent breast cancer and pregnancy, as well as the unquestioned value of therapeutic abortion, began to change. Holleb and Farrow,[72] also from Memorial Hospital, reported in 1962 on 24 patients treated with radical mastectomy, and abortion was not associated with a better survival. Reports from the mid-1980s[30,31] also do not show an advantage in survival rate after therapeutic abortion.

In a 1989 article[73] reporting on 154 pregnant patients studied between 1931 and 1985, the authors stated that therapeutic abortion is associated with decreased survival. There was a 5-year survival rate of 20% with therapeutic abortion, 28% with live birth, and 50% for those who had a spontaneous abortion. Overall, the whole group had advanced disease, with only 19% documented with negative lymph nodes, and 10% with primary tumors of less than 2 cm. However, the characteristics of the patients in the three groups are unknown. Similar findings in 100 cases of gestational breast cancer seen between 1926 and 1972 were published by the Petrov Research Institute of Oncology in Leningrad.[33]

In all these data, reported numbers are small and have been collected over long time intervals. Cases are not precisely staged. Most important, any beneficial effect of abortion would be disguised by the selection factor, because it appears that the more advanced cases are more likely to undergo therapeutic abortion. For example, in a series of 63 pregnant patients at the Mayo Clinic,[31] 5-year survival rates of 43%

were reported in the interrupted group versus 59% in the full-term delivery group. However, of the 20 stage I patients, 17 delivered and only 3 were interrupted. There was an excellent 5-year survival rate of 86% in the 17 patients who were allowed to deliver. Only one of three interrupted patients survived, for a 5-year rate of 33%. However, stage I is a broad group: Most clinicians are able to predict the ones with a poor prognosis (such as those in stage I with extensive lymphatic invasion or anaplastic tumors). The inclination is to recommend abortion to them but not to the other patients in stage I.

Therapeutic abortion is strongly recommended if the issue is fetal damage from the proposed chemotherapy or radiation treatments. Treatment is always simplified with therapeutic abortion early in pregnancy. In the end, it is the mother who must make as informed a decision as possible about the pregnancy. When combined with standard therapy, any additional benefit of routine therapeutic abortion cannot be demonstrated in the published reports. Nevertheless, because survival rates are generally equivalent between those who continue pregnancy and those who abort, and the patients with more advanced disease were preferentially aborted, abortion may be beneficial, but that fact would be disguised by patient selection.

Hormone Receptors

The accuracy and ultimate value of steroid hormone receptor status during pregnancy is not well known. Routine ligand-binding assays (without exchange techniques) depend on the availability of unbound receptor, and in pregnancy all binding sites may already be occupied by endogenous hormone. In the nonpregnant state, only up to 35% of cytosol receptor was occupied by endogenous steroid, so most is available for assay.[74]

Immunohistochemical assays should be accurate in the pregnant woman, because the occupied or unoccupied receptor should be stained. One recent report compares the receptor status by immunohistochemistry to ligand-binding assay of pregnant to nonpregnant women and presents data that some estrogen receptor–negative tumors in pregnancy-associated breast cancer have estrogen receptor–mediated protein products.[75]

SUBSEQUENT PREGNANCY AFTER BREAST CANCER TREATMENT

The issue of safety after treatment of breast cancer is of great concern for the breast cancer survivor and for the physician involved in her care. Many women are delaying childbearing for different reasons (educational, professional, and personal), and it is becoming increasingly more common for them to undergo breast cancer diagnosis and treatment before initiating or completing childbearing. The delay in childbearing to the 30s or 40s occurs concordantly with an increasing incidence of breast cancer at increasing ages. Of the 175,000 new cases of breast cancer estimated for 1999, 10% to 20% occur in women of childbearing age.[76] Physicians have stressed the complete rehabilitation of patients with breast carcinoma, including reconstruction and psychosocial aspects. It is thus natural after the completion of therapy for the patient to inquire about pregnancy and childbearing.

The hormonal influence on mammary carcinogenesis is well known. The effects of first full-term pregnancy, age at menarche/menopause, and use of postmenopausal hormone replacement are significant hormonal factors in the pathogenesis of breast cancer. In fact, the importance of the endogenous hormonal milieu on breast cancer promotion has been recognized for over 100 years. In 1896, Beatson[77] noted the regression with oophorectomy in premenopausal patients with advanced local disease. The effects of estrogen on the acceleration of the growth rate of micrometastases, stimulation of dormant micrometastases, or direct carcinogenesis of a new primary are of concern in patients with breast cancer. Retrospective studies have tried to address the effects of gestational hormones or other factors unique to pregnancy in women who become pregnant after breast cancer treatment. There are several series, each with a limited number of patients, and population-based studies have been published since the mid-1990s. The authors' current large, prospective multicenter study can help to address some of these issues. Inquiries about possible enrollment of American women younger than age 44 who have been diagnosed with breast cancer within the past 8 months can be directed to the toll-free number (877) 636-7562.

Retrospective Series

Survival of Women with Subsequent Pregnancy after Breast Cancer Treatment

The earlier literature stated that at least 7% of women who did not undergo oophorectomy had one or more pregnancies. Seventy percent of these pregnancies were to be expected in the first 5 years after cancer treatment.[78] Adjuvant cytotoxic chemotherapy depletes the number of fertile patients, but as many as 11% of patients in a short-term chemotherapy study had a deliberate or unplanned pregnancy.[79] From the scanty literature available, it has been generally observed that patients with breast cancer who subsequently become pregnant have good survival rates, often the same or sometimes better than patients with no subsequent pregnancy.[80,81]

The limited data on outcome after subsequent pregnancy in patients with breast carcinoma have been derived from retrospective series, some of which use case-matching methods in an attempt to eliminate the obvious bias of pregnancy occurring in those with the better prognosis. There have been sporadic retrospective studies from single institutions, with each comprising fewer than 100 patients. In 1954, White[14] reported that eight (67%) of the patients who became pregnant lived at least 5 years, and 58% survived 10 years. In 1962, a series of 52 patients from Memorial Hospital had an overall 5-year survival rate of 52%.[72] Another similar-sized study reported in 1969[82] included 53 patients with 5- and 10-year survival rates of 77% and 69%, respectively. In 1970, Cooper and Butterfield[83] reported a 75% 5-year survival rate in 32 patients. Fifty percent of patients in a 1973 series survived 5 years.[84]

Case-matching studies were also performed to lessen the influence of pregnancy occurring only in those with a good prognosis. In 1965, Peters and Meakin[21] matched 96 patients with subsequent pregnancy over several decades with patients with similar age and clinical stage. The patients with subsequent pregnancy had a longer disease-free and overall survival than those without subsequent pregnancy. In an analysis from 1970, Cooper and Butterfield[83] matched each of 40 patients who subsequently became pregnant with two control subjects as determined by the clinical stage, age, status of lymph node involvement, and equal survival at least to the time of pregnancy. The patients with subsequent pregnancy had a survival time superior to that of the control group.

Memorial Sloan-Kettering Cancer Center reported an 80% 5-year survival rate for stages I and II (AJC classification) patients after subsequent pregnancy. The study included 41 patients studied over 30 years. No detrimental effect was noted of subsequent pregnancy, even among patients with positive axillary lymph nodes or among those who had a pregnancy less than 2 years after mastectomy.[85] In a 1986 nationwide French study, the 10-year survival rate of 68 patients who had subsequent pregnancy was 71%. The survival of the negative-node patients was 90% at 10 years, with no difference between cases and control subjects.[86]

The largest series, by Clark and Chua,[73] of 136 patients diagnosed over 5 decades at the Princess Margaret Hospital in Toronto, is an update of the series reported by Peters and Meakin in 1965.[21] They reported an excellent overall 5-year survival rate of 78%. In 1989, Ariel and Kempner[87] found that subsequent pregnancies did not affect overall prognosis in a large private practice experience.

Data on subsequent pregnancy have also been reported in the analysis of adjuvant chemotherapy trials, showing similar recurrence rates and survival for patients who had undergone subsequent pregnancy compared to those who did not.[79] Recently, small studies from Greece[88] and New Zealand[38] were reported, with approximately 20 patients each who had a pregnancy after treatment for breast cancer. The recurrence rate and survival of the women were similar to that of patients of similar age and stage without pregnancy.

Specific Issues in Subsequent Pregnancy: Timing, Multiple Pregnancies, Breast-feeding, Abdominal Muscle Breast Reconstruction

Three groups of investigators in retrospective series have examined the question of the timing of subsequent pregnancy on breast cancer prognosis. The length of the interval between breast cancer diagnosis and pregnancy affects prognosis, because women who defer a pregnancy for many years are also those who have remained disease free for longer periods.

Clark and Chua[73] found that 72% of their patients became pregnant within 2 years of treatment. Those who became pregnant within 6 months had a comparatively poor prognosis—a 5-year survival rate of 54% compared with a 78% 5-year survival rate among those who waited 6 months to 2 years to become pregnant after breast cancer diagnosis. Those who waited 5 years or longer to become pregnant had 100% 5-year survival from that point. The data are consistent with the fact that the longer survival after diagnosis is, *per se*, an indicator of the patients' better prognosis (whether pregnancy occurs or not). The 1986 French series[86] and the Memorial Hospital series,[85] which are smaller, do not find a statistically significant difference between outcome of patients based on the interval. Among those who became pregnant, 18% and 35.3%[83] have had multiple pregnancies. Clark and Reid[25] found that 25% of those who had one pregnancy, those who had more than one, and those with multiple pregnancies appeared to have improved survival. Rissanen[82] found that 34% of patients in his series had two or more post-treatment pregnancies, and those women survived as well as those with one pregnancy. Multiple pregnancies affect prognosis for the same reason that interval affects prognosis: Women who have more than one pregnancy are also those who have remained disease free for greater periods (to have achieved the multiple pregnancies) and thereby already have demonstrated their better prognosis.

There are few data specific to nursing, except for one small report on 13 patients who had undergone breast conservation surgery and radiation.[89] All women reported little or no enlargement of the treated breast during pregnancy. Only one woman was able to nurse from the treated breast and only for a short period of 4 months. On the other hand, breast-feeding was successful from the untreated breast.

Lastly, 14 women in two reports from Brazil[90] and the United States[91] underwent successful pregnancy and birth after transverse rectus abdominis muscle flap reconstructions. A small proportion were delivered vaginally.

Possible Biases in Study Design

How much reliance can be placed on these reports to adequately advise patients on subsequent pregnancy after breast cancer treatment? Because pregnancy is not coded as a disease or in any other way by the record room or tumor registry, cases over the previous decades are found by memory, as with the Memorial Hospital series.[85] Even if a chart or tumor registry review of all premenopausal women had been undertaken, the occurrence of subsequent pregnancy might not have been noted.

The methods section of all of the retrospective series ignores the question of the denominator, the total number of patients with subsequent pregnancies. The largest series, from 1989, states simply, "We have reviewed patients whose case histories are currently available."[73] Because cases over the decades have been obtained in these reports from the many clinicians' memories, and because it is human nature to remember those who have been seen more recently, the design of these studies is predisposed to find and report on the patients who are alive, a recollection bias.

For all of these reasons, each report contains a small fraction of such patients from that institution. For example, consider a typical series, that from Memorial Sloan-Kettering Cancer Center: Over 30 years, 41 stage I and II patients were found who became pregnant after breast cancer treatment, and they had an outstanding 80% 5-year survival.[85] However, based on the numbers and ages of women seen in those 30 years, as obtained from the Memorial Hospital Tumor Registry, and assuming that only 7% of breast cancer patients younger than 40 years of age became pregnant, this study should have reported on at least 450 women. Therefore, the patients reported from Memorial Hospital represent a highly selected subset, possibly 10% or so of the total who became pregnant after breast cancer treatment.

Population-Based Reports

In an effort to avoid recollection bias, three large population-based studies have been published in the last 5 years. These three studies are similar because they all depend on the National Health Service record keeping and a unique identifying number that is assigned to each person at birth and is used for every hospitalization and reportable event, such as a cancer diagnosis.

Finland

The Finnish population-based study used the personal identification numbers of women with a breast cancer diagnosis and searched the national birth certificate for the years after their diagnosis.[92] The authors found 91 eligible case patients with subsequent deliveries and matched control subjects for stage, age, and year of breast cancer diagnosis. The control group also had to be alive for the same interval as that from diagnosis to delivery of their matched cases. Breast cancer survivors with a subsequent birth after their diagnosis had statistically better survival rates than control subjects of the same age and stage with no subsequent births. The control group had a 4.8-fold (confidence interval, 2.2 to 10.3) increased risk of death compared with those who delivered after the diagnosis of breast cancer.

The major flaw of the study design with the national cancer registry information is that only dates of diagnosis and death for patients and control subjects were available, with no information on recurrence data. It is likely that breast cancer patients who chose to become pregnant and give birth were disease free, as opposed to an unknown proportion of controls who had a recurrence at the time of matching but had not yet died. Thus, this bias probably contributed to the control group's having a poor survival rate, thereby making the cases appear to have a particularly good survival rate. The authors termed this bias a *healthy mother effect* to denote that the tumor registry matching design chosen did not overcome the fact that women without recurrence, "healthy mothers," were more likely to become pregnant.

Sweden

The next published study, from 1995, is from the Stockholm Breast Cancer Study Group.[7] The study subjects consisted of 2,119 women with primary operable breast cancer who were 49 years of age or younger treated between 1971 and 1988. The study subjects were matched to the Stockholm County Council inpatient care registry, by computerized record linkage through use of the unique personal identification number, to obtain information about the patient's pregnancy history. A total of 50 pregnancies in the 2,119 patients occurred after the diagnosis of breast cancer. The relative hazard of death adjusted for nodal status and age was 0.48 (confidence interval, 0.18 to 1.29) at a median follow-up of 7 years (range, 1 to 19 years). This was also the first study to report on estrogen-receptor status, which was recorded in 70% of the population. The women with subsequent pregnancies had better survival rates if their cancer had positive estrogen receptors, which at first seems counterintuitive. However, this finding is probably related to the mere fact that women with positive receptors have better survival rates and no micrometastatic disease.

Denmark

The last of the population-based studies is from Denmark.[93] The Danish study used computer linkage of the national records of Denmark on births, abortions, and breast cancer diagnosis. The authors identified 173 case patients out of 5,725 with breast cancer, 45 years old or younger, who became pregnant after treatment for breast cancer. Women who had a full-term pregnancy after treatment had a nonsignificantly reduced risk of dying (relative risk, 0.55; confidence interval, 0.28 to 1.06) compared with other women with no full-term pregnancy ($p = .08$).

Because virtually all women who undergo subsequent pregnancy are recurrence free, the need for appropriate recurrence-free control subjects for matching arises. In the Danish study, computer-matched linkage was accomplished on 93% of patients, and information on recurrence was available on 82% of them. However, it is unclear how carefully recurrence was sought and diagnosed. Furthermore, in an attempt to report on as many pregnancies as possible, they entered cases until 1994, and thus some had a limited follow-up of approximately one year.

The population-based studies try to avoid the recollection bias prevalent in the retrospective studies, but they add

TABLE 2. *Selected studies on subsequent pregnancy*

Author	Year	No. of patients	Study period	10-yr survival node negative (%)/ positive (%)
Harvey	1981	41	1940–1970	80/79
Ribiero	1986	57	1941–1980	64/26
Mignot	1986	68	1940–1985	71
Ariel	1989	46	1950–1980	76/56
Clark	1989	136	1931–1985	64
Sankila	1994	92	1967–1989	93
Schoultz	1995	50	1971–1988	Not given
Kroman	1997	173	1978–1995	Not given

biases perhaps in the choice of control subjects for the matching. These three population-based studies add to the retrospective studies that show no detriment to subsequent pregnancy after breast cancer treatment. However, peculiar biases to each type of study exist. Table 2 is a summary of the studies on subsequent pregnancy.

Prospective Study

Until the issue is subjected to a prospective study, the effect of subsequent pregnancy is not really known. Only a prospective study would provide comprehensive information on each patient at baseline, including clinical characteristics, treatment variables, and then a follow-up for medical status and recurrence, as well as any reproductive events. However, a prospective trial design is lengthy, and therefore expensive, with the goals obtained perhaps 10 years after its inception. The design of an ideal prospective study would include accruing breast cancer patients at diagnosis to get the extensive and comprehensive baseline data. With M. D. Anderson Cancer Center and Wake Forest University Medical Center in Winston-Salem, North Carolina, we at Memorial Sloan-Kettering Cancer Center have launched such a prospective study accruing young women within 8 months of diagnosis, with study data consisting of menstrual cycles, quality of life, and any reproductive events. The short-term goal is the study of premature menopause, addressing symptoms, and sexual dysfunction. No inpatient visits are necessary; all data are obtained by mail and phone. Patient referrals can be directed to (877) 636-7562.

Unfortunately, statistics on survival after subsequent pregnancy will be forthcoming only after the next several years, and we can only advise our patients with results based on the available studies: retrospective and population based.

MANAGEMENT SUMMARY

- Modified radical mastectomy is the preferred local management of a patient with breast cancer during pregnancy. There is much experience regarding pregnancy and general anesthesia, due to the large numbers of various surgical procedures performed annually on pregnant women.
- Radiotherapy should be avoided during any trimester because of the dose, due mainly to internal scatter, absorbed by the fetus. Limited breast resection during pregnancy and radiotherapy delayed until after delivery has been reported, but local control rates are unknown.
- Therapeutic abortion cannot be proved to be beneficial. However, the existing reports have small numbers as well as patient selection in which more patients with more advanced disease are more likely to undergo abortion. The value of therapeutic abortion is uncertain, with the exception that breast cancer treatment is greatly simplified without concern of fetal effects from the treatment modalities.
- Chemotherapy during pregnancy must be considered on a case-by-case basis because of the risk of fetal damage, particularly early in pregnancy (see Table 1).

REFERENCES

1. Moolgavkar SH, Day NE, Stevens RG. Two-stage model for carcinogenesis: epidemiology of breast cancer in females. *J Natl Cancer Inst* 1980;65:559.
2. Guinee VF, Olsson H, Moller T, et al. Effects of pregnancy on prognosis for young women with breast cancer. *Lancet* 1994;343:1587.
3. de la Rochefordiere A, Asselain B, Campana F, et al. Age as prognostic factor in premenopausal breast carcinoma. *Lancet* 1993;341:1039.
4. Adami HO, Malker B, Holmberg L, Persson I, Stone B. The relationship between survival and age at diagnosis in breast cancer. *N Engl J Med* 1986;315:559.
5. Kroman N, Wohlfahrt J, Andersen KW, Mouridsen HT, Westergaard T, Melbye M. Time since childbirth and prognosis in primary breast cancer: population based study. *BMJ* 1997;315:851.
6. Olson SH, Zauber AG, Tang J, Harlap S. Relation of time since last birth and parity to survival of young women with breast cancer. *Epidemiology* 1998;9:669.
7. Von Schoultz E, Johansson H, Wilking N, Rutqvist L. Influence of prior and subsequent pregnancy on breast cancer prognosis. *J Clin Oncol* 1995;13:430.
8. Ewertz M, Gillanders S, Meyer L, Zedeler K. Survival of breast cancer patients in relation to factors which affect the risk of developing breast cancer. *Int J Cancer* 1991;49:526.
9. Wallack MK, Wolf JA Jr, Bedwinek J, et al. Gestational carcinoma of the female breast. *Curr Probl Cancer* 1983;7:1.
10. Saunders CM, Baum M. Breast cancer and pregnancy: a review. *J R Soc Med* 1993;86:162.
11. Anderson JM. Mammary cancers and pregnancy. *BMJ* 1979;1:1124.
12. Allen HH, Nisker JA. Cancer in pregnancy: therapeutic guidelines. In: Allen HH, Nisker JA, eds. *Cancer in pregnancy: an overview*. New York: Futura, 1988;3.
13. Kilgore AR, Bloodgood JC. Tumors and tumor-like lesions of the breast in association with pregnancy. *Arch Surg* 1929;18:2079.
14. White TT. Carcinoma of the breast and pregnancy. *Ann Surg* 1954;139:9.
15. Haagensen CD, Stout AP. Carcinoma of the breast: criteria of operability. *Ann Surg* 1943;118:859.
16. Harrington SW. Carcinoma of the breast: results of surgical treatment when the carcinoma occurred in course of pregnancy or lactation and when pregnancy occurred subsequent to operation, 1910-1933. *Ann Surg* 1937;106:690.
17. Byrd BF, Bayer DS, Robertson JC, et al. Treatment of breast tumors associated with pregnancy and lactation. *Ann Surg* 1962;155:940.
18. Bunker ML, Peters MV. Breast cancer associated with pregnancy or lactation. *Am J Obstet Gynecol* 1963;85:312.
19. Montgomery TL. Detection and disposal of breast cancer in pregnancy. *Am J Obstet Gynecol* 1961;81:926.

20. Miller HK. Cancer of the breast during pregnancy and lactation. *Am J Obstet Gynecol* 1962;83:607.
21. Peters VM, Meakin JW. The influence of pregnancy in carcinoma of the breast. *Prog Clin Cancer* 1965;1:471.
22. Mickal A, Torres JE, Mule JG. Carcinoma of breast in pregnancy and lactation. *Am Surg* 1963;29:509.
23. Rosemond GP. Carcinoma of the breast during pregnancy. *Clin Obstet Gynecol* 1963;6:994.
24. DeVitt JE, Beattie WG, Stoddart TG. Carcinoma of the breast and pregnancy. *Can J Surg* 1964;7:124.
25. Clark RM, Reid J. Carcinoma of the breast in pregnancy and lactation. *Int J Radiat Oncol Biol Phys* 1978;4:693.
26. Applewhite RR, Smith LR, DeVicenti F. Carcinoma of the breast associated with pregnancy and lactation. *Am Surg* 1973;39:101.
27. Crosby CH, Barclay THC. Carcinoma of the breast: surgical management of patients with special conditions. *Cancer* 1971;28:1628.
28. Petrek JA, Dukoff R, Rogatko A. Prognosis of pregnancy-associated breast cancer. *Cancer* 1991;67:869.
29. Anderson BO, Petrek JA, Byrd DR, Senie RT, Borgen PI. Pregnancy influences breast cancer stage at diagnosis in women 30 years of age and younger. *Ann Surg Oncol* 1996;3:204.
30. Nugent P, O'Connell TX. Breast cancer and pregnancy. *Arch Surg* 1985;120:1221.
31. King RM, Welch JS, Martin JL, et al. Carcinoma of the breast associated with pregnancy. *Surg Gynecol Obstet* 1985;160:228.
32. Ribiero GG, Jones DA, Jones M. Carcinoma of the breast associated with pregnancy. *Br J Surg* 1986;73:607.
33. Deemarsky LJ, Neishtadt EL. Breast cancer and pregnancy. *Breast* 1980;7:17.
34. Tretli S, Kvalheim G, Thoresen S, Host H. Survival of breast cancer patients diagnosed during pregnancy or lactation. *Br J Cancer* 1988; 58:382.
35. Bonnier P, Romain S, Dilhuydy JM, et al. Influence of pregnancy on the outcome of breast cancer: a case-control study. Societe Francaise de Senologie et de Pathologie Mammaire Study Group. *Int J Cancer* 1997;72:720.
36. Zemlickis D, Lishner M, Degendorfer P, et al. Maternal and fetal outcome after breast cancer in pregnancy. *Am J Obstet Gynecol* 1992;166:781.
37. Ishida T, Yokoe T, Kasumi F, et al. Clinicopathologic characteristics and prognosis of breast cancer patients associated with pregnancy and lactation: analysis of case-control study in Japan. *Jpn J Cancer Res* 1992;83:1143.
38. Lethaby AE, O'Neill MA, Mason BH, Holdaway IM, Harvey VJ. Overall survival from breast cancer in women pregnant or lactating at or after diagnosis. Auckland Breast Cancer Study Group. *Int J Cancer* 1996;67:751.
39. Ezzat A, Raja MA, Berry J, et al. Impact of pregnancy on non-metastatic breast cancer: a case control study. *Clin Oncol* 1996;8:367.
40. Boice JD Jr. Fetal risk to radiotherapy and chemotherapy exposure in utero. *Cancer Bull* 1986;38:293.
41. Miller R, Mulvihill S. Small head size after atomic radiation. *Teratology* 1976;14:355.
42. Kimler BF. Prenatal irradiation: a major concern for the developing brain. *Int J Radiat Biol* 1998;73:423.
43. Miller RW. Epidemiological conclusions from radiation toxicity studies. In: *Late effects of radiation*. London: Taylor and Francis, 1970.
44. Doll R, Wakeford R. Risk of childhood cancer from fetal irradiation. *Br J Radiol* 1997;70:130.
45. Miller RW. Transplacental carcinogenesis. *Cancer Bull* 1986;38:300.
46. Brent RL. The effects of ionizing radiation, microwaves, and ultrasound on the developing embryo: clinical interpretations and applications of the data. *Curr Probl Pediatr* 1984;14:61.
47. Mossman KL, Hill LT. Radiation risks in pregnancy. *Obstet Gynecol* 1982;60:237.
48. Baker J, Ali A, Groch MW, et al. Bone scanning in pregnant patients with breast carcinoma. *Clin Nucl Med* 1987;12:519.
49. Harbert JC. Efficacy of bone and liver scanning in malignant disease: facts and options. In: *Nuclear medicine annual.* New York: Raven, 1982.
50. Kanal E. Pregnancy and the safety of magnetic resonance imaging. *Magn Reson Imaging Clin N Am* 1994;2:309.
51. Adzick NS, Harrison MR. The unborn surgical patient. *Curr Probl Surg* 1994;31:1.
52. Mattison DR, Angtuaco T. Magnetic resonance imaging in prenatal diagnosis. *Clin Obstet Gynecol* 1988;31:353.
53. National Council on Radiation Protection and Measurements. Report no 39: Basic radiation protection criteria. Washington: US Government Printing Office, 1971.
54. Woo SY, Fuller LM, Cundiff JH, et al. Radiotherapy during pregnancy for clinical stages IA-IIA Hodgkin's disease. *Int J Radiat Oncol Biol Phys* 1992;23:407.
55. Veronesi U, Luini A, Del Vecchio M, et al. Radiotherapy after breast-preserving surgery in women with localized cancer of the breast. *N Engl J Med* 1993;328:1587.
56. Kuerer HM, Cunningham JD, Bleiweiss IJ, et al. Conservative surgery for breast carcinoma associated with pregnancy. *Breast J* 1998;4:171.
57. Doll DC, Ringenberg S, Yarbro JW. Antineoplastic agents and pregnancy. *Semin Oncol* 1989;16:337.
58. Zemlickis D, Lishner M, Degendorfer P, et al. Fetal outcome after in utero exposure to cancer chemotherapy. *Arch Intern Med* 1992;152:573.
59. Glantz JC. Reproductive toxicology of alkylating agents. *Obstet Gynecol Surv* 1994;49:709.
60. Turchi JJ, Villasis C. Anthracyclines in the treatment of malignancy in pregnancy. *Cancer* 1988;61:435.
61. Berry DL, Theriault RL, Holmes FA, et al. Management of breast cancer during pregnancy using a standard protocol. *J Clin Oncol* 1999;17:855.
62. Buekers TE, Lallas TA. Chemotherapy in pregnancy. *Obstet Gynecol Clin North Am* 1998;25:323.
63. Eltorky M, Khare VK, Osborne P, et al. Placental metastasis from maternal carcinoma: a report of three cases. *J Reprod Med* 1995; 40:339.
64. Potter JF, Schoeneman M. Metastases of maternal cancer to the placenta and fetus. *Cancer* 1970;25:380.
65. Smythe AR, Underwood PB, Kreutner A. Metastatic placental tumors: report of three cases. *Am J Obstet Gynecol* 1973;125:1149.
66. Fox H. Non-trophoblastic tumors of the placenta. In: Fox H, ed. *Pathology of the placenta*. Philadelphia: WB Saunders, 1978:357.
67. Gianopoulos JG. Establishing the criteria for anesthesia and other precautions for surgery during pregnancy. *Surg Clin North Am* 1995; 75:33.
68. Pedersen H, Finster M. Anesthetic risks in the pregnant surgical patient. *Anesthesiology* 1979;51:439.
69. Mazze RI, Kallen B. Reproductive outcome after anesthesia and operation during pregnancy: a registry study of 5405 cases. *Am J Obstet Gynecol* 1989;161:1178.
70. Haagensen CD. The treatment and results in cancer of the breast at the Presbyterian Hospital, New York. *AJR Am J Roentgenol* 1949;62:328.
71. Adair FE. Cancer of the breast. *Surg Clin North Am* 1953;33:313.
72. Holleb AI, Farrow JH. The relation of carcinoma of the breast and pregnancy in 283 patients. *Surg Gynecol Obstet* 1962;115:65.
73. Clark RM, Chua T. Breast cancer and pregnancy: the ultimate challenge. *Clin Oncol* 1989;1:11.
74. Sakai F, Saez S. Existence of receptors bound to endogenous estradiol in breast cancers in premenopausal and postmenopausal women. *Steroids* 1976;27:99.
75. Elledge RM, Ciocca DR, Langone G, McGuire WL. Estrogen receptor, and her-2/neu protein in breast cancers from pregnant patients. *Cancer* 1993;71:2499.
76. Landis SH, Murray T, Bolden S, Wingo PA. Cancer statistics 1999. *Cancer J Clin* 1999;49:8.
77. Beatson GT. On the treatment of inoperable cases of carcinoma of the mamma: suggestions for a new method of treatment. *Lancet* 1896;2:104.
78. Donegan WL. Breast cancer and pregnancy. *Obstet Gynecol* 1977; 50:244.
79. Sutton R, Buzdar AU, Hortobagyi GN. Pregnancy and offspring after adjuvant chemotherapy in breast cancer patients. *Cancer* 1990; 65:847.
80. Danforth DN. How subsequent pregnancy affects outcome in women with a prior breast cancer. *Oncology* 1991;11:23.
81. Petrek JA. Pregnancy safety after breast cancer. *Cancer* 1994;74:528.
82. Rissanen PM. Pregnancy following treatment of mammary carcinoma. *Acta Radiol Ther Phys Biol* 1969;8:415.
83. Cooper DR, Butterfield J. Pregnancy subsequent to mastectomy for cancer of the breast. *Ann Surg* 1970;171:429.

84. Cheek JH. Cancer of the breast in pregnancy and lactation. *Am J Surg* 1973;126:729.
85. Harvey JC, Rosen PP, Ashikari H, et al. The effect of pregnancy on the prognosis of carcinoma of the breast following radical mastectomy. *Surg Gynecol Obstet* 1981;153:723.
86. Mignot L, Morvan F, Berdah J, et al. Pregnancy after breast cancer: results of a case-control study. *Presse Med* 1986;15:1961.
87. Ariel I, Kempner R. The prognosis of patients who become pregnant after mastectomy for breast cancer. *Int Surg* 1989;74:185.
88. Malamos NA, Stathopoulos GP, Keramopoulos A, Papadiamantis J, Vassilaros S. Pregnancy and offspring after the appearance of breast cancer. *Oncology* 1996;53:471.
89. Higgins S, Haffty BG. Pregnancy and lactation after breast-conserving therapy for early stage breast cancer. *Cancer* 1994;73:2175.
90. Carramaschi FR, Ramos MLC, Pinotti JA, Ferreira MC. Pregnancy following breast reconstruction with TRAM flaps. *Breast J* 1998; 4:258.
91. Chen L, Hartrampf CR. Successful pregnancies following TRAM flap surgery. *Plast Reconstr Surg* 1993;91:69.
92. Sankila R, Heinavaara S, Hakulinen T. Survival of breast cancer patients after subsequent term pregnancy: "healthy mother effect." *Am J Obstet Gynecol* 1994;170:818.
93. Kroman N, Jensen MB, Melby M, et al. Should women be advised against pregnancy after breast-cancer treatment? *Lancet* 1997;350:319.

Diseases of the Breast, 2nd ed.,
edited by Jay R. Harris.
Lippincott Williams & Wilkins, Philadelphia © 2000.

CHAPTER 45

Occult Primary Cancer with Axillary Metastases

Alain Fourquet, Anne de la Rochefordière, and François Campana

Breast cancer can sometimes present as an isolated axillary adenopathy without any detectable breast tumor by palpation or radiologic examination. These occult primary cancers are staged as T0, N1 (stage II in the Union Internationale Contre le Cancer/American Joint Committee classification). This staging requires that proper clinical *and* mammographic investigations be done to rule out the presence of small breast tumor. If this is accomplished, axillary metastases of occult breast primary cancer represent a rare clinical entity first described by Halsted in 1907.[1]

FREQUENCY

The incidence of an occult primary tumor with axillary metastases is low. Incidence rates ranged from 0.3% to 1.0% of operable breast cancers in the largest reported series.[2–6] Some 350 cases have been reported in the literature since the 1950s. Because these series are limited and management policies have varied widely during this period, comparing characteristics of the patients, management, and results of treatment is difficult. Many of these patients had suspicious mammograms.[2,7,8,9] Presumably, the constant improvement of the quality of mammography has decreased the rate of occult primary with axillary metastases. Interpretation of these comparisons should only be done with caution.

The characteristics of the patients with T0, N1 breast cancer are similar to those of patients with typical stage II disease. The series from the Institut Curie included 59 patients treated between 1960 and 1997. The median patient age was 57 years (range, 36 to 79 years). Thirty-four patients (58%) were postmenopausal, including two patients under hormone replacement therapy. Fifteen patients (25%) had family histories of breast cancer. Twenty-eight (47.5%) had left axillary nodes, and 31 (52.5%) had right axillary nodes.

A. Fourquet: Department of Radiation Oncology, Institut Curie, Paris, France
A. de la Rochefordière: Institut Curie, Paris, France
F. Campana: Institut Curie, Paris, France

DIAGNOSIS

Axillary Adenopathy

Isolated axillary adenopathy is a benign condition in most patients. Lymphomas are the most frequently occurring malignant tumors.[10]

Adenocarcinoma in areas other than the breast may include thyroid, lung, gastric, pancreatic, and colorectal cancer.[11] These tumors, however, probably do not have isolated axillary metastases as the only presentation of disease, and an extensive search for primary adenocarcinoma other than breast cancer is not recommended.[4,9,12] A thorough clinical examination and chest radiography may prove sufficient. Tumor markers may help in the diagnosis of metastatic colon or pancreatic cancers.

Axillary adenopathy usually consists of one or two involved nodes, sometimes with large diameters. The median axillary node size at presentation in the patients treated at the Institut Curie was 30 mm (range, 10 to 70 mm). The initial diagnosis of malignancy was achieved by node excision in 25 of 59 patients, by fine-needle aspiration in 26 patients, and by core-needle biopsy (drill biopsy) in 8 patients.

A primary breast cancer located in the axillary tail of the breast may be confounded with an axillary node. The presence of normal lymph node structure surrounding foci of carcinoma on the pathologic sample usually leads to the diagnosis of metastasis to a lymph node. The recognition of a metastatic lymph node can, however, be difficult because of massive involvement, with extension of the tumor into the axillary fat and disappearance of the lymphoid patterns.

Breast Cancer

Bilateral mammography should always be performed in the presence of metastatic adenocarcinoma in an axillary lymph node. Baron et al.[2] report an overall 44% accuracy in the diagnosis of occult breast cancer in a series of 34 patients, in which only nine mammographies were considered suspicious. Nonetheless, any suspicious image should be removed for pathologic analysis.

Studies suggest that magnetic resonance imaging (MRI) of the breast may improve the accuracy of conventional mammography in detecting breast cancer. Promising results were published of the use of MRI in characterizing nonpalpable but radiologically detectable breast lesions in patients.[13,14] In patients with T0, N1 breast cancer, studies[15–17] have shown that MRI could detect early contrast-enhanced images in the breast. Morris and colleagues[15] report on 12 patients with axillary node metastases without clinically or mammographically detectable breast tumor. Breast MRI detected early contrast-enhanced foci in 9 of the 12 patients (75%). Breast cancer was found in all but one of the nine patients who were subsequently operated on. Brenner and Rothman[16] performed MRI of the breast on four patients with occult carcinoma metastatic to the axilla: Foci of enhancement were detected in all patients, and ultrasound-guided surgical biopsies could be performed in all cases. Breast carcinoma was identified in all four patients. Similarly, Tilanus-Linthorst et al.[17] detected enhancing lesions with MRI in four patients: MRI-directed, ultrasound-guided fine-needle aspiration cytology found carcinoma cells in all four patients. Early contrast-enhanced lesions were seen in all three patients with T0, N1 tumors who had breast MRI at the Institut Curie in 1997. Two patients underwent a wide excision of the areas that were detected with MRI. In both patients, pathology was positive for invasive adenocarcinoma with associated ductal carcinoma *in situ*. The third patient, who had a small, 5-mm early contrast-enhanced image that could not be localized with sonography, was not operated on and underwent whole breast irradiation with an additional boost. The high sensitivity of breast MRI suggests that it could be used systematically in searching for a breast primary tumor. However, because of its low specificity and the difficulties in localizing small, early contrast-enhancing foci in some instances, difficult management problems may occur. Further studies on larger series are therefore necessary. Other breast-imaging procedures are under investigation, such as color Doppler sonography[18] and positron emission tomography.[19]

In patients who have nonpalpable breast masses and normal mammograms, the mammary origin of a metastatic adenocarcinoma to an axillary lymph node cannot be established with certainty. Therefore, the diagnosis of occult breast cancer can only be highly presumed based on a bundle of elements, including sex, age, isolated adenopathy, and histologic diagnosis of adenocarcinoma.

High estrogen or progesterone receptor levels found in the metastatic axillary nodes can help to confirm a primary breast tumor[20]; however, three series[2,3,21] report that 50% to 86% of occult breast cancer cases were found to be negative for estrogen receptors. Because surgical excision of the palpable node was often the first diagnostic procedure, rarely was an attempt made to analyze the receptors by biochemical methods. In the Institut Curie series, receptor analysis was done in only 14 of the 59 tumors (24%) and was positive in 6 of 14. Immunohistochemical detection of hormone receptors can now be done in paraffin-embedded tissue[22] and should therefore be carried out systematically.

TABLE 1. *Occurrence of breast cancer in the nontreated breast*

Investigators	Breast failures/ nontreated breasts	Delay (mo)
Atkins and Wolff[23]	5/9	9–17
Ellerbroek et al.[3]	7/13	11–47
Feigenberg et al.[8]	0/4	—
Feuerman et al.[24]	0/1	—
Haagensen[5]	3/5	5–64
Halsted[1]	2/3	NA
Kemeny et al.[12]	0/7	—
Klopp[25]	1/1	48
Merson et al.[21]	9/17	2–34
Van Ooijen et al.[26]	3/14	16–56
Institut Curie, present series	2/2	9, 67

NA, not available.

NATURAL HISTORY

After removal of an axillary adenopathy, a breast cancer eventually developed in the untreated breast in 32 of 76 patients (42%) described in the literature, with recurrence intervals ranging from 5 months to 67 months (Table 1). Patient samples were limited in these series, however, and follow-up periods varied widely.

The number of pathologically involved lymph nodes seen after axillary dissection is high. Rosen and Kimmel[27] report a median of three involved nodes (range, 1 to 65 nodes) in 48 patients. Merson et al.[21] report that more than three nodes were involved in 23 of 46 patients who underwent axillary dissections. Twenty-six patients in the Institut Curie series had an axillary dissection as initial treatment. The median number of involved nodes was 3 (range, 1 to 20). During follow-up, 16 of the 59 patients in the series had distant metastases: 4 (25%) in the brain, 5 (31%) in the liver, 3 (19%) as cervical nodes, and 3 in multiple sites. One patient had isolated bone metastases. Nine patients had contralateral disease, which occurred in the contralateral breast alone in five patients. Of note, four patients had isolated contralateral axillary node metastases.

TREATMENT AND RESULTS

Mastectomy with axillary node dissection has been the most commonly used treatment in patients with occult primary tumors. The combined analysis of 13 published series

TABLE 2. *Pathologic report after mastectomy*

Investigators	Years	Patients with mastectomy	*In situ* carcinoma	Invasive carcinoma	Carcinoma (%)
Ashikari et al.[7]	1946–75	34	3	20	67
Bhatia et al.[20]	1977–85	11	2	9	100
Baron et al.[2]	1975–78	28	4	16	71
Ellerbroek et al.[3]	1944–87	13	0	1	8
Feigenberg et al.[8]	1971–74	4	0	3	80
Feuerman et al.[24]	1949–61	2	0	1	50
Fitts et al.[4]	1948–63	11	0	7	70
Haagensen[5]	1916–66	13	0	12	92
Kemeny et al.[12]	1973–85	11	2	3	45
Merson et al.[21]	1945–87	33[a]	0	27	82
Owen et al.[6]	1907–50	27	0	25	92
Patel et al.[9]	1952–79	29	0	16	60
Weigenberg and Stetten[28]	1937–48	5	0	5	100

[a]Includes six patients with superolateral quadrantectomy.

has shown that breast cancer was found in the mastectomy specimen in 156 of 221 patients (71%) (Table 2). Invasive tumors were found in 145 of 221 patients (66%). These data, along with the fact that nearly 50% of the patients who received no form of breast treatment will eventually have disease recurrence in the breast, support the recommendation that the breast be treated when no tumor can be detected clinically or mammographically.

Three studies report the results of breast-conserving treatment of T0, N1 cancer. The group from the M. D. Anderson Cancer Center in Houston[3] treated 29 of 42 patients with breast preservation; the breast was irradiated in 16, and no breast treatment was given to 13. Breast recurrences occurred in 18% of the irradiated breast group and in 54% of the nonirradiated breast group. Survival did not differ between those who underwent mastectomy and those who did not. In the Memorial Sloan-Kettering series,[2] 7 of 35 patients had a breast-conserving treatment, with radiotherapy in 6. Five-year survival rates were similar between this group and patients who had a mastectomy. Merson et al.[21] reported on 29 patients who had breast conservation. Breast recurrences occurred in 9 of 17 patients who did not receive breast irradiation and in 2 of 6 patients who had breast irradiation. Of the 59 patients treated between 1960 and 1997 at the Institut Curie, 3 had mastectomies. Two patients underwent neither mastectomy nor breast irradiation. Both eventually had breast cancer, at 9 months and 67 months, respectively. Fifty-four patients received whole breast irradiation (median dose, 59 Gy; range, 50 to 70 Gy). Breast recurrence occurred in 9 of 54 patients; the 8-year risk of ipsilateral breast recurrence was 12%. All patients who had recurrences were treated by mastectomy. The 8-year breast preservation rate was 93%. The results of these studies therefore support the use of breast irradiation as an alternative to mastectomy.

After axillary node dissection, should irradiation be delivered to the remaining lymph nodes? Few data are available in the literature to support any treatment options. A substantial risk for nodal involvement of the upper axilla can be suspected, however, based on the fact that three involved nodes are expected to be found in one-half of the patients. In patients with axillary node involvement associated with an invasive breast cancer, irradiation of the upper axilla is typically delivered when four or more nodes are involved.[29] A 1997 study[30] has shown that, in patients with axillary node involvement, postmastectomy irradiation of the chest wall and regional nodes decreased the rate of long-term distant metastases and improved survival, even in patients who received adjuvant chemotherapy or hormone therapy. Therefore, by analogy with other stage II tumors, irradiation of the upper axilla can be recommended in these instances, providing that axillary dissection was performed. Fifty-eight of 59 patients treated at the Institut Curie received nodal irradiation. In most instances, only the upper axilla and supraclavicular nodes were treated after complete axillary nodal dissection, whereas the whole axilla was treated when a simple adenectomy had been performed. There were four axillary node recurrences: One was isolated, but three were associated with a breast recurrence. The indications for internal mammary node irradiation are currently much debated in patients with a breast mass and central or medial tumor or axillary involvement. Recommendations about treatment of the internal mammary nodes in patients with occult primaries and axillary adenopathy are difficult to formulate, because the evaluation of internal mammary node irradiation in this rare form of breast cancer is impossible on the basis of limited retrospective series. Because the location of the primary tumor is unknown, the Institut Curie policy supports the irradiation of the internal mammary nodes in all patients.

The reported 5-year actuarial survival rates after treatment of occult breast cancer with axillary metastases range from 36% to 79% (Table 3). The 5-year survival estimate in the 59 patients treated at the Institut Curie was 84% with a median follow-up of 89 months (range, 17 to 431 months). The survival rate was 76% at 8 years. These figures seem higher than

TABLE 3. *Five-year survival rates for patients with occult breast carcinoma*

Investigators	Patients	Follow-up (mo)	Actuarial survival rate (%)
Ashikari et al.[7]	42	NA	79
Baron et al.[2]	35	58 mean	75
Ellerbroek et al.[3]	42	131 median	72
Feuerman et al.[24]	47	NA	36[a]
Kemeny et al.[12]	18	NA	57
Merson et al.[21]	56	123 median	76.5
Institut Curie, present series	59	89 median	84

NA, not available.
[a]Crude survival rate.

those observed after treatment of patients with stage II disease and detectable breast tumor. This has been emphasized by several authors.[4,6,12,21,24] However, these survival rate estimates are derived from small series of patients with various durations of follow-up and heterogeneous treatment modalities. Rosen and Kimmel[27] attempted to evaluate the results more precisely by matching a series of 48 patients with occult breast primary and axillary node metastases with a series of patients with stage II breast cancer who presented with palpable breast tumor (T1, N1 and T2, N1). Although the difference was not statistically significant, higher overall survival and size- or node status–adjusted survival rates were observed in the group of patients with occult primary tumors.

Reliable prognostic analyses are difficult to perform because of the multiple selection biases in the retrospective series and the small sample size. Rosen and Kimmel[27] showed that survival was determined by the number of axillary nodes involved, with patients with fewer than four nodes involved doing better than those with more than four nodes involved. Baron et al.[2] showed that estrogen receptor–positive patients fared better than estrogen receptor–negative patients. Our findings corroborated those indicating that survival was longer in patients with less than four involved axillary nodes: The 5-year survival rates were 91% and 65%, respectively ($p = .03$).

Is there a role for adjuvant systemic treatment in patients with occult primary breast cancer? As mentioned previously, because of the rarity of this disease and the multiple selection biases, the efficacy of systemic therapy in patients with T0, N1 breast cancer is impossible to ascertain. By analogy with stage II node-positive breast cancer, the general tendency is to use the same criteria (i.e., axillary node involvement) to prescribe systemic chemotherapy or hormone therapy. Twenty-seven of the 59 patients treated at Institut Curie received adjuvant chemotherapy, with a regimen of cyclophosphamide, doxorubicin, and 5 fluorouracil. Patients who received chemotherapy were slightly younger and had more involved nodes than those who did not, but these differences were not statistically significant. Survival and metastases-free interval rates were not statistically different in the 27 patients who received chemotherapy and in the 32 patients who did not. This apparent lack of benefit from chemotherapy may be explained by the fact that in this particular group of patients, chemotherapy did not reverse the adverse prognostic influence of massive nodal involvement. Little is known about the effect of hormone therapy in these patients. Of 13 patients who received tamoxifen for at least 2 years in the Institut Curie series, only 1 developed distant metastases, 7 years after diagnosis. The numbers are too small to make significant statistical comparisons, but these results suggest that hormone treatment may be very effective and support its use, at least in patients who have high hormone receptor levels.

The common policy in most institutions is to give adjuvant systemic therapy to patients with involved axillary nodes. Although the outcome of patients with occult primary and axillary metastases seems slightly better than that of patients with stage II node-positive breast cancer, these findings need to be confirmed by larger series. Therefore, adjuvant systemic treatment should be given to such patients.

MANAGEMENT SUMMARY

Occult primary breast cancer presenting as an axillary lymph node is rare and represents a clinical entity with an outcome better than that found in patients with stage II breast cancer and palpable mass and axillary involvement. The heterogeneity of treatment and the limited number of patients studied in the published literature make it difficult to standardize treatment options. However, several guidelines can be used:

- After the diagnosis of adenocarcinoma has been established by surgical removal of an isolated axillary mass, extensive workup evaluation is not necessary. A thorough clinical examination, chest radiographs, bilateral mammograms, and tumor markers are sufficient to establish a high presumption of axillary metastases of mammary origin.
- The use of breast MRI to detect occult breast cancer is promising. However, its low specificity, as well as the difficulties in localizing small breast lesions with the current techniques, makes it difficult to recommend its systematic use. Further evaluation is necessary.
- An axillary dissection should be done to provide prognostic indicators (number of involved nodes) as well as sufficient material for hormone receptor dose. In addition, axillary dissection contributes to local control in the axilla.
- The breast should be treated. Breast-conserving therapy in patients with an occult breast primary by whole breast irradiation to a dose of 50 to 55 Gy limits the risk for disease recurrence and is an alternative to mastectomy.
- Irradiation of the upper axilla and supraclavicular area, to a maximum dose of 45 Gy, is recommended in patients with more than three involved axillary nodes. The whole axilla should be irradiated in patients who did not undergo axillary node dissection.

- By analogy to the indications for patients with stage II node-positive breast cancer (who always receive some type of adjuvant systemic treatment), adjuvant chemotherapy or hormone therapy should be given to those with occult primary tumors with axillary metastases, even though their outcome appears to be slightly better.

REFERENCES

1. Halsted W. The results of radical operations for the cure of carcinoma of the breast. *Ann Surg* 1907;46:1.
2. Baron PL, Moore MP, Kinne DW, et al. Occult breast cancer presenting with axillary metastases: updated management. *Arch Surg* 1990;125:210.
3. Ellerbroek N, Holmes F, Singletary T, et al. Treatment of patients with isolated axillary nodal metastases from an occult primary carcinoma consistent with breast origin. *Cancer* 1990;66:1461.
4. Fitts WT, Steiner GC, Enterline HT. Prognosis of occult carcinoma of the breast. *Am J Surg* 1963;106:460.
5. Haagensen CD. The diagnosis of breast carcinoma. In: Haagensen CD, ed. *Diseases of the breast.* Philadelphia: WB Saunders, 1971:486.
6. Owen HW, Dockerty MB, Gray HK. Occult carcinoma of the breast. *Surg Gynecol Obstet* 1954;98:302.
7. Ashikari R, Rosen PP, Urban JA, et al. Breast cancer presenting as an axillary mass. *Ann Surg* 1976;183:415.
8. Feigenberg Z, Zer M, Dinstman M. Axillary metastases from an unknown primary source: a diagnostic and therapeutic approach. *Isr J Med Sci* 1976;12:1153.
9. Patel J, Nemoto T, Rosner D, et al. Axillary lymph node metastasis from an occult breast cancer. *Cancer* 1981;47:2923.
10. Pierce EH, Gray HK, Dockerty MB. Surgical significance of isolated axillary adenopathy. *Ann Surg* 1957;145:104.
11. Copeland EM, McBride CM. Axillary metastases from unknown primary sites. *Ann Surg* 1973;178:25.
12. Kemeny MM, Rivera DE, Teri JJ, et al. Occult primary adenocarcinoma with axillary metastases. *Am J Surg* 1986;152:43.
13. Orel SG, Mendonca MH, Reynolds C, et al. MR imaging of ductal carcinoma in situ. *Radiology* 1997;202:413.
14. Gilles R, Meunier M, Trouffleau P, et al. Diagnosis of infraclinical lesions of the breast with dynamic MRI: results of a prospective and multicenter study. *J Radiol* 1997;78:293.
15. Morris EA, Schwarz LH, Dershaw DD. Imaging of the breast in patients with occult primary breast carcinoma. *Radiology* 1997;205:437.
16. Brenner RJ, Rothman BJ. Detection of primary breast cancer in women with known adenocarcinoma metastatic to the axilla: use of MRI after negative clinical and mammographic examination. *J Magn Reson Imaging* 1997;7:1153.
17. Tilanus-Linthorst MMA, Obdeijn AIM, Botenbal M, et al. MRI in patients with axillary metastases of occult breast carcinoma. *Breast Cancer Res Treat* 1997;44:179.
18. Lee WJ, Chu JS, Chang KJ, Chen KM. Occult breast carcinoma. Use of color Doppler in localization. *Breast Cancer Res Treat* 1996;37:299.
19. Block EF, Meyer MA. Positron emission tomography in diagnosis of occult adenocarcinoma of the breast. *Am Surg* 1998;64:906.
20. Bhatia SK, Saclarides TJ, Witt TR, et al. Hormone receptor studies in axillary metastases from occult metastases. *Cancer* 1987;59:1170.
21. Merson M, Andreola S, Galimberti V, et al. Breast carcinoma presenting as axillary metastases without evidence of a primary tumor. *Cancer* 1992;70:504.
22. Pertschuk LP, Kim DS, Nayer K, et al. Immunocytochemical estrogen and progestin receptor assays in breast cancer with monoclonal antibodies. Histopathologic, demographic and biochemical correlations and relationship to endocrine response and survival. *Cancer* 1990;66:1663.
23. Atkins H, Wolff B. The malignant gland in the hospital. *Guy's Hosp Rep* 1960;1:109.
24. Feuerman L, Attie JN, Rosenberg B. Carcinoma in axillary lymph nodes as an indicator of breast cancer. *Surg Gynecol Obstet* 1962;114:5.
25. Klopp CT. Metastatic cancer of axillary lymph node without a demonstrable primary lesion. *Ann Surg* 1950;131:437.
26. van Ooijen B, Bontenbal M, Henzen-Logmans, et al. Axillary nodal metastases from an occult primary consistent with breast carcinoma. *Br J Surg* 1993;80:1299.
27. Rosen PP, Kimmel M. Occult breast carcinoma presenting with axillary lymph node metastases: a follow-up study of 48 patients. *Hum Pathol* 1990;21:518.
28. Weigenberg HA, Stetten D. Extensive secondary axillary lymph node carcinoma without clinical evidence of primary breast lesion. *Surgery* 1951;29:217.
29. Harris JR, Recht A. Conservative surgery and radiotherapy. In: Harris JR, Hellman S, Henderson CI, Kinne DW, eds. *Breast diseases,* 2nd ed. Philadelphia: Lippincott, 1991:413.
30. Overgaard M, Hansen PS, Overgaard J, et al. Postoperative radiotherapy in high-risk premenopausal women with breast cancer who receive adjuvant chemotherapy. Danish Breast Cancer Cooperative Group 82b Trial. *N Engl J Med* 1997;337:949.

XI

Diseases of the Breast, 2nd ed.,
edited by Jay R. Harris.
Lippincott Williams & Wilkins, Philadelphia © 2000.

Evaluation after Primary Therapy

CHAPTER 46

Evaluation of Patients after Primary Therapy

Daniel F. Hayes

Since the 1970s, technological advances have improved the ability to detect metastatic breast cancer earlier in the course of the disease. The clinical use of screening for early relapse, and the precise strategies to do so, remain controversial. However, in this chapter, the utility of early detection in patient care is discussed, with recommendations for the most appropriate means of follow-up of patients after primary therapy. Indeed, during the mid-1990s consensus panels from the United States, Canada, and Europe issued recommendations and guidelines for follow-up after primary therapy.

CLINICAL SIGNIFICANCE OF EARLY DETECTION

In general, it has been widely assumed by patients and caregivers that early detection of any cancer, whether as a new primary malignancy or as a recurrence, leads to more effective therapy. Thus, many studies have addressed methods to improve diagnostic techniques. Moreover, investigations of the natural history of patients with breast cancer have generated data regarding risk, timing, and sites of recurrence. These data are reviewed in greater detail in Chapters 28 and 29. Studies evaluating the clinical use of ongoing routine follow up after primary therapy have only recently been reported. In this regard, potential benefits of routine follow-up might include detection of new primary cancers or improved treatment of metastatic disease. These two issues are fundamentally different and are discussed separately.

Screening for New Primary Cancers

The detection of new intraparenchymal breast tumors may be the most important indication for careful follow-up of patients with breast cancer after primary treatment. Large randomized screening trials of the general population have demonstrated that mortality from breast cancer can be reduced as a function of early detection and therapy of new primary breast cancers. The risk of a subsequent second primary breast cancer is elevated relative to the general population in women

D. F. Hayes: Breast Cancer Program, Lombardi Cancer Center, Georgetown University Medical Center, Washington, D.C.

who have had a prior breast cancer. No randomized screening trials have been performed in patients who have had a previous breast cancer. However, several studies in which patients were monitored after primary therapy for the detection of recurrent breast cancer have demonstrated that a contralateral breast cancer develops in approximately 0.5% to 1.0% per year.[1–7] Screening patients after primary therapy of a first breast cancer for the occurrence of a second breast cancer, using criteria at least as stringent as current recommendations for the general population, is indicated. Patients with an ipsilateral breast recurrence after breast-conserving therapy may have the same prognosis as patients with a new primary breast cancer, and follow-up and therapy of patients treated with breast-conserving therapy to detect such recurrences at an early stage is important[8,9] (see Chapter 47).

The incidence of colon and ovarian cancers is statistically elevated in patients with a previous history of breast cancer. However, this risk is not dramatically higher than in the general population, except in patients who have an apparent inherited genetic predisposition, such as germ-line mutations or deletions in the *BRCA1* or *BRCA2* genes, or both.[10–13] Because screening programs for these diseases are already reasonably widespread, more aggressive follow-up beyond what is recommended for the routine population is not indicated in patients who have had a primary breast cancer. Moreover, patients treated with adjuvant therapies may be at risk for treatment-related induction of second malignancies.[14] For example, uterine carcinoma is increased two- to threefold in patients who are taking adjuvant tamoxifen compared to untreated control subjects.[15,16] However, the absolute incidence of such malignancies is still low (fewer than 1% per 5-year follow-up period). Routine screening should include yearly pelvic examination and Papanicolaou smears and careful evaluation of any reported abnormal vaginal bleeding or pelvic symptoms.

Is Early Detection of Extramammary Recurrences Beneficial?

Although technological advances may permit early detection of metastases, controversy remains regarding whether such detection is clinically relevant.[17–26] The following reasons might justify early detection of metastases:

- *More effective treatment*. Metastases might be more effectively treated if they are detected earlier. "More effective treatment" of patients with recurrent disease implies that these patients are more likely to be cured, live longer, or enjoy a superior quality of life (improved palliation) as a result of earlier diagnosis of recurrent disease.
- *Emotional security*. Early detection or, perhaps more important, the lack of it, may be of emotional value to either the patient or the treating physician, or both.
- *Investigational end point*. Delay of recurrence after primary therapy is frequently used as an end point for many investigative therapies. Therefore, detection of recurrence on a consistent basis is important for research purposes.

In contrast, routine screening has at least three potential disadvantages:

- *Overtreatment*. Inappropriate application of therapy with associated morbidity and occasionally mortality in a setting in which the benefits of early treatment have not been demonstrated.
- *Emotional damage*. Increased emotional trauma for patients whose lives may be shattered by finding an asymptomatic recurrence months to years before the onset of symptoms.
- *Increased costs*. Screening patients for early detection of recurrence may lead to increased direct expense, as a result of the costs of the screening diagnostic tests, and increased indirect costs incurred by any further testing that is required to confirm suspicious findings and by early application of therapy. Further increased indirect costs may be incurred by the patient as a function of time lost from family or employment, or both, because of required clinic visits.

Routine Screening for Metastases as a Means of Providing More Effective Treatment

Cure or Prolongation of Survival

Most studies concerning long-term follow-up of patients with recurrent breast cancer suggest that few, if any, women are ever "cured," regardless of whether they receive therapy.[27–31] The success of adjuvant systemic therapy in certain subgroups of patients after primary therapy suggests that treatment of breast cancer might be more successful if administered relatively early in the clinical course.[32] However, the survival benefits of treatment of patients with metastatic disease remain unproven (see Chapter 48). Studies with historical controls suggest that certain subgroups of patients with metastatic disease may benefit from aggressive treatment, but these studies are limited by their retrospective design.[33,34] Survival benefits observed in prospectively randomized trials, in which more effective treatments are compared to less effective regimens, suggest that treatment of patients with metastases might prolong survival. However, such survival differences have been modest (see Chapter 48).[33,34]

The studies discussed in the previous paragraph pertained to patients with documented, evaluable, and usually symptomatic metastatic disease. Treatment of patients with detectable, asymptomatic, or impending but undetectable metastases might be more beneficial if given before the disease is more widespread. Several retrospective studies have addressed whether early detection results in improved survival. In general, the results of these studies suggest that long-term survival of patients is similar, regardless of whether they were diagnosed when their symptoms developed or when they were asymptomatic[1,3,35–37] (Fig. 1).

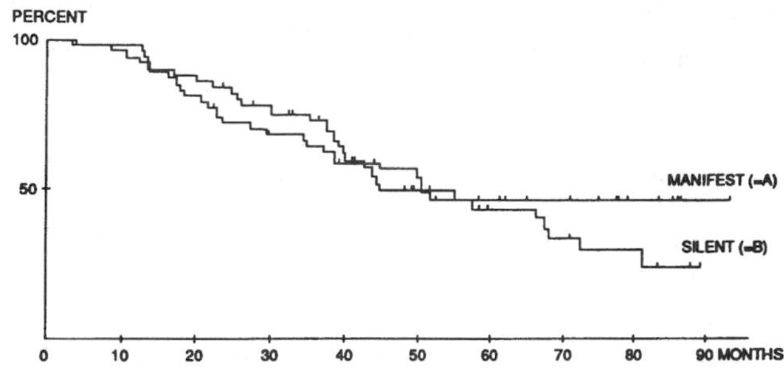

FIG. 1. Overall survival in patients with breast cancer according to whether they presented with symptomatic (manifest) or asymptomatic (silent) metastases (p = .11). (From ref. 3, with permission.)

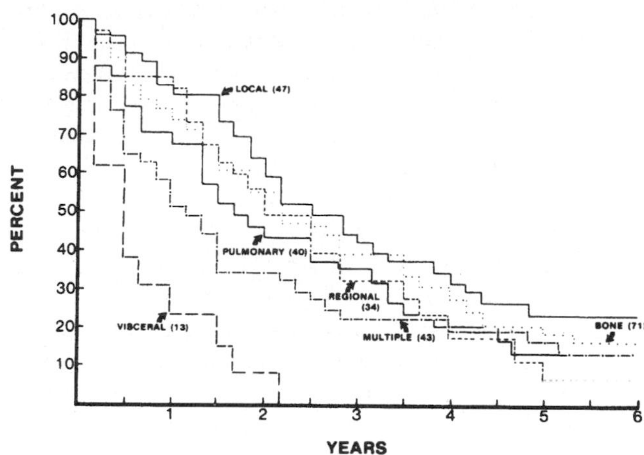

FIG. 2. Survival after recurrence in patients with breast cancer according to initial site of recurrence. (From ref. 38, with permission.)

In three retrospective studies, however, patients who presented with asymptomatic metastases had a substantially longer survival from the time of recurrence than those who presented with symptomatic recurrences.[38–40] Because routine screening might provide a lead time for patients whose metastases are detected asymptomatically, the improved survival for these patients may simply reflect lead-time bias rather than the effects of early treatment. Indeed, when measured from the time of initial diagnosis rather than first metastases, survival was identical for patients who presented with interval, symptomatic recurrences compared to those with asymptomatic metastases diagnosed at routine follow-up visits. Even when patients were diagnosed with modern diagnostic tests, such as computed tomographic (CT) imaging and assays for circulating tumor markers (CEA, CA15-3, CA27.29), overall survival for the two groups of patients (symptomatic versus asymptomatic) has been nearly identical.[39]

In addition to lead-time bias, retrospective studies may also be misleading, because survival from time of first recurrence depends on the site of the first recurrence. For example, median survival after relapse of patients who present with local chest wall recurrence after mastectomy is superior to that of patients who present with visceral metastases[38,41,42] (Fig. 2). In this regard, in one retrospective study, those patients who had asymptomatic recurrences had a prolonged overall survival compared to those with symptomatic recurrences if their first site of recurrence was on the chest wall or in bone. Patients with visceral metastases, however, had a similar survival from first recurrence regardless of whether they presented with symptoms.[36]

Only two studies have been reported in which routinely screened patients with rising tumor marker levels but no detectable disease have been prospectively randomized to immediate treatment versus observation until symptoms occur.[43,44] However, these studies are small, the results that have been presented are only preliminary, and no conclusions can be drawn.

Two large randomized trials have addressed overall survival in patients who were followed either with routine clinic visits or more intensely.[45,46] In these Italian studies, women with early-stage (nonmetastatic) newly diagnosed breast cancer were randomly assigned to undergo intensive follow-up (consisting of physician visit, bone scan, and chest x-ray) or to be followed in a less rigorous fashion (routine physician visits, other tests performed only as indicated). In one study, the intensive follow-up arm also included nontumor marker blood tests (e.g., alkaline phosphatase, transaminases) and liver echography.[46] Both studies included mammography in each arm. Therapy for patients with metastases was provided according to standard practice and was generally initiated at the time of documented recurrence.

The results of these two studies are remarkably similar. Intensive follow-up resulted in slightly increased frequency of detection of recurrence in one study[45] but not in the other.[46] However, in both studies, overall survival from randomization was identical for patients followed intensively or with physician visits only (Fig. 3).

In both studies, the percentage of patients who have relapsed accounts for fewer than 40% of the total patients enrolled. Therefore, it is possible that a small difference in survival of those who relapsed would be missed. However, both of these studies are large (more than 1,200 patients in each), and each has more than 100 relapsed patients per arm. Neither has even a trend toward overall survival benefit for the intensively screened (and therefore early-treated) patients. Thus, the results of these studies suggest that intensive follow-up with frequent radiographic evaluation is not indicated after primary and adjuvant therapy.

Excision of Isolated Metastases

Several authors have reported that, in selected groups of patients with breast cancer, surgical excision of isolated metastases to the brain, liver, or lung may result in prolonged disease-free survival (3 to 5 years).[47–56] However,

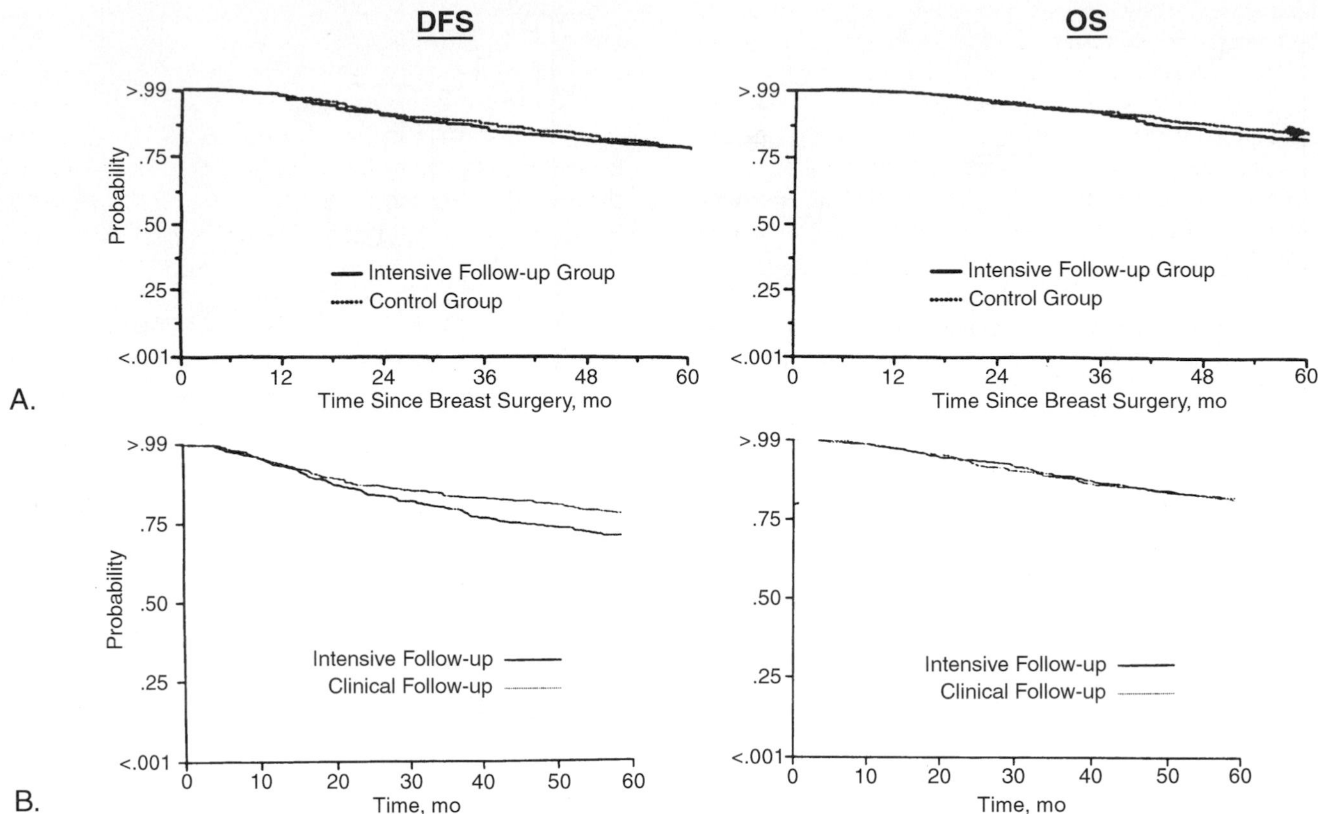

FIG. 3. Disease-free survival (DFS) and overall survival (OS) of patients in two different trials who were randomly assigned to intensive follow-up or to physician visits only after primary adjuvant therapy for carcinoma of the breast. (**A:** From ref. 46, with permission. **B:** From ref. 45, with permission.)

except for a small study in patients with brain metastases, no randomized trial of the effects of metastatectomy has ever been performed, and it is not likely to be.[49] In general, patients are selected for metastatectomy if they have a long disease-free interval from primary treatment to first relapse, have a good performance status, and exhibit relatively good prognostic factors.[57] Such patients are likely to have a prolonged survival regardless of the type of treatment they receive.[58] Although these patients may be rendered disease free, their overall survival may not be altered. Therefore, routine screening with hopes of performing metastatectomy cannot be routinely recommended and should, in general, be considered investigational (see also Chapters 52, 58, 59).

Improved Physical Palliation

In lieu of curing or prolonging survival of patients with recurrent breast cancer, improved palliation might result from earlier detection and treatment of recurrence. In this case, application of systemic therapy at the time of first relapse might delay the time until symptoms would occur. No studies have addressed whether early systemic treatment of asymptomatic patients improves palliation. Indeed, evaluation of palliation as an end point is difficult because of the subjective nature of this treatment result[21] (see Chapter 75). Nonetheless, nearly 43% of physicians who belong to the American Society of Clinical Oncology report that they believe that early detection of metastatic disease would have a positive impact on patients' quality of life.[59]

Detection of asymptomatic recurrences in certain sites might lead to therapy to prevent an impending catastrophic result of untreated tumor. For example, detection of large lytic lesions in major weight-bearing bones might allow prophylactic orthopedic stabilization to prevent a disabling fracture (see Chapter 62). However, the incidence of asymptomatic lesions that result in "catastrophic fractures" is quite small (probably less than 10%), and the value of prophylactic therapy of isolated lytic metastases is unknown.[60] Similarly, although occasionally patients present with the neurologic complications of spinal cord compression without preceding symptoms, more than 90% of patients with epidural involvement have had antecedent episodes of back pain.[61–63]

In summary, the usefulness of early detection of recurrent disease for improving palliative care is not defined. As a result, the physician and patient must assess whether treatment of asymptomatic metastases may result in improved palliation, weighing the toxicity of whatever therapy is administered versus the benefits of delaying or preventing future symptoms. Very few, if any, data exist to offer guidelines in patients with metastatic disease, although several ongoing trials of patients with metastatic disease have incorporated quality of life assessments to more objectively quantify any symptomatic benefits accrued from therapy.

Importantly, newer therapeutic agents, such as aromatase inhibitors and trastuzamab, seem to have very low toxicity profiles[64,65] (see Chapter 48). In this regard, it is possible that patients who are found to have "impending" relapse might prefer to be treated with an agent that has few side effects to delay the time to which cancer-related symptoms may develop. Studies that address this issue need to be performed. In this regard, it is reasonable to hope that as even safer treatments become available, the utility of detection of asymptomatic recurrences will increase.

Routine Screening for Metastases as a Means of Providing Emotional Support

Regular evaluation of breast cancer patients after primary therapy might provide additional emotional support to women at a time when they have suffered considerable psychological stress related to the diagnosis and treatment of their tumor. The knowledge that she remains disease free might be an important aid in returning the patient to a normal role in society. In contrast, if the treatment of asymptomatic metastases cannot be justified, then routine screenings may, in fact, have the opposite effect. The knowledge of an asymptomatic recurrence may substantially diminish the patient's quality of life during a period when she might otherwise have been emotionally secure.[66] In a survey of breast cancer patients in North Carolina, more than one-half preferred frequent (every 3 to 12 months) physician visits.[23] In a similar survey of patients being followed after primary and adjuvant therapy in England, 81% felt "reassured and less anxious" when they had their follow-up visit, and more than 75% preferred to visit a specialty clinic rather than a general practitioner.[17]

Importantly, in one of the two Italian randomized trials of intensive follow-up versus physician visits only, prospective analysis of quality of life was performed.[46] More than 70% of all patients in both arms of this trial stated that they wished to have regular and frequent physician visits, even if they were asymptomatic. However, overall quality of life perceptions, overall health perceptions, and specific measures of body image, emotional well-being, social functioning, symptoms, and satisfaction with health care were nearly identical in the two follow-up groups. Of interest, in a selected group of women in this study, quality of life was shown to decline after relapse. Thus, if early detection of asymptomatic recurrence does not lead to prolonged survival or improved palliation, it may decrease quality of life. These results suggest that, although some sort of follow-up schedule does appear to be reassuring and worthwhile, the less intense, and therefore less expensive, program may be more satisfactory.

A secondary but related issue regards the most appropriate setting in which breast cancer patients should be followed after primary and adjuvant treatment. These patients might be followed by the specialists who evaluated and treated them (surgical oncology, radiation oncology, medical oncology) or by their primary care physician, or both. Because several consensus panels have suggested very conservative approaches (see Management Summary), the need for ongoing follow-up with breast cancer specialists has been questioned.[67] Instead, it has been suggested that follow-up with primary care physicians might be preferable. The following are several possible advantages of transferring follow-up from specialists to general practitioners[67,68]:

- Enhanced continuity of care (one doctor takes care of patient)
- Decreased burden on already busy specialists, thus freeing up their time to see and care for "active patients"
- Improved quality of life for patients (fewer doctor visits, less anxiety-provoking visits)
- Reduced cost of care (primary care physician less expensive than specialist)

In contrast, others have argued that women who have had breast cancer, especially if they have had adjuvant systemic therapy, are better served by follow-up with a more highly trained specialist. The following are several possible advantages to specialist follow-up[68,69]:

- Enhanced continuity of care (the physician who treated the patient maintains ongoing follow-up)
- Improved emotional security for patients (they might prefer the security of knowing that evaluation has been performed by a highly trained specialist)
- Reduced costs of care (specialist might be more cognizant of precise conservative guidelines and might also be more efficient in evaluations of new symptoms and physical findings)

This issue has been addressed in a prospective randomized trial, in which 296 English women with breast cancer received routine follow-up either in the hospital (with specialists) or in general practice.[70] The early results of this study suggest that follow-up in general practice did not result in a delay in time to diagnosis. Indeed, formal quality of life analysis suggests that the two groups of women have similar anxiety levels and health-related quality of life scores. However, at the time of reporting, median follow-up was only 18 months, and only a small fraction (26 of 296; 9%) had relapsed. Furthermore, more than 30% of women who were offered a chance to participate in this study declined, presumably because of a preference for whom they wished to see.

When physicians are queried about who should follow breast cancer patients, surveys demonstrate that their preference is highly biased toward their own specialty.[71,72,73] In general, each group, including general practitioners, feels comfortable with and wishes to continue following patients after primary and adjuvant therapy.

TABLE 1. *Direct cost estimates for intensive follow-up of patients after primary and adjuvant therapy*[a]

Author	Reference no.	Type of follow-up	Country/state	Years	Dollars per patient per yr[b]
Shapira[c]	20		U.S.	1990	
		Intensive			$1,417
		Minimal			$250
Mapelli[c]	85		Italy	1994	
		Intensive			$489
		Minimal			$186
Tomiak[c]	86		Canada	1997	
		Surgeons[d]			$197
		Radiation oncol			$228
		Medical oncol			$226
		minimal			$113
Simon	84	Mixed (actual)	U.S./Michigan	1989–1991	$362

[a]Direct costs are costs accrued due to screening diagnostic tests and physician visits. Excludes extra diagnostic tests to evaluate suspicious screening test result.
[b]Estimated U.S. dollars at time of publication of original source.
[c]Cost estimates based on assumptions for routine practice in geographic location.
[d]Cost estimates based on tests routinely ordered by surgeons, radiation oncologists, or medical oncologists or if minimalist approach.
[e]Cost estimates based on actual practice in institution.

Direct surveys of patients' preferences have provided mixed results. Some patients have expressed "anger and distress about being discharged to their general practitioners," viewing the specialist setting "as the best defense against a recurrence."[74] Adewuyi-Dalton et al., who performed the previously mentioned prospective randomized trial,[68] concluded that "a preference for continuity of care may suggest that GP [general practitioner] follow-up would be preferred, but access to specialist service is valued and may be of particular importance during the early stages of follow up."[67] Indeed, in reporting preliminary results from another trial, in which patients were randomly assigned to follow-up on a conventional schedule or to visits only after mammography, other investigators have noted that "twice as many patients in both groups expressed a preference for reducing rather than increasing follow-up."[75]

It appears that patients are generally most interested in adequate and competent follow-up but wish to return to their normal lives as quickly and efficiently as possible. Occasional routine but unobtrusive office visits appear to be important. One suggested compromise between those in favor of frequent specialists' visits and those who recommend only general practitioner visits might be the use of specialty-trained nurse clinicians or practitioners, or both. These professionals might optimally deliver specialized advice and follow-up while freeing specialist physicians for more active consultations and treatment.[76,77]

Detection of Metastases as an Investigational End Point

An important indication for systematic follow-up is to compare the time to recurrence between patients on different arms of investigational studies. Such an end point [i.e., disease-free interval (DFI)] is important for many studies in which different forms of either primary or adjuvant systemic therapy are compared. Evaluation of DFI may allow analysis of trials earlier than when either overall survival or cure is used as an end point, and DFI differences (in lieu of overall survival differences) have served as valid criteria for early stoppage of trials and alterations in general health care policies.[78–82] However, most patients are unlikely to consider this end point sufficient to justify the more costly and potentially hazardous intensive follow-up if they derive no direct benefit.[17] Moreover, some authors have raised concern over the risk that surrogate markers may not reflect true clinical outcomes, such as quality of life or survival.[83]

Expense of Routine Screening

Potential disadvantages of early detection of metastatic disease include inappropriate application of toxic therapy for which no benefit is established and decreased emotional well-being for patients who were otherwise doing well. A third disadvantage is the additional cost of performing diagnostic tests.

The direct cost of any follow-up strategy depends on the frequency of follow-up, the precise tests performed, and the costs of the tests in that particular institution. Indirectly, intense follow-up may also generate expenses related to more extensive workup of suspicious but nondiagnostic test results. Finally, therapy-related costs may be escalated in patients who are diagnosed earlier and therefore are treated for a longer period of time than they would be if their recurrence were detected when symptoms developed.

In one analysis, it was estimated that direct costs for an intensive follow-up program in the United States in 1990 would be nearly fivefold higher than for a "minimalist" (physical examination and mammography) schedule ($5,375 versus $1,025 per 5-year follow-up period).[20] The same author projected that a universal minimalist surveillance policy in the United States would save nearly $812 million in 1995. Similar estimates have been made for follow-up costs in the United States, Canada, and Italy[84–86] (Table 1). Taken together, these data suggest that intensive follow-up programs cost roughly two- to fivefold more than minimalist approaches. Thus, intensive follow-up programs are quite expensive, especially in light of the relative lack of improved benefit. However, some follow-up does appear to be beneficial and indicated, as reflected in the Management Summary at the conclusion of this chapter.

INCIDENCE, SITES, AND TIMING OF METASTASES

Although intensive screening for metastases may not be indicated, it is worthwhile to review the available technology. Screening for metastatic disease would be most efficiently performed with a test that has 100% sensitivity and specificity for breast cancer. No such test exists. The development of monoclonal antibody technology generated optimism that a specific "cancer" scintigraphic or serologic test might be available. Unfortunately, the results of radiolabeled antibody imaging have been disappointing, although radioimmunoimaging may help to evaluate selected patients with difficult diagnostic problems.[87,88] The emergence of positron emission tomography (PET) has provided a new technology that appears to have reasonable sensitivity and specificity.[88] However, large-scale studies have not been reported to permit a precise evaluation of the true clinical use of this promising modality. Available serologic assays may suggest recurrent cancer, but none is specific either for cancer in general or breast cancer in particular.[90]

Given the uncertainties of diagnostic modalities, understanding the performance characteristics of the various tests that are available is worthwhile. The performance characteristics of any diagnostic tool determine how useful it will be in detecting early recurrences. For any screening test to be of value, it must be sufficiently sensitive to commonly detect the event in question, yet specific enough that a positive test reliably predicts that event. Sensitivity and specificity are combined with the relative incidence of having an event (in this case, recurrent cancer) to provide a measure of the "predictive value" of a given test value. A *positive predictive value* is the likelihood that a positive test is truly indicative of the presence of cancer, whereas the *negative predictive value* is the likelihood that a negative test means the patient does not have recurrent cancer.

Therefore, an exquisitely sensitive test may have a poor positive predictive value if it has poor specificity or if the patient is very unlikely to have an event. Likewise, a very specific test may have a poor negative predictive value if it has low sensitivity or if the event is very likely to occur, or both. The most frequently used tests, other than symptoms and physical examination, are bone scans, chest x-rays, liver-spleen scans, CT scans, and serologic tests. For each potential site of recurrence and for each clinical setting, having some idea of the relative positive and negative predictive values is important.

In summary, the clinician must rely on placing available information from organ-specific radiographic and scintigraphic techniques in the context of which patients are most likely to suffer recurrence and in which those recurrences are most likely to appear.

Candidates and Time Frame

Screening is most efficiently applied to those patients who are most likely to suffer an event. The risk of subsequent systemic relapse after primary therapy is related to a number of prognostic factors (see Chapter 32). Of these, the presence of histologic invasion beyond the basement membrane, the clinical stage, and the presence and number of axillary lymph node metastases are the most important determinants.[28,91,92] Other prognostic factors have been identified but are less powerful in predicting subsequent distant recurrence (see Chapter 32). Nonetheless, the likelihood of detecting recurrent disease will be greater in patients with more advanced disease at presentation than in patients with favorable clinical and pathologic prognostic factors.

Screening might be focused during a time when patients are most likely to have recurrences. Although the risks of relapse in patients in different clinical prognostic categories differ, the risk of relapse within a given category varies according to the time point of follow-up after primary therapy. The rate of recurrences after primary therapy rises to a peak during the second to fifth year of follow-up.[28,93,94] Although the yearly risk of relapse in the remaining patients decreases after the fifth year, the risk of recurrence continues for as long as 15 or more years.[28,29,95] Patients with more favorable cancers (smaller than 2 cm or negative nodes, or both) experience a smaller hazard ("lower peak") in the first 5 years, but their subsequent annual risk of recurrence in years 5 to 15 is roughly similar to that of patients with larger or node-positive cancers.[94]

The beneficial effect of adjuvant systemic therapy on the risk of relapse in certain subgroups of patients has been well documented (see Chapter 37). Nonetheless, although the treated populations relapse at a lower rate, survival curves have not yet begun to "plateau," even in the more mature studies.[31,96] These results suggest that even those patients who benefit from adjuvant systemic therapy remain at risk for recurrence throughout their lifetime. Indeed, a review of patients treated in adjuvant trials performed by the Eastern Cooperative Oncology Group demonstrated that the hazard curve pattern in these patients mimics that of untreated patients: a peak during the first 3 years with subsequent decline.[97] This pattern was observed in patients treated with

TABLE 2. *Distribution of sites of first recurrence after primary therapy for carcinoma of the breast*

			Recurrence site as percentage of all recurrences[a]			
				Distant		
Author	Reference no.	Bone scan[b]	Local-regional	Bone	Lung	Liver
Rutgers	1	No	23	62	26	22
Stierer	3, 244	NA	30	44	32	NA
Tomin	38	NA	32	28	16	5
Pedrazzini	117	Yes	29	16	NA	NA
Pandya	106	Yes	39	37		
Winchester	118	No	19	38	NA	NA
Zwaveling	35	No	19	63	29	21
Broyn	36	As needed	32	20	<1	NA
Kamby	245	Yes × 1 yr	38	35	23	6–10
Hatschek	246	Yes	36	30	22	11
Pisansky	103	No	37			
Zedeler	101	No	31	45	25	18
Crippa	102	Yes	24	42		
Hannisdal	93	Yes	29	44	23	10
Crivellari	186	Yes	17	35	NA	10

NA, not available.
[a]Site of first relapse either singly or in combination with all sites.
[b]If yes, bone scans were performed routinely. If no, bone scans performed as needed or not performed.

chemotherapy and in those given tamoxifen plus chemotherapy. Thus, follow-up practices in groups treated with adjuvant systemic therapy should probably not differ from those of other groups with similar initial risks of relapse.

In summary, patients with breast cancer may never be free from risk of relapse, even if the original prognostic factors are favorable or if they received adjuvant therapy. Frequent follow-up of "high-risk" patients during the first 1 to 5 years after primary therapy appears to be justified. The practice of gradually increasing the interval between evaluations is consistent with the decreasing hazard of relapse after primary therapy, but the clinician must be aware that no patient can ever be considered "cured."

Organ Screening

Breast cancer metastasizes to almost all, if not all, organs of the body. Autopsy studies have demonstrated that in 50% to 75% of patients who ultimately die of breast cancer, the disease is widespread, involving bone, lungs, and liver simultaneously.[98–100]

Several studies, however, have demonstrated that distribution of metastases in patients at first recurrence differs from that in patients studied at autopsy (Table 2). Fifty to seventy-five percent of patients relapse first in a single organ only, and the remaining patients suffer recurrence in multiple organs simultaneously. Fifteen to forty percent of first recurrences are local-regional, involving chest wall or axillary/supraclavicular lymph nodes, or both. An additional 30% to 60% of first recurrences are in bone, with another 10% to 15% involving bone in combination with other sites. Patients less commonly manifest pulmonary, hepatic, or central nervous system (CNS) disease as their first site of metastases. In most studies, only 5% to 15% of all first recurrences are in the lung, thorax, or both; only 3% to 10% are in the liver; and fewer than 5% are in the CNS[1,35,36,38,93,101,102] (see Table 2).

Factors Predictive of the First Site of Relapse

Although many prognostic factors have been identified to predict whether and when a patient will relapse, few provide clues regarding where a specific patient will relapse. As discussed in Chapter 47, local-regional relapse after mastectomy is higher in certain subgroups of patients. These include patients with positive nodes and those with large or locally advanced primary tumors.[103] Estrogen receptor–negative patients are more likely to have recurrences in visceral organs than are estrogen receptor–positive patients, although considerable overlap exists.[35,36,102,104–112] Of interest, lobular carcinomas may recur more commonly on serosal surfaces than ductal carcinomas, particularly in the peritoneum and meninges.[113,114]

The effect of adjuvant systemic therapy on the first site of recurrence is not well established. Scant data have been reported regarding the effect of adjuvant systemic therapy on the distribution of distant metastases. Patients who are receiving adjuvant chemotherapy may be slightly more likely to present with liver metastases as the first site of recurrence.[6,115] In one study, of those patients who did not receive adjuvant therapy and who had relapses, only 2% had initial liver metastases.[6] In contrast, 12.5% of those who received CMF (cyclophosphamide, methotrexate, 5-fluorouracil) for 6

TABLE 3. *Association of symptoms with first recurrence*

Investigators	Reference	Symptoms at recurrence (% all recur)	Bone symptoms if positive bone scan (%)	Lung symptoms if positive chest x-ray (%)	Lead time[a]
Rutgers	1	77	59	NA	None
Stierer	3, 244	60	36	82	None
Tomin	38	64	69	66	12 mo
Pandya	106	NA	69	50 ("visc.")	NA
Scanlon	5	79	NA	NA	NA
Winchester	118	91 (if not on a routine) 65 (if on protocol)	NA	NA	NA
Zwaveling	35	73	57	46	NA
Broyn	36	64	NA	NA	None
Crippa	102	NA	41	NA	NA
Hannisdal	93	66	63	84	19 mo
GIVID	46	69 (intensive)[b]	NA	NA	NA
		79 (control)	NA	NA	NA

GIVID, Interdisciplinary Group for Cancer Care Evaluation; NA, not available; visc., visceral.
[a]Median time from diagnosis by diagnostic test to onset of symptoms.
[b]Patients were randomly assigned to intensive or control follow-up schedules. See text for details.

months and 6.9% of those who received CMF for 12 months and who relapsed had initial hepatic recurrence.

The incidence of CNS metastases may be higher in patients who have received chemo- and hormonal therapy.[98,116] However, the percentage of patients with CNS as the first site of recurrence is still less than 5%.[6]

In summary, the incidence and sites of local-regional and distant relapse may be altered by various primary and adjuvant treatments. Although the time to recurrence (and ultimately survival) may be affected by the use of adjuvant therapy, the ratio of local recurrence to distant recurrence at initial sites of relapse is not substantially affected. Therefore, screening recommendations for follow-up should be based on likelihood of recurrence and the clinical utility of early detection.

DETECTION OF EARLY METASTASES

Association of Metastases with Symptoms

Several retrospective studies indicate that well over 50%, and perhaps as many as 75%, of all patients with recurrent breast cancer present with symptomatic metastases[1,3,5,35–38,106,115,117,118] (Table 3). Most of these studies are retrospective and were not designed to specifically evaluate the detection of metastases before the onset of symptoms. However, even in studies in which patients were carefully and routinely followed, only 20% to 30% of those with recurrences were detected before the onset of symptoms[1,35,45,46,93,101–103,106,115,117] (see Table 3). Those patients who have asymptomatic metastases detected by routine scanning appear to represent approximately 5% to 30% of all patients who have undergone primary and adjuvant therapy for breast cancer.[117,119] Of note, in one reported randomized trial, 31% of patients screened intensively were found to have asymptomatic recurrence, compared to 31% of those followed by physician visit only.[46]

The detection of asymptomatic metastases might be related to the first site of metastases. For example, although local recurrences can cause pain, itching, or bleeding, more commonly they are discovered by the patient or her physician as asymptomatic masses on the chest wall or in the regional lymph nodes (see Table 3). Indeed, in one study with routine follow-up, only 8% of all metastases were detected clinically, while the patient was asymptomatic.[93] However, of those whose first recurrence was local-regional, 60% were detected by the physician in asymptomatic patients. Patients with visceral metastases as their first site of recurrence may more commonly present with symptoms.[3,93] Of patients with bone as the first site of metastasis, between 35% and 70% present with bone pain as an indication of their relapse. Patients with first recurrence in other organs manifest symptoms appropriate to the organ system involved, but the percentage of asymptomatic first recurrences in these patients is not substantially different than for patients with local or bone relapses (see Table 3). Patients with intrathoracic/pulmonary metastases may present with cough, shortness of breath, chest pain, or a combination of these.[4,120] Patients with liver metastases as their first recurrence most commonly present with anorexia, weight loss, malaise, and, occasionally, right upper quadrant pain. Jaundice is usually an indication of far-advanced disease and is extremely uncommon as a sign of first relapse.[121] In the occasional patient who presents with CNS metastases as the first site of recurrence, symptoms are normally related to the specific site of involvement. These may include such nonspecific findings as headache, nausea, vomiting, or mental status changes, or they may be the result of specific neurologic damage such as cranial nerve palsies, motor dysfunction, or spinal cord compression[122] (see Chapter 52).

TABLE 4. *Occurrence of metastases as a function of number of new abnormalities on bone scintigraphy*

New abnormalities	Occurrences	With metastases (%)
1	182	20 (11%)
2	26	9 (35%)
3	9	4 (45%)
4	2	1 (50%)
5	4	4 (100%)
6	2	2 (100%)
>6	14	14 (100%)
Total	**239**	**54 (23%)**

Modified from ref. 124.

TABLE 5. *Initial radiographic characterization and diagnosis at follow-up for 236 new bone scan abnormalities in 183 patients with breast cancer*

Initial radiographic interpretation	Diagnosis at follow-up	
	Benign	Malignant[a]
Normal	92	13 (12%)
Degenerative disease	58	1 (2%)
Fracture	19	0
Other benign process	14	0
Equivocal abnormality	15	1 (6%)
Abnormality suggestive of metastasis	11	2 (15%)
Consistent with metastasis	5	5 (50%)
Total	**214**	**22 (9%)**

[a]Values in parentheses are percentages of patients with that condition in whom bone metastases developed.
Modified from ref. 127.

Symptoms are not always a reliable indicator of recurrent disease and frequently result in further evaluations that do not demonstrate metastatic cancer. For example, in one study, of all patients who presented with a symptom that was believed to be suggestive of recurrent disease, further evaluation indicated metastases in only 35%.[109] Investigators from the Netherlands have reported that as many as 40% of patients believed to be free of disease who presented with "bone pain" had normal bone scans and did not develop malignant disease during the subsequent year of follow-up.[123]

Thus, approximately 70% of all patients who have recurrences bring their relapse to the attention of their physician with specific symptoms. With the exception of local-regional relapse being more commonly asymptomatic, no commonly occurring site of relapse appears more likely than others to produce symptoms. Of the 20% to 25% of patients who are found to have asymptomatic recurrences by routine evaluation, the lead time from diagnosis to time of symptoms has been estimated to be approximately 12 months.[38] However, this figure is highly dependent on the criteria and intervals specified for obtaining scans and can be much shorter or longer.[3,35,107]

Evaluation of Specific Sites of Metastasis

Bone Metastases

Screening for Recurrence

On average, approximately 40% to 50% of all first recurrences are in bone (see Table 2). Of the available imaging modalities, bone scintigraphy is the most sensitive method of detecting skeletal metastases. Bone scan results can vary depending on technical details, such as the type of radiotracer and equipment used and the radiologist's interpretation.

Bone scintigraphy is abnormal if increased uptake is detected when compared to adjacent bone. New scintigraphic lesions in a patient who has otherwise not had a recurrence must be interpreted carefully to distinguish bone metastases from benign disorders. If such foci are changed in relation to a baseline scintigraphic study, the nature of the abnormalities requires further evaluation. Several features have been identified that help to predict whether new foci of uptake represent malignancy. These include the appearance of new lesions compared to a baseline scintigraphic image and the appearance of more than one new lesion[124,125] (Table 4). Of note, the annual hazard rate of bone scan conversion from negative to positive parallels that of the risk of metastases in general.[102] Thus, the timing of new lesions may also be helpful in interpreting the bone scan.

The site of a new lesion is also helpful in distinguishing benign from malignant findings. Abnormal radiotracer uptake in the axial skeleton (pelvis, spine, sternum) is more likely to represent metastases than is a "hot spot" in ribs, skull, or long bones.[125,126] Radiographic evaluation of new foci of scintigraphic uptake can be critical in diagnosis of bone metastasis. In one study, plain radiographs were helpful in determining the cause of uptake in nearly one-half the cases[127] (Table 5). Lytic or blastic lesions that correlate with the scintigraphic abnormality are highly suggestive of a malignant cause. Moreover, benign causes of uptake, such as degenerative joint disease, trauma, or bone infarcts can also be well defined.

In summary, new scintigraphic findings caused by bone metastases can usually be distinguished from those caused by benign processes by careful interpretation and judicious use of plain bone radiography. If indicated, CT or magnetic resonance imaging (MRI) can help to further evaluate such lesions. Indeed, MRI and CT are occasionally more sensitive and specific than bone scintigraphy in detecting bone metastases.[128–131] Therefore, in symptomatic patients with normal skeletal scintigraphy and plain radiographs, MRI evaluation is indicated. MRI may be especially helpful in distinguishing patients with vertebral body wedge collapse due to extraosseous metastases from patients with osteoporotic compression fractures, which, of course, would be treated much differently.[128] Of note, normal bone marrow T1 and T2 signal intensity ratios may change during chemotherapy treatment, especially if high doses of chemotherapy are given.[132] However, these changes can be easily distinguished from those that are known to reflect metastatic disease. Preliminary studies have suggested that fluorine 18–labeled glucose PET may also provide an effective means of diagnosing bone metastases.[130] In two small studies, fluorine 18–labeled glucose PET appeared to be more sensitive than standard technetium 99m (^{99m}Tc) bone scintigraphy, especially for lytic lesions.[133,134] Indeed, the two techniques may be complementary, because the latter may be more sensitive for sclerotic lesions.[134] The true clinical utility of this promising technology remains to be demonstrated.

Monitoring Metastatic Disease

Routine bone scanning can also be used to monitor patients with known metastatic disease who are receiving palliative therapy. Response of bone lesions can be documented by decrease or disappearance of tracer uptake in areas of previously demonstrated metastases. However, complete normalization of abnormal bone scans is unusual.[135] Responses can be further confirmed by radiographic demonstration of conversion of a lytic lesion to one of a blastic nature. A more subtle finding is the appearance of a sclerotic rim around a previously defined lytic lesion, suggesting incomplete healing.

Serial bone scans obtained during hormone- or chemotherapy may actually worsen in association with a clinical response.[135–139] This so-called scintigraphic flare is manifested by increased uptake in previously observed metastatic sites and even the appearance of new abnormal uptake in previously normal sites. Flare can be distinguished from progression by clinical history and by appearance of obvious healing (sclerosis) of a previously lytic lesion on correlative bone radiographs. Scintigraphic flare can be observed in 30% to 50% of patients who experience a response to systemic therapy (hormone- or chemotherapy). It is detectable within 1 to 2 months after initiation of therapy and may last as long as 6 or more months.[135] In one study, scintigraphic flare was frequently misinterpreted as progression, resulting in inappropriate clinical changes to an alternative regimen.[138]

The mechanism of flare is not certain, but it probably occurs from preferential adsorption of the ^{99m}Tc-phosphonate compound in foci of new hydroxyapatite crystal formation at a time of bone repair, mediated by osteoblastic activity. Scintigraphic flare should be distinguished from clinical flare, which is manifested by increased bone pain or transient hypercalcemia, often in association with initiation of a new endocrine regimen. Whether those patients who experience scintigraphic flare with response have a more prolonged time to treatment failure or overall survival is not clear.[135,136,140]

Liver Metastases

The liver is an unusual site for first metastases, especially in the absence of disease elsewhere (see Table 2). Therefore, routine liver scanning is less likely to be diagnostic for recurrence than routine bone scintigraphy. Hepatic enzyme elevation or elevations of tumor markers may serve as indications for further evaluation of the liver. CT scanning can detect more than 90% of hepatic lesions and is generally considered the evaluation of choice.[141–144] However, certain benign diseases of the liver can cause misinterpretation of an hepatic CT scan. For example, fatty liver involvement may create focal alterations of hepatic density on CT scan that mimic metastases. In patients with minor degrees of fatty infiltration, liver scanning with ^{99m}Tc-sulfur colloid is normal, because the hepatic reticuloendothelial system is not affected by this benign condition. With extensive fatty infiltration, hepatomegaly and redistribution to the spleen and bone can occur, but focal photopenic abnormalities on the radiocolloid scan have not been reported.

Hepatic hemangiomas are relatively common causes of false-positive CT scans. These can be solitary or multiple. They can be distinguished from malignant lesions with a number of modalities, including real-time sonography, MRI, and contrast-enhanced CT.[145–147] Hepatic hemangioma can also be distinguished by the observation of diminished initial flow followed by intense focal uptake in delayed images during scintigraphy after intravenous injection with ^{99m}Tc-labeled autologous red blood cells.[148–151] Single photon emission CT images may also provide high-resolution evaluation of suspicious lesions, especially if they are deep-seated.[152] Ultimately, fine-needle biopsy may be required for a definitive diagnosis. On occasion, patients may have physical or biochemical evidence, or both, of hepatic metastases in the presence of a normal CT scan. These patients may have microscopic malignant infiltration of the liver sinusoid (as opposed to focal deposits of parenchymal disease). In such cases, radiocolloid liver-spleen scintigraphy may be more sensitive than CT.[153] Although not absolutely diagnostic, heterogeneous tracer uptake is strongly suggestive of metastasis.

Pulmonary Metastases

Like the liver, the thorax is a relatively uncommon site of first recurrence, accounting for approximately 5% to 20% of all initial relapses (see Table 2). Intrathoracic metastases can be identified with the use of routine chest radiography, which may demonstrate hilar or mediastinal lymphadenopathy, pulmonary nodules, the presence of pleural-based nodules, or a pleural effusion. In fewer than 1% of patients, breast cancer metastases present as lymphangitic spread, manifested on chest x-ray as diffuse reticular nodular infiltrates that are usually bilateral.[41,154,155] Thoracic CT scanning is more sensitive than routine chest x-ray for defining metastases. However, because the incidence of intrathoracic metastases as a site of first recurrence is low and routine plain radiography is reasonably sensitive, CT scanning should be reserved for further evaluation of suspicious findings.[156–158] Similarly, MRI should be limited to evaluating patients with particularly difficult diagnostic problems.

Pleural effusions result from several etiologies, many of which are benign. Therefore, the appearance of a new pleural effusion in a patient without prior or concurrent evidence of metastatic breast cancer should be further evaluated by thoracentesis and cytologic examination (see Chapter 57). The presence of elevated tumor markers within a pleural effusion or staining of suspicious cells with monoclonal antibodies directed against tumor-associated antigens may suggest a malignant origin. These assays are not sufficiently specific to be used as an absolute indicator of metastases.[159–164] In the absence of positive cytology or evidence of recurrence elsewhere, especially in a patient with a relatively low risk of relapse, a benign etiology for a new pleural effusion should be considered.

Of particular interest is the development of pleural or pulmonary changes in patients who have undergone excisional biopsy and breast irradiation. In up to 15% of patients who receive tangential field irradiation for breast conservation, pleural-based changes develop in the anterior, upper thorax during the first 2 to 24 months after treatment.[165–167] This occurrence may be less frequent in patients treated with modern techniques.[167] These changes may mimic pulmonary metastases and may change with time.[168,169] Thoracic CT scanning may be helpful in distinguishing benign from malignant causes. The risk of secondary lung cancer may be increased in patients who have been previously treated with radiation to the chest wall.[170] Thus, full evaluation of a patient with new pulmonary changes is important to rule out a curable, new primary lung cancer.

Central Nervous System Metastases

Because the incidence of the nervous system as a site of first recurrence is extremely low (see Table 2), routine screening for recurrence in these sites is not recommended for patients with breast cancer. Evaluation of either the central or peripheral nervous system should be reserved for those patients in whom symptoms are suggestive of recurrent breast cancer. In one autopsy series, most (approximately 60%) CNS metastases were parenchymal, and the remainder were dural (approximately 25%) or leptomeningeal (approximately 15%).[114]

CT scanning provides an accurate evaluation of the brain in patients with CNS metastases. The classic finding is an enhancing ring lesion or lesion within the parenchyma, with most metastases located in the supratentorial grey-white matter junction, although cerebellar lesions are not uncommon.[116,171] Brain metastases are solitary in approximately 40% to 50% of patients with CNS parenchymal disease.[116,122,172] Other CT findings include osteolytic skull metastases with contiguous extension into the extradural and dural mater.

In patients with highly suggestive clinical symptoms and normal CT scans, the use of MRI, especially with gadolinium enhancement, provides a more sensitive test.[171,173–175] In one study of patients with small cell lung cancer, both methods detected all CNS lesions of 2 cm or larger.[173] However, gadolinium-enhanced T1-weighted images were superior in detecting smaller metastases.[173] Short repetition time, gadolinium-enhanced scans may be particularly helpful in detecting lesions of the posterior fossa.[174]

As with the evaluation of suspicious effusions, investigators have assayed cerebrospinal fluid (CSF) for the presence of tumor markers such as carcinoembryonic antigen (CEA).[176] Although CEA may be elevated in patients with carcinomatous meningitis, elevated CEA in CSF does not definitively indicate leptomeningeal involvement, because elevated peripheral CEA levels may produce high CSF levels as well.[176] The lack of 100% specificity for neoplastic cells prevents complete reliance on positive monoclonal antibody staining as an indication of malignant involvement.[177–179]

Intracranial findings may not necessarily represent metastases. For example, patients with a prior history of breast cancer have a slightly higher than expected incidence of meningiomas.[180–183] Differentiation of meningioma from metastases is not always easily performed by noninvasive techniques and may require biopsy. Furthermore, other benign diseases, such as cerebrovascular accidents or intracranial infections, must also be considered. In one study, all patients with a previous history of cancer who had CT or MRI findings suggestive of metastases were biopsied to determine eligibility for a prospectively randomized therapeutic trial. Eleven percent (6 of 54) were found to have benign conditions, and one-half of these were reversible.[49]

USE OF SEROLOGIC ASSAYS FOR SCREENING AND EVALUATION OF PATIENTS WITH BREAST CANCER

An inexpensive and accurate blood test that indicates metastases would be of great use in screening asymptomatic patients for recurrence. As with all screening modalities, such a test would be valuable only if it is sensitive and specific and if the incidence of the event for which it predicts is relatively high. Several such markers have been proposed. These include molecules that are elevated nonspecifically with any inflammatory process (so-called acute-phase reactants), substances that are elevated in the setting of abnormalities of specific organs (e.g., liver function enzymes or enzymes and proteins contained within bone), or relatively specific tumor markers, such as CEA and CA15-3.

Nonspecific Circulating Markers

Although acute-phase reactants are frequently elevated in patients with metastatic breast cancer, they are also elevated in association with many other nonmalignant processes.

TABLE 6. *Alkaline phosphatase as an indicator of recurrent breast cancer in the liver*

Study	Reference	No. of patients	Sensitivity[a]	Specificity[b]
Royal Marsden	191	287	18/51 (35%)	NA
Brigham	192	55	35/51 (67%)	(60%)
Naval	193	NA	5/8 (63%)	NA
Surrey	247	152	15/46 (32%)	77/94 (82%)
Case	194	192	18/19 (95%)	(80%)
Bowman-Gray	184	146	45/91 (49%)	37/39 (95%)
UCLA	195	109	29/50 (58%)	29/35 (83%)
Guys	196	730	NA	45/106 (42%)
IBCSG	186	4,105	127/179 (71%)	720/956 (75%)[c]

IBCSG, International Breast Cancer Study Group; NA, not available; UCLA, University of California, Los Angeles.
[a]Number of patients with positive liver-spleen scan (denominator) who had elevated alkaline phosphatase (numerator) (%).
[b]Number of patients with elevated alkaline phosphatase (denominator) who had positive liver-spleen scan (numerator) (%).
[c]Of 956 patients with elevated alkaline phosphatase, 720 were found to have cancer at some site; 127 (13%) had liver metastases.

The poor specificity of acute-phase reactants precludes reliable clinical use. In contrast, elevations of either bone-related enzymes, such as alkaline phosphatase (AP), or liver function tests (LFTs), such as AP or serum glutamic oxaloacetic transaminase (SGOT), may be predictive of recurrent metastases. Of interest, of those patients who have relapsed, few with local-regional relapse have elevated AP or transaminase levels.[93] Therefore, a rising level of either of these two enzymes (or similar bone- or liver-based enzymes), if associated with recurrence, is most likely predictive of distant metastases.

Between 30% and 60% of patients with true positive bone scans have elevated AP levels.[93,117,121,184–186] Unfortunately, a substantial number of patients with bone metastases have normal AP levels. Furthermore, an elevated AP may be secondary to etiologies other than bone metastases, including liver metastases and many benign liver and bone conditions.[115,173] For example, the Ludwig Breast Cancer Study Group observed that only 34% of 290 patients with elevated AP levels had bone metastases when they were scintigraphically or radiographically evaluated.[117] Other investigators have reported that almost 20% of patients with an elevated AP remained free of detectable metastatic disease.[184] In summary, the negative predictive value of AP for bone metastases (i.e., a negative test implies the absence of diseases) is relatively low, and many elevated AP levels represent false-positives. Nonetheless, rising serial AP levels do provide an indication for bone scintigraphy in patients with a prior history of breast cancer, especially in the setting of suspicious symptoms, because 40% to 80% of these patients have detectable bone metastases.

The specific bone isoform of AP (BAP) is rarely elevated in patients with metastases to nonbone sites. However, the sensitivity of BAP in patients with limited bone sites (one or two) is very poor.[187–190] Therefore, it seems unlikely that screening BAP levels is any more useful than screening standard AP levels, although BAP might be used to distinguish bone from liver in different diagnostic cases.

As with AP levels for bone recurrence, serial LFTs may be valuable in monitoring for liver metastases. However, as with bone tests, these tests are relatively insensitive and nonspecific. Furthermore, the low incidence of liver as a first site of recurrence further reduces the positive predictive value of AP for liver metastases (see Table 2). The frequency of LFT elevations in patients with liver metastases ranges from 32% to 95%[191–198] (Table 6). Unfortunately, as is the case in using AP to screen for bone recurrence, LFTs may be falsely elevated in 60% to 80% of patients[184,192,194,195] (see Table 6). Persistently rising AP levels, in the absence of known benign liver disease, are more predictive of recurrent breast cancer than are isolated elevations.[184] Likewise, SGOT is elevated by many nonmalignant conditions of the liver, but abnormal levels associated with elevations in other markers and LFTs may indicate hepatic metastases. Thus, serial AP and SGOT levels may, by themselves, be unreliable indicators of relapse. However, their use in combination with clinical evaluation and specific tumor markers indicates the necessity for further radiographic evaluation.

Tumor-Associated Antigens

Screening for Relapse

Ideally, monitoring of a substance in the blood that is shed specifically by the cancer for which the patient is being followed would provide a sensitive and reliable means of detecting early recurrence. Several potential circulating markers have been studied in breast cancer.[90] Of these, the two most widely investigated and commonly used have been CEA and products of the *MUC*1 gene, also known as *sialomucins*. Assays that detect the *MUC*1 gene include CA15-3,

TABLE 7. *Circulating tumor markers as indicators of impending breast cancer recurrence*

Marker	True positive		False-positive	Median lead time
	All recur	Nonlocal		
CEA	40%	55%	1–5%	4–6 mo
MUC1[a]	40%	65%	1–5%	4–6 mo
erb-b2	30%	30%	0–3%	4–6 mo

CEA, carcinoembryonic antigen.
[a]MUC1: CA15-3, CA27.29, mammary serum antigen, mammary cancer antigen, Br549.
Compiled from refs. 208, 210–212, 227, 230, 231, 248–259.

CA27.29, and CA549; mammary cancer antigen; mammary serum antigen; and breast mucin antigen.[199–204] The extracellular domain of the protein product of the HER-2/*erb*-b2/c-neu protooncogene has also been detected in human circulation, and it is frequently elevated in patients with breast cancer when compared to normal control subjects.[205–206] Although these circulating tumor markers are not commonly elevated in patients with early-stage breast cancer, several studies have demonstrated that rising levels during follow-up after primary and adjuvant therapy are highly predictive of recurrent disease (Table 7). The likelihood of having elevated levels is a function of burden of disease and the expression of the protein by the respective cancer cells.[90,207] Approximately 40% to 50% of patients who suffer non–local-regional relapse have elevated CEA levels at the time of relapse.[90] The fraction of patients with elevated CEA levels preceding documented relapse is slightly lower (20% to 50%). Of patients who are destined to suffer recurrent breast cancer, 40% to 50% have an antecedent rising *MUC*1 assay level (see Table 7). Circulating *erb*-b2 is less commonly elevated in both metastatic and antecedent disease.[90,208] However, in patients with known *erb*-b2–positive breast cancers, the sensitivity of this assay approaches or exceeds that of the *MUC*1 assays in the general breast cancer population, and studies have demonstrated that rising *erb*-b2 levels are associated with impending relapse.[208] Moreover, because expression of the three antigens (CEA, CA15-3, and *erb*-b2) appears to be complementary among patients, monitoring the three assays may detect as many as 75% of patients before the presence of detectable disease.[208]

Lead times for these markers in relation to the presence of either symptomatic or clinical or radiographically detectable metastases, or both, range from 3 to 12 months. However, the lead time depends greatly on how often the samples are collected and how often the patient is seen and radiographs are performed.[208,210–212,227,230,231,248–259] Importantly, lead times also depend on the cutoff used to designate whether a sample is elevated. The less stringent the cutoff, the longer the lead time. In general, the median lead time is approximately 6 months (see Table 7).[208,210–212,227,230,231,248–259]

The specificity of marker elevation also depends on the cutoff chosen. All of these markers are present in normal serum/plasma, and biological fluctuations may cause transient elevations.[209] The most common means of establishing a cutoff level is to determine a level that is two standard deviations above the mean level of a normal control population. In this regard, by definition, 5% of the "normal" population will be above the "cutoff." Therefore, several authors have established more stringent cutoffs to distinguish a truly rising level from a transient normal one. For example, one group of authors has proposed that only levels that exceed the normal cutoff, and that when repeated 30 or more days later have increased by 25% or more, are considered true "positives."[210] Other authors have used similar criteria. [211,212]

Marker levels can be elevated for one of many reasons not related to metastatic breast cancer (Table 8). Twenty percent of patients with benign breast conditions have elevated CEA or MUC1 antigen, or both.[213] CEA, MUC1, and *erb*-b2 levels may be elevated in malignancies of other epithelial organs (e.g., colon, lung, ovary, prostate).[199,214,215] Nonspecific, benign inflammatory conditions of epithelial organs can also cause elevated tumor marker levels. Thus, high marker levels have been reported in hepatitis, inflammatory bowel disease, and inflammatory lung disease. Smoking can

TABLE 8. *Sensitivity and specificity of circulating breast cancer tumor–associated antigens*

Antigen	Cutoff	Percentage of patients with values above cutoff									
			Breast cancer stage				Benign		Other malignancies		
		Controls	I	II	III	IV/Met	Breast	Liver	RT	GI	Other
CEA	5 ng/mL	5	10	15	35	60	20	60	55	85	50
TPA	90 U/mL		27	37	57		30				
GCDP	50 ng/mL	15	20	30	12	50	30		16	11	
CA15-3	22 U/mL	9		36		73	20	50	71	61	66
DF3	25 U/mL	9	17			68		25	7	9	58
CA549	10 U/mL	2	1		53	88	4	26	32	18	50
MCA	11 U/mL	5	20	21	35						
MSA	300 U/mL	2	72	82	75	87	18		71	60	70
erb-b2	Depends on assay	2–5	15	15	25	40	15	38	13	21	10–25

GI, gastrointestinal; Met, metastatic; RT, respiratory.
Compiled from refs. 200–203, 207, 214, 215, 260–267.

cause elevated CEA levels, in the range of 2 to 10 ng per mL. Furthermore, because these markers are cleared by the liver, they may be elevated in cirrhosis and other conditions of hepatic failure.[214,215]

Taken together, these data suggest that of those patients who are going to relapse, 50% to 75% have at least one rising circulating tumor marker preceding symptoms or detectable disease. The lead time between the identification of the marker elevation and detectable disease is, on average, approximately 6 months. However, the usefulness of monitoring tumor-associated antigens for the detection of relapse has not been established. As discussed, no data suggest that patient outcomes are improved as a result of providing a 4- to 6-month lead time of a symptomatic, impending recurrence. Therefore, at least two clinical guidelines expert panels have independently not recommended routine monitoring of any of these markers in asymptomatic patients who are otherwise free of detectable disease.[216,217] Nonetheless, if a rising marker level is identified, it is important to rule out a new malignancy arising from another organ and benign inflammatory diseases of the lung, liver, and gastrointestinal tract.

Monitoring Metastatic Disease

Although the use of tumor-associated antigens for screening for recurrence is not established, determination of serial levels of these markers can be helpful to aid in monitoring the clinical course of patients with metastatic breast cancer who are receiving palliative therapy.[216,219] Serial CA15-3 levels correlate with disease course in 60% to 70% of metastatic patients during therapy, compared with only approximately 40% correlation for CEA.[219] Serial CA15-3 levels can be particularly helpful in increasing or decreasing the clinician's inclination to change clinical course. For example, if a patient receiving therapy is believed to have a 30% chance of progressing, but the CA15-3 level increases by more than 25%, the probability of true progression (assuming that the elevation is not a spike, discussed in the next paragraph) is raised to 75%. Thus, serial CA15-3 levels can be particularly helpful as adjuncts to other clinical evaluations in patients whose disease course is difficult to determine.

Investigators have reported the occurrence of temporary antigen level "spikes" in patients who have recently begun effective therapies and in whom clinical responses eventually occur.[220–222] Spikes in CEA or CA15-3 levels, or both, have been reported from 1 to 4 months after the initiation of effective therapy in up to 48% of responding patients. The clinician must be careful not to interpret a rising tumor-associated antigen level during an early period of a new therapeutic modality to represent progression. Rather, such a spike may predict ultimate response. Distinguishing between a spike and true progression may be very difficult and may be possible only with longer follow-up of the patient.[222]

Other Uses of Circulating Tumor Markers

Other potential uses for monitoring circulating tumor markers include screening the general population for the presence of new primary breast cancers and determination of prognosis for patients with newly diagnosed cancers. In general, none of the available assays for any of the tumor-associated antigens is sufficiently sensitive or specific to be used for screening the general population. For example, CA15-3 is elevated in only approximately 30% of patients with new primary breast cancers.[199,223–227] With a specificity of approximately 90% in a "normal" population, the predictive value of a positive test would be only approximately 2%.

Likewise, circulating markers are of little value in the determination of the differential diagnosis of newly discovered suspicious lesions of the breast. Because up to 20% of patients with benign mammary diseases have elevated CA15-3 or CEA levels, the predictive value of either of these tests in this setting is unacceptably low. Moreover, none of these assays is tissue specific, although gross cystic disease protein may be restricted to only a few malignancies other than breast cancer.[214,215,228,229] Therefore, in general, circulating markers are unreliable indicators of the primary site in patients with tumors of unknown origin. However, the mucin assays are relatively specific for epithelial tissues and may be useful in distinguishing very poorly differentiated carcinomas from mesenchymal or hematologic malignancies.

Circulating tumor markers could be useful as prognostic indicators in breast cancer. Although some authors have reported that patients with primary or metastatic disease who have elevated CEA levels may have a worse prognosis,[230–232] other studies have failed to show a correlation between perioperative CEA levels and clinical outcome.[220,233–236] Immunoperoxidase and immunoblot studies have suggested that expression of the mucin antigens in primary breast tissues may be associated with prolonged disease-free intervals.[237] Because higher serum levels are linked to higher tumor burden, no studies have definitively demonstrated that circulating MUC1 levels are independently favorable or unfavorable. Of interest, a monoclonal antibody enzyme-linked immunosorbent assay has been used to detect a circulating protein related to the c-neu oncogene.[205,206] Because overproduction of c-*erb*-b2 in primary tumors predicts for a worse prognosis in patients with node-positive breast cancer, evaluation of levels of circulating neu-related protein might also have prognostic significance. At least one study has suggested that serum c-*erb*-b2 likely may be independently associated with poor prognosis.[238]

SCREENING PRACTICES AFTER PRIMARY THERAPY

Several surveys have documented patterns of care among physicians who follow breast cancer patients. These studies represent different geographic locations in

TABLE 9. *Current consensus and guideline recommendations regarding follow-up after primary therapy for breast cancer*

	Clinic visit[a] (no. of yr)			Laboratory tests			Radiographs			
Group	1–3	3–5	>5	CBC	Liver	TMs	Mammogram	Bone imaging	Lung imaging	Liver imaging
ASCO Breast Cancer Surveillance Expert Panel	q3–6m	q6–12m	q12m	prn	prn	prn	q12m	prn	prn	prn
Italian Consensus Conference	q3m × 2 yr	q6m	q12m	prn	prn	prn	q1–2 yr	prn	prn	prn
Canadian Steering Committee	1 × at 4–6 wk, then q4–6m	prn	prn	prn	prn	prn	q12m	prn	prn	prn
German Oncological Societies	q3m	q6m	NA	prn	prn	prn	Ipsi q6m × 3 yr, then q12m contra q12m	prn	prn	prn
ASCO Tumor Marker Expert Panel	NA	NA	NA	NA	NA	prn	NA	NA	NA	NA

ASCO, American Society of Clinical Oncology; CBC, complete blood cell count (white blood cell count and differential, red blood cell count and indices, platelets); Liver, liver function tests (alkaline phosphatase, transaminase, lactic dehydrogenase); NA, not addressed; prn, perform only as needed, not on routine basis;. TMs, tumor markers (CEA, CA15-3, CA27.29, c-*erb*-b2).
[a]History, physical examination, counseling, breast self-examination.

the United States as well as in Canada, Great Britain, and Europe.[59,72,86,239,240] In general, a trend toward "minimalism" is apparent, reflecting the results of the retrospective and prospective studies that have failed to demonstrate any survival advantage for early diagnosis and reflecting the general attitude of the consensus recommendations of the expert panels. These studies suggest that most physicians perform history and physical examinations every 3 to 6 months for the first 5 years, with decreasing frequency afterward. Furthermore, complete blood counts and LFTs are ordered on a similar frequency. Approximately 25% of physicians still order specific tumor marker assays (CEA and/or CA15-3), although currently published surveys were performed before publication of the American Society of Clinical Oncology guidelines.[216,217,241] Chest x-rays were ordered every 9 to 12 months by more than 50% of respondents in older studies, as was routine bone scintigraphy. However, the use of these appears to be decreasing remarkably. Other radiographs and scans were ordered much less commonly.

CONSENSUS RECOMMENDATIONS

Several consensus panels have met to develop recommendations and guidelines for follow-up of breast cancer patients after primary therapy.[26,216,217,240,242,243] These recommendations are similar and are summarized in Table 9.

MANAGEMENT SUMMARY

Intensive follow-up may be indicated for patients who participate in clinical research protocols in which disease-free survival is an end point. Furthermore, clinical trials testing innovative therapies might best be performed in patients with asymptomatic recurrence, so effective palliative therapy is not required immediately. Studies of newer tumor markers may provide longer lead times between evidence of occult recurrence and detectable metastases, although further studies are required to determine whether treatment of such patients is advantageous. In the meantime, the following recommendations are suggested for routine follow-up of patients after primary therapy for breast cancer:

1. No specific follow-up measures for detection of recurrence should be performed while patients are receiving adjuvant chemotherapy.
2. Mammography (and other screening for new malignancies, such as colorectal, ovarian, cervical, and uterine) should be performed on a yearly basis.
3. Routine clinic visits, including history and physical examination, are reasonably performed every 3 to 4 months during the first 3 years after primary therapy, every 6 months for the next 2 to 3 years, and perhaps on a yearly basis thereafter. Routine monitoring of LFTs and tumor markers may provide inexpensive indications of recurrence, but the clinical advantage of such information is uncertain. The use of bone scans, chest x-rays, or liver or CNS imaging modalities does not appear to be indicated on a routine basis, unless the patient has symptoms that suggest further evaluation is required or if serologic tests are rising in a manner strongly indicative of recurrent disease.

ACKNOWLEDGMENT

Dr. Hayes acknowledges the contributions, to this chapter and to the field, of his former coauthor and good friend, Dr.

William Kaplan, who passed away during the preparation of the prior edition of this book.

REFERENCES

1. Rutgers EJ, van Slooten EA, Muck HM. Follow-up after treatment of primary breast cancer. *Br J Surg* 1989;76:187.
2. Umbach GE. Screening for recurrent breast cancer [Letter]. *J Clin Oncol* 1987;5:1127.
3. Stierer M, Rosen HR. Influence of early diagnosis on prognosis of recurrent breast cancer. *Cancer* 1989;64:1128.
4. Chaudary MA, Maisey MN, Shaw PJ, Rubens RD, Hayward JL. Sequential bone scans and chest radiographs in the postoperative management of early breast cancer. *Br J Surg* 1983;70:517.
5. Scanlon EF, Oviedo MA, Cunningham MP, et al. Preoperative and follow-up procedures on patients with breast cancer. *Cancer* 1980;46:977.
6. Valagussa P, Tesoro Tess JD, Rossi A, Tancini G, Banfi A, Bonadonna G. Adjuvant CMF effect on site of first recurrence and appropriate follow-up intervals, in operable breast cancer with positive axillary nodes. *Breast Cancer Res Treat* 1982;1:349.
7. Adair F, Berg J, Joubert L, Robbins GF. Long-term follow-up of breast cancer patients: the 30-year report. *Cancer* 1974;33:1145.
8. Fisher B, Anderson S, Fisher E, et al. Significance of ipsilateral breast tumour recurrence after lumpectomy. *Lancet* 1991;338:327.
9. Harris JR, Connolly JL, Schnitt SJ, et al. The use of pathologic features in selecting the extent of surgical resection necessary for breast cancer patients treated by primary radiation therapy. *Ann Surg* 1985;201:164.
10. Rozen P, Fireman Z, Figer A, Ron E. Colorectal tumor screening in women with a past history of breast, uterine, or ovarian malignancies. *Cancer* 1986;57:1235.
11. Fraumeni J, Grundy G, Creagan E, Everson R. Six families prone to ovarian cancer. *Cancer* 1975;36:364.
12. Lynch H, Harris R, Guirgis H, Maloney K, Carmody L, Lynch J. Familial association of breast/ovarian carcinoma. *Cancer* 1978;41:1543.
13. Matloff E, Peshkin B. Complexities in cancer genetic counseling. breast and ovarian cancer. In: DeVita VT, Heilman S, Rosenberg S, eds. *Cancer: principles and practice of oncology. Updates*. Cedar Knolls, NJ: Lippincott–Raven Publishers, 1998:1.
14. Shapiro CL, Henderson IC. Late cardiac effects of adjuvant therapy: too soon to tell? *Ann Oncol* 1994;5:196.
15. Fornander T, Cedermark B, Mattsson A, et al. Adjuvant tamoxifen in early breast cancer: occurrence of new primary cancers. *Lancet* 1989;1:117.
16. Fisher B, Costantino JP, Redmond CK, Fisher ER, Wickerham DL, Cronin WM. Endometrial cancer in tamoxifen-treated breast cancer patients: findings from the National Surgical Adjuvant Breast and Bowel Project (NSABP) B-14. *J Natl Cancer Inst* 1994;86:527.
17. Morris S, Corder AP, Taylor I. What are the benefits of routine breast cancer follow-up? *Postgrad Med J* 1992;68:904,
18. Tomiak EM, Piccart MJ. Routine follow-up of patients following primary therapy for early breast cancer: What is useful? *Acta Clin Belg Suppl* 1993;15:38.
19. Tomiak E, Piccart M. Routine follow-up of patients after primary therapy for early breast cancer: changing concepts and challenges for the future. *Ann Oncol* 1993;4:199.
20. Schapira DV. A minimalist policy for breast cancer surveillance. *JAMA* 1991;265:380.
21. Wertheimer MD. Against minimalism in breast cancer follow-up [Editorial]. *JAMA* 1991;265:396.
22. Holli K, Hakama M. Effectiveness of routine and spontaneous follow-up visits for breast cancer. *Eur J Cancer Clin Oncol* 1989;25:251.
23. Muss HB, Tell GS, Case LD, Robertson P, Atwell BM. Perceptions of follow-up care in women with breast cancer. *Am J Clin Oncol* 1991;14:55.
24. Kagan AR, Steckel RJ. Routine imaging studies for the posttreatment surveillance of breast and colorectal carcinoma. *J Clin Oncol* 1991;9:837.
25. Loprinzi CL. It is now the age to define the appropriate follow-up of primary breast cancer patients [Editorial]. *J Clin Oncol* 1994;12:881.
26. Sauer H. Significance of tumor markers during the follow-up of women without symptoms after treatment of primary breast cancer. *Anticancer Res* 1997;17:3059.
27. Langlands A, Pocock S, Kerr G, Gore S. Long-term survival of patients with breast cancer: a study of the curability of the disease. *BMJ* 1979;2:1247.
28. Rosen P, Groshen W, Saigo P, Kinne D, Hellman S. A long-term follow-up study of survival in Stage I (TINOMO) and Stage II (TIN-IMO) breast carcinoma. *J Clin Oncol* 1989;7:355.
29. Rutqvist LE: Increasing incidence and constant mortality rates of breast cancer: time trends in Stockholm County 1961–1973. *Breast Cancer Res Treat* 1984;4:233.
30. Harris J, Hellman S: Observations on survival curve analysis with particular reference to breast cancer treatment. *Cancer* 1986;57:925.
31. Early Breast Cancer Trialist's Collaborative Group. Polychemotherapy for early breast cancer: an overview of the randomized trials. *Lancet* 1998;352:930.
32. Early Breast Cancer Trialists' Collaborative Group. Systemic treatment of early breast cancer by hormonal, cytotoxic, or immune therapy: 133 randomised trials involving 31,000 recurrences and 24,000 deaths among 75,000 women. *Lancet* 1992;339:1.
33. Hayes DF, Henderson IC. CAF in metastatic breast cancer: standard therapy or another effective regimen? *J Clin Oncol* 1987;5:1497.
34. Hayes DF, Henderson IC, Shapiro CL. Treatment of metastatic breast cancer: present and future prospects. *Semin Oncol* 1995;22:5.
35. Zwaveling A, Albers GHR, Felthuis W, Hermans J. An evaluation of routine follow-up for detection of breast cancer recurrences. *J Surg Oncol* 1987;34:194.
36. Broyn T, Froyen J. Evaluation of routine follow-up after surgery for breast carcinoma. *Acta Chir Scand* 1982;148:401.
37. Imoto S, Jitsuiki Y. Detection of the first recurrence during intensive follow-up of breast cancer patients. *Jpn J Clin Oncol* 1998;28:597.
38. Tomin R, Donegan WL. Screening for recurrent breast cancer—its effectiveness and prognostic value. *J Clin Oncol* 1987;5:62.
39. Joseph E, Hyacinthe M, Lyman GH, et al. Evaluation of an intensive strategy for follow-up and surveillance of primary breast cancer. *Ann Surg Oncol* 1998;5:522.
40. Kamby C. Routine check-ups of patients with breast cancer: significance of the referral pattern for survival after recurrence. *Ugeskr Laeger* 1991;153:2119.
41. Hietanen P. Chest radiography in the follow-up of breast cancer. *Acta Rad Oncol* 1986;25:15.
42. Karabali-Dalagama S, Souhami RL, O'Higgins NJ, Soumilas A, Clark CG. Natural history and prognosis of recurrent breast cancer. *BMJ* 1978;2:730.
43. Jager W, Kramer S, Lang N. Disseminated breast cancer: Does early treatment prolong survival without symptoms? *Breast* 1995;4:65a.
44. Kovner F, Merimsky O, Hareuveni M, Wigler N, Chaitchik S. Treatment of disease-negative but mucin-like carcinoma-associated antigen-positive breast cancer patients with tamoxifen: preliminary results of a prospective controlled randomized study. *Cancer Chemother Pharmacol* 1994;35:80.
45. Roselli Del Turco M, Palli D, Cariddi A, Ciatto S, Pacini P, Distante V. Intensive diagnostic follow-up after treatment of primary breast cancer: a randomized trial. *JAMA* 1994;271:1593.
46. GIVIO (Interdisciplinary Group for Cancer Care Evaluation) Investigators. Impact of follow-up and testing on survival and health-related quality of life in breast cancer patients: a multicenter randomized controlled trial. *JAMA* 1994;271:1587.
47. Martin EWJ, Minton JP, Carey LC. CEA-directed second-look surgery in the asymptomatic patient after primary resection of colorectal carcinoma. *Ann Surg* 1985;202:310.
48. Wilkins E, Head J, Burke J. Pulmonary resection for metastatic neoplasms in the lung. *Am J Surg* 1978;135:480.
49. Patchell R, Tibbs P, Walsh J, et al. A randomized trial of surgery in the treatment of single metastases to the brain. *N Engl J Med* 1990;322:494.
50. Livartowski A, Chapelier A, Beuzeboc P, et al. Surgical excision of pulmonary metastasis of cancer of the breast: apropos of 40 patients. *Bull Cancer* 1998;85:799.
51. Simpson R, Kennedy C, Carmalt H, McCaughan B, Gillett D. Pulmonary resection for metastatic breast cancer. *Aust N Z J Surg* 1997;67:717.
52. Staren ED, Salerno C, Rongione A, Witt TR, Faber LP. Pulmonary resection for metastatic breast cancer. *Arch Surg* 1992;127:1282.
53. Elias D, Lasser PH, Montrucolli D, Bonvallot S, Spielmann M. Hepatectomy for liver metastases from breast cancer. *Eur J Surg Oncol* 1995;21:510.

54. Raab R, Nussbaum KT, Behrend M, Weimann A. Liver metastases of breast cancer: results of liver resection. *Anticancer Res* 1998;18:2231.
55. Schneebaum S, Walker MJ, Young D, Farrar WB, Minton JP. The regional treatment of liver metastases from breast cancer. *J Surg Oncol* 1994;55:26.
56. Boogerd W, Hart AA, Tjahja IS. Treatment and outcome of brain metastasis as first site of distant metastasis from breast cancer. *J Neurooncol* 1997;35:161.
57. Hayes DF. Is there a role for pulmonary nodulectomy in urologic cancers? In: Garnick M, ed. *Genitourinary cancer*. New York: Churchill Livingstone, 1985:243.
58. Anderson J, Cain K, Gelber R. Analysis of survival by tumor response. *J Clin Oncol* 1983;1:710.
59. Simon MS, Hoff M, Hussein M, Martino S, Walt A. An evaluation of clinical follow-up in women with early stage breast cancer among physician members of the American Society of Clinical Oncology. *Breast Cancer Res Treat* 1993;27:211.
60. Ryan J, Rowe D, Salcicuolio G. Prophylactic internal fixation of the femur for neoplastic lesions. *J Bone Joint Surg* 1976;58:1071a.
61. Harrison K, Muss H, Ball M, McWhorter M, Case D. Spinal cord compression in breast cancer. *Cancer* 1985;55:2839.
62. Boogerd W, van der Sande JJ, Kröger R. Early diagnosis and treatment of spinal epidural metastasis in breast cancer: a prospective study. *J Neurol Neurosurg Psychiatry* 1992;55:1188.
63. Maranzano E, Latini P, Checcaglini F, et al. Radiation therapy of spinal cord compression caused by breast cancer. Report of a prospective trial. *Int J Radiat Oncol Biol Phys* 1992;24:301.
64. Ellis MJ, Hayes DF. Improving hormone therapy for breast cancer. *The Breast Journal* 1997[Suppl]:57.
65. Cobleigh M, Vogel C, Tripathy D, et al. Efficacy and safety of herceptin (humanized anti-HER2 antibody) as a single agent in 222 women with HER2 overexpression who relapsed following chemotherapy for metastatic breast cancer. *Proc Am Soc Clin Oncol* 1998;17:97a.
66. Mueller CB. Asymptomatic metastases: to treat or not to treat? *Surgery* 1983;93:328.
67. Dewar J. Follow up in breast cancer [Editorial]. *BMJ* 1995;310:685.
68. Adewuyi-Dalton R, Ziebland S, Grunfeld E, Hall A. Patients' views of routine hospital follow-up: a qualitative study of women with breast cancer in remission. *Psychooncology* 1998;7:436.
69. Rainsbury D. Routine follow up of breast cancer in primary care. Follow up by non-specialists should not be encouraged [Letter/comment]. *BMJ* 1996;313:1547.
70. Grunfeld E, Mant D, Yudkin P, et al. Routine follow up of breast cancer in primary care: randomised trial *BMJ* 1996;313:665.
71. Grunfeld E, Mant D, Vessey MP, Fitzpatrick R. Specialist and general practice views on routine follow up of breast cancer patients in general practice. *Fam Pract* 1995;12:60.
72. Stark ME, Crowe JP Jr. Breast cancer evaluation and follow-up: a survey of the Ohio chapter of the American College of Surgeons. *Am Surg* 1996;62:458.
73. Worster A, Wood ML, McWhinney IR, Bass MJ. Who provides follow-up care for patients with early breast cancer? *Can Fam Physician* 1995;41:1314.
74. Maher J, Bradburn J, Adewuyi-Dalton R. Follow up in breast cancer: patients prefer specialist follow up [Letter/comment]. *BMJ* 1995; 311:54.
75. Gulliford T, Opomu M, Wilson E, Hanharn I, Epstein R. Popularity of less frequent follow up for breast cancer in randomised study: initial findings from the hotline study. *BMJ* 1997;314:174.
76. Kunkler I, Tierney A, Jodrell N, Forbes J. Routine follow up of breast cancer in primary care. More use should be made of specialist nurses [Letter/comment]. *BMJ* 1996;313:1547.
77. Anonymous. The patient's point of view: results of the working group on socio-psychological implications of follow-up. *Ann Oncol* 1995;6[Suppl 2]:65.
78. Fisher B, Costantino J, Redmond C, et al. A randomized clinical trial evaluating tamoxifen in the treatment of patients with node-negative breast cancer who have estrogen-receptor-positive tumors. *N Engl J Med* 1989;320:479.
79. Fisher B, Redmond C, Dimitrov N, et al. A randomized clinical trial evaluating sequential methotrexate and fluorouracil in the treatment of patients with node-negative breast cancer who have estrogen-receptor-negative tumors. *N Engl J Med* 1989;320:473.
80. Mansour E, Gray R, Shatila A, et al. Efficacy of adjuvant chemotherapy in high-risk node-negative breast cancer. *N Engl J Med* 1989;320:485.
81. Ludwig Breast Cancer Study Group. Prolonged disease-free survival after one course of perioperative adjuvant chemotherapy for node-negative breast cancer. *N Engl J Med* 1989;320:491.
82. DeVita V. Breast cancer therapy: exercising all our options. *N Engl J Med* 1989;320:527.
83. Fleming TR, DeMets D. Surrogate end points in clinical trials: Are we being misled? *Ann Int Med* 1996;125:605.
84. Simon MS, Stano M, Severson RK, Hoff MS, Smith DW. Clinical surveillance for early stage breast cancer: an analysis of claims data. *Breast Cancer Res Treat* 1996;40:119.
85. Mapelli V, Dirindin N, Grilli R. Economic evaluation of diagnostic follow-up after primary treatment for breast cancer. Results of the working group on economic-organizational aspects of follow-up. *Ann Oncol* 1995;6:61.
86. Tomiak EM, Diverty B, Verma S, et al. Follow-up practices for patients with early stage breast cancer: a survey of Canadian oncologists. *Cancer Prev Control* 1998;2:63.
87. Lind P, Gallowitsch HJ, Mikosch P, et al. Radioimmunoscintigraphy with Tc-99m labeled monoclonal antibody 170H.82 in suspected primary, recurrent, or metastatic breast cancer. *Clin Nucl Med* 1997;22:30.
88. Dillman RO. Monoclonal antibodies for treating cancer. *Ann Int Med* 1989;111:592.
89. Wahl R. Clinical oncology update: the emerging role of positron emission tomography. In: DeVita VT, Hellman S, Rosenberg S, eds. *Cancer: principles and practice of oncology: Update 11*. Cedar Knolls, NJ: Lippincott–Raven, 1997:1.
90. Stearns V, Yamauchi H, Hayes DF. Circulating tumor markers in breast cancer: accepted utilities and novel prospects. *Breast Cancer Res Treat* 1998;52:239.
91. Fisher E, Sass R, Fisher B. Pathologic findings from the National Surgical Adjuvant Project for breast cancers (Protocol no. 4). *Cancer* 1984;53:712.
92. Osborne CK. Prognostic factors for breast cancer: Have they met their promise? [Editorial]. *J Clin Oncol* 1992;10:679.
93. Hannisdal E, Gundersen S, Kvaloy S, et al. Follow-up of breast cancer patients stage I-II: a baseline strategy. *Eur J Cancer* 1993;29a:992.
94. Dernicheli R, Abbattista A, Miceli R, Valagussa P, Bonadonna G. Time distribution of the recurrence risk for breast cancer patients undergoing mastectomy: further support about the concept of tumor dormancy. *Breast Cancer Res Treat* 1996;41:177.
95. Brinkley D, Haybittle J. The curability of breast cancer. *Lancet* 1975;2:95.
96. Early Breast Cancer Trialist's Collaborative Group. Tamoxifen for early breast cancer: an overview of the randomised trials. *Lancet* 1998; 351:1451.
97. Saphner T, Tormey DC, Gray R. Annual hazard rates of recurrence for breast cancer after primary therapy. *J Clin Oncol* 1996;14:2738.
98. Amer MH: Chemotherapy and pattern of metastases in breast cancer patients. *J Surg Oncol* 1982;19:101.
99. Cho S, Choi H. Causes of death and metastatic patterns in patients with mammary cancer. *Am J Clin Pathol* 1980;73:232.
100. Hagemeister FBJ, Buzdar AU, Luna MA, Blumenschein GR. Causes of death in breast cancer: a clinicopathologic study. *Cancer* 1980;46:162.
101. Zedeler K, Keiding N, Kamby C. Differential influence of prognostic factors on the occurrence of metastases at various anatomical sites in human breast cancer. *Stat Med* 1992;11:281.
102. Crippa F, Seregni E, Agresti R, Bombardieri E, Buraggi GL. Bone scintigraphy in breast cancer: a ten-year follow-up study. *J Nucl Biol Med* 1993;37:57.
103. Pisansky TM, Ingle JM, Schaid DJ, et al. Patterns of tumor relapse following mastectomy and adjuvant systemic therapy in patients with axillary lymph node-positive breast cancer: influence of clinical, histopathologic, and flow cytometric factors. *Cancer* 1993;72:1247.
104. Campbell FC, Blarney RW, Elston CW, Nicholson RI, Griffiths K, Haybittle JL. Oestrogen-receptor status and sites of metastasis in breast cancer. *Br J Cancer* 1981;44:456.
105. Qazi R, Chuang J-L, Drobyski W. Estrogen receptors and the pattern of relapse in breast cancer. *Arch Intern Med* 1984;144:2365.
106. Pandya KJ, McFadden ET, Kalish LA, Tormey DC, Taylor SG IV, Falkson G. A retrospective study of earliest indicators of recurrence in patients on Eastern Cooperative Group adjuvant chemotherapy trials for breast cancer: a preliminary report. *Cancer* 1985;55:202.
107. Kamby C, Dirksen H, Vejborg I, et al. Incidence and methodologic aspects of the occurrence of liver metastases in recurrent breast cancer. *Cancer* 1987;59:1524.

108. Powles TJ, Smith IE, Ford HT, Coombes RC, Jones JM, Gazet JC. Failure of chemotherapy to prolong survival in a group of patients with metastatic breast cancer. *Lancet* 1980;1:580.
109. Ormiston MC, Timoney AG, Qureshi AR. Is follow up of patients after surgery for breast cancer worthwhile? *J R Soc Med* 1985;78:920.
110. Horton J. Follow-up of breast cancer patients. *Cancer* 1984;53:790.
111. Forrest APM, Cant ELM, Roberts MM, et al. The computed tomographic findings in intracranial metastases due to breast carcinoma. *Br J Surg* 1979;66:749.
112. Kamby C, Rose C, Ejlertsen B, et al. Stage and pattern of metastases in patients with breast cancer. *Eur J Cancer Clin Oncol* 1987;23:1925.
113. Harris M, Howell A, Chrissohou M, Swendell RIC, Hudson M, Sellwood RA. A comparison of the metastatic pattern of infiltrating lobular carcinoma and infiltrating duct carcinoma of the breast. *Br J Cancer* 1984;50:23.
114. Lamovec J, Zidar A. Association of leptomeningeal carcinomatosis in carcinoma of the breast with infiltrating lobular carcinoma: an autopsy study. *Arch Pathol Lab Med* 1991;115:507.
115. Kamby C, Rose C, Ejlertsen J, et al. Adjuvant systemic treatment and the pattern of recurrences in patients with breast cancer. *Eur J Cancer Clin Oncol* 1988;24:439.
116. Boogerd W, Vos VW, Hart AAM, Baris G. Brain metastases in breast cancer; natural history, prognostic factors and outcome. *J Neurooncol* 1993;15:165.
117. Pedrazzini A, Gelber R, Isley M, Castiglione M, Goldhirsch A. First repeated bone scan in the observation of patients with operable breast cancer. *J Clin Oncol* 1986;4:389.
118. Winchester DP, Sener SF, Khandekar JD, et al. Symptomatology as an indicator of recurrent or metastatic breast cancer. *Cancer* 1979;43:956.
119. Wickerharn L, Fisher B, Cronin W. The efficacy of bone scanning in the follow-up of patients with operable breast cancer. *Breast Cancer Res Treat* 1984;4:303.
120. Heitanen P, Miettenen M, Makinen J. Survival after first recurrence in breast cancer. *Eur J Cancer Clin Oncol* 1986;22:913.
121. Arnstein NB, Harbert JC, Byrne PJ. Efficacy of bone and liver scanning in breast cancer patients treated with adjuvant chemotherapy. *Cancer* 1984;54:2243.
122. Weisberg L. The computed tomographic findings in intracranial metastases due to breast carcinoma. *Comput Radiol* 1986;6:297.
123. Schutte HE. The influence of bone pain on the results of bone scans. *Cancer* 1979;44:2039.
124. Jacobson A, Cronin E, Stomper P, Kaplan W. Bone scans with one or two new abnormalities in cancer patients with no known metastases: frequency and serial scintigraphic behavior of benign and malignant lesions. *Radiology* 1990;175:229.
125. Jacobson A, Stomper P, Jochelson M, Ascoli D, Henderson I, Kaplan W: Association between number and sites of new bone scan abnormalities and presence of skeletal metastases in patients with breast cancer. *J Nucl Med* 1990;31:387.
126. Corcoran RJ, Thrall JH, Kyle RW, Kaminski RJ, Johnson MC. Solitary abnormalities in bone scans: patients with extraosseous malignancies. *Radiology* 1976;121:663.
127. Jacobson A, Stomper P, Cronin E, Kapian W. Bone scans with one or two new abnormalities in cancer patients with no known metastases: reliability of interpretation of initial correlative radiographs. *Radiology* 1990;174:503.
128. Jones AL, Williams MP, Powles TJ, et al. Magnetic resonance imaging in the detection of skeletal metastases in patients with breast cancer. *Br J Cancer* 1990;62:296.
129. Algra PR, Bloem JL, Tissing H, Falke TH, Arndt JW, Verboom LJ. Detection of vertebral metastases: comparison between MR imaging and bone scintigraphy. *Radiographics* 1991;11:219.
130. Petren MM, Andreasson I, Nyman R, Hemmingsson A. Detection of breast cancer metastases in the cervical spine. *Acta Radiol* 1993;34:543.
131. Petren-Mallmin M. Clinical and experimental imaging of breast cancer metastases in the spine. *Acta Radiol Suppl* 1994;391:1.
132. Altehoefer C, Laubenberger J, Lange W, et al. Prospective evaluation of bone marrow signal changes on magnetic resonance tomography during high-dose chemotherapy and peripheral blood stem cell transplantation in patients with breast cancer. *Invest Radiol* 1997; 32:613.
133. Petren-Mallmin M, Andreasson I, Ljunggren O, et al. Skeletal metastases from breast cancer: uptake of I SF-fluoride measured with positron emission tomography in correlation with CT. *Skeletal Radiol* 1998;27:72.
134. Cook GJ, Houston S, Rubens R, Maisey MN, Fogelman I. Detection of bone metastases in breast cancer by 18FDG PET: differing metabolic activity in osteoblastic and osteolytic lesions. *J Clin Oncol* 1998;16:3375.
135. Janicek MJ, Hayes DF, Kaplan WD. Healing flare in skeletal metastases from breast cancer. *Radiology* 1994;192:201.
136. Alexander JL, Gillespie PJ, Edelstyn GA. Serial bone scanning using technetium 99m diphosphonate in patients undergoing cyclical combination chemotherapy for advanced breast cancer. *Clin Nucl Med* 1976;1:13.
137. Rossleigh M, Lovegrove F, Reynolds P, Byrne M, Whitney B. The assessment of response to therapy of bone metastases in breast cancer. *Aust N Z J Med* 1984;14:19.
138. Vogel CL, Shemano I, Reynolds R, Gams R. The "worsening" bone scan in breast cancer clinical trials: a potentially significant source of error in response evaluation. *Proc Am Soc Clin Oncol* 1992;11:50.
139. Schneider JA, Divgi CR, Scott AM, et al. Flare on bone scintigraphy following Taxol chemotherapy for metastatic breast cancer. *J Nucl Med* 1994;35:1748.
140. Coleman R, Mashiter G, Whitaker K, Moss D, Rubens R, Fogelman I. Bone scan flare predicts successful systemic therapy for bone metastasis. *J Nucl Med* 1988;29:1354.
141. Snow J, Goldstein H, Wallace S. Comparison of scintigraphy, sonography, and computed tomography in the evaluation of hepatic neoplasms. *Am J Radiol* 1979;132:915.
142. Knopf D, Torres W, Fajman W, Sones P. Liver lesions: comparative accuracy of scintigraphy and computed tomography. *Am J Radiol* 1982;138:623.
143. Alderson P, Adams D, McNeil B, et al. Computed tomography, ultrasound, and scintigraphy of the liver in patients with colon or breast carcinoma: a prospective comparison. *Radiology* 1983;149:225.
144. Bronskill MJ, Henkelman RM, Poon PY, et al. Magnetic resonance imaging, computed tomography, and radionuclide scintigraphy in detection of liver metastases. *Can Assoc Radiol J* 1988;39:3.
145. Bree R, Schwab R, Neiman H. Solitary echogenic spot in the liver: Is it diagnostic of a hemangioma? *Am J Radiol* 1982;140:41.
146. Itai Y, Ohtomo K, Furui S, Yamauchi T, Minami M, Yashiro N. Noninvasive diagnosis of small cavernous hemangioma of the liver: advantage of MRI. *Am J Radiol* 1985;145:1195.
147. Freeny P, Marks W. Patterns of contrast enhancement of benign and malignant hepatic neoplasms during bolus dynamic and delayed CT. *Radiology* 1986;160:613.
148. Front D, Royal H, Israel O, Parker J, Kolodny G. Scintigraphy of hepatic hemangiomas: the value of Tc-99m-labeled red blood cells—concise communication. *J Nucl Med* 1981;22:684.
149. Rabinowitz S, McKusick K, Strauss H. 99mTc red blood cell scintigraphy in evaluating focal liver lesions. *Am J Radiol* 1984;143:63.
150. Moinuddin M, Allison J, Montgomery J, Rockett J, McMurray J. Scintigraphic diagnosis of hepatic hemangioma: its role in the management of hepatic mass lesions. *Am J Radiol* 1985;145:223.
151. Watson A. Diffuse intra-sinusoidal metastatic carcinoma of the liver. *J Pathol Bact* 1955;69:207.
152. Tumeh S, Benson C, Nagel J, English R, Holman L. Cavernous hemangioma of the liver: detection with single-photon emission computed tomography. *Radiology* 1987;164:353.
153. Drum D, Beard J. Scintigraphic criteria for hepatic metastases from cancer of the colon and breast. *J Nucl Med* 1976;17:677.
154. Vestergaard A, Herrstedt J, Thomsen HS, Dombernowsky P, Zedeler K. The value of yearly chest X-ray in patients with stage I breast cancer. *Eur J Cancer Clin Oncol* 1989;25:687.
155. Ciatto S, Pacini P, Andreoli C, et al. Chest X-ray survey in the follow-up of breast cancer patients. *Br J Cancer* 1989;60:102.
156. Libshitz H, North L. Pulmonary metastases. *Radiol Clin North Am* 1982;20:437.
157. Chang A, Schaner E, Conkle D, Flye M, Doppman J, Rosenberg S. Evaluation of computed tomography in the detection of pulmonary metastases. *Cancer* 1979;43:913.
158. Mintzer R, Malave S, Neiman H, Michaelis L, Vanecko R, Sanders J. Computed vs. conventional tomography in evaluation of primary and secondary pulmonary neoplasms. *Radiology* 1979;132:653.
159. Pinto M, Bernstein L, Brogan D, Criscuolo E. Immunoradiometric assay of CA 125 in effusions: comparison with carcinoembryonic antigen. *Cancer* 1987;59:218.
160. Ghosh A, Spriggs A, Taylor-Papadimitriou J, Mason D. Immunocytochemical staining of cells in pleural and peritoneal effusions with a panel of monoclonal antibodies. *J Clin Pathol* 1983;36:1154.

161. Epenetos A, Canti G, Taylor-Papadimitriou J, Curling M, Bodmer W. Use of two epithelium-specific monoclonal antibodies for diagnosis of malignancy in serous effusions. *Lancet* 1982;2:1004.
162. Menard S, Rilke F, Della Torre G, et al. Sensitivity enhancement of the cytologic detection of cancer cells in effusions by monoclonal antibodies. *Am J Clin Pathol* 1985;83:571.
163. Martin S, Moshiri S, Thor A, Vilasi V, Chu E, Schlom J. Identification of adenocarcinoma in cytospin preparations of effusions using monoclonal antibody B72.3. *Am J Clin Pathol* 1986;86:10.
164. Johnston W, Szpak C, Lottich S, Thor A, Schlom J. Use of a monoclonal antibody (1372.3) as an immunocytochemical adjunct to diagnosis of adenocarcinoma in human effusions. *Cancer Res* 1985;45:1894.
165. Srinivasan G, Kurtz DW, Lichter AS. Pleural-based changes on chest x-ray after irradiation for primary breast cancer: correlation with findings on computerized tomography. *Int J Radiat Oncol Biol Phys* 1983;9:1567.
166. Polansky S, Ravin C, Prosnitz L. Pulmonary changes after primary irradiation of early breast cancer. *Am J Roentgenol* 1980;134:101.
167. Lingos TI, Recht A, Vicini F, Abner A, Silver B, Harris JR. Radiation pneumonitis in breast cancer patients treated with conservative surgery and radiation therapy. *Int J Radiat Oncol Biol Phys* 1991;21:355.
168. Majurin ML, Valavaara R, Varpula M, Kurki T, Kulmala J. Low-dose and conventional-dose high resolution CT of pulmonary changes in breast cancer patients treated by tangential field radiotherapy. *Eur J Radiol* 1995;20:114.
169. Svane G, Rotstein S, Lax I. Influence of radiation therapy on lung tissue in breast cancer patients. CT assessed density changes 4 years after completion of radiotherapy. *Acta Oncol* 1995;34:845.
170. Neugut AI, Robinson E, Lee WC, Murray T, Karwoski K, Kutcher GJ. Lung cancer after radiation therapy for breast cancer. *Cancer* 1993;71:3054.
171. Peretti-Viton P, Margain D, Murayama N, Kadr I, Peragut JC. Brain metastases [Review]. *J Neuroradiol* 1991;18:161.
172. Khansur T, Haick A, Patel B, Balducci L, Vance R, Thigpen JT. Preoperative evaluation with radionuclide brain scanning and computerized axial tomography of the brain in patients with breast cancer. *Am J Surg* 1988;155:232.
173. Golfieri R, Cherryman GR, Olliff JF, Husband JE. Comparative evaluation of computerized tomography/magnetic resonance (1.5 T) in the detection of brain metastasis. *Radiol Med* 1991;82:27.
174. Sze G, Milano E, Johnson C, Heier L. Detection of brain metastases: comparison of contrast-enhanced MR with unenhanced MR and enhanced CT. *Am J Neuroradiol* 1990;11:785.
175. Davis PC, Hudgins PA, Peterman SB, Hoffinan JJ. Diagnosis of cerebral metastases: double-dose delayed CT vs contrast-enhanced MR imaging. *Am J Neuroradiol* 1991;12:293.
176. Klee G, Tallman R, Goellner J, Yanagihara T. Elevation of carcinoembryonic antigen in cerebrospinal fluid among patients with meningeal carcinomatosis. *Mayo Clin Proc* 1986:61:9.
177. Garson J, Coakham H, Kemshead J, et al. The role of monoclonal antibodies in brain tumor diagnosis and CSF cytology. *J Neurooncol* 1985;3:165.
178. Coakham H, Brownell B, Harper E, et al. Use of monoclonal antibody panel to identify malignant cells in cerebrospinal fluid. *Lancet* 1984;1:1095.
179. Hancock W, Medley G. Monoclonal antibodies to identify tumor cells in CSG. *Lancet* 1983;2:739.
180. Schoenberg B, Christine B, Whisnant J. Nervous system neoplasms and primary malignancies of other sites: the unique association between meningiomas, and breast cancer. *Neurology* 1975;25:7105.
181. Smith F, Slavik M, MacDonald J. Association of breast cancer with meningioma: report of two cases and review of the literature. *Cancer* 1978;42:1992.
182. Burns P, Naresh J, Bain G. Association of breast cancer with meningioma: a report of five cases. *Cancer* 1986;58:1537.
183. Zon L, Johns W, Stomper P, et al. Breast carcinoma metastatic to a meningioma. *Arch Intern Med* 1989;149:959.
184. White DR, Maloney JJ III, Muss HB, et al. Serum alkaline phosphatase determination: value in the staging of advanced breast cancer. *JAMA* 1979;242:1147.
185. Khansur T, Haick A, Patel B, Balducci L, Vance R, Thigpen T. Evaluation of bone scan as a screening work-up in primary and local-regional recurrence of breast cancer. *Am J Clin Oncol* 1987;10:167.
186. Crivellari D, Price KN, Hagen M, et al. Routine tests during follow-up of patients after primary treatment for operable breast cancer. International (Ludwig) Breast Cancer Study Group (IBCSG). *Ann Oncol* 1995;6:769.
187. Reale MG, Santini D, Marchei GG, et al. Skeletal alkaline phosphatase as a serum marker of bone metastases in the follow-up of patients with breast cancer. *Int J Biol Markers* 1995;10:42.
188. Cooper EH, Forbes MA, Hancock AK, Parker D, Laurence V. Serum bone alkaline phosphatase and CA549 in breast cancer with bone metastases. *Biomed Pharmacother* 1992;46:31.
189. Ritzke C, Stieber P, Untch M, Nagel D, Eiermann W, Fateh-Moghadam A. Alkaline phosphatase isoenzymes in detection and follow up of breast cancer metastases. *Anticancer Res* 1998;18:1243.
190. Bombardieri E, Martinetti A, Miceli R, Mariani L, Castellani MR, Seregni E. Can bone metabolism markers be adopted as an alternative to scintigraphic imaging in monitoring bone metastases from breast cancer? *Eur J Nucl Med* 1997;24:1349.
191. DeRivas L, Coombes RC, Mccready VR, et al. Tests for liver metastases in breast cancer: evaluation of liver scan and liver ultrasound. *Clin Oncol* 1980;6:225.
192. Sugarbaker PH, Beard JO, Drum DE. Detection of hepatic metastases from cancer of the breast. *Am J Surg* 1977;133:531.
193. Sears HF, Gerber FH, Strurtz DL, Fouty WJ. Liver scan and carcinoma of the breast. *Surg Gynecol Obstet* 1975;140:409.
194. Wiener SN, Sachs SH. An assessment of routine liver scanning in patients with breast cancer. *Arch Surg* 1978;113:126.
195. Castagna J, Benfield JR, Yamada H, Johnson DE. The reliability of liver scans and function tests in detecting metastases. *Surg Gynecol Obstet* 1972;134:463.
196. Wang DY, Knyba RE, Bulbrook RD, Millis RR, Hayward JL. Serum carcinoembryonic antigen in the diagnosis and prognosis of women with breast cancer. *Eur J Cancer Clin Oncol* 1984;20:25.
197. Schreve R, Terpstra O, Ausema L, Lameris J, van Seijen A, Jeekel J. Detection of liver metastases: a prospective study comparing liver enzymes, scintigraphy, ultrasonography and computed tomography. *Br J Surg* 1984;71:947.
198. Kemeny M, Sugarbaker P, Smith T, et al. A prospective analysis of laboratory tests and imaging to detect hepatic lesions. *Ann Surg* 1982;195:163.
199. Hayes DF, Zurawski Jr VR, Kufe DW. Comparison of circulating CA 15-3 and carcinoembryonic antigen levels in patients with breast cancer. *J Clin Oncol* 1986;4:1542.
200. Beveridge R, Chan D, Bruzek D, et al. A new biomarker in monitoring breast cancer: CA 549. *J Clin Oncol* 1988;6:1815.
201. Chan D, Beveridge R, Muss H, et al. Use of Truquant BR radioimmunoassay for early detection of breast cancer recurrence in patients with stage II and stage III disease. *J Clin Oncol* 1997;15:2322.
202. Bombardieri E, Gion M, Mione R, Dittadi R, Bruscagnin G, Buraggi G. A mucinous-like carcinoma-associated antigen (MCA) in the tissue and blood of patients with primary breast cancer. *Cancer* 1989;63:490.
203. Stacker SA, Sacks NP, Golder J, et al. Evaluation of MSA as a serum marker in breast cancer: a comparison with CEA. *Br J Cancer* 1988; 57:298.
204. Molina R, Filella X, Mengual P, et al. MCA in patients with breast cancer: correlation with CEA and CA 15-3. *Int J Biol Markers* 1990;5:14.
205. Hayes DF, Carney W, Tondini C, Petit D, Henderson IC, Kufe DW. Elevated circulating c-neu oncogene product in patients with breast cancer. *Breast Cancer Res Treat* 1989;14:135a.
206. Carney W, Hamer P, Petit D, et al. Detection and quantitation of the neu oncoprotein. *J Tumor Marker Oncol* 1991;6:53.
207. Colomer R, Ruibal A, Salvador L. Circulating tumor marker levels in advanced breast carcinoma correlate with the extent of metastatic disease. *Cancer* 1989;64:1674.
208. Molina R, Jo J, Zanon G, et al. Utility of c-erbB-2 in tissue and in serum in the early diagnosis of recurrence in breast cancer patients: comparison with carcinoembryonic antigen and CA 15.3. *Br J Cancer* 1996;74:1126.
209. Gion M, Cappelli G, Mione R, et al. Variability of tumor markers in the follow-up of patients radically resected for breast cancer. *Tumour Biol* 1993;14:325.
210. Ruibal A, Colomer R, Genolla J. Prognostic value of CA 15-3 serum levels in patients having breast cancer. *Horm Metab* 1987;1:11.
211. Colomer R, Ruibal A, Genolla J, et al. Circulating CA 15-3 levels in the postsurgical follow-up of breast cancer patients and in non-malignant diseases. *Breast Cancer Res Treat* 1989;13:123.
212. Molina R, Zanon G, Filella X, et al. Use of serial carcinoembryonic antigen and CA 15.3 assays in detecting relapses in breast cancer patients. *Breast Cancer Res Treat* 1995;36:41.
213. Hayes DF. Tumor markers for breast cancer. *Ann Oncol* 1993;4:807.

214. Colomer R, Ruibal A, Genolla J, Salvador L. Circulating CA 15-3 antigen levels in non-mammary malignancies. *Br J Cancer* 1989;59:283.
215. Molina R, Jo J, Filella X, et al. Serum levels of C-erbB-2 (HER-2/neu) in patients with malignant and non-malignant diseases. *Tumour Biol* 1997;18:188.
216. American Society of Clinical Oncology (ASCO) Expert Panel. Clinical practice guidelines for the use of tumor markers in breast and colorectal cancer. Report of the ASCO expert panel. *J Clin Oncol* 1996;14:2843,
217. American Society of Clinical Oncology (ASCO) Expert Panel. 1997 update of recommendations for the use of tumor markers in breast and colorectal cancer. *J Clin Oncol* 1998;16:793.
218. Hayes DF, Tondini C, Kufe DW. Clinical applications of CA15-3. In: Snell S, ed. *Serological cancer markers*. Totowa, NJ: Humana Press, 1992:281.
219. Tondini C, Hayes DF, Gelman R, Henderson IC, Kufe DW. Comparison of CA15-3 and carcinoembryonic antigen in monitoring the clinical course of patients with metastatic breast cancer. *Cancer Res* 1988;48:4107.
220. Loprinzi CL, Tormey DC, Rasmussen P, et al. Prospective evaluation of carcinoembryonic antigen levels and alternating chemotherapeutic regimens in metastatic breast cancer. *J Clin Oncol* 1986;4:46.
221. Hayes DF, Kiang DT, Korzun A, Tondini C, Wood W, Kufe D. CA15-3 and CEA spikes during chemotherapy for metastatic breast cancer. *Proc Am Soc Clin Oncol* 1988;7:38a.
222. Yasasever V, Camlica H, Karaloglu D, Dalay N. Utility of CA15-3 and CEA in monitoring breast cancer patients with bone metastases: special emphasis on "spiking" phenomena. *Clin Biochem* 1997;30:53.
223. Colomer R, Ruibal A, Navarro M, Encabo G, Sole LA, Salvador L. Circulating CA15.3 levels in breast cancer. Our present experience. *Int J Biol Markers* 1986;1:89.
224. Gion M, Mione R, Dittadi R, Fasan S, Pallini A, Bruscagnin G. Evaluation of CA15/3 serum levels in breast cancer patients. *J Nucl Med and Allied Sciences* 1986;30:29.
225. Pons-Anicet DM, Krebs BP, Mira R, Namer M. Value of CA15:3 in the follow-up of breast cancer patients. *Br J Cancer* 1987;55:567.
226. Fujino N, Haga Y, Sakamoto K, et al. Clinical evaluation of an immunoradiometric assay for CA15-3 antigen associated with human mammary carcinomas: comparison with carcinoembryonic antigen. *Jpn J Clin Oncol* 1986;16:335
227. Kallioniemi O, Oksa H, Aaran R, Hietanen T, Lehtinen M, Koivula T. Serum CA1 5-3 assay in the diagnosis and follow-up of breast cancer. *Br J Cancer* 1988;58:213.
228. Mazoujian G, Pinkus GS, Davis S, Haagensen DE Jr. Immunohistochemistry of a gross cystic disease fluid protein (GCDFP-15) of the breast: a marker of apocrine epithelium and breast carcinomas with apocrine features. *Am J Pathol* 1983;110:105.
229. Hayes DF, Bast R, Desch CE, et al. A tumor marker utility grading system (TMUGS): a framework to evaluate clinical utility of tumor markers. *J Nat Cancer Inst* 1996;88:1456.
230. Bezwoda W, Derman D, Bothwell T. Significance of serum concentrations of carcinoembryonic antigen, ferritin and calcitonin in breast cancer. *Cancer* 1981;48:1623.
231. DeJong-Bakker M, Hart A, Persijn J. Prognostic significance of CEA in breast cancer: a statistical study. *Eur J Cancer Clin Oncol* 1981;17:1307.
232. Krebs B, Lupo R, Namer M. CEA associated with hormonotherapy in metastatic breast cancer. *Bull Cancer* 1976;63:485.
233. Doyle P, Nicholson R, Groome G. Carcinoembryonic antigen: its role as tumor marker in breast cancer. *Clin Oncol* 1981;7:53.
234. Koch M, Paterson A, McPherson T. Slope analysis of plasma carcinoembryonic antigen levels in monitoring response to treatment in patients with metastatic carcinoma of the breast. *Clin Oncol* 1980;6:323.
235. Mughal AW, Hortobagyi GN, Fritsche HA, Buzdar AU, Yap HY, Blumenschein GR. Serial plasma carcinoembryonic antigen measurements during treatment of metastatic breast cancer. *JAMA* 1983;249:1881.
236. Theriault RL, Hortobagyi GN, Fritsche HA, Frye D, Martinez R, Buzdar AU. The role of serum CEA as a prognostic indicator in stage II and III breast cancer patients treated with adjuvant chemotherapy. *Cancer* 1989;63:828.
237. Wilkinson M, Howell A, Harris M, Taylor-Papadimitriou J, Swindell R, Sellwood R. The prognostic significance of two epithelial membrane antigens expressed by human mammary carcinomas. *Int J Cancer* 1984;33:299.
238. Molina R, Jo J, Filella X, et al. C-erbB-2 oncoprotein in the sera and tissue of patients with breast cancer. Utility in progress. *Anticancer Res* 1996;16:2295.
239. Loomer L, Brockschmidt JK, Muss HB, Saylor G. Postoperative follow-up of patients with early breast cancer. *Cancer* 1991;67:55.
240. Boccardo F, Bruzzi P, Cionini L, et al. Appropriateness of the use of clinical and radiologic examinations and laboratory tests in the follow-up of surgically treated breast cancer patients. Results of the working group on the clinical aspects of follow-up. *Ann Oncol* 1995;6:57.
241. Paridaens R, Bruning P, Klijn J, et al. An EORTC crossover trial comparing single-agent Taxol and doxorubicin as first- and second-line chemotherapy in advanced breast cancer. *Proc Am Soc Clin Oncol* 1997;16:154a.
242. American Society of Clinical Oncology (ASCO) Expert Panel. Recommended breast cancer surveillance guidelines. *J Clin Oncol* 1997;15:2149.
243. Canadian Steering Committee on Clinical Practice Guidelines for the Care and Treatment of Breast Cancer. Follow-up after treatment of breast cancer. *Can Med Assoc J* 1998;158[Suppl 3]:65.
244. Stierer M, Rosen HR. [Effect of early diagnosis on the prevention of metastatic breast cancer]. *Wien Klin Wochenschr* 1989;101:138.
245. Kamby C, Rose C. Metastatic pattern response to endocrine therapy in human breast cancer. *Breast Cancer Res Treat* 1986;8:197.
246. Hatschek T, Carstensen J, Fagerber G, Stal O, Grontoft O, Nordenskjold B. Influence of s-phase fraction on metastatic pattern and post-recurrence survival in a randomized mammography screening trial. *Breast Cancer Res Treat* 1989;14:321.
247. Coombes RC, Powels TJ, Gazet JC, et al. Assessment of biochemical tests to screen for metastases in patients with breast cancer. *Lancet* 1980;1:296.
248. Lamerz R, Leonhardt A, Ehrhart H. Serial carcinoembryonic antigen determination in the management of metastatic breast cancer. *Oncol Dev Biol Med* 1980;1:123.
249. Lee YN. Carcinoembryonic antigen as a monitor of recurrent breast cancer. *J Surg Oncol* 1982;20:109.
250. Staab HJ, Ahlemann LM, Anderer FA, Zwirner M, Schindler AE. Optimizing tumor markers in breast cancer: monitoring, prognosis, and therapy control. *Cancer Detect Prev* 1985;8:35.
251. Haagensen D, Ammirata S, Dilley W, Wells S. Tumor markers for detection of occult metastasis during the disease-free interval after mastectomy. *Surg Forum* 1980;31:433.
252. Falkson HC, Flakson G, Portugal MA, VanDerWatt JJ, Schoeman HS. Carcinoembryonic antigen as a marker in patients with breast cancer receiving postsurgical adjuvant chemotherapy. *Cancer* 1982;49:1859.
253. Chatal J, Chupin F, Ricolleau G. Use of serial carcinoembryonic antigen assays in detecting relapse in breast cancer involving high risk of metastasis. *Eur J Cancer* 1981;17:233.
254. Nicolini A, Carpi A, Di MG, Giuliani L, Giordani R, Palla S. A rational postoperative follow-up with carcinoembryonic antigen, tissue polypeptide antigen, and urinary hydroxyproline in breast cancer patients. *Cancer* 1989;63:2037.
255. Nicolini A, Colombini C, Luciani L, Carpi A, Giuliani L. Evaluation of serum CA 15-3 determination with CEA and TPA in the post-operative follow-up of breast cancer patients. *Br J Cancer* 1991;64:154.
256. Gion M, Barioli P, Mione R, et al. Tumor markers in breast cancer follow-up: a potentially useful parameter still awaiting definitive assessment. Forza Operativa Nazionale sul Carcinoma Mammario (FONCaM). *Ann Oncol* 1995;6:31.
257. Molina R, Prats M, Zanon G, et al. Use of serial determinations of tumor markers (CEA, CA 15-3) in the early diagnosis of relapse in breast cancer patients. *Breast Cancer Res Treat* 1989;14:169a.
258. Thirion B, Ricolleau G, Fumoleau P. Result of a prospective study of the CA 15-3 reliability in early detection of breast cancer recurrence. In: Ceriani R, ed. Third international workshop on monoclonal antibodies and breast cancer. 1988.
259. Safi F, Kohler I, Rottinger E, Suhr P, Beger HG. Comparison of CA 15-3 and CEA in diagnosis and monitoring of breast cancer. *Int J Biol Markers* 1989;4:207.
260. Beard D, Haskell C. Carcinoembryonic antigen in breast cancer. *Am J Med* 1986;80:241.
261. Lepera P, Valtolina M, Cocciolo M. A preliminary evaluation of CEA and TPA clinical value in an ongoing trial on patients with operable breast cancer. *J Nucl Med Allied Sci* 1985;29:97.
262. Haagensen D, Mazoujian G, Holder W, Kister S, Wells S. Evaluation of a breast cyst fluid protein detectable in the plasma of breast carcinoma patients. *Ann Surg* 1977;185:279.

263. Hayes DF, Zurawski V, Kufe DW. Comparison of circulating breast cancer associated antigen CA 15-3 with CEA in patients with breast cancer. *Proc Am Soc Clin Oncol* 1986;5:12a.
264. Hayes DF, Sekine H, Ohno T, Abe M, Keefe K, Kufe DW. Use of a murine monoclonal antibody for detection of circulating plasma DF3 antigen levels in breast cancer patients. *J Clin Invest* 1985; 75:1671.
265. Kerin MJ, McAnena OJ, O'Malley VP, Grimes H, Given HF. CA 15-3: its relationship to clinical stage and progression to metastatic disease in breast cancer. *Br J Surg* 1989;76:838.
266. Eskelinen M, Kataja V, Harnalainen E, Kosma VM, Penttila I, Alhava E. Serum tumour markers CEA, AFP, CA 15-3, TPS and Neu in diagnosis of breast cancer. *Anticancer Res* 1997;17:1231.
267. Willsher PC, Beaver J, Pinder S, et al. Prognostic significance of serum c-erbB-2 protein in breast cancer patients. *Breast Cancer Res Treat* 1996;40:251.

Diseases of the Breast, 2nd ed.,
edited by Jay R. Harris.
Lippincott Williams & Wilkins, Philadelphia © 2000.

XII

Management of Recurrent Breast Cancer

CHAPTER 47

Local-Regional Recurrence after Mastectomy or Breast-Conserving Therapy

Abram Recht, Steven E. Come, Susan L. Troyan, and Norman L. Sadowsky

We define *local recurrence* as being any reappearance of cancer in the ipsilateral breast, chest wall, or skin overlying the chest wall after initial therapy. *Regional recurrence* refers to tumor involving the ipsilateral axillary lymph nodes, supraclavicular lymph nodes, infraclavicular lymph nodes, and/or internal mammary lymph nodes. An *isolated* (or *solitary*) *recurrence* refers to the reappearance on routine evaluation of breast cancer in one of these areas in the absence of other disease. In this chapter, we discuss the detection of local and regional recurrence, patient evaluation after its discovery, management, and subsequent prognosis.

A. Recht: Harvard Medical School, Department of Radiation Oncology, Beth Israel Deaconess Medical Center, Boston, Massachusetts
S. E. Come: Harvard Medical School, Hematology-Oncology Units, Beth Israel Deaconess Medical Center, Boston, Massachusetts
S. L. Troyan: Breast Care Center, Department of Surgery, Harvard Medical School, Beth Israel Deaconess Medical Center, Boston, Massachusetts
N. L. Sadowsky: Department of Radiology, Tufts University School of Medicine, Faulkner-Sagoff Breast Imaging and Diagnostic Centre, Faulkner Hospital, Boston, Massachusetts

LOCAL RECURRENCE AFTER MASTECTOMY

Presenting Signs and Symptoms

Local recurrence after mastectomy usually presents as one or more asymptomatic nodules in or under the skin of the chest wall. These nodules are usually located in or near the scar of the mastectomy or skin graft, with most others in the skin flaps.[1] Occasionally, local recurrence may take the form of an erythematous, often pruritic skin rash. Recurrences in the pectoralis muscles alone have been described but appear to be rare.[2] Asymptomatic gross and microscopic recurrences have been discovered rarely at the time of delayed reconstruction.[3] Recurrences may develop at the suture lines or remaining skin of the chest wall after reconstruction with a myocutaneous flap but only rarely are found (sometimes through mammography) under or in the flap itself.[4–6] Simultaneous recurrence in chest wall and regional nodal sites occurs in approximately 30% of patients.[1,7]

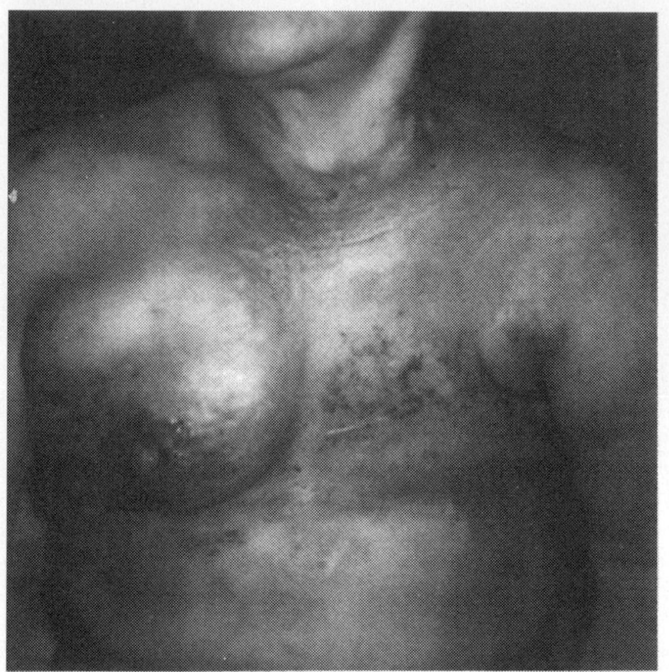

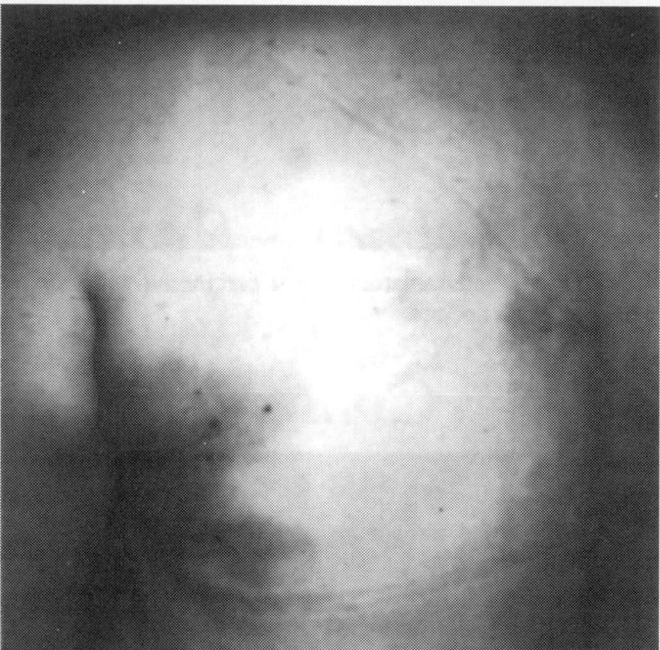

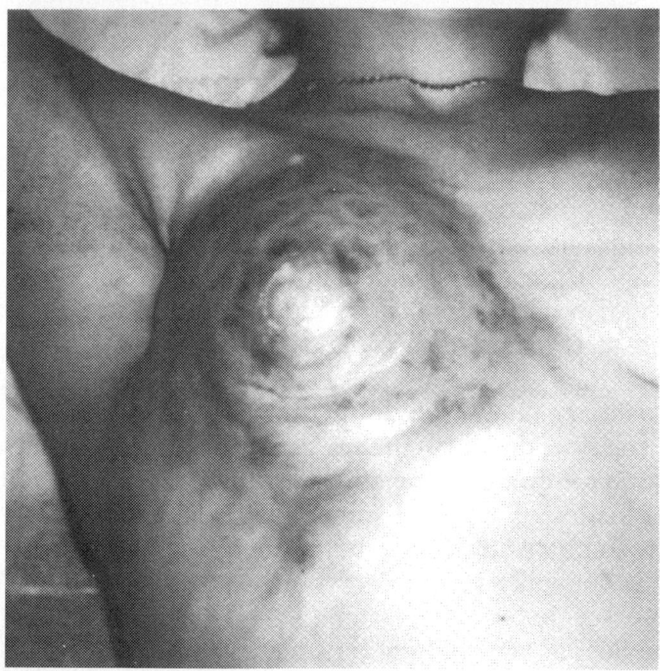

FIG. 1. Carcinoma *en cuirasse*. (Courtesy of Arthur Skarin M.D., Dana-Farber Cancer Institute, Boston.)

Carcinoma *en cuirasse* is a distinct form of diffuse infiltration of the skin or subcutaneous tissues of the chest wall, with woody induration and spread of tumor well beyond the limits of standard surgical or radiation therapy boundaries. Nodules and ulceration are often present (Fig. 1).

Approximately 80% to 90% of local recurrences appear by 5 years after mastectomy; nearly all occur by 10 years.[8–10] Local recurrences up to 50 years after initial surgery have been reported, however.[11] Many of these may actually be new primary tumors arising in breast tissue not removed by mastectomy, rather than "recurrences." For example, one patient has been described who developed an intracystic papillary ductal carcinoma *in situ* arising in a background of atypical ductal hyperplasia.[12]

Approximately one-fourth to one-third of patients with local or regional recurrence, or both, have had preceding distant metastases.[10,13,14] Another one-fourth of patients are diagnosed as having simultaneous local and distant failure or develop distant metastases within a few months of thc discovery of local recurrence.[1,7] This pattern appears to hold true regardless of the interval from initial surgery to recurrence.[15]

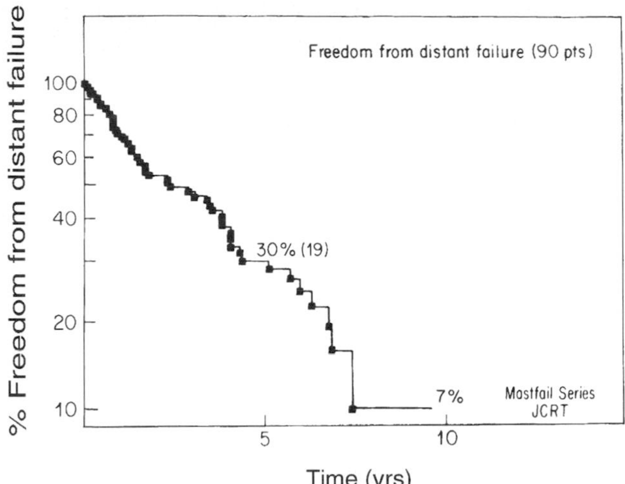

FIG. 2. Freedom from distant failure after radiotherapy for isolated local recurrence, Joint Center for Radiation Therapy (JCRT) 1968–1978. (From ref. 17, with permission.)

Subsequent Morbidity and Spread

Only 25% to 30% of patients with chest wall failure experience significant morbidity due to their local recurrence.[10,16] It is not clear to what extent this favorable outcome is the result of the treatments they receive, rather than the natural history of their illness. In a series of 100 patients with *uncontrolled* local-regional disease, however, 62 had one or more significant symptoms before death.[13] Patients with carcinoma *en cuirasse* may also have restrictive pulmonary deficits related to the bandlike subcutaneous infiltration that may circumscribe chest expansion. Local recurrence in itself may rarely be a cause of death due to infection or pneumothorax.[7,16]

Prognosis

Despite aggressive local treatment, almost all patients with an isolated local recurrence after mastectomy eventually develop distant metastases. For example, in a series of patients with local and/or regional recurrence treated from 1968 to 1978 at the Joint Center for Radiation Therapy (JCRT), Boston, Massachusetts, the 5- and 10-year actuarial rates of freedom from distant metastases were 30% and 7%, respectively (Fig. 2).[17] The corresponding rates of overall survival were 50% and 26%. Patients surviving without disease 15 years and 21 years[18] after treatment with radiation therapy have been described, however, and two patients were reported alive and without disease at 13 years[19] and 24 years[20] after radical surgical procedures.

Numerous factors have been proposed as influencing the disease-free interval and length of survival after the discovery and treatment of an isolated local and/or regional recurrence, including the interval between mastectomy and local recurrence, initial surgical stage and lymph node status at the time of mastectomy: the number of sites of recurrence, the particular site of recurrence (i.e., in the chest wall alone, in lymph nodes alone, in a combination of these, or in specific lymph nodes), tumor grade, patient age at initial diagnosis, estrogen and progesterone receptor status, and prior treatment.

Few series have been analyzed for the impact of these factors using multivariate analysis. The largest patient group in which such factors were examined using multivariate analysis was one of 230 patients with isolated local or regional, or both, recurrence treated at the Mallinckrodt Institute of Radiology, St. Louis.[21] Both the site of recurrence and the disease-free interval were statistically significant predictors for overall survival. When 116 patients with disease found *only* on the chest wall were examined, the size and extent of the recurrent disease were the only significant factors predicting the subsequent length of disease-free survival, but the only significant predictor of overall survival was the disease-free interval. In a group of 225 patients from Switzerland, the time to subsequent development of distant metastases depended on the disease-free interval, initial nodal status, and the extent of disease at the time of recurrence; however, the disease-free interval was not a statistically significant factor in predicting overall survival.[22] In a series of 163 patients from Würzburg, Germany, multivariate analysis showed only the original pathologic axillary nodal status and the presence of necrosis to have statistically significant impacts on survival after local-regional recurrence.[23] In a series of 140 patients with local-regional failure from Copenhagen, Denmark, only the number of positive nodes and the serum lactate dehydrogenase level were significant prognostic factors on multivariate analysis.[24] A disease-free interval of 24 months or longer, the ability to excise the recurrence, and the initial axillary nodal status were predictive of disease-free survival length among 128 patients treated at the University of Pennsylvania; prolonged disease-free interval, tumor excision, and achieving local control were statistically significant predictors of overall survival.[25] When all three factors were favorable (as occurred in 18% of their patient population), the 5-year rates of relapse-free and overall survival were 59% and 61%, respectively. In a study of 69 patients with local-regional failure after receiving adjuvant chemotherapy (5-fluorouracil, doxorubicin, and cyclophosphamide, FAC) with or without postoperative radiotherapy at M. D. Anderson Cancer Center in Houston, only complete response to salvage therapy and recurrence during adjuvant therapy were significant on multivariate analysis.[26] Not all possible factors were examined in each of these studies, however. Also, some of the results of these studies are contradictory. For example, disease-free interval after initial treatment was a significant predictor of outcome, such as time to relapse after recurrence, in two multivariate analyses [University of Pennsylvania[25] and JCRT (unpublished data)] but not in two others (Switzerland[22] and Würzburg[23]) that also included this factor.

There is little information about whether patients who develop a local recurrence despite postmastectomy radiotherapy have a different prognosis after local recurrence than patients never irradiated, with contradictory results from two randomized trials.[10,27] A borderline effect (p = .083) was found for this factor in multivariate analysis of the Würzburg series.[23] Prior systemic therapy did not seem to adversely affect outcome subsequent to local failure in a randomized trial[10] or in several nonrandomized series.[21,23,25,28–30] In another nonrandomized series, however, only 4% (one of 23) of such patients survived 5 years or more after local failure[31]; this may have reflected patient selection for such adjuvant therapy rather than the treatment itself. Developing local-regional failure *during* administration of adjuvant chemotherapy was a poor prognostic sign in the M. D. Anderson Cancer Center experience, with 5- and 10-year overall survival rates of 25% and 10%, respectively, for this group, compared with 80% and 60%, respectively, for patients with recurrence after the completion of chemotherapy.[26]

Pretreatment Evaluation

Occasionally, other benign or malignant conditions may mimic a local recurrence. The most common of these is a foreign body cyst around suture material. Sometimes a bony nodule develops on a rib or costal cartilage as a result of surgical trauma.[32] Patients who undergo reconstruction with a myocutaneous flap can develop areas of fat necrosis that may clinically or radiologically mimic recurrent disease.[33] Radiation-induced sarcomas of the bones or soft tissues of the chest wall appear at a median of 10 years after postoperative treatment, but this latency period is variable.[34] Therefore, a biopsy should be obtained in all cases of suspected local recurrence, both to establish the diagnosis and also to obtain tissue for estrogen and progesterone receptor assays. The estrogen receptor status of the primary tumor and that of subsequent metastases is the same in only 75% to 85% of patients.[35] Of note, a study from the Massachusetts General Hospital suggested that estrogen-receptor immunohistochemical assay may be more accurate than the dextran-coated charcoal method for chest wall biopsies.[36]

The patient should have a complete restaging to find distant metastases, as outlined in Chapter 33. In addition, 25% to 67% of patients with chest wall or nodal recurrences may have additional sites of involvement discovered only on a computed tomography (CT) scan of the chest.[37–40] Such findings appear to be more common in patients with short disease-free intervals or multiple clinically evident sites of disease.[40] The most common site of unsuspected disease (20% to 33% of patients) is the internal mammary nodes, most commonly under or near the second and third intercostal spaces.[39] Other evidence of disease sometimes detected only on CT scan includes sternal erosion, mediastinal adenopathy, ipsilateral and contralateral axillary adenopathy, rib metastasis, involvement of the brachial plexus, nonpalpable tumor in the chest wall, and lung metastases. (Of note, lymphatic drainage patterns may be substantially altered after primary treatment.[41]) No studies have compared the effectiveness of magnetic resonance imaging (MRI) with CT in this context; in practice, the two may be used interchangeably. Whole-body positron emission tomography using fluorine-18-deoxyglucose appears to detect some sites of recurrence (particularly small lymph nodes) not seen on CT or MRI[42]; however, this test also may result in false-positive and false-negative results.[42,43]

Treatment Results

Radiation Therapy

Patients with a recurrence in one portion of the chest wall or draining lymph node areas may develop a further local recurrence if treatment is not given to the entire chest wall. In the Mallinckrodt series, the 5-year chest wall failure rate was 25% when "adequate" volumes were treated, compared with 64% when small fields were treated; the respective 10-year actuarial rates were 37% and 82%.[44] In the group treated with small fields, two-thirds of the subsequent failures occurred outside the field margins. Doses of 50 Gy or higher prevented new lesions from appearing in the uninvolved chest wall in approximately 90% of patients in this series. In the Milan experience, the 5-year local recurrence rate among patients undergoing tumor excision was 15% when the entire chest wall was irradiated, compared with 36% when limited fields were used.[45] The rates were 37% and 56%, respectively, among patients irradiated without tumor excision.

Similarly, patients with chest wall lesions may subsequently have recurrences in regional nodes when only the chest wall is irradiated. The risk of recurrence in untreated supraclavicular nodes was substantial (16%) in one series,[44] but was much lower (5%) in another.[25] The risks of clinically evident recurrences in untreated axillary or internal mammary nodes appear to be small.[25,44]

When large chest wall fields and appropriate nodal irradiation are used, the majority of subsequent local failures are at the original site(s) of disease.[17] In general, the higher the dose of radiation delivered, the less likely is such in-field failure.[44,46] The volume of disease remaining at the time of irradiation is a critical determinant of the likelihood of achieving long-term local control (Table 1). If excision can be performed, the size of lesion has little impact on the likelihood of achieving local control.[25] However, gross tumor excision was possible in only one-third to two-thirds of patients treated in recent series.[17,25,44] When gross residual disease is present, giving a "boost" dose to achieve a total of more than 60 Gy is needed. Such doses achieve long-term local control in perhaps one-half of such patients.[25,44] Even when large fields are used, failures in the adjacent chest wall or other areas at the edges of the fields can occur. These "marginal misses" appear to be more likely in patients with the larger or more numerous recurrences. In the JCRT series, the incidence of marginal misses was 3% (one of 29 patients) among patients undergoing complete excision (i.e., who had small amounts of disease); the incidence was 16% (9 of 58) among the remaining patients.[17] Others have found similar results.[47]

The ability to achieve local control with radiotherapy also appears to be related to the specific sites involved. Most series

TABLE 1. *Radiation dose, extent of surgery, and chance of in-field tumor recurrence*

Dose (Gy)	Complete excision	Residual 3 cm or smaller	>3 cm/diffuse/ multiple
≤49.99	11% (1/9)	29% (2/7)	88% (7/8)
50.00–54.99	4% (1/26)	20% (1/5)	47% (7/15)
55.00–59.99	5% (1/21)	22% (2/9)	18% (2/11)
60.00–64.99	18% (4/22)	0% (0/9)	50% (10/20)
≥65	0% (0/2)	0% (0/6)	47% (7/15)

Data from ref. 44.

show higher local control rates when the chest wall or lymph nodes are involved, rather than both.[17,48–50] Recurrences in the mastectomy scar itself may be more difficult to eradicate than other chest wall recurrences.[51] Control of inflammatory-type skin recurrences may be especially difficult. In particular, carcinoma *en cuirasse* is generally resistant to both local and systemic therapy. It is not clear, however, to what degree these findings are governed by the volume or resectability of disease, rather than the specific site. Patients who suffer a local failure after mastectomy and reconstruction appear to have local control rates and outcome similar to those of patients who had not had a reconstruction.[52] One series from Erlangen-Nuremberg, Germany, found that the complete response rate to a concurrent chemoradiotherapy program was substantially lower for patients with simultaneous local regional and distant failure (none of 12 patients) compared with patients with local-regional failure only (nine of 28 patients, or 32%).[53]

To treat the internal mammary nodes adequately, one must usually include larger volumes of the lung and (for left-sided lesions) heart than are needed to treat the chest wall and supraclavicular nodes. Given the rarity of subsequent recurrence there, the value of treating the internal mammary nodes is uncertain; hence, one must carefully weigh the increased potential morbidity, especially in patients who may have received high doses of doxorubicin. Because of the potential complications, the previously dissected axilla is *not* irradiated unless clinically involved or only a minimal dissection had been performed initially, but a supraclavicular field is always used.

At the JCRT, we generally use the same techniques used for treatment of the intact breast (see Chapter 37). The lateral border of the tangential fields is usually placed at the midaxillary line, unless tumor is located close to this edge. Sometimes it is necessary to use supplementary electron-beam fields matched to the edge of the photon fields to adequately cover the extent of the tumor laterally or inferiorly. The placement of the matchline between the tangential and supraclavicular fields must also be done carefully, as it is preferable to avoid putting this in an area of gross disease. The optimal frequency with which to employ bolus is not known. At a minimum, gross lesions and biopsy scars should be covered with bolus daily, and the remainder of the chest wall treated with bolus in place at least every other day. When patients have had prior reconstruction with a myocutaneous flap, bolus needs to be applied only to the native skin. Boosts are usually done with electrons. We generally use 1.8- to 2.0-Gy fractions given five times weekly. Initial doses of 45 to 50 Gy are used, with a boost of 10 to 20 Gy to areas of gross disease and biopsy scars, yielding a minimum total dose of 60 Gy or higher. Treatment is given without planned breaks. In the past, the M. D. Anderson Cancer Center often used twice-daily fractions of 1.5 Gy to a dose of 45 Gy in 3 weeks, with a boost of 15 Gy, also given with twice-daily fractionation.[54] However, there is no clear advantage for such fractionation compared with once-daily treatment.

Treatment can also be given with electron beams alone or with mixed photon-electron beams.[54] Techniques using electron arcs or rotational motions have also been described.[55,56] A "reverse hockey stick" technique may be particularly useful for patients with extensive chest wall and nodal involvement.[57] Other radiotherapy techniques have also been used either in conjunction with conventional external-beam treatments or by themselves, such as low- or high-dose rate surface molds[58–60] and interstitial implantation.[61] There are no clear differences in local control between the different megavoltage photon or electron treatment techniques, and the selection of these is dictated by individual preference and facilities. The advantages and disadvantages of using these modalities have not been rigorously compared, however.

Complication rates from properly performed radiotherapy are low. Acute erythema and skin desquamation are nearly universal but self-limited. Telangiectasis and mild subcutaneous fibrosis commonly develop with time, but serious subacute or chronic complications are rare. In one series of 224 patients (all of whom having previously had an axillary dissection), 3% developed radiation pneumonitis, 4% soft tissue necrosis or ulceration, 3% bone necrosis, and 1% neuropathy.[44] The risk of arm edema was 11% (eight of 75 patients) when elective irradiation was given, compared with 1% (one of 109) when it was not used. All soft-tissue complications occurred among patients who received a dose of 60 Gy or higher, except one patient who received 50 Gy, in whom doxorubicin was given concurrently with radiotherapy. Bone complications occurred only among patients receiving doses of 54 Gy or higher. Chest wall ulceration or soft-tissue necrosis occurred in approximately 5% of patients treated to doses of more than 60 Gy in two other series.[55,62] The long-term impact of radiotherapy on the reconstructed or prosthetically augmented breast is described in detail in Chapter 39. Concurrent administration of chemotherapy may also increase the risk of pneumonitis, pericarditis, or brachial plexopathy,[50] as well as acute skin and hematologic reactions. However, the chemotherapy program and the details of radiotherapy administration are likely important in this regard. The Erlangen-Nuremberg group found less cutaneous and hematologic toxicity when a split-course radiotherapy was combined with cyclophosphamide, methotrexate, and 5-fluorouracil than when a conventional continuous course of radiotherapy was given with two concurrent cycles of 5-fluorouracil and mitomycin-C.[53]

Finally, does aggressive radiotherapy change the outcome in these patients? Most series suggest that patients who achieve a complete response or maintain local control after aggressive radiotherapy for an isolated local recurrence have longer survival times than patients who do not.[18,25,26,28,44,48,50,63] Whether this reflects the effects of therapy or a correlation of the likelihood of response with a less aggressive natural history is unclear. Nonetheless, all but a few patients who achieved local control in past series eventually developed distant metastases and died of breast cancer. Even if it is only rarely curative, however, effective local treatment may have an important impact on the overall quality of a patient's life.

Reirradiation

Little information exists on re-treating patients after postoperative chest wall irradiation or previous radiotherapy given for recurrence. In one series, 36 previously irradiated patients had lower rates of local control (36% versus 68%) and survival at 10 years (20% versus 35%) than 88 previously untreated patients.[51] Chen and colleagues[48] reported similar findings. Patients in these two series did not, however, undergo reirradiation of all previously treated areas because of fear of complications. In another series, no evidence of soft-tissue necrosis was seen in 13 patients receiving an additional 40 to 60 Gy in 4 to 6 weeks using electrons, after previous treatment of 40 to 50 Gy to the entire chest wall.[64] The sizes of the electron fields were not reported. Although nine of 13 patients were described as having local control for their remaining lifetime or follow-up, three of these patients had further chest wall recurrences outside the re-treated volume. Another group of seven patients who had previous postoperative radiation therapy were re-treated with electrons to small fields, given a dose of 40 to 50 Gy, sometimes with a 10- to 15-Gy boost.[65] At death or last follow-up, five of nine patients had a complete response to treatment, with full healing of the chest wall, and eight of nine patients had stable or controlled disease. One patient suffered osteomyelitis; most patients had milder complications, which were slow to resolve, however. In-field local control was achieved among nine of 11 patients re-treated with a surface mold to doses of 60 Gy in two to three applications.[58] One patient developed a superficial necrosis that healed after 8 weeks. Thus, re-treatment of limited volumes with limited radiation doses can result in meaningful palliation in selected patients, although such therapy seems very unlikely to result in cure.

Surgery

Limited local excision has been used in only a few patients.[8,63,66–68] Further local failure occurs in 60% to 75% of patients so treated. For selected patients, local control rates in excess of 75% have been obtained with very wide local excision of skin and subcutaneous tissue[69] or partial or full-thickness chest wall resection,[70–73] with some patients surviving 5 years or more. (Technical aspects of radical resection for chest wall recurrence or necrosis are discussed in Chapters 36 and 39.) The likelihood of further local recurrence appears to be higher for patients presenting with multiple nodules on the chest wall than for those with a single nodule.[74]

Some authors have advocated using chest wall resection as the initial treatment of isolated local failure. The local and distant relapse rates after this approach are high, however, and the treated-related morbidity may be substantial. In a series of 69 patients from Copenhagen, Denmark, treated in this manner, the 5-year actuarial local control rate was 50%, with a 62% rate of overall survival.[75] Among 23 such patients in Osaka, 48% had further local-regional recurrences. The 5-year relapse-free and overall survival rates were 26% and 48%, respectively.[76]

Approximately 40% of patients with breast cancer undergoing partial or full-thickness chest wall resection from 1979 to 1988 at the M. D. Anderson Cancer Center developed significant complications, although most of these did not require major interventions.[71] In a series of 18 patients treated in Milan from 1977 to 1988, only one patient required reoperation (for repair of flap necrosis).[72]

Hyperthermia

Six randomized trials have compared the results of radiotherapy with or without hyperthermia in this setting.[77,78] Four of these trials showed no difference in complete response rates between the arms, whereas in two trials (including the largest, which still included only 149 patients), there was a substantial benefit to hyperthermia. A meta-analysis that included five of these studies showed a complete response rate of 49% to radiotherapy alone, compared with 59% for thermoradiotherapy.[78] However, there was substantial heterogeneity between the patient populations, treatment parameters, and response rates among these five trials.

Tumor size and technical factors may play substantial roles in the likelihood of benefit from hyperthermia.[77,79–81] However, disappointing local control rates (approximately 40% at 5 years) have been found even in patients who achieved desired thermal parameters.[79,81]

One hope has been that hyperthermia will allow further limited-dose radiotherapy to benefit previously irradiated patients. Many or most such patients achieve complete response with acceptable complication rates.[79,82,83] Many of these responses are transient, however.

Hyperthermia may increase the risk of complications after radiotherapy. Severe thermal blisters and necrosis or poorly healing skin ulcers were observed in 16% of patients in a cooperative group study[84] and in 35% of patients treated at Stanford.[85] Many of these patients, however, had previously been irradiated. Most of these complications heal slowly with conservative management, although rarely surgery may be needed. Concomitant chemotherapy, radiotherapy, and hyperthermia were used in a study conducted at the JCRT.[86] No improvement in response rate was obtained compared with studies using radiotherapy alone or radiotherapy plus hyperthermia. Toxicity was substantial, however, particularly among previously irradiated patients.

Thus, the value of hyperthermia in combination with irradiation in the management of patients with locally recurrent breast cancer is uncertain. Substantial technical problems also remain to be solved in administering hyperthermia and in measuring its effects.

Other Local Therapies

Photodynamic therapy (using hematoporphyrin derivatives as a photosensitizing agent for treatment with high-intensity xenon arc lamps or lasers) has resulted in only a minority of patients having a complete response, which is usually transient.[87–89] However, nearly all patients included in these series were heavily pretreated and also often had very extensive disease. The long-term benefits of photodynamic therapy in untreated patients with less extensive disease are thus unknown. New agents that may increase the effectiveness of photodynamic therapy are beginning to be used.[90] Photodynamic therapy can cause considerable pain. Superficial skin necrosis is also common, although surgical repair is rarely needed.[88]

Intraarterial regional chemotherapy has been used in small series of patients with previously treated local recurrences.[91,92] A number of groups have reported using anticancer drugs topically (e.g., 5-fluorouracil[93] or hexadecyl phosphocholine, also known as *miltefosine*[94,95]) in patients with ulcerating breast tumors or subcutaneous metastases. Some responses have been produced by these approaches, but they tend to be short-lived.

Although feasible in principle, direct injection of chemotherapy drugs or biological response modifiers into chest wall recurrences has not been frequently used. One group found an objective response rate of 20% to intralesional injection of cisplatin contained in a carrier matrix allowing prolonged tumor-cell exposure.[96] Two groups have reported good response rates to interferons given either in combination with radiotherapy or by themselves.[97,98]

Electrochemotherapy, the administration of an electric pulse directly to a superficial lesion in conjunction with systemic or intralesional administration of chemotherapy, has also been shown to be effective in producing regressions in a variety of histologic tumor types.[99,100] It may be useful for local-regional recurrence after mastectomy or breast-conserving therapy also, although data in breast cancer patients is lacking.

Meticulous topical treatments may provide adequate control of local infections and pain. The use of 0.5% silver nitrate–soaked dressing with local débridement and skin grafts may substantially reduce bleeding and infection.[65] Such aggressive local management, similar to treatment of burn patients, may palliate symptoms in many patients for their remaining life. Local infections can also be vigorously treated with frequent changes of povidone-iodine or saline-wetted gauze bandages. Other aspects of the nursing care of breast cancer patients with compromise of the skin can be found in Chapter 71. Broad-spectrum oral antibiotics may also be helpful. Metronidazole has been effective in treating foul-smelling ulcerated lesions.[101]

Systemic Therapy

The only randomized trial addressing whether using "adjuvant" systemic therapy, in conjunction with other treatment at the time of local recurrence, can prolong disease-free or overall survival time was conducted in Switzerland from 1982 to 1991.[102] One hundred sixty-seven eligible patients having a positive or undetermined estrogen-receptor assay, disease-free interval of more than 1 year, and three or fewer nodules, each 3 cm or smaller in diameter without fixation, underwent complete gross tumor resection and radiotherapy. A total dose of 50 Gy in 25 fractions was given to the "involved region"; whether the entire chest wall or nodal regions were irradiated was not stated. They then were randomly allocated to receive either tamoxifen until relapse or observation. (An attempt was made to treat a "high-risk" group that did not meet these entry criteria with doxorubicin, cyclophosphamide, and vincristine; however, only 50 patients could be accrued to that portion of the study, which was not further analyzed.) With a median follow-up of 6.3 years, the 5-year relapse-free survival rates were 59% and 36% in the tamoxifen and observation arms, respectively, the difference being statistically significant. However, this difference had nearly disappeared by 8 to 9 years after randomization. Overall survival rates were the same in both groups. An update of this study reported that tamoxifen reduced local progression but was associated with increased distant failure rates in premenopausal patients, whereas both local and distant progression rates were reduced in postmenopausal patients.[103] The 5-year survival rates in the premenopausal patients on the control and tamoxifen arms were 90% and 60%, respectively; in postmenopausal patients, the respective rates were 71% and 78%. (The respective 5-year disease-free survival rates were 55% and 57% in the premenopausal patients and 29% and 60% in the postmenopausal patients.) There were 35 premenopausal patients in this study, however, compared with 132 postmenopausal patients. The detrimental effects of hormonal therapy in premenopausal patients seen in this study also stands in contradiction to the clear benefits hormonal therapy has shown for premenopausal patients in the adjuvant setting (see Chapter 38). Thus, these findings should be interpreted cautiously.

The same group has described a large retrospective series in which no apparent improvement in outcome was found for those patients who received systemic therapy compared with those who did not.[22] Another retrospective series was performed by investigators at the Mallinckrodt Institute of Radiology in St. Louis, Missouri in which a matched-pair analysis was used to compare the results in patients treated with and without systemic therapy.[21] Differences between the 53 patients in the chemotherapy-treated group and its control group with regard to local control, freedom from distant metastases, disease-free survival, and overall survival were small and did not reach statistical significance. However, these differences were statistically significant (except for local control) when comparing the 59 patients treated with hormonal therapy and irradiation to those treated with radiotherapy alone. Other investigators have also retrospectively shown some benefit from the use of systemic therapy,[25,63,104,105] but their validity is difficult to assess.

Few data exist regarding the results of very-high-dose chemotherapy with autologous marrow or peripheral stem cell support in patients with local recurrence after mastectomy. A report from the University of Chicago included nine patients who had isolated local and/or regional disease (including one patient with disease in an intact breast and lymph nodes).[106] Only one of these patients, however, did not relapse after transplant therapy. Of note, five patients did not receive radiotherapy to the sites of initial recurrence, and three failed in these sites; only one of four patients who were irradiated relapsed at a previous site of disease. No additional toxicity resulted from consolidation radiotherapy. A study performed at the Cleveland Clinic found the progression-free survival rate at 4 years was only 15% in a group of 54 patients with chest wall or regional nodal failure; however, no data regarding the use of local-regional therapy or other population characteristics were reported.[107]

Most investigators (with the exception of the Swiss study discussed above) have not found that the addition of chemotherapy or hormonal therapy markedly improves local control when compared with technically adequate radiotherapy alone.[21,108] In one study, 18 patients having gross total excision of tumor who received chemotherapy and radiotherapy had an actuarial 5-year local control rate of 78%, compared with 38% among 58 such patients treated with radiotherapy only.[25] However, there was no difference in local control rates for patients with gross residual disease or for any patients treated with hormonal therapy.

Very little information is available on the ability of systemic chemotherapy or hormonal therapy to control local disease without the use of radiotherapy or surgery. The Southwest Oncology Group treated 53 patients with local recurrence with doxorubicin or cyclophosphamide-doxorubicin-fluorouracil combinations, without irradiation.[109] Complete response was obtained in 34%, and partial response in 28% of patients. The duration of these responses was not given. Another series found a local control rate of 46% (23 of 50) in patients treated with surgical excision and similar chemotherapy.[108] Response rates (complete plus partial) of local disease to various hormonal manipulations have been reported in 30% to 40% of patients in older series, in which hormone-receptor levels were not known, with median durations of response of 8 to 19 months.[1,8,63,110] Bedwinek and colleagues[13] found that four of 11 patients had lifetime local control. One study showed a surprisingly high complete response rate of 64% and partial response rate of 21% in 42 patients treated with either chemotherapy (12 patients) or hormone therapy (30 patients), with six patients still in complete response at 3 years.[63] In general, however, systemic treatment alone is unlikely to cause local disease to regress permanently.[10]

Several other considerations are important in deciding whether systemic treatment should be used at the time of local recurrence, either as the sole therapy or as part of a combined-modality program. Adjuvant systemic therapy is now commonly used after initial diagnosis of the primary tumor. Therefore, for many patients who suffer local recurrence, questions of drug resistance and patient tolerance to further treatment must be addressed, similar to those facing patients with overt systemic relapse (see Chapter 43).

RECURRENCE IN THE BREAST AFTER CONSERVATIVE SURGERY

Presenting Symptoms and Signs

Roughly one-third to one-half of local recurrences after initial treatment of invasive cancers with conservative surgery and radiotherapy have been detected solely by follow-up mammography, with the rest divided nearly equally between those found on physical examination without any suspicious radiologic signs and those detected both by examination and mammography.[111–115] The physical and radiologic characteristics of recurrent lesions are the same in general as those of tumors that are discovered initially.

In general, the physical examination after treatment shows only mild thickening without a mass effect. Either surgery or radiotherapy may cause changes in physical examination, however, such as masslike regions of fibrosis, which may occasionally be difficult clinically to distinguish from a local recurrence.[116] The findings associated with a recurrence may be subtle, especially when the primary tumor was of infiltrating lobular histology. Recurrences of these lesions often produce only minimal thickening or retraction at the biopsy site without a mass.[117] In rare patients, the only sign of recurrence may be diffuse breast retraction or hardening, either occurring within a few years of treatment[114] or much later (16 and 17 years after radiotherapy, in the case of two patients personally followed by one of the authors of this chapter). Hence, changes in the physical examination that occur more than 1 to 2 years after the completion of radiotherapy must be viewed as suspicious. Recurrence in the nipple alone, presenting as Paget's disease, has been reported but seems rare.[118,119]

The anticipated radiologic changes in the treated breast are highly variable but usually include skin thickening,

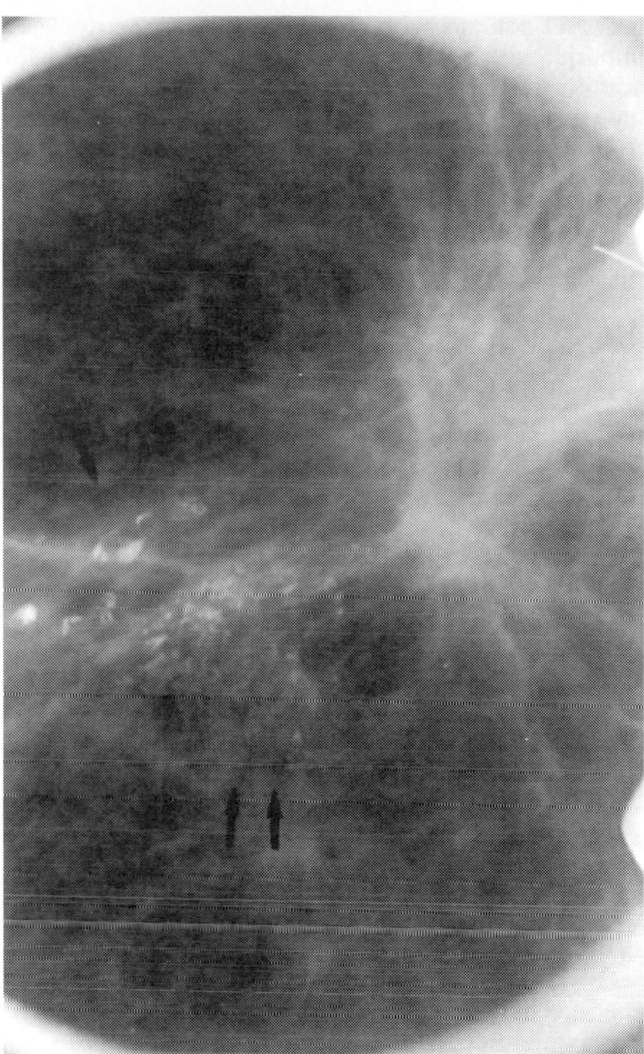

FIG. 3. Spot compression mammogram showing fibrous distortion and coarse calcifications of fat necrosis (*single arrow*) after conservative surgery and radiotherapy, with new casting-type intraductal calcifications (*double arrows*) representing recurrent carcinoma.

increased density of the fibroglandular and suspensory apparatus of the breast, the appearance of coarse calcifications, and mass and/or architectural distortion in the tumor bed.[120,121] Scarring in the tumor bed is particularly frequent in patients who had postoperative hematomas.[122] Substantial overlap in radiologic appearance may exist between benign and malignant lesions.[111,114,123–127] Benign and malignant radiologic changes may coexist (Fig. 3). Some authors have suggested that the presence of a central lucency in a mass occurring in the tumor bed is indicative of surgical scarring rather than a recurrence.[128] "Suspicious" microcalcifications that develop after treatment may be either benign or malignant histologically,[129] although ones that develop in a different quadrant from the initial tumor have a high likelihood of being malignant.[130] Recurrent lesions tend to have mammographic features similar to the original primary tumor, although concordance in this regard is not perfect.[120,131] Of note, in one series, two of six recurrences among 55 patients who had a tumor that originally could not be detected radiologically were detected solely by mammograms[132]; hence, mammography is an important part of the follow-up of all patients, regardless of the original presentation of the tumor. Recurrences of infiltrating lobular carcinomas are particularly likely to be radiographically occult.[112]

Prognosis

In most institutions' experiences, breast recurrence after conservative surgery and radiation therapy has a better prognosis than local recurrence after mastectomy. The 5-year actuarial rate of distant or further local recurrence in a group of 90 patients with breast failure from the JCRT (either before or simultaneous with the appearance of distant metastases) was 46%.[133] In other series, 35% to 70% of all patients with breast recurrences were alive at 5 years, with long-term disease-free survival in approximately 30% to 50% of patients.[134–143] In one randomized trial comparing breast-conserving therapy with mastectomy, prognosis after local relapse was very similar in the two groups.[144] However, patients often received doses of 75 Gy to the tumor bed, making early detection of recurrences difficult, according to the investigators.

Five percent to 10% of patients with local recurrence presented with concurrent distant metastases in most series,[115,133–136,138,139,143] although in one series from Guy's Hospital, London, one-third of patients had distant failure at presentation.[145] Another 5% to 10% have locally extensive recurrences that preclude surgery or concomitant inoperable regional nodal recurrences.[133,136,138,146] Patients who have recurrences in the skin alone or with an inflammatory-type picture have a very poor prognosis, more similar to patients with extensive and rapid chest wall recurrence after mastectomy than to patients with breast parenchymal failures.[146,147]

Factors that influence prognosis in operable patients (discussed further below) are not well-established. The most important variable affecting subsequent outcome in patients undergoing mastectomy in the JCRT experience was the histology of the recurrence.[148] One hundred twenty-three patients had salvage mastectomy. The median subsequent follow-up in patients without further disease was 39 months (range, 0 to 144 months). The 5-year actuarial rate of further recurrence in this group was 37%, and the 5-year cause-specific survival rate was 79% (see Fig. 2). There were no further recurrences among 14 patients with only noninvasive cancer or among 10 patients with predominantly noninvasive disease with only focal areas of invasion. In contrast, 38% of patients (38 of 99) with predominantly infiltrating tumors suffered a further recurrence. The first sites of further recurrence were the chest wall (seven patients), regional nodes (one patient), distant metastases only (25 patients), or both local-regional and distant sites simultaneously (five patients). The 5-year actuarial rate of further relapse in this subgroup was therefore 52%. Similar results regarding the impact of histology at recurrence have been reported from the University of Pennsylvania[113] and the Karolinska Hospital, Stockholm.[143] In a series from Memorial Sloan-Kettering Cancer Center, however, two of 10 patients with purely *in situ* carcinoma at recurrence subsequently relapsed after salvage surgery (compared with 11 of 36 patients with an invasive recurrence).[140]

Considerable controversy exists regarding the prognostic significance of other factors. Tumor size larger than 2 cm at recurrence[135] and diffuse involvement of the breast or dermal lymphatic involvement[115,138] have been reported to be poor prognostic signs. Axillary nodal involvement at recurrence was a prognostic factor in two series in which the effect of histology was not separately examined,[135,140,149] but was not a prognostic factor in the JCRT experience where histology was separately examined.[148] Axillary nodal status at the time of recurrence often cannot be assessed adequately, however, because axillary dissection is frequently preformed as part of the patient's initial treatment. In most,[113,134,135,138,140,141,149–151] but not all,[148] series, the longer the time to failure after initial therapy, the better the prognosis on univariate analysis. Time to recurrence, however, was not a significant prognostic factor in a multivariate analysis performed on an earlier version of the Yale University series.[152] The clinical size of the original primary tumor[138] and the original clinical stage[135,149] have had an impact on prognosis at recurrence in some series but not in others.[148] Patients who originally had pathologically positive lymph nodes who undergo salvage mastectomy do not appear to fare worse than node-negative patients.[138] In the JCRT experience, the location of the tumor with regard to the original lesion was not a significant prognostic factor,[148] although in a report from Yale University, patients with "new" primary tumors had a better prognosis than patients with a "true recurrence."[137] The results were not subdivided by the histology of the lesion at relapse, however. No information is available regarding the implications of hormone-receptor assays performed on the recurrence. Among patients in one series with operable, localized recurrences studied with flow cytometry, none of 13 patients recurred who had a "favorable" profile at relapse (i.e., diploid with low S-phase fraction), compared with 10 of 15 patients with a "poor" profile who recurred subsequently.[152] This factor was statistically significant on multivariate analysis. In an update of the Yale experience, all eight patients identified as having a germ-line mutation for the *BRCA1* or *BRCA2* gene who developed a local failure underwent salvage mastectomy and were alive without recurrence at a median follow-up of 7.7 years later.[153]

Pretreatment Evaluation

Even "highly suspicious" findings on follow-up examination or mammography may be due to benign causes. For example, in one series, 28% of patients who had suspicious radiologic masses that could also be palpated had no evidence of recurrence on biopsy.[124] The most common benign cause of suspicious findings is probably fat necrosis. This may create a mass on palpation or mimic a carcinoma on mammography[154] or on MRI.[155] Occasionally, breast abscesses or cellulitis developing after treatment may mimic an inflammatory-type recurrence,[156,157] and biopsy is sometimes required to distinguish between these possibilities. Rarely, patients may develop patches of white or yellowish well-circumscribed sclerosis and induration after radiotherapy. These may be surrounded by a more highly pigmented, bruiselike area, and sometimes may be preceded by the development of erythema. This phenomenon has been termed *postirradiation morphea* or *circumscribed scleroderma*. Such lesions may appear weeks[158] to years[159] after treatment. Again, biopsy is required to confirm the clinical impression. Sarcomas are the most dangerous of the alternative diagnoses but fortunately are rare in this patient population (see Chapter 60).

Other imaging studies may be useful in evaluating patients with abnormal findings on physical examination or mammography. Ultrasound may sometimes be helpful in distinguishing benign and malignant lesions.[125,160] Color Doppler ultrasound is not useful, however, as five of seven recurrent lesions in one series did not display increased flow.[161] Breast MRI has a high accuracy rate but still results in false-positive or false-negative findings in 10% to 20% of patients.[162–165] Contrast-enhanced CT scans,[166] positron emission tomography,[43,167] and scintimammography[168] have also demonstrated high accuracy in small series. Nonetheless, it is debatable whether these modalities should be used routinely in the evaluation of patients with suspected recurrence, especially with the ease, wide availability, higher accuracy rate, and relatively low cost of core biopsy (see below).

A study at the JCRT found that open biopsies of larger than 1 mL in volume had a false-negative rate of 3% (one of 31 cases), as opposed to 14% (two of 14) for smaller biopsies (mostly freehand core-needle biopsies).[169] Others have reported very high accuracy for fine-needle aspiration cytology,[170] especially in patients with new microcalcifications on follow-up mammograms.[171] Mammogram- or ultrasound-directed core-needle biopsy is an increasingly popular alternative to aspiration cytology, which has the advantage of producing a larger specimen for evaluation. However, the results of such biopsies must be interpreted cautiously on occasion. In a series from Memorial Sloan-Kettering Cancer Center, open surgical biopsy found ductal carcinoma *in situ* in both of two patients in whom core biopsy showed only atypical ductal hyperplasia.[172] It is also sometimes difficult to distinguish between radiation-induced cellular atypia and malignancy, even in large open biopsies.[173,174] Hence, consultation with expert pathologists may be very helpful in deciding on the management of a patient with an equivocal tissue or cytologic specimen.

Complications were rare in two series when the volume of removed tissue was less than 10 mL,[124,169] although in another series, four of 16 such biopsies resulted in a wound infection.[175] Complication rates were higher when larger biopsies are performed or, in one series, in patients with larger breasts or when skin was removed.[175] Patients with wound-healing complications may have substantial worsening of the cosmetic results of therapy.[175]

As noted, some patients present with simultaneous breast and distant failure. Hence, appropriate staging for distant metastases should be performed before definitive therapy.

Treatment Results

Mastectomy

Five-year relapse-free survival rates for patients with an isolated operable breast relapse treated with mastectomy are approximately 60% to 75%. Overall or cause-specific survival rates are 70% to 85% (Fig. 4).[138,142,148,149] Subsequent chest wall recurrences occur in fewer than 10% of patients treated with mastectomy in most series,[148,149,176] although chest wall failure rates of approximately 50% have been reported in two series of salvage mastectomy after initial treatment with conservative surgery without radiotherapy,[177,178] and a rate of 18% was reported in a series that did not separate those patients who had or had not had radiotherapy as part of their initial therapy.[143] Most patients who develop further local failure after mastectomy have progressive local-regional disease despite further treatment.[143,176] In our experience, patients with skin involvement at the time of relapse usually rapidly experience recurrences on the chest wall after mastectomy.

In an earlier review of the JCRT experience,[133] 37 patients underwent ipsilateral axillary sampling or dissection at the time of their breast recurrence. In nine cases (24%), metastatic carcinoma was found; no nodal involvement was seen in 19 patients (51%); and no nodal tissue was recovered in nine patients (24%). Axillary exploration was more likely to find some nodal tissue in patients who had not had prior dissection (10 of 11) than in patients who did (3 of 14). Although in this series there were no complications related to the exploration, such complications have been reported by others.[176] Hence, reexploration of the previously dissected axilla does not seem warranted in the absence of suspicious adenopathy. In one series, 3 of 19 patients treated initially with axillary irradiation only developed a lymphocele after complete axillary dissection performed at the time of mastectomy.[119]

Postoperative complications after mastectomy were rare in two series.[133,140] Slow wound healing, wound breakdown, and infections have been more common in other series, however.[119,176]

Many patients treated with mastectomy for local failure desire breast reconstruction. Immediate reconstruction with a myocutaneous flap at the time of mastectomy is psychologically advantageous and also promotes tissue healing (see Chapter 39). The risk of complications is slightly greater than in patients who have not had prior radiotherapy, and overall cosmetic results may not be as favorable.[179]

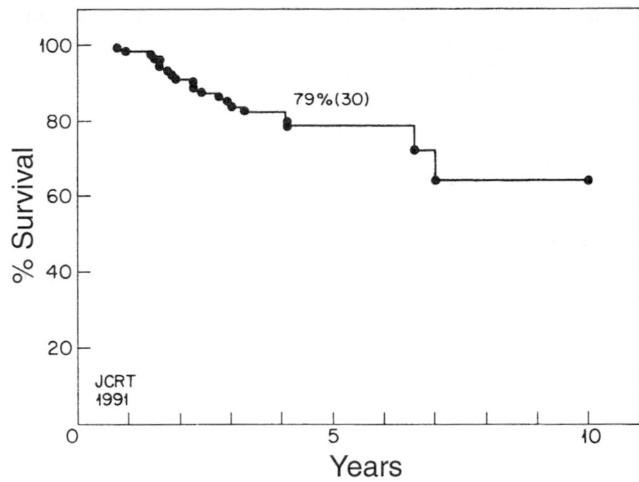

FIG. 4. Actuarial cause-specific survival rate in patients undergoing salvage mastectomy. (From ref. 148, with permission.)

Complication rates in one series were higher when latissimus flaps were used (47%) than when rectus abdominis flaps were used (25%),[179] but many of these were minor. Complete flap loss has not been reported.[179,180] Submuscularly placed tissue expanders have been poorly tolerated by previously irradiated patients.[181,182] Other types of subpectoral prostheses appear less subject to complications, at least in carefully selected individuals.[138,183]

Breast-Conserving Surgery

Whether salvage mastectomy results in superior long-term survival rates for patients with local failure after initial breast-conserving therapy compared with treatment with lesser procedures is unclear. Mastectomy specimens, however, frequently reveal substantial residual disease outside the biopsy cavity. In two series, 22% and 29% of evaluated specimens had residual tumor located in two or more quadrants of the breast.[138,173] Experience using breast-conserving surgery for the treatment of local recurrence shows patients have a substantial risk of further breast recurrence, consistent with these pathologic data. For example, 91 patients with mobile lesions smaller than 2 cm without skin involvement were treated with wedge excisions for a breast recurrence after lumpectomy and radiotherapy at the Marseilles Cancer Institute.[184] This group constituted 52% of their patients undergoing salvage procedures between 1963 and 1982. The actuarial 10-year survival rate was 65%. One-third of patients had further local failure by 5 years. However, the use of further salvage therapy resulted in an ultimate local failure rate of 9% (8 of 91 patients), compared with 9% (eight of 85) among patients whose initial salvage surgery was mastectomy. In the JCRT series, 16 patients refused mastectomy for a biopsy-proven recurrence and were treated with excision only.[148] Two of ten patients with noninvasive recurrences and three of six patients with invasive recurrences failed locally from 20 to 78 months later. In a series from Stockholm, seven of 14 patients treated with wide local excision had a subsequent breast failure, and this second recurrence could not be locally controlled with further treatment in five of the seven cases.[143] Morbidity from wide local excision as a salvage procedure has been reported as low.[185]

Few data are available regarding the chance of still preserving the breast in patients who fail initial treatment with conservative surgery alone. Rates of performing salvage breast-conserving therapy in such patients have ranged from 30% to 100%.[186–189] It is not clear what the risk of a second local recurrence is for such individuals. In a series from Women's College Hospital, Toronto, the 5-year actuarial second local recurrence rate was 69% for patients treated with further breast-conserving surgery alone and 11% for 14 patients treated with conservative surgery and radiotherapy.[190]

Reirradiation

Some patients have been re-treated with wide excision and interstitial implantation or external irradiation to a small part of the breast. In one such series, 25 patients in Marseilles who had recurrences after treatment to a dose of 70 Gy (including a boost) were re-treated with reexcision and brachytherapy between 1974 and 1992; six patients were treated with brachytherapy alone.[191] A dose of 40 Gy to 60 Gy was given. With a mean follow-up of 4 years, 7 (23%) of these 31 patients experienced further local failure (four in the same quadrant as the recurrence and three in another quadrant). One patient developed a necrosis in the tumor bed. Cosmetic results were considered "fair" in 24 of the 25 cases in which reexicision was performed. Other groups have reported similar results with excision plus brachytherapy.[192–194] At the University of Pittsburgh, 16 patients who received initial doses of 50 Gy to the breast (without a boost being used) were treated with repeat lumpectomy and reirradiation of the operative site to 50 Gy in 25 fractions with electrons.[195] Only eight patients had a minimum potential follow-up of 5 years, however; two of these patients experienced recurrences locally within that time, and another at 62 months after re-treatment. An update of this series reported similar findings.[196] No serious complications were noted from reirradiation.

Systemic Therapy

Assessing the roles of adjuvant chemotherapy or hormonal therapy after local recurrence after initial breast-conserving management poses the same problems as does assessing their roles following chest wall recurrence after mastectomy. There was no improvement in outcome in patients so treated in the JCRT[148] or Stockholm[143] experiences, but those patients receiving systemic therapy were likely those thought to have poor prognoses. Some individuals with chest wall fixation may respond sufficiently to chemotherapy or hormonal therapy to allow mastectomy.[176] Systemic therapy alone is not effective in obtaining permanent local control of inoperable disease, however.[176]

REGIONAL LYMPH NODE RECURRENCE

Presenting Signs and Symptoms

The first manifestation of nodal recurrence is usually an asymptomatic mass in the axilla or in the supraclavicular fossa. Some solitary "sternal metastases" may result from direct extension of involved internal mammary nodes.[197] Nodal failures may occur more than 5 years after primary treatment.[198,199]

Only a minority of patients present with symptoms referable to regional failure (e.g., arm edema, neurologic impairment, or pain) in addition to lymphadenopathy. In the JCRT series of patients with nodal recurrence without simultaneous breast failure,[198] such symptoms were found at presentation in 31% of patients (12 of 38). These totals included 23% of patients (five of 22) with (initially) isolated axillary failure and 44% of patients (seven of 16) with other sites of nodal failure.

Subsequent Morbidity and Spread

Significant pain or other distressing symptoms at last follow-up or death were present in 32% of patients with regional failure (12 of 38) in the JCRT experience.[198] Sixteen percent of patients (three of 19) with isolated axillary failure and 25% of patients (three of 12) with failure at other nodal sites who did not have such symptoms on presentation developed them despite treatment. In another series, 24% of patients who developed regional nodal failure after mastectomy had at least one significant symptom during follow-up.[10] Pain and/or arm edema may be more common among patients with supraclavicular recurrence; in a series from Vienna, 38% of patients (15 of 39) with isolated supraclavicular recurrences suffered such symptoms at diagnosis or before death.[200]

In one series, recurrence on the chest wall occurred in 27% of patients (7 of 26) with supraclavicular nodal failure who did not undergo elective chest wall irradiation.[44] The risk of such subclinical involvement of the chest wall when there is recurrence at other nodal sites is unknown.

Prognosis

Prognosis after nodal recurrence may be related to which site is involved. In the JCRT series, with a median follow-up of 45 months, 61% (11 of 18) of patients with isolated axillary failure were alive without disease, compared with 38% (three of eight) of patients with other involved nodal sites.[198] Median and long-term survival after recurrence in the supraclavicular lymph nodes after mastectomy are similar, in most series,[17,201,202] to those of patients with isolated chest wall recurrence, but some suggest a worse prognosis.[21,200] A few long-term survivors have been reported.[203] In one series, 19 patients with isolated internal mammary node recurrences had a better prognosis than other patients with local recurrence (median disease-free interval, 60 months)[17]; others have reported similar findings.[21] In other series, however, such patients had a worse prognosis.[31,200] Patients with asymptomatic regional failures did not survive longer than patients with symptomatic ones in a series from Milwaukee.[204]

Pretreatment Evaluation

Careful evaluation for other nodal and distant sites of failure should be conducted before therapy. Concurrent distant metastases are especially common in patients with supraclavicular disease.[142] In patients with symptoms suggestive of brachial plexopathy (see Chapter 49) or arm edema without obvious adenopathy (see Chapter 64), it may be difficult to distinguish clinically between tumor recurrence in the axilla and the effects of postoperative radiotherapy. MRI may be helpful in this regard, as focal enhancement with gadolinium suggests the presence of tumor rather than radiation-related fibrosis.[205] In patients with axillary failure following breast-conservation therapy, the presence of a simultaneous breast recurrence should be ruled out by careful physical examination and mammography.

Treatment Results

Surgery and Radiation Therapy

Radiotherapy has been roughly as effective in controlling nodal failures after mastectomy as for chest wall recurrences in most series.[17,48,50,206] For example, in a series from the JCRT, the 5-year actuarial control rate among 21 such patients was 78%.[17] Nodal control was 82% among 28 patients treated with complete gross excision at the Mallinckrodt Institute of Radiology, compared with 66% among 62 patients not undergoing excision.[44]

The results of salvage treatment in patients with nodal failure after initial breast-conserving therapy appear similar. Regional control was achieved in 78% of patients (18 of 23) in the JCRT series when gross total excision or radiotherapy, or both, were used[198]; there were no differences between different nodal sites in this regard (JCRT, unpublished data). Similar results have been reported by others.[206,207]

The risks of complications after salvage therapy for regional failure alone have not been reported in these series.

Systemic Therapy

Adjuvant chemotherapy and/or hormonal therapy was frequently given to patients after regional nodal recurrence after breast-conserving therapy in the JCRT series.[198] Its impact on the subsequent course was difficult to assess because of the heterogeneity of the population.[198] When used alone, systemic therapy was unable to control regional disease,[198] although better success has been reported by others.[206] In a retrospective study from Messina, Italy,[208] the combination of systemic therapy with surgery and/or radiotherapy appeared to be more effective than systemic therapy alone in prolonging progression-free and overall survival time after isolated supraclavicular recurrence.

Very-high-dose chemotherapy has also been used in patients with only regional failure. In one series, four of the 13 long-term disease-free survivors (of 80 patients undergoing transplant) had nodal relapses only, but the total number of patients entered with isolated regional recurrence was not reported.[209]

MANAGEMENT

The overwhelming majority of patients who experience local recurrence after mastectomy will ultimately develop distant metastases. Many patients may live for years after local recurrence, however, especially if they have favorable prognostic factors. The side effects of uncontrolled local recurrence may be highly distressing, although only rarely will they lead directly to the death of the patient. At present, there is no agreement on which patients benefit from the different available treatments or at what point in the course of the disease treatment should be instituted. Nonetheless, we believe that the more favorable the prognostic factors are, the more aggressive treatment should be. Local treatment of patients with no evidence of distant metastases will reduce morbidity for many patients and may increase survival time for a few individuals. Whenever possible, lesions should be grossly excised, and this should be followed by radiation therapy. Although the value of adjuvant systemic therapy in this situation is not established, it appears reasonable to use it for patients who have not been previously treated. However, it seems unlikely that there is much value to giving additional systemic therapy to patients who develop local failure shortly after initial adjuvant treatment.

Breast recurrence after conservative surgery and radiotherapy has a better prognosis than chest wall failure after mastectomy. Because early detection of a recurrence might lead to improved salvage results, biopsy should be used when recurrence cannot be easily excluded. We prefer a small open biopsy or ultrasound- or stereotactically guided core-needle biopsy rather than aspiration cytology; however, if these latter procedures are performed, a negative result should be interpreted cautiously. If a recurrence is detected and there is no evidence of dissemination on appropriate restaging, mastectomy is generally viewed as the standard therapy. If desired, reconstruction should be performed using a myocutaneous flap. Treatment by wide local excision, with or without further irradiation, is associated with a substantial risk of further breast failure. Whether such an approach decreases long-term survival rates is not known, however. Such an approach should probably only be used rarely (e.g., for patients who refuse mastectomy). The role of adjuvant systemic therapy after breast recurrence has not been established. If patients have not previously been treated with systemic therapy, we tend to recommend such treatment based on our current policy for a patient presenting with the same clinical-pathologic features who has not had a prior diagnosis of breast cancer (see Chapter 38). The value of re-treating patients who received prior systemic therapy is unknown.

Patients with isolated axillary recurrences can often be successfully treated with surgery or radiation therapy, with some surviving long-term. Patients with other regional nodal failure sites fare much worse. The risk of subsequent relapse in the clinically uninvolved chest wall in patients treated initially with mastectomy is sufficiently high to justify the use of comprehensive radiotherapy fields in patients not previously irradiated. No evidence exists, however, to support the requirement that mastectomy should be used in patients initially treated with breast-conserving surgery who do not have a clinically apparent simultaneous local failure. Systemic therapy alone cannot control gross nodal disease; its value in this setting in conjunction with surgery or radiotherapy is unclear.

REFERENCES

1. Gilliland MD, Barton RM, Copeland EM. The implications of local recurrence of breast cancer as the first site of therapeutic failure. *Ann Surg* 1983;197:284.
2. Scanlon EF. Local recurrence in the pectoralis muscles following modified radical mastectomy for carcinoma. *J Surg Oncol* 1985;30:149.
3. Granik MS, Bragdon RW, Hanna DC. Recurrent breast cancer at the time of breast reconstruction. *Ann Plast Surg* 1987;18:69.
4. Mund DF, Wolfson P, Gorczyca DP, Fu YS, Love SM, Bassett LW. Mammographically detected recurrent nonpalpable carcinoma developing in a transverse rectus abdominus myocutaneous flap: a case report. *Cancer* 1994;74:2804.
5. Dowden RV. Mammography after implant breast reconstruction. *Plast Reconstr Surg* 1995;96:119.
6. Salas AP, Helvie MA, Wilkins EG, et al. Is mammography useful in screening for local recurrences in patients with TRAM flap breast reconstruction after mastectomy for multifocal DCIS? *Ann Surg Oncol* 1998;5:456.
7. Andry G, Suciu S, Vico P, et al. Locoregional recurrences after 649 modified radical mastectomies: incidence and significance. *Eur J Surg Oncol* 1989;15:476.
8. Donegan WL, Perez-Mesa CM, Watson FR. A biostatistical study of locally recurrent breast carcinoma. *Surg Gynecol Obstet* 1966;122:529.
9. Zimmerman K, Montague E, Fletcher G. Frequency, anatomical distribution and management of local recurrences after definitive therapy for breast cancer. *Cancer* 1966;19:67.
10. Tennvall-Nittby L, Tenegrup I, Landberg T. The total incidence of locoregional recurrence in a randomized trial of breast cancer TNM Stage II: the South Sweden Breast Cancer Trial. *Acta Oncol* 1993;32:641.
11. Morton JJ, Morton JH. Cancer as a chronic disease. *Ann Surg* 1953; 137:683.
12. Mackarem G, Roche CA, Silverman ML, Hughes KS. The development of new, primary noninvasive carcinoma of the breast 29 years after bilateral radical mastectomy. *Breast J* 1998;4:51.
13. Bedwinek JM, Fineberg B, Lee J, Ocwieza M. Analysis of failures following local treatment of isolated local-regional recurrence of breast cancer. *Int J Radiat Oncol Biol Phys* 1981;7:581.
14. Fentiman IS, Matthews PN, Davison OW, Millis RR, Hayward JL. Survival following local skin recurrence after mastectomy. *Br J Surg* 1985;72:14.
15. Papaioannou AN, Tanz FJ, Volk H. Fate of patients with recurrent carcinoma of the breast: recurrence five years or more after initial treatment. *Cancer* 1967;20:371.
16. Marshall K, Redfern A, Cady B. Local recurrences of carcinoma of the breast. *Surg Gynecol Obstet* 1974;139:406.
17. Aberizk WJ, Silver B, Henderson IC, Cady B, Harris JR. The use of radiotherapy for treatment of isolated locoregional recurrence of breast carcinoma after mastectomy. *Cancer* 1986;58:1214.
18. Chu FCH, Lin FJ, Kim JH, Suh SH, Garmatis CJ. Locally recurrent carcinoma of the breast: results of radiation therapy. *Cancer* 1976;37:2677.
19. Snyder AF, Farrow GM, Masson JK, Payne WS. Chest-wall resection for locally recurrent breast cancer. *Arch Surg* 1968;97:246.
20. Shimkin MB, Lucia EL, Low-Beer VA, Bell HG. Recurrent cancer of the breast: analysis of frequency, distribution, and mortality at the University of California Hospital, 1918 to 1947, inclusive. *Cancer* 1954;7:29.
21. Halverson KJ, Perez CA, Kuske RR, Garcia DM, Simpson JR, Fineberg B. Locoregional recurrence of breast cancer: a retrospective comparison of irradiation alone versus irradiation and systemic therapy. *Am J Clin Oncol* 1992;15:93.
22. Brunner KW, Harder F, Greiner R, et al. Das loko-regionale Rezidiv nach operiertem Mammakarzinom: prognostische Faktoren und therapeutische Konsequenzen. *Schweiz Med Wochenschr* 1988;118:1976.
23. Willner J, Kiricuta IC, Kölbi O. Beeinflußt der Primärtumor die Prognose bei lokoregionärem Rezidiv nach Mastektomie wegen Mammakarzinom? *Strahlenther Onkol* 1994;171:18.
24. Kamby C, Senegeløv L. Pattern of dissemination and survival following isolated locoregional recurrence of breast cancer: a prospective study with more than 10 years of follow-up. *Breast Cancer Res Treat* 1997;45:181.
25. Schwaibold F, Fowble BL, Solin LJ, Schultz DJ, Goodman RL. The results of radiation therapy for isolated local regional recurrence after mastectomy. *Int J Radiat Oncol Biol Phys* 1991;21:299.
26. Mora EM, Singletary SE, Buzdar AU, Johnston DA. Agressive therapy for locoregional recurrence after mastectomy in Stage II and III breast cancer patients. *Ann Surg Oncol* 1996;3:162.
27. Baral E, Ogenstad S, Wallgren A. The effect of adjuvant radiotherapy on the time of occurrence and prognosis of local recurrence in primary operable breast cancer. *Cancer* 1985;56:2779.
28. Danoff BF, Coia LR, Cantor RI, Pajak TF, Kramer S. Locally recurrent breast carcinoma: the effect of adjuvant chemotherapy on prognosis. *Radiology* 1983;147:849.
29. Valagussa P, Rossi A, Tancini G, Bonadonna G. Is there any effective salvage treatment for relapsing operable breast cancer with N+? *Proc Am Soc Clin Oncol* 1985;4:56a(abst).
30. Buzdar A, McNeese MD, Hortobagyi GN, et al. Is chemotherapy effective in reducing the local failure rate in patients with operable breast cancer? *Cancer* 1990;65:394.
31. Deutsch M, Parsons J, Mittal BB. Radiation therapy for local-regional recurrent breast cancer. *Int J Radiat Oncol Biol Phys* 1986;12:2061.
32. Haagensen CD. *Diseases of the breast*, 3rd ed. Philadelphia: WB Saunders, 1986.
33. Lee CH, Poplack SP, Stahl RS. Mammographic appearance of the transverse rectus abdominus musculocutaneous (TRAM) flap. *Breast Dis* 1994;7:99.
34. Brady MS, Gaynor JJ, Brennan MF. Radiation-associated sarcoma of bone and soft tissue. *Arch Surg* 1992;127:1379.
35. Allegra JC, Barlock A, Huff KK, Lippman ME. Changes in multiple or sequential estrogen receptor determinations in breast cancer. *Cancer* 1980;45:792.
36. Chen Z, Hoover HC, Koerner F. Estrogen receptor determinations of cutaneous recurrences of breast cancers: reduced sensitivity of hormone binding assays. *Breast J* 1995;1:107.
37. Lindfors KK, Meyer JE, Busse PM, Kopans DB, Munzenrider JE, Sawicka JM. CT evaluation of local and regional breast cancer recurrence. *AJR Am J Roentgenol* 1985;145:833.
38. Rosenman J, Churchill CA, Mauro MA, Parker LA, Newsome J. The role of computed tomography in the evaluation of post-mastectomy locally recurrent breast cancer. *Int J Radiat Oncol Biol Phys* 1988;14:57.
39. Scatarige JC, Fishman EK, Zinreich ES, Brem RF, Almaraz R. Internal mammary lymphadenopathy in breast carcinoma: CT appraisal of anatomic distribution. *Radiology* 1988;167:89.

40. Cheng JC, Cheng SH, Lin K-J, Jian JJ, Chan K-Y, Huang AT. Diagnostic thoracic-computed tomography in radiotherapy for loco-regional recurrent breast carcinoma. *Int J Radiat Oncol Biol Phys* 1998;41:607.
41. Perre CI, Hoefnagel CA, Kroon BBR, Zoetmulder FAN, Rutgers EJT. Altered lymphatic drainage after lymphadenectomy or radiotherapy of the axilla in patients with breast cancer. *Br J Surg* 1996;83:1258.
42. Bender H, Kirst J, Palmedo H, et al. Value of [18]fluoro-deoxyglucose positron emission tomography in the staging of recurrent breast carcinoma. *Anticancer Res* 1997;17:1687.
43. Moon DH, Maddahi J, Silverman DHS, Glaspy JA, Phelps ME, Hoh CK. Accuracy of whole-body fluorine-18-FDG PET for the detection of recurrent or metastatic breast carcinoma. *J Nucl Med* 1998;39:431.
44. Halverson KJ, Perez CA, Kuske RR, Garcia DM, Simpson JR, Fineberg B. Isolated local-regional recurrence of breast cancer following mastectomy: radiotherapeutic management. *Int J Radiat Oncol Biol Phys* 1990;19:851.
45. Kenda R, Lozza L, Zucali R. Results of irradiation in the treatment of chest wall recurrent breast cancer. *Radiother Oncol* 1992;24[Suppl 1]:S41a(abst).
46. Patanaphan V, Salazar OM, Poussin-Rosillo H. Prognosticators in recurrent breast cancer: a 15-year experience with irradiation. *Cancer* 1984;54:228.
47. Stadler B, Kogelnik HD. Local control and outcome of patients irradiated for isolated chest wall recurrences of breast cancer. *Radiother Oncol* 1987;8:105.
48. Chen KK-Y, Montague E, Oswald M. Results of irradiation in the treatment of locoregional breast cancer recurrence. *Cancer* 1985; 56:1269.
49. Magno L, Bignardi M, Micheletti E, Bardelli D, Plebani F. Analysis of prognostic factors in patients with isolated chest wall recurrence of breast cancer. *Cancer* 1987;60:240.
50. Mendenhall NP, Devine JW, Mendenhall WM, Bland KI, Million RR, Copeland EM. Isolated local-regional recurrence following mastectomy for adenocarcinoma of the breast treated with radiation therapy alone or combined with surgery and/or chemotherapy. *Radiother Oncol* 1988;12:177.
51. Toonkel LM, Fix I, Jacobson LH, Wallach CB. The significance of local recurrence of carcinoma of the breast. *Int J Radiat Oncol Biol Phys* 1983;9:33.
52. Chu FCH, Kaufmann TP, Dawson GA, Kim YS, Rajaratnam S, Hoffman LA. Radiation therapy of cancer in prosthetically augmented or reconstructed breasts. *Radiology* 1992;185:429.
53. Plasswilm L, Sauer R. Simultane radiochemotherapie beim rezidivierten und metastasierten Mammakarzinom. *Strahlenther Onkol* 1995; 171:689.
54. McNeese MD, Fletcher GH, Levitt SH, Khan FM. Breast cancer. In: Levitt SH, Khan FM, Potish RA, eds. *Levitt and Tapley's technological basis of radiation therapy: practical clinical applications*, 2nd ed. Philadelphia: Lea & Febiger, 1992:232.
55. Lo TCM, Salzman FA, Wright KA, Costey GE. Megavolt electron irradiation in the treatment of recurrent carcinoma of the breast on the chest wall. *Acta Radiol Oncol* 1983;22:97.
56. McNeely LK, Jacobson GM, Leavitt DD, Stewart JR. Electron arc therapy: chest wall irradiation of breast cancer patients. *Int J Radiat Oncol Biol Phys* 1988;14:1287.
57. Pezner RD, Lipsett JA, Forell B, et al. The reverse hockey stick technique: postmastectomy radiation therapy for breast cancer patients with locally advanced tumor presentation or extensive loco-regional recurrence. *Int J Radiat Oncol Biol Phys* 1989;17:191.
58. Delanian S, Housset M, Brunel P, et al. Iridium 192 plesiocurietherapy using silicone elastomer plates for extensive locally recurrent breast cancer following chest wall irradiation. *Int J Radiat Oncol Biol Phys* 1992;22:1099.
59. Svoboda VHJ, Kovarik J, Morris F. High dose-rate MicroSelectron molds in the treatment of skin tumors. *Int J Radiat Oncol Biol Phys* 1995;31:967.
60. Fritz P, Hensley FW, Berns C, Schraube P, Wannenmacher M. First experiences with superfractionated skin irradiation using large afterloading molds. *Int J Radiat Oncol Biol Phys* 1996;36:147.
61. Weshler Z, Wygoda A, Newman R, Weinberg A, Wexler MR. The role of brachytherapy in the treatment of chest-wall recurrences of breast carcinoma. *Eur J Cancer* 1993;29A[Suppl 6]:S70a(abst).
62. Madoc-Jones H, Nelson AJ, Montague ED. Evaluation of the effectiveness of radiotherapy in the management of early nodal recurrences from adenocarcinoma of the breast. *Breast* 1976;2:31.
63. Beck TM, Hart NE, Woodard DA, et al. Local or regionally recurrent carcinoma of the breast: results of therapy in 121 patients. *J Clin Oncol* 1983;1:400.
64. Laramore GE, Griffin TW, Parker RG, Gerdes AJ. The use of electron beams in treating local recurrence of breast cancer in previously irradiated fields. *Cancer* 1978;41:991.
65. Elkort RJ, Kelly W, Mozden PJ, et al. A combined treatment program for the management of locally recurrent breast cancer following chest wall irradiation. *Cancer* 1980;46:647.
66. Tough ICK. The significance of recurrence in breast cancer. *Br J Surg* 1966;53:897.
67. Bedwinek JM, Lee J, Fineberg B, Ocwieza M. Prognostic indicators in patients with isolated local-regional recurrence of breast cancer. *Cancer* 1981;47:2232.
68. Probstfeld MR, O'Connell TX. Treatment of locally recurrent breast carcinoma. *Arch Surg* 1989;124:1127.
69. Salvadori B, Rovini D, Squicciarini P, Conti R, Cusumano F, Grassi M. Surgery for local recurrences following deficient radical mastectomy for breast cancer: a selected series of 39 cases. *Eur J Surg Oncol* 1992;18:438.
70. McCormack PM, Bains MS, Burt ME, Martini N, Chaglassian T, Hidalgo DA. Local recurrent mammary carcinoma failing multimodality therapy: a solution. *Arch Surg* 1989;124:158.
71. Kroll SS, Schusterman MA, Larson DL, Fender A. Long-term survival after chest-wall reconstruction with musculocutaneous flaps. *Plast Reconstr Surg* 1990;86:697.
72. Muscolino G, Valente M, Lequaglie C, Ravasi G. Correlation between first disease-free interval from mastectomy to second disease-free interval from chest wall resection. *Eur J Surg Oncol* 1992;18:49.
73. Faneyte IF, Rutgers EJT, Zoetmulder FAN. Chest wall resection in the treatment of locally recurrent breast carcinoma: indications and outcome for 44 patients. *Cancer* 1997;80:886.
74. Flook D, Webster DJT, Hughes LE, Mansel RW. Salvage surgery for advanced local recurrence of breast cancer. *Br J Surg* 1988;76:512.
75. Dahlstrøm KK, Andersson AP, Andersen M, Krag C. Wide local excision of recurrent breast cancer in the thoracic wall. *Cancer* 1993;72:774
76. Miyauchi K, Koyama H, Noguchi S, et al. Surgical treatment for chest wall recurrence of breast cancer. *Eur J Cancer* 1992;28A:1059.
77. Perez CA, Pajak T, Emami B, Hornback NB, Tupchong L, Rubin P. Randomized Phase III study comparing irradiation and hyperthermia with irradiation alone in superficial measurable tumors. *Am J Clin Oncol* 1991;14:133.
78. International Collaborative Hyperthermia Group. Radiotherapy with or without hyperthermia in the treatment of superficial localized breast cancer: results from five randomized controlled trials. *Int J Radiat Oncol Biol Phys* 1996;35:731
79. Kapp DS, Cox RC. Thermal treatment parameters are most predictive of outcome in patients with single tumor nodules per treatment field in recurrent adenocarcinoma of the breast. *Int J Radiat Oncol Biol Phys* 1995;33:887.
80. Sherar M, Liu F-F, Pintilie M, et al. Relationship between thermal dose and outcome in thermoradiotherapy treatments for superficial recurrences of breast cancer: data from a Phase III trial. *Int J Radiat Oncol Biol Phys* 1997;39:371.
81. Lee HK, Antell AG, Perez CA, et al. Superificial hyperthermia and irradiation for recurrent breast carcinoma of the chest wall: prognostic factors in 196 tumors. *Int J Radiat Oncol Biol Phys* 1998; 40:365.
82. Van der Zee J, Treurniet-Donker AD, The SK, et al. Low dose irradiation in combination with hyperthermia: a palliative treatment for patients with breast cancer recurring in previously irradiated areas. *Int J Radiat Oncol Biol Phys* 1988;15:1407.
83. Amicheti M, Valdagni R, Graiff C, Valentini A. Local-regional recurrences of breast cancer: treatment with radiation therapy and local microwave hyperthermia. *Am J Clin Oncol* 1991;14:60.
84. Scott R, Gillespie B, Perez CA, et al. Hyperthermia in combination with definitive radiation therapy: results of a phase I/II RTOG study. *Int J Radiat Oncol Biol Phys* 1988;15:711.
85. Kapp DS, Barnett TA, Cox RS, Lee ER, Lohrbach A, Fessenden P. Hyperthermia and radiation therapy of local-regional recurrent breast cancer: prognostic factors for response and local control of diffuse or nodular tumors. *Int J Radiat Oncol Biol Phys* 1991;20:1147.
86. Bornstein BA, Zouranjian PS, Hansen JL, et al. Local hyperthermia, radiation therapy, and chemotherapy in patients with local-regional

recurrence of breast carcinoma. *Int J Radiat Oncol Biol Phys* 1992;25:79.
87. Schuh M, Nseyo UO, Potter WR, Dao TL, Dougherty TJ. Photodynamic therapy for palliation of locally recurrent breast carcinoma. *J Clin Oncol* 1987;5:1766.
88. Sperduto PW, DeLaney TF, Thomas G, et al. Photodynamic therapy for chest wall recurrence in breast cancer. *Int J Radiat Oncol Biol Phys* 1991;21:441.
89. Khan SA, Dougherty TJ, Mang TS. An evaluation of photodynamic therapy in the management of cutaneous metastases of breast cancer. *Eur J Cancer* 1993;29A:1686.
90. Panella TJ, Wieman TJ, Dougherty S, et al. Lutecium texaphyrin (LuTEX) photodynamic therapy (PDT) of patients with refractory locally recurrent breast cancer. *Proc Am Soc Clin Oncol* 1998;17:165a(abst).
91. Görich J, Hasan I, Majdali R, et al. Previously treated, locally recurrent breast cancer: treatment with superselective with intraarterial chemotherapy. *Radiology* 1995;197:199.
92. Lewis WG, Walker VA, Ali HH, Sainsbury JRC. Intra-arterial chemotherapy in patients with breast cancer: a feasibility study. *Br J Cancer* 1995;71:605.
93. Ban T, Nistor C, Nistor V, et al. Ointments with 5-fluorouracil, used in care of patients with breast exulcerative cancers. *Ann Oncol* 1990;1[Suppl]:20a(abst).
94. David M, Sindermann H, Junge K, Peukert M. Topical treatment of skin metastases with 6% miltefosine solution (Miltex) in patients with breast cancer. A meta-analysis of 443 patients. *Proc Am Soc Clin Oncol* 1997;16:150a(abst).
95. Gad-El-Mawia N, Gaafar R, Zikri Z, Hamza MR. Improvement in quality of life using hexadecyl phosphocholine, Miltex (M), in breast cancer patients with extensive skin lesions. *Proc Am Soc Clin Oncol* 1997;16:169a(abst).
96. Fernando I, Eisenberg PD, Roshon S, Mansi J, Mills G, de Vries E. Evaluation of intratumoral cisplatin/epinephrine injectable gel for palliative treatment of metastatic breast cancer. *Ann Oncol* 1998;9[Suppl 2]:181(abst).
97. Szepesi S, Schopohl B, Böttcher HD. Combined treatment with radiation therapy and IFN-β intralesional: clinical results. *Eur J Cancer* 1991;27[Suppl 2]:S220a(abst).
98. Habif DV, Ozzello L, De Rosa CM, Cantell K, Lattes R. Regression of skin recurrences of breast carcinomas treated with intralesional injections of natural interferons alpha and gamma. *Cancer Invest* 1995;13:165.
99. Mir LM, Glass LF, Sersa G, et al. Effective treatment of cutaneous and subcutaneous malignant tumours by electrocautery. *Br J Cancer* 1998;77:2336.
100. Heller R, Jaroszeski MJ, Reintgen DS, et al. Treatment of cutaneous and subcutaneous tumors with electrochemotherapy using intralesional bleomycin. *Cancer* 1998;83:148.
101. Ashford R, Plant G, Maher J, Teare L. Double blind trial of metronidazole in malodorous ulcerating tumours [Letter]. *Lancet* 1984;1:1232.
102. Borner M, Bacchi M, Goldhirsch A, et al. First isolated locoregional recurrence following mastectomy for breast cancer: results of a Phase III multicenter trial comparing systemic treatment with observation after excision and radiation. *J Clin Oncol* 1994;12:2071.
103. Borner MM, Bacchi M, Castiglione M. Possible deleterious effect of tamoxifen in premenopausal women with locoregional recurrence of breast cancer. *Eur J Cancer* 1996;32A:2173.
104. Holmes FA, Buzdar AU, Kau S-W, et al. Combined-modality approach for patients with isolated recurrences of breast cancer (IV-NED). *Breast Dis* 1994;7:7.
105. Renner K, Renner H. Simultaneous combined radio-chemotherapy of locally recurrent or haematogeneous metastatic breast carcinoma. *Strahlenther Onkol* 1988;164:20a(abst).
106. Mundt AJ, Sibley GS, Williams S, et al. Patterns of failure of complete responders following high dose chemotherapy and autologous bone marrow transplantation for metastatic breast cancer: implications for the use of adjuvant radiation therapy. *Int J Radiat Oncol Biol Phys* 1994;30:151.
107. Overmoyer BA, Carinder J, Andresen S, et al. The efficacy of high dose chemotherapy with autologous bone marrow transplantation for the treatment of osseous metastasis from breast cancer. *Breast Cancer Res Treat* 1997;46:72a(abst).
108. Janjan NA, McNeese MD, Buzdar AU, et al. Management of locoregional recurrent breast cancer. *Cancer* 1986;58:1552.
109. Hoogstraten B, Gad-el-Mawla N, Maloney TR, et al. Combined modality therapy for first recurrence of breast cancer: a Southwest Oncology Group study. *Cancer* 1984;54:2248.
110. Helman P. Breast cancer: aspects of local recurrence. *South Afr Med J* 1961;35:197.
111. Stomper PC, Recht A, Berenberg AL, Jochelson MS, Harris JR. Mammographic detection of recurrent cancer in the irradiated breast. *AJR Am J Roentgenol* 1987;148:39.
112. Dershaw DD, McCormick B, Osborne MP. Detection of local recurrence after conservative therapy for breast carcinoma. *Cancer* 1992;70:493.
113. Orel SG, Fowble BL, Solin LJ, Schultz DJ, Conaant EF, Troupin RH. Breast cancer recurrence after lumpectomy and radiation therapy for early-stage disease: prognostic significance of detection method. *Radiology* 1993;188:189.
114. Hassell PR, Olivotto IA, Mueller HA, Kingston GW, Basco VE. Early breast cancer: detection of recurrence after conservative surgery and radiation therapy. *Radiology* 1990;176:731.
115. Haffty BG, Fischer D, Beinfield M, McKhann C. Prognosis following local recurrence in the conservatively treated breast cancer patient. *Int J Radiat Oncol Biol Phys* 1991;21:293.
116. Recht A, Sadowsky NL, Cady B. Clinical problems in follow-up of patients following conservative surgery and radiotherapy. *Surg Clin N Am* 1990;70:1179.
117. Schnitt SJ, Connolly JL, Recht A, Silver B, Harris JR. The influence of infiltrating lobular histology on local tumor control in breast cancer patients treated with conservative surgery and radiotherapy. *Cancer* 1989;64:448.
118. Markopoulos C, Gazet JC. Paget's disease of the nipple occurring after conservative management of early breast cancer. *Eur J Surg Oncol* 1988;14:77.
119. Barr LC, Phillips RH, Brunt AM, Ellis H. Salvage mastectomy after failed breast-conserving therapy for carcinoma of the breast. *Ann R Coll Surg Engl* 1991;73:126.
120. Sadowsky NL, Semine A, Harris JR. Breast imaging: a critical aspect of breast conserving treatment. *Cancer* 1990;65:2113.
121. Brenner RJ, Pfaff JM. Mammographic features after conservation therapy for malignant breast disease: serial findings standardized by regression analysis. *AJR Am J Roentgenol* 1996;167:171.
122. Orford JE, Ingram DM, Kaard AO, Sheiner HJ. Scar formation after breast-conserving surgery for cancer. *Br J Surg* 1993;80:1003.
123. Dershaw DD, McCormick B, Cox L, Osborne MP. Differentiation of benign and malignant local tumor recurrence after lumpectomy. *Radiology* 1990;155:35.
124. Solin LJ, Fowble BL, Schultz DJ, Rubenstein JR, Goodman RL. The detection of local recurrence after definitive irradiation for early stage carcinoma of the breast: an analysis of the results of breast biopsies performed in previously irradiated breasts. *Cancer* 1990;65:2497.
125. Mendelson EB. Evaluation of the postoperative breast. *Radiol Clin North Am* 1992;30:107.
126. Dershaw DD. Mammography in patients with breast cancer treated by breast conservation (lumpectomy with or without radiation). *AJR Am J Roentgenol* 1995;164:309.
127. Ciatto S, Cataliotti L, Distante V, Rontini M, Muraca MG. Diagnostic features of 225 consecutive cases of cancer recurrence in the conserved breast. *Breast* 1997;6:367.
128. Mitnick J, Roses DF, Harris MN. Differentiation of postsurgical changes from carcinoma of the breast. *Surg Gynecol Obstet* 1988;166:549.
129. Jager JJ, Langendijk JA, Dohmen JP, et al. Mammography in the follow-up after breast-conserving treatment in cancer of the breast; suitability for mammographic interpretation, validity and interobserver variation. *Br J Radiol* 1995;68:754.
130. Solin LJ, Fowble BL, Troupin RH, Goodman RL. Biopsy results of new calcifications in the postirradiated breast. *Cancer* 1989;63:1956.
131. Philpotts LE, Lee CH, Haffty BG, Lange RC, Tocino I. Mammographic findings of recurrent breast cancer after lumpectomy and radiation therapy: comparison with the primary tumor. *Radiology* 1996;201:767.
132. Samuels JL, Haffty BG, Lee CH, Fischer DB. Breast conservation therapy in patients with mammographically undetected breast cancer. *Radiology* 1992;185:425.
133. Recht A, Schnitt SJ, Connolly JL, et al. Prognosis following local or regional recurrence after conservative surgery and radiotherapy for early stage breast carcinoma. *Int J Radiat Oncol Biol Phys* 1989;16:3.
134. Fourquet A, Campana F, Zafrani B, et al. Prognostic factors of breast recurrence in the conservative management of early breast cancer: a 25-year follow-up. *Int J Radiat Oncol Biol Phys* 1989;17:719.
135. Kurtz JM, Amalric R, Brandone H, et al. Local recurrence after breast-conserving surgery and radiotherapy: frequency, time course, and prognosis. *Cancer* 1989;63:1912.

136. Leung S, Otmezguine Y, Calitchi E, Mazeron JJ, Le Bourgeois JP, Pierquin B. Locoregional recurrences following radical external beam irradiation and interstitial implantation for operable breast cancer: a twenty three year experience. *Radiother Oncol* 1986;5:1.
137. Haffty BG, Carter D, Flynn SD, et al. Local recurrence versus new primary: clinical analysis of 82 breast relapses and potential applications for genetic fingerprinting. *Int J Radiat Oncol Biol Phys* 1993;27:575.
138. Fowble B, Solin L, Schultz D, Rubenstein J, Goodman RL. Breast recurrence following conservative surgery and radiation: patterns of failure, prognosis, and pathologic findings from mastectomy specimens with implications for treatment. *Int J Radiat Oncol Biol Phys* 1990;19:833.
139. Stotter AT, McNeese MD, Ames FC, Oswald MJ, Ellerbroek NA. Predicting the rate and extent of locoregional failure after breast conservation therapy for early breast cancer. *Cancer* 1989;64:2217.
140. Osborne MP, Borgen PI, Wong GY, Rosen PP, McCormick B. Salvage mastectomy for local and regional recurrence after breast-conserving operation and radiation therapy. *Surg Gynecol Obstet* 1992;174:189.
141. Veronesi U, Marubini E, Del Vecchio M, et al. Local recurrences and distant metastases after conservative breast cancer treatments: partly independent events. *J Natl Cancer Inst* 1995;87:19.
142. Kemperman H, Borger J, Hart A, Petrse H, Bartelink H, van Dongen JA. Prognostic factors for survival after breast conserving therapy for Stage I and II breast cancer. The role of local recurrence. *Eur J Cancer* 1995;31A:690.
143. Dalberg K, Mattsson A, Sandelin K, Rutqvist LE. Outcome of treatment for ipsilateral breast tumor recurrence in early-stage breast cancer. *Breast Cancer Res Treat* 1998;49:69.
144. Van Dongen JA, Bartelink H, Fentiman IS, et al. Factors influencing local relapse and survival and results of salvage treatment after breast-conserving therapy in operable breast cancer: EORTC Trial 10801, breast conservation compared with mastectomy in TNM Stage I and II breast cancer. *Eur J Cancer* 1992;28A:801.
145. Chaudary MA, Nagadowska M, Smith P, Gregory W, Fentiman IS. Local recurrence after breast conservation treatment: outcome following salvage mastectomy. *Breast* 1998;7:33.
146. Kurtz JM, Jacquemier J, Brandone H, et al. Inoperable recurrence after breast-conserving surgical treatment and radiotherapy. *Surg Gynecol Obstet* 1991;172:357.
147. Gage I, Schnitt SJ, Recht A, et al. Skin recurrences after breast-conserving therapy for early stage breast cancer. *J Clin Oncol* 1998;16:480.
148. Abner AL, Recht A, Eberlein T, et al. Prognosis following salvage mastectomy for recurrence in the breast after conservative surgery and radiation therapy for early-stage breast cancer. *J Clin Oncol* 1993;11:44.
149. Kurtz JM, Spitalier J-M, Amalric R, et al. The prognostic significance of late local recurrence after breast-conserving therapy. *Int J Radiat Oncol Biol Phys* 1990;18:87.
150. Chauvet B, Lemseffer A, Fetissoff F, et al. Disappearance of the in situ component: a criterion predictive of metastasis in breast cancer after local relapse. *Radiother Oncol* 1992;25:181.
151. Haffty BG, Reiss M, Beinfield M, Fischer D, Ward B, McKhann C. Ipsilateral breast tumor recurrence as a predictor of distant disease: implications for systemic therapy at the time of local relapse. *J Clin Oncol* 1996;14:52.
152. Haffty BG, Toth M, Flynn S, Fischer D, Carter D. Prognostic value of DNA flow cytometry in the locally recurrent, conservatively treated breast cancer patient. *J Clin Oncol* 1992;10:1839.
153. Turner BC, Harrold E, Gumbs AA, et al. Elevated frequency of germline BRCA1/BRCA2 gene mutations in locally recurrent breast cancer patients following lumpectomy and radiation therapy: implications for breast conserving management in affected patients. *Int J Radiat Oncol Biol Phys* 1998;42[Suppl]:109a(abst).
154. Boyages J, Bilous M, Barraclough B, et al. Fat necrosis of the breast following lumpectomy and radiation therapy for early breast cancer. *Radiother Oncol* 1988;13:69.
155. Solomon B, Orel S, Reynolds C, Schnall M. Delayed development of enhancement in fat necrosis after breast conservation therapy: a potential pitfall of MR imaging of the breast. *AJR Am J Roentgenol* 1998;170:966.
156. Keidan RD, Hoffman JP, Weese JL, et al. Delayed breast abscesses after lumpectomy and radiation therapy. *Ann Surg* 1990;56:440.
157. Staren E, Klepek S, Hartsell B, et al. The dilemma of breast cellulitis after conservation surgery and radiation therapy. *Breast Cancer Res Treat* 1993;27:188a(abst).
158. Trattner A, Figer A, David M, Lurie H, Sandbank M. Circumscribed scleroderma induced by postlumpectomy radiation therapy. *Cancer* 1991;68:2131.
159. Colver GB, Rodger A, Mortimer PS, Savin JA, Neill SM, Hunter JAA. Post-irradiation morphoea. *Br J Dermatol* 1989;120:831.
160. Frazier TG, Furnay AP, Rose D, Murphy JT. Ultrasound mammography in the follow-up of the post irradiated breast. *Breast Cancer Res Treat* 1988;12:113a(abst).
161. Cosgrove DO, Bamber JC, Davey JB, McKinna JA, Sinnett HD. Color Doppler signals from breast tumors: work in progress. *Radiology* 1990;176:175.
162. Dao TH, Rahmouni A, Campana F, Laurent M, Asselain B, Fourquet A. Tumor recurrence versus fibrosis in the irradiated breast: differentiation with dynamic gadolinium-enhanced MR imaging. *Radiology* 1993;187:751.
163. Gilles R, Guinebretière J-M, Shapeero LG, et al. Assessment of breast cancer recurrence with contrast-enhanced subtraction MR imaging: preliminary results in 26 patients. *Radiology* 1993;188:473.
164. Lewis-Jones HG, Whitehouse GH, Leinster SJ. The role of magnetic resonance imaging in the assessment of local recurrent breast cancer. *Clin Radiol* 1991;43:197.
165. Mumtaz H, Davidson T, Hall-Craggs MA, et al. Comparison of magnetic resonance imaging and conventional triple assessment in locally recurrent breast cancer. *Br J Surg* 1997;84:1147.
166. Hagay C, Cherel P, De Maulmont C, Mayras C, Plantet M, Garbay JR. Contrast-enhanced CT mammography: evaluation in local breast recurrence. *Radiology* 1993;189:406a(abst).
167. Chaiken L, Rege S, Hoh C, et al. Positron emission tomography with fluorodeoxyglucose to evaluate tumor response and control after radiation therapy. *Int J Radiat Oncol Biol Phys* 1993;27:455.
168. Tierney S, Fenlon HM, Phelan N, O'Sullivan P, Ennis JT, Gorey TF. Scintimammography in the assessment of local recurrence following conservative breast surgery. *Br J Surg* 1998;85[Suppl 1]:51a(abst).
169. Recht A, Harris JR. Negative breast biopsies after primary radiation therapy: safety and accuracy. *Int J Radiat Oncol Biol Phys* 1985; 11[Suppl 1]:131a(abst).
170. Ciatto S. Letter to the editor. *Breast* 1994;3:130.
171. Mitnick JS, Vasquez MF, Roses DF, Harris MN, Schechter S. Recurrent breast cancer: stereotaxic localization for fine-needle aspiration biopsy: work in progress. *Radiology* 1992;182:103.
172. Liberman L, Dershaw DD, Durfee S, et al. Recurrent carcinoma after breast conservation: diagnosis with stereotaxic core biopsy. *Radiology* 1995;197:735.
173. Schnitt SJ, Connolly JL, Recht A, Silver B, Harris JR. Breast relapse following primary radiation therapy for early breast cancer. II. Detection, pathologic features and prognostic significance. *Int J Radiat Oncol Biol Phys* 1985;11:1277.
174. Peterse JL, Van Heerde P. Fine needle cytology of breast lesions after breast conserving treatment: cytology of radiation induced changes in normal breast epithelium. Fourth EORTC Breast Cancer Working Conference. London, September 1987.
175. Pezner RD, Lorant JA, Terz J, Ben-Ezra J, Odom-Maryon T, Luk KH. Wound-healing complications following biopsy of the irradiated breast. *Arch Surg* 1992;127:321.
176. Stotter A, Kroll S, McNeese M, Holmes F, Oswald MJ, Romsdahl M. Salvage treatment of loco-regional recurrence following breast conservation therapy for early breast cancer. *Eur J Surg Oncol* 1991;17:231.
177. Cajucom CC, Tsangaris TN, Nemoto T, Driscoll D, Penetrante RB, Holyoke ED. Results of salvage mastectomy for local recurrence after breast-conserving surgery without radiation therapy. *Cancer* 1993;71:1774.
178. McCready D, Fish E, Hiraki G, Ross T, Wall J, Lickley L. Total mastectomy is not mandatory treatment for breast recurrence following lumpectomy. *Breast Cancer Res Treat* 1990;16:173a(abst).
179. Kroll SS, Schusterman MA, Reece GP, Miller MJ, Smith B. Breast reconstruction with myocutaneous flaps in previously irradiated patients. *Plast Reconstr Surg* 1994;93:460.
180. Howrigan P, Slavin SA. Salvage mastectomy and chest wall reconstruction using myocutaneous flaps. *Breast Dis* 1991;4:39a(abst).
181. Dickson MG, Sharpe DT. The complications of tissue expansion in breast reconstruction: a review of 75 cases. *Br J Plast Surg* 1987;40:629.
182. Olenius M, Jurell G. Breast reconstruction using tissue expansion. *Scand J Plast Reconstr Hand Surg* 1992;26:83.
183. Barreau-Pouhaer L, Lê MG, Rietjens M, et al. Risk factors for failure of immediate breast reconstruction with prosthesis after total mastectomy for breast cancer. *Cancer* 1992;70:1145.
184. Spitalier J-M, Ayme Y, Brandone H, Amalric R, Kurtz JM. Treatment of mammary recurrences after breast conservation. *Breast Dis* 1991;4:20a(abst).

185. Kurtz JM, Amalric R, Brandone H, et al. Results of wide excision for mammary recurrence after breast conserving therapy. *Cancer* 1988; 61:1969.
186. Martelli G, DePalo G, Rossi N, et al. Long-term follow-up of elderly patients with operable breast cancer treated with surgery without axillary dissection plus adjuvant tamoxifen. *Br J Cancer* 1995;72:1251.
187. Schnitt SJ, Hayman J, Gelman R, et al. A prospective study of conservative surgery alone in the treatment of selected patients with Stage I breast cancer. *Cancer* 1996;77:1094.
188. Clark RM, Whelan T, Levine M, et al. Randomized clinical trial of breast irradiation following lumpectomy and axillary dissection for node-negative breast cancer: an update. *J Natl Cancer Inst* 1996;88:1659.
189. Liljegren G, Holmberg L, Adami H-O, Westman G, Graffman S, Bergh J. Sector resection with or without postoperative radiotherapy: five-year results of a randomized trial. *J Natl Cancer Inst* 1994;86:717.
190. McCready DR, Chapman J-A, Wall JL, Lickley LA. Characteristics of local recurrences following lumpectomy for breast cancer. *Cancer Invest* 1994;12:568.
191. Cowen D, Altschuler C, Blanc B, et al. Second conservative surgery and brachytherapy for isolated breast carcinoma recurrence. *Proc European Society of Mastology*. Venice, March 1994:146a(abst).
192. Maulard C, Housset M, Brunel P, Delanian S, Taurelle R, Baillet F. Use of perioperative or split-course interstitial brachytherapy techniques for salvage irradiation of isolated local recurrences after conservative management of breast cancer. *Am J Clin Oncol* 1995;18:348.
193. Jolicoeur M, Maingon P, Bône-Lepinoy MC, et al. Combined re-excision and perioperative interstitial brachytherapy for salvage of breast conservation therapy recurrences. *Int J Radiat Oncol Biol Phys* 1997;39[Suppl]:259a(abst).
194. Resch A, Mock U, Fellner C, et al. Breast conserving surgery and PDR-brachytherapy for recurrent breast cancer after primary breast conserving treatment including EBT and HDR-brachytherapy—preliminary results. *Eur J Cancer* 1997;33[Suppl 8]:S159a(abst).
195. Mullen EE, Deutsch M, Bloomer WD. Salvage radiotherapy for local failures of lumpectomy and breast irradiation. *Radiother Oncol* 1997;42:25.
196. Deutsch M. Repeat high dose partial breast irradiation after lumpectomy for in-breast tumor recurrences following initial lumpectomy and radiotherapy. *Int J Radiat Oncol Biol Phys* 1998;42[Suppl 1]:255a(abst).
197. Kwai AH, Stomper PC, Kaplan WD. Clinical significance of isolated scintigraphic sternal lesions in patients with breast cancer. *J Nucl Med* 1988;29:324.
198. Recht A, Pierce SM, Abner A, et al. Regional nodal failure after conservative surgery and radiotherapy for early-stage breast carcinoma. *J Clin Oncol* 1991;9:988.
199. Recht A, Houlihan MJ. Axillary lymph nodes and breast cancer: a review. *Cancer* 1995;76:1491.
200. Hirn-Stadler B. Das Supraklavikularrezidiv des Mammakarzinoms. *Strahlenther Onkol* 1990;166:774.
201. Fentiman IA, Lavelle MA, Caplan D, Miller N, Millis RR, Hayward JL. The significance of supraclavicular fossa node recurrence after radical mastectomy. *Cancer* 1986;57:908.
202. Kiricuta IC, Willner J, Kölbl O, Bohndorf W. The prognostic significance of the supraclavicular lymph node metastases in breast cancer patients. *Int J Radiat Oncol Biol Phys* 1993;28:387.
203. Jackson SM. Carcinoma of the breast—the significance of supraclavicular lymph node metastases. *Clin Radiol* 1966;17:107.
204. Tomin R, Donegan WL. Screening for recurrent breast cancer—its effectiveness and prognostic value. *J Clin Oncol* 1987;5:62.
205. Bonnerot V, Dao T, Campana F, Nguyen TT, Ollivier L, Neuenschwander S. Evaluation of MR imaging for detecting recurrent tumor within irradiated brachial plexus. *Radiology* 1993;189:151a(abst).
206. Gateley CA, Mansel RE, Owen A, Redford J, Sellwood RA, Howell A. Treatment of the axilla in operable breast cancer. *Br J Surg* 1991;78:750a(abst).
207. Fowble B, Solin LJ, Schultz DJ, Goodman RL. Frequency, sites of relapse, and outcome of regional node failures following conservative surgery and radiation for early breast cancer. *Int J Radiat Oncol Biol Phys* 1989;17:703.
208. Maisano R, Adamo V, Santacaterina A, et al. Supraclavicular lymph-node metastases (SLM) from breast cancer (BC) as only site of distant disease. A curable disease? *Ann Oncol* 1996;7[Suppl 5]: 22a(abst).
209. Dunphy FR, Spitzer G, Rossiter Fornoff JE, et al. Factors predicting long-term survival for metastatic breast cancer patients treated with high-dose chemotherapy and bone marrow support. *Cancer* 1994;73:2157.

Diseases of the Breast, 2nd ed.,
edited by Jay R. Harris.
Lippincott Williams & Wilkins, Philadelphia © 2000.

CHAPTER 48

Treatment of Metastatic Breast Cancer

Matthew J. Ellis, Daniel F. Hayes, and Marc E. Lippman

Since the 1970s, advances in primary and adjuvant systemic therapies have substantially improved both survival and quality of life (QOL) in patients with newly diagnosed, locally confined (stage I to III) breast cancer. In spite of these advances, 20% to 30% of patients with breast cancer suffer a systemic relapse. Furthermore, metastatic disease is diagnosed at the time of presentation in 1% to 5% of patients. The therapeutic approach to patients with advanced breast cancer is distinct from that of patients with early-stage disease. Therefore, it is important to understand the natural history of metastatic breast cancer and to appreciate what can be accomplished by treatment.

GOALS OF THERAPY

Cure

Most patients faced with a diagnosis of breast cancer consider achieving a "cure" as their most important aim. For an individual patient, breast cancer can be considered cured if the disease is eradicated, permitting a normal life span without threat of recurrence.[1–4] Most patients perceive that they are cured if they have remained disease free after initial primary and adjuvant treatment for a prolonged period of time, usually 5 to 10 years. However, even in the primary diagnosis setting, no individual with a history of an invasive breast cancer is ever completely free from the threat of recurrence. Although the annual hazard rate of relapse is highest in the initial 5 years after diagnosis, it never returns to zero, even after 30 years.[5–9] Nonetheless, a large population of patients do achieve a cure, if *cure* is defined as achieving a risk of death within a population of breast cancer survivors that is similar to individuals in an age-matched population who never had the disease.[2] For example, as many as 75% or more of patients with node-negative breast cancer may be cured.

M. J. Ellis: Departments of Medicine and Oncology, Lombardi Cancer Center, Georgetown University Medical Center, Washington, D.C.

D. F. Hayes: Breast Cancer Program, Lombardi Cancer Center, Georgetown University Medical Center, Washington, D.C.

M. E. Lippman: Departments of Pharmacology and Medicine, Lombardi Cancer Center, Georgetown University Medical Center, Washington, D.C.

In contrast to patients with early-stage disease, women with metastatic breast cancer are unlikely to be cured by any definition. Even with the most active therapies, complete remissions are uncommon, and only a fraction of those in remission remain progression free for a prolonged period. This conclusion is illustrated by the experience with FAC [5-fluorouracil (5FU), doxorubicin, and cyclophosphamide (CPA)] chemotherapy for metastatic breast cancer at the M. D. Anderson Hospital in Houston.[10] Between the mid-1960s and the mid-1980s, nearly 1,500 patients with advanced breast cancer were treated with FAC at this institution. Of these, 245 patients were rendered free of detectable disease (complete response), and 30 (12% of the patients in complete remission, 2% of the original cohort of treatable patients) remained disease and progression free after 5 to 20 years (Fig. 1).

The Eastern Cooperative Oncology Group and Cancer and Leukemia Group B also reviewed their experience of chemotherapy for advanced disease to identify long-term survivors. They examined clinical outcomes for 378 premenopausal women with metastatic disease who were entered into randomized studies in the mid-1970s in which various permutations of oophorectomy and chemotherapy were compared.[11] Median survival was 28 months, with 22% of patients alive at 5 years. With follow-up ranging from 4 to 15 years, only 14% of patients remained alive. Even in the best prognostic group, 10-year survival was no more than 10%, with only one-half of these long-term survivors still free of disease. These data therefore suggest that 5% to 10% of patients with metastatic breast cancer may survive 5 or more years, and perhaps 2% to 5% become long-term survivors and might even be considered cured.

Prolongation of Survival

Some form of active treatment for advanced breast cancer has been available for more than a century, rendering prospective randomized clinical trials of therapy versus observation unethical.[12] In the absence of untreated controls, survival benefits associated with treatment must be estimated indirectly.[13] An important confounding factor when comparing different patient populations is the extra-

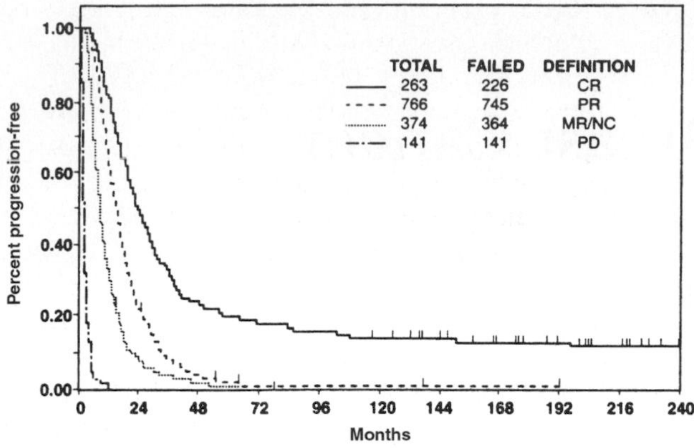

FIG. 1. Survival of patients with metastatic breast cancer after achieving complete response from treatment with cyclophosphamide (FAC): the M. D. Anderson Hospital experience. This group, which included 1,544 patients with metastatic breast cancer, was treated with 5-fluorouracil, doxorubicin, and FAC. Kaplan-Meier curve of all patients, including the 263 who achieved complete remission (CR), is shown. MR, marginal response; NC, no change; PD, progressive disease; PR, partial remission. (From ref. 10, with permission.)

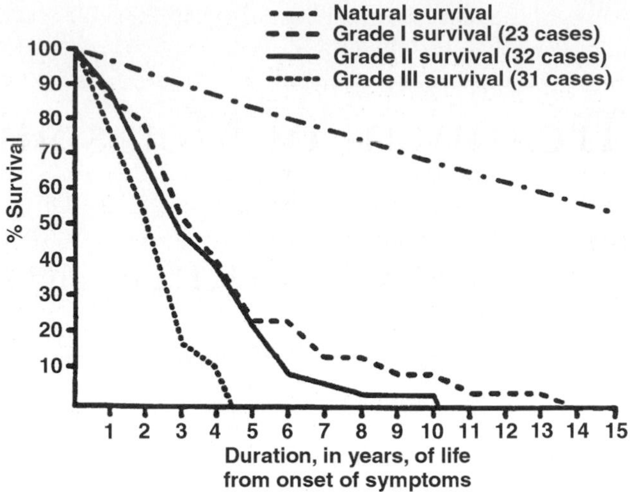

FIG. 2. Survival of patients with metastatic breast cancer: the Middlesex Hospital experience, 1805 to 1933. Two hundred fifty patients who presented to the Middlesex Hospital with what was eventually proved by autopsy to be metastatic breast cancer were followed until death. (Modified from ref. 18.)

ordinarily variable clinical course of metastatic breast cancer. The mean survival for patients with metastatic breast cancer is 18 to 24 months, but the range of survival extends from a few months to many years.[14–17] Bloom et al.[18] illustrated the remarkable heterogeneity of the untreated natural history of breast cancer by drawing on nineteenth century records from the Middlesex Hospital in London. Because the breast cancer patients described were admitted to the Middlesex for nursing and symptom management, most were, in all likelihood, suffering from locally advanced or metastatic disease. Although many of these patients died within a few months or years, some survived for 5 to 15 years, with a small group achieving survival times equivalent to those of an age-matched group of women who lived in London during the same period (Fig. 2). These observations suggest that a small population of patients with far-advanced breast cancer have very indolent disease, even without treatment.

One approach to assessing the effectiveness of therapy for breast cancer is to compare the survival of patients treated in the modern era with that of patients treated before the widespread application of chemotherapy. This approach is fraught with biases that are inherent in retrospective comparisons, including the heterogeneity of the natural and treated history of breast cancer as well as advances in medical technology. More sensitive diagnostic techniques, such as nuclear scanning, computed tomography, magnetic resonance imaging, and sensitive and specific circulating tumor markers, generate "lead time bias," also referred to as *staging drift*. These sensitive tests result in earlier identification of patients with low-volume, advanced disease who, in an earlier period, would have been considered to have disease confined to the breast. Staging drift results in an improvement of prognosis for all stages over time, independent of therapy, even if survival of the total population is unchanged. Other advances in medicine, including antibiotics, blood product support, and critical care medicine, are also likely to contribute to improved survival for contemporary patients that is independent of specific breast cancer therapies.

Many investigators have observed that patients who respond to therapy survive longer than "nonresponders." This observation has led some physicians to conclude that prolonged survival in "responders" is because of the therapy. Although this conclusion may in part be valid, factors associated with likelihood of response are also favorable prognostic factors.[19] In other words, patients who are most likely to respond are also those who are most likely to survive the longest regardless of therapeutic interventions.

Perhaps the most informative approach to assessing survival benefits is to examine prospective randomized trials in which patients were assigned a therapy that was eventually proved to be ineffective.[13] For example, in a series of randomized phase II trials, Ahmann et al.[20] compared response rates for previously untested agents with standard combination CMF (CPA, methotrexate, and 5FU) chemotherapy. Overall, the response rate to combination chemotherapy was approximately 55%. In one phase of the study, a small group of patients were assigned to methyl-CCNU, an ineffective treatment that was associated with a response rate of only 5%. Overall survival (OS) for these patients was inferior to those who received CMF, but the difference in survival between the two groups was only 6 months (mean OS, mCCNU: 11.2 months; mean OS, CMF: 18.5 months). However, because the group that received mCCNU was almost universally treated with other (presumably more effective) therapy on progression, the survival benefits for active therapy could be greater than this. More recently, at least two studies have demonstrated that estrogen deprivation therapy with a selective aromatase inhibitor (SAI) is more effective than megestrol acetate or aminoglutethimide for postmenopausal women with tamoxifen-resistant disease (see section Endocrine Therapy).[21] Several of these studies documented improved response rates for SAI therapy. Reflecting this increased activity, time to progression and OS for patients treated with an aromatase inhibitor were improved, but only by a few months.

These results suggest that systemic therapy of patients with metastatic disease probably extends survival for most patients, but only modestly so. The experiences described previously suggest that the proportional reduction in mortality from systemic therapy for metastatic breast cancer is approximately 30%. Interestingly, this relative reduction in mortality is similar to the benefit reported for adjuvant systemic therapy in the primary disease setting.[22,23] However, because the overall mortality of the group is so high (approaching or exceeding 90% at 5 years), and median OS is so short (18 to 24 months), a 30% proportional benefit is associated with only modest extensions of life for most patients.

Newly introduced therapies may further improve the odds of survival over time for patients with metastatic breast cancer. As noted, the introduction of specific and potent aromatase inhibitors appears to result in some additional survival.[21] Several new chemotherapeutic agents have now been shown to have activity in advanced disease that is resistant to standard medications; these include the taxanes, vinorelbine, and capecitabine. Moreover, studies have demonstrated that an antibody directed against *erb*-b2, designated *trastuzumab*, may also provide survival benefits when used with paclitaxel compared with paclitaxel therapy alone.[24] Finally, phase I and II clinical trials of very high dose chemotherapy, requiring bone marrow stem cell support, have frequently demonstrated that a small group of patients with metastatic disease may be rendered disease free for 2 to 5 years or more (see Chapter 38). However, it remains to be seen whether any of these therapies offers substantially prolonged survival or even higher cure rates for the large majority of patients who are currently destined to die of breast cancer within a relatively short period of time after their first recurrence.

Quality of Life

Because our current approaches to the treatment of metastatic breast cancer are not associated with dramatic survival benefits, the focus of treatment is on palliation. An improvement in QOL can often be achieved by the judicious application of both local and systemic therapies. Successful palliative therapy requires the treating physician to reduce disease-related symptoms with effective therapy without imposing excessive symptoms associated with treatment-related toxicity.

Objective documentation of palliation, unlike that of mortality or disease progression, is problematic. Most clinicians have difficulty in objectively assessing improvements in QOL. However, it is clear that patients with symptomatic metastatic disease often experience an improved sense of well-being with therapy, despite frequent toxicities. Several efforts have been made to objectively quantify QOL benefits associated with treatment for metastatic disease.[25–27] These measures require semiobjective analysis of QOL by the patient or caregiver with linear self-assessment analogue scales or other analytical tools, and it appears that QOL scores can be assigned with relatively good reproducibility. These quantitative measures permit comparisons of one type of therapy versus another. Using such scales, several investigations have now documented that despite the toxicities of therapy, chemotherapy improves QOL for a large fraction of patients, depending on the disease setting and the relative efficacy and toxicity of the agents used.[28] The issue of QOL analysis is covered in greater detail in Chapter 75.

Objective tumor response is often assumed to be a surrogate for cure, prolongation of survival, or palliation. In many clinical trials, comparison of the response rates between two treated populations is used as an end point to determine relative efficacy. By consensus, a drug is considered "active" in the metastatic setting if more than 20% of patients experience a response in a phase II trial.[29] However, response may not be a reliable surrogate for improved survival. Furthermore, more than 50% of patients with recurrent breast cancer have disease that is not considered measurable (see Chapter 46). For example, patients with bone disease or miliary pulmonary and chest wall recurrences may experience a symptomatic response, from which symptoms are reduced as a function of reduction in burden of disease. However, in these patients, response may be difficult to document. Although these women clearly benefit from treatment, they would not be scored as responders in classic clinical trial terms. Indeed, investigators have proposed that stable disease is a reasonable surrogate for successful therapy, and time to disease progression is also frequently regarded as a critical end point.[30]

In contrast, not all patients who respond to therapy benefit from that response. For example, patients with minimally symptomatic, indolent disease might respond to a given treatment, but if the treatment is fraught with considerable toxicity, the patient may not appreciate the benefit. If patient survival in this circumstance is not substantially improved, perhaps because the disease was not rapidly lethal in the first place, then the response obtained by application of that therapy is not justified.

CHOOSING THE OPTIMAL THERAPEUTIC MODALITY

The challenge to providing the best care for patients with metastatic breast cancer is to carefully weigh the odds of achieving palliation for each alternative treatment and to review treatment priorities with each patient. Some patients may be willing to accept a high burden of toxicity for small survival benefits, whereas others may only wish to be treated if toxicity is minimal and the likelihood of palliation is high.[31] To make these decisions, the clinician must (a) establish the diagnosis of advanced breast cancer, (b) estimate the patient's prognosis, (c) try to predict which therapy is most likely to be effective with the least toxicity, and (d) understand the goals of therapy for each individual.

Establish the Diagnosis of Advanced Breast Cancer and Obtain Predictive Markers for Response

Not all clinically suspicious lesions that occur after a diagnosis of breast cancer are metastases, and not all the symptoms that a patient with advanced disease experiences are due to metastases. For most patients who are not otherwise known to have suffered a recurrence, a biopsy is indicated. First, histologic confirmation reassures the clinician that he or she is treating metastatic breast cancer, because the differential diagnosis of any new lesion includes both benign processes and second malignancies. Solitary pulmonary nodules are a particularly prominent example of the need for a metastatic disease biopsy, because up to 50% of cases may actually be new primary lung cancers, especially in patients with a history of tobacco use (see Chapter 58).[32] A second reason to biopsy suspicious lesions is to obtain a more precise, and updated, characterization of relevant predictive factors. Up to 20% of measurements of estrogen receptor (ER) content between primary and metastatic lesions may be discordant, either as a function of technical assay variability or biologic heterogeneity.[33] Furthermore, with the advent of targeted therapy of *erb*-b2–positive tumors with trastuzamab, the molecular profile of metastatic disease is becoming increasingly important in selecting therapies. Skin nodules, lymph nodes, pleural effusions, and ascites can be simply evaluated by biopsy or cytology. Furthermore, important advances in transcutaneous needle aspirations and biopsies of lesions in soft tissues and even bone have made histologic confirmation of pulmonary, hepatic, and bone lesions relatively easy and safe.[34–36]

Establish Whether the Need for Successful Treatment Is Urgent (Prognosis)

In the adjuvant setting, prognostic factors such as TNM and tumor grade may help select a group of patients whose prognosis is so favorable that they might elect to forgo selected therapies, sacrificing a presumably small potential benefit to avoid associated toxicities.[37] In the metastatic setting, few patients would elect to forgo all treatments.[38,39] However, selected prognostic factors, combined with clinical judgment, might help to decide which treatment modality to apply and in what order.

Certain clinical factors predict the rate of progression and early mortality. These include the length of the interval between primary diagnosis and relapse, the number of sites of metastatic disease, and visceral organ involvement.[40,41] Favorable outcomes are most likely when a recurrence occurs 5 or more years after initial diagnosis and therapy, presumably reflecting the more indolent nature of late-relapsing breast cancers.[40–46] The site of recurrence is also important. Patients with isolated sites of metastases, especially on the chest wall or in surrounding lymph nodes, may enjoy prolonged disease-free survival after treatment (see Chapter 47). In contrast, patients with hepatic or lymphangitic pulmonary disease, or both, have shorter times to progression and OS.[40,47]

Factors that are important for prognosis in early-stage disease have been examined after relapse. Very young age (younger than 35 years) has been considered a poor prognostic factor in early-stage disease, but the effect of age on survival after recurrence is not established.[17,42,48] The original TNM stage does not provide an indication of prognosis after relapse. As in the primary setting, ER content and tumor grade are favorable prognostic factors for patients with metastatic breast cancer. In several studies, patients whose primary tumors expressed low or negative ER content and were judged to be poorly differentiated had more rapid progression and mortality after relapse when compared to patients with ER-rich and better-differentiated tumors.[17,42,48] The prognosis of patients with *erb*-b2 amplification or overexpression, or both, may also be worse in the metastatic setting, although very few, if any, studies have specifically addressed this issue.

Several prognostic indices have been proposed for metastatic breast cancer.[40,41,49] For example, a relatively simple model was developed in 1998 by investigators in the Japanese Clinical Oncology Group that incorporates history of prior adjuvant chemotherapy, presence of distant lymph node and liver metastases, elevated serum lactic dehydrogenase levels, and short disease-free interval.[50] In the initial development of this index, 233 patients with metastatic disease were stratified into three risk groups, with median survival times of 45.5, 24.6, and 10.6 months (Fig. 3). When applied to a separate set of 315 patients, the prognostic validity of this index was confirmed, with nearly identical median survival times of 49.6, 22.8, and 10 months. Individual clinicians may choose to select other prognostic indices. However, this and other studies suggest that even within the population of nearly incurable patients with metastatic breast cancer, careful selection can identify those who are relatively more likely to do well than others. One can apply this information to make rational decisions for individual patients regarding which modality, and in what order, might best be chosen to achieve optimal palliation.

Fundamentally, two classes of therapeutic modalities exist: local (e.g., surgery, radiation, hyperthermia) or systemic (e.g., endocrine therapy, chemotherapy, novel therapies). For patients who have not received any therapy for recurrent disease, the odds of response to local therapies are usually higher than for systemic therapies. However, local therapies are, of course, limited to the direct field in which the treatment can be performed or applied. Two questions must be considered when prioritizing between local and sys-

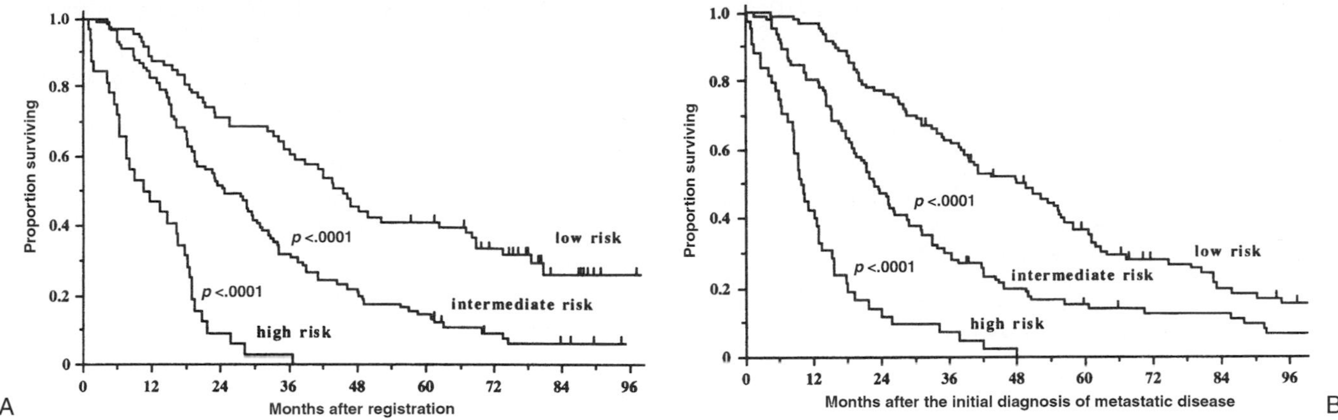

FIG. 3. Prognostic index for patients with metastatic breast cancer. These patients were categorized into one of three prognostic subgroups (low, intermediate, and high risk of death) based on prior adjuvant systemic chemotherapy, disease-free interval, sites of metastases, and lactic dehydrogenase levels. **A:** Overall surivival of 233 patients in initial study used to develop index. **B:** Overall survival of distinct set of 315 patients used for validation of index. Note that the corresponding survival curves for each category (low, intermediate, high risk) are nearly identical for each set of patients. (Modified from ref. 50.)

temic treatment: (a) Is the patient in or near a catastrophic situation locally, and (b) how widespread is the disease? For example, a patient with only local recurrence, or a patient with recurrence in a single metastatic site, might be optimally palliated with local treatment first, or perhaps even alone without systemic therapy, until she subsequently suffers relapse or progression. Likewise, a patient with a single bone lesion who is quite symptomatic or has evidence of impending fracture, or both, is better treated with surgery and radiation than with systemic therapy. On the other hand, a patient with widespread multisite disease who has minimal to moderate symptoms is better served with systemic treatment, saving the local therapy for later, more urgent events. These considerations are covered in more detail in Chapters 60, 61, and 62 (Fig. 4). Systemic therapy and local therapy can be overlapped in urgent cases. Combining modalities can be accomplished easily in some circumstances (endocrine therapy plus radiation) but may be more problematic in others (chemotherapy plus surgery).

The choice of which systemic therapy to administer should also be based on the sense of urgency related to the site of disease and its apparent relative growth rate (Fig. 5). As discussed in the following sections, predictive factors, such as ER content, may help to guide the choice of therapy by providing an indication of how likely it is that a given modality will produce a response. However, one should not base the decision as to whether to use endocrine or chemotherapy solely on predictive factors.[51] The risks and benefits for each therapy also need to be considered. For example, because palliation is more likely for a patient who experiences a response to endocrine therapy compared to similar response induced by chemotherapy, an initial trial of endocrine therapy is preferred for patients who are likely to respond (see the section Endocrine Therapy). However, for symptomatic patients whose conditions are likely to be refractory to endocrine therapy, chemotherapy is a better initial choice, despite its increased toxicity-benefit ratio. Perhaps the most compelling factor in deciding to treat a patient with endocrine therapy rather than chemotherapy is whether the patient can afford the consequences of not receiving an active therapy during the first few months after initiation of treatment should endocrine therapy not work.

Together, these considerations suggest that a patient with slowly progressive disease, no visceral organ involvement, and minimal symptom burden might be best served with a trial of endocrine therapy, even if her tumor has low ER expression. Although the chance of a response may be lower in ER-poor tumors, it is never absent. The benefit of an "endocrine therapy first" approach is that if a response occurs, it will be associated with a good QOL, given the favorable toxicity profile of most endocrine treatments. Fur-

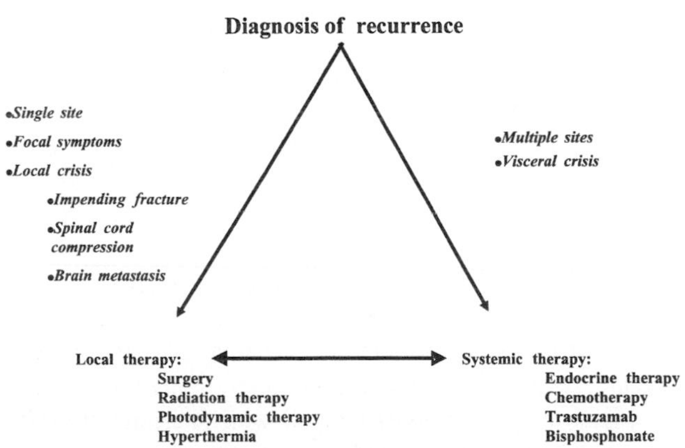

FIG. 4. Decision algorithm for patients with metastatic breast cancer: local versus systemic therapy.

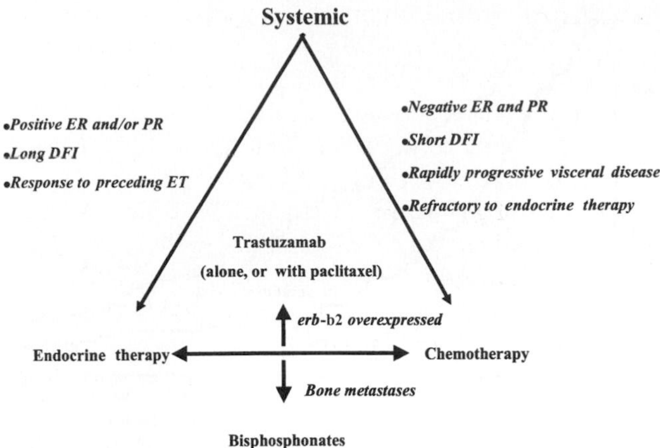

FIG. 5. Decision algorithm for patients with metastatic breast cancer. Selection of systemic modality: endocrine therapy (ET) versus chemotherapy. DFI, disease-free interval; ER, estrogen receptor; PR, progesterone receptor.

thermore, if there is no response in the "good prognosis" patient, she is not substantially less likely to respond to chemotherapy, because her performance status or visceral function will probably not have declined significantly. In contrast, a patient with rapidly growing disease, especially if it involves visceral organs such as the lung or liver, or both, is better treated with chemotherapy first, because it is almost always more likely to induce a response than is endocrine therapy under these circumstances. In cases with rapid progression, the clinician needs to avoid a period of ineffective therapy in which performance status and organ function may decline, substantially reducing the chances of a response to the next therapeutic modality.

Predictive Factors

Local Therapy

The most important factors that predict the success of local therapy are those that indicate the extent of the disease. Larger and more extensive tumors are more difficult to resect or encompass in the field of irradiation, and they are therefore more likely to recur at the site[52] (see Chapter 47). Molecular factors for response to irradiation have been investigated. Two promising factors, although still investigational, are p53 status and insulinlike growth factor I receptor (IGF-IR) expression. In several studies, patients whose tumors harbor mutations in p53 appear less likely to benefit from radiation and more likely to relapse in irradiated fields.[53,54] However, the results of at least one study do not suggest that p53 abnormalities predict higher local relapse rates after radiation.[55] IGF-IR expression may also be associated with resistance to radiation. In a small but provocative case control study, it was observed that patients who had local relapse after breast irradiation were more likely to have high tissue levels of IGF-IR than those who did not suffer local recurrence.[56] Neither p53 nor IGF-IR has been sufficiently studied to determine whether it should be used to make clinical decisions, such as forgoing radiation therapy in favor of other treatment modalities if radiation would normally be indicated.[57,58]

TABLE 1. *Response to endocrine therapy by hormone receptor status*

Estrogen receptor	Progesterone receptor	Response to endocrine therapy
Negative	Negative	<10%
Positive	Negative	20–30%
Negative	Positive	30–50%
Positive	Positive	50–75%

Modified from ref. 62.

Endocrine Therapy

Clinical features that predict responsiveness to endocrine therapy in the metastatic setting include a long relapse-free interval, metastatic sites restricted to bone and soft tissue, and previous response to endocrine therapy.[59,60] However, in all of oncology, perhaps the best example of a predictive factor for a specific systemic therapy is tumor content of ER. Measurement of tumor ER is routinely used to further assist in the decision to use endocrine therapy, as ER expression is associated with a 50% to 60% likelihood of a response, whereas ER-low tumors have a less than 10% chance of response[61] (Table 1). Progesterone receptor (PR) is an estrogen-regulated gene whose expression indicates that ER is functional. Measurement of PR expression therefore improves the predictive power of ER analysis.[62] However, fully 20% to 25% of ER-positive, PR-positive tumors remain resistant to tamoxifen. This finding implies that tamoxifen resistance occurs even when estrogen signaling is intact and that other, as yet unidentified, factors may also be required for a response to tamoxifen. The molecular basis of ER as a predictive factor, as well as newer investigational markers, such as *erb*-b2, are discussed extensively in the section Endocrine Therapy for Metastatic Breast Cancer.

As discussed previously, the decision to withhold endocrine therapy and proceed with chemotherapy is clear-cut for symptomatic patients with ER-negative, PR-negative metastatic tumors, because the response rate to endocrine therapy is unacceptably low (10% or less). However, the occasional response to endocrine therapy in ER-negative cells may in part be explained by false-negative ER analysis.[63] A trial of endocrine therapy is particularly appropriate if the patient displays other clinical features of endocrine therapy–responsive disease (long disease-free interval, bone and soft-tissue disease, and an indolent pattern of progression). It can be reasonably stated that a trial of endocrine therapy should be offered to every patient at some time during the course of her illness.

Chemotherapy

Unlike ER and endocrine therapy, no predictive test for a response to chemotherapy has been sufficiently validated to use in a standard clinical setting.[57] For patients who have not been previously treated with chemotherapy in the metastatic setting, the odds of responding, and therefore benefiting, are usually quite high, on the order of 50% to 75%. The most consistent predictors of resistance (failure to benefit) to chemotherapy are nonspecific clinical features, including progression on prior chemotherapy in the metastatic setting or relapse within 12 months after adjuvant chemotherapy, poor performance status, and increasing number of sites of disease, especially when visceral.[40,41,50,64–71]

Many efforts have been made to identify more accurate predictors of response to chemotherapy. An appealing approach is to establish short-term breast cancer cultures to directly assay chemotherapy sensitivity and resistance. Although initial investigations were met with enthusiasm, subsequent studies of the predictive use of "culture and sensitivity" for breast cancer have been disappointing, in part because of the difficulty of growing primary breast cancers in culture.[72–76] Several investigators have used more sophisticated culturing techniques to establish more reliable assays.[77–81] For example, investigators from San Antonio report that short-term cultures could be established from approximately 75% of patients who were treated with continuous-infusion 5FU.[82] The response rate overall was 24%. Of 25 patients who were evaluable, *in vitro* response was significantly correlated with clinical response ($p = .002$). Of six clinical responders, five also responded *in vitro*, for an assay sensitivity of 83%. Of 19 nonresponders, 17 were nonresponders *in vitro*, for a specificity of 89%. The positive predictive value of the test was 71% (5 of 7), and the negative predictive value was 94% (17 of 18). In other studies, it appears that *in vitro* prediction of high levels of resistance is strongly correlated with poor response to chemotherapy, but *in vitro* sensitivity is not as predictive of response.[77,81,83] Moreover, *in vitro* assay results may depend on the specific drug tested and the methods used in the assay.[77,83] Nonetheless, these encouraging results suggest that this approach may be feasible in the future for other drugs, although *in vitro* drug resistance assays remain investigational at present.[78–81,83]

Distinct molecular markers have been evaluated as potential predictive factors for chemotherapy in general or for certain specific agents. Soon after the discovery of ER as a predictive factor for response to endocrine therapy, several investigators evaluated its relative worth as a predictor of response to chemotherapy. Overall the data are mixed, but there is some suggestion that patients with ER-positive tumors are less likely to respond to chemotherapy than those with ER-negative tumors.[84–90] Because ER itself is not likely to be a target of chemotherapy, it probably serves as a surrogate of other important biological pathways that serve to render cancer cells sensitive or resistant to chemotherapy. Markers of cellular proliferation, such as flow cytometric evaluation of the fraction of cells in S phase, determination of radiolabeled thymidine uptake, and immunohistochemical staining for the proliferation antigen Ki67 are all associated with higher chemotherapy response rates.[55,91–94] However, none of these markers is sufficiently accurate to form the basis of a decision to treat or withhold therapy.

A number of gene products are currently under investigation as chemotherapy response markers, including *p*-glycoprotein (gp170), a drug efflux pump that mediates multidrug resistance (MDR), the tumor suppressor p53, and the protooncogene *erb*-b2. *p*-Glycoprotein gp170 is overexpressed in approximately 40% of breast cancers and is associated with resistance to drugs with a plant or bacterial origin.[95] However, heterogeneity in the design of the reported investigations makes it impossible to draw solid conclusions regarding the role of gp170 chemotherapy resistance in breast cancer. Likewise, preclinical and several preliminary clinical studies suggest that cancers with mutated p53 are less likely to respond to chemotherapy.[96–101] However, studies that consider response rates to individual therapies, or specific doses, are contradictory, perhaps because specific p53 mutations may predict differential effects of different classes of chemotherapeutic agents. Substantially more research is required before evaluation of p53 mutation status can be used to make clinical decisions in breast cancer.[57]

Perhaps the most exciting data relate to the protooncogene, c-*erb*-b2, also designated *HER-2* or c-*neu* (in this chapter, we designate this gene and its products as *erb*-b2). *Erb*-b2 amplification and overexpression have been implicated as a prognostic factor, independent of systemic therapy, but several investigations have also suggested that it may be a predictive factor for resistance to, or benefit from, certain systemic therapies (Table 2). In this regard, preclinical and clinical studies have suggested that *erb*-b2 amplification and overexpression are associated with resistance to endocrine therapy, although not all studies support this hypothesis (see discussion in Endocrine Therapy regarding *erb*-b2 and endocrine therapy).[102–108] *Erb*-b2 amplification

TABLE 2. *Possible roles of* erb*-b2 amplification or overexpression, or both, as a prognostic factor*

Role of *erb*-b2	Possible clinical use: hypothetic better or worse outcome if *erb*-b2 positive compared to *erb*-b2 negative
Prognosis	Worse
Predictive	—
Hormone therapy	Worse
Chemotherapy	—
CMF-like therapy	Worse
Doxorubicin-containing therapy	Equal or better
Taxanes	Data insufficient to develop hypothesis
Trastuzamab	Better

CMF, cyclophosphamide, methotrexate, 5-fluorouracil.

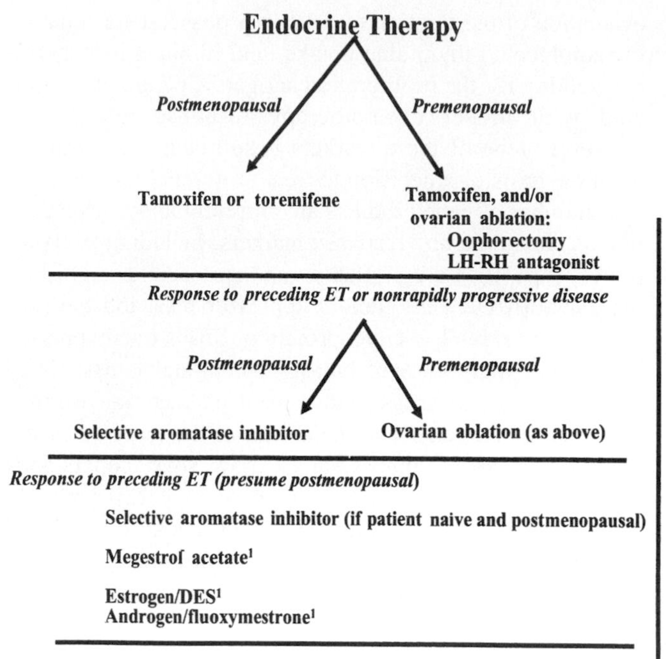

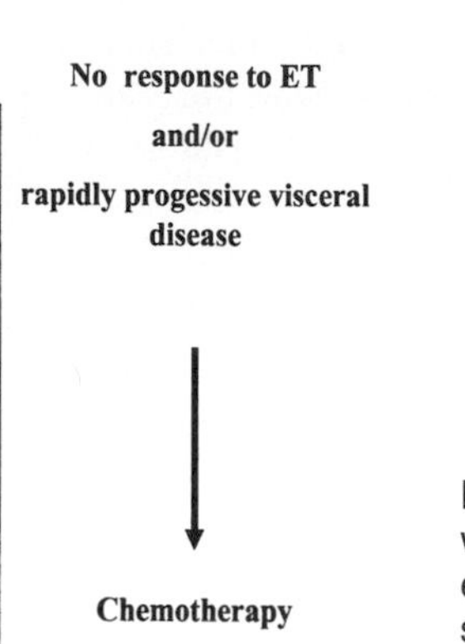

FIG. 6. Decision algorithm for patients with metastatic breast cancer: sequential endocrine therapies (ET). DES, diethylstilbestrol; LH–RH, leutenizing hormone–releasing hormone. [1]Information limited regarding response data after disease progression after tamoxifen and selective aromatase inhibitor.

and overexpression can also predict sensitivity or resistance to certain kinds of chemotherapy. For example, results of several studies have suggested that patients whose tumors overexpress *erb*-b2 are less likely to benefit from adjuvant nondoxorubicin-containing regimens—such as CMF or phenyl-alanine mustard, 5-fluorouracil (Pf)—than patients whose tumors have normal *erb*-b2 expression levels.[109–111] Furthermore, *erb*-b2–positive patients seem to benefit from the addition of doxorubicin.[111–113] Finally, although not fully evaluated, it is likely that therapies directed against *erb*-b2, such as trastuzamab, will be most effective in those patients whose tumors overexpress cell surface *erb*-b2.[24,114–116] Currently, in the metastatic setting, *erb*-b2 should be used principally to select patients for trastuzamab therapy.

TREATMENT ALGORITHMS

Determination of the diagnosis, prognosis, and predictive factor profile should permit the clinician to plan an optimal approach toward treating patients with metastatic breast cancer (see Figs. 3–7). For patients with metastases isolated to a single site, or for those patients with impending catastrophes—for example, fracture or spinal cord compression—local therapies are a reasonable first choice (see Fig. 4). If systemic therapy is indicated, and if an endocrine response is likely, endocrine therapy is the preferred first-line systemic treatment (see Figs. 5 and 6). For those patients with rapidly progressive disease, marked visceral involvement, and a high symptom burden who are unlikely to respond to endocrine therapy, or those whose disease has become refractory to endocrine therapy, chemotherapy is likely to provide improvement of QOL for some time (see Figs. 5 and 7). Trastuzamab is appropriate for *erb*-b2–positive patients, but insufficient experience is available to provide precise guidelines regarding when it should be initiated. Current indications include its use as a single agent for patients whose disease has become refractory to other therapy or in combination with paclitaxel when use of that agent is appropriate. The combination of trastuzamab with doxorubicin-containing regimens should be avoided, and the role of combinations with other chemotherapeutic agents or with endocrine therapies remains undefined. Bisphosphonate therapy is indicated for any patient with lytic, and probably blastic, bone metastases, in combination with either endocrine therapy or chemotherapy (see Chapter 61) (see Figs. 5–7).

Combining Modalities

In theory, one might increase the overall benefit from systemic therapy by combining chemotherapy and endocrine therapy. Such a strategy might be successful based on simple additive effects. Moreover, investigators have published preclinical models suggesting that endocrine therapy might be used to "synchronize" proliferating neoplastic cells so that chemotherapy is more effective, resulting in a synergistic effect.[117] Of course, combining therapies also leads to additive toxicities. Therefore, if this strategy does not substantially prolong survival, palliation will suffer. Furthermore, other preclinical models have suggested that certain combinations might be antagonistic.[118]

Several randomized trials comparing combined chemotherapy and endocrine therapy either to endocrine therapy alone or

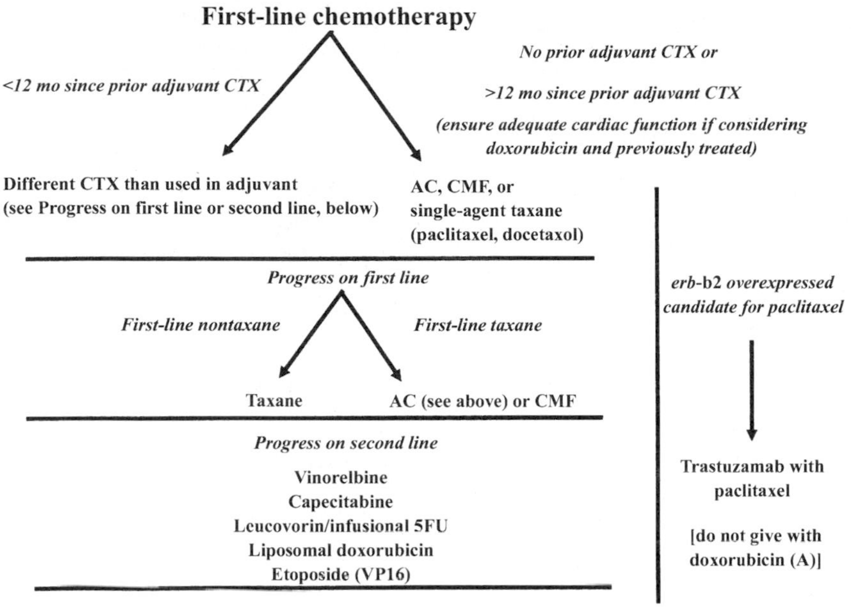

First-line chemotherapy

<12 mo since prior adjuvant CTX

No prior adjuvant CTX or
>12 mo since prior adjuvant CTX
(ensure adequate cardiac function if considering doxorubicin and previously treated)

Different CTX than used in adjuvant (see Progress on first line or second line, below)

AC, CMF, or single-agent taxane (paclitaxel, docetaxol)

Progress on first line

First-line nontaxane → **Taxane**

First-line taxane → **AC (see above) or CMF**

Progress on second line

Vinorelbine
Capecitabine
Leucovorin/infusional 5FU
Liposomal doxorubicin
Etoposide (VP16)

erb-b2 overexpressed candidate for paclitaxel

Trastuzamab with paclitaxel

[do not give with doxorubicin (A)]

FIG. 7. Decision algorithm for patients with metastatic breast cancer: sequential chemotherapies (CTX). AC, doxorubicin, cyclophosphamide; CMF, cyclophosphamide, methotrexate, 5-fluorouracil (5FU).

to chemotherapy alone have been reported. Efforts to induce higher response rates by estrogen "priming" have been unsuccessful.[117,119–121] When the intent of combining endocrine and chemotherapy has been additive, response rates for the combination of modalities are usually higher, but the OS benefits are either modest or nonexistent. In 1998, Fossati et al.[122] performed an overview of published randomized trials in patients with metastatic breast cancer. They detected no OS advantage in prospective randomized comparisons of combinations of chemotherapy plus tamoxifen, chemotherapy plus estrogen, chemotherapy plus oophorectomy, and chemotherapy plus medroxyprogesterone acetate versus chemotherapy alone (Fig. 8). One can conclude that for most patients, serial application of chemotherapy after a patient's disease has become refractory to endocrine therapy is optimal for QOL, and survival is not compromised (see Figs. 5–7).

Monitoring Therapy

Judicious serial application of therapy requires careful assessments of the success of each regimen. The optimal approach toward monitoring patients with metastatic breast cancer is not well established. One can monitor such patients by taking a careful history, performing a physical examination, serially evaluating circulating tumor markers and radiographic studies, or performing any combination of these. A more detailed discussion of the use of markers and radiographic tests for monitoring patients who are free of disease after primary and adjuvant treatment is provided in Chapter 46. The principal reason for monitoring patients with metastatic disease is to determine whether the currently applied treatment is achieving the desired goal or whether one should choose an alternative and presumably less desirable (because it was not chosen in the first place) therapeutic maneuver.

If palliation is the primary objective of therapy, one could argue that clinical history alone is sufficient to determine success of therapy. Furthermore, if the patient has easily accessible and measurable disease, such as large chest wall nodules or palpable lymphadenopathy, physical examination may provide an unequivocal indication of response or progression. In the face of dramatic reduction of symptoms that were clearly related to the metastases or a clearly demonstrable reduction in the size of palpable lesions, or both, markers and radiographic tests are likely to be irrelevant. In this case, these tests simply confirm what the clinician and patient already know: that the patient is benefiting from the therapy. However, many patients have more subtle signs and symptoms that may actually be confused with toxicity of therapy or with other conditions not related to the malignancy. Furthermore, nearly 50% of patients with newly diagnosed metastatic breast cancer have disease that is not easily measured by physical examination, such as bone-only, pleural, or miliary (multiple, smaller than 1-cm) skin metastases. In these patients, surrogate indicators of benefit or progression, such as changes in serial circulating markers or findings on radiographic evaluations, or both, can be essential in deciding whether to continue the present therapy or to proceed with whatever might be the next appropriate treatment (see Figs. 4–7). Indeed, in a set of practice guidelines proposed by an expert panel convened by the American Society of Clinical Oncology in 1997, monitoring "selected" patients with metastatic disease was the sole recommended use for circulating tumor markers.[57,58]

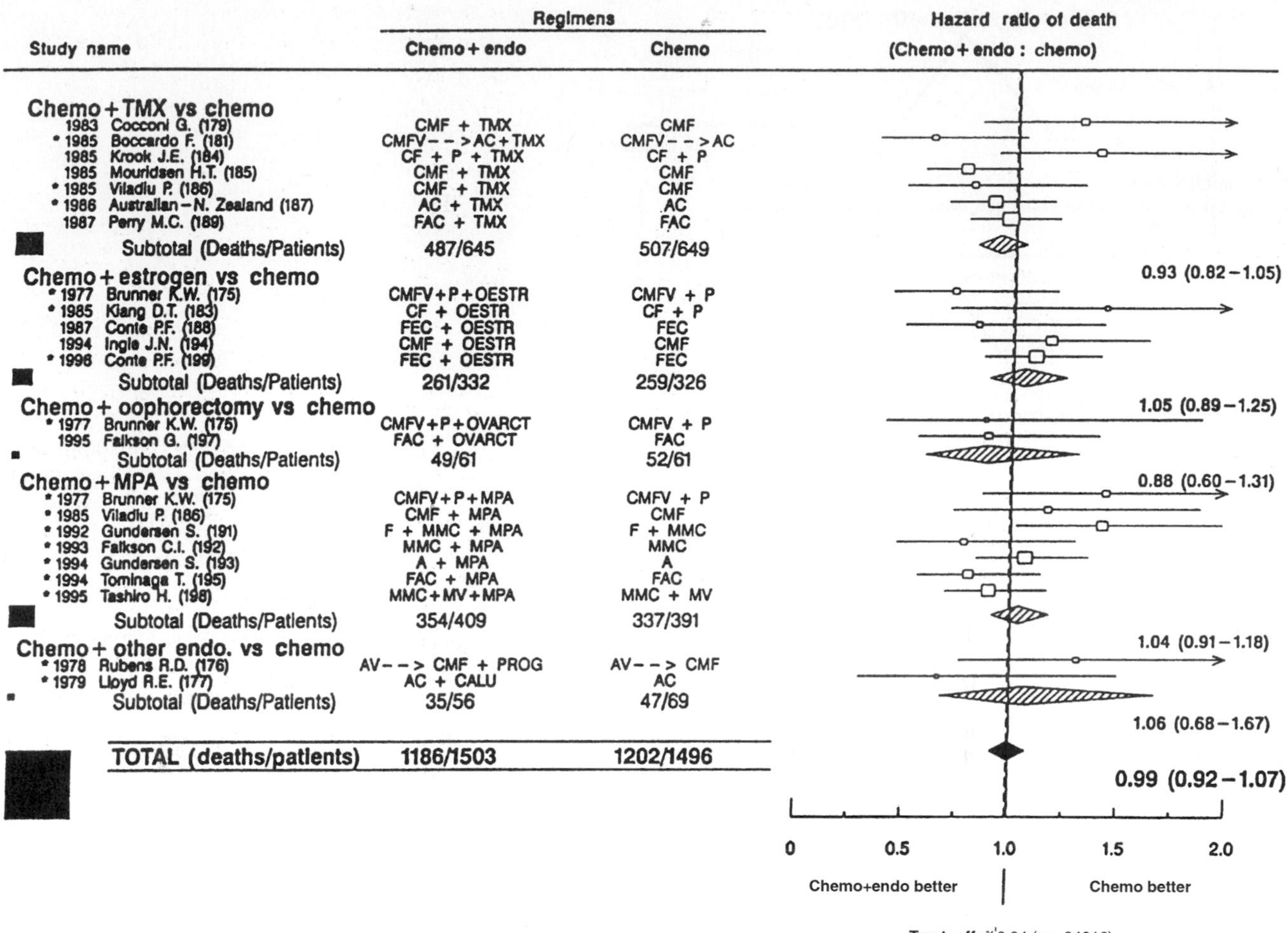

FIG. 8. Chemotherapy plus hormone therapy versus chemotherapy alone for patients with metastatic breast cancer: a systematic review. All prospective randomized studies published as of December 31, 1997, were reviewed and included in this analysis. Test for heterogeneity: X^2HetT = 28.6, df = 22, p = .15; X^2HetB = 2.45, df = 4, p = .65; X^2HetW = 26.15, df = 18, p = .09. *Hazard ratio (HR) obtained from survival curves; A, doxorubicin; C, cyclophosphamide; CALU, calusterone; E, epirubicin; F, 5-fluorouracil; M, methotrexate; MMC, mitomycin-C; MPA, medroxyprogesterone acetate; OESTR, diethylstilbestrol/conjugated estrogens; OVARCT, oophorectomy; P, prednisone/prednisolone; PROG, norethisterone acetate; TMX, tamoxifen; V, vincristine; open boxes, HR results from individual studies; cross-hatched and filled triangles, subtotal and overall HR with their 95% confidence intervals. (From ref. 122, with permission.)

Although the use of tumor markers for screening for recurrence is not established, determination of serial levels of these markers can be helpful to aid in monitoring the clinical course of patients with metastatic breast cancer who are receiving palliative therapy.[57,58,123,124] Serial MUC1 protein (e.g., CA15-3 and/or CA27.29) levels correlate with disease course in 60% to 70% of metastatic patients during therapy, compared with only approximately 40% correlation for carcinoembryonic antigen.[124,125] Serial tumor marker levels can be particularly helpful in increasing or decreasing the clinical suggestion of a change in clinical course. For example, if a patient receiving therapy is believed to have a 30% chance of progressing, but the CA15-3 level increases by more than 25%, the probability of true progression (assuming that the elevation is not a spike, discussed in the next paragraph) is raised to 75%. Thus, serial tumor marker levels can be used as an adjunct to other clinical evaluations for patients whose disease course is difficult to determine. Moreover, judicious use of serial tumor marker levels may decrease the cost of care by minimizing the need for more expensive radiographic evaluation.[126]

One must be aware of some caveats in evaluating these surrogate indicators of disease course. Up to 20% of patients treated with successful systemic therapy may experience a so-called tumor marker "spike" or "flare" during the first 1 to 2 months after initiation of treatment[127,128] (Fig. 9). This transient increase in marker levels, followed by a decline to and below baseline, is probably due to release of antigen during therapy-induced cytolysis of tumor cells. Furthermore, most circulating tumor markers, including carcinoembryonic antigen and the products of the MUC1 gene (CA15-3, CA27.29),

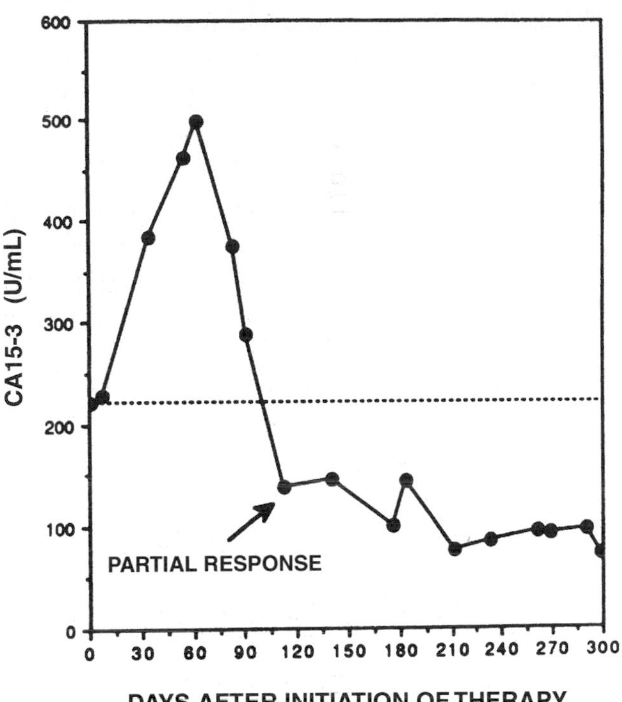

FIG. 9. Tumor marker spike. Serial CA15-3 levels were followed in a patient who responded to combination chemotherapy. (From ref. 123, with permission.)

are produced and cleared by the liver. Patients who have abnormal liver function, especially if caused by benign inflammatory processes, may have falsely elevated and rising marker levels that are easily confused with progressive cancer.[125]

Serial radiographic evaluations, using plain radiographs, computed tomography, or both; magnetic resonance imaging; and positron emission tomography (PET) scanning, can provide reliable indications of tumor response or progression. Serial bone scintigraphy results can also be helpful in monitoring patients, but if not carefully interpreted, they may be misleading. The radionuclide used in bone scintigraphy, technetium 99 phosphonate, is taken up by osteoblastic activity surrounding metastatic deposits, rather than by the cancer cells themselves. Therefore, in a patient who experiences a response to therapy, one may see a "scintigraphic healing flare" in serial bone scans that may appear as early as 2 months, peak as late as 6 months, and persist for as long as 9 to 12 months after initiation of therapy.[129,130]

Of course, a worsening bone scan, defined as increased uptake at previously known sites or the appearance of new sites of tracer uptake, or both, can also indicate progressive disease. These two circumstances (scintigraphic flare and progressive disease) can often be distinguished by placing the results of the bone scan in the clinical context (does the patient have better or worse symptoms?) or by performing ancillary testing. For example, a declining tumor marker level may indicate that the patient is responding.[125] In this situation, plain film radiographs of the scintigraphically "positive" bony areas can be very helpful. Sclerosis of previously lytic lesions is highly indicative of response, and appearance or enlargement of lysis is almost certainly associated with progression.[131] In some patients, bone metastases are principally sclerotic. In these cases, serial plain films are less helpful, because one cannot observe lytic to sclerotic changes usually associated with healing. In contrast, bone metastases in other patients may be purely lytic. In these cases, technetium 99 phosphate bone scintigraphy may be falsely negative, and plain film skeletal surveys can be quite helpful, diagnostically and for monitoring purposes.

Flare reactions can also be detected by fluorodeoxyglucose PET.[132] In a small study, seven tamoxifen responders (none of whom had a clinical flare reaction) had a significant increase in glucose uptake 7 to 10 days after starting tamoxifen, whereas the four nonresponders did not. These data suggest that metabolic flare detected by PET might predict responsiveness to tamoxifen.

When used together, clinical, biochemical, and radiographic monitoring can be carefully applied to optimize treatment of patients with metastatic breast cancer. These indicators of disease status can help the clinician decide whether to continue treatment that is likely to be of value for the patient or to proceed with the next appropriate modality (see Figs. 4–7). With a combination of clinical judgment and serial changes in monitoring studies, the clinician can serially apply surgery, radiation, hormonal, chemo-, and immunotherapies in a manner designed to achieve successful and prolonged palliation.

In summary, most patients with metastatic breast cancer can benefit from local and systemic therapies. Many experience modest survival prolongation, some live for many years longer, and a few may actually be cured. More important, a large fraction of patients will achieve palliation by thoughtful application of surgery, radiation, endocrine therapy, and chemotherapy. Many therapeutic choices are available, so that a sophisticated understanding of how and when these therapies work will help the clinician provide optimal care for patients in this setting.

ENDOCRINE THERAPY FOR METASTATIC BREAST CANCER

The favorable benefit-toxicity ratio of endocrine therapy for breast cancer, because of the selective nature of targeting of the estrogen/ER pathway, has made this modality the treatment of choice for many patients with breast cancer. Beatson's[12] historic observations on breast cancer regression after oophorectomy, published in 1896, provided the first insight into the estrogen-dependent nature of breast cancer. Further surgical research followed, initiating a century-long search for new breast cancer endocrine therapies that continues with considerable vigor. Initially, researchers focused on procedures that

TABLE 3. *Alternative endocrine therapies for breast cancer*

Endocrine therapy class	Agent
Antiestrogens with mixed agonist/antagonist profile	Tamoxifen Toremifene Idoxifene Droloxifene Raloxifene SERM3
Pure antiestrogens with no agonist properties	Faslodex EM800
Aromatase inhibitors—steroidal	Formestane Exemestane
Aromatase inhibitors—nonsteroidal	Anastrozole Letrozole Aminoglutethimide
Luteinizing hormone–releasing hormone agonists	Leuprolide Goserelin
Sex steroids—progestins	Megestrol acetate Medroxyprogesterone acetate
Sex steroids—estrogens	Diethylstilbestrol Premarin
Sex steroids—androgens	Fluoxymesterone
Retinoids	All transretinoic acid Fenretinide Targretin
erb-b2/HER-2/neu targeting antibody	Trastuzamab

SERM, selective estrogen receptor modulator.

removed other endocrine organs besides the ovaries. Twenty percent to 40% of patients experienced disease regression in response to resection of the adrenal glands and pituitary, although at considerable cost in terms of surgical morbidity and mortality.[133–135] Starting in the 1960s, ablative surgery began to be replaced by pharmacologic approaches.[136] Currently, most patients are managed with medical rather than surgical forms of endocrine therapy, which are listed in Table 3. In this discussion, breast cancer endocrine therapies that target sex hormone receptors are classified in the following way: (a) antiestrogens, (b) estrogen deprivation therapies, and (c) sex steroid therapies, including androgens, estrogens, and progestins. A separate category of "endocrine treatments" has been added, in which therapies are directed toward signal transduction pathways separate from ER. These "sex steroid receptor–independent" endocrine therapies target other steroid hormone receptors or peptide growth factor receptors that are involved in the growth, death, or differentiation of breast cancer cells. Agents in this new class of endocrine therapies include the *erb*-b2 targeting antibody, trastuzamab, and several classes of retinoids.

Endocrine Therapy Algorithm

Because palliation is the principal goal of therapy, one can be relatively pragmatic about selection of hormonal agents for individual patients. However, results from four decades of clinical trials, in which new approaches were compared with contemporary "standard therapies," provide important information regarding the optimal sequence of endocrine therapies (see Fig. 6). In general, these trials have tended to demonstrate that different endocrine therapies are equivalent in terms of efficacy, but they may differ substantially in regard to safety and tolerability. As a result, relative toxicity, rather than progressive improvements in antitumor activity, has governed the preference for particular therapies.[137] For both pre- and postmenopausal women with advanced disease, tamoxifen is usually selected as first-line endocrine therapy. Although tamoxifen does not appear to have superior activity to alternatives such as oophorectomy, high-dose estrogen, or megestrol acetate, its safety and tolerability are clearly superior.[138–140] After disease progression on tamoxifen, estrogen deprivation therapy with either luteinizing hormone– releasing hormone agonists (LHRH-A) or oophorectomy is a favored approach for premenopausal women. Consideration can also be given to combining tamoxifen with LHRH-A at the outset of treatment.[141–144]

In contrast, oophorectomy and LHRH-A are ineffective treatments for postmenopausal women.[145,146] Historically, high-dose estrogen was the first effective endocrine therapy for postmenopausal women and remained the therapy of choice for metastatic breast cancer through the mid to late 1970s.[147,148] Estrogen therapy was quickly replaced by tamoxifen for first-line treatment. Even as second-line therapy, estrogen was subsequently replaced by other, better tolerated medications, such as megestrol acetate, medroxyprogesterone acetate, aminoglutethimide, or a combination of these.[140,149,150] In the 1990s, SAIs replaced all of these alternatives for second-line therapy, because they appear to have safety and efficacy advantages over megestrol acetate and aminoglutethimide.[151–153]

Patients with disease progression after tamoxifen and an SAI are a newly defined group in whom to consider third-line endocrine therapy. For patients with a clear history of a prior response to first- or second-line treatment, or both, progestational agents, such as megestrol acetate, and even androgenic agents can be considered. The following sections expand on these conclusions, discussing each class of endocrine therapy in turn to further justify the treatment algorithm.

TAMOXIFEN: CLINICAL ASPECTS

The decline in breast cancer mortality in Western countries is considered to be in part because of tamoxifen,[154] and tamoxifen is arguably the single most useful drug in the treatment of both early- and advanced-stage disease.[63] Tamoxifen is a nonsteroidal triphenylethylene that was first synthesized in 1966. The drug was initially developed as an oral contraceptive, but instead of blocking ovarian function, it induces ovulation. Activity in metastatic breast cancer was first described in the early 1970s, and tamoxifen rapidly became

TABLE 4. *Toxicities of tamoxifen for patients at high risk from breast cancer*

Adverse event (per 1,000 women/yr)	Placebo	Tamoxifen	Excess of adverse events in tamoxifen group
Cerebrovascular accident	0.92	1.45	0.53
Transient ischemic attack	0.96	0.73	−0.23
Pulmonary embolism	0.23	0.69	0.46
Deep vein thrombosis	0.84	1.34	0.5
Cataract development	21.72	24.82	3.1
Invasive endometrial cancer	0.91	2.30	1.39
In situ endometrial cancer	0.18	0.06	−0.12
Total adverse events	**25.76**	**31.39**	**5.63**

From ref. 173, with permission.

the drug of choice for advanced disease. Response rates to tamoxifen range from 16% to 56%, and the toxicity profile is clearly superior to that of previous endocrine therapies, such as high-dose estrogen or adrenalectomy.[138–140,155–158] The favorable experience with tamoxifen in the metastatic setting led to prospective randomized clinical trials of tamoxifen as adjuvant therapy (reviewed in Chapter 37). A recent meta-analysis concluded that 5 years of adjuvant tamoxifen therapy almost halves the 10-year recurrence risk for patients with ER-positive tumors and cuts the 10-year risk of death by 26%.[23] Unfortunately, this important mortality reduction observed in the adjuvant setting is in marked contrast with the outcomes in metastatic disease, in which tamoxifen is rarely associated with irreversible remissions. Nonetheless, patients with metastatic disease may achieve excellent disease control and palliation with tamoxifen. Although the overall mean time to disease progression for patients with metastatic disease treated with tamoxifen is approximately 6 months, the duration of response (for those who do respond) is between 12 and 18 months, and responses in some patients may persist for several years.[140,158–160]

Recognition that Tamoxifen Is a Mixed Estrogen Receptor Agonist and Antagonist

Initially, tamoxifen was believed to be an "antiestrogen" in breast tissue through competitive inhibition of estrogen binding to ER. With increasing experience, clinicians observed effects of tamoxifen on several other organ systems. For example, tamoxifen is associated with the development of endometrial cancer and venous thrombosis, which are now recognized to be a result of estrogenic effects on endometrium and the coagulation system.[161–167] The paradoxic estrogenic action of tamoxifen is also associated with beneficial effects on bone and potentially the cardiovascular system, because prolonged tamoxifen use improves bone mineral density and blood lipid profile.[168–172] Furthermore, the mixed agonist/antagonist characteristics of tamoxifen explain, in part, several unusual, well-described clinical syndromes associated with treatment with the drug, including tamoxifen-induced flare reactions and tumor regressions after withdrawal of tamoxifen therapy.

Tamoxifen Toxicity

The complex risk-benefit analysis generated by the tissue-specific mixed agonist/antagonist actions of tamoxifen has to be carefully considered when prescribing tamoxifen in the adjuvant and prevention settings. These considerations are less critical in the metastatic setting, but important side effects must be considered. The tamoxifen chemoprevention trial, National Surgical Adjuvant Breast and Bowel Project (NSABP) P-01, has established one of the most accurate sources of information on tamoxifen toxicity, because the true incidence of tamoxifen side effects was not obscured by tumor-related medical problems.[173] In NSABP P-01, the excess incidence of serious adverse events (pulmonary embolus, deep venous thrombosis, cerebrovascular accident, cataract, and endometrial cancer) for patients who received tamoxifen therapy was five to six events per 1,000 patient-years of treatment. Less serious but troublesome side effects of tamoxifen included hot flashes, nausea, and vaginal discharge. Depression is also considered a side effect of tamoxifen, although there was no clear evidence of this association for women who received tamoxifen or placebo in NSABP P-01. The incidence of tamoxifen side effects from NSABP P-01 are summarized in Table 4. In summary, tamoxifen therapy is usually well tolerated, and serious toxicities occur in approximately 1 in 200 patients annually. Tamoxifen is therefore suitable for almost any patient in whom endocrine therapy for metastatic disease is being considered. Patients with a significant history of thrombosis are an exception. In this situation, estrogen deprivation therapy can be considered as an alternative initial approach (see Anastrozole and Letrozole).

Tamoxifen-Induced Tumor Flare Reactions

A transient exacerbation of symptoms or "flare reaction" was first observed during the treatment of postmenopausal women with high-dose estrogen. A clinical flare reaction is characterized by a dramatic increase in bone pain, an increase in size and number of metastatic skin nodules, and erythema.[174–176] Typically, symptoms occur from 2 days to 3 weeks after the start of treatment and can be accompanied by hypercalcemia, which occurs in approximately 5% of patients.[177] In clinical trials that compared endocrine therapies, an increase in bone pain or in skin lesions was observed in 4% to 7% of patients who received high-dose estrogen and 3% to 13% of patients receiving tamoxifen.[177,178] Flare has also been observed with fluoxymesterone and megestrol acetate.[179,180] Interestingly, flare has not been frequently documented with aromatase inhibitor treatment (aminoglutethimide, letrozole, and anastrozole). These data suggest that flare is mainly associated with endocrine therapies that exhibit agonist properties. Tumor regression may occur as the flare reaction subsides. Therefore, patients should not be considered resistant to tamoxifen therapy within the first month of starting treatment if they have flarelike symptoms. Pain and hypercalcemia should be treated aggressively. If symptoms are mild, tamoxifen therapy can be continued to determine whether the patient will respond. In more severe cases, tamoxifen can be stopped and then reintroduced once symptoms have improved. Because tamoxifen flare is a transient phenomenon, clinicians should look for objective evidence of disease progression if the patient's symptoms are not resolving after 4 to 6 weeks. Clinical flare, which appears to be relatively specific to endocrine therapy, should be distinguished from tumor marker flare and bone scintigraphic flare, which have been described previously (see section Monitoring Therapy).

Tamoxifen Withdrawal Responses

Between 25% and 35% of patients treated with estrogens have a secondary response if estrogen is stopped when disease progression is diagnosed.[139,181,182] The same phenomena can be observed on withdrawal of tamoxifen and progestins, although less frequently.[183] Convincing withdrawal responses generally occur when patients experience an initial response, followed by subsequent recurrence of tumor.[184] Some patients experience disease stability for more than 6 months, although it is usually short lived.[183] Therefore, discontinuation of tamoxifen and withholding subsequent therapy for a period of time to determine whether a withdrawal response occurs may prove to be a successful maneuver in selected patients, adding to the total time a patient receives benefit from endocrine therapy. Tamoxifen withdrawal therapy is appropriate for patients who responded well to prior tamoxifen therapy and whose symptoms are minimal at the time of progression.[137]

PHARMACOKINETIC, BIOLOGICAL, AND MOLECULAR ASPECTS OF ENDOCRINE THERAPY

For patients with advanced disease, drug resistance is the biggest limit of tamoxifen therapy. Despite the presence of ER, metastatic breast cancer frequently fails to respond to tamoxifen. Furthermore, all responding patients eventually experience disease progression. Therefore, progress in breast cancer endocrine therapy depends on our ability to understand and overcome resistance to treatment. A discussion of tamoxifen pharmacology and the complex molecular biology of ER signal transduction is therefore instructive.

Tamoxifen Pharmacokinetics

Tamoxifen has a half-life of 7 days, and steady-state levels are reached only after a month. A single daily 20-mg dose is now universally recommended, because it has been established that higher doses are no more effective and are associated with higher toxicity.[158,160,185,186] The metabolism of tamoxifen is complex, and a number of metabolites have antiestrogenic or estrogenic properties. The metabolism of tamoxifen may be affected by coadministration of medications that alter the activity of liver cytochrome P450 enzymes.[187,188] However, the clinical significance of these drug interactions is unknown. As long as a patient has a functioning alimentary tract, tamoxifen pharmocokinetics are not believed to be a major impediment to a favorable response. The tissue half-life is prolonged, and the drug may still be detected in tissues months after treatment.[189] It has been proposed that intratumoral conversion of tamoxifen to estrogenic metabolites may be one mechanism of tamoxifen resistance.[190] Certainly estrogenic metabolites can be detected in tumors, although it remains unclear whether they are present in sufficient quantities to overcome the simultaneous presence of tamoxifen and antiestrogenic tamoxifen metabolites. Long-term tamoxifen (5 years or more) might result in evolution of cancer cell clones that are resistant to tamoxifen by virtue of developing tamoxifen dependence. In other words, over time, clones may emerge with modified signal transduction pathways through which tamoxifen operates as an agonist rather than an antagonist.[190,191]

Estrogen Receptor Biology

Resistance to tamoxifen is easy to explain in the absence of ER expression. However, many ER-positive tumors are intrinsically resistant, and almost all cases of ER-positive metastatic disease ultimately become refractory to tamoxifen. From a clinical standpoint, ER-positive, tamoxifen-resistant breast cancer can be considered to exhibit either primary resistance (no response to tamoxifen) or secondary resistance (progression after disease regression or stability). Approximately one-third of patients with secondary tamoxifen resistance obtain clinical benefit from subsequent endocrine therapy. More surprisingly, other endocrine therapies may also be effective in postmenopausal women with primary tamoxifen resistance, with a response rate of approximately 15% (Table 5). Taken together, these observations suggest that tamoxifen resistance occurs in breast cancer cells that remain estrogen dependent. Therefore, improvement on tamoxifen should be possible if the ER signal transduction pathway can be targeted more effectively.

TABLE 5. *Response rates to second-line endocrine therapy for patients with primary tamoxifen resistance*

Trial	Letrozole, 0.5 mg	Letrozole, 2.5 mg	Megestrol acetate	Aminoglutethimide
Letrozole vs megestrol acetate				
No. of primary tamoxifen-resistant patients	15	21	26	—
Response rate	6.7%	28.6%	16.4%	—
Letrozole vs aminoglutethimide				
No. of primary tamoxifen-resistant patients	44	30	—	33
Response rate	15.9%	16.7%	—	9.1%

Adapted from refs. 151, 153.

Estrogen Receptor Protein Structure and Function

The molecular target for breast cancer endocrine therapies is the ER, a member of the nuclear hormone receptor family that includes the PR, androgen receptor, retinoid receptors [retinoic acid receptor (RAR) and RXR], glucocorticoid receptor, and vitamin D receptor. These receptors operate as ligand-dependent transcription factors that bind to DNA to regulate gene expression in response to lipid-soluble hormones.[192,193] ER shares many structural features with other members of the nuclear receptor superfamily, with six components or "domains," A to F (Fig. 10A). Estradiol and antiestrogens such as tamoxifen bind to the ligand-binding site in the E domain. The E domain also mediates ER dimerization, with assistance from residues in domain C. The sequence-specific DNA-binding function resides in domain C. Domain D contains a nuclear localization signal required for transfer of ER from the cytoplasm to the nucleus. Domains that promote transcription [activation functions (AF)] are present in domains A/B (AF1) and domain E (AF2).

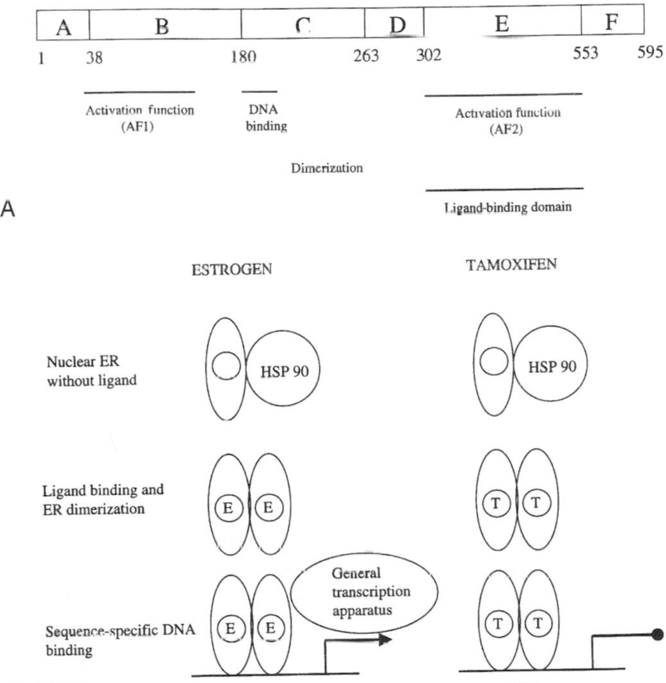

FIG. 10. Structure and function relationships in estrogen receptor (ER), with simple model of estrogen (E) and tamoxifen (T) action. **A:** Structure of ER. A to F represent different domains of ER, with text descriptions below. Numbers represent amino acids from amino to carboxy termini. **B:** Basic model in which ligand (estrogen or tamoxifen) displaces heat shock protein (HSP), resulting in binding of ligand-receptor complex to estrogen receptor element (ERE) of gene promoter region. Arrow, gene activation; circle, gene repression.

A simple model of ER function is provided in Fig. 10B. Estrogen or tamoxifen binds to the ligand-binding domain, ER is released from heat shock protein 90, and ER dimerization occurs. Sequence-specific DNA binding to a sequence referred to as an *estrogen response element* follows. In the presence of estrogen, messenger RNA (mRNA) transcription is promoted through AF2. Residues in AF1 also promote transcription; however, the function of AF1 does not require the presence of estrogen.[194] In Fig. 10B, tamoxifen-bound ER is shown as inactive, because tamoxifen inhibits AF2 function in breast cancer cells. Although providing a starting point for discussion, this simple paradigm does not reflect the complex molecular pharmacology of tamoxifen.[195] For example, the model provides no insight into the tissue-specific mixed agonist/antagonist actions of tamoxifen. In addition, the model does not explain why tamoxifen is not always effective in breast cancer, even when ER is present and functional. Therefore, more complex models are required (Fig. 11).

Corepressors and Coactivators

Figure 11A focuses on the identification of nuclear proteins that interpret the difference between estrogen-bound ER and tamoxifen-bound ER. These proteins are termed *coactivators* and *corepressors*. Coactivators increase the transcriptional activity of ER by promoting an interaction between ER and the general transcription apparatus, a protein complex that provides the machinery for mRNA transcription.[196] Corepressors restrain ER activity, maintaining ER in a protein-DNA complex that does not promote transcription.[197] ER coactivators [CBP/p300, TIF2, GRIP-1,

A Estrogen promotes coactivator (CoA) interactions which activate the general transcription apparatus (GTA)

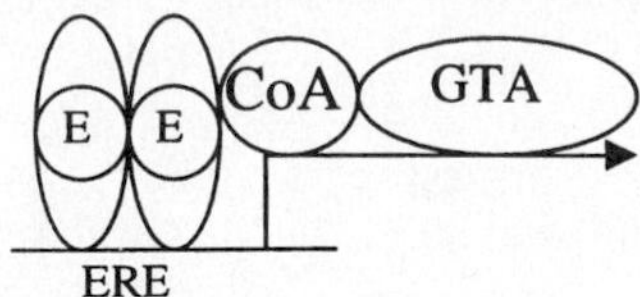

Tamoxifen promotes corepressor (CoR) interactions that prevent activation of the general transcription apparatus

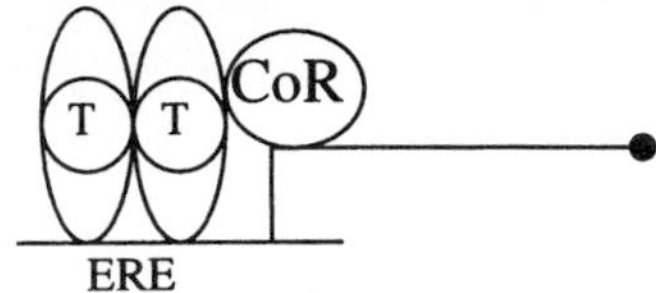

B Estrogen receptor is phosphorylated by protein kinases activated by growth factors and neurotransmitters

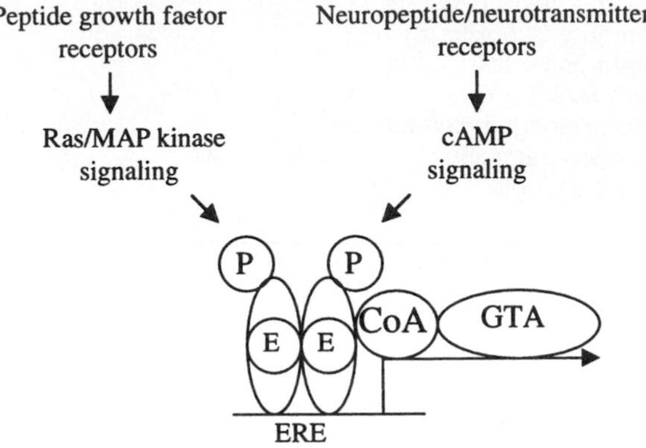

C ER interacts with other DNA-binding transcription factors to modulate the trancription of genes that do not possess an ERE

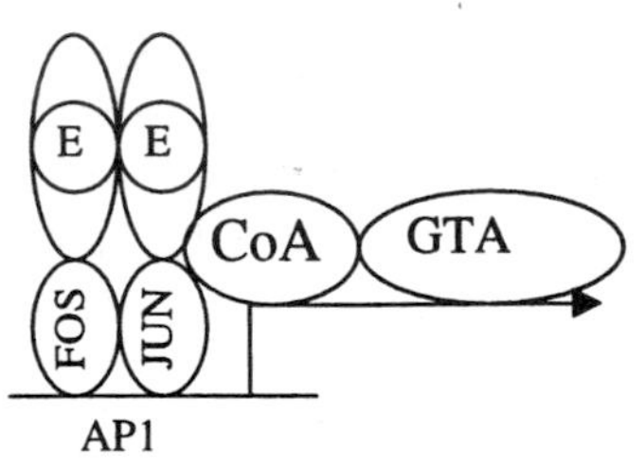

D ERβ, a second ER, interacts with classic EREs and forms complexes with AP1 transcription factors. Activities in the presence of estrogens and antiestrogens (T) differ from ERα

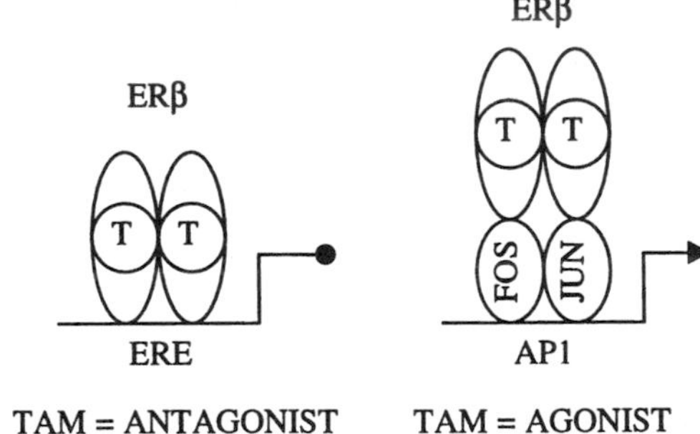

FIG. 11. More complex models of estrogen (E) and tamoxifen (T) actions through estrogen receptor (ER). cAMP, cyclic adenosine monophosphate; ERE, estrogen receptor element; MAP, mitogen-activated protein kinase; P, phosphorylated amino acid; TAM, tamoxifen.

ERAP160, SRC-1, and amplified in breast cancer 1 (AIB1)] and corepressors (N-CoR and SMRT) are exquisitely sensitive to the conformational changes that occur in the ligand-binding domain.[198–204] Tamoxifen distorts the ligand-binding domain, generating an abnormal conformation that disrupts coactivator binding.[205] Subsequently, corepressor molecules are recruited to ER, holding ER in an inactive state.[206] Because tamoxifen induces both dimerization and DNA binding, inactivation of ER depends on the net effect of tamoxifen on coactivator and corepressor interactions, which may differ between cell types and tumors. In some cells AF2 inhibition may be bypassed when enough coactivator function is recruited to the N terminal, ligand-independent domain, AF1.[207] Other cells may express a coactivator protein that can bind and activate AF2 despite the presence of tamoxifen.[203] Coactivator and corepressor proteins are therefore considered key to the molecular basis for the tissue-specific mixed agonist/antagonist profile of tamoxifen. Differences in coactivator/corepressor status between tumors may also help explain the variable response to tamoxifen in ER-positive breast cancer.[208]

Modulation of Estrogen Receptor Function through Second Messengers

ER expression and function are strongly influenced by growth factor signaling (Fig. 11B). As a result, ER expression levels correlate with distinct patterns of growth factor receptor overexpression. For example, ER-negative tumors overexpress epidermal growth factor receptor family members, in particular epidermal growth factor receptor (EGFR) and *erb*-b2.[209–212] When *erb*-b2 or EGFR is activated in experimental systems, ER expression is suppressed. Chronic activation of ER-positive, *erb*-b2–positive cell lines with heregulin, a ligand for the *erb*-b family of receptors, leads to ER down-regulation and hormone independence.[103,213] These data suggest that EGFR and *erb*-b2 signaling bypass the requirement for estrogen for breast cancer cell growth and drive breast cancer cells into an ER-negative, endocrine therapy–resistant state.[214] In contrast, signaling though the IGF-IR provides an example of a positive interaction between growth factor signaling and ER function. Several key components of the IGF system (e.g., the IGF-I receptor and the signaling intermediate IRS-1) are regulated by estrogen. As a result, IGF-I and estrogen synergistically promote the growth of breast cancer cells.[215,216] The angiogenic fibroblast growth factor family also regulates ER function. In an animal model, fibroblast growth factor stimulation of breast cancer resulted in induction of tamoxifen resistance but not ER down-regulation.[217] Finally, the neurotransmitter dopamine and the second messenger cyclic adenosine monophosphate (cAMP) also influence ER function through phosphorylation.[218–221] Interestingly, activation of cAMP leads to phosphorylation in the AF2 domain, altering the agonist/antagonist response to tamoxifen.[222] This observation suggests a role for cAMP in modulating tissue-specific effects of tamoxifen. In conclusion, ER is at the center of a complex web of signaling interactions that become deregulated as breast cancer cells evolve toward an estrogen-independent (and tamoxifen-resistant) phenotype. Insights into the cross talk between ER and other signal transduction pathways provide a rationale for novel therapeutic approaches and suggest new predictive tests for endocrine therapy sensitivity.

Estrogen Receptor Function through "Nonclassic" Estrogen Response Elements

The classic estrogen response element consists of two palindromic DNA sequences separated by a three base pair spacer sequence. ER binds most strongly to this sequence, although it is also capable of promoting transcription through sequences that have only partial homology to a classic estrogen receptor element (ERE). In these cases, nearby response elements for other transcription factors—for example, SP1—contribute to ER activity.[223,224] Clearly, the activity of any ERE is dependent on overall promoter context. In perhaps the most surprising departure from the "standard model," ER can induce transcription without direct contact with DNA (Fig. 11C). In these instances, ER operates in conjunction with a second transcription factor that provides the sequence-specific DNA-binding function. Through this indirect mechanism, ER can influence transcription through a greater variety of promoter sequences. Examples include the AP1 site (a target for many signals involved in cellular proliferation) and a polypurine tract in the transforming growth factor β promoter, referred to as a *raloxifene response element*.[225–228] Because AP1 transcription factors, such as c-fos and c-jun, are key regulators of cell growth, ER-dependent AP1 activation may be critical to estrogen-dependent cell cycle progression. Furthermore, new classes of antiestrogen do not have the same effect on AP1 activity as tamoxifen, which may help to explain differences in the clinical activity between compounds.[226]

Estrogen Receptor Beta: A Second Estrogen Receptor Gene

The identification of a second gene, *ERβ*, has provided a further layer of complexity to our understanding of estrogen-regulated gene expression[229,230] (Fig. 11D). ERβ is similar in structure to ER (now designated *ERα*) but is less important than ERα for normal reproductive organ development and function (at least in the mouse).[231] Nonetheless, ERβ mRNA is expressed by breast cancer cells and therefore has a potential role in breast cancer pathogenesis and endocrine therapy sensitivity.[232] ERα and ERβ are highly homologous in the DNA-binding domain (96%), with ERα/ERβ heterodimers readily forming on an ERE.[233] The homology in the ligand-binding domain between the two receptors is also high (58%); however, affinities for estrogens and antiestrogens vary between ERα and ERβ.[234] Consequently, responses to different ligands may be more distinct than might be anticipated from primary sequence analysis.[235] In contrast to the hormone and DNA-binding domains, ERα and ERβ are not homologous in the N terminal A/B (transactivation) domains. As a result, the transcriptional properties of ERα and ERβ are dissimilar. When the activity of an ERβ homodimer through an ERE is examined, tamoxifen is a potent antagonist with no partial agonist actions (due to a lack of an AF1-ligand–independent activation function).[236] In contrast, tamoxifen is an agonist through ERβ when signaling is through an AP1 site. This observation suggests that an increase in ERβ activity through AP1 might provide an additional explanation for the agonist effects of tamoxifen, as well as for tamoxifen resistance in ER-positive breast cancers.[226] Information on the clinical significance of ERβ expression in breast cancer is limited. However, Speirs et al.[237] have observed that breast cancers that coexpress ERα and ERβ tend to be node positive and higher grade than tumors that express ERα alone,[237] and Dotzlaw et al.[232] note that ERβ-expressing tumors are more frequently PR negative. These correlations suggest an adverse effect of ERβ expression on prognosis.

MOLECULAR CORRELATIONS WITH CLINICAL RESISTANCE TO TAMOXIFEN IN ESTROGEN RECEPTOR–POSITIVE BREAST CANCER

The complexity of ER function explains in part why patients with breast tumors that express ER do not universally respond to tamoxifen or other endocrine therapies. Possible mechanisms of resistance include mutations or alternative mRNA splicing, or both, of the *ER* genes; interaction with other growth factor signal transduction pathways (such as *erb*-b2); and abnormal expression or function of coactivators and repressors.

Estrogen Receptor Mutation and Alternative Messenger Ribonucleic Acid Splicing

The determination of the structure of the *ER* led to an early hypothesis that invoked *ER* gene mutation as a mechanism for tamoxifen resistance.[238] However, subsequent studies demonstrated that somatic mutations in *ER* are rare, occurring in fewer than 1% of either ER-positive or ER-negative

TABLE 6. *Summary of reports that investigated the relationship between endocrine therapy and* erb-*b2 status*

Study	Specimen	Technique	Number	*erb*-b2–negative response (%)	*erb*-b2–positive response (%)
Wright	Paraffin	IHC	72	37	7
Leitzel	Serum	EIA	300	41	21
Berns	Extract	PCR	359	56	17
Archer	Paraffin	IHC	92	80	19
Newby	Paraffin	IHC	155	56	0
Yamauchi	Serum	EIA	94	56	9
Elledge	Paraffin	IHC	205	57	54
			Mean response	55	18

EIA, enzyme-linked immunoassay; IHC, immunohistochemistry; PCR, polymerase chain reaction.
Compiled from refs. 106, 107, 108, 246, 559, 560, 561.

breast cancers.[239] Therefore, it seems unlikely that *ER* mutations substantially contribute to many clinical cases of tamoxifen resistance.[240]

In contrast, alternatively spliced *ER* mRNA variants have frequently been identified in normal and malignant breast tissues.[241] These mRNA variants lack one or several exons because of exon "skipping." A transcript that has received particular attention lacks exon 5; that is, exon 4 directly splices into exon 6, with preservation of the reading frame.[242] The exon 5–deleted variant (d5) binds to DNA, but not estrogen, and activates transcription in an estrogen-independent manner (a dominant positive receptor). These properties imply a role in estrogen-independent growth. However, coexpression of d5 with an intact *ER* did not alter the transcriptional response to estrogen, arguing against a critical role in breast cancer pathogenesis.[243,244] On the other hand, Gallacchi et al.[245] have found a significant increase in d5 expression in metastatic disease when compared with the respective primary tumor. *ERβ* transcripts have not yet been fully examined, and a thorough investigation of multiple ER transcripts in breast cancer could still provide important information relevant to predicting endocrine therapy sensitivity.

erb-b2 and Tamoxifen Resistance

Because ER function is strongly influenced by peptide growth factor signaling, ER-positive tumors that are resistant to endocrine therapy might be identified through analysis of the expression of these growth factors and their receptors. In this regard, *erb*-b2 expression has been extensively examined. The presence of *erb*-b2 tumor immunostaining was first shown to correlate with resistance to endocrine therapy in a small group of patients with metastatic disease. Among patients with ER-positive tumors, *erb*-b2 expression was associated with a tamoxifen response rate of only 20%, and for patients with ER-negative tumors, 0%. In contrast, patients with *erb*-b2–negative tumors had response rates of 41% for ER-positive and 27% for ER-negative tumors.[246] Since this 1992 report, several studies have produced conflicting results regarding *erb*-b2 and endocrine benefit. For example, the extracellular domain of *erb*-b2 (*erb*-b2-ECD) is shed by *erb*-b2–positive tumor cells and can be detected in human circulation with a convenient immunoassay.[247] Circulating *erb*-b2 is frequently elevated in patients with *erb*-b2 positive cancers.[248] In a study by Leitzel et al.,[248] circulating *erb*-b2 levels were analyzed from 300 patients who were enrolled in a trial of megestrol acetate or fadrozole as second-line endocrine therapy for advanced breast cancer. Patients with elevated serum *erb*-b2 levels (19% of the total) had a response rate to endocrine therapy of 20.7%, compared to 41% for patients with low serum *erb*-b2 levels. Duration of response and survival were significantly shorter in the *erb*-b2–positive group.[106] A study with a similar design reported a comparable result for patients who received the antiestrogen, droloxifene. Elevated pretreatment *erb*-b2 levels in plasma (two standard deviations above the mean for normal subjects) had a response probability of only 10%, a level generally associated with ER-negative tumors.[107] However, the relationship between endocrine therapy responsiveness and *erb*-b2 expression has not been observed in all studies.

Elledge et al.[108] have studied *erb*-b2 expression by immunohistochemistry in tissues collected in the 1980s from patients with metastatic breast cancer by the Southwest Oncology Group. These tissues were originally collected to investigate the impact of ER expression on endocrine therapy responsiveness. In this study, no difference in response rate, time to progression, or OS between *erb*-b2–positive and *erb*-b2–negative patients was demonstrated[108] (Table 6). A potential explanation for the discrepancy between studies is the possibility that *erb*-b2-ECD analysis does not exclude patients with ER-negative, *erb*-b2–positive tumors, for whom the endocrine therapy response rates are understandably low. Given the uncertainty of the clinical evidence on the relationship between endocrine therapy resistance and *erb*-b2 expression, *erb*-b2–positive, ER-positive patients should not be denied the potential benefits of tamoxifen or other endocrine therapies in either the metastatic or early disease settings.

Coactivators and Corepressors and Tamoxifen Resistance

Only limited information is available on coactivator and corepressor function in human breast cancer. However, several observations raise the possibility that these molecules may be critical determinants of the efficacy of endocrine therapy. For example, ER-positive MCF-7 breast cancer cells form tumors in nude mice that regress with tamoxifen treatment. If tamoxifen is continued, tumor growth resumes. This growth is tamoxifen dependent, because withdrawal of tamoxifen causes a second, temporary regression.[249] This animal model is reminiscent of clinical tumor regressions that may occur after tamoxifen is stopped for disease progression (withdrawal response).[183] Levels of the corepressor N-CoR are suppressed in the tamoxifen-stimulated tumors when compared to their tamoxifen-sensitive counterparts.[208] This finding suggests that prolonged tamoxifen exposure alters the coactivators and corepressor balance in favor of the agonist, growth-promoting properties of tamoxifen. Another potential player in the coactivator and corepressor profile in breast cancer cells is the gene designated *AIB1*.[250] AIB1 is located at 20q12, a region amplified in both breast and ovarian cancer. The encoded protein is an ER coactivator, and studies have shown that AIB1 is associated with ER expression in breast cancer samples.[251] More data can be expected on the relationship between tamoxifen resistance and coactivator/corepressor status in human breast cancer samples.

STRATEGIES TO OVERCOME RESISTANCE TO ENDOCRINE THERAPY IN ESTROGEN RECEPTOR–POSITIVE BREAST CANCER

New Selective Estrogen Receptor Modulators

In theory, agents that absolutely inhibit ER function might be more effective than tamoxifen. Indeed, several pure antiestrogens are under clinical development (see Development of Pure Antiestrogens). However, drugs devoid of all estrogenic activities might be problematic in the adjuvant and prevention settings, because secondary "hormone replacement therapy–like" benefits of tamoxifen are considered worthwhile for postmenopausal women. This concern has stimulated the development of alternative antiestrogens with a modified mixed agonist/ antagonist profile. Ideally, these drugs are antiestrogenic in the breast and retain beneficial effects on bone mineralization and blood lipid profile but do not exhibit adverse estrogenic effects on the endometrium. Drugs such as tamoxifen that exhibit a mixed agonist/antagonist profile have been designated as *selective ER modulators* (*SERM*) to reflect these remarkable properties. In 1998, a new SERM, raloxifene, was approved in the United States for treatment of osteoporosis.[252,253] Raloxifene appears to have the same tissue-specific ER agonistic and antagonistic characteristics as tamoxifen, except that it does not appear to stimulate endothelial proliferation. However, an early evaluation of raloxifene activity in tamoxifen-resistant breast cancer was disappointing, and little further clinical research directed toward metastatic breast cancer has been performed.[254] Consequently, it is difficult to know where to place raloxifene in the treatment of metastatic breast cancer, because it has never been compared directly to tamoxifen, and it does not appear to have activity in tamoxifen-refractory patients.

A third-generation SERM, currently designated *SERM3*, appears to have a similar profile as tamoxifen and raloxifene but with greater ER antagonist activity in breast cancer models. Preliminary results from phase I studies of SERM3 have been reported, and it appears safe and well-tolerated.[255] Results from phase II trials, as well as plans for phase III development, should be available soon.

It is important to emphasize that although new SERMs may represent a small advance in terms of safety, they are not necessarily more efficacious. Activity in advanced tamoxifen-resistant disease is considered by many clinicians to provide critical evidence that a new endocrine therapy may be more active than tamoxifen. Antiestrogens with a mixed agonist/antagonist profile, even if modified to improve tissue-specific toxicity, are likely to exhibit cross-resistance with tamoxifen, because any compound that promotes ER dimerization and DNA binding is prone to the same resistance mechanisms that limit the activity of tamoxifen.[256,257] Indeed, none of the new SERMs, including idoxifene (which, at best, has minor activity in tamoxifen-resistant disease), droloxifene, and toremifene, has been found to have substantial, or indeed any, activity in tamoxifen-refractory patients.[258–262] Nonetheless, toremifene does exhibit equivalent activity and toxicity in patients with untreated metastatic breast cancer, and it is a reasonable alternative to tamoxifen for first-line treatment of advanced breast cancer.[262,263] However, toremifene displays cross-resistance with tamoxifen and should not be used in tamoxifen-resistant disease.[254,264]

Development of Pure Antiestrogens

Because resistance to tamoxifen might be due to partial agonist effects, antiestrogens without agonist activity could be more effective. ICI 182,780 (Faslodex) is a "pure" antiestrogen at an advanced stage of clinical development. Faslodex has a steroid structure that blocks ER dimerization, inhibits DNA binding, increases ER turnover, and suppresses ER levels.[265–267] As a result, it blocks ER function before coactivator binding, theoretically overcoming resistance driven by the agonist properties of tamoxifen. Preclinical studies in models of tamoxifen-resistant disease have been promising, and clinical trials for patients with tamoxifen-resistant advanced disease are under way.[268] Faslodex is administered as a monthly intramuscular injection. Data from a small phase II trial have demonstrated activity in tamoxifen-resistant advanced disease, with 7 of 19 patients who received 250 mg a month experiencing partial responses. A further 6 of 19 patients achieved stable disease for at least 24 weeks.[269] Two large, prospective, randomized clinical trials are under way: For patients with tamoxifen-resistant disease, Faslodex is being compared to anastrozole (an SAI); for patients with advanced disease who have never received tamoxifen or have not received the drug for at least 1 year, Faslodex is being compared to tamoxifen. A second pure antiestrogen, EM800, is also being compared in a phase III trial with anastrozole. EM800 is orally active and structurally related to raloxifene.[270]

Estrogen Deprivation Therapy for Premenopausal Women

Beatson[12] demonstrated the benefits of estrogen deprivation in locally advanced breast cancer after oophorectomy. In subsequent clinical experience throughout the twentieth century, it has been demonstrated that oophorectomy results in objective responses in approximately one-third of unselected premenopausal patients.[145] Since the 1970s, tamoxifen has been favored for first-line therapy in premenopausal women, because oophorectomy and tamoxifen have similar efficacy, but tamoxifen is more convenient and arguably has less toxicity.[138,142,159,271] Nonetheless, trials with a crossover design have demonstrated that responses to oophorectomy after disease progression on tamoxifen are not uncommon, particularly when the patient had an initial response to tamoxifen.[142]

In the 1980s, LHRH-As were introduced, providing an alternative to oophorectomy. LHRH-As (goserelin and leuprolide) are peptide analogues of LHRH that are 50 to 100 times more potent than the natural hormone. Acting on the pituitary, LHRH-A treatment first stimulates follicle-stimulating hormone and luteinizing hormone secretion and then profoundly suppresses the pituitary ovarian axis, with a fall in estrogen to menopausal levels.[272,273] In patients with prostate cancer, LHRH-As may induce a transient rise in androgens with a risk of disease exacerbation. Although no large increases in estrogen levels have been detected when women with advanced breast cancer are treated with LHRH-As, breast cancer flare reactions have been reported with this treatment.[272,274,275] In these cases, flare may be due to gonadotropin release.[141] Results from prospective randomized trials have demonstrated that response rates to LHRH-A are comparable to those observed with oophorectomy. Therefore, treatment with an LHRH-A is a viable alternative for patients who do not wish to undergo surgery.[141]

Most recently, in 1995, consideration has been given to treating premenopausal women with a combination of tamoxifen and LHRH-A.[144] A meta-analysis of four trials addressing this question suggests that LHRH-A plus tamoxifen is more effective than single-agent LHRH-A. Response rates for the combination were 39% compared with 30% for LHRH-A alone. However, the combination results in only a modest improvement in progression-free survival (8.7 versus 5.4 months) and OS (2.9 versus 2.5 years).[143] Based on these results, it is reasonable to recommend a combination of LHRH-A and tamoxifen as first-line endocrine therapy to premenopausal women with metastatic breast cancer. However, because the OS gains from combination therapy are small, patients may be equally well served by sequential treatment with tamoxifen first and ovarian suppression at the time of disease progression.

Estrogen Deprivation Therapy for Postmenopausal Women

The therapeutic benefits of reducing estrogen levels by ovarian ablation or LHRH-A therapy are restricted to patients with functioning ovaries. As ovarian function declines, the relative proportion of estrogens synthesized in extragonadal sites increases, and eventually nonovarian estrogens predominate in the circulation.[276,277] Peripheral tissues depend on the aromatization of androgenic precursors of adrenal origin (testosterone and androstenedione) to generate estradiol and estrone (Fig. 12). Aromatase, the enzyme responsible for this conversion, is present in adipose tissue, liver, muscle, and brain. Aromatase activity has also been identified in the epithelial and stromal components of the breast. Therefore, local synthesis of estrogens may contribute to breast cancer growth in postmenopausal women.[278–281] In support of this theory, the decline in estrogen after menopause is less marked in breast tissue because of a combination of aromatase activity and preferential estrogen uptake from the circulation.[282–285] Furthermore, aromatase activity has been shown to correlate with a marker of breast cancer cell proliferation, and quadrants of the breast bearing a breast cancer have more aromatase expression than those that do not bear tumors.[286–288] Taken together, these observations suggest a model for postmenopausal breast cancer that focuses on intratumoral estrogen synthesis.[289–291]

Aromatase is an enzyme complex consisting of the P450 cytochrome, P450arom, and a flavoprotein, NADPH cytochrome P450 reductase, that regenerates active aromatase after completion of the aromatization reaction. The active site of aromatase contains a heme complex responsible for the nucleophilic attack on the androgenic precursor C19 methyl group that generates formic acid and an aromatized A ring characteristic of estrogenic steroids. Because estrogen production is the last step in the generation of steroidal compounds, selective inhibition of aromatase does not block the production of corticosteroids and mineralocorticoids. Aromatase is therefore a particularly appealing therapeutic target for breast cancer endocrine therapy.[292]

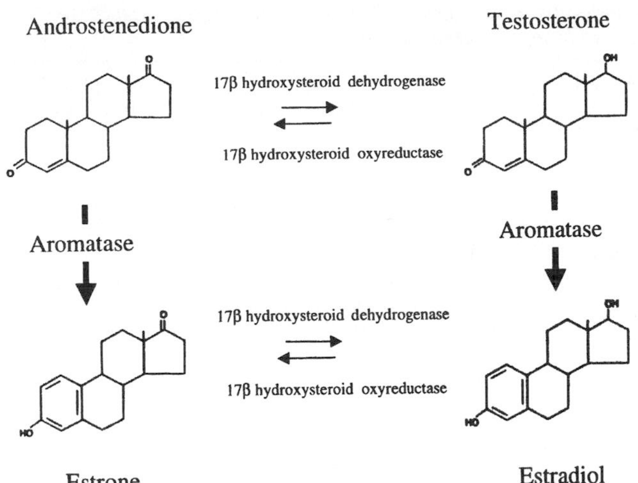

FIG. 12. The conversion of androgens to estrogens by aromatase.

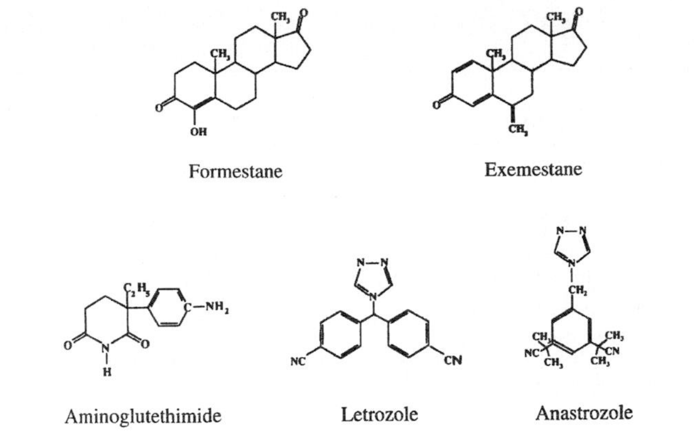

For many years, the breast cancer–promoting actions of postmenopausal estrogens have been targeted with tamoxifen. However, the development of SAIs has provided a significant and effective alternative approach. SAIs suppress postmenopausal estrogen levels by selectively inhibiting the aromatase enzyme. Two SAIs, anastrozole and letrozole, are approved in the United States and Europe for postmenopausal women with advanced breast cancer for whom tamoxifen has ceased to have a therapeutic benefit. A third SAI, exemestane, is under clinical development. Not only are these drugs safer and better tolerated than previous second-line endocrine therapy alternatives, such as progestins and aminoglutethimide, but they are more active.

Aminoglutethimide

Aminoglutethimide, the prototypic aromatase inhibitor, was first used at high doses in metastatic breast cancer as an alternative to surgical adrenalectomy. When lower doses were found to be as effective, it became appreciated that inhibition of aromatase, rather than suppression of general steroidogenesis, was key to the therapeutic action of aminoglutethimide.[293,294] Unfortunately, even at the lowest doses that are effective in breast cancer, aminoglutethimide inhibits the formation of corticosteroids by blocking multiple P450 enzymes involved in steroid biosynthesis.[295] Lack of specificity exposes patients to the risk of glucocorticoid deficiency. In addition, the value of aminoglutethimide is limited by troublesome side effects that include rash, nausea, and somnolence.[296] Despite these difficulties, clinical trials have demonstrated that aminoglutethimide has clinical activity similar to that of tamoxifen as first-line treatment for advanced breast cancer.[297,298] For patients with advanced disease who have tamoxifen resistance, the response rate is approximately 30%.[150,299] However, concern over side effects restricted the use of aminoglutethimide to the "third-line" setting of endocrine therapy–responsive patients with acquired resistance to tamoxifen and megestrol acetate. The finding that aminoglutethimide was effective after disease progression on tamoxifen provided a strong rationale for the development of more potent and selective aromatase inhibitors.[297,298]

FIG. 13. The structure of nonsteroidal and steroidal aromatase inhibitors.

Aromatase Inhibitor Development

Two distinct solutions emerged for the problem of designing more potent, specific, and safer aromatase inhibitors than aminoglutethimide. One approach was to refine the mechanism of action exhibited by aminoglutethimide. This led to a family of "nonsteroidal" inhibitors that disrupt the aromatase active-site by coordinating within the heme complex, without affecting the active sites of other steroidogenic enzymes.[292] Further studies focused on a series of imidazole and triazole derivatives with "molecular shapes" that efficiently coordinate within the aromatase heme complex (Fig. 13).

Anastrozole and Letrozole

Anastrozole was the first SAI to be approved in both North America and Europe. A daily dose of 1 mg rapidly suppresses estradiol, estrone, and estrone sulfate levels to close to assay detection limits.[300] Suppression is maintained long term with no compensatory rise in androstenedione levels. Importantly, even at higher doses (5 to 10 mg), anastrozole administration does not affect basal or adrenocorticotropic hormone–stimulated cortisol and aldosterone levels.[301] Anastrozole is rapidly absorbed, with maximum levels occurring within 2 hours after administration. Less than 10% of the drug is cleared as unchanged drug because of extensive metabolism. Two international phase III clinical trials enrolled postmenopausal women with tamoxifen-resistant

TABLE 7. *Summary of phase III clinical trials that compared selective aromatase inhibitors with megestrol acetate in patients with tamoxifen-resistant advanced breast cancer*

End point	Letrozole (2.5 mg)	Megestrol acetate (160 mg)	Anastrozole (1 mg)	Megestrol acetate (160 mg)
Complete response	6.9%	4.2%	2%	2%
Partial response	16.7%	12.2%	8%	6%
Stable disease >24 wk	11.4%	15.6%	25%	26%
Overall response rate	35%	32%	35%	34%
Median time to progression	5.6 mo	5.5 mo	5.3 mo	5.3 mo
Median overall survival	25.3 mo	21.5 mo	26.7 mo	22.5 mo
2-yr survival	51%	44%	56.1%	46.3%

Adapted from refs. 151, 152.

disease to compare the activity of anastrozole with megestrol acetate (40 mg four times a day; Table 7). Two doses of anastrozole, 1 mg and 10 mg, were examined in these trials. Both doses were known to suppress circulating estrogens to the limit of assay detection. However, a 10-mg dose was included to address the possibility that efficient inhibition of intratumoral aromatase might require a higher dose. Both trials were restricted to postmenopausal patients with ER-positive tumors, unless a response to tamoxifen treatment had been previously documented in the case of an ER-negative or unknown tumor. Progressive disease developed in approximately one-half of the patients during or after adjuvant tamoxifen treatment. Tamoxifen resistance developed in the rest during treatment for metastatic disease. Very few patients with advanced disease who did not have a history of a response to tamoxifen were entered into either trial.

The results of an overview of both trials, incorporating data from 764 patients, were published in 1996.[21] Patient and tumor characteristics were evenly distributed in the three arms of the trials. Objective response rates were low: Compete response plus partial response were 10.3% in the 1-mg anastrozole group, 8.9% in the 10-mg anastrozole group, and 7.9% in the megestrol acetate group. However, 25.1%, 22.6%, and 26.1% of patients, respectively, had stable disease at 24 weeks suggesting benefit even without objective response.[30,302] Therefore, overall, approximately one-third of patients benefited from therapy, with no differences in disease-free survival emerging between the three treatment arms. Despite this, patients who received 1 mg anastrozole experienced a longer median survival than those on megestrol acetate (26.7 months versus 22.5 months, p = .02; Fig. 14). There was also a higher 2-year survival for patients treated with 1 mg anastrozole than for those who received megestrol acetate (56.1% versus 46.3%, respectively). A trend for significant improvement in median survival was also seen with the 10-mg dose (25.5 months, p = .10) versus megestrol acetate.[152]

Although the extension of life with anastrozole is relatively small, these results are significant, because it is very uncommon for endocrine therapy trials in the metastatic setting to demonstrate any improvement in OS. In both trials, anastrozole was well tolerated. Of note, anastrozole was associated with less weight gain than megestrol acetate, which will be considered a major advantage over progestins by many physicians and patients. In contrast, nausea and vomiting were more common with anastrozole. However, gastrointestinal side effects are less troublesome with the 1-mg dose, and gastrointestinal problems rarely lead to interruption of therapy (Table 8).

Letrozole has a similar profile as anastrozole, combining high potency, selectivity, and promising activity against advanced breast cancer in phase I/II trials.[303–306] Both letrozole doses examined in phase III trials, 0.5 mg and 2.5 mg, suppress estrogen levels more than 90% (less than 0.5 pmol/L).[307] As with anastrozole, liver metabolism is the major elimination pathway, and the half-life of 50 hours allows a once-a-day dosing schedule. Because only 5% is excreted in the urine, letrozole can be safely prescribed in patients with renal insufficiency. However, letrozole should be used with caution when patients have severe liver impairment. Also, like anastrozole, letrozole has been compared to megestrol acetate in a prospective randomized trial, in which 551 patients were randomly assigned to take daily doses of letrozole, 0.5 mg; letrozole, 2.5 mg; or megestrol acetate, 160 mg[151] (see Table 7). Letrozole, 2.5 mg, produced a significantly higher overall response rate (24%) compared with megestrol acetate (16%)

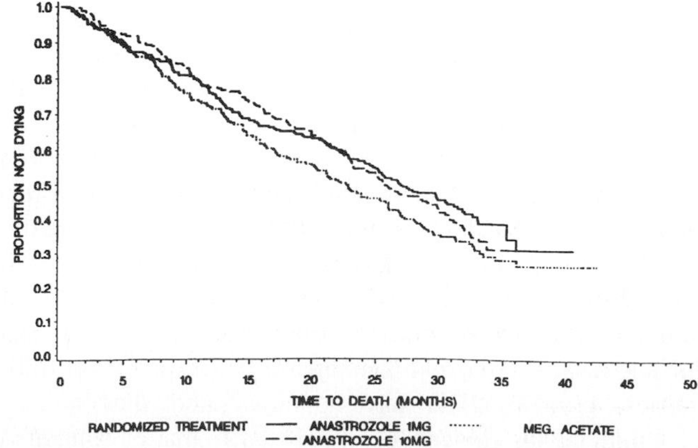

FIG. 14. Combined survival analysis from two trials comparing 1 mg and 10 mg of anastrozole with 40 mg four times per day of megestrol acetate. (From ref. 152, with permission.)

TABLE 8. *Side effect profile (%) of anastrozole, letrozole, and megestrol acetate*

Side effect	Letrozole	Megestrol acetate	Anastrozole	Megestrol acetate	Significance
Nausea	10.9	9	16[a]	11	Yes
Dyspnea	9.2	16.4	9	21	Yes
Headache	12.6	9	13	10	—
Peripheral edema	8.6	7.9	5	11	—
Weight gain	4	16	2	12	Yes
Hot flashes	5	4	12	8	—
Thromboembolic events	0	8	3	5	Yes

[a]Significant for anastrozole only.
Adapted from refs. 151, 152.

and letrozole, 0.5 mg (13%). Letrozole, 2.5 mg, was also superior to letrozole, 0.5 mg, and megestrol acetate for time to treatment failure. Although not statistically significant, a trend in OS benefit was observed for letrozole compared to megestrol acetate (median time OS, 25.3 months for letrozole, 2.5 mg, and 21.5 months for megestrol acetate). In a manner similar to that observed for anastrozole, letrozole was significantly better tolerated than megestrol acetate with respect to serious adverse experiences, discontinuation due to poor tolerability, cardiovascular side effects, and weight gain. Nausea appeared to be less problematic (see Table 8).

Letrozole has also been examined in a nonblinded study, in comparison with aminoglutethimide, 250 mg twice a day.[153] Five hundred fifty-five women with tamoxifen-resistant breast cancer were entered. Response rates were highest for 2.5 mg letrozole (19.5%), compared with 0.5 mg (16.7%) and aminoglutethimide (12.4%). Both doses of letrozole were significantly superior to aminoglutethimide in time to disease progression. In addition, a significant survival benefit emerged in favor of letrozole, 2.5 mg (median survival, 30 months) against aminoglutethimide (19 months, $p = .02$; Fig. 15). The 0.5-mg dose did not produce a significant survival benefit over aminoglutethimide, despite estrogen suppression that is nearly indistinguishable from that seen with letrozole, 2.5 mg. Nonetheless, an improvement in breast cancer outcomes is probably associated with the profound decrease in estrogen levels associated with the use of letrozole, because response, time to progression, and median duration of response were significantly superior for both letrozole doses.

These findings support the assumption that clinical outcomes for estrogen-deprivation therapies are related to the degree of estrogen suppression. This important conclusion is relevant to the adjuvant setting, in which estrogen deprivation to improve breast cancer outcomes must outweigh the possible detrimental effects of estrogen deficiency on other organ systems. Importantly, letrozole treatment was associated with very few serious adverse events, was better tolerated than aminoglutethimide, and does not require steroid support.

Taken together, the results from these phase III studies with nonsteroidal SAIs represent the largest clinical trial experience in second-line breast cancer endocrine therapy for advanced disease. It is reasonable to conclude that letrozole and anastrozole are the new standard in endocrine therapy for tamoxifen-resistant metastatic breast cancer. Although megestrol acetate may still play a small role in the third-line setting, aminoglutethimide should now be considered obsolete.

Steroidal Aromatase Inhibitors: Exemestane and Formestane

An alternative strategy to nonsteroidal inhibition of aromatase is the development of "steroidal" aromatase inhibitors, resistant to aromatase action, that bind aromatase and block conversion of androgenic substrates. Two compounds, formestane (4-hydroxyandrostenedione) and exemestane, emerged from preclinical studies as drugs suitable for clinical development.[308] As can be appreciated from the structures in Fig. 13, both compounds retain androgenic properties, but side chain substitutions prevent conversion to estrogenic metabolites. It has been proposed that formestane and exemestane (or modified forms of these drugs) exhibit tight or even irreversible binding to the aromatase active site.[309] Steroidal aromatase inhibitors are therefore considered "mechanism based" or "suicide" inhibitors, because they permanently inactivate aro-

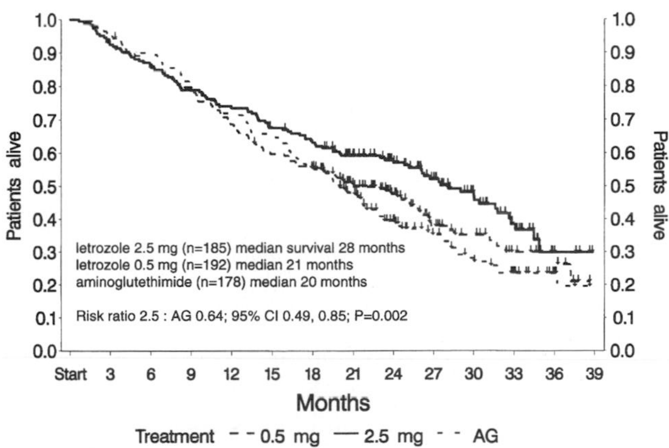

FIG. 15. Survival analysis from a trial comparing 2.5 mg and 0.5 mg letrozole with 500 mg twice a day of aminoglutethimide. AG, aminoglutethimide; CI, confidence interval. (From ref. 153, with permission.)

matase.[310] As a result, recovery of aromatase requires synthesis of new aromatase molecules. *In vivo*, suicide inhibition is characterized by persistently low aromatase activity despite complete drug clearance. Because suicide inhibition prolongs drug action, intermittent dosing should be possible, potentially improving the side effect–benefit ratio.

Formestane was the first steroidal aromatase inhibitor to be assessed in the clinic and, before anastrozole and letrozole, was the most widely studied. It is 60-fold more potent than aminoglutethimide and suppresses 65% of estrogen production with, on average, a 40% decrease in serum estrone levels.[311,312] A series of phase II trials of 250 mg formestane given every 2 weeks has shown response rates of 23% to 39%, with stabilization of disease in a further 14% to 29% of patients.[313–316] Predictably, responses were more frequent for patients with ER-positive tumors and a history of a response to tamoxifen. In phase III studies, formestane produced response rates equivalent to those of tamoxifen (33% versus 37%). However, responses to formestane were less durable.[317] In the second-line setting, formestane proved to have antineoplastic activity similar to that of megestrol acetate.[318] Formestane side effects are mild and include hot flashes, rash, facial swelling, and sterile abscesses at the injection site. Bioavailability of oral formestane is limited, and the current formulation is for parenteral injection.[311] Formestane has been approved in many countries (Lentaron), although not in the United States. Its use is restricted to patients whose disease has progressed on tamoxifen therapy.

Exemestane has significant advantages over formestane, because it is more potent and is efficiently absorbed orally.[319] A daily 25-mg dose suppresses serum estradiol and estrone to between 60% and 74% of control.[320,321] In a recently reported phase II trial involving 134 women with tamoxifen-resistant disease, the overall response rate was 22%. In addition, a further 31% had no change in disease for at least 24 weeks. Median duration of objective response was 68 weeks, and time to progression was 29 weeks. Interestingly, with other SAIs, responses were observed in visceral disease and in patients who never responded to tamoxifen, with a 25% overall response rate for patients with primary tamoxifen resistance.[322–325] These observations challenge the dogma that further endocrine therapy should not be offered to patients who do not show an initial response to tamoxifen and that visceral metastases are resistant to endocrine therapy. A preliminary report also exists on the efficacy of exemestane for patients in whom resistance has developed to nonsteroidal aromatase inhibitors (aminoglutethimide, letrozole, and anastrozole). If a stable disease category was included, the overall success rate was 25% (complete response plus partial response, 7%; stable disease, 18%), indicating that exemestane may be active in the third-line endocrine therapy setting.[326] A phase III trial has been completed in tamoxifen-resistant advanced disease in which patient treatment was randomly assigned to either exemestane or megestrol acetate. The results from this trial were made available in 1999. Exemestane was found to be superior to megestrol acetate for time to progression and overall survival.[327]

First-Line Endocrine Therapy for Postmenopausal Patients: Tamoxifen versus a Selective Aromatase Inhibitor

Tamoxifen remains first-line endocrine therapy for advanced breast cancer. Retreatment with tamoxifen is also the standard approach for patients who relapse after completing adjuvant tamoxifen, as long as the relapse is at least a year since they last took the drug.[328] However, the safety and efficacy of anastrozole and letrozole have encouraged clinical trials that directly compare SAI therapy with tamoxifen for advanced disease. These studies include tamoxifen-naive patients and patients who have taken tamoxifen in the adjuvant setting but who have not received the drug for at least a year. Two principal clinical hypotheses could favor SAI therapy over tamoxifen: (a) SAIs may be active for patients who never respond to tamoxifen, or (b) responses to aromatase inhibitors might be more durable than those with tamoxifen. The potential size of the "aromatase inhibitor–sensitive, tamoxifen-resistant" population can be estimated from the response rate to aromatase inhibitors in primary tamoxifen-resistant disease, which is approximately 15% (see Table 5). Based on these data, trials are powered to detect between a 10% and 20% difference in study end points in favor of aromatase inhibition. However, these estimates assume that the size of tamoxifen-sensitive, aromatase inhibitor–resistant cancer populations is insignificant. The actual size of this population is unknown, although patients who cross over to tamoxifen after initial treatment with aminoglutethimide have been shown to have a low chance of a response.[297]

Selective Aromatase Inhibitor Therapy for Premenopausal Women

The success of SAI therapy in postmenopausal women has raised the issue of whether this approach might be successful in premenopausal women. Unfortunately, inhibition of ovarian aromatase activity is associated with polycystic ovaries and androgen excess caused by activation of the pituitary-ovarian axis. The clinical consequences of ovarian aromatase deficiency are best illustrated by the occurrence of hypergonadotrophic hypogonadism, multicystic ovaries, virilism, and bone demineralization in individuals with hereditary aromatase deficiency.[329,330] Furthermore, although polycystic ovary syndrome in women has a less well-defined etiology, low aromatase activity is thought to play a part.[331] Thus, SAI therapy is contraindicated in premenopausal women. However, consideration is being given to treating premenopausal women who have advanced breast cancer with combinations of LHRH analogues and SAIs. In a small pharmacokinetic study, the SAI vorozole suppressed estrogen levels beyond those achieved by goserelin alone. The combination was well tolerated, and there was no significant rise in androgens.[332] The data supporting a combination of LHRH-A plus tamoxifen for postmenopausal women suggest that a trial of LHRH-A plus tamoxifen versus LHRH-A plus SAI might be the optimal phase III design.[143] However, given the lack of data concerning the safety and efficacy of an SAI/LHRH-A combination, it should be stressed that outside of a clinical trial, SAI treatment should be reserved for postmenopausal patients. Until more information becomes available, premenopausal patients with metastatic breast cancer that is resistant to tamoxifen and LHRH-A should be treated with megestrol acetate. The alternative is to offer oophorectomy, followed by an SAI (see Fig. 6). This latter approach is the most likely to be effective in view of the advantage of SAI therapy over megestrol acetate for postmenopausal women.

ENDOCRINE THERAPIES USING SEX STEROIDS

Progestins

Patients who have low-volume disease that is restricted to bone or soft tissue, few symptoms, and a history of a response to either tamoxifen or an SAI (or both) can be considered candidates for further endocrine therapy. The optimal approach to third-line endocrine therapy needs to be redefined. Sex steroid therapy with progestins, androgens, and estrogens presents alternatives. Of these, megestrol acetate (160 mg a day) is the most likely to be considered. Although early studies suggested that higher doses were more active, subsequent randomized controlled trials did not confirm these findings.[333–335] Higher doses of megestrol acetate are clearly associated with more weight gain, fluid retention, vaginal bleeding, and a decline in QOL. Progestins are also associated with an increased risk of thromboembolic events (see Table 8) and should be avoided in patients who have cardiac or thromboembolic disorders. Medroxyprogesterone acetate, which requires intramuscular dosing, has also been studied extensively but offers no clear advantages in terms of efficacy or safety.[336]

The mechanisms of action of megestrol acetate and medroxyprogesterone acetate are unclear. They may inhibit aromatase activity or increase estrogen turnover, because estrogen levels fall during progestin therapy.[336] If suppression of circulating estrogen is key, one would predict a low response rate after disease progression on an SAI. However, these drugs may act through the glucocorticoid receptor, androgen receptor, or PR. If so, progestins may be active despite SAI resistance. Unfortunately, trials that compared SAI therapy with megestrol acetate did not use "crossover" designs to systematically study the activity of megestrol acetate after SAI failure. Therefore, megestrol acetate should not be abandoned until activity has been reevaluated in appropriate patients with SAI and tamoxifen-resistant disease. Because it is unlikely that future phase III designs will include a megestrol acetate control arm, new information will probably be limited to uncontrolled patient series.

Androgens

Androgens, including testosterone, fluoxymesterone, and the less virilizing testolactone, are associated with response rates in the range of 20%.[328] Major side effects include virilization and jaundice. Furthermore, androgens are one of the few agents that have been shown to be inferior to another endocrine agent (high-dose estrogen).[337] The weak androgen danazol has also been studied because of an additional action on pituitary gonadotropin secretion. Again, the single-agent response rate was approximately 20%, with side effects that include edema and hot flashes.[338] Androgens are rarely used to treat metastatic breast cancer. If considered, fluoxymesterone (Halotestin), 10 mg orally twice a day, is as effective and nontoxic as any other.[339]

High-Dose Estrogen

Before the advent of contemporary endocrine therapy options, administration of high doses of estrogen was the treatment of choice for breast cancer. This option should only be considered in postmenopausal women, because high-dose estrogens are ineffective before the menopause.[148] Although the mechanism of action is largely unknown, estrogens have been shown to induce breast cancer regressions in animal models associated with suppression of insulinlike growth factor signaling.[340] Patients with prior heavy exposure to endocrine therapy (tamoxifen, megestrol acetate, and an aromatase inhibitor) may still respond to diethylstilbestrol, 5 mg three times a day.[341] Unfortunately, pharmacologic doses of estrogen will always be limited by a high burden of side effects that include breast tenderness, vaginal discharge, and, more seriously, congestive cardiac failure and venous thrombosis. As with progestins, estrogens are contraindicated if the patient has a thromboembolic or cardiac disorder. Obtaining diethylstilbestrol is difficult in the United States, and therefore alternative estrogens, including formulations that are normally used for hormone replacement therapy, may have to be considered.[147]

COMBINATION ENDOCRINE THERAPIES VERSUS SEQUENTIAL SINGLE-AGENT THERAPY

Antiestrogen/Estrogen Deprivation Therapy Combinations

A discussion of endocrine therapies for breast cancer would be incomplete without consideration of data concerning endocrine therapy combinations. From a mechanistic point of view, combinations can be classified as antiestrogen and estrogen deprivation combinations or antiestrogen and sex steroid combinations. Antiestrogen and estrogen deprivation combinations continue to intrigue investigators. The improvements in response rate, progression-free survival, and OS associated with the combination of LHRH-A plus tamoxifen when compared with LHRH-A alone were discussed in the section Estrogen Deprivation Therapy for Premenopausal Women.[143] These data contrast with studies in postmenopausal women in whom the combination of tamoxifen and estrogen deprivation with aminoglutethimide is no more active than tamoxifen alone, and considerably more toxic.[298,342–344] Interestingly, the potential of combining an aromatase inhibitor and tamoxifen has been extensively reexamined in a trial in which the adjuvant treatment of 9,000 postmenopausal patients was randomly assigned to tamoxifen, anastrozole, or the combination (ATAC trial). The results of this trial will take several years to mature. Currently, there are no data available on the combination of an SAI with tamoxifen in the metastatic setting. Therefore, tamoxifen and SAIs should be used in sequence and not in combination until the efficacy and toxicity of the combination have been carefully examined. It is particularly important to avoid treating patients with a letrozole-tamoxifen combination, as tamoxifen may impair the efficacy of letrozole by accelerating letrozole clearance through the liver.[345]

Antiestrogen–Sex Steroid Combinations

Tamoxifen has been examined in combination with androgens, estrogens, and progestins.[346–349] Although gains in response rates were observed, time to progression and OS were not affected. The broad conclusion from these studies is that the addition of sex steroids adds toxicity to tamoxifen therapy without any clear gain in clinical outcomes. Combining sex steroids with tamoxifen is therefore not recommended.

Combinations with Other Noncytotoxic Drugs

The use of bisphosphonate therapy for patients with bone metastases is discussed in Chapter 61. In brief, bisphosphonates are routinely combined with endocrine therapy or chemotherapy, because pamidronate has been shown to reduce skeletal morbidity for patients with breast cancer metastatic to bone.[350,351] In the future, bisphosphonates may be combined with adjuvant SAI therapy to abrogate the skeletal effects of estrogen deficiency. The combination of an SAI with bisphosphonates in the adjuvant setting is particularly intriguing because of reports that prophylactic bisphosphonates may reduce the incidence of bone metastasis.[352,353]

NOVEL ENDOCRINE THERAPIES DIRECTED TOWARD SIGNAL TRANSDUCTION PATHWAYS OTHER THAN THOSE INDUCED BY SEX STEROIDS

Classically, "endocrine therapy" for breast cancer has implied interference with the signal transduction pathway mediated by the ER. Several investigational approaches toward disruption of other signal transduction pathways have been pursued. These approaches offer promise for development of therapies with toxic-therapeutic ratios that mimic those seen with tamoxifen and other classic endocrine therapies.

Retinoids

Retinoic acid and its derivatives interact with a family of receptors that have similar structural motifs as those described previously for ER and PR (see Fig. 10A). The receptors for retinoids are designated *retinoic acid receptors*. One RAR agonist, all transretinoic acid (ATRA), has not been found to have substantial single-agent activity in metastatic disease. However, a study of the combination of ATRA and tamoxifen suggests that ATRA might reverse tamoxifen resistance.[354] Among 20 patients with tamoxifen-resistant disease, one response and 6 patients with stable disease were observed when further tamoxifen therapy was combined with ATRA. In another small study, fenretinide, an ATRA prodrug, although inactive as a single agent, also had activity in combination with tamoxifen.[355,356] Further research on fenretinide has been focused on prevention and adjuvant settings.[357] Interest has shifted to a new class of retinoids, designated *rexinoids*. Rexinoids interact with a second family of retinoid receptor, RXR, in preference to RAR. In preclinical models, an RXR agonist, targretin, was active and synergistic with tamoxifen.[358] Targretin has been well tolerated in phase I trials, and it is being examined in a phase II clinical trial, both as a single agent and in combination with tamoxifen.

Trastuzamab

The results of completed clinical trials released in 1998 and 1999 have demonstrated that the *erb*-b2 targeting antibody trastuzamab has antitumor activity in *erb*-b2 overexpressing malignancies (see Future Prospects for Metastatic Breast Cancer, later in text). Because resistance to endocrine therapy in ER-positive breast cancers may be associated with overexpression of *erb*-b2, trials of the combination of trastuzamab with endocrine therapy are appealing. Tumors that coexpress ER and *erb*-b2 are relatively common and are therefore a logical target for the trastuzamab–endocrine therapy combination treatment.[108] However, no clinical data are available regarding responses to a trastuzamab–endocrine therapy combination. A trial examining the activity of a combination of tamoxifen and trastuzamab is being conducted.

SUMMARY OF ENDOCRINE TREATMENT FOR METASTATIC BREAST CANCER

We are now entering a new phase of endocrine therapy development, in which the choice of treatment is driven by

TABLE 9. *Ongoing endocrine therapy trials*

Class of agent	Agents in trial
Nonsteroidal SAI vs progestin	Letrozole vs megestrol acetate
Steroidal SAI vs progestin	Exemestane vs megestrol acetate
Nonsteroidal SAI vs same	Letrozole vs anastrozole
Nonsteroidal SAI vs tamoxifen	Letrozole vs tamoxifen Anastrozole vs tamoxifen
Pure antiestrogen vs nonsteroidal SAI	Faslodex vs anastrozole EM800 vs anastrozole
Pure antiestrogen vs tamoxifen	Faslodex vs tamoxifen
Rexinoid plus tamoxifen	Targretin plus tamoxifen (phase 2)
HER-2 targeting antibody plus tamoxifen	Trastuzamab plus tamoxifen (phase 2)

SAI, selective aromatase inhibitor.

improvements in efficacy rather than reduced toxicity. It is likely that the treatment algorithm in Fig. 6 will quickly become outdated. Table 9 provides a summary of the pending clinical trials discussed in this chapter that will mature during the life of this edition. Although new endocrine therapies will target ER ever more efficiently, perhaps the greatest hope for the future lies in new agents that target non–sex steroid–mediated signal transduction pathways so that breast cancers without an intact ER pathway can be targeted with specific molecular therapies. Trastuzamab is just the first step on this new road.

CHEMOTHERAPY FOR METASTATIC BREAST CANCER

Principles of Chemotherapy

Breast cancer is one of the most chemosensitive of the common solid malignancies. Most previously untreated patients, and even many previously treated patients, are likely to benefit from chemotherapy in the metastatic setting. However, this benefit comes at the cost of increased toxicity, especially in comparison to that usually experienced with endocrine therapy. Response rates higher than 20% have been reported for several single agents, including alkylating agents, anthracyclines and anthraquinones, antimetabolites, vinca alkyloids, and the taxanes (Table 10). Therefore, fundamental properties of each class of agents, combinations of agents, increasing doses, and various schedules are reviewed.

Anthracyclines/Anthraquinones

Before the advent of the taxanes, the anthracyclines, especially doxorubicin, and anthracycline-like drugs were believed to be the most active agents in breast cancer, with single-agent response rates in untreated patients of 35% to 50%.[20,359–361] Of note, overall efficacy of mitoxantrone appears to be slightly lower than for either doxorubicin or epirubicin, whether compared as single agents or in combination with other drugs, although this observation has not been made consistently in all trials.[359,361–365]

Like most chemotherapeutic agents, members of this class cause nausea, vomiting, hair loss, and bone marrow suppression. The risk of these side effects appears to be sim-

TABLE 10. *Commonly used doses and schedules of frequently administered chemotherapeutic agents for breast cancer*

Agent	Usual doses	Usual route	Usual schedule
Capecitabine	1.0–2.0 g/m²	po	Daily × 14 d every 21 d
Cyclophosphamide	400–600 mg/m²	i.v.	Every 21 d
	100 mg/m² (max, 150 mg)	po	Daily × 14 d every 21 d
Docetaxel	80–100 mg/m²	i.v.	Every 21 d
	30–35 mg/m²	i.v.	Every 7 d
Doxorubicin	40–75 mg/m²	i.v.	Every 21 d
Epirubicin	60–90 mg/m²	i.v.	Every 21 d
Etoposide	50 mg	po	Daily × 14 d every 21 d
Fluorouracil	400–600 mg/m²	i.v.	Day 1, 8 every 28 d
	500 mg/m²	Continuous infusion	Day 1–3, with leucovorin, every 21 d
Methotrexate	40–60 mg/m²	i.v.	Day 1, 8 every 28 d
Mitoxantrone	10–15 mg/m²	i.v.	Every 21 d
Mitomycin C	10 mg/m²	i.v.	Day 1 every 42 d
Paclitaxel	175–200 mg/m²	i.v.	Every 21 d
	80–100 mg/m²	i.v.	Every 7 d
Vinblastine	3–4 mg/m²	i.v.	Day 1, 8 every 21 d
Vinorelbine	20–25 mg/m²	i.v.	Day 1, 8 every 21 d

Doses are ranged based on whether agent is used as single agent or in combination and on degree of prior treatment, performance status, and bone marrow function of patient. None of these suggestions is meant to be absolute, and for each agent, other alternative doses and schedules have been reported. Max, maximum.

ilar for doxorubicin and epirubicin but is less common with mitoxantrone.[359–361] Myocardial damage resulting in clinical congestive heart failure (CHF) is a major class-specific toxicity of the anthracyclines and anthracycline-like agents. The incidence of CHF is directly related to cumulative total dose, increasing sharply above 450 mg per m^2 for doxorubicin.[365] Epirubicin and mitoxantrone are less cardiotoxic, on a dose basis, than doxorubicin.[359,361–363,367] However, it appears that epirubicin is also less effective than doxorubicin on a dose basis, and therefore the curves for both efficacy and CHF may simply be shifted to the right.[360,368–371]

Investigators have tried several strategies to reduce the risk of CHF related to doxorubicin. For example, it appears that in addition to total cumulative dose, total peak dose/infusion is also a risk factor. Prolonged infusions (6 to 96 hours) or more frequent infusions of lower doses of doxorubicin are associated with less risk of cardiotoxicity than when the drug is delivered by bolus.[372–374] A second approach has been to incorporate doxorubicin into liposomes. This strategy appears to permit higher cumulative doses with a much lower incidence of CHF.[375–380] A third means of reducing the risk of CHF is to coadminister cardioprotectant agents, such as dexrazoxane.[381] Although these strategies have been effective in reducing the risk of clinically important heart failure, there are important caveats to each. For example, longer or more frequent infusions of doxorubicin are less convenient for the patient, and the costs of liposomal doxorubicin and dexrazoxane are considerable.[382] Moreover, there has been concern that these approaches may result in less efficacy. If given at appropriate doses, infusional doxorubicin appears to be as active as bolus therapy every 3 weeks.[372,373,383] Insufficient data regarding liposomal doxorubicin versus free doxorubicin are available to make valid conclusions, although 1998 results from a randomized trial suggest that the two are equally efficacious.[378] In two randomized trials of doxorubicin with or without dexrazoxane, response rates were slightly worse for the group that received the cardioprotectant.[381] More important, because most patients develop resistance to doxorubicin before they reach cumulative doses that place them at high risk for CHF, this concern is often not relevant. However, it is reasonable to convert to one of these strategies in selected patients who continue to benefit from the drug after cumulative doses of 300 mg per m^2, especially if other options are not as satisfactory as continuing with doxorubicin. In this regard, dexrazoxane exerts a protective effect even after a cumulative dose of 300 mg per m^2 doxorubicin.[381] In the randomized trials of this agent, the cardioprotective effect of dexrazoxane either was observed whether the drug was started initially or after 300 mg per m^2 doxorubicin compared to patients who receive only placebo.[381]

Because of their high rates of activity, agents from this class have served as the bases for several combination chemotherapeutic regimens. Perhaps the most widely used of these combinations is FAC (or CAF),[384–389] epirubicin with CPA and 5-fluorouracil, commonly designated *FEC*,[365,390,391] or both. In general, the response rates to these regimens in previously untreated patients with metastatic disease range from 20% to 60%, and the combination seems slightly more active but also more toxic than the previously existing "standard," CMF.[386] Doxorubicin, epirubicin, and mitoxantrone have been tested in combinations with almost every other active agent, as doublets, triplets, or more. Although several phase I and II studies suggest that the combinations may be more active than the individual drugs alone, prospective randomized trials have failed to support this notion. Each of these is discussed in the context of the different chemotherapeutic agents below.

Alkylating Agents

Alkylating agents have long been one of the cornerstones of therapy for breast cancer in the adjuvant and metastatic settings. Of these, CPA is the most widely used. In a number of studies, single-agent CPA induced responses in 10% to 60% of patients.[392] In addition to the common chemotherapy side effects frequently seen with chemotherapy, such as nausea, vomiting, alopecia, and bone marrow depression, CPA is associated with a small risk of urinary bladder hemorrhage, although this toxicity is almost completely eliminated by adequate hydration and frequent urination. Alkylating agents are also associated with an increased risk of myelogenous leukemias. The excess risk is related to both the individual drugs and the cumulative dose. Because even modest cumulative doses of oral L-phenylalanine mustard (melphalan) confer an increased risk of leukemia of 30-fold or higher, it is rarely used to treat breast cancer.[393,394] In contrast, the additional risk of leukemia related to CPA is very low (threefold) and is probably less than that at cumulative doses below 20,000 mg per m^2.[395,396]

Ifosfamide (IFF) appears to have little activity as a single agent in breast cancer, with response rates of 7% to 15% in previously treated or chemotherapy-naive patients.[397,398] Although IFF has been incorporated into combination chemotherapy regimens, it is not clear that this agent adds benefit to the other drugs with which it is combined. The added toxicities and costs of IFF make it an unappealing choice for the average patient with metastatic breast cancer.[399–405]

The activity of cisplatin and its congener, carboplatin, in metastatic breast cancer remains controversial. Both of these drugs have become mainstays in very high dose regimens that require bone marrow stem cell support (see Chapter 38). Reported response rates of these drugs as single agents, when administered at nonmyeloablative doses, range from 0 to 25%.[392,406–410] Like ifosfamide, cisplatin and carboplatin have frequently been included in combinations with other agents that have known activity. It is not clear that these combinations have superior efficacy to what one might expect from the use of the partner drugs if given as single agents.[392]

In summary, outside of clinical trials, little role exists for either cisplatin or carboplatin in patients with metastatic breast cancer. However, *in vitro* data suggest that the parent antibody of trastuzamab may reverse resistance to cisplatin by modulating *erb*-b2 activity.[411] In a small phase II study, the response rate of trastuzamab and cisplatin in patients with doxorubicin-refractory disease was 24%, with minor response or stabilization of disease in an additional 24% of patients.[116] Studies of trastuzamab and carboplatin in breast cancer patients are now under way. This combination must be considered promising but investigational.

Antimetabolites

Like alkylating agents, antimetabolites have served as fundamental components of chemotherapeutic regimens for breast cancer. Of the inhibitors of dihydrofolate reductase, methotrexate has been most widely used, although derivatives such as trimetrexate also have single-agent activity.[412] However, the ease of administration and favorable toxicity profile of methotrexate have maintained it as the antifol of choice for this disease. Small studies of high-dose methotrexate (2 to 3 g/m^2) did not indicate evidence of increased activity; the higher cost and toxicities suggest that there is no role for this modality in the treatment of patients with metastatic breast cancer.[413–415] For the most part, methotrexate is used in the standard "oral" CMF regimen, which consists of oral CPA (100 mg/m^2/day; days 1 to 14), intravenous methotrexate (40 mg/m^2, days 1 and 8), and intravenous 5FU (600 mg/m^2, days 1 and 8).[416]

5FU and its derivatives have continued to be widely used for metastatic breast cancer. Importantly, activity of this class of drugs appears to be highly dependent on schedule, with frequent or prolonged infusions being superior to single-bolus administration. Furthermore, the activity of 5FU may be enhanced by modulation with leucovorin.[417–426] Response rates of 20% to 40% have been reported, even in patients who have previously progressed on 5FU-containing regimens, such as CMF. Several regimens have been suggested, but most include either daily bolus or continuous infusions of 5FU at 200 to 500 mg per m^2 per day for 1 to 3 days or weekly 5FU at higher doses (1,000 to 2,000 mg/m^2/day), with or without leucovorin. Recently, orally active derivatives of 5FU have been studied, including tegafur and capecitabine. In general, recommended dosage schedules include daily therapy for several days, sometimes weeks, and may or may not include oral leucovorin.[427–430] Response rates to these drugs are reported to be 20% to 35%, even in patients who have received heavy pretreatment for metastatic disease, often including 5FU-containing regimens.[427–430]

5FU and its derivatives tend not to induce alopecia to the extent seen with doxorubicin, alkylating agents, or the taxanes, and nausea and vomiting are uncommon, appearing in fewer than 10% of patients who are treated. The effects of 5FU plus leucovorin on bone marrow are also less toxic, and it is rare to witness grade 3/4 neutropenia or thrombocytopenia. However, other gastrointestinal side effects, including diarrhea and mucositis, are common, with grade 1 and 2 symptoms seen in up to 90% and grade 3/4 toxicities occurring in 20% or more of patients. Perhaps the most bothersome side effect, and often the dose-limiting toxicity for the oral agents, is hand-foot syndrome, which has been reported in up to 20% of patients.[427–430] Although the etiology of this syndrome is not entirely established, it appears to occur as a function of cumulative dose and prolonged concentrations during single cycles. Therefore, manipulation of either the total dose per day or the number of days that the patient takes the drug can minimize these symptoms. If mucositis, diarrhea, and hand-foot syndrome can be avoided, single-agent infusional 5FU or its oral derivatives can often result in effective palliation for patients whose disease has become refractory to other regimens.

Prolonged infusional and daily 5FU, or daily oral tegafur, with or without leucovorin, have each been studied in combination with other active agents. In particular, the combination of mitoxantrone (Novantrone), 5FU, and leucovorin (designated *NFL*) has proved to be an effective and well-tolerated regimen for patients with metastatic disease. Response rates to this regimen range from 27% to 65%, again even in patients whose disease has previously been refractory to 5FU-containing regimens.[431–435] Tegafur has also been incorporated in a combination with leucovorin and mitoxantrone, with a similarly high response rate (62%) and acceptable toxicity profile. A randomized trial comparing NFL to CMF in previously untreated patients with metastatic disease demonstrated that response rates were statistically significantly higher for NFL (45% versus 26%), although time to progression was only a few months longer and OS was nearly identical.[436] From these studies, one can conclude that it is reasonable to recommend NFL to patients in the metastatic setting, especially given the relative lack of alopecia, although it is probably otherwise not substantially superior to other choices.

Tubular-Acting Agents: Vinca Alkaloids and Taxanes

Vinca Alkaloids and Derivatives

Early in the experience of combination chemotherapy for breast cancer, vincristine was incorporated into CMF-type regimens. However, phase II studies of vincristine as a single agent suggest that its activity is not very high, with response rates often less than 10%.[392] Given the low activity and frequent neurotoxicity of vincristine, coupled with the availability of better agents in this class, there is little reason to continue to use it in patients with breast cancer.

In contrast, three other agents in this class, vindesine, vinblastine, and vinorelbine, are all reasonably active and much better tolerated, due in part to more selective microtubular protein binding. Vindesine, vinblastine, and vinorelbine have become widely used drugs in the treatment of metastatic breast cancer. Each of these has reported response rates as high as 40%.[437–448] Of these, vinorelbine has gained increasing acceptance. When delivered intravenously at 25 to 35 mg per m^2 on days 1 and 8 of a 3-week cycle, vinorelbine induces single-agent response rates of 30% to 40%, even in patients whose disease is refractory to anthracyclines, with an acceptable neurotoxicity profile.[437–441,449] Because earlier studies suggested that the activity and toxicity of vinblastine may be dose and schedule dependent, at least one phase I study was conducted to test vinorelbine on a day 1 to 3 schedule, but gastrointestinal and neurotoxicities were prohibitive.[450] In addition to the anticipated hematologic toxicities and neurotoxicities, these agents can occasionally induce acute, severe peritumoral pain.[449] This reaction, which occurs in fewer than 5% of patients, can begin during or immediately after the infusion and may last several minutes to hours, requiring narcotic analgesic relief. However, it is self-limiting and does not seem to result in long-term disability. The etiology of this phenomenon is not clear, but in the few patients who have been retreated, it has occasionally been recurrent.

As expected, these agents have been included in multiple combination regimens with alkylating agents (CPA, IFF, cisplatin, carboplatin, mitomycin-C), antimetabolites (5FU/leucovorin), anthracyclines (doxorubicin, epirubicin, mitoxantrone), taxanes (paclitaxel, docetaxel), or a combination of these. In each case, the combinations are reported to be active, but toxicities are usually additive. In the absence of randomized trial data, it is very difficult to ascertain whether anything is to be gained from using these combinations as opposed to applying the agents singly in a serial fashion. Of note, the combination of mitomycin-C and vinblastine was shown to be active in anthracycline-resistant metastatic breast cancer and became quite popular as second-line therapy before the widespread use of the taxanes.[451,452] However, mitomycin-C/vinblastine has been proved to be inferior to single-agent docetaxel alone in a prospective randomized trial.[453] This combination seems to have very little role in modern therapy, given the high incidence of thrombocytopenia and life-threatening hemolytic-uremic syndrome.

Taxanes

The taxanes are derived from bark (paclitaxel) or needles (docetaxel) of the Pacific Western and European yew trees, although both are now produced via chemical synthesis. Whereas vinca alkaloids prevent microtubule assembly, the taxanes stabilize microtubules and induce G_2-cycle arrest.[454] Initial phase I efforts to deliver paclitaxel were hampered by its poor solubility and an unacceptable rate of life-threatening allergic and anaphylactoid reactions. These problems are probably related to hypersensitivity to the obligate solute carrier, polyoxyethylated castor oil and alcohol (Cremaphor EL). However, these reactions can be minimized, and nearly eliminated, by pre- and posttreatment with dexamethasone, diphenhydramine, and cimetidine or ranitidine, and by decreasing the rate of infusions of the drug.[455] Indeed, experience with weekly infusions of paclitaxel at moderate doses infused over 1 hour has suggested that treatment with steroids is unnecessary for most patients, although they have been included in weekly docetaxel regimens.[456,457]

Paclitaxel has engendered considerable enthusiasm for metastatic breast cancer treatment because of its high activity in doxorubicin-naive and refractory patients. All studies reported to date have documented response rates of at least 20% in previously treated patients, and several have reported responses as high as 35% to 55%.[458–467] The precise dose and schedule of paclitaxel have not been determined. In initial investigations, paclitaxel was delivered at doses of 135 to 250 mg per m^2 over 3 to 24 hours every 3 weeks.[468] A single prospective randomized trial in patients with metastatic disease, some of whom had been pretreated and some of whom had not, has suggested a slight advantage for 175 mg per m^2 over 135 mg per m^2.[469] In this study, response rates were 29% versus 22% ($p = .11$), times to progression were 4.2 months versus 3.0 months ($p = .027$), and OS was 11.7 months versus 10.5 months ($p = .32$), respectively, for the higher and lower doses. In a 1998 randomized study performed by the Cancer and Leukemia Group B, doses of 175 mg per m^2, 210 mg per m^2, and 250 mg per m^2 were compared.[470] Response rates were 21%, 28%, and 22% ($p = .64$); times to treatment failure were 3.8 months, 4.1 months, and 4.8 months ($p = .03$); and OS was 9.8 months, 11.8 months, and 11.9 months ($p = .48$), respectively, for the three arms. Investigators have also reported that paclitaxel can be administered weekly at doses of 80 to 100 mg per m^2 for several weeks, and sometimes without cessation, with a remarkable lack of hematologic or neurotoxicity.[471] In a single phase II experience at Memorial Sloan-Kettering, the response rate was more than 50%, even in patients whose disease was refractory to anthracyclines.[471] A prospective randomized trial comparing paclitaxel using this schedule to the more standard every-3-week schedule is now under way.

Toxicities of paclitaxel are relatively predictable and, for most patients, reasonably tolerable. Paclitaxel induces very little nausea or vomiting, but, when delivered every 3 weeks, alopecia occurs in nearly 100% of patients. In 5% to 15% of patients, a syndrome of myalgias and arthralgias develops, ranging from very mild and requiring only occasional nonnarcotic analgesia to incapacitating pain. This syndrome normally begins 24 to 72 hours after infusion and lasts from 2 to 4 days.[461,472] For those patients with severe symptoms, continuation of dexamethasone from the day of treatment through the expected time of myalgias can be quite effective. However, because this syndrome is relatively rare, extension of dexamethasone is only indicated for those who experience it during the first cycle, thus avoiding the toxicities of steroid use in the remaining, unaffected patients. As with the vinca alkaloids, peripheral neuropathy is reasonably common, although grade 3 or 4 neuropathy occurs in only 10% to 15% of treated patients.[472] Peripheral neuropathy appears to be associated with higher doses or shorter infusions, or both, and after multiple cycles of administration. Early experiences with weekly infusions of lower doses suggest that this strategy may reduce peripheral neuropathy, despite the much larger cumulative doses.[471,473]

Although docetaxel is structurally similar to paclitaxel and also appears to exert its antitumor activity by stabilizing microtubular assemblies, the two drugs are not identical.[474] Preclinical studies suggest that docetaxel may be less susceptible to resistance because of MDR mechanisms, in particular that mediated by MDR protein.[475] Several phase II studies of docetaxel in metastatic breast cancer have demonstrated that, like paclitaxel, it is remarkably effective even in patients whose disease has become refractory to nontaxane therapies, with response rates frequently between 35% and 60%.[476–492]

No studies have been reported in which docetaxel and paclitaxel have been directly compared in patients with breast cancer. In general, response rates reported from phase II studies of docetaxel appear higher than those from studies of paclitaxel, but these trials differ widely in design, patient selection, dose, and schedules. In a phase II study, 25% of patients who had previously progressed while receiving paclitaxel experienced a subsequent response to docetaxel.[493] However, all of the responses were observed in patients who had previously been treated with 3-hour paclitaxel infusions, and no responses were seen in patients who had previously progressed after receiving paclitaxel for 24 hours. In this regard, investigators from Memorial Sloan-Kettering Cancer Center reported a similar response rate to paclitaxel administered as a 96-hour infusion in patients who had previously progressed after 3-hour infusions of the same drug.[494] In separate randomized trials in which either paclitaxel or docetaxel has been compared with doxorubicin, little if any benefit was observed between paclitaxel and doxorubicin, whereas docetaxel induced higher response rates.[495–497] Prospective randomized trials in adjuvant and metastatic settings of paclitaxel versus docetaxel are under way.

Fewer studies of dose and schedule of docetaxel have been performed than for paclitaxel. For the most part, the drug has been delivered as a 1-hour infusion at 100 mg per m^2, every 3 weeks. A few studies of weekly docetaxel have been reported, and the recommended dose appears to be 30 to 40 mg per m^2 per week by 1-hour infusion.[457] As with paclitaxel, weekly docetaxel appears to remain quite active and may have less neuro- and hematologic toxicity.[498–500] Although occasional hypersensitivity reactions are seen with docetaxel, they are less common than with paclitaxel. Like paclitaxel, docetaxel rarely causes nausea and vomiting, and it induces alopecia almost universally. Similarly, cumulative doses of docetaxel result in peripheral neuropathies. Unlike paclitaxel, docetaxel induces fluid retention, resulting in peripheral edema and pleural effusions. In early phase II studies, fluid retention was cumulative after several cycles in as many as 95% of treated patients and was often the dose-limiting toxicity.[476,501,502] However, with appropriate premedication using 3 to 5 days of corticosteroids, the cumulative doses of docetaxel associated with fluid retention are much higher, although refractory pleural effusions can occur.[491] Docetaxel is also associated with cumulative dose-related nail changes, although the precise incidence is not entirely clear.[503,504]

Paclitaxel and docetaxel can cause profound hematologic depression, resulting in neutropenia and leukopenia.[505,506] These are usually transient and noncumulative. However, because both drugs are cleared by the hepatobiliary system, patients with hepatic dysfunction should be treated especially cautiously, with dose reductions and careful blood count monitoring. Indeed, weekly schedules of lower doses might be ideal for such patients, because the drug can be titrated against white blood cell counts.[471]

Paclitaxel and docetaxel have been included in a number of combinations with other active agents. Regimens containing taxanes and anthracyclines have appeared particularly active in phase II trials. However, combinations of paclitaxel and doxorubicin may be associated with development of CHF at cumulative doxorubicin doses much lower than are of usual concern. Although not seen in all studies, heart failure has occurred in as many as 20% of patients treated with this combination.[507–510] Because paclitaxel can alter doxorubicin pharmacokinetics, investigators have suggested that CHF may be reduced by administering the doxorubicin before the paclitaxel.[507,511] Other strategies include limiting cumulative doxorubicin to less than 350 mg per m^2 or using cardioprotectants, or both.[512] Paclitaxel has been combined with other nondoxorubicin, anthracycline-like agents without excess cardiac toxicities.[513,514] Thus far, docetaxel-doxorubicin combinations have not produced higher than expected rates of CHF.[515]

As with many of the combination chemotherapies discussed previously, it is not clear that the added toxicities of combining taxanes with other drugs are justified by increased benefits. Led by the Eastern Cooperative Oncology Group, the U.S. Intergroup performed a prospective randomized trial that compared paclitaxel alone versus doxorubicin alone versus a combination of the two in patients with previously untreated metastatic disease.[495] Patients who received the single-agent arms were treated with the other drug at the time of progression on the first drug. Although response rates and times to first treatment failure for the combination were higher than for either drug alone, OS for all three groups was similar. Cardiac toxicity was equivalent for patients in either the doxorubicin or the combination arms.

It is possible that single-agent taxane therapy may be superior to combination chemotherapeutic regimens that do not contain a taxane. At least two studies have directly addressed this issue. In one, patients with metastatic breast cancer received either paclitaxel or CMF plus prednisone (CMFP) as first-line therapy.[516] The two groups had nearly identical response rates and times to treatment failure. Patients treated with paclitaxel had a 6-month survival advantage compared to those who received CMFP (17.3 months versus 11.3 months), but this difference was not statistically significant. Formal QOL analysis suggested that patients favored the single-agent paclitaxel treatment. In a multicenter prospectively randomized European trial, docetaxel has been compared with mitomycin-C and vinblastine in patients who had anthracycline-resistant disease.[453] Response rates (48% versus 33%, $p = .008$), times to progression (19 months versus 11 months, $p = .001$), and OS

(11.4 months versus 8.7 months, $p = .009$) were all significantly superior for patients who received docetaxel compared to those treated with mitomycin-C–vinblastine.

Early experiences with the combination of paclitaxel and trastuzamab (see previous discussion) are very encouraging. In a 1998-reported randomized trial, the response rates, times to progression, and even OS for patients with doxorubicin-refractory disease treated with a combination of paclitaxel and trastuzamab were nearly double those treated with paclitaxel alone.[24] This exciting observation is discussed in greater detail below, but these data suggest that when chemotherapy is appropriate in *erb*-b2–positive patients, this combination should be strongly considered.

In summary, the taxanes have rapidly become cornerstones of treatment for patients with hormone-refractory metastatic breast cancer. These drugs appear to lack cross-resistance with commonly used agents in breast cancer, including alkylating agents, doxorubicin, and the antimetabolites. Furthermore, if used judiciously, they are reasonably well tolerated. Moreover, in some trials, taxanes appear to provide a small but potentially important survival advantage. It is clear that these agents have fundamentally changed the approach toward the patient with metastatic breast cancer. However, the question of the precise agent or combination of agents, dose, and schedule of administration is still unanswered for both drugs and remains the objective of ongoing clinical investigations.

Etoposide

Etoposide (VP16) is a semisynthetic podophyllotoxin that has excellent oral availability. Although early studies of this agent suggested that it had little or no activity in metastatic breast cancer, more recent phase II trials have indicated response rates or at least stabilization of disease in 25% to 50% of patients, even if they were heavily pretreated.[517–523] When given orally at 50 mg per m^2 per day, the agent can be titrated to toxicities, which are principally hematologic and gastrointestinal. Because of its ease of administration, relatively low toxicity profile, and reasonable activity rate, oral VP16 is an attractive agent as third- or fourth-line chemotherapy in metastatic disease.

Specific Issues regarding Chemotherapy

Combination versus Serial Single Agents

The principle of nonoverlapping mechanisms of resistance and toxicities has been the basis for applying combination chemotherapy. This strategy resulted in cures for human malignancies such as Hodgkin's disease, non-Hodgkin's lymphoma, certain leukemias, and germ cell carcinoma of the testicle.[524] Although combination chemotherapy has been widely embraced, the validity of this concept has not been confirmed in breast cancer. In several randomized trials comparing combination chemotherapy to single-agent therapy, response rates are higher in the combination arms, and times to first progression are longer. However, OS has only been minimally improved at best, in the groups that received combination therapy first. Fossati et al.[122] estimate that the proportional reduction in overall mortality for combinations versus single agents is only 18%, translating to an absolute benefit in survival of 9% at 1 year, 5% at 2 years, and only 3% after 5 years (Fig. 16). When combination chemotherapy is compared to single agents other than anthracyclines, the survival benefit is higher, with proportional mortality reductions approaching 30%. The absolute reduction in mortality remains modest, as described previously for the study performed by Ahmann et al.,[20] comparing CFP and CCNU. Indeed, if an anthracycline is the single agent against which combinations are compared, the proportional reduction in mortality was only 13%.[122] Moreover, in two randomized trials of combination versus single-agent therapy in patients with metastatic disease (CMFP versus paclitaxel; CEF versus epirubicin), formal QOL analyses favored the single-agent arms even though response rates were slightly lower.[516,525]

Dose

The issue of dose response and chemotherapy is discussed in great detail in Chapter 38. It is not known whether delivery of very high doses of chemotherapy, requiring bone marrow stem cell support, adds benefit above that achieved with standard doses.[526] Therefore, very-high-dose chemotherapy is not recommended outside of a clinical trial. However, results of prospective randomized trials performed in the 1980s suggested that decreasing doses below what would be considered standard levels today does result in suboptimal response rates, shorter time to progression, and inferior palliation. For example, Tannock et al.[527] compared treatment of patients with metastatic breast cancer with CMF at doses of (C)600/(M)40/(F)600 mg per m^2, respectively, to doses of (C)300/(M)20/(F)300 mg per m^2. Response rates were substantially higher in the higher-dose arm, although survival was only marginally improved. Importantly, in a subset of patients, QOL assessments were performed and suggested a trend toward health improvement in spite of the toxicities associated with higher doses. Similarly, other randomized trials have confirmed the relative benefit of dose escalation within ranges that do not require growth factor or hematopoietic stem cell support for anthracyclines (epirubicin, 90 better than 60 mg/m^2) and taxanes (paclitaxel, 175 better than 135 mg/m^2).[369,528] The concept of extending doses to levels that require growth factor or hematopoietic stem cell support has not been supported by the results of randomized trials, either for anthracyclines (epirubicin, 90 mg/m^2 or more) or paclitaxel (175 mg/m^2 or more).[369,470] The dose-limiting toxicities for these drugs are

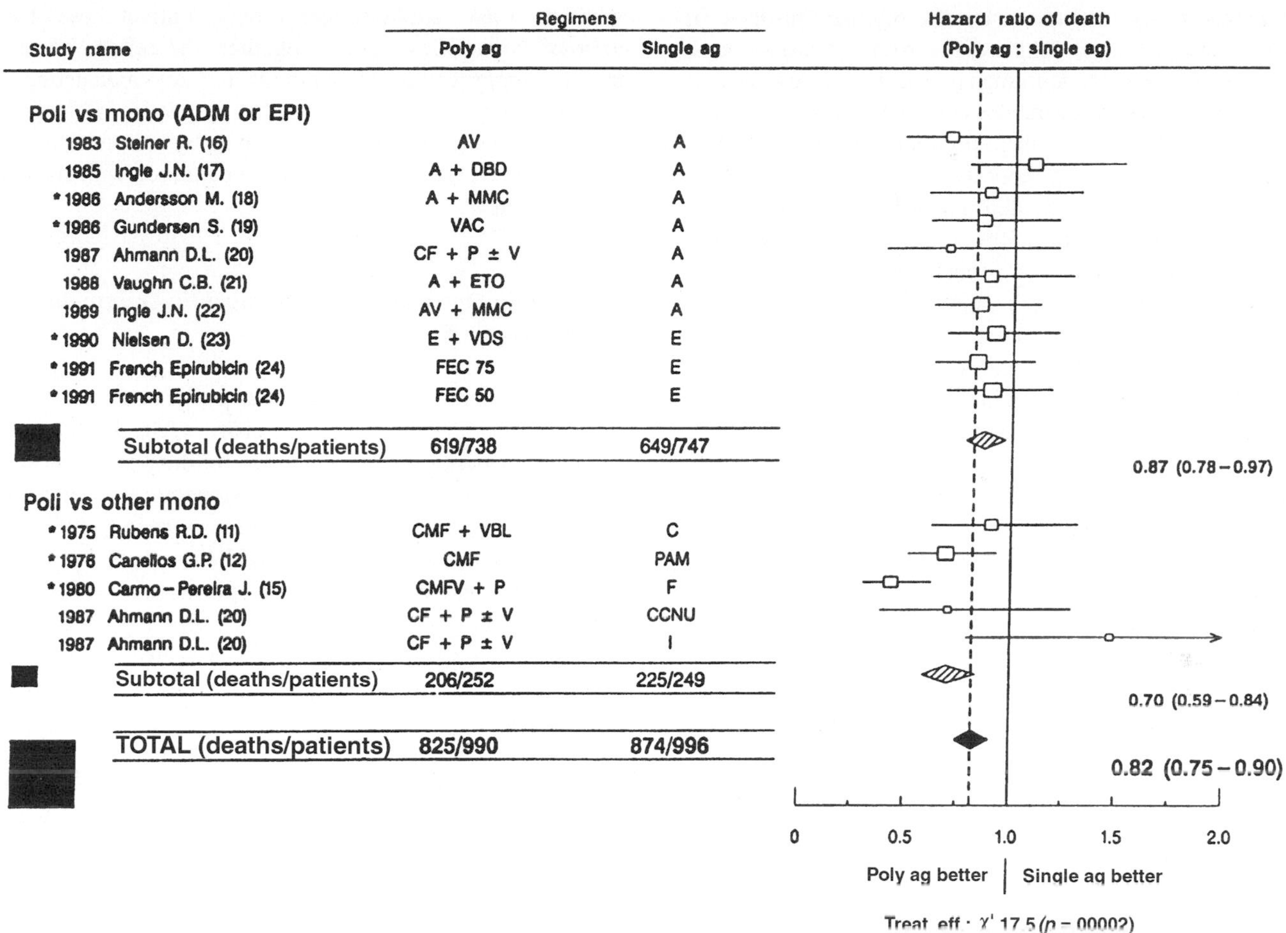

FIG. 16. Combination (poly) chemotherapy versus single-agent chemotherapy as first-line chemotherapy for patients with metastatic breast cancer: a systematic review. All prospective randomized studies published as of December 31, 1997, were reviewed and included in this analysis. Test for heterogeneity: X^2HetT = 22.19, df = 14, p = .07; X^2HetB = 4.09, df = 1, p = .04; X^2HetW = 18.1, df = 13, p = 0.15. A, doxorubicin; ag, aminoglutethimide; c, continuous; C, cyclophosphamide; CCNU, lomustine; D, doxorubicin; DBD, mitolactol; E, epirubicin; eff., efficacy; ETO, etoposide; F, 5-fluorouracil; i, intermittent; I, ifosfamide; M, methotrexate; mono, monochemotherapy; MMC, mitomycin-C; P, epirubicin; PAM, melphalan; Poli, polychemotherapy; Treat., treatment; V, vincristine; VBL, vinblastine; VDS, vindesine; open boxes, HR results from individual studies; cross-hatched and filled triangles, subtotal and overall HR with their 95% confidence intervals; *, Hazard ratio (HR) obtained from survival curves. (From ref. 122, with permission.)

nonhematopoietic (cardiac and neurologic, respectively). Therefore, it may be impossible to dose escalate to more myelosuppressive doses anyway.

Schedule

The relative value of different schedules of chemotherapy for metastatic breast cancer is less well studied than for dose. Several preliminary, uncontrolled studies have suggested that doxorubicin, 5FU, and the taxanes can be delivered at reasonably high doses with less toxicity when administered weekly rather than every 3 or 4 weeks.[425,456,529–531] In theory, the delivery of these drugs at higher "dose densities" might result in enhanced activity either because of more frequent exposure to drug or higher cumulative drug delivered, or both. These benefits might be achieved at little or no expense of toxicity. However, few randomized trials have been performed addressing the issue of schedule. In a large randomized trial, classic "oral CMF" (C for 14 days, intravenous MF on day 1 and day 8), delivered every 4 weeks was compared to intravenous CMF delivered every 3 weeks. Response rates, time to progression, and OS were all statistically (although only modestly) better in the oral CMF.[532] It is difficult to ascribe this apparent benefit to schedule, because several factors differed between the two treatment groups, only one of which was a schedule of CPA (100 mg/m^2/day orally for 14 days versus 600 mg/m^2 i.v. day 1 only). In another study of chemotherapy schedule, weekly CMF was compared with CMF delivered every 4 weeks.[530] Overall, the scheduled dose delivery of the two regimens was identical. Although the weekly schedule was associated with less toxicity, the every-4-week regimen resulted in higher response rates, longer time to progression, and, remarkably, nearly a doubling in survival (median OS: weekly, 11.8 months; every 4 weeks, 21.2 months). Likewise, FEC (5FU, 500 mg/m^2; epirubicin, 60 mg/m^2; CPA, 500 mg/m^2) administered monthly was more effective than the same doses of FEC divided into weekly administration (response rates, 47% versus 30%, p = .02; times to progression, 9.2 months versus 5.4 months, p = .005; OS, 21.2 months versus 11.8 months, p = .01).[391] These studies suggest that the monthly administration of chemotherapy is superior to weekly if the same total cumulative doses are achieved. However, the principal theoretical advantage of weekly doses, besides less toxicity, is the ability to achieve much higher cumulative doses of drug in a denser schedule.[533] As noted, a prospective randomized trial of dose-dense, weekly paclitaxel versus standard, every-3-week administration is under way.

In summary, the concepts of escalating dose above "standard" levels and of shortening the interval for chemotherapeutic agents are appealing. However, neither of these approaches has been supported by data from prospective randomized trials. Importantly, randomized trials have indicated that lowering doses below an "optimal" level may have deleterious effects, not only on QOL but also on survival. Although strict guidelines are not widely accepted, the doses listed in Table 9 are reasonably well supported in the literature and do not routinely require either growth factor or hematopoietic stem cell support.

Continuous versus Intermittent Therapy

Because QOL and palliation are principal objectives of therapy in the metastatic setting, several investigators have addressed the issue of offering "drug holidays" to patients who have achieved response after several cycles of chemotherapy. At least four randomized trials have addressed potential benefits of continuous chemotherapy when compared to "induction" for a set number of cycles, followed by a drug holiday until progression.[26,399,534,535] Although trial designs differed, no survival advantage was observed in any of the three for either continuous or intermittent therapy. However, in one study, treatment with only *three* cycles of induction was associated with a worse QOL when compared to continuous therapy.[26] In contrast, in a study by Muss et al.,[534] six cycles of induction therapy were compared to continuous therapy. Although QOL was not strictly measured in this study, surrogate measures of QOL, such as changes in performance status and toxicities of chemotherapy, seem to favor the intermittent approach.[534] Likewise, in a 1996 study from Germany, patients randomly assigned to intermittent therapy after a response to epirubicin and ifosfamide had a superior QOL to those who continued the same therapy.[399]

It must be noted that these studies were performed before the availability of taxanes, and it is not known whether the addition of paclitaxel or docetaxel might affect these observations. Nonetheless, taken together, the results of these studies suggest that intermittent therapy, consisting of induction with an optimal number of cycles of standard chemotherapy (probably six), followed by a drug holiday, is appropriate for patients who achieve palliation with standard chemotherapy.

Is There an Optimal Chemotherapeutic Treatment for Metastatic Breast Cancer?

From the preceding discussions, one can conclude that although chemotherapy may improve QOL in hormone-refractory patients, the impact on OS for most patients can be measured in terms of a few months. However, there are some hints that suboptimal treatments might result in significantly, and perhaps substantially, shortened life spans for certain patients. In this regard, several single agents clearly have activity in breast cancer at reasonably tolerable levels, including alkylating agents (CPA), antimetabolites (fluorouracil, capecitabine), antifols (methotrexate), anthracyclines and related anthraquinones (doxorubicin, mitoxantrone, epirubicin), vinca alkyloids (vinblastine, vinorelbine), the taxanes (paclitaxel, docetaxel), and etoposide (see Table 10). Several newer agents have been reported to be active, including liposomal-encapsulated doxorubicin, gemcitabine, and perhaps inhibitors of topoisomerase II. From the results of several randomized trials, one can conclude that initial treatment with either combinations of CPA, methotrexate, fluorouracil, and an anthracycline, or single-agent treatment with either an anthracycline or a taxane, is likely to result in a reasonable chance (30% to 60%) of response and palliation. These studies also suggest that survival will be roughly identical, regardless of which regimen is chosen.[70,122,389,453,495,516] If the initial regimen chosen is not effective, or when it ultimately becomes ineffective (as most do), then switching the patient's care to an alternative therapy is reasonable and appropriate (see Fig. 7).

Few studies have directly compared the choice of one member of a class of chemotherapeutic agents to another member of the same class. Mitoxantrone has been compared directly with doxorubicin and found to be slightly less effective but also less toxic.[361] In two studies in which direct comparisons of doxorubicin with epirubicin were performed in the metastatic setting, clinical outcomes were essentially identical.[360,363] No reported studies compare paclitaxel with docetaxel. In the absence of such studies, it is reasonable to choose the agent with which the clinician has the most experience and trust.

Clearly, anthracyclines and taxanes are very active as single agents. Phase II studies of combination chemotherapy of these two types of therapies (for example, AT) appear to result in very high response rates.[536] However, routine first-line use of these combinations is not yet indicated, given the equivalent survival results and increased toxicity, especially

TABLE 11. *New strategies to treat breast cancer*

Mechanisms of action	Examples
Agents that disrupt estrogen/estrogen receptor pathway	SERM III Faslodex
New chemotherapeutic agents	Gemcitabine
Modulation of established chemotherapeutic agents	Leucovorin/5FU ? Trastuzamab/paclitaxel
Agents with novel mechanisms of action	
Angiogenesis inhibitors	TNP 470 Matrix metalloproteinase inhibitors
Immunotherapies/vaccines	Mono- and bispecific antibodies against *erb*-b2, CEA, and MUC-1 Vaccine strategies targeted toward same antigens
Peptide growth hormone signal transduction inhibitors	Trastuzamab Farnesyl transferase inhibitors
Gene therapy	Antisense against *erb*-b2, Bcl-2 Strategies to reintroduce wild-type p53

5FU, 5-fluorouracil; CEA, carcinoembryonic antigen; SERM, selective estrogen receptor modulator.

cardiac, observed thus far.[460,495,537] Nonetheless, there may be a small group of patients who have rapidly progressive visceral metastases for whom expected survival is very short in the absence of effective therapy. For these patients, the combination of an anthracycline and a taxane "up front" is appropriate, because the patient's performance status may degenerate too quickly to permit a second regimen to be tested if the first is not successful. In this case, consideration must be given to *erb*-b2 (HER-2/neu) status. Some studies have suggested that therapy with trastuzamab (see discussion of trastuzamab in the following section) is additive, if not synergistic, with paclitaxel in patients whose tumors overexpress this oncoprotein (see the following section). However, because of concerns about CHF, trastuzamab should be avoided with anthracyclines.

PROSPECTS FOR METASTATIC BREAST CANCER

Clearly, more effective treatments are necessary for metastatic breast cancer, a common, highly debilitating, and frequently lethal disease. Basically, four different strategies have been pursued in development of new agents for treatment of metastatic breast cancer (Table 11). First, as discussed in the section Endocrine Therapy, new agents that might interfere with the estrogen-ER axis are being studied. Several agents are either in clinical trials or are being developed that further decrease estrogen production, disrupt the estrogen-ER interaction, bind ER but induce deleterious (for the cancer cell) results, or perturb downstream, ER-induced pathways that lead to cellular growth and survival.

Second, new therapies that act via mechanisms that are classically believed to be in the domain of "chemotherapy" continue to be generated. These include derivatives of already accepted agents, such as anthracyclines, antimetabolites, antifols, and taxanes. These agents might have enhanced therapeutic-toxic ratios by virtue of increased tissue specificity, higher binding affinity constants for their targets, alternative methods of delivery, or other innovations. However, although these agents may slightly improve the therapeutic-toxic ratio of chemotherapy, it seems unlikely that they will have a major impact on survival.

Novel chemotherapeutic agents have also been derived from classes of compounds that have not typically been very active in breast cancer, such as agents that effect pyrimidine synthesis (gemcitabine) or agents that inhibit topoisomerase I (camptothecins). Representatives of these classes are now in phase II clinical trials. Reported response rates for these agents appear to be in the same range as those for more classic breast cancer chemotherapeutic drugs.[538–540] Therefore, it is similarly unlikely that they will substantially change the very poor potential for cure of most patients with metastatic breast cancer.

A third approach to improving cancer chemotherapy is with agents that, by themselves, have little if any antineoplastic activity but alter or "modulate" cellular or metabolic pathways that are responsible for chemotherapeutic resistance. Few examples of successful chemomodulation have been reported for breast cancer treatment. Perhaps the most successful experience with chemomodulation is the use of leucovorin to enhance the uptake of 5FU into the quaternary complex of thymidylate synthase. Addition of leucovorin to 5FU has been shown to clearly improve outcomes in colon cancer.[541] As noted previously, several phase II studies of this approach in metastatic breast cancer have appeared favorable, although the only randomized trial reported so far failed to demonstrate any benefit over 5FU alone when delivered in the same dose and schedule.[417,420,422,542,543] Another approach toward modulation is interruption of MDR function, which may be an important factor in mediating resistance to chemotherapy in breast cancer.[95] Clinical trials of modulation of MDR have been reported, using a number of agents that bind to and inhibit gp170 activity, including verapamil, dexverapamil, lonidamine, toremifene, and megestrol acetate.[544–555] Phase I studies have suggested that the combinations can be delivered safely, but so far the results from phase II and III studies have been disappointing.[544,545,547]

Finally, and perhaps most exciting, are completely novel approaches that seem to work via mechanisms that were not previously exploited (see Table 11). These include agents that inhibit angiogenesis, sophisticated immunotherapies (including vaccines against tumor-associated antigens), small molecules that interfere with cell signal transduction pathways, and various approaches toward

TABLE 12. *Trastuzamab in combination with chemotherapy: randomized trial in metastatic disease*

Treatment	Response rate	Time to progression	Overall survival	Congestive heart failure[a]
CTX	36	5.5	20.9	NA
CTX + trastuzamab	62	8.6	25.4	NA
AC	42	6.5	24.5	3
AC + trastuzamab	65	9.0	33.4	18
Paclitaxel	25	4.2	18.4	4
Paclitaxel + trastuzamab	57	7.1	22.1	0

AC, doxorubicin and cyclophosphamide; CTX, chemotherapy.
[a]Grade III or IV.
Adapted from refs. 24, 562.

gene therapy. These are described in greater detail in Chapters 49, 50, and 51.

Of these novel approaches, arguably the first real success to be observed has been the experience with trastuzamab. This humanized monoclonal antibody binds with a specific epitope of the *erb*-b2 protein. The parent antibody, monoclonal antibody 4D5, induces a specific biologic response through activation of *erb*-b2; this response includes autophosphorylation of the tyrosine kinase internal domain, leading to inhibition of cellular growth, decreased malignant potential, and perhaps reversal of resistance to endocrine therapy and certain chemotherapies.[103,556–558] Phase I and II clinical trials with a humanized form of the monoclonal antibody 4D5, designated *trastuzamab*, have demonstrated that multiple doses of the antibody can be given safely alone and in combination with certain chemotherapeutic agents. In these studies, development of human antihuman antibody responses was not identified. Antibody treatment as a single agent induced responses in 15% to 20% of patients with *erb*-b2 overexpressing cancers. Trastuzamab in combination with cisplatin induced responses in nearly 25% of heavily pretreated patients.[114–116] Moreover, the results of a large randomized trial have demonstrated that trastuzamab is at least additive, and perhaps synergistic, with other chemotherapeutic agents.[24] In combination with first-line doxorubicin and CPA (AC) chemotherapy, trastuzamab modestly increased response rates and time to progression when compared to AC alone. In a second part of this same clinical trial, patients with doxorubicin-refractory metastatic breast cancer were randomly assigned to treatment with either trastuzamab and paclitaxel or paclitaxel alone. The patients treated with the combination experienced nearly a doubling in response, time to progression, and even survival when compared to those treated with paclitaxel alone[24] (Table 12).

These studies also suggest that trastuzamab is reasonably well tolerated. Only a few patients suffered allergic-type reactions, although some were severe. Of note, several patients were retreated without recurrent allergic episodes. Trastuzamab does not appear to enhance hematopoietic, hepatic, or renal toxicities of standard chemotherapeutic agents. However, a worrisome increase in CHF was observed in all three of the large trials. In the study in which trastuzamab was delivered concurrently with AC, the CHF rate was six times that observed with AC alone.[24] Furthermore, CHF was also observed in 2% of patients treated with trastuzamab and paclitaxel, whereas none was detected in patients who received paclitaxel alone. Importantly, 3% of patients who were treated in a separate trial with trastuzamab alone developed CHF.[115] However, the latter study was not randomized, and therefore it is difficult to ascertain whether this rate of CHF was greater than background in this heavily treated population.

Regardless, it appears that trastuzamab will become an accepted part of the therapeutic armamentarium for treating patients with metastatic breast cancer. Entry into these early studies was restricted to patients whose tumors overexpressed *erb*-b2, as determined by immunohistochemistry with either the parent antibody (4D5) or another antibody that also recognizes the external domain. The optimal means of determining *erb*-b2 overexpression has not been established, including preferable assays or cutoffs to distinguish "positive" from "negative." Furthermore, the effects of trastuzamab in patients whose tumors do not highly overexpress *erb*-b2 have not been tested. It is anticipated that phase II and III trials of such patients with trastuzamab with concurrent chemotherapy will start soon.

Many questions remain unanswered regarding this exciting agent, including the precise toxicities associated with trastuzamab therapy, the best schedule and dose, the optimal combination with various chemotherapeutic agents, and whether trastuzamab can enhance the beneficial effects of endocrine therapy. However, it is clear that this agent works in a fundamentally different way than other drugs that are active against breast cancer. At the least, it is reasonable to offer trastuzamab to patients whose tumors overexpress *erb*-b2 and whose disease has become refractory to standard endocrine and chemotherapeutic agents. Moreover, trastuzamab is a reasonable choice in combination with paclitaxel for *erb*-b2–positive patients. Nonetheless, one must be very cautious in prescribing trastuzamab in combination with doxorubicin-containing regimens or in any patient who has previously had doxorubicin or has evidence of cardiac dysfunction because of the risk of associated CHF.

It is likely that trastuzamab is merely a first step toward our efforts to develop true "molecular therapies" that target novel pathways of signal transduction. Several phase I and II, and even III, studies are under way investigating the effects of inhibitors of the angiogenesis process. None of these agents has been found to have remarkable antitumor activity in the classic sense (reduction of tumor burden), but it is anticipated that they may work by inhibiting tumor growth rather than by inducing tumor lysis. In that regard, studies of these agents either in association with or following effective chemotherapy are under way.

SUMMARY

For women with metastatic breast cancer, progress toward substantially increasing the odds of cure or prolonged survival has been painstakingly slow. Nonetheless, many patients achieve satisfactory to excellent palliation of cancer-related symptoms by judicial application of local and systemic therapies. In that regard, several new effective agents have become available for treatment of metastatic breast cancer, including drugs that work by disrupting the estrogen/ER pathway and drugs that have relatively nonspecific cytolytic actions. Trastuzamab represents the first agent in a class of anticipated therapies that seem to work by inhibiting signal transduction induced by peptide growth factors and their associated receptors. Taken together, these therapies offer most patients with metastatic breast cancer a series of treatments that should at the least improve QOL and also modestly prolong survival.

MANAGEMENT SUMMARY

1. Confirm the presence of metastastic disease by biopsy if possible, and perform predictive factor assays (ER, PR, *erb*-b2).
2. Determine the current morbidity that a patient is experiencing from metastatic breast cancer.
3. Assess the relative prognosis of the patient (disease-free interval from end of primary and adjuvant systemic therapy, presence or absence of visceral disease, number of sites of disease, performance status).
4. Decide the relative benefits and risks of applying local versus systemic therapies (see Fig. 4).
5. If systemic therapy is chosen, decide the relative benefits and risks of applying endocrine therapy versus chemotherapy (see Fig. 5).
6. If endocrine therapy is chosen, decide the relative benefits and risks of sequence of therapies (see Fig. 6).
7. For hormone-refractory patients, select the sequence of chemotherapeutic agents that is most likely to work with the fewest side effects (see Fig. 7).
8. Follow the patient using history, physical, radiographic, and serologic data to decide whether to continue with selected regimen or change to alternative.

REFERENCES

1. Fentiman I, Cuzick J, Millis R, Hayward J. Which patients are cured of breast cancer? *BMJ* 1984;289:1108.
2. Haybittle J. The evidence for cure in female breast cancer. *Comments Res Breast Dis* 1983;3:181.
3. Halsted WS. The results of operations for the cure of cancer of the breast performed at the Johns Hopkins Hospital from June, 1889, to January, 1894. *Johns Hopkins Hosp Rep* 1894–1895;iv:297.
4. Harris JR, Henderson IC. Natural history and staging of breast cancer. In: Harris JR, Hellman S, Henderson IC, et al, eds. *Breast diseases*. Philadelphia: JB Lippincott, 1987:233.
5. Rutqvist L, Wallgren A, Nilsson B. Is breast cancer a curable disease? *Cancer* 1984;53:1793.
6. Rutqvist LE. Increasing incidence and constant mortality rates of breast cancer: time trends in Stockholm County 1961–1973. *Breast Cancer Res Treat* 1984;4:233.
7. Rutqvist L, Wallgren A. Long-term survival of 458 young breast cancer patients. *Cancer* 1985;55:658.
8. Rosen P, Groshen W, Saigo P, Kinne D, Hellman S. A long-term follow-up study of survival in Stage I (TINOMO) and Stage II (TINIMO) breast carcinoma. *J Clin Oncol* 1989;7:355.
9. Rosen PP, Groshen S, Kinne DW. Prognosis in T2N0M0 Stage I breast cancer: a 20-year follow-up study. *J Clin Oncol* 1991;9:1650.
10. Greenberg P, Hortobagyi G, Smith T, Ziegler L, Frye K, Buzdar A. Long-term follow-up of patients with complete remission following combination chemotherapy for metastatic breast cancer. *J Clin Oncol* 1996;14:2197.
11. Falkson G, Gelman RS, Leone L, Falkson CI. Survival of premenopausal women with metastatic breast cancer. Long-term follow-up of Eastern Cooperative Group and Cancer and Leukemia Group B studies. *Cancer* 1990;66:1621.
12. Beatson GW. On the treatment of inoperable cases of carcinoma of the mamma: suggestions for a new method of treatment with illustrative cases. *Lancet* 1896;2:104.
13. Henderson IC. Chemotherapy for advanced disease. In: Harris J, Hellman S, Henderson I, et al, eds. *Breast diseases*. Philadelphia. JB Lippincott, 1987:428.
14. Aaltomaa S, Lipponen P, Eskelinen M, et al. Prediction of outcome after first recurrence of breast cancer. *Eur J Surg* 1992;158:13.
15. Crowe JP Jr, Gordon NH, Hubay CA, et al. Estrogen receptor determination and long-term survival of patients with carcinoma of the breast. *Surg Gynecol Obstet* 1991;173:273.
16. Lee CG, McCormick B, Mazumdar M, Vetto J, Borgen PI: Infiltrating breast carcinoma in patients age 30 years and younger. Long term outcome for life, relapse, and second primary tumors. *Int J Radiat Oncol Biol Phys* 1992;23:969.
17. Vogel CL, Azevedo S, Hilsenbeck S, East DR, Ayub J. Survival after first recurrence of breast cancer. The Miami experience. *Cancer* 1992;70:129.
18. Bloom H, Richardson W, Harrier EJ. Natural history of untreated breast cancer. *BMJ* 1962;2:213.
19. Anderson J, Cain K, Gelber R. Analysis of survival by tumor response. *J Clin Oncol* 1983;1:710.
20. Ahmann DL, Schaid DJ, Bisel HF, Hahn RG, Edmonson JH, Ingle JN. The effect on survival of initial chemotherapy in advanced breast cancer: polychemotherapy versus single drug. *J Clin Oncol* 1987;5:1928.
21. Buzdar A, Jonat W, Howell A, et al. Anastrozole, a potent and selective aromatase inhibitor, versus megestrol acetate in postmenopausal women with advanced breast cancer: results of overview analysis of two phase III trials. *J Clin Oncol* 1996;14:2000.
22. Early Breast Cancer Trialist's Collaborative Group. Polychemotherapy for early breast cancer: an overview of the randomized trials. *Lancet* 1998;352:930.
23. Early Breast Cancer Trialist's Collaborative Group. Tamoxifen for early breast cancer: an overview of the randomised trials. *Lancet* 1998; 351:1451.
24. Slamon D, Leyland-Jones B, Shak S, et al. Addition of Herceptin (humanized anti-HER2 antibody) to first line chemotherapy for HR2 overexpressing metastatic breast cancer (HER2+/MBC) markedly increases anticancer activity: a randomized multinational controlled phase III trial. *Proc Am Soc Clin Oncol* 1998;17:98a.
25. Weeks J. Quality-of-life assessment: performance status upstaged? [Editorial]. *J Clin Oncol* 1992;10:1827.

26. Coates A, Gebski V, Bishop JF, et al. Improving the quality of life during chemotherapy for advanced breast cancer. *N Engl J Med* 1987;317:1490.
27. Donovan K, Sanson-Fisher RW, Redman S. Measuring quality of life in cancer patients. *J Clin Oncol* 1989;7:959.
28. Osoba D. Health-related quality of life as a treatment endpoint in metastatic breast cancer. *Can J Oncol* 1995;1[Suppl 5]:47.
29. Simon R. Design and conduct of clinical trials. In: DeVita VT Jr, Hellman S, Rosenberg SA, eds. *Cancer: principles and practice of oncology*, 4th Edition. Philadelphia: JB Lippincott, 1993:418.
30. Robertson J, Lee D. Static disease of long duration (greater than 24 weeks) is a important remission criterion in breast cancer patients treated with the aromatase inhibitor "Arimadex" (anastrozole). *Breast Cancer Res Treat* 1997;46:214(abst).
31. McQuellon RP, Muss HB, Hoffman SL, Russell G, Craven B, Yellen SB. Patient preferences for treatment of metastatic breast cancer: a study of women with early-stage breast cancer. *J Clin Oncol* 1995;13:858.
32. Wilkins E, Head J, Burke J. Pulmonary resection for metastatic neoplasms in the lung. *Am J Surg* 135:480,1978
33. Hull DF III, Clark GM, Osborne CK, Chamness GC, Knight WA III, McGuire WL. Multiple estrogen receptor assays in human breast cancer. *Cancer Res* 1983;43:413.
34. Armstrong DN, King P, Ross AH, Foubister G, Griffiths JM. Multiple fine needle liver aspiration cytology in the diagnosis of liver metastases: a prospective comparison with ultrasound and radionuclide scanning. *J R Coll Surg Edinb* 1988;33:244.
35. Pedersen L, Guldhammer B, Kamby C, Aasted M, Rose C. Fine needle aspiration and Tru-Cut biopsy in the diagnosis of soft tissue metastases in breast cancer. *Eur J Cancer Clin Oncol* 1986;22:1045.
36. Pedersen L, Balslev I, Guldhammer B, Rose C. Repeated fine needle aspirations in the diagnosis of soft tissue metastases in breast cancer. *Eur J Cancer Clin Oncol* 1988;24:1039.
37. Hayes DF, Trock B, Harris A. Assessing the clinical impact of prognostic factors: when is "statistically significant" clinically useful? *Breast Cancer Res Treat* 1998;52:305.
38. Lindley C, Vasa S, Sawyer T, Winer E. Quality of life and preferences for treatment following systemic adjuvant therapy for early stage breast cancer. *J Clin Oncol* 1998;16:380.
39. Ravdin P, Siminoff I, Harvey J. Survey of breast cancer patients concerning their knowledge and expectations of adjuvant therapy. *J Clin Oncol* 1998;16:515.
40. Swenerton KD, Legha SS, Smith T, et al. Prognostic factors in metastatic breast cancer treated with combination chemotherapy. *Cancer Res* 1979;39:1552.
41. Hortobagyi GN, Smith TL, Legha SS, et al. Multivariate analysis of prognostic factors in metastatic breast cancer. *J Clin Oncol* 1983;1:776.
42. Clark G, Sledge G, Osborne CK, McGuire W. Survival from first recurrence: relative importance of prognostic factors in 1,015 breast cancer patients. *J Clin Oncol* 1987;5:55.
43. Harris J, Hellman S. Observations on survival curve analysis with particular reference to breast cancer treatment. *Cancer* 1980;57:925.
44. Heitanen P, Miettenen M, Makinen J. Survival after first recurrence in breast cancer. *Eur J Cancer Clin Oncol* 1986;22:913.
45. Powles TJ, Smith IE, Ford HT, Coombes RC, Jones JM, Gazet JC. Failure of chemotherapy to prolong survival in a group of patients with metastatic breast cancer. *Lancet* 1980:580.
46. Ross MB, Buzdar AU, Smith TL, et al. Improved survival of patients with metastatic breast cancer receiving combination chemotherapy: comparison of consecutive series of patients in 1950s, 1960s, and 1970s. *Cancer* 1985;55:341.
47. Tomin R, Donegan WL. Screening for recurrent breast cancer—its effectiveness and prognostic value. *J Clin Oncol* 1987;5:62.
48. Leivonen MK, Kalima TV. Prognostic factors associated with survival after breast cancer recurrence. *Acta Oncol* 1991;30:583.
49. Robertson JF, Dixon AR, Nicholson RI, Ellis IO, Elston CW, Blamey RW. Confirmation of a prognostic index for patients with metastatic breast cancer treated by endocrine therapy. *Breast Cancer Res Treat* 1992;22:221.
50. Yamamoto N, Watanabe T, Katsumata N, et al. Construction and validation of a practical prognostic index for patients with metastatic breast cancer. *J Clin Oncol* 1998;16:2401.
51. Hayes DF, Bast R, Desch CE, et al. A tumor marker utility grading system (TMUGS): a framework to evaluate clinical utility of tumor markers. *J Natl Cancer Inst* 1996;88:1456.
52. Harris JR, Recht A, Amalric R, et al. Time course and prognosis of local recurrence following primary radiation therapy for early breast cancer. *J Clin Oncol* 1984;2:37.
53. Turner BC, Glazer PM, Gumbs AA, et al. The regulation of ipsilateral breast tumor recurrence after lumpectomy and radiation therapy by the transcription factors p53 and AP2. *Proc Am Soc Therapeutic Radiat Oncol* 1997;39:135a.
54. Zellars RC, Clark GM, Allred DC, Herman TS, Elledge R. Prognostic value of p53 for local failure in mastectomy treated breast cancer patients. *Proc Am Soc Clin Oncol* 1998;17:104a.
55. Rozan S, Vincent-Salomon A, Zafrani B, et al. No significant predictive value of c-erbB-2 or p53 expression regarding sensitivity to primary chemotherapy or radiotherapy in breast cancer. *Int J Cancer* 1998;79:27.
56. Turner BC, Haffty BG, Narayanan L, et al. Insulin-like growth factor–1 receptor overexpression mediates cellular radioresistance and local breast cancer recurrence after lumpectomy and radiation. *Cancer Res* 1997;57:3079.
57. ASCO Expert Panel. 1997 update of recommendations for the use of tumor markers in breast and colorectal cancer. *J Clin Oncol* 1998;16:793.
58. ASCO Expert Panel. Clinical practice guidelines for the use of tumor markers in breast and colorectal cancer: report of the American Society of Clinical Oncology Expert Panel. *J Clin Oncol* 1996;14:2843.
59. Santen RJ, Manni A, Harvey H, Redmond C. Endocrine treatment of breast cancer in women. *Endocr Rev* 1990;11:221.
60. Epstein RJ. The clinical biology of hormone-responsive breast cancer. *Cancer Treat Rev* 1988;15:33.
61. Clark G, Osborne C, McGuire W. Correlations between estrogen receptor, progesterone receptor, and patient characteristics in human breast cancer. *J Clin Oncol* 1984;2:1102.
62. Clark GM, McGuire WL. Steroid receptors and other prognostic factors in primary breast cancer. *Semin Oncol* 1988;15:20.
63. Osborne CK. Tamoxifen in the treatment of breast cancer. *N Engl J Med* 1998;339:1609.
64. Valagussa P, Tancim G, Bonadonna G. Salvage treatment of patients suffering relapse after adjuvant CMF chemotherapy. *Cancer* 1986; 58:1411.
65. Perez JE, Machiavelli M, Leone BA, et al. Bone-only versus visceral-only metastatic pattern in breast cancer: analysis of 150 patients. A GOCS study: Grupo Oncologico Cooperativo del Sur. *Am J Clin Oncol* 1990;13:294.
66. Ahmann DL, Schaid DJ, Ingle JN, et al. A randomized trial of cyclophosphamide, doxorubicin, and prednisone versus cyclophosphamide, 5-fluorouracil, and prednisone in patients with metastatic breast cancer. *Am J Clin Oncol* 1991;14:179.
67. Falkson G, Gelman R, Falkson CI, Glick J, Harris J. Factors predicting for response, time to treatment failure, and survival in women with metastatic breast cancer treated with DAVTH: a prospective Eastern Cooperative Oncology Group study. *J Clin Oncol* 1991;9:2153.
68. Rabinovich M, Vallejo C, Bianco A, et al. Development and validation of prognostic models in metastatic breast cancer: a GOCS study. *Oncology* 1992;49:188.
69. Pronzato P, Bertelli G, Gardin G, Rubagotti A, Conte PF, Rosso R. Analysis of time to response to chemotherapy in 316 metastatic breast cancer patients. *Oncology* 1993;50:460.
70. Aisner J, Cirrincione C, Perloff M, et al. Combination chemotherapy for metastatic or recurrent carcinoma of the breast: a randomized phase III trial comparing: cyclophosphamide, doxorubicin, thiotepa, and halotestin (VATH) versus VATH alternating with cyclophosphamide, methotrexate, 5-fluorouracil, vinblastine, and prednisone (CMFVP): Cancer and Leukemia Group B Study 8281. *J Clin Oncol* 1995;13:1443.
71. Rahman Z, Frye D, Buzdar A, et al. Impact of selection process on response rate and long-term survival of potential high-dose chemotherapy candidates treated with standard-dose doxorubicin-containing chemotherapy in patients with metastatic breast cancer. *J Clin Oncol* 1997;15:3171.
72. Hoffman RM. In vitro assays for chemotherapy sensitivity. *Crit Rev Oncol Hematol* 1993;15:99.
73. Salmon SE. Human tumor colony assay and chemosensitivity testing. *Cancer Treat Rep* 1984;68:117.
74. Furukawa T, Kubota T, Hoffman RM. Clinical applications of the histoculture drug response assay. *Clin Cancer Res* 1995;1:305.

75. Von Hoff DD, Kronmal R, Salmon SE, et al. A Southwest Oncology Group study on the use of a human tumor cloning assay for predicting response inpatients with ovarian cancer. *Cancer* 1991;67:20.
76. Jones SE, Dean JC, Young LA, Salmon SE. The human tumor clonogenic assay in human breast cancer. *J Clin Oncol* 1985;3:92.
77. Fruehauf J, Bosanquet A. In vitro determination of drug response: a discussion of clinical applications. In: DeVita VT, Hellman S, Rosenberg S, eds. *Cancer: principles and practice of oncology/PPO updates*. Philadelphia: JB Lippincott, 1993:1.
78. Eltabbakh GH, Piver MS, Hempling RE, et al. Correlation between extreme drug resistance assay and response to primary paclitaxel and cisplatin in patients with epithelial ovarian cancer. *Gynecol Oncol* 1998;70:392.
79. Weisenthal LM, Kern DH. Prediction of drug resistance in cancer chemotherapy: the Kern and DiSC assays [see comments]. *Oncology (Huntingt)* 1991;5:93.
80. Tavassoli FA, Cook CB, Pestaner JP. A comparison of two commercially available in vitro chemosensitivity assays. *Oncology* 1995;52:411.
81. Mechetner E, Kyshtoobayeva A, Zonis S, et al. Levels of multidrug resistance (MDRI) P-glycoprotein expression by human breast cancer correlate with in vitro resistance to taxol and doxorubicin. *Clin Cancer Res* 1998;4:389.
82. Elledge RM, Clark GM, Hon J, et al. Rapid in vitro assay for predicting response to fluorouracil in patients with metastatic breast cancer. *J Clin Oncol* 1995;13:419.
83. Kern DH. Heterogeneity of drug resistance in human breast and ovarian cancers [see comments]. *Cancer J Sci Am* 1998;4:41.
84. Hilf R, Feldstein M, Gibson S, Savlov E. The relative importance of estrogen receptor analysis as a prognostic factor for recurrence or response to chemotherapy in women with breast cancer. *Cancer* 1980;45:1993.
85. Kiang D. Correlation between estrogen-receptor proteins and response to chemotherapy in patients with breast cancer. *Cancer Treat Rep* 1984;68:577.
86. Levine R, Lippman M. Relationship between estrogen-receptor proteins and response to chemotherapy in breast cancer. *Cancer Treat Rep* 1984;68:573.
87. Lippman ME, Allegra JC, Thompson EB, et al. The relation between estrogen receptors and response rate to cytotoxic chemotherapy in metastatic breast cancer. *N Engl J Med* 1978;298:1223.
88. Livingston R. Breast cancer and response to chemotherapy: a possible relationship between hormone receptors and doxorubicin. *Cancer Treat Rev* 1982;9:229.
89. Rubens R, Hayward J. Estrogen receptors and response to endocrine therapy and cytotoxic chemotherapy in advanced breast cancer. *Cancer* 1980;46:2922.
90. Kiang DT, Frenning DH, Goldman AI, Ascensao VF, Kennedy BJ. Estrogen receptors and responses to chemotherapy and hormonal therapy in advanced breast cancer. *N Engl J Med* 1978;299:1330.
91. Hatschek T, Carstensen J, Fagerber G, Stal O, Grontoft O, Nordenskjold B. Influence of s-phase fraction on metastatic pattern and post-recurrence survival in a randomized mammography screening trial. *Br Cancer Res Treat* 1989;14:321.
92. Krajewski S, Blomqvist C, Franssila K, et al. Reduced expression of proapoptotic gene BAX is associated with poor response rates to combination chemotherapy and shorter survival in women with metastatic breast adenocarcinoma. *Cancer Res* 1995;55:4471.
93. Tsai CM, Chang KT, Wu LH, et al. Correlations between intrinsic chemoresistance and HER-2/neu gene expression, p53 gene mutations, and cell proliferation characteristics in non-small cell lung cancer cell lines. *Cancer Res* 1996;56:206.
94. Amadori D, Volpi A, Maltoni R, et al. Cell proliferation as a predictor of response to chemotherapy in metastatic breast cancer: a prospective study. *Breast Cancer Res Treat* 1997;43:7.
95. Trock B, Leonessa F, Clarke R. Multidrug Resistance in Breast Cancer: a meta-analysis of MDR1/gp170 expression and its possible functional significance. *J Natl Cancer Inst* 1997;89:917.
96. Clahsen PC, van de Velde CJ, Duval C, et al. p53 protein accumulation and response to adjuvant chemotherapy in premenopausal women with node-negative early breast cancer. *J Clin Oncol* 1998;16:470.
97. Formenti SC, Dunnington G, Uzieli B, et al. Original p53 status predicts for pathological response in locally advanced breast cancer patients treated preoperatively with continuous infusion 5-fluorouracil and radiation therapy. *Int J Radiat Oncol Biol Phys* 1997;39:1059.
98. FujiWara T, Grimm EA, Mukhopadhyay T, Zhang WW, Owen-Schaub LB, Roth JA. Induction of chemosensitivity in human lung cancer cells in vivo by adenovirus-mediated transfer of the wild-type p53 gene. *Cancer Res* 1994;54:2287.
99. Lenz H, Danenberg KD, Leichman C, et al. p53 status, thymidylate synthase levels are predictors of chemotherapy efficacy in patients with advanced colorectal cancer. *Proc Amer Soc Clin Oncol* 1996;15:504.
100. Lowe SW, Ruley HE, Jacks T. p53-dependent apoptosis modulates the cytotoxicity of anticancer agents. *Cell* 1993;74:957.
101. Lowe SW, Bodis S, McClatchey A. p53 status and the efficacy of cancer therapy in vivo. *Science* 1994;266:807.
102. Benz CC, Scott GK, Sarup JC, et al. Estrogen-dependent, tamoxifen-resistant turnorigenic growth of MCF-7 cells transfected with HER2/neu. *Breast Cancer Res Treat* 1992;24:85.
103. Pietras R, Arboleda J, Reese D, et al. HER-2 tyrosine kinase pathway targets estrogen receptor and promotes hormone-independent growth in human breast cancer cells. *Oncogene* 1995;10:2435.
104. Wright C, Angus B, Nicholson S, et al. Expression of c-erbB-2 oncoprotein: a prognostic indicator in human breast cancer. *Cancer Res* 1989;49:2087.
105. Carlomagno C, Perrone F, Gallo C, et al. c-erbB2 overexpression decreases the benefit of adjuvant tamoxifen in early-stage breast cancer without axillary lymph node metastases. *J Clin Oncol* 1996;14:2702.
106. Leitzel K, Teramoto Y, Konrad K, et al. Elevated serum c-erbB-2 antigen levels and decreased response to hormone therapy of breast cancer. *J Clin Oncol* 1995;13:1129.
107. Yamauchi H, O'Neill A, Gelman R, Carney W, Hosch S, Hayes DF. Prediction of response to antiestrogen therapy in advanced breast cancer patients by pretreatment circulating levels of extracellular domain of the HER-2/c-neu protein. *J Clin Oncol* 1997;15:2518.
108. Elledge RM, Green S, Ciocca D, et al. HER-2 expression and response to tamoxifen in estrogen receptor-positive breast cancer: a Southwest Oncology Group Study. *Clin Cancer Res* 1998;4:7.
109. Allred DC, Clark G, Tandon A, et al. HER-2/neu in node-negative breast cancer: prognostic significance of overexpression influenced by the presence of in situ carcinoma. *J Clin Oncol* 1992;10:599.
110. Gusterson BA, Gelber RD, Goldhirsch A, et al. Prognostic importance of c-erbB-2 expression in breast cancer. *J Clin Oncol* 1992;10:1049.
111. Paik S, Bryant J, Park C, et al. erbB-2 and response to doxorubicin in patients with axillary lymph node-positive, hormone receptor negative breast cancer. *J Natl Cancer Inst* 1998;90:1361.
112. Muss HB, Thor A, Berry DA, et al. c-erbB-2 expression and S-phase activity predict response to adjuvant therapy in women with node-positive early breast cancer. *N Engl J Med* 1994;330:1260.
113. Thor AD, Berry DA, Budman DR, et al. erbB-2, p53, and adjuvant therapy interactions in lymph node-positive breast cancer. *J Natl Cancer Inst* 1998;90:1346.
114. Baselga J, Tripathy D, Mendelsohn J, et al. Phase II study of weekly intravenous recombinant humanized anti-p185HER2 monoclonal antibody in patients with HER2/neu-overexpressing metastatic breast cancer. *J Clin Oncol* 1996;14:737.
115. Cobleigh M, Vogel C, Tripathy D, et al. Efficacy and safety of herceptin (humanized anti-HER2 antibody) as a single agent in 222 women with HER2 overexpression who relapsed following chemotherapy for metastatic breast cancer. *Proc Am Soc Clin Oncol* 1998;17:97A.
116. Pegram M, Lipton A, Hayes DF, et al. Phase II study of receptor-enhanced chemosensitivity using recombinant humanized anti-p185HER2/neu monoclonal antibody plus cisplatin in patients with HER 2/neu-overexpressing metastatic breast cancer refractory to chemotherapy treatment. *J Clin Oncol* 1998;16:2659.
117. Lippman ME. Efforts to combine endocrine and chemotherapy in the management of breast cancer: do two and two equal three? *Breast Cancer Res Treat* 1983;3:117.
118. Osborne CK, Kitten L, Arteaga CL. Antagonism of chemotherapy-induced cytotoxicity for human breast cancer cells by antiestrogens. *J Clin Oncol* 1989;7:710.
119. Lippman ME, Cassidy J, Wesley M, Young RC. A randomized attempt to increase the efficacy of cytotoxic chemotherapy in metastatic breast cancer by hormonal synchronization. *J Clin Oncol* 1984;2:28.

120. Conte PF, Baldini E, Gardin G, et al. Chemotherapy with or without estrogenic recruitment in metastatic breast cancer. A randomized trial of the Gruppo Oncologico Nord Ovest (GONO). *Ann Oncol* 1996;7:487.
121. Ingle IN, Foley JF, Mailliard JA. Randomized trial of cyclophosphamide, methotrexate, and 5-fluorouracil with or without estrogenic recruitment in women with metastatic breast cancer. *Cancer* 1994;73:2337.
122. Fossati R, Confalonieri C, Tom V, et al. Cytotoxic and hormonal treatment for metastatic breast cancer: a systematic review of published randomized trials involving 31,510 women. *J Clin Oncol* 1998; 16:3439.
123. Hayes DF, Tondini C, Kufe DW. Clinical applications of CA15-3. In: Sell S, eds. *Serological cancer markers*. Totowa, NJ: Humana Press, 1992:281.
124. Tondini C, Hayes DF, Gelman R, Henderson IC, Kufe DW. Comparison of CA15-3 and carcinoembryonic antigen in monitoring the clinical course of patients with metastatic breast cancer. *Cancer Res* 1988;48:4107.
125. Steams V, Yarnauchi H, Hayes DF. Circulating tumor markers in breast cancer: accepted utilities and novel prospects. *Breast Cancer Res Treat* 1998;52:239.
126. Robertson JFR, Whynes D, Dixon A, Blarney R. Potential for cost economies in guiding therapy in patients with metastatic breast cancer. *Br J Cancer* 1995;72:174.
127. Kiang DT, Greenberg U, Kennedy BJ. Tumor marker kinetics in the monitoring of breast cancer. *Cancer* 1990;65:193.
128. Hayes DF, Kiang DT, Korzun A, Tondini C, Wood W, Kufe D. CA15-3 and CEA spikes during chemotherapy for metastatic breast cancer. *Proc Am Soc Clin Oncol* 1988;7:38a.
129. Janicek MJ, Hayes DF, Kaplan WD. Healing flare in skeletal metastases from breast cancer. *Radiology* 1994;192:201.
130. Vogel CL, Schoenfelder J, Shemano I, Hayes DF, Gams RA. Worsening bone scan in the evaluation of antitumor response during hormonal therapy of breast cancer. *J Clin Oncol* 1995;13:1123.
131. Jacobson A, Stomper P, Cronin E, Kaplan W. Bone scans with one or two new abnormalities in cancer patients with no known metastases: reliability of interpretation of initial correlative radiographs. *Radiology* 1990;174:503.
132. Dehdashti F, Flanagan FL, Mortimer JE, Katzenellenbogen J, Welch MJ, Siegel BA. Positron emission tomographic assessment of "metabolic flare" to predict response of metastatic breast cancer to antiestrogen therapy. *Euro J Nuclear Med* 1999;26:51.
133. Sarfaty G, Tallis M. Probability of a woman with advanced breast cancer responding to adrenalectomy or hypophysectomy. *Lancet* 1970;2:685.
134. Harvey HA, Santen RJ, Osterman J, Samojlik E, White DS, Lipton A. A comparative trial of transsphenoidal hypophysectomy and estrogen suppression with aminoglutethimide in advanced breast cancer. *Cancer* 1979;43:2207.
135. Nomura Y, Tashiro H, Osaki A. Long term survival and the prognostic factors of advanced breast cancer patients treated with adrenooophorectomy. *Breast Cancer Res Treat* 1995;33:47.
136. Hayward J. Cancer of the breast. Treatment of the advanced disease. *BMJ* 1970;1:469.
137. Hayes DF, Henderson IC, Shapiro CL. Treatment of metastatic breast cancer: present and future prospects. *Semin Oncol* 1995;22[Suppl 5]:5.
138. Ingle JN, Krook JE, Green SJ, et al. Randomized trial of bilateral oophorectorny versus tamoxifen in premenopausal women with metastatic breast cancer. *J Clin Oncol* 1986;4:178.
139. Ingle JN, Ahmann DL, Green SJ, et al. Randomized clinical trial of diethylstilbestrol versus tamoxifen in postmenopausal women with advanced breast cancer. *N Engl J Med* 1981;304:16.
140. Muss FIB, Case LD, Atkins JN, et al. Tamoxifen versus high-dose oral medroxyprogesterone acetate as initial endocrine therapy for patients with metastatic breast cancer: a Piedmont Oncology Association study. *J Clin Oncol* 1994;12:1630.
141. Taylor CW, Green S, Dalton WS, et al. Multicenter randomized clinical trial of goserelin versus surgical ovariectomy in premenopausal patients with receptor-positive metastatic breast cancer: an intergroup study. *J Clin Oncol* 1998;16:994.
142. Crump M, Sawka CA, DeBoer G, et al. An individual patient-based meta-analysis of tamoxifen versus ovarian ablation as first line endocrine therapy for premenopausal women with metastatic breast cancer. *Breast Cancer Res Treat* 1997;44:201.
143. Klijn JGM, Blarney RW, Boccardo F, et al. Combination LHRH-agonist plus tamoxifen treatment is superior to medical castration alone in premenopausal metastatic breast cancer. *Breast Cancer Res Treat* 1998;50:227(abst).
144. Jonat W, Kaufmann M, Blamey RW, et al. A randomised study to compare the effect of the luteinising hormone releasing hormone (LHRH) analogue goserelin with or without tamoxifen in pre- and perimenopausal patients with advanced breast cancer. *Eur J Cancer* 1995;2:137.
145. Veronesi U, Pizzocaro G, Rossi A. Oophorectomy for advanced carcinoma of the breast. *Surg Gynecol Obstet* 1975;141:569.
146. Saphner T, Troxel AB, Tormey DC, et al. Phase II study of goserelin for patients with postmenopausal metastatic breast cancer. *J Clin Oncol* 1993;11:1529.
147. Smith IE, Ford HT, Gazet JC, Powles TJ. Premarin in the management of metastatic breast carcinoma in post-menopausal patients. *Clin Oncol* 1979;5:159.
148. Kennedy BJ. Massive estrogen administration in premenopausal women with metastatic breast cancer. *Cancer* 1962;15:641.
149. Ingle JN, Ahmann DL, Green SJ, et al. Randomized clinical trial of megestrol acetate versus tamoxifen in perimenopausal or castrated women with advanced breast cancer. *Am J Clin Oncol* 1982;5:155.
150. Baufman G, Biran S. Second line hormonal therapy with aminoglutethimide in metastatic breast cancer. *Acta Oncol* 1990;29:717.
151. Dombernowsky P, Smith I, Falkson G, et al. Letrozole, a new oral aromatase inhibitor for advanced breast cancer: double-blind randomized trial showing a dose effect and improved efficacy and tolerability compared with megestrol acetate [see comments]. *J Clin Oncol* 1998;16:453.
152. Buzdar AU, Jonat W, Howell A, et al. Anastrozole versus megestrol acetate in the treatment of postmenopausal women with advanced breast carcinoma: results of a survival update based on a combined analysis of data ftom two mature phase III trials. Arimidex Study Group. *Cancer* 1998;83:1142.
153. Gershanovich M, Chaudri HA, Campos D, et al. Letrozole, a new oral aromatase inhibitor: randomised trial comparing 2.5 mg daily, 0.5 mg daily and aminoglutethimide in postmenopausal women with advanced breast cancer. Letrozole International Trial Group (AR/BC3). *Ann Oncol* 1998;9:639.
154. Hermon C, Beral V. Breast cancer mortality rates are levelling off or beginning to decline in many western countries: analysis of time trends, age-cohort and age-period models of breast cancer mortality in 20 countries. *Br J Cancer* 1996;73:955.
155. Westerberg H, Nordenskjold B, de Schryver A, Notter G. Anti-oestrogen therapy of advanced mammary carcinoma. *Acta Radiol Ther Phys Biol* 1976;15:513.
156. Morgan LR Jr, Schein PS, Woolley PV, et al. Therapeutic use of tamoxifen in advanced breast cancer: correlation with biochemical parameters. *Cancer Treat Rep* 1976;60:1437.
157. Manni A, Trujillo JE, Marshall JS, Brodkey J, Pearson OH. Antihormone treatment of stage IV breast cancer. *Cancer* 1971;43:444.
158. Rose C, Mouridsen HT. Treatment of advanced breast cancer with tamoxifen. *Recent Results Cancer Res* 1984;91:230.
159. Sawka CA, Pritchard KI, Shelley W, et al. A randomized crossover trial of tamoxifen versus ovarian ablation for metastatic breast cancer in premenopausal women: a report of the National Cancer Institute of Canada Clinical Trials Group (NCIC CTG) trial MA.1. *Breast Cancer Res Treat* 1997;44:211.
160. Bratherton DG, Brown CH, Buchanan R, et al. A comparison of two doses of tamoxifen (Nolvadex) in postmenopausal women with advanced breast cancer: l0 MG BD versus 20 MG BD. *Br J Cancer* 1984;50:199.
161. Fornander T, Cedermark B, Mattsson A, et al. Adjuvant tamoxifen in early breast cancer: occurrence of new primary cancers. *Lancet* 1989;1:117.
162. Jordan VC, Assikis VJ. Endometrial carcinoma and tamoxifen: clearing up a controversy. *Clin Cancer Res* 1995;1:467.
163. Rutqvist LE, Mattsson A. Cardiac and thromboembolic morbidity among postmenopausal women with early-stage breast cancer in a randomized trial of adjuvant tamoxifen. The Stockholm Breast Cancer Study Group. *J Natl Cancer Inst* 1993;85:1398.
164. Gorodeski GI, Beery R, Lunenfeld B, Geier A. Tamoxifen increases plasma estrogen-binding equivalents and has an estradiol agonistic effect on histologically normal premenopausal and postmenopausal endometrium. *Fertil Steril* 1992;57:320.

165. Uziely B, Lewin A, Brufman G, Dorembus D, Mor-Yosef S. The effect of tamoxifen on the endometrium. *Breast Cancer Res Treat* 1993;26:101.
166. Enck RE, Rios CN. Tamoxifen treatment of metastatic breast cancer and antithrombin III levels. *Cancer* 1984;53:2607.
167. Love RR, Surawicz TS, Williams EC. Antithrombin III level, fibrinogen level, and platelet count changes with adjuvant tamoxifen therapy. *Arch Intern Med* 1992;152:317.
168. Turken S, Siris E, Seldin D, Flaster E, Hyman G, Lindsay R. Effects of tamoxifen on spinal bone density in women with breast cancer. *J Natl Cancer Inst* 1989;81:1086.
169. Fornander T, Rutqvist LE, Sjoberg HE, Blomqvist L, Mattsson A, Glas U. Long-term adjuvant tamoxifen in early breast cancer: effect on bone mineral density in postmenopausal women. *J Clin Oncol* 1990;8:1019.
170. Love RR, Mazess RB, Barden HS, et al. Effects of tamoxifen on bone mineral density in postmenopausal women with breast cancer. *N Engl J Med* 1992;326:852.
171. Schapira, DV, Kumar NB, Lyman GH. Serum cholesterol reduction with tamoxifen. *Breast Cancer Res Treat* 1990;17:3.
172. Love RR, Newcomb PA, Wiebe DA, et al. Effects of tamoxifen therapy on lipid and lipoprotein levels in postmenopausal patients with node-negative breast cancer. *J Natl Cancer Inst* 1990;82:1327.
173. Fisher B, Costantino JP, Wickerham DL, et al. Tamoxifen for prevention of breast cancer: report of the National Surgical Adjuvant Breast and Bowel Project P-1 Study. *J Natl Cancer Inst* 1998; 90:1371.
174. McIntosh IH, Thynne GS. Tumour stimulation by antioestrogens. *Br J Surg* 1977;64:900.
175. Clarysse A. Hormone induced tumor flare. *Eur J Cancer Clin Oncol* 1985;21:585.
176. Plotkin D, Lechner JJ, Jung WE, Rosen PJ. Tamoxifen flare in advanced breast cancer. *JAMA* 1978;240:2644.
177. Beex L, Pieters G, Smals A, Koenders A, Benraad T, Kloppenborg P. Tamoxifen versus ethinyl estradiol in the treatment of postmenopausal women with advanced breast cancer. *Cancer Treat Rep* 1981;65:179.
178. Stewart HJ, Forrest AP, Gunn JM, et al. The tamoxifen trial—a double-blind comparison with stilboestrol in postmenopausal women with advanced breast cancer. *Eur J Cancer* 1980;[Suppl 1]:83.
179. Tormey DC, Simon RM, Lippman ME. Evaluation of tamoxifen dose in advanced breast cancer: a progress report. *Cancer Treat Rep* 1976;60:1451.
180. Ettinger DS, Allegra J, Bertino JR, et al. Megestrol acetate v tamoxifen in advanced breast cancer: correlation of hormone receptors and response. *Semin Oncol* 1986;13:9.
181. Kaufman RJ, Escher GC. Rebound regression in advanced mammary carcinoma. *Surg Gynec Obstet* 1961;113:635.
182. Nesto R, Cady B, Oberfield R, Pazianos A, Salzman F. Rebound response after estrogen therapy for metastatic breast cancer. *Cancer* 1976;38:1834.
183. Howell A, Dodwell DJ, Anderson H, Redford J. Response after withdrawal of tamoxifen and progestogens in advanced breast cancer. *Ann Oncol* 1992;3:611.
184. Taylor SG, Gelman RS, Falkson G, Cummings FJ. Combination chemotherapy compared to tamoxifen as initial therapy for stage IV breast cancer in elderly women. *Ann Intern Med* 1986;104:455.
185. Ward HWC. Anti-oestrogen therapy for breast cancer: a trial of tamoxifen at two dose levels. *BMJ* 1973;1:13.
186. Goldhirsch A, Joss RA, Leuenberger U, Cavalli F, Ryssel HJ, Brunner KW. An evaluation of tamoxifen dose escalation in advanced breast cancer. *Am J Clin Oncol* 1982;5:501.
187. Dehal SS, Kupfer D. CYP2D6 catalyzes tamoxifen 4-hydroxylation in human liver. *Cancer Res* 1997;57:3402.
188. Crewe HK, Lennard MS, Tucker GT, Woods FR, Haddock RE. The effect of selective serotonin re-uptake inhibitors on cytochrome P4502D6 (CYP2136) activity in human liver microsomes. *Br J Clin Pharmacol* 1992;34:262.
189. Furr BJ, Jordan VC. The pharmacology and clinical uses of tamoxifen. *Pharmacol Ther* 1984;25:127.
190. Osborne CK, Coronado E, Allred DC, Wiebe V, DeGregorio M. Acquired tamoxifen resistance: correlation with reduced breast tumor levels of tamoxifen and isomerization of trans-4-hydroxytamoxifen. *J Natl Cancer Inst* 1991;83:1477.
191. Fisher B, Dignam J, Bryant J, et al. Five versus more than five years of tamoxifen therapy for breast cancer patients with negative lymph nodes and estrogen receptor–positive tumors. *J Natl Cancer Inst* 1996;88:1529.
192. Evans R. The steroid and thyroid hormone receptor superfamily. *Science* 1988;240:889.
193. Beato M. Gene regulation by steroid hormones. *Cell* 1989;56:335.
194. Parker MG. Transcriptional activation by oestrogen receptors. *Biochem Soc Symp* 1998;63:45.
195. MacGregor JI, Jordan VC. Basic guide to the mechanisms of antiestrogen action. *Pharmacol Rev* 1998;50:151.
196. Beato M, Sanchez-Pacheco A. Interaction of steroid hormone receptors with the transcription initiation complex. *Endocr Rev* 1996;17:587.
197. Beato M, Candau R, Chavez S, Mows C, Truss M. Interaction of steroid hormone receptors with transcription factors involves chromatin remodelling. *J Steroid Biochem Mol Biol* 1996;56:47.
198. Kamei Y, Xu L, Heinzel T, et al. A CBP integrator complex mediates transcriptional activation and AP-1 inhibition by nuclear receptors. *Cell* 1996;85:403.
199. Voegel JJ, Heine MJ, Zechel C, Chambon P, Gronemeyer H. TIF2, a 160 kDa transcriptional mediator for the ligand-dependent activation function AF-2 of nuclear receptors. *EMBO J* 1996;15:3667.
200. Hong H, Kohli K, Garabedian MJ, Stallcup MR. GRIP1, a transcriptional coactivator for the AF-2 transactivation domain of steroid, thyroid, retinoid, and vitamin D receptors. *Mol Cell Biol* 1997;17:2735.
201. Halachini S, Marden E, Martin G, MacKay H, Abbondanza C, Brown M. Estrogen receptor-associated proteins: possible mediators of hormone-induced transcription. *Science* 1994;264:1455.
202. Onate SA, Tsai SY, Tsai MJ, O'Malley BW. Sequence and characterization of a coactivator for the steroid hormone receptor superfamily. *Science* 1995;270:1354.
203. Jackson TA, Richer JK, Bain DL, Takimoto GS, Tung L, Horwitz KB. The partial agonist activity of antagonist-occupied steroid receptors is controlled by a novel hinge domain-binding coactivator L7/SPA and the corepressors N-CoR or SMRT. *Mol Endocrinol* 1997;11:693.
204. Chen JD, Evans RM. A transcriptional co-repressor that interacts with nuclear hormone receptors [see comments]. *Nature* 1995;377:454.
205. Shiau AK, Barstad D, Loria PM, et al. The structural basis of estrogen receptor/coactivator recognition and the antagonism of this interaction by tamoxifen. *Cell* 1998;95:927.
206. Shibata H, Spencer TE, Onate SA, et al. Role of co-activators and corepressors in the mechanism of steroid/thyroid receptor action. *Recent Prog Horm Res* 1997;52:141.
207. McInerney EM, Katzenellenbogen BS. Different regions in activation function-1 of the human estrogen receptor required for antiestrogen- and estradiol-dependent transcription activation. *J Biol Chem* 1996;271:24172.
208. Lavinsky RM, Jepsen K, Heinzel T, et al. Diverse signaling pathways modulate nuclear receptor recruitment of N-CoR and SMRT complexes. *Proc Natl Acad Sci U S A* 1998;95:2920.
209. Harris AL, Nicholson S, Sainsbury R, Wright C, Farndon J. Epidermal growth factor receptor and other oncogenes as prognostic markers. *J Natl Cancer Inst: Monographs* 1992;11:181.
210. Nicholson S, Richard J, Sainsbury C, et al. Epidermal growth factor receptor (EGFr); results of a 6 year follow-up study in operable breast cancer with emphasis on the node negative subgroup. *Br J Cancer* 1991;63:146.
211. Zeillinger R, Kury F, Czerwenka K, et al. HER-2 amplification, steroid receptors and epidermal growth factor receptor in primary breast cancer. *Oncogene* 1989;4:109.
212. Tetu B, Brisson J. Prognostic significance of HER-2/neu oncoprotein expression in node-positive breast cancer. The influence of the pattern of immunostaining and adjuvant therapy. *Cancer* 1994;73:2359.
213. Mueller H, Kueng W, Schoumacher F, Herzer S, Eppenberger U. Selective regulation of steroid receptor expression in MCF-7 breast cancer cells by a novel member of the heregulin family. *Biochem Biophys Res Commun* 1995;217:1271.
214. El-Ashry D, Miller DL, Kharbanda S, Lippman ME, Kern FG. Constitutive Raf-1 kinase activity in breast cancer cells induces both estrogen-independent growth and apoptosis. *Oncogene* 1997;15:423.
215. Ellis MJ, Jenkins S, Hanfelt J, et al. Insulin-like growth factors and breast cancer prognosis. *Breast Cancer Res Treat* 1998;52:175.
216. Ellis MJ. The insulin-like growth factor network and breast cancer. In AM Bowcock (ed). *Breast cancer. Molecular genetics, pathogenesis and therapeutics*. Totowa, NJ: Humana Press, 1999.

217. McLeskey SW, Zhang L, El-Ashry D, et al. Tamoxifen-resistant fibroblast growth factor-transfected MCF-7 cells are cross-resistant in vivo to the antiestrogen ICI 182,780 and two aromatase inhibitors. *Clin Cancer Res* 1998;4:697.
218. Smith CL, Conneely OM, O'Malley BW. Modulation of the ligand-independent activation of the human estrogen receptor by hormone and antihormone. *Proc Natl Acad Sci U S A* 1993;90:6120.
219. Aronica SM, Katzenellenbogen BS. Stimulation of estrogen receptor-mediated transcription and alteration in the phosphorylation state of the rat uterine estrogen receptor by estrogen, cyclic adenosine monophosphate, and insulin-like growth factor-1. *Mol Endocrinol* 1993;7:743.
220. Le Goff P, Montano MM, Schodin DJ, Katzenellenbogen BS. Phosphorylation of the human estrogen receptor. Identification of homone-regulated sites and examination of their influence on transcriptional activity. *J Biol Chem* 1994;269:4458.
221. El-Tanani MK, Green CD. Two separate mechanisms for ligand-independent activation of the estrogen receptor. *Mol Endocrinol* 1997;11:928.
222. Katzenellenbogen BC, Montano MM, Ekena K, Herman ME, McInerney EM. Antiestrogens: mechanisms of action and resistance in breast cancer. *Breast Cancer Res Treat* 1997;44:23.
223. Porter W, Wang F, Wang W, Duan R, Safe S. Role of estrogen receptor/Sp1 complexes in estrogen-induced heat shock protein 27 gene expression. *Mol Endocrinol* 1996;10:1371.
224. Porter W, Saville B, Hoivik D, Safe S. Functional synergy between the transcription factor Sp1 and the estrogen receptor. *Mol Endocrinol* 1997;11:1569.
225. Barsalou A, Gao W, Anghel SI, Carriere J, Mader S. Estrogen response elements can mediate agonist activity of anti-estrogens in human endometrial Ishikawa cells. *J Biol Chem* 1998;273:17138.
226. Paech K, Webb P, Kuiper GG, et al. Differential ligand activation of estrogen receptors ERalpha and ERbeta at AP1 sites. *Science* 1997;277:1508.
227. Yang NN, Venugopalan M, Hardikar S, Glasebrook A. Identification of an estrogen response element activated by metabolites of 17beta-estradiol and raloxifene. *Science* 1996;273:1222.
228. Yang NN, Venugopalan M, Hardikar S, Glasebrook A. Correction: raloxifene response needs more than an element [letter]. *Science* 1997;275:1249.
229. Kuiper GG, Enmark E, Pelto-Huikko M, Nilsson S, Gustafsson JA. Cloning of a novel receptor expressed in rat prostate and ovary. *Proc Natl Acad Sci U S A* 1996;93:5925.
230. Mosselman S, Polman J, Dijkema R. ER beta: identification and characterization of a novel human estrogen receptor. *FEBS Lett* 1996;392:49.
231. Krege JH, Hodgin JB, Couse JF, et al. Generation and reproductive phenotypes of mice lacking estrogen receptor beta. *Proc Natl Acad Sci U S A* 1998;95:15677.
232. Dotzlaw H, Leygue E, Watson PH, Murphy LC. Expression of estrogen receptor-beta in human breast tumors. *J Clin Endocrinol Metab* 1997;82:2371.
233. Pace P, Taylor J, Suntharalingam S, Coombes RC, Ali S. Human estrogen receptor beta binds DNA in a manner similar to and dimerizes with estrogen receptor alpha. *J Biol Chem* 1997;272:25832.
234. Kuiper GG, Carlsson B, Grandien K, et al. Comparison of the ligand binding specificity and transcript tissue distribution of estrogen receptors alpha and beta. *Endocrinology* 1997;138:863.
235. Barkhem T, Carlsson B, Nilsson Y, Enmark E, Gustafsson J, Nilsson S. Differential response of estrogen receptor alpha and estrogen receptor beta to partial estrogen agonists/antagonists. *Mol Pharmacol* 1998;54:105.
236. McInerney EM, Weis KE, Sun J, Mosselman S, Katzenellenbogen BS. Transcription activation by the human estrogen receptor subtype beta (ER beta) studied with ER beta and ER alpha receptor chimeras. *Endocrinology* 1998;139:4513.
237. Speirs V, Parkes AT, Kerin MJ, et al. Coexpression of Estrogen Receptor alpha and beta: poor prognostic factors in human breast cancer? *Cancer Res* 1999;59:525.
238. Fuqua SA, Chamness GC, McGuire WL. Estrogen receptor mutations in breast cancer. *J Cell Biochem* 1993;51:135.
239. Roodi N, Bailey LR, Kao WY, et al. Estrogen receptor gene analysis in estrogen receptor-positive and receptor-negative primary breast cancer. *J Natl Cancer Inst* 1995;87:446.
240. Karnik PS, Kulkarni S, Liu XP, Budd GT, Bukowski RM. Estrogen receptor mutations in tamoxifen-resistant breast cancer. *Cancer Res* 1994;54:349.
241. Pfeffer U, Fecarotta E, Arena G, Forlani A, Vidall G. Alternative splicing of the estrogen receptor primary transcript normally occurs in estrogen receptor positive tissues and cell lines. *J Steroid Biochem Mol Biol* 1996;56:99.
242. Zhang QX, Borg A, Fuqua SA. An exon 5 deletion variant of the estrogen receptor frequently coexpressed with wild-type estrogen receptor in human breast cancer. *Cancer Res* 1993;53:5882.
243. Rea D, Parker MG. Effects of an exon 5 variant of the estrogen receptor in MCF-7 breast cancer cells. *Cancer Res* 1996;56:1556.
244. Pfeffer U, Fecarotta E, Vidall G. Coexpression of multiple estrogen receptor variant messenger RNAs in normal and neoplastic breast tissues and in MCF-7 cells. *Cancer Res* 1995;55:2158.
245. Gallacchi P, Schoumacher F, Eppenberger-Castori S, et al. Increased expression of estrogen-receptor exon-5-deletion variant in relapse tissues of human breast cancer. *Int J Cancer* 1998;79:44.
246. Wright C, Nicholson S, Angus B, et al. Relationship between c-*erb*B-2 protein product expression and response to endocrine therapy in advanced breast cancer. *Br J Cancer* 1992;65:118.
247. Carney W, Hamer P, Petit D, et al. Detection and quantitation of the neu oncoprotein. *J Tumor Marker Oncol* 1991;6:53.
248. Leitzel K, Teramoto Y, Sampson E, et al. Elevated soluble c-erbB-2 antigen levels in the serum and effusions of a proportion of breast cancer patients. *J Clin Oncol* 1992;10:1436.
249. Gottardis MM, Jordan VC. Development of tamoxifen-stimulated growth of MCF-7 tumors in athymic mice after long-term antiestrogen administration. *Cancer Res* 1988;48:5183.
250. Anzick SL, Kononen J, Walker RL, et al. AIB1, a steroid receptor coactivator amplified in breast and ovarian cancer. *Science* 1997;277:965.
251. Bautista S, Valles H, Walker RL, et al. In breast cancer, amplification of the steroid receptor coactivator gene AIB1 is correlated with estrogen and progesterone receptor positivity. *Clin Cancer Res* 1998;4:2925.
252. Lufkin EG, Whitaker MD, Nickelsen T, et al. Treatment of established postmenopausal osteoporosis with raloxifene: a randomized trial. *J Bone Miner Res* 1998;13:1747.
253. Balfour JA, Goa KL. Raloxifene. *Drugs Aging* 1998;12:335.
254. Buzdar AU, Hortobagyi G. Update on endocrine therapy for breast cancer. *Clin Cancer Res* 1998;4:527.
255. Hudis C, Buzdar A, Munster P, et al. Phase I study of a third-generation selective estrogen receptor modulator (SERM3, LY353381, HCL) in refractory, metastatic breast cancer. *Breast Cancer Res Treat* 1998;50:306(abst).
256. O'Regan RM, Cisneros A, England GM, et al. Effects of the antiestrogens tamoxifen, toremifene, and ICI 182,780 on endometrial cancer growth. *J Natl Cancer Inst* 1998;90:1552.
257. Gradishar WJ, Jordan VC. Clinical potential of new antiestrogens. *J Clin Oncol* 1997;15:840.
258. Coombes RC, Haynes BP, Dowsett M, et al. Idoxifene: report of a phase I study in patients with metastatic breast cancer. *Cancer Res* 1995;55:1070.
259. Grasser WA, Pan LC, Thompson DD, Paralkar VM. Common mechanism for the estrogen agonist and antagonist activities of droloxifene. *J Cell Biochem* 1997;65:159.
260. Haarstad H, Lonning PE, Gundersen S, Wist E, Raabe N, Kvinnsland S. Influence of droloxifene on metastatic breast cancer as first-line endocrine treatment. *Acta Oncol* 1998;37:365.
261. Buzdar AU, Hortobagyi GN. Tamoxifen and toremifene in breast cancer: comparison of safety and efficacy. *J Clin Oncol* 1998;16:348.
262. Hayes DF, Van Zyl JA, Hacking A, et al. Randomized comparison of tamoxifen and two separate doses of toremifene in postmenopausal patients with metastatic breast cancer. *J Clin Oncol* 1995;13:2556.
263. Vogel CL. Phase II and III clinical trials of toremifene for metastatic breast cancer. *Oncology (Huntingt)* 1998;12:9.
264. Vogel CL, Shemano I, Schoenfelder J, Gams RA, Green MR. Multicenter Phase II efficacy trial of toremifene in tamoxifen-refractory patients with advanced breast cancer. *J Clin Oncol* 1993;11:345.
265. Dauvois S, Danielian PS, White R, Parker MG. Antiestrogen ICI 164,384 reduces cellular estrogen receptor content by increasing its turnover. *Proc Natl Acad Sci U S A* 1992;89:4037.

266. Dauvois S, White R, Parker MG. The antiestrogen ICI 182780 disrupts estrogen receptor nucleocytoplasmic shuttling. *J Cell Sci* 1993;106:1377.
267. DeFriend D, Howell A, Nicholson R. Investigation of a new pure antiestrogen ICI 182780 in women with primary breast cancer. *Cancer Res* 1994;54:408.
268. Osborne CK, Coronado-Heinsohn EB, Hilsenbeck SG, et al. Comparison of the effects of a pure steroidal antiestrogen with those of tamoxifen in a model of human breast cancer. *J Natl Cancer Inst* 1995;87:746.
269. Howell A, DeFriend D, Robertson J, Blamey R, Walton P. Response to a specific antioestrogen (ICI 182780) in tamoxifen-resistant breast cancer. *Lancet* 1995;345:29.
270. MacGregor J, Jordan VC. Classification of the antiestrogen EM-800 using a novel assay system. *Proc Am Acad Cancer Res* 1999;40:639a.
271. Buchanan RB, Blamey RW, Durrant KR, et al. A randomized comparison of tamoxifen with surgical oophorectomy in premenopausal patients with advanced breast cancer. *J Clin Oncol* 1986;4:1326.
272. Dowsett M, Jacobs S, Aherne J, Smith IE. Clinical and endocrine effects of leuprorelin acetate in pre- and postmenopausal patients with advanced breast cancer. *Clin Ther* 1992;14:97.
273. Nicholson RI, Walker KJ, Turkes A, et al. Endocrinological and clinical aspects of LHRH action (ICI 118630) in hormone dependent breast cancer. *J Steroid Biochem* 1985;23:843.
274. Robertson JF, Walker KJ, Nicholson RI, Blamey RW. Combined endocrine effects of LHRH agonist (Zoladex) and tamoxifen (Nolvadex) therapy in premenopausal women with breast cancer. *Br J Surg* 1989;76:1262.
275. Lissoni P, Barni S, Crispino S, Cattaneo G, Tancini G. Endocrine and clinical effects of an LHRH analogue in pretreated advanced breast cancer. *Tumori* 1988;74:303.
276. Longcope C. Metabolic clearance and blood production rates of estrogens in postmenopausal women. *Am J Obstet Gynecol* 1971;111:778.
277. MacDonald P, Rombaut R, Siliteri P. Plasma precursors of estrogen. I. Extent of conversion of plasma alpha-4 androstenedione to estrone in normal males and nonpregnant normal, castrate and adrenalectomized females. *J Clin Endocrinol Metab* 1967;27:1103.
278. Santen R, Santner S, Pauley R, et al. Estrogen production via the aromatase enzyme in breast carcinoma: which cell type is responsible? *J Steroid Biochem Mol Biol* 1997;61:267.
279. Santner SJ, Pauley RJ, Tait L, Kaseta J, Santen RJ. Aromatase activity and expression in breast cancer and benign breast tissue stromal cells. *J Clin Endocrinol Metab* 1997;82:200.
280. Abul-Hajj Y, Iverson R, Kiang D. Aromatization of androgens by human breast cancer. *Steroids* 1979;33:205.
281. Dowsett M, Lee K, Macaulay VM, Detre S, Rowlands M, Grimshaw R. The control and biological importance of intratumoral aromatase in breast cancer. *J Steroid Biochem Mol Biol* 1996;56:145.
282. Pasqualini JR, Chetnite G, Nestour EL. Control and expression of oestrone sulphatase activities in human breast cancer. *J Endocrinol* 1996;150:S99.
283. de Jong P, van de Ven J, Nortier H, et al. Inhibition of breast cancer tissue aromatase activity and estrogen concentrations by the third-generation aromatase inhibitor vorozole. *Cancer Res* 1997;57:2109.
284. Thorsen T, Tangen M, Stoa K. Concentrations of endogenous estradiol as related to estradiol receptor sites in breast tumor cytosol. *Eur J Cancer Clin Oncol* 1982;18:333.
285. Masamura S, Santer S, Gimotty P, George J, Santen R. Mechanism for maintenance of high breast tumor estradiol concentrations in the absence of ovarian function: role of very high affinity tissue uptake. *Breast Cancer Res Treat* 1997;42:215.
286. Lu Q, Nakmura J, Savinov A, et al. Expression of aromatase protein and messenger ribonucleic acid in tumor epithelial cells and evidence of functional significance of locally produced estrogen in human breast cancers. *Endocrinology* 1996;137:3061.
287. Bulun S, Price T, Aitken J, Mahendroo M, Simpson E. A link between breast cancer and local estrogen biosynthesis suggested by quantification of breast adipose tissue aromatase cytochrome P450 transcripts using competitive polymerase chain reaction after reverse transcription. *J Clin Endocrinol Metab* 1993;77:1622.
288. Bulun S, Mahendroo M, Simpson E. Aromatase gene expression in adipose tissue: relationship to breast cancer. *J Steroid Biochem Mol Biol* 1994;49:319.
289. Yeu W, Wang J-P, Hamilton C, Demers L, Santen R. In situ aromatization enhances breast tumor estradiol levels and cellular proliferation. *Cancer Res* 1998;58:927.
290. Dowsett M. Endocrine treatment of advanced breast cancer. *Acta Oncol* 1996;35:68.
291. Miller WR, Mullen P, Telford J, Dixon JM. Clinical importance of intratumoral aromatase. *Breast Cancer Res Treat* 1998;49:S27.
292. Brodie A, Njar V. Aromatase inhibitors and breast cancer. *Semin Oncol* 1996;23:10.
293. Samojlik E, Santen R, Wells S. Adrenal suppression with aminoglutethimide II. Differential effects of aminoglutethimide on plasma androstenedione and estrogen levels. *J Clin Endocrinol Metab* 1977;45:480.
294. Bonneterre J, Coppens H, Mauriac L, et al. Aminoglutethimide in advanced breast cancer: clinical results of a French multicenter randomized trial comparing 500 mg and 1 g/day. *Eur J Cancer Clin Oncol* 1985;21:1153.
295. Carella MJ, Dimitrov NV, Gossain VV, Srivastava L, Rovner DR. Adrenal effects of low-dose aminoglutethimide when used alone in postmenopausal women with advanced breast cancer. *Metabolism* 1994;43:723.
296. Goldhirsch A, Gelber RD. Endocrine therapies of breast cancer. *Semin Oncol* 1996;23:494.
297. Smith I, Ham's A, Morgan M, et al. Tamoxifen versus aminoglutethimide in advanced breast carcinoma: a randomized cross-over trial. *BMJ* (*Clin Res Ed*) 1981;283:1432.
298. Smith I, Harris A, Morgan M, Gazet J, McKinna J. Tamoxifen versus aminoglutethimide versus combined tamoxifen and aminoglutethimide in the treatment of advanced breast carcinoma. *Cancer Res* 1982;42:3430s.
299. Harris A, Powles T, Smith I, et al. Aminoglutethimide for the treatment of advanced postmenopausal breast cancer. *Eur J Cancer Clin Oncol* 1983;19:11.
300. Dowsett M, Vorobiof D, Kleeberg U, Carrion R, Dodwell D, Robertson J. A randomized comparison assessing oestrogen suppression with arimadex (anastrozole) and formestane in postmenopausal advanced breast cancer patients. *Eur J Cancer* 1996;32A[Suppl 2]:49.
301. Plourde PV, Dyroff M, Dowsett M, Demers L, Yates R, Webster A. Arimidex: a new, oral once-a-day aromatase inhibitor. *J Steroid Biochem Mol Biol* 1995;53:175.
302. Robertson JF, Willsher PC, Cheung KL, Blamey RW. The clinical relevance of static disease (no change) category for 6 months on endocrine therapy in patients with breast cancer. *Eur J Cancer* 1997;33:1774.
303. Iveson T, Smith I, Ahern J, Smithers D, Trunet P, Dowsett M. Phase I study of the oral nonsteroidal aromatase inhibitor CGS 20267 in postmenopausal patients with advanced breast cancer. *Cancer Res* 1993;53:266.
304. Bisagni G, Coccom G, Scaglione F, Fraschini F, Pfister C, Trunet P. Letrozole, a new oral non-steroidal aromastase inhibitor in treating postmenopausal patients with advanced breast cancer. A pilot study. *Ann Oncol* 1996;7:99.
305. Tominaga T, Ohashi Y, Abe R. Phase II trial of letrozole (a novel oral nonsteroidal aromatase inhibitor) in postmenopausal patients with advanced or recurrent breast cancer. *Eur J Cancer* 1995;31A[Suppl 5]:S81(abst).
306. Lipton A, Demers L, Harvey H, et al. Letrozole (CGS 20267). A phase I study of a new potent oral aromatase inhibitor of breast cancer. *Cancer* 1995;75:2132.
307. Klein KO, Demers LM, Santner SJ, Baron J, Cutler GBJ, Santen RJ. Use of ultrasensitive recombinant cell bioassay to measure estrogen levels in women with breast cancer receiving the aromatase inhibitor, letrozole. *J Clin Endocrinol Metab* 1995;80:2658.
308. Banting L. Inhibition of aromatase. *Prog Med Chem* 1996;33:147.
309. Sjoerdsma A. Suicide inhibitors as potential drugs. *Clin Pharm Ther* 1981;30:3.
310. Brodie A, Hendrickson J, Tsai-Morris C. Inactivation of aromatase in vitro by 4-OHA and 4-acetoxyandrostenedione and sustain effects in vivo. *Steroids* 1981;38:696.
311. Dowsett M, Cunningham D, Stein R, et al. Dose-related endocrine effects and pharmacokinetics of oral and intramuscular 4-hydroxyandrostenedione in postmenopausal breast cancer patients. *Cancer Res* 1989;49:1306.

312. Dowsett M, Mehta A, King N, et al. An endocrine and pharmacokinetic study of four oral doses of formestane in postmenopausal breast cancer patients. *Eur J Cancer* 1992;28:415.
313. Brodie AM, Santen RJ. Aromatase and its inhibitors in breast cancer treatment—overview and perspective. *Breast Cancer Res Treat* 1994;30:1.
314. Brodie A. Aromatase inhibitors in the treatment of breast cancer. *J Steroid Biochem Mol Biol* 1994;49:281.
315. Goss PE, Gwyn KM. Current perspectives on aromatase inhibitors in breast cancer. *J Clin Oncol* 1994;12:2460.
316. Bajetta E, Zilembo N, Barni S, et al. A multicentre, randomized, pharmacokinetic, endocrine and clinical study to evaluate formestane in breast cancer patients at first relapse: endocrine and clinical results. The Italian Trials in Medical Oncology (I.T.M.O.) group. *Ann Oncol* 1997;8:649.
317. Perez Carrion R, Alberola Candel V, Calabresi F, et al. Comparison of the selective aromatase inhibitor formestane with tamoxifen as first-line hormonal therapy in postmenopausal women with advanced breast cancer. *Ann Oncol* 1994;7[5 Suppl]:S19.
318. Thurlimann B, Castiglione M, Hsu-Schmitz S, et al. Formestane versus megestrol acetate in postmenopausal breast cancer patients after failure of tamoxifen: a phase III prospective randomised cross over trial of second-line hormonal treatment (SAKK 20/90). Swiss Group for Clinical Cancer Research (SAKK). *Eur J Cancer* 1997;33:989.
319. Lonning P, Paridaens R, Thurlimann B, Piscitelli G, di Salle E. Exemestane experience in breast cancer treatment. *J Steroid Biochem Mol Biol* 1997;61:151.
320. Evans T, Di Salle E, Ornati G, et al. Phase I and endocrine study of exemestane (FCE 24304), a new aromatase inhibitor, in postmenopausal women. *Cancer Res* 1992;52:5933.
321. Zilembo N, Noberasco C, Bajetta E, et al. Endocrinological and clinical evaluation of exemestane, a new steroidal aromatase inhibitor. *Br J Cancer* 1995;72:1007.
322. Noberasco C, Bajetta E, Zilembo N, et al. Activity of formestane in de novo tamoxifen-resistant patients with metastatic breast cancer. *Oncology* 1995;52:454.
323. Gershanovich M, Chaudri H, Hornberger U, Lassus M. Comparison of letrozole 2.5mg (Femara) with megestrol acetate and with aminoglutethimide in patients with visceral disease. *Breast Cancer Res Treat* 1997;46:212(abst).
324. Howell A, Buzdar A, Jonat W. Arimidex (anastrozole)—effective in advanced breast cancer patients with visceral and liver metastases. *Breast Cancer Res Treat* 1998;50:304(abst).
325. Kvinnsland S, Anker G, Dirix L, et al. Antitumor efficacy of exemestane, a novel, irreversible, oral, aromatase inhibitor in postmenopausal patients with metastatic breast cancer failing tamoxifen. *Breast Cancer Res Treat* 1997;46:Abstract 217.
326. Lonning PE, Bajetta E, Murray R, et al. A phase II study of exemestane in metastatic breast cancer (MBC) patients failing non steroidal aromatase inhibitors. *Breast Cancer Res Treat* 1998;50:304(abst).
327. Kaufmann M, Bajetta E, Dirix LY. Survival advantage of exemestane (EXE, Dromasin) over megestrol acetate (MA) in postmenopausal women with advanced breast cancer refractory to tamoxifen (TAM): results of a phase III randomized double-blind study. *Proc Am Soc Clin Oncol* 1999;18:42a.
328. Muss HB. Endocrine therapy for advanced breast cancer: a review. *Breast Cancer Res Treat* 1992;21:15.
329. Ito Y, Fisher C, Conte F, Grumbach M, Simpson E. Molecular basis of aromatase deficiency in an adult female with sexual infantilism and polycystic ovaries. *Proc Natl Acad Sci U S A* 1993;90:11673.
330. Conte F, Grumbach M, Ito Y, Fisher C, Simpson E. A syndrome of female pseudohermaphrodism, hypergonadotropic hypogonadism, and multicystic ovaries associated with missense mutations in the gene encoding aromatase (P450arom). *J Clin Endocrinol Metab* 1994;78:1287.
331. Agarwal S, Judd H, Magoffin D. A mechanism for the suppression of estrogen production in polycystic ovary syndrome. *J Clin Endocrinol Metab* 1996;81:3686.
332. Dowsett M, Doody D, Miall S, Howes A, English J, Coombes RC. Vorozole results in greater estrogen suppression than formestane in postmenopausal women and when added to goserelin in premenopausal women with advanced cancer. *Breast Cancer Res Treat* 1999 (*in press*).
333. Muss HB, Case LD, Capizzi RL, et al. High- versus standard-dose megestrol acetate in women with advanced breast cancer: a phase III trial of the Piedmont Oncology Association. *J Clin Oncol* 1990;8:1797.
334. Tchekmedyian NS, Tait N, Abrams J, Aisner J. High-dose megestrol acetate in the treatment of advanced breast cancer. *Semin Oncol* 1988;15:44.
335. Komblith AB, Hollis DR, Zuckerrnan E, et al. Effect of megestrol acetate on quality of life in a dose-response trial in women with advanced breast cancer. The Cancer and Leukemia Group B. *J Clin Oncol* 1993;11:2081.
336. Mattsson W. Current status of high dose progestin treatment in advanced breast cancer. *Breast Cancer Res Treat* 1983;3:231.
337. Anonymous. Results of studies of the cooperative breast cancer group—1961–63. *Cancer Chemother Rep* 1964;41:1.
338. Coombes RC, Dearnaley D, Humphreys J, et al. Danazol treatment of advanced breast cancer. *Cancer Treat Rep* 1980;64:1073.
339. Henderson IC. Endocrine therapy of metastatic breast cancer. In: Harris JR, Hellman S, Henderson IC, et al., eds. *Breast diseases*. Philadelphia: JB Lippincott, 559;1991.
340. Brunner N, Spang-Thomsen M, Cullen K. The T61 human breast cancer xenograft: an experimental model of estrogen therapy of breast cancer. *Breast Cancer Res Treat* 1996;39:87.
341. Lonning PE, Anker G, Taylor PD, et al. High dose estrogen treatment in postmenopausal patients heavily exposed to endocrine treatment for advanced breast cancer. *Breast Cancer Res Treat* 1998;50:305(abst).
342. Rose C, Kamby C, Mouridsen HT, et al. Combined endocrine treatment of postmenopausal patients with advanced breast cancer. A randomized trial of tamoxifen vs. tamoxifen plus aminoglutethimide and hydrocortisone. *Breast Cancer Res Treat* 1986;7:S45.
343. Corkery J, Leonard RC, Henderson IC, et al. Tamoxifen and aminoglutethimide in advanced breast cancer. *Cancer Res* 1982;42:3409s.
344. Ingle JN, Green SJ, Ahmarin DL, et al. Randomized trial of tamoxifen alone or combined with aminoglutethimide and hydrocortisone in women with metastatic breast cancer. *J Clin Oncol* 1986;4:958.
345. Ingle JN, Suman VJ, Johnson PA, et al. Elevation of tamoxifen plus letrozole with assessment of pharmacokinetic interaction in postmenopausal women with metastatic breast cancer. *Clin Cancer Res* 1999;5:1642.
346. Bishop JF, Smith JG, Jeal PN, et al. The effect of danazol on tumour control and weight loss in patients on tamoxifen therapy for advanced breast cancer: a randomised double-blind placebo controlled trial. *Eur J Cancer* 1993;6:814.
347. Ingle JN, Twito DI, Schaid DJ, et al. Combination hormonal therapy with tamoxifen plus fluoxymesterone versus tamoxifen alone in postmenopausal women with metastatic breast cancer. An updated analysis. *Cancer* 1991;67:886.
348. Mouridsen HT, Salmitschik M, Dombernowsky P, et al. *Therapeutic effect of tamoxifen versus combined tamoxifen and diethylstilboestrol in advanced breast cancer in postmenopausal women*. Elmsford, NY: Pergamon, 1980.
349. Mouridsen HT, Palshof T, Rose C. Therapeutic effect of tamoxifen alone versus tamoxifen in combination with gestagen and oestrogen in advanced breast cancer. In: Henningsen B, Linder F, Steichele C, eds. *Endocrine treatment of breast cancer. A new approach*. New York: Springer, 1980.
350. Hortobagyi GN, Theriault RL, Lipton A, et al. Long-terrn prevention of skeletal complications of metastatic breast cancer with pamidronate. Protocol 19 Aredia Breast Cancer Study Group. *J Clin Oncol* 1998;16:2038.
351. Body JJ, Bartl R, Burckhardt P, et al. Current use of bisphosphonates in oncology. International Bone and Cancer Study Group. *J Clin Oncol* 1998;16:3890.
352. Diel IJ, Solomayer EF, Costa SD, et al. Reduction in new metastases in breast cancer with adjuvant clodronate treatment. *N Engl J Med* 1998;339:357.
353. Powles TJ, Paterson AHG, Nevantaus A, et al. Adjuvant clodronate reduces the incidence of bone metastasis in patients with primary breast cancer. *Proc ASCO* 1998;17:123a(abst).
354. Budd GT, Adamson PC, Gupta M, et al. Phase I/II trial of all-trans retinoic acid and tamoxifen in patients with advanced breast cancer. *Clin Cancer Res* 1998;4:635.
355. Modiano MR, Dalton WS, Lippman SM, Joffe L, Booth AR, Meyskens FL Jr. Phase II study of fenretinide (N-[4-hydroxyphenyl]retinamide) in advanced breast cancer and melanoma. *Invest New Drugs* 1990;8:317.
356. Cobleigh MA, Dowlatshahi K, Deutsch TA, et al. Phase I/II trial of tamoxifen with or without fenretinide, an analog of vitamin A, in women with metastatic breast cancer. *J Clin Oncol* 1993;11:474.

357. De Palo G, Camerini T, Marubim E, et al. Chemoprevention trial of contralateral breast cancer with fenretinide. Rationale, design, methodology, organization, data management, statistics and accrual. *Tumori* 1997;83:884.
358. Bischoff ED, Gottardis MM, Moon TE, Heyman RA, Lamph WW. Beyond tamoxifen: the retinoid X receptor-selective ligand LGD1069 (TARGRETIN) causes complete regression of mammary carcinoma. *Cancer Res* 1998;58:479.
359. Neidhart JA, Gochnour D, Roach R, Hoth D, Young D. A comparison of mitoxantrone and doxorubicin in breast cancer. *J Clin Oncol* 1986;4:627.
360. Hortobagyi GN, Yap HY, Kau SW, et al. A comparative study of doxorubicin and epirubicin in patients with metastatic breast cancer. *Am J Clin Oncol* 1989;12:57.
361. Henderson IC, Allegra JC, Woodcock T, et al. Randomized clinical trial comparing mitoxantrone with doxorubicin in previously treated patients with metastatic breast cancer. *J Clin Oncol* 1989;7:560.
362. Bennett JM, Muss HB, Doroshow JH, et al. A randomized multicenter trial comparing mitoxantrone, cyclophosphamide, and fluorouracil with doxorubicin, cyclophosphamide, and fluorouracil in the therapy of metastatic breast carcinoma. *J Clin Oncol* 1988;6:1611.
363. Heidemann E, Steinke B, Hartlapp J, et al. Randomized clinical trial comparing mitoxantrone with epirubicin and with doxorubicin, each combined with cyclophosphamide in the first-line treatment of patients with metastatic breast cancer. *Onkologie* 1990;13:24.
364. Hausmaninger H, Lehnert M, Steger G, et al. Randomised phase II study of epirubicin-vindesine versus mitoxantrone-vindesine in metastatic breast cancer. *Eur J Cancer* 1995;31A:2169.
365. Pavesi L, Preti P, Da Prada G, Pedrazzoli P, Poggi G, Robustelli della Cuna G. Epirubicin versus mitoxantrone in combination chemotherapy for metastatic breast cancer. *Anticancer Res* 1995;15:495.
366. von Hoff DD, Layard MW, Basa P, et al. Risk factors for doxorubicin-induced congestive heart failure. *Ann Intern Med* 1979;91:710.
367. Ryberg M, Nielsen D, Skovsgaard T, Hansen J, Jensen BV, Dombernowsky P. Epirubicin cardiotoxicity: an analysis of 469 patients with metastatic breast cancer. *J Clin Oncol* 1998;16:3502.
368. Ejlertsen B, Pfeiffer P, Pedersen D, et al. Diminished efficacy by reducing duration of CEF from 18 to 6 months in the treatment of metastatic breast cancer. *Proc Am Soc Clin Oncol* 1990;9:23.
369. Bastholt L, Dalmark M, Gjedde SB, et al. Dose-response relationship of epirubicin in the treatment of postmenopausal patients with metastatic breast cancer: a randomized study of epirubicin at four different dose levels performed by the Danish Breast Cancer Cooperative Group. *J Clin Oncol* 1990;14:1146.
370. Brufman G, Colajori E, Ghilezan N, et al. Doubling epirubicin dose intensity (100 mg/m^2 versus 50 mg/m^2) in the FEC regimen significantly increases response rates. An international randomised phase III study in metastatic breast cancer. The Epirubicin High Dose (HEPI 010) Study Group [see comments]. *Ann Oncol* 1997;8:155.
371. Findlay BP, Walker-Dilks C. Epirubicin, alone or in combination chemotherapy, for metastatic breast cancer. Provincial Breast Cancer Disease Site Group and the Provincial Systemic Treatment Disease Site Group [in process citation]. *Cancer Prev Control* 1998;2:140.
372. Legha SS, Benjamin RS, Mackay B, et al. Reduction of doxorubicin cardiotoxicity by prolonged continuous intravenous infusion. *Ann Intern Med* 1982;96:133.
373. Speyer JL, Green MD, Dubin N, et al. Prospective evaluation of cardiotoxicity during a six-hour doxorubicin infusion regimen in women with adenocarcinoma of the breast. *Am J Med* 1985;78:555.
374. Bielack S, Erttmann R, Winkler K, Landbeck G. Doxorubicin: effect of different schedules on toxicity and anti-tumor efficacy. *Eur J Cancer Clin Oncol* 1989;25:873.
375. Rahman A, Fumagalli A, Barbieri B. Antitumor and toxicity evaluation of free doxorubicin and doxorubicin entrapped in cardiolipin liposomes. *Cancer Chemo Pharmacol* 1986;16:22.
376. Rahman A, White G, More N. Pharmacological, toxicological and therapeutic evaluation in mice of doxorubicin entrapped in cardiolipin liposomes. *Cancer Res* 1985;45:796.
377. Cowens JW, Creaven PJ, Green WR, et al. Initial clinical (Phase I) trial of TLC D-99 (doxorubicin encapsulated in liposomes). *Cancer Res* 1993;53:2796.
378. Harris L, Winer E, Batist G, Rovira D, Navari R, Lee L. Phase III study of TLC D-99 (liposome encapsulated doxorubicin) vs. free doxorubicin in patients with metastatic breast carcinoma. *Proc Am Soc Clin Oncol* 1998;17:124a.
379. Ranson MR, Carmichael J, O'Byrne K, Stewart S, Smith D, Howell A. Treatment of advanced breast cancer with sterically stabilized liposomal doxorubicin: results of a multicenter phase II trial [see comments]. *J Clin Oncol* 1997;15:3185.
380. Moore M, Srinivasiah J, Feinberg B, et al. Phase II randomized trial of doxorubicin plus paclitaxel versus doxorubicin HCL liposome plus paclitaxel in metastatic breast cancer. *Proc Am Soc Clin Oncol* 1998;17:160a.
381. Swain SM. Adult multicenter trials using dexrazoxane to protect against cardiac toxicity. *Semin Oncol* 1998;25:43.
382. Bates M, Lieu D, Zagari M, Spiers A, Williamson T. A pharmacoeconomic evaluation of the use of dexrazoxane in preventing anthracycline-induced cardiotoxicity in patients with stage IIIB or IV metastatic breast cancer. *Clin Ther* 1997;19:167.
383. Buzdar AU, Marcus C, Smith TL, Blumenschein GR. Early and delayed clinical cardiotoxicity of doxorubicin. *Cancer* 1985;55:2761.
384. Hortobagyi GN, Bodey GP, Buzdar AU, et al. Evaluation of high-dose versus standard FAC chemotherapy for advanced breast cancer in protected environment units: a prospective randomized study. *J Clin Oncol* 1987;5:354.
385. Buzdar AU, Kau SW, Smith TL, Hortobagyi GN. Ten-year results of FAC adjuvant chemotherapy trial in breast cancer. *Clin Oncol* 1989;12:123.
386. Hayes DF, Henderson IC. CAF in metastatic breast cancer: standard therapy or another effective regimen. *J Clin Oncol* 1987;5:1497.
387. Aisner J, Weinberg V, Perloff M, et al. Chemotherapy versus chemoimmunotherapy (CAF v CAFVP v CMF each ± MER) for metastatic carcinoma of the breast: a CALGB study. *J Clin Oncol* 1987;5:1523.
388. Smalley RV, Lefante J, Bartolucci A, Carpenter J, Vogel C, Krauss S. A comparison of cyclophosphamide, Adriamycin, and 5-fluorouracil (CAF) and cyclophosphamide, methotrexate, 5-fluorouracil, vincristine and prednisone (CMFVP) in patients with advanced breast cancer. *Breast Cancer Res Treat* 1983;3:209.
389. Falkson G, Tormey DC, Carey P, Witte R, Falkson HC. Long-term survival of patients treated with combination chemotherapy for metastatic breast cancer. *Eur J Cancer* 1991;27:973.
390. Coombes RC, Bliss JM, Marty M, et al. Randomised trial comparing adjuvant FEC with CNIF in premenopausal patients with node positive resectable breast cancer. *Proc Am Soc Clin Oncol* 1991;10.41.
391. Blomqvist C, Elomaa I, Rissanen P, Hietanen P, Nevasaari K, Helle L. Influence of treatment schedule on toxicity and efficacy of cyclophosphamide, epirubicin, and fluorouracil in metastatic breast cancer: a randomized trial comparing weekly and every-4-week administration. *J Clin Oncol* 1993;11:467.
392. Honig S. Treatment of metastatic disease. In: Harris JR, Lippman M, Morrow M, et al, eds. *Diseases of the breast*. Philadephia: Lippincott–Raven, 1996:667.
393. Greene MH, Harris EL, Gershenson DM, et al. Melphalan may be a more potent leukemogen than cyclophosphamide. *Ann Intern Med* 1986;105:360.
394. Curtis RE, Boice JD Jr, Moloney WC, Ries LG, Flannery JT. Leukemia following chemotherapy for breast cancer. *Cancer Res* 1990;50:2741.
395. Bonadonna G, Valagussa P, Moliterni A, Zambetti M, Terenziani M. Risk of acute leukemia and other malignancies following CMF-based adjuvant chemotherapy. *Proc Am Soc Clin Oncol* 1993;12:61.
396. Curtis RE, Boice JD Jr, Stovall M, et al. Risk of leukemia after chemotherapy and radiation treatment for breast cancer. *N Engl J Med* 1992;326:1745.
397. Ingle JN, Krook JE, Mailliard JA, Hartmann LC, Wieand HS. Evaluation of ifosfamide plus mesna as first-line chemotherapy in women with metastatic breast cancer. *Am J Clin Oncol* 1995;18:498.
398. Walters RS, Holmes FA, Valero V, Esparza-Guerra L, Hortobagyi GN. Phase II study of ifosfamide and mesna in patients with metastatic breast cancer. *Am J Clin Oncol* 1998;21:413.
399. Becher R, Kloke O, Hayungs J, et al. Epirubicin and ifosfamide in metastatic breast cancer. *Semin Oncol* 1996;23:28.
400. Campisi C, Fabi A, Papaldo P, et al. Ifosfamide given by continuous-intravenous infusion in association with vinorelbine in patients with anthracycline-resistant metastatic breast cancer: a phase I–II clinical trial. *Ann Oncol* 1998;9:565.
401. Drinkard L, Hoffman P, Bitran J, et al. Ifosfamide in combination with Navelbine or Taxol and granulocyte colony stimulating factor support in advanced non-small cell lung cancer: 2 parallel Phase I–II trials. 7th World Conference on Lung Cancer, Denver, Colorado, 1994.

402. Ghavamzadeh A. Treatment of metastatic breast cancer with the combination of ifosfamide, epirubicin and 5-fluorouracil. *Cancer Chemother Pharmacol* 1990;26:S66.
403. Hoffmann W, Weidmann B, Migeod F, Konner J, Seeber S. Epirubicin and ifosfamide in patients with refractory breast cancer and other metastatic solid tumours. *Cancer Chemother Pharmacol* 1990;26:S69.
404. Leone BA, Vallejo CT, Romero AO, et al. Ifosfamide and vinorelbine as first-line chemotherapy for metastatic breast cancer. *J Clin Oncol* 1996;14:2993.
405. Pronzato P, Queirolo P, Landucci M, et al. Phase II study of vinorelbine and ifosfamide in anthracycline resistant metastatic breast cancer. *Breast Cancer Res Treat* 1997;42:183.
406. Vermorken JB, Gundersen S, Smyth JF, et al. Randomized Phase II trial of iproplatin and carboplatin in advanced breast cancer. *Proc Am Soc Clin Oncol* 1986;5:73.
407. Booth BW, Weiss RB, Korzun AH, Wood WC, Carey RW, Panasci LC. Phase II trial of carboplatin in advanced breast carcinoma: a Cancer and Leukemia Group B study. *Cancer Treat Rep* 1985;69:919.
408. Kolaric K, Vukas D. Carboplatin activity in untreated metastatic breast cancer—a Phase II trial. *Proc Am Soc Clin Oncol* 1990;9:26.
409. Sledge GW, Rothe BJ. Cisplatin in the management of breast cancer. *Semin Oncol* 1989;16:110.
410. Rozencweig M, Nicasie C, Beer M. Phase I study of carboplatin given on a five-day intravenous schedule. *J Clin Oncol* 1983;1:621.
411. Pegram MD, Finn RS, Arzoo K, Beryt M, Pietras RJ, Slamon DJ. The effect of HER-2/neu overexpression on chemotherapeutic drug sensitivity in human breast and ovarian cancer cells. *Oncogene* 1997;15:537.
412. Dawson NA, Costanza ME, Korzun AH, et al. Trimetrexate in untreated and previously treated patients with metastatic breast cancer: a Cancer and Leukemia Group B study. *Med Pediat Oncology* 1991;19:283.
413. Boarman DM, Baram J, Allegra CJ. Mechanism of leucovorin reversal of methotrexate cytotoxicity in human MCF-7 breast cancer cells. *Biochem Pharmacol* 1990;40:2651.
414. Frei Ed, Blum RH, Pitman SW, et al. High dose methotrexate with leucovorin rescue. Rationale and spectrum of antitumor activity. *Am J Med* 1980;68:370.
415. Benz C, Silverberg M, Cadman E. Use of high-dose oral methotrexate sequenced at 24 hours with 5-FU: a clinical toxicity study. *Cancer Treat Rep* 1983;67:297.
416. Canellos GP, Pocock SJ, Taylor SG, Sears W, Klaasen DJ, Band PR. Combination chemotherapy for metastatic breast carcinoma. Prospective comparison of multiple drug therapy with L-phenylalanine mustard. *Cancer* 1976;38:1882.
417. Doroshow JH, Leong L, Margolin K, et al. Refractory metastatic breast cancer: salvage therapy with fluorouracil and high-dose continuous infusion leucovorin calcium. *J Clin Oncol* 1989;7:439.
418. Lokich JJ, Ahlgren JD, Gullo JJ, Philips JA, Fryer JG. A prospective randomized comparison of continuous infusion fluorouracil with a conventional bolus schedule in metastatic colorectal carcinoma. A Mid-Atlantic Oncology Program study. *J Clin Oncol* 1989;7:425.
419. Loprinzi CL. 5-Fluorouracil with leucovorin in breast cancer. *Cancer* 1989;63:1045.
420. Swain AM, Lippman ME, Egan EF, Drake JC, Steinberg SM, Allegra CJ. Fluorouracil and high-dose leucovorin in previously treated patients with metastatic breast cancer. *J Clin Oncol* 1989;7:890.
421. Hansen RM. 5-Fluorouracil by protracted venous infusion: a review of recent clinical studies. *Cancer Invest* 1991;9:637.
422. Margolin KA, Doroshow JH, Akman SA, et al. Effective initial therapy of advanced breast cancer with fluorouracil and high-dose, continuous infusion calcium leucovorin. *J Clin Oncol* 1992;10:1278.
423. Ng JSY, Cameron DA, Lee L, Dixon JM, Leonard RCF. Infusional 5-fluorouracil given as a single agent in relapsed breast cancer: its activity and toxicity. *Breast* 1994;3:87.
424. Regazzom S, Pesce G, Marini G, Cavalli F, Goldhirsch A. Low-dose continuous intravenous infusion of 5-fluorouracil for metastatic breast cancer [see comments]. *Ann Oncol* 1996;7:807.
425. Nieto Y, Martin M, Alonso JL, et al. Weekly continuous infusion of 5-fluorouracil with oral leucovorin in metastatic breast cancer patients with primary resistance to doxorubicin. *Breast Cancer Res Treat* 1998;50:167.
426. Wilke H, Klaassen U, Achterrath W, et al. Phase I/II study with a weekly 24-hour infusion of 5-fluorouracil plus high-dose folinic acid (HD-FU/FA) in intensively pretreated patients with metastatic breast cancer. *Ann Oncol* 1996;7:55.
427. Alonso V, Santader C, Florian J, et al. Phase II trial of oral tegafur and folinic acid with mitoxantrone as first-line regimen in patients with metastatic breast cancer. *Tumori* 1996;82:61.
428. Blum JL, Jones SE, Buzdar AU, et al. Multicenter phase II study of capecitabine in paclitaxel-refractory metastatic breast cancer. *J Clin Oncol* 1999;17:485.
429. Kajanti MJ, Pyrhonen SO, Maiche AG. Oral tegafur in the treatment of metastatic breast cancer: a phase II study. *Eur J Cancer* 1993;6:863.
430. Sole LA, Albanell J, Bellmunt J, Ribas A, Gallego OS, Carulla J. Phase II trial of an all-oral regimen of tegafur and folinic acid in patients with previously treated metastatic breast cancer. *Cancer* 1995;75:831.
431. Hainsworth JD, Andrews MB, Johnson DH, Greco FA. Mitoxantrone, fluorouracil, and high-dose leucovorin: an effective, well-tolerated regimen for metastatic breast cancer. *J Clin Oncol* 1991;9:1731.
432. Jones SE, Mennel RG, Brooks B, et al. Phase II study of mitoxantrone, leucovorin, and infusional fluorouracil for treatment of metastatic breast cancer. *J Clin Oncol* 1991;9:1736.
433. Louvet C, de Gramont A, Demuynck B, et al. Folinic acid, 5-fluorouracil bolus and infusion and mitoxantrone with or without cyclophosphamide in metastatic breast cancer. *Eur J Cancer* 1993;29A:1835.
434. Bascioni R, Giorgi F, Silva RR, et al. Mitoxantrone, fluorouracil, and L-folinic acid in anthracycline-pretreated metastatic breast cancer patients. *Breast Cancer Res Treat* 1997;45:205.
435. Ingle JN, Kardinal CG, Suman VJ, et al. Mitoxantrone dose augmentation utilizing filgrastim support in combination with fixed-dose 5-fluorouracil and leucovorin in women with metastatic breast cancer. *Breast Cancer Res Treat* 1997;43:193.
436. Hainsworth JD. Mitoxantrone, 5-fluorouracil and high-dose leucovorin (NFL) in the treatment of metastatic breast cancer: randomized comparison to cyclophosphamide, methotrexate and 5-fluorouracil (CMF) and attempts to improve efficacy by adding paclitaxel. *Eur J Cancer Care (Engl)* 1997;6:4.
437. Fumoleau P, Delgado FM, Delozier T, et al. Phase II trial of weekly intravenous vinorelbine in first-line advanced breast cancer chemotherapy. *J Clin Oncol* 1993;11:1245.
438. Bruno S, Lira-Puerto V, Teixeira L, Mickiewecz E, Fernandez O, Martinez L. Phase II trial with vinorelbine, (Navelbine, NVB) in the treatment of advanced breast cancer (ABC). *Ann Oncol* 1992;3[Suppl 1]:268A(abst).
439. Romero A, Rabinovich MG, Vallejo CT, et al. Vinorelbine as first-line chemotherapy for metastatic breast cancer. *J Clin Oncol* 1994;12:336.
440. Tresca P, Fumoleau P, Roche H, Pinon G, Serin D, Marie FN. Vinorelbine, a new active drug in breast carcinoma: results of an ARTAC Phase II trial. *Breast Cancer Res Treat* 1990;16:161.
441. Marty M, Leandri S, Extra JM, Espie M, Besenval M. A Phase II study of vinorelbine in patients with advanced breast cancer. *Proc Am Assoc Cancer Res* 1989;30:256.
442. Bezwoda WR, de Moor NG, Derman D, Lange M, Saner R, Dando R. Combination chemotherapy of metastatic breast cancer: a randomized trial comparing the use of adriamycin to that of vinblastine. *Cancer* 1979;44:392.
443. Yap HY, Blumenschein GR, Keating MJ, Hortobagyi GN, Tashima CK, Loo TL. Vinblastine given as a continuous 5-day infusion in the treatment of refractory advanced breast cancer. *Cancer Treat Rep* 1980;64:279.
444. Carter S. Single and combination nonhormonal chemotherapy. *Cancer* 1972;30:1543.
445. Cobleigh MA, Williams SD, Einhorn LH. Phase II study of vindesine in patients with metastatic breast cancer. *Cancer Treat Rep* 1981;65:659.
446. DiBella NJ, Berris R, Garfield D, Fink K, Speer I, Sakamoto A. Vindesine in advanced breast cancer, lymphoma and melanoma. A Colorado Clinical Oncology Group study. *Invest New Drugs* 1984;2:323.
447. Smith IE, Coombes RC, Evans BD, et al. Vindesine as a single agent and in combination with adriamycin in the treatment of metastatic breast carcinoma. *Eur J Cancer* 1980;[Suppl 1]:271.
448. Robins HI, Tormey DC, Skelley MJ, et al. Vindesine. A phase II trial in advanced breast cancer patients. *Cancer Clin Trials* 1981;4:371.
449. Terenziani M, Demicheli R, Brambilla C, et al. Vinorelbine: an active, non cross-resistant drug in advanced breast cancer. Results from a phase II study. *Breast Cancer Res Treat* 1996;39:285.

450. Havlin KA, Ramirez MJ, Legler CM, et al. Inability to escalate vinorelbine dose intensity using a daily ×3 schedule with and without filgrastim in patients with metastatic breast cancer. *Cancer Chemother Pharmacol* 1999;43:68.
451. Sedlacek SM. First-line and salvage therapy of metastatic breast cancer with mitomycin/vinblastine. *Oncology* 1993;50[Suppl 1]:10.
452. Perrone F, De Placido S, Carlomagno C, et al. Chemotherapy with mitomycin C and vinblastine in pretreated metastatic breast cancer. *Tumori* 1993;79:254.
453. Nabholtz JM, Crown J. Phase III studies of single-agent docetaxel in patients with metastatic breast cancer who have progressed despite previous chemotherapy regimens: preliminary results. *Semin Oncol* 1998;25:4.
454. Gelmon K. The taxoids: paclitaxel and docetaxel. *Lancet* 1994;344:67.
455. Rowinsky EK, Cazenave LA, Donehower RC. Taxol: a novel investigational antimicrotubule agent. *J Natl Cancer Inst* 1990;82:1247.
456. Seidman A, Murphy B, Hudis C. Activity of Taxol by weekly 1h infusion in patients with metastatic breast cancer. *Proc Am Soc Clin Oncol* 1997;16:148a.
457. Hainsworth J, Burris H, Erland J, Thomas M, Greco F. Phase I trial of docetaxel administered by weekly infusion in patients with advanced refractory cancer. *J Clin Oncol* 1998;16:2164.
458. Reichman BS, Seidman AD, Crown JPA, et al. Paclitaxel and recombinant human granulocyte colony-stimulating factor as initial chemotherapy for metastatic breast cancer. *J Clin Oncol* 1993;11:1943.
459. Seidman AD, Reichman BS, Crown JP, et al. Taxol plus recombinant human granulocyte-colony stimulating factor as initial and as salvage chemotherapy for metastatic breast cancer: a preliminary report. *J Natl Cancer Inst Monogr* 1993;15:171.
460. Holmes FA. Combination chemotherapy with Taxol (paclitaxel) in metastatic breast cancer. *Ann Oncol* 1994;5:S23.
461. Davidson NG. Single-agent paclitaxel as first-line treatment of metastatic breast cancer: the British experience. *Semin Oncol* 1996;23:6.
462. Michael M, Bishop JF, Levi JA, et al. Australian multicentre phase II trial of paclitaxel in women with metastatic breast cancer and prior chemotherapy [see comments]. *Med J Aust* 1997;166:520.
463. Geyer CE Jr, Green SJ, Moinpour CM, et al. Expanded phase II trial of paclitaxel in metastatic breast cancer: a Southwest Oncology Group study. *Breast Cancer Res Treat* 1998;51:169.
464. Gianni L, Munzone E, Capri G, et al. Paclitaxel in metastatic breast cancer: a trial of two doses by a 3-hour infusion in patients with disease recurrence after prior therapy with anthracyclines [see comments]. *J Natl Cancer Inst* 1995;87:1169.
465. Vermorken JB, ten Bokkel Huinink WW, Mandjes I, et al. High dose paclitaxel with granulocyte colony-stimulating factor in patients with advanced breast cancer refractory to16–22 anthracycline therapy: a European cancer center trial. *Semin Oncol* 1995;22[Suppl 8]:16.
466. Fontzilas G, Athanassiades A, Giannakakis T, et al. A phase II study of paclitaxel in advanced breast cancer resistant to anthracyclines. *Eur J Cancer Clin Oncol* 1997;32a:47.
467. Vici P, Conti F, Di Lauro L, et al. Paclitaxel in anthracycline-resistant breast cancer patients. *Proc Am Soc Clin Oncol* 1997;16:196a.
468. Rowinsky EK, Chaudhry V, Forastiere AA, et al. Phase I and pharmacologic study of paclitaxel and cisplatin with granulocyte colony-stimulating factor: neuromuscular toxicity is dose-limiting. *J Clin Oncol* 1993;11:2010.
469. Nabholtz JM, Gelmon K, Bontenbal M, et al. Multicenter, randomized comparative study of two doses of paclitaxel in patients with metastatic breast cancer [see comments]. *J Clin Oncol* 1996;14:1858.
470. Winer E, Berry D, Duggan D, et al. Failure of higher dose paclitaxel to improve outcome in patients with metastatic breast cancer. *Proc Am Soc Clin Oncol* 1998;17:101a.
471. Seidman AD, Hudis CA, Albanel J, et al. Dose-dense therapy with weekly 1-hour paclitaxel infusions in the treatment of metastatic breast cancer. *J Clin Oncol* 1998;16:3353.
472. Seidman A. The emerging role of paclitaxel in breast cancer therapy. *Clin Cancer Res* 1995;1:247.
473. Gelmon KA, Tolcher A, O'Reilly S, et al. A phase I–II study of biweekly paclitaxel as first-line treatment in metastatic breast cancer. *Ann Oncol* 1998;9:1247.
474. Von Hoff DD. The taxoids: same roots, different drugs. *Semin Oncol* 1997;24:S13.
475. Vanhoefer U, Cao S, Harstrick A, Seeber S, Rustum YM. Comparative antitumor efficacy of docetaxel and paclitaxel in nude mice bearing human tumor xenografts that overexpress the multidrug resistance protein (MRP) [see comments]. *Ann Oncol* 1997;8:1221.
476. Valero V, Holmes FA, Walters RS, et al. Phase II trial of docetaxel: a new, highly effective antineoplastic agent in the management of patients with anthracycline-resistant metastatic breast cancer [see comments]. *J Clin Oncol* 1995;13:2886.
477. Shapiro JD, Millward MJ, Rischin D, et al. Activity and toxicity of docetaxel (Taxotere) in women with previously treated metastatic breast cancer. *Aust N Z J Med* 1997;27:40.
478. Chevalier B, Fumoleau P, Kerbrat P, et al. Docetaxel is a major cytotoxic drug for the treatment of advanced breast cancer: a phase II trial of the Clinical Screening Cooperative Group of the European Organization for Research and Treatment of Cancer. *J Clin Oncol* 1995;13:314.
479. Erazo-Valle A, Lira-Puerto V, Cervantes G, et al. Docetaxel in advanced breast cancer: a phase II study. *Proc Am Soc Clin Oncol* 1995;14:136a.
480. Dieras V, Chevallier B, Kerbrat P, et al. A multicentre phase II study of docetaxel 75 mg/m2 as first line chemotherapy for patients with advanced breast cancer: a report of the Clinical Screening Group of the EORTC. *Br J Cancer* 1996;74:650.
481. Fumoleau P, Chevallier B, Kerbrat P. A multicentre phase II study of the efficacy and safety of docetaxel as first-line treatment of advanced breast cancer: report of the Clinical Screening Group of the EORTC. *Ann Oncol* 1996;7:165.
482. Alexopoulos C, Rigatos G, Efremidou A, et al. Phase II study of taxotere monotherapy in previously treated patients with advanced breast cancer. *Eur J Cancer* 1997;33[Suppl 8]:153.
483. Borisova T. Taxotere in the treatment of patients with advanced breast cancer. *Eur J Cancer* 1997;33[Suppl 8]:154a.
484. Ravdin P, Burris H, Cook G, et al. Phase II trial of docetaxel in advanced anthracycline-resistant or anthracenedione-resistant breast cancer. *J Clin Oncol* 1995;13:2879.
485. ten Bokkel Huinink WW, Prove A, Piccart M, et al. A phase II trial with docetaxel in second line treatment with chemotherapy for advanced breast cancer. *Ann Oncol* 1994;5:527.
486. Vorobiof D, Chasen M, Moeken R. Phase II trial of single agent docetaxel in previously treated patients with advanced breast cancer. *Proc Am Soc Clin Oncol* 1996;15:130a.
487. Terzoli E, Nistico C, Garufi C, et al. Docetaxel in advanced breast carcinoma patients pretreated with anthracyclines. *Proc Am Soc Clin Oncol* 1998;17:177a.
488. Li W, Sun Y, Zhang X. Phase II study of docetaxel in Chinese patients with advanced/metastatic breast cancer. *Proc Am Soc Clin Oncol* 1998;17:176a.
489. Trandafir L, Chahine A, Spielman M, et al. Efficacy of taxotere in advanced breast cancer patients not eligible for further anthracyclines. *Proc Am Soc Clin Oncol* 1996;15:105a.
490. Adachi I, Watanabe T, Takashima S, et al. A late phase II study of RP56976 (docetaxel) in patients with advanced or recurrent breast cancer. *Br J Cancer* 1996;73:210.
491. Piccart MJ, Klijn J, Paridaens R, et al. Corticosteroids significantly delay the onset of docetaxel-induced fluid retention: final results of a randomized study of the European Organization for Research and Treatment of Cancer Investigational Drug Branch for Breast Cancer. *J Clin Oncol* 1997;15:3149.
492. vanOosterom A, Dieras VT-H, Tubiana-Hulen M, et al. Taxotere in previously treated patients with metastatic breast cancer: stratification for anthracycline resistance. *Proc Am Soc Clin Oncol* 1996;15:141a.
493. Valero V, Jones SE, Von Hoff DD, et al. A phase II study of docetaxel in patients with paclitaxel-resistant metastatic breast cancer. *J Clin Oncol* 1998;16:3362.
494. Seidman AD, Hochhauser D, Gollub M, et al. Ninety six-hour paclitaxel infusion after progression during short taxane exposure: a phase II pharmacokinetic and pharmacodynamic study in metastatic breast cancer. *J Clin Oncol* 1996;14:1877.
495. Sledge G, Neuberg D, Ingle J, Martino S, Wood W. Phase III trial of doxorubicin vs. paclitaxel vs. doxorubicin + paclitaxel as first line therapy for metastatic breast cancer: an Intergroup trial. *Proc Am Soc Clin Oncol* 1997;16:1a.
496. Gamucci T, Piccart M, Bruning P, et al. Single agent taxol versus doxorubicin as first-line chemotherapy in advanced breast cancer. Final results of an EORTC randomized study with crossover. *Proc Am Soc Clin Oncol* 1998;17:111a.

497. Chan S. Docetaxel vs doxorubicin in metastatic breast cancer resistant to alkylating chemotherapy. *Oncology (Huntingt)* 1997;11:19.
498. Loffler T, Freund W, Droge C, Hausamen T. Activity of weekly taxotere in patients with metastatic breast cancer. *Proc Am Soc Clin Oncol* 1998;17:113a.
499. Tomiak E, Piccart MJ, Kerger J, et al. Phase I study of docetaxel administered as a 1-hour intravenous infusion on a weekly basis. *J Clin Oncol* 1994;12:1458.
500. Burris H. Weekly schedules of docetaxel. *Semin Oncol* 1998;25:21.
501. Hudis CA, Seidman AD, Crown JP, et al. Phase II and pharmacologic study of docetaxel as initial chemotherapy for metastatic breast cancer. *J Clin Oncol* 1996;14:58.
502. Trudeau ME, Eisenhauer EA, Higgins BP, et al. Docetaxel in patients with metastatic breast cancer: a phase II study of the National Cancer Institute of Canada-Clinical Trials Group. *J Clin Oncol* 1996;14:422.
503. Llombart-Cussac A, Pivot X, Spielmann M. Docetaxel chemotherapy induces transverse superficial loss of the nail plate [letter]. *Arch Dermatol* 1997;133:1466.
504. Obermair A, Binder M, Barrada M, Bancher-Todesca D, Asseryanis E, Kubista E. Onycholysis in patients treated with docetaxel [letter]. *Ann Oncol* 1998;9:230.
505. Ravdin PM. The international experience with docetaxel in the treatment of breast cancer. *Oncology (Huntingt)* 1997;11:38.
506. Eisenhauer EA, Vermorken JB. The taxoids. Comparative clinical pharmacology and therapeutic potential. *Drugs* 1998;55:5.
507. Martin M, Lluch A, Ojeda B, et al. Paclitaxel plus doxorubicin in metastatic breast cancer: preliminary analysis of cardiotoxicity. *Semin Oncol* 1997;24:S17.
508. Hortobagyi GN, Willey J, Rahman Z, Holmes FA, Theriault RL, Buzdar AU. Prospective assessment of cardiac toxicity during a randomized phase II trial of doxorubicin and paclitaxel in metastatic breast cancer. *Semin Oncol* 1997;24:S17.
509. Gianni L, Munzone E, Capri G, et al. Paclitaxel by 3-hour infusion in combination with bolus doxorubicin in women with untreated metastatic breast cancer: high antitumor efficacy and cardiac effects in a dose-finding and sequence-finding study [see comments]. *J Clin Oncol* 1995;13:2688.
510. Dombernowsky P, Gehl J, Boesgaard M, Paaske T, Jensen BV. Doxorubicin and paclitaxel, a highly active combination in the treatment of metastatic breast cancer. *Semin Oncol* 1996;23:23.
511. Holmes FA, Madden T, Newman RA, et al. Sequence-dependent alteration of doxorubicin pharmacokinetics by paclitaxel in a phase I study of paclitaxel and doxorubicin in patients with metastatic breast cancer. *J Clin Oncol* 1996;14:2713.
512. Hortobagyi GN, Holmes FA. Optimal dosing of paclitaxel and doxorubicin in metastatic breast cancer. *Semin Oncol* 1997;24:S4.
513. Hainsworth JD, Jones SE, Mennel RG, Blum JL, Greco FA. Paclitaxel with mitoxantrone, fluorouracil, and high-dose leucovorin in the treatment of metastatic breast cancer: a phase II trial. *J Clin Oncol* 1996;14:1611.
514. Luck HJ, Thomssen C, du Bois A, et al. Phase II study of paclitaxel and epirubicin as first-line therapy in patients with metastatic breast cancer. *Semin Oncol* 1997;24:S17.
515. Dieras V. Review of docetaxel/doxorubicin combination in metastatic breast cancer. *Oncology (Huntingt)* 1997;11:31.
516. Bishop J, Dewar J, Tattersall M, et al. Taxol alone is equivalent to CMFP combination chemotherapy as frontline treatment in metastatic breast cancer. *Proc Am Soc Clin Oncol* 1997;16:153a.
517. Sledge GW Jr. Etoposide in the management of metastatic breast cancer. *Cancer* 1991;67:266.
518. Atienza DM, Vogel CL, Trock B, Swain SM. Phase II study of oral etoposide for patients with advanced breast cancer. *Cancer* 1995;76:2485.
519. Bezwoda WR, Seymour L, Ariad S. High-dose etoposide in treatment of metastatic breast cancer. *Oncology* 1992;49:104.
520. Calvert AH, Lind MJ, Millward MM, et al. Long-term oral etoposide in metastatic breast cancer: clinical and pharmacokinetic results. *Cancer Treat Rev* 1993;19:27.
521. Martin M, Lluch A, Casado A, et al. Clinical activity of chronic oral etoposide in previously treated metastatic breast cancer [see comments]. *J Clin Oncol* 1994;12:986.
522. Neskovic-Konstantinovic ZB, Bosnjak SM, Radulovic SS, Mitrovic LB. Daily oral etoposide in metastatic breast cancer. *Anticancer Drugs* 1996;7:543.
523. Pusztai L, Walters RS, Valero V, Theriault PL, Hortobagyi GN. Daily oral etoposide in patients with heavily pretreated metastatic breast cancer. *Am J Clin Oncol* 1998;21:442.
524. DeVita VT. Principles of chemotherapy. In: DeVita V, Hellman S, Rosenberg S, eds. *Principles and practice of oncology*. Philadelphia: JB Lippincott, 1989:276.
525. Joensuu H, Holli K, Heikkinen M, et al. Combination chemotherapy versus single-agent therapy as first- and second-line treatment in metastatic breast cancer: a prospective randomized trial. *J Clin Oncol* 1998;16:3720.
526. Zujewski J, Nelson A, Abrams J. Much ado about not . . . enough data: high-dose chemotherapy with autologous stem cell rescue for breast cancer. *J Natl Cancer Inst* 1998;90:200.
527. Tannock I, Boyd N, DeBoer G, et al. A randomized trial of two dose levels of cyclophosphamide, methotrexate, and fluorouracil chemotherapy for patients with metastatic breast cancer. *J Clin Oncol* 1988;6:1377.
528. Nabholtz JM, Gelmon K, Bontenbal M, et al. Randomized trial of two doses of taxol in metastatic breast cancer. *Proc Am Soc Clin Oncol* 1993;12:60.
529. Ellis GK. Alternating weekly doxorubicin and 5-fluorouracil/leucovorin followed by weekly doxorubicin and daily cyclophosphamide in Stage IV breast cancer. *Cancer* 1991;68:934.
530. Blomqvist C, Elomaa I, Rissanen P, Hietanen P, Nevasaani K, Helle L. Influence of treatment schedule on toxicity and efficacy of cyclophosphamide, epirubicin, and fluorouracil in metastatic breast cancer: a randomized trial comparing weekly and every-4-week administration. *J Clin Oncol* 1993;11:467.
531. Hainsworth J. Weekly docetaxel: safety, efficacy, and feasibility. *Proc Chemo Foundation Symp XV*. 1997.
532. Engelsman E, Klijn JCM, Rubens RD, et al. "Classical" CMF versus a 3-weekly intravenous CMF schedule in postmenopausal patients with advanced breast cancer: an EORTC Breast Cancer Co-Operative Group Phase III trial (10808). *Eur J Cancer* 1991;27:966.
533. Seidman AD, Hudis CA, McCaffrey J, et al. Dose-dense therapy with paclitaxel via weekly 1-hour infusion: preliminary experience in the treatment of metastatic breast cancer. *Semin Oncol* 1997;24:S17.
534. Muss HB, Case LD, Richards F II, et al. Interrupted versus continuous chemotherapy in patients with metastatic breast cancer. *N Engl J Med* 1991;325:1342.
535. Cocconi G, Bisagni G, Bacchi M, et al. A comparison of continuation versus late intensification followed by discontinuation of chemotherapy in advanced breast cancer. A prospective randomized trial of the Italian Oncology Group for Clinical Research (GOIRC). *Ann Oncol* 1990;1:36.
536. Gianni L, Capri G. Experience at the Istituto Nazionale Tumori with paclitaxel in combination with doxorubicin in women with untreated breast cancer. *Semin Oncol* 1997;24:S1.
537. Gianni L, Capri G, Mezzelani A, et al. HER-2/neu amplification and response to doxorubicin/paclitaxel (AT) in women with metastatic breast cancer. *Proc Am Soc Clin Oncol* 1997;16:139a.
538. Chang AY. The potential role of topotecan in the treatment of advanced breast cancer. *Semin Oncol* 1997;24:S20.
539. Cersosimo RJ. Topotecan: a new topoisomerase I inhibiting antineoplastic agent. *Ann Pharmacother* 1998;32:1334.
540. Fleming GF, Kugler JW, Hoffman PC, et al. Phase II trial of paclitaxel and topotecan with granulocyte colony-stimulating factor support in stage IV breast cancer. *J Clin Oncol* 1998;16:2032.
541. O'Connell MJ, Mailliard JA, Kahn MJ, et al. Controlled trial of fluorouracil and low-dose leucovorin given for 6 months as postoperative adjuvant therapy for colon cancer. *J Clin Oncol* 1997;15:246.
542. Loprinzi CL, Ingle JN, Schaid DJ, Buckner JC, Edmonson JH, Allegra CJ. 5-fluorouracil plus leucovorin in women with metastatic breast cancer: a Phase II study. *Am J Clin Oncol* 1991;14:30.
543. Parnes H, Berry D, Aisner J, et al. A randomized phase III study of cyclophosphamide (C), doxorubicin (A) and 5-fluorouracil (F) (CAF) with and without Leucovorin for metastatic breast cancer: Cancer and Leukemia Group B Study (CALGB) 9140. *Proc Am Soc Clin Oncol* 1998;17:110A.
544. Lehnert M, Mross K, Schueller J, Thuerlimann B, Kroeger N, Kupper H. Phase II trial of dexverapamil and epirubicin in patients with non-responsive metastatic breast cancer. *Br J Cancer* 1998;77:1155.
545. Mross K, Bohn C, Edler L, et al. Randomized phase II study of single-agent epirubicin +/– verapamil in patients with advanced meta-

static breast cancer. An AIO clinical trial. Arbeitsgemeinschaft Internistische Onkologle ofthe GenTian Cancer Society [see comments]. *Ann Oncol* 1993;4:45.
546. Salama ZB, Dilger C, Czogalla W, Otto R, Jaeger H. Quantitative determination of verapamil and metabolites in human serum by high-performance liquid chromatography and its application to biopharmaceutic investigations. *Arznelmittelforschung* 1989;39:210.
547. Tolcher AW, Cowan KH, Solomon D, et al. Phase I crossover study of paclitaxel with r-verapamil in patients with metastatic breast cancer. *J Clin Oncol* 1996;14:1173.
548. Lippo K, Ellmen J, Vanttinen E, Anttila M. Toremifene concentration and multidrug resistance in lung tumors. *Cancer Chemother Pharmacol* 1997;39:212.
549. DeGregorio MW, Ford JM, Benz CC, Wiebe VJ. Toremifene: pharmacologic and pharmacokinetic basis of reversing multidrug resistance. *J Clin Oncol* 1989;7:1359.
550. Chatterjee M, Harris AL. Enhancement of Adriamycin cytotoxicity in a multidrug resistant Chinese hamster ovary (CHO) subline, CHO-Adrr, by toremifene and its modulation by alpha I acid glycoprotein. *Eur J Cancer* 1990;26:432.
551. Baker WJ, Maenpaa JU, Wurz GT, et al. Toremifene enhances cell cycle block and growth inhibition by vinblastine in multidrug resistant human breast cancer cells. *Oncol Res* 1993;5:207.
552. Fleming GF, Amato JM, Agresti M, Safa AR. Megestrol acetate reverses multidrug resistance and interacts with P-glycoprotein. *Cancer Chemother Pharmacol* 1992;29:445.
553. Wood L, Palmer M, Hewitt J, et al. Results of a phase III, double-blind, placebo-controlled trial of megestrol acetate modulation of P-glycoprotein-mediated drug resistance in the first-line management of small-cell lung carcinoma. *Br J Cancer* 1998;77:627.
554. Chang AY. Megestrol acetate as a biomodulator. *Semin Oncol* 1998;25:58.
555. Wang L, Yang CP, Horwitz SB, Trail PA, Casazza AM. Reversal of the human and murine multidrug-resistance phenotype with megestrol acetate. *Cancer Chemother Pharmacol* 1994;34:96.
556. Pietras R. Antibody to HER-2/neu receptor blocks DNA repair after cisplatin in human breast and ovarian cancer cells. *Oncogene* 1994;9,1829.
557. Pietras R. HER-2/neu signaling regulates estrogen receptor in breast cancer (Meeting Abstract). *Proc Annu Meet Am Assoc Cancer Res* 1995;15:36a.
558. Shepard HM, Lewis GD, Sarup JC, et al. Monoclonal antibody therapy of human cancer: taking the HER2 protooncogene to the clinic. *J Clin Immunol* 1991;11:117.
559. Berns EMJJ, Foekens JA, van Staveren IL, et al. Oncogene amplification and prognosis in breast cancer: relationship with systemic treatment. *Gene* 1995;159:11.
560. Archer SG, Eliopoulos A, Spandidos D, et al. Expression of ras p2l, p53 and c-erbB-2 in advanced breast cancer and response to first line hormonal therapy. *Br J Cancer* 1995;72:1259.
561. Newby JC, Johnston SR, Smith IE, Dowsett M. Expression of epidermal growth factor receptor and c-erbB2 during the development of tamoxifen resistance in human breast cancer. *Clin Cancer Res* 1997;3:1643.
562. Norton L, Slamon D, Leyland-Jones B, et al. Overall survival advantage to simultaneous chemotherapy plus the humanized anti-HER2 monoclonal antibody herceptin in HER2-overexpressing metastatic breast cancer. *Proc Am Soc Clin Oncol* 1999;18:127a.

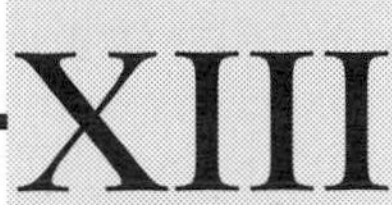

Diseases of the Breast, 2nd ed.,
edited by Jay R. Harris.
Lippincott Williams & Wilkins, Philadelphia © 2000.

New Breast Cancer Therapeutic Approaches

CHAPTER 49

Angiogenesis as a Diagnostic and Therapeutic Target

Stephen B. Fox and Adrian L. Harris

Angiogenesis is the generation of new vessels from the existing vasculature and is essential for tumor growth and metastasis.[1] It is a complex, dynamic process involving endothelial cell migration, proliferation, tube formation, and anastomosis, events controlled by angiogenic factors.[2] Endothelial cells may also vascularize tumors by intussusception. Although orchestrated by the neoplastic cell, successful angiogenesis involves coordination of other tumor elements, such as accessory cells and the extracellular matrix.

ANGIOGENIC SWITCH

To initiate the neovascularization, the tumor must switch to an angiogenic phenotype. This may be a result of genetic change but can also be a response to local stresses such as hypoxia (see Regulation by Hypoxia-Regulated Transcription Factors). Evidence, mostly from transgenic models with reproducible histologically distinct tumor stages, suggests that the acquisition of this phenotype occurs early in tumor development and that it is rate limiting with regard to tumor progression.[3,4] Evidence from human breast tissues supports this early transformation model,[5] with 30% of hyperplastic and 66% of neoplastic breast being angiogenic, compared with only 3% of normal breast.[6] Furthermore, angiogenesis induced by morphologically normal lobules from malignant breast is twice that derived from nonneoplastic breast,[7] an observation being clarified by genetic analysis.[8,9]

ANGIOGENIC STIMULATORS

The angiogenic promoters and inhibitors that underlie the initiation of the angiogenic program can originate from the neoplastic cell or from other tumor elements, or both. Thus,

S. B. Fox: Department of Anatomical Pathology, Christchurch Hospital, Christchurch, New Zealand
A. L. Harris: Imperial Cancer Research Fund, Medical Oncology Unit, Churchill Hospital, Headington, Oxford, United Kingdom

TABLE 1. *Tumor angiogenic promoters and inhibitors*

Angiogenic promotors
Vascular endothelial growth factor-A/B/C/D
Placenta growth factor
Angiopoietin 1, 2 and 4
Thymidine phosphorylase
Acidic and basic fibroblast growth factor (FGF)
CXC ELR chemokines (peptide motifs)
Pleiotrophin/midkine
Prostaglandins
Eicosanoids
Transforming growth factor (TGF) α and β
Platelet-derived growth factor
Scatter factor
Angiogenic inhibitors
Thrombospondin 1 and 2
Angiostatin
Endostatin
16-kd prolactin fragment
PEX (a metalloprotease domain)
CXC ELR-negative chemokines

the neoplastic cell can recruit inflammatory cells, such as macrophages[10] and mast cells,[11] both rich sources of angiogenic factors and cytokines, or release sequestered growth factors[12,13] or their receptors[14] from the extracellular matrix.[15] Endothelium itself can also secrete autocrine and paracrine factors that amplify these responses.[16] Platelets, also a rich source of angiogenic factors that are often elevated in malignancy, can be activated by tumor endothlieum or epithelium.

Many of the angiogenic factors that regulate physiologic angiogenesis have been shown to be important in tumors. Vascular endothelial growth factor (VEGF) has emerged as a central regulator not only in breast cancer angiogenesis but also in a wide spectrum of neoplasms (reviewed in ref. 17). VEGF is one of a family of polypeptides currently comprising VEGF-A, VEGF-B, VEGF-C, VEGF-D, and placenta growth factor, which exist in a number of isoforms. These bind variably to three high-affinity endothelial cell tyrosine kinase receptors, flt-1, KDR, and flt-4, the latter of which might be restricted to lymphatic endothelia[18]; an isoform-specific receptor, neuropilin-1, has also been identified.[19] Further modulation is achieved by heparin, which is not only required for binding of VEGF [and basic fibroblast growth factor (FGF)] but can also compete for receptor sites. This complex pathway enables the VEGFs to have numerous effects, including enhancing vascular permeability (thereby augmenting tumor stroma formation) and increasing endothelial cell proliferation and tube formation[20] through regulation of endothelial integrins. Integrins are necessary for vascular remodeling,[21,22] migration, and up-regulation of urokinase.

Whereas many angiogenic factors such as VEGF result in classic endothelial cell responses such as proliferation, others, including thymidine phosphorylase (TP)[23] and the angiopoietins,[24] are chemotactic for endothelium. TP catalyses the metabolism of thymidine to thymine and 2-deoxyribose phosphate, the active metabolite. Although its enzymatic action is essential for its angiogenic activity, the mechanism of action of the angiogenic sugar is unknown, with a receptor yet to be identified. Nevertheless, when it is transfected into MCF-7 breast cancer cells and implanted into nude mice, there is increased tumor growth but not vascular density,[25] in accordance with its migratory but nonmitogenic effect on endothelium. The enzyme is up-regulated 10- to 50-fold in a range of human tumor types including breast cancers (see Acquisition of an Angiogenic Phenotype and Angiogenesis as a Prognostic Marker).

The mechanism(s) by which the newly identified angiopoietin-Tie2 receptor pathway regulates angiogenesis has yet to be elucidated fully. Although angiopoietin-1 (but not angiopoietin-2) has been shown to be migratory for endothelium, targeted mutations suggest that this pathway has additional roles, including the recruitment and stabilization of the vessel wall.[26] In human breast tumors, up-regulation of the angiopoietin receptor, Tie2, has been demonstrated on endothelium, and in 1998 several members of the ephrin signaling pathway, in addition to its numerous neural patterning functions, were also shown to dictate the differentiation of vessels into arteries and veins, possibly by interplaying with the Tie2 pathway.[27] Although many angiogenic factors are known (Table 1), their role in human tumor angiogenesis has yet to be fully unraveled.

ANGIOGENESIS INHIBITORS AND TUMOR DORMANCY

It is now recognized that the balance of angiogenic stimulators and inhibitors determines the net angiogenic activity of a tumor. Thus, up-regulation of the previously mentioned positive factors or suppression of several naturally occurring inhibitors, or both, can result in angiogenesis. Inhibitors tend to be either large multimodular proteins such as thrombospondin-1[28] or SPARC,[29] which contain inhibitory domains, or, like angiostatin,[30] endostatin,[31] PEX,[32] 14-kd prolactin fragment,[33] laminin,[34] and fibronectin,[35] are proteolytically cleaved from larger noninhibitory molecules of varying classes during tumor angiogenesis. Although the generation of inhibitors such as angiostatin and thrombospondin-1 (which is higher in tumors than in normal breast tissues[36]) appears paradoxic, their appropriate spatial and temporal expression is necessary for successful neovascularization. Thus, to prevent excessive leakiness and hemorrhage around vessels, inhibitors such as the urokinase plasminogen activator inhibitor-1[37] might be required to terminate proteolysis, which, if excessive, would result in capillary autodestruction.

The suppression of angiogenesis by inhibitors may also be responsible for tumor dormancy, with high apoptosis due to hypoxia balancing cell proliferation. Loss of inhibitors may then result in angiogenesis and increased cell survival but without a concomitant increase in cell division[38]; angiostatin and endostatin seem particularly potent in this effect.

CAPILLARY RESPONSE TO ANGIOGENIC FACTORS

Angiogenic factors have numerous effects on the target capillary.[2,39] The stroma around the capillary is proteolytically degraded by plasmin[40] and the matrix metalloproteinases.[41] This enables endothelial cells to proliferate[42] and migrate to form sprouts, which fuse to form a new vascular network.[2] During this process, interactions with the surrounding stroma and adjacent cells via cell adhesion molecules of the notch,[43] selectin,[44] integrin,[45] and immunoglobulin families[46] play an important role not only in physical interactions but also in signal transduction.

ACQUISITION OF AN ANGIOGENIC PHENOTYPE

Common oncogenes and tumor-suppressor genes associated with neoplastic cell transformation also appear to play a central role in activating the angiogenic switch. *Ras*, raf, and src transformed cells exhibit a strong angiogenic phenotype,[47,48] partly through up-regulation of VEGF.[49–51] Wild-type p53 appears to have a powerful suppressor role, both reducing stimulators, such as VEGF,[51] and increasing inhibitors[52,53]; mutant p53 is reported to up-regulate VEGF expression.[54] The von Hippel–Lindau tumor-suppressor gene not only modulates growth factor levels[55] but also affects the hypoxic responsiveness of tumors (see Regulation by Hypoxia-Regulated Transcription Factors). This is convincing genetic evidence that oncogenes may dually regulate angiogenesis and that angiogenesis is a key process in tumor transformation. The transfection of retinoblastoma, another tumor-suppressor gene, is also associated with an increase in inhibitory activity.[56]

It is likely that different tumor types use different genetic mechanisms to elicit a blood supply. This is not surprising, because each vascular bed has unique characteristics and phenotypes that distinguish each organ. This may be reflected in the angiogenic phenotype of different tumors at different stages of development. Thus, TP is preferentially expressed in *in situ*[57] and T1 breast tumors[58] and in invasive rather than superficial transitional cell bladder carcinomas; conversely, VEGF expression is associated with superficial, not invasive, bladder tumors.[59] No matter which pathways are activated to elicit the tumor neovasculature, the resultant vessels are architecturally and structurally abnormal, features that are mirrored functionally by aberrant tumor blood flow,[60] vascular permeability, shunting, and hypoxic characteristics.

REGULATION BY HYPOXIA-REGULATED TRANSCRIPTION FACTORS

Once a tumor vasculature has been established, remodeling of vessels continues.[61] This is determined by a combination[62] of the molecular pathways activated at the particular stage of tumor development and by environmental factors, such as tumor site, blood flow, glucose, and hypoxia,[63,64] with some stimuli acting synergistically with oncogenes.[65] These changes result in amplification of the normal tissue response to stress.

A key pathway by which hypoxia enhances angiogenesis through factors such as VEGF and inducible nitric oxide synthase[66] is by activating the transcription factor hypoxia-inducible factor 1a [(HIF-1α) this pathway is also present in other hypoxia-responsive genes, including those involved in glycolysis (LDHa) and glucose transport (glut1)]. HIF-1α binds to the aryl-hydrocarbon nuclear translocator, which then binds a specific DNA hypoxia response element, resulting in increased messenger ribonucleic acid (mRNA) transcription[67] (for VEGF, a 3' adenylate-rich element also enhances mRNA stability; in tumors, there is also an additional mechanism to potentiate translation[68]). Hypoxia, via another hypoxia-inducible transcription factor [endothelial paraaminosalicylic acid domain protein-1 (EPAS)[69] also known as HIF-2a], selectively present in endothelium, can also control the response of the angiogenic factor angiopoietin via up-regulation of its receptor Tie2.[69] The importance of the HIF-1α pathway, even in fully transformed cells, has been demonstrated *in vivo*, with tumors of HIF-1α mutants growing significantly more slowly and with reduced angiogenesis. This shows that the hypoxic signaling is intact *in vivo* and suggests that its inhibition may be of therapeutic value (gene therapy can be targeted to hypoxic areas using constructs, with multiple hypoxia response elements regulating a therapeutic gene).

ANGIOGENESIS AS A PROGNOSTIC MARKER

Although the vascular nature of tumors has been recognized for many centuries, it is only in the last decade, with the advent of specific endothelial markers, that quantitation of tumor angiogenesis has been performed. Most studies have used variations of the method of Weidner et al.,[70] who demonstrated that mean tumor microvessel density in breast cancers highlighted by immmunohistochemistry from the most vascular field gave independent prognostic information. Since these initial reports in breast cancer, numerous studies of many tumor types have demonstrated that quantitation by microvessel as a measure of angiogenesis is a powerful prognostic tool.[71] It has also been suggested that angiogenesis quantitation might help predict the likelihood of *in situ* cancers' progressing[72,73] or a tumor's responding to treatment[74–78] and has been shown to correlate directly with the presence of bone marrow micrometastases.[79]

Not all studies, however, have been able to show that microvessel number gives independent prognostic information (Table 2). The discrepancies are likely due to differences in one or more of the following methodologic variables: (a) the selection of antibody to highlight the capillaries, (b) the vascular parameter quantified (i.e., microvessel number, area, perimeter), (c) the area of tumor to be assessed, (d) the measuring technique, (e) the experience of the observer, and (f) the statistical analysis used (reviewed in refs. 71 and 109). To overcome these problems and to help

TABLE 2. *Summary of published series reporting the relationship between quantitative tumor angiogenesis and prognosis in breast cancer*

Author (ref.)	Year	No.	Follow-up (mo)	Magnification	Field area (mm^2)	Antibody
For						
Weidner et al.[70]	1992	165	51	×200	0.7386	FVIII
Horak et al.[80]	1992	103	30	×400	0.196	CD31
Bosari et al.[81]	1992	120	108 min	×200	—	FVIII
Toi et al.[82]	1993	125	62	×200	—	FVIII/CD31
Visscher et al.[a83]	1993	58	—	×50	—	Collagen IV
Fox et al.[84]	1994	109 (N–)	25	×250	0.196	CD31
Lipponen et al.[85]	1994	173	**120**	×40	0.49	Collagen IV
Fregene et al.[86]	1994	316	**94**	×400	0.19	FVIII
Toi et al.[c87]	1995	328	—	×200	—	FVIII
Fox et al.[88]	1995	211	42	×250	0.196	CD31
Bevilacqua et al.[89]	1995	211 (N–)	78	×200	0.74	CD31
Ogawa et al.[90]	1995	155	82	×200	0.785	FVIII
Obermair et al.[91]	1995	230	**74**	×200	0.25	FVIII
Barbareschi et al.[a92]	1995	91	66.3	×200	0.74	CD31
Kohlberger et al.[a93]	1996	60	79	×200	0.25	FVIII
Simpson et al.[a94]	1996	178	71	×20	0.74	CD34
Heinmann et al.[95]	1996	167	184	×400	0.145	CD34
Karelia et al.[e96]	1997	51	>60	×200	0.74	FVIII
Acenero et al.[97]	1998	112	>60	×200	0.74	FVIII
Narita et al.[98]	1998	100	88	×200	0.25	FVIII
Gasparini et al.[99]	1998	531	76	×200	0.74	CD31
Kumar et al.[135]	1999	106	60	×400	—	CD105
Against						
Hall et al.[100]	1992	87	—	×400	0.126	FVIII
Van Hoef et al.[101]	1993	93 (N–)	151	×200	0.123	FVIII
Siitonen et al.[102]	1995	77 (N–)	84 max	×200	0.739	CD34/FVIII
Axelsson et al.[103]	1995	220	136	×250	0.37	FVIII
Goulding et al.[104]	1995	141	144 min	×250	0.37	CD31
Costello et al.[105]	1995	87	114 max	×200	0.22	FVIII
Morphopoulos et al.[d106]	1996	160	61.2	×200	0.785	FVIII
Kato et al.[107]	1997	109	168	×200	—	FVIII
Tan et al.[108]	1997	66	200	×200	—	FVIII
Clahsen et al.[77]	1998	346 (N–)	49	×250	0.384	CD31

The number of vessels/mm and follow-up times are median; bold indicates mean.
—, not stated in paper; CC, Chalkley count (a CC of 6 equates to 100 vessels/mm^2 at ×250); Max, maximal; min, minimal; N–/+, node negative/positive; NS, not significant; OS, overall survival; RFS, relapse-free survival.
[a]Image analysis.
[b]Per field area.
[c]An update of the 1993 paper.
[d]Lobular carcinomas.
[e]Advanced stage.
Modified from ref. 109.

determine the reliability of the technique, a discussion paper with a consensus methodology has been proposed.[110]

Nevertheless, because of the described limitations of methods used to exploit tumor angiogenesis as a prognostic marker, several groups have investigated other measures of angiogenesis. Thus, angiogenic factors,[111] proteases,[112] and cell adhesion molecules[113,114] in patient tumor[111] or fluid samples, or both,[115] have been measured to assess their potential use. Although some studies have demonstrated a significant relationship of microvessel number to VEGF[116,117] or TP, or both,[118] in breast cancer, not all studies have shown a relationship with survival.[58,116,119,120] Nevertheless, analyzing VEGF, acidic and basic FGF, transforming growth factor β1, placenta growth factor, TP, and pleiotrophin in series of pri-

Cut-off	No. of fields	Vessels/ mm²	Univariate analysis RFS	Univariate analysis OS	Multivariate analysis RFS	Multivariate analysis OS
<34; 34–67; 68–100; >100	1	76	p <.001	p <.001	p <.001	p <.001
Median	3	100	—	p = .04	—	—
Mean node and recurrence	3	84[b]	p <.004	p <.008	p <.028	—
100/150	3	99[b]	p <.01	—	p = .0226	—
—	All tumor	19	p = .001	—	—	—
Median	3	5.3 (CC)	p = .01	p = .028	p = .039	p = .019
40	6	86.3	NS	p = .0054	NS	p = .009
<25; 25–75; >75 centiles	1	—	p = .02	—	Significant in some models	—
100	3	84	p = .00001	—	p = .0000011	—
Thirds	3	5.7 (CC)	—	—	—	—
Continuous variable	3	—	p = .0001	p = .018	p = .0033	p = .044
Mean	3	67.5	p <.025	p <.01	p = .002	p = .001
40	1	51	p <.0001	—	p = .004	—
66	3	84	p = .002	—	—	—
Median	4	52.5	p = .024	—	—	—
Vessel area and no.	1	142	NS	p = .023	p = .002 (N+)	p = .002 (N+)
<15/field	3 (<10)	138	p = .018	—	p = .04	—
>34	3	34	p <.02	p <.001	—	—
Highest: >48	3	54	p <.05	—	p <.05	—
120	5	—	p <.0001	p <.0001	p <.05	p <.05
Continuous variable	3	80	p <.00001	p <.00001	p <.00001	p <.00001
Continuous/quartiles	4	3–7 (CC)	p <.0431	p <.0017	p <.001	p <.001
—	5	13	—	—	p >.05	—
<68; 68–100; >100	4	245	p = .92	p = .99	—	—
Highest/upper tertile	3	44/64	NS	—	—	—
Median	3	184 (N–/N+)	—	—	p = .65	p = .67
Median	3	64	NS	NS	NS	NS
Median	3	186	p = .6	p = .5	—	—
≤75: 76–100: >101–125: >126	3	139	NS	NS	—	
Highest/64	3	70	—	p = .03	—	p = .46
Median	3	50	—	p = .4	—	p = .12
Highest/75	3	—	p = .1	—	—	—

mary breast cancer, it was observed that although all tumors variably expressed each factor and that levels varied by at least tenfold, only VEGF related to relapse,[117] suggesting that these studies are valuable in identifying the most important factors involved in human cancer. Further, it might be possible to predict the likely response of patients to particular treatments; TP may be directly related to effectiveness of therapy, because this enzyme activates the prodrug capecitabine to 5-fluorouracil.

Several noninvasive imaging techniques, including thermography, color Doppler, and magnetic resonance, are also being assessed.[121] These should be considered research tools to investigate tumor biology rather than methods of selection of poor-risk patients. Because angiogenesis is a contin-

TABLE 3. *Antiangiogenesis agents in current trials and those likely to be tested once formulated*[a]

Agent	Description
Protease inhibitors[b]	
Marimastat	Synthetic
Neovastat(49)	Shark cartilage
Ag3340	Synthetic, more selective than marimastat
Bay 12-9566	Synthetic, more selective than marimastat CGS 27023A Less soft-tissue toxicity
PEX	Peptide fragment of metalloprotease blocks binding to integrins
Titanocene dichloride	Type IV collagenase inhibitor (MKT-4)
(Other targets include urokinase and its receptor)	
Methionine aminopeptidase 2 inhibitor[b]	
AGM1470 (TP470)	Synthetic fumagillin analogue
VEGF receptor antagonism	
Anti-VEGF antibody	VEGF neutralizing antibody
CGP41251	VEGF kinase and PKC inhibitor
SU-5416	flk-1 (KDR, VEGF-R2) inhibitor
(Most large companies have VEGF-R kinase inhibitors due to go into study)	
Heparinlike molecules	
Suramin(38)	
Pentosan polysulphate	Inhibits binding of angiogenic factors to:
Tecogulan DS-4152	Heparin
(GM 06, GM1474)	Heparin analogues blocking bFGF
Other signaling pathways	
CT-2584	Phospholipase-D modulation
Carboxyaminotriazole (CA1)	Inhibition of calcium channel signaling
Leflunomide SU-101	PDGF receptor kinase inhibitor
Bryostatin-1	PKC inhibitor
Cytokine pathways	
IL12	Induces interferon
Interferon α	Inhibits basic FGF production
Thalidomide	Inhibits TNF-α production
Platelet factor 4	Inhibits VEGF binding
Cytran IM	
Linomide	Inhibits macrophage migration
(COX-2 inhibitors are also being studied)	
Antiplatelet and anticoagulant	
Fragmin	Anticoagulant inhibits release of VEGF
Vascular targeting	
LM609	Antibody to $\alpha_v\beta_3$ integrin[133]
CM101	Streptococcal group B toxin inflames tumor endothelium[134]
Angiomab	Antibody to fibronectin splice variant in tumor endothelium
Vitaxin	$\alpha_v\beta_3$ integrin antagonist
TNT	Tumor necrosis therapy I^{131} targeted to a nuclear antigen leaking from necrotic areas
Peptide inhibitors from larger molecules	
Endostatin	From plasminogen
Angiostatin	From collagen type XVIII
(Neither is in trial due to formulation problems)	
Microtubule inhibitors	
Paclitaxel (Taxol)	Has some antivascular effects
2-Methoxyestradiol	Tubulin inhibitor
Others	
Razoxane	Topoisomerase II inhibitor
Desrazoxane	
Squalamine	Sodium exchange inhibitor aminosterol from shark cartilage
BioMedica p450	Hypoxia-regulated gene therapy
Captopril	Angiotensin-converting enzyme inhibitor
CS-994	Dinaline derivative, unknown mechanism

KDR, kinase inert domain–containing receptor; VEGF, vascular endothelial growth factor.
[a]Reviewed in ref. 132.
[b]The drugs most widely assessed.

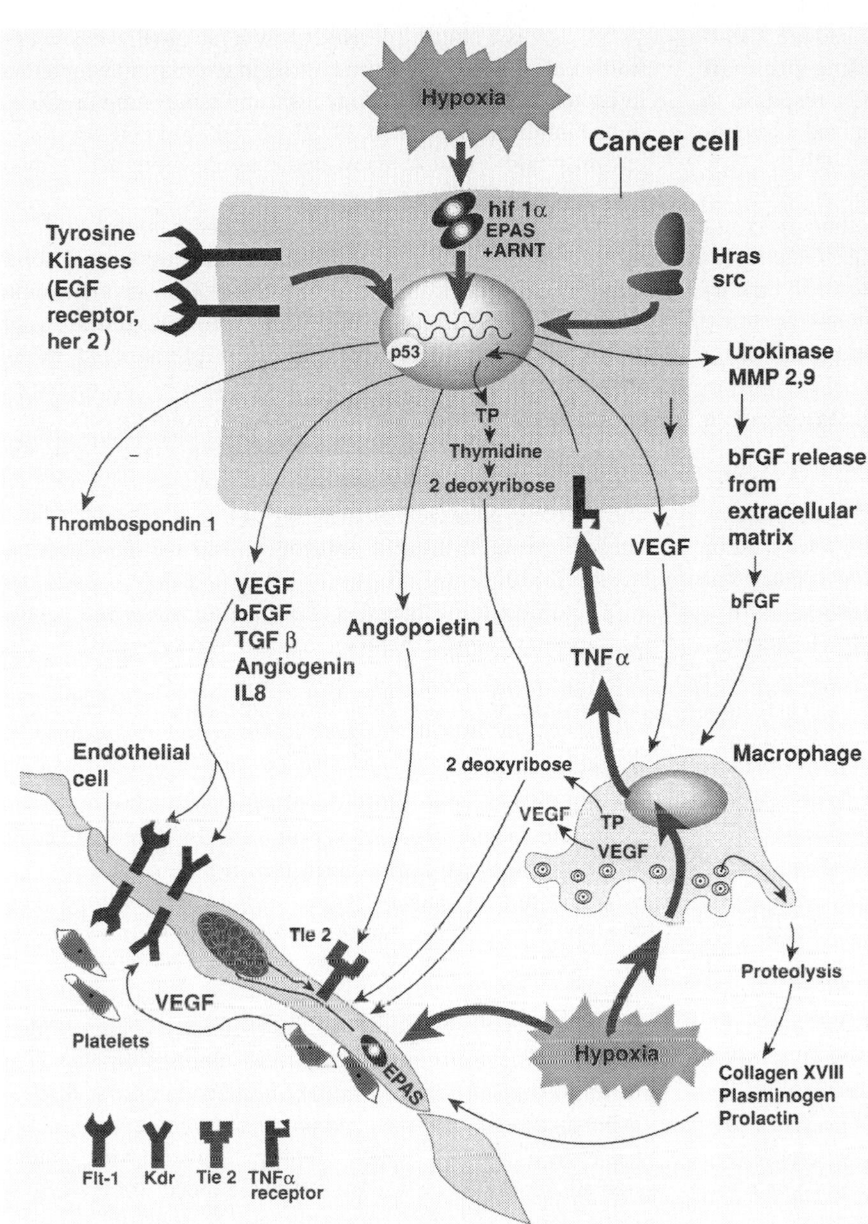

FIG. 1. Summary of angiogenic factors and cellular interactions in breast cancer. Hypoxia can activate gene transcription via hypoxia-inducible factor (HIF)-1α and endothelial paraaminosalicylic acid domain protein (EPAS)-1 (HIF-2α) transcription factors in tumor cells, macrophages, and endothelium, inducing vascular endothelial growth factor (VEGF). Platelets also release VEGF on aggregation. Various oncogenes activate angiogenesis and synergize with hypoxia. Macrophages are attracted by VEGF and can proteolytically release basic fibroblast growth factor from stroma, as well as producing VEGF and thymidine phosphorylase (TP). Inhibitory breakdown products are also made by macrophages. Tumor necrosis factor α (TNF-α) induced in macrophages by hypoxia is a potent stimulus to TP production in tumor cells. Tumor cells release a wide range of angiogenic factors and proteases. Hypoxia also up-regulates the Tie2 receptor on endothelial cells, and angiopoietin-1 binds the receptor, synergizing with VEGF. TP catalyses the breakdown of thymidine intracellularly to a diffusable angiogenic sugar, 2-deoxyribose. p53 induces the angiogenesis suppressor thrombospondin-1, and therefore mutations result in loss of the angiogenesis suppressor. Kdr, kinase inert domain–containing receptor; TGF-β, transforming growth factor β.

uous risk factor, patients should not be excluded from future antiangiogenic therapies.

ANGIOGENESIS AS A THERAPY TARGET

The clinical importance of tumor angiogenesis has raised hopes that specific therapies directed against the tumor vasculature will be developed and effective. The parallel advances in our understanding of the mechanisms of angiogenesis have produced a plethora of targets and drugs (Table 3, Fig. 1).

Two basic approaches should be distinguished: *vascular targeting*[122] and *antiangiogenesis*.[123] In the former, therapies are used to actively destroy the established tumor vasculature, often in a matter of hours, whereas antiangiogenesis aims to prevent the generation of new vessels. Vascular targeting, which affects both growing and quiescent endothelium, has been based on the selective delivery of potent toxins to tumor endothelium or has used the susceptibility of the tumor vasculature to apoptosis in response to cytokines—for example, tumor necrosis factor–alpha. Antiangiogenesis is just as effective, with significant inhibition of tumor growth being induced by interfering with as little as one component of the angiogenic process. Nevertheless, it is apparent that the two approaches are complementary and attack different aspects of the tumor vasculature. Because endothelial cells are the first to come into contact with any anticancer agent, major efforts to target the vasculature or exploit the hypoxic microenvironment using gene therapy have been pursued. Examples include the KDR (VEGF-R2)[124] promoter and hypoxia response elements regulated by HIF-1α or EPAS-1.[125]

In clinical trials, the drugs most widely studied are metalloprotease inhibitors. Marimastat is completing phase III randomized trials as maintenance therapy after response to chemotherapy is obtained. This is a randomized placebo-controlled design favored by many companies with this type of agent (Ag3340, Bay12-9566). The problem with this design is that potential synergy with chemotherapy is not detected, and at least one-half of the patients treated with chemotherapy may not enter the trial because of lack of response; still, there is no reason to suppose cross-resistance to the metalloprotease inhibitor, and synergy has been shown with concomitant medication.

The major side effects have been musculoskeletal, with frozen shoulder and Dupuytren's contractures typically occurring after 2 to 3 months. These effects are reversible, and lower doses of drugs are used as maintenance therapy. Inhibition of type I collagenase may be a contributory factor to the connective tissue problems, and newer analogues that do not block this enzyme have fewer side effects.

Neovastat is an extract of shark cartilage that has been investigated and prepared in a rational pharmacologic approach from frozen cartilage. It is completing well-organized trials in benign and malignant disease (e.g., psoriasis and rheumatoid arthritis).

The synthetic fumagillin analogue AGM1470 is being widely studied, but the optimum schedule needs to be determined because of its rapid metabolism, and it has yet to be properly assessed with adequate drug exposure. The target is methionine–amino peptidase II, but why this should give such specificity to endothelial inhibition is not known.

Genentech (San Francisco, California) is conducting trials of a blocking anti-VEGF antibody in solid tumors. It may be possible to assess effects *in vivo* by measuring vascular permeability with magnetic resonance imaging. This approach is being developed for several drugs that interfere with VEGF signaling, because VEGF is the major growth factor causing vascular permeability. Assessment of short-term changes in permeability can help complete phase I trials with a relevant end point to use the appropriate drug dosing in earlier-stage tumors.

Several companies are testing inhibitors of VEGF receptor kinases, usually the VEGF-R type 2 (KDR, flk-1). Oral (CGP41251) and intravenous (Sugen, San Francisco, California) compounds are in trial and may have advantages of tissue penetration compared to blocking antibody.

Heparinlike drugs have a broad spectrum of antiangiogenic activity, because most vascular growth factors have heparin-binding domains needed for optimum interactions with their receptors—for example, basic FGF and VEGF. Suramin has been studied for many years and has a very narrow therapeutic ratio; despite some activity in hormone-resistant prostatic cancer, it has not established a place in standard therapy. Other heparinlike molecules have proved inactive or toxic; for example, tecogulan caused coagulation abnormalities—a predictable side effect for heparinlike drugs.

Other signaling pathways besides angiogenic factors include calcium channels. CA1 (carboxyaminotriazole) is under study in combination with chemotherapy.

SU-101 is a platelet-derived growth factor (PDGF) receptor kinase inhibitor in phase III trial in gliomas, in which this receptor has a role in angiogenesis and tumor growth. Combined inhibitors that block PDGF, VEGF, and FGF receptors are in phase I trial (Sugen) and may be more active than those that inhibit one pathway.

Interferon alpha is the best-established cytokine with an antiangiogenic effect, but this is clearly modest in most solid tumors. A broader spectrum of activity than in melanoma and renal cancer would be expected if antiangiogenesis were the main mechanism. Thalidomide is pleiotrophic in its effects but does reduce cytokine production by macrophages and has produced response in a range of solid tumors.

Of the agents in trials, those with direct toxic effects on the vasculature, inducing endothelial inflammation or apoptosis, have produced the clearest evidence of tumor response. These include the $\alpha_v\beta_3$ integrin antagonists and the streptococcal toxin, CM101.

The different mechanisms of antiangiogenesis and vascular targeting suggest that they may be used synergistically in the future. For small micrometastases without established vasculature, inhibition of new vessel formation would be a prime target. On the other hand, larger metastases with established vessels would be more effectively managed by vascular destruction initially and then preventing regrowth of vessels. These approaches remain to be developed once the role of these drugs has been established.

Potent antiangiogenic agents, such as angiostatin[126] and endostatin,[31,127] cause tumor regression in animal models. However, although there are many agents in phase I and II, and a few in phase III, trials, regression appears to occur more rarely, with only occasional cases of regression being reported on antiangiogenic therapy.[128] This has important implications for the design of future clinical trials. Although stable disease is not a generally accepted end point in chemotherapy trials, it has been shown to be beneficial for patients receiving tamoxifen and thus may be a more justifiable model for antiangiogenic drugs. Therefore, in some clinical trials of advanced cancers, alternative end points, including tumor blood flow and vascular permeability, have been measured to detect a biological effect. Plasma, serum, or urine measurements of vascular growth factors, their receptors, or other endothelial markers may also be helpful but remain to be validated.[71] In the management of breast cancer, in which neoadjuvant or primary chemotherapy represents an important clinical situation, antiangiogenesis therapy can be assessed using serial biopsies and imaging. Vascular targeting is less of a problem in assessing response because of acute vessel destruction.

An important issue is to maximize and maintain responses—for example, using conventional and antiangiogenesis agents. Thus, akin to the development of hyperthermia in combination with radiotherapy, antiangiogenesis agents can be similarly assessed. Antiangiogenic agents have been shown to demonstrate synergy with radiotherapy and many conventional anticancer drugs,[129] including tamoxifen. Several studies are currently using groups randomized to chemotherapy versus chemotherapy and antiangiogenesis as a maintenance therapy versus placebo after maximal response to chemotherapy.

The duration of therapy is presently unclear, but many propose long-term maintenance. This should not be problematic, as with conventional chemotherapeutic agents, because endothelium, being genetically stable, should not become refractory to treatment. However, potential mechanisms of antiangiogenic resistance might arise. Indeed, studies of lung tumors have demonstrated a novel nonangiogenic mechanism of tumor growth, with tumor cells colonizing existing vessels without angiogenesis.[130]

Inhibition of angiogenesis is likely to be important in management of all stages of breast cancer but might be most effective in small primary tumors or metastases that are developing a blood supply. Integration with existing modalities using innovative trial designs may be needed to ensure optimal use of these agents, which may also be better in combination, thereby blocking multiple targets.[131] A detailed review of drugs in trial has been published by Zhang and Harris.[132]

WEB SITES FOR ANGIOGENESIS TRIALS

http://207.121.187.155/NCI_CANCER_TRIALS/zones/Pressinfo/Angio/, for information from NCI on antiangiogenesis and new clinical trials.

Visit ASCO OnLine (http://www.asco.org/), a searchable Web site, for trial results represented at 1998 (34th) meeting of American Society of Clinical Oncology (ASCO), which was held in May 1998. These ASCO proceedings can also be used as reference material, for example, anti-VEGF mAB, SU-5416, and vitaxin, etc.

Try http://www.angio.org/index2.htm or http://www.angio.org for the Angiogenesis Foundation.

REFERENCES

1. Folkman J. What is the evidence that tumours are angiogenesis dependent? *J Natl Cancer Inst* 1990;82:4.
2. Paweletz N, Knierim M. Tumor-related angiogenesis. *Crit Rev Oncol Hematol* 1989;9:197.
3. Hanahan D, Christofori G, Naik P, et al. Transgenic mouse models of tumor angiogenesis: the angiogenic switch, its molecular controls, and prospects for preclinical therapeutic models. *Eur J Cancer* 1996;32A:2386.
4. Skobe M, Rockwell P, Goldstein N, et al. Halting angiogenesis suppresses carcinoma cell invasion. *Nat Med* 1997;3:1222.
5. Heffelfinger S, Yassin R, Miller M, et al. Vascularity of proliferative breast disease and carcinoma in situ correlates with histological features. *Clin Cancer Res* 1996;2:1873.
6. Brem SS, Jensen HM, Gullino PM. Angiogenesis as a marker of preneoplastic lesions of the human breast. *Cancer* 1978;41:239.
7. Jensen HM, Chen I, De VM, et al. Angiogenesis induced by "normal" human breast tissue: a probable marker for precancer. *Science* 1982;218:293.
8. Deng G, Lu Y, Zlotnikov G, et al. Loss of heterozygosity in normal tissue adjacent to breast carcinomas. *Science* 1996;274:2057.
9. Larson PS, de las Morenas A, Cupples LA, et al. Genetically abnormal clones in histologically normal breast tissue. *Am J Pathol* 1998;52:159.
10. Polverini PJ. How the extracellular-matrix and macrophages contribute to angiogenesis-dependent diseases. *Eur J Cancer* 1996;32A:2430.
11. Ribatti D, Nico B, Vacca A, et al. Do mast cells help to induce angiogenesis in B-cell non-Hodgkin's lymphomas? *Br J Cancer* 1998;77:1900.
12. Vlodavsky I, Fuks Z, Ishai MR, et al. Extracellular matrix-resident basic fibroblast growth factor: implication for the control of angiogenesis. *J Cell Biochem* 1991;45:167.
13. Czubayko F, Liaudet-Coopman ED, Aigner A, et al. A secreted FGF-binding protein can serve as the angiogenic switch in human cancer. *Nat Med* 1997;3:1137.
14. Hanneken A, Maher P, Baird A. High affinity immunoreactive FGF receptors in the extracellular matrix of vascular endothelial cells—implications for the modulation of FGF-2. *J Cell Biol* 1995;128:1221.
15. Senger D. Molecular framework for angiogenesis. *Am J Pathol* 1996;149:1.
16. Franck-Lissbrant I, Haggstrom S, Damber JE, et al. Testosterone stimulates angiogenesis and vascular regrowth in the ventral prostate in castrated adult rats. *Endocrinology* 1998;139:451.
17. Nicosia RF. What is the role of vascular endothelial growth factor-related molecules in tumor angiogenesis? *Am J Pathol* 1998; 153:11.
18. Jeltsch M, Kaipainen A, Joukov V, et al. Hyperplasia of lymphatic vessels in VEGF-C transgenic mice. *Science* 1997;276:1423.
19. Soker S, Takashima S, Miao HQ, et al. Neuropilin-1 is expressed by endothelial and tumor cells as an isoform-specific receptor for vascular endothelial growth factor. *Cell* 1998;92:735.
20. Pepper MS, Ferrara N, Orci L, Montesano R. Potent synergism between vascular endothelial growth factor and basic fibroblast growth factor in the induction of angiogenesis in vitro. *Biochem Biophys Res Commun* 1992;189:824.
21. Friedlander M, Brooks PC, Shaffer RW, et al. Definition of two angiogenic pathways by distinct alpha v integrins. *Science* 1995;270:1500.
22. Koolwijk P, van Erck M, de Vree W, et al. Cooperative effect of TNF-α, βFGF, and VEGF on the formation of tubular structures of human microvascular endothelial cells in a fibrin matrix, role of urokinase activity. *J Cell Biol* 1996;132:1177.
23. Haraguchi M, Kazutaka M, Uemura K, et al. Angiogenic activity of enzymes. *Nature* 1994;168:198.
24. Witzenbichler B, Maisonpierre PC, Jones P, et al. Chemotactic properties of angiopoietin-1 and -2, ligands for the endothelial-specific receptor tyrosine kinase Tie2. *J Biol Chem* 1998;273:18514.
25. Moghaddam A, Zhang HT, Fan TP, et al. Thymidine phosphorylase is angiogenic and promotes tumor growth. *Proc Natl Acad Sci U S A* 1995;92:998.
26. Hanahan D. Signalling vascular morphogenesis and maintenance. *Science* 1997;277:48.
27. Peters K, Coogan A, Berry D, et al. Expression of Tie2/Tek in breast tumour vasculature provides a new marker for evaluation of tumour angiogenesis. *Br J Cancer* 1998;77:51.
28. Tolsma SS, Volpert OV, Good DJ, Frazier WA, Polverini PJ, Bouck N. Peptides derived from 2 separate domains of the matrix protein thrombospondin-1 have anti-angiogenic activity. *J Cell Biol* 1993;122:497.
29. Sage EH. Terms of attachment: SPARC and tumorigenesis. *Nat Med* 1997;3:144.
30. O'Reilly MS, Holmgren L, Shing Y, et al. Angiostatin: a novel angiogenesis inhibitor that mediates the suppression of metastases by a Lewis lung carcinoma. *Cell* 1994;79:315.
31. O'Reilly MS, Boehm T, Shing Y, et al. Endostatin: an endogenous inhibitor of angiogenesis and tumor growth. *Cell* 1997;88:277.
32. Brooks PC, Silletti S, von Schalscha TL, Friedlander M, Cheresh DA. Disruption of angiogenesis by PEX, a noncatalytic metalloproteinase fragment with integrin binding activity. *Cell* 1998;92:391.
33. Ferrara N, Clapp C, Weiner R. The 16K fragment of prolactin specifically inhibits basal or fibroblast growth factor stimulated growth of capillary endothelial cells. *Endocrinology* 1991;129:896.
34. Sakamoto N, Iwahana M, Tanaka NG, et al. Inhibition of angiogenesis and tumor growth by a synthetic laminin peptide, CDPGYIGSR-NH2. *Cancer Res* 1991;51:903.
35. Grant MB, Caballero S, Bush DM, et al. Fibronectin fragments modulate human retinal capillary cell proliferation and migration. *Diabetes* 1998;47:1335.
36. Bertin N, Clezardin P, Kubiak R, et al. Thrombospondin-1 and -2 messenger RNA expression in normal, benign, and neoplastic human breast tissues: correlation with prognostic factors, tumor angiogenesis, and fibroblastic desmoplasia. *Cancer Res* 1997;57:396.
37. Bajou K, Noel A, Gerard RD, et al. Absence of host plasminogen activator inhibitor 1 prevents cancer invasion and vascularization. *Nat Med* 1998;4:923.
38. Holmgren L, O'Reilly MS, Folkman J. Dormancy of micrometastases: balanced proliferation and apoptosis in the presence of angiogenesis suppression. *Nat Med* 1995;1:149.

39. Warren B, Greenblatt M, Kommineni V. Tumor angiogenesis: ultrastructure of endothelial cells in mitosis. *Br J Exp Pathol* 1972;53:216.
40. Pepper M, Montesano R. Proteolytic balance and capillary morphogenesis. *Cell Diff Devel* 1990;32:319.
41. Fisher C, Gilbertson BS, Powers EA, et al. Interstitial collagenase is required for angiogenesis in vitro. *Dev Biol* 1994;162:499.
42. Fox SB, Gatter K, Bicknell R, et al. Relationship of endothelial cell proliferation to tumor vascularity in human breast cancer. *Cancer Res* 1993;53:9161.
43. Zimrin AB, Pepper MS, McMahon GA, et al. An antisense oligonucleotide to the notch ligand jagged enhances fibroblast growth factor-induced angiogenesis in vitro. *J Biol Chem* 1996;271:32499.
44. Bischoff J. Cell adhesion and angiogenesis. *J Clin Invest* 1997; 100:S37.
45. Brooks PC. Role of integrins in angiogenesis. *Eur J Cancer* 1996;32A:P:2423.
46. DeLisser HM, Christofidou-Solomidou M, Strieter RM, et al. Involvement of endothelial PECAM-1/CD31 in angiogenesis. *Am J Pathol* 1997;151:671.
47. Kallinowski F, Wilkerson R, Moore R, et al. Vascularity, perfusion rate and local tissue oxygenation of tumors derived from ras-transformed fibroblasts. *Int J Cancer* 1991;48:121.
48. Grugel S, Finkenzeller G, Weindel K, et al. Both v-Ha-Ras and v-Raf stimulate expression of the vascular endothelial growth factor in NIH 3T3 cells. *J Biol Chem* 1995;270:25915.
49. Arbiser JL, Moses MA, Fernandez CA, et al. Oncogenic H-ras stimulates tumor angiogenesis by two distinct pathways. *Proc Natl Acad Sci U S A* 1997;94:861.
50. Okada F, Rak JW, Croix BS, et al. Impact of oncogenes in tumor angiogenesis: mutant K-ras up-regulation of vascular endothelial growth factor/vascular permeability factor is necessary, but not sufficient for tumorigenicity of human colorectal carcinoma cells. *Proc Natl Acad Sci U S A* 1998;95:3609.
51. Mukhopadhyay D, Tsiokas L, Sukhatme VP. Wild-type p53 and v-Src exert opposing influences on human vascular endothelial growth factor gene expression. *Cancer Res* 1995;55:6161.
52. Dameron KM, Volpert OV, Tainsky MA, et al. The p53 tumor suppressor gene inhibits angiogenesis by stimulating the production of thrombospondin. *Cold Spring Harb Symp Quant Biol* 1994;59:483.
53. Van Meir EG, Polverini PJ, Chazin VR, et al. Release of an inhibitor of angiogenesis upon induction of wild type p53 expression in glioblastoma cells. *Nat Genet* 1994;8:171.
54. Kieser A, Weich HA, Brandner G. Mutant p53 potentiates protein kinase C induction of vascular endothelial growth factor expression. *Oncogene* 1994;9:963.
55. Knebelmann B, Ananth S, Cohen HT, et al. Transforming growth factor alpha is a target for the von Hippel-Lindau tumor suppressor. *Cancer Res* 1998;58:226.
56. Dawson D, Tolsma S, Volpert O, et al. Retinoblastoma gene expression alters angiogenic phenotype. *Proc Am Assoc Cancer Res* 1995;63:88(abst).
57. Engels K, Fox SB, Whitehouse RM, et al. Up-regulation of thymidine phosphorylase expression is associated with a discrete pattern of angiogenesis in ductal carcinomas in situ of the breast. *J Pathol* 1997;182:414.
58. Fox SB, Westwood M, Moghaddam A, et al. The angiogenic factor platelet-derived endothelial cell growth factor/thymidine phosphorylase is up-regulated in breast cancer epithelium and endothelium. *Br J Cancer* 1996;73:275.
59. O'Brien T, Fox SB, Dickinson A, et al. Expression of the angiogenic factor thymidine phosphorylase/platelet derived endothelial cell growth factor in primary bladder cancers. *Cancer Res* 1996;56:4799.
60. Vaupel P, Kallinowski F, Okunieff P. Blood flow, oxygen and nutrient supply, and metabolic microenvironment of human tumors: a review. *Cancer Res* 1989;49:6449.
61. Fox SB, Kakolyris S, Taylor M, et al. Vascular remodelling in breast cancer angiogenesis assessed by LH39 basement membrane antigen and CD31. *Proc Am Assoc Cancer Res* 1997;38:54(abst).
62. Levy AP, Levy NS, Iliopoulos O, et al. Regulation of vascular endothelial growth factor by hypoxia and its modulation by the von Hippel-Lindau tumor suppressor gene. *Kidney Int* 1997;51:575.
63. Shweiki D, Neeman M, Itin A, et al. Induction of vascular endothelial growth factor expression by hypoxia and by glucose deficiency in multicell spheroids: implications for tumor angiogenesis. *Proc Natl Acad Sci U S A* 1995;92:768.
64. Carmeliet P, Dor Y, Herbert JM, et al. Role of HIF-1alpha in hypoxia-mediated apoptosis, cell proliferation and tumour angiogenesis. *Nature* 1998;394:485.
65. Mazure NM, Chen EY, Yeh P, et al. Oncogenic transformation and hypoxia synergistically act to modulate vascular endothelial growth factor expression. *Cancer Res* 1996;56:3436.
66. Gallo O, Masini E, Morbidelli L, et al. Role of nitric oxide in angiogenesis and tumor progression in head and neck cancer. *J Natl Cancer Inst* 1998;90:587.
67. Damert A, Ikeda E, Risau W. Activator-protein-1 binding potentiates the hypoxia-inducible factor-1-mediated hypoxia-induced transcriptional activation of vascular-endothelial growth factor expression in C6 glioma cells. *Biochem J* 1997;327:419.
68. Scott PA, Smith K, Poulsom R, et al. Differential expression of vascular endothelial growth factor mRNA vs protein isoform expression in human breast cancer and relationship to eIF-4E. *Br J Cancer* 1998;77:2120.
69. Tian H, McKnight SL, Russell DW. Endothelial PAS domain protein 1 (EPAS1), a transcription factor selectively expressed in endothelial cells. *Genes Dev* 1997;11:72.
70. Weidner N, Folkman J, Pozza F, et al. Tumor angiogenesis: a new significant and independent prognostic indicator in early-stage breast carcinoma. *J Natl Cancer Inst* 1992;84:1875.
71. Fox SB, Harris AL. Markers of tumor angiogenesis: clinical applications in prognosis and anti-angiogenic therapy. *Invest New Drugs* 1997;15:15.
72. Guidi A, Fischer L, Harris J, Schnitt S. Microvessel density and distribution in ductal carcinoma in situ of the breast. *J Natl Cancer Inst* 1994;86:614.
73. Engels K, Fox SB, Whitehouse RM, et al. Distinct angiogenic patterns are associated with high-grade in situ ductal carcinomas of the breast. *J Pathol* 1997;181:207.
74. Protopapa E, Delides GS, Revesz L. Vascular density and the response of breast carcinomas to mastectomy and adjuvant chemotherapy. *Eur J Cancer* 1993;29A:1141.
75. Paulsen T, Aas T, Borresen AL, et al. Angiogenesis does not predict clinical response to doxorubicin monotherapy in patients with locally advanced breast cancer [letter]. *Int J Cancer* 1997;74:138.
76. Gasparini G, Fox SB, Verderio P, et al. Angiogenesis adds information to estrogen receptor status in predicting the efficacy of adjuvant tamoxifen in node-positive breast cancer patients. *Clin Cancer Res* 1996;2:1191.
77. Clahsen PC, van de Velde CJ, Duval C, et al. p53 protein accumulation and response to adjuvant chemotherapy in premenopausal women with node-negative early breast cancer. *J Clin Oncol* 1998;16:470.
78. Jacquemier JD, Penault-Llorca FM, Bertucci F, et al. Angiogenesis as a prognostic marker in breast carcinoma with conventional adjuvant chemotherapy: a multiparametric and immunohistochemical analysis. *J Pathol* 1998;184:130.
79. Fox SB, Leek RD, Bliss J, et al. Association of tumor angiogenesis with bone marrow micrometastases in breast cancer patients. *J Natl Cancer Inst* 1997;89:1044.
80. Horak ER, Leek R, Klenk N, et al. Angiogenesis, assessed by platelet/endothelial cell adhesion molecule antibodies, as indicator of node metastases and survival in breast cancer. *Lancet* 1992;340:1120.
81. Bosari S, Lee AK, DeLellis RA, et al. Microvessel quantitation and prognosis in invasive breast carcinoma. *Hum Pathol* 1992;23:755.
82. Toi M, Kashitani J, Tominaga T. Tumor angiogenesis is an independent prognostic indicator in primary breast carcinoma. *Int J Cancer* 1993;55:371.
83. Visscher D, Smilanetz S, Drozdowicz S, Wykes S. Prognostic significance of image morphometric microvessel enumeration in breast carcinoma. *Anal Quant Cytol* 1993;15:88.
84. Fox SB, Leek R, Smith K, et al. Tumor angiogenesis in node negative breast carcinomas—relationship to epidermal growth factor receptor and survival. *Breast Cancer Res Treat* 1994;29:109.
85. Lipponen P, Ji H, Aaltomaa S, Syrjanen K. Tumour vascularity and basement membrane structure in breast cancer as related to tumour histology and prognosis. *J Cancer Res Clin Oncol* 1994;120:645.
86. Fregene TA, Khanuja PS, Gimotty PA, et al. The relationship of microvessel counts to tumor size, estrogen receptor status, lymph node metastasis, and disease-free survival in patients with stage I and II breast cancer. *Int J Oncol* 1994;5:1437.
87. Toi M, Inada K, Suzuki H, et al. Tumor angiogenesis in breast cancer: its importance as a prognostic indicator and the association with vas-

cular endothelial growth factor expression. *Breast Cancer Res Treat* 1995;36:193.
88. Fox SB, Leek RD, Weekes MP, et al. Quantitation and prognostic value of breast cancer angiogenesis: comparison of microvessel density, Chalkley count and computer image analysis. *J Pathol* 1995;177:275.
89. Bevilacqua P, Barbareschi M, Verderio P, et al. Prognostic value of intratumoral microvessel density, a measure of tumor angiogenesis, in node-negative breast carcinoma: results of a multiparametric study. *Breast Cancer Res Treat* 1995;36:205.
90. Ogawa Y, Chung Y, Nakata B, et al. Microvessel quantitation in invasive breast cancer by staining for factor VIII-related antigen. *Br J Cancer* 1995;71:1297.
91. Obermair A, Kurz C, Czerwenka K, et al. Microvessel density and vessel invasion in lymph-node-negative breast cancer: effect on recurrence-free survival. *Int J Cancer* 1995;62:126.
92. Barbareschi M, Weidner N, Gasparini G, et al. Microvessel quantitation in breast carcinomas. *Appl Immunochem* 1995;3:75.
93. Kohlberger P, Obermair Sliutz G, Heinzl H, et al. Quantitative immunohistochemistry of factor VIII-related antigen in breast carcinoma. *Am J Clin Pathol* 1996;105:705.
94. Simpson JF, Ahn C, Battifora H, et al. Endothelial area as a prognostic indicator for invasive breast carcinoma. *Cancer* 1996;77:2077.
95. Heinmann R, Ferguson D, Powers C, Recant W, Weichselbaum R, Hellman S. Angiogenesis as a predictor of long term survival for patients with node-negative breast cancer. *J Natl Cancer Inst* 1996;88:1764.
96. Karelia NH, Patel DD, Balar DB, et al. Prognostic significance of tumor angiogenesis in advanced breast carcinoma: an Indian experience. *Neoplasma* 1997;44:163.
97. Acenero MJ, Gallego MG, Ballesteros PA, et al. Vascular density as a prognostic indicator for invasive ductal breast carcinoma. *Virchows Arch* 1998;432:113.
98. Narita M, Nakao K, Ogino N, et al. Independent prognostic factors in breast cancer patients. *Am J Surg* 1998;175:73.
99. Gasparini G, Toi M, Verderio P, et al. Prognostic significance of p53, angiogenesis, and other conventional features in operable breast cancer: subanalysis in node-positive and node-negative patients. *Int J Oncol* 1998;12:1117.
100. Hall NR, Fish DE, Hunt N, et al. Is the relationship between angiogenesis and metastasis in breast cancer real? *Surg Oncol* 1992;1:223.
101. Van Hoef ME, Knox WF, Dhesi SS, et al. Assessment of tumour vascularity as a prognostic factor in lymph node negative invasive breast cancer. *Eur J Cancer* 1993;29A:1141.
102. Siitonen S, Haapasalo H, Rantala I, Helin H, et al. Comparison of different immunohistochemical methods in the assessment of angiogenesis: lack of prognostic value in a group of 77 selected node-negative breast carcinomas. *Mod Pathol* 1995;8:745.
103. Axelsson K, Ljung BM, Moore DH II, et al. Tumor angiogenesis as a prognostic assay for invasive ductal breast carcinoma. *J Natl Cancer Inst* 1995;87:997.
104. Goulding H, Abdul RN, Robertson JF, et al. Assessment of angiogenesis in breast carcinoma: an important factor in prognosis? *Hum Pathol* 1995;26:1196.
105. Costello P, McCann A, Carney DN, et al. Prognostic significance of microvessel density in lymph node negative breast carcinoma. *Hum Pathol* 1995;26:1181.
106. Morphopoulos G, Pearson M, Ryder WD, et al. Tumour angiogenesis as a prognostic marker in infiltrating lobular carcinoma of the breast. *J Pathol* 1996;180:44.
107. Kato T, Kimura T, Miyakawa R, et al. Clinicopathologic study of angiogenesis in Japanese patients with breast cancer. *World J Surg* 1997;21:49.
108. Tan P, Cady B, Wanner M, et al. The cell cycle inhibitor p27 is an independent prognostic marker in small (T1a,b) invasive breast carcinomas. *Cancer Res* 1997;57:1259.
109. Fox SB. Tumour angiogenesis and prognosis. *Histopathology* 1997;30:294.
110. Vermeulen PB, Gasparini G, Fox SB, et al. Quantification of angiogenesis in solid human tumors: an international consensus on the methodology and criteria of evaluation. *Eur J Cancer* 1996;32A:2474.
111. Toi M, Taniguchi T, Yamamoto Y, et al. Clinical-significance of the determination of angiogenic factors. *Eur J Cancer* 1996;32A:2513.
112. Fox SB, Stuart N, Smith K, et al. High levels of uPA and PAI-1 are associated with highly angiogenic breast carcinomas. *J Pathol* 1993;170 [Suppl]:388A(abst).
113. Fox SB, Turner GD, Gatter KC, et al. The increased expression of adhesion molecules ICAM-3, E- and P-selectins on breast cancer endothelium. *J Pathol* 1995;177:369.
114. Schadendorf D, Heidel J, Gawlik C, et al. Association with clinical outcome of expression of VLA-4 in primary cutaneous malignant melanoma as well as P-selectin and E-selectin on intratumoral vessels. *J Natl Cancer Inst* 1995;87:366.
115. Nguyen M. Angiogenic factors as tumor markers. *Invest New Drugs* 1997;15:29.
116. Toi M, Kondo S, Suzuki H, et al. Quantitative analysis of vascular endothelial growth factor in primary breast cancer. *Cancer* 1996; 77:1101.
117. Relf M, LeJeune S, Scott PA, et al. Expression of the angiogenic factors vascular endothelial cell growth factor, acidic and basic fibroblast growth factor, transforming growth factor beta-1, platelet-derived endothelial cell growth factor, placenta growth factor, and pleiotrophin in human primary breast cancer and its relation to angiogenesis. *Cancer Res* 1997;57:963.
118. Toi M, Hoshina S, Taniguchi T, et al. Expression of platelet derived endothelial cell growth factor/thymidine phosphorylase in human breast cancer. *Int J Cancer* 1995;64:79.
119. Gasparini G, Toi M, Gion M, et al. Prognostic-significance of vascular endothelial growth factor protein in node-negative breast-carcinoma. *J Natl Cancer Inst* 1997;89:139.
120. Linderholm B, Tavelin B, Grankvist K, et al. Vascular endothelial growth factor is of high prognostic value in node-negative breast carcinoma. *J Clin Oncol* 1998;16:3121.
121. Passe TJ, Bluemke DA, Siegelman SS. Tumor angiogenesis: tutorial on implications for imaging. *Radiology* 1997;203:593.
122. Huang X, Molema G, King S, et al. Tumor infarction in mice by antibody-directed targeting of tissue factor to tumor vasculature. *Science* 1997;275:547.
123. Brem S. Angiogenesis antagonists: current clinical trials. *Angiogenesis* 1998;2:9.
124. Jaggar RT, Chan HY, Harris AL, et al. Endothelial cell-specific expression of tumor necrosis factor alpha from the KDR or E-selectin promoters following retroviral delivery. *Hum Gene Ther* 1997;8:2239.
125. Dachs GU, Patterson AV, Firth JD, et al. Targeting gene expression to hypoxic tumor cells. *Nat Med* 1997;3:515.
126. O'Reilly MS, Holmgren L, Chen C, et al. Angiostatin induces and sustains dormancy of human primary tumors in mice. *Nat Med* 1996;2:689.
127. Boehm T, Folkman J, Browder T, et al. Antiangiogenic therapy of experimental cancer does not induce acquired drug resistance. *Nature* 1997;390:404.
128. Kudelka AP, Verschraegen CF, Loyer E. Complete remission of metastatic cervical cancer with the angiogenesis inhibitor TNP-470 [letter]. *N Engl J Med* 1998;338:991.
129. Herbst RS, Takeuchi H, Teicher BA. Paclitaxel/carboplatin administration along with antiangiogenic therapy in non-small-cell lung and breast carcinoma models. *Cancer Chemother Pharmacol* 1998;41: 497.
130. Pezzella F, Pastorin OU, Tagliabue E, et al. Non-small-cell lung carcinoma tumor growth without morphological evidence of neo-angiogenesis. *Am J Pathol* 1996;151:1417.
131. Nelson NJ. Inhibitors of angiogenesis enter phase III testing. *J Natl Cancer Inst* 1998;90:960.
132. Zhang HT, Harris AL. Anti-angiogenic therapies in cancer clinical trials. *Exp Opin Invest Drugs* 1998;7:1629.
133. Sipkins DA, Cheresh DA, Kazemi MR, et al. Detection of tumor angiogenesis in vivo by alpha$_V$beta$_3$-targeted magnetic resonance imaging. *Nat Med* 1998;4:623.
134. DeVore RF, Hellerqvist CG, Wakefield GB, et al. Phase I study of the antineovascularization drug CM101. *Clin Cancer Res* 1997;3:365.
135. Kumar S, Ghellal A, Li C, et al. Breast carcinoma: vascular density determined using CD105 antibody correlates with tumor prognosis. *Cancer Res* 1999;59:856.

CHAPTER 50

Diseases of the Breast, 2nd ed.,
edited by Jay R. Harris.
Lippincott Williams & Wilkins, Philadelphia © 2000.

Immunology and Immunotherapy

Martin A. Cheever and Mary L. Disis

Breast cancer expresses multiple antigens that can be recognized by the human immune system. These antigens allow the immune system to discriminate breast cancer cells from normal breast epithelial cells. Some patients with breast cancer have an ongoing immune response to breast cancer antigens. The ongoing immune response may have the potential to destroy breast cancer cells. Breast cancer–specific immunotherapies, including vaccines and antibodies, are in clinical development and in human clinical trials. The enthusiasm for breast cancer–specific immunotherapy is a reflection of the current state of immunologic science. At the molecular level, T-cell and antibody interactions with antigens are understood well enough to allow intelligent engineering of specific immunotherapies. The potential for rational development and testing of specific immunotherapies in breast cancer is immense.

IMMUNE SYSTEM AND BREAST CANCER

Breast cancer antigens are derived from aberrant proteins expressed by breast cancer–related genes. The progression of breast cancer from *in situ* to invasive to metastatic forms is the result of progressive changes in the genes of cancer cells that facilitate increased growth, invasion, and metastasis. Many of the altered cancer-related genes code for synthesis of proteins that have altered primary amino acid sequence, increased levels of synthesis, or other modifications, such as changes in shape and associated lipids and carbohydrates. Any protein, lipid, or carbohydrate changed in this way can potentially function as a target for immunotherapy.

The great theoretical advantage of immunotherapy is specificity. The specificity of immunity is engendered by antibodies and T cells. Antibodies are produced by B cells in response to immune stimulation by specific antigens. An antigen is defined simply as any substance that reacts with an antibody or T-cell receptor. Classically, antibodies are thought to be most adept at binding to and clearing bacteria and viruses from extracellular fluids. Antibodies can also mediate lysis of cancer cells by several distinct mechanisms (Fig. 1). Formation of antigen-antibody immune complexes can activate the complement cascade (see Fig. 1A). The terminal cytolytic pathway of the complement cascade can result in lysis and destruction of the antibody-coated targets. The activated complement components also can profoundly amplify inflammation and phagocytosis. Antibody-coated target cancer cells have an antibody Fc portion free to bind to the Fc receptor on cytolytic effector cells, such as macrophages and NK cells. Macrophages and NK cells can kill cancer cells, especially when activated and held in close apposition to cancer cells by antibodies bridging from the cancer cell to the killer cells via interactions between the Fc portion of antibodies and Fc receptors on killer cells (see Fig. 1B).

The inhibition of cancer cell growth by antibodies binding to growth factor receptors at the surface of cancer cells has been recognized as an effective therapeutic use of antibodies. The importance of growth factor receptors for breast cancer is well established. Growth factor receptors, such as epidermal growth factor receptor and HER-2/neu, include an extracellular domain that receives a growth signal and an intracellular domain that conveys that signal to the cell nucleus for cell division. Antibodies specific for a particular growth factor receptor may bind to the extracellular domain and mediate an antitumor effect by altering the ability of the growth factor receptor to function (see Fig. 1C).

The T-cell arm of the immune system is critically important for the generation of robust immunity against an antigen. Antibodies are most adept against cell surface molecules, including growth factor receptors. By marked contrast, T cells are adept against both cell surface and intracellular molecules. Comprehension and appreciation of T-cell responses to breast cancer antigens requires the understanding that T cells primarily recognize peptide fragments of antigens bound in the cleft of major histocompatibility complex (MHC) molecules. The peptides recognized by T cells are small, usually 9 to 12 amino acids in length. As a consequence, T cells recognize primary protein amino acid structure and are quite adept at recognizing small

M. A. Cheever: Department of Medicine, University of Washington School of Medicine, Seattle, Washington; Corixa Corporation, Seattle, Washington

M. L. Disis: Department of Medicine, Division of Oncology, University of Washington School of Medicine, Seattle, Washington

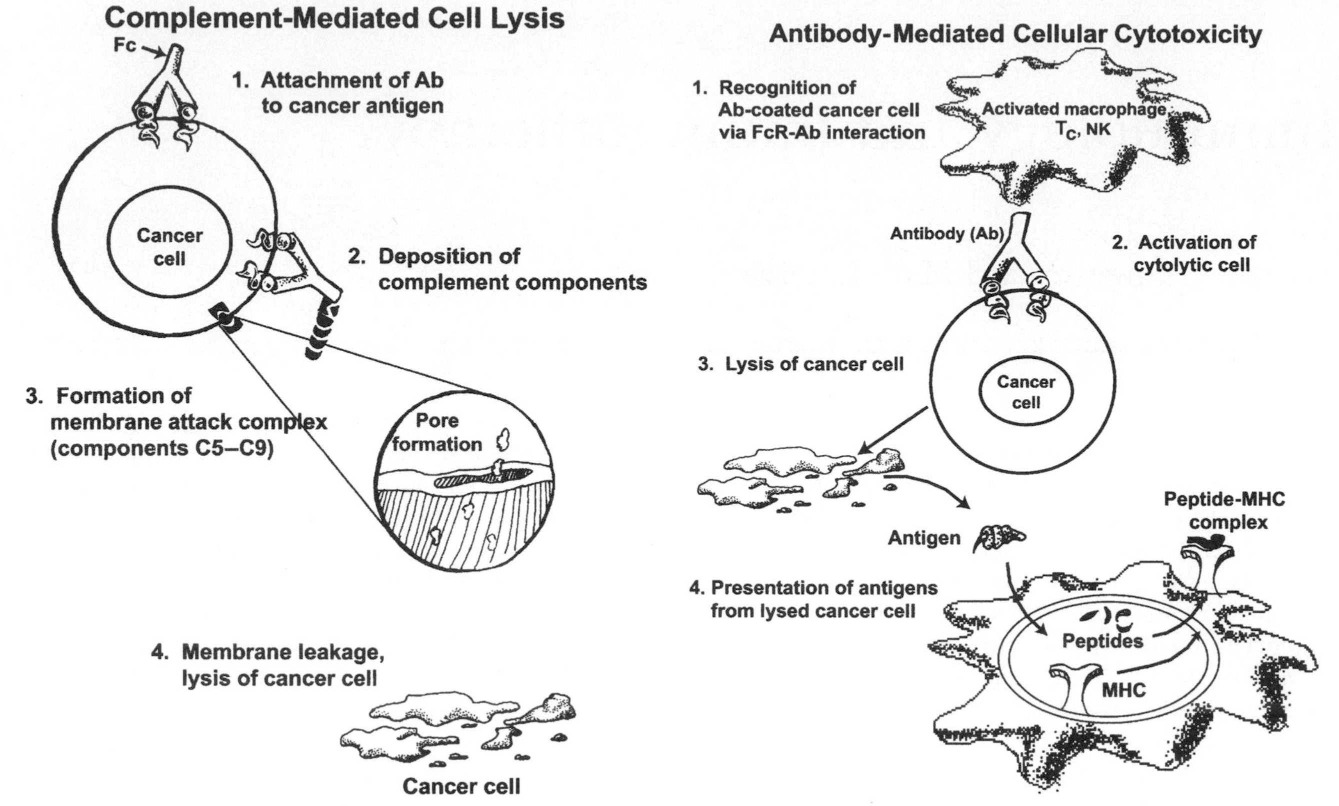

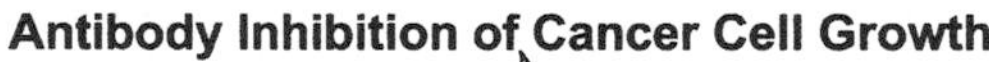

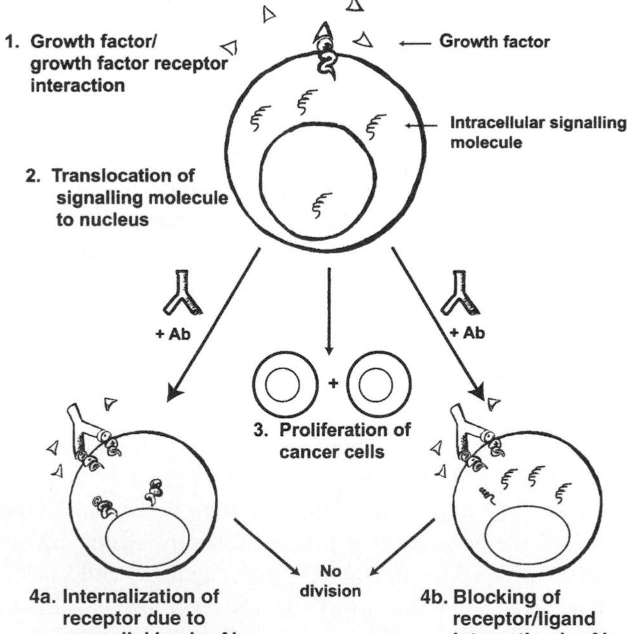

FIG. 1. Antibody (Ab) responses can mediate anticancer effects via multiple mechanisms. **A:** In complement-mediated cell lysis, Ab binds to a cancer antigen present on the cell surface of a breast cancer cell. Attachment of the Ab to the cell surface breast cancer antigen results in deposition of complement components and activation of the complement cascade, a series of enzymatic proteins, resulting in pore formation and cancer cell death. **B:** In Ab-mediated cellular cytotoxicity, Ab binds to a cell surface cancer antigen and is cross-linked via interaction of Fc receptor (FcR) and Ab to cells with a cytotoxic potential. Cross-linking between cancer cells and cytotoxic cells, such as macrophages, cytotoxic T cells (T_c cells), and NK cells, via Fc receptor interactions can activate the cytolytic cells and result in lysis of cancer cells. In addition, activated antigen-presenting cells may take up antigens from lysed cancer cells and display processed cancer antigen peptides to T cells as complexes of peptides and major histocompatibility complex (MHC) molecules, further facilitating and enhancing specific T-cell responses. **C:** Abs can inhibit cancer cell growth by binding to growth factor receptors at the surface of cancer cells. Ab may block cancer cell proliferation by causing receptor internalization or by blocking growth factor–growth factor receptor interaction.

changes in proteins, even single amino acid substitutions. The binding of peptide to MHC molecules takes place inside the cell (Fig. 2). The peptide-MHC complex is then shuttled to the cell surface. The peptides bound to MHC molecules and recognized by T cells are derived from degraded internal, extracellular, or cell surface proteins. Indeed, T cells can target proteins that have never been present at the cell surface except as degraded fragments in the cleft of MHC molecules. Any aberrantly expressed internal protein is a potential breast cancer antigen for T-cell responses.

The type of immune response elicited is influenced by the cellular location of the antigenic protein (see Fig. 2). In gen-

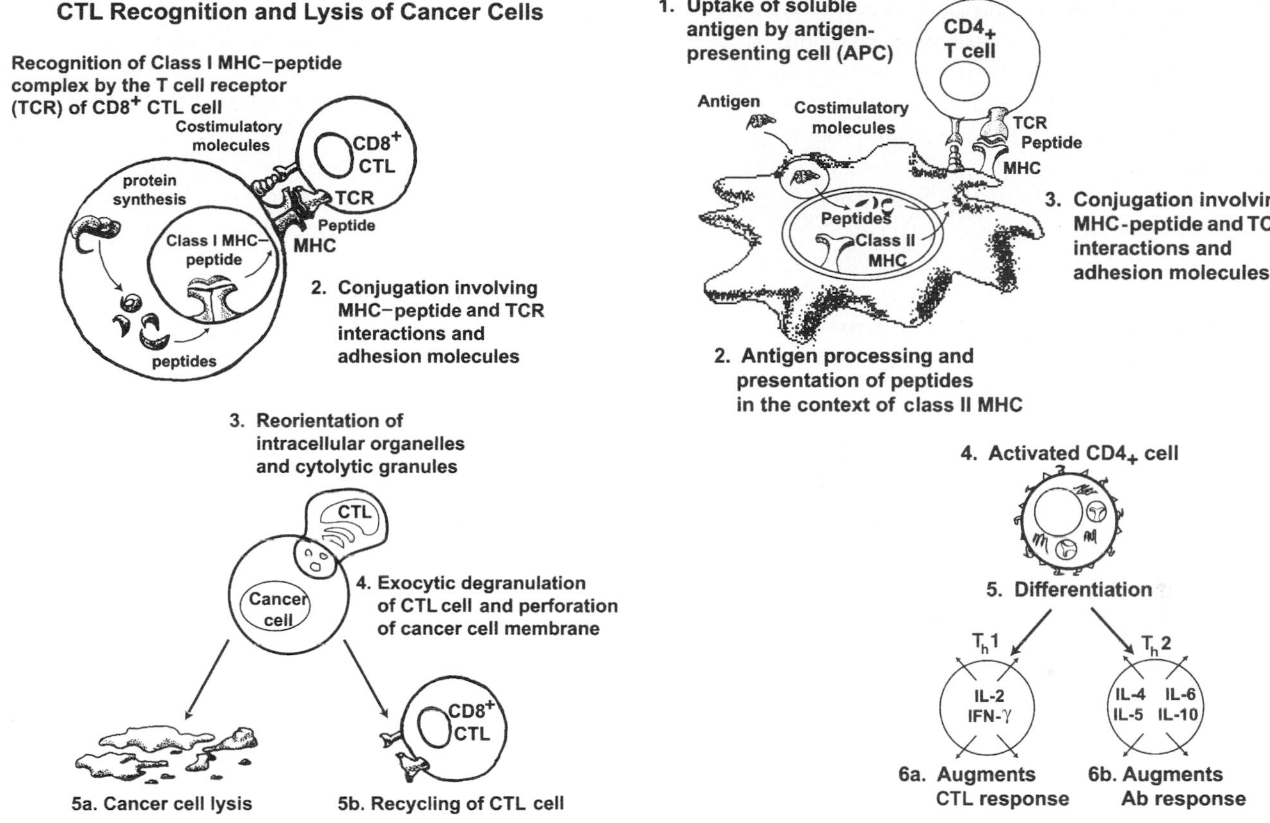

FIG. 2. T cells recognize peptide fragments of immunogenic proteins presented by major histocompatibility complex (MHC) molecules. **A:** An intercellular protein is processed into peptides. The processed peptides are presented as class I MHC–peptide complexes to cytotoxic T cells (CTL cells). Such CTL cells are activated, and the activated CTL cells lyse cancer cells. The peptides bound to class I MHC molecules and recognized by CTL cells are derived from degraded proteins synthesized by the cancer cell itself. **B:** An extracellular protein is processed into peptides by an antigen-presenting cell (APC). The peptides are presented as class II MHC–peptide complexes to helper T cells (T_h cells). Such T_h cells are activated, and subsequently T_h cells are activated and differentiated to secrete cytokines. Depending on the character of various differentiation signals elicited by the peptide-MHC complexes, the T_h secretes cytokines for augmentation of either an antibody (Ab) or a CTL-immune response. The peptides bound to class II MHC molecules of APC and recognized by T_h are derived primarily from degraded proteins present in the extracellular environment. IFN, interferon; IL, interleukin; TCR, T-cell antigen receptor.

eral, intercellular proteins are displayed as peptides bound in the cleft of class I MHC molecules to elicit responses from cytotoxic T cells (CTL cells) that express the cell marker CD8 ($CD8^+$ cells). $CD8^+$ CTL cells can kill cells that synthesize an antigen (see Fig. 2A). In contrast to the way endogenously synthesized proteins are handled, extracellular proteins are brought inside the cells through another antigen-processing pathway and are displayed as peptides bound in the cleft of class II MHC molecules to elicit responses from helper T cells (T_h cells) that express the cell marker CD4 ($CD4^+$ cells) (see Fig. 2B). $CD4^+$ T_h cells have the potential to augment the antigen-specific immune response via cytokine secretion. Subsets of $CD4^+$ T cells, T_h1 cells, secrete cytokines such as interleukin-2 and interferon-γ that stimulate the proliferation and activity of CTL cells. Subsets of $CD4^+$ T cells, T_h2, secrete cytokines such as interleukin-4, interleukin-5, interleukin-6, and interleukin-10 that result in more effective antibody formation.

Antibodies and T cells can recognize entirely different types of antigens. Because T cells recognize peptides, T cells do not ordinarily recognize carbohydrate or lipid moieties. Antibodies, on the other hand, are adept at recognizing carbohydrates and lipids. T cells recognize changes in primary amino acid sequence. Antibodies recognize changes in the tertiary structure of complex proteins resulting from changes in primary amino acid sequence. Perhaps more important, changes in the level of expression and timing of expression of enzymes involved in posttranslational modification of proteins, such as folding, glycosylation, phosphorylation, and lipidation, can yield changes in tertiary structure recognizable by antibodies. Any cell surface molecule with an altered tertiary structure or altered posttranslational modification is a potential breast cancer antigen for antibody responses.

Multiple mutated genes and resultant aberrant proteins are found in cancer cells.[1] Each aberrant protein represents a potential breast cancer antigen. Chromosomal alterations are primary events in the initiation and evolution of cancer. Many carcinogens are mutagens. As cancers progress, mutations compound. Alterations occur in genes that normally function to maintain genomic integrity, such as caretaker genes, giving rise to increased genetic aberrations.[1] *BRCA1* and *BRCA2* breast cancer susceptibility genes are examples of caretaker genes.[2]

The extent to which mutagenic carcinogens play a role in the development of breast cancer is debatable,[3] but most patients are exposed to mutagenic chemotherapy. In animal models, the mutagenic effect of chemotherapy readily gives rise to new cancer antigens. The new cancer antigens are difficult to detect in the primary host and are usually detected only by using tumor transplantation experiments that are not possible to perform in humans. Exact extrapolation to humans is impossible. However, chemotherapy is known to induce chromosomal aberrations in peripheral blood lymphocytes. Presumably, mutations in peripheral blood lymphocytes are a reflection of mutations in cancer cells.[4,5] Chemotherapy is likely to induce antigens recognizable by the immune system.

BREAST CANCER ANTIGENS

Breast cancer antigens can be unique or shared.[6–9] Randomly mutated genes give rise to antigens unique to each individual. Nonrandom gene alterations, such as mutations in p53 hot spots, give rise to shared tumor antigens that occur in multiple patients. Many alterations in cancer-related genes are nonsense mutations, deletions, or insertions. Each can give rise to cancer-associated proteins and thus cancer-associated antigens. If mutations result in a lack of protein expression, cancer antigens do not occur except as the result of changes in downstream proteins.

Commonly overexpressed oncogenic proteins are another category of shared breast cancer antigen. The immune response to normal self-proteins is generally dampened by the phenomenon of immunologic tolerance. Protein overexpression, however, can increase the concentration of peptide-MHC complexes above the threshold necessary for T-cell recognition and allow T-cell responses that otherwise might not occur. Examples of overexpressed oncogenic proteins that are in current or contemplated immunotherapy trials include HER2, mammaglobin, and carcinoembryonic antigen.[10–13] Trials are also targeting differentiation proteins that are not normally expressed by breast tissue or adult tissue, including prostate specific antigen, MAGE, and SSX-expressed proteins.[14–17]

The number of breast cancer antigens identified is likely to increase substantially over the next several years. Publicly and commercially sponsored genomic approaches are identifying virtually all of the genes transcribed in normal and cancerous cells. By extrapolation, all cancer antigens will be known or knowable. The important question of whether breast cancer antigens exist has been answered. Breast cancer antigens do exist. The most important questions now and for some time in the future are "Which antigens are the best targets?" and "How can an effective immune response best be elicited?"

IMMUNE RESPONSES TO BREAST CANCER ANTIGENS

The identification of multiple breast cancer antigens begs the question of whether an immune response occurs to such antigens in patients with breast cancer and, as a corollary, whether the immune response is effective and beneficial. Accumulated evidence that immune responses occur has invigorated efforts to develop breast cancer vaccines and other specific immunotherapies.

Immune responses to shared breast cancer antigens are measurable in many breast cancer patients.[10,17–22] The best studied antigens are p53, MUC1, and HER-2/neu. Immunity to HER-2/neu is discussed in this section. MUC1 and p53 are discussed in the Breast Cancer Vaccines section.

The extent to which immune responses occur to unique breast cancer antigens is not known. Detection of immune response to unique cancer antigens in the autochthonous host is exceedingly difficult. In animal models, transplantation experiments are used. Human studies of tumor-infiltrating T cells are the best substitute for transplantation experiments. Tumor-infiltrating T cells have been used in some nonbreast cancers to identify both unique and shared cancer antigens.[23] Less work on tumor-infiltrating T cells has been performed for breast cancer than for melanoma. Tumor-infiltrating T cells can be grown out of primary breast cancer tumors.[20,24–27] In a large study of many tumor types, although T cells from breast cancer could be grown *in vitro*, specific cytolysis of breast cancer was not observed.[26] The majority of T cells expanded by culture were $CD4^+$ T_h cells and not $CD8^+$ CTL cells. Accordingly, tumor-infiltrating T cells from several breast cancer patients have been shown to recognize and secrete cytokines in response to autologous breast cancer.[27,28] The antigens recognized on autologous cancers have not been reported. However, T cells from peripheral blood of breast cancer patients have been shown in some cases to recognize shared breast cancer antigens, including HER2 and MUC1.[10,19]

Relatively few such studies have examined immune responses to autologous breast cancer, in part because of the difficulty of obtaining adequate cancer biopsy material from primary breast cancer and the relative rarity of therapeutic metastatic tumor resection in breast cancer. The experience with breast cancer tumor-infiltrating T cells may be too small to draw conclusions as to the presence or absence of breast cancer–specific T cells. The general lack of reactivity in breast cancer tumor-infiltrating T cells may be related to suppressive factors secreted by breast cancer (see section Mechanisms of Escape from Breast Cancer Immunity) and may be more profound at the primary site. T cells at the site of primary breast cancer have been observed to be in a state of partial activation but lack interleukin-2 cytokine expression.[29,30] CTL cells specific for breast cancer, however, have been elicited from pleural effusions[31] and peripheral blood of patients with breast cancer.

Once an ongoing specific immune response is identified in breast cancer patients, determining whether the immune response is beneficial is an even more difficult proposition, especially in patients destined to die of their cancers. Extrapolating from studies in chronic infectious diseases, many patients die of progressive disease in the face of a vigorous ongoing immune response. The immune responses can be beneficial in prolonging survival but ineffective in preventing death. Within any individual with progressive disease, determining the extent to which the immune response is impacting survival is difficult, if not impossible.

The difficulty in determining the role of specific immunity in breast cancer is highlighted by studies of the HER2 antigen system. Some patients with breast cancer have detectable immunity to HER2.[10,32–34] Antibody responses are detectable in approximately 10% of patients with breast cancer and correlate with the presence of breast cancer that overexpresses HER2.[35] The strong implication is that immunity develops as a result of exposure of patients to HER-2/neu protein overexpressed by autochthonous cancer. T_h cell responses also occur[32] but are more difficult to detect or less frequent.[10,36] CTL responses have been detected in some patients with cancer overexpressing HER2, but the frequency and level of response has not been well quantified.[34,37]

Determining the role of immunity to HER2 in patients with HER2-positive cancer is complicated by multiple interrelated variables. Overexpression of HER2 is associated with aggressive disease and a poor outcome for patients with invasive ductal cancer.[38] This is not true for all categories of patients, however.[39,40] Among patients with HER-positive invasive ductal cancer, outcome is improved for patients receiving high-dose anthracycline-containing chemotherapy.[39] Chemotherapy is given to kill cancer cells, but it can also have either positive or negative effects on immune responses depending on regimen and timing. High-dose chemotherapy and radiation therapy regimens can be profoundly immunosuppressive.[41–44] In animal models, immunity to cancer has a substantial synergistic effect with many chemotherapy regimens,[45] and the effect is highly dependent on timing.[46] The extent to which the synergistic animal chemotherapy data can be extrapolated to human breast cancer is speculative at best.

Lymphoplasmacytic infiltration in small primary tumors is also associated with a favorable prognosis for patients with stage I breast cancers that show HER2 overexpression.[40] HER2 gene amplification is linked to dense lymphocyte infiltration. Whether the infiltration is the result of HER2 expression, immunity to HER2, or unrelated factors is not known.[47] The favorable prognosis of patients with localized invasive ductal carcinoma leads to speculation that immunity to HER2 might exist and might be responsible for the infiltration and improved outcome. Other studies of breast cancer–infiltrating lymphocytes, however, have observed a preponderance of macrophages in tumors that overexpress HER2 and a preponderance of T cells in tumors that do not overexpress HER2.[48,49] The presence of a predominant macrophage infiltrate versus a T-cell infiltrate could mean that specific immune responses are not operative. Studies correlating the character of the infiltrate with specific immune responses might resolve the issue.

The character of the immune response to HER2 might impact outcome more than the presence or absence of immunity. Both antibody and T-cell responses occur and can have either positive or negative effects. HER2 is a growth factor receptor. Monoclonal antibodies can have either inhibitory or stimulatory effects.[50] T_h-cell response can be skewed toward T_h1 or T_h2 responses. In some model systems, T_h1 responses can have greater therapeutic effects. CTL cells are likely to be beneficial, but CTL cells can kill only cancers positive for class I MHC molecules. Some breast cancers have loss and down-regulation of class I MHC.[51–54] The presence of a dominant CTL response in the face of a class I MHC–negative cancer can divert and render useless the immune response.[55,56]

INFLAMMATION AND PROGNOSIS

One of the most fascinating issues is whether inflammation and lymphocyte infiltration are of benefit or detriment to breast cancer outcome. It makes intuitive sense that an ongoing specific immune response against cancer cells would benefit patients. Countervailing is the strong and often-voiced hypothesis that inflammation and lymphocyte infiltration are associated with a worsened prognosis.[57,58]

Studies of the prognostic significance of inflammation in breast cancer have yielded conflicting results.[57,59] One problem in analyzing the significance of inflammation for the outcome of breast cancer is that inflammation and specific immune responses are not synonymous. Inflammation can result from specific immune responses, but other possible causes exist that are less likely to be associated with benefit. As an example, "inflammatory" breast cancer has a poor prognosis and is associated with substantial inflammation, often including lymphocyte infiltration. The inflammation is thought to be due largely to infiltration of lymphatics by aggressive cancer cells and not to a specific immune response. In a similar vein, invasive ductal carcinoma with extensive tumor necrosis can be associated with intense inflammation.[59] Immune response possibly could be the cause of necrosis, but the necrosis is much more likely to be due to too rapid tumor growth and the inflammatory response to be secondary to the aggressive nature of the cancer.

Inflammation and lymphocyte infiltration in breast cancer have been the focus of a profusion of articles for decades. Of the multitude of studies of inflammation in breast cancer, none has correlated inflammation with the presence or absence of specific immune responses. The assays for specific immunity are new and are just beginning to be assessed. The extent to which specific immune responses and inflammation can be separately defined and evaluated is unknown, but the study of immunity and inflammation as separate variables would be useful.

Another factor confounding the assessment of immunity and inflammation is that the most aggressive cancers are likely to be the most antigenic. The most aggressive cancers have the greatest quantity of aberrant genes and proteins and thus potential antigens. The least aggressive cancers are closest to normal "self" breast tissue and thus the least antigenic. The most aggressive cancers might be accompanied by a greater degree of inflammation, because they are the most antigenic. Thus, even if immunity is found to correlate with poor prognosis, the immune response in and of itself might not be detrimental. Parenthetically, the cancers that are the most aggressive and thus the most antigenic might also be the most able to evolve mechanisms to escape from immune destruction.

A negative role for immunity and inflammation in breast cancer is implied by the observation that the incidence of *de novo* breast cancer is decreased in women chronically immunosuppressed after organ transplant.[60] The implied conclusion is that immunity and inflammation are directly involved in worsening the prognosis and that the immunosuppression overcomes the negative effect of immunity and inflammation. By contrast, skin cancers associated with human papillomavirus infection and lymphomas associated with Epstein-Barr virus infection are both clearly increased by immunosuppression associated with organ transplantation. The implied conclusion is that suppressed immunity allows human papillomavirus and Epstein-Barr virus infection and subsequent cancer induction to progress. The major difference in the incidence of breast cancer among organ transplant recipients is seen in the first year, which suggests the alternative hypothesis that breast examination before transplantation may have excluded some patients who would otherwise have been shortly diagnosed as having cancer.

If inflammation does worsen breast cancer prognosis, several possible mechanisms exist. Macrophages are a major component of breast cancer infiltration. Activated macrophages can kill cancer cells, but activated macrophages can also secrete immunosuppressive substances to suppress specific immune responses in the face of an inflammatory infiltrate. Alternatively, inflammation might directly stimulate breast cancer through the function of cytokines and growth factors such as interleukin-6, colony-stimulating factor, tumor necrosis factor α, epidermal growth factor–like growth factor, basic fibroblast growth factor, and factors capable of affecting angiogenesis and digestion of matrix.[48,61–65] As examples, tumor-infiltrating lymphocytes have been shown to produce heparin-binding epidermal growth factor–like growth factor and basic fibroblast growth factor, both of which can have stimulatory effects on breast cancer cells.[66] Tumor necrosis factor α has been shown to promote progression from premalignancy to malignancy in animals[65] and may also promote tumor angiogenesis.[64] In addition to stimulating cancer cell growth, macrophages can also profoundly prevent activation of T cells by a variety of mechanisms, such as suppressing expression of the zeta chain of the CD3–T-cell receptor complex.[67]

Too many interacting and competing variables may exist to allow realistic expectations of determining the role of existent immune responses to breast cancer antigens. Ultimately, the extent to which immunity can provide benefit will be determined by vaccine trials.

STRESS, BREAST CANCER, AND IMMUNITY

Several intriguing areas exist in which immunity to breast cancer has been conjectured to provide substantial benefit, including immunity augmented by psychosocial factors, immunity induced by pregnancy, and immunity induced by preexisting *in situ* cancer. Each is discussed below.

Psychosocial Factors

Several trials of psychosocial intervention show clear benefit in terms of disease-free survival and overall survival.[68–70] The reasons for improved outcome are not known. One hypothesis is that stress has a negative impact on the immune system and that psychosocial intervention can reverse the effect.[68] Immune responses are under the influence of neuroendocrine mediators. Animal experiments have shown associations between stress, depletion of neurotransmitters, suppression of immunity, and ability to prevent growth of transplanted cancers.[71]

Among the mechanisms by which the nervous system can impact the immune system are responsivity to the neuroendocrine peptide β-endorphin and to glucocorticosteroid hormones. Lymphocytes have receptors for both, and cytokines produced by lymphocytes can influence the production of neuroendocrine hormones. Exogenous opiates can have a suppressive effect on specific immune effector mechanisms.[72] Similarly, NK- and T-cell function can be reduced by elevated concentrations of β-endorphin.[73] Endogenous β-endorphin is elevated after experimentally induced stress.[74] The power of β-endorphin on the immune system is demonstrated by skin allograft experiments showing that grafts are less likely to be rejected at increased concentrations of β-endorphin. Corticosteroids can also be strongly immunosuppressive at concentrations induced by stress. Corticosteroids can interrupt normal signal transduction, induce secretion of transforming growth factor β—a potent inhibitor of T cells, NK cells, and other effector cells of the immune system—and decrease interleukin-2 production. β-Endorphin and glucocorticosteroids can alter the ratio of T_h1 to T_h2 to accentuate T_h2 responses, which might be less effective against cancer than T_h1 responses.[72,75]

Cancer-related stress has been correlated with decreased NK and nonspecific mitogen-induced T-cell proliferative responses.[76] The extent to which NK cells are important in outcome is unknown. The level of NK cells can be low in cancer patients with large tumor burdens,[77] and NK levels may be inversely related to lymph node metastasis at the time of diagnosis.[71] Specific immune responses may be initiated and maintain NK responses, however, and may, in and of themselves, be more powerful and longer-lasting than NK responses. No studies have attempted to correlate changes in stress with changes in specific immune responses. NK responses and mitogen responses are nonspecific measures of immune response. These measures may be surrogates of tumor-specific responses, but no studies have been done to demonstrate that nonspecific immune responses are paralleled by changes in specific immune responses.

Despite the attractiveness of the hypothesis that psychosocial factors may influence the tumor-specific immune response, proving a role for immune response in the phenomenon is very difficult. Too many variables may exist to allow the key determinants to be identified. In the end, intervention with vaccines or other immunotherapeutic manipulations might more consistently perturbate the immune response.

Pregnancy

An even more central role for immunity has been suggested by the theory that immunity to breast cancer antigens is generated by pregnancy. Multiparity protects against the development of breast cancer. One hypothesis is that the fetus or the developing breast carries antigens that are similar to antigens on breast cancer cells and that pregnancy can induce immunity to such antigens. Supporting the hypothesis is the observation that antibodies reactive with breast cancer proteins are present in the sera of multiparous women.[78,79] Also, T cells specific for MUC1 are more numerous in multiparous women.[80,81] The issue of the effect of immunity on pregnancy-associated decrease in breast cancer incidence might best be resolved by studies measuring specific immune responses to breast cancer antigens.

In Situ Breast Cancer

Studies using population-based data from the Survival, Epidemiology, and End Results (SEER) Program of the National Cancer Institute demonstrated that patients with an invasive breast cancer who had a prior or simultaneous *in situ* breast cancer have a significantly better survival rate.[82,83] One explanation is that an immune response to breast cancer antigens occurs and is beneficial. Inflammation can occur with DCIS early in the evolution of breast cancer. In DCIS, clusters of B cells and T cells can be situated either adjacent to involved ducts or in the interductal stroma.[63] Whether immunity to breast cancer antigens is a component of DCIS-associated inflammation is an open experimental question.

MECHANISMS OF ESCAPE FROM BREAST CANCER IMMUNITY

Perhaps the most compelling evidence that immunity plays a role in the evolution of breast cancer is the observation that breast cancers evolve multiple sophisticated mechanisms of escape from immune destruction. Why would mechanisms to escape immunity evolve without immunologic pressure?

Mechanisms of escape include decrease in MHC molecules and secretion of immunosuppressive factors, including cytokines, placental immunosuppressive proteins, and mucins that can block T-cell lysis.[84–86] The expression of class I MHC molecules by cancer cells is mandatory for CTL recognition and killing. Many advanced breast cancers have decreased or absent class I MHC.[51,52,54] The loss of MHC molecules is thought to provide a "footprint" of previous CTL responses. Some have proposed that the best place to look for cancer antigens may be in patients with class I MHC–negative cancer cells. The absence of class I MHC molecules is an indicator that antigen is present and that cancer-specific CTL cells are also present and have been operative. As an aside, although T cells cannot recognize cancer cells with a complete loss of class I MHC molecules, loss of class I MHC molecules does not preclude effective immunotherapy mediated by antibodies and T_h cells. In fact, a substantial body of evidence shows that loss of class I MHC molecules predisposes to increased susceptibility to NK-mediated killing.[87–89]

Breast cancer can induce a general immunoincompetence, most probably mediated by secretion of immunosuppressive factors that can prevent the generation of immunity and the ability of immune T cells to function. Factors secreted by breast cancer and capable of suppressing immune responses include transforming growth factor β, interleukin-6, interleukin-10, tumor necrosis factor α, and histamine as well as unidentified substances that can mediate or otherwise cause signaling defects in T cells.[90–92] Substances like transforming growth factor β can produce a shieldlike effect around breast cancer, preventing the induction of an adequate immune response. If an immune response is generated, soluble factors can cause deficiencies in the ability of immune T cells, NK cells, and antigen-presenting cells to transmit and interpret activation signals, producing profound immunosuppression.[67,93–96] In advancing cancer, drastic reductions can occur in expression of specific phosphotyrosine kinases that participate in signal transduction.[97–99] As a consequence, immune cells are unable to proliferate and unable to synthesize and secrete cytokines. Signaling defects in breast cancer patients can be detected early in the course of the disease and need not necessarily be related to decreased zeta chain expression.[100] The effect of cytokines is also complex. Despite the effect of transforming growth factor β on immunity, one study has shown that favorable outcome of breast cancer is positively correlated with levels of transforming growth factor β1; the speculation is that the favorable outcome is caused by the breast cancer growth–inhibitory effects of transforming growth factor β.[101,102]

BREAST CANCER VACCINES

Proposals to test therapeutic vaccines to augment breast cancer immunity require an explanation as to why existing immune response to breast cancer is inadequate. The immune system is most effective at eliminating invading microorganisms. Invading microorganisms present a large concentration of foreign antigen and provoke an immediate innate immune response composed of NK cells and macrophages. Bacterial lipopolysaccharide and viral-induced interferon activate the nonspecific innate immune system, recruiting phagocytic cells and NK cells to the site of infection and raising an inflammatory site. The inflammatory site supplies cytokines and other inflammatory mediators that provide essential activation signals for facilitating antigen-specific immune responses and may direct antigen-specific immune responses.[103,104]

In cancer, the majority of proteins expressed are normal. The abnormal proteins evolve slowly and are presented without the context of bacterial products. Activated NK cells and macrophages are capable of killing cancer cells *in vitro*. With the slow growth and evolution of cancer cells to a more antigenic or "foreign" phenotype, however, what signals would activate NK cells and macrophages to a cytolytic state capable of killing cancer cells is not clear. Thus, cancer cannot be expected to induce the same type of vigorous response as do invading microorganisms. Accordingly, vaccination regimens with cancer antigens often use bacterial products as adjuvants to mimic the stimulus of invading microorganisms.

Vaccines can be constructed to induce immune responses to either unique or shared cancer antigens. Immunization against unique cancer antigens requires that patients be vaccinated with their own cancer material. Clinical trials to induce an immune response to unique antigens have been performed primarily in cases of melanoma but are increasingly being proposed for breast cancer cases. Autologous cellular vaccines are difficult to generate for breast cancer. Often, limited tumor is available, and primary breast cancer is difficult to propagate in culture. New methods focusing on the generation of total tumor RNA may allow surrogates for autologous tumor to be created using autologous antigen-presenting cells expressing tumor antigens.[105] However, clinical trials involving shared breast cancer antigens are easier to contemplate and their results are easier to interpret. Among the breast cancer antigens being used in current clinical trials are mucins, HER2, MAGE, and carcinoembryonic antigen.

HER-2/neu Vaccines

The presence of existing immune responses to HER2[32,33] provides assurance that immune tolerance can be overcome and that some vaccine formulations can elicit an immune response. Antibody therapy studies in animals and humans confirm that immunity to HER2 can improve survival[106,107] and underscore the power of an appropriately directed specific immune response in breast cancer. HER2 is a cell surface molecule that is shed and, as such, can be recognized by T_h cells, antibodies, and CTL cells. Preclinical data confirm that antibodies, T_h cells, and CTL cells can recognize HER2 and can have cytolytic or therapeutic effects.[37,108] One goal of designing HER2 vaccines is to develop a strategy for inducing all three effector mechanisms.

Much discussion has been given to whether antibodies, T_h cells, or CTL cells mediate the best anticancer immune responses. The discussion is specious: Each can mediate effective immune responses, and most effective immune responses involve the interplay of multiple effector mechanisms. Which immune response is best depends entirely on the cellular location of the proposed target. CTL cells can potentially recognize any protein synthesized by the target cell, including intracellular proteins, provided processed peptide fragments of the protein are presented by class I MHC molecules. T_h cells recognize proteins exogenous to cancer cells that are taken up and presented by class II MHC molecules on macrophages and dendritic cells. For T_h cells to function, cancer cells need not express class II MHC molecules. Antibodies can potentially recognize any protein, but they need to bind to cell surface antigens to be effective against cancer. Antibody responses against internal breast cancer proteins, such as p53, are often observed but are unlikely to be beneficial.

Methods of generating immunity to "self" oncogenic proteins, such as HER2, are not well established. Vaccines can induce immunity to self-proteins, but immunologic tolerance can profoundly dampen immune response vigor. One method to overcome tolerance is to immunize to peptide fragments rather than to whole proteins. When this method was used, immunity to rat neu protein could be elicited in rats.[109] Rat neu is highly homologous to human HER2. Accordingly, several vaccine trials have been initiated with peptides from the natural sequence of HER2.[110,111] In one ongoing trial, patients are being immunized with groups of HER2 peptides of 15 amino acids in length designated to elicit T_h- and CTL-cell responses.

Conclusions after analysis of the first patients[110] are that vaccination is feasible and that immunity to HER2 protein can be elicited. In a second study, immunization with a single peptide of nine amino acids designated to elicit CTL responses induced CTL cells specific for the peptide but failed to induce CTL cells that could lyse HER2-positive cancer cells.[111] The results point out a major problem with peptide-based vaccines. T cells elicited by immunizing to peptides often have T-cell receptor affinities too low for recognizing and killing tumor cells. Moreover, MHC molecules present only a minority of peptide fragments of any protein.

Additional HER2 vaccine strategies in preclinical development include the use of additional peptide combinations, whole HER2 protein, and alternative adjuvants, including autologous dendritic cells. Adjuvants are critical for circumventing tolerance to self. Other contemplated trials will test immunization with recombinant HER2 expressed by viral vectors and "naked" plasmid DNA.[112,113] Each allows expression of HER2 in a more immunogenic context than by the autochthonous cancer cells, and each allows the expression of encoded cytokines and costimulatory molecules with the target antigen.[114]

Mucin Vaccines

Mucins are heavily glycosylated high–molecular-weight proteins on the surface of normal epithelium. One member of the mucin family receiving substantial attention as a breast cancer vaccine is MUC1.[115] MUC1 is a cell surface mucin with a transmembrane domain and polar expression on the apical surface of epithelium. In breast cancer, MUC1 is expressed in a nonpolar fashion and is underglycosylated, exposing otherwise hidden epitopes. T cells usually recognize peptide-MHC complexes and are activated to kill cancer cells by cross-linking of the T-cell receptor by the peptide-MHC complexes on cancer cells. T-cell recognition of MUC1 is unusual in that MUC1 has multiple reiterative exposed epitopes that can themselves cross-link the T-cell receptor. MUC1-specific T cells can recognize and kill MUC1-positive cancer cells by direct recognition of MUC1 without the normal requirement that the target antigen be processed and presented by MHC molecules.[19] In addition, MUC1 can be presented by certain MHC molecules as a processed peptide.[116]

MUC1 vaccine development is encouraged by the presence of existing immune responses to MUC1. T cells and antibodies specific for the exposed epitopes can be detected in breast cancer patients. CTL cells against MUC1 were first observed in patients with pancreatic cancer. The same CTL cells were shown to recognize MUC1 on breast cancer cells.[117] MUC1-specific CTL cells can be found in patients with advanced breast cancer, but they are neither potent nor numerous. In early breast cancer, the frequency of CTL cells is higher, but it diminishes with tumor progression. MUC1 T_h-cell responses are usually not found in breast cancer patients; this leads to the assumption that little processing and presentation of MUC1 occur or, more likely, that tolerance to MUC1 occurs at the T_h-cell level. T_h cells are necessary for immunoglobulin class switch from IgM to IgG. Without T_h cells, very few B cells are activated. When detected, antibody to MUC1 is primarily IgM.[118] In some patients, low-level IgG and IgA have been detected in early breast cancer, a finding that indicates that helper cell activity can be operative, but the levels diminish with tumor progression.[19] In one study, circulating immune complexes containing MUC1 were measured in sera from 25% of breast cancer patients before treatment. An inverse correlation was seen between positivity for immune complexes and extent of disease; the inference is that immunity to MUC1 protects against disease progression.[119]

The several MUC1 vaccines in clinical trials have been designed to elicit either classic MHC-restricted responses or nonclassic MUC1-specific CTL responses, as well as T_h-cell and antibody responses. Immunization to a synthetic MUC1 peptide with bacille Calmette-Guérin as an adjuvant induced delayed-type hypersensitivity responses, but only in a minority of patients.[120] Immunization with synthetic MUC1 peptide linked to keyhole-limpet hemocyanin elicited CTL cells in more than one-half of metastatic breast cancer patients. IgG MUC1-specific responses were detected, but levels were low and were present in only a few patients.[121] The detection of CTL responses is encouraging, but the low level antibody response implies a lack of T_h-cell responses that might be essential for maintaining a CTL response. In another study, immunization with MUC1, linked to mannan to increase uptake by antigen-presenting cells, induced IgG antibody in one-half of the patients[122] but only very low CTL responses.[123] A MUC1 formulation capable of inducing T_h cell responses is probably needed to induce and maintain adequate levels of CTL and IgG antibody immunity.[124]

Abnormal glycosylation of MUC1 by breast cancer cells also results in expression of a mucin-associated carbohydrate moiety, sialyl-Tn (STn). STn is expressed in the majority of breast cancers.[125] Vaccination of metastatic breast cancer patients with synthetic STn linked to keyhole-limpet hemocyanin induces IgG antibody in some patients, and survival of vaccinated patients correlates with the level of IgG antibody responses elicited.[126] One potential problem with carbohydrate-based vaccines is that carbohydrates rarely induce T_h-cell responses, and T_h-cell responses are necessary for long-term immunologic memory. Induction of IgG antibody by STn vaccines, however, implies that the T_h cells necessary for immunoglobulin class switch from IgM to IgG are present. STn-specific T_h cells have been observed in vaccinated patients.[127] The level of immune response elicited in vaccine studies commonly correlates with survival, because less-sick patients respond better than patients in poor health. Thus, the presence of a correlation between level of immunity obtained and outcome does not necessarily indicate that immunity caused the improved outcome. Results are quite encouraging, however, and have led to the initiation of a large phase III randomized trial of STn vaccination in patients with minimal residual disease.

p53 Vaccines

The p53 proteins are expressed in breast cancer in a wide variety of mutant and truncated forms. Antibody to p53 is found in approximately 25% of breast cancer patients and correlates with the presence of mutant p53.[18] The strong implication is that immunity to p53 develops as a result of expression of aberrant p53. Although antibody to p53 is found primarily in patients with cancers expressing mutant p53, the predominant antibody response is directed to regions uninvolved by mutations—that is, areas of "self."[128] The majority of p53 antibodies detected are IgG, which predicts coexistent T_h-cell responses. Due to the heterogeneity of p53 mutations, T-cell responses to the mutant region are difficult to evaluate. However, T_h-cell immunity to wild-type p53 protein has been detected in several breast cancer patients with antibody responses to p53.[129]

The p53 protein is an intracellular protein; thus, antibody responses to p53 are not expected to have much impact on outcome. The presence of immunity, however, might serve as a marker for general immunogenicity and prognosis. In one study, patients were evaluated for the presence of p53 antibodies at the time of new recurrence. The recurrence-free interval was almost the same for antibody-positive and antibody-negative patients.[130] Isolating all appropriate variables for such studies is problematic. Given that p53 expression can impact outcome and possibly response to therapy, information is needed regarding not only whether antibody is present but also whether mutant p53 is present. Outcome in relation to immunity can be most accurately assessed by treating all patients with the same regimen.

Vaccines for inducing CTL immunity to mutant p53 are in clinical trials. CTL cells specific for the mutant segment of p53 peptide can lyse transformed cells[131] and function in therapy in murine models.[132] A major problem in developing p53 CTL vaccines is that the mutations are complex. CTL cells can be effective only if the mutant segment binds to MHC molecules during the normal p53 protein degradative process. Moreover, p53 is a suppressor gene. A lack of p53 function is responsible for oncogenicity. If CTL responses to p53 result in p53-negative variants, the malignant phenotype might not change. Vaccines and T-cell therapy directed against normal p53 are also being considered[133–136] but must deal with the issue of a presumed high level of immunologic tolerance to a protein expressed in every cell and the reciprocal problem that a vigorous immune response might cause undue toxicity.

MAGE Vaccines

MAGE proteins are encoded by members of a family of genes expressed during fetal development and often in cancer. In the adult, MAGE proteins are present only in cancer and testes. The role of MAGE in cancer is unknown, but members of the family are expressed so commonly in cancer that they probably play a role in malignant transformation or maintenance of the transformed state. MAGE-1 was first identified as the target antigen of CTL cells specific for autologous malignant melanoma.[137] However, members of the MAGE family are also expressed in a significant fraction of breast cancers and in melanoma.[15] Moreover, MAGE-specific precursors have been found to be present among tumor-infiltrating lymphocytes from a patient with breast cancer.[20] Vaccines specific for MAGE peptides and protein are being tested in melanoma and breast cancer.

Prostate Antigen Vaccines

Several proteins expressed by normal breast in small amounts, and by male prostate in larger amounts, are also expressed by breast cancer. These include prostate-specific antigen and prostate-specific membrane antigen.[138,139] Expression of prostate proteins in breast cancer may be dependent on the presence of androgen receptors.[140] Expression is not static and can be perturbed by changes in hormonal environment; the presence of synthetic progestins, for example, can induce expresssion.[141] Vaccines and immunotoxins targeting prostate antigens, such as prostate-specific antigen and prostate-specific membrane antigen, are being developed for prostate cancer.[14,141–143] The same immunotherapies have been proposed for use in breast cancer.

FUTURE CLINICAL TRIALS

New molecular approaches will soon allow identification of virtually all proteins expressed by each individual's breast cancer. By identifying all proteins expressed by breast cancer and by focusing on proteins with limited expression in other tissues, researchers will be able to generate many additional vaccine candidates. Mammaglobin, for example, is a vaccine candidate identified by isolating differentially expressed human breast cancer genes.[11] Expression of mammaglobin is tightly restricted to adult mammary gland, and thus is a marker of metastatic breast cancer.[144] Mammaglobin is overexpressed in many primary breast cancers and expression is increased in metastasis, which implies that expression is linked to breast tissue growth.[145] Mammaglobin will be tested as a vaccine candidate. Many other vaccine candidates will be identified by similar methods.

The major roadblock to developing breast cancer vaccines is immunologic tolerance to self-antigens, which dampens the ability to induce immunity to self-proteins. Gene therapy techniques are being evaluated as a ploy to circumvent tolerance. Transfection of genes encoding stimulatory cytokines and costimulatory molecules can overcome many of the reasons for poor immunogenicity of cancer cells.

The use of dendritic cell vaccines might accomplish the same vaccine goals as gene therapy. Dendritic cells are the most effective stimulator cells for priming T-cell responses and already express the appropriate stimulatory cytokines and costimulatory molecules necessary for inducing T-cell responses. Dendritic cells are powerful vaccine adjuvants for inducing immunity to shared cancer antigens or autologous cancer cells. In mice, immunization using dendritic cells mixed with tumor cells can inhibit the growth of breast cancer.[146] Dendritic cells can be cultured from patients after bone marrow transplantation and thus will be tested as vaccine adjuvants to prevent recurrence of breast cancer in that setting.[147]

T-cell therapy is substantially more effective than the use of vaccines for the treatment of established disease. Vaccination to induce T-cell responses, followed by *in vitro* expansion of immune T cells and T-cell therapy, is cumbersome but is more effective than vaccination alone when cancer is already established.[148] The use of nonspecifically activated regional lymph node cells is being tested in phase I clinical trials.[149] Combining this approach with prior specific vaccination is likely to be more effective. Immunologic tolerance operates by depleting T cells with high affinity for self-antigens. Gene transfer methods are also being used to introduce high-affinity T-cell receptors into autologous T cells and even to introduce antibodies with high affinity tumor reactivity into T cells.

The most effective form of specific immunotherapy in clinical practice is allogeneic donor T-cell therapy for leukemia as part of bone marrow transplantation regimens.[150] The antileukemia effect of allogeneic T cells is so striking and profound that studies to invoke a similar graft versus tumor effects in breast cancer will be attempted.[151,152] The major problem encountered in using allogeneic T cells in therapy is graft-versus-host toxicity. Successful use of this method in breast cancer depends on whether the powerful antihost immune response can be directed against breast cancer to the exclusion of normal tissues.

Specific immunotherapy probably will work best early in the course of disease, when there is lower tumor burden, less evolution of escape mechanisms, and less immunoincompetence from accumulated effects of chemotherapy. Methods for early diagnosis and for detection of early relapse may be essential for the most effective application of specific immunotherapies.[153,154] Immunotherapies will probably have the greatest effect when applied early in the disease and in conjunction with other modalities.

REFERENCES

1. Hussain SP, Harris CC. Molecular epidemiology of human cancer: contribution of mutation spectra studies of tumor suppressor genes. *Cancer Res* 1998;58:4023.
2. Kinzler KW, Vogelstein B. Cancer-susceptibility genes. Gatekeepers and caretakers. *Nature* 1997;386:761.
3. Laden F, Hunter DJ. Environmental factors and female breast cancer. *Annu Rev Public Health* 1998;19:101.
4. Frenkel K, Klein CB. Methods used for analyses of "environmentally" damaged nucleic acids. *J Chromatogr* 1993;618:289.
5. Hagmar L, Bonnassi S, Stromberg U, et al. Chromosomal aberrations in lymphocytes predict human cancer. A report from the European Study Group on Cytogenetic Biomarkers and Health (ESCH). *Cancer Res* 1998;58:4117.
6. Mumberg D, Wick M, Schreiber H. Unique tumor antigens redefined as mutant tumor-specific antigens. *Semin Immunol* 1996;8:289.
7. Hollstein M, Shomer B, Greenblatt M, et al. Somatic point mutations in the p53 gene of human tumors and cell lines: updated compilation. *Nucleic Acids Res* 1996;24:141.
8. Sasa M, Kondo K, Komaki K, Morimoto T, Monden Y. p53 alteration correlates with negative ER, negative PgR, and high histologic grade in breast cancer. *J Surg Oncol* 1994;56:46.
9. Tsuda H, Iwaya K, Fukutomi T, Hirohashi S. p53 mutations and c-erbB-2 amplification in intraductal and invasive breast carcinomas of high histologic grade. *Jpn J Cancer Res* 1993;84:394.
10. Disis ML, Cheever MA. HER-2/neu protein. A target for antigen specific immunotherapy of human cancer. *Adv Cancer Res* 1997;71:343.
11. Watson MA, Fleming TP. Mammaglobin, a mammary-specific member of the uteroglobin gene family, is overexpressed in human breast cancer. *Cancer Res* 1996;56:860.
12. Bhattacharya-Chatterjee M, Foon KA. Anti-idiotype antibody vaccine therapies of cancer. *Cancer Treat Res* 1998;94:51.
13. Schlom J. Strategies for the development of recombinant vaccines for the immunotherapy of breast cancer. *Breast Cancer Res Treat* 1996;38:27.
14. Xue BH, Zhang Y, Sosman JA, Peace DJ. Induction of human cytotoxic T lymphocytes specific for prostate-specific antigen. *Prostate* 1997;30:73.
15. Brasseur F, Marchand M, Vanwijck R, et al. Human gene MAGE-1, which codes for a tumor-rejection antigen, is expressed by some breast tumors. *Int J Cancer* 1992;52:839.
16. Tureci O, Chen YT, Sahin U, et al. Expression of SSX genes in human tumors. *Int J Cancer* 1998;77:19.
17. Henderson RA, Finn OJ. Human tumor antigens are ready to fly. *Adv Immunol* 1996;62:217.
18. Davidoff AM, Iglehart JD, Marks JR. Immune response to p53 is dependent upon p53/HSP70 complexes in breast cancers. *Proc Natl Acad Sci U S A* 1992;89:3439.
19. Finn OJ, Jerome KR, Henderson RA, et al. MUC-1 epithelial tumor mucin-based immunity and cancer vaccines. *Immunological Rev* 1995;145:61.
20. Toso JF, Oei C, Oshidari F, et al. MAGE-1-specific precursor cytotoxic T-lymphocytes present among tumor-infiltrating lymphocytes from a patient with breast cancer: characterization and antigen-specific activation. *Cancer Res* 1996;56:16.
21. Conroy SE, Sasieni PD, Amin V, et al. Antibodies to heat-shock protein 27 are associated with improved survival in patients with breast cancer. *Br J Cancer* 1998;77:1875.
22. Albert ML. Tumor specific killer cells in paraneoplastic cerebellar degeneration. *Nat Med* 1998;4:1321.
23. Rosenberg SA. The immunotherapy of solid cancers based on cloning the genes encoding tumor-rejection antigens. *Annu Rev Med* 1996;47:481.
24. Baxevanis CN, Dedoussis GV, Papadopoulos NG, Missitzis I, Stathopoulos GP, Papamichail M. Tumor specific cytolysis by tumor infiltrating lymphocytes in breast cancer. *Cancer* 1994;74:1275.
25. Crannage KE, Rogers K, Jacob G, et al. Factors influencing the establishment of tumour-infiltrating lymphocyte cultures from human breast carcinoma and colon carcinoma tissue. *Eur J Cancer* 1991;27:149.
26. Yannelli JR, Hyatt C, McConnell S, et al. Growth of tumor-infiltrating lymphocytes from human solid cancers: summary of a 5-year experience. *Int J Cancer* 1996;65:413.

27. Dadmarz R, Sgagias MK, Rosenberg SA, Schwartzentruber DJ. CD4+ T lymphocytes infiltrating human breast cancer recognise autologous tumor in an MHC-class-II restricted fashion. *Cancer Immunol Immunother* 1995;40:1.
28. Schwartzentruber DJ, Solomon D, Rosenberg SA, Topalian SL. Characterization of lymphocytes infiltrating human breast cancer: specific immune reactivity detected by measuring cytokine secretion. *J Immunother* 1992;12:1.
29. Coventry BJ, Weeks SC, Heckford SE, Sykes PJ, Bradley J, Skinner JM. Lack of IL-2 cytokine expression despite Il-2 messenger RNA transcription in tumor-infiltrating lymphocytes in primary human breast carcinoma: selective expression of early activation markers. *J Immunol* 1996;156:3486.
30. Wong PY, Staren ED, Tereshkova N, Braun DP. Functional analysis of tumor-infiltrating leukocytes in breast cancer patients. *J Surg Res* 1998;76:95.
31. Linehan DC, Goedegebuure PS, Peoples GE, Rogers SO, Eberlein TJ. Tumor-specific and HLA-A2-restricted cytolysis by tumor-associated lymphocytes in human metastatic breast cancer. *J Immunol* 1995; 155:4486.
32. Disis ML, Calenoff E, Murphy AE, et al. Existent T-cell and antibody immunity to HER2/neu protein in patients with breast cancer. *Cancer Res* 1994;54:16.
33. Pupa SM, Menard S, Andreola S, Colnaghi MI. Antibody response against the c-erbB-2 oncoprotein in breast carcinoma patients. *Cancer Res* 1993;53:5864.
34. Ioannides CG, Whiteside TL. T cell recognition of human tumors: implications for molecular immunotherapy of cancer. *Clin Immunol Immunopathol* 1993;66:91.
35. Disis ML, Pupa SM, Gralow JR, Dittadi R, Menard S, Cheever MA. High-titer HER-2/neu protein-specific antibody can be detected in patients with early-stage breast cancer. *J Clin Oncol* 997;15:3363.
36. Tuttle TM, Anderson BW, Thompson WE, et al. Proliferative and cytokine responses to class II HER-2/neu-associated peptides in breast cancer patients. *Clin Cancer Res* 1998;4:2015.
37. Peoples GE, Goedegebuure PS, Smith R, Linehan DC, Yoshino I, Eberlein TJ. Breast and ovarian cancer-specific cytotoxic T lymphocytes recognize the same HER2/neu-derived peptide. *Proc Natl Acad Sci U S A* 1995;92:432.
38. Slamon DJ, Clark GM, Wong SG, Levin WJ, Ullrich A, McGuire WL. Human breast cancer: correlation of relapse and survival with amplification of the HER-2/neu oncogene. *Science* 1987;235:177.
39. Thor AD, Berry DA, Budman DR, et al. erbB-2, p53, and efficacy of adjuvant therapy in lymph node-positive breast cancer. *J Natl Cancer Inst* 1998;90:1346.
40. Rilke F, Colnaghi M, Cascinelli N, et al. Prognostic significance of HER-2/neu expression in breast cancer and its relationship to other prognostic factors. *Int J Cancer* 1991;49:44.
41. Stewart TH, Retsky MW, Tsai SC, Verma S. Dose response in the treatment of breast cancer. *Lancet* 1994;343:402.
42. Beitsch P, Lotzova E, Hortobagyi G, Pollock R. Natural immunity in breast cancer patients during neoadjuvant chemotherapy and after surgery. *Surg Oncol* 1994;3:211.
43. Berger M, Irschick E, Fritsch E, et al. Influence of local radiotherapy of breast cancer patients on the frequency of cytotoxic T-lymphocyte precursor cells. *Immunobiology* 1990;180:261.
44. Mackall CL, Fleisher TA, Brown MR, et al. Distinctions between CD8+ and CD4+ T-cell regenerative pathways result in prolonged T-cell subset imbalance after intensive chemotherapy. *Blood* 1997; 89:3700.
45. Apostolopoulos V, Popovski V, McKenzie IF. Cyclophosphamide enhances the CTL precursor frequency in mice immunized with MUC1-mannan fusion protein (M-FP). *J Immunother* 1998;21:103.
46. Zielinski CC, Stuller I, Dorner F, Potzi P, Muller C, Eibl MM. Impaired primary, but not secondary, immune response in breast cancer patients under adjuvant chemotherapy. *Cancer* 1986;58:1648.
47. Tang R, Kacinski B, Validire P, et al. Oncogene amplification correlates with dense lymphocyte infiltration in human breast cancers: a role for hematopoietic growth factor release by tumor cells? *J Cell Biochem* 1990;44:189.
48. Lee AH, Happerfield LC, Bobrow LG, Millis RR. Angiogenesis and inflammation in invasive carcinoma of the breast. *J Clin Pathol* 1997;50:669.
49. Pupa SM, Bufalino R, Invernizzi AM, et al. Macrophage infiltrate and prognosis in c-erbB-2-overexpressing breast carcinomas. *J Clin Oncol* 1996;14:85.
50. Hurwitz E, Stancovski I, Sela M, Yarden Y. Suppression and promotion of tumor growth by monoclonal antibodies to ErbB-2 differentially correlate with cellular uptake. *Proc Natl Acad Sci U S A* 1995;92:3353.
51. Kaklamanis L, Leek R, Koukourakis M, Gatter KC, Harris AL. Loss of transporter in antigen processing 1 transport protein and major histocompatibility complex class I molecules in metastatic versus primary breast cancer. *Cancer Res* 1995;55:5191.
52. Vitale M, Rezzani R, Rodella L, et al. HLA class I antigen and transporter associated with antigen processing (TAP1 and TAP2) down-regulation in high-grade primary breast carcinoma lesions. *Cancer Res* 1998;58:737.
53. Cabrera T, Angustias Fernandez M, Sierra A, et al. High frequency of altered HLA class I phenotypes in invasive breast carcinomas. *Hum Immunol* 1996;50:127.
54. Hicklin DJ, Marincola FM, Ferrone S. HLA class I antigen downregulation in human cancers: T-cell immunotherapy revives an old story. *Mol Med Today* 1999;4:178.
55. Seung S, Urban JL, Schreiber H. A tumor escape variant that has lost one major histocompatibility complex class I restriction element induces specific CD8+ T cells to an antigen that no longer serves as a target. *J Exp Med* 1993;178:933.
56. Van Waes C, Monach PA, Urban JL, Wortzel RD, Schreiber H. Immunodominance deters the response to other tumor antigens thereby favoring escape: prevention by vaccination with tumor variants selected with cloned cytolytic T cells in vitro. *Tissue Antigens* 1996;47:399.
57. O'Sullivan C, Lewis CE. Tumour-associated leucocytes: friends or foes in breast carcinoma? *J Pathol* 1994;172:229.
58. Stewart TH, Heppner GH. Immunological enhancement of breast cancer. *Parasitol* 1997;115(Suppl):S141.
59. Lee AH, Happerfield LC, Millis RR, Bobrow LG. Inflammatory infiltrate in invasive lobular and ductal carcinoma of the breast. *Br J Cancer* 1996;74:796.
60. Stewart T, Tsai SC, Grayson H, Henderson R, Opelz G. Incidence of de-novo breast cancer in women chronically immunosuppressed after organ transplantation. *Lancet* 1995;346:796.
61. Basolo F, Calvo S, Fiore L, Conaldi PG, Falcone V, Toniolo A. Growth-stimulating activity of interleukin 6 on human mammary epithelial cells transfected with the int-2 gene. *Cancer Res* 1993;53:2957.
62. Scholl SM, Crocker P, Tang R, Pouillart P, Pollard JW. Is colony-stimulating factor-1 a key mediator of breast cancer invasion and metastasis? *Mol Carcinog* 1993;7:207.
63. Lee AH, Happerfield LC, Bobrow LG, Millis RR. Angiogenesis and inflammation in ductal carcinoma in situ of the breast. *J Pathol* 1997;181:200.
64. Vukanovic J, Isaacs JT. Linomide inhibits angiogenesis, growth, metastasis, and macrophage infiltration within rat prostatic cancers. *Cancer Res* 1995;55:1499.
65. Heppner GH, Miller BE. Enhanced tumor progression following TNF or interferon treatment of mice bearing preneoplastic lesions. *Proc Am Assoc Cancer Res* 1996;37:157.
66. Peoples GE, Blotnick S, Takahashi K, Freeman MR, Klagsbrun M, Eberlein TJ. T lymphocytes that infiltrate tumors and atherosclerotic plaques produce heparin-binding epidermal growth factor–like growth factor and basic fibroblast growth factor: a potential pathologic role. *Proc Natl Acad Sci U S A* 1995;92:6547.
67. Otsuji M, Kimura Y, Aoe T, Okamoto Y, Saito T. Oxidative stress by tumor-derived macrophages suppresses the expression of CD3 zeta chain of T-cell receptor complex and antigen-specific T-cell responses. *Proc Natl Acad Sci U S A* 1996;93:13119.
68. Spiegel D, Sephton SE, Terr AI, Stites DP. Effects of psychosocial treatment in prolonging cancer survival may be mediated by neuroimmune pathways. *Ann N Y Acad Sci* 1998;840:674.
69. Spiegel D. Psychosocial aspects of breast cancer treatment. *Semin Oncol* 1997;24:S1.
70. Finn OJ. Assessing the important effector mechanisms in the immune response against cancer. In Baum A, Anderson B, eds. *Psychosocial interventions in cancer.* 1999 (*in press*).
71. Levy SM, Herberman RB, Maluish AM, Schlien B, Lippman M. Prognostic risk assessment in primary breast cancer survival may be mediated by neuroimmune pathways. *Health Psychol* 1985;4:99.

72. Panerai AE, Sacerdote P. Beta-endorphin in the immune system: a role at last? *Immunol Today* 1997;18:317.
73. Sacerdote P, di San Secondo VE, Sirchia G, Manfredi B, Panerai AE. Endogenous opioids modulate allograft rejection time in mice: possible relation with Th1/Th2 cytokines. *Clin Exp Immunol* 1998;113:465.
74. Wilckens T, De Rijk R. Glucocorticoids and immune function: unknown dimensions and new frontiers. *Immunol Today* 1997;9:418.
75. Blotta MH, DeKruyff RH, Umetsu DT. Corticosteroids inhibit IL-12 production in human monocytes and enhance their capacity to induce IL-4 synthesis in CD4+ lymphocytes. *J Immunol* 1997;158:5589.
76. Andersen BL, Farrar WB, Golden-Kreutz D, et al. Stress and immune responses after surgical treatment for regional breast cancer. *J Natl Cancer Inst* 1998;90:30.
77. Whiteside TL, Herberman RB. Role of human natural killer cells in health and disease. *Clin Diagn Lab Immunol* 1994;1:125.
78. Forsman LM, Jouppila PI, Andersson LC. Sera from multiparous women contain antibodies mediating cytotoxicity against breast carcinoma cells. *Scand J Immunol* 1984;19:135.
79. Janerich DT. The fetal antigen hypothesis for breast cancer, revisited. *Med Hypotheses* 1994;43:105.
80. Botelho F, Clark DA. How might pregnancy immunize against breast cancer? *Am J Reprod Immunol* 1998;39:279.
81. Agrawal B, Reddish MA, Krantz MJ, Longenecker BM. Does pregnancy immunize against breast cancer? *Cancer Res* 1995;55:2254.
82. Naresh KN, Borges AM. Prognostic significance of in situ carcinoma associated with invasive breast carcinoma: a natural experiment in cancer immunology? *Cancer* 1997;79:1846.
83. Black MM, Zachrau RE, Hankey BF, Feuer EJ. Prognostic significance of in situ carcinoma associated with invasive breast carcinoma. A natural experiment in cancer immunology? *Cancer* 1996;78:778.
84. Rosen HR. Placental isoferritin-associated p43 in pregnancy and breast cancer. Minireview. *Neoplasma* 1996;43:354.
85. Rosen HR, Ausch C, Reinerova M, et al. Activated lymphocytes from breast cancer patients express the characteristics of type 2 helper cells—a possible role for breast cancer-associated p43. *Cancer Lett* 1998;127:129.
86. Hilkens J, Vos HL, Wesseling J, et al. Is episialin/MUC1 involved in breast cancer progression? *Cancer Lett* 1995;90:27.
87. Ruiz-Cabello F, Garrido F. HLA and cancer: from research to clinical impact. *Immunol Today* 1998;19:537.
88. Lanier LL. NK cell receptors. *Annu Rev Immunol* 1998;16:359.
89. Garrido F, Ruiz-Cabello F, Cabrera T, et al. Implications for immunosurveillance of altered HLA class I phenotypes in human tumours. *Immunol Today* 1997;18:89.
90. Dolo V, Pizzurro P, Ginestra A, Vittorelli ML. Inhibitory effects of vesicles shed by human breast carcinoma cells on lymphocyte 3H-thymidine incorporation, are neutralised by anti TGF-beta antibodies. *J Submicrosc Cytol Pathol* 1995;27:535.
91. Merendino RA, Arena A, Capozza AB, Chillemi S, Mesiti M. Serum levels of interleukin-10 in patients affected by breast cancer. *Immunol Lett* 1996;53:59.
92. Camp BJ, Dyhrman ST, Memoli VA, Mott LA, Barth RJ Jr. In situ cytokine production by breast cancer tumor-infiltrating lymphocytes. *Ann Surg Oncol* 1996;3:176.
93. Zea AH, Curti BD, Longo DL, et al. Alterations in T cell receptor and signal transduction molecules in melanoma patients. *Clin Cancer Res* 1995;1:1327.
94. Finke JH, Zea AH, Stanley J, et al. Loss of T-cell receptor zeta chain and $p56^{lck}$ in T cells infiltrating human renal cell carcinoma. *Cancer Res* 1993;53:5613.
95. Nagacomi H, Petersson M, Magnusson I, et al. Decreased expression of the signal-transducing zeta chain in tumor-infiltrating T cells, and NK cells of patients with colorectal carcinoma. *Cancer Res* 1993;53:5610.
96. Lai P, Rabinowich H, Crowley-Nowick PA, Bell MC, Mantovani G, Whiteside TL. Alterations in expression and function of signal-transducing proteins in tumor-associated T and natural killer cells in patients with ovarian carcinoma. *Clin Cancer Res* 1996;2:161.
97. Alberola-Ila J, Takaki S, Kerner JD, Perlmutter R. Differential signaling by lymphocyte antigen receptors. *Ann Rev Immunol* 1997;15:125.
98. Ochoa AC, Longo DL. Alteration of signal transduction in T cells from cancer patients. *Important Adv Oncol* 1995;43.
99. Gunji Y, Hori S, Aoe T, et al. High frequency of cancer patients with abnormal assembly of the T cell receptor-CD3 complex in peripheral blood T lymphocytes. *Jpn J Cancer Res* 1994;85:1189.
100. Nieland JD, Loviscek K, Kono K, et al. PBLs of early breast carcinoma patients with a high nuclear grade tumor unlike PBLs of cervical carcinoma patients do not show a decreased TCR zeta expression but are functionally impaired. *J Immunother* 1998;21:317.
101. Marrogi AJ, Munshi A, Merogi AJ, et al. Study of tumor infiltrating lymphocytes and transforming growth factor-beta as prognostic factors in breast carcinoma. *Int J Cancer* 1997;74:492.
102. Murray PA, Barrett-Lee P, Travers M, Luqmani Y, Powles T, Coombes RC. The prognostic significance of transforming growth factors in human breast cancer. *Br J Cancer* 1993;67:1408.
103. Paul WE, Seder RA. Lymphocyte responses and cytokines. *Cell* 1994;76:241.
104. Fearon DT, Locksley RM. The instinctive role of innate immunity in the acquired immune response. *Science* 1996;272:50.
105. Gilboa E, Nair SK, Lyerly HK. Immunotherapy of cancer with dendritic-cell-based vaccines. *Cancer Immunol Immunother* 1998;46:82.
106. Katsumata M, Okudaira T, Samanta A, et al. Prevention of breast tumour development in vivo by downregulation of the p185neu receptor. *Nat Med* 1995;1:644.
107. Pegram MD, Lipton A, Hayes DF, et al. Phase II study of receptor-enhanced chemosensitivity using recombinant humanized anti-p185HER2/neu monoclonal antibody plus cisplatin in patients with HER2/neu-overexpressing metastatic breast cancer refractory to chemotherapy treatment. *J Clin Oncol* 1998;16:2659.
108. Fisk B, Blevins TL, Wharton JT, Ioannides CG. Identification of an immunodominant peptide of HER-2/neu protooncogene recognized by ovarian tumor-specific cytotoxic T lymphocyte lines. *J Exp Med* 1995;181:2109.
109. Disis ML, Gralow JR, Bernhard H, Hand SL, Rubin WD, Cheever MA. Peptide based, but not whole protein, vaccines elicit immunity to HER-2/neu, an oncogenic self protein. *J Immunol* 1996;156:3151.
110. Disis ML, Grabstein KH, Sleath PR, Cheever MA. Generation of immunity to the HER-2/neu oncogenic protein in patients with breast and ovarian cancer using a peptide based vaccine. *Clin Cancer Res* 1999; 6:1289.
111. Zaks TZ, Rosenberg SA. Immunization with a peptide epitope (p369–377) from HER-2/neu leads to peptide-specific cytotoxic T lymphocytes that fail to recognize HER 2/neu + tumors. *Cancer Res* 1998;58:4902.
112. Concetti A, Amici A, Petrelli C, Tibaldi A, Provinciali M, Venanzi FM. Autoantibody to p185erbB2/neu oncoprotein by vaccination with xenogenic DNA. *Cancer Immunol Immunother* 1996;43:307.
113. Chen Y, Hu D, Eling DJ, Robbins J, Kipps TJ. DNA vaccines encoding full-length or truncated Neu induce protective immunity against Neu-expressing mammary tumors. *Cancer Res* 1998;58:1965.
114. Emtage PC, Wan Y, Bramson JL, Graham FL, Gauldie J. A double recombinant adenovirus expressing the costimulatory molecule B7 1 (murine) and human IL-2 induces complete tumor regression in a murine breast adenocarcinoma model. *J Immunol* 1998; 160:2531.
115. Abe M, Kufe D. Characterization of cis-acting elements regulating transcription of the human DF3 breast carcinoma-associated antigen (MUC1) gene. *Proc Natl Acad Sci U S A* 1993;90:282.
116. Apostolopoulos V, Karanikas V, Haurum JS, McKenzie IF. Induction of HLA-A2-restricted CTLs to the mucin 1 human breast cancer antigen. *J Immunol* 1997;159:5211.
117. Jerome KR, Barnd DL, Bendt KM, et al. Cytotoxic T-lymphocytes derived from patients with breast adenocarcinoma recognize an epitope present on the protein core of a mucin molecule preferentially expressed by malignant cells. *Cancer Res* 1991;51:2908.
118. Kotera Y, Fontenot JD, Pecher G, Metzgar RS, Finn OJ. Humoral immunity against a tandem repeat epitope of human mucin MUC-1 in sera from breast, pancreatic, and colon cancer patients. *Cancer Res* 1994;54:2856.
119. von Mensdorff-Pouilly S, Gourevitch MM, Kenemans P, et al. Humoral immune response to polymorphic epithelial mucin (MUC-1) in patients with benign and malignant breast tumours. *Eur J Cancer* 1996;32A:1325.
120. Goydos JS, Elder E, Whiteside TL, Finn OJ, Lotze MT. A phase I trial of a synthetic mucin peptide vaccine. Induction of specific immune reactivity in patients with adenocarcinoma. *J Surg Res* 1996;63:298.
121. Reddish M, MacLean GD, Koganty RR, et al. Anti-MUC1 class I restricted CTLs in metastatic breast cancer patients immunized with a synthetic MUC1 peptide. *Int J Cancer* 1998;76:817.

122. Karanikas V, Hwang LA, Pearson J, et al. Antibody and T cell responses of patients with adenocarcinoma immunized with mannan-MUC1 fusion protein. *J Clin Invest* 1997;100:2783.
123. Apostolopoulos V, Osinski C, McKenzie IF. MUC1 cross-reactive Gal alpha(1,3)Gal antibodies in humans switch immune responses from cellular to humoral. *Nat Med* 1998;4:315.
124. Hiltbold EM, Ciborowski P, Finn OJ. Naturally processed class II epitope from the tumor antigen MUC1 primes human CD4+ T cells. *Cancer Res* 1998;58:5066.
125. Thor AD, Ohuchi N, Szpak CA, Johnston WW, Schlom J. Distribution of oncofetal antigen tumor-associated glycoprotein-72 defined by monoclonal antibody B72.3. *Cancer Res* 1986;46:3118.
126. MacLean GD, Reddish MA, Koganty RR, Longenecker BM. Antibodies against mucin-associated sialyl-Tn epitopes correlate with survival of metastatic adenocarcinoma patients undergoing active specific immunotherapy with synthetic STn vaccine. *J Immunother Emphasis Tumor Immunol* 1996;19:59.
127. Sandmaier BM, Oparin DV, Holmberg LA, Reddish MA, MacLean GD, Longenecker BM. Evidence of a cellular immune response against sialyl-Tn in breast and ovarian cancer patients after high-dose chemotherapy, stem cell rescue, and immunization with Theratope STn-KLH cancer vaccine. *J Immunother* 1999;1:54.
128. Schlichtholz B, Legros Y, Gillet D, et al. The immune response to p53 in breast cancer patients is directed against immunodominant epitopes unrelated to the mutational hot spot. *Cancer Res* 1992;52:6380.
129. Tilkin AF, Lubin R, Soussi T, et al. Primary proliferative T-cell response to wild-type p53 protein in patients with breast cancer. *Eur J Immunol* 1995;25:1765.
130. Regidor PA, Regidor M, Callies R, Schindler AE. Detection of p53 auto-antibodies in the sera of breast cancer patients with a new recurrence using an ELISA assay. Does a correlation with the recurrence free interval exist? *Eur J Gynaecol Oncol* 1996;17:192.
131. Yanuck M, Carbone DP, Pendleton CD, et al. A mutant p53 tumor suppressor protein is a target for peptide-induced CD8+ cytotoxic T cells. *Cancer Res* 1993;53:3257.
132. Noguchi Y, Richards EC, Chen YT, Old LJ. Influence of interleukin 12 on p53 peptide vaccination against established Meth A sarcoma. *Proc Natl Acad Sci U S A* 1995;92:2219.
133. Theobald M, Biggs J, Hernandez J, Lustgarten J, Labadie C, Sherman LA. Tolerance to p53 by A2.1-restricted cytotoxic T lymphocytes. *J Exp Med* 1997;185:833.
134. Gnjatic S, Cai Z, Viguier M, Chouaib S, Guillet JG, Choppin J. Accumulation of the p53 protein allows recognition by human CTL of a wild-type p53 epitope presented by breast carcinomas and melanomas. *J Immunol* 1998;160:328.
135. Ropke M, Regner M, Claesson MH. T cell-mediated cytotoxicity against p53-protein derived peptides in bulk and limiting dilution cultures of healthy donors. *Scand J Immunol* 1995;42:98.
136. Nijman HW, Van-der-Burg SH, Vierboom MP, Houbiers JG, Kast WM, Melief CJ. p53, a potential target for tumor-directed T cells. *Immunol Lett* 1994;40:171.
137. van der Bruggen P, Traversari C, Chomez P, et al. A gene encoding an antigen recognized by cytolytic T lymphocytes on a human melanoma. *Science* 1991;254:1643.
138. Uria JA, Velasco G, Santamaria I, Ferrando A, Lopez-Otin C. Prostate-specific membrane antigen in breast carcinoma. *Lancet* 1997;349:1601.
139. Diamandis EP, Yu H. Prostate-specific antigen and lack of specificity for prostate cells. *Lancet* 1995;345:1186.
140. Hall RE, Clements JA, Birrell SN, Tilley WD. Prostate-specific antigen and gross cystic disease fluid protein-15 are co-expressed in androgen receptor-positive breast tumours. *Br J Cancer* 1998;78:360.
141. Essand M, Pastan I. Anti-prostate immunotoxins: cytotoxicity of E4 antibody-Pseudomonas exotoxin constructs. *Int J Cancer* 1998;77:123.
142. Liu K-J, Chatta GS, Twardzik DR, et al. Identification of rat prostatic steroid binding protein as a target antigen of experimental autoimmune prostatitis: implication for prostate cancer therapy. *J Immunol* 1997;159:472.
143. Fong L, Ruegg CL, Brockstedt D, Engleman EG, Laus R. Induction of tissue-specific autoimmune prostatitis with prostatic acid phosphatase immunization: implications for immunotherapy of prostate cancer. *J Immunol* 1997;159:3113.
144. Min CJ, Tafra L, Verbanac KM. Identification of superior markers for polymerase chain reaction detection of breast cancer metastases in sentinel lymph nodes. *Cancer Res* 1998;58:4581.
145. Watson MA, Darrow C, Zimonjic DB, Popescu NC, Fleming TP. Structure and transcriptional regulation of the human mammaglobin gene, a breast cancer associated member of the uteroglobin gene family localized to 11q13. *Oncogene* 1998;16:817.
146. Coveney E, Wheatley GHI, Lyerly HK. Active immunization using dendritic cells mixed with tumor cells inhibits the growth of primary breast cancer. *Surgery* 1997;122:228.
147. Fisch P, Kohler G, Garbe A, et al. Generation of antigen-presenting cells for soluble protein antigens ex vivo from peripheral blood CD34+ hematopoietic progenitor cells in cancer patients. *Eur J Immunol* 1996;26:595.
148. Cheever MA, Chen W. Therapy with cultured T cells: principles revisited. *Immunological Rev* 1997;157:177.
149. Lind DS, Tuttle TM, Bethke KP, Frank JL, McCrady CW, Bear HD. Expansion and tumour specific cytokine secretion of bryostatin-activated T-cells from cryopreserved axillary lymph nodes of breast cancer patients. *Surg Oncol* 1993;2:273.
150. Collins RH Jr, Shpilberg O, Drobyski WR, et al. Donor leukocyte infusions in 140 patients with relapsed malignancy after allogeneic bone marrow transplantation. *J Clin Oncol* 1997;15:433.
151. Eibl B, Schwaighofer H, Nachbaur D, Marth C, et al. Evidence for a graft-versus-tumor effect in a patient treated with marrow ablative chemotherapy and allogeneic bone marrow transplantation for breast cancer. *Blood* 1996;88:1501.
152. Morecki S, Yacovlev E, Diab A, Slavin S. Allogenic cell therapy for a murine mammary carcinoma. *Cancer Res* 1998;58:3891.
153. Racila E, Euhus D, Weiss AJ, et al. Detection and characterization of carcinoma cells in the blood. *Proc Natl Acad Sci U S A* 1998;95:4589.
154. Eaton MC, Hardingham JE, Kotasek D, Dobrovic A. Immunobead RT-PCR: a sensitive method for detection of circulating tumor cells. *Biotechniques* 1997;22:100.

CHAPTER 51

Diseases of the Breast, 2nd ed.,
edited by Jay R. Harris.
Lippincott Williams & Wilkins, Philadelphia © 2000.

Biological Therapy

Neal Rosen, Laura Sepp-Lorenzino, and Marc E. Lippman

Progress in combined modality-therapy has not been sufficient to cure patients with advanced-stage breast cancer. The hope for future major advances that could achieve cure of these patients has been placed in what has been broadly called *biological therapy*. This term has not been rigorously defined. It tends to be used to denote any therapy designed to directly interfere with the molecular pathways responsible for tumorigenesis, to stimulate host resistance to the tumor, or to restore the normal, nonmalignant phenotype to the cancer cell. The common feature of these therapies is their selective action on targets required for tumor viability and progression, unlike radiation therapy and traditional forms of chemotherapy.[1–6] For example, retinoids are remarkably effective in treating acute promyelocytic leukemia, a cancer dependent on a fusion protein containing part of retinoic acid receptor α.

This distinction between biological and traditional therapy is artificial. Taxanes were discovered and are considered to be traditional cytotoxics with selective activity against some tumors. They were found later to be natural products that bind to a specific site in tubulin and prevent microtubule depolymerization.[7] Selective toxicity to tumors may be a result of tumor cell–specific alterations in mitotic checkpoint pathways. Yet, these drugs are not considered to be biological therapies.

The use of this term reflects the idea that inhibition of pathways required for tumor growth or metastasis is more effective and less toxic than chemotherapy. In some sense, the effectiveness and tolerability of antiestrogen and antiandrogen therapy in breast and prostate cancer is proof of this principle. The identification and molecular characterization of signaling pathways responsible for abnormal growth, inhibition of apoptosis, cellular invasion and metastasis, and angiogenesis have generated a plethora of targets for new therapeutic agents. Advances in medicinal and combinatorial chemistry, antibody manufacture, and biotechnology have made possible the rapid development of potent selective agents that affect these pathways. Over the next several years, a major proportion of clinical research will be devoted to testing new biological therapies. The challenge now is to identify the best targets and to develop effective ways for testing the clinical efficacy of their inhibitors.

TARGETS FOR BIOLOGICAL THERAPY

A revolution in the understanding of the molecular basis for oncogenesis has occurred since the early 1950s. Work in this area has shown that mutations in genes that encode proteins involved in the regulation of cellular proliferation, differentiation, apoptosis, and invasion are responsible for the phenotype of the cancer cell.[8–13] This body of work has allowed the elucidation in more or less detail of the molecular pathways responsible for these phenomena. Much of the current work on the development of biological therapies is aimed at devising strategies for the return of these pathways to the normal state, inhibiting dysregulated processes and replacing normal pathways that have been inactivated.

The decision as to whether a particular process represents a valid target is based on whether it is altered in a significant number of tumors and whether this alteration is required for their growth, viability, or invasion.[4,14] Some molecular lesions may be required for tumor development but exert no effect in late, established cancers.

REGULATORS OF PROLIFERATION

Much attention has been given to pathways required for proliferation. As outlined in Chapters 15 and 19, many of the components of the intrinsic cell cycle machinery have been identified. Furthermore, the signaling pathways whereby extracellular factors regulate proliferation have been delineated to some degree.[15] Most of the protooncogene and suppressor-gene products that have been identified function normally as elements of these pathways. Thus, the retinoblastoma and p16 suppressor oncogenes are frequently inactivated by mutations, and the cyclin D family is often overexpressed early in the development of breast cancer.[8,9] In

N. Rosen: Department of Medicine, Cell Biology, and Genetics, Memorial Sloan-Kettering Cancer Center, New York, New York

L. Sepp-Lorenzino: Memorial Sloan-Kettering Cancer Center, New York, New York

M. E. Lippman: Departments of Pharmacology and Medicine, Lombardi Cancer Center, Georgetown University Medical Center, Washington, D.C.

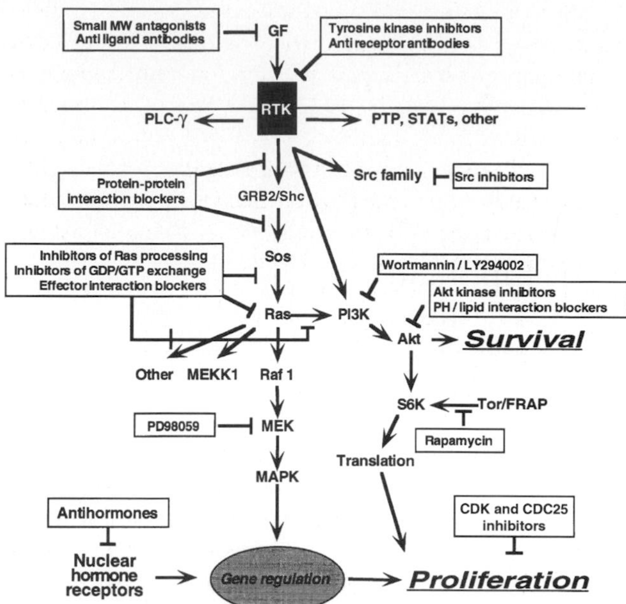

FIG. 1. Biological therapies targeting the signal transduction pathway of growth factor receptors. CDK, cyclin-dependent kinase; GF, growth factor; GDP, guanosine diphosphate; GTP, guanosine triphosphate; MAPK, mitogen-activated protein kinase; MEK, MAPK-kinase; MEKK1, MAPK-kinase-kinase 1; MW, molecular weight; PH, pleckstrin homology domain; PI3K, phosphatidylinositol 3'-kinase; PLC, phospholipase C; PTP, protein tyrosine phosphatase; RTK, receptor tyrosine kinase; S6K, ribosomal S6 kinase; STATs, signal transduction- and transcription-activating transcription factors.

tumors with wild-type retinoblastoma protein, the activity of the complex of cyclin D and the cyclin-dependent kinases (CDKs) CDK4 and CDK6 is almost always activated, either by cyclin D overexpression or by loss of the p16 cyclin kinase inhibitor.[16–18] Therefore, inhibitors of CDK4 are being developed because of their potential usefulness in many cancers. Other cyclin kinases are being targeted as well.

Similarly, growth factors bind to receptors activating complex ramified pathways that transduce the mitogenic signal, in part by stimulating the cell cycle machinery (Fig. 1). Ligand activation of receptor tyrosine kinases leads to receptor autophosphorylation and engagement of second messenger molecules that activate distinct pathways.[19–21] These include the Ras/Raf/mitogen-activated protein (MAP) kinase pathway, the phosphatidylinositol 3'-kinase (PI3-kinase)/Akt pathway, phospholipases, and the STAT transcription factors.[22–27] In breast cancer, overexpression of growth factors and several of the receptor tyrosine kinases is a common event. Prominent among the latter are members of the HER kinase family, including HER-2.[28,29] Amplification of the HER-2 gene occurs in 20% to 30% of human breast cancers and is associated with poor prognosis, although its biological consequences are not really understood.[30,31] Antibodies directed against HER-2 have antitumor activity in animals and humans (see HER2 section). This work may be considered as proof of the principle that selective inhibition of particular signal transduction pathways can be useful therapeutically.

Mutations in the *ras* gene family have been found in approximately 30% of human tumors, but no mutations in *ras* or *raf* have been described in breast cancers.[32,33] Nevertheless, activation of the growth factor or receptor that initiates the cascade ought to lead to and require activation of the downstream signaling molecules to maintain cell growth. Thus, these molecules have also become targets for development of therapies.

The *PTEN* tumor-suppressor gene has been shown to be inactivated in a significant number of breast cancers.[34–36] The protein product of this gene is both a protein and a phospholipid phosphatase. One of its preferred substrates is phosphatidylinositol 3'-phosphate (PI(3')P).[37] This phospholipid is generated when PI3-kinase is activated as a result of receptor tyrosine kinase activation. PI(3')P activates another protein kinase, Akt, that causes both induction of cyclin D expression and inhibition of programmed cell death.[38–40] PTEN dephosphorylates PI(3')P and inactivates this pathway. One would predict that the activation of receptor tyrosine kinases and the inactivation of PTEN in breast cancers would lead to marked, unregulated increases in PI(3')P and activation of Akt. Inhibitors of Akt would block this pathway and cause growth inhibition and apoptosis.[6]

THERAPEUTIC INDEX

Results in cellular model systems strongly suggest that effective inhibition of any of the key elements of the cell cycle machinery or mitogenic signal transduction pathways blocks the growth of cancer cells. Most or all of these proteins, however, are thought to play a central role in the normal physiologic regulation of proliferation and other processes. Potent inhibitors of these processes would be expected to have profound effects on the host. Preliminary data with the first generation of signal transduction inhibitors show that this is not necessarily the case. Farnesyl transferase inhibitors, drugs that inhibit the processing of wild-type Ras, and MEK inhibitors that prevent MAP kinase activation are both relatively nontoxic at doses that inhibit tumor growth in mice.[41,42] The outstanding question is why these drugs have a therapeutic index. These data suggest that the understanding of these pathways is at best incomplete and does not allow valid prediction of the consequences of their inhibition. At this time, *a priori* deductions as to whether a particular therapeutic strategy selectively affects the tumor at any dose are probably not warranted. The task of choosing targets for drug development is therefore that much more difficult.

NUCLEAR RECEPTORS

Activation of signal transduction pathways by growth factors leads in part to functional activation of DNA-binding proteins that regulate the transcription of ensembles of genes. Other hormones (steroids, retinoids, vitamin D) bind directly to nuclear transcription factors and alter their activity. These hormones have complex effects on cells and may alter function and stimulate growth or differentiation.

Therapies based on preventing the hormone-dependent growth of breast cancers, either by removing the ovaries or by treating with hormone antagonists that bind to the receptor, are described extensively elsewhere in this volume. These therapies may be considered as among the first useful "biological therapies." They are rationally designed strategies to selectively inhibit a particular protein required for breast cancer growth.[43] They are effective and relatively nontoxic.[44,45] Interest continues in the development of tissue-specific antiestrogens and agents that inhibit estrogen-independent activation of the estrogen receptor.

Other hormones that bind to nuclear receptors cause growth inhibition and sometimes differentiation of breast cancer cells. These include retinoids and vitamin D. In experimental systems for breast and other cancers, these agents can induce varying degrees of differentiation and tumor regression. Clinical trials are now in progress with a variety of vitamin D and retinoid analogues.[46–48] The oral availability and predicted low toxicity of these compounds have led to the suggestion that they could be given over the long term to healthy, high-risk women to prevent cancer.[49–50] Retinoids have been effective when used in this way in patients at high risk for development of head and neck cancer.

APOPTOSIS

The past decade has brought recognition that both normal development and tumorigenesis represent a balance between the regulated proliferation and death of cells.[39,51,52] Programmed cell death, or *apoptosis*, is an induced, regulated suicide of the cell resulting from the activation of a cascade of proteases called *caspases*.[53,54] Apoptosis is required for normal development and tissue remodeling, and in metazoan cells is a fundamental response to various forms of cellular damage.[51,52,55] Radiation therapy and many forms of cytotoxic chemotherapy cause the apoptotic death of cancer cells.

Mutations that cause unregulated stimulation of cell growth or unbalanced activation of the cell cycle lead to apoptosis.[39,51] Oncogenic transformation therefore must be associated with inhibition or suppression of the apoptotic pathway. Several antiapoptotic proteins are overexpressed in tumor cells.[12,13] At least one, Bcl-2, acts as an oncogene.[56] Several growth factors, notably type I insulinlike growth factor (IGF-I), activate Akt kinase–mediated antiapoptotic pathways.[57–59] The p53 tumor-suppressor gene mediates apoptosis in response to DNA damage; this pathway is attenuated or lost in many of the tumors in which p53 is inactivated.[60–62]

Thus, suppression of the apoptotic response is a fundamental property of cancer cells. An ancillary consequence of this suppression is resistance to radiation and chemotherapy.[12,13] Targeting of antiapoptotic pathways is an attractive therapeutic strategy for at least two reasons. First, inhibitors of these pathways should lead to the death of tumor cells with aberrantly regulated growth. Second, such inhibitors should enhance the effectiveness of DNA-damaging agents and other drugs that induce apoptosis.

Active programs exist for the identification of inhibitors of Akt and IGF-I receptor expression and function.[2,6,63–65] A phase I clinical trial of an antisense inhibitor of Bcl-2 expression has been completed, and the inhibitor has shown clinical activity in lymphoma patients. Bcl-2 prevents apoptosis by binding to and sequestering certain proapoptotic proteins, such as Bad.[56] Overexpression of Bcl-2 is associated with oncogenesis and decreased apoptosis in response to cytotoxics.[13,66,67] These properties suggest that an antisense compound to Bcl-2 would be useful when given in combination with chemotherapeutic agents. Several trials addressing this issue are now in progress, including one in breast cancer patients in which the antisense compound is given together with a taxane.

Another therapeutic strategy involves the activation of apoptotic pathways. Such activation could involve introduction into the cell of proapoptotic tumor-suppressor genes, such as the p53 gene,[68–71] or the activation of intact physiologic pathways, such as those regulated by tumor necrosis factor or ceramide.[72]

INVASION, METASTASIS, AND ANGIOGENESIS

Loss of normal interactions with surrounding cells and extracellular matrix, invasion through the basement membrane, and the potential to metastasize to distant organs are fundamental properties of cancer cells.[73–77] Furthermore, significant growth of the tumor mass probably requires the new blood vessel formation induced by the tumor cell.[76,78] Although much of molecular cancer research has concentrated on the pathways responsible for dysregulated growth, patient mortality is almost invariably due to metastasis. Metastatic processes are therefore attractive targets for therapy. Loss of adhesion molecules required for interactions with stroma and neighboring epithelial cells, constitutive activation of growth pathways that normally require integrin interactions, activation of the proteolysis of basement membrane components, and expression of angiogenic factors are common properties of cancer cells.[73–77] A variety of metalloproteinases, collagenase, and other neutral proteinases are overexpressed in invasive breast cancer, and the metalloproteinase inhibitor proteins are often dysregulated.[75,77] Thus, multiple processes are probably necessary for systemic dissemination of cancer that provide targets amenable to inhibition.[79,80] The development of selective inhibitors of tumor invasion or angiogenesis is generating a great deal of activity and excitement.[78,81–84] These are discussed elsewhere in this book.

Several representative strategies are mentioned here for their heuristic value. Cellular invasion and metastasis depend on altered adhesion to normal cells and proteolytic degradation of the basement membrane.[74] Degradation of the extracellular matrix involves the concerted action of a number of proteolytic systems and safeguarding inhibitors expressed by the tumor and surrounding stromal cells. These include the urokinase-type plasminogen activator (uPA) system, matrix metalloproteinases (MMPs), and other extracellular proteases.[77] MMPs and uPA are highly expressed by some tumors, and their levels can serve as prognostic and predictive factors.[85] Studies of breast cancer patients demonstrated that the levels of uPA and neu in tumors were correlated with relapse rate.[86–88] Moreover, thrombospondin 1 was shown to up-regulate the uPA system and promote breast cancer invasion.[89,90] The uPA system regulates the production of plasmin from plasminogen. The activator uPA is secreted by tumor and normal cells and binds to the uPA receptor on the cell surface. Its extracellular activity is regulated by specific inhibitors, serpin a2 antiplasmin and plasminogen activator inhibitors types 1 and 2 (PAI-1 and PAI-2).[91,92] As with uPA, the level of expression of PAI-1 has been found to have predictive value.[93]

Preclinical studies have demonstrated that targeting of MMPs and of the uPA system are valid strategies for affecting tumor growth.[85,94] Tressler et al. identified urokinase receptor peptide antagonists by a combination of phage display libraries and synthesis of peptide analogues. These antagonists were effective in blocking the growth of MDA-MB-231 breast cancer cells grafted in nude mice.[95] Moreover, a noncatalytic fragment of uPA fused to the CH_2 and CH_3 regions of the mouse immunoglobulin IgG1 was shown to specifically bind to human uPA receptor, to prevent binding of uPA, and to inhibit tumor growth *in vivo*.[96] Anti-uPA monoclonal antibodies are also being developed that exhibit potent cytolytic effects against human breast cancer cells.[97] Other strategies being tested include enzymatic cleavage of the uPA receptor with glycosylphosphatidylinositol-specific phospholipase C, antisense oligonucleotide targeting of the uPA receptor, and inhibition of plasminogen binding.[90]

Adhesion molecules—the integrin system, in particular—are also being targeted for therapy. The integrin family is composed of heterodimeric $\alpha\beta$ transmembrane receptors involved in establishing cell-matrix interactions. Integrins recognize the Arg/Gly/Asp (RGD) sequences present in extracellular matrix components such as fibronectin, vitronectin, vascular cell adhesion molecules, etc. Specific integrins mediate organ-specific interactions. For example, the vitronectin receptor ($\alpha_v\beta_3$ integrin), which mediates bone attachment for osteoclasts, is overexpressed in bone breast cancer metastasis.[98,99] Possibly, then, inhibiting the vitronectin receptor might prevent bone metastasis in breast cancer patients. Several RGD-based peptidomimetic inhibitors and antiintegrin antibodies (LM609 and Vitaxin) are being tested as potential chemotherapeutic drugs.[100–102] An alternative approach involves naturally occurring RGD-containing peptides called *disintegrins*.[103] These proteins were originally identified in snake venoms and were shown to prevent adhesion by interfering with integrin binding. Disintegrins may be useful not only in prevention of platelet aggregation and as antiangiogenesis agents, by preventing endothelial cell attachment, but also as antimetastatic agents.[104]

The microvasculatures of different tissues can be distinguished from one another on the basis of specific surface markers and biological properties. Furthermore, the neovasculature induced by tumors has different characteristics than that of the tissue of origin.[74,76] These differences can be used as tools for directing toxic therapy to the tumor or its blood vessels.[105] Ruoslahti and his coworkers used phage display libraries to isolate peptides that target the blood vessels in a tissue-specific manner.[106,107] They linked cytotoxic drugs to these peptides and caused the selective death of tumor cells, which resulted in marked antitumor response in animals.[108] Whether this sort of strategy works by killing the tumor vasculature and thus the tumor, or whether it serves to concentrate the cytotoxic drug at the tumor site and thus kill tumor cells directly, is not clear. In either case, these results provide proof of principle that targeting therapy to the tumor endothelium can be effective.

Several major unanswered questions remain regarding this approach. The details of the complex interplay of cellular receptors, matrix components, proteinases, and protein inhibitors responsible for cellular migration are poorly understood. Furthermore, the normal function and potential redundant relationships among these proteins is undefined. Choosing the appropriate target is difficult. The best clinical setting for the use of such drugs is also unclear.[84,109–111] They might be cytostatic and effective only as adjuvant therapy or for minimal disease. One is then faced with the prospect of performing large-scale adjuvant studies on drugs that show no hint of activity in preliminary trials in advanced disease. This may be a general problem in the testing of biological agents, many of which may be most useful against micrometastases or less advanced disease.

THERAPEUTIC STRATEGIES

Most of the therapeutic strategies described here involve the inhibition or replacement of the function of specific proteins. The efficient development of modalities that can accomplish these goals has been made possible by rapid advances in molecular biology, nucleic acid and peptide chemistry, combinatorial chemistry, and antibody generation. Gene therapy and immunotherapy are described in other chapters. These technical advances have allowed the development of specific potent reagents for the inhibition or modulation of the targeted protein.[4–6] Whereas in the past, the major impediment to progress was the development of such compounds, the likely problem in the future is how to choose the most promising strategies and how to test them.[4,14] The remainder of this chapter is devoted to a more detailed discussion of the development of inhibitors of mitogenic signal transduction. These are the most well-delineated pathways and are probably farthest along in terms of development of clinical inhibitors. Furthermore, the successful use of anti–HER-2 antibodies in the treatment of metastatic breast cancer provides validation of this approach.

GROWTH FACTOR RECEPTORS

Multiple transmembrane growth factor receptors have been found to be highly expressed or activated in human tumors.[30,31,112] Mutational or ligand-induced activation of these receptors is required for malignant transformation in many experimental animal and tissue culture systems and is presumed to play an equally important role in a substantial fraction of human tumors. HER family and IGF family kinases transduce mitogenic growth factor signals,[113–116] activation of IGF-I receptor strongly inhibits apoptosis,[57,117,118] and Met and fibroblast growth factor (FGF) and vascular endothelial growth factor (VEGF) receptor kinases play important roles in stimulating invasion, metastasis, and angiogenesis.[76,78,83,119]

For a variety of reasons, receptor tyrosine kinases were among the first targets for the development of biological therapy.[3,120] First, they are of clear importance for both carcinogenesis and tumor progression. Second, fairly straightforward strategies exist for receptor kinase inhibition. Monoclonal antibodies directed against the extracellular domain of several of these receptors have been isolated.[121] Some of these block receptor action by preventing ligand binding or receptor dimerization or by altering receptor internalization. Previous difficulties with immune response to the antibody have been solved, for the most part, with the advent of humanized antibodies.[122] However, efficient delivery of these large molecules to all tissue spaces remains problematic.

Other means of inhibiting receptor tyrosine kinases are possible. The biological function of these proteins is dependent on their enzymatic activity. Potent small-molecule tyrosine kinase inhibitors should effectively inhibit receptor tyrosine kinase function, perhaps more efficiently than antibodies. The problem is specificity; hundreds of cellular tyrosine kinases exist, and they are involved in regulating most cellular processes. The techniques of combinatorial and synthetic chemistry, together with rapid robotic screening of libraries of compounds, have allowed the identification of selective small-molecule inhibitors.[120,123–125] Most of these interact with the catalytic or adenosine triphosphate–binding site of the enzyme. Inhibitors that selectively inhibit the activity of HER family, platelet-derived growth factor receptor, VEGF receptor, and Src family tyrosine kinases have been identified, and all but the last are in early clinical trial.[76,84,110,123,125–127]

Small molecules that bind to the extracellular domain of growth factor receptors and prevent ligand binding without activating the receptor are also being studied.[128–131] The potential advantages of such molecules compared with antibodies are ease of manufacture and increased bioavailability. Other therapeutic strategies take advantage of these receptors as overexpressed or mutated proteins at the surface of the cancer cell. These therapies target the immune response or toxic substances to the tumor. Liposome-encapsulated toxins or plasmids may be directed to cancer cells with antireceptor antibodies.[105,132–134] Biological toxins and radionuclides can be covalently linked or chelated with these antibodies. Finally, mutated receptors with an altered extracellular domain are true tumor-specific antigens that could be used in the development of vaccines or other immunotherapy.[135]

In breast cancer, the receptors that have been studied most intensely as therapeutic targets are members of the HER kinase family, epidermal growth factor receptor (EGFR), and HER-2.

Epidermal Growth Factor Receptor

Epidermal growth factor receptor (EGFR) is a transmembrane receptor tyrosine kinase that is the archetype of the HER kinase family. This family contains four closely related members (HER-1 through HER-4) that transduce the mitogenic signal of several extracellular growth factors.[28,136] Growth factor binding to an HER kinase induces homodimerization or heterodimerization of the kinase with other members of the family, tyrosine kinase activation, and receptor auto- or transphosphorylation with attendant transduction of the growth signal. Several families of ligands bind to these receptors, including the heregulins (or neu differentiating factors, NDFs) that bind to HER-3 and HER-4 and seven different ligands that bind to EGFR. These latter include members of the epidermal growth factor (EGF) family.

Almost all breast cancers express one or more members of the HER kinase family. EGF and transforming growth factor α (TGF-α) are mitogenic for many breast cancer cells, and EGFR is overexpressed in many tumors and amplified in some.[30,31,114,137,138] Furthermore, EGFR and EGFR ligands are coexpressed in many breast cancer cell lines, so that they contain a potential autocrine growth loop.[114] These findings led to the hypothesis that inhibition of EGFR would be useful as antitumor therapy. Mendelsohn and his colleagues developed a monoclonal antibody (225) directed against the extracellular domain of EGFR and pioneered the development of antigrowth factor therapy in their studies of this reagent.[139,140] Antibody 225 binds to EGFR and blocks its activation by ligand.[141] The antibody itself has little or no agonist activity.[141] Addition of the antibody to most cancer cell lines that express high levels of EGFR causes only modest growth inhibition. However, the antibody has much greater inhibitory activity against mouse xenografts of human cancer cells that overexpress EGFR.[140]

These include MDA-MB-468, a breast cancer cell line. The reason for the discrepancy between the *in vitro* and animal data is not known. Although the antibody is presumed to work by blocking signaling, an immune mechanism has not been completely ruled out. Fab fragments of the antibody do have some activity *in vivo*.[142,143] The antibody might exert its effects on tumor stroma or in a paracrine fashion. Tumors treated with 225 have decreased blood vessel density, and inhibition of angiogenesis has been invoked as the mechanism of tumor inhibition in animals.[121] Mendelsohn's group tested in animal models whether blockade of the EGF receptor could be usefully combined with chemotherapy. They found that antibody 225 acted synergistically with doxorubicin (doxorubicin hydrochloride), cisplatin, or taxanes in its ability to kill breast cancer xenografts in mice.[144] Similar data were obtained with trastuzumab (Herceptin), an antibody directed against HER-2.[145]

The mechanism whereby blockade of HER kinase signaling acts synergistically with toxic drugs is not yet understood. Activation of transmembrane tyrosine kinases, notably IGF-I receptor, inhibits apoptosis[57,117,118] through Akt kinase and NFkB-dependent pathways. These signals may also directly regulate DNA repair. These findings suggest that some antireceptor antibodies may be effective when given in combination with radiation and chemotherapeutic agents.[145–147] This suggestion has been confirmed in a trial in which trastuzumab and Taxol (semisynthetic paclitaxel) showed benefit in advanced breast cancer.[148,149]

The 225 antibody has been tested clinically, and some activity has been seen in head and neck cancer. Its use in breast cancer has been limited by the low frequency of EGF receptor amplification or overexpression observed in this disease. In phase I trials of 225 and doxorubicin in breast cancer, the dose-limiting toxicity was a marked folliculitis not seen with either drug alone.[150]

HER-2

Another member of the HER kinase family seems to play a more prominent role in the development of breast cancer. HER-2 is a transmembrane kinase closely related to EGFR. No ligand that binds to HER-2 with high affinity has been isolated. Rather, the binding of ligand to EGFR or especially to HER-3 or HER-4 causes these receptors to heterodimerize with HER-2. This activates the HER-2 tyrosine kinase and is associated with transphosphorylation and autophosphorylation of the members of the heterodimer and the initiation of signals that lead to mitogenesis and inhibition of apoptosis.[28,29,136]

HER-2 was originally identified as amplified in several human mammary carcinoma cell lines. It was subsequently shown to be amplified and overexpressed in many human tumors and has been most intensely investigated in mammary carcinomas.[151] HER-2 is overexpressed in 50% to 60% of ductal carcinomas *in situ*, in almost all comedo-type carcinomas, and in 20% to 30% of infiltrating ductal carcinomas.[30,31] Amplification or overexpression of HER-2/neu is associated with poor prognosis in breast cancer patients. Patients bearing tumors with elevated HER-2/neu levels have a shorter disease-free survival and increased relapse rates.[30,31] These tumors tend to be resistant to certain forms of chemotherapy, including cyclophosphamide (Cytoxan), methotrate, and 5-fluorouracil, perhaps because of decreased induction of apoptosis.[152]

Overexpression of HER-2 probably plays a role in the development of the tumors in which it is present. Overexpression is often secondary to gene amplification, which usually occurs and is maintained because of positive selective pressure. Expression of mutationally activated HER-2 and overexpression of wild-type HER-2 when other HER family kinases are also expressed cause the malignant transformation of immortalized fibroblast and mammary epithelial cell lines.[28,29,136] Furthermore, transgenic mice that express high levels of or activated HER-2 in the mammary gland develop breast tumors at a high frequency.[153] These data and the association of overexpression with poor prognosis in human tumors suggest that HER-2 is a logical target for the development of biological therapies. The high frequency of HER-2 overexpression in ductal carcinoma *in situ* remains to be explained, however.

Several strategies are being used for inhibition of HER-2 function or expression. The first of these uses monoclonal antibodies directed against the extracellular domain of HER-2.[154,155] Studies in animals have shown that such antibodies are effective in inhibiting the growth of tumor xenografts that overexpress HER-2. Like the anti-EGFR antibodies, the anti–HER-2 antibodies have been demonstrated to have much greater inhibitory activity against xenografts than tumor cells grown in tissue culture. Activity seems to be confined to tumors in which HER-2 is overexpressed.[156] Finally, these antibodies also synergize with cytotoxic drugs, such as Taxol and doxorubicin, to inhibit tumor growth in mice.[144,145,156] These findings led to the development and testing of a humanized monoclonal antibody that binds to HER-2 (rhuMAb HER-2 or trastuzumab).[154,155,157] Phase I studies of this antibody showed that therapeutic serum concentrations were achievable and toxicity was low, consisting of low-grade fevers in a minority of patients. In phase II studies, in which the antibody alone was administered to women with previously treated metastatic breast cancer whose tumors overexpressed HER-2, a 10% to 15% response rate was achieved.[158] The responses lasted for an average of 5 months, although some were more durable. These encouraging data, the minimal toxicity of the antibody, and the preclinical data showing synergy with cytotoxic drugs led to several combination studies. Phase II studies showed the feasibility of giving the drug in combination with cisplatin, doxorubicin, or Taxol. A randomized phase III study, in which trastuzumab was used in combination with first-line chemotherapy (adriamycin-cyclophosphamide or paclitaxel), extended the disease-free survival period and increased the response rate achieved by the cytotoxic drug alone.[157] The incidence of cardiotoxicity with the trastuzumab-doxorubicin combination, however, was significantly greater than that seen with doxorubicin alone.

These studies provide the first convincing evidence that blockade of activated signaling pathways can be useful in the treatment of human tumors. They also corroborate the *in vitro* and animal data that show synergistic activity of anti-receptor antibodies and cytotoxic agents. The frequency and duration of response to the antibody when given alone or in combination are modest, however. Several possible reasons for this result can be cited. First, the HER-2 pathway may not be activated or may not be required for the growth of most tumors in which HER-2 is overexpressed. If this is the case, other methods for inhibiting HER-2 function will not be any more effective than trastuzumab. The other possibility is that trastuzumab does not optimally inhibit transduction of the growth signal initiated by HER-2. The antibody may not fully penetrate tumor tissue and may not efficiently or durably inhibit receptor function. Furthermore, trastuzumab is a partial agonist of the HER-2 receptor, which may limit its effectiveness. Finally, the possibility exists that HER-2 exerts a growth signal together with other receptors and that inhibition of HER-2 alone has only marginal effects on tumor cell growth.

An intense search is therefore under way for alternative methods of inhibiting the HER family of receptors. Other anti–HER-2 antibodies are being sought that more efficiently block signaling or receptor dimerization and do not act as partial agonists.[159] Small molecules are also being developed that bind to the extracellular domain of the receptor and thus mimic antibody action by preventing ligand binding and receptor dimerization and activation. Such small molecules would be less likely to cause allergic reactions and would probably have greater tissue penetration.

Another strategy is therapeutic inhibition of receptor function rather than blockade of receptor activation. Many commercial and academic laboratories have been successful in synthesizing selective tyrosine kinase inhibitors.[3,120,123–125] Most of these are small molecules that bind to the adenosine triphosphate–binding site of the kinase. Specificity is conferred by the portion of the molecule that binds to nearby amino side chains that are peculiar to the specific kinase. In this way, inhibitors of the platelet-derived growth factor receptor and the VEGF receptor tyrosine kinases have been isolated and are presently in early clinical trial.[76,84,110,160,161] Similarly, several groups have isolated potent and relatively specific inhibitors of the HER family of tyrosine kinases. For the most part, these inhibitors are not selective for individual members of the family.[124,125] The advantages of such inhibitors are that, in tissue culture systems, they can completely suppress HER kinase activity and presumably signaling, and that as small molecules they are more likely to penetrate the tumor tissue efficiently. The theoretical disadvantage is decreased specificity compared with that of monoclonal antibodies, which react to a particular tyrosine kinase. An inhibitor of the entire family of HER kinases is likely to be more effective in suppressing tumor growth than a more selective drug. HER kinases work as heterodimers, and a pan-HER kinase inhibitor is less likely to be defeated by redundancy within the system. For the same reason, it is more likely to have toxic effects on normal tissues secondary both to inhibition of its postulated targets and inhibition of other, perhaps unknown, tyrosine kinases. Thus, the therapeutic index of such drugs in the treatment of different tumors cannot be deduced and probably can be determined only in phase I and phase II human studies.

Several such inhibitors have been developed and are in early trial. For example, PD168393, developed by Fry et al., binds irreversibly to and inactivates the catalytic activity of EGFR and HER-2/neu.[162] It is active at nontoxic doses in xenograft models of tumors that overexpress either HER-2 or EGFR. This compound is unique because it is an irreversible inhibitor; it will be tested in humans soon. Another Parke-Davis compound, PD153035, is a reversible inhibitor of EGFR and, to a lesser degree, HER-2/neu, and suppresses the proliferation and clonogenicity of a wide panel of EGFR-overexpressing human cancer cell lines and xenografts.[163]

Another strategy for suppressing signaling pathways that are essential for cancer cell growth is to inhibit the expression of key signaling proteins rather than to inhibit their activity. This might be achieved with antisense or ribozyme agents that prevent messenger RNA (mRNA) translation, with agents that interfere with transcription of the gene encoding the signaling protein, or with drugs that induce the selective destruction of the protein.[164–166] All of these strategies are in development for HER-2 and for several other important signaling proteins.

Antisense vectors or oligonucleotides can inhibit the expression of particular genes by hybridizing to the mRNA encoding the targeted gene and preventing the translation or inducting the instability of the mRNA.[166] In the past, a great deal of skepticism existed regarding the feasibility of this approach, especially the ability to achieve adequate serum and cellular concentrations. This methodology has also been applied to growth factor receptors. HER-2 antisense vectors were shown to be somewhat effective in reducing the expression of HER-2/neu in breast and ovarian cancer cells.[167–169] Treatment of HER-2/neu–overexpressing cell lines with antisense oligonucleotides for HER-2/neu, but not with sense or scrambled oligonucleotides, specifically down-regulated mRNA expression and reduced pp185 protein expression.[167]

The E1A adenoviral gene product represses HER-2/neu expression by interfering with the activity of its promoter.[170] Several gene transfer protocols were investigated in animal models, and expression of E1A resulted in tumor suppression of HER-2/neu–driven tumors. A liposome delivery system has been tested in a phase I multicenter study, which showed effective reduction of HER-2/neu levels in the tumors of patients with metastatic breast and ovarian cancer.[171]

A novel method for reducing levels of HER-2 expression involves drugs that induce its degradation. Ansamycin antibiotics are natural products that bind to the chaperone protein Hsp90.[172–174] This binding causes the proteasomal degradation of a subset of proteins that require Hsp90 function, including certain transmembrane tyrosine kinases, steroid receptors, and the Raf serine kinase.[175–177] HER family tyrosine kinases are the most sensitive targets of the drug so far identified. Addition of geldanamycin, one of these antibiotics, to cancer cells causes their G_1 arrest and subsequent apoptosis. Breast cancer cell lines with amplified HER-2 kinase are especially sensitive to this drug. A derivative of geldanamycin is currently in Phase I trial.

Other Growth Factor Receptors

Although the HER kinase family has become the prototypic target for development of selective therapies in breast cancer, other growth factor receptors are also involved in maintaining malignant transformation. IGF-I receptor, the FGF family of receptors, and the Met tyrosine kinase have all been implicated in the induction and progression of breast cancer, and strategies for their inhibition, including production of monoclonal antibodies and selective tyrosine kinase inhibitors, are in development.

Several ideas for inhibiting activation of the IGF-I receptor have been put forward.[178–180] Multiple circulating IGF-binding proteins exist that act to sequester IGF-I and IGF-II and also to modulate their function.[181] In addition, IGF-II receptor binds IGF-I with high affinity and targets it for lysosomal degradation.[182] IGF-binding proteins or extracellular domain of the IGF-II receptor could potentially be administered intravenously and used to lower the concentrations of free serum IGF-I and IGF-II and abrogating autocrine or paracrine loops involving these factors. The feasibility of this strategy is under investigation.[182,183] Activation of the IGF receptor is mitogenic but also transduces a powerful antiapoptotic signal.[57–59] Inhibition of this receptor might therefore be quite useful in conjunction with cytotoxic chemotherapy.[13,52]

The Met and FGF receptors supply a growth signal, but these receptors are also integrally involved in transducing the signals for cell motility and invasion as well as angiogenesis.[74,76,78,119] A variety of similar agents (antibodies, tyrosine kinase inhibitors) are being developed for inhibition of the receptors.[76,78,83] If potent drugs are developed and their primary effects are on invasion and the tumor cell–stroma interaction, investigators will have to learn how to assess whether they worked biochemically or as anticancer agents.[84,109–111] Such drugs may be static or effective only in the setting of adjuvant therapy or minimal disease. Prolonged drug administration may be required to achieve a tumor response. To test such drugs, clear ideas must be developed regarding the type and stage of tumor in which they are most likely to be useful and intermediate markers that will allow evaluation of whether the targeted process is affected.

INTRACELLULAR SIGNALING MOLECULES

Ras and Farnesyl Transferase Inhibitors

The Ras protein undergoes a posttranslational modification consisting of covalent attachment of a 15-carbon prenyl (farnesyl) residue to its C-terminal cysteine.[184] Farnesylation is required for the anchorage of Ras in the plasma membrane and for its transforming activity. This reaction is catalyzed by an enzyme, farnesyl transferase, that has a limited set of substrate proteins, including members of the Ras family.[185,186] Most prenylated proteins in the cell are linked to the 20-carbon geranylgeranyl group by a different enzyme. Therefore, farnesyl transferase inhibitors (FTIs) would be expected to inhibit the membrane anchorage and function of a restricted set of cellular proteins, including Ras. FTIs would be expected to inhibit the growth of tumor cells that require Ras function.[41,185]

Potent specific FTIs have been synthesized by a number of groups.[41,187–189] They inhibit Ha-Ras processing and cause the reversion of Ha-Ras–transformed cells in culture and the regression of the tumors that occur in Ha-Ras transgenic mice.[190,191] Many of the effects of the FTIs were unexpected, however. They are much less effective in inhibiting Ki-Ras–induced tumors[192,193] because, in the presence of the inhibitor, Ki-Ras undergoes the alternate modification, geranygeranylation.[194–197] The molecular significance of this "bypass" mechanism remains unclear.[190,191] Geranylgeranylated Ha mutant Ras can transform cells, but wild-type geranylgeranylated Ras has growth-inhibitory properties.[198]

FTIs were designed to be inhibitors of tumors containing mutations in the Ras gene. Results in cellular and animal model systems showed that its effects were much more complex. Tumors with activated wild-type Ras, such as breast cancer, can be quite sensitive.[199] Yet toxicity was limited, despite the central role played by the Ras protein in multiple physiologic processes. Furthermore, although Ki-Ras processing is relatively unaffected,[194,197] some pancreatic and colorectal tumors with Ki-Ras mutation are very sensitive.[199,200] Further studies showed that the drug causes growth inhibition by multiple mechanisms. Whereas Ha-Ras is probably the target in cells in which this gene is mutated, other farnesylated proteins, such as RhoB, are probably more important in other tumors.[201,202] In breast cancer cells with wild-type p53, FTI induces p21 expression and G_1 block. If p53 is mutated, however, G_1 block does not occur, and cells undergo endoreduplication of DNA and apoptosis in M phase.[203]

The low toxicity of FTI in preclinical models suggested that it might be useful when given in combination with cytotoxic agents. Tissue culture and animal studies show that FTI acts additively with radiation and several chemotherapeutic agents.[204–206] Tissue culture studies give some suggestion that FTI acts synergistically with taxanes to inhibit the growth of breast cancer cells. FTI seems to sensitize tumor cells to the mitotic block caused by taxanes.[205,206]

FTIs are now in early clinical trial. What lessons can be learned from the preclinical results? First, despite the successful development of a potent selective inhibitor of a specific oncoprotein, its effects on tumor cells are complex and were not predicted. They depend in large part on which particular genetic mutations gave rise to the tumor. Second, because of this, determining *a priori* which tumors are the preferred targets is very difficult. Breast cancer and other tumors with wild-type Ras were not originally thought to be appropriate targets for FTI, but empiric data and the Taxol interaction suggest otherwise. Third, the therapeutic index of the drug is not predicable from its postulated mechanism of action.

The cautionary conclusion is that the investigator must be wary of deductions made from mechanistic data obtained in model systems and must not allow them to prejudice the design of clinical trials. The current clinical trials of FTI presume it is a static drug and must be given continuously, and therefore orally, to patients with tumors containing Ras mutation. The challenge with FTIs and other similar functional antagonists is to determine how and in which tumors they are most likely to work so they can be tested most efficiently.

Other approaches that antagonize Ras function by inhibiting its expression are also being developed. Anti-Ras antisense and ribozyme drugs are at different stages of preclinical development. Antisense oligonucleotides directed at point mutations in Ki-Ras genes have been successfully used in colon, lung, and pancreatic cancer cell culture systems and animal models to selectively inhibit the proliferation of cells expressing the point-mutated *ras*.[207–211] Similarly, ribozymes have been designed to target mutated *ras* mRNAs.[212]

Targets Downstream of Ras

Breast cancer has a very low incidence of *ras* mutation, so strategies to selectively inhibit the expression of mutant Ras are unlikely to be useful. Other strategies under development that affect targets downstream of Ras are more likely to be applicable.[2] Ras exerts its effects by physically interacting with several target proteins, including PI3-kinase and the Raf serine kinase.[213,214] Activation of Raf initiates a cascade of activated serine kinases, including MEK and MAP kinase.[27] MAP kinase has multiple substrates involved in the initiation of growth and other aspects of the transformed phenotype. These include a variety of transcription factors that induce the expression of multiple regulatory genes.

One proposed strategy for inhibiting this cascade is the development of peptides that block the binding of Raf to the effector domain of activated Ras.[215,216] Thus far, this approach has not led to the development of useful drugs, probably because of the difficulty in preventing protein-protein interactions with peptides and in creating peptide drugs that are transported into cells in adequate amounts. Another approach being developed is reduction of Raf expression with antisense techniques. Phosphorothioate antisense Raf oligonucleotides reduce raf mRNA and protein expression in human tumor cell lines and inhibit tumor growth *in vitro* and *in vivo*.[217–220]

Selective small-molecule inhibitors of the Ras→MAP kinase cascade are also being developed. One such inhibitor is a flavonoid that selectively inhibits activation of mitogen-activated protein kinase kinase 1 (MEK1) by Ras or MEK kinase.[42,221] PD098059 ([2-(2'-amino-3'-methoxyphenyl)-oxanaphthalen-4-1]) exerts its effect by binding to the inactive form of MEK1 and preventing its activation by Raf or MEK kinase *in vitro* and *in vivo*. In human breast cancer cells, it inhibited the activation of MAP kinase by heregulin[222] and insulin,[223] and exerted potent antiproliferative effects at concentrations in the micromolar range. This class of inhibitors has been shown to inhibit tumor growth in animals at doses that do not cause toxicity.[42] MAP kinase has been demonstrated to be a key component of pathways that are important to many normal physiologic processes, and most would have predicted that such an inhibitor would be inordinately toxic. Why this drug is not is unclear, but these data again emphasize the point that therapeutic index is very difficult to deduce from the mechanism of action of the agent.

Another key signal intermediate is the enzyme PI3-kinase.[26,224] This enzyme catalyzes the phosphorylation of phosphatidyl inositol. The product of this reaction, PI(3')P, then binds to and activates a series of targets, including the Akt protein kinase.[225] PI3-kinase may be activated either by phosphorylation and binding to activated transmembrane tyrosine kinase growth factor receptors or by binding to activated Ras. Several lines of evidence suggest that PI3-kinase is essential for induction of growth or transformation by growth factor receptors. Mutations in receptors that selectively abrogate their ability to activate PI3-kinase are defective in their ability to cause transformation. The suppressor oncogene *PTEN*—which is inactivated in a large proportion of tumors, including breast tumors, prostate tumors, and glioblastomas—encodes a lipid phosphatase that dephosphorylates PI(3')P.[37] A target of PI(3')P, Akt, is a protooncogene, the activation of which inhibits apoptosis and stimulates the cell cycle by increasing cyclin D expression.

These data suggest that either PI3-kinase or Akt are extremely attractive targets for drug development. Two drugs that inhibit PI3-kinase inhibit the growth and activate apoptosis of a wide spectrum of tumor cell lines but are not usable *in vivo*.[226–228] These results point out the complex array of potential targets for new cancer drugs and the difficulty in choosing which are the most promising for focused development.

INHIBITORS OF COMPONENTS OF THE CELL CYCLE MACHINERY

Activation of growth factor signal pathways has pleiotropic effects and results in stimulation of the cell division cycle, inhibition of apoptosis and terminal differentiation, and changes in the interaction of the cell with its local environment. The mechanisms by which the cascade of signals induced by growth factors affects these processes are being worked out and represent a complex set of interactions that can be targeted by therapeutic strategies. Most strategies directed at these mechanisms are currently in the basic development or preclinical stage, so they are not discussed here in detail. The centrality of regulators of the cell division cycle to the cancer process, however, has made these regulators the focus of much current drug development, so some mention is made of the current state of this research.

Over the last several years, great strides have been made in understanding how the cell cycle is regulated. Activation of a series of serine kinases (cyclin-dependent kinases, or CDKs) is required for progression through the important cell cycle regulatory points: early G_1, the G_1-S transition, and passage from G_2 into mitosis. The temporal control of individual CDKs is accomplished by the timed increase in expression of a series of proteins, cyclins, that bind to and activate individual CDKs.[15,229–231] Other regulatory proteins are required for cyclin-CDK activation, such as the CDC25 CDK phosphatases, or function to inhibit cyclin CDK function (p16, p21, p27, p57). Activators and inhibitors of cell division, such as growth factors and DNA-damaging agents, work in large part by engaging pathways that regulate CDKs and their substrates.[232]

Two reasons can be put forward for focusing on the development of agents that interfere with CDK activity or restore its normal regulation in cancer cells. First, as outlined above, the most commonly identified mutated oncogenes and suppressor genes in human cancers encode components of the cell cycle machinery. Second, the identification of activated CDKs in cancers offers obvious targets for the development of inhibitory drugs.[10]

The cyclin D–CDK4 kinase pathway is required for early progression through the G_1 phase of the cell cycle and is activated in most human cancers, either through loss of its inhibitor, p16, through amplification or overexpression of CDK4 or cyclin D, or through loss of its substrate, the Rb protein.[8,9] Cyclin D and CDK4 are often amplified or overexpressed in breast cancer.[233] Moreover, overexpression appears to be associated with specific disease phenotypes, altered responsiveness to therapeutic intervention, and patient survival.[234,235]

Development of selective inhibitors of CDK4 kinase are therefore the subject of large-scale efforts by many investigators and are currently in preclinical development. Other less selective inhibitors have been identified and are already being tested in patients. Flavopiridol (HMR 1275, L86-8275), an *N*-methylpiperidinyl, chlorophenyl flavone, was identified by the National Cancer Institute as a novel antineoplastic agent with activity toward a variety of human tumor cell lines. These effects correlate with its ability to potently inhibit the activity of CDC2 (CDK1), CDK4, and CDK2 and to induce either G_1 or G_2 cell cycle arrest. Phase I studies yielded positive results that led to currently ongoing phase II trials. A chlorinated derivative of flavopiridol ((-)-*cis*-5,7-dihydroxyphenyl-8-[4-(3-hydroxy-1-methyl) piperidinyl]-4H-1-benzopyran-4-1 hydrochloride hemihydrate (L86-8276)), is currently in phase I clinical trials as a drug against breast tumors.[236,237]

Another inhibitor currently in clinical trials is 7-hydroxystaurosporine (UCN-1). UCN-1 was originally identified as a protein kinase C inhibitor but was later shown to inhibit several Ser-Thr and Tyr kinases. It suppresses growth of cancer cells at nanomolar concentrations and potentiates the antiproliferative activity of DNA-damaging agents, including ionizing radiation in p53-deficient cells.[238,239] This potentiation resides in the ability of UCN-1 to induce loss of the G_2 checkpoint after DNA damage. Specifically, UCN-1 abrogates G_2 arrest after DNA damage by affecting a protein kinase that regulates the activation of CDK1, the CDK responsible for the G_2-M transition. DNA damage prevents activation of CDK1 and allows the cell to arrest in G_2 and undergo repair. UCN-1 blocks this inhibitory pathway, so that cells with damaged DNA enter mitosis and undergo apoptosis.[238,239]

These approaches represent novel strategies that take advantage of what has been learned about cell cycle regulation to induce the growth arrest and apoptosis of tumor cells. This area is in its infancy; many new strategies are currently in development. The issues, as with all of these strategies, are to identify the best setting in which to use and test these modalities and to determine whether inhibitors of pathways fundamental to normal cellular physiology have acceptable toxicity.

REFERENCES

1. Alessandro R, Spoonster J, Wersto RP, Kohn EC. Signal transduction as a therapeutic target. *Curr Top Microbiol Immunol* 1996;213:67.
2. Levitzki A. Targeting signal transduction for disease therapy. *Curr Opin Cell Biol* 1996;8:239.
3. McInnes C, Sykes BD. Growth factor receptors structure, mechanism, and drug discovery. *Biopolymers* 1997;43:339.
4. Chabner BA, Boral AL, Multani P. Translational research: walking the bridge between idea and cure—seventeenth Bruce F. Cain Memorial Award lecture. *Cancer Res* 1998;58:4211.
5. Dillon DA, Howe CL, Bosari S, Costa J. The molecular biology of breast cancer: accelerating clinical applications. *Crit Rev Oncog* 1998;9:125.
6. Heimbrook DC, Oliff A. Therapeutic intervention and signaling. *Curr Opin Cell Biol* 1998;10:284.
7. Horwitz SB. Taxol (paclitaxel): mechanisms of action. *Ann Oncol* 1994;5[Suppl 6]:S3.
8. Kaelin WG Jr. Alterations in G1/S cell-cycle control contributing to carcinogenesis. *Ann N Y Acad Sci* 1997;833:29.
9. Bartkova J, Lukas J, Bartek J. Aberrations of the G1- and G1/S-regulating genes in human cancer. *Prog Cell Cycle Res* 1997;3:211.
10. Giordano A, Rustum YM, Wenner CE. Cell cycle: molecular targets for diagnosis and therapy: tumor suppressor genes and cell cycle progression in cancer. *J Cell Biochem* 1998;70:17.
11. Nojima H. Cell cycle checkpoints, chromosome stability and the progression of cancer. *Hum Cell* 1997;10:221.
12. LaCasse EC, Baird S, Korneluk RG, MacKenzie AE. The inhibitors of apoptosis (IAPS) and their emerging role in cancer. *Oncogene* 1998;17:3247.
13. Haq R, Zanke B. Inhibition of apoptotic signaling pathways in cancer cells as a mechanism of chemotherapy resistance. *Cancer Metastasis Rev* 1998;17:233.
14. Boral AL, Dessain S, Chabner BA. Clinical evaluation of biologically targeted drugs: obstacles and opportunities. *Cancer Chemother Pharmacol* 1998;42[Suppl]:S3.

15. Assoian RK. Control of the G1 phase cyclin-dependent kinases by mitogenic growth factors and the extracellular matrix. *Cytokine Growth Factor Rev* 1997;8:165.
16. Parry D, Bates S, Mann DJ, Peters G. Lack of cyclin D-Cdk complexes in Rb-negative cells correlates with high levels of pl6lNK4/MTS1 tumor suppressor gene product. *EMBO J* 1995;14:503.
17. Lukas J, Parry D, Aagaard L, et al. Retinoblastoma-protein-dependent cell-cycle inhibition by the tumour suppressor p16. *Nature* 1995;375:503.
18. Jarrard DF, Bova GS, Ewing CM, et al. Deletional, mutational, and methylation analyses of CDKN2 (p16/MTS1) in primary and metastatic prostate cancer. *Genes Chromosomes Cancer* 1997;19:90.
19. Ullrich A, Schlessinger J. Signal transduction by receptors with tyrosine kinase activity. *Cell* 1990;61:203.
20. Weiss FU, Daub H, Ulirich A. Novel mechanisms of RTK signal generation. *Curr Opin Genet Dev* 1997;7:80.
21. Lemmon MA, Schlessinger J. Transmembrane signaling by receptor oligomerization. *Methods Mol Biol* 1998;84:49.
22. Pawson T, Scott JD. Signaling through scaffold, anchoring, and adaptor proteins. *Science* 1997;278:2075.
23. Pawson T. Protein modules and signaling networks. *Nature* 1995;373:573.
24. Medema RH, Bos JL. The role of p2l ras in receptor tyrosine kinase signaling. *Crit Rev Oncog* 1993;4:615.
25. Marshall MS. Ras target proteins in eukaryotic cells. *FASEB J* 1995;9:1311.
26. Wymann MP, Pirola L. Structure and function of phosphoinositide 3-kinases. *Biochim Biophys Acta* 1998;1436:127.
27. Schaeffer HJ, Weber MJ. Mitogen-activated protein kinases: specific messages from ubiquitous messengers. *Mol Cell Biol* 1999;19:2435.
28. Alroy I, Yarden Y. The ErbB signaling network in embryogenesis and oncogenesis: signal diversification through combinatorial ligand-receptor interactions. *FEBS Lett* 1997;410:83.
29. Tzahar E, Yarden Y. The ErbB-2/HER2 oncogenic receptor of adenocarcinomas: from orphanhood to multiple stromal ligands. *Biochim Biophys Acta* 1998;1377:M25.
30. Ross JS, Fletcher JA. The HER-2/neu oncogene in breast cancer: prognostic factor, predictive factor, and target for therapy. *Stem Cells* 1998;16:413.
31. Revillion F, Bonneterre J, Peyrat JP. ERBB2 oncogene in human breast cancer and its clinical significance. *Eur J Cancer* 1998;34:791.
32. Bos JL. *ras* oncogenes in human cancer: a review. *Cancer Res* 1989;49:4682.
33. Clark GJ, Der CJ. Aberrant function of the Ras signal transduction pathway in human breast cancer. *Breast Cancer Res Treat* 1995;35:133.
34. Teng DH, Hu R, Lin H, et al. MMAC1/PTEN mutations in primary tumor specimens and tumor cell lines. *Cancer Res* 1997;57:5221.
35. Li J, Yen C, Liaw D, et al. PTEN, a putative protein tyrosine phosphatase gene mutated in human brain, breast, and prostate cancer. *Science* 1997;275:1943.
36. Steck PA, Pershouse MA, Jasser SA, et al. Identification of a candidate tumour suppressor gene, MMAC1, at chromosome 10q23.3 that is mutated in multiple advanced cancers. *Nat Genet* 1997;15:356.
37. Maehama T, Dixon JE. The tumor suppressor PTEN/MMAC1, dephosphorylates the lipid second messenger, phosphatidylinositol 3,4,5-trisphosphate. *J Biol Chem* 1998;273:13375.
38. Alessi DR, Cohen P. Mechanism of activation and function of protein kinase B. *Curr Opin Genet Dev* 1998;8:55.
39. Nunez G, del Peso L. Linking extracellular survival signals and the apoptotic machinery. *Curr Opin Neurobiol* 1998;8:613.
40. Muise-Helmericks RC, Grimes HL, Bellacosa A, Maistrom SE, Tsichlis PN, Rosen, N. Cyclin D expression is controlled post-transcriptionally via a phosphatidylinositol 3-kinase/Akt-dependent pathway. *J Biol Chem* 1998;273:29864.
41. Gibbs JB, Oliff A. The potential of farnesyltransferase inhibitors as cancer chemotherapeutics. *Ann Rev Pharmacol Toxicol* 1997;37:143.
42. Alessi DR, Cuenda A, Cohen P, Dudley DT, Saltiel AR. PD 098059 is a specific inhibitor of the activation of mitogen-activated protein kinase kinase in vitro and in vivo. *J Biol Chem* 1995;270:27489.
43. Favoni RE, de Cupis A. Steroidal and nonsteroidal oestrogen antagonists in breast cancer: basic and clinical appraisal. *Trends Pharmacol Sci* 1998;19:406.
44. Fisher B, Costantino JP, Wickerham DL, et al. Tamoxifen for prevention of breast cancer: report of the National Surgical Adjuvant Breast and Bowel Project P-1 study. *J Natl Cancer Inst* 1998;90:1371.
45. Buzdar AU, Hortobagyi GN. Tamoxifen and toremifene in breast cancer: comparison of safety and efficacy. *J Clin Oncol* 1998;16:348.
46. Kude JM, Soo Lee J, Griffin T, et al. Phase I trial of 9-cis retinoic acid in adults with solid tumors. *Clin Cancer Res* 1996;2:287.
47. Gulliford T, English J, Colston KW, Menday P, Moller S, Coombes RC. A phase I study of the vitamin D analogue EB 1089 in patients with advanced breast and colorectal cancer. *Br J Cancer* 1998;78:6.
48. Budd GT, Adamson PC, Gupta M, et al. Phase I/II trial of all-trans retinoic acid and tamoxifen in patients with advanced breast cancer. *Clin Cancer Res* 1998;4:635.
49. Mehta RG, Moriarty RM, Mehta RR, et al. Prevention of preneoplastic mammary lesion development by a novel vitamin D analogue, 1alpha-hydroxyvitamin D5. *J Natl Cancer Inst* 1997;89:212.
50. De Palo G, Camerini T, Marubini E, et al. Chemoprevention trial of contralateral breast cancer with fenretinide. Rationale, design, methodology, organization, data management, statistics and accrual. *Tumori* 1997;83:884.
51. Green DR. Apoptotic pathways: the roads to ruin. *Cell* 1998;94:695.
52. Jarpe MB, Widmann C, Knall C, et al. Anti-apoptotic versus pro-apoptotic signal transduction: checkpoints and stop signs along the road to death. *Oncogene* 1998;17:1475.
53. Thornberry NA. Caspases: key mediators of apoptosis. *Chem Biol* 1998;5:R97.
54. Nunez G, Benedict MA, Hu Y, Inohara N. Caspases: the proteases of the apoptotic pathway. *Oncogene* 1998;17:3237.
55. Milligan CE, Schwartz LM. Programmed cell death during animal development. *Br Med Bull* 1997;53:570.
56. Reed JC. Bcl2 family proteins. *Oncogene* 1998;17:3225.
57. Kulik G, Klippel A, Weber MJ. Antiapoptotic signalling by the insulin-like growth factor I receptor, phosphatidylinositol 3-kinase, and Akt. *Mol Cell Biol* 1997;17:1595.
58. Dafta SR, Dudek H, Tao X, et al. Akt phosphorylation of BAD couples survival signals to the cell-intrinsic death machinery. *Cell* 1997;91:231.
59. Cardone MH, Roy N, Stennicke HR, et al. Regulation of cell death protease caspase-9 by phosphorylation. *Science* 1998;282:1318.
60. Chen X, Ko LJ, Jayaraman L, Prives C. p53 levels, functional domains, and DNA damage determine the extent of the apoptotic response of tumor cells. *Genes Dev* 1996;10:2438.
61. Polyak K, Waldman T, He TC, Kinzler KW, Vogelstein B. Genetic determinants of p53-induced apoptosis and growth arrest. *Genes Dev* 1996;10:1945.
62. Asschert JG, Velienga E, De Jong S, de Vries EG. Mutual interactions between p53 and growth factors in cancer. *Anticancer Res* 1998;18:1713.
63. Kiess W, Haskell JF, Lee L, et al. An Ab that blocks insulin-like growth factor (IGF) binding to the type II receptor is neither an agonist nor an inhibitor of IGF-stimulated biological responses in L6 myoblasts. *J Biol Chem* 1987;262:12745.
64. Burfeind P, Chernicky CL, Rininsiand F, Ilan J, Ilan J. Antisense RNA to the type I insulin-like growth factor receptor suppresses tumor growth and prevents invasion by rat prostate cancer cells in vivo. *Proc Natl Acad Sci U S A* 1996;93:7263.
65. Parrizas M, Gazit A, Levitzki A, Wertheimer E, LeRoith D. Specific inhibition of insulinlike growth factor-1 and insulin receptor tyrosine kinase activity and biological function by tyrphostins. *Endocrinology* 1997;138:1427.
66. van Brussel JP, Mickisch GH. Circumvention of multidrug resistance in genitourinary tumors. *Int J Urol* 1998;5:1.
67. Yang D, Ling Y, Almazan M, Guo RAM, Brown B, Lippman ME. Tumor regression of human breast carcinomas by combination therapy of anti-bcl2 antisense oligonucleotide and chemotherapeutic drugs. *Proc Am Assoc Cancer Res* 1999;40:4814.
68. Nielsen LL, Dell J, Maxwell E, Armstrong L, Maneval D, Catino JJ. Efficacy of p53 adenovirus-mediated gene therapy against human breast cancer xenografts. *Cancer Gene Ther* 1997;4:129.
69. Li P, Bui T, Gray D, Klamut HJ. Therapeutic potential of recombinant p53 overexpression in breast cancer cells expressing endogenous wild-type p53. *Breast Cancer Res Treat* 1998;48:273.
70. Seth P, Brinkmann U, Schwartz GN, et al. Adenovirus-mediated gene transfer to human breast tumor cells: an approach for cancer gene therapy and bone marrow purging. *Cancer Res* 1996;56:1346.
71. Seth P, Katayose D, Li Z, et al. A recombinant adenovirus expressing wild type p53 induces apoptosis in drug-resistant human breast can-

cer cells: a gene therapy approach for drug-resistant cancers. *Cancer Gene Ther* 1997;4:383.
72. Szumiel I. Monitoring and signaling of radiation-induced damage in mammalian cells. *Radiat Res* 1998;150:S92.
73. St. Croix B, Kerbel RS. Cell adhesion and drug resistance in cancer. *Curr Opin Oncol* 1997;9:549.
74. Woodhouse EC, Chuaqui RF, Liofta LA. General mechanisms of metastasis. *Cancer* 1997;80:1529.
75. Noel A, Gilles C, Bajou K, et al. Emerging roles for proteinases in cancer. *Invasion Metastasis* 1997;17:221.
76. Harris SR, Thorgeirsson UP. Tumor angiogenesis: biology and therapeutic prospects. *In Vivo* 1998;12:563.
77. Benaud C, Dickson RB, Thompson EW. Roles of the matrix metalloproteinases in mammary gland development and cancer. *Breast Cancer Res Treat* 1998;50:97.
78. Jones A, Harris AL. New developments in angiogenesis: a major mechanism for tumor growth and target for therapy. *Cancer J Sci Am* 1998;4:209.
79. Yu AE, Hewitt RE, Connor EW, Stetier-Stevenson WG. Matrix metalloproteinases. Novel targets for directed cancer therapy. *Drugs Aging* 1997;11:229.
80. Gomez DE, Alonso DF, Yoshiji H, Thorgeirsson UP. Tissue inhibitors of metalloproteinases: structure, regulation and biological functions. *Eur J Cell Biol* 1997;74:111.
81. Gastl G, Hermann T, Steurer M, et al. Angiogenesis as a target for tumor treatment. *Oncology* 1997;54:177.
82. Harris AL, Zhang H, Moghaddam A, et al. Breast cancer angiogenesis—new approaches to therapy via antiangiogenesis, hypoxic activated drugs, and vascular targeting. *Breast Cancer Res Treat* 1996;38:97.
83. Siemeister G, Martiny-Baron G, Marme D. The pivotal role of VEGF in tumor angiogenesis: molecular facts and therapeutic opportunities. *Cancer Metastasis Rev* 1998;17:241.
84. Harris AL. Anti-angiogenesis therapy and strategies for integrating it with adjuvant therapy. *Recent Results Cancer Res* 1998;152:341.
85. Stephens RW, Brunner N, Janicke F, Schmitt M. The urokinase plasminogen activator system as a target for prognostic studies in breast cancer. *Breast Cancer Res Treat* 1998;52:99.
86. Look MP, Foekens JA. Clinical relevance of the urokinase plasminogen activator system in breast cancer. *APMIS* 1999;107:150.
87. Duffy MJ, Duggan C, Mulcahy HE, McDermott EW, O'Higgins NJ. Urokinase plasminogen activator: a prognostic marker in breast cancer including patients with axillary node-negative disease. *Clin Chem* 1998;44:1177.
88. Duffy MJ, O'Grady P, Devaney D, O'Siorain L, Fennelly JJ, Lijnen HJ. Urokinase-plasminogen activator, a marker for aggressive breast carcinomas. Preliminary report. *Cancer* 1988;62:531.
89. Gao AG, Lindberg FP, Dimitry JM, Brown E, Frazier WA. Thrombospondin modulates alpha v beta 3 function through integrin-associated protein. *J Cell Biol* 1996;135:533.
90. Albo D, Berger DH, Rothman VL, Tuszynski GP. Role of urokinase plasminogen activator receptor in thrombospondin 1-mediated tumor cell invasion. *J Surg Res* 1999;82:331.
91. Reuning U, Magdolen V, Wilhelm O, et al. Multifunctional potential of the plasminogen activation system in tumor invasion and metastasis (review). *Int J Oncol* 1998;13:893.
92. Andreasen PA, Kjoiler L, Christensen L, Duffy MJ. The urokinase-type plasminogen activator system in cancer metastasis: a review. *Int J Cancer* 1997;72:1.
93. de Wifte JH, Sweep CG, Klijn JG, et al. Prognostic impact of urokinase-type plasminogen activator (uPA) and its inhibitor (PAI-1) in cytosols and pellet extracts derived from 892 breast cancer patients. *Br J Cancer* 1999;79:1190.
94. Rabbani SA. Metalloproteases and urokinase in angiogenesis and tumor progression. *In Vivo* 1998;12:135.
95. Tressler RJ, Pitot PA, Stratton JR, et al. Urokinase receptor antagonists: discovery and application to in vivo models of tumor growth. *APMIS* 1999;107:168.
96. lgnar DM, Andrews JL, Witherspoon SM, et al. Inhibition of establishment of primary and micrometastatic tumors by a urokinase plasminogen activator receptor antagonist. *Clin Exp Metastasis* 1998; 16:920.
97. Abaza MS, Narayan RK, Atassi MZ. Anti-urokinase-type plasminogen activator monoclonal antibodies inhibit the proliferation of human breast cancer cell lines in vitro. *Tumour Biol* 1998;19:229.
98. Davies J, Warwick J, Totty N, Philip R, Helfrich M, Horton M. The osteoclast functional antigen implicated in the regulation of bone-resorption is biochemically related to the vitronectin receptor. *J Cell Biol* 1989;109:1817.
99. Liapis H, Flath A, Kitazawa S. Integrin avb3 expression by bone-residing breast cancer metastasis. *Diagn Mol Pathol* 1996;5:127.
100. Sheu JR, Lin CH, Peng HC, Huang TF. Triflavin, an Arg-Gly-Asp-containing peptide, inhibits the adhesion of tumor cells to matrix proteins via binding to multiple integrin receptors expressed on human hepatoma cells. *Proc Soc Exp Biol Med* 1996;213:71.
101. Smit JW, van der Pluijm G, Vloedgraven HJ, Lowik CW, Goslings BM. Role of integrins in the attachment of metastatic follicular thyroid carcinoma cell lines to bone. *Thyroid* 1998;8:29.
102. Brooks PC, Stromblad S, Klemke R, Visscher D, Sarkar FH, Cheresh DA. Antiintegrin alpha v beta 3 blocks human breast cancer growth and angiogenesis in human skin. *J Clin Invest* 1995;96:1815.
103. McLane MA, Marcinkiewicz C, Vijay-Kumar S, Wierzbicka-Patynowski I, Niewiarowski S. Viper venom disintegrins and related molecules. *Proc Soc Exp Biol Med* 1998;219:109.
104. Yeh CH, Peng HC, Huang TF. Accutin, a new disintegrin, inhibits angiogenesis in vitro and in vivo by acting as integrin alphavbeta3 antagonist and inducing apoptosis. *Blood* 1998;92:3268.
105. Panchal RG. Novel therapeutic strategies to selectively kill cancer cells. *Biochem Pharmacol* 1998;55:247.
106. Pasqualini R, Ruoslahti E. Organ targeting in vivo using phage display peptide libraries. *Nature* 1996;380:364.
107. Rajofte D, Arap W, Hagedorn M, Koivunen E, Pasqualini R, Ruoslahti E. Molecular heterogeneity of the vascular endothelium revealed by in vivo phage display. *J Clin Invest* 1998;102:430.
108. Arap W, Pasqualini R, Ruoslahti E. Cancer treatment by targeted drug delivery to tumor vasculature in a mouse model. *Science* 1998;279:377.
109. Augustin HG. Antiangiogenic tumour therapy: will it work? *Trends Pharmacol Sci* 1998;19:216.
110. Molema G, Meijer DK, de Leij LF. Tumor vasculature targeted therapies: getting the players organized. *Biochem Pharmacol* 1998;55: 1939.
111. Voest EE. Inhibitors of angiogenesis in a clinical perspective. *Anticancer Drugs* 1996;7:723.
112. Cohen BD, Siegall CB, Bacus S, et al. Role of epidermal growth factor receptor family members in growth and differentiation of breast carcinoma. *Biochem Soc Symp* 1998;63:199.
113. de Jong JS, van Diest PJ, van der Valk P, Baak JP. Expression of growth factors, growth-inhibiting factors, and their receptors in invasive breast cancer. II: Correlations with proliferation and angiogenesis. *J Pathol* 1998;184:53.
114. de Jong JS, van Diest PJ, van der Valk P, Baak JP. Expression of growth factors, growth inhibiting factors, and their receptors in invasive breast cancer. I: An inventory in search of autocrine and paracrine loops. *J Pathol* 1998;184:44.
115. Sepp-Lorenzino L. Structure and function of the insulin-like growth factor receptor. *Breast Cancer Res Treat* 1998;47:235.
116. Rasmussen AA, Cullen KJ. Paracrine/autocrine regulation of breast cancer by the insulin-like growth factors. *Breast Cancer Res Treat* 1998;47:219.
117. Baserga R, Resnicoff M, D'Ambrosio C, Valentinis B. The role of the IGF-I receptor in apoptosis. *Vitam Horm* 1997;53:65.
118. Wu X, Fan Z, Masui H, Rosen N, Mendelsohn J. Apoptosis induced by an anti-epidermal growth factor receptor monoclonal antibody in a human colorectal carcinoma cell line and its delay by insulin. *J Clin Invest* 1995;95:1897.
119. Vande Woude GF, Jeffers M, Cortner J, Alvord G, Tsarfaty I, Resau J. Met-HGF/SF: tumorigenesis, invasion and metastasis. *Ciba Found Symp* 1997;212:119(discussion 130,148).
120. Levitzki A, Gazit A. Tyrosine kinase inhibition: an approach to drug development. *Science* 1995;267:1782.
121. Fan Z, Mendelsohn J. Therapeutic application of anti-growth factor receptor antibodies. *Curr Opin Oncol* 1998;10:67.
122. Farah RA, Clinchy B, Herrera L, Vitetta ES. The development of monoclonal antibodies for the therapy of cancer. *Crit Rev Eukaryot Gene Expr* 1998;8:321.
123. Traxler P, Furet P, Mett H, Buchdunger E, Meyer T, Lydon N. Design and synthesis of novel tyrosine kinase inhibitors using a pharmacophore model of the ATP-binding site of the EGF-R. *J Pharm Belg* 1997;52:88.

124. Fry DW, Nelson JM, Slintak V, et al. Biochemical and antiproliferative properties of 4-[ar(alk)ylamino]pyridopyrimidines, a new chemical class of potent and specific epidermal growth factor receptor tyrosine kinase inhibitor. *Biochem Pharmacol* 1997;54:877.
125. Singh J, Dobrusin EM, Fry DW, Haske T, Whitty A, McNamara DJ. Structure-based design of a potent, selective, and irreversible inhibitor of the catalytic domain of the erbB receptor subfamily of protein tyrosine kinases. *J Med Chem* 1997;40:1130.
126. Levitzki A. SRC as a target for anti-cancer drugs. *Anticancer Drug Des* 1996;11:175.
127. Lawrence DS, Niu J. Protein kinase inhibitors: the tyrosine-specific protein kinases. *Pharmacol Ther* 1998;77:81.
128. Blanco-Aparicio C, Molina MA, Fernandez-Salas E, et al. Potato carboxypeptidase inhibitor, a T-knot protein, is an epidermal growth factor antagonist that inhibits tumor cell growth. *J Biol Chem* 1998;273:12370.
129. Date K, Matsumoto K, Kuba K, Shimura H, Tanaka M, Nakamura T. Inhibition of tumor growth and invasion by a four-kringle antagonist (HGF/NK4) for hepatocyte growth factor. *Oncogene* 1998;17:3045.
130. Matthews JM, Hammacher A, Howlett GJ, Simpson RJ. Physicochemical characterization of an antagonistic human interleukin-6 dimer. *Biochemistry* 1998;37:10671.
131. Lowman HB, Chen YM, Skelton NJ, et al. Molecular mimics of insulin-like growth factor 1 (IGF-1) for inhibiting IGF-1: IGF-binding protein interactions. *Biochemistry* 1998;37:8870.
132. Pastan I. Targeted therapy of cancer with recombinant immunotoxins. *Biochim Biophys Acta* 1997;1333:C1.
133. Rihova B. Targeting of drugs to cell surface receptors. *Crit Rev Biotechnol* 1997;17:149.
134. Goren D, Horowitz AT, Zalipsky S, Woodle MC, Yarden Y, Gabizon A. Targeting of stealth liposomes to erbB-2 (Her/2) receptor: in vitro and in vivo studies. *Br J Cancer* 1996;74:1749.
135. Brossart P, Stuhler G, Flad T, et al. Her-2/neu-derived peptides are tumor-associated antigens expressed by human renal cell and colon carcinoma lines and are recognized by in vitro induced specific cytotoxic T lymphocytes. *Cancer Res* 1998;58:732.
136. Earp HS, Dawson TL, Li X, Yu H. Heterodimerization and functional interaction between EGF receptor family members: a new signaling paradigm with implications for breast cancer research. *Breast Cancer Res Treat* 1995;35:115.
137. Naidu R, Yadav M, Nair S, Kutty MK. Expression of c-erbB3 protein in primary breast carcinomas. *Br J Cancer* 1998;78:1385.
138. Cance WG, Liu ET. Protein kinases in human breast cancer. *Breast Cancer Res Treat* 1995;35:105.
139. Ennis BW, Valverius EM, Bates SE, et al. Anti-epidermal growth factor receptor antibodies inhibit the autocrine-stimulated growth of MDA-468 human breast cancer cells. *Mol Endocrinol* 1989;3:1830.
140. Goldstein NI, Prewett M, Zuklys K, Rockwell P, Mendelsohn J. Biological efficacy of a chimeric antibody to the epidermal growth factor receptor in a human tumor xenograft model. *Clin Cancer Res* 1995;1:1311.
141. Brown PM, Debanne MT, Grothe S, et al. The extracellular domain of the epidermal growth factor receptor. Studies on the affinity and stoichiometry of binding, receptor dimerization and a binding-domain mutant. *Eur J Biochem* 1994;225:223.
142. Fan Z, Baselga J, Masui H, Mendelsohn J. Antitumor effect of anti-epidermal growth factor receptor monoclonal antibodies plus cis-diamminedichloroplatinum on well-established A431 cell xenografts. *Cancer Res* 1993;53:4637.
143. Fan Z, Masui H, Altas I, Mendelsohn J. Blockade of epidermal growth factor receptor function by bivalent and monovalent fragments of 225 anti-epidermal growth factor receptor monoclonal antibodies. *Cancer Res* 1993;53:4:322.
144. Baselga J, Norton L, Masui H, et al. Antitumor effects of doxorubicin in combination with anti-epidermal growth factor receptor monoclonal antibodies. *J Natl Cancer Inst* 1993;85:1327.
145. Baselga J, Norton L, Albanell J, Kim YM, Mendelsohn J. Recombinant humanized anti-HER2 antibody (Herceptin) enhances the antitumor activity of paclitaxel and doxorubicin against HER2/neu overexpressing human breast cancer xenografts. *Cancer Res* 1998;58:2825.
146. Pietras RJ, Poen JC, Gailardo D, Wongvipat PN, Lee HJ, Slamon DJ. Monoclonal antibody to HER-2/neureceptor modulates repair of radiation-induced DNA damage and enhances radiosensitivity of human breast cancer cells overexpressing this oncogene. *Cancer Res* 1999;59:1347.
147. Pietras RJ, Pegram MD, Finn RS, Maneval DA, Slamon DJ. Remission of human breast cancer xenografts on therapy with humanized monoclonal antibody to HER-2 receptor and DNA-reactive drugs. *Oncogene* 1998;17:2235.
148. Slamon D, Leyland-Jones B, Shak S, et al. Addition of herceptin TM (humanized anti-HER2 antibody) to first line chemotherapy for HER2 overexpression metastatic breast cancer (HER2+/MBC) markedly increases anticancer activity: a randomized multinational controlled phase III trial. *Proc Ann Meet Am Soc Clin Onc* 1998;17:A377.
149. Goldenberg MM. Trastuzumab, a recombinant DNA-derived humanized monoclonal antibody, a novel agent for the treatment of metastatic breast cancer. *Clin Ther* 1999;21:309.
150. Modjtahedi H, Hickish T, Nicolson M, et al. Phase I trial and tumour localisation of the anti-EGFR monoclonal antibody ICR62 in head and neck or lung cancer. *Br J Cancer* 1996;73:228.
151. Slamon DJ, Clark GM, Wong SG, Levin WJ, Ullrich A, McGuire WL. Human breast cancer: correlation of relapse and survival with amplification of the HER-2/neu oncogene. *Science* 1987;235:177.
152. Pegram MD, Paulefti G, Slamon DJ. HER-2/neu as a predictive marker of response to breast cancer therapy. *Breast Cancer Res Treat* 1998;52:65.
153. Guy CT, Webster MA, Schaller M, Parsons TJ, Cardiff RD, Muller WJ. Expression of the neu protooncogene in the mammary epithelium of transgenic mice induces metastatic disease. *Proc Natl Acad Sci U S A* 1992;89:10578.
154. Shepard HM, Lewis GD, Sarup JC, et al. Monoclonal antibody therapy of human cancer: taking the HER2 protooncogene to the clinic. *J Clin Immunol* 1991;11:117.
155. Lewis GD, Figari I, Fendly B, et al. Differential responses of human tumor cell lines to anti-p185HER2 monoclonal antibodies. *Cancer Immunol Immunother* 1993;37:255.
156. Baselga J, Seidman AD, Rosen PP, Norton L. HER2 overexpression and paclitaxel sensitivity in breast cancer: therapeutic implications. *Oncology (Huntingt)* 1997;11:43.
157. Pegram MD, Lipton A, Hayes DF, et al. Phase II study of receptor enhanced chemosensitivity using recombinant humanized anti-p185HER2/neu monoclonal antibody plus cisplatin in patients with HER2/neu-overexpressing metastatic breast cancer refractory to chemotherapy treatment. *J Clin Oncol* 1998;16:2659.
158. Baselga J, Tripathy D, Mendelsohn J, et al. Phase II study of weekly intravenous recombinant humanized anti-p185HER2 monoclonal antibody in patients with HER2/neu-overexpressing metastatic breast cancer. *J Clin Oncol* 1996;14:737.
159. Klapper LN, Vaisman N, Hurwitz E, Pinkas Kramarski R, Yarden Y, Sela M. A subclass of tumor-inhibitory monoclonal antibodies to ErbB-2/HER2 blocks crosstalk with growth factor receptors. *Oncogene* 1997;14:2099.
160. Shawver LK, Schwartz DP, Mann E, et al. Inhibitior of platelet-derived growth factor-mediated signal transduction and tumor growth by N-[4-(trifluoromethyl)-phenyl]5-methylisoxazole-4-carboxamide. *Clin Cancer Res* 1997;3:1167.
161. Boschelli DH, Wu Z, Klutchko SR, et al. Synthesis and tyrosine kinase inhibitory activity of a series of 2- amino-8H-pyrido[2,3-d]pyrimidines: identification of potent, selective platelet-derived growth factor receptor tyrosine kinase inhibitors. *J Med Chem* 1998;41:4365.
162. Fry DW, Bridges AJ, Denny WA, et al. Specific, irreversible inactivation of the epidermal growth factor receptor and erbB2, by a new class of tyrosine kinase inhibitor. *Proc Natl Acad Sci U S A* 1998;95:12022.
163. Bos M, Mendelsohn J, Kim YM, Albanell J, Fry DW, Baselga J. PD153035, a tyrosine kinase inhibitor, prevents epidermal growth factor receptor activation and inhibits growth of cancer cells in a receptor number-dependent manner. *Clin Cancer Res* 1997;3:2099.
164. Persidis A. Ribozyme therapeutics. *Nat Biotechnol* 1997;15:921.
165. Gewirtz AM, Sokol DL, Ratajczak MZ. Nucleic acid therapeutics: state of the art and future prospects. *Blood* 1998;92:712.
166. Ho PT, Parkinson DR. Antisense oligonucleotides as therapeutics for malignant diseases. *Semin Oncol* 1997;24:187.
167. Roh H, Pippin J, Boswell C, Drebin JA. Antisense oligonucleotides specific for the HER2/neu oncogene inhibit the growth of human breast carcinoma cells that overexpress HER2/neu. *J Surg Res* 1998;77:85.

168. Sacco MG, Barbieri O, Piccini D, et al. In vitro and in vivo antisense-mediated growth inhibition of a mammary adenocarcinoma from MMTV-neu transgenic mice. *Gene Ther* 1998;5:388.
169. Porumb H, Gousset H, Letellier R, et al. Temporary ex vivo inhibition of the expression of the human oncogene HER2 (NEU) by a triple helix-forming oligonucleotide. *Cancer Res* 1996;56:515.
170. Yu D, Hung MC. The erbB2 gene as a cancer therapeutic target and the tumor- and metastasis-suppressing function of E1A. *Cancer Metastasis Rev* 1998;17:195.
171. Hortobagyi GN, Hung MC, Lopez-Berestein G. A Phase I multicenter study of E1A gene therapy for patients with metastatic breast cancer and epithelial ovarian cancer that overexpresses HER-2/neu or epithelial ovarian cancer. *Hum Gene Ther* 1998;9:1775.
172. Whitesell L, Mimnaugh EG, De CB, Myers CF, Neckers LM. Inhibition of heat shock protein HSP90-pp60v-src heteroprotein complex formation by benzoquinone ansamycins: essential role for stress proteins in oncogenic transformation. *Proc Natl Acad Sci U S A* 1994;91:8324.
173. Stebbins CE, Russo AA, Schneider C, Rosen N, Hartl FU, Pavietich NP. Crystal structure of an Hsp90-geldanamycin complex: targeting of a protein chaperone by an antitumor agent. *Cell* 1997;89:239.
174. Prodromou C, Roe SM, Piper PW, Pearl LH. A molecular clamp in the crystal structure of the N-terminal domain of the yeast Hsp90 chaperone. *Nat Struct Biol* 1997;4:477.
175. Sepp-Lorenzino L, Ma Z, Lebwohl DE, Vinitsky A, Rosen N. Herbimycin A induces the 20S proteasome- and ubiquitin-dependent degradation of receptor tyrosine kinases. *J Biol Chem* 1995;270:16580.
176. Schulte TW, An WG, Neckers LM. Geldanamycin-induced destabilization of Raf-1 involves the proteasome. *Biochem Biophys Res Commun* 1997;239:655.
177. Stancato LF, Silverstein AM, Owens-Grillo JK, Chow YH, Jove R, Pratt WB. The hsp90-binding antibiotic geldanamycin decreases Raf levels and epidermal growth factor signaling without disrupting formation of signaling complexes or reducing the specific enzymatic activity of Raf kinase. *J Biol Chem* 1997;272:4013.
178. Yee D. The insulin-like growth factor system as a target in breast cancer. *Breast Cancer Res Treat* 1994;32:85.
179. Yee D. The insulin-like growth factors and breast cancer—revisited. *Breast Cancer Res Treat* 1998;47:197.
180. Pollak MN. Endocrine effects of IGF-I on normal and transformed breast epithelial cell: potential relevance to strategies for breast cancer treatment and prevention. *Breast Cancer Res Treat* 1998;47:209.
181. Oh Y. IGF-independent regulation of breast cancer growth by IGF binding proteins. *Breast Cancer Res Treat* 1998;47:283.
182. Oates AJ, Schumaker LM, Jenkins SB, et al. The mannose 6-phosphate/insulin-like growth factor 2 receptor (M6P/IGF2R), a putative breast tumor suppressor gene. *Breast Cancer Res Treat* 1998;47:269.
183. Van den Berg CL, Cox GN, Stroh CA, et al. Polyethylene glycol conjugated insulin-like growth factor binding protein 1 (IGFBP-1) inhibits growth of breast cancer in athymic mice. *Eur J Cancer* 1997;33:1108.
184. Zhang FL, Casey PJ. Protein prenylation: molecular mechanisms and functional consequences. *Ann Rev Biochem* 1996;65:241.
185. Gelb MH, Scholten JD, Sebolt LJ. Protein prenylation: from discovery to prospects for cancer treatment. *Curr Opin Chem Biol* 1998;2:40.
186. Dunten P, Kammloft U, Crowther R, Weber C , Palermo R, Birktoft J. Protein farnesyltransferase: structure and implications for substrate binding. *Biochemistry* 1998;37:7907.
187. Sebti SM, Hamilton AD. Inhibition of Ras prenylation: a novel approach to cancer chemotherapy. *Pharmacol Ther* 1997;74:103.
188. Aoyama T, Satoh T, Yonemoto M, et al. A new class of highly potent farnesyl diphosphate-competitive inhibitors of farnesyltransferase. *J Med Chem* 1998;41:143.
189. Augeri DJ, O'Connor SJ, Janowick D, et al. Potent and selective non-cysteine-containing inhibitors of protein farnesyltransferase. *J Med Chem* 1998;41:4288.
190. Cox AD, Der CJ. Farnesyltransferase inhibitors and cancer treatment: targeting simply Ras? *Biochim Biophys Acta* 1997;1333:F51.
191. Gibbs JB, Graham SL, Hartman GD, et al. Farnesyltransferase inhibitors versus Ras inhibitors. *Curr Opin Chem Biol* 1997;1:197.
192. Sun J, Qian Y, Hamilton AD, Sebti SM. Ras CAAX peptidomimetic FTI 276 selectively blocks tumor growth in nude mice of a human lung carcinoma with K-Ras mutation and p53 deletion. *Cancer Res* 1995;55:4243.
193. Liu M, Bryant MS, Chen J, et al. Effects of SCH 59228, an orally bioavailable farnesyl protein transferase inhibitor, on the growth of oncogene-transformed fibroblasts and a human colon carcinoma xenograft in nude mice. *Cancer Chemother Pharmacol* 1999;43:50.
194. Lerner EC, Zhang TT, Knowles DB, Qian Y, Hamilton AD, Sebti SM. Inhibition of the prenylation of K-Ras, but not H- or N-Ras, is highly resistant to CAAX peptidomimetics and requires both a farnesyltransferase and a geranylgeranyltransferase I inhibitor in human tumor cell lines. *Oncogene* 1997;15:1283.
195. Zhang FL, Kirschmeier P, Carr D, et al. Characterization of Ha-ras, N-ras, KiRas4A, and Ki-Ras4B as in vitro substrates for farnesyl protein transferase and geranylgeranyl protein transferase type 1. *J Biol Chem* 1997;272:10232.
196. Whyte DB, Kirschmeier P, Hockenberry TN, et al. K- and N-Ras are geranylgeranylated in cells treated with farnesyl protein transferase inhibitors. *J Biol Chem* 1997;172:14459.
197. Rowell CA, Kowalczyk JJ, Lewis MD, Garcia AM. Direct demonstration of geranylgeranylation and farnesylation of Ki-Ras in vivo. *J Biol Chem* 1997;272:14093.
198. Cox AD, Hisaka MM, Buss JE, Der CJ. Specific isoprenoid modification is required for function of normal, but not oncogenic, Ras protein. *Mol Cell Biol* 1992;12:2606.
199. Sepp-Lorenzino L, Ma Z, Rands E, et al. A peptidomimetic inhibitor of farnesyl:protein transferase blocks the anchorage-dependent and -independent growth of human tumor cell lines. *Cancer Res* 1995;55:5302.
200. Nagasu T, Yoshimatsu K, Rowell C, Lewis MD, Garcia AM. Inhibition of human tumor xenograft growth by treatment with the farnesyl transferase inhibitor B956. *Cancer Res* 1995;55:5310.
201. Du W, Lebowitz PF, Prendergast GC. Cell growth inhibition by farnesyltransferase inhibitors is mediated by gain of geranylgeranylated RhoB. *Mol Cell Biol* 1999;19:1831.
202. Lebowitz PF, Prendergast GC. Non-Ras targets of farnesyltransferase inhibitors: focus on Rho. *Oncogene* 1998;17:1439.
203. Sepp-Lorenzino L, Rosen N. A farnesyl:protein transferase inhibitor induces p2l expression and G1 block in p53-wild type tumor cells. *J Biol Chem* 1998;273:20243.
204. Bernhard EJ, McKenna WG, Hamilton AD, et al. Inhibiting Ras prenylation increases the radiosensitivity of human tumor cell lines with activating mutations of ras oncogenes. *Cancer Res* 1998; 58:1754.
205. Moasser MM, Sepp-Lorenzino L, Kohl NE, et al. Farnesyl transferase inhibitors cause enhanced mitotic sensitivity to taxol and epothilones. *Proc Natl Acad Sci U S A* 1998;95:1369.
206. Sepp-Lorenzino L, Balog A, Su D-S, et al. The microtubule-stabilizing agents epothilones A and B and their desoxyderivatives induce mitotic arrest and apoptosis in human prostate cancer cells. *Prostate Cancer Prostatic Dis* 1999;2:41.
207. Schwab G, Chavany C, Duroux I, et al. Antisense oligonucleotides adsorbed to polyalkylcyanoacrylate nanoparticles specifically inhibit mutated Ha-ras-mediated cell proliferation and tumorigenicity in nude mice. *Proc Natl Acad Sci U S A* 1994;91:10460.
208. Sakakura C, Hagiwara A, Tsujimoto H, et al. Inhibition of colon cancer cell proliferation by antisense oligonucleotides targeting the messenger RNA of the Ki-ras gene. *Anticancer Drugs* 1995;6:553.
209. Aoki K, Yoshida T, Sugimura T, Terada M. Liposome-mediated in vivo gene transfer of antisense K-ras construct inhibits pancreatic tumor dissemination in the murine peritoneal cavity. *Cancer Res* 1995;55:3810.
210. Kita K, Saito S, Morioka CY, Watanabe A. Growth inhibition of human pancreatic cancer cell lines by anti-sense oligonucleotides specific to mutated K-ras genes. *Int J Cancer* 1999;80:553.
211. Alemany R, Ruan S, Kataoka M, et al. Growth inhibitory effect of anti-K-ras adenovirus on lung cancer cells. *Cancer Gene Ther* 1996;3:296.
212. Li M, Lonial H, Citarelia R, Lindh D, Colina L, Kramer R. Tumor inhibitory activity of anti-ras ribozymes delivered by retroviral gene transfer. *Cancer Gene Ther* 1996;3:221.
213. Campbell SL, Khosravi-Far R, Rossman KL, Clark GJ, Der CJ. Increasing complexity of Ras signaling. *Oncogene* 1998;17:1395.
214. Wiftinghofer A. Signal transduction via Ras. *Biol Chem* 1998;379:933.
215. Fridman M, Tikoo A, Varga M, Murphy A, Nur EKMS, Maruta H. The minimal fragments of c-Raf-1 and NF1 that can suppress v-Ha-Ras-induced malignant phenotype. *J Biol Chem* 1994;269:30105.

216. Clark GJ, Drugan JK, Terrell RS, et al. Peptides containing a consensus Ras binding sequence from Raf-1 and the GTPase activating protein NF1 inhibit Ras function. *Proc Natl Acad Sci U S A* 1996;93:1577.
217. Monia BP, Johnston JF, Geiger T, Muller PA, Fabbro D. Antitumor activity of a phosphorothioate antisense oligodeoxynucleotide targeted against C-raf kinase. *Nat Med* 1996;2:668.
218. Monia BP. First- and second-generation antisense inhibitors targeted to human c-raf kinase: in vitro and in vivo studies. *Anticancer Drug Des* 1997;12:327.
219. Geiger T, Muller M, Monia BP, Fabbro D. Antitumor activity of a C-raf antisense oligonucleotide in combination with standard chemotherapeutic agents against various human tumors transplanted subcutaneously into nude mice. *Clin Cancer Res* 1997;3:1179.
220. Gokhale PC, Soldatenkov V, Wang FH, Rahman A, Dritschilo A, Kasid U. Antisense raf oligodeoxyribonucleotide is protected by liposomal encapsulation and inhibits Raf-1 protein expression in vitro and in vivo: implication for gene therapy of radioresistant cancer. *Gene Ther* 1997;4:1289.
221. Dudley DT, Pang L, Decker SJ, Bridges AJ, Saltiel AR. A synthetic inhibitor of the mitogen-activated protein kinase cascade. *Proc Natl Acad Sci U S A* 1995;92:7686.
222. Fiddes RJ, Janes PW, Sivertsen SP, Sutherland RL, Musgrove EA, Daly RJ. Inhibition of the MAP kinase cascade blocks heregulin-induced cell cycle progression in T-47D human breast cancer cells. *Oncogene* 1998;16:2803.
223. Dufourny B, Albias J, van Teeffelen HA, et al. Mitogenic signaling of insulin-like growth factor I in MCF-7 human breast cancer cells requires phosphatidylinositol 3-kinase and is independent of mitogen activated protein kinase. *J Biol Chem* 1997;272:31163.
224. Toker A, Cantley LC. Signalling through the lipid products of phosphoinositide-3-OH kinase. *Nature* 1997;387:673.
225. Klippel A, Kavanaugh WM, Pot D, Williams LT. A specific product of phosphatidylinositol 3-kinase directly activates the protein kinase Akt through its pleckstrin homology domain. *Mol Cell Biol* 1997;17:338.
226. Vlahos CJ, Matter WF, Hui KY, Brown RF. A specific inhibitor of phosphatidylinositol 3-kinase, 2-(4-morpholinyl)-8-phenyl-4H-1-benzopyran-4-one (LY294002). *J Biol Chem* 1994;269:5241.
227. Wymann MP, Bulgarelli LG, Zvelebil MJ, et al. Wortmannin inactivates phosphoinositide 3-kinase by covalent modification of Lys-802, a residue involved in the phosphate transfer reaction. *Mol Cell Biol* 1996;16:1722.
228. Norman BH, Shih C, Toth JE, et al. Studies on the mechanism of phosphatidylinositol 3-kinase inhibition by wortmannin and related analogs. *J Med Chem* 1996;39:1106.
229. Morgan DO. Cyclin-dependent kinases: engines, clocks, and microprocessors. *Annu Rev Cell Dev Biol* 1997;13:261.
230. Morgan DO, Fisher RP, Espinoza FH, et al. Control of eukaryotic cell cycle progression by phosphorylation of cyclin-dependent kinases. *Cancer J Sci Am* 1998;4[Suppl 1]:S77.
231. Roussel MF. Key effectors of signal transduction and G1 progression. *Adv Cancer Res* 1998;74:1.
232. Russell P. Checkpoints on the road to mitosis. *Trends Biochem Sci* 1998;23:399.
233. An HX, Beckmann MW, Reifenberger G, Bender HG, Niederacher D. Gene amplification and overexpression of CDK4 in sporadic breast carcinomas is associated with high tumor cell proliferation. *Am J Pathol* 1999;154:113.
234. Tsihiias J, Kapusta L, Slingerland J. The prognostic significance of altered cyclin-dependent kinase inhibitors in human cancer. *Annu Rev Med* 1999;50:401.
235. Steeg PS, Zhou Q. Cyclins and breast cancer. *Breast Cancer Res Treat* 1998;52:17.
236. Carlson BA, Dubay MM, Sausville EA, Brizuela L, Worland PJ. Flavopiridol induces G1 arrest with inhibition of cyclin-dependent kinase (CDK) 2 and CDK4 in human breast carcinoma cells. *Cancer Res* 1996;56:2973.
237. De Azevedo WF Jr, Mueller-Dieckmann HJ, Schulze-Gahmen U, Worland PJ, Sausville E, Kim SH. Structural basis for specificity and potency of a flavonoid inhibitor of human CDK2, a cell cycle kinase. *Proc Natl Acad Sci U S A* 1996;93:2735.
238. Seynaeve CM, Stetier-Stevenson M, Sebers S, Kaur G, Sausville EA, Worland PJ. Cell cycle arrest and growth inhibition by the protein kinase antagonist UCN-01 in human breast carcinoma cells. *Cancer Res* 1993;53:2081.
239. Wang Q, Fan S, Eastman A, Worland PJ, Sausville EA, O'Connor PM. UCN-01: a potent abrogator of G2 checkpoint function in cancer cells with disrupted p53. *J Natl Cancer Inst* 1996;88:956.

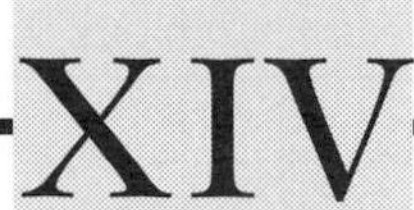

Diseases of the Breast, 2nd ed.,
edited by Jay R. Harris.
Lippincott Williams & Wilkins, Philadelphia © 2000.

Site-Specific Therapy of Metastatic Breast Cancer

CHAPTER 52

Brain Metastases

Patrick Y. Wen and Timothy D. Shafman

Brain metastases are the most common neurologic complication in patients with breast cancer. In the 1990s, there have been important advances in the diagnosis and management of this condition. These include the widespread availability of magnetic resonance imaging (MRI), enabling of detection of small metastases, and studies that have clarified the role of surgery, radiotherapy, and radiosurgery in the management of these tumors. As a result, most patients receive effective palliation, and the majority do not die from their brain metastases.

INCIDENCE AND EPIDEMIOLOGY

It is estimated that between 97,800 and 170,000 new cases of brain metastases occur each year in the United States.[1,2] This number may be increasing as a result of the increased ability of MRI to detect small metastases and as systemic therapy improves and cancer patients live longer.[3–9]

Breast cancer is the second most common cause of brain metastases after lung cancer, accounting for 14% to 20% of the total (Table 1).[7,8–15] The overall incidence of brain metastases in patients with breast cancer varies between series. Estimates of the incidence of clinically apparent metastases range from 5.9% to 16.2% of breast cancer patients,[5,16] whereas the incidence of metastases in autopsy studies ranges from 18% to 30%.[5,17,18]

Brain metastases are more likely to occur in premenopausal women with aggressive, widely disseminated disease.[19] There is no relationship between the size or site of the primary tumor or the number of positive lymph nodes and the development of brain metastases. However, estrogen receptor–negative tumors are more likely to metastasize to the brain than are estrogen receptor–positive tumors.[20] The development of brain metastases is delayed in patients who received adjuvant chemotherapy or hormonal therapy, but overall survival is not affected.[16,19,20]

P. Y. Wen: Department of Neurology, Harvard Medical School, Boston, Massachusetts; Department of Neurology, Division of Neuro-oncology, Brigham and Women's Hospital, Boston, Massachusetts

T. D. Shafman: Department of Radiation Oncology, Harvard Medical School, Brigham and Women's Hospital, Boston, Massachusetts

TABLE 1. *Frequency of brain metastases by primary tumor type*

Primary tumor	No. of patients	Percent
Lung	270	48
Breast	82	15
Melanoma	50	9
Colon	26	5
Other known primary	72	13
Unknown primary	61	11
Total	**561**	**100**

From ref. 6, with permission.

TABLE 2. *Symptoms of brain metastasis in 392 patients*

Symptom	No. of patients	Percent
Headache	163	42
Focal weakness	107	27
Mental change	121	31
Seizure	80	20
Gait ataxia	65	17
Sensory disturbance	24	6
Speech problems	40	10

From ref. 6, with permission.

METHOD OF SPREAD AND DISTRIBUTION

The most common mechanism of metastases to the brain is hematogenous spread.[6] These metastases are usually located directly beneath the grey-white junction.[13] Brain metastases tend to occur at this site because the blood vessels decrease in size at this point and act as a trap for clumps of tumor cells. Brain metastases also tend to be more common at the terminal "watershed areas" of arterial circulation (the zones on the border of or between the territories of major cerebral vessels).[6,13] The distribution of metastases roughly follows the relative weight of (and blood flow to) each area. Approximately 80% of brain metastases are located in the cerebral hemispheres, 15% in the cerebellum, and 5% in the brain stem.[3,13]

Brain metastases from breast cancer are often single, in contrast to malignant melanoma and lung cancer, which have a greater tendency to produce multiple lesions.[13,21] In one study using computed tomography (CT) scan data, 56% of brain metastases from breast cancer were single, and 44% were multiple.[13] However, studies using MRI suggest that the percentage of single metastases is generally lower than was previously believed, accounting for only one-third to one-fourth of patients with cerebral metastases.[6,22]

CLINICAL MANIFESTATIONS

The majority of brain metastases (more than 80%) in breast cancer patients are discovered after the diagnosis of systemic cancer has been made (metachronous presentation).[8] It is estimated that more than two-thirds of patients with cerebral metastases have some neurologic symptoms during the course of their illness.[3,6]

The signs and symptoms caused by brain metastases are extremely variable, and the presence of brain metastases should be suspected in any breast cancer patients in whom new neurologic symptoms develop. The majority of patients present with progressive neurologic dysfunction resulting from a gradually expanding tumor mass and the associated edema or, rarely, the development of obstructive hydrocephalus. Approximately 10% to 20% of patients present acutely with seizures, whereas another 5% to 10% present acutely as a result of strokes caused by embolization of tumor cells or invasion or compression of an artery by tumor, or hemorrhage into a metastasis.[3,8,23] The latter is relatively uncommon, as brain metastases in breast cancer patients tend not to bleed, unlike metastases from tumors such as melanoma or choriocarcinoma.[8]

The clinical presentation of brain metastases is similar to that of other brain tumors (Tables 2 and 3) and includes headaches, focal neurologic dysfunction, cognitive dysfunction, and seizures.

Headaches occur in approximately 40% to 50% of patients with brain metastases. These headaches are usually dull, nonthrobbing, and indistinguishable from tension headaches.[24] The headaches are commonly on the same side as the tumor, although they can be diffuse. Supratentorial metastases typically produce headaches with a frontal location, because the majority of supratentorial pain-sensitive structures are supplied by the trigeminal nerve. The posterior fossa is supplied by cranial nerves IX and X, and the upper cervical nerves and metastases in this area tend to result in pain in the occipital region or neck, although these tumors can occasionally produce pain in the retroorbital region or vertex.[25] Headaches characteristic of increased intracranial pressure, such as early-morning headaches or headaches exacerbated by coughing, bending, and straining, are present in fewer than one-half of patients with brain metastases.[6] These headaches may be associated with nausea, vomiting, transient visual obscurations, and, rarely, syncope. Patients with multiple metastases and metastases in the posterior fossa have a higher frequency of headaches.[6] Because patients are increasingly diagnosed earlier in the course of their disease as a result of the widespread availability of neuroimaging studies, papilledema is now present in fewer than 10% of patients at the time of presentation.[25]

TABLE 3. *Signs of brain metastasis in 392 patients*

Sign	No. of patients	Percent
Altered mental status	139	35
Hemiparesis	174	44
Hemisensory loss	36	9
Papilledema	36	9
Gait ataxia	49	13

From ref. 6, with permission.

Focal neurologic dysfunction is the presenting symptom of 20% to 40% of patients. Hemiparesis is the most common complaint, but the precise symptom varies depending on the location of the metastases.[6,25]

Cognitive dysfunction, including memory problems and mood or personality changes, is the presenting symptom in one-third of patients. However, cognitive dysfunction can be detected in up to 75% of patients if the mental status is examined. The discrepancy in the frequency of signs and symptoms may be explained by the slowness with which the signs develop, by frank denial, or by neglect when the symptoms involve the nondominant hemisphere.[6]

Seizures are the presenting symptom in 10% to 20%[26] of patients with brain metastases, and they eventually develop in an additional 10% to 20% during the course of their illness.[27–29] These patients generally have partial seizures that may secondarily generalize.

DIAGNOSIS

When a breast cancer patient presents with multiple brain lesions, there is usually little doubt about the diagnosis. However, metastases must be distinguished from primary brain tumors (benign or malignant), abscesses, demyelination, cerebral infarctions or hemorrhages, progressive multifocal leukoencephalopathy, and effects of treatment including radiation necrosis. The diagnosis of brain metastases in patients with a single lesion is more difficult. In a study by Patchell et al.,[30] 11% of patients who were initially believed to have a single brain metastasis were given a different diagnosis after the lesion was biopsied. One-half of the nonmetastatic lesions were primary brain tumors, whereas the other half were infections. The false-positive rate for diagnosis of multiple metastases is probably significantly less than the 11% for single metastases. However, in any patient in whom the diagnosis of brain metastases is in doubt, a biopsy should be performed, because this is the only reliable method of establishing the diagnosis.

A single dural-based lesion in a patient with breast cancer poses a particular diagnostic dilemma. The incidence of meningiomas is increased in patients with breast cancer, so it is important to differentiate a dural-based metastasis from a meningioma.[31–33] Frequently, imaging studies are inconclusive, and these patients need to have a biopsy or surgical resection of the lesion to establish the diagnosis.

In addition to diagnosing the brain metastases, it is important to differentiate those patients with single or solitary metastases from those with multiple brain metastases, because their subsequent treatment will be different. The term *single brain metastasis* refers to a single cerebral lesion, and no implication is made regarding the extent of extracranial disease. In contrast, the term *solitary brain metastasis* describes the relatively rare occurrence of a single brain metastasis that is the only known site of metastatic cancer in the body.[6,13]

Although CT scans detect the majority of brain metastases, the best diagnostic test for brain metastases is contrast-enhanced MRI.[22,34–36] This test is more sensitive than enhanced CT scanning (including double-dose delayed-contrast) or nonenhanced MRI in detecting lesions in patients suspected of having cerebral metastases and in differentiating these metastases from other central nervous system (CNS) lesions.[22,34–36] Radiographic features that help differentiate brain metastases from other CNS lesions include the presence of multiple lesions (which helps distinguish metastases from gliomas or other primary tumors), localization of the lesion at the grey-white junction, more circumscribed margins, and relatively large amounts of vasogenic edema compared to the size of the lesion.[6,37] Most metastases appear on T2-weighted MRI images as a result of the peritumoral edema associated with metastases. However, T2-weighted MRI images may miss small metastases (smaller than 5 mm) that do not have much edema and small lesions lying within the edema of a larger lesion. Therefore, contrast-enhanced T1-weighted MRI images are usually necessary. Angiography is now rarely performed. Functional imaging studies, such as single-photon emission computed tomography, positron emission tomography, functional MRI, and magnetic resonance spectroscopy, do not have a role in diagnosing brain metastases but may occasionally be helpful in differentiating tumor recurrence from necrosis in patients who have been treated with stereotactic radiosurgery.[38]

MANAGEMENT

The management of patients with brain metastases can be divided into symptomatic and definitive therapy. Symptomatic therapy includes the use of corticosteroids for the treatment of peritumoral edema and anticonvulsants for control of seizures, whereas definitive therapy includes treatments such as surgery, radiotherapy, and chemotherapy directed at eradicating the tumor itself.

SYMPTOMATIC THERAPY

Corticosteroids

Corticosteroids were first used for treating peritumoral edema by Kofman et al.[39] in 1957 in patients with breast cancer. Subsequently, Galicich et al.[40] in 1961 introduced the use of dexamethasone, and this has remained the standard treatment for peritumoral edema ever since. Corticosteroids are usually indicated in any patient with symptomatic edema. The mechanism of action is not well understood. They may produce their antiedema effect by reducing the permeability of tumor capillaries[41–43] and increasing the clearance of peritumoral edema by facilitating the transport of fluid into the ventricular system, from which it is cleared by cerebrospinal fluid bulk flow.[44]

Most patients are started on dexamethasone, which has the advantage over other corticosteroids of having relatively little mineralocorticoid activity, reducing the potential for fluid retention. In addition, dexamethasone may be associated with a lower risk of infection and cognitive impairment.[45] The usual starting dose is a 10-mg load, followed by 4 mg four times a day, although there is some evidence that lower doses may be as effective.[46] Dexamethasone is often given in four divided doses, but its biological half-life is sufficiently long to allow the medication to be administered twice a day.[47] Most patients improve symptomatically within 24 to 72 hours, although neuroimaging studies may not show a decrease in the amount of edema for up to 1 week.[47] In general, headaches tend to respond better than focal deficits. If 16 mg dexamethasone is insufficient, the dose can be increased up to 100 mg per day.

Despite their usefulness, corticosteroids are associated with a large number of well-known side effects, including myopathy, weight gain, fluid retention, hyperglycemia, insomnia, gastritis, acne, and immunosuppression.[48] The frequency of these complications can be reduced by using the lowest possible dose of corticosteroids.[47] Increasing evidence exists that patients with brain tumor who are receiving corticosteroids are at increased risk of developing *Pneumocystis carinii* pneumonitis.[49–51] This complication can be prevented by treating patients, especially those older than age 50, who are receiving prolonged courses of corticosteroid with trimethoprim-sulfamethoxazole prophylaxis.[6]

Anticonvulsants

As discussed in the section Clinical Manifestations, seizures are the presenting symptom in approximately 10% to 20% of patients with brain metastases and are present at some stage of the illness in another 10% to 20% of patients.[25,27–29,52,53] The treatment of patients with brain metastases who present with seizures is straightforward and involves the use of standard anticonvulsants. To minimize toxicity, patients should be treated with the lowest effective dose of medication, and polytherapy should be avoided whenever possible. Electroencephalography may be useful if the diagnosis of seizures is in doubt, but it is not routinely needed for patients who give a clear history of seizures or do not have symptoms suggestive of seizures.

In addition to the usual complications of anticonvulsants, patients with brain tumor experience an increased incidence of certain side effects, especially drug rashes. Approximately 20% of brain tumor patients treated with phenytoin and undergoing cranial irradiation develop a morbilliform rash, and a small percentage develop Stevens-Johnson syndrome.[54,55] Stevens-Johnson syndrome has also been described in brain tumor patients who receive carbamazepine,[56] whereas patients who receive phenobarbital have an increased incidence of shoulder-hand syndrome.[57]

In addition to producing adverse effects, anticonvulsants have clinically significant interactions with other drugs commonly used in patients with brain metastases. Phenytoin induces the hepatic metabolism of dexamethasone and significantly reduces the half-life and bioavailability of this corticosteroid.[58] Conversely, dexamethasone may reduce phenytoin levels.[59] A number of chemotherapeutic agents commonly used in patients with breast cancer interact with phenytoin, causing the levels to fall and potentially leading to breakthrough seizures,[60] whereas hepatic enzyme–inducing anticonvulsants, such as phenobarbital and phenytoin, may interfere with chemotherapeutic agents such as taxol.[61]

Because the risk of seizures in patients with infratentorial metastases is very small, anticonvulsant therapy is usually not indicated. The role of anticonconvulsant therapy in patients with supratentorial brain metatases who have not had a seizure is unknown. Cohen et al.[27] retrospectively reviewed 160 patients with brain metastases who have not had a seizure and found that those who received prophylactic anticonvulsant therapy with phenytoin had the same frequency of late seizures (10%) as patients who received no treatment.[27] Glantz et al.[28] conducted a small, prospective, placebo-controlled randomized study involving 74 patients that evaluated the efficacy of valproic acid in protecting patients with newly diagnosed brain metastases from seizures.[28] No significant difference was found in the incidence of seizures between patients who received valproic acid (35%) or placebo (24%) after a median follow-up of 7 months, suggesting that prophylactic anticonvulsants may not be effective in these patients. More recently, Weaver et al.[29] completed a prospective randomized study of prophylactic anticonvulsants in 100 patients with brain tumor, including 60 with metastases who have not had seizures.[29] Overall, 26% of patients had seizures. No difference was found in the seizure rate between patients who took anticonvulsants and those who were on no medications. Although this study was limited by a small number of patients and a high noncompliance rate (45% of patients had subtherapeutic anticonvulsant levels), it also did not support the use of prophylactic anticonvulsants in patients with brain metastases. Glantz et al.[62] reviewed the evidence concerning the efficacy of prophylactic anticonvulsants. Because the number of patients in these studies was small, the authors also performed a meta-analysis of the four randomized clinical trials addressing this issue. They concluded that there was no statistical evidence showing a significant benefit of prophylactic anticonvulsant.

Because of the increased incidence of allergic reactions in patients with brain metastases who receive anticonvulsant therapy, and the lack of clear evidence that anticonvulsant therapy reduces the incidence of seizures, routine anticonvulsant therapy is probably unnecessary in breast cancer patients with brain metastases who have not experienced a seizure. Possible exceptions to this are patients with brain metastases in areas of high epileptogenicity (e.g., motor cortex) and patients with both brain metastases and leptomeningeal metastases.[8,63] These patients have a higher incidence of seizures and may benefit from prophylactic anticonvulsant therapy.

Venous Thromboembolic Disease

Venous thromboembolic disease is common in patients with brain metastases, occurring in approximately 20% of patients.[64] The optimal therapy is unknown. These patients are often perceived to be at increased risk of intracranial hemorrhage with anticoagulation because of the vascularity of the tumors and anecdotal case reports of hemorrhage. As a result, the majority of brain metastases patients with venous thromboembolic disease are managed with inferior vena cava (IVC) filtration devices rather than anticoagulation. However, a study by Levin et al.[65] suggests that brain tumor patients with venous thromboembolic disease treated with IVC filters experience a high percentage of complications. Moreover, several retrospective studies suggest that the risk of intracranial hemorrhage in patients with primary brain tumors who are anticoagulated outside the immediate postoperative period may not be significantly increased.[25,66] In 1994, Schiff and DeAngelis[67] reviewed the experience at Memorial Sloan-Kettering Cancer Center with anticoagulation in patients with brain metastases in whom venous thromboembolic disease developed. Of the 42 patients who received anticoagulation at some stage of their treatment, three patients (7%) experienced cerebral hemorrhage. In two of these patients, the bleeding occurred in the setting of supratherapeutic anticoagulation. These studies suggest that anticoagulation may be more effective than IVC filter placement and is acceptably safe when the prothrombin time is maintained in the therapeutic range, especially in patients with brain metastases from breast cancer, because these tumors generally do not hemorrhage.

DEFINITIVE TREATMENT

The management of brain metastases is directed at relieving neurologic symptoms and achieving long-term control of the tumors. The therapeutic modalities available include surgery, radiotherapy, chemotherapy, and hormonal therapy. The optimal combination of therapies for each patient depends on careful evaluation of numerous factors, including the location, size, and number of brain metastases; the patient's age, general condition, and neurologic status; the extent of the systemic cancer, as well as the tumor's response to past therapy and its potential response to future treatments; and possible damage to other organ systems from previous treatment.[6]

SURGERY

The role of surgery in patients with brain metastases is to provide immediate relief of symptoms resulting from the mass effect of the tumor, to establish a histologic diagnosis, and to improve local control of the tumor. Advances in neuroanesthesia and neurosurgery, including the use of computer-assisted stereotactic techniques, cortical mapping, intraoperative ultrasound, and functional and intraoperative MRI, have significantly improved the safety of surgical resection of brain metastases.[6,68,69]

For surgical candidates, the most important factor to consider is the extent of the extracranial disease (Fig. 1). Patients with extensive systemic disease generally have a very limited prognosis and only rarely benefit from surgery. Other important factors influencing the decision concerning surgery include the presence of single or multiple metastases, the location of the tumor, the neurologic status of the patient, and the interval between diagnosis of the primary neoplasm and the brain metastasis.[6,70–73]

SINGLE BRAIN METASTASES

Until the late 1990s, the optimal treatment for patients with a single brain metastasis was controversial. A number of uncontrolled retrospective studies suggested that patients with a single brain metastasis who underwent surgical resection in addition to radiotherapy generally had better outcomes than patients treated with radiotherapy alone. However, these studies were limited by the inevitable selection bias resulting from the inclusion of patients in better condition in surgical series.[71–74] Three randomized prospective studies have now evaluated the role of surgery as an adjunct to whole brain radiotherapy for patients with a single brain metastasis.[30,75–77]

Patchell et al.[30] were the first to address this issue in a prospective randomized study. Fifty-four patients with or without active systemic cancer and a single brain metastasis were randomized to receive either biopsy of the metastases followed by whole brain radiotherapy (36 Gy in 12 fractions) or surgical resection followed by radiotherapy. Six of the 54 patients (11%) did not have a metastasis and were excluded from the study, leaving 48 patients. The patients treated with surgery and whole brain radiotherapy had fewer local recurrences (20% versus 52%), improved survival (40 weeks versus 15 weeks), and a better quality of life, as measured by the Karnofsky performance status (KPS), than patients who received whole brain radiotherapy alone. The median time to recurrence for patients who received surgery and radiotherapy was more than 59 weeks, compared to 21 weeks for patients receiving whole brain radiotherapy alone. A multivariate analysis showed that the factors that correlated significantly with increased survival were surgical treatment of the metastasis, the absence of extracranial disease, longer time to the development of the brain metastasis, and younger age.

A second prospective randomized trial evaluating the role of surgery for patients with single brain metastasis was reported by Vecht et al.[75] and by Noordijk et al.[76] In this study, 63 patients with a single brain metastasis documented by CT scanning were randomized to receive either surgery and whole brain radiotherapy or whole brain radiotherapy

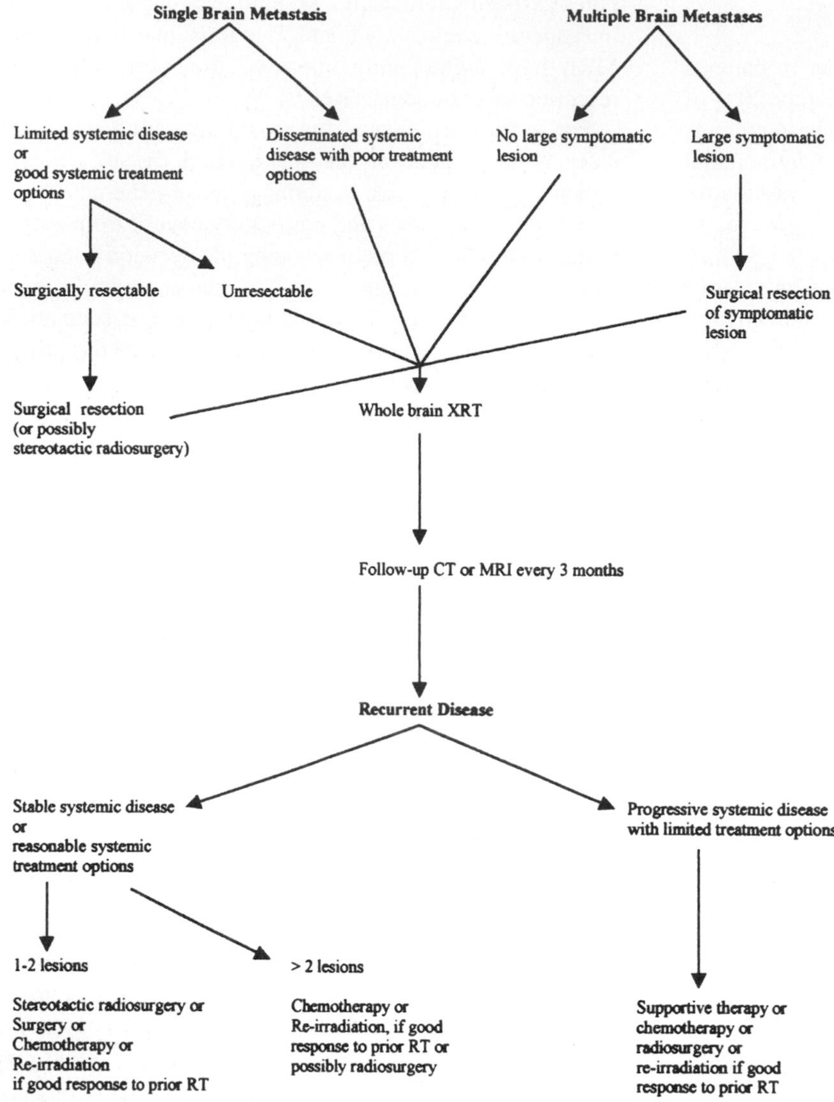

FIG. 1. Management summary for the treatment of breast cancer patients with brain metastases. CT, computed tomography; MRI, magnetic resonance imaging; RT, radiation therapy, XRT, radiotherapy.

alone. The radiotherapy dose was a nonconventional scheme of two fractions a day of 2 Gy each, for a total of 40 Gy given over 2 weeks. Unlike Patchell's study, patients randomized to radiotherapy alone did not undergo a stereotactic biopsy to confirm the diagnosis of metastases, and MR imaging was not performed to exclude multiple small metastases that might have been missed by CT imaging. The overall survival of patients treated with surgery and radiotherapy was significantly longer than that of patients treated with radiotherapy alone (10 months versus 6 months, p = .04). In addition, combined treatment also resulted in significantly increased functionally independent survival [(FIS) 7.5 months versus 3.5 months, p = .06]. The greatest benefit was seen in patients with stable extracranial disease (median survival, 12 months versus 7 months; median FIS, 9 months versus 4 months). Patients with active extracranial disease had a median survival of only 5 months and an FIS of 2.5 months and did not appear to benefit from the addition of surgery. This is consistent with the concept that the extent of systemic disease largely determines the survival of the patient and overcomes any potential advantage that the addition of surgery might have provided in controlling the brain metastasis.[6] Patients older than 60 years had decreased survival rates compared to younger patients (hazard ratio of dying, 2.74; p = .001), consistent with the general importance of age as an adverse prognostic factor for brain tumors.

In contrast to these two studies, a 1997 multicentered, randomized study from Canada failed to detect a difference in survival or quality of life between patients who underwent surgery plus radiotherapy and those who had radiotherapy alone.[77] In this study, the 43 patients randomized to radiotherapy alone had a median survival of 6.3 months, whereas the 41 patients randomized to surgery and radiotherapy had a median survival of only 5.6 months. The failure of this study to demonstrate that the addition of surgery to radiotherapy improved the outcome of patients may be due to the fact that it included patients with a lower baseline median KPS and a higher proportion of extracranial disease.[77,78]

In 1997, two retrospective studies specifically evaluated the role of surgery for brain metastases in breast cancer patients. Pieper et al.[79] reviewed the results of 63 breast cancer patients with newly diagnosed brain metastases who underwent surgery. These patients had a median survival of 16 months. Recurrent metastases developed in 28 of the patients at a median interval of 15 months. Of these, 11 were local, 10 were distal, and 7 developed leptomeningeal disease. Significant favorable prognostic factors included young age, postoperative radiotherapy, good preoperative neurologic status, and limited extracranial disease. Wronski et al.[80] reviewed the experience from Memorial Sloan-Kettering Cancer Center of breast cancer patients with brain metastases who underwent surgery. Of the 70 patients reported, 56 had a single brain metastasis. These patients had a median survival of 16.2 months after the diagnosis of the brain metastases (very similar to the results of Pieper et al.[79]) and an overall median survival of 54 months after the diagnosis of the primary breast tumor. Surprisingly, no difference in survival was found for patients who had single or multiple lesions. Favorable prognostic factors included positive hormone receptors, age younger than 50 years, lesions less than 4 cm in diameter, postoperative radiotherapy, and the absence of leptomeningeal disease. Overall, these studies, together with those of Patchell et al.,[30] Vecht et al.,[75] and Noordijk et al.,[76] provide support for the use of surgery in addition to whole brain radiotherapy for patients with a single brain metastasis and stable extracranial disease.

MULTIPLE BRAIN METASTASES

The role of surgery in patients with multiple brain metastases is usually limited to resection of a large, symptomatic, or life-threatening lesion; to obtain tissue for diagnosis in patients without a known primary tumor; to differentiate a brain metastasis from other cerebral lesions, such as a meningioma; or to resection two or more lesions that can be removed through the same craniotomy.[6] However, as surgical techniques have improved, the ability to resect multiple lesions is becoming more feasible. In one study, Bindal et al.[81] evaluated the efficacy of surgery in 56 patients with multiple brain metastases. These patients were divided into those who had one or more lesions remaining after surgery (group A, n = 30), and those who had all lesions removed (group B, n = 26). In addition, the patients in group B were matched by tumor type, presence or absence of extracranial disease, and time from diagnosis of primary tumor to diagnosis of brain metastases to a group of patients undergoing surgery for a single metastasis (group C, n = 26). The median survivals for patients in groups A, B, and C were 6, 14, and 14 months, respectively. These results suggest that if all the lesions can be removed surgically in patients with multiple brain metastases, the outcome is significantly improved and comparable to the outcome of patients who underwent surgery for a single lesion. However, in contrast to this study, Hazuka et al.[82] found that surgery was of little benefit in patients with multiple brain metastases. They report a series consisting of 28 patients with a single metastasis and 18 patients with multiple metastases. The patients with multiple metastases who underwent surgery and radiation therapy had a median survival of only 5 months, compared to 12 months for those with single brain metastases. In both studies, the surgical morbidity and mortality for patients with multiple brain metastases were low and comparable to those reported for patients with a single metastasis undergoing surgery. However, these conflicting results make it difficult to draw firm conclusions regarding the value of surgical resection in patients with multiple brain metastases. It seems likely that the results of the study by Bindal et al.[81] can only be achieved in highly selected patients treated at a major brain tumor center and are unlikely to have widespread application.

RECURRENT METASTATIC BRAIN TUMORS

For patients in whom recurrent disease develops after standard treatment for brain metastases, surgery may have a role, especially if there is a single symptomatic lesion. In an early study, Sundaresan et al.[83] reported the results of reoperation in 21 patients with brain metastasis. Two-thirds of the patients experienced neurologic improvement, and the median duration of the improvement was 6 months. There was no mortality, and only one patient developed increased neurologic deficits after surgery. More recently, Sawaya[6] reviewed the experience from the M. D. Anderson Cancer Center of 48 patients who underwent reoperation for recurrent brain metastasis. The median interval between the first craniotomy and the diagnosis of recurrence was 6.7 months, and the median survival after craniotomy was 21.9 months. Multivariate analysis revealed that survival was negatively affected by the presence of systemic disease (p = .008), KPS 70 (p = .008), time to recurrence less than 4 months (p = .008), age 40 years (p = .051), and primary tumor type of breast or melanoma (p = .028). Thirty patients had local recurrence, 16 had distant recurrence, and two had both. At the time of recurrence, six (12.5%) patients had two lesions; all the others harbored a single lesion. Four patients were asymptomatic before and after reoperation. Thirty-three (75%) of the 44 symptomatic patients improved after reoperation, and 11 (25%) were stabilized. There was no operative mortality. New or increased neurologic deficits developed in five patients (10.4%) after surgery. In three of these patients, the deficits completely resolved within 30 days of surgery.

These results provide support for surgical resection of recurrent brain metatases in selected patients with symptomatic lesions. Factors that should be considered include the length of time since the initial operation, location of the recurrent tumor, age and performance status of the patient, extent of extracranial disease, and radiosensitivity of the tumor.[6,84] In general, the sooner the metastasis recurs after initial resection, the less likely that reoperation will provide a significant period of palliation.[6,84]

RADIATION THERAPY

Radiation therapy is the mainstay of treatment for patients with brain metastases due to breast cancer. Radiation is effective in the palliation of neurologic symptoms and also significantly decreases the likelihood of death due to neurologic causes. In most patients, overall survival is more likely to be determined by the activity and extent of extracranial disease than by the success or failure of radiotherapy or surgery to control brain metastases.

The main goal of radiation therapy for the treatment of brain metastases is to improve neurologic deficits caused by the tumor deposit. The published overall response rate of neurologic symptoms ranges from 70% to 90%.[85] In one study, 74% of patients had improvement of neurologic symptoms, and 65% maintained this for the duration of their lives or for at least 9 months.[86] Deficits of cranial nerves improve in approximately 40% of patients. However, the potential for improvement is directly related to the time from diagnosis to the time until the start of radiation therapy.[85] Any patient with known metastatic breast cancer and new cranial nerve deficits should rapidly undergo a contrast-enhanced MRI. If metastatic disease is discovered at the skull base or on the meninges, corticosteroids should be administered promptly and radiation therapy initiated as soon as possible.

The optimal dose fractionation schedules for patients with brain metastases has been evaluated with randomized trials conducted by the Radiation Therapy Oncology Group (RTOG). The RTOG completed two trials of several dose/fraction schedules that were subsequently reported together.[87] In the first trial, patients were randomized to 40 Gy in 4 weeks, 40 Gy in 3 weeks, 30 Gy in 3 weeks, or 30 Gy in 2 weeks. The second trial randomized patients to 40 Gy in 3 weeks, 30 Gy in 2 weeks, or 20 Gy in 1 week. The overall response rate and median survival were equivalent in all arms of these studies. Patients treated in the shortest time, with larger fractions, responded more quickly, but the duration of the clinical response and the time to progression were similar in each treatment arm. Symptoms were palliated in 75% to 80% of the patients in all treatment arms of these protocols.[88] The studies of the RTOG failed to identify the best dose and fractionation schedule for the treatment of brain metastasis but did allow for the identification of clinical factors associated with better survival.[89,90] Patients with breast cancer and no soft-tissue metastases were among a group of patients with a favorable prognosis who had a median survival of 28 weeks versus 11 weeks for the remaining patients. The standard treatment regimen for brain metastasis now includes all of these dose ranges and is dependent on issues such as the severity of CNS symptomology, extent of systemic disease, and physician preference.

POSTOPERATIVE RADIATION THERAPY

The goal of postoperative whole brain radiation therapy in patients with solitary brain metastasis is to destroy microscopic residual cancer cells at the site of resection and at other locations within the brain. Theoretically, this should reduce the recurrence rate and prolong survival. A 1998 randomized trial examined the role of postoperative whole brain radiation therapy in patients with single metastasis.[91] Patients received surgical resection of the metastasis and were then randomly assigned to treatment with whole brain radiation therapy or no further treatment. Patients who received radiation were less likely to fail in the brain (18% versus 70%), and this was true both at the original site of disease (10% versus 46%) and other areas of the brain (14% versus 37%). Treated patients were also less likely to die of neurologic causes (14% versus 44%), but no difference was seen in overall survival or duration of functional independence between the treated and untreated groups. The results of this study suggest that postoperative whole brain radiation therapy in patients with a resected solitary metastasis significantly reduces the incidence of neurologic death but has little impact on the overall survival of the patient, which is mainly dependent on the extent of systemic disease.

An important benefit of aggressive treatment for solitary brain metastasis is the likelihood that some patients will become long-term survivors. In one review of 28 breast cancer patients with solitary brain metastasis as the first site of disease recurrence, the median overall survival was 16 months.[92] In a patient with an expected survival of more than 1 year, the neurocognitive impairment that can occur with whole brain radiation therapy can potentially diminish the value of aggressive treatment. Daily fraction size is thought to be related to long-term CNS toxicity, and a retrospective review of 70 patients treated with postoperative radiation therapy using fractions of 300 cGy or greater revealed that 11% showed evidence of dementia.[93] Therefore, patients with a solitary CNS metastasis from breast cancer with no or controlled systemic disease are best treated with daily fractions of 250 cGy or less to decrease the likelihood of long-term CNS toxicity.

LATE TOXICITY

For long-term survivors after whole brain radiation therapy, late complications can be debilitating. Leukoencephalopathy and brain atrophy can lead to neurocognitive deterioration and dementia, whereas brain necrosis can result in more specific neurologic sequelae, depending on the site of necrosis.[93] Neuroendocrine dysfunction can also be serious.[48,93] The risk for late complications from whole brain radiation is related to total dose, fraction size, patient age, extent of disease, and neurologic impairment at presentation.[94] Prior or concurrent chemotherapy may also affect the occurrence of late CNS toxicity. If whole brain radiotherapy is to be given, a dose-fraction schedule should be used that takes into account the overall clinical status of the patient while maximizing the palliation of symptoms and, if appropriate, minimizing the risk of long-term complications.

REIRRADIATION

The number of patients who receive reirradiation of brain metastasis is quite small, because most have progressive disease elsewhere in the body and should be treated with supportive care measures. However, there are times when recurrence of brain metastasis develops in a patient with controlled systemic disease. Patients with a solitary or a few (three or less) metastases are candidates for treatment with radiosurgery, as this produces less toxicity than repeating whole brain radiation therapy (see the following section, Stereotactic Radiosurgery) and is likely to be more effective than systemic therapy.[95] Other patients should be considered for treatment with systemic chemotherapy or hormonal therapy, as discussed in other sections of this chapter. For patients not eligible for radiosurgery or systemic therapy, treatment with whole or partial brain radiation may be indicated. A 1992 review evaluated 189 patients from three separate studies who were reirradiated.[85] The overall clinical response rate was 42% to 75%, and the median survival from the time of reirradiation was between 3.5 and 5 months. The published techniques of reirradiation include doses from 8.0 Gy in 2 weeks to 30.6 Gy in 3 weeks, with a median of approximately 20 Gy in 2 weeks, but there is no consensus on which dose fractionation schedule is appropriate or how long after the initial course of radiation therapy it is appropriate to reirradiate.[96] The tolerance of the brain is more than likely to be exceeded by reirradiation, but with the limited survival of these patients, data are inadequate to evaluate the consequences of this treatment.[97]

STEREOTACTIC RADIOSURGERY

Stereotactic radiosurgery is a technique that delivers a high single dose of radiation to a radiographically discrete treatment volume. Radiosurgery can be performed with high-energy x-rays produced by linear accelerators, with gamma rays from the gamma knife, and less frequently with charged particles, such as protons produced by cyclotrons.[98] All of the stereotactic radiation techniques result in rapid falloff of dose at the edge of the target volume, resulting in a clinically insignificant radiation dose to normal nontarget tissue. Metastases are usually small, radiographically discrete lesions that are noninvasive, making them ideal targets for radiosurgery.[99] The results of radiosurgery used for the treatment of 248 patients with 421 metastatic lesions were reported in 1995.[95] Only 48 of 421 (11%) lesions have progressed within the radiosurgery volume after a median follow-up of 26 months. The median survival for this group of patients was 9.4 months, measured from the time of radiosurgery. A total of 6% of the patients in this series required reoperation for increasing mass effect and steroid dependency due to radiation necrosis. In a multivariate analysis, the absence of systemic disease (relative risk, 4.4; p = .0001) and age younger than 60 years (relative risk, 1.6; p = .002) were factors associated with improved survival. Histology had no influence on local control or toxicity, indicating that breast cancer metastases are appropriate targets for radiosurgery.

The Patchell study[30] and the Vecht study[75,76] indicate that patients with a single brain metastasis who are treated with surgery and radiotherapy have a survival advantage compared to those treated with radiotherapy alone. Many clinical investigators believe that radiosurgery can act as an alternative to surgical resection.[100,101] Although there are no completed randomized trials comparing radiosurgery to surgery, Auchter et al.[102] identified 122 patients who met the selection criteria used by Patchell et al.[30] and were treated with whole brain radiotherapy (median, 37.5 Gy) followed by a radiosurgery boost (median, 17 Gy). The overall local control rate was 86%, with an actuarial median survival of 56 weeks and a neurologic median survival of KPS greater than 70% of 44 weeks. These results are comparable to the surgery and radiation therapy arms of the Patchell,[30] Vecht,[75] and Noordijk[76] studies and are better than the whole brain treatment alone arms.

Evidence suggests that aggressive local therapy (surgery and whole brain radiation therapy) for patients with a single brain metastasis can produce superior survival compared to treatment with whole brain radiation therapy alone. Radiosurgery can be used as a substitute for surgery, and this likely will result in comparable outcomes. For patients with a small asymptomatic or mildly symptomatic lesion, radiosurgery appears to be an excellent alternative to operation. Radiosurgery may also be useful in patients with recurrence of brain metastasis after whole brain radiation therapy (Fig. 2). The study by Patchell et al.[91] reveals that 37% of patients had recurrences in other sites within the brain if they did not receive whole brain radiation, and, in addition, other investigators have shown that better local control is obtained in patients who received whole brain radiation therapy in addition to radiosurgery.[101] Therefore, the use of up-front radiosurgery alone should be limited to cases in which no alternatives are available, such as prior high-dose radiation to the head and neck area or when the patient refuses whole brain radiation therapy. Finally, radiosurgery cannot be justified as an adjunct to whole brain radiotherapy in patients with multiple brain metastasis or progressive systemic disease.

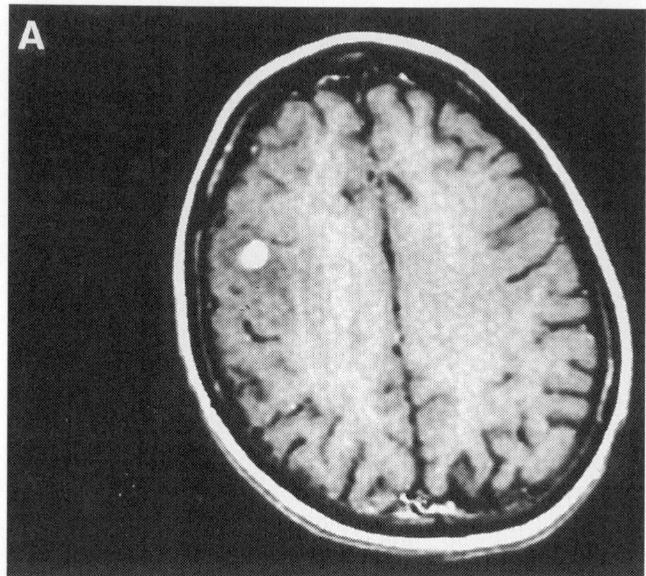

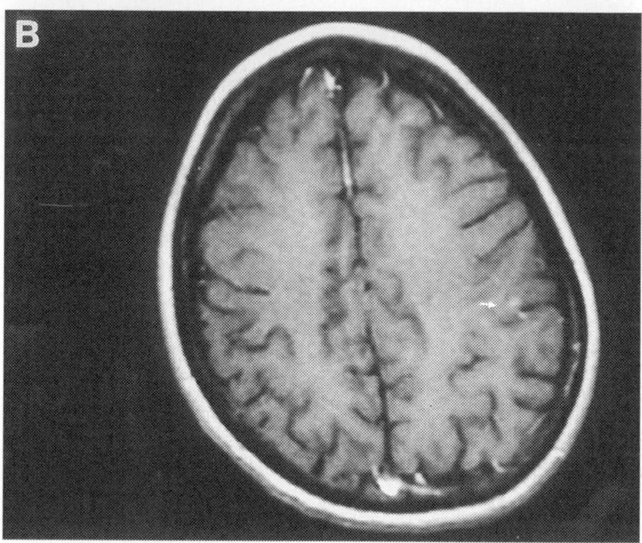

FIG. 2. Forty-two-year-old woman with breast cancer with a recurrent brain metastasis treated with stereotactic radiosurgery. **A:** Axial T1-weighted magnetic resonance image (MRI) of the brain enhanced with gadolinium showing a metastasis in the right frontal lobe. The patient had received whole brain radiation therapy 2 years previously for a cerebellar metastasis. An 18-Gy dose was administered with a 12.5-mm collimator using two noncoplanar arcs for a tumor volume of 0.58 cc. **B:** Axial T1-weighted MRI 6 months later showing resolution of the original metastasis. There is now a small metastasis in the left frontal lobe (*arrow*) that was also treated successfully with radiosurgery.

CHEMOTHERAPY

The role of chemotherapy for the treatment of patients with brain metastases has not been defined. Chemotherapy is rarely used as part of the overall management of brain metastases. Traditionally, it has generally been assumed that the blood–brain barrier prevented chemotherapeutic agents from entering the CNS. However, evidence exists that the blood–brain barrier is in fact disrupted within brain tumors.[103] This suggests that other factors may be more important in determining the generally disappointing results of chemotherapy for brain metastases, such as the intrinsic resistance to chemotherapy of many tumors that metastasize to the brain.[104]

Patients with metastatic breast cancer have been treated with chemotherapy since 1970, and the results have been generally more promising than chemotherapy for brain metastases from less chemosensitive tumors. In the largest series to date, Rosner et al.[105] treated 100 consecutive breast cancer patients with brain metastases with several chemotherapy regimens. Of note, these patients had not received prior chemotherapy for their systemic disease. Overall, 50% of patients had an objective response [10% had a complete response (CR), and 40% had a partial response (PR)]. In addition, 9% had stable disease. The median duration of remission for complete responders was 10 months, and for partial responders it was 7 months. Twenty-seven of 52 (52%) patients treated with cyclophosphamide (C), 5-fluorouracil (F), and prednisone (P) (CFP); 19 of 35 (54%) patients treated with CFP-methotrexate (M) and vincristine (V); 3 of 7 (43%) patients treated with methotrexate, vincristine, and prednisone; and 1 of 6 (17%) who received cyclophosphamide and doxorubicin (A) responded. Rosner et al.[106] subsequently treated an additional 26 patients with progressive brain metastases from breast cancer with four different chemotherapeutic regimens: CFP, CFPMV, CA, and mitomycin and vinblastine sulfate (Velban). Objective responses were seen in 61% of patients, and another 15% had stable disease. The median survival for responders was 12 months, compared with 2.4 months for nonresponders. Prior systemic chemotherapy did not affect the response of the brain metastases, arguing against the concept of the brain as a pharmacologic sanctuary.

Cocconi et al. treated 22 consecutive patients with brain metastases from breast cancer with cisplatin and etoposide every 3 weeks.[107] Five (23%) had a complete response and seven (32%) had a partial response, giving an overall response rate of 55%. Median duration of response was 40 weeks, and median survival was 58 weeks.

Boogerd et al.[108] treated 20 patients with CMF or cyclophosphamide, adriamycin, and 5-fluorouracil (CAF). Seven patients had recurrent disease after whole brain radiotherapy. Objective tumor regression occurred in 76% of patients after two cycles of chemotherapy. The median duration of neurologic remission was 30 weeks, with a median survival of 25 weeks (range 2 to 83 weeks). When the results of these chemotherapy patients were compared to those of 29 historical control subjects treated with whole brain radiotherapy, the neurologic response rate, duration of response, and median survival were found to be better in the patients treated with chemotherapy.

In 1997, Kaba et al.[109] treated 115 patients with progressive or recurrent brain metastases with a combination of drugs, including thioguanine, procarbazine, dibromodulcitol, CCNU, 5-fluorouracil, and hydroxyurea (TPDC-FuHu), designed to improve the efficacy of CCNU. Twenty-eight of the patients had breast cancer; in these patients the overall response rate (CR + PR) was 66%, and the median time to progression was 26 weeks.

Lange et al.[110] treated 61 patients with brain metastases from breast cancer with radiotherapy and concurrent chemotherapy with ifosfamide and BCNU. Twenty percent of patients had a CR, 45% had a PR, and the overall median survival was 8 months.[110] Whether the chemotherapy produced any additional benefit is unclear. Reports also exist of patients responding to intraarterial carmustine[111] and cisplatin.[112]

Overall, these studies suggest that chemotherapy has some activity against brain metastases from breast cancer and may have a role as palliative therapy in patients with recurrent disease after radiotherapy.

HORMONAL THERAPY

Hormonal agents such as tamoxifen have small lipophilic molecules that readily cross the blood–brain barrier. In one study by Lien et al.,[113] the concentration of tamoxifen and its metabolites was found to be 46-fold higher in brain metastases than in blood. No formal studies have evaluated the therapeutic efficacy of hormonal therapy for brain metastases, but there are several anecdotal reports of brain metastases from breast cancer responding to tamoxifen[114,115] and megestrol acetate.[116]

PROGNOSIS

The median survival of patients with untreated brain metastases is approximately 1 month.[14] The addition of steroids increases survival to 2 months,[13] and whole brain radiation therapy further improves survival to 3 to 6 months.[15,87] Patients with single brain metastases and limited extracranial disease who are treated with surgery and whole brain radiotherapy have a median survival of approximately 10 to 16 months.[30,75,79,88] Breast cancer patients with brain metastases generally have a more favorable prognosis than do brain metastases patients with other types of primary tumor.[88] Favorable prognostic factors include the absence of systemic disease, young age (younger than 60 years), good performance status (KPS of 70 or greater), long time to development of metastasis, surgical resection, and, possibly, positive hormone receptors.[6,29,74,85,86,114,117,118.]

Brain metastases represent an increasingly important problem in patients with breast cancer. A number of advances, including the introduction of stereotactic radiosurgery, have allowed a greater percentage of patients to receive effective palliation. However, more effective treatments are needed. In addition, as patients survive longer, neurologic complications of radiation are seen with increasing frequency.

REFERENCES

1. Posner JB. Management of brain metastases. *Rev Neurol* 1992;148:477.
2. Sawaya R, Bindal RK. Metastatic brain tumors. In: Kaye AH, Laws ER, eds. *Brain tumors*. Edinburgh, UK: Churchill Livingstone, 1995:923.
3. Cairncross JG, Posner JB. The management of brain metastases. In Walker MD, eds. *Oncology of the nervous system*. Boston: Nijhoff, 1983:341.
4. Walker AE, Robins M, Weinfeld FD. Epidemiology of brain tumors: the national survey of intracranial neoplasms. *Neurology* 1985;35:219.
5. Takakura K, Sano K, Hojo S, et al. *Metastatic tumors of the central nervous system*. Tokyo: Igaku-Shoin, 1982:113.
6. Loeffler JS, Patchell RA, Sawaya R. Metastatic brain cancer. In: DeVita VT, Hellman S, Rosenberg SA, eds. *Cancer: principles and practice of oncology*. Philadelphia: Lippincott–Raven, 1997:2523.
7. Pickren JW, Lopez G, Tsukada Y, et al. Brain metastases: an autopsy study. *Cancer Treat Symp* 1983;2:295.
8. Posner JB. *Neurologic complications of cancer*. Philadelphia: FA Davis, 1995.
9. Boogerd W, Voss VW, Hart AAM, Baris G. Brain metastases in breast cancer: natural history, prognostic factors and outcome. *J Neurooncol* 1993;15:165.
10. Flowers A, Levin VA. Management of brain metastases from breast carcinoma. *Oncology* 1993;7:21.
11. Posner JB, Chernick NL. Intracranial metastases from systemic cancer. *Adv Neurol* 1978;19:579.
12. Zimm S, Wampler GL, Stablein D, Hazra T, Young HF. Intracerebral metastases in solid tumor patients: natural history and results of treatment. *Cancer* 1981;48:384.
13. Delattre JY, Krol G, Thaler HT, Posner JB. Distribution of brain metastases. *Arch Neurol* 1988;45:741.
14. Markesbery WR, Brooks WH, Gupta GD, et al. Treatment for patients with cerebral metastases. *Arch Neurol* 1978;35:754.
15. Cairncross JG, Kim JH, Posner JB. Radiation therapy for brain metastases. *Ann Neurol* 1980;7:529.
16. DiStefano A, Yap HY, Hortobagyi GN, et al. The natural history of breast cancer patients with brain metastases. *Cancer* 1979;44:1913.
17. Tsukada Y, Fouad A, Pickren JW, et al. Central nervous system metastases from breast carcinoma: autopsy study. *Cancer* 1983;52:2349.
18. Lee Y. Breast carcinoma: pattern of metastatic spread at autopsy. *J Surg Oncol* 1983;23:175.
19. Sparrow GEA, Rubens RD. Brain metastases from breast cancer: clinical course, prognosis, and influence on treatment. *Clin Oncol* 1981;7:291.
20. Stewart JF, King RJ, Sexton SA, et al. Oestrogen receptors, sites of metastatic disease, and survival in recurrent breast disease. *Eur J Cancer Clin Oncol* 1981;17:449.
21. Dropcho EJ. Management of multiple brain metastases. In: Hachinski VC, ed. *Challenges in neurology*. Philadelphia: FA Davis, 1992: 269.
22. Sze G, Milano E, Johnson C, et al. Detection of brain metastases: comparison of contrast-enhanced MR with unenhanced MR and contrast CT. *Am J Neuroradiol* 1990;11:785.
23. Nutt SH, Patchell RA. Intracranial hemorrhage associated with primary and secondary tumors. *Neurosurg Clin N Am* 1992;3:591.
24. Forsyth PA, Posner JB. Headaches in patients with brain tumors: a study of 111 patients. *Neurology* 1993;43:1678.
25. Wen PY. Diagnosis and management of brain tumors. In: Black PM, Loeffler JS, eds. *Cancer of the nervous system*. Cambridge, UK: Blackwell Science, 1997:106.
26. Coia LR, Aaronson N, Linggood R, et al. A report of the consensus workshop panel on the treatment of brain metastases. *Int J Radiat Oncol Biol Phys* 1992;23:223.
27. Cohen N, Strauss G, Lew R, et al. Should prophylactic anticonvulsants be administered to patients with newly-diagnosed cerebral metastases? A retrospective analysis. *J Clin Oncol* 1988;6:1621.

28. Glantz M, Cole B, Friedberg M, et al. A randomized, blinded, placebo-controlled trial of divalproex sodium prophylaxis in adults with newly diagnosed brain tumors. *Neurology* 1996;46:985.
29. Weaver S, Deangelis LM, Fulton D, et al. A prospective randomized study of prophylactic anticonvulsants in patients with primary or metastatic brain tumors and without seizures. *Ann Neurol* 1997; 42:430.
30. Patchell RA, Tibbs PA, Walsh JW, et al. A randomized trial of surgery in the treatment of single metastases to the brain. *N Engl J Med* 1990;322:494.
31. Smith FP, Savik M, McDonald JS. Association of breast cancer with meningioma: report of two cases and review of the literature. *Cancer* 1978;42:1992.
32. Schoenberg BS, Christine BW, Whisnant JO. Nervous system neoplasms and primary malignancy of other sites: the unique association between meningiomas and breast cancer. *Neurology* 1975;25:705.
33. Rubinstein AB, Schein M, Reichenthal E. The association of carcinoma of the breast with meningioma. *Surg Gynecol Obstet* 1989;169: 334.
34. Yuh WTC, Engelken JD, Muhonen MG, et al. Experience with high-dose gadolinium MR imaging in the evaluation of brain metastases. *AJNR Am J Neuroradiol* 1992;13:335.
35. Davis PC, Hudgins PA, Peterman SB, et al. Diagnosis of cerebral metastases: double-dose delayed CT vs contrast-enhanced MR imaging. *AJNR Am J Neuroradiol* 1991;12:293.
36. Runge VM, Kirsch JE, Burke VJ, et al. High-dose gadoteridol in MR imaging of intracranial neoplasms. *J Magn Reson Imaging* 1992;2:9.
37. Williams AL. Tumors. In: Williams AL, Haughton VM, eds. *Cranial computed tomography: a comprehensive text.* St. Louis: Mosby, 1985:17.
38. Schwartz RB. Functional imaging of CNS tumors. In: Black PB, Loeffler JS, eds. *Cancer of the nervous system.* Cambridge, UK: Blackwell Science, 1997:98.
39. Kofman S, Garvin JS, Nagamani, et al. Treatment of cerebral metastases from breast cancer with prednisone. *JAMA* 1957;163:1473.
40. Galicich JH, French LA, Melby JC. Use of dexamethasone in the treatment of cerebral edema associated with brain tumors. *Lancet* 1961; 81:46.
41. Hedley-Whyte ET, Hsu DW. Effect of dexamethasone in blood–brain barrier in the normal mouse. *Ann Neurol* 1986;19:373.
42. Fishman RA. *Cerebrospinal fluid in diseases of the nervous system*, 2nd ed. Philadelphia: WB Saunders, 1992.
43. Nakagawa H, Groothuis DR, Patlak CS, et al. Dexamethasone reduces brain tumor extracellular space capillary permeability: implications for diagnosis and therapy. *Neurology* 1984;34:184.
44. Eidelberg D. Neurological effects of steroid treatment. In: Rottenberg DA, ed. *Neurological complications of cancer treatment.* Boston: Butterworth–Heinemann, 1991:173.
45. Batchelor T, DeAngelis LM. Medical management of cerebral metastases. *Neurosurg Clin North Am* 1996;7:435.
46. Vecht CJ, Hovestadt A, Verbiest HBC, et al. Dose-effect relationship of dexamethasone on Karnofsky performance in metastatic brain tumors: a randomized study of doses of 4, 8, and 16 milligrams per day. *Neurology* 1994;44:675.
47. Vecht CJ, Verbiest HBC. Use of glucocorticoids in neuro-oncology. In: Wiley RG, ed. *Neurological complications of cancer*. New York: Marcel Dekker, 1995:199.
48. Delattre JY, Posner JB. Neurological complications of chemotherapy and radiation therapy. In: Aminoff MJ, ed. *Neurology and general medicine*. New York: Churchill Livingstone, 1994:421.
49. Henson JW, Jalaj JK, Walker RW, et al. Pneumocystis carinii pneumonia in patients with primary brain tumors. *Arch Neurol* 1991;48:406.
50. Slivka A, Wen PY, Shea WM, Loeffler JS. *Pneumocystis carinii* pneumonia during steroid taper in patients with primary brain tumors. *Am J Med* 1993;94:216.
51. Schiff D. Pneumocystis pneumonia in brain tumor patients: risk factors and clinical features. *J Neurooncol* 1996;27:235.
52. Morris HH, Estes ML. Brain tumors and chronic epilepsy. In: Wyllie E, ed. *The treatment of epilepsy: principles and practice*. Philadelphia: Lea & Febiger, 1993:659.
53. Cascino GD. Epilepsy and brain tumors: implications for treatment. *Epilepsia* 1990;3:S37.
54. Delattre JY, Safai B, Posner JB. Erythema multiforme and Stevens-Johnson syndrome in patients receiving cranial irradiation and phenytoin. *Neurology* 1988;38:194.
55. Mamon H, Wen PY, Loeffler JS. Allergic skin reactions to anticonvulsant medications in patients receiving cranial radiation. *Epilepsia* 1999;40:341.
56. Khe HX, Delattre J-Y, Poisson M. Stevens-Johnson syndrome in a patient receiving cranial irradiation and carbamazepine. *Neurology* 1990;40:1144.
57. Taylor LP, Posner JB. Phenobarbital rheumatism in patients with brain tumor. *Ann Neurol* 1989;25:92.
58. Werk EE, Choi Y, Sholiton Z, et al. Interference in the effect of dexamethasone by diphenylhydantoin. *N Engl J Med* 1969;281:32.
59. Lawson LA, Blouin RA, Smith RB, et al. Phenytoin-dexamethasone interaction: a previously unreported observation. *Surg Neurol* 1981; 16:23.
60. Grossman SA, Sheidler VR, Gilbert MR. Decreased phenytoin levels in patients receiving chemotherapy. *Am J Med* 1989;87:505.
61. Fetell MR, Grossman SA, Fisher JD, et al. Preirradiation paclitaxel in glioblastoma multiforme: efficacy, pharmacology, and drug interactions. New Approaches to Brain Tumor Therapy Central Nervous System Consortium. *J Clin Oncol* 1997;15:3121.
62. Glantz MJ, Cole BF, Forsyth PA, et al. Anticonvulsant prophylaxis in patients with brain tumors: a systematic review of the evidence (*in press*).
63. Jacobs M, Phuphanich S. Seizures in brain metastasis and meningeal carcinomatosis. *Proc Am Soc Clin Oncol* 1990;96:A373.
64. Sawaya R, Zuccarello M, Elkalliny M, Nishiyama H. Postoperative venous thromboembolism and brain tumors: part 1. Clinical profile. *J Neurooncol* 1992;14:119.
65. Levin JM, Schiff D, Loeffler JS, et al. Complications of therapy for venous thromboembolic disease in patients with brain tumors. *Neurology* 1993;43:1111.
66. Ruff RL, Posner JB. The incidence and treatment of peripheral venous thrombosis in patients with glioma. *Ann Neurol* 1983;13:334.
67. Schiff D, DeAngelis LM. Therapy of venous thromboembolism in patients with brain metastases. *Cancer* 1994;73:493.
68. Kelly PJ, Abe H, Aida T, et al. Results of computed tomography-based computer-assisted stereotactic resection of metastatic intracranial tumors. *Neurosurgery* 1988;22:7.
69. Ebeling U, Schmid UD, Ying H, et al. Safe surgery of lesions near the motor cortex using intraoperative mapping techniques: a report on 50 patients. *Acta Neurochir* (*Wein*) 1992;119:23.
70. Sundaresan N, Galicich J. Surgical treatment of brain metastases: clinical and computerized tomography evaluation of the results of treatment. *Cancer* 1985;55:1382.
71. Galicich JH, Sundaresan N, Arbit E, et al. Surgical treatment of single brain metastasis: factors associated with survival. *Cancer* 1980;45:381.
72. Winston KR, Walsh JW, Fischer EG. Results of operative treatment of intracranial metastatic tumors. *Cancer* 1980;45:2639.
73. White K, Fleming T, Laws E. Single metastasis to the brain. Surgical treatment in 122 consecutive patients. *Mayo Clin Proc* 1981;56:424.
74. Ransohoff J. Surgical management of metastatic tumors. *Semin Oncol* 1975;2:21.
75. Vecht CJ, Haaxma-Reiche EM, Noordijk GW, et al. Treatment of single brain metastasis: radiotherapy alone or combined with neurosurgery? *Ann Neurol* 1993;83:583.
76. Noordijk EM, Vecht CJ, Haaxma-Reiche H, et al. The choice of treatment of single brain metastasis should be based on extracranial tumor activity and age. *Int J Radiat Oncol Biol Phys* 1994;29:711.
77. Mintz AP, Kestle J, Rathbone MP, et al. A randomized trial to assess the efficacy of surgery in addition to radiotherapy in patients with a single brain metastasis. *Cancer* 1996;78:1470.
78. Mintz AP, Cairncross JG. Treatment of a single brain metastasis. The role of radiation following surgical resection. *JAMA* 1998;280:1527.
79. Pieper DR, Hess KR, Sawaya RE. Role of surgery in the treatment of brain metastases in patients with breast cancer. *Ann Surg Oncol* 1997;4:481.
80. Wronski M, Arbit E, McCormick B, Wronski M. Surgical treatment of 70 patients with brain metastases from breast carcinoma. *Cancer* 1997;80:1746.
81. Bindal RK, Sawaya R, Leavens ME, et al. Surgical treatment of multiple brain metastases. *J Neurosurg* 1993;79:210.
82. Hazuka MB, Burleson W, Stroud DN, et al. Multiple brain metastases are associated with poor survival in patients treated with surgery and radiotherapy. *J Clin Oncol* 1993;11:369.
83. Sundaresan N, Sachdev V, DiGiacinto G. Reoperation for brain metastases. *J Clin Oncol* 1988;6:1625.

84. Kaye A. Malignant brain tumors. In: Little J, Awad I, eds. *Reoperative neurosurgery*. Baltimore: Williams & Wilkins, 1992:49.
85. Coia LR. The role of radiation therapy in the treatment of brain metastases. *Int J Radiat Oncol Biol Phys* 1992;23:22.
86. Cairncross JG, Kim JH, Posner JB. Radiation therapy for brain metastasis. *Ann Neurol* 1980;7:529.
87. Borgelt B, Gelber R, Kramer S, et al. The palliation of brain metastases. Final results of the first two studies by the Radiation Therapy Oncology group. *Int J Radiat Oncol Biol Phys* 1980;6:1.
88. Berk L. An overview of radiotherapy trials for the treatment of brain metastases. *Oncology* 1995;9:1205.
89. Gelber R, Larson M, Borgelt B, et al. Equivalence of radiation schedules for the palliative treatment of brain metastases in patients with favorable prognosis. *Cancer* 1981;48:1749.
90. Diener-West M, Dobbins TW, Phillips TL, et al. Identification of an optimal subgroup for treatment evaluation of patients with brain metastases using RTOG study 7916. *Int J Radiat Oncol Biol Phys* 1989; 16:669.
91. Patchell RA, Tibbs PA, Regine WF, et al. Postoperative radiotherapy in the treatment of single brain metastases to the brain. *JAMA* 1998;280:1485.
92. Boogerd W, Hart AA, Tjahja IS. Treatment and outcome of brain metastasis as first site of distant metastasis from breast cancer. *J Neurooncol* 1997;35:161.
93. DeAngelis L, Delattre J-Y, Posner JB. Radiation-induced dementia in patients cured of brain metastases. *Neurology* 1989;39:789.
94. Schultheiss TE, Kun LE, Ang KK, et al. Radiation response of the central nervous system. *Int J Radiat Oncol Biol Phys* 1995;31:1093.
95. Alexander E III, Moriarty TM, Davis RB, et al. Stereotactic radiosurgery for the definitive, noninvasive treatment of brain metastases. *J Natl Cancer Inst* 1995;87:34.
96. Cooper JS, Steinfield A, Lerch IA. Cerebral metastases: value of reirradiation in selected patients. *Radiology* 1990;174:883.
97. Schultheiss TE, Kun LE, Ang KK, et al. Radiation response of the central nervous system. *Int J Radiat Oncol Biol Phys* 1995;31:1093.
98. Phillips MH, Stelzer KJ, Griffin TW, et al. Stereotactic radiosurgery: a review and comparisons of methods. *J Clin Oncol* 1994;12:1085.
99. Loeffler JS, Kooy HM, Wen PY, et al. The treatment of recurrent brain metastases with stereotactic radiosurgery. *J Clin Oncol* 1990;8:576.
100. Mehta MP, Rozental JM, Levin AB, et al. Defining the role of radiosurgery in the management of brain metastases. *Int J Radiat Oncol Biol Phys* 1992;24:619.
101. Flickinger JC, Kondziolka D, Lunsford LD, et al. A multi-institutional experience with stereotactic radiosurgery for solitary brain metastasis. *Int J Radiat Oncol Biol Phys* 1994;28:797.
102. Auchter RM, Lamond JP, Alexander E III, et al. A multi-institutional outcome and prognostic factor analysis of radiosurgery for resectable single brain metastasis. *Int J Radiat Oncol Biol Phys* 1996;35:27.
103. Vick NA, Khandekar JD, Bigner DD. Chemotherapy of brain tumors: the blood-brain barrier is not a factor. *Arch Neurol* 1977;34:523.
104. Buckner JC. The role of chemotherapy in the treatment of patients with brain metastases from solid tumors. *Cancer Metastasis Rev* 1991; 10:335.
105. Rosner D, Nemoto T, Lane WW. Chemotherapy induces regression of brain metastases in breast carcinoma. *Cancer* 1986;58:832.
106. Rosner D, Flowers A, Lane WW. Chemotherapy induces regression of brain metastases in breast carcinoma patients: update study. *Proc Ann Meet Am Soc Clin Oncol* 1993;12:A508.
107. Cocconi G, Lottici R, Bisagni G, et al. Combination therapy with platinum and etoposide of brain metastases from breast carcinoma. *Cancer Invest* 1990;8:327.
108. Boogerd W, Dalesio O, Bais EM, et al. Response of brain metastases from breast cancer to systemic chemotherapy. *Cancer* 1992;69:972.
109. Kaba SE, Kyritsis AP, Hess K, et al. TPDC-FuHu chemotherapy for the treatment of recurrent metastatic brain tumors. *J Clin Oncol* 1997;15:1063.
110. Lange OF, Scheef W, Haase KD. Palliative radio-chemotherapy with ifosfamide and BCNU for breast cancer patients with cerebral metastases. A 5-year experience. *Cancer Chemother Pharmacol* 1990;26:S78.
111. Madajewicz S, West CR, Park MC, et al. Phase II study of intraarterial BCNU therapy for metastatic brain tumors. *Cancer* 1981;47:653.
112. Lehane DE, Bryan RN, Horowitz B, et al. Intra-arterial cisplatin chemotherapy for patients with primary and metastatic brain tumors. *Cancer Drug Deliv* 1983;1:69.
113. Lien EA, Wester K, Lonning PE, et al. Distribution of tamoxifen and metabolites into brain tissue and brain metastases in breast cancer patients. *Br J Cancer* 1991;63:641.
114. Colomer R, Casas D, del Campo JM, et al. Brain metastases from breast cancer may respond to endocrine therapy. *Breast Cancer Res Treat* 1986;12:83.
115. Pors H, Edler von Eyben F, Sorensen OS, et al. Long-term remission of multiple brain metastases with tamoxifen. *J Neurooncol* 1991;10:173.
116. Van der Gaast A, Alexieva-Figusch J, Vecht C, et al. Complete remission of a brain metastasis to third line hormonal treatment with megestrol acetate. *Am J Clin Oncol* 1990;13:507.
117. Swift P, Phillips T, Martz K, et al. CT characteristics of patients with brain metastases treated in RTOG study 79-16. *Int J Radiat Oncol Biol Phys* 1993;25:209.
118. Gaspar L, Scott C, Rotman M, et al. Recursive partitioning analysis (RPA) of prognostic factors in three Radiation Therapy Oncology Group (RTOG) brain metastases trials. *Int J Radiat Oncol Biol Phys* 1997;37:745.

Diseases of the Breast, 2nd ed.,
edited by Jay R. Harris.
Lippincott Williams & Wilkins, Philadelphia © 2000.

CHAPTER 53

Epidural Metastases

Craig D. McColl and Ronnie J. Freilich

Epidural spinal cord compression (ESCC) is one of the true neurologic emergencies that arises in the management of patients with breast cancer. As the prognosis for good functional outcome is primarily dependent on the degree of impairment at the commencement of treatment, it is important that clinicians who care for patients with breast cancer remain vigilant about the possible presence of ESCC. More than 91% of patients with ESCC have symptoms for longer than 1 week before a diagnosis is made,[1] with a mean duration of pain of 6 weeks.[2] This should allow the clinician adequate time to investigate patients with symptoms and signs that are suggestive of epidural metastasis and to institute appropriate therapy. Compromise of the conus medullaris and cauda equina by epidural metastasis is generally included in a discussion of ESCC, as the natural history and management of these problems are similar to those of compression of the spinal cord itself.

PATHOLOGY

Epidural metastases most commonly arise from metastases to the vertebral column (85%). They arise less commonly from metastases to the paravertebral space (5% to 10%) that either secondarily invade bone and then grow into the epidural space or invade the epidural space directly through the intervertebral foramen. In rare instances, direct hematogenous spread to the epidural space or to the parenchyma of the spinal cord occurs,[3,4] but this presentation is more likely with lymphoma than with breast cancer, and if ESCC develops as the first manifestation of cancer, the absence of bony or skeletal metastases makes breast cancer an unlikely diagnosis.[5]

The vertebral column is the most frequent site of metastases to bone. Vertebral metastases occur in up to 41% of all patients with cancer[6] and in 60% of patients with breast cancer.[7] The incidence in patients with advanced breast cancer may be as high as 84%.[3] This high incidence relates to the fact that cancers of the breast (as well as cancers of the lung and pelvis) are in communication with Batson's vertebral plexus,[8] a low-pressure, valveless venous system that fills when thoracoabdominal pressure is raised (e.g., by maneuvers such as coughing, straining, and lifting). The presence of growth factors in bone marrow may also be a contributing factor.[9] Of patients with breast cancer and ESCC, 93% have known bone metastases at the onset of their neurologic deficit, with a median time from the first bone metastasis to ESCC of 11 months (range, 0 to 7.5 years). Breast cancer is commonly associated with multilevel vertebral metastases, as compared with lung cancer, in which a single level is usually involved.[10] Stark et al.[10] demonstrated noncontiguous vertebral involvement in 50% of patients with breast cancer who had abnormal plain spine radiography, and epidural tumor was multifocal in 29%. As would be anticipated from their origin in the vertebral bodies, the majority of epidural metastases are situated anterior or anterolateral to the spinal cord,[11] which has important implications for their surgical management.

Spinal cord damage in ESCC is due primarily to direct compression of the spinal cord by tumor and rarely to compression of radicular arteries that pass through the intervertebral foramen.[3] Axonal swelling and white matter edema occur early in animal models of ESCC, whereas grey matter damage occurs later.[12] Prolonged cord compression results in necrosis of both grey and white matter. Early spinal cord damage is likely due to venous stasis, whereas arteriolar compression by tumor is probably responsible for the late stage of tissue necrosis.[12]

INCIDENCE

The overall incidence of ESCC in patients with cancer is approximately 5%.[13,14] A similar incidence (4%) has been reported in patients with breast cancer.[1] Breast cancer accounts for 7% to 32% of all cases of ESCC in patients with cancer.[10,11,15–20] The median time from the diagnosis of breast cancer to the onset of ESCC is 42 months, with a range of 0 to 28 years.[1] ESCC may be the initial presentation of cancer; this occurs more frequently in a general hospital than in a specialized cancer center.[10,11] In some instances, biopsy of an epidural metastasis is required to establish the diagnosis of cancer.

C. D. McColl: Department of Neurosciences, Monash Medical Centre, Clayton, Victoria, Australia
R. J. Freilich: Department of Neurosciences, Monash Medical Centre, Clayton, Victoria, Australia

TABLE 1. *Symptoms and signs of epidural spinal cord compression in 130 patients who presented to a large cancer hospital*

Symptom/ sign	First symptom (%)	Symptoms at diagnosis (%)	Signs at diagnosis (%)
Pain	96	96	—
Weakness	2	76	87
Autonomic dysfunction	0	57	—
Sensory loss	0	51	78
Ataxia	2	3	7
Herpes zoster	0	2	2
Flexor spasms	0	1	1

From ref. 10, with permission.

CLINICAL SYMPTOMS AND SIGNS

ESCC due to breast cancer occurs most commonly in the thoracic spine,[10,11,21] in part because this is the longest section of the vertebral column but also because of the pattern of drainage from Batson's plexus and the proximity of the primary tumor to the thoracic vertebrae. The principal symptom of ESCC is pain (Table 1). It is the initial symptom in 96% of patients and precedes other symptoms by a mean of 6 weeks.[2] Pain is of three types: local, radicular, and referred. Local back pain is usually a constant ache and occurs in almost all patients. Radicular pain is caused by involvement of nerve roots by the tumor mass and is typically described as a shooting pain. It is more common with cervical and lumbosacral lesions than with thoracic lesions.[11] With cervical or lumbosacral epidural metastases, radicular pain is typically unilateral. With thoracic disease, however, radicular pain is commonly bilateral, producing a bandlike pain or tightness that may be felt more at the lateral or anterior chest wall than in the back itself. Referred pain occurs at a distant site from the lesion and does not radiate. For example, T12–L1 vertebral lesions may be referred to both iliac crests or both sacroiliac joints, whereas C7–T1 lesions may be referred to the interscapular region or to both shoulders.[22]

The pain of epidural metastasis is worsened by lying supine, possibly because of filling of vertebral veins in this position. Patients typically report that they are unable to sleep lying down and need to sleep sitting up; this information is often not volunteered by patients but must be sought by direct questioning. The Valsalva maneuver (coughing, sneezing, or straining at stool) exacerbates the pain of epidural metastases, as it fills vertebral veins and also raises intracranial pressure, which is then transmitted to the already compromised spinal canal. Pain is also worsened by stretching maneuvers, such as neck flexion in the case of cervical or upper thoracic tumors and straight leg raising with lumbosacral or thoracic lesions. Escalating back pain in patients with cancer is a particularly ominous indicator of the possibility of ESCC. Tenderness may be present over the vertebral column at the site of the lesion, and there may be referred tenderness at the site of referred or radicular pain.

Myelopathy is the other characteristic clinical finding in ESCC. Myelopathic symptoms include limb weakness, numbness and paresthesias, and sphincter disturbance (urinary retention, urinary urgency, constipation, or fecal urgency). At the time of diagnosis, 76% of patients complain of weakness, 87% are weak on examination, 57% have autonomic dysfunction, 51% have sensory symptoms, and 78% have sensory deficits on examination.[11] In many series, fewer than 50% of patients are ambulant at diagnosis, and up to 25% are paraplegic[1,2,11]; these figures are significant because prognosis is related to clinical deficit at presentation. Outcomes might be improved if patients were encouraged to present earlier.

Signs of a myelopathy include paraparesis or quadriparesis, increased tone, clonus, hyperreflexia, extensor plantar responses, a distended bladder, or a sensory level. A patch of hyperesthesia may be present at the upper aspect of the sensory level. The sensory, motor, and reflex levels are only an approximate indication of the site of pathology; because sensory fibers retain their somatotopic organization as they ascend in the cord, the actual site of cord compression may be several segments above the apparent sensory level. Furthermore, there may be multiple sites of epidural disease. The entire spinal cord should therefore be imaged in all patients with myelopathy.

The myelopathy may be incomplete, and it is a serious error to dismiss the possibility of ESCC on the basis that any particular sign is absent. Neither a sensory level nor an extensor plantar response is necessary to make the clinical diagnosis of ESCC. Dorsal column sensation (vibration and proprioception) and spinothalamic sensation (pain and temperature) need to be assessed independently in all cancer patients with back pain. Because the subjective appreciation of light touch involves both sensory pathways, light touch sensation may be reasonably well preserved, even in the presence of a clear-cut sensory level for pain or vibration sense when these are tested separately. A hemicord or Brown-Séquard's syndrome may occur, although this is rare in ESCC[10,11] and, in an oncologic population, is more typical of intramedullary cord metastasis or radiation myelopathy.[23] Involvement of spinocerebellar tracts in the spinal cord can lead to lower extremity ataxia out of proportion to the degree of weakness. Dorsal column involvement can lead to a sensory ataxia with positive rhombergism while sparing power and reflexes. Both of these clinical presentations may focus the attention of the unwary examiner on the cerebellum, thereby delaying diagnosis.[24] Patients may also present with herpes zoster, presumably as a result of reactivation of latent virus by compression of the dorsal root ganglion by tumor.[11]

ESCC at the conus medullaris and cauda equina produces different neurologic symptoms and signs, although pain is still a prominent feature, particularly with cauda equina lesions. Conus lesions typically present with early and marked sphincter disturbance and perineal sensory loss. Anal sphincter tone may be lax, and there may be an absent

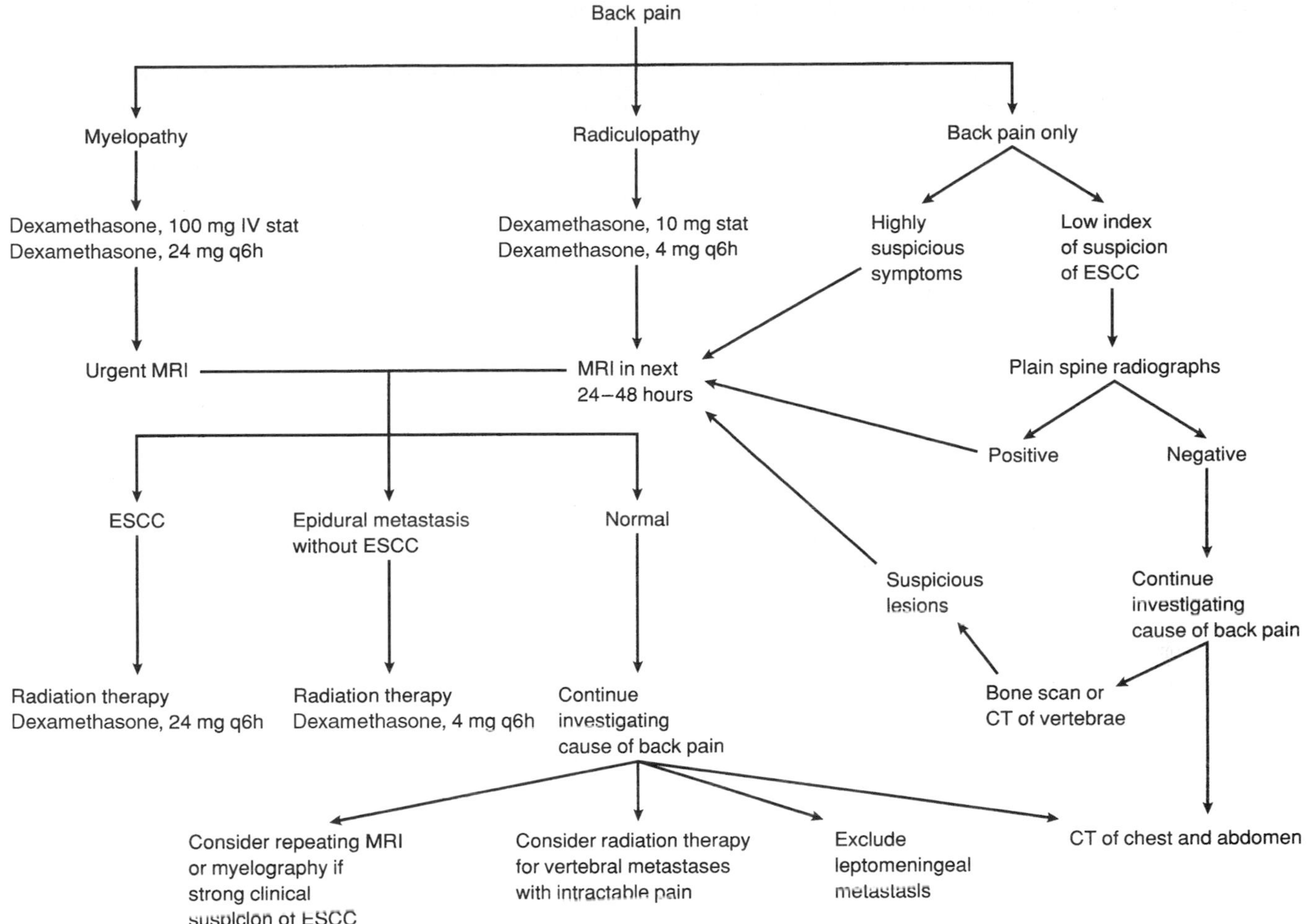

FIG. 1. Algorithm for the investigation and treatment of patients with breast cancer and back pain. CT, computed tomography; ESCC, epidural spinal cord compression; IV, intravenously; MRI, magnetic resonance imaging; stat, immediately.

anal wink. Cauda equina lesions produce patchy lower motor neuron signs related to the lumbar and sacral nerve roots—hyporeflexia or areflexia, myotomal leg weakness, and dermatomal sensory loss; sphincter disturbance tends to occur late and to be less marked than in conus lesions. When the signs include a mixture of upper and lower motor neuron features or dermatomal sensory loss as well as a sensory level, the possibility of coexistent nerve root involvement and cord compression should be considered.

INVESTIGATIONS

The serious consequences of untreated ESCC, paraplegia or quadriplegia, necessitate an orderly and expeditious investigation of all patients in whom this diagnosis is suspected. The imaging modalities that have been used in the investigation of ESCC include plain spine radiographs, radionuclide bone scans, and computed tomography (CT) of the spine, as well as techniques that definitively image the epidural space: myelography (with or without CT) and magnetic resonance imaging (MRI). As most patients with ESCC present with back pain, the investigation of ESCC can be regarded as the investigation of patients with cancer and back pain. It is not practical or appropriate to perform definitive imaging of the epidural space in every patient with cancer who has back pain, and this has led to the development of algorithms for the investigation and treatment of these patients,[3,25–28] as shown in Figure 1. When discussing the available investigational tools, it is useful to consider the following clinical presentations: isolated back pain with a normal neurologic examination, radiculopathy, plexopathy, and myelopathy.

Isolated Back Pain

Plain Spine Radiographs

Several studies have demonstrated the clinical usefulness of plain radiographs in the assessment of possible epidural disease. Of patients with epidural metastases, 85% have a vertebral body metastasis seen on plain radiography at the appropriate level.[10,11] This figure varies depending on the type of tumor: Epidural disease due to breast cancer has been associated with visible vertebral metastases in 94% to 98% of cases,[10,29] whereas only 32% of patients with lymphoma and ESCC have bony abnormalities on plain radiographs.[30] Plain radiographs may be less sensitive in detecting bony disease at certain sites, particularly the C7–T1 vertebrae (which are commonly involved in breast cancer), as overlying bone and mediastinal shadows may obscure the image of these vertebrae. Rodichok et al.[31] found epidural metastases in 25 of 34 (74%) patients with isolated back pain, no neurologic abnormalities, and an abnormal plain radiograph. In contrast, Graus et al.[32] found ESCC in only 12 of 35 (34%) patients in this setting. When Graus classified the x-ray abnormalities by the types of changes seen, however, it was found that epidural metastases were present in 7 of 8 (87%) patients with more than 50% vertebral collapse and 4 of 13 (31%) patients with isolated pedicle destruction but only 1 of 14 (7%) patients with metastasis restricted to the vertebral body without severe collapse. Both studies demonstrated an incidence of epidural metastasis of 3% or less in patients with normal plain radiographs. If plain radiographs of the spine are abnormal, more definitive imaging needs to be arranged on an urgent basis (see Fig. 1).

Radionuclide Bone Scans

Bone scintigraphy is more sensitive than plain radiography in the detection of epidural metastasis.[33] On occasion, however, scintigraphy fails to detect metastatic breast cancer if the metastases produce purely lytic bone lesions.[34] Scintigraphy may also be insensitive after radiotherapy.[28] Furthermore, scintigraphy is less specific than radiography.[33] In patients with an abnormal bone scan but a normal plain radiograph, Portenoy et al.[33] found epidural metastases in only 1 of 9 (12%) symptomatic segments (defined as vertebral segments that produce pain or neurologic signs) and 0 of 22 (0%) asymptomatic segments. It was concluded that bone scans may, however, play a role in the assessment of back pain: For example, normal findings on bone scan may confirm that an epidural metastasis is unlikely in patients with normal findings on radiography. In the study of Rodichok et al.,[31] epidural metastases were demonstrated in 15 of 26 (58%) patients with back pain, no neurologic signs, and abnormal findings on bone scan, compared to 2 of 10 (20%) patients with normal findings on bone scan.[31] Bone scans were not performed in many cases, because the clinical picture and plain radiographs led immediately to myelography. The authors determined that bone scans do not contribute significantly to the information obtained from plain radiographs. Portenoy et al.[33] recommend that asymptomatic spinal metastases discovered on staging bone scans should be characterized further with plain radiography.

Computed Tomographic Scanning

CT scanning without the instillation of myelographic dye is more sensitive than plain radiographs in detecting vertebral and paravertebral metastases, and it has been demonstrated that cortical disruption adjacent to the epidural space is a useful marker of epidural metastasis.[26,35] CT does not visualize the epidural space adequately, however. Furthermore, CT produces axial images, and thus only a limited area of the spine can be imaged by this technique. CT scans may be useful in differentiating vertebral collapse due to tumor from that due to osteoporosis.

Summary

In patients with breast cancer and isolated back pain without neurologic abnormalities, plain spine radiographs are the appropriate first line of investigation. Definitive imaging of the epidural space should be performed if plain films are abnormal. In patients with a clinical picture that is strongly suggestive of epidural metastasis (e.g., back pain that is significantly exacerbated by lying flat and worsened by the Valsalva maneuver), definitive imaging of the epidural space should still be performed even if a plain radiograph is normal; in fact, it is reasonable to proceed straight to MRI in this situation. The potential difficulties in interpreting changes at the C7–T1 vertebrae should be considered if this is the site of clinical suspicion. In patients with local back pain with characteristics that are not strongly suggestive of epidural metastasis, definitive imaging of the epidural space is not indicated if a plain radiograph is normal. Investigations must proceed, however, to determine the cause of the back pain. Bone scan and CT scan of the vertebrae may be performed; if suspicious lesions are seen, particularly on CT scan, then definitive imaging of the epidural space should be considered. Other investigations that may be performed include CT scan of the chest or abdomen to exclude lesions such as paravertebral or visceral metastases. The differential diagnosis of back pain also includes leptomeningeal metastases, but there are usually other clinical clues to suggest this diagnosis.

Radiculopathy

Radiculopathy is associated with a high incidence of epidural metastases. In the series of cancer patients with back pain by Rodichok et al.,[31] 27 of 43 (63%) patients with radiculopathy and without signs of spinal cord involvement were found to have epidural metastases, compared with 27 of 61 (44%) patients with local back pain alone. When plain radiographs were abnormal, epidural metastases were found in 20 of 22 (91%) patients with radiculopathy. Similarly, in patients with abnormal findings on plain radiographs, Graus et al.[32] found epidural metastases in 47 of 67 (70%) patients with radiculopathy, as compared with 12 of 35 (34%)

patients with local back pain alone. Importantly, in the series of Graus and of Rodichok, epidural metastases were found in 9% to 33% of patients with radiculopathy and normal findings on plain radiographs.[31,32]

Given the high incidence of epidural metastases in patients with radiculopathy, even in those with normal findings on plain radiographs, it is reasonable to proceed straight to definitive imaging of the epidural space in all patients with breast cancer and radiculopathy. It is important to remember that in the thoracic spine, which is the most common site of ESCC in breast cancer, radiculopathy commonly presents as bilateral, bandlike dermatomal pain and that, in some situations, lateral or even anterior chest pain may be more prominent than back pain.

Plexopathy

The possibility of epidural metastasis must be considered in patients with breast cancer and a malignant brachial plexopathy, as tumor may infiltrate directly along the plexus to the epidural space. Brachial plexus lesions present with pain (usually in the shoulder girdle and radiating to the elbow, medial side of the forearm, and medial two digits) as well as weakness and sensory symptoms in a segmental distribution. Clinical clues to the presence of epidural metastases in the setting of brachial plexopathy include a panplexopathy (as compared to the more usual lower plexopathy with involvement of C7, C8, and T1 nerve roots) and the presence of Horner's syndrome (indicating more proximal involvement).[36] The presence of back pain also suggests that the tumor has grown proximally, but back pain may be absent with epidural extension. Patients with brachial plexopathy require imaging of the brachial plexus with CT or MRI and, if vertebral body collapse or erosion is present at the C7–T1 levels or if a paraspinal mass is seen, then definitive imaging of the epidural space should be performed. It should be noted that epidural tumor is present in approximately one-third of patients with paraspinal lesions and a normal plain radiograph.[32] If MRI is used to image the brachial plexus, the cervical and upper thoracic spine can be imaged at the same time.

Myelopathy

Definitive Imaging of the Epidural Space: Magnetic Resonance Imaging and Myelography

Definitive imaging of the epidural space is required in patients with myelopathy and in other patients in whom the clinical presentation or investigations strongly suggest the presence of epidural metastases. Myelography was the traditional mainstay of investigation of ESCC, but MRI is now the investigation of choice.

Myelography is performed by the instillation of a contrast agent into the subarachnoid space through a lumbar spinal puncture (Fig. 2). Water-soluble contrast agents, such as iohexol (Omnipaque), are used rather than the older lipid-soluble agents, such as iophendylate (Pantopaque), which produced complications such as arachnoiditis. CT can be performed after myelography to provide axial images through abnormal regions. If a complete spinal block is present on myelography, a cisternal C1–C2 puncture must be performed to identify the upper border of the block to allow for adequate treatment planning. CT scanning after myelography may assist in the delineation of this upper border, as enough contrast material may get past the block to be seen on CT; however, this occurs in fewer than 50% of cases with complete block.[37] Cerebrospinal fluid should be collected when myelography is performed to exclude leptomeningeal metastasis. Myelography may be contraindicated in patients with a coagulopathy and in individuals with raised intracranial pressure from intracerebral metastases. A spinal tap performed in patients with a complete block may worsen the neurologic deficit as a result of the creation of a pressure differential between the spinal canal above and below the block.[38]

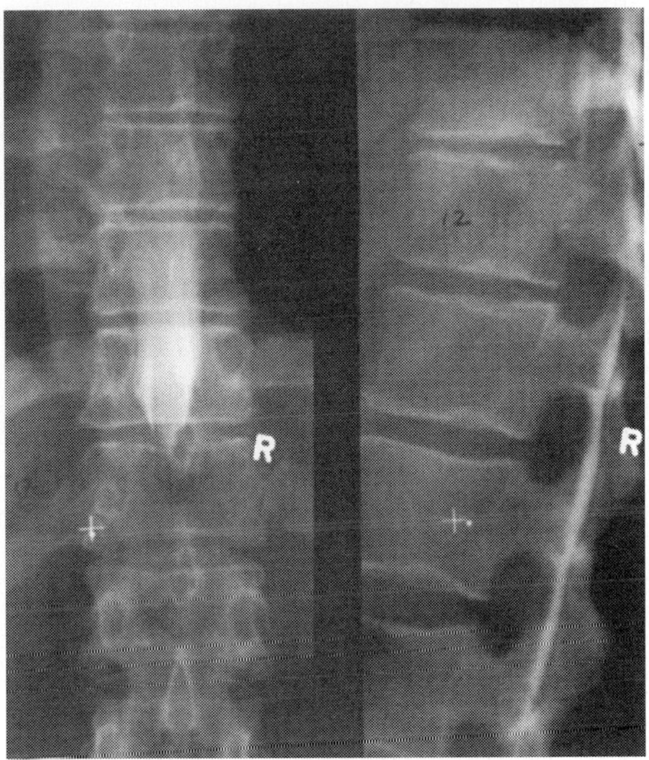

FIG. 2. Myelogram showing a complete block to the flow of contrast material. The upper level of the block at T11–T12 is delineated by a C1–C2 injection (*left*), whereas the lower level of the block at T12–L1 is demonstrated by a lumbar injection (*right*). Note the right T12 pedicle erosion seen on the left side of the diagram.

MRI has a number of advantages: It is noninvasive, it produces excellent delineation of soft-tissue planes, it is

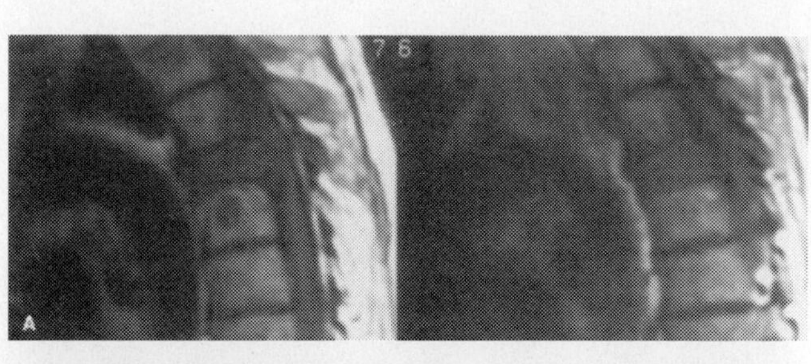

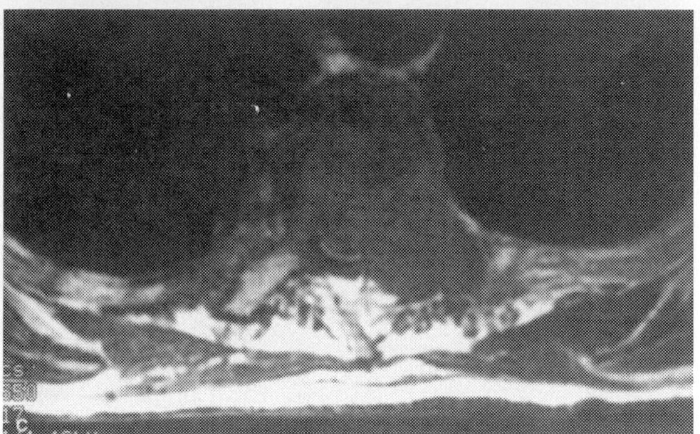

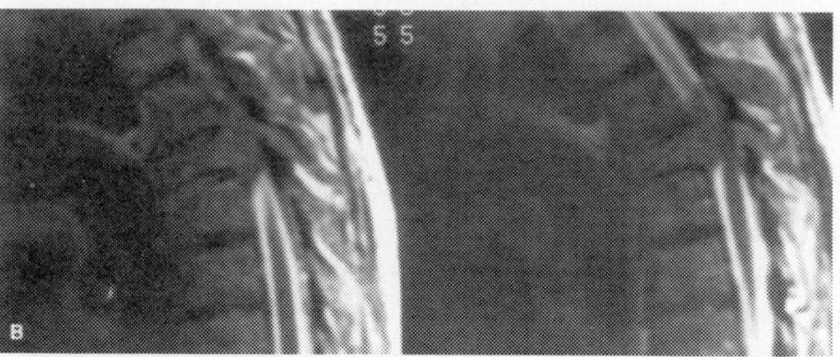

FIG. 3. A: Sagittal T1-weighted magnetic resonance imaging (MRI) scans demonstrating epidural spinal cord compression. The vertebral body is completely replaced by tumor and appears hypodense. Tumor extends posteriorly from the vertebral body to compress the spinal cord from its anterior aspect; this is the most common pathology encountered with epidural metastases. The two scans shown are 4 mm apart; the degree of spinal cord compression appears less severe on the scan on the right, emphasizing the inadequacy of a single midline sagittal image as a "screening test" for epidural metastasis. Note the hypodense signal in multiple vertebral bodies indicative of diffuse bony metastases in this patient. **B:** In this sagittal T2-weighted MRI sequence, cerebrospinal fluid is white and the spinal cord is grey; pathology is better demonstrated on T2-weighted than on T1-weighted images. **C:** This axial T1-weighted image shows the vertebral canal to be almost completely obliterated by tumor extending posteriorly from the vertebral body.

very sensitive in the detection of vertebral and paravertebral metastases, and it provides imaging in three planes (sagittal, coronal, and axial; Fig. 3). Furthermore, MRI is useful in discriminating between benign and malignant vertebral collapse.[39] Several early studies that compared MRI with myelography in the evaluation of patients with suspected ESCC suggested that MRI was not as sensitive as myelography.[40,41] The scanning protocols for these studies did not, however, routinely include axial images; sagittal images (with or without coronal images) may easily miss a small or laterally placed metastasis. Other investigators, on the other hand, have shown MRI to be as sensitive as myelography in the detection of epidural metastases, including the detection of small lesions and metastases that produce nerve root compression.[42,43] In some instances, MRI has been shown to be superior to myelography: in being more sensitive in the detection of epidural metastases, in accurately determining the upper border of a complete block, in imaging multiple sites of spinal block, and in the detection of paravertebral and vertebral metastases.[41–43] Furthermore, the quality of MRI technology has continued to improve since its introduction,[39] casting doubt on original estimates of its utility. A retrospective cost-effectiveness study concluded that, when the results of incorrect or delayed diagnoses were taken into account, the cost of diagnosing ESCC in an American institution was 65% higher in the pre-MRI era than since MRI became available in 1985.[44] The use of MRI was calculated to produce a similar saving (40%) in a British context.[45] Although MRI is recommended as the investigation of choice in ESCC, it is important to remember that, in some situations, MRI scanning may give a false-negative result, and repeat MRI or myelography may be indicated if a strong clinical suspicion of epidural metastases remains, particularly if the MRI scan was degraded by artifact. Furthermore, if MRI is not readily available or cannot be performed (e.g., in patients with pacemakers or the occasional patient with severe claustrophobia), myelography should be performed.

An unenhanced MRI scan can establish the diagnosis of ESCC. If this is normal, then a contrast-enhanced scan using gadolinium-DTPA should be obtained to look for leptomeningeal metastasis, which may mimic the presentation of ESCC. The entire spine should be imaged, as epidural disease may be present at multiple levels, and the spinal level indicated by clinical examination may be several segments below the level of the lesion.[46] It is important to obtain axial scans in addition to sagittal images. A "screening" midline sagittal scan is inadequate; multiple sagittal scans using thin slices should be performed. Coronal images of the spine are not required routinely. Adequate analgesia (including corticosteroids) should be administered before the MRI is performed, as the patient must lie motionless for the scan, and lying flat may worsen the back pain. If the patient cannot tolerate the full procedure, or if there is not enough time to perform an MRI of the entire spine, then the area of interest should be imaged first, followed at a later time by imaging of the remainder of the spine. When ordering radiologic investigations, a clear distinction should be made between the suspected neurologic level of involvement and the suspected vertebral level; the discrepancy between these is greatest at the inferior end of the spinal cord. Because the spinal cord terminates at the first lumbar vertebra, all of the lumbar segments and some of the sacral segments of the cord are usually situated within the thoracic spine.

TREATMENT

Corticosteroids

Corticosteroids, usually in the form of dexamethasone, are used routinely in the management of ESCC, because they reduce pain and sometimes stabilize or improve neurologic deficits.[3,18] Although one animal model of ESCC showed no effect of high-dose glucocorticoids on spinal cord water content,[47] other models have shown that these drugs do reduce the vasogenic edema associated with ESCC, primarily by decreasing capillary permeability.[48–50] The effect on vasogenic edema was found to be dose-dependent when intramuscular dexamethasone was given to animals in doses equivalent to human doses of 1.5 mg, 15 mg, and 150 mg twice a day.[50] The clinical signs of ESCC in the animals were stabilized or improved by the high-dose dexamethasone regimen,[48,49] and this effect has been shown to be dose-dependent.[50]

Extrapolating the experimental data to humans suggests a role for the use of high-dose dexamethasone in acute ESCC. One 1980 study demonstrated that a bolus dose of 100 mg dexamethasone intravenously, followed by a tapering schedule starting with 96 mg a day in four divided doses for 3 days, has a significant and rapid effect on the pain associated with ESCC.[51] In a 1989 study, no difference in pain, ambulation, or bladder function was seen in 37 patients with ESCC who received either a 10- or 100-mg bolus of dexamethasone intravenously.[52] A randomized controlled trial in 1994, however, showed that, in 57 patients with ESCC who proceeded to radiotherapy, high-dose dexamethasone significantly increased the proportion of patients who remained ambulant after treatment.[53] Although it has been suggested that it might be feasible to withhold steroids in patients with good motor function who are proceeding directly to radiotherapy, this approach has only been assessed in one small, uncontrolled study.[54]

A bolus dose of 100 mg dexamethasone is recommended for patients with ESCC, followed by a taper of steroids over 2 to 3 weeks while the patient receives definitive therapy. The bolus dose of steroids is given once the clinical diagnosis is made and before an MRI is performed. An increase in steroid dose during the taper may be required if pain worsens. Patients with radicular pain receive a bolus of 10 mg dexamethasone, followed by a dose of 4 mg four times a day that is subsequently tapered, pending the results of neuroimaging. If MRI demonstrates cord compression (or if myelography shows a block of greater than 80%), the high-dose regimen is used, whereas the low-dose regimen is used for patients with epidural disease without cord compression (or a block on myelography of less than 80%).

The only difference between oral and intravenous administration of dexamethasone is that systemic availability is slowed by approximately 30 minutes when it is given by the oral route. Intravenous dexamethasone is recommended for the initial bolus to provide analgesia quickly, but, unless the patient has a nonfunctioning gut, oral dexamethasone is generally used at other times. Prolonged use of high-dose dexamethasone is associated with more side effects than low-dose dexamethasone, but, for short-term use, the toxicity of the doses is similar.[3] In areas in which *Pneumocystis carinii* infection is common, patients who are receiving steroids should be on prophylaxis against this opportunistic pathogen.[55] The recommended regimen is trimethoprim-sulfamethoxazole, one double-strength tablet twice a day, three consecutive days a week (Monday to Wednesday). Some authors recommend H_2 blockers, such as ranitidine, to reduce the risk of peptic ulceration during steroid therapy.[56]

Surgery and Radiation Therapy

Decompressive laminectomy (with or without radiation therapy) was the mainstay of treatment for ESCC until the mid-1980s with clinical improvement noted in 30% to 40% of cases.[57] Several studies have demonstrated that the outcome achieved by radiation alone is as good as that of laminectomy and radiation combined; this applies not only to radiosensitive tumors, such as breast cancer, but also to more radioresistant tumors.[1,11,58,59] The outcome for radiosensitive tumors, however, is better than that for radioresistant tumors, regardless of the treatment modality used.[11] The poor response to laminectomy is due, at least in part, to the anterior or anterolateral location of most epidural metastases; epidural metastases are difficult to remove using the posterior approach of a laminectomy, and a posterior decompression does not relieve the anterior spinal cord compession. Laminectomy may further weaken a spine that is already compromised by vertebral destruction. Overall, surgery is associated with a higher complication rate than radiation therapy, particularly in the setting of steroid use.[11,59] Considering all tumor types, one review concluded that surgery for ESCC was associated with a mortality of 6% to 24% and a nonneurologic complication rate of approximately 10%.[60] These observations have led to the use of radiation therapy as the initial treatment of choice for the majority of patients with ESCC.

To circumvent the problems associated with laminectomy, an anterolateral surgical approach to ESCC has been developed using vertebral body resection and stabilization of the spine with methylmethacrylate.[61–64] Bone grafts have been used for stabilization and are recommended in cases in which survival beyond 6 months is anticipated, but the grafts may not tolerate subsequent radiation therapy, particularly in the first 3 to 6 weeks after grafting.[65,66] Several nonrandomized studies have indicated that vertebral body resection (with or without radiation therapy) is superior to radiation alone in terms of ambulation and sphincter control, with some studies showing significant recovery of ambulation in paraplegic patients.[62–64,67–70] It has also been claimed that, in patients with a variety of tumor types, aggressive surgery can improve long-term survival.[70] These studies have used surgery in highly selected patients, however, and have often used historical controls for comparison. Furthermore, surgical morbidity with this approach may be considerable, with postoperative complication rates of 10% to 48% reported for vertebral body resection.[64,70] No well-controlled, randomized, prospective trial has compared radiation therapy with vertebral body resection, and the conduction of such a study may be difficult, in part because the decision for the type of treatment depends on the individual patient.

A posterolateral approach has been proposed as a less aggressive alternative to vertebral body resection, with removal of the lamina, facet joint, and pedicle on the involved side, followed by instrumentation to achieve stability.[71] Only small series of patients treated in this manner have been reported, with limited follow-up, but the technique may find a role in the palliation of patients with advanced disease.[70]

Despite these refinements in surgical technique, focal radiation therapy is recommended as first-line treatment for ESCC in patients with breast cancer, using a dose of up to 3,000 cGy (30 Gy). Short-course radiotherapy involving two doses of 800 cGy has also been proposed, producing results comparable to those obtained with higher doses in one uncontrolled study.[72] No dose fractionation schedule has proved to be significantly more efficacious than others.[23] Radiation therapy should be begun on an urgent basis. In situations in which patients present in the middle of the night, when it is logistically difficult to obtain neuroimaging or commence radiation therapy, the high-dose steroid regimen may be commenced; the radiation therapists can be notified about the patient and an MRI performed the first thing the following morning. The use of radiation therapy for recurrent ESCC, when this involves re-irradiating a previously treated segment of spinal cord, poses a significant risk of producing radiation myelopathy[73] and is generally not recommended. Re-irradiation has been used with some success by Schiff et al.,[74] however, who suggest that myelopathy is unlikely to occur within the limited life expectancy of this population. Radiotherapy is also recommended for asymptomatic patients with radiologic evidence of cord compression.[75]

Surgery is recommended for patients whose disease progresses or relapses despite radiation therapy, for those with unstable spines due to fracture-dislocation of the vertebrae, and for patients in whom the spinal cord compression is largely caused by bony fragments in the epidural space rather than tumor. In view of the favorable results reported with vertebral body resection during the 1990s, this option should be considered in paraplegic patients.[75] Surgery may also be indicated in patients with an unknown primary malignancy, although a percutaneous needle biopsy (usually under radiologic guidance) will be informative in most cases and will have fewer complications than an open procedure.[76,77] The surgical approach used (vertebral body resection or laminectomy) is dictated by the site of the epidural metastasis in relation to the spinal cord. One retrospective study in 1996 showed significantly better functional outcomes with emergency surgery than with surgery postponed to the next elective operating list within 24 hours.[78] This finding may have reflected selection bias, but, nevertheless, it is generally recommended that surgery be performed as soon as possible.

Chemotherapy

Chemotherapy does not play a significant role in the treatment of ESCC due to metastatic breast cancer, although Boogerd et al.[79] describe protracted remission of epidural metastases in four patients with breast cancer who received chemotherapy and hormonal therapy. Chemotherapy may be a more important treatment modality in highly chemosensitive tumors, such as germ cell tumors and neuroblastoma.[80,81]

Supportive Therapy

Patients with myelopathy due to ESCC require close attention to analgesia, bowel and bladder care, and the prevention of pressure sores. Prophylaxis against venous thromboembolism should always be considered in bed-bound patients.

PROGNOSIS

The outcome of ESCC is directly related to the patient's clinical condition at the commencement of treatment (Table 2). Patients who are ambulant are far more likely to remain ambulant after treatment: 79% to 100% of patients who are ambulant before treatment remain so, whereas only 18% to 69% of nonambulant patients regain the ability to walk.[1,2,11,82–84] In most series, fewer than 10% of patients who are paraplegic or quadriplegic before treatment regain the ability to walk,[1,2,11,82–84] although vertebral body resec-

TABLE 2. *Treatment outcome as influenced by pretreatment ambulatory status*

			Patients ambulant after treatment				
				Nonambulant before treatment			
Study	No. of patients	Tumor type	Ambulant before treatment	Overall	Paretic	Plegic	Treatment modality
1	70	Breast	96% 22/23	45% 13/29	—	—	RT = laminectomy
2	59	All	100% 13/13	26% 12/46	35% 11/31	7% 1/15	RT ± laminectomy
10	235	All	75% 60/80	35% 54/155	45% 52/116	5% 2/39	RT = laminectomy + RT
60	158	All	79% 33/42	14% 16/116	18% 16/89	0% 0/27	Radiotherapy
64	72	All	81% 34/42	62% 21/32	62% 21/32	—	Vertebral body resection
70	110	All	≥94% ≥58/62	84% 32/48	—	—	Vertebral body resection
72	49	All	91% 21/23	38% 10/26	50% 10/20	0% 0/6	RT ± surgery
82	345	All	79% 103/131	18% 38/214	21% 35/165	6% 3/49	RT = laminectomy ± RT
83	105	All	96% 48/50	47% 26/55	56% 25/45	10% 1/10	RT
84	56	Breast	97% 29/30	69% 18/26	74% 17/23	33% 1/3	RT
85	153	All	91% 72/79	28% 21/74	—	—	RT ± laminectomy

RT, radiotherapy; =, treatments are equally effective; ±, with or without.

tion has been associated with ambulation rates of up to 24% in initially paraplegic patients,[75] and, in one study, 6 of 13 paraplegic patients became ambulant after receiving vertebral body resection and radiotherapy.[62]

The prognosis for breast cancer patients treated with radiotherapy alone has been characterized by Maranzano et al.[84] The likelihood of responding to radiation therapy is dependent on the pretreatment ambulatory status, whereas duration of response is dependent on the posttreatment ambulatory status.[84] In Maranzano's study, 18 of 26 (69%) patients who were nonambulant before treatment became at least partially ambulant with treatment (walking alone or with support). Only 1 ambulant patient of 30 (3%) became nonambulant despite treatment, underscoring the value of early diagnosis. The median duration of response was 12 months for all patients, 15 months for patients who were ambulant after treatment, and only 2 months for those who were nonambulant after treatment.[84] Bladder control was regained in 67% of patients with sphincter dysfunction.

The mean survival of patients with breast cancer in whom ESCC develops is 5 to 14 months, and the median survival is 4 to 13 months.[1,20,82,84] The time from diagnosis of breast cancer to the development of ESCC has been found to be a predictor of survival, with patients who develop ESCC after 3 or more years having a better survival.[1] One study suggests a longer survival in patients treated with both laminectomy and radiation therapy compared with patients treated by either laminectomy or radiation alone, but these differences may be explained by selection bias.[82] One study has demonstrated no survival difference in patients treated with surgery or radiation.[1] Although proponents of vertebral body resection have claimed that this technique may prolong survival,[70] controlled studies have not been performed. Posttreatment ambulatory status is the most important factor influencing survival in patients with breast cancer.[1,84] In the study by Maranzano et al.,[84] the median survival was 13 months for all patients, 17 months for patients who were ambulant after treatment, and only 2 months for those who were nonambulant after treatment. The 1-year survival of posttreatment ambulant patients in this study was 66%, versus 10% for nonambulant patients. Local control of the breast cancer at the site of spinal metastasis did not appear to be responsible for the improved survival in ambulant patients, however, as most deaths were due to progression of systemic disease rather than relapse in the irradiated spine.[84] In another series reported by Maranzano et al.,[83] which included patients with ESCC due to other cancer types, median survival was better in patients with breast cancer (12 months) than in patients with other tumor types (3 to 7 months). This relatively long survival, in association with the fact that early diagnosis may preserve ambulatory status, underscores the potential value of prompt investigation and treatment of ESCC in patients with breast cancer.

REFERENCES

1. Hill ME, Richards MA, Gregory WM, Smith P, Rubens RD. Spinal cord compression in breast cancer: a review of 70 cases. *Br J Cancer* 1993;68:969.
2. Kim RY, Spencer SA, Meredith RF, et al. Extradural spinal cord compression: analysis of factors determining functional prognosis—prospective study. *Radiology* 1990;176:279.
3. Posner JB. Back pain and epidural spinal cord compression. *Med Clin North Am* 1987;71:185.
4. Byrne TN. Spinal cord compression from epidural metastases. *N Engl J Med* 1992;327:614.
5. Dethy S, Piccart MJ, Paesmans M, et al. History of brain and epidural metastases from breast cancer in relation with the disease evolution outside the central nervous system. *Eur Neurol* 1995;35:38.
6. Byrne TN, Waxman SG. Spinal cord compression: diagnosis and principles of management. *Contemporary Neurology Series*, vol 33. Philadelphia: F.A. Davis, 1990.
7. Fornasier VL, Horne JG. Metastases to the vertebral column. *Cancer* 1975;36:590.
8. Batson OV. The vertebral venous system: Caldwell Lecture, 1956. In: Weiss L, Gilbert HA, eds. *Bone metastasis*. Boston: GK Hall, 1981:21.
9. Arguello F, Baggs RB, Duerst RE, Johnstone L, McQueen K, Frantz CN. Pathogenesis of vertebral metastasis and epidural spinal cord compression. *Cancer* 1990;65:98.
10. Stark RJ, Henson RA, Evans SWJ. Spinal metastases: a retrospective survey from a general hospital. *Brain* 1982;105:189.
11. Gilbert RW, Kim J-H, Posner JB. Epidural spinal cord compression from metastatic tumor: diagnosis and treatment. *Ann Neurol* 1978;3:40.
12. Kato A, Ushio Y, Hayakawa T, Yamada K, Ikeda H, Mogami H. Circulatory disturbance of the spinal cord with epidural neoplasm in rats. *J Neurosurg* 1985;63:260.
13. Barron KD, Hirano A, Araki S, Terry RD. Experiences with metastatic neoplasms involving the spinal cord. *Neurology* 1959;9:91.
14. Bach F, Larsen BH, Rohde K, et al. Metastatic spinal cord compression: occurrence, symptoms, clinical presentations and prognosis in 398 patients with spinal cord compression. *Acta Neurochir (Wien)* 1990;107:37.
15. Torma T. Malignant tumors of the spine and spinal extradural space. *Acta Chir Scand Suppl* 1957;225:1.
16. White WA, Patterson RH, Bergland RM. Role of surgery in the treatment of spinal cord compression by metastatic neoplasm. *Cancer* 1971;27:558.
17. Fornasier VL, Horne JG. Metastases to the vertebral column. *Cancer* 1975;36:590.
18. Greenberg HS, Kim JH, Posner JB. Epidural spinal cord compression from metastatic tumor: results with a new treatment protocol. *Ann Neurol* 1980;8:361.
19. Dunn RC, Kelly WA, Wohns RNW, Howe JF. Spinal epidural neoplasia: a 15-year review of the results of surgical therapy. *J Neurosurg* 1980;52:47.
20. Constans JP, de Divitiis E, Donzelli R, Spaziante R, Meder JF, Haye C. Spinal metastases with neurological manifestations: review of 600 cases. *J Neurosurg* 1983;59:111.
21. Sundaresan N, Digiacinto GV, Hughes JE, Cafferty M, Vallejo A. Treatment of neoplastic spinal cord compression: results of a prospective study. *Neurosurgery* 1991;29:645.
22. Foley KM. Pain syndromes in patients with cancer. In: Bonica JJ, Ventafridda V, eds. *Advances in pain research and therapy*, vol. 2. New York: Raven Press, 1979:59.
23. Schiff D, Batchelor T, Wen P. Neurologic emergencies in cancer patients. *Neurol Clin North Am* 1998;16:449.
24. Hainline B, Tuszynski MH, Posner JB. Ataxia in epidural spinal cord compression. *Neurology* 1992;42:2193.
25. Lewis DW, Packer RJ, Raney B, Rak IW, Belasco J, Lange B. Incidence, presentation, and outcome of spinal cord disease in children with systemic cancer. *Pediatrics* 1986;78:438.
26. O'Rourke T, George CB, Redmond J, et al. Spinal computed tomography and computed tomographic metrizamide myelography in the early diagnosis of metastatic disease. *J Clin Oncol* 1986;4:576.
27. Portenoy RK, Lipton RB, Foley KM. Back pain in the cancer patient: an algorithm for evaluation and management. *Neurology* 1987;37:134.
28. Redmond JR, Friedl KE, Cornett P, Stone M, O'Rourke T, George CB. Clinical usefulness of an algorithm for the early diagnosis of spinal metastatic disease. *J Clin Oncol* 1988;6:154.
29. Harrison KM, Muss HB, Ball MR, McWhorter M, Case D. Spinal cord compression in breast cancer. *Cancer* 1985;55:2839.
30. Haddad P, Thaell JF, Kiely JM, Harrison EG, Miller RH. Lymphoma of the spinal extradural space. *Cancer* 1976;38:1862.
31. Rodichok LD, Ruckdeschel JC, Harper GR, et al. Early detection and treatment of spinal epidural metastases: the role of myelography. *Ann Neurol* 1986;20:696.
32. Graus F, Krol G, Foley KM. Early diagnosis of spinal epidural metastasis (SEM): correlation with clinical and radiological findings [Abstract]. *Proc Am Soc Clin Oncol* 1985;4:269.
33. Portenoy RK, Galer BS, Salamon O, et al. Identification of epidural neoplasm: radiography and bone scintigraphy in the symptomatic and asymptomatic spine. *Cancer* 1989;64:2207.
34. Tryciecky EW, Gottschalk A, Ludema K. Oncologic imaging: interactions of nuclear medicine with CT and MRI using the bone scan as a model. *Semin Nucl Med* 1997;2:142.
35. Weissman DE, Gilbert M, Wang H, Grossman SA. The use of computed tomography of the spine to identify patients at high risk for epidural metastases. *J Clin Oncol* 1985;3:1541.
36. Kori SH, Foley KM, Posner JB. Brachial plexus lesions in patients with cancer: 100 cases. *Neurology* 1981;31:45.
37. Kori SH, Shah CP. Efficacy of metrizamide CT in delineating upper level of epidural metastatic disease [Abstract]. *Neurology* 1987;37[Suppl 1]:337.
38. Hollis PH, Malis LI, Zappulla RA. Neurological deterioration after lumbar puncture below complete spinal subarachnoid block. *J Neurosurg* 1986;64:253.
39. Traill Z, Richards MA, Moore NR. Magnetic resonance imaging of metastatic bone disease. *Clin Orthop* 1995;312:76.
40. Krol G, Heier L, Becker R, Sundaresan N, Watson R, Deck M. MRI and myelography in the evaluation of epidural extension of primary and metastatic tumors. In: Valk J, ed. *Neuroradiology 1985/1986*. Amsterdam: Elsevier Science, 1986:91.
41. Heier LA, Krol G, Sundaresan N, Watson RC, Deck MDF. MR imaging in evaluation of epidural lesions: comparison with myelography [Abstract]. *Radiology* 1985;157:150.
42. Carmody RF, Yang PJ, Seeley GW, Seeger JF, Unger EC, Johnson JE. Spinal cord compression due to metastatic disease: diagnosis with MR imaging versus myelography. *Radiology* 1989;173:225.
43. Williams MP, Cherryman GR, Husband JE. Magnetic resonance imaging in suspected metastatic spinal cord compression. *Clin Radiol* 1989;40:286.
44. Jordan JE, Donaldson SS, Enzmann DR. Cost effectiveness and outcome assessment of magnetic resonance imaging in diagnosing cord compression. *Cancer* 1995;75:2579.
45. Podd TJ, Walkden SE. The use of MRI in the investigation of spinal cord compression [Letter]. *Br J Radiol* 1992;65:187.
46. Cook AM, Lau TN, Tomlinson MJ, et al. Magnetic resonance imaging of the whole spine in suspected malignant spinal cord compression: impact on management. *Clin Oncol* 1998;10:39.
47. Siegal T, Shohami E, Shapira Y, Siegal T. Indomethacin and dexamethasone treatment in experimental neoplastic spinal cord compression: part 2. Effect on edema and prostaglandin synthesis. *Neurosurgery* 1988;22:334.
48. Ushio Y, Posner R, Posner JB, Shapiro WR. Experimental spinal cord compression by epidural neoplasm. *Neurology* 1977;27:422.
49. Ushio Y, Posner R, Kim JH, Shapiro WR, Posner JB. Treatment of experimental spinal cord compression caused by extradural neoplasms. *J Neurosurg* 1977;47:380.
50. Delattre JY, Arbit E, Thaler HT, Rosenblum MK, Posner JB. A dose-response study of dexamethasone in a model of spinal cord compression caused by epidural tumor. *J Neurosurg* 1989;70:920.
51. Greenberg HS, Kim JH, Posner JB. Epidural spinal cord compression from metastatic tumor: results with a new treatment protocol. *Ann Neurol* 1980;8:361.

52. Vecht CJ, Haaxma-Reiche H, van Putten WLJ, de Visser M, Vries EP, Twijnstra A. Initial bolus of conventional versus high-dose dexamethasone in metastatic spinal cord compression. *Neurology* 1989;39:1255.
53. Sorensen S, Helweg-Larsen S, Mourisden H, et al. Effect of high-dose dexamethasone in carcinomatous metastatic spinal cord compression treated with radiotherapy: a randomised trial. *Eur J Cancer* 1994;1:22.
54. Maranzano E, Latini P, Beneventi S, et al. Radiotherapy without steroids in selected metastatic spinal cord compression patients. *Am J Clin Oncol* 1996;19:179.
55. Sepkowitz KA, Brown AE, Telzak EE, Gottlieb S, Armstrong D. Pneumocystis carinii pneumonia among patients without AIDS at a cancer hospital. *JAMA* 1992;267:832.
56. Ciezki J, Macklis RM. The palliative role of radiotherapy in the management of the cancer patient. *Semin Oncol* 1995;2[Suppl 3]:82.
57. Gorter K. Results of laminectomy in spinal cord compression due to tumours. *Acta Neurochir (Wien)* 1978;42:177.
58. Young RF, Post EM, King GA. Treatment of spinal epidural metastases: randomized prospective comparison of laminectomy and radiotherapy. *J Neurosurg* 1980;53:741.
59. Findlay GF. Adverse effects of the management of malignant spinal cord compression. *J Neurol Neurosurg Psychiatry* 1984;47:761.
60. Podd TJ, Carpenter DS, Baughan CA, et al. Spinal cord compression: prognosis and implications for treatment fractionation. *Clin Oncol* 1992;6;341.
61. Siegal T, Siegal T, Robin G, Lubetzki KI, Fuks Z. Anterior decompression of the spine for metastatic epidural cord compression: a promising avenue of therapy? *Ann Neurol* 1982;11:28.
62. Harrington KD. Anterior cord decompression and spinal stabilization for patients with metastatic lesions of the spine. *J Neurosurg* 1984;61:107.
63. Siegal T, Siegal T. Surgical decompression of anterior and posterior malignant epidural tumors compressing the spinal cord: a prospective study. *Neurosurgery* 1985;17:424.
64. Sundaresan N, Galicich JH, Lane JM, Bains MS, McCormack P. Treatment of spinal metastases by vertebral body resection. *J Neurosurg* 1985;63:676.
65. Bell GR. Surgical treatment of spinal tumours. *Clin Orthop* 1997;335:54.
66. Gokaslan ZL. Spine surgery for cancer. *Curr Opin Oncol* 1996;8:178.
67. Sundaresan N, DiGiacinto GV, Hughes JEO et al. Treatment of neoplastic spinal cord compression: results of a prospective study. *Neurosurgery* 1991;29:645.
68. Sundaresan N, Scher H, DiGiacinto GV, et al. Surgical treatment of spinal cord compression in kidney cancer. *J Clin Oncol* 1986,4:1851.
69. Saengnipanthkul S, Jirarattanaphochai K, Rojviroj S, et al. Metastatic adenocarcinoma of the spine. *Spine* 1992;17:427.
70. Sundaresan N, Sachdev VP, Holland JF, et al. Surgical treatment of spinal cord compression from epidural metastasis. *J Clin Oncol* 1995;13:2330.
71. Shaw B, Mansfield FL, Borges L. One-stage posterolateral decompression and stabilization for primary and metastatic vertebral tumors in the thoracic and lumbar spine. *J Neurosurg* 1989;70:405.
72. Maranzano E, Latini P, Perucci E, et al. Short–course radiotherapy (8 Gy × 2) in metastatic spinal cord compression: an effective and feasible treatment. *Int J Radiat Oncol Biol Phys* 1997;38:1037.
73. Janjan NA. Radiotherapeutic management of spinal metastases. *J Pain Symptom Manage* 1996;1:47.
74. Schiff D, Shaw EG, Cascino TL. Outcome after spinal reirradiation for malignant epidural spinal cord compression. *Ann Neurol* 1995;37:583.
75. Loblaw DA, Laperriere NJ. Emergency treatment of malignant extradural spinal cord compression: an evidence–based guideline. *J Clin Oncol* 1998;16:1613.
76. Fyfe I, Henry A, Mulholland R. Closed vertebral biopsy. *J Bone Joint Surg* 1983;65:140.
77. Findlay GF, Sandeman DR, Buxton P. The role of needle biopsy in the management of malignant spinal compression. *Br J Neurosurg* 1988;2:479.
78. Harris JK, Sutcliffe JC, Robinson NE. The role of emergency surgery in malignant spinal extradural compression: assessment of functional outcome. *Br J Neurosurg* 1996;10:27.
79. Boogerd W, van der Sande JJ, Kröger R, Bruning PF, Somers R. Effective systemic therapy for spinal epidural metastases from breast carcinoma. *Eur J Cancer Clin Oncol* 1989;25:149.
80. Sanderson IR, Pritchard J, Marsh HT. Chemotherapy as the initial treatment of spinal cord compression due to disseminated neuroblastoma. *J Neurosurg* 1989;70:688.
81. Cooper K, Bajorin D, Shapiro W, Krol G, Sze G, Bosl GJ. Decompression of epidural metastases from germ cell tumors with chemotherapy. *J Neurooncol* 1990;8:275.
82. Sørensen PS, Børgesen SE, Rohde K, et al. Metastatic epidural spinal cord compression: results of treatment and survival. *Cancer* 1990;65:1502.
83. Maranzano E, Latini P, Checcaglini F, et al. Radiation therapy in metastatic spinal cord compression: a prospective analysis of 105 consecutive patients. *Cancer* 1991;67:1311.
84. Maranzano E, Latini P, Checcaglini F, et al. Radiation therapy of spinal cord compression caused by breast cancer: report of a prospective trial. *Int J Radiat Oncol Biol Phys* 1992;24:301
85. Helweg-Larsen S. Clinical outcome in metastatic spinal cord compression: a prospective study in 153 patients. *Acta Neurol Scand* 1996:94;26.

Diseases of the Breast, 2nd ed.,
edited by Jay R. Harris.
Lippincott Williams & Wilkins, Philadelphia © 2000.

CHAPTER 54

Leptomeningeal Metastasis

Lisa M. DeAngelis, Lisa R. Rogers, and Kathleen M. Foley

Leptomeningeal metastasis occurs when tumor spreads to the leptomeninges that surround the brain and spinal cord. It has emerged as an important diagnostic and therapeutic problem in patients with solid tumors and in patients with leukemia and lymphoma. Prolonged patient survival and enhanced clinical detection contribute to the increased frequency of leptomeningeal metastasis observed in these patients.

The frequency of leptomeningeal metastasis in clinical series of breast cancer patients is estimated to be 2% to 5%[1–3]; autopsy series provide a similar estimate of 3% to 6%.[4,5] Leptomeningeal metastasis usually coexists with disseminated systemic disease, but it can also occur as an isolated site of relapse in patients with a history of breast cancer. Determining the diagnosis is often difficult, because the presenting neurologic signs can be confused with other central nervous system complications of breast cancer. Neuroimaging and laboratory tests aid in establishing the diagnosis but are limited by a lack of sensitivity, specificity, or both. Optimal therapy has not been defined; difficulties of drug distribution in the cerebrospinal fluid (CSF) and neurotoxicity are two important factors that impede the success of standard therapies. Nevertheless, in some patients, an aggressive approach is rewarding. This chapter reviews the clinical presentation of this disorder, the methods of diagnosis, and the recommended therapeutic approaches.

CLINICAL SETTING

Although the histologic subtype of breast cancer is not described in most series of leptomeningeal metastasis, lobular carcinoma has a predilection for spread to the subarachnoid space. In a clinical series, Harris et al.[6] report that leptomeningeal metastasis occurred in 9 of 56 patients (16%) with lobular carcinoma but in only 1 of 309 patients (0.3%) with ductal carcinoma, a statistically significant difference. Conversely, parenchymal brain metastasis occurred more commonly in patients with ductal carcinoma, although the difference was not statistically significant. Autopsy studies have confirmed the propensity for lobular carcinoma to spread to the leptomeninges.[5,7] The reason that lobular carcinoma metastasizes to the leptomeninges is not clear, but the pattern of systemic metastasis also differs between these subtypes.[5–7]

A wide interval between the diagnosis of breast cancer and the occurrence of leptomeningeal metastasis has been reported; in large series, it ranges from a few weeks to more than 15 years.[8,9] In rare instances, leptomeningeal metastasis is the initial manifestation of breast cancer. Many patients with solid tumor have widespread metastatic disease when leptomeningeal metastasis is diagnosed, but in patients with breast cancer, the tumor may be inactive or responding to chemotherapy. Of 40 breast cancer patients with leptomeningeal metastasis reported by Yap et al.,[3] the systemic disease was responding or stable in 14 (35%), and no evidence of active systemic tumor was present in 12 (30%) when leptomeningeal metastasis was diagnosed. In the remainder, leptomeningeal metastasis was concurrent with systemic relapse.

PATHOPHYSIOLOGY OF LEPTOMENINGEAL METASTASIS

The cerebral and spinal meninges are composed of the dura mater, arachnoid, and pia mater (Fig. 1). The leptomeninges include the arachnoid and pia mater. The pia is a thin lining, closely adherent to the surface of the brain and spinal cord, separated from the arachnoid by fine trabeculae. It follows the sulci of the cerebral cortex and penetrates the parenchyma of the central nervous system in association with arterioles. The associated parenchymal perivascular space is termed the *Virchow-Robin space* (see Fig. 1). Pathologic evidence suggests several methods by which tumor cells reach the leptomeninges, including hematogenous spread to the vessels of the arachnoid or to the choroid plexus of the ventricles (the latter produces dissemination of

L. M. DeAngelis: Department of Neurology, Memorial Sloan-Kettering Cancer Center, New York, New York

L. R. Rogers: Department of Neurology, Wayne State University School of Medicine, Detroit, Michigan

K. M. Foley: Departments of Neurology, Neuroscience, and Clinical Pharmacology, Joan and Sanford I. Weill Medical College, New York Presbyterian Hospital - Cornell University, New York, New York; Pain and Palliative Care Service, Department of Neurology, Memorial Sloan-Kettering Cancer Center, New York, New York

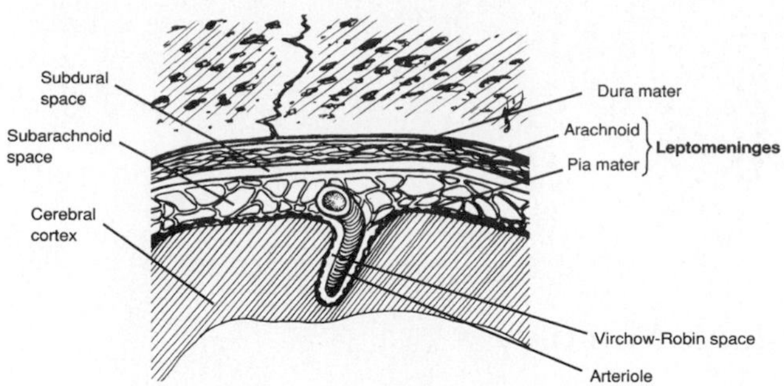

FIG. 1. Relation of the cerebral meninges to the brain.

TABLE 1. *Presenting symptoms and signs of leptomeningeal metastases*

Symptoms and signs	Percentage
Spinal radiculopathy	48
Cranial nerves	45
III, IV, VI	22
VII	23
Headache	40
Cerebral	38
Limb weakness	38
Mental change	29
Difficulty walking	26
Cerebellar signs	24
Sensory abnormalities	23
Seizures	6

Modified from ref. 12.

malignant cells to the leptomeninges by normal CSF flow) and from direct extension of adjacent metastasis in the cerebral parenchyma or dura or lymphatic paraspinal region.

Autopsy studies demonstrate that, when tumor reaches the leptomeninges, it grows in a sheetlike fashion along the surface of the brain, spinal cord, and nerve roots.[10] It usually disseminates widely but may be limited to portions of the cerebral or spinal leptomeninges. A less common pattern of tumor growth is the formation of multifocal nodules, which typically develop on the cauda equina and on the ventricular surface of the brain. Leptomeningeal metastasis usually is accompanied by a fibroblastic proliferation of the meninges. A significant inflammatory response is rarely seen pathologically in the leptomeninges, but occasionally reactive lymphocytes accompany malignant cells in a CSF specimen. When tumor enters the subarachnoid space from a parenchymal or dural metastasis, a fibrotic reaction often develops that walls off the tumor, and diffuse leptomeningeal dissemination does not occur.[10] Tumor can ensheath meningeal arteries and veins within the subarachnoid space and extend into the Virchow-Robin spaces, resulting in perivascular tumor cuffing and parenchymal invasion. Tumor also can encase or invade the spinal and cranial nerves.

The clinical symptoms and signs of leptomeningeal metastasis reflect the pathologic process of subarachnoid tumor infiltration. Cerebral symptoms often result from hydrocephalus, caused by tumor cells proliferating in the basal cisterns and obstructing CSF flow. Cerebral symptoms also can be caused by interference of local cortical function caused by direct competition for blood flow and essential metabolites between metabolically active tumor and the underlying cortical tissue, or direct parenchymal invasion.[11] Cranial and spinal nerve symptoms result from neoplastic compression or destruction of the nerves.

CLINICAL MANIFESTATIONS

A clue to the clinical diagnosis of leptomeningeal metastasis is the simultaneous occurrence of multifocal abnormalities at more than one level of the neuraxis (cerebral, cranial nerve, and spinal).[12] Characteristically, a careful neurologic examination often reveals more signs than are suggested by the clinical symptoms. In a study of 90 patients with leptomeningeal metastasis from solid tumors (one-half had breast carcinoma), Wasserstrom et al.[9] found that 47 patients complained of symptoms referable to one area of the neuraxis only, but on examination signs were restricted to one area of the neuraxis in only 17 patients; 50 had abnormalities in two areas, and 23 patients in all had involvement in three areas. A study of leptomeningeal metastasis in 33 patients with breast cancer confirmed these findings; 16 complained of symptoms in only one area, but on examination 27 had involvement of two or three areas.[8]

Spinal symptoms are the most common presentation of leptomeningeal metastasis (Table 1). The most common complaint is limb weakness, typically involving the legs, which may be accompanied by paresthesias of the extremities and pain in the spine or limbs. Neurologic examination may reveal asymmetric depression of deep tendon reflexes, radicular limb weakness, and sensory loss. Signs of meningeal irritation, such as nuchal rigidity, are rare. Cerebral symptoms of leptomeningeal metastasis result, in large part, from the obstruction of CSF flow and include headache, changes in mentation (lethargy, confusion, and memory loss), nausea and vomiting, and ataxia. Seizures occur in fewer than 10% of patients and are rare as the presenting symptom. The most common finding of cerebral dysfunction on neurologic examination is a change in mentation. The most common cranial nerve symptom is diplopia. Hearing loss, vision loss, and facial numbness also occur. Paresis of the extraocular muscles is the most common cranial nerve abnormality, followed by facial weakness and diminished hearing.[8,9]

METHODS OF DIAGNOSIS

The definitive method to diagnose leptomeningeal metastasis is to demonstrate malignant cells in CSF, typically obtained by lumbar puncture. Malignant cells are not identified in the CSF of patients with parenchymal, dural, or epidural metastasis, and they indicate metastasis to the subarachnoid space.[13] The initial lumbar CSF cytologic examination gives negative results in up to 46% of patients with leptomeningeal metastasis.[9] The detection of malignant cells depends partly on the amount of CSF available for analysis, and the yield increases with additional spinal taps. In some patients, an alternate site for spinal puncture also increases the yield. Rogers et al.[14] found that cytologic examination of cisternal CSF was more sensitive than lumbar CSF in 3 of 12 patients with documented leptomeningeal metastasis. In some instances, the failure to detect malignant cells in CSF reflects adherence of the cells to central nervous system structures without exfoliation into the CSF. Finally, the failure to detect malignant cells may indicate that the tumor is localized. In an autopsy study of 30 cases of leptomeningeal metastasis, Glass et al.[13] found that 76% of patients with multifocal or disseminated leptomeningeal tumor had a positive CSF cytologic evaluation, versus only 58% of patients who had focal disease. Immunohistochemical staining and fluorescence *in situ* hybridization occasionally enhance the detection of carcinoma by cytologic examination.[15,16] However, flow cytometry can be a useful adjunct in some cases of leptomeningeal metastasis,[17] although it has not been well studied in patients with breast cancer. If CSF results are repeatedly negative, a definitive diagnosis can also be obtained by leptomeningeal biopsy.

The CSF of most patients with leptomeningeal metastasis has abnormalities of the routine chemistries and white blood cell count.[9] Elevated protein is the most common abnormality but is usually less than 100 mg per dL. Up to one-half of patients have a pleocytosis, usually mononuclear. Approximately one-third of patients have depressed CSF glucose; CSF glucose less than 70% of simultaneous serum glucose is pathologic. CSF tumor markers also can be useful to detect leptomeningeal tumor when the cytologic examination gives negative results, but they are limited by a low sensitivity and specificity. β-Glucuronidase is elevated in more than one-half of patients with leptomeningeal metastasis, but it is also elevated in patients with acute and chronic infectious meningitis.[18] CSF carcinoembryonic antigen (CEA) is elevated in some cases of breast carcinoma metastatic to the leptomeninges.[19] CSF CEA must be compared with serum CEA, because extremely elevated serum levels can cross the blood–brain barrier. Elevation of the total lactic acid dehydrogenase (LDH) or the percentage of the LDH-5 isoenzyme can also indicate leptomeningeal metastasis.[20] However, CSF LDH can be elevated in infections and other disorders of the central nervous system. The CSF β-2-microglobulin level can be elevated in leptomeningeal carcinoma,[21] but it is also elevated with central nervous system infection and after intrathecal methotrexate administration. A combination of markers can be useful.[22] Elevations of CSF tumor markers must be interpreted cautiously in patients with other sites of central nervous system metastasis in close proximity to the ventricles or leptomeningeal surfaces. Tumor marker values are lower in the ventricular than lumbar CSF, making interpretation from this region difficult. Other CSF markers that have been reported to aid in the diagnosis of leptomeningeal metastasis include HMFG1 antigen,[23] glucosephosphate isomerase,[24] creatine kinase-BB,[25] and tissue polypeptide antigen.[26]

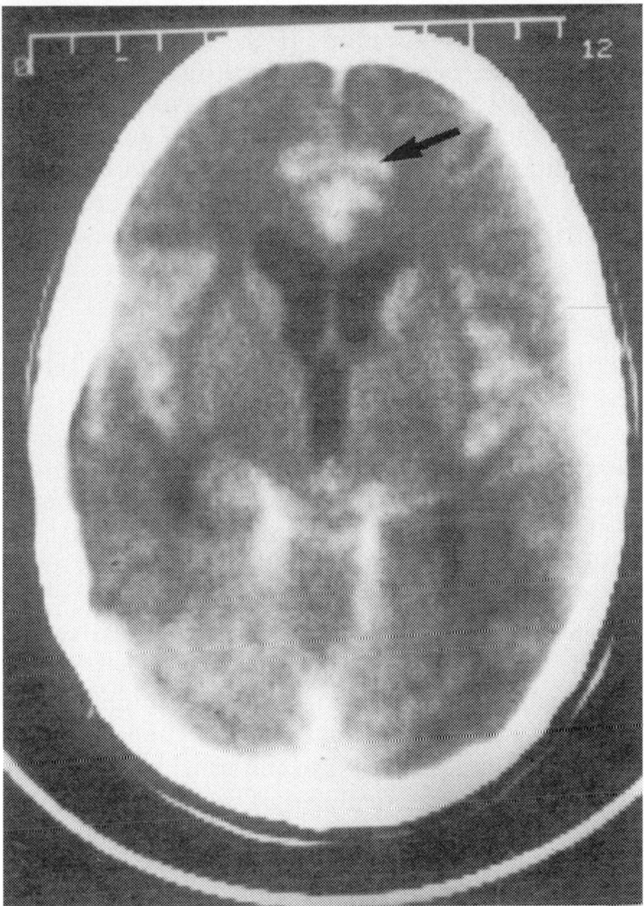

FIG. 2. Axial contrast-enhanced brain computed tomographic scan reveals abnormal diffuse enhancement of the leptomeninges, sulci, cisterns, and tentorium. The arrow demonstrates leptomeningeal and sulcal enhancement. The lateral and third ventricles are enlarged, which is consistent with hydrocephalus.

Neuroimaging procedures are indicated in patients who are thought or proved to have leptomeningeal metastasis to exclude parenchymal brain or spinal epidural lesions, which can produce a similar clinical picture, and to determine the extent of disease. Typically, neuroimaging is obtained before lumbar puncture, and gadolinium-enhanced magnetic resonance scanning is the best technique for either cranial or spinal imaging, although computed tomographic scanning can occasionally reveal leptomeningeal tumor[27,28] (Fig. 2). Indirect or suggestive evidence of leptomeningeal metastasis may present on cranial imaging, such as hydrocephalus or small superficial metastases deep in sulci. There may be very specific findings, such as enhancement of the tentorium, basal cisterns, ependyma, or leptomeninges over the convexities (Fig. 3). Spinal magnetic resonance imaging (MRI) may reveal tumor nodules or diffuse enhancement of the cauda

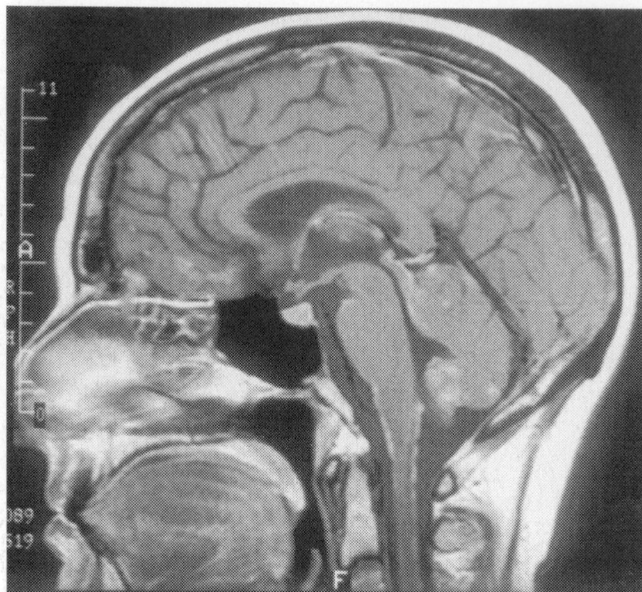

FIG. 3. Leptomeningeal metastases from breast cancer. Sagittal gadolinium-enhanced brain magnetic resonance imaging reveals diffuse linear enhancement of the tectum, ventral and dorsal medulla, and upper cervical cord. Patchy enhancement can also be seen coating the cerebellum and inferior frontal lobe.

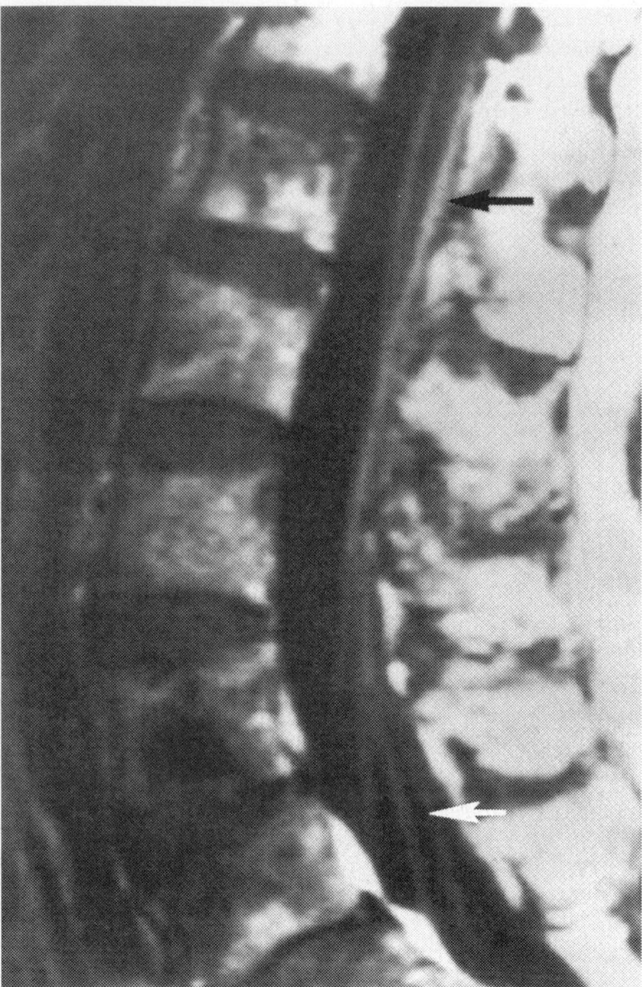

FIG. 4. Sagittal gadolinium-enhanced spine magnetic resonance imaging reveals thickening and linear enhancement of the leptomeninges adjacent to the distal spinal cord (*dark arrow*) and on the lumbosacral nerve roots (*white arrow*).

equina (Fig. 4). Nodules may stud the surface of the spinal cord. In a patient with known cancer, these specific findings are sufficient to diagnose leptomeningeal metastases. In these circumstances, CSF documentation is unnecessary to initiate treatment, and a lumbar puncture may be harmful if a substantial bulky tumor is present in the distal thecal sac.[29] Despite the sensitivity of MRI, it is negative in 25% to 30% of all patients with a positive CSF cytology, but it is negative in only 10% of patients with solid tumors, compared to 55% in patients with hematologic malignancies.[27–29] However, these radiographic findings in patients who are not known to have systemic cancer cannot automatically be attributed to metastasis, because primary leptomeningeal tumors, infection, postoperative, or even postlumbar puncture changes can mimic subarachnoid metastases.[30]

The diagnosis of leptomeningeal metastasis usually requires a high index of suspicion. Initial testing may not reveal the diagnosis, and the physician often must resort to a variety of tests combined with clinical findings to establish the diagnosis. Occasionally, a presumptive diagnosis is made if the clinical picture is suggestive, other diagnoses are excluded, and the CSF is abnormal despite a negative CSF cytologic examination.

TREATMENT

Vigorous treatment of leptomeningeal metastasis can improve neurologic function and prevent further deterioration; however, sustained remissions are rare, and patients usually succumb to their neurologic disease. Treatment often involves radiotherapy plus chemotherapy—intrathecal, systemic, or both. Interpretation of published treatment results is difficult because of a nonuniform selection of patients and treatment design. Most studies have used whole-brain or involved-field radiation therapy to bulky disease and symptomatic sites.

Patients with leptomeningeal metastasis should undergo enhanced MRI of the entire neuraxis to search for bulky disease. Radiation should be administered to symptomatic areas—that is, cranial irradiation for cranial neuropathies—and to bulky disease, because intra-CSF chemotherapy penetrates only a short distance into bulky tumor deposits. In addition, bulky tumor deposits impair CSF flow, causing an accumulation of drug proximal to the flow obstruction.[31] The use of complete spine radiotherapy is discouraged, because it is associated with acute morbidities, such as esophagitis, and can result in severe myelosuppression, particularly in patients who are receiving or have received systemic chemotherapy. Whole-brain radiation can enhance the neurotoxicity of chemotherapy administered into the CSF and should be used only when there are symptoms from the brain or cranial nerves or a cranial CSF flow obstruction is present. Data do not suggest that systemic or intra-CSF administration of corticosteroids is effective in treating leptomeningeal metastasis, but steroids are indicated if intracranial pressure is raised.

Leptomeningeal metastasis involves the entire neuraxis, and therefore treatment must encompass the entire CSF volume. Radiotherapy is used focally, and chemotherapy is usually used to treat the whole CSF compartment. Leptomeningeal tumor develops its own vascular supply, which lacks a blood–brain barrier, but it is often difficult to obtain high levels of drug in the CSF with standard intravenous chemotherapy. For this reason, treatment usually involves administration of chemotherapy directly into the CSF. Direct CSF instillation achieves a higher concentration of chemotherapy in the subarachnoid space, because the initial volume of distribution is smaller than the vascular compartment, and the clearance half-life is longer in the spinal fluid for some agents.[32] In addition, intra-CSF instillation often reduces or spares systemic toxicity, although the CSF can act as a reservoir for methotrexate, which can slowly leak into the peripheral circulation, causing mucositis and myelosuppression. A disadvantage to chemotherapy instillation into the CSF is the frequent occurrence of CSF flow abnormalities, which can result in nonuniform distribution of the drug throughout the CSF pathways, reducing efficacy and increasing local toxicity.[33,34]

CSF flow studies often demonstrate abnormalities of CSF flow, which result in compartmentalization of CSF pathways.[31,33,34] Flow abnormalities usually correlate with bulky disease identified by neuroimaging[31]; however, impairment of CSF flow can occasionally develop in the absence of obvious structural disease. CSF block prevents homogeneous distribution of chemotherapy and may be an important factor in the failure of intra-CSF chemotherapy to eradicate leptomeningeal tumor. Furthermore, it may contribute to neurotoxicity, particularly leukoencephalopathy.[31,35] Areas of bulky tumor that cause CSF flow impairment may respond to involved-field radiotherapy, permitting intra-CSF chemotherapy to distribute throughout the CSF. Patients with bulky tumor can be presumed to have disrupted CSF flow; however, patients with normal neuroimaging should have a CSF flow study performed before intrathecal chemotherapy is administered.

Chemotherapy can be instilled directly into the lumbar subarachnoid space or the ventricular system via an Ommaya reservoir (Heyer-Schulte NeuroCare Group, Pleasant Prairie, Wisconsin). Intraventricular administration usually is recommended, because this assures delivery of drug into the CSF; lumbar punctures result in inadvertent epidural or subdural injection in 10% of procedures. In addition, a lumbar puncture may be contraindicated if an epidural mass is present. Most important, delivery of drug into the ventricular system ensures a more uniform drug distribution. Shapiro et al.[36] performed a pharmacokinetic study of methotrexate injection into the ventricular system and the lumbar thecal sac; intraventricular injection was more reliable and ensured better distribution of drug throughout the subarachnoid space (Fig. 5). In addition, the use of a ventricular reservoir allows for simple repetitive administration. If the patient requires a ventriculoperitoneal shunt for hydrocephalus, a subcutaneous reservoir with an on-off device can be considered; however, it often functions poorly. Alternatively, when a shunt is necessary, chemotherapy can be administered by lumbar puncture.

Only three drugs are conventionally instilled into the CSF: methotrexate, cytarabine, and thiotepa. Only methotrexate and thiotepa have intrinsic activity against breast cancer. Intra-CSF administration of methotrexate usually is performed twice a week initially, and the frequency is gradually tapered. The dose is fixed at 12 to 15 mg per dose, because the volume of CSF is identical for all patients regardless of size. Some[37] advocate a "concentration time" approach in which 2 mg methotrexate is given every day for 5 days; this gives a more sustained concentration of drug with a reduced total dose. This approach also allows monitoring of methotrexate levels, but it is demanding on the patient, requiring frequent trips to the physician's office. Alternatively, a high-dose intrathecal methotrexate regimen may give a higher response rate and longer survival.[38]

Response criteria in leptomeningeal metastasis are not standardized. Most reported studies define *complete response* as the normalization of CSF and improvement of clinical symptoms. Sixty percent to 80% of patients show response after intra-CSF methotrexate, with or without radiation.[3,8] Response may be durable, even if only a partial response is obtained.[39] Methotrexate seems to provide an improved survival compared with no therapy in most studies, with a median survival ranging from 3 to 6 months[3,8,40–42] and a median survival of 15 months in those who respond.[3,8] Boogerd et al.,[41] however, report similar survivals among patients with similar pretreatment characteristics who were not treated or who were treated with intraventricular methotrexate.

Intra-CSF thiotepa has been studied in small numbers of patients with leptomeningeal metastasis from solid tumors, including breast carcinoma. The dosage is usually 10 mg twice a week to start, and the frequency is decreased over 1 to 3 months. In a comparative randomized study of intraventricular methotrexate versus thiotepa in 52 patients with solid tumors, 25 of whom had breast carcinoma, Grossman et al.[42] found a slight survival advantage with methotrexate. Thiotepa has a rapid half-life in the CSF, which may limit its effectiveness. No evidence shows that combination intra-CSF chemotherapy is better than single agent, and toxicity is additive.[43] Investigational agents available in protocol settings for treating leptomeningeal metastasis from solid tumors include liposomal cytarabine,[44] diaziquone,[45] interleukin-2,[46] radioactively tagged monoclonal antibodies,[47] nitrosoureas,[48] and 4-hydroperoxycyclophosphamide.[49]

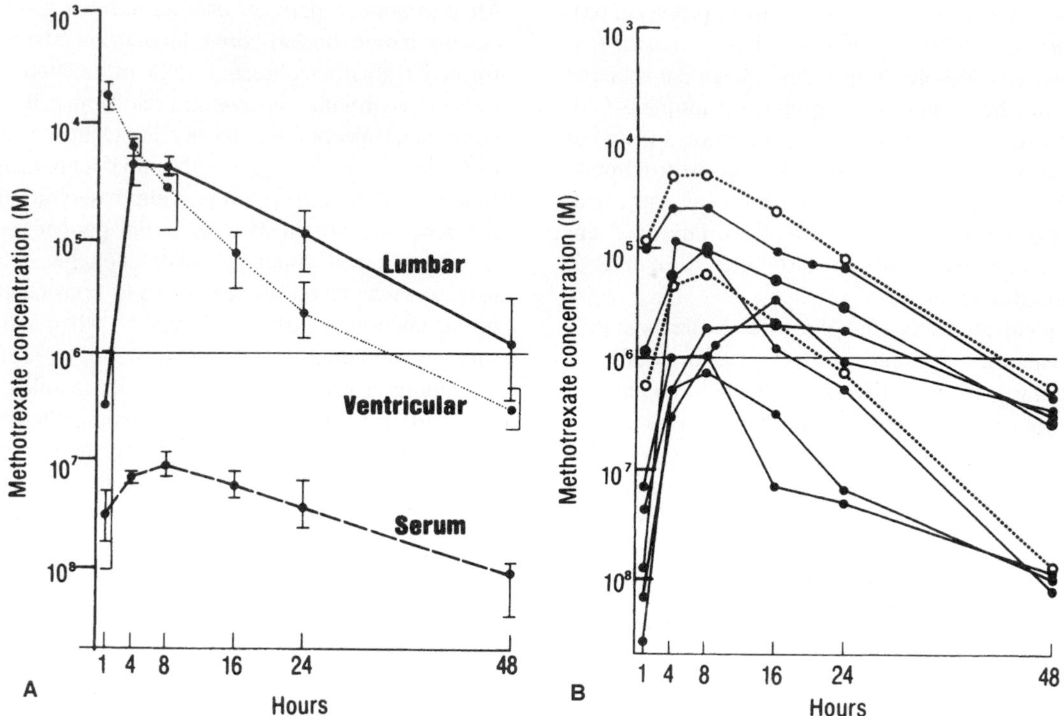

FIG. 5. A: Methotrexate distribution (mean range) in five studies after administration of 6.25 mg per m^2 through the Ommaya reservoir. **B:** Intraventricular methotrexate concentration in nine studies after lumbar administration. Solid circles represent seven studies at a methotrexate dose of 6.25 mg per m^2. Open circles represent two studies at a dose of 12.5 mg per m^2. (From ref. 36, with permission.)

A new approach to the chemotherapeutic treatment of leptomeningeal metastasis is to use systemic drugs, which are either lipophilic and can penetrate into the subarachnoid space or are administered in high doses to reach the leptomeninges.[50,51] This has the theoretical benefits of reaching the entire CSF regardless of CSF flow dynamics and treating both bulky and microscopic disease. However, it subjects patients to the systemic toxicities of intravenous chemotherapy. This has been studied with high-dose methotrexate and is reported to give a median survival of 13.8 months, far superior to standard intrathecal chemotherapy, which has a median survival of only 2.3 months.[50] This study included only one patient with breast cancer and needs to be substantiated before this regimen can be recommended.

Neurotoxicity after irradiation of the nervous system and intra-CSF and systemic chemotherapy is a significant obstacle to aggressively treating patients with leptomeningeal metastasis. The most common neurologic complication of intra-CSF chemotherapy is a transient aseptic meningitis, which develops within hours of injection and produces headache, fever, stiff neck, and confusion. It does not necessarily recur on subsequent injections, and corticosteroids can prevent or ameliorate the reaction.[9] The most significant neurologic complication of intra-CSF methotrexate is necrotizing leukoencephalopathy. The risk of leukoencephalopathy rises with increasing total methotrexate dose, prolonged CSF methotrexate levels, and concurrent cranial radiotherapy.[52,53] Leukoencephalopathy can often be identified first on cranial MRI, in which increased signal, predominantly in the periventricular white matter, can be seen on T2 or FLAIR images. Patients develop apathy, memory loss, gait disturbance, and, later, urinary incontinence. Clinical abnormalities correlate loosely with the severity of changes seen radiographically. Focal leukoencephalopathy can result from high local cerebral concentrations of methotrexate around the Ommaya reservoir catheter, particularly if inadvertent separation of the catheter occurs.[54,55] Systemic complications of methotrexate include stomatitis and myelosuppression. Low-dose oral leucovorin protects against these toxicities in patients who are receiving intrathecal methotrexate. Thiotepa can cause myelosuppression, particularly when concurrent systemic chemotherapy is administered. Any drug can also cause a myelopathy after lumbar injection.[56] Clinically significant complications related to the Ommaya reservoir system are rare and include bacterial meningitis and intracerebral hemorrhage.

CSF from the Ommaya reservoir and periodic lumbar punctures are necessary for determining CSF response. If neurologic decline occurs, the possibility of treatment-related toxicity or progressive leptomeningeal tumor must be evaluated. If the latter occurs, the chemotherapy agent should be changed, radiation administered to bulky areas, or both. Patients must also be monitored for progression of their systemic disease, although in large series[3,41] most patients with breast cancer died of progressive leptomeningeal disease.

Leptomeningeal metastasis remains one of the most intractable complications of systemic cancer. Early diagnosis and novel treatments with reduced potential for neurotoxicity are sorely needed. Furthermore, if one could identify patients at highest risk for leptomeningeal metastasis, prophylactic therapy might be beneficial, as with lymphoma. However, some patients, especially those with breast cancer, respond to existing treatment and can have prolonged survival.

REFERENCES

1. Sondak V. Leptomeningeal spread of breast cancer: report of case and review of the literature. *Cancer* 1981;48:395.
2. Hitchins RN, Bell DR, Woods RL, et al. A prospective randomized trial of single-agent versus combination chemotherapy in meningeal carcinomatosis. *J Clin Oncol* 1987;5:1655.
3. Yap HY, Yap BS, Rasmussen S, et al. Treatment for meningeal carcinomatosis in breast cancer. *Cancer* 1982;49:219.
4. Tsukada Y, Fouad A, Pickren JW, et al. Central nervous system metastasis from breast carcinoma: autopsy study. *Cancer* 1983;52:2349.
5. Lamovec J, Zidar A. Association of leptomeningeal carcinomatosis in carcinoma of the breast with infiltrating lobular carcinoma: an autopsy study. *Arch Pathol Lab Med* 1991;115:507.
6. Harris M, Howell A, Chrissohou M, et al. A comparison of the metastatic pattern of infiltrating lobular carcinoma and infiltrating duct carcinoma of the breast. *Br J Cancer* 1984;50:23.
7. Smith DB, Howell A, Harris M, et al. Carcinomatous meningitis associated with infiltrating lobular carcinoma of the breast. *Eur J Surg Oncol* 1985;11:33.
8. Ongerboer de Visser BW, Somers R, Nooyen WH, et al. Intraventricular methotrexate therapy of leptomeningeal metastasis from breast carcinoma. *Neurology* 1983;33:1565.
9. Wasserstrom WR, Glass JP, Posner JB. Diagnosis and treatment of leptomeningeal metastases from solid tumors: experience with 90 patients. *Cancer* 1982;49:759.
10. Olson ME, Chernik NL, Posner JB. Infiltration of the leptomeninges by systemic cancer. *Arch Neurol* 1974;30:122.
11. Siegal T, Mildworf B, Stein D, et al. Leptomeningeal metastasis: reduction in regional cerebral blood flow and cognitive impairment. *Ann Neurol* 1985;17:100.
12. Jayson GC, Howell A. Carcinomatous meningitis in solid tumors. *Ann Oncol* 1996;7:773.
13. Glass JP, Melamed M, Chernik NL, et al. Malignant cells in cerebrospinal fluid (CSF): the meaning of a positive CSF cytology. *Neurology* 1979;29:1369.
14. Rogers LR, Duchesneau PM, Nunez C, et al. Comparison of cisternal and lumbar CSF examination in leptomeningeal metastasis. *Neurology* 1992;42:1239.
15. Jorda M, Ganjei-Azar P, Nadji M. Cytologic characteristics of meningeal carcinomatosis. *Arch Neurol* 1998;55:181.
16. van Oostenbrugge RJ, Hopman AHN, Lenders MH, et al. Detection of malignant cells in cerebrospinal fluid using fluorescence in situ hybridization. *J Neuropathol Exp Neurol* 1997;56:743.
17. Cibas ES, Malkin MG, Posner JB, et al. Detection of DNA abnormalities by flow cytometry in cells from cerebrospinal fluid. *Am J Clin Pathol* 1987;88:570.
18. Schold SC, Wasserstrom WR, Fleisher M, et al. Cerebrospinal fluid biochemical markers of central nervous system metastases. *Ann Neurol* 1980;8:597.
19. Twijnstra A, Nooyen WJ, van Zanten AP, et al. Cerebrospinal fluid carcinoembryonic antigen in patients with metastatic and nonmetastatic neurological diseases. *Arch Neurol* 1986;43:269.
20. Twijnstra A, van Zanten AP, Hart AAM, et al. Serial lumbar and ventricle cerebrospinal fluid lactate dehydrogenase activities in patients with leptomeningeal metastases from solid and haemotological tumors. *J Neurol Neurosurg Psychiatry* 1987;50:313.
21. Twijnstra A, vanZanten AP, Nooyen WJ, et al. Cerebrospinal fluid 2-microglobulin: a study in controls and patients with metastatic and nonmetastatic neurological diseases. *Eur J Cancer Clin Oncol* 1986;22:387.
22. Ongerboer de Visser BW, van Zanten AP, Twijnstra A, et al. Sensitivity and specificity of cerebrospinal fluid biochemical markers of central nervous system metastases. *Prog Exp Tumor Res* 1985;29:105.
23. Moseley RP, Oge K, Shafqat S, et al. HMFG1 antigen: a new marker for carcinomatous meningitis. *Int J Cancer* 1989;44:440.
24. Newton HB, Fleisher M, Schwartz MK, et al. Glucosephosphate isomerase as a CSF marker for leptomeningeal metastasis. *Neurology* 1991;41:395.
25. Bach F, Bach FW, Pedersen G, et al. Creatine kinase-BB in the cerebrospinal fluid as a marker of CNS metastases and leptomeningeal carcinomatosis in patients with breast cancer. *Eur J Cancer Clin Oncol* 1989;25:1703.
26. Bach F, Soletormos G, Dombernowsky P. Tissue polypeptide antigen activity in cerebrospinal fluid: a marker of central nervous system metastases of breast cancer. *J Natl Cancer Inst* 1991;83:779.
27. Chamberlain MC, Sandy AD, Press GA. Leptomeningeal metastasis: a comparison of gadolinium-enhanced MR and contrast-enhanced CT of the brain. *Neurology* 1990;40:435.
28. Sze G, Soletsky S, Bronen R, et al. MR imaging of the cranial meninges with emphasis on contrast enhancement and meningeal carcinomatosis. *AJNR Am J Neuroradiol* 1989;10:965.
29. Freilich RJ, Kro G, DeAngelis LM. Neuroimaging and cerebrospinal fluid cytology in the diagnosis of leptomeningeal metastasis. *Ann Neurol* 1995;38:51.
30. Buff BL, Schnick RM, Norregaard T. Meningeal metastasis of leiomyosarcoma mimicking meningioma: CT and MR findings. *J Comput Assist Tomogr* 1991;15:166.
31. Mason WP, Yeh SDJ, DeAngelis LM. Indium-diethylenetriamine pentaacetic acid cerebrospinal fluid flow studies predict distribution of intrathecally administered chemotherapy and outcome in patients with leptomeningeal metastases. *Neurology* 1998;50:438.
32. Poplack DG, Bleyer WA, Horowitz ME. Pharmacology of antineoplastic agents in cerebrospinal fluid. In: Wood JH, ed. *Neurobiology of cerebrospinal fluid*. New York: Plenum Publishing, 1980:561.
33. Chamberlain MC, Corey-Bloom J. Leptomeningeal metastasis: 111 indium-DTPA CSF flow studies. *Neurology* 1991;41:1765.
34. Grossman SA, Trump DL, Chen DCP, et al. Cerebrospinal fluid flow abnormalities in patients with neoplastic meningitis. *Am J Med* 1982;73:641.
35. Glantz MJ, Hall WA, Cole BF, et al. Diagnosis, management, and survival of patients with leptomeningeal cancer based on cerebrospinal fluid-flow status. *Cancer* 1995;75:2919.
36. Shapiro WR, Young DF, Mehta BM. Methotrexate: distribution in cerebrospinal fluid after intravenous, ventricular and lumbar injections. *N Engl J Med* 1975;293:161.
37. Bleyer WA, Poplack DG, Simon RM. "Concentration X time" methotrexate via a subcutaneous reservoir: a less toxic regimen for intraventricular chemotherapy of central nervous system neoplasms. *Blood* 1978;51:835.
38. Fizazi K, Asselain B,Vincent-Salomon A, et al. Meningeal carcinomatosis in patients with breast carcinoma. *Cancer* 1996;77:1315.
39. Siegal T, Lossos A, Pfeffer MR. Leptomeningeal metastasis: analysis of 31 patients with sustained off-therapy response following combined-modality therapy. *Neurology* 1994;44:1463.
40. Trump DL, Grossman SA, Thompson G, et al. Treatment of neoplastic meningitis with intraventricular thiotepa and methotrexate. *Cancer Treat Rep* 1982;66:1599.
41. Boogerd W, Hart AAM, van der Sande JJ, et al. Meningeal carcinomatosis in breast cancer: prognostic factors and influence of treatment. *Cancer* 1991;67:1685.
42. Grossman SA, Finkelstein DM, Ruckdeschel JC, et al. Randomized prospective comparison of intraventricular methotrexate and thiotepa in patients with previously untreated neoplastic meningitis. *J Clin Oncol* 1993;11:561.
43. Giannone L, Greco FA, Hainsworth JD. Combination intraventricular chemotherapy for meningeal neoplasia. *J Clin Oncol* 1986;4:68.
44. Chamberlain MC, Khatibi S, Kim JC, et al. A phase I study of DepoFoam/Ara-C in the treatment of carcinomatous meningitis. *Arch Neurol* 1993;50:261.
45. Berg SL, Balis FM, Zimm S, et al. Phase I/II trial and pharmacokinetics of intrathecal diaziquone in refractory meningeal malignancies. *J Clin Oncol* 1992;10:143.

46. Moser RP, Black JB, London WG, et al. Pilot study of intraventricular interleukin-2 for the treatment of leptomeningeal cancer [Abstract]. *Proc Annu Meet Am Soc Clin Oncol* 1991;10:384.
47. Moseley RP, Benjamin JC, Ashpole RD, et al. Carcinomatous meningitis: antibody-guided therapy with I-131 HMFg1. *J Neurol Neurosurg Psychiatry* 1991;54:260.
48. Levin VA, Chamberlain M, Silver P, et al. Phase I/II study of intraventricular and intrathecal ACNU for leptomeningeal neoplasia. *Cancer Chemother Pharmacol* 1989;23(5):301.
49. Arndt CAS, Colvin OM, Balis FM, et al. Intrathecal administration of 4-hydroperoxycyclophosphamide in rhesus monkeys. *Cancer Res* 1987;47:5932.
50. Glantz MJ, Cole BF, Recht L, et al. High-dose intravenous methotrexate for patients with nonleukemic leptomeningeal cancer: is intrathecal chemotherapy necessary? *J Clin Oncol* 1998;16:1561.
51. Grant R, Naylor B, Greenberg HS, et al. Clinical outcome in aggressively treated meningeal carcinomatosis. *Arch Neurol* 1994;51:457.
52. Bleyer WA. Neurological sequelae of methotrexate and ionizing radiation: a new classification. *Cancer Treat Rep* 1981;65:89.
53. Shapiro WR, Chernik NL, Posner JB. Necrotizing encephalopathy following intraventricular instillation of methotrexate. *Arch Neurol* 1973;28:96.
54. Lemann W, Wiley RG, Posner JB. Leukoencephalopathy complicating intraventricular catheters: clinical, radiographic and pathologic study of 10 cases. *J Neurooncol* 1988;6:77.
55. de Waal R, Algra PR, Heimans JJ, et al. Methotrexate induced brain necrosis and severe leukoencephalopathy due to disconnection of an Ommaya device. *J Neurooncol* 1993;15:269.
56. Hahn AF, Feasby TE, Gilbert JJ. Paraparesis following intrathecal chemotherapy. *Neurology* 1983;33:1032.

Diseases of the Breast, 2nd ed.,
edited by Jay R. Harris.
Lippincott Williams & Wilkins, Philadelphia © 2000.

CHAPTER 55

Brachial Plexopathy

Nathan I. Cherny and Bella Kaufman

In patients with cancer, symptoms and signs of brachial plexopathy may be attributable to acute brachial neuritis, trauma to the plexus during surgery or anesthesia, metastatic spread of tumor, transient or permanent radiation injury, or radiation-induced plexus tumors. In patients with breast cancer, metastatic spread of tumor, radiation injury to the plexus, and second primaries are the most common causes of such signs. Careful evaluation of the clinical history, symptoms, and signs, as well as the results of electrodiagnostic and imaging studies, are helpful in diagnosing the cause of a brachial plexopathy.

TUMOR INFILTRATION OF THE BRACHIAL PLEXUS (METASTATIC BRACHIAL PLEXOPATHY)

Tumor infiltration of the plexus is common because of its proximity to the draining axillary lymph nodes. Yet this was the diagnosis in only 5% of case referrals evaluated by one neurologic consultation unit[1] and 4% of patients referred to a cancer pain unit.[2] Early and accurate diagnosis is critical to prevent irreversible nerve damage and chronic neuropathic pain, and to determine the prognosis and treatment of tumors.

Clinical Symptoms and Signs

Pain

Eighty-five percent of patients with tumor infiltration present with pain that is moderate to severe and often precedes neurologic signs or symptoms by up to 9 months.[3–7]

The pain distribution depends on the site of plexus involvement. Typically, the pain radiates in the sensory distribution of the lower plexus, usually involving the shoulder girdle and radiating to the elbow, medial side of the forearm, and the fourth and fifth fingers (consistent with involvement of the lower plexus C-7, C-8, T-1).[3–5]

Other, less common clinical presentations are occasionally observed, including pain localized to the posterior aspect of the arm or to the elbow, a burning or freezing sensation and hypersensitivity of the skin along the ulnar aspect of the arm, or pain referred to either the shoulder girdle or the tip of either the index finger or thumb (consistent with infiltration of the upper plexus C5-6 by tumor rising in the supraclavicular nodes).

By the time of diagnosis of a brachial plexus lesion, 98% of patients have pain, which is most often reported as severe. In the series of Kori et al.,[3] 2 of 78 patients with malignant brachial plexopathy had pain as the only symptom or sign of tumor recurrence and required exploration and biopsy of the plexus to establish the diagnosis.

Paresthesias

Paresthesias occur as a presenting symptom in 15% of patients with tumor. They are seen in an ulnar distribution with infiltration of the lower plexus, or in a median nerve distribution with lesions of the upper plexus.

Lymphedema

Lymphedema is rarely a presenting symptom of tumor infiltration of the brachial plexus,[3,4] but it does occur in approximately 10% of patients, most often in patients who have had previous radiation therapy to the plexus and who subsequently develop recurrent tumor.

Weakness

Focal weakness, atrophy, and sensory changes in the distribution of the C-7, C-8, and T-1 roots occur in more than 75% of patients. In one series of patients with brachial plexopathy arising from any tumor type, 25% of patients presented with whole-plexus motor weakness (panplexopathy).[3]

N. I. Cherny: Department of Medical Oncology, Shaare-Zedek Medical Center, Jerusalem, Israel
B. Kaufman: Department of Medical Oncology, Shaare-Zedek Medical Center, Jerusalem, Israel

Horner's Syndrome

Patients with panplexopathy or Horner's syndrome have a higher likelihood of epidural extension and should undergo imaging of the epidural space as part of their evaluation.

Palpable Masses

Careful physical examination commonly reveals palpable supraclavicular or axillary lymphadenopathy. Occasionally, tumor infiltration in the distal plexus is associated with a palpable mass or fullness in the clavipectoral triangle. In all cases, these areas need to be carefully evaluated.

Relationship to Natural History

In 12 of 78 patients with tumor infiltration of the brachial plexus included in the series of Kori et al., the plexus lesion was the only evidence of tumor, and other metastases appeared only after several months.[3] In two patients, the plexus lesion was the only sign of recurrence for 4 years. In one patient, surgical exploration after 2 years of plexopathy signs proved to be normal, but because of progressive worsening of neurologic signs, a second exploration was carried out, and it confirmed tumor recurrence.

RADIATION INJURY TO THE BRACHIAL PLEXUS

Pathophysiology of Radiation Injury

Sensitivity to a given dose of radiation is dependent on several factors, including age, the radiation dose, the size of the port, and especially the premorbid state of the irradiated nerve.[8] In cases of radiation injury to the brachial plexus, the predominant findings are in the upper plexus. When the anatomic relationship of the brachial plexus to the surrounding lymph nodes is considered, these findings are not surprising. This is because the divisions of the lower trunk run a shorter course through the radiation port, are partially protected by the clavicle, and are less likely to be damaged by irradiation than are the divisions of the upper trunk.

Three types of peripheral nerve damage after radiation therapy are possible[9]:

1. A very high dose of radiation may cause severe vascular damage to the blood vessels supplying a segment of a nerve. This type of peripheral nerve damage occurs within months to years after irradiation.
2. Extensive fibrosis of the adjacent and overlying connective tissues may damage a peripheral nerve trunk situated within intact tissue. This tends to be a very late phenomenon, occurring many years after radiation.
3. Extensive fibrosis of the adjacent and overlying connective tissues may damage a peripheral nerve trunk situated within tissues previously subjected to surgical dissection. The microvascular disruption caused by the previous dissection makes these tissues more vulnerable, and consequently fibrosis may develop more rapidly, after a few months to years.

Irrespective of the assumed predominant mechanism, the trauma of surgical removal of subcutaneous and connective tissues, irradiation, and the subsequent decreased vascularity are contributing factors in facilitating the development of early and extensive fibrosis of the adjacent connective tissues around the nerve trunk. This fibrosis and decreased vascularity, over a period of months to years, may destroy peripheral nerves and prevent the regeneration of their proximal normal portions. The degree of connective tissue injury at the time of or preceding radiation therapy may be important in influencing the subsequent development of connective tissue fibrosis.

Three distinct clinical syndromes of brachial plexopathy related to radiation therapy have been reported in patients with breast cancer: (a) reversible or transient brachial plexopathy, (b) radiation fibrosis or radiation injury to the brachial plexus, and (c) acute ischemic brachial plexopathy.[3,6,10,11] All three are uncommon clinical entities, each with a characteristic clinical presentation and course.

Transient Radiation Injury

A transient brachial plexopathy has been described in breast cancer patients immediately after radiotherapy to the chest wall and adjacent nodal areas. In retrospective studies, the incidence of this phenomenon has been variably estimated as 1.4% to 20%[5,10]; clinical experience suggests that lower estimates are more accurate. In a review of 565 patients who were treated with moderate doses of supervoltage radiation therapy (5,000 cGy in 5 weeks), Salner identified eight cases (1.4%) of transient brachial plexopathy.[10] The onset of symptoms occurred 3 to 14 months after irradiation (a median of 4.5 months). The clinical symptoms included paresthesias in the arm and hand and, less commonly, weakness and pain. Seven of the eight patients received adjuvant chemotherapy; in six patients, symptoms began after drug treatment. These cases showed a temporal clustering, possibly suggesting a neurotropic viral component. The symptoms and signs of paresthesias and weakness did not conform to any anatomic pattern but most commonly affected the distribution of the lower plexus. Weakness occurred in five of eight patients and was profound in two of them. All patients regained full strength. In three patients, residual paresthesias persisted.

Fulton[5] retrospectively evaluated 63 patients with breast cancer treated with radiation therapy to the chest wall and adjacent nodal areas, including the brachial plexus, and reported radiation-induced plexopathies in 19. Fourteen had transient plexopathy and five had a permanent plexopathy.

He suggested that transient plexopathy did not appear to predispose patients to the development of a radiation-induced permanent plexopathy. In a long-term follow-up of 1,624 patients, Pierce et al. found that radiation-induced plexopathy was transient in 16 of the 20 cases they identified. Mild symptoms, with minimal pain and weakness, were predictive of resolution.[12]

Radiation Fibrosis

Radiation fibrosis of the brachial plexus results in progressive and irreversible neurologic dysfunction of the brachial plexus. This entity has been well described in the literature.[3,5,6,8,13–18] The risk of developing chronic brachial plexopathy has been variably estimated as 0.6% to 14.0%.[3,6,10,13,15,19–22]

Time Course and Natural History

Symptoms usually develop months to years after radiotherapy,[6,13,15,23] although in many cases no latency is apparent.[17,24] In the series of Kori et al., the interval from the last dose of radiation to the first symptoms of plexus disorder in patients with radiation fibrosis ranged from 3 months to 26 years, with a median of 4 years.[3] Kori et al. observed that 5 of the 7 patients who received radiation therapy because of local disease developed radiation damage within 1 year, whereas 13 of 15 patients who received radiation therapy to the plexus as prophylaxis developed symptoms after 1 year. No good explanation exists for this finding.

Dose and Schedule Relationship

Scheduling factors associated with an increased relative risk of subsequent plexopathy include high total dose[16] and larger fraction size (more than 1,900 cGy per day).[17,21,25–27] Powell et al. examined the incidence of radiation-induced brachial plexopathy in 449 patients who had been randomized to receive either 4,600 cGy in 15 fractions or 5,400 cGy in 27 to 30 fractions. The incidence of radiation plexopathy was only 1% in the high dose–small fraction group compared with 5.9% in the low dose–large fraction cohort; these investigators concluded that fractional dose is the major scheduling risk factor.[23] Other factors associated with an increased relative risk include younger age at treatment[17,24] and concurrent cytotoxic therapy.[5,12,17]

Symptoms and Signs

Pain

Although pain is a presenting symptom in less than 20% of patients with radiation injury to the brachial plexus, its prevalence increases with time.[3,17,18,24] The pain is commonly described as mild discomfort associated with aching pain in the shoulder or hand. At the time of diagnosis, 65% of patients report discomfort or pain in the arm; in 35% it is severe.[3]

Paresthesias

In more than 50% of affected patients, paresthesias are a prominent symptom.[3] They are commonly reported to occur in the thumb and forefinger but often involve the entire hand. These symptoms are often confused with carpal tunnel syndrome, but they can be differentiated clinically and by electrodiagnostic studies.

Weakness

Proximal weakness of the arm in the deltoid distribution is observed in all patients.[3] Motor weakness typically involves the muscles innervated by the upper plexus alone or the upper and lower plexus.[3–6,15,17,20,24] Weakness in a distribution of the lower plexus is uncommon.[17,24]

Lymphedema

Lymphedema of the ipsilateral arm was observed in 16 of 22 of patients with radiation fibrosis in the series of Kori et al.[3] and in a substantial proportion of those reported by others.[4] Olsen et al. found that lymphedema was a common late consequence of radiation therapy that occurred in approximately 25% of patients, and that it was not predictive of brachial plexus fibrosis.[21]

Radiation Skin Changes

Radiation skin changes were noted in approximately one-third of the patients with radiation injury, but these changes were not predictive of an underlying plexopathy.[3]

Uncommon Signs

Horner's syndrome is rarely observed.[4,17,20,24] Occasionally, osteoradionecrosis of the ribs and, rarely, of the humeral head can be noted on plain radiographs.[14]

Natural History

The natural history of brachial plexus fibrosis is variable. Sensorimotor dysfunction may be incomplete or may progress to a severe paresis.[17,18,24] Even with advanced radiation fibrosis, severe pain is relatively uncommon, and its presence should prompt an evaluation of the patient for recurrent tumor.[3]

OTHER CAUSES OF BRACHIAL PLEXOPATHY AND NEUROPATHIC ARM PAIN

Second Primaries

Uncommonly, a malignant peripheral nerve tumor or a second primary tumor in a previously irradiated site can account for pain recurring late in the disease course.[28,29] Primary tumors of the brachial plexus are uncommon,[30–33] and nerve sheath tumors that occur years after radiation therapy are generally thought to be a late effect of the therapy.[28] This condition must be differentiated from recurrence of breast cancer, which may also occur in a plexus previously damaged by radiation fibrosis.[34]

Carpal Tunnel Syndrome

Among patients with a past medical history of breast cancer who were referred for evaluation of arm pain, 4 of 30 were found to have carpal tunnel syndrome.[4] Although electrophysiologic abnormalities that are consistent with carpal tunnel syndrome occur twice as frequently ipsilateral to the resection among women who have undergone mastectomy,[35] it is an infrequent cause of arm pain in this population, and the diagnosis requires demonstration of a prolonged sensory latency that is greater than that recorded for the median and ulnar nerves.[36,37]

Lymphedematous Brachial Plexus Compression

Some authors have suggested that lymphedema alone can produce a compression injury of the brachial plexus.[4,35] Ganel et al. performed a series of electromyographic studies on women who had undergone mastectomies with or without subsequent radiation therapy. On the basis of an increased prevalence of F-wave latency abnormalities ipsilateral to previous mastectomy in women with lymphedema, they proposed that the lymphedema may indeed cause an entrapment brachial plexopathy.[35] Vecht inferred this diagnosis in 1 of 28 patients evaluated for arm pain on the basis of negative imaging studies and a nonprogressive neurologic deficit in a patient with lymphedema.[4] In the absence of demonstrable reversibility of the neurologic deficit with effective management of the lymphedema, or surgical evaluation of the plexus to exclude recurrent tumor or radiation fibrosis, this diagnosis should be approached with clinical skepticism.

Radiation-Induced Acute Ischemic Brachial Plexopathy

Gerard et al. have reported a case of subclavian artery occlusion occurring 19 years after a patient with breast cancer was treated with 4,000 cGy irradiation to the breast and axillary area after a radical mastectomy.[11] The patient's symptoms occurred acutely after carrying a heavy object and holding her left arm outstretched above the shoulder. The lesion appeared to be acute in onset, nonprogressive, and painless. These features are in contrast to those in most cases of radiation fibrosis, in which the fibrosis typically is progressive and is associated with pain in up to 35% of patients.

DIAGNOSTIC INVESTIGATIONS

Plexopathy has many potential causes in cancer patients, the most common of which are tumor infiltration and radiation fibrosis. Often, patients with symptoms suggestive of plexopathy have received prior radiotherapy; in these patients, distinguishing between tumor infiltration and radiation-induced fibrosis is important. When radiologic findings are nondiagnostic, electrophysiologic studies may assist in making the distinction.

Cross-sectional imaging is essential in all patients with symptoms or signs compatible with plexopathy. Magnetic resonance imaging (MRI) and computed tomography (CT) are commonly used in these settings. Very little data exist comparing the sensitivity and specificity of these techniques in this setting.[38] MRI has the theoretical advantage of reliably assessing the integrity of the adjacent epidural space.[39,40] This is particularly important when clinical or radiologic features are seen that are suggestive of epidural encroachment through the intervertebral foramina.

Computed Tomographic Scan

CT scanning techniques to image the brachial plexus should include bone and soft-tissue windows and should be contrast enhanced to give clear definition of vascular structures. Because thicker slices miss subtle anatomic changes, Cooke et al.[41,42] advocate the use of narrow section (4-mm) CT with bolus intravenous enhancement to examine the root of the neck and axilla. Adequate imaging requires scanning from C-4 to T-6 vertebral bodies using a large gantry aperture to include both axillary fossae,[43] so the symptomatic plexus may be compared with the asymptomatic one. Vascular enhancement allows for identification of vascular structures that relate to the plexus. Because a high concentration of contrast can produce a streaking artifact, some experts recommend that intravenous contrast should be administered contralateral to the suspected lesion.[43] The elements of the brachial plexus are depicted as nodular or linear areas of soft-tissue density that can be difficult to identify (Figs. 1 and 2).

In a group of 42 breast cancer patients, Cooke et al.[41] evaluated 28 who had neurologic symptoms affecting the arm or hand; CT changes were seen in 96%. Among 19 postoperative patients with breast cancer and suspected local or regional recurrence, CT correctly identified the recurrence in all 15 biopsy-proven cases. Of interest, in two cases, suspicious areas on the CT scans proved to be residual pectoralis muscle.

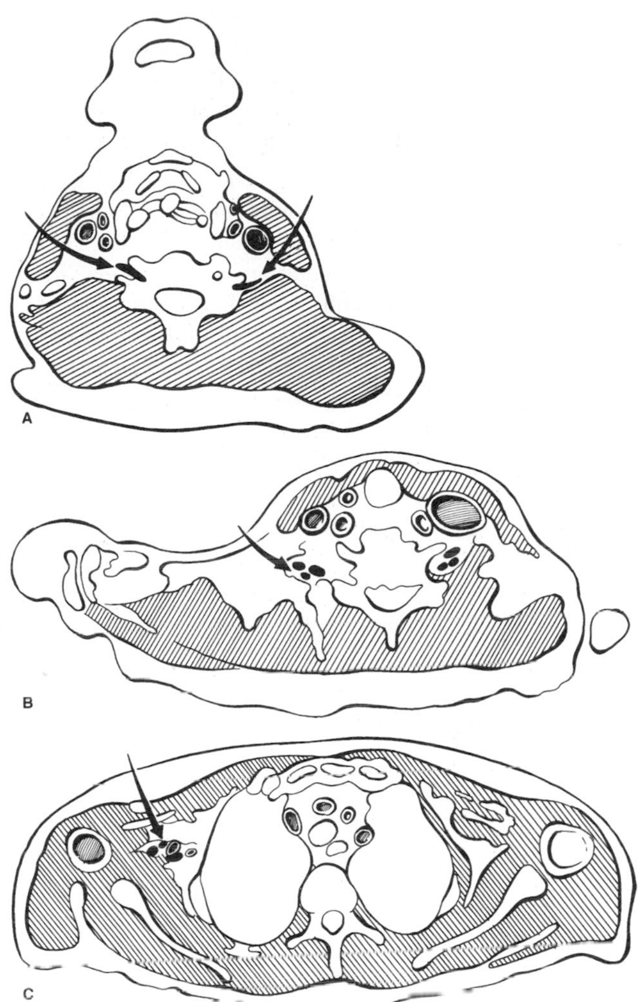

FIG. 1. Diagrams of tomographic anatomy of the normal brachial plexus. **A:** Upper cervical level. Cervical roots exit via neural foramina and proceed anterolaterally, behind major blood vessels, to form the plexus. **B:** Lower cervical level. Brachial plexus components lie between anterior and medial scalene muscles. **C:** Axillary fossa. Brachial plexus accompanies axillary arteries and veins. Neurovascular bundle, surrounded by fat tissue, lies in a triangle outlined by chest wall medially, pectoralis minor anteriorly, and subscapularis muscle posteriorly. (Adapted from ref. 43.)

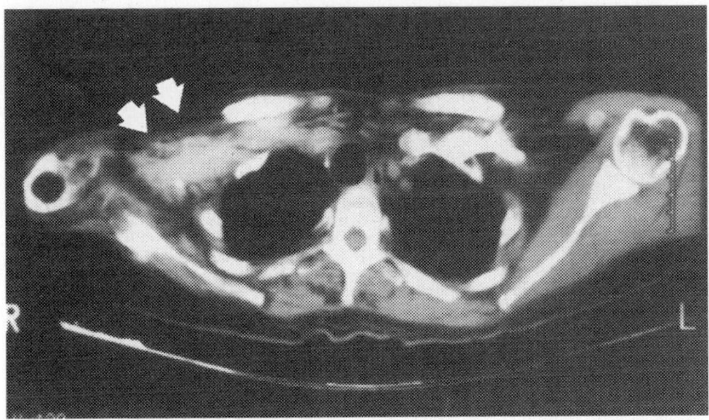

FIG. 2. Contrast-enhanced computed tomographic scan of the brachial plexus in a 57-year-old woman who had a history of breast cancer and presented with right arm and hand pain. A mass is apparent in the right brachial plexus (*arrows*). (From Cherny NI, Portenoy RK. Cancer pain: principles of assessment and syndromes. In: Wall PD, Melzack R, eds. *Textbook of Pain*, 3rd ed. Edinburgh, UK: Churchill Livingstone, 1994:787.)

In a study by Cascino et al. of patients with known tumor involving the brachial plexus, the CT scan was abnormal in 89% of patients; all but one had a circumscribed mass in the region of the brachial plexus.[19] Paravertebral extension and tumor erosion of bone were frequently demonstrated, although plain radiographs and bone scans showed normal results. In fact, plain radiographs of the spine revealed abnormalities in only 4 of 39 patients, whereas CT scanning detected spine abnormalities in 13 of 41 patients. Similarly, bone scans were not helpful and were falsely negative, especially in patients who had received prior radiation therapy. In this study,[19] CT scans were reviewed for four abnormalities: soft-tissue density changes in the region of the brachial plexus, paravertebral extension of soft-tissue masses, bony erosion, and epidural extension. Forty-one of 46 patients with metastatic plexopathy had abnormalities in the region of the symptomatic brachial plexus. Five patients had a completely normal CT scan despite proven metastatic plexopathy. In four of these patients, all other diagnostic studies (bone scans, myelograms, and cervical spine radiographs) were negative as well. One patient had an epidural tumor at C-7, detected on myelography, which was found during surgery to extend out and invade the plexus. Two patients had negative surgical explorations of the brachial plexus through an anterior approach. Postoperative CT scans demonstrated a mass deep in the brachial plexus that was confirmed to be tumor on reexploration.

The typical appearance of radiation fibrosis of the plexus on CT studies is of a diffuse infiltration and loss of tissue planes without a mass lesion.[19] Associated lymphedema in the arm is often present that is evident on CT, and occasionally radiation necrosis of the clavicle or rib or humeral head occurs at the adjacent level.[14] Tumor infiltration of the plexus cannot be differentiated from radiation fibrosis by CT studies when diffuse infiltration is noted. In such cases, CT-guided biopsy of the brachial plexus mass may be helpful.[44]

Magnetic Resonance Imaging

Although data comparing the sensitivity and specificity of MRI and CT in evaluating lesions of the brachial plexus are not available, MRI is a clinically useful test that may replace CT and myelography.[45] MRI is a noninvasive procedure that can assess the integrity of the vertebral bodies and may differentiate tumor from radiation fibrosis and fully visualize the adjacent epidural space.[46,47] Clinical experience suggests that full evaluation for brachial plexopathy requires the use

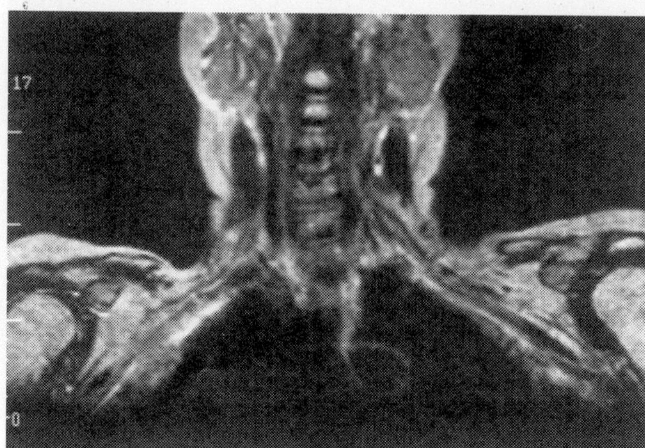

FIG. 3. Magnetic resonance image demonstrating a mass in the axilla involving the brachial plexus and invading the chest wall.

of a modified sagittal view (with 15 degrees of angulation) to assess the contents of the cervical foramina and the cervical and upper thoracic spinal cord, axial views to define a paraspinal mass, and coronal views to evaluate the peripheral components of the brachial plexus.[45]

T1-weighted images best define the relationship of tumor to the surrounding structures (Fig. 3).[48] Tumor and radiation fibrosis generate intense images. Contrary to initial reports, increased T2 signal in or near the plexus is commonly seen in radiation plexopathy and tumor infiltration and is not useful in making this distinction.[39,49] Some data suggest that dynamic gadolinium-enhanced T1-weighted imaging can help to differentiate tumor from radiation fibrosis: Recurrent tumors demonstrate early increased signal intensity of the lesion within 3 minutes after bolus injection, whereas fibrosis generates no substantial enhancement on postcontrast T1-weighted images.[50]

Because patients with brachial plexus lesions are at high risk for developing epidural cord compression from direct tumor infiltration along the plexus into the epidural space or from hematogenous spread of tumor to the vertebral body,[3,46,51] imaging should include the adjacent epidural space. Imaging of the epidural space is essential if spinal cord compression is suspected and if patients have any of the clinical findings that are commonly associated with this complication, including panplexopathy, Horner's syndrome, vertebral body erosion or collapse at the C-7 to T-1 levels, or a paraspinal mass detected on CT scanning. Accurate imaging with MRI determines the extent of epidural encroachment (which influences prognosis and may alter the therapeutic approach) and defines the appropriate radiation portals.[52]

Ultrasonography

Ultrasonographic examination of the axilla is a useful technique for the identification of metastatic axillary nodes.[53,54] Although brachial plexus anatomy is identifiable by ultrasonography,[55] the role of this technique in the evaluation of malignant brachial plexopathy has not been defined. In the evaluation of the axilla for nodal disease, ultrasonography has been observed to be more sensitive than mammography[56] and digital subtraction angiography[57] but less sensitive than CT scanning.[57] Hypoechoic masses frequently indicate tumor. Hyperechoic lesions are much less specific and may be either malignant or benign.[57] Color Doppler ultrasonography can detect alterations in blood flow around axillary nodes infiltrated with tumor. In a prospective study involving 75 patients who subsequently underwent axillary dissection,[54] this technique demonstrated a sensitivity of 70%, specificity of 98%, and positive predictive value of 96%. These impressive results are substantially better than those observed using other imaging modalities and suggest a potential use of this technique in the assessment of patients with brachial plexopathy that is worthy of further evaluation.

Positron Emission Tomography

Positron emission tomography (PET) scanning, although not widely available, may be a useful technique for the evaluation of axillary nodes.

Several prospective studies of patients who subsequently underwent axillary dissection have demonstrated a very high degree of sensitivity (90% to 95%) and negative predictive value (90% to 97%).[54,58–60] Experience is inadequate to draw conclusions regarding the specificity of this approach. In two studies, the specificity was only approximately 70%, and false-positive findings were commonplace.[54,60]

Electrophysiologic Studies

Electrophysiologic studies may be useful in distinguishing tumor infiltration from radiation fibrosis. Electrodiagnostic studies in patients with radiation fibrosis have been demonstrated to show signs of fibrillation and positive waves associated with denervation. Widespread myokymia is strongly suggestive of radiation-induced plexopathy.[20,61–64] Roth et al.[64] assessed electrodiagnostically a patient with radiation fibrosis after radiation therapy for breast cancer who had clinical myokymia, cramps, and pain. They related the myokymia to the existence of a persistent conduction block of several years' duration. Streib et al.[65] also reported conduction blocks in two patients treated for breast cancer. Plexus exploration in one of the patients did not reveal constrictive connective tissue or other sources of nerve entrapment. The exact cause of conduction block is not fully understood. A study comparing H-reflexes of the flexor carpi radialis muscle among 52 controls and 25 patients with radiation-induced brachial plexopathy found decreased conduction velocity in 13 of the affected patients.[66]

In malignant plexopathy, electromyography typically reveals fibrillation potentials and positive waves characteristic of denervation in the distribution of the brachial plexus that is consistent with plexus signs and symptoms.[19,20,61,67] A

TABLE 1. *Causes of brachial plexopathy in patients with breast cancer and distinguishing clinical features*

Feature	Tumor infiltration	Radiation fibrosis	Transient radiation injury	Acute ischemic injury
Incidence of pain	80%	18%	40%	Painless
Location of pain	Shoulder, upper arm, elbow, 4th and 5th fingers	Shoulder, wrist, hand	Hand, forearm	Hand, forearm
Nature of pain	Dull ache in shoulder, lancinating pains in elbow and ulnar aspect of hand; occasional paresthesias and dysesthesias	Ache in shoulder; prominent paresthesias in C-5/C-6 distribution of hand and arm	Ache in shoulder; prominent paresthesias in C-5/C-6 distribution of hand and arm	Paresthesias in C-5/C-6 distribution of hand and arm
Severity	Moderate to severe (severe in 98%)	Usually mild to moderate (severe in 20%–35%)	Mild	Mild
Course	Progressive neurologic dysfunction: atrophy and weakness in C-7/T-1 distribution, persistent pain; occasional Horner's syndrome	Progressive weakness; panplexus or upper plexus distribution; Horner's syndrome uncommon	Transient weakness with complete resolution	Acute nonprogressive weakness and sensory loss
Study findings				
Magnetic resonance imaging	High–signal-intensity mass on T2-weighted images; may enhance with gadolinium	Low–signal-intensity lesion on T2-weighted images; generally nonenhancing with gadolinium	No data	Normal
Computed tomography	Mass: circumscribed or diffuse tissue infiltration	Diffuse tissue infiltration	Normal	Angiography demonstrates subclavian artery segmental obstruction
Electromyography	Segmental slowing	Diffuse myokymia	Segmental slowing	Segmental slowing

normal electromyograph in the cervical paraspinal muscles is usually adequate to exclude the presence of root disease. In the rare instances that myokymia is observed in patients with tumor infiltration of the brachial plexus, it is localized and may be isolated to one muscle group alone[61]; widespread myokymic discharges are strongly suggestive of radiation-induced plexopathy.[20,61–63]

Median somatosensory evoked potentials may be helpful in differentiating between radiculopathy and brachial plexus injury. In a series of studies of 49 patients with suspected unilateral brachial plexus problems, median somatosensory evoked potentials were always normal in injuries of upper trunk and root avulsions confined to one or two root levels and were abnormal in generalized plexopathies, multiple trunk lesions, and multiple root avulsions.[68] This test may be useful in patients with pain but without evidence of neurologic abnormalities who are at risk for tumor infiltration of the brachial plexus. Indeed, exploration of the plexus should be considered for select patients who have suggestive clinical findings and abnormal median somatosensory evoked potentials.

Surgical Exploration

The differential diagnosis of tumor infiltration from radiation injury to the plexus may be made in the majority of cases using the clinical criteria, imaging, and electrophysiologic studies (Table 1). If these diagnostic approaches fail to define the nature of the neurologic disorder, however, exploration of the plexus should be considered. Such exploration should be undertaken only under the following circumstances:

1. The CT scan and MRI are normal or show no evidence of change from before the onset of symptoms.
2. The site of neurologic involvement is certain (for example, a lesion that can be localized to either the upper or lower plexus). This factor is important in determining the appropriate surgical approach. Upper plexus dysfunction may best be assessed through a supraclavicular approach, whereas involvement of the lower plexus is best assessed through a posterior scapular approach or a high posterior thoracotomy, commonly used to explore apical tumors of the lung.[69]
3. A work-up including tumor marker assays to establish the full extent of disease has been completed and shows no evidence of diffuse metastatic disease.
4. The onset of symptoms and signs occurs several years after completion of successful antitumor therapy, or treatment for the presumed primary tumor does not appear to be effective.

In a study to assess the role of brachial plexus exploration in defining the cause of the patient's pain and neurologic deficit, Payne and Foley[29] reported on a patient with breast cancer who had been previously irradiated to the brachial plexus for extraneural disease and who developed pain and weakness in her left upper extremity. Radiographic studies demonstrated evidence of radiation fibrosis in the apex of the lung, but all other studies demonstrated no evidence of breast tumor recurrence. Biopsy of the area of radiation fibrosis revealed adenocarcinoma of the lung as the cause of the patient's progressive plexopathy.[29]

In a second patient with pain and progressive plexopathy and negative radiologic studies, exploration of the plexus revealed no evidence of tumor. Approximately 3 months later, the patient developed evidence of a chest wall recurrence and ultimately died of widely metastatic breast cancer. At autopsy, diffuse infiltration of the brachial plexus was found to be the cause of the patient's symptoms and signs.

In the study of Kori et al.,[3] no adverse effects of surgical exploration of the plexus were noted, but the procedure requires an expert surgeon who can carefully distinguish fibrous tissue from nerve tissue using intraoperative neurophysiologic techniques.

TREATMENT OF BRACHIAL PLEXOPATHY

The care of patients with brachial plexopathy requires an integrated approach involving primary therapy appropriate to the specific diagnosis along with symptomatic treatment of pain.

Primary Therapies

Treatment of Radiation Fibrosis

The management of patients with radiation fibrosis begins with the establishment of an accurate diagnosis to rule out metastatic disease. No proven methods of reversing neurologic damage exist. Splinting the arm at the chest wall, preventing subluxation of the shoulder joint, and using intensive physical therapy to manage lymphedema[70,71] are common approaches to managing the musculoskeletal pain syndromes associated with this disorder.

Some authors have suggested the use of neurolysis with pedicle omentoplasty to treat radiation fibrosis.[72–75] Cumulative anecdotal data suggest that this procedure frequently results in reduction of pain and that progression of neurologic deficit can be arrested in some cases.[18,72–75] In the largest series, LeQuang reported on 60 patients followed from 2 to 9 years and advocated early surgery as soon as possible after the onset of paresthesias.[72] Surgical exploration of the brachial plexus is difficult, and further injury to the nerve may be associated with a worsening pain syndrome after surgically induced nerve injury.[76] Further studies are necessary to assess the usefulness of this technique to preserve neurologic function and to treat pain.

Treatment of Tumor Infiltration

The treatment of tumor infiltration of the brachial plexus depends on the status of the patient's disease, the extent of neurologic involvement, and any prior history of radiation therapy to the brachial plexus. In patients with tumor infiltration of the brachial plexus with evidence of metastatic disease in other sites, systemic chemotherapy is a reasonable approach. In those who have undergone previous radiation therapy to the region, systemic therapies involving either cytotoxic or hormonal therapies may offer the only reasonable antitumor treatment. In a patient who has not received radiation therapy previously, however, if the neurologic signs are rapidly progressive or if evidence of epidural spinal cord compression is seen, radiation therapy is the procedure of choice. As stated in Diagnostic Investigations, MRI or myelography should be used to define the exact radiation ports in these cases.

The dose of radiation therapy used varies. In the reported series, a dose of 3,000 cGy delivered over a 3-week period and a dose of 5,000 cGy delivered over a period of 5 weeks represent the most commonly used dose levels.[3,10,67,77] Clinical evidence suggests that the use of steroids provides pain relief in patients with tumor infiltration of the brachial plexus, and these drugs are often used to provide analgesia during therapy.[78] If the diagnosis of brachial plexus tumor infiltration is made early and effective therapy is instituted, the patient's neurologic symptoms should resolve, and a marked reduction in pain should be noted.

Data are conflicting on the likelihood of benefit from palliative radiotherapy for malignant brachial plexopathy in breast cancer. In a review of the published, as well as his own, experience to date, Ampil reported that the total delivered dose, rather than the width of the therapy port, was the most important factor in achieving optimal symptomatic palliation.[77] In his series of 23 patients, significant pain relief was achieved in 77.2% of patients for a median of 3 months; the observed objective response rate was 46%. In the series by Nisce and Chu, 12 of 47 patients (25.5%) with metastatic brachial plexopathy and breast cancer had complete pain relief for a mean duration of 15 months, and 23 (49%) had partial pain relief for a mean duration of 6 months.[79] These researchers suggested that higher doses of irradiation (5,000 cGy) were more effective than lower doses. In the retrospective review of Kori et al., results of the treatment of metastatic plexopathy were disappointing.[3] Radiation therapy in doses of 2,000 to 5,000 cGy delivered to the plexus relieved pain in only 46% of cases.[3] Neurologic improvement was minimal, and persistent, chronic pain was the most significant problem. In Fulton's experience with 44 breast cancer patients with definite (n = 31) or probable (n = 13) brachial plexopathy, 9 of the 17 patients treated with radiation therapy improved.[5] Among patients for whom radiation therapy was no longer a therapeutic option because of prior radiation therapy, the yield from systemic therapies was low: Two of seven patients responded to hormonal therapy, and only one of six patients responded to chemotherapy.

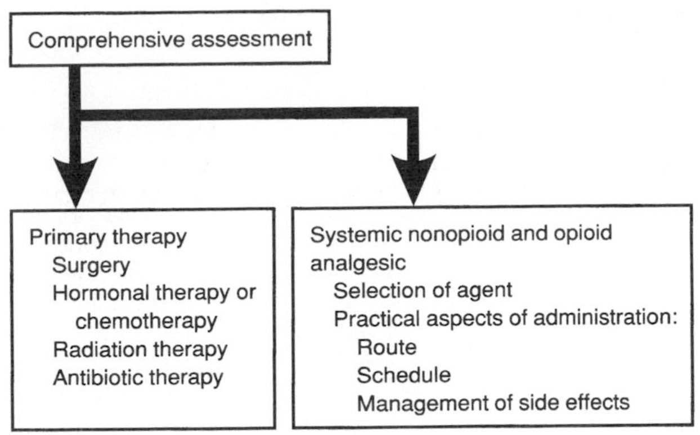

If balance between pain relief and side effects is suboptimal, consider

Noninvasive strategies to improve balance between analgesia and side effects

Reduce opioid requirements
- Appropriate primary therapy
- Addition of nonopioid analgesic
- Addition of an adjuvant analgesic
- Use of cognitive or behavioral techniques
- Use of an orthotic device or other physical medicine approach

Switch to another opioid

If balance between pain relief and side effects is suboptimal, consider

Invasive strategies to improve balance between analgesia and side effects

Regional analgesic techniques (spinal opioids)
Neural blockade
Neuroablative techniques

If balance between pain relief and side effects is suboptimal, consider

Role of sedating pharmacotherapy

FIG. 4. Approach to the management of pain associated with brachial plexopathy.

No reports have been published on the specific effects of chemotherapy or hormonal therapy on malignant brachial plexopathy. Anecdotally, clinical experience indicates that patients with malignant infiltration of the plexus who respond to systemic therapy generally have substantial relief of plexopathy-related pain. Because most responses are partial and subsequently followed by relapse, pain often returns when disease recurs. Indeed, worsening pain is often the earliest indicator of recurrence or progression.

Management of Pain

Analgesic Pharmacotherapy

An approach to the management of brachial plexus pain is illustrated in Fig. 4. Primary antitumor therapies should be considered for patients with tumor invasion of the brachial plexus. All patients with pain should initially be treated with analgesic pharmacotherapy in accordance with the "Three-Step Analgesic Ladder" of the World Health Organization.[80,81]

Opioids in the Management of Brachial Plexus Pain

A trial of opioid therapy should be given to all patients with pain of moderate or greater severity, irrespective of the pathophysiologic mechanism underlying the pain.[82–86] Patients who present with severe pain are usually treated with an opioid customarily used in step 3 of the analgesic ladder. Patients with moderate pain have been conventionally treated with a combination product containing acetaminophen or aspirin plus codeine, dihydrocodeine tartrate, hydrocodone bitartrate, oxycodone hydrochloride, and propoxyphene hydrochloride. The doses of these combination products can be increased until the maximum dose of the nonopioid coanalgesic is attained (e.g., 4,000 mg acetaminophen); beyond this dose, the opioid contained in the combination product can be increased as a single agent, or the patient can be switched to an opioid conventionally used for strong pain. Recent years have witnessed the proliferation of new opioid formulations that may improve the convenience of drug administration for patients with moderate pain. These include controlled-release formulations of codeine, dihydrocodeine tartrate, oxycodone hydrochloride, morphine sulfate, and tramadol hydrochloride in dosages appropriate for moderate pain.

Opioids should be administered by the least invasive and most convenient route able to provide adequate analgesia for the patient. In routine practice, the oral route is usually the most appropriate. Parenteral routes of administration should be considered for patients who have impaired swallowing or gastrointestinal obstruction, those who require the rapid onset of analgesia, and highly tolerant patients who require doses that cannot otherwise be conveniently administered.

Patients with continuous or frequently recurring pain generally benefit from scheduled around-the-clock dosing. All patients who receive an around-the-clock opioid regimen should also be offered a "rescue dose," a supplemental dose given as needed to treat pain that breaks through the regular schedule. The rescue drug is typically identical to that administered on a continuous basis, except in the case of transdermal fentanyl and methadone hydrochloride; the use of an alternative short-half-life opioid is recommended for the rescue dose when these drugs are used. Patient-controlled analgesia is a technique of parenteral drug administration in

TABLE 2. *Opioids conventionally used in the management of severe pain (step 3 of the analgesic ladder)*

Drug	Dose (mg) equianalgesic to 10 mg i.m. morphine		Half-life (hr)	Duration of action (hr)	Comments
	i.m.	p.o.			
Morphine sulfate	10	30 (repeated dose) 60 (single dose)	2–3	3–4	M6G accumulation in renal failure may predispose to additional toxicity; wide range of formulations; on WHO essential drug list
Oxycodone hydrochloride	15	30	2–3	2–4	Formulated as single agent; can be used for severe pain
Hydromorphone hydrochloride	1.5	7.5	2–3	2–4	Wide range of formulations; useful in the elderly
Methadone hydrochloride	10	20	15–190	4–8	Plasma accumulation may lead to delayed toxicity; dosing should be initiated on a PRN basis
Meperidine hydrochloride	75	300	2–3	2–4	*Not recommended for cancer pain*; normeperidine toxicity limits use; contraindicated in patients with renal failure and those receiving MAO inhibitors
Oxymorphone hydrochloride	1	10 (p.r.)	2–3	3–4	No oral formulation available; less histamine release than other opioids
Levorphanol tartrate	2	4	12–15	4–8	Plasma accumulation may lead to delayed toxicity
Fentanyl transdermal system	[a]	—	—	48–72	Patches available to deliver 25, 50, 75, and 100 µg/hr

MAO, monoamine oxidase; PRN, as needed; WHO, World Health Organization.
[a]Transdermal fentanyl, 100 µg/hr.
Adapted from Cherny NI, Portenoy RK. Cancer pain management: current strategy. *Cancer* 1993;72[Suppl]:3393.

which the patient controls a pump that delivers bolus doses of an analgesic according to parameters set by the physician.

Patients in severe pain who are opioid naive should generally begin with one of the opioids conventionally used for severe pain at a dose equivalent to 5 to 10 mg of intramuscular morphine sulfate every 3 to 4 hours. If a switch from one opioid drug to another is required, an equianalgesic dose table (Table 2) is used as a guide to the starting dose. The persistence of inadequate pain relief should be addressed through a stepwise escalation of the opioid dose until adequate analgesia is reported or unmanageable side effects supervene. The severity of the pain should determine the rate of dose titration. An understanding of the strategies used to prevent or manage common opioid toxicities is needed to optimize the balance between analgesia and side effects.

Adjuvant Analgesics

Even with optimal management of adverse effects, some patients do not attain an acceptable balance between pain relief and side effects. Several types of noninvasive interventions, including adjuvant analgesics, a switch to another opioid, and the use of psychological, physiatric, or noninvasive neurostimulatory techniques, should be considered for their potential to improve this balance by reducing the opioid requirement. Adjuvant analgesics are drugs that have a primary indication other than pain but have analgesic effects in some painful conditions. The use of adjuvant analgesics can contribute substantially to the successful management of pain caused by brachial plexopathy. Numerous drugs are used empirically for this indication, including selected antidepressants, oral local anesthetics, anticonvulsants, and others. For the purpose of drug selection, distinguishing between continuous and lancinating (shooting) neuropathic pain based on the patient's history is useful (Table 3).

Corticosteroids

Corticosteroids are frequently used in the management of neuropathic pain due to infiltration or compression of neural structures by tumor.[87] Patients with advanced cancer who experience pain and other symptoms that may respond to steroids are usually given relatively small doses (e.g., dexamethasone, 1 to 2 mg, twice daily). A very short course of relatively high doses (e.g., dexamethasone, 100 mg intravenously, followed initially by 96 mg per day in divided doses) can be used to manage a severe exacerbation of pain associated with malignant brachial plexopathy. The dosage should be gradually lowered after pain reduction to the minimum needed to sustain relief.

TABLE 3. *Guide to the selection of adjuvant analgesics for neuropathic pain based on clinical characteristics*

- Continuous pain
  - Antidepressants
    - Amitriptyline hydrochloride
    - Doxepin hydrochloride
    - Imipramine hydrochloride
    - Desipramine hydrochloride
    - Nortriptyline hydrochloride
    - Trazodone hydrochloride
    - Maprotiline hydrochloride
    - Paroxetine hydrochloride
  - Oral local anesthetics
    - Mexiletine hydrochloride
  - Clonidine
- Lancinating pain
  - Anticonvulsant drugs
    - Carbamazepine
    - Phenytoin
    - Clonazepam
    - Valproate sodium
    - Baclofen

Adapted from Cherny NI, Portenoy RK. Cancer pain management: current strategy. *Cancer* 1993;72[Suppl]:3393.

Antidepressants

The tricyclic antidepressants are typically used to manage continuous dysesthesias that have not responded adequately to an opioid and lancinating neuropathic pains that are refractory to other specific adjuvant drugs.[88] These compounds are also useful in patients with pain complicated by depression and insomnia. Although the evidence for analgesic efficacy is greatest for the tertiary amine tricyclic drugs, such as amitriptyline hydrochloride, doxepin hydrochloride, and imipramine hydrochloride,[88] the secondary amine drugs, such as desipramine hydrochloride and nortriptyline hydrochloride, may be preferred when concern about sedation, anticholinergic effects, or cardiovascular toxicity is high. The selective serotonin uptake inhibitor antidepressants are less effective in the management of neuropathic pain.[88] The starting dose of a tricyclic antidepressant should be low (e.g., amitriptyline hydrochloride, 10 mg in the elderly and 25 mg in younger patients). Doses can be increased every few days by increments the same size as the starting dose. The usual effective dosage for the most widely used of these drugs, amitriptyline hydrochloride, is 50 to 150 mg per day. Continuing upward dose titration beyond this range is reasonable, however, when patients do not achieve benefit and have no limiting side effects. Plasma drug concentration, if available, may provide useful information and should be followed during the course of therapy. Very low levels in nonresponders suggest either poor compliance or an unusually rapid metabolism. In the latter case, dosages can be increased while the plasma drug level is repeatedly monitored. Likewise, nonresponders whose plasma concentration is not very low but is lower than the antidepressant range should be considered for a trial of higher dosages if side effects are not a problem.

Anticonvulsants

Anticonvulsant drugs appear to be analgesic for diverse types of lancinating neuropathic pain.[89,90] Although carbamazepine is often preferred because of the high response rate observed in cases of trigeminal neuralgia,[89] caution is required in using this drug for cancer patients with thrombocytopenia, those at risk for marrow failure (e.g., after chemotherapy), and those whose blood counts must be monitored to determine disease status. If carbamazepine is used, a complete blood count should be obtained before the start of therapy, after 2 and 4 weeks, and then every 3 to 4 months thereafter. A leukocyte count below 4,000 is usually considered to be a contraindication to treatment, and a decline to less than 3,000 or an absolute neutrophil count of less than 1,500 during therapy should prompt discontinuation of the drug. Published reports and clinical experience also support trials with other anticonvulsant drugs, including gabapentin, phenytoin, clonazepam, and valproate. Dosing guidelines for the use of these drugs as adjuvant analgesics are customarily identical to those used in the treatment of seizures. Low initial dosages are appropriate for carbamazepine, valproate sodium, and clonazepam. The administration of phenytoin often begins with the presumed therapeutic dose (e.g., 300 mg per day) or a prudent oral loading regimen (e.g., 500 mg twice, separated by hours). When low initial dosages are used, dose escalation should ensue until a favorable effect occurs, intolerable side effects supervene, or the plasma drug concentration has reached a predetermined level, which is customarily at the upper end of the therapeutic range for seizure management.

Baclofen

Baclofen, a γ-aminobutyric acid agonist effective for trigeminal neuralgia,[91] is often used in the management of lancinating pain due to neural injury of any type. A starting dosage of 10 mg three times per day is gradually escalated until analgesia is achieved or adverse effects of sedation or confusion emerge.

Oral Local Anesthetics

Local anesthetic drugs may be useful in the management of neuropathic pains characterized by either continuous or lancinating dysesthesias. Controlled trials have demonstrated the efficacy of tocainide hydrochloride[92] and mexiletine hydrochloride,[93] and clinical evidence suggests similar effects from flecainide acetate[93] and subcutaneous lidocaine.[94] Experience with the use of oral local anesthetics in the cancer population is still limited,[93] and recommendations are largely empiric. It is reasonable to undertake a trial with an oral local anesthetic in patients with continuous dysesthesias who fail to respond adequately or who cannot tolerate the tricyclic antidepressants and in patients with lancinating pains refractory to trials of anticonvulsant drugs and baclofen. Mexiletine hydrochloride is the safest of the oral local anesthetics[95,96] and is preferred. Dosing with mexiletine hydrochloride should usually start at 100 to 150 mg per day. If intolerable side effects do not occur, the dose can be increased by a like amount every few days, until the usual maximum dose of 300 mg three times per day is reached. Monitoring the electrocardiogram before therapy and periodically during treatment in high-risk groups (e.g., the elderly, those with heart disease, those receiving drugs with known cardiac effects, and those who require relatively large dosages) is recommended.

Other Agents

Experience with other drugs in the treatment of cancer-related neuropathic pain is very limited. Clonidine, an α_2-adrenergic agonist available in oral or transdermal formulations, has antinociceptive effects in the management of diverse pains but, like the tricyclic antidepressants, is conventionally used for continuous neuropathic pain in the cancer population.[97] Calcitonin (200 IU per day) has been shown to be an active analgesic in the management of some neuropathic pains, and pimozide, a phenothiazine neuroleptic, has activity against lancinating neuropathic pain. The latter drug is not preferred because of the high incidence of adverse effects, including physical and mental slowing, tremor, and parkinsonian symptoms.

Lymphedema Management

Physiatric techniques can be used to enhance analgesia and optimize the function of the patient with chronic cancer pain. The treatment of lymphedema by use of wraps, pressure stockings, or pneumatic pump devices may improve function and relieve pain and heaviness.[70,98]

Some investigators suggested that benzopyrene drugs, which stimulate proteolysis, can remove excess protein and its consequent edema.[99] Initially encouraging reports of efficacy[99] were not replicable in a placebo-controlled trial involving 140 women.[100] This approach is not recommended.[101]

Anesthetic and Neurosurgical Techniques

Invasive anesthetic and neurosurgical techniques should be considered only for patients who are unable to achieve a satisfactory balance between analgesia and side effects using systemic analgesic therapies. Techniques such as intraspinal opioid and local anesthetic administration, locoregional infusion of local anesthetic,[102] intrapleural administration of local anesthetic,[103,104] or intraventricular opioid administration[105] can potentially achieve this end without compromising neurologic integrity. The use of neurodestructive procedures, such as brachial plexus blockade,[106,107] chemical or surgical rhizotomy,[108] or a dorsal root entry zone lesion,[109] should be based on an evaluation of the likelihood and duration of analgesic benefit, the immediate and long-term risks, the likely duration of survival, and the anticipated length of hospitalization. Rarely, patients have been treated with a forequarter amputation of the limb for relief of the discomfort of a lymphedematous, functionless arm. However, this approach is not successful in providing significant pain relief, although it does improve patient complaints of a heavy, lymphedematous, useless extremity.[110–112]

MANAGEMENT SUMMARY

- Early diagnosis of tumor infiltration of the brachial plexus is important to prevent the development of chronic neuropathic pain and neurologic dysfunction.
- Evaluation consists of a careful history, a detailed neurologic examination, and MRI or CT imaging. Electrodiagnostic studies should be performed if the radiographic studies are negative for both soft-tissue and bony disease. An evaluation for evidence of metastatic disease should follow and, if findings are negative, surgical exploration should be considered to allow biopsy of adjacent lymph nodes and soft tissue.
- For patients presenting with brachial plexopathy after previous radiation therapy, the history and physical findings and follow-up using CT and MRI may be helpful in distinguishing tumor recurrence from radiation fibrosis, but none of these may be definitive. Surgical exploration should be considered if the diagnosis will affect the treatment decision—for example, in a patient with progressive symptoms of brachial plexopathy but without other evidence of distant metastases for whom documentation of recurrent disease will result in a decision to initiate anticancer treatment.

REFERENCES

1. Clouston PD, DeAngelis LM, Posner JB. The spectrum of neurological disease in patients with systemic cancer. *Ann Neurol* 1992;31:268.
2. Gonzales GR, Elliott KJ, Portenoy RK, Foley KM. The impact of a comprehensive evaluation in the management of cancer pain. *Pain* 1991;47:141.
3. Kori SH, Foley KM, Posner JB. Brachial plexus lesion in patients with cancer: 100 cases. *Neurology* 1981;13:45.
4. Vecht CJ. Arm pain in the patient with breast cancer. *J Pain Symptom Manage* 1990;15:109.
5. Fulton DS. Brachial plexopathy in patients with breast cancer. *Dev Oncol* 1987;51:249.
6. Bagley FH, Walsh JW, Cady B, Salzman FA, Oberfield RA, Pazianos AG. Carcinomatous versus radiation-induced brachial plexus neuropathy in breast cancer. *Cancer* 1978;41:2154.
7. Tsairis P, Dyck PJ, Mulder DW. Natural history of brachial plexus neuropathy. Report on 99 patients. *Arch Neurol* 1972;27:109.
8. Maruyama Y, Mylrea MM, Logothetis J. Neuropathy following irradiation. An unusual late complication of radiotherapy. *AJR Am J Roentgenol Radium Ther Nucl Med* 1967;1101:216.

9. Cavanagh JB. Effects of x-irradiation on the proliferation of cells in peripheral nerve during Wallerian degeneration in the rat. *Br J Radiol* 1968;141:275.
10. Sainer AL, Botnick LE, Herzog AG, et al. Reversible brachial plexopathy following primary radiation therapy for breast cancer. *Cancer Treat Rep* 1981;65:797.
11. Gerard JM, Franck N, Moussa Z, Hildebrand J. Acute ischemic brachial plexus neuropathy following radiation therapy. *Neurology* 1989;139:450.
12. Pierce SM, Recht A, Lingos TI, et al. Long-term radiology complications following conservative surgery (CS) and radiation therapy (RT) in patients with early stage breast cancer [see comments]. *Intl J Radiat Oncol Biol Phys* 1992;23:915.
13. Bates T, Evans RG. Audit of brachial plexus neuropathy following radiotherapy. *Clin Oncol (R Coll Radiol)* 1995:7:236.
14. Schulte RW, Adamietz IA, Renner K, Falkenreck I. Humeral head necrosis following irradiation of breast carcinoma. A case report. *Radiologe* 1989;29:252.
15. Thomas JE, Colby MY Jr. Radiation-induced or metastatic brachial plexopathy. A diagnostic dilemma. *JAMA* 1972;222:1392.
16. Basso-Ricci S, della Costa C, Viganotti G, Ventafridda V, Zanolla R. Report on 42 cases of postirradiation lesions of the brachial plexus and their treatment. *Tumori* 1980;66:117.
17. Olsen NK, Pfeiffer P, Johannsen L, Schroder H, Rose C. Radiation-induced brachial plexopathy: neurological follow-up in 161 recurrence-free breast cancer patients. *Intl Radiat Oncol Biol Phys* 1993;26:43.
18. Killer RE, Hess K. Natural history of radiation-induced brachial plexopathy compared with surgically treated patients. *J Neurol* 1990;237:247.
19. Cascino TL, Kori S, Krof G, Foley KM. CT of the brachial plexus in patients with cancer. *Neurology* 1983;133:1553.
20. Lederman RJ, Wilbourn AJ. Brachial plexopathy: recurrent cancer or radiation? *Neurology* 1984;34:1331.
21. McDermot RS. Cobalt 60 beam therapy: post-radiation effects in breast cancer patients. *J Can Assoc Radiol* 1971;122:195.
22. Uematsu M, Bornstein BA, Recht A, et al. Long-term results of post-operative radiation therapy following mastectomy with or without chemotherapy in stage I-III breast cancer. *Int J Radiat Oncol Biol Phys* 1993;25:765.
23. Powell S, Cooke J, Parsons C. Radiation-induced brachial plexus injury: follow-up of two different fractionation schedules. *Radiother Oncol* 1990;18:213.
24. Olsen NK, Pfeiffer P, Mondrup K, Rose C. Radiation-induced brachial plexus neuropathy in breast cancer patients. *Acta Oncol* 1990;129:885.
25. Svensson H, Westling P, Larsson LG. Radiation-induced lesions of the brachial plexus correlated to the dose-time-fraction schedule. *Acta Radiol Ther Phys Biol* 1975;14:228.
26. Cohen L, Svensson H. Cell population kinetics and dose time relationships for post-irradiation injury of the brachial plexus in man. *Acta Radiol Oncol Radiat Phys Biol* 1978;17:161.
27. Gillette EL, Mahler PA, Powers BE, Gillette SM, Vujaskovic Z. Late radiation injury to muscle and peripheral nerves. *Int J Radiat Oncol Biol Phys* 1995;131:1309.
28. Gorson KC, Musaphir S, Lathi ES, Wolfe G. Radiation-induced malignant fibrous histiocytoma of the brachial plexus. *J Neurooncol* 1995;126:73.
29. Payne R, Foley KM. Exploration of the brachial plexus in patients with cancer. *Neurology* 1986;36[Suppl 1]:329.
30. Zbaren P, Becker M. Schwannoma of the brachial plexus. *Ann Otol Rhinol Laryngol* 1996;105:748.
31. Sell PJ, Semple JC. Primary nerve tumours of the brachial plexus. *Br J Surg* 1987;74:73.
32. Sharma BS, Banerjee AK, Kak VK. Malignant schwannoma of brachial plexus presenting as spinal cord compression. *Neurochirurgia (Stuttg)* 1989;32:189.
33. Horowitz J, Kline DC, Keller SM. Schwannoma of the brachial plexus mimicking an apical lung tumor. *Ann Thorac Surg* 1991;52:555.
34. Brennan MJ. Breast cancer recurrence in a patient with a previous history of radiation injury of the brachial plexus: a case report. *Arch Phys Med Rehabil* 1995;76:974.
35. Ganel A, Engel J, Sela M, Brooks M. Nerve entrapments associated with postmastectomy lymphedema. *Cancer* 1979;44:2254.
36. Dawson DM. Entrapment neuropathics of the upper extremities [see comments]. *N Engl J Med* 1993;329:2013.
37. de Araujo MP. Electrodiagnosis in compression neuropathies of the upper extremities. *Orthop Clin North Am* 1996;27:237.
38. Taylor BV, Kimmel DW, Krecke KN, Cascino TL. Magnetic resonance imaging in cancer-related lumbosacral plexopathy. *Mayo Clin Proc* 1997:72:823.
39. Thyagarajan D, Cascino T, Harms G. Magnetic resonance imaging in brachial plexopathy of cancer. *Neurology* 1995:45:421.
40. Sherrier RH, Sostman HD. Magnetic resonance imaging of the brachial plexus. *J Thorac Imaging* 1993;8:27.
41. Cooke J, Powell S, Parsons C. The diagnosis by computed tomography of brachial plexus lesions following radiotherapy for carcinoma of the breast. *Clin Radiol* 1988;39:602.
42. Cooke J, Cooke D, Parsons C. The anatomy and pathology of the brachial plexus as demonstrated by computed tomography. *Clin Radiol* 1988;39:595.
43. Krol G. Evaluation of neoplastic involvement of brachial and lumbar plexus: imaging aspects. *J Back Musculoskel Rehab* 1993;13:25.
44. Cole JW, Quint DJ, McGillicuddy JE, Murphy KP. CT-guided brachial plexus biopsy. *AJNR Am J Neuroradiol* 1997;118:1420.
45. de Verdier HJ, Colletti PM, Terk MR. MRI of the brachial plexus: a review of 51 cases. *Comput Med Imaging Graph* 1993;117:45.
46. Hagen N, Stulman J, Krol G, et al. The role of myelography and magnetic resonance imaging in cancer patients with symptomatic and asymptomatic epidural disease. *Neurology* 1989;39:309.
47. Hagenau C, Grosh W, Currie M, Wiley RG. Comparison of spinal magnetic resonance imaging and myelography in cancer patients. *J Clin Oncol* 1987;5:1663.
48. Posniak HV, Olson MC, Dudiak CM, Wisniewski R, O'Malley C. MR imaging of the brachial plexus. *AJR Am J Roentgenol* 1993;161:373.
49. Wouter van Es H, Engelen AM, Witkamp TD, Ramos LM, Feldberg MA. Radiation-induced brachial plexopathy: MR imaging. *Skeletal Radiol* 1997;26:284.
50. Dao TH, Rahmouni A, Campana F, Laurent M, Asselain B, Fourquet A. Tumor recurrence versus fibrosis in the irradiated breast: differentiation with dynamic gadolinium-enhanced MR imaging. *Radiology* 1993;1187:751.
51. Kanner R, Martini N, Foley KM. Nature and incidence of postthoracotomy pain. *Proc Am Soc Clin Oncol* 1982;1:590.
52. Portenoy RK, Lipton RB, Foley KM. Back pain in the cancer patient: an algorithm for evaluation and management. *Neurology* 1987;37:134.
53. Yang WT, Ahuja A, Tang A, Suen M, King W, Metreweli C. High resolution monographic detection of axillary lymph node metastases in breast cancer [published erratum appears in *J Ultrasound Med* 1996;15:644]. *J Ultrasound Med* 1996;115:241.
54. Walsh JS, Dixon JM, Chetty U, Paterson D. Colour Doppler studies of axillary node metastases in breast carcinoma. *Clin Radiol* 1994;49:189.
55. Sheppard DG, Iyer RB, Fenstermacher MJ. Brachial plexus: demonstration at US. *Radiology* 1998,208:402.
56. Rissanen TJ, Makarainen HP, Mattila SI, Lindholm EL, Heikkinen MI, Kiviniemi HO. Breast cancer recurrence after mastectomy: diagnosis with mammography and US. *Radiology* 1993;188:463.
57. Tohnosu N, Okuyama K, Koide Y, et al. A comparison between ultrasonography and mammography: computed tomography and digital subtraction angiography for the detection of breast cancers. *Surg Today* 1993;23:704.
58. Smith IC, Ogston KN. Whitford P, et al. Staging of the axilla in breast cancer: accurate in vivo assessment using positron emission tomography with 2-(fluorine-18)-fluoro-2-deoxy-D-glucose. *Ann Surg* 1998;228:220.
59. Noh DY, Yun IJ, Kim JS, et al. Diagnostic value of positron emission tomography for detecting breast cancer. *World J Surg* 1998:22:223; discussion 7–8.
60. Adler LP, Faulhaber PF, Schnur KC, Al-Kasi NL, Shenk PR. Axillary lymph node metastases: screening with [F-18]2-deoxy-2-fluoro-d-glucose (FDG) PET. *Radiology* 1997;203:323.
61. Harper CM Jr, Thomas JE, Cascino TL, Litchy WJ. Distinction between neoplastic and radiation-induced brachial plexopathy, with emphasis on the role of EMG. *Neurology* 1989;139:502.
62. Albers JW, Allen AA, Bastron JA, Daube JR. Limb myokymia. *Muscle Nerve* 1981;4:494.
63. Flaggman PD, Kelly JJ Jr. Brachial plexus neuropathy. An electrophysiologic evaluation. *Arch Neurol* 1980;137:160.
64. Roth G, Magistris MR, Le Fort D, Desjacques P, Della Santa D. Post-radiation bronchial plexopathy. Persistent conduction block. Myokymic discharges and cramps. *Rev Neurol (Paris)* 1988;144:173.
65. Streib EW, Sun SF, Leibrock L. Brachial plexopathy in patients with breast cancer: unusual electromyographic findings in two patients. *Eur Neurol* 1982;21:256.

66. Ongerboer de Visser BW, Schimsheimer RJ, Hart AA. The H-reflex of the flexor carpi radialis muscle; a study in controls and radiation-induced brachial plexus lesions. *J Neurol Neurosurg Psychiatry* 1984;47:1098.
67. Son YH. Effectiveness of irradiation therapy in peripheral neuropathy caused by malignant disease. *Cancer* 1967;20:1447.
68. Synek VM. Validity of median nerve somatosensory evoked potentials in the diagnosis of supraclavicular brachial plexus lesions. *Electroencephalogr Clin Neurophysiol* 1986;165:27.
69. Dubuisson AS, Kline DG, Weinshcl SS. Posterior subscapular approach to the brachial plexus. Report of 102 patients. *J Neurosurg* 1993;79:319.
70. Brennan MJ. Lymphedema following the surgical treatment of breast cancer: a review of pathophysiology and treatment. *J Pain Symptom Manage* 1992;7:110.
71. Daane S, Poltoratszy P, Rockwell WB. Postmastectomy lymphedema management: evolution of the complex decongestive therapy technique. *Ann Plast Surg* 1998;40:128.
72. Le-Quang C. Post-radiotherapy lesions of the brachial plexus. Classification and results of surgical treatment. *Chirurgie* 1993;119:243.
73. Narakas AO. Operative treatment for radiation-induced and metastatic brachial plexopathy in 45 cases, 15 having an omentoplasty. *Bull Hosp Jt Dis Orthop Inst* 1984;44:354.
74. Terzis JK, Maragh H. Strategies in the microsurgical management of brachial plexus injuries. *Clin Plast Surg* 1989;16:605.
75. Brunelli G, Brunelli F. Surgical treatment of actinic brachial plexus lesions: free microvascular transfer of the greater omentum. *J Reconstr Microsurg* 1985;1:197.
76. Match RM. Radiation-induced brachial plexus paralysis. *Arch Surg* 1975;110:384.
77. Ampil FL. Radiotherapy for carcinomatous brachial plexopathy. A clinical study of 23 cases. *Cancer* 1985;56:2185.
78. Ettinger AB, Portenoy RK. The use of corticosteroids in the treatment of symptoms associated with cancer. *J Pain Symptom Manage* 1988;3:99.
79. Nisce LZ, Chu FC. Radiation therapy of brachial plexus syndrome from breast cancer. *Radiology* 1968;91:1022.
80. World Health Organization. *Cancer pain relief*, 2nd ed. Geneva: World Health Organization, 1996.
81. World Health Organization. *Cancer pain relief*. Geneva: World Health Organization, 1986.
82. Cherny NI, Thaler HT, Friedlander-Klar H, Lapin J, Portenoy RK. Opioid responsiveness of neuropathic cancer pain: combined analysis of single-dose analgesic trials (meeting abstract). *Proc Annu Meet Am Soc Clin Oncol* 1992.
83. McQuay HJ, Jadad AR, Carroll D, et al. Opioid sensitivity of chronic pain: a patient-controlled analgesia method. *Anaesthesia* 1992;47:757.
84. Jadad AR, Carroll D, Glynn CJ, Moore RA, McQuay HJ. Morphine responsiveness of chronic pain: double-blind randomised crossover study with patient-controlled analgesia [see comments]. *Lancet* 1992;339:1367.
85. Portenoy RK, Foley KM, Inturrisi CE. The nature of opioid responsiveness and its implications for neuropathic pain: new hypotheses derived from studies of opioid infusions [see comments]. *Pain* 1990;143:273.
86. Hanks GW, Forbes K. Opioid responsiveness. *Acta Anaesthesiol Scand* 1997;41:154.
87. Watanabe S, Bruera E. Corticosteroids as aduvant analgesics. *J Pain Symptom Manage* 1994;9:442.
88. McQuay HJ, Tramer M, Nye BA, Carroll D,Wiffen PJ, Moore RA. A systematic review of antidepressants in neuropathic pain. *Pain* 1996;68:217.
89. McQuay H, Carroll D, Jadad AR, Wiffen P, Moore A. Anticonvulsant drugs for management of pain: a systematic review. *BMJ* 1995;311:1047.
90. Swerdlow M. The use of anticonvulsants in the management of cancer pain. In: Erdmann W, Oyama T, Pernak MJ (eds): *The Pain Clinic I. Proceedings of the first international symposium*. Utrecht, The Netherlands: Vnu Science Press, 1985.
91. Fromm GH. Baclofen as an adjuvant analgesic. *J Pain Symptom Manage* 1994;9:500.
92. Lindstrom P, Lindblom U. The analgesic effect of tocainide in trigeminal neuralgia. *Pain* 1987;28:45.
93. Chong SF, Bretscher ME, Mailliard JA, et al. Pilot study evaluating local anesthetics administered systemically for treatment of pain in patients with advanced cancer. *J Pain Symptom Manage* 1997;13:112.
94. Brose WG, Cousins MJ. Subcutaneous lidocaine for treatment of neuropathic cancer pain. *Pain* 1991;45:145.
95. Rusidn JN. The cardiac arrhythmia suppression trial (CAST). *N Engl J Med* 1989;321:386.
96. (CAST) Cardiac Arrhythmia Suppression Trial Investigators. Preliminary report: effect of encainide and flecainide on mortality in a randomized trial of arrhythmia suppression after myocardial infarction. *N Engl J Med* 1989;321:406.
97. Owen MD, Fibuch EE, McQuillan R, Millington WR. Postoperative analgesia using a low-dose, oral-transdermal clonidine combination: lack of clinical efficacy. *J Clin Anesth* 1997;9:8.
98. Kirshbaum M. The development, implementation and evaluation of guidelines for the management of breast cancer related lymphoedema. *Eur J Cancer Care (Engl)* 1996;5:246.
99. Casley-Smith JR, Morgan RG, Piller NB. Treatment of lymphedema of the arms and legs with 5,6-benzo-[alpha]-pyrone. *N Engl J Med* 1993;329:1158.
100. Loprinzi CL, Kugler JW, Sloan JA, et al. Lack of effect of coumarin in women with lymphedema after treatment for breast cancer. *N Engl J Med* 1999;340:346.
101. Ganz PA. The quality of life after breast cancer—solving the problem of lymphedema [editorial]. *N Engl J Med* 1999;340:383.
102. Fischer HB, Peters TM, Fleming IM, Else TA. Peripheral nerve catheterization in the management of terminal cancer pain. *Reg Anesth* 1996;21:482.
103. Myers DP, Lema MJ, de Leon-Casasola OA, Bacon DR. Interpleural analgesia for the treatment of severe cancer pain in terminally ill patients. *J Pain Symptom Manage* 1993;8:505.
104. Dionne C. Tumour invasion of the brachial plexus: management of pain with intrapleural analgesia [letter]. *Can J Anaesth* 1992;39:520.
105. Cramond T, Stuart G. Intraventricular morphine for intractable pain of advanced cancer. *J Pain Symptom Manage* 1993;8:465.
106. Mullin V. Brachial plexus block with phenol for painful arm associated with Pancoast's syndrome. *Anesthesiology* 1980;53:431.
107. Cooper MG, Keneally JP, Kinchington D. Continuous brachial plexus neural blockade in a child with intractable cancer pain. *J Pain Symptom Manage* 1994;9:277.
108. Sindou M, Fobe YL. Rhizotomies and dorsal route entry zone lesions in the management of cancer related pain. In: Arbit E, ed. *Management of cancer-related pain*. Mount Kisko, Finland: Futura, 1993:341.
109. Zeidman SM, Rossitch EJ, Nashold BS Jr. Dorsal root entry zone lesions in the treatment of pain related to radiation-induced brachial plexopathy. *J Spinal Disord* 1993;6:44.
110. Fanous N, Didolkar MS, Holyoke ED, Elias EG. Evaluation of forequarter amputation in malignant diseases. *Surg Gynecol Obstet* 1976;142:381.
111. Merimsky O, Kollender Y, Inbar M, Chaitchik S, Meller I. Palliative major amputation and quality of life in cancer patients. *Acta Oncol* 1997;36:151.
112. Soucacos PN, Dailiana ZH, Beris AE, Xenakis TH, Malizos KN, Chrisovitsinos J. Major ablative procedures in orthopaedic surgery. *Bull Hosp Jt Dis* 1996:55:46.

Diseases of the Breast, 2nd ed.,
edited by Jay R. Harris.
Lippincott Williams & Wilkins, Philadelphia © 2000.

CHAPTER 56

Ocular Metastases

Beryl A. McCormick and David H. Abramson

The most common malignant lesion of the human eye is metastatic cancer. In most series of ocular metastases, the primary lesion with the highest incidence of spread to this site is breast carcinoma.[1–7] Through 1976, the question of whether metastatic disease or primary cancer represented the most common ocular malignancy was still a subject of debate.[8] As autopsy studies[2,9] and results of systematic ocular examinations[1] in cancer patients replaced series of case reports in the ophthalmic literature, however, the predominance of metastatic cancer eventually became evident.

INCIDENCE

In an autopsy study confined to examination of the globe in patients dying of cancer, Bloch and Garner[2] found that 37% of the 52 patients in their series with breast cancer had ocular metastases. In studies reviewing the incidence of breast cancer metastases to both the orbital soft tissues and the globe, a slight but consistent trend was found in favor of more frequent metastases to the choroid or middle layer of the globe than to other areas of the orbit.[1–5,10]

Table 1 shows the percentage of breast cancer cases in a series of patients with ocular metastases. The first four studies cited list the incidence for both orbital soft-tissue disease and intraocular disease, which occur in a ratio of approximately 4 to 5. The last three studies confine themselves to the globe only. With the exception of the study by Nelson et al.,[9] the incidence ranges from 40% to 70%. Unlike the others, Nelson et al. included patients with leukemia and lymphomas as well as solid tumors.

Stephens and Shields,[7] in a study of 70 patients referred with ophthalmologic symptoms, made special mention of the multiple lesions observed in patients with breast cancer primary tumors. The observation of bilateral ocular metastatic involvement also is not surprising; bilateral involvement ranges from 22% in the Stephens and Shields series[7] to 41% in the observations of Mewis and Young[11] and Rottinger et al.[12]

Frequently, the choroid is diffusely filled in with hundreds of metastatic deposits. Simultaneous metastatic involvement of both the central nervous system (CNS) and the eye is common. Because of the therapeutic implications, once ocular metastasis has been diagnosed, computed tomography (CT) or magnetic resonance imaging (MRI) should be performed to rule out concomitant CNS involvement. Maor et al.[13] documented that 3 of 42 patients with choroidal metastases from breast cancer also had brain metastases; Mewis and Young[11] found that 30 patients (41%) had CNS involvement. Of the 30 patients in their series, 15 patients had concurrent involvement, 13 had subsequent involvement, and just 2 had prior involvement.

Breast cancer is also the most likely tumor to metastasize to the eyelids. In a series by Riley[14] that combined his results and Mayo Clinic data, 38% of all metastatic lesions in the eyelids were found to be from breast cancer.

DIAGNOSIS

The median time from diagnosis of a primary breast cancer to the development of choroidal metastasis is between 3 and 4 years[10,15,16]; choroidal metastasis is the first sign of metastatic spread in approximately 20% of patients.[10,15]

The symptoms of choroidal metastasis that bring the woman to the ophthalmologist include decreased visual acuity, metamorphopsia (image distortion), a notable blind spot, diplopia, and, less frequently, pain, headache, and photophobia.[4–7,15,16] The most important test in establishing the diagnosis is indirect funduscopic examination. According to Reese,[17] findings include detachment of the retina, usually posteriorly. The detachment itself is described as having a pinkish-white color fading "off into the surrounding normal-appearing retina. Frequently, the surface of the tumor [has] a mottled appearance. Occasional hemorrhage and some pigmentary changes may occur over the involved area." Reese noticed a greyish or yellowish color to the

B. A. McCormick: Department of Radiation Oncology, Memorial Sloan-Kettering Cancer Center, New York, New York

D. H. Abramson: Department of Ophthalmology, Joan and Sanford I. Weill Medical College, New York Presbyterian Hospital - Cornell University, New York, New York

TABLE 1. *Percentage of breast cancer cases among patients with ocular metastases*

Study	Breast cancer in series (%)	Patient base	Sites
Glasburn et al.[5]	49	Radiation referrals	Orbit + globe
Freedman and Folk[4]	49	Ophthalmic referrals	Orbit + globe
Albert et al.[1]	70	Ophthalmic screen	Orbit + globe
Ferry[3]	40	Pathologic ophthalmic registry	Orbit + globe
Stephens and Shields[7]	65	Ophthalmic referrals	Uveal tract
Nelson et al.[9]	10	Autopsy	Globe
Bloch and Garner[2]	68	Autopsy	Globe

TABLE 2. *Results of external-beam radiation therapy for choroid metastases from breast cancer*

Study	No response or stable (%)	Partial response (PR) (%)	Complete response (CR) (%)
Chu et al.[15]	37	28	35
Mewis and Young[11]	67	27 (PR + CR)	
Rottinger et al.[12]	11	8	62
Thatcher and Thomas[22]	20	51	26

lesions and, on occasion, multiple foci. For single lesions, the appearance is similar to that of a primary ocular melanoma. Ultrasonography is useful in distinguishing the two: Malignant melanomas characteristically show low reflectivity in A-mode scan, whereas metastatic tumors lack this pattern. Fluorescein angiograms are useful in evaluating retinal disturbance that may not be clinically evident. Shields[18] also finds fluorescein angiography valuable for differentiating choroidal metastases from benign processes, such as hemorrhage, inflammation, and neovascular membranes. Because of the small size of the lesions and the nonspecific character of detachments, MRI[19] and CT[20] are not as useful in establishing a differential diagnosis but are helpful in treatment planning.

For patients with metastatic disease in the orbital soft tissues, the most common presenting symptoms are proptosis, ptosis, pain, diplopia, and clinical evidence of a mass.[4–6,16] Rarely a scirrhous carcinoma may cause retraction of the soft tissues and enophthalmos.[20] Imaging of the orbits by contrast-enhanced CT[20] or MRI is essential in the workup of orbital metastases.

TREATMENT AND PROGNOSIS

Appropriate treatment for most ocular metastases is a course of external-beam radiation therapy. This treatment is noninvasive and well tolerated by patients.

Treatment planning for patients with choroidal metastases consists of careful review of the ophthalmologist's examination notes and CT or MRI of the head. The presence or absence of brain metastases and bilateral disease must be established before treatment planning. Because of the multifocal nature of breast cancer in the eye, the goal of treatment planning is to design a field that encompasses all of the choroid from the equator posteriorly, with a margin. Except in unusual cases of more anteriorly located metastases, radiation to the lens can be avoided by using a lateral field with half-beam, D-shaped blocks similar to that used in retinoblastoma. Bilateral fields are appropriate for bilateral disease; for unilateral disease, a single lateral field is effective in delivering the dose to the eye while avoiding multiple entry and exit beam pathways that may compromise a course of palliative radiation at a later time to adjacent anatomic sites. For patients with concurrent CNS disease, shaped opposed fields that encompass the posterior halves of the globes, as well as the brain, are used.[21] Photon devices with some skin sparing are appropriate for this treatment. In departments in which only high-energy photon devices are available, the CT or MRI scan must be evaluated for globe location to ensure that the lateral choroid region is beyond the buildup region of the beam.

In the short term, the patient's vision may deteriorate during or just after the radiation treatments because of shifting subretinal fluid and retinal detachment at this time. Table 2 shows the results of external-beam radiation therapy in four series of choroid metastases from breast cancer. In the Chu et al. series,[15] doses ranged from 2,000 cGy in 2 weeks to 5,000 cGy in 5 weeks. In the Mewis and Young series,[11] doses delivered were consistent, ranging from 2,500 to 3,000 cGy in 10 fractions. The Thatcher and Thomas series[22] examined dose-response and documented a threshold dose equivalent of 3,250 cGy associated with a complete response. In that series, the median time for improvement was 4 weeks from the start of radiation (range, 4 days to 10 weeks). A fifth series by Maor et al.[13] also demonstrated a dose-response curve. In that study, three fraction schemes were used (2,500 cGy in 5 fractions, 2,500 cGy in 10 fractions, or 3,000 cGy in 10 fractions). A response was seen in all patients treated, but those treated at the lower doses later relapsed in the eye.[13] In a series by Rudoler et al., which reported on all histologic types but included 53% breast primaries, stable or improved vision, as defined with visual acuity testing, was observed in 57% of patients with tumors smaller than 15 mm; those who had good vision pretreatment and were younger than 55 years of age were most likely to benefit from treatment. Complications included cataracts, retinopathy, exposure keratopathy, optic neuropathy, iris neovascularization, and narrow-angle glaucoma. Two percent of the 233 eyes treated in the series required enucleation for intractable pain.[23]

For patients with orbital soft-tissue metastases, a wedged-pair arrangement of photon beams is appropriate in almost all instances. The target volume should include the contents of the bony orbit. Patients with orbital metastases tend to live longer than those with choroid metastases. Freedman and Folk[4] documented a median survival time for breast cancer patients with choroid metastases of 314 days, compared with 794 days for those with orbital metastases; however, in a small study, Ratanatharathorn et al.[10] found the opposite. In another small series of six patients, average survival after breast cancer metastasis to the eye was 32 months.[24]

The anticipated side effects of orbital external-beam radiation include periorbital edema, excessive tearing, and radiation-related inflammation of the conjunctiva. Corneal irritation and dry eye rarely are seen at the doses used in this palliative setting. Radiation-induced cataracts develop late in the lens because, when a wedged-pair field arrangement is used, this structure cannot be shielded without introducing a lens block that also shields the target. Because of the increased normal tissue complications and the longer survival time of these patients, a dose of 4,000 cGy in 3.5 to 4.0 weeks is recommended for this group.

Gragoudas[25] recommends using proton-beam therapy to treat selected patients with metastatic disease to the choroid. With limited follow-up, results seem equal, but not superior, to those of conventional external-beam therapy. Response of choroidal metastases also has been documented in patients receiving endocrine therapy or chemotherapy. Most of these reports are in patients with multiple sites of metastases that require systemic treatment. If a patient can be carefully observed by the ophthalmologist and exhibits no progression of disease, such treatment is appropriate.[26–28] In patients with limited sites of metastases or in whom visual deterioration is noted, however, external-beam therapy remains the treatment of choice to stabilize and improve the symptoms.

MANAGEMENT SUMMARY

The most common site of ocular metastasis is the choroid. The diagnosis is made by indirect funduscopic examination by an ophthalmologist.

Patients with ocular metastases should be given a workup for brain involvement as well before local treatment is planned.

Although systemic therapy may influence the rate of growth of ocular disease, external-beam radiation is the treatment of choice for patients with deteriorating vision from brain metastases.

REFERENCES

1. Albert DM, Rubenstein RA, Scheie HG. Tumor metastasis to the eye. Part 1. Incidence in 213 adult patients with generalized malignancy. *Am J Ophthalmol* 1967;63:723.
2. Bloch RS, Garner S. The incidence of ocular metastatic carcinoma. *Arch Ophthalmol* 1971;85:673.
3. Ferry AP. The biological behavior and pathological features of carcinoma metastatic to the eye and orbit. *Trans Am Ophthalmol Soc* 1973;71:373.
4. Freedman MI, Folk JC. Metastatic tumors to the eye and orbit. *Arch Ophthalmol* 1987;105:1215.
5. Glasburn JR, Klionsky M, Brady LW. Radiation therapy for metastatic disease involving the orbit. *Am J Clin Oncol* 1984;7:145.
6. Reddy S, Saxena VS, Hendrickson F, et al. Malignant metastatic disease of the eye: management of an uncommon complication. *Cancer* 1981;47:810.
7. Stephens RF, Shields JA. Diagnosis and management of cancer metastatic to the uvea: a study of 70 cases. *Ophthalmology* 1979; 86:1336.
8. Francois J, Hanssens H, Verbraeken H. Intraocular metastasis as first sign of generalized carcinomatosis. *Ann Ophthalmol* 1973;8:405.
9. Nelson CC, Hertzberg BS, Klintworth GK. A histopathologic study of 716 unselected eyes in patients with cancer at the time of death. *Am J Ophthalmol* 1983;95:788.
10. Ratanatharathorn V, Powers WE, Grimm J, et al. Eye metastasis from carcinoma of the breast: diagnosis, radiation treatment and results. *Cancer Treat Rev* 1991:18:261.
11. Mewis L, Young SE. Breast carcinoma metastatic to the choroid: analysis of 67 patients. *Ophthalmology* 1982;89:147.
12. Rottinger EM, Heckemann R, Scherer E, et al. Radiation therapy of choroidal metastases from breast cancer. *Arch Ophthalmol* 1976;200:243.
13. Maor M, Chan RC, Young SE. Radiotherapy of choroidal metastases: breast cancer as a primary site. *Cancer* 1977;40:2081.
14. Riley FG. Metastatic tumors of the eyelids. *Am J Ophthalmol* 1970;69:259.
15. Chu FCH, Huh SH, Nisce LZ, et al. Radiation therapy of choroid metastases from breast cancer. *Int J Radiat Oncol Biol Phys* 1977;2:273.
16. Dobrowsky W. Treatment of choroid metastases. *Br J Radiol* 1988;61:140.
17. Reese AB. Neoplastic metastasis to the eye and orbit. In: *Tumors of the eye*, 2nd ed. New York: Harper & Row, 1963:496.
18. Shields JA. Metastatic tumors of the uvea and retina. In: Shields JA, ed. *Diagnosis and management of intraocular tumors*. St. Louis: CV Mosby, 1983:278.
19. Wilms G, Marchal G, Van Fraeyenhoven L, et al. Shortcomings and pitfalls of ocular MRI. *Neuroradiology* 1991;33:320.
20. Hesselink JR, Davis KR, Weber AL, et al. Radiological evaluation of orbital metastases, with emphasis on computed tomography. *Radiology* 1980;137:363.
21. McCormick B, Ellsworth RE, Abramson D, et al. Radiation therapy for retinoblastoma: comparison of results with lens sparing versus lateral beam techniques. *Int J Radiol Oncol Biol Phys* 1988;15:567.
22. Thatcher N, Thomas PRM. Choroidal metastases from breast carcinoma: a survey of 42 patients and the use of radiation therapy. *Clin Radiol* 1975;26:549.
23. Rudoler SB, Shields CL, Corn BW, et al. Functional vision is improved in the majority of patients treated with external-beam radiotherapy for choroid metastases: a multivariate analysis of 188 patients. *J Clin Oncol* 1997;15,1244.
24. Merrill CF, Kaufman DI, Dimitrov NY. Breast cancer metastatic to the eye is a common entity. *Cancer* 1991;68:623.
25. Gragoudas ES. Current treatment of metastatic tumors. *Oncology* 1989;3:103.
26. MacMichael IM. Management of choroidal metastases from breast cancer. *Br J Ophthalmol* 1969;53:782.
27. Letson AD, Davidorf FH, Bruce RA. Chemotherapy for treatment of choroidal metastases from breast carcinoma. *Am J Ophthalmol* 1982;93:102.
28. Brinkley JA. Response of a choroidal metastasis to multiple-drug chemotherapy. *Cancer* 1980;45:1538.

Diseases of the Breast, 2nd ed.,
edited by Jay R. Harris.
Lippincott Williams & Wilkins, Philadelphia © 2000.

CHAPTER 57

Malignant Effusions

Lawrence N. Shulman and David J. Sugarbaker

Malignant effusions from breast cancer occur in the pleural space, pericardial space, and peritoneum. In all three cases, the cause of the effusion is directly related to serosal involvement with metastatic deposits; the exception is ascites resulting from extensive hepatic metastases. Because patients with breast cancer frequently develop metastatic disease and these locations often are involved with metastases, malignant effusions in these areas are common clinical problems.

PLEURAL EFFUSIONS

Normal Physiology

The pleural space is between the parietal pleura, lining the inside of the chest wall, and the visceral pleura, lining the outside of each lung. This space is normally lubricated to allow smooth and comfortable movement of the lung and chest wall during respiration. In the physiologic state, the pleural space contains 5 to 20 mL of fluid, the content of which reflects the plasma concentrations of glucose and electrolytes, with a similar pH.[1,2] The protein concentration usually is lower than that of plasma, however, and is generally below 2 g per dL. The fluid is produced by hydrostatic pressure from the parietal pleura and is reabsorbed by the venous and lymphatic channels of the visceral pleura. Estimates are that 5 to 50 L of fluid is produced and reabsorbed by these mechanisms each day.

Characteristics of Malignant Pleural Effusions

Malignant effusions occur when the pleura is involved with metastatic disease, which causes increased capillary leaking that results in increased fluid production and blockage of the normal vascular channels responsible for fluid reabsorption. A hallmark of malignant effusion is a high protein level (more than 3 g/dL), which classifies it as an exudative fluid. In addition, the glucose level usually is low, possibly reflecting glucose consumption by the malignant cells.[3] The pH of the malignant effusion can be normal or low (below 7.3); approximately one-third of patients with effusions have effusions with low pH.[4] The effusions with low pH may have low glucose levels and are more likely to have positive cytologic findings on the first fluid evaluation. Breast cancer patients with pleural effusions of low pH also have a mean survival time that is shorter than that of patients with effusions of normal pH (3.5 versus 16.6 months, respectively).[4] This suggests that low pH is an indication of involvement with more aggressive, metabolically active tumor, and the shorter survival for patients in this category has been confirmed by others for both breast cancer patients and patients with other tumor types.[5]

Cytologic Evaluation

Thoracentesis can provide fluid for cytologic diagnosis, and closed pleural biopsy also can be performed. The cellular component of pleural fluid is concentrated and prepared for cytologic evaluation by either filtration or centrifugation. In either case, cells are stained with Papanicolaou's stain or other appropriate stains for histologic review. Generally, volumes of 100 mL or more are optimal for evaluation. The more fluid that is processed by concentration methods, the more likely that malignant cells will be seen, although positive results sometimes can be obtained with only a few milliliters of fluid.

In one series, 81% of breast cancer patients had malignant cells identified on cytologic analysis, and an additional 6% of patients had a malignant diagnosis made with pleural biopsy, for a total diagnostic rate of 87%.[6]

Other techniques of fluid analysis, such as carcinoembryonic antigen determination, have been used to increase diagnostic accuracy of thoracentesis in this patient population; however, none has added substantially to the value of standard cytologic analyses and protein determination, and they add to the cost of the procedure.

L. N. Shulman: Department of Medicine, Harvard Medical School, Boston, Massachusetts; Department of Adult Oncology, Dana-Farber Cancer Institute, Brigham and Women's Hospital, Boston, Massachusetts

D. J. Sugarbaker: Department of Surgery, Harvard Medical School, Boston, Massachusetts; Department of Surgery/Thoracic Surgery, Brigham and Women's Hospital, Boston, Massachusetts

Malignant Pleural Effusions in Breast Cancer Patients

Overall, lung cancer is the most frequent cause of malignant pleural effusion, but breast cancer is the second most frequent cause; for women, breast cancer is the most common cause of malignant effusion. In a compilation of studies covering a total of 811 patients with malignant effusion, 23% of effusions resulted from breast cancer and 35% were from lung cancer.[2] In another series analyzing women separately, 37% of malignant effusions were found to be caused by breast cancer, whereas 20% were the result of genitourinary malignancy (mostly ovarian cancer), and 15% were from lung cancer.[7]

Effusions can be ipsilateral or contralateral to the original breast cancer, and this distinction might give insight into the mechanism of the effusion. Contralateral effusions are likely to be due to hematogenous tumor spread, whereas ipsilateral effusions might be caused by hematogenous spread or direct invasion through the chest wall by tumor resulting from chest wall or nodal recurrence. In one series, 83% of effusions were ipsilateral, 9% were contralateral, and 6% were bilateral.[8] In another series, 48% were ipsilateral, 42% were contralateral, and 10% were bilateral.[9] Despite these discrepant numbers, clearly some patients with breast cancer have chest wall recurrences, and on radiologic evaluation, tumor is seen infiltrating through the chest wall into the pleural space, resulting in malignant effusion. Likewise, gross involvement of the internal mammary nodes occasionally is associated with an ipsilateral effusion.

Malignant pleural effusion rarely occurs as a component of the initial presentation of breast cancer; more commonly, it occurs some time after the initial diagnosis of primary breast cancer, at a time when disseminated metastatic disease has developed. Time between initial diagnosis and occurrence of pleural effusion has been reported to be between 20 and 42 months, and in as many as 20% of patients, it is the only initial site of metastatic disease.[8,9] The median survival of patients with malignant effusions is the same as for patients with metastatic breast cancer in general—between 1 and 2 years.

Treatment

Malignant effusions are troublesome because of the symptoms they cause, most notably shortness of breath, cough, and pain. Shortness of breath occurs primarily because of a ventilation-perfusion mismatch. The affected lung continues to receive deoxygenated blood from the pulmonary arterial vasculature, but because of the presence of the effusion, the lung may not expand with inspiration and ventilate.

Because effusions in these patients result from the presence of pleural metastases, successful systemic treatment of the breast cancer, either with hormonal therapy or chemotherapy, results in disappearance of the effusion. The ability to accomplish this depends on the effectiveness of the therapy. Even if the therapy is effective, improvement with hormonal therapy or chemotherapy is slow, and the patient must be able to wait for this effect to occur and to understand that a beneficial effect may not be seen. Overall, in patients with newly diagnosed metastatic disease, response to systemic chemotherapy is approximately 70%; response to chemotherapy in patients with previously treated metastatic disease is variable, but in the range of 10% to 40%. Hormonal therapy can be expected to produce responses in 70% of patients with estrogen receptor–positive tumors and 10% of patients with estrogen receptor–negative tumors. These statistics should be taken into account when evaluating systemic therapy as a component of the treatment of a malignant effusion. The decision to use systemic treatment or local treatment is based on the size of the effusion, the degree of compromise of the patient, and the likelihood that systemic therapy will result in a rapid response.

Local treatment of the effusion consists of either intermittent drainage via percutaneous thoracentesis, chest tube placement, and sclerosis, or thoracotomy and sclerosis. Intermittent drainage is effective only if systemic therapy has a simultaneous beneficial impact on the pleural metastases; otherwise, pleural fluid reaccumulates quickly, often at a rate of 1 to 3 L per day.

Chest tube drainage and sclerosis involve draining the effusion dry, so that the parietal and visceral pleurae are once again in contact with each other, and instilling a sclerosing agent. Most sclerosing agents are designed to cause fusion of the parietal and visceral pleurae by chemical irritation. If the pleural surfaces become fused, the potential pleural space is obliterated, preventing reaccumulation of fluid. Chemotherapeutic agents such as thiotepa have been used in the hope that a direct antineoplastic effect would be seen and this effect would prevent reaccumulation of the effusion; however, most agents work by chemical irritation of the pleura with resultant pleural fusion.

The success of pleural sclerosis depends on the ability to keep the pleural space dry so the parietal and visceral pleurae are in contact during the instillation of the sclerosing agent, and on the irritative properties of the sclerosing agent. In practice, a chest tube is placed and attached to suction, and drainage continues until the daily fluid output falls below 100 to 200 mL. This often takes several days. In the experience of the authors, modest intravascular depletion with the aid of diuretics occasionally decreases chest tube output to the desired level. Follow-up chest radiographs are taken to evaluate the completeness of the drainage, particularly to determine whether loculated areas of effusion persist that may require chest tube repositioning or placement of additional chest tubes.

The success of pleural sclerosis is also dependent on the ability of the lung to reexpand so that the visceral and parietal pleurae come together. Lung entrapment can cause failure of lung reexpansion and may result when tumor or fibrosis encases the lung and restricts it in its collapsed state. At the time of chest tube placement, whether lung entrapment exists may not be clear. Lan et al. measured the change in pleural pressure as a function of volume of pleural fluid removed and determined a cut-off value that could be used to predict success or failure of sclerosis for patients with lung entrapment.[10] Although this technique has not been used frequently, it does confirm the pathophysiology of malignant effusions and is an option for those who are concerned about an individual patient. For the patient with trapped lung, for whom pleurodesis is not likely to be successful, pleuroperitoneal shunting has frequently been able to alleviate symptoms.[11]

Many drugs have been used as sclerosing agents, including tetracycline or similar antibiotic agents, nitrogen mustard, bleomycin sulfate, and talc. Reports in the literature of response rates for different agents vary, so it is difficult to determine which agent is most effective. These variations are probably the result of differences in techniques, differences in the tumor characteristics in various patient populations, and differences in the length of follow-up of the patients, because longer follow-up is associated with an increased failure rate. In some series, patients with various tumors are included; even when breast cancer patients are examined as a separate group, patients can be at various stages of their disease, which might affect response rates.

Nitrogen mustard, for instance, has been reported to achieve successful sclerosis in between 25% and 87% of patients.[12–14] In practice, nitrogen mustard is rarely used.

Tetracycline also has been used widely, although it is not available in the necessary formulation in the United States. Reported response rates for tetracycline vary widely. In one report, only 15% of patients receiving tetracycline had a complete response, and an additional 40% achieved partial responses (defined as patients' having reaccumulation of some pleural fluid but not requiring repeated drainage).[15] Another study reported a complete response rate of 69%.[16] These authors suggest that the acid pH of the tetracycline solution might be responsible for the beneficial effects of sclerosis, rather than the tetracycline itself; they conducted a randomized trial comparing tetracycline and a placebo solution with a similar pH (2.8). Patients sclerosed with tetracycline had a complete response rate of 69%, whereas patients sclerosed with the acid solution had an 11% response rate, suggesting that the acid pH of the tetracycline solution was not the major contributing factor for control of pleural effusions in these patients.

Because tetracycline is no longer available in the United States in the form necessary for sclerosis, doxycycline has been used in its place. Complete response rates at 1 month after sclerosis of 88% and 78% have been reported for patients treated with chest tube drainage and doxycycline instillation, respectively.[17,18] This seems to be an acceptable replacement for tetracycline.

Bleomycin sulfate has also been used extensively as a sclerosing agent. One series reported a 69% complete response rate and a 12% partial response rate 30 days after bleomycin sulfate instillation.[19] At 90 days, 54% of patients showed complete response, and 4% showed partial response. Among patients with malignant effusions from breast cancer only, 81% showed response at 30 days and 63% at 90 days. Several other studies have reported similar results, suggesting that this is one of the more effective agents available.[20,21] In a randomized comparison of bleomycin sulfate and tetracycline, 30% of the group treated with bleomycin sulfate and 53% of the group treated with tetracycline showed recurrence of pleural fluid at 90 days after sclerosis; these results suggest more prolonged control of the malignant effusion by bleomycin sulfate–induced sclerosis than by tetracycline-induced sclerosis.[22]

Talc, which causes an intense pleuritis, has also been widely used as a sclerosing agent, and some believe it to be the most effective agent available.[2] Most of the studies involving talc used more extensive surgical procedures, instilling the talc during pleuroscopy or thoracotomy under general or local anesthesia, making for a more cumbersome and risky procedure. A thoracoscopic approach, however, has the advantage of allowing the surgeon to be certain of complete fluid drainage, lysis of adhesions, and even distribution of the talc during insufflation. Weissburg et al.[23] reported a 90% success rate using pleuroscopic instillation. Other studies have suggested control rates of 90% or more, also using either pleuroscopy or open thoracotomy with talc instillation.[24] In one trial in which patients were randomized to sclerosis using either talc or nitrogen mustard, the group sclerosed with talc showed a 90% response rate compared with 56% for the group treated with nitrogen mustard The same researchers studied compared talc with tetracycline, reporting a 92% response rate to talc and a 48% response rate to tetracycline.[26] Another case control study compared sclerosis induced by talc instilled through thoracoscopic guidance with chest tube drainage and sclerosis induced by bleomycin sulfate and tetracycline, showing superiority for talc pluradesis.[27] Some centers are using talc instillation through percutaneous chest tube rather than during pleuroscopy or thoracotomy.

Other attempts to induce sclerosis using chemotherapeutic agents instilled within the pleura have had only modest success. One such report by the Lung Cancer Study Group investigated administration of a combination of cisplatin and cytarabine in the management of malignant pleural effusions in patients with various primary tumors.[28] Systemic toxicity was modest, but the complete plus partial response rate was only 49%; the median duration of response was 9 months for the complete responders and 5 months for the partial responders.

Summary

As shown in Table 1, several options exist for managing malignant pleural effusions from metastatic breast cancer. A review of the English-language literature evaluating reports on 1,168 patients suggests that talc insufflation has the highest response rate (93%), but acceptable rates were also found for tetracycline (67%), doxycycline (72%), minocycline hydrochloride (86%), and bleomycin sulfate (54%).[29] As a general recom-

TABLE 1. *Therapeutic options for the management of malignant pleural effusion*

Percutaneous drainage (thoracentesis)
Rapid and transiently effective, but unless the underlying tumor is controlled with systemic therapy, the effusion recurs rapidly.
Thoracoscopic instillation of talc
This method has the highest success rate of all procedures. It allows direct visualization of the pleural space, assuring complete drainage of the effusion and lysis of any adhesions. It also ensures relatively even distribution of the talc throughout the pleural space. The procedure can be performed under general anesthesia or local anesthesia with sedation.
Chest tube drainage and sclerosis with doxycycline or bleomycin sulfate
This procedure is relatively easy but requires chest tube drainage until the pleural fluid output falls below 100 to 200 mL per day. The success rate is lower than for talc-induced sclerosis, but the procedure does not require general anesthesia or operating room time.

TABLE 2. *Symptoms and signs of pericardial tamponade*

Symptoms
Dyspnea on exertion
Orthopnea
Tachycardia
Chest pain
Clinical signs
Tachycardia
Distant heart sounds
Decreased or absent cardiac impulse
Pericardial friction rub
Hypotension and peripheral vascular constriction
Jugular venous distention
Paradoxic movement of the jugular venous pulse
Pulsus paradoxus
Pulsus alternans
Laboratory findings
Low voltage on electrocardiogram
Electrical alternans
Enlarged globular cardiac silhouette on chest radiograph
Pericardial effusion or thickened pericardium on echocardiography
Diastolic collapse of the right atrium and ventricle on echocardiography
Pericardial effusion or thickened pericardium on computed tomography

mendation, thoracoscopic insufflation with talc or chest tube drainage with sclerosis using doxycycline, minocycline hydrochloride, or bleomycin sulfate are reasonable alternatives for the management of malignant pleural effusions.

PERICARDIAL EFFUSIONS

Breast cancer patients can develop pericardial effusions because of tumor involvement or radiation pericarditis. Pericardial involvement with tumor can lead to constrictive or effusive pericardial tamponade, either of which can result in cardiovascular collapse and death if not recognized and treated promptly.

Hemodynamics and Pathophysiology of Pericardial Tamponade

Increased intrapericardial pressure results in reduced ventricular expansion and diastolic filling.[30] This further leads to early closure of the atrioventricular valves. Myocardial muscle fiber length is shortened and stroke volume is reduced. Mean ventricular, left and right atrial, pulmonary venous, and arterial and vena caval pressures increase. As cardiac output drops, heart rate and peripheral vasoconstriction increase to maintain arterial perfusion and venous return to the heart.

Clinical Signs of Pericardial Tamponade

Because of the pathophysiology of pericardial tamponade, a number of important signs may be observed in early and later stages of pericardial tamponade, as outlined in Table 2. One of the most important and early signs is dyspnea on exertion; exertion can unmask deficits in early tamponade, because the heart is unable to increase cardiac output in response to the increased oxygen demand of the exercised muscles. As part of this phenomenon, dyspnea on exertion can be severe, although the patient can be reasonably comfortable at rest. In most study series, dyspnea is the most common complaint and is present in approximately 75% of patients with tamponade.[31] Arterial blood gases obtained at rest often show normal oxygenation, which sometimes causes the clinician to wonder about the cause of the dyspnea on exertion. Because of peripheral vasoconstriction, the patient's extremities may be cool and cyanotic.

A number of physical examination findings have been associated with tamponade, including tachycardia, decreased or absent cardiac impulse, pericardial friction rub, paradoxic movement of the jugular venous pulse, pulsus paradoxus, atrial fibrillation, and pulsus alternans. Tachycardia can become more pronounced with minimal exertion; as mentioned earlier, this results from the heart's inability to increase cardiac output with increasing muscle oxygen demand. With significant tamponade, the cardiac impulse is almost always absent. The heart, pumping with reduced stroke volume within a tense pericardial sac, transmits no discernible impulse. Pericardial friction rub sometimes is heard in the early stages of malignant pericardial involvement but may disappear when the effusion becomes larger, and causes complete separation of the pericardium and myocardium. Jugular venous distention may be more pronounced because of increased right atrial pressure. Paradoxic movement of the jugular venous pulse may be seen, increasing rather than decreasing with inspiration; presumably, this occurs because of stretching of the heart and pericardium on downward movement of the diaphragm, which results in increased intrapericardial pressure. Pulsus paradoxus, defined as a drop of 10 mm Hg or more in systolic blood pressure with inspiration, occurs by the same pathophysiologic route as paradoxic movement of the jugular venous pulse. Atrial fibrillation occurs, most probably because of the direct electrical irritative effects of pericardial metastases. Pulsus alternans and electrical alternans are seen in a few cases, and the pathophysiologic processes they represent are unclear.[32,33] Low voltage also can be seen on electrocardiogram because of reduced electrical transmission through the fluid-filled pericardial sac.

None of these clinical signs is seen universally in cases of malignant pericardial tamponade; except for tachycardia and absence of cardiac impulse, most are seen in only a few patients, so that the clinician must maintain a high degree of suspicion of pericardial involvement and, when appropriate, proceed with more definitive testing.[34] In addition, the clinician must distinguish between malignant pericardial tamponade, idiopathic tamponade, and radiation-induced pericarditis. The clinical scenario often is helpful in this differential diagnosis; for instance, radiation-induced pericarditis occurs only in patients who received radiation therapy to the pericardium.

Diagnosis

Pericardial tamponade from pericardial effusion or constrictive pericarditis is suggested by the presence of the clinical signs outlined above. Chest radiography sometimes reveals the typical enlarged globular cardiac shadow. In cases of constrictive pericardial tamponade, however, the cardiac shadow may not be enlarged. Pleural effusion is a frequent finding in patients with pericardial tamponade but obviously is not specific.[28]

Echocardiography has been a mainstay in the diagnosis of pericardial effusion and cardiac tamponade. In the case of effusive pericarditis, a fluid-filled pericardial sac can be demonstrated. Fluid often initially collects posteriorly, but as the amount of fluid increases, it usually fills the entire sac. Collapse of the right atrium and right ventricle during diastole is one of the cardinal signs of tamponade physiology and is important in determining clinical compromise in the patient with a pericardial effusion.[35] As pericardial fluid increases and intrapericardial pressure rises, right atrial collapse occurs first.[36] With increasing intrapericardial pressure, right ventricular collapse during diastole occurs; such collapse has been shown to be highly predictive of tamponade physiology, with a sensitivity of 92% and a specificity of 100% in the series of Singh et al.[36] Once right ventricular collapse occurs, drainage of pericardial fluid is likely to improve cardiac function. Dynamic studies have shown that, with removal of pericardial fluid, as intrapericardial pressure decreases a major improvement in cardiac function occurs at the same time that right ventricular collapse disappears.

Computed tomography is also useful in determining the presence of pericardial effusion and pericardial thickening, which is often present in malignant pericardial disease.[37] On occasion, it demonstrates pericardial abnormalities that are not seen on echocardiographic examination. It does not provide physiologic information, however, because it is a static study.

Pericardial Disease in Breast Cancer Patients

Breast cancer, along with lung cancer and non-Hodgkin's lymphoma, is one of the leading causes of malignant pericardial disease.[34] Pericardial involvement by breast cancer is present in approximately 25% of patients with metastatic disease by the time of death, but it is responsible for death in fewer than 5% of breast cancer patients.[38] In a large series from the Mayo Clinic, breast cancer patients were divided into three groups: those with effusions discovered incidentally on echocardiography, those without any evidence of metastatic breast cancer with symptoms suggestive of pericardial tamponade, and those with known metastatic breast cancer and signs or symptoms of pericardial tamponade.[39] Of the patients whose effusions were discovered incidentally, all had small effusions. Only 1 of the 20 patients had clinical signs of pericardial tamponade late in the course of disease; these were believed to result from malignant involvement of the pericardium, but there was no histologic confirmation. Of the patients without known metastatic disease but with symptomatic pericardial effusion, 20% required surgical treatment of tamponade, but none had definitive evidence of a malignant cause of their effusion. All cases were thought to result from radiation pericarditis. Of 38 patients with known metastatic breast cancer, 15 (39%) had large effusions and 19 (50%) had certain malignant diagnosis; others may also have had malignant causes of their effusions that were not histologically documented. In this group of patients, surgical therapy was essential for the successful management of the pericardial disease. The use of pericardiocentesis alone was associated with a high relapse rate, even when the patient was undergoing concurrent chemotherapy. Treatment with systemic chemotherapy only was associated with a high failure rate and sudden death in several patients. The median survival of patients with known malignant pericardial involvement was 17 months; median survival was 20 months for patients who had surgical management of their effusions.

Treatment

Pericardial tamponade is a medical emergency that is associated with severe symptoms and can result in sudden death. Most cases seem to result primarily from effusive pericarditis, but some are due to constrictive pericarditis, and the treatment approaches may be different for the two groups. Patients with symptomatic tamponade should not be treated with systemic therapy alone. The failure rate is high, as is the incidence of sudden cardiac death. Therapeutic options include percutaneous pericardial catheter drainage, surgical placement of a pericardial window, and pericardial stripping.

Simple catheter drainage can be lifesaving by rapidly relieving critical tamponade, for removal of even small amounts of pericardial fluid can result in substantial improvement in cardiac dynamics. This procedure has not demonstrated lasting success in most cases, however, because effusions frequently recur and sudden death can result.[39]

Tetracycline sclerosis was also used as a therapy in one study.[40] Pericardial catheters were placed into the pericardial sac and allowed to drain for 12 to 24 hours, after which lidocaine hydrochloride (Xylocaine) and tetracycline were instilled. One to five instillations were performed. The authors reported a 68% control rate with no evidence of development of constrictive pericardial compromise. In a prospective study comparing doxycycline and bleomycin sulfate as pericardial sclerosing agents, both were found to be successful in a majority of patients, although repeat sclerosis was sometimes necessary.[41] Use of bleomycin sulfate was associated with fewer symptoms and was therefore preferred in this study. In practice, sclerosis is not widely used, in part because patients require continued close monitoring and multiple treatments are often necessary, whereas pericardiotomy usually is successful in a single procedure.

Most patients are treated with surgical placement of a pericardial window, often using the subxiphoid approach.[42,43] This method can be accomplished quickly and safely, and it has a high success rate. More extensive surgical approaches using an anterior thoracotomy approach to allow removal of more of the pericardium also have been used. In one nonrandomized study comparing these two techniques, subxiphoid pericardiotomy was as effective as anterior thoracotomy and had a far lower complication rate.[44] No difference in survival was found between patients treated with subxiphoid pericardiotomy and those treated with anterior thoracotomy, and no patients undergoing subxiphoid pericardiotomy required further treatment of the pericardial effusion. In addition, no patients undergoing subxiphoid pericardiotomy had major complications, whereas one-half of the patients undergoing anterior thoracotomy sustained major complications, including pulmonary embolism, arterial embolism with gangrene, disseminated intravascular coagulation, acute renal failure, pneumonia, sepsis, pleural effusion requiring drainage, and recurrent pericardial effusion. Although this was not a randomized study, patient characteristics before treatment were similar, which suggests that the difference in complication rate was probably not because of selection of patients with more advanced disease for anterior thoracotomy.

Thoracoscopic approaches to pericardiectomy using a video-assisted thoracoscopic three-cannula technique have also been reported. This method allows for a more extensive pericardiectomy than the subxiphoid approach but is a less invasive procedure than thoracotomy. Mack et al.[45] reported on 22 patients, all of whom experienced relief of pericardial effusion without morbidity or mortality. The ability to open both the anterior and posterior pericardial cavity appears to make this approach superior to the subxiphoid approach, and morbidity and mortality are lower than with thoracotomy.

The presence of pericardial fluid allows for a safer thoracoscopic pericardiectomy. Therefore, use of catheter drainage in patients for whom a surgical approach is contemplated is not advised unless hemodynamic compromise is present. Pericardial fluid protects the myocardium during incision of the pericardium through the thoracoscopic approach. Selection of the right or left side for the thoracoscopic pericardiectomy may be dictated by the presence of a pleural effusion, because a talc pleurodesis can be performed during the same procedure if desired.

Summary

Options for the management of pericardial effusion are shown in Table 3. A review of the English-language publications addressing management of malignant pericardial effusions suggests that pericardial drainage by percutaneous catheter is effective at relieving the physiologic features causing tamponade, and for patients with tumors expected to respond rapidly to systemic therapy, this may be all that is needed.[46] When the underlying tumor cannot be expected to

TABLE 3. *Management of malignant pericardial tamponade*

Percutaneous catheter drainage
This method has the advantage of ease, can be performed rapidly and relatively safely under ultrasonic guidance, and can effectively reverse tamponade physiology. Unless a sclerosing agent is instilled or the underlying tumor is controlled rapidly with systemic therapy, the effusion is likely to recur.
Subxiphoid pericardial window placement
This procedure has low morbidity and mortality and is effective in most patients with malignant pericardial tamponade. The recurrence of effusion and tamponade is uncommon.
Video-assisted thoracoscopic surgery
This procedure, performed with a three-cannula technique, has a high success rate, low morbidity, and low mortality. It is safer when performed with pericardial effusion present, because the effusion separates the pericardium from the myocardium during the initial incision. Therefore, catheter drainage of the pericardial effusion should not be done unless hemodynamic compromise is present.
Thoracotomy and pericardial stripping
This procedure is associated with a higher complication rate than subxiphoid pericardial window placement but may be required for patients who have extensive tumor involvement of the pericardium that results in either loculated pericardial fluid or constrictive pericarditis.

respond rapidly to systemic therapy, as might be the case for patients with disseminated breast cancer, placement of a pericardial window by the subxiphoid approach is relatively safe and has a high chance of success. Video-assisted thoracoscopic surgery has a high success rate with low morbidity and mortality. For patients in whom this approach is planned, catheter drainage of the pericardial fluid should not be performed unless hemodynamic compromise occurs, because the presence of pericardial fluid protects the myocardium and makes the technique safer. Patients with extensive constrictive pericardial involvement may require open thoracotomy and pericardial stripping. These patients represent a minority of patients with breast cancer and pericardial involvement.

ASCITES

Ascites in patients with breast cancer can occur either from peritoneal serosal implants or from extensive hepatic metastases and resultant portal hypertension. Extensive hepatic metastases with portal hypertension usually occur as a terminal event, and unless systemic chemotherapy is rapidly effective in reducing the tumor burden, fatal hepatic failure ensues. In this circumstance, ascites is of secondary concern.

Ascites from peritoneal tumor implants is uncommon in breast cancer patients. The abdominal bloating is uncomfortable in itself and often causes early satiety, resulting in decreased oral intake and upward pressure on the diaphragm, which prevents full expansion of the lungs and can cause shortness of breath and dyspnea on exertion. The ascites itself is not life threatening, because the peritoneal implants are usually only one manifestation of disseminated metastatic disease, with other sites of involvement often being of more immediate concern. This situation is different from that in ovarian cancer, in which isolated intraabdominal disease is common and often is the major clinical problem for the patient.

In patients with metastatic breast cancer and ascites, the most effective therapy is systemic chemotherapy or hormonal therapy directed at reducing tumor mass, which results in a reduced amount of ascites. If this is not feasible or the ascites is particularly uncomfortable, then paracentesis can be performed and transiently improves comfort. Without control of the basic tumor, however, ascitic fluid reaccumulates. The rate of reaccumulation varies from patient to patient. Some patients experience relief of their symptoms for several days and benefit from repeated paracenteses.

Intraabdominal chemotherapy has been widely used in patients with ovarian cancer, because the peritoneum frequently is the only site of disease, and in these patients it can clearly have a palliative role. Breast cancer patients usually have other sites of metastatic disease that are frequently more troublesome to them, making intraabdominal chemotherapy an inappropriate option for most breast cancer patients.

Peritoneovenous shunts have been described as therapy for patients with malignant ascites and have been shown to reduce abdominal girth and number of paracenteses in selected groups of patients.[47–49] Complications can be serious, however, with a significant number of patients developing disseminated intravascular coagulation, sepsis, and congestive heart failure. Shunts frequently clot, and the theoretical concern exists that shunts will seed peritoneal tumor cells into the pulmonary circulation, resulting in the development of pulmonary metastases. In practice, peritoneovenous shunts are rarely used to relive ascites in patients with metastatic breast cancer.

REFERENCES

1. Leff A, Hopewell PC, Costello J. Pleural effusion from malignancy. *Ann Intern Med* 1978;88:532.
2. Hausheer FH, Yarbro JW. Diagnosis and treatment of malignant pleural effusion. *Semin Oncol* 1985;12:54.
3. Silverberg I. Management of effusions. *Oncology* 1970;24:26.
4. Sahn SA, Good JT. Pleural fluid pH in malignant effusions: diagnostic, prognostic, and therapeutic implications. *Ann Intern Med* 1988; 108:345.
5. Sanchez-Armengol A, Rodriguez-Panadero F. Survival and talc pleurodesis in metastatic pleural carcinoma revisited: report of 125 cases. *Chest* 1993;104:1482.
6. Prakash UBS, Reiman HM. Comparison of needle biopsy with cytologic analysis for the evaluation of pleural effusion: analysis of 414 cases. *Mayo Clin Proc* 1985;60:158.
7. Johnston WW. The malignant pleural effusion: a review of cytopathologic diagnoses of 584 specimens from 472 consecutive patients. *Cancer* 1985;56:905.
8. Raju RN, Kardinal CG. Pleural effusion in breast carcinoma: analysis of 122 cases. *Cancer* 1981;48:2524.
9. Fentiman IS, Millis R, Sexton S, et al. Pleural effusion in breast cancer: a review of 105 cases. *Cancer* 1981;47:2087.
10. Lan RS, Lo SK, Chuang ML, et al. Elastance of the pleural space: a predictor for the outcome of pleurodesis in patients with malignant pleural effusion. *Ann Int Med* 1997;126:768.
11. Petrou M, Kaplan D, Goldstraw P. Management of recurrent malignant pleural effusions: the complementary role of talc pleurodesis and pleuroperitoneal shunting. *Cancer* 1995;75:801.
12. Weisberger AS, Levine B, Storaasli JP. Use of nitrogen mustard in the treatment of serous effusions of neoplastic origin. *JAMA* 1955;159:1704.
13. Fracchia AA, Knapper WH, Carey JT, et al. Intrapleural chemotherapy for effusions from metastatic breast carcinoma. *Cancer* 1970;26:626.
14. Kinsey DL, Carter D, Klassen KP. Simplified management of malignant pleural effusion. *Arch Surg* 1964;89:389.
15. Gravelyn TR, Michelson MK, Gross BH, et al. Tetracycline pleurodesis for malignant pleural effusions: a 10-year retrospective study. *Cancer* 1987;59:1973.
16. Zaloznik AJ, Oswald SG, Langin M. Intrapleural tetracycline in malignant pleural effusions: a randomized study. *Cancer* 1983;51:752.
17. Robinson LA, Fleming WH, Galbraith TA. Intrapleural doxycycline control of malignant pleural effusions. *Ann Thorac Surg* 1993; 55:1115.
18. Heffner JE, Standerfer RJ, Torstveit J, et al. Clinical efficacy of doxycycline for pleurodesis. *Chest* 1994;105:1743.
19. Ostrowski MJ. An assessment of the long-term results of controlling reaccumulation of malignant effusions using intracavity bleomycin. *Cancer* 1986;57:721.
20. Bitran JD, Brown C, Desser RK, et al. Intracavitary bleomycin for the control of malignant effusions. *J Surg Oncol* 1981;16:273.
21. Paladine W, Cunningham TJ, Sponzo R, et al. Intracavitary bleomycin in the management of malignant effusions. *Cancer* 1976;38:1903.
22. Ruckdeschel JC, Moores D, Lee JY, et al. Intrapleural therapy for malignant pleural effusions: a randomized comparison of bleomycin and tetracycline. *Chest* 1991;100:1528.
23. Weissburg D, Kaufman M, Zurkowski Z. Pleuroscopy in patients with pleural effusions and pleural masses. *Ann Thorac Surg* 1980;29:205.
24. Pearson FG, Macgregor DC. Talc poudrage for malignant pleural effusion. *J Thorac Cardiovasc Surg* 1966;51:732.

25. Fentiman IS, Rubens RD, Hayward JL. Control of pleural effusions in patients with breast cancer: a randomized trial. *Cancer* 1983;52:737.
26. Fentiman IS, Rubens RD, Hayward JL. A comparison of intracavitary talc and tetracycline for the control of pleural effusions secondary to breast cancer. *Eur J Cancer Clin Oncol* 1986;22:1079.
27. Hartman DL, Gaither JM, Kesler KA, et al. Comparison of insufflated talc under thoracoscopic guidance with standard tetracycline and bleomycin pleurodesis for control of malignant pleural effusion. *J Thorac Cardiovasc Surg* 1993;105:743.
28. Rusch VW, Figlin R, Godwin D, et al. Intrapleural cisplatin and cytarabine in the management of malignant pleural effusions: a lung Cancer Study Group trial. *J Clin Oncol* 1991;9:313.
29. Walker-Renard PB, Vaughan LM, Sahn SA. Chemical pleurodesis for malignant pleural effusions. *Ann Intern Med* 1994;120:56.
30. Theologides A. Neoplastic cardiac tamponade. *Semin Oncol* 1978;5:181.
31. Cham WC, Freiman AH, Carstens PHB, et al. Radiation therapy of cardiac and pericardial metastases. *Ther Radiol* 1975;114:701.
32. Lawrence LT, Cronin JF. Electrical alternans and pericardial tamponade. *Arch Intern Med* 1963;112:415.
33. Spodick DH. Electrical alternation of the heart: its relation to the kinetics and physiology of the heart during cardiac tamponade. *Am J Cardiol* 1962;10:155.
34. Posner MR, Cohen GI, Skarin AT. Pericardial disease in patients with cancer: the differentiation of malignant from idiopathic and radiation-induced pericarditis. *Am J Med* 1981;71:407.
35. Gillam LD, Guyer DE, Gibson TC, et al. Hydrodynamic compression of the right atrium: a new echocardiographic sign of cardiac tamponade. *Circulation* 1983;68:294.
36. Singh S, Wann S, Schuchard GH, et al. Right ventricular and right atrial collapse in patients with cardiac tamponade: a combined echocardiographic and hemodynamic study. *Circulation* 1984; 70:966.
37. Isner JM, Carter BL, Bankoff MS, et al. Computed tomography in the diagnosis of pericardial heart disease. *Ann Intern Med* 1982;97:473.
38. Hagemeister FB, Buzdar AU, Luna MA, et al. Causes of death in breast cancer. *Cancer* 1980;46:162.
39. Buck M, Ingle JN, Giuliani ER, et al. Pericardial effusion in women with breast cancer. *Cancer* 1987;60:263.
40. Shepherd FA, Ginsberg JS, Evans WK, et al. Tetracycline sclerosis in the management of malignant pericardial effusion. *J Clin Oncol* 1985;3:1678.
41. Liu G, Crump M, Goss PE, Dancey J, Shepherd FA. Prospective comparison of the sclerosing agents doxycycline and bleomycin for the primary management of malignant pericardial effusion and cardiac tamponade. *J Clin Oncol* 1996;14:3141.
42. Snow N, Lucas A. Subxiphoid pericardiotomy: a safe, accurate, diagnostic and therapeutic approach to pericardial and intrapericardial disease. *Am Surg* 1983;49:249.
43. Osuch JR, Khandekar JD, Fry WA. Emergency subxiphoid pericardial decompression for malignant pericardial effusion. *Am Surg* 1985;51:298.
44. Park JS, Rentschler R, Wilbur D. Surgical management of pericardial effusion in patients with malignancies. *Cancer* 1991;67:76.
45. Mack MJ, Landreneau RJ, Hazelrigg SR, et al. Video thoracoscopic management of benign and malignant pericardial effusions. *Chest* 1993;103:390S.
46. Vaitkus PT, Herrmann HC, LeWinter MM. Treatment of malignant pericardial effusion. *JAMA* 1994;272:59.
47. Qazi R, Savlov ED. Peritoneovenous shunt for palliation of malignant ascites. *Cancer* 1982;49:600.
48. Cheung DK, Raaf JH. Selection of patients with malignant ascites for a peritoneovenous shunt. *Cancer* 1982;50:1204.
49. Souter RG, Wells C, Tarin D, et al. Surgical and pathologic complications associated with peritoneovenous shunts in management of malignant ascites. *Cancer* 1985;55:1973.

Diseases of the Breast, 2nd ed.,
edited by Jay R. Harris.
Lippincott Williams & Wilkins, Philadelphia © 2000.

CHAPTER 58

Management of Discrete Pulmonary Nodules

Steven J. Mentzer and David J. Sugarbaker

Discrete tumors of 3 cm or less in the peripheral lung are commonly referred to as *solitary pulmonary nodules*. The nodules are typically asymptomatic and are identified by routine radiographic examination. Solitary pulmonary nodules are not associated with atelectasis or hilar adenopathy. If the nodule is new, based on comparisons with previous chest radiographs, the solitary pulmonary nodule most likely represents either a cancer or a benign granuloma.[1,2]

In patients with a history of breast cancer, solitary pulmonary nodules may represent recurrent breast cancer. The lung is a common site for breast cancer metastases.[3–5] The lung is the first site of recurrence in 15% to 25% of patients with metastatic breast cancer.[6–8] Clinical series have demonstrated that the lung is second only to bone as a site of recurrent breast cancer. In more than one-half of the patients with a lung recurrence, a solitary pulmonary nodule is the presenting sign. Other common intrathoracic sites of metastatic disease include the pleura and mediastinal and internal mammary lymph nodes.[6,8]

Alternatively, the solitary pulmonary nodule may represent a primary lung cancer. Lung cancer in women is both common and frequently fatal. Lung cancer represents 13% of all cancers in women and 23% of all cancer deaths in women.[9] Radiographic appearance and clinical risk factors are generally not useful in excluding the possible diagnosis of lung cancer. Some 10% to 15% of patients with lung cancer present with a solitary pulmonary nodule; 20% of these patients are nonsmokers. The current data suggest that a solitary pulmonary nodule represents a primary lung cancer in more than 50% of patients with a history of breast cancer[10–13] (Table 1).

The most common benign pathologic diagnosis of a solitary pulmonary nodule is a granuloma. Granulomas can occur in response to inhaled particular matter or a variety of infectious pathogens. The histopathologic evaluation of granulomatous lesions typically involves special histochemical studies to exclude acid-fast bacilli, fungal forms, or inhaled particulates. Although granulomatous lesions can be routinely cultured, most granulomas are sterile and do not require further therapy.

DIAGNOSIS

Pulmonary nodules are commonly evaluated by chest computed tomography (CT). The CT scan is particularly useful in identifying benign characteristics. Granulomas can be totally calcified or can have central or laminar calcification. The presence of these features virtually excludes the diagnosis of malignant disease.[1]

When malignant disease is a possibility, CT scans provide important staging information. The chest CT of a patient with a potential malignancy routinely includes examination of the liver and adrenal glands, because these organs are frequently sites of metastatic spread. A complete chest CT also provides important anatomic information about other common metastatic sites for breast cancer: specifically, the lung, liver, intrathoracic lymph nodes, and pleura.[6–8,14] Common metastatic sites for lung cancer are intrathoracic lymph nodes, pleura, liver, and adrenal glands.

Chest CT is more sensitive than chest radiography in detecting pulmonary metastases.[15,16] Chest CT scans can detect peripheral nodules as small as 2 to 3 mm. In patients with a discrete nodule on chest radiography and a history of extrathoracic malignancy, CT may detect additional nodular lesions.[14,17] A limitation of chest CT scans is that many of these nodules are benign. [14,16,17] Furthermore, the chest CT scan cannot distinguish between primary and metastatic nodules. Although the specificity of chest CT is limited, the specificity can be enhanced with attention to other clinical factors. In addition, chest CT scans can be used for surgical planning.

Magnetic resonance imaging (MRI) has been used to evaluate lung nodules. Preliminary work suggests that conventional MRI does not have sufficient spatial resolution to provide any information beyond that provided by CT. The additional time and expense of chest MRI has precluded its routine use.

Cytologic studies to confirm a malignant diagnosis have limited value in evaluating a solitary pulmonary nodule. Cytologic specimens typically are obtained from sputum, bronchoscopic

S. J. Mentzer: Division of Thoracic Surgery, Department of Surgery, Harvard Medical School, Brigham and Women's Hospital, Boston, Massachusetts

D. J. Sugarbaker: Department of Surgery, Harvard Medical School, Boston, Massachusetts; Department of Surgery/Thoracic Surgery, Brigham and Women's Hospital, Boston, Massachusetts

TABLE 1. *Histopathologic findings after resection of pulmonary nodules*

		Histopathologic diagnosis (%)		
Study	*n*	Lung cancer	Breast cancer	Benign
Cahan et al.[12a]	78	63	30	5
Casey et al.[11]	42	52	43	5
Mentzer et al.[52b]	59	47	34	8

The patients in these series had histories of breast cancer and pulmonary nodules (typically solitary) on chest radiograph.

[a]Reported series of solitary pulmonary nodules. This report follows previous report from Cahan et al.[12]

[b]Four patients in this series had metastatic lesions identified from nonbreast occult primary tumors.

washing, and transthoracic needle biopsy. Specimens for cytologic sputum study should be obtained from sputum obtained in early morning on 3 consecutive days. Specimens should be appropriately collected to prevent oral contamination and carefully preserved to facilitate interpretation.[18] Sputum cytology can yield a malignant diagnosis in 80% of patients with a large central tumor.[19] The yield of cytologic study of sputum decreases to less than 25% with more peripheral lesions and diminishing size of the malignancy.[19] In patients undergoing bronchoscopic examination, endoscopic brushings and airway lavage of a peripheral lesion improve the cytologic yield to more than 70%.[20] The accuracy of both sputum and bronchial cytology is limited by small sample size. In addition, inflammatory exudates, excessive blood, or poor preservation decrease the tumor detection rate. Cytologically atypical cells in the lung often are associated with inflammatory disorders, further complicating the cytologic diagnosis of malignancy.

Transthoracic needle biopsy performed under fluoroscopic or CT guidance provides a cytologic specimen directly from the peripheral lung nodule. Needle-aspiration cytology provides a positive diagnosis of malignancy in 80% to 90% of patients with a malignant nodule.[21–23] The procedure is performed on an outpatient basis and carries a small risk of pneumothorax (approximately 10%).[23,24] The major problem with transthoracic needle biopsy is the appreciable false-negative rate.[25] For example, Charig et al.[21] found that, of 38 patients for whom no malignant cells were identified by the technique, 25 were subsequently confirmed to have a lung malignancy. Furthermore, the needle-aspiration cytology can differ from that of the resected specimens in as many as 35% of cases.[26] Another problem is that rarely does cytologic study positively establish a benign diagnosis. Even when bacterial or fungal forms are identified in a cytologic specimen, the possibility of a coexistent malignant disease is difficult to exclude.

Bronchoscopy also has a limited role in evaluation of a solitary pulmonary nodule. Bronchoscopy can facilitate cytologic diagnosis by airway washing, cytologic brushings, or bronchoalveolar lavage. These diagnostic approaches may be useful in establishing a diagnosis of infection caused by pulmonary pathogens such as *Mycobacterium tuberculosis*. Although infections with *M. tuberculosis* commonly result in nodular lesions, the patient must be carefully monitored to exclude coexistent carcinoma. Another bronchoscopic approach is fluoroscopically directed transbronchial biopsy. Transbronchial biopsies are useful in documenting diffuse parenchymal disease, such as lymphangitic carcinoma of the lung. The diagnostic yield of transbronchial biopsy in peripheral lung nodules is between 20% and 50%, depending on the size and location of the lesion.[1,10,27] Other limitations in the use of transbronchial biopsy to evaluate solitary pulmonary nodules are the small sample size (approximately 300 alveoli), the small risk of pneumothorax, and the potential delay in establishing a definitive diagnosis.

The most reliable approach to establishing a diagnosis in a patient with a solitary pulmonary nodule is surgery. Surgery provides adequate tissue for cytomorphologic, immunohistochemical, and protein receptor studies. In contrast to other diagnostic approaches, surgery avoids the sampling and interpretative errors that might delay definitive therapy. In the past, the major limitation with surgery was the morbidity associated with a standard thoracotomy. This limitation has been resolved with the development of videothoracoscopic surgery.

THORACOSCOPY

The thoracoscope provides an opportunity to diagnose and treat diseases of the chest with minimal morbidity. Thoracoscopic surgery involves a videothoracoscope and generally two working ports to facilitate manipulation of the lung and other intrathoracic structures[28–30] (Fig. 1). Working through two to three access ports, the surgeon can perform a variety of procedures. These minimally invasive procedures are generally referred to as *thoracoscopic operations*. The advantages of thoracoscopic video optics and miniaturized instrumentation have led to their incorporation into a variety of thoracic surgical procedures. Because these procedures are performed with variable incision lengths, this spectrum of surgical procedures has been referred to by the more inclusive term of *video-assisted thoracic surgery* (VATS).[31]

Videothoracoscopy is a surgical approach that requires the use of general anesthesia and a fully equipped operating room. Bronchoscopy is routinely performed at the beginning of the procedure to confirm placement of the double-lumen endotracheal tube or the bronchial blocker. Bronchoscopy also provides an opportunity to identify any potential occult endobronchial lesions.[32] Because bronchoscopy is routinely performed at the time of surgery, outpatient bronchoscopy is rarely indicated.

The morbidity of thoracoscopy is minimized by the small incisions used in the procedure. When pulmonary resections

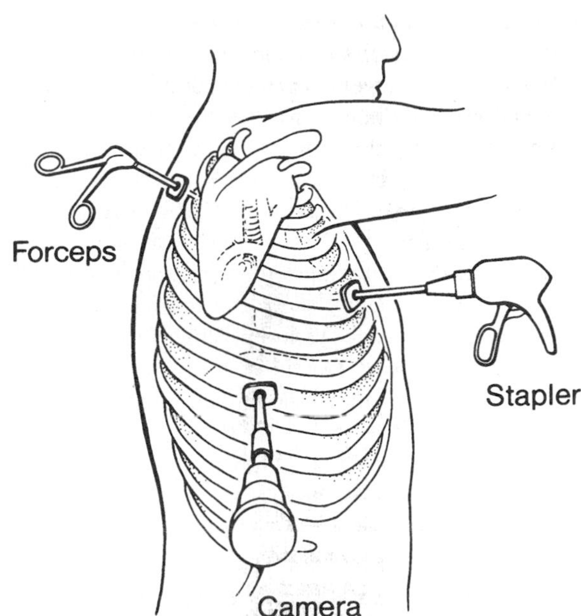

FIG. 1. Videothoracoscopy is performed with the patient in the lateral thoracotomy position. Thoracoscopy access ports are positioned to triangulate the area of interest and to facilitate the manipulation of intrathoracic structures. With single-lung ventilation, deflation of the ipsilateral lung provides an opportunity to examine the contents of the hemithorax. A solitary pulmonary nodule can be identified and resected to facilitate the histopathologic diagnosis. If the preliminary frozen section diagnosis is consistent with a primary lung metastasis, the thoracoscope can be used to surgically stage the ipsilateral hemithorax.

are performed, a chest tube drain is used to evacuate residual air and facilitate lung expansion. Depending on the extent of the resection and the condition of the remaining lung, the tube may be indwelling for less than an hour or for more than a few days.

Patients do experience some discomfort at the site of the access ports. This bruising pain can persist for several weeks. In addition, patients may complain of some numbness of the anterior chest wall. Both of these symptoms presumably are secondary to intraoperative compression of the intercostal nerve at the site of the access port. Localized discomfort is minimized by the application of intercostal nerve blocks using local anesthetics at the time of the procedure. More invasive analgesic techniques, such as the use of epidural analgesics, rarely are necessary after videothoracoscopic procedures. The typical thoracoscopic resection requires only an overnight hospitalization.

The primary benefit of thoracoscopy is the enhanced flexibility it provides in illuminating difficult diagnostic problems. Videothoracoscopy provides a panoramic view of the ipsilateral hemithorax. This view includes the visceral and parietal pleural surfaces, the internal chest wall, and the internal mammary, hilar, and paratracheal lymph nodes. In the patient with a history of breast cancer, videothoracoscopy provides an opportunity to examine the pleural surfaces for any evidence of malignancy. Small amounts of pleural fluid can be sent for cytologic examination, and biopsy can be performed directly on pleural nodules. Internal mammary, hilar, and paratracheal lymph nodes can be inspected and biopsies performed. In most cases, a solitary pulmonary nodule can be identified if it is within several centimeters of the visceral pleural surface of the lung. Adequate margins are obtained to ensure local control of a metastatic nodule and adequate sampling of a benign nodule.

Intraoperative frozen section histologic study of the lung nodule is routinely performed. If the nodule has special cytomorphologic features characteristic of the primary breast cancer, then no further staging is necessary. A benign appearance of the granulomatous lesions suggests that culturing of the nodule for mycobacterial and fungal pathogens may be appropriate. Alternatively, the frozen section histopathologic study may suggest the possibility of a primary lung cancer. For example, squamous cell differentiation, a small cell carcinoma appearance, or bronchoalveolar morphologic features would indicate a primary lung cancer. When these histopathologic characteristics are noted, a careful staging of hilar (N1) and ipsilateral paratracheal (N2) lymph nodes should be performed.

The clinical context and patient risk factors dictate whether a complete lobectomy is useful at the time of videothoracoscopy. In the case of a primary lung cancer, growing evidence suggests that only limited resection of a primary lung nodule is associated with a greater risk of local recurrence than is anatomic lobectomy.[33] Although definitive evidence is lacking, survival seems to be impacted as well.[33] The cumulative evidence at this time suggests that lobectomy is the standard cancer operation for patients with primary TX N0 or TX N1 lung cancers.

In a patient with staged disease and a definitive diagnosis of lung cancer, VATS anatomic resections often can be performed while the patient is still under anesthesia. Anatomic resection of a segment or lobe of the lung can be performed with significantly less morbidity than is associated with a standard thoracotomy. The development of improved thoracoscopic instruments should make VATS anatomic resections commonplace in the future. If an accurate histopathologic diagnosis cannot be established at the time of the thoracoscopic procedure, any further resection should be delayed. An advantage of videothoracoscopy is that it is minimally invasive. After the final pathologic specimen has been obtained, patients are physically capable of undergoing subsequent thoracotomy or VATS lobectomy.

The aggressive natural history of primary lung cancer underscores the importance of establishing a definitive histopathologic diagnosis of lung carcinoma. A definitive diagnosis, however, may be difficult to establish with peripheral adenocarcinomas. Peripheral adenocarcinomas can be ambiguous lesions, presenting a challenge to the pathologist and clinician in discriminating breast metastases from primary lung cancer.

In patients with a solitary breast metastasis, resecting the nodule may have some therapeutic value. Staren et al.[34] reported a mean survival of 58 months after resection of a solitary pulmonary nodule. Lanza et al.[35] reviewed 37 cases of surgical resection of a solitary nodule and found a 49.5% actuarial 5-year survival rate. These authors[35] and others[36,37] have found a correlation between a longer disease-free interval and improved survival after metastasectomy. This relationship is consistent with studies of metastases of other histologic types.[35,38,39] Although these retrospective studies are preliminary, the results suggest that the surgical resection of solitary pulmonary nodules may result in long-term survival benefit for selected patients.

A potential benefit for multiple metastasectomies has been proposed for sarcoma, germ cell tumors, and other selected tumors.[35,38,39] These tumors, however, are unique in their tropism for the lung. In contrast to these diseases, breast cancer does not demonstrate a selective pattern of pulmonary metastasis. The resection of multiple metastases in breast cancer is unlikely to have therapeutic value.[36]

PATHOLOGY

Primary tumors of the lung have a pathologic diagnosis of adenocarcinoma in 60% to 70% of cases.[9] Similarly, 80% of the metastatic lesions in the lung are adenocarcinoma.[3] Because of their histologic similarity, distinguishing between primary lung adenocarcinoma and metastatic breast cancer can be difficult. The combination of peripheral location, pleural retraction, anthracotic pigment, and central scarring was previously thought to be characteristic of primary lung tumors. These features, however, can be mimicked by metastatic adenocarcinoma of the breast.[40]

Occasionally, the morphologic features of the lung lesion may be identical to those of the primary breast tumor. Characteristic features, such as comedo differentiation or characteristic ductal pattern, may permit a definitive diagnosis of metastatic breast cancer. More commonly, cytomorphologic dissimilarity exists between the primary and the metastatic breast cancer lesions. This potential discrepancy is one of the primary limitations of diagnostic approaches based on cytologic studies alone.

The characteristic morphologic features of primary lung adenocarcinoma occasionally can be used to establish a diagnosis of primary lung cancer. Lung adenocarcinomas are commonly heterogeneous and can demonstrate areas of bronchoalveolar differentiation. Another characteristic of a primary lung tumor is the presence of mixed histologic features. Examples of mixed histologic types are adenosquamous differentiation and adenocarcinoma with small cell carcinoma elements. Although mixed histology can confirm a diagnosis of lung cancer, mixed histologic features are only observed in approximately 10% of non–small cell cancers.

Special studies occasionally can be helpful in distinguishing primary lung carcinoma from metastatic breast cancer. A problem with immunohistochemical or receptor protein studies is that breast cancer metastases can lose the expression of these distinguishing features. In addition, recurrent breast cancers in the lung are estrogen-receptor positive in only 25% of cases.[41] Confounding this observation is the finding that primary lung cancers can express a variety of unexpected proteins. For example, estrogen receptors are expressed in approximately 30% of primary lung adenocarcinomas.[42] Similarly, progesterone receptors have been described in approximately 15% of primary lung cancers.[42]

In addition to diagnostic cytomorphologic features, the most distinguishing pathologic feature of breast metastases to the lung is immunohistochemical staining for gross cystic disease fluid protein (GCDFP).[43–45] GCDFP is a small-molecular-weight protein that is associated with apocrine differentiation. It has not been reported in primary lung carcinomas and can effectively exclude the diagnosis of a lung primary.[44–46] The limitation of staining for GCDFP is that the antigen is present in only 30% to 50% of breast cancer metastases.[46–48] Furthermore, primary breast cancers that express this protein may lose antigen expression when they recur systemically. Although the frequency with which lung nodules express the protein is low, it is the only marker that seems to distinguish lung primaries from breast metastases.

Several new approaches are likely to help in distinguishing primary and metastatic cancers in the future. The development of new monoclonal antibodies suggests that immunohistochemical studies may contribute to the definitive diagnosis of lung cancer.[49–51] Examining the cytogenetic features of the tumor also may be helpful. Lung cancers such as small cell carcinoma seem to express characteristic chromosomal deletions. Small cell carcinoma, for example, typically demonstrates a deletion of the short arm of chromosome 3 (3p). This deletion is rarely seen in patients with breast cancer. Although uniform cytogenetic abnormalities have not been identified for adenocarcinoma of the lung or breast, this is an area that has the potential to contribute to the discrimination of primary lung carcinoma and metastatic breast cancer.

MANAGEMENT SUMMARY

Patients with a history of breast cancer and discrete pulmonary nodules need a tissue diagnosis to exclude benign disease or primary lung cancer.

Lung cancer is the most common cause of death in women with cancer. The diagnosis of a primary lung tumor must be considered in a patient with pulmonary adenocarcinoma.

A cytologic diagnosis of malignancy is rarely sufficient to exclude a primary lung cancer, and a benign cytologic diagnosis is at risk for sampling error. Thoracoscopy provides a minimally invasive approach to obtain definitive tissue for histopathologic study and staging information regarding the pleura, ipsilateral paratracheal, and internal mammary lymph nodes.

REFERENCES

1. Swensen SJ, Silverstein MD, Ilstrup DM, Schleck CD, Edell ES. The probability of malignancy in solitary pulmonary nodules. Application to small radiologically indeterminate nodules. *Arch Intern Med* 1997;157:849.
2. Anderson RW, Arentzen CE. Carcinoma of the lung. *Surg Clin North Am* 1980;60:793.
3. Abrams HL, Spiro R, Goldstein N. Metastases in carcinoma. Analysis of 1000 autopsied cases. *Cancer* 1950;3:74.
4. Warren S, Witham EM. Studies on tumor metastasis. 2. The distribution of metastases in cancer of the breast. *Surg Gynecol Obstet* 1933;57:81.
5. Saphir O, Parker ML. Metastasis of primary carcinoma of the breast with special reference to spleen, adrenal glands and ovaries. *Arch Surg* 1941;42:1003.
6. Kamby C, Vejborg I, Kristensen B, Olsen LO, Mouridsen HT. Metastatic pattern in recurrent breast cancer. Special reference to intrathoracic recurrences. *Cancer* 1988;62:2226.
7. Kamby C, Rose C, Ejlertsen B, Andersen J, Birkler NE, Rytter L, Andersen KW, Zedeler K. Stage and pattern of metastases in patients with breast cancer. *Eur J Cancer Clin Oncol* 1987;23:1925.
8. Nikkanen TA. Recurrence of breast cancer. A retrospective study of 569 cases in clinical stages I–III. *Acta Chir Scand* 1981;147:239.
9. Boring CC, Squires TS, Tong T, Montgomery S. Cancer statistics. *CA Cancer J Clin* 1994;44:7.
10. Swensen SJ, Jett JR, Payne WS, Viggiano RW, Pairolero PC, Trastek VF. An integrated approach to evaluation of the solitary pulmonary nodule. *Mayo Clin Proc* 1990;65:173.
11. Casey JJ, Stempel BG, Scanlon EF, Fry WA. The solitary pulmonary nodule in the patient with breast cancer. *Surgery* 1984;96:801.
12. Cahan WG, Castro EB, Huvos AG. Primary breast and lung carcinoma in the same patient. *J Thorac Cardiovasc Surg* 1974;68:546.
13. Cahan WG, Castro EB. Significance of a solitary lung shadow in patients with breast cancer. *Ann Surg* 1975;181:137.
14. Scott WW Jr, Fishman EK. Detection of internal mammary lymph node enlargement: comparison of CT scans and conventional roentgenograms. *Clin Imaging* 1991;15:268.
15. Chalmers N, Best JJ. The significance of pulmonary nodules detected by CT but not by chest radiography in tumour staging. *Clin Radiol* 1991;44:410.
16. Davis SD. CT evaluation for pulmonary metastases in patients with extrathoracic malignancy. *Radiology* 1991;180:1.
17. Fernandez EB, Colon E, McLeod DG, Moul JW. Efficacy of radiographic chest imaging in patients with testicular cancer. *Urology* 1994;44:243(discussion 248).
18. Walts AE. Cytologic techniques for the diagnosis of pulmonary neoplasms. In: Marchevsky AM, ed. *Lung biology in health and disease. Surgical pathology of lung neoplasms*. New York: Marcel Dekker, 1990:29.
19. Ng AB, Horak GC. Factors significant in the diagnostic accuracy of lung cytology in bronchial washing and sputum samples. II. Sputum samples. *Acta Cytol* 1983;27:397.
20. Ng AB, Horak GC. Factors significant in the diagnostic accuracy of lung cytology in bronchial washing and sputum samples. I. Bronchial washings. *Acta Cytol* 1983;27:391.
21. Charig MJ, Stutley JE, Padley SP, Hansell DM. The value of negative needle biopsy in suspected operable lung cancer. *Clin Radiol* 1991; 44:147.
22. Zakowski MF, Gatscha RM, Zaman MB. Negative predictive value of pulmonary fine needle aspiration cytology. *Acta Cytol* 1992;36:283.
23. Cristallini EG, Ascani S, Farabi R, Paganelli C, Peciarolo A, Bolis GB. Fine needle aspiration biopsy in the diagnosis of intrathoracic masses. *Acta Cytol* 1992;36:416.
24. Collins CD, Breatnach E, Nath PH. Percutaneous needle biopsy of lung nodules following failed bronchoscopic biopsy. *Eur J Radiol* 1992;15:49.
25. Veale D, Gilmartin JJ, Sumerling MD, Wadehra V, Gibson GJ. Prospective evaluation of fine needle aspiration in the diagnosis of lung cancer. *Thorax* 1988;43:540.
26. Horrigan TP, Bergin KT, Snow N. Correlation between needle biopsy of lung tumors and histopathologic analysis of resected specimens. *Chest* 1986;90:638.
27. Wang KP, Haponik EF, Britt EJ, Khouri N, Erozan Y. Transbronchial needle aspiration of peripheral pulmonary nodules. *Chest* 1984;86:819.
28. DeCamp MM Jr, Jaklitsch MT, Mentzer SJ, Harpole DH Jr, Sugarbaker DJ. The safety and versatility of video-thoracoscopy: a prospective analysis of 895 consecutive cases. *J Am Coll Surg* 1995; 181:113.
29. Mentzer SJ, Sugarbaker DJ. Thoracoscopy and video-assisted thoracic surgery. In Brooks DC, ed. *Current techniques in laparoscopy*. Philadelphia: Current Medicine, 1994;20.1–20.12.
30. Landreneau RJ, Mack MJ, Hazelrigg SR, et al. Video-assisted thoracic surgery: basic technical concepts and intercostal approach strategies. *Ann Thorac Surg* 1992;54:800.
31. McKneally MF, Lewis RJ, Anderson RJ, et al. Statement of the AATS/STS Joint Committee on Thoracoscopy and Video Assisted Thoracic Surgery. *J Thorac Cardiovasc Surg* 1992;104:1.
32. King DS, Castleman B. Bronchial involvement in metastatic pulmonary malignancy. *J Thorac Surg* 1943;12:305.
33. Ginsberg RJ, Rubinstein LV. Randomized trial of lobectomy versus limited resection for T1 N0 non-small cell lung cancer. Lung Cancer Study Group [see comments]. *Ann Thorac Surg* 1995;60:615(discussion 622).
34. Staren ED, Salerno C, Rongione A, Witt TR, Faber LP. Pulmonary resection for metastatic breast cancer. *Arch Surg* 1992;127:1282.
35. Lanza LA, Natarajan G, Roth JA, Putnam JB Jr. Long-term survival after resection of pulmonary metastases from carcinoma of the breast. *Ann Thorac Surg* 1992;54:244(discussion 248).
36. Friedel G, Linder A, Toomes H. The significance of prognostic factors for the resection of pulmonary metastases of breast cancer. *Thorac Cardiovasc Surg* 1994;42:71.
37. Schlappack OK, Baur M, Steger G, Dittrich C, Moser K. The clinical course of lung metastases from breast cancer. *Klin Wochenschr* 1988;66:790.
38. Brandt B, Ehrenhaft JL. Surgical management of pulmonary metastasis. *Curr Probl Cancer* 1980;4:1.
39. Mentzer SJ, Antman KH, Attinger C, Shemin R, Corson JM, Sugarbaker DJ. Selected benefits of thoracotomy and chemotherapy for sarcoma metastatic to the lung. *J Surg Oncol* 1993;53:54.
40. Marchevsky AM. Metastatic tumors of the lung. In: Marchevsky AM, ed. *Lung biology in health and disease. Surgical pathology of lung neoplasms*. New York: Marcel Dekker, 1990:231.
41. Johnson FE, Rosen PP, Menendez-Botet C, Schwartz MK, Ashikari R, Kinne DW. Estrogen receptor protein in visceral metastases from breast carcinoma. *Am J Surg* 1981;142:252.
42. Beattie CW, Hansen NW, Thomas PA. Steroid receptors in human lung cancer. *Cancer Res* 1985;45:4206.
43. Wick MR, Lillemoe TJ, Copland GT, Swanson PE, Manivel JC, Kiang DT. Gross cystic disease fluid protein-15 as a marker for breast cancer: immunohistochemical analysis of 690 human neoplasms and comparison with alpha-lactalbumin. *Hum Pathol* 1989;20:281.
44. Brown RW, Campagna LB, Dunn JK, Cagle PT. Immunohistochemical identification of tumor markers in metastatic adenocarcinoma. A diagnostic adjunct in the determination of primary site. *Am J Clin Pathol* 1997;107:12.
45. Pagani A, Sapino A, Eusebi V, Bergnolo P, Bussolati G. PIP/GCDFP-15 gene expression and apocrine differentiation in carcinomas of the breast. *Virchows Arch* 1994;425:459.
46. Chaubert P, Hurlimann J. Mammary origin of metastases. Immunohistochemical determination. *Arch Pathol Lab Med* 1992;116:1181.
47. Monteagudo C, Merino MJ, LaPorte N, Neumann RD. Value of gross cystic disease fluid protein-15 in distinguishing metastatic breast carcinomas among poorly differentiated neoplasms involving the ovary. *Hum Pathol* 1991;22:368.
48. Fiel MI, Cernaianu G, Burstein DE, Batheja N. Value of GCDFP-15 (BRST-2) as a specific immunocytochemical marker for breast carcinoma in cytologic specimens. *Acta Cytol* 1996;40:637.
49. Ioachim HL, Pambuccian S, Giancotti F, Dorsett B. Reactivity of lung tumors with lung-derived and non-lung-derived monoclonal antibodies. *Int J Cancer Suppl* 1994;8:132.
50. Kawai T, Torikata C, Suzuki M. Immunohistochemical study of pulmonary adenocarcinoma. *Am J Clin Pathol* 1988;89:455.
51. Souhami RL, Beverley PC, Bobrow LG, Ledermann JA. Antigens of lung cancer: results of the second international workshop on lung cancer antigens. *J Natl Cancer Inst* 1991;83:609.
52. Mentzer SJ, DeCamp MM, Harpole DH, et al. Thorascopic evaluation of intrathoracic malignancy in patients with breast cancer. 1999 (*in preparation*).

Diseases of the Breast, 2nd ed.,
edited by Jay R. Harris.
Lippincott Williams & Wilkins, Philadelphia © 2000.

CHAPTER 59

Management of Discrete Liver Metastasis

Mark S. Talamonti

More than 50% of patients who develop metastatic breast cancer ultimately manifest some degree of liver involvement.[1] Hepatic failure secondary to metastatic disease is a major cause of death in approximately 20% of patients with breast cancer.[2] In general, hepatic metastases occur in the setting of widely disseminated disease. The presence of metastatic disease isolated to the liver is an uncommon finding. Estimates are that only 2% to 12% of patients develop metastatic disease limited to the liver.[3,4] Only a small fraction of these patients have disease so limited that they are considered candidates for liver-directed therapy.

Accordingly, the principle of treatment for patients with visceral metastases, and specifically liver tumors, is to consider them part of widely disseminated disease and to treat appropriately with systemic forms of therapy, such as endocrine manipulation and systemic chemotherapy. In light of the advances made since 1980 in the treatment of patients with isolated liver metastases from colorectal and neuroendocrine tumors, consideration has now been given to identifying a subset of patients with limited metastases from breast cancer who might be considered viable candidates for liver resection. This chapter focuses on the criteria for selecting patients who may be candidates for resection and the results when resection is applied to patients with isolated liver metastases from primary breast cancer.

GENERAL PRINCIPLES OF PATIENT SELECTION FOR LIVER SURGERY

The incidence of breast cancer continues to increase throughout the United States. At the time of diagnosis, 5% to 10% of patients have hepatic metastases, and another 30% to 40% develop metastatic liver tumors subsequent to the resection of their primary tumors.[2] As noted, only 2% to 12% of these patients have limited, isolated liver metastases.[3,4] Therefore, before patients are selected for liver-directed therapies, they must undergo an extensive evaluation to rule out the presence of extrahepatic metastatic disease. In general, patients who have undergone liver resection for colorectal cancers experience a significant improvement in overall survival if they have first undergone a highly selective process to exclude extrahepatic disease. The selection of patients for liver resection is therefore largely a process of exclusion. Patients presenting with limited liver disease do not, in general, present with any severe loss of performance status.[5] The patient with an isolated liver metastasis usually does not manifest any significant weight loss or deterioration in normal daily performance status. These patients are usually asymptomatic, and the first manifestation of their liver disease may be an incidental discovery of elevated values on liver function studies or the presence of a mass lesion on routine ultrasonography or computed tomographic (CT) scan of the abdomen. The patient with a liver metastasis who demonstrates significant weight loss, weakness, and loss of performance status is unlikely to have disease limited to the liver. A routine metastatic evaluation in such a patient is likely to demonstrate pronounced pulmonary metastases or disseminated bone metastases. Thus, when a patient is considered for liver resection, the first criterion that should be met is the absence of any systemic complaints or findings that would suggest disseminated cancer or an inability to physically tolerate a major abdominal procedure. Clinical findings such as ascites, jaundice, and pain associated with large or rapidly growing hepatic tumors are usually a sign of late, advanced disease. Laboratory measurements of various tumor markers and liver enzymes may be elevated, but they are usually nonspecific in terms of defining the extent of liver disease. A patient with a discrete liver metastasis is unlikely to have a markedly elevated serum bilirubin level or alkaline phosphatase level, or high levels of the various transaminases.[5]

Precise radiographic staging of patients with a discrete liver metastasis is absolutely crucial. A CT scan of the chest, abdomen, and pelvis should be performed to exclude the presence of pulmonary metastases, pleural effusions, or significant mediastinal adenopathy. The CT scan of the abdomen and the pelvis should exclude the presence of significant extrahepatic adenopathy, ascites, and omental or peritoneal nodules. The presence of any of these findings in either the chest or the abdomen would remove the patient as a candidate for formal liver surgery. Confirmation of the

M. S. Talamonti: Department of Surgery, Gastrointestinal Oncology Program, Northwestern University School of Medicine, Chicago, Illinois

metastatic nature of these findings should be performed by radiographically guided fine-needle aspiration. In addition, adequate radiographic imaging of the liver is necessary to define the extent of liver disease and the anatomic location of any identified liver tumors. The presence of multiple, bilobar liver nodules would exclude a patient from liver surgery. The most favorable candidate for liver resection of a discrete liver metastasis is a patient with a solitary metastasis located in such a position that the surgical margin would exceed 1 to 2 cm and would not involve any major intrahepatic vascular structures. Thus, the ideal candidate for a liver resection is a patient with a solitary liver metastasis located in the periphery of the liver and in whom extensive staging studies have failed to reveal any evidence of extrahepatic metastasis. To the contrary, the patient with a large, centrally located lesion deep within the parenchyma of the liver and in close proximity to the deep hepatic veins or inferior vena cava might not be considered the most favorable candidate for such a procedure.

In addition to the anatomic and physiologic criteria used to select patients for liver resection, consideration must also be given to prognostic characteristics of the patient's primary tumor. Patients who present with simultaneous liver metastases and aggressive primary tumors should be considered for primary systemic chemotherapy. Patients with large, biologically aggressive tumors or patients with multiple axillary lymph node metastases who also have limited hepatic disease at the time of presentation should not initially be considered candidates for liver-directed therapy. In these patients, liver disease is probably only a manifestation of already widely disseminated cancer. In general, liver resection for tumors in these patients should be considered only if the tumor demonstrates a sustained response to systemic chemotherapy. Conversely, the patient who develops a solitary liver metastasis several years after having received multimodal therapy for a relatively early stage cancer would more likely be a candidate for surgical resection.

In summary, patients considered for liver resection must have experienced sustained control of the primary tumor and show sufficient performance status to withstand the rigors of surgical resection. In addition, an exhaustive metastatic evaluation, including a bone scan and CT scans of the chest, abdomen, and pelvis, should exclude extrahepatic metastases. Finally, the disease within the liver should be limited preferably to a solitary tumor located in a position not compromised by any of the major intrahepatic vascular structures.

RESULTS OF SURGICAL RESECTION

Refinements in surgical technique for the resection of metastatic tumors have significantly improved the safety of these operations. Liver resection for metastases from colorectal cancers can now be performed with an operative mortality of less than 5%.[6–19] The improvement in operative morbidity and mortality is attributed to several different factors. Improved understanding of the segmental anatomy of the liver, and specifically its intrahepatic blood supply, has allowed safer hepatic resections with minimized blood loss. In addition, improved preoperative diagnostic imaging has excluded from operation patients for whom the operative risks caused by major vascular involvement would have resulted in major complications. Resection techniques incorporating vascular inflow occlusion, minimized parenchymal destruction, decreased intraoperative blood loss, and successful management of postoperative complications have improved the safety of this operation. As a result, the operative morbidity and mortality associated with hepatic surgery has significantly decreased, with most studies reporting operative mortality rates between 2% and 7%.[6–19]

In highly selected patients, the 5-year survival rate after liver resection for metastatic colon cancer now approaches 25% to 30%.[6–19] Because of improved operative mortality rates and reasonable expectations for long-term survival after resection for colorectal metastases, several centers have begun to examine survival rates after liver resection for metastases from noncolorectal primary sites. Reports of hepatectomy for liver metastases from breast cancer have been small in number and frequently presented with results of resection for other noncolon primary tumors. In those series with strict patient selection criteria and adequate follow-up, the operative mortality rate was less than 5%, and the overall survival rate was usually significantly better than for similar patients treated with systemic chemotherapy. Most patients still succumbed to their disease, and the liver was frequently a site of recurrent cancer.

Raab et al. reported on 35 liver resections in 34 patients with liver metastases from breast cancer.[20] The median age of patients was 47 years. The median interval between the primary operation and the liver resection was 27.3 months. A solitary metastasis was present in approximately 60% of the patients. A curative resection was possible in 86% of the patients explored, and the operative mortality rate was 3%. The overall 5-year survival rate was 18.4%; median survival was 27 months. The prognosis was significantly better after a complete resection in which all gross disease was removed and the margins of resection were microscopically negative. Other factors, such as stage of the primary tumor and number and size of the metastases, had no prognostic significance. Recurrence rates within the liver were not reported.

Elias et al. of the Institut Gustav Roussy in Villejuif, France, reported on 21 patients undergoing hepatic resection for metastatic breast cancer.[21,22] Nineteen of the patients underwent combined treatment with preoperative and postoperative chemotherapy. After the liver resection, the median survival was 26 months; the 2-year and 5-year survival rates were 50% and 9%, respectively. The mean time to recurrence after hepatectomy was 14.8 months, and the liver was involved in 75% of the cases in which recurrence was seen. The liver was the first site of recurrence in 56% of these patients. In this limited series, the number of liver metastases, the number of positive lymph nodes, and a response to preoperative chemotherapy were not significant prognostic factors. Patients with negative lymph nodes in the porta hepatis tended to have a better prognosis, however, as did those in whom the liver was the first and only site of relapse.

Stehlin et al. reported on a series of 71 patients with liver metastasis treated by regional chemotherapy.[23] In nine cases, a liver resection was performed in addition to the regional therapy. These patients had a significantly better survival rate than those undergoing regional therapy alone. Median survival of the resected patients was 28 months, with an estimated 5-year survival rate of 16%. Nevertheless, the majority of these patients died with recurrent disease in the liver.

Harrison et al. described seven liver resections performed at the Memorial Sloan-Kettering Cancer Center for metastatic breast cancer.[24] Although one patient died of disease 118 months after resection, three patients died within 1 year of resection.

Because up to 75% of patients have recurrences with the liver as the initial site of relapse after resection, Schneebaum et al. combined adjuvant regional chemotherapy with liver resection.[25] A total of 40 patients were treated with regional therapy consisting of surgical resection with or without regional chemotherapy via hepatic artery or portal vein catheters. The 18 patients receiving combined regional therapy and surgery had a median survival of 27 months, compared with 5 months for a similar control group treated with systemic chemotherapy. Although the selection criteria were not completely elucidated in this report and the series is small, the data suggest a possible role for liver resection when combined with aggressive regional chemotherapy.

Because of the limited number of patients who present with an isolated or solitary liver metastasis amenable to surgical resection, other forms of liver-directed therapy have been applied for patients with liver metastases from breast cancer. Cryosurgical tumor ablation has been used to treat a variety of primary and metastatic liver tumors. Cryosurgery refers to the *in situ* freezing and devitalization of neoplastic tissue using a device that circulates liquid nitrogen within the tumor mass. Subzero temperatures of –195°C can be obtained. The general advantage is *in situ* destruction of the tumor with minimal blood loss and no significant loss of normal hepatic parenchyma.[26]

Bilchik et al. have reported their experience with cryosurgery for breast cancer metastases.[27] Their initial series of patients with noncolorectal hepatic metastases included six patients with metastatic breast tumors. The size, extent, and number of hepatic lesions were not described. At the time of the report, four of the six patients remained alive after treatment, with a mean survival of 30 months. No deaths or significant complications resulted from the procedure.

Other forms of liver-directed therapy that have been described in the treatment of patients with metastatic breast tumors include regional hepatic artery chemotherapy and chemoembolization. Neither of these methods has been subjected to a randomized controlled study comparing these modalities to systemic chemotherapy. Response rates of 20% to 40% have been reported. Overall survival rates have not been significantly greater that those for patients undergoing systemic forms of therapy, a finding that probably reflects the disseminated nature of the cancer and the advanced stage of disease at the time of treatment.

MANAGEMENT SUMMARY

Hepatic resection for metastatic breast cancer is a procedure with limited applicability but with the potential to prolong survival in highly selected patients. In properly selected patients, the limited series that have been reported suggest a median survival of 25 to 30 months, with an occasional long-term survival and cure. Patients considered for surgical resection of a discrete liver metastasis should have adequate performance status and acceptable hepatic function. Patients with poor hepatic function have a higher morbidity and mortality rate after hepatic resection and should be excluded from surgical exploration. A thorough and precise metastatic evaluation should be performed before considering patients for liver surgery. This evaluation should include a bone scan and CT scans of the chest, abdomen, and pelvis. Percutaneous biopsy should be performed on suspicious fluid collections or mass lesions outside of the liver to rule out the presence of extrahepatic metastatic disease. Precise imaging of the liver should be accomplished with helical CT scan or MRI. The presence of multiple lesions or bilobar lesions should exclude patients from surgical exploration for resection. Cryosurgery is a feasible alternative to resection for patients with bilobar, multiple metastases. Whether this technique offers any survival advantage relative to systemic treatments remains to be determined.

Finally, patterns of failure after liver resection suggest frequent relapse within the liver and at extrahepatic sites. Metastatic liver disease is usually an indication of systemic disease. Surgical excision, therefore, should be used as an adjuvant treatment to preoperative and postoperative systemic chemotherapy. Other treatments for liver metastases include hepatic artery infusional chemotherapy, radiation therapy, chemoembolization, and a variety of experimental regional perfusion procedures. None of these treatments has been shown to definitely improve the survival of patients with liver metastases from breast cancer.

REFERENCES

1. Jardines L, Callans LS, Torosian MH. Recurrent breast cancer: presentation, diagnosis and treatment. *Semin Oncol* 1993;20:538.
2. Zinser JW, Hortobagyi GN, Buzdar AU, Smith TL, Fraschini G. Clinical course of breast cancer patients with liver metastases. *J Clin Oncol* 1987;5:773.
3. Viadana E, Bross IDJ, Pickren JW. An autopsy study of some routes of dissemination of cancer of the breast. *Br J Cancer* 1973;27:336.
4. Lee Y. Breast carcinoma: patterns of metastasis at autopsy. *J Surg Oncol* 1983;23:175.

5. Foster JH, Lundy J. Liver metastases. *Curr Probl Surg* 1981;8:160.
6. Adson MA, van Heerden JA, Adson MH, et al. Resection of hepatic metastases from colorectal cancer. *Arch Surg* 1984;119:647.
7. Ringe B, Bechstein WO, Raab R, et al. Leberresektion bei 157 Patienten mit colorectalen Metastasen. *Chirurg* 1990;61:272.
8. Doci R, Gennari L, Bignami P, et al. One hundred patients with hepatic metastases from colorectal cancer treated by resection: analysis of prognostic determinants. *Br J Surg* 1991;78:797.
9. Herfarth C, Hohenberger P. Synchrone Resektion von Lebermetastasen kolorektaler Karzinome. *Langenbecks Arch Chir* (*Kongressbericht 1992*) 1992;72:66.
10. Rosen CB, Nagorney DM, Taswell HF, et al. Perioperative blood transfusion and determinants of survival after liver resection for metastatic colorectal carcinoma. *Ann Surg* 1992;216:493.
11. Sugihara K, Hojo K, Moriya Y, et al. Pattern of recurrence after hepatic resection for colorectal metastases. *Br J Surg* 1993;80:1032.
12. Gozzetti G, Mazziotti A, Grazi GL, et al. Undici anni di esperienza nella terapia chirurgica delle metastasi epatiche da tumori colo-rettali. *Chirurg Ital* 1994;46:30.
13. Gayowski TJ, Iwatsuki S, Madariaga JR, et al. Experience in hepatic resection for metastatic colorectal cancer: analysis of clinical and pathologic risk factors. *Surgery* 1994;116:703.
14. Scheele J, Altendorf-Hofmann A, Stangl R, Schmidt K. Chirurgische Resektion kolorektaler Lebermatastasen: gold-standard fur solitare und resektable Herde. *Swiss Surg Suppl* 1996;4:4.
15. Hughes KS, Simon RM, Songhorabodi S, et al. Resection of the liver for colorectal carcinoma metastases: a multi-institutional study of indications for resection. *Surgery* 1988;103:278.
16. Nordlinger B, Jaeck D, Guiguet M, et al. Surgical resection of hepatic metastases. Multicentric retrospective study by the French Association of Surgery. In: Nordlinger B, Jaeck D, eds. *Treatment of hepatic metastases of colorectal cancer*. Paris: Springer France, 1992: 129.
17. Van Ooigen B, Wiggers T, Meijer S, et al. Hepatic resections for colorectal metastases in the Netherlands, a multi-institutional 10-year study. *Cancer* 1992;70:28.
18. Fong Y, Blumgart LH, Cohen A, et al. Repeat hepatic resection for metastatic colorectal cancer. *Ann Surg* 1994;220:657.
19. Wanebo HJ, Chu LD, Vezeridis MP, et al. Patient selection for hepatic resection of colorectal metastases. *Arch Surg* 1996;131:322.
20. Raab R, Nussbaum K-T, Behrend M, Weimann A. Liver metastases of breast cancer: results of liver resection. *Anticancer Res* 1998;18:2231.
21. Elias D, Lasser PH, Montrucolli D, Bonvallot S, Spielmann M. Hepatectomy for liver metastases from breast cancer. *Eur J Surg Oncol* 1995;21:510.
22. Elias D, Lasser P, Spielmann M, et al. Surgical and chemotherapeutic treatment of hepatic metastases from carcinoma of the breast. *Surg Gynecol Obstet* 1991;172:461.
23. Stehlin JS, de Ipolyi PD, Greef PJ, McGaff CJ, Davis BR, McNary L. Treatment of cancer of the liver—twenty years' experience with infusion and resection in 414 patients. *Ann Surg* 1988;208:23.
24. Harrison LE, Brennan MF, Newman E, et al. Hepatic resection for noncolorectal, nonneuroendocrine metastases: a fifteen-year experience with ninety-six patients. *Surgery* 1997;121:625.
25. Schneebaum S, Walker MJ, Young D, Farrar WB, Minton JP. The regional treatment of liver metastases from breast cancer. *J Surg Oncol* 1994;55:26.
26. Staren E, Sabel MS, Gianakakis LM, et al. Cryosurgery of breast cancer. *Arch Surg* 1997;132:28.
27. Bilchik AJ, Sarantou T, Wardlaw JC, Ramming KP. Cryosurgery causes a profound reduction in tumor markers in hepatoma and noncolorectal hepatic metastases. *Am Surg* 1997;63:796.

Diseases of the Breast, 2nd ed.,
edited by Jay R. Harris.
Lippincott Williams & Wilkins, Philadelphia © 2000.

CHAPTER 60

Biology of Bone Metastases

Gregory R. Mundy, Theresa A. Guise, and Toshiyuki Yoneda

Cancer affects the skeleton in multiple ways. The effects of cancer cells on bone, however, are predominantly indirect and are mediated by alterations in the activities of osteoclasts and osteoblasts, the major bone-resorbing and bone-forming cells. Of all the malignancies that alter bone cell function, breast cancer is predominant. Between 70% and 100% (probably close to 100%) of patients with advanced breast cancer have skeletal involvement, and this involvement is a major cause of morbidity in these patients. This chapter reviews the mechanism by which breast cancer affects the skeleton, its clinical consequences, and potential mechanisms for treatment.

CLASSIFICATION OF BONE METASTASES

Tumors such as breast cancer that frequently involve the skeleton cause two distinct types of skeletal lesions. Breast cancer usually causes a destructive or osteolytic lesion. In this type of metastatic bone lesion, tumor products distort the normal remodeling sequence so that an increase is seen primarily in osteoclast activity. The secondary osteoblast response, seen in normal bone remodeling, is almost always impaired to a varying degree, so that the lesion is predominantly lytic. Less common is the osteoblastic response, which may occur without previous resorption. This latter response, however, is very complex and less well understood. The mechanisms that are responsible for the distinctive and discrete effects of metastatic breast cancer cells on osteoblasts and osteoclasts involved in normal bone remodeling remain obscure.

FREQUENCY OF BONE METASTASES

The most common malignant tumors that affect humankind involve the skeleton. Approximately 700,000 people die of cancer in the United States each year,[1] and at least two-thirds of these have bone metastases. More than 220,000 people die with lung and breast cancer, and the frequency of bone metastases in these patients is even greater. Although bone metastasis occurs frequently with nearly all tumors, special types of cancers have a special predilection for the skeleton. In particular, breast cancer and prostate cancer almost always metastasize to the skeleton, and other common solid tumors, such as lung cancer, frequently do. Patients with these cancers probably account for 80% or more of patients with metastatic bone disease.[2] Bone metastases also occur commonly in thyroid and renal cancers.

These estimates of the frequency of metastasis are dependent on the sensitivity of the diagnostic techniques used. The techniques that have been used most frequently are bone scanning, radiography, and histologic examination of autopsy specimens. Both radiologic and histologic assessments are limited by the extent of the sample evaluated. Bone scans survey the whole body, but because isotope accumulation depends on osteoblast activity, lesions with very low osteoblastic component may not be detected.

The natural history of skeletal metastases in patients with breast cancer is probably different from that in patients with other common malignancies, such as lung cancer. Although bone metastases occur in the majority of dying patients with each of these malignancies, the presence of bone metastases has a very different prognostic implication in breast cancer than in lung cancer. In lung cancer, the prognosis for patients with metastatic disease in any site is poor, irrespective of the histologic type. Most patients with metastatic disease are dead within a few months. In contrast, in patients with breast cancer, metastases in bone do not necessarily mean a poor short-term prognosis. The median duration of survival in patients with bone metastases alone (i.e., no metastases in other soft-tissue sites) is 24 months; 20% of patients are alive at 5 years. The duration of survival of patients with visceral involvement is much shorter, usually a matter of a few months.[3] As in women with breast cancer, the median duration of survival in men with prostate cancer is 48 months. Thus, patients with bone metastases due to breast and prostate cancer have skeletal morbidity for a significant portion of their remaining years.

G. R. Mundy: Department of Medicine, University of Texas Health Science Center at San Antonio, San Antonio, Texas

T. A. Guise: Departments of Medicine and Endocrinology, University of Texas Health Science Center at San Antonio, San Antonio, Texas

T. Yoneda: Division of Endocrinology and Metabolism, Department of Medicine, University of Texas Health Science Center at San Antonio, San Antonio, Texas

FAVORED SITES OF SKELETAL INVOLVEMENT BY MALIGNANT DISEASE

Tumor cells most frequently affect those parts of the skeleton that are the most heavily vascularized, and in particular the red bone marrow of the axial skeleton and the proximal ends of the long bones, the ribs, and the vertebral column. This is true both for hematologic malignancies and for all solid tumors, of which breast cancer is the most obvious example. Although metastases to the appendicular skeleton occur less frequently, they may be seen especially in patients with melanoma and renal cancer. Breast cancer cells sometimes metastasize to the posterior clinoid processes. The precise reasons for these unusual distributions of bone lesions are not clear. Galasko[4,5] has reviewed in detail the distribution of skeletal metastases from various solid tumors. The major, but not the sole, determinant of the site of metastasis is blood flow from the primary site. Because prostate cancer frequently metastasizes to the vertebral column, the suggestion was made 50 years ago that access through the vertebral-venous plexus of veins (Batson's plexus) is important. However, venous blood from the breast also flows into the vertebral-venous plexus, as well as the vena cava. Batson's plexus is a low-pressure, high-volume system of vertebral veins that can communicate with the intercostal veins and runs up the spine. The suggestion has been made that Batson's vertebral plexus is responsible for the distribution of prostate tumor cell metastasis to the spine. This plexus has extensive intercommunications that apparently function independently of other major venous systems, such as the pulmonary, caval, and portal systems.[6] It has been studied by the injection of dye into the dorsal vein of the penis in cadavers and experimental animals.[6] A number of workers have suggested that this system may be important for the spread of tumor cells to the axial skeleton.[4,5,7,8] Dodds et al.,[9] however, have questioned whether prostate cancer cells do in fact spread preferentially through this paravertebral plexus to the spine.

CLINICAL CONSEQUENCES

The consequences of skeletal involvement by cancer are catastrophic for the patient. Patients frequently develop intractable bone pain, which may be either constant or intermittent. It is almost always severe, however, and represents a considerable cause of morbidity in patients with advanced cancer. The causes remain obscure. Skeletal involvement also causes other complications, such as marrow suppression with leukopenia (but occasionally leukocytosis, for reasons that are not entirely clear), hypercalcemia, and pathologic fracture after trivial injury, a major problem in patients with myeloma, breast cancer, and lung cancer. The most common fractures are those of the vertebrae, which may in the older woman with breast cancer be misdiagnosed as caused by osteoporosis. Hypercalcemia occurs in approximately 30% of patients with advanced myeloma, lung cancer, and breast cancer. It occurs probably less frequently now that pamidronate (pamidronate disodium) is widely used in patients with osteolytic disease. More rarely, nerve compression syndromes occur, the most serious of which is spinal cord compression. This condition is fortunately uncommon. It is usually due to posterior displacement of the vertebral column after vertebral collapse as a consequence of pathologic fracture; more rarely, it can be due to enlarging extradural or intradural metastases that impact the spinal cord.

The pathophysiology of tumor cell metastasis to the skeleton has received more attention in the 1990s. Tumors that metastasize to the skeleton undergo a multistep process that depends not only on blood flow to specific areas of the skeleton, but also on specific properties of the tumor cells as well as host factors and molecules that favor metastasis. It is the latter that is becoming better understood. The suggestion has been made that the distribution of metastasis to distant organs can be predicted by the anatomic distribution of blood flow from the primary site in approximately 30% of cases; in the majority, however, it is the specific properties of the tumor cells at the metastatic site that determine whether the metastasis can become established.[10] This "seed and soil" concept of tumor cell spread to distant organs was first suggested in 1889 by Stephen Paget.[11]

Tumor cells have long been known to have varying capacity for metastasis. Primary tumors comprise heterogeneous populations of cells that have been shown in many studies to have differing invasive properties and different metastatic potential.[12–16] Tumor cells are unstable phenotypically for reasons that are not completely understood, although this instability has been the subject of many studies.[17,18] As tumors increase in size, the proliferating cells undergo rapid clonal diversification.[19] This diversity may be due to a host selection process, with some cells possibly having a survival advantage because of their ability to escape naturally occurring immune defense mechanisms or because of the effects of treatment with anticancer drugs or radiation therapy, which may lead to acquired genetic variability. Research has now shown that the genetic makeup of individual tumor cells can greatly influence their metastatic potential and their invasive capabilities and tumorigenicity.[10,20] In breast cancers, expression of the *HER-2/neu* oncogene occurs in parallel with aggressive behavior of the cells.[21] In some tumors, particularly melanoma, expression of the *nm23* oncogene appears to inhibit the capability of individual tumor cells to metastasize.[22,23] The expression of laminin receptors on tumor cells may cause enhanced metastatic capabilities.[24] Deletions of chromosomal material on 11p has been noted in aggressive breast cancers,[25] and deletions of chromosomes 17 and 18 may be found in colon carcinomas that arise from colonic polyps.[26,27] The downstream events that are responsible for these effects are obviously important to understand.

Multiple mechanisms are present to protect against tumor metastasis. Current evidence suggests that fewer than 1% of all tumor cells survive in the systemic circulation.[10] Tumor cells probably have a survival advantage when they circulate as aggregates, which helps prevent the destruction of individual cells from mechanical shear forces or from anoxia in the circulation.

The events that are involved in tumor cell metastasis to bone can be divided into two major types: general steps involved in tumor cell metastasis to any distant organ, such as liver, brain, or lungs, and specific steps involved in metastasis to bone. The general steps include escape of the tumor cells from the primary site and entry into the circulation. This event presumably involves the production of proteolytic enzymes by the tumor cells, because the tumor cells must invade the connective tissue at the primary site to enter the bloodstream and get into the systemic circulation. Once they enter the systemic circulation, tumor cells need to escape the normal host immune defense mechanisms, which in most cases are very effective in clearing the malignant invaders from the circulation. Once at the metastatic site, the tumor cells travel through wide-channeled marrow sinusoids. These marrow sinusoids have now been studied in some detail and probably contain wide pores, through which tumor cells can readily migrate toward bone surfaces. Tumor cells in these sites are then attracted toward the bone surface by chemotactic mechanisms that are still not clearly identified. There, they interact with this local microenvironment and change their phenotype in many cases to produce peptides that are responsible for bone destruction. One of the most notable of these peptides is the tumor product parathyroid hormone–related peptide (PTH-rP).

GENERAL STEPS IN TUMOR CELL METASTASIS

Role of Cell Adhesion Molecules

Attachment of tumor cells to other cells and to extracellular structures is an essential step in tumor cell metastasis. This tumor cell attachment is mediated by cell adhesion molecules such as laminin and E-cadherin. Cell adhesion molecules mediate not only cell-to-cell but also cell-to-substrate communications. Thus, cell adhesion molecules mediate cancer cell adhesion to normal host cells as well as to extracellular matrix and thereby regulate tumor cell invasiveness and proliferation.[28]

Decreased expression of specific cell adhesion molecules at the primary site causes disruption of the interconnections between cancer cells and promotes the detachment of cancer cells from the primary tumor. This results in initiation of local invasion and eventually in the development of metastasis. On the other hand, increased expression of cell adhesion molecules at the metastatic site might be a prerequisite for cancer cells to arrest at specific sites through the attachment to extracellular matrix. Some reports have shown that metastatic breast and ovarian cancers show enhanced expression of E-cadherin.[29] E-cadherin expression in these cancer cells may be reversibly modulated by culture conditions *in vitro*[30] and, possibly more important, by environmental factors *in vivo*.[31] Therefore, cancer cells may express either decreased or increased levels of cell adhesion molecules depending on both the stage of metastasis development and the sites of metastasis. Data suggest that the cell adhesion molecules E-cadherin and laminin are important in bone metastasis.[24,32] The most abundant cell adhesion molecules on tumor cells are integrins, which are responsible for a variety of cell-cell and cell-matrix interactions[33] and have been implicated in hematogenous dissemination.[34] Integrins mediate cancer cell attachment to vascular endothelial cells and to matrix proteins such as laminin and fibronectin, as well as to other cell adhesion molecules. Because these proteins underlie endothelium, this attachment process is a key initial step in tumor colonization.[28] A375 human melanoma cells have been found to express high levels of the $\alpha_v\beta_3$ integrin (vitronectin receptor) on the cell surface when they bind to and invade the basement membrane matrix Matrigel.[35] Synthetic antagonists to laminin have been found to inhibit osteolytic bone metastasis caused by A375 cells in nude mice.[24] At least several integrins are likely to be involved in the development of bone metastases, and this is an important area of current research.

E-cadherin (uvomorulin) is a 120-kd cell surface glycoprotein responsible for calcium-dependent epithelial cell–specific cell adhesion. E-cadherin is a homophilic cell-cell adhesion molecule and thus causes homotypic cell aggregation, which may be important in embryogenesis and morphogenesis.[36] E-cadherin is now known also to play a role in cancer invasion and metastasis. Treatment of epithelial noninvasive Madin-Darby canine kidney (MDCK) cells with monoclonal antibodies to E-cadherin renders these cells more invasive.[37] Overexpression of the E-cadherin gene in highly invasive cancer cells dramatically suppresses their invasiveness; conversely, introduction of E-cadherin–specific antisense RNA renders noninvasive epithelial cells invasive.[38] E-cadherin expression is increased in populations of MCF-7 breast cancer cells with reduced invasiveness, whereas relatively low levels of E cadherin can be detected in the highly invasive human breast cancer cells, MDA-MB-231.[39]

The capacity of the human breast cancer cell lines with varying E-cadherin expression to form metastases has been examined,[32] and MDA-MB-231 cells (low E-cadherin expression) have been found to form osteolytic bone lesions more readily *in vivo*. Whereas MDA-MB-231 cells form obvious osteolytic lesions by 4 weeks after inoculation into the left ventricle, MCF-7 cells (high E-cadherin expression) take more than 8 weeks to form similar lesions. At 4 weeks, no lesions are apparent in mice inoculated with MCF-7 cells. When transfected with E-cadherin complementary DNA (cDNA), however, MDA-MB-231 cells have markedly reduced capacity to form osteolytic bone lesions.[32]

Secretion of Proteolytic Enzymes

Tumor cells produce proteolytic enzymes to degrade basement membranes and traverse the sinusoids and capillaries through which they travel. They also use proteolytic mechanisms to invade the tissue stroma. This migration process may involve direct production of proteolytic enzymes, such as type IV collagenase by tumor cells, or even production of proteolytic enzymes by host cells. Garbisa et al.[20] suggested that production of type IV collagenase by tumor cells may be responsible for degradation of the capillary basement membrane. Basset et al.[40] showed that host cells, such as fibroblasts and stromal cells, associated with some invasive breast carcinomas express a metalloproteinase that may be involved in the invasive process. Inhibitors of matrix metalloproteinases (MMPs) have proven to be effective inhibitors of the metastatic process,[41] although their site of action is unclear. Possibly, they are important in cancer invasiveness[42,43] and bone resorption. Overexpression of the tissue inhibitor of MMP-2 (TIMP-2) in MDA-MB-231 cells by transfection has been found to markedly reduce their bone metastatic capacity.[44]

Cell Motility

Tumor cells migrate from the vasculature toward bone surfaces presumably in response to a number of chemotactic factors. Bone matrix itself contains multiple factors with chemotactic potential for tumor cells, and these are presumably released locally as a consequence of bone remodeling and bone resorption. These include fragments of type I collagen, which have been shown to cause unidirectional migration of tumor cells,[45] and fragments of the bone protein osteocalcin, which may also cause chemotaxis of tumor cells and monocytes.[46] The conditioned media harvested from resorbing or remodeling bones have chemotactic activity that stimulates the unidirectional migration of rat and human tumor cells.[47,48] The nature of the factor responsible has not been identified, but the potential candidates transforming growth factor β (TGF-β) and platelet-derived growth factor, both of which are present in abundant amounts in bone[49] and released in active form during bone resorption,[50] may play an important role.

SPECIFIC STEPS IN TUMOR CELL METASTASIS TO BONE

Cellular Mechanism of Bone Destruction

Although the precise cellular mechanism responsible for local destruction of bone by tumor cells has been a controversial issue for many years, it appears likely that the osteoclast is primarily responsible. Tumors cause bone osteolysis by producing local factors that stimulate osteoclasts, which in turn are responsible for the resorption of bone. Also, tumor cells may themselves destroy bone directly. The evidence is overwhelming that osteoclastic bone resorption is the predominant mechanism. First, when techniques such as scanning electron microscopy are used, active osteoclasts are invariably found to be present on endosteal bone surfaces adjacent to tumor deposits,[51] and distinctive osteoclast resorption lacunae are present on the bone surface. These studies have shown no evidence of smaller resorption lacunae corresponding to the size of the tumor cells. Second, drugs that effectively (and specifically) inhibit osteoclast activity, such as the bisphosphonates, plicamycin, and gallium nitrate, work very effectively in treating hypercalcemia of malignancy, which is due predominantly to increased bone resorption caused by tumors, as well as osteolytic bone disease without hypercalcemia.[52–54] Because, as far as is known, these drugs work solely through the inhibition of osteoclast function, these data indicate that osteoclasts are responsible for the bone destruction. *In vitro* evidence also suggests, however, that breast cancer cells have the capacity to cause bone resorption *in vitro*. When breast cancer cells have been added to devitalized bone, they cause both mineral release and matrix degradation.[55]

Factors Responsible for Osteoclast Stimulation at the Metastatic Site

Because the major cellular mechanism for bone destruction in osteolytic bone disease is osteoclastic, determining the mechanism by which tumor cells cause an increase in osteoclast activity has generated great interest. Studies suggest that osteoclasts are stimulated by PTH-rP, the tumor peptide that has been associated with humoral hypercalcemia of malignancy. Although many of the patients with osteolytic bone disease do not have increased plasma PTH-rP levels or increased levels of nephrogenous cyclic adenosine monophosphate, the hallmarks of humoral hypercalcemia of malignancy, this does not mean that PTH-rP is unimportant. Immunohistochemical studies have shown that expression of PTH-rP is greater in bone sites than in either soft-tissue metastases or primary tumors in patients with carcinoma of the breast.[56] The human breast cancer cell line MDA-MB-231, when inoculated into the left cardiac ventricle of nude mice, has been found to cause the development of osteolytic lesions over the following 4 to 6 weeks. In this model, PTH-rP expression is increased in those tumor cells that have metastasized to bone and cause the typical osteolytic bone lesions seen in patients with the disease.[57] When tumor-bearing nude mice are inoculated with neutralizing antibodies to PTH-rP, not only does the development of osteolytic bone lesions decrease, but the tumor burden in bone also decreases.[58] The most likely explanation for the increase in PTH-rP production in the bone microenvironment is that bone not only provides a fertile soil for the growth of tumor cells, but it also enhances the production of PTH-rP. Studies have shown that the likely mechanism for this effect is the production of TGF-β, which is released from bone in active form when bone resorbs.[50] Yin et al.[59] showed that when MDA-MB-231 cells were transfected with a dominant-negative type II TGF-β receptor subunit that made the cells unresponsive to TGF-β, PTH-rP production was not enhanced in the bone microenvironment, and osteolytic bone lesions were markedly reduced. Reversal of the dominant-negative blockade by expression of a constitutively active TGF-β type I receptor in the breast cancer cells increased tumor production of PTH-rP, enhanced osteolytic bone metastases, and decreased survival. Finally, transfection of the MDA-MB-231 cells that expressed the dominant-negative TGF-β type II receptor with the cDNA for PTH-rP resulted in constitutive tumor PTH-rP production and accelerated bone metastases. These data demonstrate an important role for TGF-β in the development of breast cancer metastasis to bone and suggest that the bone destruction is mediated by PTH-rP. Other mechanisms responsible for osteoclast stimulation and bone destruction associated with bone metastasis are likely to exist. These may involve production by the tumor cells or by host immune cells in the bone microenvironment of mediators such as transforming growth factor α, interleukin-1α, tumor necrosis factor, and interleukin-6, each of which, acting alone or in combination with PTH-rP, represents a strong stimulus to increase bone resorption.[60] Interleukin-6 markedly enhances the actions of PTH-rP on osteoclastic bone resorption both *in vitro* and *in vivo*, presumably by increasing the numbers of available osteoclast progenitors.[60]

Role of Bone-Derived Growth Factors at the Metastatic Site

Bone provides a very favorable medium for the growth of tumor cells, and clearly many tumors grow very well in this microenvironment. The reason may be that bone is a large repository or storehouse for growth-regulatory factors.[49] Bone is particularly rich in TGF-β, but it also contains other growth-regulatory factors that may act as tumor growth factors. These include bone morphogenetic proteins, heparin-binding fibroblast growth factors, platelet-derived growth factors, and insulinlike growth factors I and II. These factors may be responsible for the particularly aggressive behavior of some tumor cells in bone. They may be made available in active form as a consequence of bone resorption.[50] This has been shown for TGF-β.[59] TGF-β may alter the behavior of many tumor cells—and breast cancer cells, in particular—and cause enhanced production of PTH-rP.[61,62] Other of these bone-derived growth factors, however, may also have proliferative effects on the tumor cells. The model described by Sasaki et al.[52] provides a very useful approach for studying osteolytic bone metastasis due to breast cancer. The bone lesions in this model are typical of those in patients with the disease. The tumor cells can be modified by transfection with genes that are probably involved in the metastatic process or, to determine whether a specific mechanism is responsible, by transfection with genes that interfere with this function, such as TIMP-2 genes[44] or genes for dominant-negative type II TGF-β receptors.[59] These approaches can provide considerable insights into the molecular mechanisms responsible for

Osteolytic Metastasis

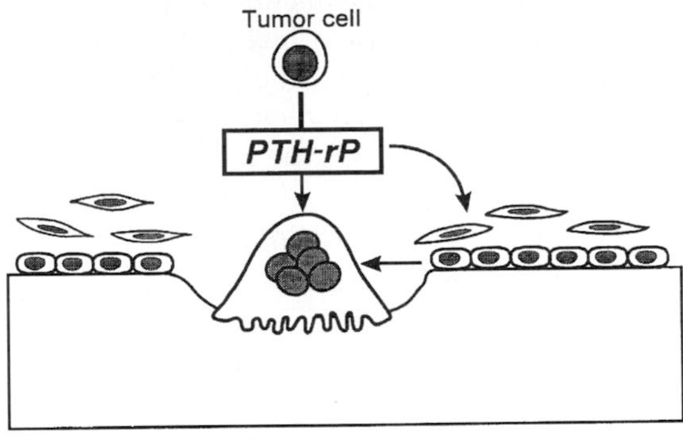

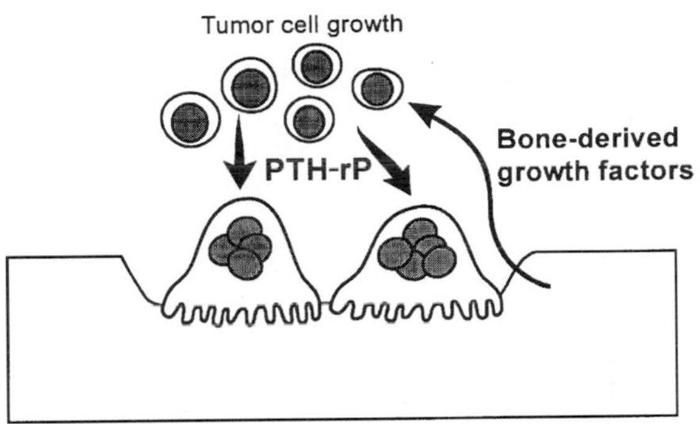

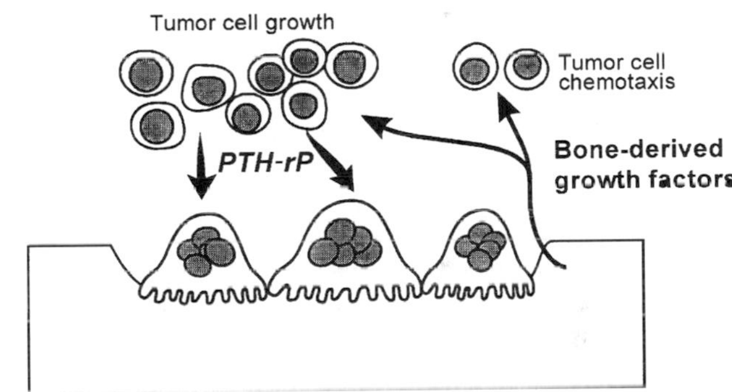

FIG. 1. Schematic illustration of a proposed mechanism of local bone destruction in osteolytic bone metastasis mediated by parathyroid hormone–related peptide (PTH-rP). Other osteolytic factors may mediate this process as well. In the top panel, tumor cell arrives in bone and stimulates osteoclastic bone resorption via secretion of PTH-rP, an effect that is mediated through the osteoblast and stromal cells. In the middle panel, osteoclastic bone resorption results in release and activation of growth factors present in bone matrix, including transforming growth factor β (TGF-β) and insulinlike growth factors (IGFs) I and II. Such factors may increase tumor production of PTH-rP (in the case of TGF-β) or increase tumor cell growth (in the case of the IGFs). The lower panel illustrates the end result of this cycle, in which increased tumor-stimulated osteoclastic bone resorption results in increased local concentration of bone-derived growth factors. Such factors increase PTH-rP production, tumor cell growth, and chemotaxis. (From ref. 57, with permission.)

osteolytic bone metastasis. Figure 1 illustrates one potential mechanism for the avidity with which breast cancer grows in bone.[57] The mechanism by which active TGF-β is released from bone is still unclear. One possibility is that it is released in active form as a consequence of osteoclastic resorption of bone.[50] Another is that tumor cells directly cause cleavage of TGF-β from its matrix-associated binding proteins, as has been shown *in vitro* (S. Dallas, *personal communication*, July 1999).

INTERACTIONS BETWEEN BONE AND TUMOR

Although loss of TGF-β receptor function[63] or its signaling molecules[64–66] has been associated with malignant progression,[67] evidence is growing that TGF-β may enhance tumor growth and invasion. TGF-β has been shown to induce an epithelial-mesenchymal transdifferentiation to an invasive phenotype.[68,69] Oft et al., using the same dominant-negative TGF-β type II receptor approach, demonstrated that TGF-β blockade decreased invasion and metastases in a mouse colon carcinoma[70,71] and that several human carcinoma cell lines lost *in vitro* invasiveness when treated with neutralizing TGF-β antibodies. Thus, TGF-β signaling appears to be required for both induction and maintenance of *in vitro* invasiveness and metastasis during late-stage tumorigenesis.

Another factor that may be important in tumor cell behavior in the bone microenvironment is calcium. Calcium released by resorbing bone may alter tumor cell proliferation[72] and subsequent behavior and growth of the metastatic tumor cells. Little information exists on this topic.

One of the major difficulties that has limited the study of bone metastasis is the lack of suitable animal models. Although this has retarded the accumulation of knowledge in the pathophysiology of bone metastasis, it has not been a problem in investigation of other types of metastases and lung metastases, in particular.[15] Arguello et al.[73] devised a technique in which tumor cells are injected directly into the left ventricle of mice. This inoculation leads to the colonization of bone in regions containing hematopoietic bone marrow by appropriate tumor cells with potential to metastasize to bone. Multiple lytic lesions arise, resembling those seen in patients with cancer. In these models, bone metastasis occurs when tumor cells have ready access to the arterial circulation. This model has been modified by the use of human tumor cells in nude mice.[24,52] Inoculation of human breast cancer cells into the left ventricle of nude mice has enabled characterization of a number of steps involved in osteolytic bone metastasis. Treating the animals with antagonists or antibodies to specific molecules involved in the process (e.g., E-cadherin, PTH-rP), transfecting the tumor cells with specific genes (e.g., those coding for E-cadherin, TIMP-2, Src, and PTH-rP) and showing their role in this process, and treating the animals with agents that regulate normal bone cell function (e.g., bisphosphonates, growth factors) has made it possible to determine the interaction between bone cells and tumor cells in the bone microenvironment. Some of the molecular mechanisms likely to be involved in the process of breast cancer metastasis to bone have been identified using this technique. Using a special modification of this technique, Yoneda et al.[74] have developed a method for specifically examining metastasis to the calvarium to give a better picture of the progressive development of bone metastasis.

Shevrin et al.[75] used prostate cancer cells to induce bone metastases after intravenous injection and occlusion of the inferior vena cava. Pollard and Luckert[76] and Pollard et al.[77] studied rat prostate adenocarcinoma cells in Lobund-Wistar rats and showed that these tumors cause a profound local change in bone formation. When this tumor is injected adjacent to a bone surface, in which the periosteum is often mildly damaged by scratching with a needle tip, the tumor stimulates adjacent new woven bone formation.

EXPERIMENTAL THERAPY

The best form of treatment for metastatic bone disease is ablative therapy for the tumor. As already indicated, in the vast majority of patients this procedure is not feasible. At the present time, most attention is being focused on drugs that inhibit osteoclast activity, such as the bisphosphonates. Since the mid-1970s, many studies have examined the effects of bisphosphonate use in patients with osteolytic bone metastases, and evidence is accumulating that treatment with bisphosphonates is extremely effective at inhibiting skeleton-related events (pathologic fractures, need for radiation or surgery for osteolytic bone disease, spinal cord compression due to vertebral collapse, and episodes of hypercalcemia). The more recent of these studies have used a double-blind randomized and controlled design. In most of them, pamidronate has been infused intravenously every month. Pamidronate therapy clearly reduces the number of skeleton-related events and also delays the onset of the first skeleton-related event in breast cancer patients with osteolytic bone metastases.[53] Reports of the effects of pamidronate on tumor mass in soft tissue or bone show variable results. Findings in the model described above, in which MDA-MB-231 cells were inoculated into the left ventricle of nude mice, suggest that bisphosphonates not only reduce osteolytic bone lesions, but also markedly reduce tumor burden in bone.[52] This is probably due to the decreased production of growth factors in the bone microenvironment by inhibition of bone remodeling. It remains unclear whether bisphosphonates also increase or alter tumor burden in other metastatic sites, although this seems unlikely from other studies (T. Yoneda and T. Michigami, *unpublished observations*, June 1998).

Although clinical studies indicate that bisphosphonates may alter metastases to soft-tissue sites,[54] no experimental evidence currently exists to show that bisphosphonates have any direct effect on tumor mass.[78,79] The hope is that a new generation of bisphosphonates that are orally active may be useful not only to treat patients with established metastases but also to prevent the development of new metastases. Although information is not currently available in this regard, inhibitors of osteoclastic bone resorption are likely to be even more effective in the prevention of new metastases than in the treatment of established metastases. Theoretically, inhibition of continued resorption would leave the patient with a residual lytic lesion in bone (although occasional patients may show some sclerosis of the healing lesion). On the other hand, in those patients who have malignancies with a predilection for the skeleton, such as breast cancer, preventive treatment with an inhibitor of osteoclastic bone resorption may prevent the initial development of an osteolytic metastasis.

As indicated under General Steps in Tumor Cell Metastasis, attention should not be focused solely on the osteoclasts. Drugs that prevent binding of tumor cells to basement membranes, such as laminin antagonists, and inhibitors of proteolytic enzyme disruption of the basement membrane or tumor cell chemotaxis may also turn out to be useful in the prevention of metastases or treatment of established metastases. Laminin antagonists prevented tumor metastasis in an experimental model[24]. Neutralizing antibodies to PTH-rP have been used to prevent progression of osteolytic bone lesions in animal models of human metastatic breast cancer.[57,58] Also, transfection of human tumor cells with inhibitors of the matrix metalloproteinases, namely TIMP-2, has led to a decrease in osteolytic bone lesions.[80]

Models such as these may have predictive value before the initiation of clinical trials with experimental therapies, such as laminin antagonists and inhibitors of proteolytic enzyme digestion.

OSTEOBLASTIC METASTASIS

Some tumors cause metastatic bone lesions that are characterized by the formation of new bone around the tumor cell deposits in the marrow cavity. Radiographs show characteristic sclerotic lesions. These occur most frequently in patients with prostate cancer, a very common tumor in elderly men that is almost always associated with osteoblastic bone metastases, if patients with this disease live long enough. Such lesions are also seen occasionally, however, in patients with other types of tumor of the urinary tract, particularly transitional cell carcinomas of the bladder, as well as in patients with a number of other types of tumor, including breast cancer, rare lung tumors, and occasionally lymphoma and myeloma. No information exists to suggest that osteoblastic metastases in breast cancer differ from those that occur in other malignancies, so this discussion reviews this topic in general.

Less is known about the mechanisms responsible for osteoblastic metastases than about those responsible for osteolytic bone lesions. Evidence is now beginning to accumulate, however, that such lesions are not due just to the formation of new bone on trabecular bone surfaces without preceding bone resorption. Biochemical markers of bone resorption are almost always increased in patients with osteoblastic bone metastases. Morphology shows that in some patients resorption increases preceding formation, although in some the new bone formation also occurs directly on sites of previous resorption.[81] This is a very interesting effect of tumors on the skeleton. It is of great interest not only to those studying the biology of tumor metastasis but also to those interested in normal bone remodeling. It probably represents an aberration in a normal physiologic mechanism, so clarification of the peptides involved in stimulating bone formation may lead not only to better understanding of the normal process of bone remodeling, but also to the development of potential therapies for the common diseases of bone loss.

A number of factors have been suggested as potential mediators of the osteoblastic metastasis associated with prostate cancer. These include fibroblast growth factors,[82–88] plasminogen activator sequence,[89–92] TGF-β,[93,94] bone morphogenetic proteins,[95] prostate-specific antigen,[96] and endothelin-1.[97] Proteases such as prostate-specific antigen and urokinase-type plasminogen activator may act by cleaving PTH-rP into inactive fragments.[96] Endothelin-1 is not only a powerful mitogenic factor for osteoblasts,[98,99] but it is also produced in large amounts by the prostatic epithelium.[100] Circulating concentrations are increased in patients with metastatic prostate cancer.[97] One of the authors has found that it may be produced in relatively large amounts by certain breast cancers *in vitro* (T.A.G., *unpublished data*, 1999). Its role in osteoblastic metastasis remains to be established. These breast cancer cell lines cause osteoblastic metastases when inoculated into the left cardiac ventricle of female nude mice.[101] Figure 2 is a schematic model based on available data from the literature that identify potential tumor-bone interactions.[57]

The presence of osteoblastic metastases is obvious from radiology of the skeleton and from measurement of serum alkaline phosphatase level, which is often markedly increased in these patients.[102] These patients suffer bone pain, which in some cases is relieved by administration of bisphosphonates such as pamidronate. However, the rationale for using pamidronate is not as clear-cut in patients with metastatic prostate cancer as it is in patients in whom osteolysis predominates. Patients with metastatic prostate cancer frequently have a marked increase in serum alkaline phosphatase levels, and radionuclide scanning may confirm the presence of predominantly osteoblastic lesions. A few

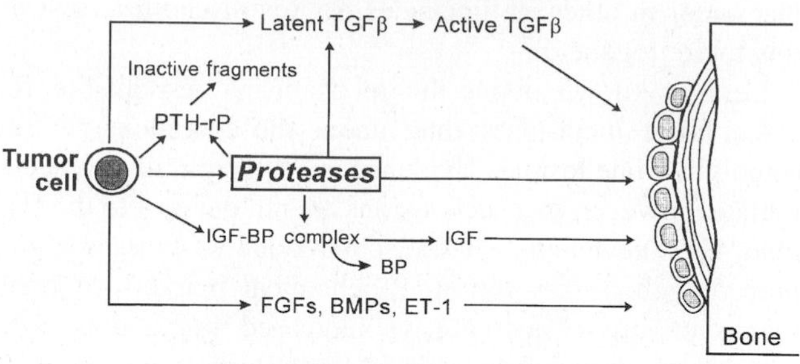

FIG. 2. Model of the formation of osteoblastic bone metastases in prostate cancer. Tumor production of factors such as transforming growth factor β (TGF-β), fibroblast growth factors (FGFs), bone morphogenetic proteins (BMPs), and endothelin-1 (ET-1) may directly stimulate osteoblastic activity and subsequent bone formation. Proteases such as prostate-specific antigen, urokinase-type plasminogen activator, and cathepsin D may activate latent TGF-β, release insulinlike growth factors (IGFs) from inhibitory binding proteins (BPs), and inactivate PTH-rP. (From ref. 57, with permission.)

patients with severe osteoblastic lesions may develop hypocalcemia, presumably because of uptake of calcium by the blastic lesions.

ACKNOWLEDGMENTS

The authors are grateful to Nancy Garrett for her expert secretarial assistance and to the National Institutes of Health for grants CA-40035, R29-CA-69158, and R01-CA-63628 for support for some of the studies reported here.

REFERENCES

1. Wingo PA, Tong T, Bolden S. Cancer statistics. *CA Cancer J Clin* 1995;45:8.
2. Rubens RD. Bone metastases—the clinical problem. *Eur J Cancer* 1998;34:210.
3. Coleman RE, Rubens RD. The clinical course of bone metastases from breast cancer. *Br J Cancer* 1987;55:61.
4. Galasko CSB. Skeletal metastases. *Clin Orthop* 1986;210:18.
5. Galasko CSB. *Skeletal metastases.* London: Butterworth–Heinemann, 1986.
6. Batson OV. The function of the vertebral veins and their role in the spread of metastases. *Ann Surg* 1940;112:138.
7. Coman DR, DeLong RP. The role of the vertebral venous system in the metastasis of cancer to the spinal column; experiments with tumour cell suspension in rats and rabbits. *Cancer* 1951;4:610.
8. van den Brenk HAS, Burch WM, Kelley H, Orton C. Venous diversion trapping and growth of blood-borne cancer cells en route to the lungs. *Br J Cancer* 1975;31:46.
9. Dodds PR, Caride VJ, Lytton B. The role of vertebral veins in the dissemination of prostatic carcinoma. *J Urol* 1981;126:753.
10. Liotta LA, Kohn E. Cancer invasion and metastases. *JAMA* 1990;263:1123.
11. Paget S. The distribution of secondary growths in cancer of the breast. *Lancet* 1889;1:571.
12. Carr I, Orr FW. Current reviews: invasion and metastasis. *CMAJ* 1983;128:1164.
13. Heppner G. Tumor heterogeneity. *Cancer Res* 1984;214:2259.
14. Poste G. Pathogenesis of metastatic disease: implications for current therapy and for the development of new therapeutic strategies. *Cancer Treat Rep* 1986;70:183.
15. Fidler IJ, Poste G. The cellular heterogeneity of malignant neoplasms: implications for adjuvant chemotherapy. *Semin Oncol* 1985;12:207.
16. Fidler IJ. Tumor heterogeneity and the biology of cancer invasion and metastasis. *Cancer Res* 1978;38:2651.
17. Nowell PS. The clonal evolution of tumor cell subpopulations. *Science* 1976;194:23.
18. Miller FR. Tumor subpopulation interactions in metastasis. *Invasion Metastasis* 1983;3:234.
19. Reedy AL, Fialkow PJ. Multicellular origin of fibrosarcomas in mice induced by the chemical carcinogen 3-methylcholanthrene. *J Exp Med* 1980;150:878.
20. Garbisa S, Pozzatti R, Muschel RJ, et al. Secretion of type IV collagenolytic protease and metastatic phenotype: induction by transfection with c-Ha-ras but not c-Ha-ras plus AD2-Ela. *Cancer Res* 1987;47:1523.
21. Slamon DJ, Clark GM, Wong SG, Levin WJ, Ullrich A, McGuire WL. Human breast cancer: correlation of relapse and survival with amplification of the HER-2/neu oncogene. *Science* 1987;235:177.
22. Liotta LA, Steeg PS. Clues to the function of Nm23 and Awd proteins in development, signal transduction, and tumor metastasis provided by studies of Dictyostelium discoideum. *J Natl Cancer Inst* 1990;82:1170.
23. Steeg PS, Bevilacqua G, Kopper L, et al. Evidence for a novel gene associated with low tumor metastatic potential. *J Natl Cancer Inst* 1988;80:200.
24. Nakai M, Mundy GR, Williams PJ, Boyce B, Yoneda T. A synthetic antagonist to laminin inhibits the formation of osteolytic metastases by human melanoma cells in nude mice. *Cancer Res* 1992;52:5395.
25. Ali IU, Lidereau R, Theillet C, Callahan R. Reduction to homozygosity of genes on chromosome 11 in human breast neoplasia. *Science* 1987;238:185.
26. Vogelstein B, Fearon ER, Hamilton SR, et al. Genetic alterations during colorectal tumor development. *N Engl J Med* 1988;319:525.
27. Baker SJ, Fearon ER, Nigro JM, et al. Chromosome 17 deletions and p53 gene mutations in colorectal carcinomas. *Science* 1989;244:217.
28. Albelda SM, Buck CA. Integrins and other cell adhesion molecules. *FASEB J* 1990;4:2868.
29. Oka H, Shiozaki H, Kobayashi K, et al. Expression of E-cadherin cells adhesion molecules in human breast cancer tissues and its relationship to metastasis. *Cancer Res* 1993;53:1696.
30. Hashimoto M, Niwa O, Nitta Y, Takeichi M, Yokoro K. Unstable expression of E-cadherin adhesion molecules in metastatic ovarian tumor cells. *Jpn J Cancer Res* 1989;80:459.
31. Mareel MM, Behrens J, Birchmeier W, et al. Down-regulation of E-cadherin expression in Madin-Darby canine kidney (MDCK) cells inside tumors of nude mice. *Int J Cancer* 1991;47:922.
32. Mbalaviele G, Dunstan CR, Sasaki A, Williams PJ, Mundy GR, Yoneda T. E-cadherin expression in human breast cancer cells suppress the development of osteolytic bone metastases in experimental metastasis model. *Cancer Res* 1996;56:4063.
33. Haynes RO. Integrins: versatility, modulation, and signaling in cell adhesion. *Cell* 1992;69:11.
34. Nip J, Shibata H, Loskutoff DJ, Cheresh DA, Brodt P. Human melanoma cells derived from lymphatic metastases use integrins alpha v beta 3 to adhere to lymph node vitronectin. *J Clin Invest* 1992;90:1406.
35. Seftor REB, Seftor EA, Gehlsen KR, et al. Role of the alpha v beta 3 integrin in human melanoma cell invasion. *Proc Natl Acad Sci U S A* 1992;89:1557.
36. Takeichi M. Cadherin cell adhesion receptors as a morphogenetic regulator. *Science* 1991;251:1451.
37. Behrens J, Mareel MM, Van Roy FM, Birchmeier W. Dissecting tumor cell invasion: epithelial cells acquire invasive properties after the loss of uvomorulin-mediated cell-cell adhesion. *J Cell Biol* 1989;108:2435.
38. Vleminckx K, Vakaet L, Mareel M, Fiers W, van Roy F. Genetic manipulation of E-cadherin expression by epithelial tumor cells reveals an invasion suppressor role. *Cell* 1991;66:107.
39. Sommers CL, Thompson EW, Torri JA, Kemler R, Gelmann EP, Byers SW. Cell adhesion molecule uvomorulin expression in human

breast cancer cell lines: relationship to morphology and invasive capacities. *Cell Growth Differ* 1991;2:365.

40. Basset P, Bellocq JP, Wolf C, et al. A novel metalloproteinase gene specifically expressed in stromal cells of breast carcinomas. *Nature* 1990;348:699.
41. Sledge WG, Qulahi M, Goulet R, Bone EA, Fife R. Effect of matrix metalloproteinase inhibitor batimastat on breast cancer regrowth and metastasis in athymic mice. *J Natl Cancer Inst* 1995;87:1546.
42. Lewin DJ. Evolutions: metastasis. *J NIH Res* 1996;9:85.
43. MacDougall JR, Matrisian LM. Contributions of tumor and stromal matrix metalloproteinases to tumor progression, invasion and metastasis. *Cancer Metastasis Rev* 1995;14:351.
44. Yoneda T, Sasaki A, Dunstan C, et al. Inhibition of osteolytic bone metastasis of breast cancer by combined treatment with the bisphosphonate ibandronate and tissue inhibitor of the matrix metalloproteinase-2. *J Clin Invest* 1997;99:2509.
45. Mundy GR, DeMartino S, Rowe DW. Collagen and collagen-derived fragments are chemotactic for tumor cells. *J Clin Invest* 1981;68:1102.
46. Mundy GR, Poser JW. Chemotactic activity of the gamma-carboxyglutamic acid containing protein in bone. *Calcif Tissue Int* 1983;35:164.
47. Orr W, Varani J, Gondek MK, Ward PA, Mundy GR. Chemotactic responses of tumor cells to products of resorbing bone. *Science* 1979; 203:176.
48. Orr FW, Varani J, Gondek MK, Ward PA, Mundy GR. Partial characterization of a bone derived chemotactic factor for tumor cells. *Am J Pathol* 1980;99:43.
49. Hauschka PV, Mavrakos AE, Iafrati MD, et al. Growth factors in bone matrix. *J Biol Chem* 1986;261:12665.
50. Pfeilschifter J, Mundy GR. Modulation of transforming growth factor beta activity in bone cultures by osteotropic hormones. *Proc Natl Acad Sci U S A* 1987;84:2024.
51. Boyde A, Maconnachie E, Reid SA, Delling G, Mundy GR. Scanning electron microscopy in bone pathology: review of methods. Potential and applications. *Scan Electron Microsc* 1986;4:1537.
52. Sasaki A, Boyce BF, Story B, et al. Bisphosphonate risedronate reduces metastatic human breast cancer burden in bone in nude mice. *Cancer Res* 1995;55:3551.
53. Hortobagyi GN, Theriault RL, Porter L, et al. Efficacy of pamidronate in reducing skeletal complications in patients with breast cancer and lytic bone metastases. *N Engl J Med* 1996;335:1785.
54. Diel IJ, Solomayer EF, Costa SD, et al. Reduction in new metastases in breast cancer with adjuvant clodronate treatment. *N Engl J Med* 1998;339:357.
55. Eilon G, Mundy GR. Direct resorption of bone by human breast cancer cells in vitro. *Nature* 1978;276:726.
56. Powell GJ, Southby J, Danks JA, et al. Localization of parathyroid hormone-related protein in breast cancer metastases—increased incidence in bone compared with other sites. *Cancer Res* 1991;51:3059.
57. Guise TA, Mundy GR. Cancer and bone. *Endocr Rev* 1998,19.18.
58. Guise TA, Yin JJ, Taylor SD, et al. Evidence for a causal role of parathyroid hormone-related protein in the pathogenesis of human breast cancer-mediated osteolysis. *J Clin Invest* 1996;98:1544.
59. Yin JJ, Selander K, Chirgwin JM, et al. TGF-beta signaling blockade inhibits PTHrP secretion by breast cancer cells and bone metastases development. *J Clin Invest* 1999;103:197.
60. DeLaMata J, Uy HL, Guise TA, et al. Interleukin-6 enhances hypercalcemia and bone resorption mediated by parathyroid hormone-related protein in vivo. *J Clin Invest* 1995;95:2846.
61. Kiriyama T, Gillespie MT, Glatz JA, Fukumoto S, Moseley JM, Martin TJ. Transforming growth factor beta stimulation of parathyroid hormone-related protein (PTHrP): a paracrine regulator? *Mol Cell Endocrinol* 1993;92:55.
62. Southby J, Murphy LM, Martin TJ, Gillespie MT. Cell-specific and regulator-induced promoter usage and messenger ribonucleic acid splicing for parathyroid hormone-related protein. *Endocrinology* 1996;137:1349.
63. Markowitz S, Wang J, Myeroff L, et al. Inactivation of the type II TGF-beta receptor in colon cancer cells with microsatellite instability. *Science* 1995;268:1336.
64. Hahn SA, Schutte M, Hoque ATMS, et al. DPC4, a candidate tumor suppressor gene at human chromosome 18q21.1. *Science* 1996;271:259.
65. Zhu Y, Richardson JA, Parada LF, Graff JM. Smad3 mutant mice develop metastatic colorectal cancer. *Cell* 1998;94:703.
66. Takaku K, Oshima M, Miyoshi H, Matsui M, Seldin MF, Taketo MM. Intestinal tumorigenesis in compound mutant mice of both Dpc4 (Smad4) and Apc genes. *Cell* 1998;92:645.
67. Massagué J. TGF-beta signal transduction. *Annu Rev Biochem* 1998;67:753.
68. Caulin C, Scholl SG, Frontelo P, Gamallo C, Quintanilla M. Chronic exposure of cultured transfected mouse epidermal cells to transforming growth factor-beta 1 induces an epithelial-mesenchymal transdifferentiation and a spindle tumoral phenotype. *Cell Growth Differ* 1995;6:1027.
69. Miettinen PJ, Ebner R, Lopez AR, Derynck R. TGF-beta induced transdifferentiation of mammary epithelial cells to mesenchymal cells: involvement of type I receptors. *J Cell Biol* 1994;127:2021.
70. Oft M, Peli J, Rudaz C, Schwarz H, Beug H, Reichmann E. TGF-beta 1 and Ha-Ras collaborate in modulating the phenotypic plasticity and invasiveness of epithelial tumor cells. *Genes Dev* 1996;10:2462.
71. Oft M, Heider K-H, Beug H. TGF beta signaling is necessary for carcinoma cell invasiveness and metastasis. *Curr Biol* 1998;8:1243.
72. Rizzoli R, Bonjour JP. High extracellular calcium increases the production of a parathyroid hormone-like activity by cultured Leydig tumor cells associated with humoral hypercalcemia. *J Bone Miner Res* 1989;4:839.
73. Arguello F, Baggs RB, Frantz CN. A murine model of experimental metastasis to bone and bone marrow. *Cancer Res* 1988;48:6876.
74. Yoneda T, Williams P, Dunstan C, Chavez J, Niewolna M, Mundy GR. Growth of metastatic cancer cells in bone is enhanced by bone derived insulin-like growth factors (IGFs). *J Bone Miner Res* 1995;10:[Suppl 1]:269(abst).
75. Shevrin D, Kukreja SC, Ghosh L, Lad TE. Development of skeletal metastasis by human prostate cancer in athymic nude mice. *Clin Exp Metastasis* 1988;6:401.
76. Pollard M, Luckert PH. Transplantable metastasizing prostate adenocarcinoma in rats. *J Natl Cancer Inst* 1975;54:643.
77. Pollard M, Luckert MS, Scheu J. Effects of diphosphonate and x-rays on bone lesions induced in rats by prostate cancer cells. *Cancer* 1988;61:2027.
78. Wingen F, Schmahl D. Distribution of 3-amino-1-hydroxypropane-1, 1-diphosphonic acid in rats and effects on rat osteosarcoma. *Arzneimittelforschung* 1985;35:1565.
79. Krempien B, Wingen F, Eichmann T, Muller M, Schmahl D. Protective effects of a prophylactic treatment with the bisphosphonate 3-amino-1-hydroxypropane-1, 1-bisphosphonic acid on the development of tumor osteopathies in the rat: experimental studies with the Walker carcinosarcoma 256. *Oncology* 1988;45:41.
80. Williams P, Mbalaviele G, Sasaki A, et al. Multi-step inhibition of breast cancer metastasis to bone. *J Bone Miner Res* 1995;10:[Suppl 1]:121(abst).
81. Charhon SA, Chapuy MC, Devlin EE, Valentin-Opran A, Edouard CM, Meunier PJ. Histomorphometric analysis of sclerotic bone metastases from prostatic carcinoma special reference to osteomalacia. *Cancer* 1983;51:918.
82. Matuo Y, Nishi N, Matsui S, Sandberg AA, Isaacs JT, Wada F. Heparin binding affinity of rat prostate growth factor in normal and cancerous prostate: partial purification and characterization of rat prostate growth factor in the Dunning tumor. *Cancer Res* 1987;47:188.
83. Mansson PE, Adams P, Kan M, McKeehan WL. Heparin-binding growth factor gene expression in normal rat prostate and two transplantable rat prostate tumors. *Cancer Res* 1989;49:2485.
84. Canalis E, Lorenzo J, Burgess WH, Maciag T. Effects of endothelial cell growth factor on bone remodeling in vitro. *J Clin Invest* 1987;79:52.
85. Canalis E, Centrella M, McCarthy T. Effects of basic fibroblast growth factor on bone formation in vitro. *J Clin Invest* 1988;81:1572.
86. Mayahara H, Ito T, Nagai H, et al. In vivo stimulation of endosteal bone formation by basic fibroblast growth factor in rats. *Growth Factors* 1993;9:73.
87. Dunstan CR, Garrett IR, Adams R, et al. Systemic fibroblast growth factor (FGF-1) prevents bone loss, increases new bone formation, and restores trabecular microarchitecture in ovariectomized rats. *J Bone Miner Res* 1995;10:[Suppl 1]:279(abst).
88. Izbicka E, Dunstan C, Esparza J, Jacobs C, Sabatini M, Mundy GR. Human amniotic tumor which induces new bone formation in vivo produces a growth regulatory activity in vitro for osteoblasts identified as an extended form of basic fibroblast growth factor (bFGF). *Cancer Res* 1996;56:633.

89. Rabbani SA, Desjardins J, Bell AW, et al. An amino-terminal fragment of urokinase isolated from a prostate cancer cell line (PC-3) is mitogenic for osteoblast-like cells. *Biochem Biophys Res Commun* 1990;173:1058.
90. Rabbani SA, Desjardins J, Bell AW, Banville D, Goltzman D. Identification of a new osteoblast mitogen from a human prostate cancer cell line, PC-3. *J Bone Miner Res* 1990;5:549(abst).
91. Achbarou A, Kaiser S, Tremblay G, et al. Urokinase overproduction results in increased skeletal metastasis by prostate cancer cells in vivo. *Cancer Res* 1994;54:2372.
92. Rabbani SA, Mazar AP, Bernier SM, et al. Structural requirements for the growth factor activity of the amino-terminal domain of urokinase. *J Biol Chem* 1992;267:14151.
93. Dallas SL, Park-Snyder S, Miyazono K, Twardzik D, Mundy GR, Bonewald LF. Characterization and autoregulation of latent transforming growth factor beta (TGF beta) complexes in osteoblast-like cell lines: production of a latent complex lacking the latent TGF beta-binding protein (LTBP). *J Biol Chem* 1994;269:6815.
94. Dallas SL, Miyazono K, Skerry TM, Mundy GR, Bonewald LF. Dual role for the latent transforming growth factor-beta binding protein in storage of latent TGF-beta in the extracellular matrix and as a structural matrix protein. *J Cell Biol* 1995;131:539.
95. Harris SE, Bonewald LF, Harris MA, et al. Effects of transforming growth factor beta on bone nodule formation and expression of bone morphogenic protein 2, osteocalcin, osteopontin, alkaline phosphatase, and type 1 collagen mRNA in long-term cultures of fetal rat calvarial osteoblasts. *J Bone Miner Res* 1994;9:855.
96. Cramer SD, Chen Z, Peehl DM. Prostate specific antigen cleaves parathyroid hormone-related protein in the PTH-like domain: inactivation of PTH-rP stimulated cAMP accumulation in mouse osteoblasts. *J Urol* 1996;156:526.
97. Nelson JB, Hedican SP, George DJ, et al. Identification of endothelin-1 in the pathophysiology of metastatic adenocarcinoma of the prostate. *Nat Med* 1995;1:944.
98. Takuwa Y, Ohue Y, Takuwa N, Yamashita K. Endothelin-1 activates phopholipase C and mobilizes Ca2+ from extra- and intracellular pools in osteoblastic cells. *Am J Physiol* 1989;257:E797.
99. Takuwa Y, Masaki T, Yamashita K. The effects of the endothelin family peptides on cultured osteoblastic cells from rat calvariae. *Biochem Biophys Res Commun* 1990;170:998.
100. Langenstroer P, Tang R, Shapiro E, Divish B, Opgenorth T, Lepor H. Endothelin-1 in the human prostate: tissue levels, source of production and isometric tension studies. *J Urol* 1993;150:495.
101. Yin JJ, Grubbs BG, Cui Y, et al. Role of endothelin-1 (ET-1) in osteoblastic metastases to bone. Paper presented at: American Society for Bone and Mineral Research Meeting; December 1998; San Francisco.
102. Tofe AJ, Francis MD, Harvey WJ. Correlation of neoplasms with incidence and localization of skeletal metastases. An analysis of 1355 diphosphonate bone scans. *J Nucl Med* 1975;16:986.

Diseases of the Breast, 2nd ed.,
edited by Jay R. Harris.
Lippincott Williams & Wilkins, Philadelphia © 2000.

CHAPTER 61

Medical Treatment of Bone Metastases

Richard L. Theriault

The osteotropism of breast cancer, although clinically well documented, has not yet lent itself to precise mechanistic explanations in *in vitro* or *in vivo* models.

Bone is the most common site of breast cancer metastasis. Up to 90% of patients dying with breast disease have bone metastasis. Bone is also the most frequent site of disease recurrence after treatment for primary breast cancer.[1–3]

Breast cancer metastases to bone may manifest radiographically as osteolytic, osteoblastic, mixed osteolytic and osteoblastic, or osteoporotic lesions.[4] Although all disease patterns can result in pain, osteolytic and osteoporotic disease are most likely to lead to catastrophic clinical complications such as pathologic fracture, especially of weight-bearing bones, or spinal cord compression.[4] Neurologic compromise may manifest as paralysis due to spinal cord compression or may manifest more subtly as radicular nerve root pain due to tumor impingement on neural foramina or as cranial nerve palsies, also due to neural foraminal encroachment in the base of the skull.

Breast cancer bone metastases most commonly occur in marrow-rich trabecular bone; as the disease progresses, involvement of cortical bone becomes clinically and radiographically evident.

Bone metastasis most commonly occurs in the pelvis (55%) and lumbar spine (54%), followed in decreasing frequency by thoracic spine (45%), ribs (43%), long bones (39%), skull (29%), and cervical spine (22%). The clinical course of breast cancer bone metastases is often that of a slowly evolving chronic condition, thus putting the patient at risk of prolonged pain and disability.[5–7]

Detection of osseous metastasis has generally been accomplished by radionuclide bone scan. The abnormalities on scan are associated with osteoblastic activity at metastatic sites. Purely lytic disease may not visualize on scan. Radiographic confirmation of bone scan abnormalities defines the pattern of disease. Magnetic resonance imaging has been shown to be a good screening approach for the detection of early trabecular metastasis.[8–10] Occasionally, computerized tomographic scanning of cortical bone is necessary to clearly define the nature and extent of disease.[11]

Regardless of radiographic appearance, bone metastasis is associated with bone loss and excess excretion of calcium as well as bone-derived proteins such as pyridinoline, deoxypyridinoline, and *N* telopeptide.[12–14] These findings implicate osteoclast activation and uncoupling of the bone remodeling unit as the final pathway to bone destruction by cancer. Although tumor-derived products—parathyroid hormone–like protein, for example—may directly activate osteoclasts, bone- and marrow-derived cytokines also play a role. These include interleukin-1, interleukin-6, and transforming growth factors.[15–17]

BONE MARROW METASTASIS

Breast cancer bone metastasis is frequently accompanied by marrow disease, although marrow involvement without apparent cortical disease has been reported.[18] Marrow disease may manifest as myelophthisic anemia with circulating nucleated red blood cells seen on a peripheral blood smear or selective cytopenia. The presence of tumor cells in marrow in patients with obvious metastatic disease may be demonstrated by marrow biopsy, which has been reported to be more accurate than marrow aspirate or clot.[19,20] Up to 60% of patients with metastatic breast cancer have been reported to have bone marrow involvement when marrow biopsies have been performed. Advances in technology, however, have resulted in detection of tumor cells in marrow in a larger proportion of breast cancer patients, even those with clinical early-stage disease. Fields et al., using a polymerase chain reaction for detection of cytokeratin 19, demonstrated cytokeratin-positive marrow cells in 52% of patients with stage II breast cancer, 57% of those with stage III disease, and 82% of those with stage IV disease.[21] Using an immunohistochemistry technique, one multicenter study reported that tumor cells were detected in the marrow of 23% of primary breast cancer patients, and that the presence of tumor cells correlated with an increase in relapse frequency. Janni et al. reported

R. L. Theriault: Department of Breast Medical Oncology, University of Texas M. D. Anderson Cancer Center, Houston, Texas

that 31% of primary breast cancer patients, including 25% of patients with stage I disease, had immunocytochemistry-positive tumor cells in marrow.[22] In a study evaluating node-positive and node-negative primary breast cancer, bone marrow positive results for tumor cells were seen in 55% of patients with positive axillary lymph nodes and in 31% of patients with negative axillary lymph nodes. A finding of marrow positive for tumor cells has been reported to have a negative impact on disease-free and overall survival by many investigators,[21–25] but others have reported no significant impact on disease-free or overall survival.[26,27]

TREATMENT OF BONE METASTASIS

Conventional treatment for bone metastasis includes systemic therapy, chemotherapy, and hormone therapy, as well as local therapies usually directed at site-specific problems. Although some reports suggest that systemic therapy is less effective for bone metastasis than for disease at other sites, this perception probably results from the limited ability to accurately measure clinical response in bone either radiographically or by radionuclide scan.[6] Average response rates for all patients and for those with bone metastases alone are reported to be 60% and 53%, respectively, in studies covering more than 850 patients.[28–33] These include one study in which a response rate of 0% was reported for bone metastases treated with chemotherapy. Whitehouse reported on a survey of site-dependent response to chemotherapy for breast cancer in which response rates for bone ranged from 0% to 30%.[34] Careful clinical interpretation of radiographs in accordance with the guidelines of the International Union Against Cancer is the most accurate method of response assessment at present.[35] Local therapy for bone morbidity includes surgery for fracture, impending fracture, or spinal cord compression, and external-beam radiation therapy, generally for the same indications and for relief of bone pain.[36,37]

SYSTEMIC THERAPY FOR MARROW METASTASIS

Marrow metastasis should not preclude chemotherapy if it is otherwise clinically indicated. Although patients with existing marrow involvement documented by biopsy or myelophthisic anemia have greater hematologic toxicity and require more intensive hematologic support during treatment, response duration and survival for such patients do not appear to be different from those of patients without obvious marrow disease.[38] A report by Rodriguez-Kraul et al. suggests that using less than full-dose chemotherapy is associated with inferior response to chemotherapy.[39]

EVOLVING APPROACH TO TREATMENT OF BONE METASTASIS

A change in the approach to treating bone disease has been evolving since the 1968 development of the bisphosphonate class of drugs. Bisphosphonates are analogues of pyrophosphate. They possess a carbon substitution for the oxygen of the pyrophosphate molecule and therefore are resistant to hydrolysis by endogenous phosphatase.[40] They have been shown *in vitro* and *in vivo* to inhibit osteoclast-mediated bone destruction. Their exact mechanism of action is not completely understood. However, they appear to preferentially localize at sites of active bone remodeling and osteolysis. They inhibit the activity of mature osteoclasts, interfering with lyzosomal enzymes and impeding recruitment and maturation of osteoclast precursors from parental monocyte-macrophage cell lines. They inhibit dissolution of hydroxyapatite crystals.[41] In addition to inhibiting malignant bone disease, they have been shown to have a salient effect on Paget's disease of bone, osteoporosis due to estrogen deficiency, and hypercorticoidism. Since demonstration of the effectiveness of etidronate (etidronate disodium) for the treatment of hypercalcemia of malignancy in the 1970s, a number of new bisphosphonates have been made available in clinical trials and medical practice. The long-term administration of etidronate in Paget's disease results in osteomalacia, which indicates inhibition of cell function for osteoblasts and osteoclasts. Newer agents have demonstrated greater osteoclast inhibition and relatively minor osteoblast inhibition, and therefore are more suited to long-term clinical use. The relative osteoclast inhibition potency ranges from 1 for etidronate disodium to 100 for pamidronate (pamidronate disodium), 1,000 for alendronate (alendronate sodium), and approximately 20,000 for the investigational agent zoledronate (Table 1).

HYPERCALCEMIA

Hypercalcemia associated with malignancy is most often due to bone metastasis; however, it may occur with visceral

TABLE 1. *Relative potency of osteoclast inhibition in the rat observed for various bisphosphonates studied in humans*

Alendronate sodium[a]	100–1,000	Neridronate	100
Cimadronate	100–1,000	Olpadronate	100–1,000
Clodronate disodium	10	Pamidronate disodium[a]	100
EB-1053	100–1,000	Risidronate	1,000–10,000
Etidronate disodium[a]	1	Tiludronate disodium	10
Ibandronate sodium	1,000–10,000	YH-529	>10,000
		Zoledronate	~20,000

[a]Commercially available in United States.

disease only, as a consequence of elevated levels of tumor-produced parathyroid hormone–related protein.[42] Treatment of hypercalcemia by bisphosphonate has had a dramatic impact on clinical care.

The efficacy of many bisphosphonates in treating hypercalcemia has been assessed in clinical trials. Etidronate, the prototype of this class of agents, has been shown to be effective in 40% to 70% of hypercalcemia patients treated. Etidronate is less effective than other agents and is no longer frequently used.[43] Clodronate (clodronate disodium), pamidronate, ibandronate (ibandronate sodium), alendronate, tiludronate (tiludronate disodium), and zoledronate have all been reported to be effective in restoring normocalcemia in cancer patients.

Dose-response effects in the treatment of hypercalcemia have been reported for ibandronate, pamidronate, and alendronate.[44–46] In comparative trials, pamidronate has been reported to be either more effective or longer lasting in its hypocalcemic effect than etidronate or clodronate.[47,48] Comparisons of alendronate with either etidronate or clodronate show an advantage for alendronate.[49,50]

Infusion rates of bisphosphonates have been examined in a few trials. Rapid infusion in a few hours of alendronate and pamidronate have been reported to be effective.[51,52] Zoledronate has the fastest reported infusion time (5 to 30 minutes).[53]

The standard treatment for hypercalcemia includes restoration of intravascular volume with normal saline and correction of other electrolyte deficits, such as hypokalemia and hypomagnesemia. Pamidronate in a single dose of 60 to 90 mg administered intravenously over 2 to 4 hours is the bisphosphonate treatment of choice in the United States. Clodronate 1,500 mg intravenously as a single dose is available in some countries. A 90-mg dose of pamidronate has been reported to be 100% effective in moderate to severe hypercalcemia. The hypocalcemic effect of bisphosphonate may not be observed for 48 to 72 hours; therefore, in emergent clinical situations, adding calcitonin to the treatment program may provide a more rapid hypocalcemic effect.[54] Bisphosphonates have become the treatment of choice for malignancy-induced hypercalcemia because of their success in achieving normocalcemia and favorable toxicity profile.[55–57] In general, oral doses are poorly assimilated, with only 1% to 10% of an oral dose absorbed through the small intestine. Increasing the oral dosage often results in gastrointestinal toxicity.

BISPHOSPHONATE TREATMENT FOR BONE METASTASIS

The concept of treating the organ affected by metastasis to preserve organ integrity and function has developed from the use of bisphosphonate to treat osteolysis and hypercalcemia due to metastatic bone disease. Two agents, clodronate and pamidronate, have been tested in several randomized trials in osteolytic disease.

Clodronate

Clodronate is a first-generation bisphosphonate with two chlorines bonded to the central carbon. It is reported to be approximately ten times more potent than etidronate in inhibiting osteoclastic activity.[58]

In 1987, Elomaa et al.[59] reported on a placebo-controlled clinical trial of oral clodronate use in breast cancer skeletal metastasis. They demonstrated a decrease in frequency of fractures, hypercalcemia, and new bone metastasis development, as well as an apparent survival advantage at 2 years (11 patients alive in clodronate group versus 4 in placebo group, $p < .004$). Seven deaths caused by hypercalcemia of malignancy occurred in the placebo group compared with only one in the clodronate group. Table 2 summarizes the results of randomized trials of bisphosphonates.

A randomized, blinded, controlled trial in which treatment with clodronate 1,600 mg per day was compared with placebo has been reported by Paterson et al.[60] In this study, patients with skeletal disease from breast cancer received systemic chemotherapy or hormonal therapy at the discretion of the attending oncologist. One hundred seventy-three patients were randomly assigned to treatment with clodronate or placebo. At a median follow-up of 14 months, patients in the clodronate-treated group showed a 46% reduction in hypercalcemia episodes, a 32% reduction in vertebral fractures, and a 20% reduction in the need for radiation therapy. Overall, significant reductions were noted in the frequency of all morbid skeletal events; hypercalcemia episodes, including terminal hypercalcemic events; vertebral fractures; and vertebral deformity in the clodronate-treated group. No impact of clodronate treatment on survival was reported.

Pamidronate

Pamidronate is an amino disodium bisphosphonate analogue. It is reported to be 100 times more potent than etidronate, with substantially more antiosteoclast activity and minimal antiosteoblast activity *in vitro* and *in vivo*.[40]

In 1987, van Holten-Verzantvoort et al. published the results of long-term bisphosphonate treatment of lytic metastasis of breast cancer.[61] This open, randomized, multicenter trial enrolled 131 patients, 70 of whom were treated with oral pamidronate, 300 mg per day. Specific cancer treatment was at the discretion of the attending physician. The study skeletal end points included hypercalcemia, bone pain warranting radiation or surgery, and pathologic or impending pathologic fracture. Reduction in skeletal morbidity was approximately 50% when cumulative complications were analyzed over time. Significant reductions in hypercalcemia, bone pain, pathologic fractures, and need for radiation therapy were noted ($p < .002$, $< .003$, $< .001$, and $< .002$, respectively). Treatment with oral pamidronate was assessed as safe and

TABLE 2. *Results of prospective randomized trials of bisphosphonate therapy for bone metastasis from breast cancer*

Study	Date	*n*	Placebo control	Agent/ route	Fracture risk	Radiation	Surgery	HCM	Pain	Survival
Elomaa et al.[59]	1987	34	Yes	Clodronate disodium p.o.	↓	NR	NR	↓	↓	Better
Paterson et al.[60]	1993	173	Yes	Clodronate disodium p.o.	↓	↓		↓	↓	No diff.
van Holten-Verzant-voort et al.[61]	1987	131	No	Pamidronate disodium p.o.	No diff.	↓	No diff.	↓	↓	No diff.
Conte et al.[83]	1996	161	No	Pamidronate disodium i.v.	No diff.	No diff.	No diff.	↓	↓	No diff.
[a]Hortobagyi et al.[63]	1996	382	Yes	Pamidronate disodium i.v.	↓	↓	↓	↓	↓	No diff.
[a]Theriault et al.[64]	1996	372	Yes	Pamidronate disodium i.v.	↓	↓	No diff.	↓	↓	No diff.
[b]Hortobagyi et al.[65]	1998	382	Yes	Pamidronate disodium i.v.	↓	↓	↓	↓	↓	No diff.
[b]Theriault et al.	1999	372	Yes	Pamidronate disodium i.v.	↓	↓	No diff.	↓	↓	No diff.

↓ decreased; HCM, hypercalcemia; No diff., no difference; NR, not reported.
[a]12-Month analysis.
[b]24-Month analysis.

effective in reducing skeletal morbidity for breast cancer patients with osteolytic metastases.

In a subsequent open, randomized study of pamidronate, van Holten-Verzantvoort et al. treated patients with breast cancer–related osteolytic bone metastases with oral pamidronate, 600 mg per day.[62] The dosage was subsequently reduced to 300 mg per day because of gastrointestinal toxicity. One hundred sixty-one patients were randomly assigned to treatment groups. Clinical cancer care and treatment were at the discretion of the attending physician. An analysis of treatment intentions showed reductions in hypercalcemia, severe bone pain, and requirements for radiotherapy (p = .003, .004, and .002, respectively). Although substantial reductions in skeletal morbidity were noted with oral pamidronate use, no survival advantage was seen.[62]

Short-term and long-term results of two large, randomized trials of the use of intravenous pamidronate for the adjunctive treatment of lytic skeletal metastasis have been reported.[63–66] In the first trial, patients with osteolytic metastasis from breast cancer who were being treated with chemotherapy were randomly assigned to receive pamidronate, 90 mg, administered intravenously over 2 hours every 3 to 4 weeks, or placebo. Three hundred eighty-two patients were assigned randomly to treatment groups, 185 to pamidronate and 197 to placebo. The patients in each group were well matched for clinically relevant factors that may impact breast cancer outcome, including age, extent of metastatic disease, presence of visceral disease, number and type of prior chemotherapies, time from diagnosis of breast cancer to development of bone metastasis, and duration of bone metastasis before clinical trial enrollment. At the 12-month analysis point, significant reductions in all skeletal complications were seen in the pamidronate-treated group.[63] These included significant reductions in risk of nonvertebral pathologic fracture, reduced frequency of radiation therapy and surgery for bone complications, and reduction in incidence of hypercalcemia. The time to first skeletal event was substantially and significantly longer in the pamidronate-treated group (13.1 months) than in the placebo group (7.0 months). In addition to the skeletal benefits, significant reductions were seen in Radiation Therapy Oncology Group (RTOG) pain and analgesic scores at the 9-month and 12-month analysis points.

Decreases in the ratio of urinary hydroxyproline to creatinine and the ratio of urinary calcium to creatinine were substantially and significantly greater in the pamidronate-treated group, confirming the inhibition of bone osteolytic activity. Clinical toxicity caused by pamidronate use was limited. Fever, transient myalgias, and increase in bone pain were seen, generally with the first infusion. Only one episode of symptomatic hypocalcemia occurred.[63]

In a parallel placebo-controlled trial, Theriault et al. reported on a group of 372 patients with osteolytic bone metastasis who were treated with hormone therapy.[64] One hundred eighty-two patients were randomly assigned to monthly infusions of pamidronate. Skeletal events—defined as fracture, spinal cord compression, radiation therapy to bone, hypercalcemia, or surgery to bone—were recorded for all participants. Results were also reported as skeletal morbidity rates, the number of skeletal events per patient per time in the study. At the 12-month analysis, a significant reduction was seen in the skeletal morbidity rate in the pamidronate-treated group compared with the nontreated group. Fewer patients receiving pamidronate required radiation, and substantial improvement in pain scores was noted (p = .009). The time to first skeletal event was 10.9 months for the pamidronate-treated group, compared with 6.9

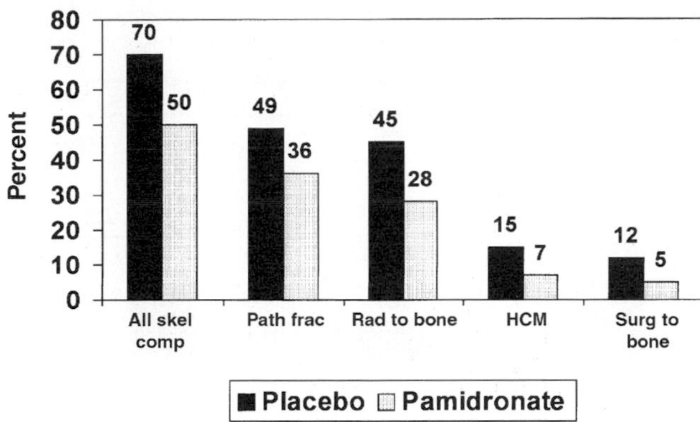

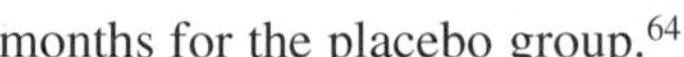

FIG. 1. Proportion of patients experiencing various skeletal events at 24 months after treatment with pamidronate disodium and chemotherapy. All skel comp, all skeletal complications; HCM, hypercalcemia; Path frac, pathological fracture; Rad to bone, radiation to bone; Surg to bone, surgery to bone.

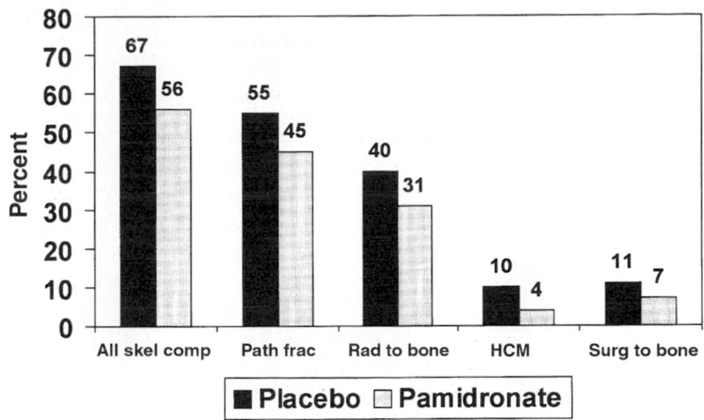

FIG. 2. Proportion of patients experiencing various skeletal events at 24 months after treatment with pamidronate disodium and hormone therapy. All skel comp, all skeletal complications; HCM, hypercalcemia; Path frac, pathological fracture; Rad to bone, radiation to bone; Surg to bone, surgery to bone.

months for the placebo group.[64]

Long-term (24-month) results of the trials reported by Hortobagyi and Theriault demonstrated sustained clinical benefit for patients continuing on a 3- to 4-week schedule of pamidronate by intravenous infusion for 24 months.[65,66] The overall skeletal complication rate in the chemotherapy trial was reduced from 70% for the group receiving placebo to 50% for the pamidronate-treated group; pathologic fracture risk was decreased from 49% to 36%, and radiation to bone was decreased from 45% to 28%. A similar, but less striking, clinical benefit was observed in the hormone therapy breast cancer trial (Figs. 1 and 2). Pooled data from these trials demonstrated consistent positive effects for pamidronate treatment of skeletal disease with regard to the proportion of patients with skeleton-related events and the skeletal morbidity rate (Figs. 3 and 4).

RTOG pain and analgesic scores remained significantly better for the pamidronate-treated group among patients undergoing both chemotherapy and hormonal therapy.[65,66] In the stratification analysis of the trial reported by Hortobagyi et al., patients with good performance status (Eastern Cooperative Oncology Group 0,1) derived the greatest skeletal benefit from pamidronate, a result suggesting that earlier, rather than later, initiation of bisphosphonate therapy is clinically appropriate.

BISPHOSPHONATE PREVENTION OF SKELETAL DISEASE

Laboratory and *in vivo* data have shown that bisphosphonate treatment may reduce the incidence or prevent the development of bone metastasis.[67–71] Kanis et al. reported on a trial in which 133 women with breast cancer metastasis but without existing bone disease were randomly assigned to treatment with oral clodronate, 1,600 mg per day, or placebo.[72] The end

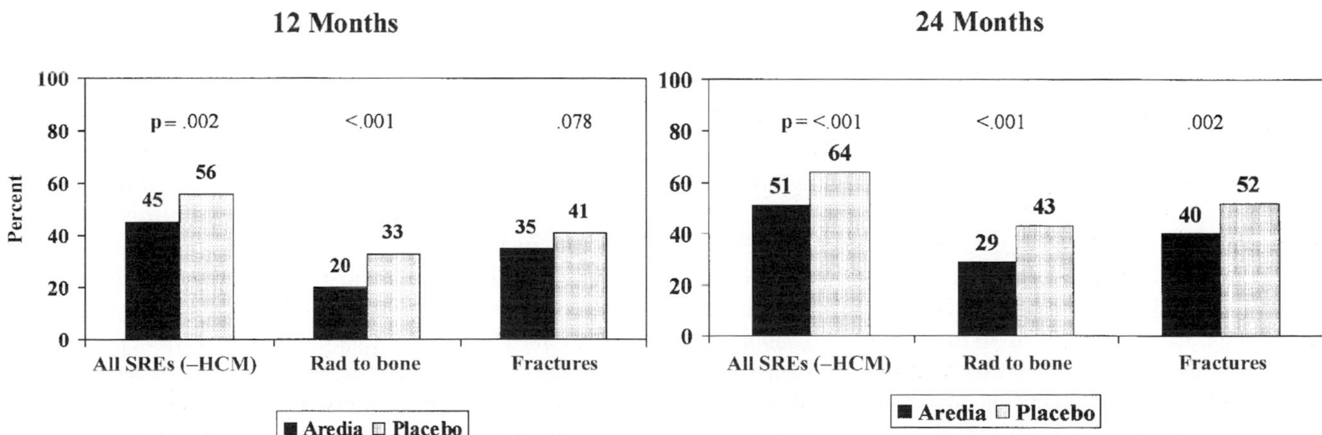

FIG. 3. Proportion of patients experiencing various skeleton-related events after treatment with intravenous pamidronate disodium (Aredia). Data are from pooled breast cancer clinical trials that included 754 patients. HCM, hypercalcemia; Rad to bone, radiation to bone; SRE, skeleton-related event.

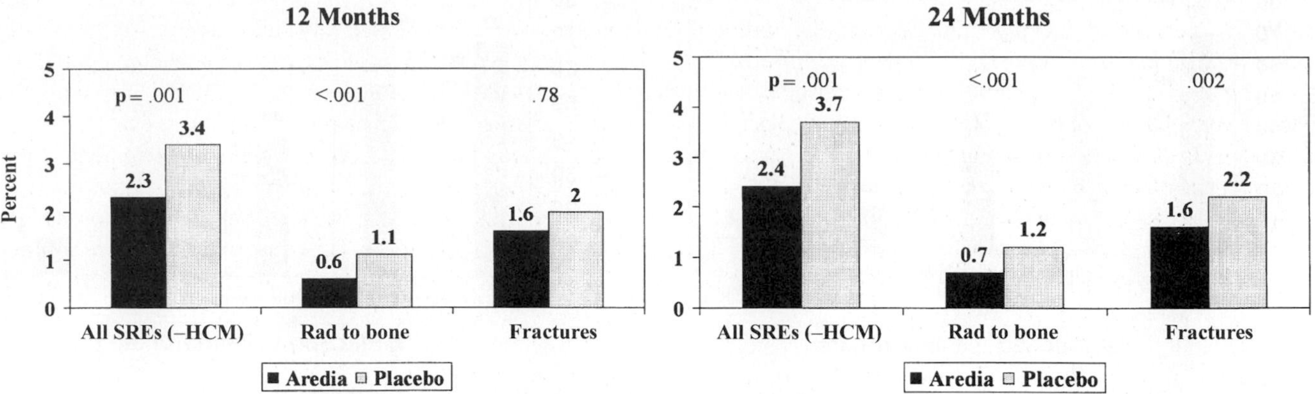

FIG. 4. Mean skeletal morbidity rate of patients treated with intravenous pamidronate disodium (Aredia). Data are from pooled breast cancer clinical trials that included 754 patients. Skeletal morbidity rate is calculated as the number of skeletal events per patient divided by the time on trial. HCM, hypercalcemia; Rad to bone, radiation to bone; SRE, skeleton-related event.

point was the frequency of development of bone metastasis, as determined by sequential radiographs and bone scans. Although skeletal metastasis developed less frequently in the clodronate-treated group than in the placebo-treated group (15 cases versus 19 cases), this difference was not statistically significant. This study had limited power to show a significant difference because of the small number of patients. Nevertheless, the clodronate-treated patients experienced fewer skeletal metastases and skeleton-related complications.[72]

Data on bisphosphonate protection from bone metastasis has been presented by Powles et al. These researchers randomly assigned 1,079 patients with primary operable breast cancer to 1,600 mg per day of clodronate or placebo for 2 years. Preliminary results showed a significant decrease in the development of bone metastases in the clodronate-treated group. Bone metastases were confirmed in 5.2% of clodronate-treated patients, compared with 8.1% of the placebo-treated group. The effect was most pronounced in postmenopausal women: 3.3% of such women in the clodronate-treated group and 7.3% in the placebo-treated group developed definite bone disease ($p = .4$).[73]

Diel et al. had previously reported on the prognostic significance of tumor cells detected in the bone marrow.[23] In a clinical trial of the use of clodronate as an adjuvant treatment in primary operable breast cancer, Diel et al.[74] randomly assigned 302 patients with primary breast cancer shown to have tumor cells in marrow (a high-risk group for metastasis development) to receive oral clodronate, 1,600 mg per day, for 2 years in addition to standard adjuvant therapy or standard adjuvant therapy only. After a median of 36 months of observation, 42 patients in the control group had developed metastases, whereas only 21 patients in the clodronate group were shown to have distant disease ($p < .001$). Visceral and osseous metastases were significantly reduced, and the number of bone metastases in those who did develop bone disease was decreased in the clodronate-treated group. A significant early survival advantage was shown for the clodronate-treated group: 22 deaths occurred in the placebo-treated group, compared with only 6 deaths in the clodronate-treated group. Saarto et al.[75] report not only no benefit from oral clodronate but also a negative effect on survival of patients receiving clodronate in the adjuvant setting. This randomized study involved 299 women with primary breast cancer given clodronate, 1,600 mg orally, daily for three years or none. The clodronate group had a higher frequency of bone and visceral metastases and poorer survival than the nonclodronate group. This is the totally opposite effect of the reports of Powles et al.[73] and Diel et al.[74] No rational hypothesis for these observations has been postulated. Additional studies of adjuvant treatment with bisphosphonate in primary breast cancer are under way or in development with the intent of not only preventing skeletal metastasis but also improving overall survival of breast cancer patients.

BONE-TARGETED RADIATION THERAPY

External-beam radiation therapy has been used in cases of bone metastasis primarily for pain relief, prevention of impending pathologic fracture, and treatment of spinal cord compression. Questions about the dosage, schedule, disease response, duration of response, and use of multidisciplinary approaches remain areas of active clinical investigation.[76,77]

Therapy with bone-seeking radioactive agents is an alternative to external-beam radiation therapy and has been used primarily for relief of bone pain. Strontium chloride 89 and samarium 153 ethylenediaminetetramethylenephosphonate (EDTMP) are commercially available for use in clinical practice. Strontium is preferentially taken up at sites of active bone tumor and has greater uptake in metastatic disease than in normal bone. Robinson et al. reported clinical response for relief of pain in 80% of breast cancer patients.[78] Twenty percent became pain free. Baziotis et al. reported on 64 breast cancer patients with painful bone metastases treated with a single injection of strontium chloride 89. Thirty-five percent of the patients experienced "dramatic decrease in bone pain," whereas 40% showed a "satisfactory" response.[79] Most studies of strontium use in breast cancer have included only 8 to 15 patients; large comparative trials of the efficacy of strontium compared with external-beam radiation therapy have not been performed.[80]

The advantages of samarium 153 EDTMP are reported to be its ease of manufacture, reasonable shelf life, and the ability to monitor the distribution of the agent. Efficacy studies are limited in size. Pain relief has been reported to occur in 60% to 80% of patients. As with strontium, hematologic toxicity is dose limiting. Alberts et al. have completed a study of dose relationship and multiple dose efficacy and toxicity for samarium. They failed to show a clear dose-response relationship for bone pain relief; however, "adequate" pain control was reported for 78% to 95% of treated patients.[81]

A randomized dose-controlled study of samarium 153 EDTMP demonstrated that treatment resulted in decreased pain, decreased levels of daytime discomfort, and improved quality of sleep. Female breast cancer patients were reported to show the most notable improvements.[82]

CONCLUSION

Bone metastases from primary breast cancer remain a substantial clinical problem. The development of bone-targeted therapeutic interventions, especially bisphosphonate treatment, that significantly impact osteoclast activation can provide palliation of pain, decrease the risk of fracture and episodes of hypercalcemia, and reduce the need for bone surgery. Their use may preclude the need for radiation therapy to bone. Bisphosphonates must be used in conjunction with conventional antitumor therapy, including systemic chemotherapy and hormonal therapy, because they have no known antitumor effect on cancer cells. Early intervention with bisphosphonates appears to provide the greatest potential for bone-sparing benefit and palliation of bone-related symptoms. The optimal schedule and duration of treatment has not yet been defined. Studies of bone-derived urinary markers may provide some insight by indicating a therapeutic end point that demonstrates the time and duration of osteoclast inhibition.[14] Additional studies combining bisphosphonates such as pamidronate and clodronate with radiopharmaceutical targeting of bone metastases may demonstrate substantial benefit over the use of either agent alone, and clinical trials using this strategy have begun.

Current Recommendations for Medical Management of Bone Metastases

Once a diagnosis of bone metastasis has been established by means of bone scan, radiography, magnetic resonance imaging, or computed tomographic scan, careful assessment for the clinical presentation of osteolytic, osteoblastic, or mixed disease should be undertaken. Serial clinical examinations for bone-related episodes and potential morbid events are warranted, especially for impending or pathologic fracture and spinal cord or nerve root compression. Systemic antineoplastic treatment with hormone therapy or chemotherapy depends on the previous treatment history and clinical situation. The new paradigm of treating the recipient organ of metastases (i.e., bone) and the potential to maintain the integrity of the organ will lead to new studies of the potential for inhibiting or preventing metastases by the use of bisphosphonates in the primary breast cancer setting. Treatment with bisphosphonates, such as intravenous administration of pamidronate, 90 mg over 2 hours on a 3- to 4-week schedule, is appropriate in patients with bone metastases. Clodronate, 1,600 mg per day by mouth, may be used in a similar fashion, although this formulation is not commercially available in all countries.

Treatment Summary for Bone Metastasis

- Clinically appropriate systemic chemotherapy or hormone therapy
- Bisphosphonate therapy initiated when bone metastases documented
  - Pamidronate disodium, 90 mg intravenously over 2 hours every 3 to 4 weeks; or
  - Clodronate disodium, 1,600 mg per day by mouth*
- Bisphosphonate therapy continued for 2 years or as long as systemic therapy is continued

Treatment Summary for Hypercalcemia

- Assess fluid balance.
- Hydrate with normal saline.
- Correct other electrolyte abnormalities—hypokalemia, hypomagnesemia.
- Administer calcitonin for immediate hypocalcemic effect (for severe hypercalcemia), minimum of 15 mg per dL or any level with central nervous system depression.
- Give pamidronate disodium, 60 to 90 mg intravenously over 2 hours.

REFERENCES

1. Viadana E, Cotter R, Picksen JW, et al. An autopsy study of metastatic sites of breast cancer. *Cancer Res* 1973;33:179.
2. Vallagusa P, Tesoro-Tess JD, Rossi P, et al. Adjuvant CMF: effect on site of first recurrence in appropriate follow-up intervals in operable breast cancer with positive axillary lymph nodes. *Breast Cancer Res Treat* 1982;1:349.
3. Galasko CSB. Skeletal metastases and mammary cancer. *Ann R Coll Surg Treat* 1972;50:3.
4. Scheid V, Buzdar AU, Smith TL, et al. Clinical course of breast cancer patients with osseous metastasis treated with combination chemotherapy. *Cancer* 1986;58:2589.

*Not available in some countries.

5. Sherry MM, Greco FA, Johnson DH, Hainsworth JD. Metastatic breast cancer confined to the skeletal system. An indolent disease. *Am J Med* 1986;81:381.
6. Coleman RE, Rubens RD. The clinical course of bone metastases from breast cancer. *Br J Cancer* 1987;55:61.
7. Coleman RE, Smith P, Rubens RD. Clinical course and prognostic factors following bone recurrence from breast cancer. *Br J Cancer* 1998;77:336.
8. Jones AL, Williams MP, Powles TJ, et al. Magnetic resonance imaging in the detection of bone metastases in breast cancer patients. *Br J Cancer* 1990;62:296.
9. Gosfield E, Alavi A, Kneeland B. Comparison of radionuclide bone scans and magnetic resonance imaging in detecting spinal metastases. *J Nucl Med* 1993;34:2191.
10. Sanal SM, Flickinger FW, Caudell MJ, et al. Detection of bone marrow involvement in breast cancer with magnetic resonance imaging. *J Clin Oncol* 1994;12:1415.
11. Vandemark RM, Shpall EJ, Affronti ML. Bone metastases from breast cancer: value of CT bone windows. *J Comput Assist Tomog* 1992;16:608.
12. Coleman RE, Houston S, James I, et al. Preliminary results of the use of urinary excretion of pyridinium crosslinks for monitoring metastatic bone disease. *Br J Cancer* 1992;65:766.
13. Demers L, Lipton A, Harvey H, et al. The measurement of pyridinium cross-links in serum of patients with metastatic bone disease. *Proc Annu Meet Am Soc Clin Oncol* 1993;12:A243.
14. Lipton A, Demers L, Curley E, et al. Markers of bone resorption in patients treated with pamidronate. *Eur J Cancer* 1998;34:2021.
15. Lowik CW, van der Pluijm G, Bloys H, et al. Parathyroid hormone and PTH-like protein stimulate interleukin-6 production by osteogenic cells: a possible role of interleukin-6 in osteoclastogenesis. *Biochem Biophys Res Commun* 1989;162:1546
16. Hauschka PV, Chen TL, Mavrakos AE. Polypeptide growth factors in bone matrix. *Ciba Found Symp* 1988;136:207.
17. Mundy GR, Bonewald LF. Role of TGFb in bone remodeling. *Ann N Y Acad Sci* 1990;593:91.
18. DiStefano A, Tashima CK, Yap HY, Hortobagyi GN. Bone marrow metastases without cortical bone involvement in breast cancer patients. *Cancer* 1979;44:196.
19. Ingle JN, Tormey DC, Tan HK. The bone marrow examination in breast cancer: diagnostic considerations and clinical usefulness. *Cancer* 1978;41:670.
20. Landys K. Prognostic value of bone marrow biopsy in breast cancer. *Cancer* 1982;49:513.
21. Fields KK, Elfenbein GJ, Trudeau WL, Perkins JB, Janssen WE, Moscinski LC. Clinical significance of bone marrow metastases as detected using the polymerase chain reaction in patients with breast cancer undergoing high-dose chemotherapy and autologous bone marrow transplantation. *J Clin Oncol* 1996;14:1868.
22. Janni W, Braun S, Hepp F, Pantel KI. Detection of isolated tumor cells in bone marrow of breast cancer patients at the time of primary diagnosis, locoregional recurrence, or metastatic disease. *Proc Am Soc Clin Oncol* 1997;38:A1797.
23. Diel IJ, Kaufmann M, Costa SD, et al. Micrometastatic breast cancer cells in bone marrow at primary surgery: prognostic value in comparison to nodal status. *J Natl Cancer Inst* 1996;88:1652.
24. Colnaghi MI. Correlation between the presence of breast tumor cells in bone marrow at the time of surgery and disease progression. *Dev Oncol* 1990;58:187.
25. Mansi JL, Powles TJ, Coombes RC. The detection and evaluation of bone marrow micrometastases in primary breast cancer. *Dev Oncol* 1987;51:299.
26. Vredenburgh JJ, Peters WP, Rosner G, et al. Detection of tumor cells in the bone marrow of stage IV breast cancer patients receiving high-dose chemotherapy: the role of induction chemotherapy. *Bone Marrow Transplant* 1995;16:815.
27. Singletary SE, Larry L, Tucker SL, Spitzer G. Detection of micrometastatic tumor cells in bone marrow of breast carcinoma patients. *J Surg Oncol* 1991;47:32.
28. George SL, Hoogstraten B. Prognostic factors in the initial response to therapy by patients with advanced breast cancer. *J Natl Cancer Inst* 1978;60:731.
29. Abeloff MD, Ettinger DS. Treatment of metastatic breast cancer with adriamycin-cyclophosphamide induction followed by alternating combination therapy. *Cancer Treat Rep* 1977;61:1685.
30. Kennealey GT, Boston B, Mitchell M, et al. Combination chemotherapy for advanced breast cancer: two regimens containing adriamycin. *Cancer* 1978;42:27.
31. Swenerton KD, Legha S, Smith T, et al. Prognostic factors in metastatic breast cancer treated with combination chemotherapy. *Cancer Res* 1979;39:1552.
32. Smalley RV, Carpenter J, Bartolucci A, et al. A comparison of cyclophosphamide, adriamycin, 5-fluorouracil (CAF) and cyclophosphamide, methotrexate, 5-fluorouracil, vincristine, prednisone (CMFVP) in patients with metastatic breast cancer. *Cancer* 1977;40:625.
33. Jones SE, Durie B, Salmon S. Combination chemotherapy with adriamycin and cyclophosphamide for advanced breast cancer. *Cancer* 1975;36:90.
34. Whitehouse JMA. Site dependent response to chemotherapy for carcinoma of the breast. *J R Soc Med* 1985;78:18.
35. Hayward JL, Carbone PP, Heuson JC, et al. Assessment of response to therapy in advanced breast cancer: a project of the programme on clinical oncology of the International Union Cancer, Geneva, Switzerland. *Cancer* 1977;39:1289.
36. Friedl W. Indication management and results of surgical therapy for pathologic fractures in patients with bone metastases. *Eur J Surg Oncol* 1990;16:380.
37. Tong D, Gillick L, Hendrickson F. The palliation of symptomatic osseous metastases: final results of the Study by the Radiation Therapy Oncology Group. *Cancer* 1982;50:893.
38. Ingle JN, Tormey DC, Bull JM, Simon RM. Bone marrow involvement in breast cancer: effect on response and tolerance to combination chemotherapy. *Cancer* 1977;39:104.
39. Rodriguez-Kraul R, Hortobagyi GN, Buzdar AU, Blumenschein GR. Combination chemotherapy for breast cancer metastatic to bone marrow. *Cancer* 1981;48:227.
40. Fleish H. Bisphosphonates: pharmacology and use in the treatment of tumour-induced hypercalcaemic and metastatic bone disease. *Drugs* 1991;42:919.
41. Fitton A, McTavish D. Pamidronate: a review of its pharmacological properties and therapeutic efficacy in resorptive bone disease. *Drugs* 1991;41:289.
42. Theriault RL, Sellin RV. Hypercalcemia of malignancy as a presenting manifestation of hepatic metastases from breast cancer. *Cancer Bull* 1991;43:588.
43. Ryzen E, Martodam RR, Troxell M, et al. Intravenous etidronate in the management of malignant hypercalcemia. *Arch Intern Med* 1985;145:449.
44. Pecherstorfer M, Herrmann Z, Body JJ, et al. Randomized phase II trial comparing different doses of the bisphosphonate ibandronate in the treatment of hypercalcemia of malignancy. *J Clin Oncol* 1996;14:268.
45. Nussbaum SR, Younger J, Vandepol CJ, et al. Single-dose intravenous therapy with pamidronate for the treatment of hypercalcemia of malignancy: comparison of 30-, 60-, and 90-mg dosages. *Am J Med* 1993;95:297.
46. Nussbaum SR, Warrell RP Jr, Rude R, et al. Dose-response study of alendronate sodium for the treatment of cancer-associated hypercalcemia. *J Clin Oncol* 1993;11:1618.
47. Purohit OP, Radstone CR, Anthony C, Kanis JA, Coleman RE. A randomised double-blind comparison of intravenous pamidronate and clodronate in the hypercalcaemia of malignancy. *Br J Cancer* 1995;72:1289.
48. Warrell RP, Mullane M, Bilezikian J, et al. Treatment of cancer associated hypercalcemia with alendronate sodium: a randomized double-blind comparison with etidronate. *Proc Am Soc Clin Oncol* 1993;12:A1514.
49. Rizzoli R, Buchs B, Bonjour JP. Effect of a single infusion of alendronate in malignant hypercalcaemia: dose dependency and comparison with clodronate. *Int J Cancer* 1992;50:706.
50. Gucalp R, Ritch P, Wiernik PH, et al. Comparative study of pamidronate disodium and etidronate disodium in the treatment of cancer-related hypercalcemia. *J Clin Oncol* 1992;10:134.
51. Gucalp R, Theriault RL, Gill I, et al. Treatment of cancer-associated hypercalcemia. Double-blind comparison of rapid and slow intravenous infusion regimens of pamidronate disodium and saline alone. *Arch Intern Med* 1994;154:1935.
52. Zysset E, Ammann P, Jenzer A, et al. Comparison of a rapid (2-h) versus a slow (24-h) infusion of alendronate in the treatment of hypercalcemia of malignancy. *Bone Miner* 1992;18:237.

53. Body JJ. Clinical research update zoledronate. Review. *Cancer* 1997; 80:1699.
54. Sekine M, Takami H. Combination of calcitonin and pamidronate for emergency treatment of malignant hypercalcemia. *Oncol Rep* 1998;5:197.
55. Gulcalp R, Theriault RL, Gill I, et al. Treatment of hypercalcemia of malignancy: double-blind comparison of rapid and slow intravenous infusion regimens of pamidronate and saline alone. *Arch Intern Med* 1994;154:1935.
56. Ralston SH, Thiebaud D, Herrmann Z, et al. Dose-response study of ibandronate in the treatment of cancer-associated hypercalcemia. *Br J Cancer* 1997;75:295.
57. Pecherstorfer M, Herrmann Z, Body JJ, et al. Randomized phase II trial comparing different doses of the bisphosphonate ibandronate in the treatment of hypercalcemia of malignancy. *J Clin Oncol* 1996;14:268.
58. Plosker GL, Goa KL. Clodronate. A review of its pharmacological properties and therapeutic efficacy in resorptive bone disease. *Drugs* 1994;47:945.
59. Elomaa I, Blomqvist C, Porkka L, et al. Treatment of skeletal disease in breast cancer: a controlled clodronate trial. *Bone* 1987;8:S53.
60. Paterson AHG, Popwles TJ, Kanis JA, et al. Double-blind controlled trial of oral clodronate in patients with bone metastases from breast cancer. *J Clin Oncol* 1993;11:59.
61. van Holten-Verzantvoort AT, Bijvoet OLM, Hermans J, et al. Reduced morbidity from skeletal metastases in breast cancer patients during long-term bisphosphonate treatment. *Lancet* 1987;2:983.
62. van Holten-Verzantvoort AT, Kroon HM, Bijvoet OLM, et al. Palliative pamidronate treatment in patients with bone metastases from breast cancer. *J Clin Oncol* 1993;11:491.
63. Hortobagyi GN, Theriault RL, Porter L, et al. Efficacy of pamidronate in reducing skeletal complications in patients with breast cancer and lytic bone metastases. Protocol 19 Aredia Breast Cancer Study Group. *N Engl J Med* 1996;335:1785.
64. Theriault RL, Lipton A, Leff R, et al. Reduction of skeletal related complications in breast cancer patients with osteolytic bone metastases receiving hormone therapy, by monthly pamidronate sodium infusion. *Proc Am Soc Clin Oncol* 1996;15:122(abst), 152(abst).
65. Hortobagyi GN, Theriault RL, Lipton A, et al. Long-term prevention of skeletal complications of metastatic breast cancer with pamidronate. *J Clin Oncol* 1998;16:2038.
66. Theriault RL, Lipton A, Hortobagyi GN, et al. Pamidronate reduces skeletal morbidity in women with advanced breast cancer and lytic bone lesions: a randomised, placebo-controlled trial. *J Clin Oncol* 1999;17:846.
67. Tamura H, Ishii S, Ikeda T, et al. Therapeutic efficacy of pamidronate in combination with chemotherapy to bone metastasis of breast cancer in a rat model. *Surg Oncol* 1996;5:141.
68. Tamura H, Ishii S, Enomoto K, et al. Evaluation of the therapeutic efficacy of bisphosphonate (BP) to bone metastasis of breast cancer in a rat model. *Proc Annu Meet Am Assoc Cancer Res* 1994;35:A2787.
69. Sasaki A, Boyce BF, Story B, et al. Bisphosphonate risedronate reduces metastatic human breast cancer burden in bone in nude mice. *Cancer Res* 1995;55:3551.
70. Wada N, Ishii S, Tamura H, et al. The prophylactic and early therapeutic effects of bisphosphonate (BP) against bone metastasis (BM) of breast cancer. *Proc Annu Meet Am Assoc Cancer Res* 1995;36:A1855.
71. Hall DG, Stoica G. Effect of the bisphosphonate risedronate on bone metastases in a rat mammary adenocarcinoma model system. *J Bone Miner Res* 1994;9:221.
72. Kanis JA, Powles T, Paterson AHG, McCloskey EV, Ashley S. Clodronate decreases the frequency of skeletal metastases in women with breast cancer. *Bone* 1996;19:663.
73. Powles TJ, Paterson AHG, Nevantaus A, et al. Adjuvant clodronate reduces the incidence of bone metastases in patients with primary operable breast cancer. *Proc Am Soc Clin Oncol* 1998;17:123a.
74. Diel IJ, Solomayer EF, Costa SD, et al. Reduction in new metastases in breast cancer with adjuvant clodronate treatment. *N Engl J Med* 1998;339:357.
75. Saarto T, Blomqvist C, Virkkuenen P. Elomaa I. No reduction of bone metastases with adjuvant Clodronate treatment in node-positive breast cancer patients. *Proc Am Soc Clin Oncol* 1999;18:128a (abst 489).
76. Bates T. A review of local radiotherapy in the treatment of bone metastases and cord compression. *Int J Radiat Oncol Biol Phys* 1990;23:217.
77. Bates T, Yarnold JR, Blitzer P, et al. Bone metastasis consensus statement. *Int J Radiat Oncol Biol Phys* 1991;23:215.
78. Robinson RG, Blake GM, Preston DF, et al. Strontium-89: treatment results and kinetics in patients with painful metastatic prostate and breast cancer in bone. *Radiographics* 1989;9:271.
79. Baziotis N, Yakoumakis E, Zissimopoulos A, et al. Strontium-89 chloride in the treatment of bone metastases from breast cancer. *Oncology* 1998;55:377.
80. Lee CK, Aeppli DM, Unger J, Boudreau RJ, Levitt SH. Strontium-89 chloride (Metastron) for palliative treatment of bony metastases. The University of Minnesota experience. *Am J Clin Oncol* 1996;19:102.
81. Alberts AS, Smit BJ, Louw WK, et al. Dose response relationship and multiple dose efficacy and toxicity of samarium-153-EDTMP in metastatic cancer to bone. *Radiother Oncol* 1997;43:175.
82. Resche I, Chatal JF, Pecking A, et al. A dose-controlled study of 153 Sm-ethylenediaminetetramethylenephosphonate (EDTMP) in the treatment of patients with painful bone metastases. *Eur J Cancer* 1997;33:1583.
83. Conte PF, Latreille J, Mauriac L, et al. Delay in progression of bone metastases in breast cancer patients treated with intravenous pamidronate: results from a multinational randomized controlled trial. The Aredia Multinational Cooperative Group. *J Clin Oncol* 1996; 14:2552.

Diseases of the Breast, 2nd ed.,
edited by Jay R. Harris.
Lippincott Williams & Wilkins, Philadelphia © 2000.

CHAPTER 62

Local Treatment of Bone Metastases

Alan D. Aaron and Christine D. Berg

Bone metastases are a significant problem for a large number of cancer patients. Bone metastases can often be the first presentation of previously undiagnosed carcinoma. Bone is the third most common site, after lung and liver, for distant metastases from adenocarcinoma. Although the bone metastasis is often clinically silent, up to 85% of patients dying from breast, prostate, or lung carcinoma primaries show bone involvement at autopsy.[1,2] At some time during the clinical course of the disease, radionuclide imaging demonstrates bone metastases in 63% of patients diagnosed with primary adenocarcinoma; 85% of adenocarcinomas metastasizing to bone are secondary to breast, lung, or prostate carcinomas.[3] The most frequent sites of bone metastases are the vertebrae, pelvis, ribs, femur, and skull. Survival can vary widely in patients with metastatic bone disease and often depends on the histology of the primary carcinoma. On average, patient survival is 24 months for prostate carcinoma, 18 months for cervical carcinoma, 13 months for colorectal carcinoma, less than 12 months for lung carcinoma, and 3.5 months for melanoma.[4,5] Patients with metastatic breast disease to bone survive 34 months on average (range, 1 to 90 months) after detection of the first metastasis.[5]

CLINICAL PRESENTATION AND DIAGNOSIS

Pain is the most frequent clinical symptom reported by patients with metastatic bone disease and ranks second only to death as the most feared aspect of cancer for patients.[6,7] An extensive review of 54 studies of cancer pain identified pain as being secondary to cancer in 7,067 of 9,007 patients diagnosed with metastatic adenocarcinoma.[8] Cancer pain is characteristically described as dull in character, gradually progressive in intensity, and constant in presentation. Night pain and pain not relieved by rest are especially worrisome. Assessing the source of pain in elderly patients is often difficult. Concomitant conditions, such as degenerative osteoarthritis of either the spine or hips, infection, or an inflammatory disease, may sometimes masquerade as cancer pain.[9] In a study by Galasko and Sylvester, 11 of 31 patients with back pain and a primary carcinoma were identified as having a nontumor cause for their pain.[10]

The etiology of cancer pain is not fully understood. Proposed causes include the stimulation of nerve endings in the endosteum resulting from release of chemical agents from destroyed bone tissue, stretching of the periosteum by increasing tumor size, fractures, and tumor growth that causes inflammation in the surrounding soft-tissue envelope.[11] The activation of both nociceptors and mechanoreceptors in the endosteum and periosteum by metastatic tumor in the bone has been hypothesized.[12–14] Direct pressure from the tumor may result in the release of several chemical mediators of pain, including substance P, prostaglandins, growth factors, bradykinin, and histamine.[14,15]

Patients may also present with pathologic fractures as the first indication of metastatic disease or at some time during their disease course. The overall incidence of pathologic fracture has been reported to be between 8% and 29%, depending on the location of lesions.[16–19] In a study of 1,800 patients with metastatic cancer to bone, 165 patients sustained a pathologic fracture.[17] In another study, Schurman and Amstutz reported on 700 patients with breast cancer, among whom 63 patients demonstrated femoral metastases.[18] Of those patients with femoral metastases, 18 patients (29%) progressed to fracture.[18] Metastases from four primary carcinomas account for approximately 80% of all fractures. Fifty percent of all pathologic fractures result from breast carcinoma metastases, whereas 10% result from kidney carcinoma metastases, 10% from lung carcinoma metastases, 5% from thyroid carcinoma metastases, and an additional 5% from metastases from other, less common adenocarcinomas.[20] The majority of these lesions appear to be osteolytic on plain radiographs; breast carcinoma metastases have been reported to appear osteoblastic in approximately 78 of 516 metastatic bone lesions (15%) (Fig. 1).[21,22] A strong relationship is seen between osteolytic lesions and the risk of fracture, whereas the primarily osteoblastic metastatic deposits such as are found in metastases from

A. D. Aaron: Department of Orthopaedic Surgery, Georgetown University Hospital, Washington, D.C.

C. D. Berg: Lung and Upper Aerodigestive Cancer Research Group, Division of Cancer Prevention, National Cancer Institute, Bethesda, Maryland

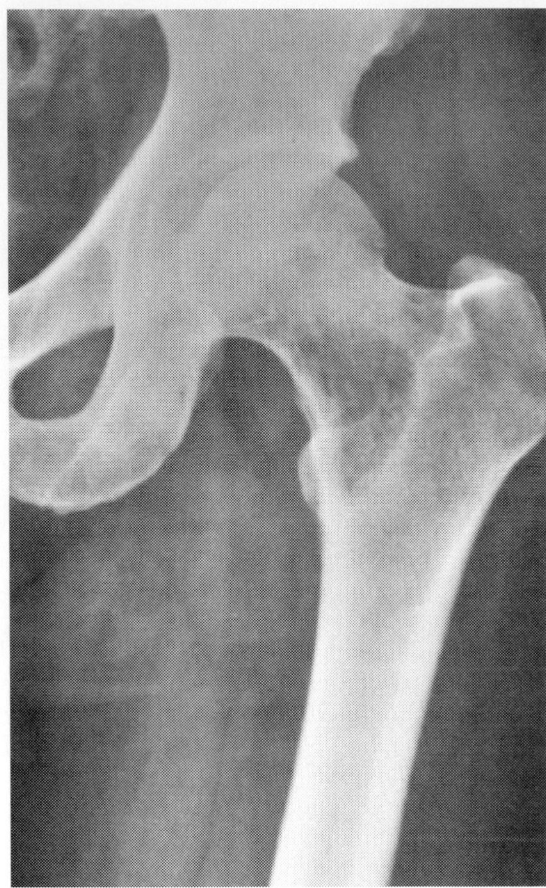

FIG. 1. Lytic breast carcinoma metastasis residing in the proximal femur. Local bone destruction without sclerotic bone production and absence of periosteal reaction are characteristic of osseous metastasis.

prostate carcinoma rarely result in pathologic fracture. In a study of 306 primary cancers metastatic to the femur, only 11 fractures (3.6%) were secondary to prostate carcinoma.[23] The most common sites of pathologic fracture are the proximal ends of the long bones; the proximal femur is the most common location. Harrington reported that 258 of 399 fractures (65%) occurred in the femur, whereas fractures of the humerus accounted for only 68 (17%) of the pathologic fractures in that series.[24]

WORKUP AND DIAGNOSIS

The majority of patients present to clinicians with pain, which often directs the patient's diagnostic workup. Plain radiographs of the affected region are often obtained and usually identify local pathology. Metastatic lesions are generally radiolucent, with a minimal periosteal reaction. Their epicenter is often located within the intramedullary canal; intracortical or juxtacortical locations are uncommon. Axial and proximal appendicular locations are common sites for metastases. Metastatic lesions are rarely located in the foot or hand. In one review of 41,833 cases, only three (0.007%) were osseous metastases to the hand.[25] When lesions are encountered in the distal extremities, clinicians should consider the possibility that metastases have occurred from primary carcinomas of the lung or kidney or that the patient is in the terminal stages of widespread metastatic disease from another primary carcinoma.[26] Bone lesions in patients older than 40 years of age are most likely to be secondary to either metastatic adenocarcinoma or myeloma. In patients younger than age 40, the likelihood of a metastatic adenocarcinoma decreases, and the probability of either bone infection or primary sarcoma of bone correspondingly increases. Once a skeletal lesion has been identified, a bone scan should be performed to define whether it is an isolated site or whether multiple bones are involved.

Radionuclide scanning with technetium (Tc) 99 methylenediphosphonate is an extremely sensitive, yet nonspecific, method of identifying associated lesions. Estimates are that a tumor must reach a size of 1 cm and destroy up to 30% to 50% of the bone before it can be detected on a plain bone radiograph.[27–30] As a more sensitive radiographic imaging mode, radionuclide scanning has been reported to detect lesions 3 months earlier than plain radiographs and has an estimated detection threshold of 2 mm in tumor size.[22,31] In a study by Galasko encompassing 50 women with metastatic breast carcinoma, only 25 lesions (50%) were apparent on plain radiographs, whereas 42 (84%) were identified with radionuclide scanning.[31] In a later study, Galasko reported that a period of 2 to 18 months was necessary before lesions identified on radionuclide scanning could be visualized on plain radiographs.[32] Although sensitive, radionuclide scanning is not specific, especially in the case of a solitary lesion. In a cumulative series of 273 patients with known primary carcinomas and abnormal bone scans at the time of diagnosis, biopsy-proven metastatic disease was identified in only 55% of patients.[33] Additional, benign causes for radionuclide uptake included trauma in 25% of cases, infection in 10% of cases, and miscellaneous factors in the remaining 10% of cases. Anatomic site was noted to be important, with the majority of metastatic lesions residing in the vertebral bodies (80%).[33]

Given that lesions identified on radionuclide scanning may be secondary to either degenerative disease or trauma, in most cases a biopsy of at least one osseous site should be considered to assist in patient staging and treatment. Patients with evidence of multiple sites of involvement on radionuclide scanning, and without impending pathologic fracture, should undergo biopsy of the most accessible lesion. Needle biopsy is generally preferred over open techniques. In cases of monostotic disease, further evaluation of the lesion is necessary before biopsy. Evaluation by computerized axial tomography (CAT) or magnetic resonance imaging (MRI) should be considered before biopsy, given the possibility that a sarcoma might be identified. Once the diagnosis of metastatic bone disease has been established, subsequent sites do not require biopsy before treatment.

The high sensitivity of radionuclide imaging for the detection of metastatic disease has led to the testing of the hypothesis that screening of asymptomatic women with a history of primary breast carcinoma may lead to the earlier detection of metastatic disease, allowing prompt treatment and perhaps improving survival rates. Two randomized trials testing the results of intensive screening revealed earlier detection of metastatic disease but showed no impact on overall 5-year survival rates.[34,35] The American Society of Clinical Oncology reviewed the available evidence and issued Breast Cancer Surveillance Guidelines that did not recommend routine use of bone scanning.[36]

Serum assays to diagnose and monitor patients with metastatic bone disease are under investigation. Although lacking specificity, serum alkaline phosphatase level has been reported by Shaffer and Pendergrass to be elevated in the majority of patients with metastatic prostate carcinoma; 77% of 158 patients with bone metastases were found to have an elevated serum alkaline phosphatase level.[37] An elevated serum alkaline phosphatase level has also been reported in patients with metastatic breast carcinoma to bone. One study of 47 patients reported elevated levels in 32% of patients, whereas another involving 167 patients reported that 53% of patients presented with elevated serum alkaline phosphatase.[38,39] Although the tests are costly and relatively insensitive, levels of urinary calcium and hydroxyproline have been used as a measure of bone resorption, with decreased levels being associated with a clinical response to treatment.[40,41]

Newer biochemical markers of bone metabolism have become available and have been evaluated for their specificity in monitoring metastatic bone disease. These immunoassays have included markers of osteoblastic activity (bone Gla protein and procollagen I carboxyterminal peptide) and osteoclastic activity (deoxypyridinoline and pyridinoline–cross-linked carboxyterminal telopeptide).[41] Bone Gla protein is a noncollagenous protein produced and deposited by osteoblasts in bone matrix and is measurable in the circulation. Its level in the sera is considered to be a measure of osteoblast function.[41] Procollagen I carboxyterminal peptide is a trimetric, globular protein cleaved from type I collagen molecules before their assembly into fibers. Its serum concentration is directly related to the activity of bone formation.[42] Deoxypyridinoline is associated with collagen cross links, found exclusively in bone and excreted in the urine; urine levels reflect bone resorption.[43,44] Pyridinoline–cross-linked carboxyterminal telopeptide, another degradation peptide of type I collagen, is also considered to reflect bone resorption.[45] In a prospective study of 388 patients, 150 patients with bone metastases were evaluated with respect to the predictability of bone involvement based on several bone metabolic markers (bone Gla protein, procollagen I carboxyterminal peptide, deoxypyridinoline, and pyridinoline–cross-linked carboxyterminal telopeptide).[41] Osteoblastic markers were elevated primarily in patients with osteoblastic metastases, whereas the majority of those with osteolytic or mixed lesions demonstrated elevated levels of osteoclastic markers.[41]

The identification of a bone alkaline phosphatase isozyme has enabled researchers to quantitate bone metastases more accurately. In a study of 44 patients with skeletal metastases, the specificity for predicting bone metastases was much greater for the bone alkaline phosphatase isozyme (90.5%) than for total alkaline phosphatase (57.2%).[46] Another study using an immunoradiometric assay of serum bone alkaline phosphatase reported a high specificity (86.5%) and sensitivity (78.6%) for demonstrating the early progression of bone metastases.[47]

BIOMECHANICAL CONSIDERATIONS

The primary indications for operative treatment of a metastatic bone lesion are alleviation of pain, prevention of neurologic compromise secondary to spinal cord compression from collapsed bone, and maintenance of the patient's ambulatory status. The decision as to whether to intervene operatively is clear in medically stable patients who sustain a pathologic fracture. In the case of impending pathologic fractures, however, decision making can become more difficult. Orthopedic surgeons are often left to predict fracture risk in patients with large metastatic bone deposits based on their size on plain radiographs. Options for treatment of a metastatic bone lesion include local radiation or surgical stabilization of an impending pathologic fracture followed by radiation.

The weakening of cortical bone by lytic metastasis is profound, even with small cortical defects. Cortical perforations are divided into two categories: stress risers and open-section defects (Fig. 2).[48] *Stress risers* are defined as perforations measuring less than the cross-sectional diameter of the bone,

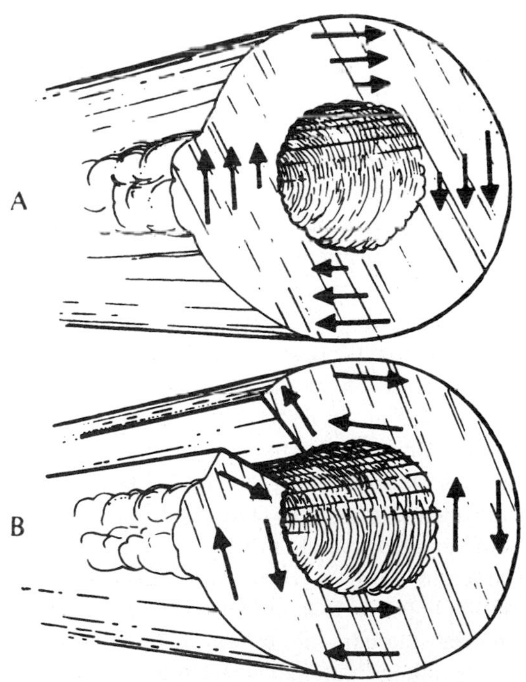

FIG. 2. A: Under torsional loading, the distribution of shear stress in a cross section of intact bone is symmetric and a linear function of the radius. **B:** An open-section defect causes a redistribution of stresses. Only the stress vectors at the periphery of the cross section are able to resist the applied torsional load. Thus, an open-section defect severely reduces the ability of the bone to carry the torsional load. (From ref. 48, with permission.)

TABLE 1. *Quantification of fracture risk*

Variable	Score 1	2	3
Site	Upper limb	Lower limb	Peritrochanter
Pain	Mild	Moderate	Functional
Lesion	Blastic	Mixed	Lytic
Size[a]	<⅓	⅓–⅔	>⅔

[a]Expressed as a fraction of bone diameter.
From ref. 58, with permission.

whereas *open-section defects* are larger than the cross-sectional bone diameter. Stress risers decrease torsional rigidity by 60%, whereas open-section defects compromise bone strength by almost 90%.[48] These results have been confirmed in *in vitro* studies.[49–51] One study using canine femora reported a 62% reduction in bending strength with small cortical defects, whereas open-section defects reduced cortical strength by 86.5%.[51] Even endosteal defects, which do not involve the entire cortex, reduce strength by 60% for a 50% reduction in cross-sectional area.[49] When endosteal defects are located at the point of maximal bending stress, the strength reduction is greater than 90%.[49]

A cortical perforation results in a concentration of forces at the edge of the defect caused by an asymmetric redistribution of the stresses experienced during loading. Pathologic fractures result if these forces overcome the fatigue strength of the cortex.[48] Available data suggest that lytic defects reduce the stiffness and strength of bone, whereas blastic metastases reduce its stiffness but not its strength.[52] Unfortunately, these observations may not relate directly to the clinical setting. Other factors may play a role in reduction of bone strength. The presence of viable tumor may impede the body's ability to repair bone defects. The bone surrounding osteolytic lesions may be weaker in older patients, who may suffer from either osteomalacia or osteoporosis. In addition, patients with a higher activity level may be at increased risk for injury. Additional cancer therapy, such as local radiation therapy or systemic chemotherapy, may slow bone repair of osteolytic lesions or adversely affect the surrounding bone. The effect of adjuvant treatment on fracture risk has been reported in a study by Tong et al. of 1,016 patients with metastatic adenocarcinoma.[53] Two groups of patients undergoing fractionated radiation therapy were compared; a higher fracture rate was reported in the group receiving doses of 40 Gy (18%) than in those receiving 20 Gy (4%).[53]

The current radiographic criteria for the operative treatment of impending fracture have been generated from retrospective studies. These often-quoted criteria are the presence of lesions that involve more than 50% of the cortex, a defect that is 2.5 cm in size, lesions of the peritrochanteric region, and lesions that continue to be painful after radiation therapy. Parrish and Murray originally proposed the idea that 50% cortical involvement demonstrates a high risk of pathologic fracture.[54] Of the 96 patients in their study series, only 4 patients presented before fracture and underwent prophylactic fixation; the remaining patients presented after fracture. A study by Fidler provided further support for the use of this parameter to predict risk of sustaining a pathologic fracture.[55] In this study of 100 bone metastases in 66 patients, the author concluded that fracture risk was low when less than 50% of the cortex was destroyed, because only one fracture occurred in 43 metastatic deposits (2.3%) in lesions of this kind.[55] Fracture risk was reported as high when more than 75% of the cortical bone was destroyed, because 19 patients (79%) of the 24 patients in this group went on to sustain fracture.[55] Unfortunately, the radiographic criterion of 50% cortical destruction comes into question because of the large overlap between those groups of patients who did and did not fracture.[55]

The premise that bone lesions larger than 2.5 cm indicate increased risk for fracture was originally proposed in a study of 338 patients, 94 of whom presented with femoral metastasis.[56] However, 8 of the 19 patients who sustained fractures were patients with lesions smaller than 2.5 cm, so the false-negative rate was 42%.[56] In a retrospective analysis by Cheng et al. of 97 bone lesions in 59 patients, evaluations made using the above radiographic criterion failed to predict any difference in fracture risk for groups of patients receiving radiation therapy who did and did not sustain fractures.[57] A 1986 attempt to objectively evaluate these criteria was undertaken by Keene et al., who focused only on breast cancer patients with proximal femoral lesions.[21] In their study, critical parameters predicting fracture risk based on lesion size and percentage of cortical involvement could not be determined, because ranges of values were similar for patients who experienced fracture and those who did not. The reliability of radiographic evaluation was questioned because lesion size could vary on any two radiographs of the same patient. Bone pain unresponsive to radiation was also evaluated and found not to correlate with fracture risk.[21]

In an attempt to address these inconsistencies, Mirels proposed a scoring system for quantifying the risk of pathologic fracture (Table 1).[58] He examined 78 lesions in 38 patients who had undergone radiation without a previous fracture. The system assigned a numeric score to four variables, which included lesion location, degree of pain, radiographic appearance, and lesion size. Twenty-two of the 25 patients with scores of 9 and above sustained fractures, whereas only 1 of the 41 patients with scores of 7 or lower sustained fractures. Four of 12 patients with a score of 8 demonstrated a fracture. Based on these data, Mirels recommended irradiating and then following lesions with a score of 7 or less and providing operative treatment for lesions with a score of 8 or higher.[58]

The central problem in the clinical evaluation of patients with impending pathologic fractures is the inaccuracy of radiographic assessment. Estimates are that between 30% and 50% bone destruction must occur before a lesion can be identified on radiography. CAT scanning, although it provides better cortical resolution, has not proven itself to be any better in the radiographic assessment of bone lesions compared with other methods. In a study using cadavers in which ten pairs of human proximal femurs were given simulated intertrochanteric metastatic bone defects, orthopedic surgeons evaluated bone strength using plain radiographs and CAT scans.[59] Their estimates of lesion size and bone strength were then analyzed for intraobserver error and compared against biomechanical testing data. No relationship was found between the measured load-bearing capacity of the femurs and the capacity estimated by the surgeons from the radiographic studies.[59]

Clearly, estimates of fracture risk based on radiographic criteria can be highly inaccurate. More qualitative measurements of fracture risk, such as those proposed by Mirels, which are easy to apply and incorporate several variables, hold promise for providing orthopedic surgeons with a better means to predict which patients are at risk for pathologic fracture.

TREATMENT

Treatment of bone metastasis is aimed at relieving pain, preventing development of pathologic fractures, enhancing mobility and function, and thereby improving the quality of life and contributing to improvement in survival. A multidisciplinary integration of the available treatment modalities should be coordinated at the time the patient presents with bony metastatic disease. Attention to adequate analgesia using the "Three-Step Analgesic Ladder" of the World Health Organization is of utmost importance.[60] The difficulty with analgesia is not lack of response but the serious side effects that can occur in the attempt to achieve pain control. Therefore, other modalities must be implemented to afford more permanent pain control. Radiation is particularly efficacious in this regard. Systemic therapies including hormonal or chemotherapeutic agents may be used. Accumulating evidence points to the role of bisphosphonates in ameliorating disease progression and is discussed in Chapter 61. The need for orthopedic intervention because of fracture risk or actual pathologic fracture and the role of radiation for pain relief or long-term tumor control to avoid fracture should be assessed clinically and radiographically.

Radiation Therapy

Radiation therapy is effective in alleviating bone pain from tumor progression. Radiation generally is the first treatment used, especially for a solitary metastasis. Typically, 80% to 90% of patients experience at least minimal relief of pain, and 40% to 60% obtain complete relief.[53,61–66] The onset of pain relief usually occurs within 4 weeks, and 70% of patients who experience some relief do not have a relapse of pain before they die. The reason for this response is unknown but has been hypothesized to occur because of tumor shrinkage or inhibition of the release of chemical pain mediators from normal bone cells. The speed with which patients respond to radiation therapy varies from days to weeks and does not adhere to a dose-response curve. Early responders (i.e., those who respond in less than 2 weeks) probably gain most of their pain relief from a rapid reduction in perosseous inflammation. Late responders may exhibit symptomatic relief because of ossification of weakened regions of bone.[53]

In determining how best to deliver radiation, a number of factors must be considered.[67] These factors include the clinical status of the patient (performance status and life expectancy) and the site of metastases, their number, and their fracture risk. Concerns arise regarding the acute tolerance of the regimen used—that is, risk of nausea, vomiting, diarrhea, and potential hematologic toxicity—as well as the late effects, especially normal tissue tolerance in patients with longer life expectancies. In addition, one wishes to know anticipated response rate, rapidity and durability of response, and subsequent need for analgesia. Information is needed on the risk of fracture after radiation and also on the potential need for reradiation and its usefulness and safety.

The radiobiologic effectiveness of radiation is highly dependent on time, dose, and fractionation. Tumor control is generally enhanced with higher total dose delivery and higher dose per fraction. The tolerance of the patient to treatment, however, is based on acute tolerance—that is, nausea and vomiting, which increase with higher dose per fraction and increased field size—and long-term normal tissue tolerance—that is, risk of radiation myelitis, which increases with higher dose per fraction and higher total dose. In general, for palliative treatment, shorter treatment courses are used to minimize patient inconvenience and cost, because the risks of long-term morbidity are lower in patients with limited life expectancy. Conversely, for curative treatment, for which long-term morbidities need to be minimized, prolonged courses to higher doses are used.

Which treatment regimen is considered optimal for the patient with bone metastases? When reviewing the available literature, one must keep in mind the difficulty of controlling for the multiplicity of factors mentioned earlier.[68] Most trials include a wide variety of primary tumor types, and the results are pooled; this pooling affects the analysis, because patients with metastases from certain tumor types, such as breast and prostate, may experience better pain relief than others.[53] Also, the assessment of pain control is not standardized across studies. Frequently, pain control is evaluated by the physician, who typically reports higher response rates than are seen in patient self-reports. In this generally ailing group, however, patients' self-report of response may be low.[61]

The Radiation Therapy Oncology Group (RTOG) performed the largest prospective randomized trial addressing the issue of dose and fractionation in the United States. A total of 1,016 patients (266 with solitary and 750 with multiple bone metastases) were entered into the trial.[53] Overall, 90% of patients who received radiation therapy experienced

TABLE 2. *Radiation Therapy Oncology Group bone metastases protocol: comparison of final results and reanalysis*

	Dose/ fraction (Gy)	Total dose (Gy)	Complete relief[a] (%)	
			Final	Reanalysis
Solitary	2.7	40.5	61	55
	4.0	20.0	53	37
			$p = .42$	$p < .0003$
Multiple	3.0	30.0	57	46
	3.0	15.0	49	36
	4.0	20.0	56	40
	5.0	25.0	49	28
			$p = .026$	$p < .0003$

[a]Definition: Final = pain disappeared with or without narcotic use; Reanalysis = absence of pain and cessation of narcotic use.

TABLE 3. *Palliative radiation for bone metastases: prospective randomized trials of single fraction versus multiple fractions*

	No. of patients	Dose/ fraction no.	Overall response (%)
Price et al.[62]	288	8 Gy/1	82
		30 Gy/10	71
Cole[63]	29	8 Gy/1	88
		24 Gy/6	85
Kagei et al.[64]	27	8, 10, 12, 15 Gy/1	86
		5 Gy/×4, ×5, ×6	92
Gaze et al.[65]	265	10 Gy/1	84
		22.5 Gy/5	89
Nielsen et al.[66]	241	8 Gy/1	72
		5 Gy/4	82

some relief of pain, and 54% achieved eventual complete pain relief. Of the 90% of patients who experienced some pain relief, 70% had no recurrence of this pain before death. The risk of fracture subsequent to radiation was low, only 8% overall. An initial analysis revealed no differences among the different radiation schedules; however, when the data were reanalyzed and complete pain relief was defined as no pain without analgesic use, a difference emerged, as shown in Table 2. The two high-dose protracted programs achieved the best results.[61] A survey of patterns of care among United States radiation oncologists revealed that 30 Gy in 10 fractions is the most common schedule in use.[69]

For patients with short life expectancies, especially those with poor performance status, in whom long-term toxicities are less of a concern, the use of short-course palliative treatments could be considered.[70] A number of prospective randomized trials have compared single-fraction treatment with a variety of more prolonged fractionated dose schedules to assess efficacy. The rationale for the single-fraction treatment is to minimize patient inconvenience and cost of therapy. All studies have shown no appreciable difference in pain relief rates between these two approaches, as demonstrated in Table 3.[62–66] The optimal single dose has not been determined. In a prospective randomized trial involving 270 patients, Hoskin et al. compared doses of 4 Gy and 8 Gy; at 4 weeks, the response rates were 44% and 69%, respectively. These researchers concluded that 8 Gy was the recommended dose for a single-fraction regimen.[71] The United Kingdom Multicentre Bone Pain Trial is a prospective randomized study comparing use of a single 8-Gy fraction with use of any multifraction regimen; the goal is to provide further data to enhance the reliability of the current evidence.[72] With additional information, modeling of cost-benefit ratios for a single fraction scheme versus more prolonged fractionation schedules that accounted for both short-term and long-term results would be helpful.[73]

Women with breast cancer metastatic to bone have relatively long life expectancies. Although the initial response to radiation is high, 30% go on to have a painful relapse at the initially treated site. Reradiation has been used in this situation to good effect. Mithal et al. performed a retrospective review of consecutively treated patients who received palliative radiotherapy and identified 57 who were re-treated once and 8 who were re-treated twice.[74] Sixty percent of both groups had breast cancer. Fractionation schemas varied. Complete and partial response was high—48 of 57 who were re-treated once (84%) and 7 of 8 who were re-treated twice (87.5%). Unfortunately, treatment morbidity was not analyzed.

Pain related to widespread metastatic disease requires a different approach. The use of systemic radionuclides is reviewed in Chapter 52. External-beam radiotherapy using a technique known as *half-body irradiation* (*HBI*) has been developed and has been found to be useful. HBI is usually applied by administering 6 to 10 Gy in one fraction to fields that encompass the upper, middle, or lower body. Response rates are high, with 60% to 80% of patients gaining pain relief rapidly, within 2 days of treatment. The mean duration of pain relief is 15 weeks. Acute toxicity, usually manifested as nausea, vomiting, or diarrhea, is common. Hematologic toxicity peaks at 2 to 3 weeks and can be life-threatening, particularly in patients with low marrow reserve from prior intensive chemotherapy. Dose-escalation studies have shown that the safest and most effective doses are 6 Gy for upper HBI and 8 Gy for lower or middle HBI.[75] Fractionated HBI is not superior.[76] Hospitalization is frequently required for upper torso HBI. Ondansetron hydrochloride has been shown in a randomized trial to be superior to chlorpromazine with dexamethasone in treating the symptoms of toxicity; its use should be considered, and it may reduce the need for hospitalization.[77]

A randomized RTOG study involving 499 patients conducted by Poulter et al. compared HBI (single 8-Gy fraction) after local field radiation (30 Gy in 10 fractions) with local field radiation alone.[78] An increase in time to disease progression and a decrease in the need for subsequent palliative radiation were seen in the group receiving HBI. Concern regarding visceral toxicities, permanent effects on bone marrow reserve if chemotherapy is subsequently required, difficulties in treatment setup, and the potential need for hospitalization have limited the use of HBI. However, it may still play a role in treating patients with diffuse lytic disease for whom radionuclides are not useful or in treating those refractory to other therapies.

Operative Treatment

Patients presenting with either a complete or impending pathologic fracture of the lower extremity should undergo operative stabilization or reconstruction in the majority of cases. The goals and benefits of rigid fixation of pathologic fractures include pain relief, resumption of ambulation, enhancement of survival, and improved fracture healing. Patients who are unstable medically or who have a life expectancy of less than 4 weeks are not considered candidates for operative treatment.[79] In a study series of 303 patients, Habermann found that 264 of 292 patients with pathologic fractures (90%) who survived the initial postoperative period reported good to excellent pain relief after internal fixation or prosthetic replacement.[23] Although operative treatment has little impact on the neoplastic process, regaining ambulatory status is imperative for patient survival. Harrington et al. reported successfully returning 281 of 297 patients with pathologic fractures (95%) to their prefracture ambulatory status after operative intervention.[80] Using prosthetic devices or internal fixation augmented with methylmethacrylate, Harrington reported that patient survival improved from 11.6 months to 24.6 months because of restoration of patient ambulatory ability and avoidance of the risks of extended bed rest.[79,80]

Rapid return to ambulation has been reported in several reviews. Ryan et al. reported that 15 of 18 patients (83%) returned to ambulation within 4 days after treatment with prophylactic intramedullary fixation of femur fractures.[81] Pain relief and improved mobility in patients treated operatively was clearly demonstrable in a study comprised of 366 patients with pathologic fractures.[80] Ninety-five percent of the patients (346 patients) who were ambulatory before fracture regained the ability to walk.[80] In the same study, excellent or good pain relief was achieved in 160 of 186 patients studied (85%).[80]

In the operative approach to pathologic fracture fixation, several factors must be taken into consideration when selecting either internal fixation or prosthetic reconstruction for patients suffering from metastatic bone disease. First, these patients often have a limited life expectancy, so rapid recovery is imperative both for maintaining quality of life and for accommodating the need to provide adjuvant treatment. Second, successful fracture healing is often unpredictable because of several factors, such as continued local tumor growth, poor bone quality, poor nutritional status, and the effects of chemotherapy and radiation therapy on bone healing. One study showed that patients who survived less than 6 months demonstrated a poor ability to heal pathologic fractures; patients who survived longer than 6 months achieved fracture union in 22 of 25 cases (88%) with surgical stabilization and a radiation dose of no more than 30 Gy.[82] The use of methylmethacrylate to reconstitute large bone defects permits immediate weight bearing in most cases. Methylmethacrylate maintains excellent rigidity, especially when compressively loaded, and is not adversely affected by radiation.[83] Biomechanical data promoting the use of methylmethacrylate was reported in a study by Ryan and Begeman.[84] In this study, 2.5-cm defects were created in cadaveric femoral shafts and either filled with methylmethacrylate or left open. Axial load and torsional strength were increased by 50% and 70%, respectively, in the methylmethacrylate-treated defects.[81]

A retrospective study by Yazawa et al. of the surgical treatment of 166 metastatic lesions of the humerus and femur in 147 patients illustrates the difficulty in dealing with pathologic fractures.[85] Proximal femoral implants included endoprostheses (28 patients), total joint arthroplasties (13 patients), screws and side plates (9 patients), and intramedullary devices (18 patients). Failure of femoral fixation or prosthetic replacement was reported in 11 of 119 patients (9.2%), whereas failure was reported in only 2 of 46 cases (4.3%) involving the upper extremity. The failure rate was high for proximal femoral lesions treated with a compression screw, with failure reported in three of nine patients (23%). Intramedullary fixation and prosthetic replacement augmented with methylmethacrylate were the most successful means used. Common reasons for failure included poor initial fixation, improper implant selection, and progression of tumor-induced bone destruction around the implant resulting in failure of fixation.[85] In addition, of the five patients with diaphyseal lesions that progressed at the operative site, four had had no postoperative radiotherapy.

In contrast to lower extremity lesions, isolated upper extremity lesions without fracture may be amenable to bracing, and operative treatment can often be avoided. For patients who depend on upper arm support to ambulate (i.e., who use a walker) or who present with bilateral upper or lower extremity involvement, however, operative stabilization should be strongly considered. Once a pathologic fracture has occurred, operative intervention should be performed. The poor results of nonoperative treatment of pathologic humerus fractures have been previously reported. In one study of 29 pathologic humerus fractures in 27 patients, 9 were treated with radiation therapy, 8 with internal fixation, and 12 by other means.[86] Of the patients treated with radiation, five had relief of pain, but four were left with a functionless extremity.[86] In contrast, patients treated with internal fixation fared better, with seven of eight patients achieving improvement in pain control and function.[86] Flemming and Beals reported on eight pathologic humerus fractures treated nonoperatively with very poor results.[87] Four fractures went on to nonunion, and pain relief was rated as poor to fair in seven patients.[87]

Operative choices for treatment of pathologic fractures of the upper extremity include compression plating, flexible intramedullary nailing augmented with methylmethacrylate, rigid intramedullary nailing with or without methylmethacrylate, and prosthetic replacement. The results of internal fixation for the treatment of pathologic humerus fractures have been evaluated in a retrospective study of 54 patients with established or impending pathologic fractures who were treated with rush rod intramedullary fixation with and without the use of methylmethacrylate.[88,89] All patients had initial relief of their preoperative pain after the procedure. However, pain was subsequently a problem in four patients because of acromial impingement from rod protrusion and in three patients because of loosening of rod fixation.[88,89] In a 1991 study of 22 pathologic humerus fractures, 17 patients who were included in the series were treated with intramedullary fixation. Postoperatively, 14 patients (82%) reported only mild to moderate pain.[90] Complications included fixation failure in 5 of 21 patients (24%) treated operatively, with compression plating failing in the 2 patients in which it was used.[90] In one study in which pathologic lesions of the humeral diaphysis were treated with a locked intramedullary nail, union was radiographically apparent in all 7 of 11 patients who survived at least 3 months and had radiographs available.[91] The recommendation has been made that this technique be reserved for those fractures occurring between the proximal one-sixth and distal one-fourth of the humerus, so that sufficient bone is available for fixation with interlocking screws.[91] Prosthetic reconstruction of humerus fractures is recommended for lesions of the proximal humerus that involve the humeral head and lesions in which there is substantial segmental diaphyseal involvement.[92,93]

Reconstruction of proximal femoral and acetabular lesions is often the most technically demanding; the implant is placed at risk for failure because the forces about the hip are extremely high for most normal activities. Forces on the proximal femur have been estimated to be 3.5 times body weight during the midstance phase of gait and to increase to 7.7 times body weight during stair climbing.[94,95] Options for operative reconstruction of the diseased proximal femur include internal fixation with either a sliding hip screw and side plate or a Zickel or reconstruction nail, prosthetic replacement with a long-stemmed femoral component, or proximal femoral replacement. The majority of authors recommend prosthetic reconstruction for femoral neck fractures, with either an endoprosthesis or total hip replacement. Intertrochanteric femur fractures can be treated with either internal fixation or a prosthetic replacement. Although internal fixation is reported to have the highest complication rate, it is still advocated by some authors.[85,96–98] Use of the Zickel nail for the treatment of proximal femoral pathologic fractures has been reported in two studies.[97,98] In one study of 21 patients treated in this way, femoral shortening secondary to disease progression occurred in 24% of the patients.[97] In the second series of 50 patients, up to 4 cm of shortening was reported.[98] Although methylmethacrylate was not used to augment internal fixation in either study, these results underscore the problems of internal fixation in the face of continued bone destruction.

Options for prosthetic replacement include a long-stemmed standard or calcar-replacing femoral component and proximal femoral replacement. The advantages of using standard or calcar-replacing femoral prostheses are ease of insertion and maintenance of both the hip flexor and abductor muscle attachments. Disadvantages include the dependence on distal femoral fixation and the possibility of disease progression, which could destabilize the femoral component. For this reason, indications for proximal femoral replacement include either failure of internal fixation or continued disease progression in patients who are unable to undergo radiation therapy. Because resection of the proximal femur to implant a proximal femoral endoprosthesis results in the sacrifice of hip abductor and flexor muscle attachments to bone, a walker or cane is usually required for efficient ambulation.

The treatment of proximal femoral lesions with prosthetic replacement has been proposed by some authors.[99] Lane et al. reported on a series of 167 consecutive pathologic or impending fractures of the hip treated with either a long-stemmed femoral endoprosthesis or a total hip arthroplasty.[99] Of the 78 patients who were able to walk before treatment, 56 (72%) were independent or used walkers after the prosthetic replacement. Of the 85 patients who were nonambulatory for 2 weeks or more before treatment, 40 patients (47%) were independent of walkers or walked with assistive devices afterward.

Several series, although small, have concentrated on proximal femoral replacement for pathologic fractures. Sim and Chao reported on 82 patients with either metastatic disease (33 patients) or a primary malignant bone tumor (49 patients) who underwent segmental replacement of the proximal femur.[100] Of this combined group of 84 patients, at least 38 (46%) had at least one complication. The most common complication was overlengthening of the extremity secondary to the use of an oversized implant, which occurred in 11 of 84 hips (13%). Hip instability was the second most frequently encountered complication and was reported in 10 hips (12%).

Acetabular insufficiency secondary to bone metastasis has been classified by Harrington according to the location and extent of tumor or amount of bone destruction.[101] In class I lesions, the lateral cortices and superior and medial acetabular walls are structurally intact. In class II lesions, deficiencies are found in the medial wall. In class III lesions, the medial and superior walls are deficient. Class I lesions can be successfully reconstructed with conventional cemented total hip arthroplasty. Class II lesions require a reconstructive technique that transfers the stress of weight bearing away from the deficient wall and onto the intact acetabular rim through the use of a protrusio ring. Class III bone loss necessitates the reconstruction of the acetabular columns with implants and methylmethacrylate to successfully fix the protrusio ring in place (Fig. 3).[101]

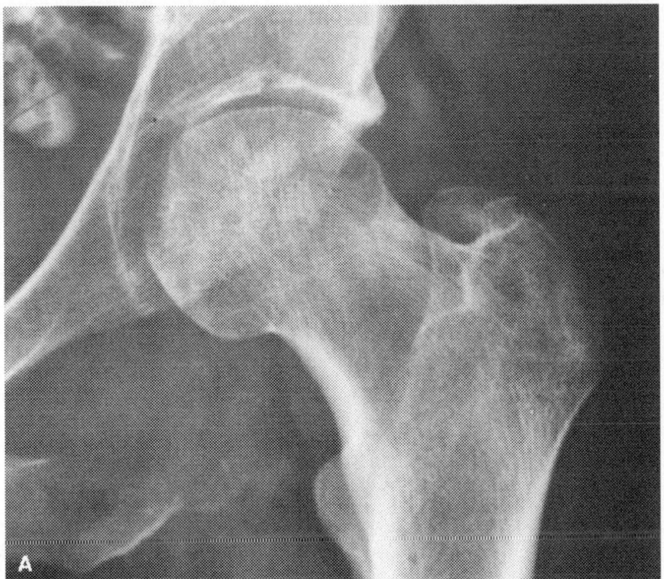

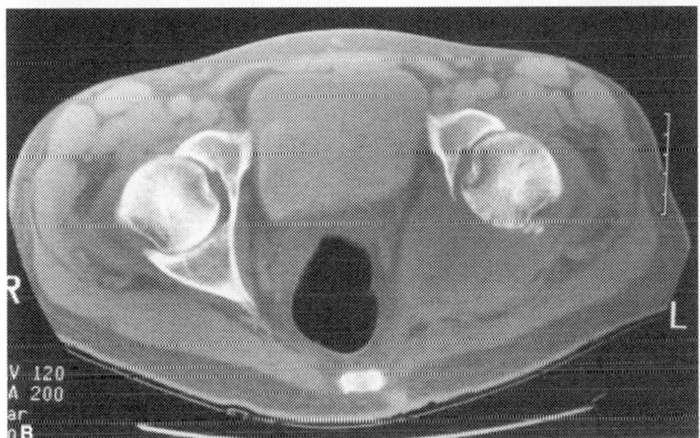

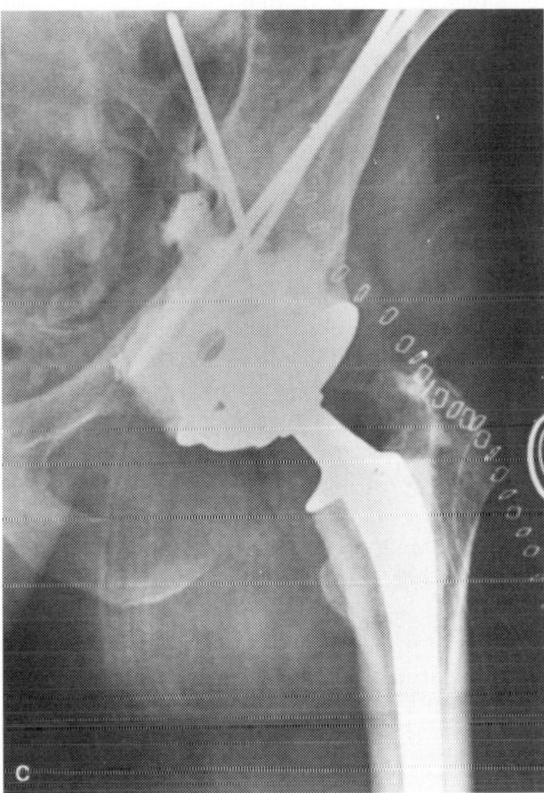

FIG. 3. A: Patient, who complained of severe pain and inability to ambulate, presented with a large lytic metastasis residing in the left ischium and posterior acetabulum. **B:** Computed tomographic scan shows a large soft-tissue mass and extensive bone involvement with disruption of the acetabular wall. **C:** A cemented total hip arthroplasty with methylmethacrylate and Steinmann pin reconstruction of the acetabulum successfully alleviated the patient's pain and permitted ambulation with a cane.

In a series reported by Harrington, 58 patients underwent acetabular reconstruction and joint replacement for metastatic periacetabular fractures.[96] This total included 37 patients with class III bone deficiency. Thirty-seven patients who survived longer than 6 months described their pain as minimal or nonexistent; all 24 patients surviving longer than 2 years had minimal or no pain. Thirty-nine of the 51 patients were ambulatory and required either no walking aids (20 patients) or a single cane (19 patients) at 6 months. Complications included loosening of the acetabular reconstruction in four patients because of progressive bone destruction after their operative procedure, with two of these being successfully revised.[96]

Radiation treatment alone for pathologic fractures is not advised. When radiation alone is used, the healing process is delayed and bone union does not occur. Combining radiation with orthopedic fixation is useful. Very few retrospective studies are available on which to base recommendations regarding the beneficial effect of postfixation radiation or to determine optimal dose and duration of radiation. One retrospective direct comparison by Townsend et al. examined 64 orthopedic stabilization procedures in 60 patients and compared treatment with surgery and radiation to treatment with surgery alone. Patients receiving radiation were found to have a higher likelihood of normal functional status than those that did not receive radiation (53% versus 11.5%, $p < .01$), as well as a decreased need for reoperation (3% versus 15%, $p = .035$).[102] Another retrospective series by Gainor and Buchert reported successful fracture healing in 90% of patients who survived longer than 6 months, who were surgically stabilized, and who received a radiation dose of no more than 30 Gy.[82]

SPINAL INVOLVEMENT

The spine is the most common site for skeletal metastasis. Seventy percent of patients who die from cancer show vertebral metastasis on postmortem examination.[103] Neurologic signs such as paraplegia, paraparesis, or sensory level abnormalities can raise suspicion for spine involvement but are not considered reliable indicators. Initial radiographic evaluation generally includes plain radiography and bone scintigraphy. MRI is superior to CAT and bone scan in detecting bone and epidural involvement. It is frequently recommended for patients who present with neurologic involvement.[104]

Once the workup is complete, patients can generally be divided into five categories, depending on the extent of neurologic involvement or bone destruction.[103] Category I patients demonstrate no significant neurologic involvement; in category II patients, the bone is involved without collapse or instability; category III patients present with major neurologic compromise without bone involvement; in category IV patients, bony collapse without neurologic involvement is demonstrated; and in category V patients, major neurologic impairment is combined with vertebral collapse. Patients in categories I and II can be treated with systemic therapies. Progression of pain or disease would merit radiation therapy. For patients in category III, who have major neurologic compromise without bone involvement, radiation therapy is warranted. Operative treatment is reserved for patients with either bony collapse and instability (category IV) or with vertebral body collapse that results in retropulsion of bone and disk fragments directly into the cord (category V).[103]

Determination of the involved spinal levels is critical to radiation treatment planning. A sagittal screening MRI of the vertebral column localizes the initial suspected area of involvement and determines the presence of additional areas of cord compression. More detailed images of the involved levels can then be made. For treatment planning purposes, the upper and lower extent of the lesion and the extent of paravertebral tumor should be determined. Planning should take into consideration the potential need for subsequent courses of radiation and therefore should minimize the exposure of normal structures and uninvolved marrow to maintain as much marrow reserve as possible for systemic therapies. Corticosteroid therapy should be initiated immediately on detection of the neurologic compromise.[105] A randomized, placebo-controlled trial has been carried out using high-dose dexamethasone (96 mg intravenously for loading; 96 mg orally, three times per day, and then a taper over 10 days). Six months after therapy, 59% of the patients treated with dexamethasone were ambulatory, compared with 33% in the placebo-treated group.[106] This high-dose regimen has toxicity, however, and a more standard dosage of 4 mg dexamethasone four times per day gradually tapered to zero is probably equally efficacious.[107] If progressive neurologic deficit occurs, the dose can be increased to a maximum of 100 mg per day. To avoid long-term steroid toxicity, the dexamethasone should be gradually tapered and discontinued, unless neurologic symptoms recur. Tapering may start during the course of radiation if the patient is stable. Radiation therapy should commence after steroids have been instituted.

In a prospective analysis by Maranzano and Latini, 209 patients with spinal cord compression who were treated with radiation and steroids were followed for a median of 49 months. Median survival was 6 months. Back pain responded to this therapy in 82% of patients. Among patients with sphincter dysfunction, 44% showed improvement.[108] Little information is available that directly compares these results with those that can be obtained with laminectomy. A prospective randomized trial by Young et al. comparing laminectomy to radiation therapy showed no difference in the effectiveness of the two treatments with regard to pain relief, improvement in ambulation, or improvement in sphincter function. Those with a complete block fared poorly regardless of treatment.[109] Further study is needed, particularly for the latter, more impaired group, to find better approaches to restoring neurologic function.

The spinal cord is sensitive to the effects of radiation. The risk of myelitis increases with total dose and also with dose per fraction. As a consequence, hyperfractionated schedules are used infrequently, and the most common treatment schema is 30 Gy in 10 fractions. For patients with poor performance status and short life expectancy, however, shorter-course radiation has been assessed. Maranzano et al. treated 45 patients with an 8-Gy fraction, which was repeated in 1 week for responders. Pain relief occurred in 67%. No late toxicity was recorded.[110]

Reradiation has been used only infrequently in patients who progress in a previously radiated spinal field because of concerns about the risk of myelitis. A series of 55 patients with recurrent spinal cord compression was analyzed by Schiff et al.; of these, 40 (74%) were ambulatory at the onset of radiation, and 42 (78%) were ambulatory at the end. The treatment was tolerated reasonably well.[111]

Only one patient, who received three courses of radiation, may have developed radiation myelitis; however, this low overall risk may be affected by the short median survival duration of 4.2 months after reradiation.

When operative treatment is needed, the treatment of choice is anterior resection of the diseased vertebral body and reconstruction with bone graft, or methylmethacrylate and spinal instrumentation as needed (Fig. 4).[103] Advances in spinal instrumentation have resulted in better methods for the stabilization of vertebral body collapse secondary to metastatic disease. Anterior cervical plates, titanium cages, and distraction rods, when used in conjunction with bone graft or cementation, have found a wide applicability in cervical and thoracic reconstructions. Occasionally, posterior instrumentation is necessary in cases in which extreme instability is apparent. The goal of surgery is to prevent neurologic compromise and restore ambulatory ability. In general, radiation therapy is delivered postoperatively. At least 62% of initially paraplegic patients regain enough neurologic recovery to walk after surgical decompression. Patients who present with

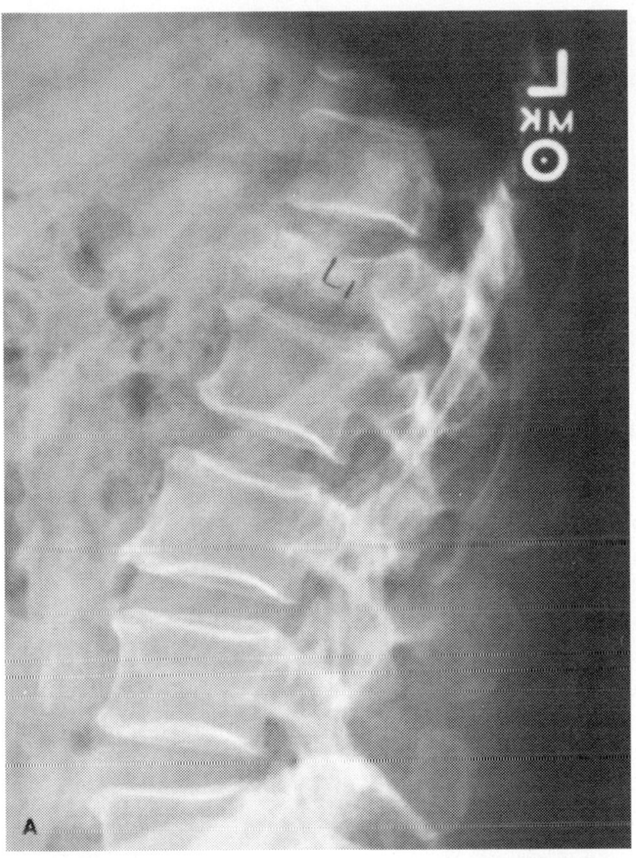
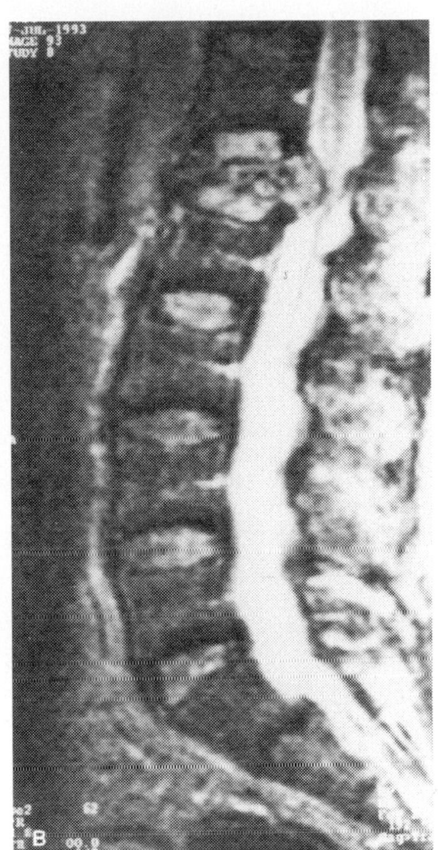
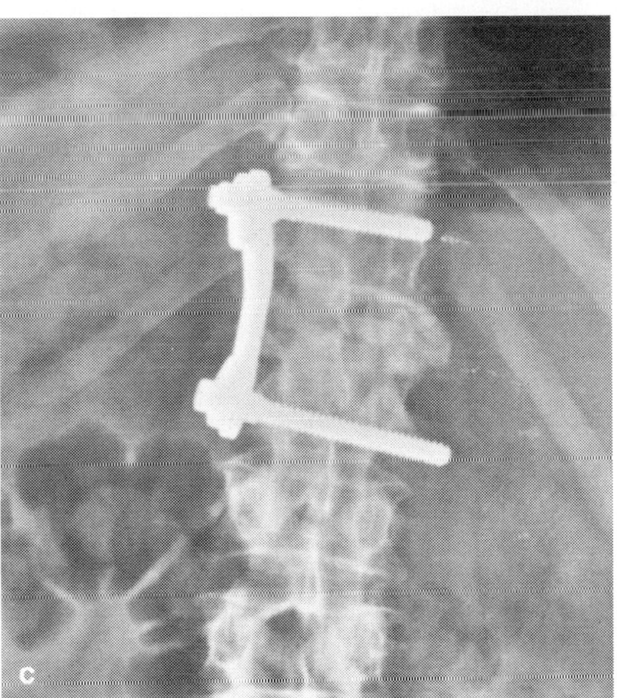

FIG. 4. A: Patient experienced back pain and lower extremity paraparesis; a lateral radiograph demonstrates bone collapse with severe compression of the first lumbar vertebral body. **B:** Sagittal magnetic resonance image reveals nerve root compression resulting from retropulsed tumor and bone fragments. **C:** Anterior vertebral corpectomy was performed, with spinal instrumentation and fusion using an iliac crest bone graft.

rapid, as opposed to chronic, spinal cord compromise and paraplegia exhibit a poor prognosis for recovery of function.[103] Most patients do not present with this degree of neurologic compromise, however, and respond well to radiation or chemotherapy without surgery.

MANAGEMENT SUMMARY

In breast cancer patients with bone metastases, radiation treatment and systemic therapy can often provide patients with excellent pain relief and potentially slow local tumor growth. Surgery and postoperative radiation should be considered in patients with bone lesions at risk for fracture. Although further clarification of current guidelines is necessary, these criteria can aid the clinician in selecting the most appropriate course of treatment. The operative management of pathologic fractures can be challenging and often is best reserved for orthopedic surgeons familiar with current techniques of pathologic fracture fixation. This is particularly true in cases of extensive acetabular and spinal involvement.

REFERENCES

1. Lote K, Walloe A, Bjersand A. Bone metastasis: prognosis, diagnosis and treatment. *Acta Radiol Oncol* 1986;25:227.
2. Stall DA. Natural history, prognosis, and staging of the bone metastases. In: Stoll BA, Parbhoo S, eds. *Bone metastases: monitoring and treatment*, 1st ed. New York: Raven Press, 1983:1.
3. Tofe AJ, Francis MD, Harvey WJ. A correlation of neoplasms with incidence and localization of skeletal metastases: an analysis of 1,355 diphosphonate bone scans. *J Nucl Med* 1975;16:986.
4. Koenders PG, Beex LVAM, Kloppenborg PWC, Smals AGH, Benraad TJ. Human breast cancer: survival from first metastasis. *Breast Cancer Res Treat* 1992;21:173.
5. Namer M. Clinical consequences of osteolytic bone metastases. *Bone* 1991;12:7.
6. Tursky B. The development of a pain perception profile: a psychophysical approach. In: Weisenberg M, Tursky B, eds. *Pain: new perspectives in therapy and research*, 1st ed. New York: Plenum Publishing, 1976:171.
7. Twycross RG. Analgesics and relief of bone pain. In: Stoll BA, Parbhoo S, eds. *Bone metastasis: monitoring and treatment.* New York: Raven Press, 1983:289.
8. Bonica JJ, Ventafridda V, Twycross RG. Cancer pain. In: Bonica JJ, ed. *The management of pain*. Philadelphia: Lea & Febiger, 1990:400.
9. Twycross RG. Management of pain in skeletal metastases. *Clin Orthop* 1995;312:187.
10. Galasko CSB, Sylvester BS. Back pain in patients treated for malignant tumours. *Clin Oncol* 1978;4:273.
11. Nielsen OS, Munro AJ, Tannock IF. Bone metastases: pathophysiology and management policy. *J Clin Oncol* 1991;9:509.
12. Byrne TN. Spinal cord compression from epidural metastases. *N Engl J Med* 1992;327:614.
13. Foley KM. The management of cancer pain. *N Engl J Med* 1986;313:84.
14. Galasko CSB. Development of skeletal metastases. In Galasko CSB, ed. *Skeletal metastases*. London: Butterworth, 1986:22.
15. Scher HI, Yagoda A. Bone metastases: pathogenesis, treatment, and rationale for use of resorption inhibitors. *Am J Med* 1987;82:6.
16. Albright JA, Gillespie TE, Butaud TR. Treatment of bone metastases. *Semin Oncol* 1980;7:418.
17. Higinbotham NL, Marcove RC. The management of pathological fractures. *J Trauma* 1965; 5:792.
18. Schurman DJ, Amstutz HC. Orthopedic management of patients with metastatic carcinoma of the breast. *Surg Gynecol Obstet* 1973;137: 831.
19. Sim FH, Edmonson JH, Mcleod RA, Unni KK. Metastatic bone disease. In: Sim FH, ed. *Diagnosis and treatment of bone tumors: a team approach*. Thorofare, NJ: Slack, 1983:259.
20. Oda MAS, Shurman DJ. Monitoring of pathological fracture. In: Stoll BA, Parbhoo S, eds. *Bone metastases: monitoring and treatment*. New York: Raven Press, 1983:271.
21. Keene JS, Sellinger DS, McBeath AA, Engber WD. Metastatic breast cancer in the femur: a search for the lesion at risk for fracture. *Clin Orthop* 1986;203:282.
22. Wilner D. Cancer metastasis to bone. In: Wilner D, ed. *Radiology of bone tumors and allied disorders*. Philadelphia: WB Saunders, 1982:3641.
23. Habermann ET. The pathology and treatment of metastatic disease of the femur. *Clin Orthop* 1982;169:70.
24. Harrington KD. The management of malignant pathologic fractures. *Instr Course Lect* 1977;26:147.
25. Wu K, Guise E. Metastatic tumors of the hand: a report of six cases. *J Hand Surg* 1978;3:271.
26. Healey JH, Turnbull AD, Miedema B, Lane JM. Acrometastases: a study of twenty-nine patients with osseous involvement of the hands and feet. *J Bone Joint Surg Am* 1986;68:743.
27. Adams JE, Isherwood I. Conventional and new techniques in radiological diagnosis. In: Stoll BA, Parbhoo S, eds. *Bone metastases: monitoring and treatment*. New York: Raven Press, 1983;107.
28. Edelstyn GA, Gillespie PJ, Grebbell FS. The radiological demonstration of osseous metastases: experimental observations. *Clin Radiol* 1967;18:158.
29. Fournasier VL, Horne JG. Metastases to the vertebral column. *Cancer* 1975;36:590.
30. Goris ML, Bretille J. Skeletal scintigraphy for the diagnosis of malignant metastatic disease to the bones. *Radiother Oncol* 1985;3:319.
31. Galasko CSB. The detection of skeletal metastases from mammary cancer by gamma camera scintigraphy. *Br J Surg* 1969;56:757.
32. Galasko CSB. Skeletal metastases and mammary cancer. *Ann R Coll Surg Engl* 1972;50:3.
33. McNeil BJ. Value of bone scanning in neoplastic disease. *Semin Nucl Med* 1984;14:277.
34. Del Turco MR, Palli D, Cariddi A, et al. Intensive diagnostic follow-up after treatment of primary breast cancer: a randomized trial. National Research Council project on breast cancer follow-up. *JAMA* 1994;271;1593.
35. Anonymous. Impact of follow-up testing on survival and health-related quality of life in breast cancer patients. The GIVIO investigators. *JAMA* 1994;271:1587.
36. Anonymous. Recommended breast cancer surveillance guidelines. American Society of Clinical Oncology. *J Clin Oncol* 1997;15:2149.
37. Schaffer DL, Pendergrass HP. Comparison of enzyme, clinical, radiographic, and radionuclide methods of detecting bone metastases from carcinoma of the prostate. *Radiology* 1976;121:431.
38. Coombes RC, Gazet JC, Ford HT, et al. Assessment of biochemical tests to screen for metastases in patients with breast cancer. *Lancet* 1980;1:296.
39. Perez DJ, Milan J, Ford HT, et al. Detection of breast carcinoma metastases in bone: relative merits of x-rays and skeletal scintigraphy. *Lancet* 983;2:613.
40. Hopkins SC, Nissenkorn I, Palmieri GM, et al. Serial spot hydroxyproline/creatinine ratios in metastatic prostate cancer. *J Urol* 1983;129:319.
41. Koizumi M, Yamada Y, Takiguchi T, et al. Bone metabolic markers in bone metastases. *J Cancer Res Clin Oncol* 1995;121:542.
42. Melkko J, Niemi S, Risteli L, Risteli J. Radioimmunoassay of carboxyterminal propeptide of human type I procollagen. *Clin Chem* 1990;36:1328.
43. Coleman RE, Houston S, James I, et al. Preliminary results of the use of urinary excretion of pyridium crosslinks for monitoring metastatic bone disease. *Br J Cancer* 1992;65:766.
44. Eyre DR, Koob TJ, Van Ness KP. Quantitation of hydroxypyridium crosslinks in collagen by high-performance liquid chromatography. *Anal Biochem* 1984;137:380.
45. Risteli J, Elomaa I, Niemi S, Novamo A, Risteli L. Radioimmunoassay for the pyridinoline cross-linked carboxy-terminal telopeptide of type I collagen. *Clin Chem* 1993;39:635.
46. Zaninotto M, Secchiero S, Rubin D, et al. Serum bone alkaline phosphatase in the follow-up of skeletal metastases. *Anticancer Res* 1995;15:2223.
47. Reale MG, Santini GG, Marchei A, et al. Skeletal alkaline phosphatase as a serum marker of bone metastases in the follow-up of patients with breast cancer. *Int J Biol Markers* 1994;10:42.
48. Pugh J, Sherry HS, Futterman B, Frankel VH. Biomechanics of pathologic fractures. *Clin Orthop* 1982;169:109.
49. Hipp JA, McBroom RJ, Cheal EJ, Hayes WC. Structural consequences of endosteal metastatic lesions in long bones. *J Orthop Res* 1989;7:828.
50. Hipp JA, Edgerton BC, An KN, Hayes WC. Structural consequences of transcortical holes in long bones loaded in torsion. *J Biomech* 1990;23:1261.
51. McBroom RJ, Cheal EJ, Hayes WC. Strength reductions from metastatic cortical defects in long bones. *J Orthop Res* 1988;6:369.

52. Hipp JA, Rosenberg AE, Hayes WC. Mechanical properties of trabecular bone within and adjacent to osseous metastases. *J Bone Miner Res* 1992;7:1165.
53. Tong D, Gillick L, Hendrickson FR. The palliation of symptomatic osseous metastases: final results of the Radiation Therapy Oncology Group. *Cancer* 1982;50:893.
54. Parrish FF, Murray JA. Surgical treatment for secondary neoplastic fractures: a retrospective study of ninety-six patients. *J Bone Joint Surg Am* 1970;52:665.
55. Fidler M. Incidence of fracture through metastases in long bones. *Acta Orthop Scand* 1981;52:623.
56. Beals RK, Lawton GD, Snell WE. Prophylactic internal fixation of the femur in metastatic breast cancer. *Cancer* 1971;28:1350.
57. Cheng DS, Seitz CB, Eyre HJ. Nonoperative management of femoral, humeral and acetabular metastasis in patients with breast carcinoma. *Cancer* 1980;45:1533.
58. Mirels H. Metastatic disease in long bones. *Clin Orthop* 1989; 249:256.
59. Hipp JA, Springfield DS, Hayes WC. Predicting pathologic fracture risk in the management of metastatic bone defects. *Clin Orthop* 1995;312:120.
60. World Health Organization. Cancer pain relief and palliative care: report of a WHO expert committee. Technical report series no. 804. Geneva: World Health Organization, 1990.
61. Blitzer PH. Reanalysis of the RTOG study of the palliation of symptomatic osseous metastasis. *Cancer* 1985;55:1468.
62. Price P, Hoskin PJ, Easton D, et al. Prospective randomized trial of single and multifraction radiotherapy schedules in the treatment of painful bony metastases. *Radiother Oncol* 1986;6:247.
63. Cole DJ. A randomized trial of a single treatment versus conventional fractionation in the palliative radiotherapy of painful bone metastases. *Clin Oncol* 1989;1:59.
64. Kagei K, Suzuki K, Shirato H, et al. A randomized trial of single and multifraction radiation therapy for bone metastasis: a preliminary report (article in Japanese). *Gan No Rinsho* 1990;36:2553.
65. Gaze MN, Kelly CG, Kerr GR, et al. Pain relief and quality of life following radiotherapy for bone metastases: a randomised trial of two fractionation schedules. *Radiother Oncol* 1997;45:109.
66. Nielsen OS, Bentzen SM, Sandberg E, et al. Randomized trial of single dose versus fractionated palliative radiotherapy of bone metastases. *Radiother Oncol* 1998;47:233.
67. Janjan NA. Radiation for bone metastases. *Cancer* 1997;80:1628.
68. McQuay HJ, Carroll D, Moore RA. Radiotherapy for painful bone metastases: a systematic review. *Clin Oncol* 1997;9:150.
69. Ben-Josef E, Shamsa F, Williams AO, et al. Radiotherapeutic management of osseous metastases: a survey of current patterns of care. *Int J Radiat Oncol Biol Phys* 1998;40:915.
70. Rose CM, Kagan AR. The final report of the expert panel for the radiation oncology bone metastasis work group of the American College of Radiology. *Int J Radiat Oncol Biol Phys* 1998;40:1117.
71. Hoskin PJ, Price P, Easton D, et al. A prospective randomised trial of 4-Gy or 8-Gy single doses in the treatment of metastatic bone pain. *Radiother Oncol* 1992;23:74.
72. Barton R, Hoskin P, Yarnold J. Radiotherapy for bone pain: is a single fraction good enough? UK Multicentre Bone Pain Trail Collaborators. *Clin Oncol* 1994;6:354.
73. Dale RG, Jones B. Radiobiologically based assessments of the net costs of fractionated radiotherapy. *Int J Radiat Oncol Biol Phys* 1996;36:739.
74. Mithal NP, Needham PR, Hoskin PJ. Retreatment with radiotherapy for painful bone metastases. *Int J Radiat Oncol Biol Phys* 1994;29:1011.
75. Salazar OM, Rubin P, Hendrickson FR, et al. Single-dose half-body irradiation for palliation of multiple bone metastases from solid tumors. *Cancer* 1986;58:29.
76. Scarantino CW, Caplan R, Rotman M, et al. A phase I/II study to evaluate the effect of fractionated hemibody irradiation in the treatment of osseous metastases—RTOG 88-22. *Int J Radiat Oncol Phys* 1996;36:37.
77. Sykes AJ, Kiltie AE, Stewart AL. Ondansetron versus chlorpromazine and dexamethasone combination for the prevention of nausea and vomiting: a prospective, randomised study to assess efficacy, cost effectiveness and quality of life following single-fraction radiotherapy. *Support Care Cancer* 1997;5:500.
78. Poulter CA, Cosmatos D, Rubin P, et al. A report of RTOG 8206: a phase III study of whether the addition of single dose hemibody irradiation to standard fractionated local field irradiation is more effective than local field irradiation alone in the treatment of symptomatic osseous metastases. *Int J Radiat Oncol Biol Phys* 1992;23:207
79. Harrington KD. Introduction. In: Harrington KD, ed. *Orthopaedic management of metastatic bone disease*. St. Louis: Mosby, 1988:1.
80. Harrington KD, Sim FH, Enis JE, Johnston JO, Dick HM, Gristina AG. Methylmethacrylate as an adjunct in internal fixation of pathological fractures. *J Bone Joint Surg Am* 1976;58:1047.
81. Ryan JR, Rowe DF, Salciccioli GG. Prophylactic internal fixation of the femur for neoplastic lesions. *J Bone Joint Surg Am* 1976; 58:1071.
82. Gainor BJ, Buchert P. Fracture healing in metastatic bone disease. *Clin Orthop* 1983;178:297.
83. Murray JA, Bruels MC, Lindberg RD. Irradiation of polymethylmethacrylate. *J Bone Joint Surg Am* 1974;56:311.
84. Ryan JR, Begeman PC. The effects of filling experimental large cortical defects with methylmethacrylate. *Clin Orthop* 1984;185:306.
85. Yazawa Y, Frassica FJ, Chao EYS, Pritchard DJ, Sim FH, Shives TC. Metastatic bone disease: a study of the surgical treatment of 166 pathologic humeral and femoral fractures. *Clin Orthop* 1990;251:213.
86. Douglas HO, Shukla SK, Mindell, E. Treatment of pathological fractures of long bones excluding those due to breast cancer. *J Bone Joint Surg [Am]* 1976;58:1055.
87. Flemming JE, Beals RK. Pathologic fracture of the humerus. *Clin Orthop* 1986;203:258.
88. Lewallen RP, Pritchard DJ, Sim FH. Treatment of pathologic fractures or impending fractures of the humerus with Rush rods and methylmethacrylate: experience with 55 cases in 54 patients, 1968–1977. *Clin Orthop* 1982;166:193.
89. Sim FH, Pritchard DJ. Metastatic disease in the upper extremity. *Clin Orthop* 1982;169:83.
90. Vail TP, Harrelson JM. Treatment of pathologic fracture of the humerus. *Clin Orthop* 1991;268:197.
91. Redmond BJ, Biermann JS, Blasier RB. Interlocking intramedullary nailing of pathological fractures of the shaft of the humerus. *J Bone Joint Surg* 1996;78:891.
92. Chin H, Frassica FJ, Hein TJ, et al. Metastatic diaphyseal fractures of the shaft of the humerus: the structural strength evaluation of a new method of treatment with a segmental defect prosthesis. *Clin Orthop* 1989;248:231.
93. Sim FH, Frassica FJ, Chao EYS. Orthopaedic management using new devices and prostheses. *Clin Orthop* 1995;312:160.
94. Crowninshield RD, Johnston RC, Andrews JG, Brand RA. A biomechanical investigation of the human hip. *J Biomech* 1978;11:75.
95. Patriarco AG, Mann RW, Simon SR, Mansour JM. An evaluation of the approaches of optimization models in the prediction of muscle forces during human gait. *J Biomech* 1981;14:513.
96. Harrington KD. Orthopaedic management of extremity and pelvic lesions. *Clin Orthop* 1995;312:136.
97. Mickelson MR, Bonfiglio M. Pathological fractures in the proximal part of the femur treated by Zickel-nail fixation. *J Bone Joint Surg Am* 1976;58:1067.
98. Zickel RE, Mouradian, WH. Intramedullary fixation of pathological fractures and lesions of the subtrochanteric region of the femur. *J Bone Joint Surg Am* 1976;58:1061.
99. Lane JM, Sculco TP, Zolan S. Treatment of pathological fractures of the hip by endoprosthetic replacement. *J Bone Joint Surg Am* 1980; 62:954.
100. Sim FH, Chao EYS. Bone loss in the proximal femur: proximal femoral replacement. In: Morrey B, ed. *Joint replacement arthroplasty*. New York: Churchill Livingstone, 1991:820.
101. Harrington KD. The management of acetabular insufficiency secondary to metastatic malignant disease. *J Bone Joint Surg Am* 1981; 63:653.
102. Townsend PW, Smalley SR, Cozad SC, et al. Role of postoperative radiation therapy after stabilization of fractures caused by metastatic disease. *Int J Radiat Oncol Biol Phys* 1995;31:43.
103. Harrington KD. Metastatic disease of the spine. *J Bone Joint Surg Am* 1986;68:1110.
104. Smoker WRK, Godersky JC, Knutzon R, et al. The role of MR imaging in evaluating metastatic spinal disease. *AJR Am J Roentgenol* 1987;149:1241.

105. Weissman DE. Glucocorticoid treatment for brain metastases and epidural spinal cord compression: a review. *J Clin Oncol* 1988;6:543.
106. Sorensen PS, Helweg-Larsen S, Mouridsen H, et al. Effect of high-dose dexamethasone in carcinomatous metastatic spinal cord compression treated with radiotherapy: a randomised trial. *Eur J Cancer* 1994;30A:22.
107. Heimdal K, Hirschberg H, Slettebo H, et al. High incidence of serious side effects of high-dose dexamethasone treatment in patients with epidural spinal cord compression. *J Neurooncol* 1992;12:141.
108. Maranzano E, Latini P. Effectiveness of radiation therapy without surgery in metastatic spinal cord compression: final results from a prospective trial. *Int J Radiat Oncol Biol Phys* 1995;32:959.
109. Young RF, Post EM, King GA. Treatment of spinal cord epidural metastases: randomized prospective comparison of laminectomy and radiotherapy. *J Neurosurg* 1980;53:741.
110. Maranzano E, Latini P, Perrucci E, et al. Short-course radiotherapy (8 Gy × 2) in metastatic spinal cord compression: an effective and feasible treatment. *Int J Radiat Oncol Biol Phys* 1997;38:1037.
111. Schiff D, Shaw EG, Cascino TL. Outcome after spinal reirradiation for malignant epidural spinal cord compression. *Ann Neurol* 1995;37:583.

XV

Diseases of the Breast, 2nd ed.,
edited by Jay R. Harris.
Lippincott Williams & Wilkins, Philadelphia © 2000.

Breast Cancer in Special Populations

CHAPTER 63

Breast Cancer in Older Women

Gretchen G. Kimmick and Hyman B. Muss

Age is a major risk factor for breast cancer. According to 1998 cancer statistics, 1 in 15 women aged 60 to 79 years developed breast cancer between 1992 and 1994, compared with 1 in 25 women aged 40 to 59 years and 1 in 227 women younger than age 39 years.[1] The increasing incidence of breast cancer with age has been seen predominantly in women older than 50 years.[2] The number of women in the age groups of 65 to 74 years, 75 to 84 years, and 85 and older is predicted to nearly double by 2050 (Fig. 1). These data portend a significant increase in breast cancer cases in the geriatric population.

Several studies have indicated that breast cancer survival is poorer for older women.[3–6] Overall 10-year disease-specific survival was 51% for breast cancer cases listed in the National Swedish Cancer registry, but only 44% for older women.[3] Among cases in the Finnish Cancer Registry, increasing age was associated with decreased 10-year survival in women with node-positive disease (49% for women aged 46 to 50 years versus 35% for women older than age 75 years; $p < .001$) but not those with node-negative or localized breast cancer.[4] United States statistics on breast cancer mortality also show an increasing mortality rate with increasing age.[7]

Age-related differences in breast cancer survival may be related to differences in disease stage at diagnosis. Stage-specific relative survival was worse only for patients aged 85 years and older in an analysis of data from the Surveillance, Epidemiology, and End Results (SEER) Program.[8] Older and younger women with localized and regional stages of breast cancer fared equally well, but older women were diagnosed with metastatic disease more frequently and fared worse. Other retrospective analyses report higher rates of localized disease in older women with similar 10-year actuarial breast cancer–specific survival and disease-free survival after adjustment for TNM stage.[9,10]

In general, poor prognostic factors are less common in breast tumors of older women. Postmenopausal women have lower breast cancer cell proliferation rates as measured

G. G. Kimmick: Department of Internal Medicine—Hematology/Oncology, Wake Forest University School of Medicine, Winston-Salem, North Carolina

H. B. Muss: Department of Medicine, University of Vermont, Fletcher Allen Health Care, Vermont Cancer Center, Burlington, Vermont

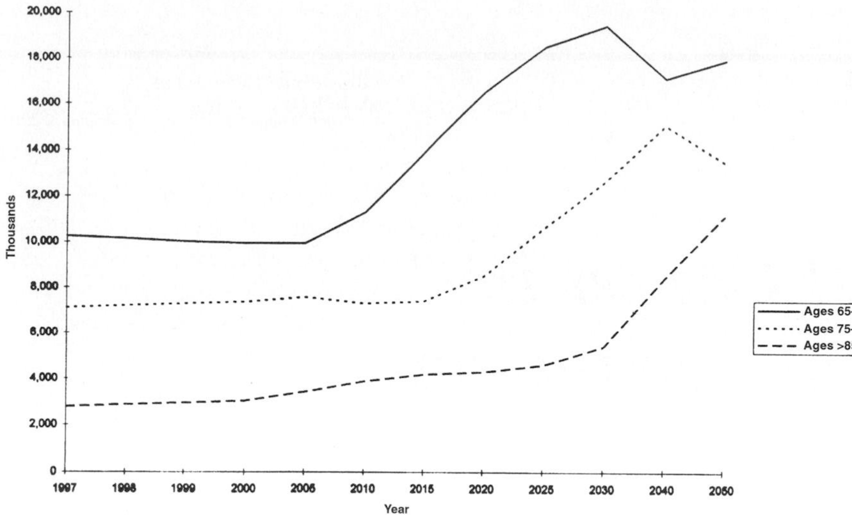

FIG. 1. Population projections for women in the United States (in thousands). (Data from U.S. Bureau of the Census. *Statistical Abstracts of the United States*, 117th ed. Washington: U.S. Government Printing Office; 1997; and *The National Data Book*. Washington: Hoover's Business Press, 1997.)

by the thymidine-tritium labeling index[11] and a higher frequency of hormone receptor–positive tumors.[12,13] Also, more indolent histologies, such as mucinous and papillary carcinomas, are more frequent in older-age women.[8] Lyman et al. studied 274 women aged 65 and older with locoregional breast cancer who were part of a cohort of 1,267 women treated at a single center.[14] The older women had more early-stage cancers, lower histologic grades, higher hormone-receptor levels, lower S-phase fractions, and longer recurrence-free and overall survival.

COMORBIDITY, SURVIVAL, AND TREATMENT PREFERENCE

In Western societies, life expectancy is approximately 15.5 years at age 70 and 9.2 years at age 80[7] (Table 1). The number of coexisting illnesses increases with advancing age. These comorbid conditions have great influence on screening for and treatment of breast cancer.[15] In fact, deaths unrelated to breast cancer are more likely in breast cancer patients older than age 65 than in those younger than 65 years (20% versus 3%, $p < .001$).[16]

TABLE 1. *Average remaining lifetime at various ages*

Age (yr)	Life expectancy, males and females (yr)	Life expectancy, females (yr)
55–60	25.1	27.2
60–65	21.1	23.1
65–70	17.5	19.2
70–75	14.2	15.5
75–80	11.2	12.2
80–85	8.5	9.2
≥85	6.2	6.6

Table shows average number of years of life remaining at the beginning of the age interval.
From ref. 7, with permission.

In a series of studies, Satariano and others explored the association of comorbid illness and mortality in women with breast cancer.[17–19] Two years after an assessment of comorbidity by interviews of 463 breast cancer patients aged 55 to 84 years, the women who had died were more likely to have reported one or more comorbid conditions than were the survivors (62% versus 38%).[17] Furthermore, the greater the number of comorbid conditions, the higher the risk of death from all causes, including breast cancer, independent of age and stage of disease. Compared to women with no comorbid conditions, women reporting one comorbid condition were 2.5 times more likely to die, and those reporting two or more comorbid conditions were 3.4 times more likely to die. After 4 years of follow-up, women with two or more concurrent conditions were 2.2 times more likely to die from breast cancer (95% confidence interval, 1.13 to 4.18) after adjustment for other factors.[18] Heart disease was a major risk factor; women with symptomatic heart disease that limited daily activity were 2.4 times more likely to die of breast cancer (95% confidence interval, 1.07 to 5.52). In addition, an interaction was found between comorbidity and stage at diagnosis.[19] Among patients with three or more comorbid conditions, stage of disease had little additional effect on survival; early breast cancer diagnosis in women with a high level of comorbidity conferred no survival disadvantage.

Two studies have shown that age is an independent predictor of management. Newschaffer et al. linked cancer registry records of a cohort of 2,252 women aged 66 years and older who had early breast cancer to Medicare provider and reimbursement data files and *International Classification of Diseases* (ninth edition) codes.[20] Even after controlling for comorbidity, increasing age was associated with a decrease in any surgical treatment, non–breast-conserving procedures, and radiation therapy after breast-conserving surgery. Similarly, Greenfield et al. found that, among 420 women with breast cancer, 81% of those older than 50 years with "no" or "mild" comorbidity were treated aggressively, compared with 59% with "severe" comorbidity.[21] When comorbidity, stage, and hospital location were controlled for, age still remained an independent factor that significantly affected treatment practices. This age effect was evident in patients aged 65 years and older.

Poor social support, limited access to transportation, and impaired cognition are associated with delays in diagnosis and increased risk of inadequate treatment of cancer patients aged 65 and older.[22] Measures of health status—including the presence of other medical diagnoses and comorbidities, functional status, level of physical activity, socioeconomic status, cognitive status, type of treatment (definitive or other), and the availability of social support—all predicted 10-year survival.

As women age, their values and preferences for treatment change, and these changes may not be discerned by family or health care providers. In a prospective, longitudinal, multicenter study, Tsevat et al. explored the priorities of 1,438 seriously ill patients.[23] Patients who had a projected overall 6-month mortality rate of 50%, their surrogates, and their physicians were interviewed serially over a 6-month period. Time trade-off utilities and health ratings were used to assess health values, determinants of health values, and any change in health values over time. Health values varied widely among patients, which limited the use of identifying "average preferences" in decisions for individual patients. Moreover, patients' values for their current state of health could not be predicted. The health values and ratings of participating patients varied inversely with depression but were generally higher than their surrogates or their physicians realized. Thus, substituting a surrogate's preference for that of a patient who cannot or will not participate in decision making may be inappropriate, unless the patient prefers family decision making to alternative strategies, such as advanced planning. In addition, patients' health values changed over time, a finding that suggests that the preferences of seriously ill patients may need to be obtained serially.

PREVENTION

Prevention of breast cancer has been reviewed in Chapter 19. Three breast cancer prevention trials studying treatment with tamoxifen (tamoxifen citrate) versus placebo have been reported.[24–26] The largest of these trials, the National Surgical Adjuvant Breast and Bowel Project Prevention trial (NSABP P-1), was the only trial to show a dramatic reduction in invasive and noninvasive breast cancer.[24] All women aged 60 years and older were eligible to participate, regardless of other risk factors; 30% of trial participants were older than 60 years, and 6% were older than 70 years. The impressive early results of this trial must be tempered with caution, as tamoxifen use was associated with a significantly higher incidence of endometrial cancer and thromboembolic events in postmenopausal women. Nevertheless, the preventive benefits of tamoxifen may outweigh the risks for many older patients.

A second prevention trial comparing tamoxifen with raloxifene (raloxifene hydrochloride), NSABP P-2 (also called the Study of Tamoxifen and Raloxifene, or STAR, trial), is underway. Raloxifene lacks estrogen agonist effects on the uterus; preliminary data suggest that raloxifene may prevent breast cancer without increasing endometrial cancer risk.[27]

SCREENING

Breast cancer screening (Chapter 11) involves mammography, clinical breast examination, and breast self-examination. Large randomized trials have shown that routine annual or biannual mammography in women aged 50 to 75 years is associated with a reduction in breast cancer–related mortality of 25% to 30% within 5 to 6 years of initiation.[28] Because many of these trials did not include women older than 75 years, the optimal upper age limit for mammographic screening is still a matter of debate. Recommendations, therefore, are based on retrospective data and results of small studies with surrogate end points. A number of retrospective reviews suggest that, in older women, tumors detected by mammography are smaller and earlier in stage than tumors detected by other means.[29–32] Comparing mammographic results of women aged 50 to 64 (n = 21,226) and of women aged 65 and older (n = 10,914), Faulk et al. found that mammography had a higher positive predictive value, a higher yield of positive biopsies, and a greater cancer detection rate per 1,000 studies in older women.[31]

A forum on breast cancer screening in older women, jointly funded by the National Cancer Institute and the National Institute of Aging in 1990, recommended breast self-examination monthly, breast physical examination yearly, and mammography every 2 years for women aged 65 years and older.[33] Issues that could not be resolved completely were the proper interval for screening (12 versus 24 versus 36 months) and the extent to which clinical breast examination contributed to a decrease in mortality. A retrospective study of Field et al. supports the use of annual mammography in this age group; smaller, earlier-stage tumors were found by annual mammography than by biennial screening.[34]

Another widely debated issue is the age at which mammography ceases to offer benefit. Some experts recommend mammography for healthy women up to age 85 years.[35] Because the average 85-year-old woman in the United States is expected to live 9.2 more years and survival benefit is evident after 5 to 6 years of follow-up in large randomized screening trials, an age cutoff based on life expectancy should be used.[18] In fact, in a decision analysis constructed to compare the utility of breast cancer screening using mammography with that of physical breast examination in older women, the benefits of screening mammography outweighed the financial costs for older women, irrespective of age, but the magnitude of benefit decreased with increasing age and comorbidity.[36]

Mammography rates decrease with increasing age, continuing to decline into the ninth decade of life.[37–42] Rates as low as 26.7% in a 2-year period for women 75 and older have been reported.[41] Poor level of function; limitations in activities of daily living; poor general health; a history of stroke, hip fracture, or dementia; older age; low income; low education level; fewer primary care visits; lack of a place to go for health care; and failure of physicians to recommend or discuss mammography are directly associated with lower screening rates.[38,39,41,43–45] Interestingly, a history of hypertension, diabetes mellitus, or myocardial infarction was not associated with mammography use.[41] Attention to factors associated with lower mammography use improves screening rates. The physician's recommendation is probably the most important stimulus for obtaining screening mammography in older women. Emphasizing the reassurance that mammography brings recipients may also be helpful.[46]

MANAGEMENT OF THE PRIMARY LESION

Standard Management

Advanced age is also found to be a risk factor for undertreatment, even after control for comorbidity, cognitive status, social support, and functional status.[21,47–49] Yancik et al. found surgery to be performed less frequently for breast cancer in women older than age 85 years.[8] Bergman et al. found that older women had less extensive surgical procedures and less adjuvant radiation; as a result, a decrease was seen in disease-related 10-year survival of such women compared with younger patients—32% versus 57%, respectively.[6] Other authors have also documented omission of adjuvant radiation after breast conservation and less breast-preserving procedures in older women.[8,48,50,51]

Management of a primary breast tumor is discussed in Section 9. Older women tolerate breast surgery well,[52] with operative mortality rates of 1% to 2% consistently reported.[53,54] The main factor influencing surgical morbidity is not age but the presence of coexistent disease.[6,8] Older women also tolerate breast irradiation[55,56] and should be offered the option of breast preservation, as body image and the loss of a breast are important issues regardless of age. Given a choice, women aged 70 and older were more likely to choose breast-conserving surgery than mastectomy.[57]

Standard treatment for breast cancer has similar outcomes in older and younger women.[58,59] When older women were compared with women younger than age 65 years, breast-conserving surgery plus definitive breast irradiation was found to yield 10-year rates of local failure of 4% versus 13%, disease-free survival of 72% versus 72%, and overall survival of 84% versus 82%, respectively.[58] Results were similar in a study of Solin et al., but the older women had more deaths from intercurrent disease in that study (11% versus 2%; $p = .0006$).[59]

Nonstandard Management

Tamoxifen Alone as Primary Treatment

The use of tamoxifen instead of surgery for operable breast cancer may delay the need for surgical intervention. Despite good initial response rates of 30% to 60%, high relapse rates are found during follow-up, necessitating additional local treatment. Nevertheless, tamoxifen as a first-line treatment is of value in older breast cancer patients who are unable to tolerate surgery.

The use of tamoxifen alone as initial treatment for localized breast cancer was first studied in women who were not candidates for or refused surgery.[60] In this 4-year pilot study, 67 women aged 75 years and older with clinically localized breast cancer were treated with tamoxifen. Seventy-three percent responded sufficiently to continue treatment; almost all the tumors that eventually responded showed signs of response after 1 month of treatment. Actuarial 5-year survival rate was 49.4% and was highest for those showing an initial complete response (92%).[61] Since that report, similar response rates with limited response durations, ranging from 10 to 50 months, have been reported.[62–67] Responses have been best in patients with estrogen receptor–rich tumors.[64]

Studies comparing the efficacy of tamoxifen therapy and surgery with or without tamoxifen therapy found similar survival rates overall but higher local control rates with surgery[68–71] (Table 2). Response rates to tamoxifen alone ranged from 28% to 67%, with one-third to two-thirds of patients developing progressive local disease. In contrast, wide excision alone in older women resulted in local control rates ranging from 71% to 97%.[51,72–74]

Two randomized trials examined the effect of surgery in addition to tamoxifen.[75,76] The British Cancer Research Campaign trial found that further surgery was necessary in 35 patients treated with tamoxifen and 15 patients managed with surgery and tamoxifen ($p = .001$).[75] In the randomized, multicenter trial conducted by the Group for Research on Endocrine Therapy in the Elderly, significantly less local recurrence was also seen in those treated with surgery and tamoxifen than in those treated with tamoxifen alone ($p = .00045$).[76] In the group treated with tamoxifen alone, 7.6% had a complete response, 29.3% had a partial response, and 50.4% had stable disease.

Overall, 63% of patients treated with tamoxifen alone as a first-line treatment may have tumor regression.[77] This regression can persist up to 5 years in 90% of patients who

TABLE 2. *Survival and local control rates after treatment with tamoxifen citrate alone and surgery with or without tamoxifen*

			Overall survival (%)		Local recurrence (%)	
	n	Median follow-up	Tamoxifen	Surgery	Tamoxifen	Surgery
Retrospective review						
van Dalsen and deVries[68]	171	41 mo	68	72	27	6
Tamoxifen vs surgery without tamoxifen						
Nottingham group[71]	135	2 yr	85	74.6	44	24
St. George Hospital[69]	116	3 yr	78.3	80.3	25	37.5
St. George Hospital[70]	200	6 yr	66	72	56	44
Tamoxifen vs surgery and tamoxifen						
British Cancer Research Campaign[75]	381	34 mo	82.5	84.8	23	7.5
Group for Research on Endocrine Therapy in the Elderly[76]	473	36 mo	82.6	79.7	25.4	6.3

respond initially to treatment.[61] The median time to response to tamoxifen is 13.5 weeks (range, 5 to 124 weeks). Although women who have a complete response to tamoxifen have a very good 5-year survival, clinical prediction of response is inaccurate unless immunocytochemical assay of fine-needle aspirates is used to assess estrogen-receptor status.[78] Surgery, however, consistently results in better local control; as many as 60% of patients treated with tamoxifen alone for localized disease eventually have local tumor progression requiring further local therapy, such as radiation or surgery. When local disease progresses or recurs, patients managed initially with surgery are always fit to take tamoxifen, irrespective of the state of the patient or disease; patients initially treated with tamoxifen alone, however, may be unfit for surgery on progression.

Other Nonstandard Combinations of Tumor Excision, Tamoxifen, and Radiation

Addition of tamoxifen or radiation therapy to local excision results in better local tumor control in older women[70,73] and may improve survival.[79–81] In a decision analysis using the Markov process, radiation and tamoxifen provided the optimal postlumpectomy therapy for a stage I (T1b NX M0) mammographically detected breast cancer in a 74-year-old woman without comorbidities.[82]

In older women who are unable to tolerate anesthesia and find it difficult to attend daily adjuvant radiation treatments, breast-sparing surgery performed under local anesthesia, followed by tamoxifen therapy—without axillary dissection or adjuvant radiation—may be considered.[83,84] A retrospective study of patients treated in this manner demonstrated that, 5 and 10 years from initial surgery, local relapse rates in the breast were 5.4% and 8.7%, relapse rates in the ipsilateral axilla were 4.3% and 5.9%, and incidences of distant metastases were 6.2% and 13.4%, respectively.[84] Low local relapse rates (3.8%) at a median follow-up of 39 months in patients not receiving radiation therapy were also found in a controlled clinical trial comparing quadrantectomy versus quadrantectomy plus radiotherapy in treatment of postmenopausal women older than 55 years with breast cancers smaller than 2.5 cm.[85] Two other studies addressing the same issue, however, showed higher local recurrence rates in women who did not receive adjuvant radiation.[51,74]

The use of tamoxifen alone after lumpectomy has been investigated as a means of obviating the need for radiation therapy. Results of retrospective studies raise skepticism, because local recurrence rates may be higher without radiation.[86] The Cancer and Leukemia Group B has implemented a prospective randomized trial (CALGB 9343) for women aged 70 and older with stage T1 estrogen receptor–positive or progesterone receptor–positive primary tumors to resolve this issue. After lumpectomy, all women are placed on tamoxifen and then randomized to receive breast radiation or not.

The role of axillary lymph node dissection is coming under increasing scrutiny for women of all ages because of its major associated morbidity, lymphedema (see Chapter 69). Three small retrospective reports examining the benefits and outcomes related to axillary dissection in older women suggest that this procedure might be avoided.[52,87,88] Newer procedures associated with minimal morbidity, such as sentinel lymph node surgery, may be helpful for assessing nodal status in older women.

The schedule and duration of adjuvant radiation may be an obstacle for older persons. Two retrospective analyses examined the use of weekly radiation schedules.[89,90] Rostom et al. reported the use of once-weekly irradiation for 84 older patients with breast cancer (stages I–IV).[89] Treatment was well tolerated: Reactive fibrosis, skin thickening, or both occurred in 25 patients, symptomatic pneumonitis was reported in four patients, and brachial plexopathy in one. Among patients with stage I and II tumors, local control and cosmetic results were encouraging. Maher et al. evaluated a regimen that included tamoxifen use and once-weekly radiation therapy, for a total of seven fractions, in a group of women with a mean age of 81 years (range, 64 to 91).[90] At a median follow-up of 36 months, the overall survival rate was 87%, the disease-specific survival rate was 88%, and the local recurrence rate was 14%. With the high dose per frac-

TABLE 3. *Benefit of tamoxifen citrate adjuvant therapy in women 70 years and older*

Approximate duration of tamoxifen use (yr)	Reduction in risk of relapse (%)	Reduction in risk of death (%)
1	22 (9)	8 (8)
2	42 (8)	36 (7)
5	54 (13)	34 (13)

Numbers in parentheses are standard deviations.
From ref. 91, with permission.

tion, 39% of patients experienced moderate fibrosis at the primary site. No rib fractures, radiation pneumonitis, or brachial plexopathy were seen. Studies exploring brachytherapy to the surgical bed after lumpectomy are in progress.

Adjuvant Therapy

The 1998 updated meta-analyses of adjuvant therapy trials by the Early Breast Cancer Trialists' Collaborative Group clearly show the benefit of adjuvant tamoxifen therapy and adjuvant chemotherapy in improving relapse-free and overall survival in women with early-stage breast cancer.[91,92] Tamoxifen therapy offers marked benefit to women aged 70 years and older[91] (Table 3). The proportional reduction in breast cancer relapse and mortality were similar for women with node-negative and node-positive tumors. Patients with estrogen receptor–positive tumors benefited from tamoxifen, as did women with unrecorded estrogen-receptor status; women with tumors devoid of estrogen receptor derived no benefit from tamoxifen therapy regardless of age.

In the 47 adjuvant chemotherapy trials included in the meta-analysis, involving 18,000 women, only approximately 600 women (3%) were 70 years and older.[92] This sample size was insufficient to determine the benefits of chemotherapy in this age group. However, the proportional benefits of chemotherapy for patients aged 70 years and older are unlikely to be different than those for postmenopausal women 50 to 69 years old. For patients aged 50 to 69 years, the proportional risk reductions were 20% (standard deviation, 3%) for recurrence and 11% (standard deviation, 3%) for overall mortality. This mortality reduction translates into 2% and 3% net gains in 10-year survival for women with node-negative and node-positive breast cancer, respectively.

The overview analyses also clearly showed that, in women with hormone receptor–positive tumors, the combination of tamoxifen and chemotherapy was significantly better than the use of either modality alone.[91,92] The proportional reductions in recurrence and death were 22% (standard deviation, 4%) versus 12% (standard deviation, 4%) for chemotherapy versus no adjuvant therapy; 19% (standard deviation, 3%) versus 11% (standard deviation, 4%) for chemotherapy and tamoxifen versus tamoxifen alone; and 52% versus 47% for chemotherapy and tamoxifen versus chemotherapy alone.[91,92] Anthracycline-containing chemotherapy was associated with a small but significant further reduction in the risk of recurrence (12%; standard deviation, 4%) and a marginal reduction in mortality (11%; standard deviation, 5%; $p = .02$) compared with chemotherapy using cyclophosphamide, methotrexate, and 5-fluorouracil. Although these differences are significant, they are small; non–anthracycline-containing regimens might be preferable in older patients, in whom the risk of anthracycline cardiac toxicity is higher than in younger patients.[93]

TABLE 4. *Recommendations for adjuvant therapy for women older than 70 years*

Risk category	Definition	Treatment
Node negative		
Minimal/low	≤1cm, ER and/or PR positive, grade I	No treatment or tamoxifen
Moderate	>1 cm and ≤2 cm, grade I or II, ER and/or PR positive	Tamoxifen ± chemotherapy
High	>2 cm, ER and/or PR negative or grade II or III	Tamoxifen; chemotherapy if ER/PR negative
Node positive		
ER positive	Any	Tamoxifen
ER negative	Any	Chemotherapy

ER, estrogen receptor; PR, progesterone receptor.
Grades: I, well differentiated; II, moderately differentiated; III, poorly differentiated.
Modified from ref. 94.

The consensus of experts participating in the St. Gallen Breast Cancer Conference in 1998 regarding adjuvant therapy for women older than 70 years of age are presented in Table 4.[94] In women older than 70, particularly women aged 75 and older and those with significant comorbid illness, toxicities of adjuvant therapy must be considered carefully. Clinical trials addressing the role of adjuvant chemotherapy in older women are greatly needed.

Major issues to consider in determining the benefit of adjuvant therapy for older women are anticipated survival and comorbid illness. Using a Markov model, Extermann et al. studied the threshold risk of relapse at which adjuvant tamoxifen and chemotherapy offered benefit to women up to age 85, including those with and without comorbidity.[95] Using data from the 1992 overview analysis,[96] they examined the threshold risk for a 1% benefit in 5-year or 10-year relapse rate or survival; the assumption was that the tumor was estrogen receptor–positive and that 5 years of tamoxifen therapy, standard chemotherapy, or both was used. For tamoxifen, the threshold risks of relapse were 11% and 20% for a 1% benefit in 10-year survival for healthy and sick women at age 65, respectively. At age 85, the threshold risks of relapse were 28% and 35% for a 1% benefit in 5-year survival for healthy and sick women, respectively (no 10-year survival benefit was seen in this age group). For chemotherapy, the threshold risk of relapse was 19% for a healthy 65-year-old and 62% for a sick 85-year-old. Overall, comorbidity increased the threshold risk of relapse by approximately 10% for tamoxifen therapy and 20% for chemotherapy.

Cost is also pertinent. Desch et al. reported that the cost-benefit ratio of adjuvant chemotherapy in women with estrogen receptor–negative, node-negative breast cancer who were between 60 and 80 years of age was high but within the range of other commonly reimbursed procedures.[97]

TREATMENT OF METASTATIC DISEASE

Metastatic breast cancer is incurable. All women, regardless of age, should be managed using the principles outlined in Chapter 48. Treatment should be focused on maintaining the highest quality of life while controlling symptoms. Endocrine manipulation is the mainstay of treatment for metastatic breast cancer in older women. Older patients should be offered chemotherapy when metastases become refractory to endocrine treatment. The response rates to and toxicity profiles of the standard chemotherapy regimens for metastatic breast cancer are similar in younger and older women who are in reasonable general health.[98–102] A detailed review of the pharmacology of chemotherapeutic agents in older patients has been published.[103] Most cytotoxic agents are metabolized in the liver, and only patients with major liver function abnormalities have increased risk of toxicity. Caution should be exercised and dose modification considered for patients with liver dysfunction selected for treatment with anthracyclines or taxanes. Methotrexate excretion is dependent on renal function; before methotrexate is administered to older women, creatinine clearance should be measured. Gelman and Taylor modified methotrexate dosage on the basis of renal function in older women with advanced breast cancer without compromise of its therapeutic effect.[99] The risk of anthracycline-related cardiotoxicity is no higher in otherwise healthy older women than in younger women. In one series, deaths due to cardiopulmonary causes were noted in 6% of women older than 65 years, compared with 5% of women aged 50 to 64 years receiving chemotherapy.[101] The severity and duration of myelosuppression is increased in older patients but has not resulted in major differences in mortality related to neutropenia, sepsis, or bleeding.[100,101] Nausea and vomiting may be less frequent in older patients,[104] and psychosocial adjustment to chemotherapy appears better for older than for younger women.[105] The response rates to subsequent "salvage" chemotherapy regimens are generally poor; however, taxanes have shown substantial activity even in heavily pretreated patients.[106,107] Data concerning the use of taxanes in older patients are needed. The use of vinorelbine tartrate has been studied in women older than 65 years; the drug has similar pharmacokinetics and a favorable toxicity profile in older women and in younger women.[108] Liposome-encapsulated doxorubicin hydrochloride (Doxil and others) is being tested in older patients because of its minimal cardiac toxicity and ease of administration.[109] Capecitabine (Xeloda), an oral fluorouracil prodrug, has been approved for use in metastatic breast cancer. Capecitabine is well tolerated, although hand-foot syndrome is frequent and can be dose limiting.[110] Trials in older patients are warranted.

Trastuzumab (Herceptin), a humanized monoclonal antibody, has been approved for use in patients with metastatic breast cancer whose tumors express HER-2/neu (c-*erb*-b2).[111] The favorable toxicity profile of this compound suggests that it should be considered for use in older women with metastatic disease.

MANAGEMENT SUMMARY

Screening

Yearly clinical breast examination and monthly breast self-examination are recommended for all women. Yearly mammography is recommended up to age 75 years and should be continued after age 75 years in women who have one or no limiting comorbid condition. Compliance with mammography is best if recommended by the primary physician. In women with multiple comorbidities, the benefit of screening mammography should be weighed against the estimated life expectancy.

Local Definitive Therapy

Standard treatment options, including modified radical mastectomy or lumpectomy followed by breast radiation therapy, should be offered to all women who are fit and willing to undergo surgery. Axillary dissection should be considered for most patients. Other nonstandard treatment approaches should be offered only within the context of an established research endeavor or if the patient is medically unfit or unwilling to undergo general anesthesia.

Systemic Adjuvant Therapy

Adjuvant hormonal therapy with tamoxifen should be considered in all postmenopausal women with hormone receptor–positive tumors. Only older women with a very low risk of distant metastases (less than 10%) or severe comorbid illness should not be offered tamoxifen. Adjuvant systemic chemotherapy should be considered for older women whose risk of systemic breast cancer recurrence is sufficiently high—that is, women whose tumors are hormone receptor–negative and larger than 1 cm and women who have large (larger than

4 cm) tumors (regardless of hormone-receptor status) or who have axillary lymph node involvement (regardless of tumor size). For women aged 75 and older, life expectancy and comorbidity must be factored into the treatment decision.

Treatment of Metastatic Disease

Endocrine therapy is the standard front-line treatment for women with hormone receptor–positive metastatic breast cancer. Patients with hormone receptor–negative metastatic breast cancer whose metastases are not rapidly progressive or life threatening should have at least one trial of an endocrine agent. The sequence of endocrine therapy should be tamoxifen → an aromatase inhibitor → megestrol acetate → estrogens or corticosteroids (in selected patients). Systemic chemotherapy for metastatic breast cancer should be reserved for women with symptomatic disease who have progression of metastases on endocrine therapy. Adjunct therapies for metastatic breast cancer involving bone include bisphosphonates, strontium chloride 89, and radiation therapy.

REFERENCES

1. Landis SH, Murray T, Bolden S, Wingo PA. Cancer statistics, 1998. *CA Cancer J Clin* 1998;48:6.
2. Kessler LG. The relationship between age and incidence of breast cancer. Population and screening program data. *Cancer* 1992;69:1896.
3. Adami HO, Malker B, Holmberg L, Persson I, Stone B. The relation between survival and age at diagnosis in breast cancer. *N Engl J Med* 1986;315:559.
4. Holli K, Isola J. Effect of age on the survival of breast cancer patients. *Eur J Cancer* 1997;33:425.
5. Host H, Lund E. Age as a prognostic factor in breast cancer. *Cancer* 1986;57:2217.
6. Bergman L, Kluck HM, van Leeuwen FE, et al. The influence of age on treatment choice and survival of elderly breast cancer patients in south-eastern Netherlands: a population-based study. *Eur J Cancer* 1992;28A:1475.
7. US Department of Health and Human Services. Health United States 1996-7 and injury chartbook; 1997. DHHS Publication no (PHS) 97-1232. Hyattsville, Maryland: National Center for Health Statistics, 1997.
8. Yancik R, Ries LG, Yates JW. Breast cancer in aging women. A population-based study of contrasts in stage, surgery, and survival. *Cancer* 1989;63:976.
9. Herbsman H, Feldman J, Seldera J, Gardner B, Alfonso AE. Survival following breast cancer surgery in the elderly. *Cancer* 1981;47:2358.
10. Masetti R, Antinori A, Terribile D, et al. Breast cancer in women 70 years of age or older. *J Clin Oncol* 1996;13:2722.
11. Gentili C, Sanfilippo O, Silvestrini R. Cell proliferation and its relationship to clinical features and relapse in breast cancers. *Cancer* 1981;48:974.
12. McCarty KS, Silva JS, Cox EB, Leight GS, Wells SA. Relationship of age and menopausal status to estrogen receptor content in primary carcinoma of the breast. *Ann Surg* 1983;197:123.
13. von Rosen A, Gardelin A, Auer G. Assessment of malignancy potential in mammary carcinoma in elderly patients. *Am J Clin Oncol* 1987;10:61.
14. Lyman GH, Lyman S, Balducci L, et al. Age and the risk of breast cancer recurrence. *Cancer Control* 1996;3:421.
15. Satariano WA. Comorbidity and functional status in older women with breast cancer: implications for screening, treatment, and prognosis. *J Gerontol* 1992;47:24.
16. Fish EB, Chapman JA, Link MA. Competing causes of death for primary breast cancer. *Ann Surg Oncol* 1998;5:368.
17. Satariano WA, Ragheb NE, Dupuis MA. Comorbidity in older women with breast cancer: an epidemiologic approach. In: Yancik R, Yates J, eds. *Cancer in the elderly: approaches to early detection and treatment.* New York: Springer, 1989:71.
18. Satariano WA. Aging, comorbidity, and breast cancer survival: an epidemiologic view. *Adv Exp Med Biol* 1993;330:1.
19. Satariano WA, Ragland DR. The effect of comorbidity on 3-year survival of women with primary breast cancer. *Ann Intern Med* 1994;120:104.
20. Newschaffer CJ, Penberthy L, Desch CE, Retchin SM, Whittemore M. The effect of age and comorbidity in the treatment of elderly women with nonmetastatic breast cancer. *Arch Intern Med* 1996;156:85.
21. Greenfield S, Blanco DM, Elashoff RM, Ganz PA. Patterns of care related to age of breast cancer patients. *JAMA* 1987;257:2766.
22. Goodwin JS, Hunt WC, Samet JM. Determinants of cancer therapy in elderly patients. *Cancer* 1993;72:594.
23. Tsevat J, Cook EF, Green ML, et al. Health values of the seriously ill. *Ann Intern Med* 1995;122:514.
24. Fisher B, Costantino JP, Wickerham L, et al. Tamoxifen for prevention of breast cancer: report of the National Surgical Adjuvant Breast and Bowel Project P-1 study. *J Natl Cancer Inst* 1998;90:1371.
25. Powles T, Eeles R, Ashley S, et al. Interim analysis of the incidence of breast cancer in the Royal Marsden Hospital tamoxifen randomised chemoprevention trial. *Lancet* 1998;352:98.
26. Veronesi U, Maisonneuve P, Costa A, et al. Prevention of breast cancer with tamoxifen: preliminary findings from the Italian randomised trial among hysterectomised women. Italian Tamoxifen Prevention Study. *Lancet* 1998;352:93.
27. Cummings SR, Norton L, Eckert S, et al. Raloxifene reduces the risk of breast cancer and may decrease the risk of endometrial cancer in post-menopausal women. Two-year findings from the Multiple Outcomes of Raloxifene Evaluation (MORE) Trial. *Proc Am Soc Clin Oncol* 1998;17:2a.
28. Kerlikowske K, Grady D, Rubin SM, Sandrock C, Ernster VL. Efficacy of screening mammography. A meta-analysis. *JAMA* 1995;273:149.
29. Hwang ES, Cody HS III. Does the proven benefit of mammography extend to breast cancer patients over age 70? *South Med J* 1998; 91:522.
30. Wilson TE, Helvie MA, August DA. Breast cancer in the elderly patient: early detection with mammography. *Radiology* 1994;190:203.
31. Faulk RM, Sickles EA, Sollitto RA, Ominsky SH, Galvin HB, Frankel SD. Clinical efficacy of mammographic screening in the elderly. *Radiology* 1995;194:193.
32. Peer PG, Holland R, Hendriks JH, Mravunac M, Verbeek AL. Age-specific effectiveness of the Nijmegen population-based breast cancer-screening program: assessment of early indicators of screening effectiveness. *J Natl Cancer Inst* 1994;86:436.
33. Costanza ME. Breast cancer screening in older women. Synopsis of a forum. *Cancer* 1992;69:1925.
34. Field LR, Wilson TE, Strawderman M, Gabriel H, Helvie MA. Mammographic screening in women more than 64 years old: a comparison of 1- and 2-year intervals. *AJR Am J Roentgenol* 1998;170:961.
35. van Dijck JA, Broeders MJ, Verbeek AL. Mammographic screening in older women. Is it worthwhile? *Drugs Aging* 1997;10:69.
36. Mandelblatt JS, Wheat ME, Monane M, Moshief RD, Hollenberg JP, Tang J. Breast cancer screening for elderly women with and without comorbid conditions. A decision analysis model. *Ann Intern Med* 1992;116:722.
37. Anda RF, Sienko DG, Remington PL, Gentry EM, Marks JS. Screening mammography for women 50 years of age and older: practices and trends, 1987. *Am J Prev Med* 1990;6:123.
38. Burg MA, Lane DS, Polednak AP. Age group differences in the use of breast cancer screening tests. *J Aging Health* 1990;2:514.
39. Burns RB, McCarthy EP, Freund KM, et al. Variability in mammography use among older women. *J Am Geriatr Soc* 1996;44:922.
40. Blustein J. Medicare coverage, supplemental insurance, and the use of mammography by older women. *N Engl J Med* 1995;332:1138.
41. Blustein J, Weiss LJ. The use of mammography by women aged 75 and older: factors related to health, functioning, and age. *J Am Geriatr Soc* 1998;46:941.
42. Weinberger M, Saunders AF, Samsa GP, et al. Breast cancer screening in older women: practices and barriers reported by primary care physicians. *J Am Geriatr Soc* 1991;39:22.

43. Mor V, Pacala JT, Rakowski W. Mammography for older women: who uses, who benefits? *J Gerontol* 1992;47:43.
44. Coleman EA, Feuer EJ. Breast cancer screening among women from 65 to 74 years of age in 1987-88 and 1991. NCI Breast Cancer Screening Consortium. *Ann Intern Med* 1992;117:961.
45. Fox SA, Siu AL, Stein JA. The importance of physician communication on breast cancer screening of older women. *Arch Intern Med* 1994;154:2058.
46. Thomas LR, Fox SA, Leake BG, Roetzheim RG. The effects of health beliefs on screening mammography utilization among a diverse sample of older women. *Women Health* 1996;24:77.
47. Schwaibold F, Fowble BL, Solin LJ, Schultz DJ, Goodman RL. The results of radiation therapy for isolated local regional recurrence after mastectomy. *Int J Radiat Oncol Biol Phys* 1991;21:299.
48. Silliman RA, Guadagnoli E, Weitberg AB, Mor V. Age as a predictor of diagnostic and initial treatment intensity in newly diagnosed breast cancer patients. *J Gerontol* 1989;44:M46.
49. Mohle-Boetani J. Age at breast cancer diagnosis as a predictor of subsequent survival. In: Macieira-Coehlo A, Nordenskjold B, eds. *Cancer and aging*. Boca Raton, FL: CRC Press, 1990:245.
50. Lazovich DA, White E, Thomas DB, Moe RE. Underutilization of breast-conserving surgery and radiation therapy among women with stage I or II breast cancer. *JAMA* 1991;266:3433.
51. Kantorowitz DA, Poulter CA, Sischy B, et al. Treatment of breast cancer among elderly women with segmental mastectomy or segmental mastectomy plus postoperative radiotherapy. *Int J Radiat Oncol Biol Phys* 1988;15:263.
52. Wazer DE, Erban JK, Robert NJ, et al. Breast conservation in elderly women for clinically negative axillary lymph nodes without axillary dissection. *Cancer* 1994;74:878.
53. Amsterdam E, Birkenfeld S, Gilad A, Krispin M. Surgery for carcinoma of the breast in women over 70 years of age. *J Surg Oncol* 1987;35:180.
54. Svastics E, Sulyok Z, Besznyak I. Treatment of breast cancer in women older than 70 years. *J Surg Oncol* 1989;41:19.
55. Lindsey AM, Larson PJ, Dodd MJ, Brecht ML, Packer A. Comorbidity, nutritional intake, social support, weight, and functional status over time in older cancer patients receiving radiotherapy. *Cancer Nurs* 1994;17:113.
56. Wyckoff J, Greenberg H, Sanderson R, Wallach P, Balducci L. Breast irradiation in the older woman: a toxicity study. *J Am Geriatr Soc* 1994;42:150.
57. Sandison AJ, Gold DM, Wright P, Jones PA. Breast conservation or mastectomy: treatment choice of women aged 70 years and older. *Br J Surg* 1996;83:994.
58. Merchant TE, McCormick B, Yahalom J, Borgen P. The influence of older age on breast cancer treatment decisions and outcome. *Int J Radiat Oncol Biol Phys* 1996;34:565.
59. Solin LJ, Schultz DJ, Fowble BL. Ten-year results of the treatment of early-stage breast carcinoma in elderly women using breast conserv ing surgery and definitive breast irradiation. *Int J Radiat Oncol Biol Phys* 1995;33:45.
60. Preece PE, Wood RA, Mackie CR, Cuschieri A. Tamoxifen as initial sole treatment of localized breast cancer in elderly women: a pilot study. *BMJ* 1982;284:869.
61. Horobin JM, Preece PE, Dewar JA, Wood RA, Cuschieri A. Long-term follow-up of elderly patients with locoregional breast cancer treated with tamoxifen only. *Br J Surg* 1991;78:213.
62. Bradbeer JW, Kyngdon J. Primary treatment of breast cancer in elderly women with tamoxifen. *Clin Oncol (R Coll Radiol)* 1983;9:31.
63. Allan SG, Rodger A, Smyth JF, Leonard RC, Chetty U, Forrest AP. Tamoxifen as primary treatment of breast cancer in elderly or frail patients: a practical management. *BMJ* 1985;290:358.
64. Akhtar SS, Allan SG, Rodger A, Chetty UD, Smyth JF, Leonard RC. A 10-year experience of tamoxifen as primary treatment of breast cancer in 100 elderly and frail patients. *Eur J Surg Oncol* 1991;17:30.
65. Ciatto S, Bartoli D, Iossa A, Grazzini G, Cirillo A. Response of primary breast cancer to tamoxifen alone in elderly women. *Tumori* 1991;77:328.
66. Ciatto S, Cirillo A, Confortini M, Cardillo C. Tamoxifen as primary treatment of breast cancer in elderly patients. *Neoplasma* 1996;43:43.
67. Bergman L, van Dongen JA, van Ooijen B, van Leeuwen FE. Should tamoxifen be a primary treatment choice for elderly breast cancer patients with locoregional disease? *Breast Cancer Res Treat* 1995; 34:77.
68. van Dalsen AD, de Vries JE. Treatment of breast cancer in elderly patients. *J Surg Oncol* 1995;60:80.
69. Gazet JC, Markopoulos C, Ford HT, Coombes RC, Bland JM, Dixon RC. Prospective randomized trial of tamoxifen versus surgery in elderly patients with breast cancer. *Lancet* 1988;1:679.
70. Gazet JC, Ford HT, Coombes RC, et al. Prospective randomized trial of tamoxifen vs surgery in elderly patients with breast cancer. *Eur J Surg Oncol* 1994;20:207.
71. Robertson JF, Todd JH, Ellis IO, Elston CW, Blamey RW. Comparison of mastectomy with tamoxifen for treating elderly patients with operable breast cancer. *BMJ* 1988;297:511.
72. Clark RM, McCulloch PB, Levine MN, et al. Randomized clinical trial to assess the effectiveness of breast irradiation following lumpectomy and axillary dissection for node-negative breast cancer. *J Natl Cancer Inst* 1992;84:683.
73. Reed MW, Morrison JM. Wide local excision as the sole primary treatment in elderly patients with carcinoma of the breast. *Br J Surg* 1989;76:898.
74. Veronesi U, Luini A, Del Vecchio M, et al. Radiotherapy after breast-preserving surgery in women with localized cancer of the breast. *N Engl J Med* 1993;328:1587.
75. Bates T, Riley DL, Houghton J, Fallowfield L, Baum M. Breast cancer in elderly women: a Cancer Research Campaign trial comparing treatment with tamoxifen and optimal surgery with tamoxifen alone. The Elderly Breast Cancer Working Party. *Br J Surg* 1991;78:591.
76. Mustacchi G, Milani S, Pluchinotta A, De Matteis A, Rubagotti A, Perrota A. Tamoxifen or surgery plus tamoxifen as primary treatment for elderly patients with operable breast cancer: the G.R.E.T.A. Trial. Group for Research on Endocrine Therapy in the Elderly. *Anticancer Res* 1994;14:2197.
77. Margolese RG, Foster RS Jr. Tamoxifen as an alternative to surgical resection for selected geriatric patients with primary breast cancer. *Arch Surg* 1989;124:548.
78. Gaskell DJ, Hawkins RA, de Carteret S, Chetty U, Sangster K, Forrest AP. Indications for primary tamoxifen therapy in elderly women with breast cancer. *Br J Surg* 1992;79:1317.
79. Yeh S, Tan LR, O'Connell TX. Segmental mastectomy and tamoxifen alone provide adequate locoregional control of breast cancer in elderly women. *Am Surg* 1997;63:854.
80. Dunser M, Haussler B, Fuchs H, Margreiter R. Tumorectomy plus tamoxifen for the treatment of breast cancer in the elderly. *Eur J Surg Oncol* 1993;19:529.
81. von Rueden DG, Sessions SC. Alternative therapy for elderly patients with breast cancer. *Am Surg* 1994;60:72.
82. Carter KJ, Ritchey NP, Castro F, et al. Treatment of early-stage breast cancer in the elderly: a health-outcome-based approach. *Med Decis Making* 1998;18:213.
83. Martelli G, Moglia D, Boracchi P, Del Prato I, Galante E, De Palo G. Surgical resection plus tamoxifen as treatment of breast cancer in elderly patients: a retrospective study. *Eur J Cancer* 1993;29A:2080.
84. Martelli G, DePalo G, Rossi N, et al. Long-term follow-up of elderly patients with operable breast cancer treated with surgery without axillary dissection plus adjuvant tamoxifen. *Br J Cancer* 1995;72: 1251.
85. Veronesi U, Luini A, Del Vecchio M, et al. Radiotherapy after breast-preserving surgery in women with localized cancer of the breast. *N Engl J Med* 1993;328:1587.
86. Cooke AL, Perera F, Fisher B, Opeitum A, Yu N. Tamoxifen with and without radiation after partial mastectomy in patients with involved nodes. *Int J Radiat Oncol Biol Phys* 1995;31:777.
87. Feigelson BJ, Acosta JA, Feigelson HS, Findley A, Saunders EL. T1 breast carcinoma in women 70 years of age and older may not require axillary lymph node dissection. *Am J Surg* 1996;172:487.
88. Naslund E, Fernstad R, Ekman S, Schultz I, Hjalmar ML, Askergren J. Breast cancer in women over 75 years: is axillary dissection always necessary? *Eur J Surg* 1996;162:867.
89. Rostom AY, Pradhan DG, White WF. Once weekly irradiation in breast cancer. *Int J Radiat Oncol Biol Phys* 1987;13:551.
90. Maher M, Campana F, Mosseri V, et al. Breast cancer in elderly women: a retrospective analysis of combined treatment with tamoxifen and once-weekly irradiation. *Int J Radiat Oncol Biol Phys* 1995;31:783.
91. Anonymous. Tamoxifen for early breast cancer: an overview of the randomised trials. Early Breast Cancer Trialists' Collaborative Group. *Lancet* 1998;351:1451.

92. Anonymous. Polychemotherapy for early breast cancer: an overview of the randomized trials. Early Breast Cancer Trialists' Collaborative Group. *Lancet* 1998;352:930.
93. Von Hoff DD, Layard MW, Basa P, et al. Risk factors for doxorubicin-induced congestive heart failure. *Ann Intern Med* 1979;91:710.
94. Goldhirsch A, Glick JH, Gelber RD, Senn H-J. Meeting highlights: International Consensus Panel on the treatment of primary breast cancer. *J Natl Cancer Inst* 1998;90:1601.
95. Extermann M, Balducci L, Lyman GH. What threshold for adjuvant therapy in older breast cancer patients? *Proc Am Soc Clin Oncol* 1998;17:102a.
96. Anonymous. Systemic treatment of early breast cancer by hormonal, cytotoxic, or immune therapy. 133 randomized trials involving 31,000 recurrences and 24,000 deaths among 75,000 women. Early Breast Cancer Trialists' Collaborative Group. *Lancet* 1992; 339:1.
97. Desch CE, Hillner BE, Smith TJ, Retchin SM. Should the elderly receive chemotherapy for node-negative breast cancer? A cost-effectiveness analysis examining total and active life-expectancy outcomes. *J Clin Oncol* 1993;11:777.
98. Begg CB, Elson PJ, Carbone PP. A study of excess hematologic toxicity in elderly patients treated on chemotherapy protocols. In: Yancik R, Yates J, ed. *Cancer in the elderly: approaches to early detection and management*. New York: Springer-Verlag, 1989.
99. Gelman RS, Taylor SG. Cyclophosphamide, methotrexate, and 5-fluorouracil chemotherapy in women more than 65 years old with advanced breast cancer: the elimination of age trends in toxicity by using doses based on creatinine clearance. *J Clin Oncol* 1984;2:1404.
100. Christman K, Muss HB, Case LD, Stanley V. Chemotherapy of metastatic breast cancer in the elderly. The Piedmont Oncology Association experience. *JAMA* 1992;268:57.
101. Ibrahim NK, Frye DK, Buzdar AU, Walters RS, Hortobagyi GN. Doxorubicin-based chemotherapy in elderly patients with metastatic breast cancer. Tolerance and outcome. *Arch Intern Med* 1996;156:882.
102. Giovanazzi-Bannon S, Rademaker A, Lai G, Benson AB III. Treatment tolerance of elderly cancer patients entered onto phase II clinical trials: an Illinois Cancer Center study. *J Clin Oncol* 1994;12:2447.
103. Kimmick GG, Fleming R, Muss HB, Balducci L. Cancer chemotherapy in older adults—a tolerability perspective. *Drugs Aging* 1997;10:34.
104. Begg CB, Cohen JL, Ellerton J. Are the elderly predisposed to toxicity from cancer chemotherapy? An investigation using data from the Eastern Cooperative Oncology Group. *Cancer Clin Trials* 1980;3:369.
105. Nerenz DR, Love RR, Leventhal H, Easterling DV. Psychosocial consequences of cancer chemotherapy for elderly patients. *Health Serv Res* 1986;20:961.
106. Ravdin PM, Valero V. Review of docetaxel (Taxotere), a highly active new agent for the treatment of metastatic breast cancer. *Semin Oncol* 1995;22(Suppl 4):17.
107. Hortobagyi GN, Holmes FA. Single-agent paclitaxel for the treatment of breast cancer: an overview [Review]. *Semin Oncol* 1996;23:4.
108. Sorio R, Robieux I, Galligioni E, et al. Pharmacokinetics and tolerance of vinorelbine in elderly patients with metastatic breast cancer. *Eur J Cancer* 1997;33:301.
109. Ranson MR, Carmichael J, O'Byrne K, Stewart S, Smith D, Howell A. Treatment of advanced breast cancer with sterically stabilized liposomal doxorubicin: results of a multicenter phase II trial. *J Clin Oncol* 1997;15:3185.
110. Blum JL, Buzdar AU, LoRusso PM, Kuter I, Vogel C, Burger HU, et al. A multicenter phase II trial of XelodaTM (capecitabine) in paclitaxel-refractory metastatic breast cancer. *Proc Am Soc Clin Oncol* 1998;17:125a.
111. Cobleigh MA, Vogel CL, Tripathy D, Robert NJ, Scholl S, Fehrenbacher L, et al. Efficacy and safety of HerceptinTM (humanized anti-HER2 antibody) as a single agent in 222 women with HER2 overexpression who relapsed following chemotherapy for metastatic breast cancer. *Proc Am Soc Clin Oncol* 1998;17:97a.

Diseases of the Breast, 2nd ed.,
edited by Jay R. Harris.
Lippincott Williams & Wilkins, Philadelphia © 2000.

CHAPTER 64

Breast Cancer in Minority Women

Jon F. Kerner, Bruce J. Trock, and Jeanne S. Mandelblatt

In 1986, 15 years after the war on cancer was declared by President Nixon, the National Cancer Institute published its cancer control objectives for the nation to reduce age-adjusted cancer mortality by 50% by the year 2000.[1] Included were three goals related to breast cancer: (a) dietary objectives to reduce the total fat consumption of the U.S. population from 38% of total calories from fat in 1980 to less than 35% by 1990 and less than 25% by the year 2000, (b) screening prevalence objectives to increase the use of clinical breast examinations (CBE) from 43% in 1980 to 70% in 1990 and 80% by the year 2000 and to increase the use of mammography (among women 50 to 70 years of age) from 14% in 1980 to 45% in 1990 and 80% by the year 2000, and (c) treatment objectives to increase the application of state-of-the-art treatment for selected cancer sites, including breast cancer. The projected reductions in breast cancer mortality, which would be achieved if these objectives were met, were estimated to be 25% from reducing fat, 16% from expanding use of breast cancer screening services, and 14.3% from expanding access to state-of-the-art breast cancer treatment.

During the same decade that the National Cancer Institute's year 2000 objectives were formulated and published, the U.S. population became significantly more ethnically diverse. For example, the U.S. African-American female resident population grew by 14.4% from 1980 to 1990. The U.S. Hispanic female resident population grew 49.6%, and the U.S. Asian or Pacific Islander female resident population increased by 111%. The U.S. white female resident population increased by only 6.7%.[2] This increasing diversity was accompanied by high rates of poverty among African-American and Hispanic minorities. Thus, although the majority of poor people are white, only 7% of white people fell below the poverty level in 1990. In contrast, 26.3% of African-Americans, 22.3% of Latin-Americans, 27% of Native Americans, and 11.6% of Asian- and Pacific Island–Americans fell below the poverty level in 1990.[3] Census reports indicate that this trend of increasing ethnic diversity and disproportional poverty among U.S. minority populations continued through the 1990s.

As we reach the twenty-first century, little progress has been observed with respect to reducing age-adjusted breast cancer incidence and mortality. From 1973 to 1995, age-adjusted mortality declined by a modest 6.3% among all women combined. The majority of this mortality reduction was experienced by white women, who had an 8.5% reduction in age-adjusted breast cancer mortality from 1973 to 1995, while at the same time experiencing a 36.3% increase in age-adjusted breast cancer incidence. African-American women also experienced a large increase in age-adjusted breast cancer incidence from 1973 to 1995 (37%). However, they had a 26.3% increase in breast cancer mortality.[4]

Although older women in general have higher incidence and higher mortality rates from breast cancer than younger women, older women are also more likely to develop and die from competing disease causes. Moreover, older minority women also experience higher mortality from these competing causes of death. Thus, the absolute risk of dying from breast cancer declines with increasing age as a result of competing mortality risks. Mor et al.[5] point out that, in 1987, 2.9% of all deaths among women aged 65 to 74 were from breast cancer, whereas for women aged 75 to 84 the figure is 1.7%. However, should the incidence and mortality of competing diseases (e.g., cardiovascular disease) continue to decline through the year 2000, then the percentage of disease and death attributed to breast cancer will rise.

How do endemic poverty and increasing cultural diversity within society interact with tumor biology and individual behavior with respect to the achievement of national breast cancer control objectives? With respect to our understanding of the epidemiology of breast cancer in the United States, national cancer incidence and mortality data do not adequately capture information on the cultural or socioeconomic diversity within at-risk minority populations. Disease data are largely limited to African-American–white racial comparisons that, although informative, may mask large ethnic group and socioeconomic status (SES) variations that are important to our understanding of the public health prob-

J. F. Kerner: Department of Oncology, Lombardi Cancer Center, Georgetown University Medical Center, Washington, D.C.

B. J. Trock: Departments of Human Oncology and Biostatistics and Epidemiology, Lombardi Cancer Center, Georgetown University Medical Center, Washington, D.C.

J. S. Mandelblatt: Department of Medicine, Lombardi Cancer Center, Georgetown University Medical Center, Washington, D.C.

lem represented by breast cancer. Regional and local cancer data provide some insights into ethnic group variation. However, socioeconomic data are lacking at all levels, and investigators are often left having to estimate the impact of SES using ecologic analyses of census tract information.[6–8] Furthermore, data on income or education alone are not sufficient to capture the influence on health outcomes of relative socioeconomic disparities of disadvantaged populations.

In recent years, considerable attention has been directed to the meaning of racial and ethnic variation in cancer research, particularly focusing on the question of whether race represents a biological construct. Recently, the President's Cancer Panel convened a meeting called "The Meaning of Race in Science—Considerations for Cancer Research." Among the conclusions reached by this panel were the concepts that race is a social construct and that biologically distinct races do not exist.[9] Although a purely biological definition of race based on genetics—that is, a group with a major proportion of genotypes derived from a shared genetic background—is not scientifically justified, the way that this conclusion is interpreted by researchers has important implications for breast cancer research. Research continues to explore whether differences of phenotype or genotype, or both, contribute in part to the disparity in mortality and survival rates between African-American and white women. Quite apart from the question of race as a biological construct, there are also methodologic difficulties in trying to parse the "biologic effect of race" from environmental and system determinants of breast cancer outcomes. Race and ethnicity are composite terms that encompass historical, biological, sociocultural,[10] and environmental factors, including exposure to racism.[11,12]

Turning to behavior, data do exist for certain breast cancer risk factors that may vary by race/ethnicity (e.g., reproductive factors, diet), and some surveys have even oversampled African-American and Hispanic populations to explore in more depth risk factors among these historically underrepresented groups. However, national and state budgetary limitations often reduce needed sample sizes, limit efforts to provide for bilingual interviewers, and preclude rigorously translated interview instruments. This, in turn, fails to ensure full participation by minorities who may be at high risk.[13] Case control and cohort studies that attempt to identify risk factors that could lead to new prevention initiatives for underserved minorities are rare.[14–16]

Turning to early detection of breast cancer, the literature is replete with behavioral studies documenting that older, low-income, less educated, and ethnic minority populations make less use of available mammography and clinical breast examination services than their younger, better-educated, white, middle-class counterparts. However, why these differences persist is rarely examined or explained.[9] Several intervention studies have been designed and implemented to promote the use of mammography and CBEs, with some early success displayed. However, the key health care system factors that deter medically underserved women from seeking breast cancer screening have neither been eliminated nor overcome.[17]

Much less studied are the consequences of the medically underserved having to seek diagnostic resolution of an abnormal mammogram or abnormal clinical breast examination in a health care system with insufficient resources to address their needs. These women are more likely to be without insurance, on Medicaid, or otherwise financially compromised by the process. In addition, few studies have examined the variation in access to state-of-the-art treatment services for underserved minority breast cancer patients in the United States. In this updated review, we reassess what is known about minority and medically underserved women at risk for development of breast cancer. In particular, we examine the epidemiology, tumor biology, and sociology of breast cancer in relation to race and ethnicity and to state-of-the-art breast cancer prevention, early detection, diagnosis, and treatment services.

EPIDEMIOLOGY AND TUMOR BIOLOGY

Breast cancer incidence rates among medically underserved minorities vary considerably by population and geographic level of data. Nationally, although African-American women experience lower overall breast cancer incidence (101 per 100,000) than white women (115 per 100,000),[18] a consistent age dependence has been noted for several decades.[19] At very young ages, incidence rates in African-American women exceed those in whites, but the excess decreases with age. The ratio of rates in African-American compared to white women is 3.1 at ages 20 to 24, 1.4 at ages 30 to 34, and 1.04 at ages 40 to 44, with a crossover to higher rates in white women at age 50.[18] This crossover has been increasing over time, occurring at age 40 in 1969 to 1971,[19] age 45 in 1986 to 1990,[20] and age 50 in 1991 to 1995.[18]

The reasons for this crossover are not entirely clear. A recent review of case control studies of breast cancer in African-American women found that risk factors and the relative risks associated with these factors were similar to those in white women.[21] However, there are differences in the prevalence of these risk factors that could contribute to the observed crossover. Compared to white women, African-American women have earlier age at menarche, earlier age at first full-term pregnancy, and earlier age at menopause.[22] Earlier age at menarche increases risk, and some, but not all, studies have found this effect to be greater for premenopausal breast cancer.[23] Three case control studies in African-American women that were stratified by menopausal status found slightly stronger effects of early menarche on premenopausal breast cancer.[24–26] Although earlier age at first full-term pregnancy reduces breast cancer risk, a number of studies have suggested that this effect is preceded by a transient increase in risk for approximately 10 years after the last full-term pregnancy.[27–29] Earlier age at menopause reduces risk of postmenopausal breast cancer. Thus, all three of these reproductive risk factors could influence the crossover in risk observed in African-American compared to white women.

Limited data are collected on a federal, state, or local basis and are irregularly published on breast cancer incidence among other underserved minorities.[30–32] Native Hawaiians have the highest age-adjusted breast cancer incidence rates, with Mexican-Americans from New Mexico, residents of Puerto Rico, and Native Americans reporting the lowest rates.[33] A significant problem in tracking cancer incidence among certain minority groups, such as Hispanics, is that of ethnic group identification in both numerator (i.e., cancer incidence registry) and denominator (i.e., census) data. Thus, ethnic group variation among Hispanics is virtually impossible to assess, because the quality of the ethnicity and country of origin identification in the cancer incidence registries and the census is widely variable from one region of the United States to another.[34]

Returning to breast cancer risk factors, the well-established risk factors include older age, family history of breast cancer, early menarche, late age at birth of first child, late age at menopause, history of benign breast disease, and exposure to ionizing radiation.[35] These established risk factors share two things in common: (a) Except for radiation, the increased relative risk of developing breast cancer associated with them is modest (relative risk, 1.5 to 2.0), and (b) none lend themselves to simple preventive interventions.[18] Although diet,[36,37] alcohol,[38,39] and cigarette smoking[40] have all been reported as potential risk factors for breast cancer and lend themselves to breast cancer prevention interventions, the analytic epidemiologic data suggest weak associations, no association, or contradictory associations.[41] Also, few studies have examined variation in cancer risk factors among medically underserved populations,[11] although some have speculated about how differential exposure to risk factors may explain racial and ethnic group variation in cancer incidence.[15,42]

Fewer studies have examined etiologically relevant molecular markers in African-American women. No significant racial differences have been observed in the prevalence of p53 mutations.[43–46] In addition to overall mutation prevalence, specific p53 mutations are of interest, because the type of mutation may vary according to the carcinogenic exposure.[47] Two studies evaluated mutation spectra and found potential differences between African-American and white women.[44,46] However, the type of mutation that differed was not the same in the two studies, the numbers were very small, and in one of the studies,[46] the area of residence differed by race in a manner that could give rise to exposure differences. In contrast to these studies of somatic mutations, studies examining inherited polymorphisms in p53 haplotypes have not found consistent racial differences or associations with breast cancer risk,[48,49] but the numbers of African-American women in these studies have again been very small. Because differences in p53 mutation patterns have potential clinical and etiologic importance, further studies of somatic and germ-line mutation are needed, with sufficient numbers within mutation categories.

Other molecular markers have received even less study in multiethnic populations. No racial difference was found in the prevalence of *erb*-B2 overexpression.[43,45,50] Two studies found a similar small excess of high S-phase tumors in African-American women[43,50]; the difference was not statistically significant in the latter study, but the number of African-American women was small. No significant difference in Ki67, another measure of proliferative status, was observed in two studies,[45,50] although a nonsignificant higher value was observed for African-American women in the study by Weiss.[50] Two studies have examined polymorphisms in the *CYP1A1* gene, which produces an enzyme that metabolizes some environmental carcinogens (e.g., polyaromatic hydrocarbons). One study found a significant increase in risk associated with the homozygous variant of the *MspI* polymorphism among African-American women (odds ratio, 9.7) but no association among white women.[51] However, a second study found no association with this polymorphism among either group.[52] This study also found no associations with *GSTT1* and *GSTM1* polymorphisms, which have also been implicated in carcinogen activation. A study of polymorphisms in the *CYP1B1* found significant differences by race in two variants of the gene but no associations with breast cancer risk in either race group.[53] In this study, the homozygous variant of the *m1* Val allele was associated with an increased frequency of estrogen receptor (ER)–positive tumors in white, but not African-American, women. However, this variant was significantly more common among African-American women, and therefore it is unlikely to explain their higher incidence of ER-negative tumors.

The influence of the *BRCA1* susceptibility gene has received little study in African-American women. No African-American women with *BRCA1* mutations were identified in a population-based case control study, but the number of African-American women was small.[54] In a study of nine African-American families with clustering of breast cancer, *BRCA1* mutations were associated with apparent inherited susceptibility in five of the families (56%).[55] The authors of this study point out that the ancestral genetic background for most African-Americans is West African, a population in which, in contrast to populations of European descent, breast cancer is rare, occurs predominantly in younger women, and has an aggressive phenotype.[55] Thus, a great need for more studies of inherited predisposing mutations in African-American women clearly exists.

Of importance to medically underserved minority populations is the fact that the epidemiologic research on which these interventions are based usually fails to include the medically underserved. Moreover, research to test prevention interventions has had enormous difficulty in recruiting these populations to participate. Thus, poor women, less educated women, women of color, women who do not speak English, and older women are often severely underrepresented, if represented at all, in these studies. This is particularly a concern for molecular and genetic epidemiologic studies, in which the failure to involve underserved minorities may limit the biological variability observed and may compromise the external validity of study conclusions. Prevention trials based on new markers of breast cancer risk may be similarly compromised.

Part of the difficulty in involving medically underserved minorities stems from the fact that many of these studies focus on convenience samples recruited through the academic medical centers in which the investigator's research is supported. Reaching out to involve underserved minority communities can pose significant practical, as well as methodologic, difficulties (e.g., difficulty in completing follow-up in cohort studies). Moreover, many underserved minority communities are reluctant to participate in these observational studies, given a history of being studied for decades with little or no evidence that individual participation contributes to the health or well-being of their communities and some particularly notorious evidence that participation is synonymous with exploitation.[56] The effect is that the underserved are understudied, and the benefits that may occur from epidemiologic research leading to primary prevention are not experienced by those who may need them most.

To involve medically underserved minorities in descriptive epidemiologic studies may require linking these types of research to intervention research that evaluates health services (e.g., cancer screening) that are desired and appreciated by the underserved population of interest. Thus, collecting molecular markers from medically underserved patients recruited for a cancer screening trial,[57] with full informed consent, can provide an excellent opportunity to study biological variation in a high-risk population that would be unlikely to consent to a strictly observational study design. Also, remuneration for time involved in study participation may be critical in low-income communities.

EARLY DETECTION AND CLINICAL FOLLOW-UP OF BREAST CANCER

Overall breast cancer mortality is higher in African-American women (31.5 per 100,000) than in white women (25.7 per 100,000), and age-specific mortality is also higher at every age except 85 and older.[18] As with incidence, the relative excess among African-Americans decreases with age; the excess is 50% at ages 45 to 49 but decreases to 10% by ages 65 to 69.[18] Although incidence rates have increased since 1973 for African-American and white women, regardless of age, during the same period mortality has increased only among African-American women aged 50 and older, with a 29% change.[18]

The higher mortality among African-American women despite lower overall incidence is a reflection of their poorer survival experience. Although 5-year relative survival rates for African-American women have increased by 54% since 1973, these rates are still lower than those for white women. A major contributor to this disparity is more advanced stage at diagnosis among African-Americans. Although increased use of mammography has improved the stage distribution for African-American women, they are still diagnosed with more advanced tumors, with 45.5% above stage I, compared to 36.6% among white women.[18] Hispanics are also less likely than whites to be diagnosed with early-stage breast cancer.[58]

Later stage of breast cancer at diagnosis among medically underserved female populations can be explained by two principal factors. The first factor is limited access to and less use of baseline (prevalence screening) and routine (incidence screening) CBEs and mammography.[59,60] Second, even when breast cancer screening use increases, or perhaps because it increases, more delay in diagnostic resolution and higher rates of incomplete clinical follow-up of abnormal breast cancer screening test findings may be observed. Lower screening use rates and inadequate or delayed clinical follow-up among the medically underserved can, in turn, be explained by patient behavior, clinician behavior, and health care system barriers and inequities.

With respect to the use of breast cancer screening services, baseline and routine mammography use are generally lower than routine CBE, with virtually all adult women having had at least one CBE in their lifetime.[61] Although guidelines for annual CBEs are relatively clear and agreed on by providers, the elderly,[62] patients with low income, and ethnic and racial minorities have lower use rates,[63] with the rate-limiting barrier among many of the medically underserved being the absence of a regular source of primary care.[64,65] In the absence of a regular primary care provider, public education campaigns are particularly important and have focused on making women (a) aware of the importance of routine screening, (b) knowledgeable about sources of screening, (c) active initiators of the screening process, and (d) adherent to recommended screening guidelines.[64]

In contrast to CBE, the use picture for mammography is far less clear. In general, national prevalence estimates of breast cancer screening may report "ever screened" or "screened within the past year." The former estimate is usually higher than the latter, indicating that some women in any screening program are being screened for the first time (i.e., the prevalence screen). Reports tend to group these women with those who have been previously screened when trying to determine who gets screened and who does not.[66] Factors that predict individual mammographic screening include the individual and joint effects of age, education, and income, as well as urban versus rural residence. Reasons reported for not being screened continue to show physician failure to recommend a mammogram as the most prevalent reason (30.7%), followed by the patient's not thinking it was needed (22.3%) or not having a problem (14.3%).[67] In addition to income, inconvenience and the price of mammography have been shown to be barriers to use.[68,69]

Although baseline and routine mammography utilization rates have increased over time,[70] elderly, low-income, and racial and ethnic minority populations remain at particularly high risk for mammography underuse,[71] particularly with respect to regular incidence screening.[72] Whereas for CBE, having a regular source of care increased the likelihood that a medically underserved woman would be screened, for mammography, this is not necessarily the case. A number of studies have focused on psychosocial factors that may contribute to a lower uptake of mammography screening among African-American women.[73–76] One review of qualitative research studies has identified a number of cultural barriers to cancer screening among African-American women.[77] These included a core set of beliefs that place cancer prevention practices as a low priority in women's lives, the perceived association of breast cancer and physical injury, and a value system that equates biopsy with exposure of the tumor to air and a poorer prognosis. It should be noted, however, that reports that adjust for SES differences among racial and ethnic groups suggest that there be more variability in breast screening practices within groups.[78] For example, factors that influence mammography behavior among African-Americans have been reported to differ significantly by age.[79] Women aged 40 to 49 were most influenced by knowledge of screening guidelines and exposure to information about breast screening on radio or television. Having health insurance and the level of education were most important for African-American women 50 to 64 years of age, and having a physician recommendation and confidence in being able to obtain a mammogram were most important for African-American women aged 65 and older.

In a study of women at higher risk because they had a first-degree relative with breast cancer, Lerman et al.[80] showed that psychological distress about breast cancer had a significant impact on reducing annual mammography adherence among those first-degree relatives of breast cancer patients with less than a high school education. Adherence among first-degree relatives with more than a high school education appeared unaffected by their level of breast cancer worries. Thus, the response to perceiving oneself at risk for breast cancer appears to vary based on one's educational background, and those medically underserved populations with less than a high school education may avoid seeking breast cancer screening services when they perceive themselves to be at risk.

Gemson et al.[81] report that physician practices with 50% or higher African-American patient populations are less likely to follow mammography guidelines than are physician practices in which 50% or more of the patients are white, and within the same practice physicians are more likely to order mammograms for white than for African-American patients. African-American and Hispanic women are most likely to have ever had a mammogram when their regular source of care was a hospital emergency room or an outpatient clinic, compared with white, non-Hispanic women, who were most likely to have ever had a mammogram if they were part of a prepaid health plan.[82]

Women may come in for early detection with or without a symptom. Although cancer screening is differentiated from case finding, in part, on the basis of this distinction,[83] many women go to a breast cancer screening program because of a perceived problem. This is particularly true in low-income and ethnically diverse communities, in which specialized programs for the early detection of cancer may be more user-friendly than the usual public hospital clinic programs. In addition, before increased health insurance coverage of screening mammography, recording a symptom to justify billing a diagnostic procedure was a common practice.

Among some populations, particularly low-income and minority populations, fatalism about cancer and negativism about cancer therapy are widespread.[84] Although knowledge of cancer symptoms and belief in the possibility of early detection and cure may lead to prompter action, the experience among medically underserved populations of reduced cancer survival in general and reduced breast cancer survival in particular[10] may lead them to be more pessimistic about the efficacy of early detection and treatment and cause them to delay seeking care. Other factors that may contribute to delay in seeking care include a woman's social role (i.e., worker versus homemaker), fear about the impact of diagnosis and treatment, health care access, and perceived consequences of delay.[85]

What are the implications of the combination of health care system barriers and differential risk perception among low-income and medically underserved populations? Before screening, low-income women may be anxious about being at risk for development of the disease, fatalistic about breast cancer outcomes, and facing considerable financial and health care system barriers. Thus, they are less likely to seek breast screening. If, on obtaining a first breast screening examination, a medically underserved woman's findings are negative for cancer, and her perception of risk goes down,[86] she appears less likely to return for a routine annual or biannual screening follow-up examination than a woman who maintains a certain level of concern and views routine breast cancer screening as part of her overall health priorities. For a disadvantaged woman with a finding that is suspicious for cancer or that requires more immediate follow-up, or both, the barriers to obtaining a definitive diagnosis combined with fatalism about outcomes may lead to delayed or discontinued follow-up of abnormal findings.

Turning to clinical follow-up, relatively limited attention has been paid to a problem that occurs in the interval between screening for, and treatment of, breast cancer: delays or incomplete clinical follow-up, or both, of abnormal mammographic and clinical breast findings. As noted at the beginning of this chapter, in 1986, the National Cancer Institute set 45% as its target for annual mammogram prevalence and 70% as its target for CBEs among women 50 years of age and older.[1] By the year 2000, these targets were to be 80% prevalence for both procedures. Assuming 20% of these women would have an abnormality that required some clinical follow-up, almost 3.5 million women in 1990 would have required clinical follow-up if the 45% mammography goal alone had been achieved. Official public health attention to this matter has been largely limited to recommendations for the development of breast (and cervical) cancer clinical follow-up practice guidelines for physicians and the development of office-based clinical follow-up systems.[87]

There are several steps from the discovery of an abnormal breast screening finding through the diagnostic resolution and treatment for cancer. These include (a) what happens in the interval between the screening encounter and the notification of an abnormal finding, (b) what transpires between patient notification and patient action, (c) what the patient brings to the diagnostic encounter, (d) what happens during the diagnostic encounter, and (e) what transpires from diagnosis through treatment. Although, on average, two procedures are performed to evaluate each abnormal breast screening examination,[88] the appropriate time span from notification of abnormal results to diagnostic resolution has not been established, and the end point of this period is variously defined in the literature as time to first diagnostic test, time to biopsy, time to completion of workup, or time to diagnostic resolution.[89]

In a survey of a 10% random sample of U.S. mammography facilities,[90] only 27.1% of the facilities reported having complete clinical follow-up information on all patients, and an additional 46.5% of the facilities reported having such information on 50% or more of their patients. In a study of procedures to improve follow-up for referrals of patients at risk for cancer,[91] standardized communication from a nurse after examination, combined with one written and one telephone reminder, and a patient form to be returned after compliance improved complete follow-up from 68.2% in the control group to 89.0% in the experimental group. However, one-half of the patients who were eligible for the intervention were not included in the study because of direct physician referral, a missed opportunity by the nurses to see the patient, or because the nurses were too busy.

Perhaps as important as *when* feedback about abnormal findings is provided to patients is *how* it is provided. Little is known about how women differ in their reactions to abnormal cancer screening test results.[92] Ideally, no screening program should be initiated without a specific plan for effectively communicating abnormal results and procedures for follow-up.[49] Cancer prevention and control intervention research have begun to test some mechanisms for improving patient willingness to complete follow-up. The perception of the health care system by patients with abnormal cancer screening findings can be affected by prior experience with the system and by their experience in trying to set up a diagnostic follow-up appointment. For medically underserved patients, the time and effort entailed in negotiating public health systems may be prohibitive. Likewise, the psychological consequences of waiting for weeks or even months for an initial appointment can be profound. System barriers may promote delay or denial, or both, because (a) the "cure" may be seen as worse than the disease[46] and (b) any slowness in the system to respond to the patient's need for clinical follow-up may communicate a lack of urgency.

Results of large-scale surveys that focus on African-American–white differences in cancer knowledge and behaviors[93] and in access to care[94] point to a need for further research to address the unique experiences of African-American patients that give rise to negative perceptions and attitudes regarding health care delivery. Underlying this concern is the question of whether these attitudes are associated with lower SES or whether they constitute a pattern common to most African-Americans, regardless of their SES. Although a review conducted by the American Cancer Society concluded that income rather than race was responsible for African-American–white differences in knowledge and behaviors,[95] income alone may not account for the differences.

Findings that African-Americans continue to face repeated incidents of racial discrimination[96] suggest that attitudes of minority groups toward health care may be shaped by such experiences and that an understanding of these attitudes may be essential to addressing the reluctance or inability of some women to pursue diagnostic resolution after an abnormal CBE or mammogram. Support for this assertion can be found in the results of a national survey that revealed significant race differences in the use of health care even after controlling for the effects of income, health status, age, and sex.[55] Societal-level determinants (e.g., racism) of stage of disease at diagnosis may place important limitations on individual-level interventions designed to promote prompt follow-up of symptoms or abnormal screening findings. For example, Catalano and Satariano demonstrated that breast tumors registered in San Francisco from 1983 to 1993 were less likely to be diagnosed at a local stage of development during periods of unexpectedly high unemployment.[97] Moreover, African-American women were three times more likely to be diagnosed with late-stage breast cancer than non-Hispanic white women during periods of high unemployment. Above and beyond poverty, there has been a 30-year trend of disproportionate job losses among African-Americans.[98] Structural changes in the job market combined with racial or ethnic discrimination may have a powerful and unanticipated impact on stage of disease at diagnosis for low-income and minority breast cancer patients.

African-Americans often live segregated in areas of poverty and "urban blight." Living in such a socioeconomically deprived area, with high unemployment and crime, can lead to a life view focused on day-to-day survival and an erosion of social cohesion, community participation, and trust (i.e., "social capital").[99] Such perspectives can represent a barrier to seeking cancer screening services, follow-up of any abnormal test results, or, when symptoms develop, to a delay in obtaining needed care.[100] Area-level indicators of low social class and deprivation have been consistently noted to be associated with poor cancer outcomes. For example, in one study of determinants of breast cancer stage at diagnosis in New York City, Mandelblatt et al. found that the effects of race and public hospital care on stage were attributable to area indicators of poverty, in which individuals who lived in neighborhoods with high poverty or unemployment rates were more likely to have their cancer diagnosed at late stage than were the nonpoor.[101,102] Neighborhood resources, such as number of mammography facilities per female population, have also been noted to influence breast cancer stage at diagnosis. Many "safety net" hospitals serving African-American populations have also closed because of large financial losses and cutbacks in public funding. Many nonprofit hospitals with large portions of uncompensated care have been forced to close or reduce services as well.[103] Such hospital closures have occurred disproportionately in inner city and rural areas, seriously decreasing already limited access for the populations that depend on those institutions.[103]

DISEASE PRESENTATION, DIAGNOSIS, AND TREATMENT

In addition to later stage of disease at diagnosis, which clearly contributes to poorer treatment outcomes among African-Americans, within tumor stage categories survival is worse for African-American women, and the disparity increases with disease stage. Among women diagnosed with localized disease, 5-year relative survival rates are only 10% higher among white women, but this relative advantage increases to 25% for regional disease and 61% for distant disease.[18] Several reasons explain why stage alone does not eliminate the racial disparity in survival. First, variation in tumor behavior exists within tumor stage categories, and within these categories, African-American women are probably diagnosed with more advanced tumors.[1043,105] Second, socioeconomic and cultural factors contribute to reduced access to state-of-the-art adjuvant treatment, follow-up, and supportive care and also contribute to a higher prevalence of other chronic diseases and obesity.[106] These factors are all likely to have a greater impact on survival for women with regional or metastatic disease.

Data from a number of studies suggest that tumors in African-American women may have a more aggressive phenotype. African-American women exhibit a number of adverse breast cancer pathology attributes more frequently than white women. Most studies have found a significantly higher prevalence of poorly differentiated tumors,[107–113] high-grade nuclear atypia,[108,127] and ER-negative[43,108–110,112–122] and progesterone receptor–negative tumors[43,113,120,122,123] among African-American women. However, some studies have not found significant differences in tumor grade[50,117,124] or hormone receptors.[43] Few of the studies that considered hormone receptor status adjusted for differences in age or menopausal status. In the three studies that did adjust for age,[43,45,122] differences remained in two studies.[41,120] However, in the study by Elledge et al.,[43] among women younger than age 35 there was a nonsignificantly higher prevalence of hormone receptor–positive tumors among African-American women than among white or Hispanic women. Racial differences have also been noted in the frequency of lobular and medullary histologies. However, these histologies occur in only a small percentage of patients regardless of race, and absolute differences between racial groups are small; thus, these differences are unlikely to contribute to a significant portion of the survival differential.[21] The fact that African-American and white patient tumors on average may vary phenotypically does not mean that, with equivalent access to state-of-the-art diagnostic and treatment technologies, outcomes could not be comparable between African Americans and whites.[125] Rather, if individual patients from any race or ethnic group could obtain the best possible care for their particular type of breast disease, stage-specific outcomes would be much more likely to be equivalent.

Experiences that transcend lines of social class among African-Americans emerge as potentially significant in contributing to reduced access to state-of-the art care and differences in perceptions of the quality of care received. For example, Hunter et al.[126] found that factors associated with stage of disease at diagnosis were expressed differently among African-American and white breast cancer patients. Among African-Americans, indicators of access to health care, lack of mammography use, and increased body mass index contributed significantly to stage differences, whereas income was marginally associated with stage among whites. In addition, having a CBE by a physician, a history of patient delay, and nuclear grade of the tumor explained up to 50% of the excess risk of stage III to IV tumors versus stage I to II N0 among African-American compared to white women.

The context of the diagnostic encounter may play an important role in determining subsequent patient behavior.[127] Whether screened by a primary care physician or through an inreach or outreach cancer screening program, the breast cancer screening patient who requires clinical follow-up has a limited, if any, prior relationship with clinical follow-up service providers to whom she is referred. In the absence of such a personal relationship, and without the advocacy role of a personal physician, previous experience with the health care system helps to determine the response of the patient to the diagnostic encounter as well as any follow-up recommendations made.

When low-income and ethnically diverse patients receive care, what does the health care system convey to them? The following statement was often made by cancer patients and their families in a series of national hearings held by the American Cancer Society in 1989[128]: "When I went into the system (with an abnormality) I knew I was poor, but then the system made me feel poor." Scheduling clinical follow-up for weeks or months after a sign or symptom of cancer is detected, onerous financial and medical clearances for diagnostic and subsequent treatment procedures, and the inability to communicate with the provider are all significant barriers. These quality of care barriers are all too common in the underresourced health care systems that serve many low-income and culturally diverse populations.

In a 1998 seminal article, Lannin et al.[129] examined the predictors of late stage at diagnosis for women with breast cancer and a matched population control group. Being African-American was significantly associated with having later-stage disease at diagnosis, although this effect diminished after controlling for SES. Most striking was the finding that after considering SES and cultural beliefs (e.g., folk beliefs, religious beliefs, relationships with men, fatalism, beliefs about treatment, and knowledge), the race effect was no longer significant.[129] This study is the first of which we are aware that measures and segregates the intertwined effects of race, social class, and cultural beliefs and demonstrates that beliefs held by certain vulnerable groups are actually the important determinants of outcome.

When African-American breast cancer patients are compared with white breast cancer patients, many differences emerge that could contribute to poorer survival (overall and within stage of disease at diagnosis).[130] African-American breast cancer patients are less likely to be married, have a lower SES, have less education, and are more likely to list a publicly funded facility as a usual source of care than white breast cancer patients. African-American breast cancer patients have more comorbid illnesses, are more likely to be overweight, and are more likely to be current smokers. With respect to their prognosis and treatment, African-American breast cancer patients are diagnosed with more advanced disease, are more likely to have poorly differentiated and ER-negative tumors, and are less likely to have undergone therapeutic surgery or to have received radiation therapy as compared to white breast cancer patients.

Many of these factors are interrelated and, based on the fact that 40% of African-American–white differences in overall survival were explained by more advanced disease at diagnosis, and another 15% were explained by histologic-pathologic differences, the authors concluded[86] that public health resources should focus primarily on promoting the early detection of breast cancer. Although treatment differences explained no new additional survival variance after controlling for stage and tumor characteristics, treatment was measured crudely (as present or absent), and stage-specific African-American–white survival differences were not examined because of reduced sample sizes. Thus, variation in the quality of multidisciplinary breast cancer patient management in relation to stage-specific survival differences among African-Americans and whites has not yet been examined.

Although various guidelines for the optimal treatment of breast cancer have been published[131] and promoted, variation in access to and patterns of therapeutic surgical, radiation therapy, and systemic therapy persist.[132] A variety of pattern of care studies of regional and hospital variation in treatment for breast cancer have documented that substantial variation exists and that this variation is related in part to geographic locale (urban versus rural), type of hospital (teaching versus nonteaching), physician characteristics (years in practice, solo practice), and patient characteristics (age, health insurance).[133–136] Assuming that medically underserved populations are more likely to be seen in "resource-limited" health care institutions, in which access to state-of-the-art care may be more limited, then physician and patient alike may be handicapped in providing and receiving the best that multidisciplinary breast cancer management has to offer.

Beyond geographic and institutional variation in available breast cancer treatment resources, a better understanding of patient and physician interactions during treatment decision making is important,[63,64] particularly as it relates to the medically underserved. From the provider's perspective, family practice residents believe that poor patients are more likely to miss appointments than others, more likely to be late for appointments, and less knowledgeable about their illnesses.[137] One in four residents believed that poor patients did not appreciate the work of their physicians and nurses, and 43% claimed that the poor are more difficult patients. Finally, many of these residents indicated that the poor are unlikely to practice preventive health behaviors (72%), are unlikely to be compliant with their medical regimens (60%), and cared less than others about their health (41%).

Poor and ethnically diverse patients tend to view the health care system as cold, unfriendly, and insensitive to their particular cultural needs. Providers regard these patients as noncompliant and unappreciative. Given these views, the prospects of ensuring clinical follow-up and access to state-of-the art care for many of these patients would appear dim. Distrust of the health care system is linked with noncompliance.[138] Thus, building a community's confidence in its medical providers may be as important for breast cancer control as improving access to primary care and ensuring adequate early-detection facilities. Likewise, educating providers about the different health beliefs held by African-Americans[139] and other minorities and the unique problems and barriers that all poor people face in adhering to providers' advice is important. Improving the image of community health care can be achieved by directing new and expanded resources toward community-based and culturally appropriate disease detection and clinical follow-up programs that also ensure that the promise of early detection leading to cure can be kept for all patients.[140]

DISCUSSION

With respect to breast cancer, as well as many other cancers, the medically underserved are understudied, not well understood by many in the medical and academic research communities, and attended by health care institutions that are underfunded and often do not have the resources necessary to ensure access to state-of-the-art cancer screening, clinical follow-up, diagnosis, and treatment. At the same time, medically underserved women are more likely to be diagnosed with late-stage breast cancer, and some groups (e.g., African-American women) bear the greatest breast cancer mortality burden in the nation. Although the short-term emphasis on increasing the use of existing breast cancer screening resources has contributed somewhat to downstaging breast cancer in these high-risk women, the inaccessibility of screening services for many women combined with the barriers to prompt and effective clinical follow-up, diagnosis, and treatment suggest that the long-term burden of breast cancer will continue to grow for the medically underserved.

The complex underlying biological, psychological, behavioral, and sociocultural processes and pathways whereby race and ethnicity exert their influence on breast cancer outcomes remains poorly understood.[10,141] Phinney[142] suggests that ethnicity is made up of three component parts: (a) culture, (b) ethnic identity, and (c) minority status. Rather than focusing on racial and ethnic groups as discrete categories defined largely by visible phenotypic characteristics (e.g., skin color), viewing race and ethnicity as multidimensional psychological and social constructs may help to move our understanding of how culture, ethnic identity, and minority status influence individual risks of developing and dying from breast cancer. Furthermore, examining the biological aspects that either result from or are expressed within sociocultural determinants of race and ethnicity can provide valuable information to shape prevention, detection, and treatment strategies.

Evidence in support of differences in tumor biology between African-Americans and whites rests primarily on higher incidence of ER and progesterone receptor–negative tumors and poor tumor grade. Studies of differences in other prognostic markers and inherited mutations or polymorphisms with potential impact on susceptibility are too few and too small for any clear conclusions. However, data from a number of studies suggest the existence of differences between races or ethnic groups in gene frequencies for a number of genes; therefore, it is plausible that such differences may exist for polymorphisms relevant to breast cancer.

When considering the evidence for differences in tumor biology in racial or ethnic groups (e.g., African-American women), it is important to clarify the context. Race and ethnicity, as they are used in cancer research, are sociocultural rather than biological constructs.[143] Defining race and ethnicity on the basis of sharing a majority of genetic background is not scientifically justified. Genetic variation within currently defined racial groups is approximately 85%, far exceeding the amount of variation between groups.[144] Nevertheless, genetic variation between racial groups exists, and therefore it is almost certain that differences in biological behavior also exist. However, these biological differences are not a reflection of a genetic background intrinsic to the characteristics that define a specific racial or ethnic group, such as a pattern of "African" genotypes. Rather, they reflect differences in gene frequencies, which are a by-product of historical patterns of reproduction within populations that result largely from geographic, social, and cultural factors.

Typically, when race or ethnicity is used in clinical and epidemiologic cancer research to stratify groups with *definably different* patterns of risk or outcome, the racial and ethnic groups are defined according to external characteristics (i.e., physical appearance, self-report) that incorporate great heterogeneity in genetic background. To the extent that biological differences are noted between racial and ethnic groups, the import of such differences depends on the degree of overlap between the racial or ethnic group defined as a sociocultural community or entity and the inheritance patterns in germ-line mutations or the selective environmental exposures impacting somatic mutations that give rise to the biology.

Thus, if the frequency of a particular polymorphism relevant to cancer is found to truly differ significantly among racial or ethnic groups, it may be wise to broadly tailor prevention or research protocols to address this racial or ethnic distinction. For example, in evaluating an individual pedigree to determine whether testing is warranted for a *BRCA1* mutation, different criteria can be used for Ashkenazi Jews compared to other ethnic groups. Furthermore, if significant racial or ethnic differences in risk or survival persist after a comparison has been adjusted for known prognostic, socioeconomic, and health care access measures, tailoring clinical practices or research to this residual difference may be prudent.

When resources are limited, triaging and tailoring research and service resources to those patients and communities with greatest breast cancer burden would appear to be a logical first step. However, in the absence of any serious progress toward health care reform, and in the absence of a sustainable infrastructure for community-based research, those who need the most will undoubtedly continue to receive the least. Efforts to involve these high-risk populations in cutting-edge cancer research should play a role in improving access to state-of-the-art prevention, early detection, and treatment trials for breast cancer. However, if this is to be accomplished, more serious efforts must be made to provide sufficient resources to sustain a community-based research infrastructure and to involve medically underserved community leaders in the design and implementation of this research. Only this can ensure that the research will be accepted by the community and that the interventions tested have a reasonable chance of proving themselves cost-effective and maintaining themselves after the initial research grant funding has ended.

Solutions to the inclusion problems in breast cancer prevention and treatment trials are not likely to be facilitated by the National Institutes of Health–imposed requirement for "proportional representation" in publicly funded research. On the contrary, in situations in which class, race, ethnic, or age differences are of potential scientific importance, overrepresentation of medically underserved minorities will be required to ensure sufficient statistical power to explore and test group differences. Conversely, in situations in which being a member of an underserved minority is unlikely to contribute to variation in the risk markers of interest, then proportional representation becomes an arbitrary evaluation standard with no internal or external validity. This will require a scientific judgment call, in which the evidence will often be limited and usually insufficient. Nevertheless, the effort made to consider the alternatives, and specifically to address the mechanisms for obtaining minority oversampling where necessary, will be superior to the current system of "rubber-stamping" all research in which underserved minorities are proportionately represented in the proposed design but are rarely accrued in the actual study.

For all breast cancer intervention research involving, from the very beginning of the study design, community, medical, and, if available, scientific leaders, reflecting the sociocultural background of the study populations of interest will help to ensure acceptance when field accrual begins. Formative research (e.g., focus groups) and qualitative research to explore community attitudes toward the intervention can also help to identify potential trouble spots before the trials begin. Of equal importance is the need to develop mechanisms by which the community being studied is provided feedback about the final results of the study in an educationally and culturally appropriate manner. Such community debriefings are extremely rare, given the pressure to get study findings into the professional literature. However, in the long run, efforts to provide the study subjects with the findings of the study in a user-friendly format greatly contribute to the trust necessary for individuals to volunteer and participate fully.

Whether focused on service delivery or inclusion in research, academic health centers must take the lead in forging partnerships with the medically underserved communities in their regional service areas.[145] Of the 126 academic health centers in the United States, 75% have medically underserved minority populations in their local area.[146] Essential characteristics of these partnerships include community-based leadership and ownership of specific programs, training and use of community health workers, joint planning for research, and services targeted to meet community health problems.[146] In the absence of such joint efforts to collaborate, initiatives to study racial and ethnic variation in breast cancer risks and biology and to reduce breast cancer mortality among medically underserved minorities remain unlikely to be effective.

REFERENCES

1. Greenwald P, Sondik E, eds. Cancer control. Objectives for the nation: 1985–2000. *J Natl Cancer Inst Monogr* 1986;2:105.
2. National Center for Health Statistics. Health: United States, 1992. Hyattsville, MD: Public Health Service; 1993.
3. US Bureau of the Census. 1990 census of population, social and economic characteristics. Washington: Government Printing Office; 1990.
4. Miller BA, Kolonel LN, Bernstein L, et al (eds). Racial/ethnic patterns of cancer in the United States. 1988–1992. NIH Pub No. 96–4104. Bethesda, MD: National Cancer Institute; 1996.
5. Mor V, Pacala JT, Rakowski W. Mammography for older women: who uses, who benefits? *J Gerontol* 1992;47:43–49.
6. Baquet CR, Horm JW, Gibbs T, Greenwald P. Socioeconomic factors and cancer incidence among blacks and whites. *J Natl Cancer Inst* 1991;83:551–557.
7. Krieger N. Social class and the black/white crossover in the age-specific incidence in breast cancer: a study linking census-derived data to population-based registry records. *Am J Epidemiol* 1990;131:804–814.
8. Michalski TA, Nattinger AB. The influence of black race and socioeconomic status on the use of breast conserving surgery for medicare beneficiaries. *Cancer* 1997;79:314–319.
9. National Cancer Institute. Report of the President's cancer panel: the meaning of race in science—considerations for cancer research. New York: National Institutes of Health, 1997.
10. Meyerowitz BE, Richardson J, Hudson S, Leedham B. Ethnicity and cancer outcomes: behavioral and psychosocial considerations. *Psych Bull* 1998;123:47–70.
11. Freeman H. Race, poverty, and cancer. *J Natl Cancer Inst* 1991;83 :526–527.
12. Freeman HP. Poverty, race, racism, and survival. *Ann Epidemiol* 1993;3:145–149.
13. Kerner JF, Breen N, Tefft M, Silsby J. Tobacco use among multi-ethnic Latino populations. *Ethn Dis* 1998;8:167–183.
14. Brinton LA, Benichou J, Gammon MD, Brogan DR, Coates R, Schoenberg JB. Ethnicity and variation in breast cancer incidence. *Int J Cancer* 1997;73:349–355.
15. Krieger N, Wolff MS, Hiatt RA, Rivera M, Vogelman J, Orentreich N. Breast cancer and serum organochlorines: a prospective study among white, black, and Asian women. *J Natl Cancer Inst* 1994;86:589–599.
16. Mayberry PM, Stoddard-Wright C. Breast cancer risk factors among black women and white women: similarities and differences. *Am J Epidemiol* 1992;136:1445–1456.
17. Preston JA, Scinto JD, Ni W, et al. Mammography underutilization among older women in Connecticut. *J Am Geriatr Soc* 1997;45: 1310–1314.
18. Ries LAG, Kosary CL, Hankey BF, Miller BA, Edwards BK, eds. SEER cancer statistics review 1973–1995. Bethesda, MD: National Cancer Institute, 1998.
19. Gray GE, Henderson BE, Pike MC. Changing ratio of breast cancer incidence rates with age of black females compared with white females in the United States. *J Natl Cancer Inst* 1980;64:461–63.
20. Miller BA, Ries LAG, et al. SEER cancer statistics review 1973–1990. Bethesda, MD: US Department of Health and Human Services, 1993.
21. Trock BJ. Breast cancer in African-American women: epidemiology and tumor biology. *Breast Cancer Res Treat* 1996;40:11–24.
22. Moormeier J. Breast cancer in black women. *Ann Intern Med* 1996;124:897–905.
23. Kelsey JL, Gammon MD, John EM. Reproductive factors and breast cancer. *Epidemiol Rev* 1993;15:36–47.
24. Austin H, Cole P, Wynder E. Breast cancer in black American women. *Int J Cancer* 1979;24:541–544.
25. Schatzkln A, Palmer JR, et al. Risk factors for breast cancer in black women. *J Natl Cancer Inst* 1987;78:213–217.
26. Laing AE, Demenais FM, Williams R, et al. Breast cancer risk factors in African–American women: the Howard University tumor registry experience. *J Natl Med Assoc* 1993;85:931–939.
27. Bruzzi P, Negri E, La Vecchia C, et al. Short term increase in risk of breast cancer after full term pregnancy. *BMJ* 1988;297:1096–1098.
28. Williams EMI, Jones L, Vessey MP, et al. Short term increase in risk of breast cancer associated with full term pregnancy. *BMJ* 1990;300:578–579.
29. Lambe M, Hsieh C, Trichopoulos D, et al. Transient increase in the risk of breast cancer after giving birth. *N Engl J Med* 1994;331:5–9.
30. Trapido EJ, Chen F, Davis K, et al. Cancer in south Florida Hispanic women: a 9-year assessment. *Arch Intern Med* 1994;154:1083–1088.
31. Polednak AP. Cancer incidence in the Puerto Rican–born population of Connecticut. *Cancer* 1992;70:1172–1176.
32. Wolfgang PE, Semeiks PA, Burnett WS. Cancer incidence in New York City Hispanics, 1982–85. *Ethn Dis* 1991;1:263–272.
33. Baquet CR, Ringen K, Pollack ES, et al. Cancer among blacks and other minorities: statistical profiles. Bethesda, MD: National Cancer Institute, 1986.
34. Trapido EJ, Obeso JL, Stein NS, Rotger A. Unidos por la salud para vivir bien cancer: data report. Washington: National Hispanic Leadership Initiative on Cancer of the National Coalition of Hispanic Health and Human Service Organizations, 1995.
35. Harris JR, Lippman ME, Veronesi U, Willett W. Breast cancer (part 1). *N Engl J Med* 1992;327:319–328.
36. Wynder EL, Cohen LA, Rose DP, Stellman SI. Dietary fat and breast cancer: where do we stand on the evidence? *J Clin Epidemiol* 1994:47:217–222.
37. Hargreaves MK, Buchowski MS, Hardy RE, Rossi SR, Rossi JS. Dietary factors and cancers of the breast, endometrium, and ovary: strategies for modifying fat intake in African-American women. *Am J Obstet Gynecol* 1997:176:S255-S264.
38. Gapstur SM, Potter JD, Sellers TA, Folsom AP. Increased risk of breast cancer with alcohol consumption in postmenopausal women. *Am J Epidemiol* 1992;136:1221–1231.

39. Friedenreich CM, Howe GR, Miller AB, Jain MG. A cohort study of alcohol consumption and risk of breast cancer. *Am J Epidemiol* 1993;137:512–520.
40. Calle EE, Miracle-McMahill HL, Thun M, Heath CW. Cigarette smoking and risk of fatal breast cancer. *Am J Epidemiol* 1994;139:1001–1007.
41. Willett W. Response to Wynder et al's paper on dietary fat and breast cancer. *J Clin Epidemiol* 1994;47:223–226.
42. Anonymous. Cancer incidence among New York City Hispanics. *N Y State J Med* 1990;90:44–45.
43. Elledge RM, Clark GM, et al. Tumor biologic factors and breast cancer prognosis among white, Hispanic, and black women in the United States. *J Natl Cancer Inst* 1994;86:705–712.
44. Shiao YH, Chen VW, Scheer WD, et al. Racial disparity in the association of p53 gene alterations with breast cancer survival. *Cancer Res* 1995;55(7):1485–1490.
45. Krieger N, van den Eden SK, Zava D, Okamoto A. Race/ethnicity, social class, and prevalence of breast cancer prognostic biomarkers: a study of white, black, and Asian women in the San Francisco bay area. *Ethn Dis* 1997;7:137–149.
46. Blaszyk H, Vaughn CB, et al. Novel pattern of p53 gene mutations in an American black cohort with high mortality from breast cancer. *Lancet* 1994;343:1195–1197.
47. Hussain SP, Harris CC. Molecular epidemiology of human cancer: contribution of mutation spectra studies of tumor suppressor genes. *Cancer Res* 1998;58:4023–4037.
48. Weston A, Pan CF, Ksieski HB, et al. P53 haplotype determination in breast cancer. *Cancer Epidemiol Biomarkers Prev* 1997;6:105–112.
49. Weston A, Godbold JH. Polymorphisms of H-ras-1 and p53 in breast cancer and lung cancer: a meta-analysis. *Environ Health Perspect* 1997;105[Suppl 4]:919–926.
50. Weiss S, Tartter P, et al. Ethnic difference in risk and prognostic factors for breast cancer. *Cancer* 1995;76:268–274.
51. Taioll E, Trachman J, et al. A CYP1A1 restriction fragment length polymorphism is associated with breast cancer in African-American women. *Cancer Res* 1995;55:3757–3758.
52. Bailey LR, Roodi N, Verrier CS, Yee CJ, Dupont WD, Parl FF. Breast cancer and CYP1A1, GSTM1, and GSTT1 polymorphisms: evidence of a lack of association in Caucasians and African-Americans. *Cancer Res* 1998;58:65–70.
53. Bailey LR, Roodi N, Dupont WD, Parl FF. Association of cytochrome p4501B1 (CYP1B1) polymorphism with steroid receptor status in breast cancer. *Cancer Res* 1998;58:5038–5041.
54. Newman B, Mu H, Butler LM, Millikan RC, Moorman PG, King MC. Frequency of breast cancer attributable to BRCA1 in a population-based series of American women. *JAMA* 1998;279:915–921.
55. Gao Q, Neuhausen S, Cummings S, Luce M, Olopade OI. Recurrent germ-line BRCA1 mutations in extended African-American families with early-onset breast cancer. *Am J Hum Genet* 1997;60:1233–1236.
56. Thomas SB, Quinn SC. Public health then and now: the Tuskegee syphilis study, 1932 to 1972. *Am J Public Health* 1991;81:1498–1505.
57. Mandelblatt J, Traxter M,. Lakin P, et al. Breast and cervical cancer screening of poor, elderly, black women: clinical results and implications. *Am J Prev Med* 1993;9(3):133–138.
58. Chen F, Trapido EJ, Davis K. Differences in stage at presentation of breast and gynecologic cancers among whites, blacks, and Hispanics. *Cancer* 1994;73:2838–2842.
59. McCarthy EP, Bums PB, Coughlin SS, et al. Mammography use helps to explain differences in breast cancer stage at diagnosis between older black and white women. *Ann Intern Med* 1998;128:729–736.
60. Burns RB, McCarthy EP, Freund KM, Marwill SL, Schwartz M, Ash A, Moskowitz MA. Black women receive less mammography even with similar use of primary care. *Ann Intern Med* 1996;125:173–182.
61. Breen N, Kessler L. Trends in cancer screening—United States, 1987 and 1992. *Oncology (Huntingt)* 1996;10(3):328–330.
62. King EU, Resch N, Rimer B, et al. Breast cancer screening practices among retirement community women. *Prev Med* 1993;22:1–19
63. US Department of Health and Human Services. The national strategic plan for the early detection and control of breast and cervical cancer. Centers for Disease Control, Food and Drug Administration, National Cancer Institute; 1994.
64. Mandelblatt JS. Breast and cervical cancer screening in elderly poor women. In: DeVita VT, Hellman S, Rosenburg SA, eds. *Oncology: principles and practice of cancer prevention update*. Philadelphia: JB Lippincott, 1993.
65. O'Malley AS, Mandelblatt J, Gold K, Cagney KA, Kerner J. Continuity of care and the use of breast and cervical cancer screening services in a multi-ethnic community. *Arch Intern Med* 1997;157:1462–1470.
66. Breen N, Kessler L. Changes in use of screening mammography: evidence from the 1987 and 1990 national health interview surveys. *Am J Public Health* 1994;84:62–67.
67. Mammography and breast examination—results from the behavioral risk factor surveillance system, 1992 [commentary]. *Oncology (Huntingt)* 1993;7:48-53.
68. Urban N, Anderson GL, Peakcock S. Mammography screening: how important is cost as a barrier to use? *Am J Public Health* 1994;84:50–55.
69. Taylor VM, Thompson B, Montano DE, Machloch J, Johnson K, Li S. Mammography use among women attending an inner-city clinic. *J Cancer Educ* 1998;13:96–101.
70. Anonymous. Mammography and breast examination for older women—results from the behavioral risk factor surveillance system, 1992 [Commentary]. *Oncology (Huntingt)* 1993;7:48–53.
71. Whitman S, Ansell D, Lacey L, et al. Patterns of breast and cervical cancer screening at three public health centers in an inner city urban area. *Am J Public Health* 1991;81:1651–53.
72. Mandelblatt J, Traxler M, Lakin P, et al. Mammography and Papanicolaou smear use by elderly poor black women. *J Am Geriatr Soc* 1992;40:1001–1007.
73. Bowen D, Hickman KM, Powers D. Importance of psychological variables in understanding risk perceptions and breast cancer screening in African-American women. *Womens Health* 1997;3:227–42.
74. Miller AM, Champion VL. Attitudes about breast cancer and mammography: racial, income and educational differences. *Womens Health* 1997;26:41–63.
75. Champion V, Menon U. Predicting mammography and breast self-examination in African-American women. *Cancer Nurs* 1997;20:31.
76. Glanz K, Resch N, Lerman C, Rimer BK. Black-white differences in factors influencing mammography use among employed female health maintenance organization members. *Ethn Health* 1996;1:207–220.
77. Hoffman–Goetz L, Mills SL. Cultural barriers to cancer screening among African-American women: a critical review of the qualitative literature. *Womens Health* 1997;3:183–201.
78. Hiatt RA, Pasick RJ. Unsolved problems in early breast cancer detection: focus on the underserved. *Breast Cancer Res Treat* 1996;40: 37–51.
79. Danigelis NL, Worden JK, Mickey RM. The importance of age as a context for understanding African-American women's mammography screening behavior. *Am J Prev Med* 1996;12:358–366.
80. Lerman C, Daly M, Sands C, et al. Mammography adherence and psychological distress among women at risk for breast cancer. *J Natl Cancer Inst* 1993;85:1074–1080.
81. Gemson DH, Elinson J, Messeri P. Differences in physician prevention practice patterns for white and minority patients. *J Community Health* 1988;13:53–64.
82. Fox SA, Stein JA. The effect of physician-patient communication on mammography utililization by different ethnic groups. *Med Care* 1991;29:1065–1082.
83. Winawer SJ, Kemer JF. Sigmoidoscopy: case finding versus screening [Editorial]. *Gastroenterology* 1988;95:527–530.
84. American Cancer Society. Cancer and the poor: a report to the nation. Findings of regional hearings conducted by the American Cancer Society. Atlanta: American Cancer Society, 1989.
85. Facione NC, Dodd MJ, Holzemer W, Meleis AI. Helpseeking for self-discovered breast symptoms. *Cancer Prac* 1997;5:220–227.
85. Lerman C, Trock B, Rimer BK, et al. Psychological and behavioral implications of abnormal mammograms. *Ann Int Med* 1991;114:657–661.
87. US Department of Health and Human Services. The national strategic plan for the early detection and control of breast and cervical cancers. 1994:30–31.
88. Kerlikowski K, Grady D, Barclay J, et al. Positive predictive value of screening mammography by age and family history of breast cancer. *JAMA* 1993;270:2444–2450.
89. Kerlikowski K. Timelines of follow-up after abnormal screening mammography. *Breast Cancer Res Treat* 1996;90:53–64.
90. Houn F, Brown ML. Current practice of screening mammography in the United States: data from the National Survey of Mammography Facilities. *Radiology* 1994;190:209–215.
91. Manfredi C, Lacey L, Warnecke R. Results of an intervention to improve compliance with referrals for evaluation of suspected malig-

nancies at neighborhood public health centers. *Am J Public Health* 1990;80:85–87.
92. Lerman CE, Rimer BK. Psychosocial impact of cancer screening. *Oncology* 1993; 7:67–72.
93. Jepson C, Kessler LG, Portnoy B, Gibbs T. Black-white differences in cancer prevention knowledge and behavior. *Am J Public Health* 1991;81:501–504.
94. Blendon RJ, Aiken LH, Freeman HE, Corey CR. Access to medical care for black and white Americans: a matter of continuing concern. *JAMA* 1989;261:278–281.
95. American Cancer Society. Cancer and the poor: a report to the nation. Findings of regional hearings conducted by the American Cancer Society. Atlanta, GA: American Cancer Society, 1989.
96. Feagin JR. The continuing significance of race: anti-black discrimination in public places. *Am Soc Rev* 1991;56:101–116.
97. Catalano RA, Satariano WA. Unemployment and the likelihood of detecting early-stage breast cancer. *Am J Public Health* 1998;88:586–589.
98. Williams DR. African-American health: the role of the social environment. *J Urban Health* 1998;75:300–321.
99. Kawachi I, Kennedy BP, Lochner K, Prothrow-Stith D. Social capital, income inequality, and mortality. *Am J Public Health* 1997;87:1491–1498.
100. Womeodu RJ, Bailey JE. Barriers to cancer screening. *Med Clin North Am* 1996;80:115–133.
101. Mandelblatt J, Andrews H, Kerner J, Zauber A, Burnett W. Determinants of late stage of diagnosis of breast and cervical cancer: the impact of age, race, social class, and hospital type. *Am J Public Health* 1991;81:646–649.
102. Mandelblatt J, Andrews H, Kao R, Wallace R, Kerner J. The late-stage diagnosis of colorectal cancer: demographic and socioeconomic factors. *Am J Public Health* 1996;86:1794–1797.
103. Rice MF. Inner-city hospital closures/relocations: race, income status, and legal issues. *Soc Sci Med* 1987;24:889–896.
104. Dansev RD, Hessel P, Browde S, et al. Lack of significant independent effect of race on survival in breast cancer. *Cancer* 1988;61:1908–1912.
105. Jones B, Kasl S, et al. Can mammography screening explain the race difference in stage at diagnosis of breast cancer? *Cancer* 1995;75: 2103–2113.
106. Coates RL, Clark WS, Eley JW, et al. Race, nutritional status, and survival from breast cancer. *J Natl Cancer Inst* 1990;82:1684–1691.
107. Ownby HE, Frederick J, Russo J, et al. Racial differences in breast cancer patients. *J Natl Cancer Inst* 1985;75:55–60.
108. Hunter C, Redmond C, et al. Breast cancer: factors associated with stage at diagnosis in black and white women. *J Natl Cancer Inst* 1993;85:1129–1137.
109. Eley W, Hill HA, et al. Racial differences in survival from breast cancer: results of the National Cancer Institute black/white survival study. *JAMA* 1994;272:947–954.
110. Mohla S, Sampson CC, Khan T, et al. Estrogen and progesterone receptors in breast cancer in Black Americans. *Cancer* 1982;50:552–559.
111. Valanis B, Wirman J, Hertzberg VS. Social and biological factors in relation to survival among black vs. white women with breast cancer. *Breast Cancer Res Treat* 1987;9:135–143.
112. Kovi J, Mohla S, et al. Breast lesions in black women. *Pathol Annu* 1989;24:199–218.
113. Simon MS, Severson RK. Racial differences in breast cancer survival: the interaction of socioeconomic status and tumor biology. *Am J Obstet Gynecol* 1997;176:S233–S239.
114. Natarajan N, Nismoto T, Mettlin C, Murphy EP. Race–related differences in breast cancer patients: results of the 1982 national survey of breast cancer by the American College of Surgeons. *Cancer* 1985;56:1704–1709.
115. Gordon N, Joseph C, et al. Socioeconomic factors and race in breast cancer recurrence and survival. *Am J Epidemiol* 1992;135:609–618.
116. Muss HB, Hunter CP, Wesley M, et al. Treatment plans for black and white women with stage II node-positive breast cancer: the national cancer institute black/white cancer survival study experience. *Cancer* 1992;70:2460–2467.
117. Freeman H, Wasfie T. Cancer of the breast in poor black women. *Cancer* 1989;63:2562–2569.
118. Pegoraro RJ, Nirmul D, Reinach SG, et al. Breast cancer prognosis in three different racial groups in relation to steroid hormone receptor status. *Breast Cancer Res Treat* 1986;7:111–118.
119. Pegoraro RJ, Karnan V, Nirmul D, et al. Estrogen and progesterone receptors in breast cancer among women of different racial groups. *Cancer Res* 1986;46:2117–2120.
120. Beverly LN, Flanders WD, Go RC, et al. A comparison of estrogen and progesterone receptors in black and white breast cancer patients. *Am J Public Health* 1987;77:351–353.
121. Stanford J, Greenberg R. Breast cancer incidence in women by estrogen receptor status and race. *Am J Public Health* 1989;79:71–77.
122. Gapstur SM, Dupuis J, Gann P, Collila S, Winchester DP. Hormone receptor status of breast tumors in black, Hispanic and non-Hispanic white women: an analysis of 13,239 cases. *Cancer* 1996;77:1465–1471.
123. Dignan JJ, Redmond CK, Fisher B, Costantino JP, Edwards BK. Prognosis among African American women and white women with lymph node negative breast carcinoma. Findings from two randomized clinical trials of the National Surgical Adjuvant Breast and Bowel Project (NSABP). *Cancer* 1997;80:80–97.
124. Shiao YH, Chen VW, Scheer WD, et al. Racial disparity in the association of p53 gene alterations with breast cancer survival. *Cancer Res* 1995;55:1485–1490.
125. Heimann R, Ferguson D, Powers C, Suri D, Weichselbaum RR, Hellman S. Race and clinical outcome in breast cancer in a series with long-term follow-up evaluation. *J Clin Oncol* 1997;15:2329–2337.
126. Hunter C, Redmond CK, Chen VW, et al. Breast cancer associated with stage at diagnosis in black and white women. *J Natl Cancer Inst* 1993;85:1129–1137.
127. Celantano D. The Lerman/Rimer article reviewed. *Oncology* 1993; 7:72–75.
128. Testimony given at American Cancer Society Hearings on Cancer in the Poor. Atlanta, GA: 1989.
129. Lannin DR, Mathews HF, Mitchell J, Swanson MS, Swanson FH, Edwards MS. Influence of socioeconomic and cultural factors on racial differences in late-stage presentation of breast cancer. *JAMA* 1998;279:1801–1807.
130. Eley JW, Hill HA, Chen VW, et al. Racial differences in survival from breast cancer. *JAMA* 1994;272:947–954.
131. National Institutes of Health Consensus Conference. Treatment of early-stage breast cancer. *JAMA* 1991;265:391–395.
132. Ayanian JZ, Guadagnoli E. Variations in breast cancer treatment by patient and provider characteristics. *Breast Cancer Res Treat* 1996;40(1):65–74.
133. Samet JM, Hunt WC, Farrow DC. Determinants ot receiving breast conserving surgery. *Cancer* 1994;13:2344–2351.
134. Ayanian JZ, Kohler BA, Abe T, Epstein AM. The relation between health insurance coverage and clinical outcomes among women with breast cancer. *N Engl J Med* 1993;329:326–331.
135. Iscoe NA, Goel V, Wu K, et al. Variation in breast cancer surgery in Ontario. *Can Med Assoc J* 1994;150:345–352.
136. Whelan T, Marcellus D, Clark R, Levine M. Adjuvant radiotherapy for early breast cancer: patterns of practice in Ontario. *Can Med Assoc J* 1993;149:1273–1277.
137. Price JH, Desmond SM, Snyder FF, Kimmel SR. Perceptions of family practice residents regarding health care and poor patients. *J Fam Prac* 1988;27:615–621.
138. Greenwald HP, Becker SW, Nevift MC. Delay and noncompliance in cancer detection: a behavioral perspective for health planners. *Milbank Mem Fund Q Health Soc* 1978;56:212–230.
139. Pierce RL. African-American cancer patients and culturally competent practice. *J Psych Soc Oncol* 1997;15:1–17.
140. Kerner JF, Dusenbury L, Mandelblatt JS. Poverty and cultural diversity: challenges for health promotion among medically underserved populations. *Annu Rev Publ Health* 1993;14:355–377.
141. Adler NE, Boyce WT, Chesney MA, Folkman S, Syme SL. Socioeconomic inequalities in health: no easy solution. *JAMA* 1993;269: 3140–3145.
142. Phinney JS. When we talk about American ethnic groups, what do we mean? *Am Psych* 1996;51:918–927.
143. Freeman HF. The meaning of race in cancer of the breast. *Cancer J Sci Am* 1997;3:76–77.
144. Freeman H. The meaning of race in science—considerations for cancer research. Report of the President's Cancer Panel. Bethesda, MD: National Institutes of Health, National Cancer Institute, 1998.
145. Levine DM, Becker DM, Bone LR, et al. Community–academic health center partnerships for underserved minority populations. *JAMA* 1994;272:309–311.
146. The Pew Health Professions Commission. Health professions education for the future: schools in service to the nation. Report of the Pew Health Professions Commission. Durham, NC: The Pew Health Professions Commission, 1993.
147. Commentary. Mammography and breast examination—results from Behavioral Risk Factor Surveillance System, 1992. *Oncology* 1993; 7(12): 48–53.

Diseases of the Breast, 2nd ed.,
edited by Jay R. Harris.
Lippincott Williams & Wilkins, Philadelphia © 2000.

CHAPTER 65

End-of-Life Considerations in Breast Cancer Patients

Jane M. Ingham

Although remarkable advances have been made in the prevention, early diagnosis, and treatment of breast cancer, it remains a disease associated with significant mortality. The health professionals who are responsible for the provision of oncologic care for breast cancer patients are frequently faced with providing care for individuals who are approaching the end of life. The problems faced by these patients and by their caregivers present unique and important challenges for these individuals, for health care professionals, and for health systems. Although the focus of medical intervention and research has largely been on life-sustaining treatments, increasing attention has been directed toward strategies that have the potential to have a positive impact on quality of life. Within this context, it is important to consider the end-of life experience for breast cancer patients.

This chapter addresses the epidemiology of the end-of-life experience for breast cancer patients, including the spectrum of problems faced by these individuals and their caregivers. The components of optimal end-of-life care are addressed, in addition to some approaches to optimizing this care. Although it must be acknowledged that there is a wide variability in the cancer experience for individuals living in different countries, much of the epidemiologic data reported in this chapter relate to the experiences of breast cancer patients in the United States. Nonetheless, much of the discussion, particularly the aspects that address the components of optimal end-of-life care, has broad applicability worldwide. Finally, although discussion about the end-of-life components of the illness experience has increased, both the experience itself and interventions that may be specific to the end-of-life period have not been given high priority in oncology educational initiatives, health care delivery, or research. Given the paucity of data pertaining to this subject, areas that are in need of further research are highlighted throughout the chapter.

J. M. Ingham: Department of Medicine, Division of Palliative Care, Lombardi Cancer Center, Georgetown University Medical Center, Washington, D.C.

EPIDEMIOLOGIC ASPECTS OF THE BREAST CANCER END-OF-LIFE EXPERIENCE

To develop appropriate strategies for optimal end-of-life care, we must have some understanding of the end-of-life experiences of cancer patients. Although some data are available to illuminate the experiences of breast cancer patients as they approach the end of their lives, it is difficult to describe with accuracy "when," "how," and "where" patients with breast cancer die. These issues have only been explored in part, and much more information is needed. The data that are available come from epidemiologic studies that describe survival and mortality; from "sociologic" studies that explore place of death, medical involvement toward the end of life, and the caregiver experience; and from studies of the symptoms experienced by patients who are nearing the end of life.

Breast Cancer Mortality

In 1990, there were 5 million deaths from cancer worldwide, with cancer being proportionately more common as a cause of death in developed countries.[1] In 1995 in the United States, it was estimated that there were just over 1.25 million new cases of cancer (excluding basal and squamous cell skin cancer and *in situ* carcinomas except urinary bladder)[2] and almost 538,000 deaths. This figure represents almost one-fourth of the total deaths that occurred that year in the United States.[3] Also in the United States, 184,300 new cases of breast cancer were expected to be diagnosed in 1998, with 43,900 breast cancer–related deaths. These deaths represent 7.8% of all deaths from cancer and 16% of deaths from cancer in women.[4]

Some of the statistics relating to cancer deaths in the United States show encouraging trends, particularly those that relate to cancer mortality and 5-year relative cancer survival rates. With specific regard to breast cancer, the mortality for breast cancer in women decreased by 1.8% per year between 1990 and 1994,[5] and the 5-year relative survival rates (%) for white women with breast cancer improved from 63% to 86%; for African-American women, they increased from 46% to 70% between the periods 1960 to 1963 and 1986 to 1993.[4] Nonetheless, despite these statistics, death from breast cancer remains common, with mortality and 5-year survival figures varying and influenced by many factors, including age, race, stage at diagnosis, and treatment strategies.

Although between 1988 and 1992 the median age at death for all cancers in the United States was 71 years,[6] the median age at death for breast cancer was slightly younger (67 years). Clear differences exist among races, with the median age at death being 68 years for white women and 61 years for African-American women. Of the deaths caused by breast cancer, 26.0% occurred between the ages of 64 and 74 years, 21.0% between 75 and 84 years, 20.5% between 55 and 64 years, 13.5% between 45 and 54 years, 9.9% older than 85 years, and 7.6% between 35 and 44 years.[6] In 1994, the most common cancer to cause death in females between the ages of 15 and 54 was breast cancer.[4]

The impact of various factors, including race and ethnicity, on breast cancer has been explored in some detail.[7] This has been addressed in more detail elsewhere in this text. For example, again in the United States, it is known that higher percentages of African-American women have advanced disease at diagnosis than white women. Using staging according to Surveillance, Epidemiology, and End Results historical categories rather than the American Joint Committee on cancer staging system,[4] it has been documented in white women that 60% of newly diagnosed breast cancers represent localized disease, 31% regional, and 6% distant. The respective figures for African-American women are, in contrast, 49%, 37%, and 9%. Similarly, 5-year survival rates demonstrate significant differences among races. Five-year survival, based on stage at diagnosis between 1986 and 1993, was 97% for white women with localized disease, 77% for regional disease, and 21% for distant disease.[4] For African-American women, the corresponding figures were 90%, 61%, and 17%. Aside from the clear impact on the length of illness, little is known about the more global impact of these statistics on the end-of-life experience for individual patients and caregivers.

More complex analyses have explored other aspects of survival.[8,9] For example, it has been demonstrated that women with stage IV breast cancer have longer survival times as they move further in time from their diagnosis.[9] Further, survival from time of first recurrence depends on site of first recurrence, with visceral recurrence having the shortest length of survival, after multiple-site recurrence, pulmonary metastases, and local disease recurrence (see Chapter 46). The experience of living with advanced breast cancer, of living within these "survival times," is clearly likely to be impacted by new therapies and, consequently, is constantly changing and dependent on access to these treatments. Therapies directed at the disease itself and those directed at palliation alone have the potential to change this experience. Survival time could potentially be lengthened by new therapies, but quality of survival also may be impacted by treatment strategies. For example, the impact of therapy with bisphosphonates on the incidence of bone fractures could potentially have a dramatic impact on the day-to-day survival experience of patients with bony metastases.

Although the previously mentioned statistics give information about the trends and timing of death relative to age, stage of disease, and race, they provide little information to illuminate the experience of patients who are nearing the end of life. Furthermore, given that these data relate predominantly to the United States, they may not reflect the experiences of patients in other countries, especially those in developing nations, in which patterns of disease and access to health care vary. Clearly, survival times and time from diagnosis to death are factors that are likely to have an impact on the end-of-life experience for individuals, their families, and other caregivers. In addition, race and ethnicity and associated socioeconomic factors, including education and poverty levels, are likely to influence the physical, psychological, and social aspects of the end-of-life experience. Data that specifically explore the particular impact of these issues on aspects of the end-of-life experience of breast cancer patients are not available.

Aspects of the End-of-Life Experience Related to Extent of Disease at Time of Death

An important aspect of breast cancer that relates to the end-of-life experience is the extent of disease and the extent and nature of concurrent disease processes in the weeks before and at the time of death. Much of the information obtained about this aspect of the breast cancer experience is derived from the information on death certificates and from reports to cancer registries. Although at the time of death most patients dying from breast cancer have metastatic disease, disease extent is often poorly documented on death certificates. The use of autopsy data may provide more accurate information, but the rate of autopsies is low, particularly for cancer deaths (autopsies were performed in only 2.5% of the 1993 U.S. cancer deaths[10]), and the most recent autopsy data specific to breast cancer are from the early 1980s. These studies reported that between 50% and 75% of patients die with widespread disease involving bone, lung, and liver.[11–13]

In summary, although antemortem investigations in patients with cancer often clarify the diagnosis and extent of disease, the approach to documentation of this information is poorly systematized and, when combined with the very low autopsy rate for cancer-related deaths, does not facilitate the detailed evaluation of the nature of the dying process. In particular, more detailed and accurate information about the extent and nature of the disease processes present at the end of life could potentially foster the advancement of medical understanding of the pathophysiology of symptoms and distress at this time and also foster the development of symptom-specific palliative interventions.[14]

Aspects of the End-of-Life Experience Related to Place of Residence

Further insight into the end-of-life experience of breast cancer patients is provided by information that relates to the places of residence of patients as they approach the end of life. In developed countries, most patients die in institutions, yet clinical experience suggests that most patients in these countries express a preference to be in their home toward the end of life. In a small survey exploring this matter that was undertaken in 98 patients with a spectrum of cancer diagnoses in the United Kingdom, 58% of participating patients expressed a preference to die at home, 20% preferred the hospital, and 20% preferred an inpatient hospice.[15] Several social and disease-related factors have been shown to influence the likelihood of cancer patients' dying in particular locations, and these include age, the type of cancer, time from diagnosis, symptoms, and hospice participation. Furthermore, access to care and the goals of care likely influence place of death, although few data are available to illuminate this aspect of the end-of-life experience. For example, it would seem probable that those patients who are focused on life-sustaining interventions would be more likely to seek hospitalization toward the end of life.

Despite the preferences of patients, most deaths in developed countries occur in medical institutions. High rates for institutionalized death are evident, for example, in the United States (78%), Finland (75%), Sweden (79%), and Iceland (80%), whereas lower rates are recorded in other parts of Europe, including Bulgaria (25%), Spain (30%), and Italy (37%).[16] Of the approximately 2.2 million deaths that occur annually in the United States, 1990 death certificate data indicate that approximately 62% occurred in hospitals, 16% in nursing homes, and 17% in homes.[17] The rate of inhospital deaths varies with age and in 1990 was reported as ranging from 48% to 91%.[17] Particularly in older age groups, many patients die in nursing homes.

In the United States, cancer is the disease process most commonly associated with a home death.[17] In comparison to deaths in the overall population, home death is more common for patients with malignant neoplasms, with 25.8% of cancer patients dying at home, 58.2% in hospitals, and 13.3% in nursing homes.[17] Little information is available to quantify the proportion of patients in the United States who die at home with specific cancers, and the breast cancer statistics appear to be similar to the statistics for other cancer patients.[18,19] It has been demonstrated, however, that death from breast cancer is more likely to occur in the home setting in the United States than death that occurs as a consequence of lymphoma or leukemia.[18,20]

Length of time from diagnosis to death has been shown to influence place of death, with death being more likely to occur in the hospital for patients with a recent cancer diagnosis. Although not quantified, this trend may reflect an early focus on life-sustaining treatments, with shifts in goals over time. In a study of 2,989 cancer deaths in New York State between 1976 and 1978, 90% of patients whose cancer had been diagnosed for less than 1 month died in acute care hospitals, compared with 65% to 70% of those whose diagnosis had been made 1 month or more before death.[20] Short time from diagnosis to death and advanced age are factors that are likely to be associated with institutional death, but evidence exists that admission to a hospice overrides this tendency.[21]

Hospice participation is associated with a higher likelihood of death at home,[19] with one U.S. survey demonstrating that hospice patients were 2.8 times as likely to die at home as nonhospice patients and an Italian survey demonstrating that home death was twice as frequent among patients who used the services of a palliative care team when compared with those who did not use such services.[22] The availability of inpatient hospice beds has been demonstrated in one U.S. study to be the variable that most significantly determined site of death—those who were enrolled in a hospice program with access to inpatient beds were more likely to die in the inpatient setting.[22]

Several other factors have been explored with regard to their impact on place of death. In a 1981 National Hospice Study, a survey of U.S. hospice patients reported that those who were younger, married, more educated, and in higher income groups were more likely to die at home.[23] The same survey reported that patients whose primary caregivers were were employed were less likely to die at home. Patients' symptom profiles were also shown to influence site of death. For example, in this survey the presence of disorientation increased the likelihood of death occurring in the inpatient setting.[23,24]

The economics of health care delivery and geographic factors have an impact on differences in sites of death among nations and within specific countries. In developing countries, where access to health care may be limited, death is far less likely to occur in an institution. Variability within a country may reflect variations in the availability and reimbursability of hospice and home health care services in rural and urban areas. Economic factors that influence place of death are complex. Aside from clear national differences in the availability of health services and national health care priorities, economic factors at the family level are also likely to be highly significant. In the United States, although Mor and Hiris[23] found that higher income was associated with increased likelihood of death occurring at home, McCusker[20] demonstrated that although this held true for the highest four socioeconomic groups, the lowest socioeconomic group had a pattern of a relatively high percentage of home deaths and a low percentage of deaths in chronic care facilities. The moderate increase in the proportion of deaths occurring in homes or in hospices between 1970 and the late 1980s in the United States, which has been particularly evident in patients with cancer, has been driven in part by the development of the Medicare hospice benefit.[25] The increase in the rate of nursing home deaths, particularly among the very elderly, may be related to changes in hospital reimbursement policies, such as prospective payment, utilization review, and preadmission screening.[25,26]

Although death certificate–based statistics provide data relating to the moment of death, they do not give information to clarify the place of residence or site of treatment during the hours, weeks, and months before death, and they do not shed any light on quality of life and quality of care in each setting. Clinical experience suggests that moves between hospitals, homes, subacute facilities, and hospices are not infrequent. Supporting this observation are data from the 1986 National Mortality Followback Survey, a survey of the experiences of more than 16,000 decedents in the United States.[27] This survey reported that 81% of decedents received some institutional care during the last year of life, with 44% receiving between 1 week and 1 month of this care. Another study of 1,227 elderly patients dying in Connecticut reported that almost 70% of patients resided at more than one site during the last 90 days of life.[28] No comparable data are available to describe the experiences of breast cancer patients or to explain the impact of various therapeutic approaches on this experience.

Much has been speculated, but very little information is available about the variation in the quality of life before death among different sites. Although the National Hospice Study, which assessed 1,754 terminal cancer patients in the United States, found little difference between sites, some indicators suggested that pain and symptom control may have been better in the inpatient hospice setting.[23,24,29] Each environment—home, hospital, and nursing home—presents its own particular challenges in the care of the dying as well as potential advantages. For example, the nursing home is an environment that, in comparison to acute care hospitals, is characterized by low levels of physician involvement, relatively low ratios of registered nurses to patients and residents, and staff who may not have been trained in caring for dying patients.[30] Yet this environment may be the place that some individuals define as their home. Although methodologic challenges exist in the assessment of the quality of care toward the end of life, more information is needed to quantify the experiences of patients and their caregivers in different environments so that strategies can be implemented to improve and optimize care.

An example of a study that has provided significant insight into the inhospital experiences of patients at the end of life and the quality of care in that setting is the SUPPORT study (Study to Understand Prognoses and Preference for Outcomes and Risks of Treatment), in which the experiences of 4,301 seriously ill medical inpatients hospitalized in one of five teaching hospitals were documented.[31] The data from this study were combined with the information from another study of elderly patients to further explore the end-of-life experiences associated with medical illness.[32] Although a subpopulation in this study had lung and colon cancer, there were no data directly relating to breast cancer. Nonetheless, the study raised concerns about pain management practices and other important aspects of the end-of-life experience. For example, relatives reported that more than one-third of conscious patients were perceived to be in moderate to severe pain for more than one-half of the time during the last 3 days of life.[31] In addition, there was evidence that physicians were often unaware of patient preferences for cardiopulmonary resuscitation. Although these data cannot be extrapolated to directly reflect the experience of patients with breast cancer, they do provide some insights into the end-of-life inpatient experience in the United States.

In summary, the impact of the place of death on quality of life and numerous aspects of the quality of care toward the end of life remain largely unquantified. Information specific to the needs and experiences of the breast cancer population is not available. The availability of a spectrum of facilities to meet the needs of patients and families is clearly optimal. For example, home care nursing supports are important for patients who wish to be at home toward the end of life, and inpatient beds are also often needed for intensive management of certain symptoms or for situations in which patient or family needs, or both, are such that home-based care is not possible. Although health care professionals who care for patients with advanced illness should optimally have some understanding of the quality of care in various environments, such information is, most frequently, unavailable. When care is planned, each patient's case must be considered with an awareness of many factors, including patient goals and needs, the availability of caregivers, family structure, cultural preferences, and the availability of home care and hospice services.

Aspects of the End-of-Life Experience Related to Medical Involvement in Patient Care

In developed countries, chronic illness is usually associated with significant contact with health care professionals, particularly before death. Information is not available that is specific to the medical interactions between breast cancer patients and health professionals during the last weeks of life. Neither is information available about the proportions of these patients who receive particular treatment interventions, such as palliative therapies, cardiopulmonary resuscitation, and mechanical ventilation. Some data are available that pertain to the more general experience of cancer patients.

In a retrospective study of cancer deaths in New York State, investigators found that although all of the patients surveyed had seen a doctor in the 6 months before death, a lack of face-to-face contact with the physicians was evident as death approached. More than one-half of the patients surveyed spent at least 1 of the last 2 weeks at home; 17% had no contact, although 31% had telephone contact with their physician during this period.[33] It must be noted, however, that physicians, and specifically oncologists, in the United States are commonly involved in the care of patients with breast cancer who are approaching the end of life, although this contact is often indirectly facilitated through hospice nurse contact with patients.[34,35]

In addition to the involvement of individual health care professionals, the "system of care" must be considered when evaluating the medical involvement in end-of-life care. In 1996, the National Hospice Organization estimated that 390,000 patients were treated by hospices in the United States.[35] It has been estimated that 40% of cancer patients who die are enrolled in hospice programs, and 58% of those in hospice care have cancer as their primary diagnosis.[34,35] In the United States, the hospice is usually, from a practical perspective, a system of care distinct from the system that exists within the acute care hospital system. In other countries it is a more flexible system, defined broadly as a philosophy of care, and available to individuals with life-threatening illness who may still seek some life-sustaining treatments. Hospice programs usually offer an array of services delivered through a team approach and aim to ensure quality of life for the patient and his or her family, most commonly in the home.

In the United States, patients who enroll in hospice programs usually elect to focus on comfort and quality of life without pursuing life-prolonging interventions. Data extracted from Medicare records in the United States suggest that patients spend only short periods as hospice patients, despite eligibility criteria that allow enrollment when the prognosis is younger than age 6 months. In a survey of 6,451 hospice patients, 80.2% of whom had cancer, Christakis and Escarce[36] found that the median survival after enrollment was only 36 days, with 15.5% of the patients dying within 7 days and 14.9% living longer than 180 days. Patients with breast cancer represented 5.6% of this population and had a median survival of 43.5 days, with 13.5% dying within 7 days of enrollment and 9% living longer than 180 days. These statistics demonstrate a pattern of late referral of breast cancer patients to hospice programs. The factors that influence this pattern have not been quantified, although there are likely many contributing factors, including patient preferences for life-sustaining therapies, the occurrence of unexpected and sudden deterioration in health status and prognosis, and patient, family, or physician reluctance to consider hospice care.

PHYSICAL SYMPTOMS AND SIGNS AND THE END-OF-LIFE EXPERIENCE

Despite growing interest in quality of life outcomes, very few surveys have described the "physical" experience of the last weeks, days, or hours of patients with cancer. End-of-life care must be responsive to individual needs and distress; nonetheless, it is helpful for physicians, patients, and health care providers to have some understanding of the common sources of patient and family distress. In addition to facilitating the optimization of individual care plans, the development of an understanding of expected and common outcomes is essential if standards of care and quality monitoring are to be implemented in the end-of-life setting.

A number of factors must be considered when interpreting the data that relate to the end-of-life experience of breast cancer patients. Among the factors that limit our understanding of the experience of this group of patients is the fact that most studies focusing on the end-of-life experience have been undertaken in the hospice or palliative care setting, although, as noted, most deaths in developed countries occur in the hospital setting. Furthermore, the majority of the surveys of cancer patients have been conducted in the United Kingdom, Europe, and Canada, and few contain information specific to the breast cancer experience. Most surveys of advanced cancer patients have been undertaken at various points during the course of the disease, such as at admission to hospice or the palliative care unit,[37–42] or have represented attempts to quantify the prevalence and impact of particular symptoms in the setting of advanced disease,[43–60] with a paucity of longitudinal information available to quantify the development or the resolution of symptoms over time. Several investigations have focused specifically on the dying process or the last weeks of life,[29,61–75] and others have highlighted aspects of the dying process by characterizing the differences in the quality of care provided by inpatient and home care services.[24,76–80] The interpretation of these surveys is rendered more complex by the wide variability in the quality of the methodologies used in these studies. For example, two aspects of the "physical experience," symptom distress and mental state before death, have been the focus of a number of investigations, yet the investigations of these have been hampered by the (not uncommon) failure of investigators to use validated instruments for assessment and the methodologic difficulties that arise when assessing symptoms and distress in the very ill. Many surveys have been conducted without patient self-report providing the basis of the report of distress. Moreover, especially in the weeks before death, a proportion of patients are usually unable to complete outcome measures; in such cases, reports are often provided by a caregiver, usually a family member. Although family and health professional perceptions are important and may, in part, reflect the patient experience, retrospective "third party" assessments have been demonstrated to correlate poorly with the patient's perception of pain and other symptoms.[81,82] Numerous other methodologic issues must be considered when interpreting data pertaining to symptom distress, not the least of which is that many surveys do not document pain syndromes or treatments, and therefore the impact of undertreatment on symptom distress cannot be ascertained.

Methodologic difficulties notwithstanding, the array of available surveys demonstrates that there is a degree of commonality in the end-of-life experience. A spectrum of symptoms are commonly in need of intervention, symptoms are frequently undertreated, and the variability in the experience and in patient preferences and goals is significant and implies that no one model of care suffices to address the needs of all individuals.[30]

TABLE 1. *Symptom prevalence in 70 patients with breast cancer*

Symptom	Prevalence (%)
Lack of energy	80.0
Worrying	75.0
Feeling sad	68.6
Pain	60.0
Feeling nervous	68.6
Feeling drowsy	68.1
Dry mouth	62.9
Difficulty sleeping	48.6
Feeling irritable	48.6
Lack of appetite	51.4
Nausea	44.9
Difficulty concentrating	44.3
Numbness/tingling in hands/feet	33.8
Feeling bloated	43.5
Change in taste	37.1
Constipation	30.0
Cough	37.1
"I don't look like myself"	36.8
Itching	26.5
Weight loss	30.9
Swelling of arms or legs	32.9
Problems with sexual interest or activity	20.3
Dizziness	31.9
Diarrhea	25.7
Shortness of breath	25.7
Vomiting	27.1
Problems with urination	15.7
Hair loss	23.2
Mouth sores	20.0
Difficulty swallowing	14.5

Adapted from ref. 60.

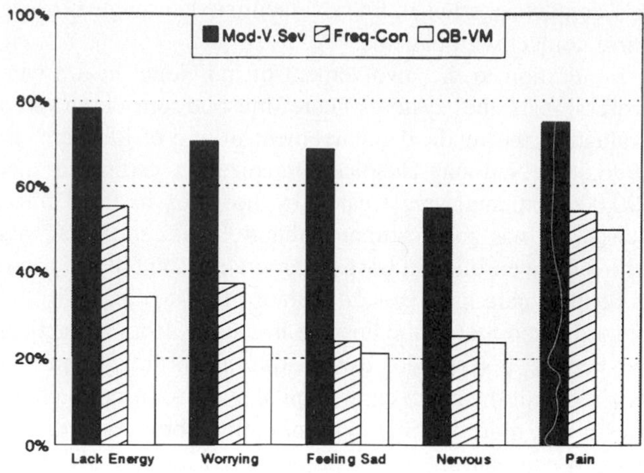

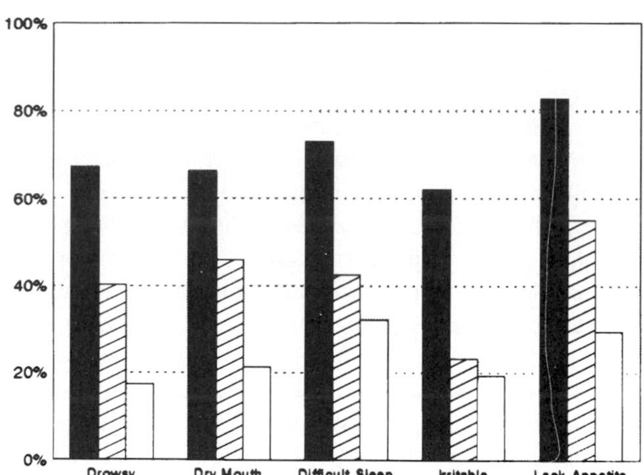

FIG. 1. This figure illustrates the frequency, severity, and distress associated with symptoms in a cancer population. The *solid bar* indicates the proportion of patients who described the symptom as "moderate," "severe," or "very severe." The *hatched bar* indicates the proportion who described the frequency of the symptom as "frequent" or "almost constant." The *open bar* indicates the proportion who described the distress associated with the symptom as "quite a bit" or "severe." (From ref. 60, with permission.)

Spectrum of Symptom Distress in Patients with Advanced Cancer

Given that few studies provide specific information about breast cancer, the information that exists must be interpreted, recognizing that it reflects the "advanced cancer" experience in general. The common symptoms that have been reported in this population include fatigue, pain, anxiety, and anorexia, each with prevalence rates reported to be higher than 50%.[38,41,55,56,60,67,68,72,79] In addition, most patients with advanced cancer experience multiple symptoms.[41,60,68] Although the sources of distress are generally reported as "physical" symptoms (e.g., pain or anorexia), this finding more likely reflects survey methodology that has not addressed "psychological" symptoms, particularly anxiety and depression. Studies that have specifically explored these symptoms have reported them to be common.[40,44,47,49,60,83]

Instruments have now been developed to assess symptoms in a manner that facilitates a more comprehensive assessment of their impact and burden. Symptom prevalence, when reported alone, provides only minimal insight into the degree of distress caused by symptoms. The mere presence of a symptom cannot be viewed as a measure of distress; however, distress itself is a measurable entity, as is the impact of symptoms on function. In a study of 243 cancer patients, of whom 62.6% had metastatic disease and 28.8% had breast cancer, the severity, frequency, and distress associated with each symptom were explored.[60] Table 1 documents the symptom prevalence rates for the breast cancer subpopulation in this study. The most common symptoms reported in the subgroup of patients with breast cancer were fatigue, worrying, feeling sad, nervousness, and drowsiness. The study did not document the severity, frequency, and distress associated with each specific cancer, but Fig. 1 demonstrates these dimensions for the most prevalent symptoms overall. As this figure illustrates, although the symptom characteristics were variable, the proportion of patients who described a symptom as relatively intense or frequent always exceeded the proportion who reported it as highly distressing. Pain, although somewhat less prevalent than other symptoms, was more commonly rated as highly distressing. The mean number of symptoms per patient was 11.5 (±6.0) per patient, with inpatients reporting more symptoms than outpatients (13.5 ± 5.4 versus 9.7 ± 6.0, $p = .002$). Also, those patients with a Karnofsky performance score of less than 80 had more symptoms than those with a score of greater than 80 (14.8 ± 5.5 versus 9.2 ± 4.9, $p = .0001$). Moreover, this study also demonstrated that the number of symptoms per patient was highly associated with heightened psychological distress and poorer quality of life. Although numerous studies could be cited to address symptom prevalence in advanced cancer, this investigation, unlike others, contains information specific to the breast cancer population and is also one of the few studies that has addressed the prevalence of symptoms in addition to symptom distress.[55,60,84]

Coyle et al.[68] also focused on multiple symptoms in an attempt to explore the progression of the symptoms toward the end of life. These investigators reviewed the records of 90 cancer outpatients from the 4 weeks before their deaths. The patients ranged in age from 23 to 82 years, and two-thirds had cancers of lung, colon, or breast. All patients were cared for at home during this period, but only 19% were able to engage in some form of limited activity outside the home. Although the common symptoms at 4 weeks before death (fatigue, pain, weakness, sleepiness, and cognitive impairment) remained common at 1 week before death, there were changes in prevalence. The prevalence of sleepiness, for example, increased from 24% to 57%, whereas pain prevalence decreased from 54% to 34%.

Specific Symptoms in Patients with Advanced Cancer

With regard to the breast cancer experience toward the end of life, several symptoms warrant particular mention, including pain, dyspnea, and anxiety or depression. Large surveys have repeatedly documented that pain is experienced by 70% to 90% of patients with advanced cancer.[85–88] The National Hospice Study (n = 1,754) documented that pain became more prevalent in cancer patients during the last weeks of life, and, of the patients enrolled in this study who could provide self-report data, 25% indicated that persistent or severe pain was present within 2 days of death.[51] This proportion had increased from 17% in the previous 6 days. In the SUPPORT study, 40% to 46% of patients with cancer who had been conscious were perceived by their relatives to have had moderate to severe pain for more than one-half of the time during the last 3 days of life.[31,32]

The interpretation of the data relating to pain at the end of life is complicated by several factors, including the methodologic factors discussed previously and others relating to clinical practice issues. It is further complicated by the widely acknowledged problem of undertreatment of pain, a problem that exists despite the fact that numerous approaches are available to effectively treat pain.[89] The commonly accepted approach to cancer pain relief, outlined in the World Health Organization Cancer Pain Guidelines,[90,91] uses a comprehensive pain assessment and a combination of opioid, nonopioid, and adjuvant drugs titrated to the individual needs of the patient according to the severity of the pain. These guidelines have been tested in numerous studies, which have confirmed that this approach can provide adequate pain relief for 70% to 90% of cancer patients who experience cancer pain.[89,92–96] Other, somewhat more complex, interventions are available to address pain that is not responsive to the simple "guideline" interventions.[89] Nonetheless, a wealth of data indicate that pain is undertreated. For example, in the United States, a survey of 1,308 oncology outpatients being treated by the physician members of the Eastern Cooperative Oncology Group reports that 67% of patients described recent pain, and 36% reported pain that was severe enough to impair function.[97] Forty-two percent of the patients who reported pain were not given adequate analgesia, and 86% of the physicians believed that the majority of cancer patients with pain were undermedicated.[98] Similar findings have been reported in a survey undertaken in France.[99] As a consequence of these findings, it is not possible to ascertain whether the high prevalence of pain in advanced disease reflects worsening pathology, undertreatment, or both.

Another symptom commonly reported toward the end of life is dyspnea. Variable prevalence rates have been described in advanced cancer, ranging from 20% to 78%.[53,57,59,66] Methodologic inconsistencies between studies likely account, at least in part, for this wide variation. Two studies have reported that dyspnea increases at the end of life. The National Hospice Study reported that dyspnea was present in 70% of 1,754 patients during the final 6 weeks of life,[53] and a study by Higginson and McCarthy[57] of 86 cancer patients found that dyspnea was a severe symptom near death. The SUPPORT study reported dyspnea as being moderate to severe for the last few days of life in 70% and 30% of lung and colon cancer patients, respectively. Of note, the prevalence of dyspnea in breast cancer patients in the study by Portenoy et al.,[60] described previously, was 25.7%. Dyspnea, although not a symptom that has been studied as intensively as pain, is treatable, and management guidelines exist that describe effective strategies to minimize patient distress.[100] As with the data on pain, these studies do not contain details of symptom management strategies, and prevalence likely reflects, in part, undertreatment.

Anxiety, worry, nervousness, and sadness have commonly been reported in patients with advanced cancer.[40,44,47,49,60,83] In an interview-based study of 44 patients with metastatic breast cancer undertaken between 1 and 7 weeks before their death, 66% scored in the case range for anxiety, and 50% were in the range for depression.[101] As with the symptoms discussed above, effective treatment guidelines have been described for these conditions.[102]

Symptoms in the Last Hours of Life

The data describing the experience of cancer patients in the last hours of life come from descriptive surveys and, most commonly, from hospice and palliative care settings.

Most deaths in these settings are reported to have been "peaceful."[65,69] Most studies reporting the experiences of cancer patients during the last hours of life incorporate methodology based on observer reports, with the observers including family members, other caregivers, and nursing or medical staff.[29,65–70,72–74,103] The difficulties encountered in the assessment of the imminently dying population have led clinicians and investigators to rely on such reports despite concerns about the validity of this approach. Observer-based reports, especially those describing the clinical status of uncommunicative patients, describe clinical situations, and, although such reports may imply that distress was present, it cannot be concluded with certainty that the observed patient was aware of distress. Methodologic difficulties notwithstanding, the most frequently reported symptoms present in the last hours of life include pain, dyspnea, congestion, and restlessness.[29,65–70,72–74,103] Saunders[65] documented the hospice inpatient experiences of 98 of 100 consecutive patients with terminal cancer and reported that 60% of patients were "peaceful" for 24 hours or longer, 27% had some "transient distress" in the period between 4 and 24 hours before death, and 13% had "transient distress" present only in the 4-hour period immediately before death. Considerable discussion and controversy exist in the palliative care literature about the role of sedative medications in the management of "unendurable" symptoms at the end of life. A 1991 survey of 100 cancer patients in the last days of life observed that only 18% of them required sedating treatment for pain or delirium, although 57% of patients were unresponsive by the day of death.[72] The proportion of patients who have intolerable symptoms remains unresolved, and, of the few studies that exist, even fewer have included any analysis of the interaction between symptoms and palliative interventions with such medication use.

The routine use of simple measures to quantify self-reported distress, along with the implementation of existing treatment guidelines, has the potential to greatly improve the end-of-life experience for patients. Nonetheless, as discussed previously, the assessment of distress in the imminently dying continues to pose significant methodologic challenges. If the dimensions of apparent distress in the dying are to be quantified and the impact of treatments on apparent distress in this population is to be assessed, the development of instruments to facilitate the comparison of observations made by health care professionals, families, and other caregivers is also important. At the bedside, the relief of apparent distress remains contingent on skilled and attentive nursing care and medical care that is reactive to reported, observed, and apparent distress by means of careful physical assessment and the skilled use of nursing and pharmacologic interventions.

Performance Status, Mental Status, and Consciousness toward the End of Life

Epidemiologic surveys have rarely focused on detailed descriptions of either performance status or mental status toward the end of life. In a 1974 British study of 279 deaths occurring in patients with a variety of cancers (17 breast cancer deaths), 69% of the patients who died at home and 77% of those who died in the hospital spent fewer than 3 weeks unable to get out of bed without assistance before death. Fifteen percent of the homebound patients and 5% of the hospital patients were reported as "never" being bedfast before death.[63] Although these data cannot be extrapolated to draw conclusions about the experience of patients in the late 1990s or the experience of patients with specific cancers, such as breast cancer, this report suggests that although patients may not be able to undertake work activities close to the end of life, it is possible for the majority of cancer patients to maintain a high performance status until close to death. Of note, this study also reflects a population and time period in which treatment strategies were not as effective as those implemented in the 1990s.

Level of consciousness toward the end of life is influenced by a diverse range of factors, including extent of disease, coexisting organ failure, and medication use. Specific breast cancer data are, again, not available. The SUPPORT study describes the experiences of lung cancer patients (n = 409) and documents that 80% were reported by family members to be conscious for the 3 days before death, with 55% reported as being able to communicate effectively at this time.[32] In the colon cancer population (n = 148), these figures were 70% and 40%, respectively. A survey of cancer patients who died at St. Christopher's Hospice in the United Kingdom describes 10% as alert, 67% as drowsy or semiconscious, and 23% as unarousable or unconscious during the 24 hours before death.[65] Another small survey of inpatient and home care cancer deaths found that one-third of these patients were able to interact 24 hours before death; this decreased to one-fifth at 12 hours before death and one-tenth in the hour before death.[104]

Although most cancer patients appear to remain alert until close to death, delirium has been found to be highly prevalent in this population, particularly in the days immediately before death. Massie et al.[48] report that delirium developed in 11 (85%) of 13 terminally ill cancer patients before death, with the early symptoms often misdiagnosed as anxiety, anger, depression, or psychosis. Posner defined the potential etiologies of delirium as "direct effects" related to tumor involvement and "indirect effects"; the latter category includes drugs, electrolyte imbalance, cranial irradiation, organ failure, nutritional deficiencies, vascular complications, paraneoplastic syndromes, and other factors.[105–111] In a survey of 94 cancer patients referred for neurologic assessment of encephalopathy, a multifactorial etiology of this problem was demonstrated in most patients, with metabolic causes, drugs, and central nervous system metastases being the most common etiologic factors.[112] Bruera et al.[113] studied 66 episodes of cognitive failure in 39 patients admitted to a palliative care service and demonstrated that this condition is often reversible during the last weeks of life. Drugs, sepsis, and brain metastasis were found to be the most frequently detected etiologic factors, and 22 (33%) of the 66 episodes improved, 10 spontaneously and 12 as a

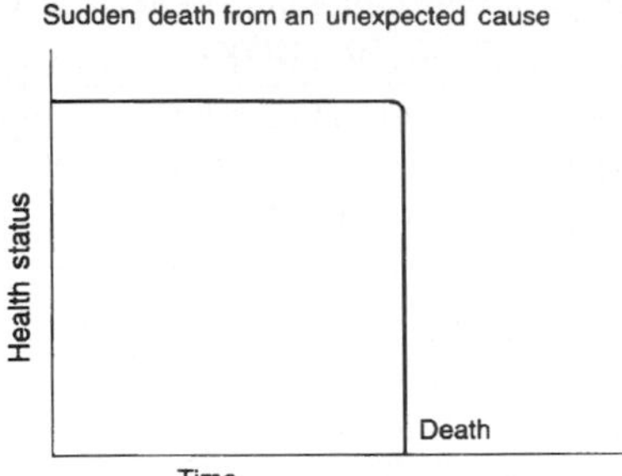

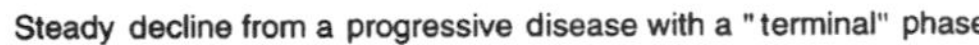

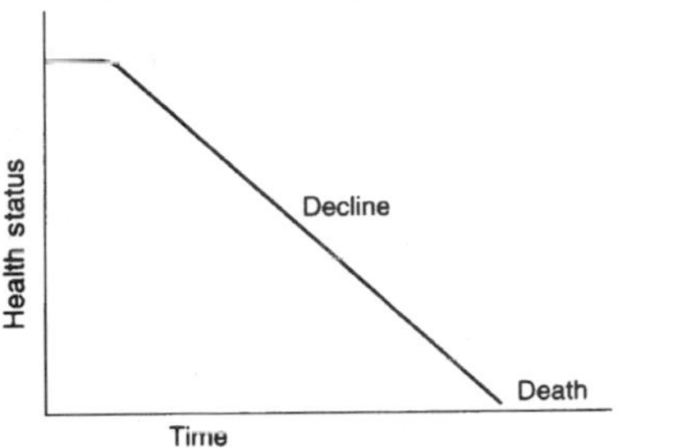

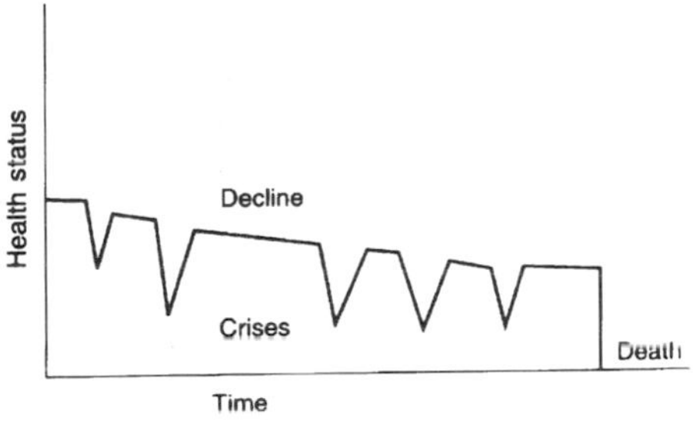

FIG. 2. Death trajectories. This figure represents greatly simplified examples of three possible trajectories toward death. (From ref. 30, with permission.)

result of treatment. The treatment interventions in this study included strategies that treated the cognitive impairment itself in addition to those that focused on addressing etiologic factors. For example, neuroleptic drugs were used to treat agitation, *and* if an electrolyte disturbance or a particular medication was identified as being a contributing factor, an attempt was made to remove it or to minimize its impact.

Performance status and level of consciousness contribute to the concept of a "trajectory of dying," which has been used to describe the similarities and differences in patient experiences over the course of illness that leads to death[30,114–117] (Fig. 2). Little, if any, information is available to accurately describe the common breast cancer trajectory, but the clinical perception of the experience reflects a combination of the trajectories B and C described in Fig. 2. Clearly, the trajectory of illness is an individual experience, and new treatment strategies, with an intensified focus on quality of life and maintenance of function, have the potential to affect this trajectory through impact on disease progression, performance status, symptom distress, and overall quality of life. It is feasible, for example, that the common trajectory of disease could begin to reflect more of a combination of trajectories A and C. The trajectory is an important consideration for a variety of reasons. First, the preference of most individuals with breast cancer is to maintain function and quality of life for the maximum length of time, and the trajectory of illness is reflective, in part, of the outcome of interventions. In addition, an understanding of the "common trajectory" is important in facilitating planning for expected contingencies. For example, if the trajectory A is to begin to reflect the more common course of disease progression, patients and families may need to be aware that precipitous functional decline and sudden death are a possibility, whereas trajectory B is likely to be associated with higher needs for physical assistance and support toward the end of life. Furthermore, these issues are highly relevant when consideration is being given to health system–related interventions for patients and families. For example, the role and functioning of hospice programs most likely needs to be reconsidered if new treatments result in disease trajectories that differ significantly from those that have traditionally been expected.

Treatment Interventions for Symptom Management toward the End of Life

It is beyond the scope of this chapter to address the specific strategies that exist to address each of the symptoms that may occur toward the end of life. The fields of pain management and palliative care have evolved to such a degree that extensive literature addresses the palliation of each of the many common symptoms that arise in patients with advanced cancer-related disease. Although more research-based data would be optimal to quantify the end-of-life experience, it is apparent from the hospice literature and the clinical experience of palliative care clinicians and oncologists that comfort can be achieved in almost all patients. Comprehensive textbooks are available that address many aspects of palliative care,[118,119] and included in these texts are extensive reviews of the assessment and treatment of specific symptoms, such as pain,[88,89,120] dyspnea,[100,121] confusion,[122–124] anxiety and depression,[102] and sleep disturbance.[125] As discussed, despite the existence of an array of symptom-specific treatment strategies, evidence remains that these treatment strategies are underused or are not optimally implemented, or both.[32,97,98,126,127]

Finally, although palliative care is a growing field of both clinical and research endeavor, the scientific basis on which treatment decisions are made regarding the implementation of symptom relief strategies varies greatly in depth and quality. For example, pain research has evolved as a field of endeavor, with an extensive and rapidly evolving research base that addresses a myriad of aspects of this symptom. Major advances have been made in the understanding of pain-related basic pathophysiologic mechanisms, assessment methodologies, treatment interventions, societal barriers to effective pain relief, and effective educational strategies for health professionals. Although research that focuses on other aspects of distress is evolving, in comparison to pain, there is far less information relating to other symptoms, including, for example, confusion, restlessness, and dyspnea.

These concerns notwithstanding, significant advances have been made in this field. For example, validated tools have been developed to assess distress associated with common symptoms in the cognitively intact patient, and, consequently, the impact of treatment interventions directed toward the palliation of these common symptoms can now be accurately assessed.[60,84,128–130] In addition, assessment instruments have been developed that can facilitate the assessment of delirium and cognitive impairment.[122,131] Numerous aspects of palliative care remain in need of further research—including, for example, the development of instruments for the assessment of distress in cases in which self-report is not feasible, interventions to minimize the distress associated with less common but distressing symptoms, and the barriers to symptom relief and approaches to eliminating those barriers.

CAREGIVER EXPERIENCES TOWARD THE END OF LIFE

Although most caregivers (primarily family members) are highly motivated and committed to providing care, the caregivers of cancer patients experience substantial burdens.[132–138] Not only is the caregiver called on to provide emotional support for the patient through periods of stress, but, with shifts in care occurring from inpatient to outpatient settings, caregivers also are increasingly being required to provide medical and nursing care in the home. Moreover, particularly in developing countries where patients may have little or no access to health care professionals, the family caregiver may be the *only* caregiver toward the end of a patient's life.

In a survey of 492 caregivers of cancer patients, the caregivers reported needs in a variety of categories: informational, household, physical, psychological, spiritual, legal and financial, respite care, and others.[132] The needs that these caregivers most frequently defined as important and unsatisfied are listed, in order of frequency, in Table 2.[132] The needs of, and burdens experienced by, caregivers impact on patients and caregivers and, although little has been documented that is specific to the breast cancer population, this impact can be substantial toward the end of life. Most attempts at quantifying the impact of caregiving have focused on negative aspects of caregiving, and few investigators have explored the positive aspects of providing care.[139] The impact of increasing caregiver burden on patients has been demonstrated. Unmet patient needs occur more frequently in settings in which the burden of care on caregivers is greater—for example, in situations in which patients are greatly debilitated or financial resources are limited.[133,134] Data also exist to quantify aspects of the impact of caregiving on caregivers. Although the SUPPORT study did not report on data specific to the breast cancer experience,[135] the investigators reported that 34% of patients nearing the end of life required "considerable assistance" from a family member. In 20% of cases, the family caregiver had to quit work or make a major life change to provide care. Loss of most or all of the family savings was reported by 31% of families. In the families in which increased economic hardship was present, a preference for comfort care over life-extending care was more commonly expressed by patients.[137] Numerous aspects of the health and sense of well-being of caregivers can be affected by the experience of living with a family member who is nearing the end of life.[136,138] Moreover, the period of bereavement after the loss of a family member can have a significant physical and psychological impact.[136]

Some investigators have explored the factors that place caregivers at greater risk for experiencing the negative outcomes associated with caregiving. For example, a study of 302 cancer patients explored the predictors of anxiety in family members or caregivers in the last 4 weeks of life.[140] The diagnosis of breast cancer, younger age, low patient mobility, and shorter time from diagnosis to death were all cited as predictors of family anxiety. The SUPPORT study reported that the families that were more likely to experience significant impact were those of the younger, poorer, and more functionally dependent patients.[137]

Further information is needed that is specific to the impact of caring on the caregivers of patients with breast cancer.

TABLE 2. *Top 25 barrier needs reported by 492 caregivers of cancer patients*

1. Information about the underlying reasons for symptoms
2. Information about what symptoms to expect
3. Information about what to expect in the future
4. Information about treatment of side effects
5. Information about community resources
6. Honest and updated information
7. Ways to reassure my patient
8. Ways to deal with my patient's decreased energy
9. Ways to deal with the unpredictability of the future
10. Information about medications (side effects and scheduling)
11. Ways to encourage my patient
12. Information about my patient's psychological needs
13. Methods to decrease my stress
14. Ways of coping with my patient's diagnosis of cancer
15. Information about the type and extent of my patient's illness
16. Ways to cope with role changes
17. Information about the physical needs of my patient
18. Activities that will make my patient feel purposeful
19. Ways to be more patient and tolerant
20. Ways to deal with my depression
21. Ways to maintain a normal family life
22. Ways to discuss death with my patient
23. Ways to deal with my fears
24. Ways to combat fatigue
25. Ways to provide my patient with adequate nutrition

From ref. 132, with permission.

Likewise, controlled clinical trials should be undertaken of family-based interventions designed to minimize caregiver burden and optimize caregiver health. The absence of data notwithstanding, it is apparent that significant stresses on caregivers exist and that caregivers are extremely important in the lives of patients with cancer. It is therefore imperative that health care professionals pay heed to assessment of caregiver needs and explore and implement strategies that aim to assist in minimizing caregiver burden.[141,142] From a policy perspective, a need exists for increasing attention to be given to the provision of assistance to caregivers who are instrumental in the provision of medical and nursing care for patients with cancer. This is occurring in a number of countries, and, in an attempt to further encourage such initiatives, the World Health Organization has made recommendations that suggest the implementation of policies that address formal systems of recompense for principal family caregivers and the implementation of medical and nursing programs to back up and support home care.[91,143]

TABLE 3. *American Medical Association Institute for Ethics elements of quality of end-of-life care for patients in the last phase of life*

1. The opportunity to discuss and plan end-of-life care
2. Trustworthy assurance that physical and mental suffering will be carefully attended to and comfort measures intently secured
3. Trustworthy assurance that preferences for withholding or withdrawing life-sustaining intervention will be honored
4. Trustworthy assurance that there will be no abandonment by the physician
5. Trustworthy assurance that dignity will be a priority
6. Trustworthy assurance that burden to family and others will be minimized
7. Attention to the personal goals related to the dying process
8. Trustworthy assurance that caregivers will assist the bereaved through the early stages of mourning and adjustment

Adapted from ref. 145.

OPTIMAL END-OF-LIFE CARE FOR PATIENTS WITH BREAST CANCER

Optimal end-of-life care is inseparable from optimal care throughout the course of illness. The care of breast cancer patients and their families during the last phase of life requires a commitment on the part of individual oncologists and families to assisting patients through this time of life and a broader commitment to fostering optimal care from the institutions involved in care delivery and from those responsible for the shaping of health policy. The perception of optimal care varies, but it can be broadly defined as follows: "Optimal care for each patient depends upon determination of the most appropriate and realistic goals of medical treatment and implementing appropriate treatment measures designed to achieve those goals."[144] Such goals can only be determined by ongoing interactions between physicians, patients, and families. Physicians in this setting should optimally be compassionate, considerate, and skilled and knowledgeable in areas related to patient and family assessment and options for interventions. Although the appropriate health professional for a specific intervention may not be the oncologist or even a physician, physicians are commonly the "gatekeepers" of the health system and therefore need to have an understanding of the assessment of distress to facilitate appropriate referral. In addition, in such assessments, physicians and other professionals should be attuned to, and respectful of, patient and family needs, preferences, and cultural priorities.

In 1998, the American Society for Clinical Oncology (ASCO)[145] published guidelines that address cancer care toward the end of life. These guidelines address the components of care that are considered essential to a humane system of cancer care and the barriers that must be addressed if such a system is to be fully implemented. The section that follows addresses those elements and barriers and provides some information about a practical approach to the assessment of patients who are experiencing increasingly burdensome illness or are nearing the end of life, or both.

Components of Optimal End-of-Life Care

The ASCO statement on cancer care during the last phase of life defines the components of optimal care at the end of life.[145] This statement suggests that cancer care should be centered around the long-standing and continuous relationship between the patient and primary oncologist or other physician with training and interest in end-of-life care. Furthermore, cancer care should be responsive to the patient's wishes and based on truthful, sensitive, and empathic communication with the patient. Cancer care should, throughout the course of illness, focus on and optimize quality of life with "meticulous attention to the myriad of physical, spiritual, and psychosocial needs of the patient and family." To elaborate, the ASCO statement supported and reiterated the American Medical Association Institute for Ethics statement that defined eight elements of quality end-of-life care[145] (Table 3). Essentially, the ASCO statement embraced and firmly endorsed the concept of integrating the principles of palliative care throughout the course of illness. Such an approach, as represented figuratively by the Canadian Palliative Care Association in Fig. 3,[146] represents a proactive approach to end-of-life distress and an attempt to optimize care through the course of cancer.

Practical Aspects of Optimal End-of-Life Care

From a practical perspective, end-of-life care involves a series of assessments that result in a care plan. The "palliative care" components of such an assessment, in nearly all

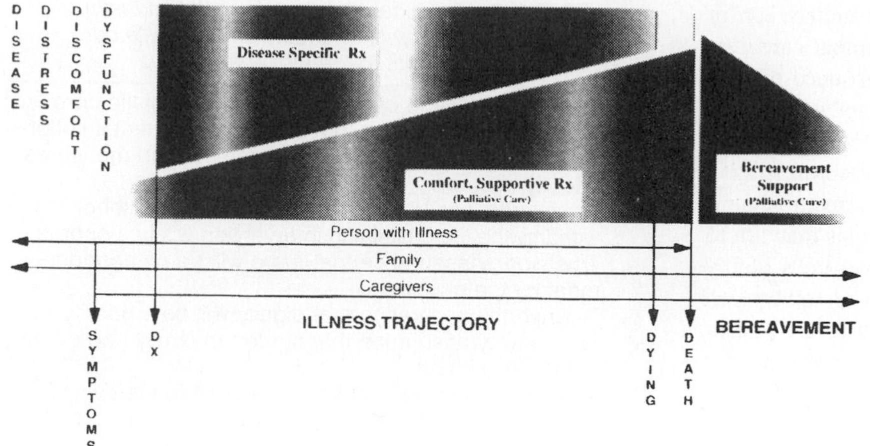

FIG. 3. The continuum of palliative care: figurative representation of the incorporation of palliative care throughout the course of illness. Dx, diagnosis; Rx, medication. (From ref. 146, with permission.)

cases, overlaps with the components that are focused on the therapeutic interventions directed toward the oncologic problem. The assessment and plan, by necessity, must therefore reflect an understanding of both of these aspects of care.

A complete assessment must include assessment of disease status and prognosis; patient and family preferences and goals, including advanced care plans; patient emotional status and spiritual needs; family functioning and needs; patient functional status; therapeutic options and their relative benefits and burdens; and available resources[30] (Table 4). The plan should reflect an understanding of the patient and family goals, which themselves may need to be repeatedly addressed as disease progresses. Recognizing that the choices that a patient or family makes in the last days or hours of life may be the same or different from their previously expressed preferences is important. In each individual case, health care professionals must be attentive to the goals and needs of patients and families and seek to assist in decision making with an understanding of the available resources. In developing the plan of care, from a practical point of view with respect to the delivery of patient care and from a more global care perspective, it is important to consider the patient *and* family (or caregivers) as the "unit" around which the care plan should be centered. As discussed in the section Caregiver Experiences toward the End of Life, not only are family caregivers often those who are responsible for the delivery of direct patient care, but they also represent a population that is likely to benefit from interventions directed toward their own health and well-being.

The plan of care should incorporate an approach to plan reassessment in the setting of new problems or clinical changes. Oncologists who provide care for cancer patients with advanced disease are in a position to recognize changes in disease suggesting that the care plan should be reviewed. Transitions in disease status that necessitate a change in the care plan can be either subtle or dramatic. Often, such transitions occur around a hospitalization, with the diagnosis of disease in a new site, or with the failure of a particular therapeutic approach to control the disease. Transitions should be responded to with a review and update of the care plan.

After an assessment of the disease status and the patient and family needs, and consideration of the problems that are expected to occur in the future, it can be helpful to consider some specific questions about the care plan. These questions,

TABLE 4. *Assessment components of a comprehensive oncology care management plan (including palliative care assessments)*

1. *Disease status and symptom assessment.* Consider treatment options, prognosis, and anticipated symptoms. An understanding of the extent of disease and concurrent disease is essential in planning appropriate interventions.
2. *Assessment of functional status.* Assessment of the patient's function should be undertaken with consideration given to the need for assistance or special assessment; for example, physical therapy assessment.
3. *Emotional and spiritual assessment.* Consider these issues and the role of referral to social work, psychological, pastoral, or spiritual counselor for either assessment or intervention.
4. *Assessment of patient/family goals and preferences.* Initiate discussion of these and consider issues related to identification of surrogate decision maker and documentation of preferences.
5. *Family assessment.* Specific attention should be given to family coping, needs, family understanding of the disease and likely developments, and the support systems (specific providers and nonprofessional supports) that are in place.
6. *Therapy review and evaluation.* Regular and event-driven reviews should be planned with assessment of medications, nonpharmacologic therapies, and the benefits and burdens of therapies.
7. *Resource review and evaluation.* Regular and event-driven reviews should be planned with assessment of support systems (specific providers and nonprofessional supports) and physical supports. Consideration should be given to available resources and whether these could be used more efficiently or effectively. Particular attention should be given to whether resources will be adequate to address any anticipated patient and/or family crises or distress.

Adapted from ref. 30.

which relate broadly to the "system of care," include the following: Whom will the family call if something becomes problematic? Are increased patient or family supports needed? Have the patient and family needs been fully defined and all available resources accessed? With regard to the latter, oncologists should develop an understanding of other resources available and question whether the patient or family, or both, would be likely to benefit from specialized review to either assist in the defining of needs or to deliver care. Such assessments or interventions could, for example, be undertaken by a palliative care physician or nurse, a social worker, a counselor, a physical therapist, a nurse with special expertise in pain or wound management, or a chaplain. Other specific questions that can be helpful in planning care include the following: Does the system of care represent that which is most expert in meeting the needs of the patient and family? Will the system of care be capable of meeting the *anticipated* needs? Would this patient benefit from a proactive system of home care or a system that has the capacity to facilitate a visit by a nurse or another health professional to the home in an emergency, or both?

The need for care at the end of life often intensifies, rather than lessens, and an expansion of the team of caregivers is often important if needs are to be addressed. In this process, physicians should be cognizant of the stresses that advanced disease can cause and aware that patients may benefit from the system of care being made less unwieldy. Easy access to care by the patient and caregivers is imperative in the setting of far-advanced illness, regardless of goals of care. A comfort-related intervention may require as urgent a response as a life-sustaining intervention. To facilitate access, it can be helpful to have one point of access to the "system of care" for the patient and family, such as a dedicated nurse to assist in triaging the patient's concerns. Furthermore, patients and families may benefit from a proactive approach to their concerns; for example, a proactive telephone call from a physician or nurse may detect and avert an impending crisis.

The expert knowledge of a physician who has an understanding of the physiology of disease, distress, and pharmacologic interventions can be invaluable in the care of patients who are nearing the end of life. Most important, however, in devising a practical plan, it should be recognized that, although the expertise of a physician is important, patient care is likely to be optimized through a team approach to care that incorporates the specialized input of a number of professionals. Numerous practical issues often need to be assessed, and frequently the team is most appropriately coordinated by a nurse who can anticipate and assess patient problems in the home and triage accordingly. Roles vary within the team and often overlap. For example, social workers, who are frequently charged with devising a hospital discharge plan that can be responsive to patient and family needs, cannot be expected to have the same depth of understanding as an oncologist of likely disease progression and the medical problems that may arise. Similarly, an oncologist may not have the same array of counseling skills as a social worker or counselor. Community-based nurses may not have the same knowledge of therapeutic options as an oncologist, but an oncologist may not be able to assess all patients in their homes. Through collaborative efforts that recognize the importance of the skills of each team member and foster effective communication within the team, plans can be shaped and responsive care delivered.

The available systems for end-of-life care vary among regions and nations. In the United States and in many other countries, hospice and palliative care teams are available to assist oncology health professionals in the delivery of care. Some of these teams focus solely on patients who seek only comfort measures, and others participate in the delivery of care to those who are living with advanced illness and yet are still seeking life-sustaining therapies. If the goals, as defined by the patient and family, fit with the philosophy of care of a hospice or palliative care team, then the system of care can often be both intensified and optimized by a referral to this team. In most cases, such teams foster continued involvement by the oncologist as the primary physician and therefore truly reflect an intensification of the system of care rather than a major shift in care delivery. Many of these teams also offer specialized physician services to complement the oncology expertise through the availability of specialized symptom management input.

Optimal end-of-life care is contingent on many factors. In delivering such care, physicians, nurses, and other health care professionals need to be skilled and knowledgeable, compassionate and humane. The spectrum of problems encountered in the period before death reflects the breadth of problems that patients and families experience during the course of a lifetime. Consequently, it is not possible to address all aspects of end-of-life care in this chapter. Toward the end of life, intensified skill and expertise are not infrequently needed by health professionals around a number of aspects of care. The assessment and management of individual symptoms can be challenging, communication may need to reflect an understanding of a myriad of personal and cultural issues, and any array of complex issues may arise relating to family conflicts, existential concerns, physician-assisted suicide, and euthanasia. Focused, detailed, and extensive analysis would be required to effectively address each of these topics and to provide clinicians with an understanding of how to address each of these matters with their patients. Although it is beyond the scope of this chapter to address each of these topics, specialized texts are now available that address these and many other specific issues that arise in palliative care settings.[118,119]

Finally, an important component of optimal end-of-life care is the evaluation of that care. Although measures have been developed to assess an array of specific symptoms and quality of life, the development of much-improved information systems and tools for measuring outcomes at this time of life is critical to the creation of effective and accountable systems of care and to the effective functioning of internal and external systems of quality monitoring and improvement.[30] Although many efforts are being made within the United

States and other countries to improve end-of-life care, when encountering a patient in need of end-of-life care, physicians often find a health care system that is not structured in a way that fosters the provision of optimal end-of-life care. Much potential exists for the improvement of care toward the end of life, and the challenge for all physicians involved in care of the dying is to explore the options available in their practice environment and, in collaboration with others, to slowly build a system that ultimately improves the care of the dying in their community.

Barriers to Optimal Symptom Management and End-of-Life Care

Numerous barriers exist that interfere with optimal symptom management and end-of-life care.[130,145,147] Through the development of an understanding of these barriers, physicians and other health professionals can proceed to address and minimize the problems that hinder the delivery of optimal end-of-life care. These barriers can be found at the level of the patient and family, among the health care professionals, and within health care systems.

The barriers to symptom management are linked to the symptom itself and to the broader concepts that influence end-of-life care. For example, frequently encountered barriers to effective pain management include fears among patients, family members, and physicians about the use of opioids for pain; patient stoicism related to the reporting of pain; problems related to caregiver burden and its impact on the administration of pain relief; economic barriers that impede access to pain medicines and physician care; limited physician knowledge about pain management; and numerous other factors.[147]

The guidelines published by ASCO[145] defined several significant, broad areas in which barriers to high-quality end-of-life care exist. Clinical barriers included attitudinal issues related to death that were viewed as "inappropriate," ineffective communication between patients and physicians, fragmentation of health care, and lack of availability, or lack of access to, high-quality end-of-life care. To address these concerns, the ASCO Task Force suggested an intensified focus on education, a recognition of the need to incorporate palliative care principles throughout the course of cancer treatment, the broader establishment of palliative care programs, and an increased focus on the patient and family dynamic within the context of cancer care. In particular, the development of training programs, formal curricula, and other educational initiatives was encouraged, with the aim of addressing educational deficits. Economic barriers were defined, and an emphasis was placed on encouraging those responsible for reimbursement systems to address policy matters that relate to many issues, including, for example, disincentives that hinder optimal end-of-life care and standards that would ensure more uniform coverage for the provision of opioids. Research initiatives were suggested that would foster an increased focus on outcomes, predictors, and interventions during the last phase of life. The report also suggested that, in the United States, hospice services need to be used more effectively. Finally, the task force addressed the complex problem of physician-assisted suicide and, although neither condoning nor condemning the practice, stated that the intensity of the national debate in the United States was obscuring the essential problem that many patients do not receive optimal end-of-life care.

From an organizational perspective, it has been suggested that care can be improved through the development of cancer programs that commit to embracing four essential components of cancer treatment: the prevention of cancer, the early diagnosis of cancer, treatments to cure and prolong the lives of patients with cancer, and the prevention and treatment of suffering.[148] An extensive report produced by the U.S. Institute of Medicine (IOM) addressed, in detail, similar concerns as those addressed by ASCO and made similar recommendations.[30] An additional recommendation by the IOM related to the need for continued public discussion to develop a better understanding of the modern experience of dying and of the obligation of communities to those who are approaching death.

Although the ASCO and the IOM reports address the care of patients within the United States,[30,145] they have broad applicability worldwide. Within many health systems, practical barriers exist related to inadequate access to health care, particularly for the poor, the elderly, and minorities. Laws that relate to the prescribing of opioid analgesics impede effective pain management, and, in some countries, the availability of opioids for medical use continues to be extremely limited. Worldwide, access and economic barriers are major impediments to optimal end-of-life care. Although the poor in developed countries, such as the United States, often experience such problems, the most dramatic access-related disparities exist between those who live in developed nations and those who reside in developing nations.[143] Globally, the major barrier that impedes the improvement of end-of-life care relates to unevenly distributed resources. Almost 60% of the world's new cancer patients present in developing countries, with at least 80% of these individuals presenting with incurable cancer at the time of diagnosis.[143] Only 5% of the world's total resources for cancer control are in developing countries, in which the large part of the resources is being spent on strategies directed toward cure, with minimal allocation to palliation.[143] To begin to address these concerns, the World Health Organization has been attempting to foster an increased focus on pain relief and palliative care in health care education and in national health policy development.[90,91]

CONCLUSION

This chapter has reviewed some of the experiences that breast cancer patients encounter during the last phase of life associated with this disease. In addition, the crucial elements of optimal end-of-life care have been discussed. Physicians and nurses who care for breast cancer patients are in a unique and important position to assist these individuals and their families in minimizing distress at this most challenging time of life. Furthermore, through the delivery of optimal end-of-life care, health professionals are in a position to foster positive experiences at the end of life for patients and caregivers.[149] Notwithstanding the many questions that remain unanswered and the research opportunities that abound, the care of breast cancer patients and families should embrace the principles of optimal care described in this chapter to minimize distress and optimize quality of life at the end of life.

REFERENCES

1. World Health Organization: Global health situation. *Weekly Epidemiol Record* 1993;68(6):33–36.
2. Wingo PA, Tong T, Bolden S. Cancer statistics, 1995. *CA Cancer J Clin,* 1995;45:8–30.
3. Rosenberg HM, Ventura SJ, Maurer JD, et al. Births and deaths: United States, 1995. In: National Center for Health Statistics. *Monthly vital statistics report.* Hyattsville, MD: National Center for Health Statistics 1996;45[Suppl 2]:1–40.
4. Landis SH, Murry T, Bolden S, Wingo PA. Cancer statistics, 1998. *CA Cancer J Clin* 1998;48(1):6–30.
5. Ries LAG, Kosary CL, Hankey BF, et al. SEER Cancer Statistics Review, 1973–1994. Bethesda, MD: US Department of Health and Human Services, Public Health Services, National Institutes of Health, National Cancer Institute, 1997.
6. Kosary CL, Gloeckler Ries MS, Miller BA, Hankey BF, Harras A, Edwards BK. SEER Cancer Statistics Review, 1973–1992. Bethesda, MD: US Department of Health and Human Services, Public Health Services, National Institutes of Health, National Cancer Institute, 1996.
7. Parker SL, Davis KJ, Wingo PA, Ries LAG, Heath CW. Cancer statistics by race and ethnicity. *Ca Cancer J Clin* 1998;48(1):31–48.
8. Chu KC. Mortality rates by stage-at-diagnosis. *Semin Surg Oncol* 1994;10:7–11.
9. Henson DE, Ries L, Carriaga MT. Conditional survival of 56,268 patients with breast cancer. *Cancer* 1995;76:237–242.
10. Gardner P, Hudson BL. Advance report of final mortality statistics, 1993. *Mon Vital Stat Rep* 1996;44[Suppl 7]:72.
11. Amer MH. Chemotherapy and pattern of metastases in breast cancer patients. *J Clin Oncol* 1982;19:101.
12. Cho S, Choi H. Causes of death and metastatic patterns in patients with mammary cancer. *Am J Clin Pathol* 1980;73:232.
13. Hagemeister FBJ, Buzdar AU, Luna MA, et al. Causes of death in breast cancer: a clinicopathologic study. *Cancer* 1980;46:162.
14. McGinnis JM, FoegeWH. Real, true and genuine causes of death in the United States—what are they? [Reply]. *Mod Pathol* 1994;7(5):527–528.
15. Townsend J, Frank AO, Fermont D, Dyer S, Karran O, Walgrove A, et al. Terminal cancer care and patients' preference for place of death: a prospective study. *BMJ* 1990;301(6749):415–417.
16. World Health Organization.World health statistics annual 1992. Geneva: World Health Organization, 1992.
17. National Center for Health Statistics. General mortality, 1990. Hyattsville, MD: National Center for Health Statistics, 1994. Data on file.
18. Polissar L, Severson RK, Brown NK. Factors affecting place of death in Washington State, 1968–1981. *J Community Health* 1987;12(1):40–55.
19. Moinpour CM, Polissar L. Factors affecting place of death of hospice and non-hospice cancer patients. *Am J Public Health* 1989;79: 1549–1551.
20. McCusker J. Where cancer patients die: an epidemiologic study. *Public Health Rep* 1983;98:170–177.
21. Moinpour CM, Polissar L, Conrad DA. Factors associated with length of stay in hospice. *Med Care* 1990;28:363–368.
22. Costantini M, Camoirano E, Madeddu L, Bruzzi P, Verganelli E, Henriquet F. Palliative home care and place of death among cancer patients: a population-based study. *Palliat Med* 1993;7:323–331.
23. Mor V, Hiris J. Determinants of site of death among hospice cancer patients. *J Health Soc Behav* 1983;24:375–85.
24. Greer DS, Mor V, Morris JN, Sherwood S, Kidder D, Birnbaum H. An alternative in terminal care: results of the National Hospice Study. *J Chronic Dis* 1986;39:9–26.
25. McMillan A, Mentnech RM, Lubitz J, McBean AM, Russell D. Trends and patterns in place of death for Medicare enrollees. *Health Care Financ Rev* 1990;12:1–7.
26. Sager MA, Easterling DV, Kindig DA, Anderson OW. Changes in the location of death after passage of Medicare's prospective payment system. *N Engl J Med* 1989;320:433–439.
27. Seeman I. National mortality followback survey: 1986. Summary, United States National Center for Health Statistics. *Vital Health Stat* 1992;20:entire issue.
28. Brock DB, Foley DJ. Demography and epidemiology of dying in the US with emphasis on deaths of older persons. *Hosp J* 1998;13(1–2):49–60.
29. Morris JN, Suissa S, Sherwood S, Wright SM, Greer D. Last days: a study of the quality of life of terminally ill cancer patients. *J Chronic Dis* 1986;39(1):47–62.
30. Committee on Care at the End of Life. Approaching death: improving care at the end of life. Field MJ, Cassel CK, eds. Washington: Institute of Medicine, 1997.
31. The SUPPORT Principal Investigators. A controlled trial to improve care for seriously ill hospitalized patients. *JAMA* 1995;274:1591–1598.
32. Lynn J, Teno JM, Phillips RS, Wu AW, Desbiens N, Harrold J, et al. Perceptions by family members of the dying experience of older and seriously ill patients. *Ann Intern Med* 1997;126(2):97–106.
33. McCusker J. The terminal period of cancer: definition and descriptive epidemiology. *J Chronic Dis* 1984;37(5):377–385.
34. Haupt BJ. Characteristics of patients receiving hospice care services: United States, 1994. *Adv Data* 1997;282:1–14.
35. National Hospice Organization (NHO): NHO Statistics. Arlington, VA: National Hospice Organization, 1996.
36. Christakis NA, Escarce JJ. Survival of Medicare patients after enrollment in hospice programs. *N Engl J Med* 1996;335:172–178.
37. Wilkes E. Some problems in cancer management. *Proc Roy Soc Med* 1974;67:1001–1005.
38. Brescia FJ, Adler D, Gray G, Ryan MA, Cimino J, Mamtani R. Hospitalized advanced cancer patients: a profile. *J Pain Symptom Manage* 1990;5:221–227.
39. Brescia F. Approaches to palliative care: notes of a deathwatcher. In: Foley KM, Bonica JJ, Ventafridda V, eds. *Advances in pain research and therapy second international congress on cancer pain,* vol 16. New York: Raven Press, 1990:393–397.
40. McCarthy M. Hospice patients: a pilot study in 12 services. *Palliat Med* 1990;4:93–104.
41. Curtis EB, Krech R, Walsh TD. Common symptoms in patients with advanced cancer. *J Palliat Care* 1991;7:25–29.
42. Donnelly S, Walsh D. The symptoms of advanced cancer. *Semin Oncol* 1995;22[Suppl 3]:67–72.
43. Twycross RG. The use of narcotic analgesics in terminal illness. *J Med Ethics* 1975;1:10–17.
44. Plumb MM, Holland J. Comparative studies of psychological function in patients with advanced cancer. I. Self–reported depressive symptoms. *Psychosom Med* 1977;39:264–276.
45. Levine PM, Silberfarb PM, Lipowski ZJ. Mental disorders in cancer patients: a study of 100 psychiatric referrals. *Cancer* 1978;42:1385–1391.
46. McKegney FP, Bailey LR, Yates JW. Prediction and management of pain in patients with advanced cancer. *Gen Hosp Psychiatry* 1981;3:95–101.
47. Plumb M, Holland J. Comparative studies of psychological function in patients with advanced cancer. II. Interviewer-rated current and past psychological symptoms. *Psychosom Med* 1981;43:243–254.
48. Massie MJ, Holland J, Glass E. Delirium in terminally ill cancer patients. *Am J Psychiatry* 1983;140:1048–1050.
49. Bukberg J, Penman D, Holland JC. Depression in hospitalized cancer patients. *Psychosom Med* 1984;46:199–212.
50. Heyse-Moore L, Baines MJ. Control of other symptoms. In: Saunders C, ed. *The management of terminal malignant disease.* London: Edward Arnold, 1984:100–132.
51. Morris JN, Mor V, Goldberg RJ, Sherwood S, Greer DS, Hiris J. The effect of treatment setting and patient characteristics on pain in ter-

minal cancer patients: a report from the National Hospice Study. *J Chronic Dis* 1986;39:27–35.
52. Reuben DB, Mor V. Nausea and vomiting in terminal cancer patients. *Arch Intern Med* 1986;146:2021–2023.
53. Reuben DB, Mor V. Dyspnea in terminally ill cancer patients. *Chest* 1986;89:234–236.
54. Goldberg RJ, Mor V, Weimann M, Greer DS, Hiris J. Analgesic use in terminal cancer patients: report from the national hospice study. *J Chronic Dis* 1986;39:37–45.
55. Dunlop GM. A study of the relative frequency and importance of gastrointestinal symptoms and weakness in patients with far advanced cancer. *Palliat Med* 1989;4:37–43.
56. Grosvenor M, Bulcavage L, Chlebowski RT. Symptoms potentially influencing weight loss in a cancer population. Correlations with primary site, nutritional status, and chemotherapy administration. *Cancer* 1989;63:330–334.
57. Higginson I, McCarthy M. Measuring symptoms in terminal cancer: are pain and dyspnoea controlled? *J R Soc Med* 1989;82:264–267.
58. Ventafridda V, DeConno F, Ripamonti C, Gamba A, Tamburini M. Quality-of-life assessment during a palliative care programme. *Ann Oncol* 1990;1:415–420.
59. Heyse-Moore LH. How much of a problem is dyspnoea in advanced cancer? *Palliat Med* 1991;5:20–26.
60. Portenoy RK, Thaler HT, Kornblith AB, Lepore JM, Friedlander KH, Coyle N, et al. Symptom prevalence, characteristics and distress in a cancer population. *Qual Life Res* 1994;3:183–189.
61. Exton-Smith AN. Terminal illness in the aged. *Lancet* 1961;2: 305–308.
62. Hinton JM. The physical and mental distress of the dying. *Q J Med* 1963;32:1–21.
63. Ward AWM. Terminal care in malignant disease. *Soc Sci Med* 1974;8:413–420.
64. Witzel L. Behavior of the dying patient. *BMJ* 1975;2:81–82.
65. Saunders C. Pain and impending death. In: Wall P, Melzack R, eds. *Textbook of pain*. New York: Churchill Livingstone, 1984:472–478.
66. Hockley JM, Dunlop R, Davies RJ. Survey of distressing symptoms in dying patients and their families in hospital and the response to a symptom control team. *BMJ (Clin Res Ed)* 1988;296:1715–1717.
67. Reuben DB, Mor V, Hiris J. Clinical symptoms and length of survival in patients with terminal cancer. *Arch Intern Med* 1988;148: 1586–1591.
68. Coyle N, Adelhardt J, Foley KM, Portenoy RK. Character of terminal illness in the advanced cancer patient: pain and other symptoms during the last four weeks of life. *J Pain Symptom Manage* 1990;5:83–93.
69. Lichter I, Hunt E. The last 48 hours of life. *J Palliat Care* 1990;6: 7–15.
70. Ventafridda V, Ripamonti C, De CF, Tamburini M, Cassileth BR. Symptom prevalence and control during cancer patients' last days of life. *J Palliat Care* 1990;6:7–11.
71. Bedard J, Dionne L. The experience of La Maison Michel Sarrazin (1985–1990): profile analysis of 952 terminal cancer patients. *J Palliat Care* 1991;7:48–53.
72. Fainsinger R, Miller MJ, Bruera E, Hanson J, MacEachern T. Symptom control during the last week of life on a palliative care unit. *J Palliat Care* 1991;7:5–11.
73. Brock DB, Holmes MB, Foley DJ, Holmes D. Methodological issues in a survey of the last days of life. In: Wallace RB and Woolson RF, eds. *The epidemiologic study of the elderly*. New York: Oxford University Press, 1992:315–332.
74. Foley DJ, Miles TP, Brock DB, Phillips C. Recounts of elderly deaths: endorsements for the patient self-determination act. *Gerontologist* 1995;35:119–121.
75. Ingham JM, Layman-Goldstein M, Derby S, Hawke W, Hicks J, Portenoy R, et al. Characteristics of the dying process in cancer patients in a hospice and a cancer center. *Proc Am Soc Clin Oncol* 1994;13:172.
76. Kane RL, Wales J, Bernstein L, Leibowitz A, Kaplan S. A randomised controlled trial of hospice care. *Lancet* 1984;1:890–894.
77. Vinciguerra V, Degnan TJ, Sciortino A, O'Connell M, Moore T, Brody R, et al. A comparative assessment of home versus hospital comprehensive treatment for advanced cancer patients. *J Clin Oncol* 1986;4:1521–1528.
78. Ventafridda V, De CF, Vigano A, Ripamonti C, Gallucci M, Gamba A. Comparison of home and hospital care of advanced cancer patients. *Tumori* 1989;75:619–625.
79. Dunphy KP, Amesbury BDW. A comparison of hospice and homecare patients: patterns of referral, patient characteristics and predictors on place of death. *Palliat Med* 1990;4:105–111.
80. Searle C. A comparison of hospice and conventional care. *Soc Sci Med* 1991;32:147–152.
81. Higginson I, Priest P, McCarthy M. Are bereaved family members a valid proxy for a patient's assessment of dying? *Soc Sci Med* 1994;38:553–557.
82. Clipp EC, George LK. Patients with cancer and their spouse caregivers: perceptions of the illness experience. *Cancer* 1992;69:1074–1079.
83. Holland JC, Rowland J, Plumb M. Psychological aspects of anorexia in cancer patients. *Cancer Res* 1977;37:2425–2428.
84. Portenoy RK, Thaler HT, Kornblith AB, Lepore JM, Friedlander KH, Kiyasu E, et al. The Memorial Symptom Assessment Scale: an instrument for the evaluation of symptom prevalence, characteristics and distress. *Eur J Cancer* 1994;30A:1326–1336.
85. Portenoy RK. Cancer pain: epidemiology and syndromes. *Cancer* 1989;63:2298–2307.
86. Bonica JJ. Treatment of cancer pain: current status and future needs. In: Fields HL, Dubner R, Cervero F, eds. *Advances in pain research and therapy*. New York: Raven Press, 1985:589–616.
87. Stjernsward, J, Teoh N. The scope of the cancer pain problem. In: Foley KM, Bonica JJ, Ventafridda V, eds. *Advances in pain research and therapy, Second International Congress on Cancer Pain*, vol 16. New York: Raven Press, 1990:7–12.
88. Foley KM. The treatment of cancer pain. *N Engl J Med* 1985;313: 84–95.
89. Cherny NI. Cancer pain: principles of assessment and treatment. In: Berger A, Portenoy R, Weissman DE, eds. *Principles and practice of supportive oncology*; 1st ed. Philadelphia: Lippincott–Raven, 1998:3–42.
90. World Health Organization. Cancer pain relief. Geneva: World Health Organization, 1986.
91. World Health Organization. Cancer pain relief and palliative care. Geneva: World Health Organization, 1990.
92. Walker VA, Hoskin PJ, Hanks GW, White ID. Evaluation of WHO analgesic guidelines for cancer pain in a hospital-based palliative care unit. *J Pain Symptom Manage* 1988;3:145–149.
93. Ventafridda V, Tamburini M, Caraceni A, De CF, Naldi F. A validation study of the WHO method for cancer pain relief. *Cancer* 1987;59:850–856.
94. Takeda F. Results of field-testing in Japan of WHO draft interim guidelines on relief of cancer pain. *Pain Clin* 1986;1:83–89.
95. Grond S, Zech D, Lynch J, Diefenbach C, Schug SA, Lehmann KA. Validation of World Health Organization guidelines for pain relief in head and neck cancer: a prospective study. *Ann Otol Rhinol Laryngol* 1993;102:342–348.
96. Schug SA, Zech D, Dorr U. Cancer pain management according to WHO analgesic guidelines. *J Pain Symptom Manage* 1990;5:27–32.
97. Cleeland CS, Gonin R, Hatfield AK, Edmonson JH, Blum RH, Stewart JA, et al. Pain and its treatment in outpatients with metastatic cancer. *N Engl J Med* 1994;330:592–596.
98. VonRoenn JH, Cleeland CS, Gonin R, Hatfield AK, Pandya KJ. Physician attitudes and practice in cancer pain management: a survey from the Eastern Cooperative Oncology Group. *Ann Intern Med* 1993;119:121–126.
99. Larue F, Colleau SM, Brasseur L, Cleeland CS. Multicentre study of cancer pain and its treatment. *BMJ* 1995;310:1034–1037.
100. Bruera E, Ripamonti C. Dyspnea in patients with advanced cancer. In: Berger A, Portenoy R, Weissman DE, eds. *Principles and practice of supportive oncology*, 1st ed. Philadelphia: Lippincott–Raven, 1998:295–309.
101. Hopwood P, Howell P, Maguire P. Psychiatric morbidity in patients with advanced cancer of the breast: prevalence measured by two self rating questionnaires. *Br J Cancer* 1991;64:349–352.
102. Payne D, Massie MJ. Depression and anxiety. In: Berger A, Portenoy R, Weissman DE, eds. *Principles and practice of supportive oncology*, 1st ed. Philadelphia: Lippincott–Raven, 1998:497–512.
103. Ingham JM, Layman-Goldstein M, Coyle N, Derby S, Adelhardt J, Hicks J, et al. Abstract presented at: International conference on the care of the terminally ill. Montreal, Quebec, Canada, September 1994.
104. Ingham JM, Layman-Goldstein M, Derby S, et al. The characteristics of the dying process in cancer patients in a hospice and cancer center. *Proc Am Soc Clin Oncol* 1994;13:172.

105. Posner JB. Neurologic complications of systemic cancer. *Dis Mon* 1979;25:1–60.
106. Silberfarb PM, Philibert D, Levine PM. Psychosocial aspects of neoplastic disease: II. Affective and cognitive effects of chemotherapy in cancer patients. *Am J Psychiatry* 1980;137:597–601.
107. Oxman TE, Silberfarb PM. Serial cognitive testing in cancer patients receiving chemotherapy. *Am J Psychiatry* 1980;137:1263–1265.
108. Silberfarb PM. Chemotherapy and cognitive defects in cancer patients. *Annu Rev Med* 1983;34:35–46.
109. Patchell RA, Posner JB. Cancer and the nervous system. In: Holland JC, Rowland JH, eds. *Handbook of psychooncology*. New York: Oxford University Press, 1989:327–341.
110. Meyers CA, Abbruzzese JL. Cognitive functioning in cancer patient: effect of previous treatment. *Neurology* 1992;42:434–436.
111. Barbato M. Thiamine deficiency in patients admitted to a palliative care unit. *Palliat Med* 1994;8:320–324.
112. Tuma R, DeAngelis L. Acute encephalopathy in patients with systemic cancer. *Ann Neurol* 1992;32:288.
113. Bruera E, Miller L, McCallion J, Macmillan K, Krefting L, Hanson J. Cognitive failure in patients with terminal cancer: a prospective study. *J Pain Symptom Manage* 1992;7:192–195.
114. Glaser BG, Strauss AL. *Awareness of dying*. Chicago: Aldine Publishing, 1965.
115. Glaser BG, Strauss AL. *Time for dying*. Chicago: Aldine Publishing, 1968.
116. Pattison EM. *The experience of dying*. Englewood Cliffs, NJ: Prentice-Hall, 1977.
117. McCormick TR, Conley BJ. Patients' perspectives on dying and on the care of dying patients. *West J Med* 1995;163:236–243.
118. *Principles and practice of supportive oncology*, 1st ed. Berger A, Portenoy R, Weissman DE, eds. Philadelphia: Lippincott–Raven, 1998.
119. Doyle D, Hanks GWC, MacDonald N, eds. *Oxford textbook of palliative medicine*, 2nd ed. Oxford, UK: Oxford University Press, 1998.
120. Cherny NI, Portenoy RK. Practical issues in the management of cancer pain. In: Wall PD, Melzack R, eds. *Textbook of pain*, 3rd ed. Edinburgh, UK: Churchill-Livingstone, 1994:1437–1467.
121. Ajemian I. Palliative management of dyspnea. *J Palliat Care* 1991;7:44–45.
122. Ingham J, Caraceni A. Delirium. In: Berger A, Portenoy R, Weissman DE, eds. *Principles and practice of supportive oncology*, 1st ed. Philadelphia: Lippincott–Raven, 1998:477–498.
123. Lipowski ZJ. Update on delirium. *Psychiatr Clin North Am* 1992;15:335–346.
124. Fainsinger RL, Tapper M, Bruera E. A perspective on the management of delirium in terminally ill patients on a palliative care unit. *J Palliat Care* 1993;9:4–8.
125. Sateia MJ, Silberfarb PM. Sleep in palliative care. In: Doyle D, Hanks G, MacDonald N, eds. *Oxford textbook of palliative medicine*. Oxford, UK: Oxford University Press, 1993:472–486.
126. Vortherms R, Ryan P, Ward S. Knowledge of, attitudes toward, and barriers to pharmacologic management of cancer pain in a statewide random sample of nurses. *Res Nurs Health* 1992;15:459–466.
127. Cherny NI, Ho MN, Bookbinder M, Fahey TJ, Portenoy RK, Foley KM. Cancer pain: knowledge and attitudes of physicians at a cancer center. *Proc Am Soc Clin Oncol* 1994;13:434.
128. Ingham JM, Portenoy RK. The measurement of pain and other symptoms. In: Doyle D, Hanks GWC, MacDonald N, eds. *Oxford textbook of palliative medicine*, 2nd ed. Oxford, UK: Oxford University Press, 1998;203–221.
129. Daut RL, Cleeland CS, Flanery RC. Development of the Wisconsin Brief Pain Questionnaire to assess pain in cancer and other diseases. *Pain* 1983;17:197–210.
130. Bruera E, Kuehn N, Miller MJ, Selmser P, Macmillan K. The Edmonton Symptom Assessment System (ESAS): a simple method for the assessment of palliative care patients. *J Palliat Care* 1991;7:6–9.
131. Smith MJ, Breitbart WS, Platt MM. A critique of instruments and methods to detect, diagnose, and rate delirium. *J Pain Symptom Manage* 1995;10:35–77.
132. Hileman JW, Lackey NR, Hassanein RS. Identifying the needs of home caregiver of patients with cancer. *Oncol Nurs Forum* 1992;19:771–777.
133. Seigal K, Raveis VH, Houts P, Mor V. Caregiver burden and unmet patient needs. *Cancer* 1991;68:1131–1140.
134. Mor V, Masterson-Allen S, Houts P, Seigal K. The changing needs of patients with cancer at home. *Cancer* 1992;69:829–838.
135. Covinsky KE, Goldman L, Cook F, Oye R, Desbiens N, Reding D, et al. The impact of serious illness on patient's families. *JAMA* 1994;272:1839–1844.
136. Kristjanson LJ, Ashcroft T. The family's cancer journey: a literature review. *Cancer Nurs* 1994;17:1–17.
137. Covinsky KE, Landerfeld S, Teno J, Connors AF, Dawson N, Youngner S, et al. Is economic hardship on the families of the seriously ill associated with patient and surrogate care preferences? *Arch Intern Med* 1996;156:1737–1741.
138. Manne S. Cancer in the marital context: a review of the literature. *Cancer Invest* 1998;16:188–202.
139. Swensen C, Fuller S. Expression of love, marriage problems, commitment and anticipatory grief in the marriages of cancer patients. *J Marriage Fam* 1992;54:191–196.
140. Higginson I, Priest P. Predictors of family anxiety in the weeks before death. *Soc Sci Med* 1996;43:1621–1625.
141. Loscalzo MJ, Zobora J. Care of the cancer patient: response of family and staff. In: Bruera E, Portenoy RK, eds. *Topics in palliative care*, vol 2. New York: Oxford University Press, 1999:209–245.
142. Katz L, Chochinov H. The spectrum of grief in palliative care. In: Bruera E, Portenoy RK, eds. *Topics in Palliative Care*, vol 2. New York: Oxford University Press, 1998;295–310.
143. Stjernsward J, Pampallona S. Palliative medicine—a global perspective. In: Doyle D, Hanks GWC, MacDonald N, eds. *Oxford textbook of palliative medicine*. Oxford, UK: Oxford University Press, 1998:1227–1245.
144. The American Academy of Neurology Ethics and Humanities Subcommittee. Palliative care in neurology. *Neurology* 1996;46:870–872.
145. ASCO Task Force on Cancer Care at the End of Life. Cancer care during the last phase of life. *J Clin Oncol* 1998;16:1986–1996.
146. Ferris FD. *Palliative care: towards a consensus in standardized principles of practice*. Ontario, Canada: The Canadian Palliative Care Association, 1995.
147. Ingham JM, Foley KM. Pain and the barriers to its relief at the end of life: a lesson for improving end of life health care. *Hosp J* 1998;13(1/2):89–100.
148. MacDonald N. A proposed matrix for organizational changes to improve quality of life in oncology. *Eur J Cancer* 1995;31A[Suppl 6]:S18–S21.
149. Byock I. *Dying well: the prospect for growth at the end of life*. New York: Riverhead Books, 1997.

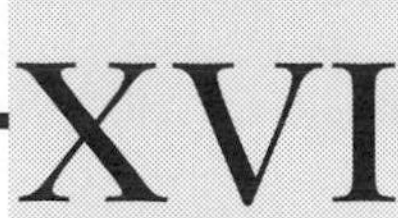

Diseases of the Breast, 2nd ed.,
edited by Jay R. Harris.
Lippincott Williams & Wilkins, Philadelphia © 2000.

Issues in Breast Cancer Survivorship

CHAPTER 66

Nursing Care in Patient Management and Quality of Life

Karen Hassey Dow and Barbara Hansen Kalinowski

Nursing care in patient management is an integral part of interdisciplinary oncology care from the time of the patient's diagnosis through treatment, recurrence, and survival. Nurses have an enormous influence on patient care, decision making, and symptom management. In this chapter, we recognize that several common concerns and issues occur across the disease trajectory and at particular points during treatment. Thus, this chapter is divided into patient care management during early-stage disease, with particular attention to surgery, radiation therapy, and chemotherapy, and patient care management during advanced disease. Each section emphasizes patient management issues related to education, symptom management, and psychosocial support.

K. H. Dow: School of Nursing, College of Health and Public Affairs, University of Central Florida, Orlando, Florida
B. H. Kalinowski: Brigham and Women's Hospital, Dana-Farber Cancer Institute, Boston, Massachusetts

PATIENT CARE MANAGEMENT IN EARLY-STAGE BREAST CANCER

Education

The available options for breast cancer treatment and the choices facing women today can be overwhelming and confusing.[1–3] Decisions about primary treatment, adjuvant therapy, and hormonal therapy are made at a time when patients are facing a potentially life-threatening disease. Patients who are best able to make decisions about treatment are those who can express and communicate their beliefs, feelings, and preferences; actively listen to information that their oncology team is sharing with them; and search out additional information or second opinions from trusted and respected sources. Likewise, clinicians who are best able to assist their patients in making reasonable decisions about treatment are those who recognize that decision making is a process that occurs over time, acknowledge their patients' vulnerabilities and difficulties in making decisions, translate confusing statistics and data into meaningful and personal forms, and encourage questions no matter how simple they seem.[1]

Enormous amounts of lay teaching materials are available in written (e.g., books, pamphlets, and brochures), audiovisual (e.g., tapes and audiocassettes), computer-assisted, and Web-based formats. In addition, internet groups, support groups, counselors, and individual networking efforts help patients find information. The volume of information available can be overwhelming and can sometimes hinder decision making. Clinicians need to take the time to carefully assess their patients' developmental stages, educational levels, amounts of anxiety, energy levels, personal coping styles, past experiences, and family histories in guiding them through the information to help make a decision.[4–6] Nurses can help patients and their families discern what is useful during this stressful time and what can be used at a later date by knowing what resources are available in their institution, in the community, regionally, and nationally.

The number of nonpalpable detected lesions has increased in the past several years. Tissue sampling of a nonpalpable lesion or mammographic abnormality can be accomplished in a variety of ways via needle localization, ultrasound-guided localization, core and stereotactic fine-needle aspiration, or any combination of these. Patients commonly ask for information about the specific procedure, available technology, expertise of the clinicians who will perform the biopsy, expectation of discomfort, and time frame for receiving biopsy results. Because these procedures are performed on an outpatient basis, institution-specific teaching guides and brochures can help to enhance patients' understanding. During the procedure, patients may find it helpful to use relaxation and distraction techniques to aid in allaying anxiety and decreasing discomfort.

Teaching related to surgery should include a discussion of the variability in length of hospital stay, wound care, pain management, prosthesis, and time to healing.[7] For example, the length of stay for lumpectomy and mastectomy with or without reconstruction can range from several hours to several days. Likewise, wound care and pain management differ between a lumpectomy and mastectomy. Nurses are generally the oncology providers who can help ensure that patients receive specific instructions on postsurgical care management.

Because length of stay is relatively short, preoperative teaching should ideally begin in the surgeon's office and can be tailored to the specific health care facility and surgical procedure. Orientation to the surgical facility, waiting areas, patients' rooms, and methods of communication between surgeon and patients and family is an important part of preparation for breast surgery. Verbally walking through the surgical experience—admission, anesthesia consult, operating room waiting or holding area, recovery room, and discharge home or admission to the hospital—can be reassuring for patients and can help to correct misconceptions and decrease anxiety on the day of the procedure. Teaching at this time also includes information about postoperative routines (e.g., respiratory exercises, use of intravenous lines, pain relief, and postoperative mobility) and can help to individualize postoperative care for preexisting conditions that may have an impact on the immediate postoperative period (e.g., arthritis, chronic obstructive pulmonary disease). Discharge teaching begins before surgery and can be reinforced after the operation.

Symptom Management after Surgery

Surgical Wound Care

Approaches to wound management include providing information about dressing changes, measurement and recording of drainage, watching for signs and symptoms of infection, and personal hygiene. Patients prefer some expectation of what their surgical incision will look like. In certain instances, an appropriate visual diagram or photograph of similar surgery can illustrate the results. Patient anxiety about viewing the incision, particularly the mastectomy scar, can be lessened by having a time to look at the incision with the surgeon or nurse, or both, as part of the postoperative plan. Normal postoperative sensations and pain are to be expected. However, unusually painful sensations may occur, particularly in the axilla or the upper arm.[8] Drains may be used in the mastectomy site and in the axilla to help decrease swelling. However, patients find them uncomfortable and difficult to manage or empty. Thus, arrangements for having a visiting nurse in the home are useful in providing patients with assistance with physical care, personal hygiene, and monitoring of postoperative complications (i.e., seroma, hematoma, increased pain or discomfort, and fever). Finally, a plan for postoperative follow-up appointments, radiation oncology, and medical oncology consultations should be in place.

Pain Management

The experience of postoperative pain varies widely, depending on individual and cultural characteristics, the surgical procedure, and pain medication relief. Some patients experience relatively little discomfort with lumpectomy, whereas others have major pain after mastectomy and reconstruction that requires large doses of narcotic relief. A plan for postsurgical pain management is imperative. Clinicians and patients need to engage in discussions about the usual range of experiences with postoperative pain and discomfort and their trajectory and institute an individualized plan of effective pain relief strategies, such as a patient-controlled analgesia pump, progressive stepladder approach of oral analgesic use, and adjuvant nonpharmacologic approaches, such as breathing, relaxation, and distraction exercises. The plan needs to be tailored for patients who are in the inpatient, ambulatory, or home care settings.

Hand and Arm Care: Prevention of Lymphedema

Factors that place patients at higher risk of developing lymphedema include the extent of axillary node dissection, obesity, increased age, and postoperative wound complications.[9] Patients at higher risk require meticulous instruction about care of the affected hand and arm in an effort to prevent lymphedema.[10] Generally, patients should be encouraged to develop and maintain a regular exercise plan tailored to their physical capabilities and to avoid activities that present new challenges to their body (e.g., lifting of heavy objects, such as suitcases or grocery bags) that can create a challenge to the lymphatic system in the arm. Prevention of infection is also very important. Patients need to protect their hands by preventing burns while cooking, avoiding cutting or injuring cuticles, and using emollients or creams to avoid chapped skin. They need specific instructions to call or notify the appropriate health care provider if swelling or infection develops. Once lymphedema occurs, treatment includes a combination of manual lymphatic therapy, compression with bandages and garments, mechanical compression pumps, and, in certain instances, exercise.[9]

Exercise and Mobility

Limited mobility of the arm and shoulder as a result of discomfort, swelling, and the surgical defect are expected, particularly after axillary surgery. Gentle stretching exercises can usually begin soon after surgery (usually 48 hours postoperatively) and should be individualized by the surgeon to reflect the extent of the operation, presence of drains, and preoperative capabilities of the patient. Table 1 lists postmastectomy exercises to improve mobility. For patients who will receive radiation therapy as part of their treatment, regaining adequate range of motion is extremely important, because the radiation treatment position requires the arm to be abducted at a 160-degree angle. Referral to physical therapy after breast surgery may be needed to reinforce the exercise plan, improve range of motion, and strengthen areas weakened after surgical procedures such as autogenous flap reconstruction.

TABLE 1. *Suggestions for exercises after breast surgery*

Getting started

Start slowly, 5 to 10 minutes two or three times a day. Work up to one-half hour every day for several weeks, then increase to two sessions a day. Do 10 to 15 repetitions of each exercise. Warm up before exercising—it relieves stress and makes it easier.

Loosening up

Usually may start when drains and/or stitches are out. Check with your physician if you have questions about when to start.

- Arm swings: Stand up, put hand (unaffected side) on chair (to the side), bend forward at the waist, and swing other arm back and forth, side to side.
- Side raises: Raise arm up from side, hold four counts, and stretch.
- Back reach (stretches muscle in chest): Grab wrist behind back with unaffected hand, bend at elbow, pull arm up gently, hold for four counts.

Stretching

Do these exercises slowly and gently. Hold the positions for five counts, relax, and breathe.

- Stick raises: Lie on back (on bed or mat), hold stick (broom handle, cane) in both hands, raise arms over head, let gravity do the work. Hold five counts.
- Snow angel: Lie on back (on bed or mat), raise arms over head, reach as high as you can (do not let it hurt). Hold five counts, lower arms slowly.
- Wall crawls: Stand in front of wall. With both hands walk fingers up the wall until you feel a pull, hold five counts. Slide hand down the wall, make sure you keep shoulders square with the wall. Step closer to increase the stretch.

Adapted from Webb S. *Back in the swing: stretch and strengthen after breast surgery.* Boston: Boston Group for Medical Education, 1995; and ref. 10.

Prosthesis

Prosthetic fitting for women who have had a mastectomy and reconstruction with tissue expanders should be done around the time of the first postoperative follow-up appointment or when the incision has healed. However, women benefit from receiving specific information about how, when, and where to purchase a prosthesis and having a temporary prosthesis in hand before discharge from the hospital. Nurses use a variety of resources to provide this necessary information, such as brochures, audiotapes, and videocassettes. Another strategy is to have a professional prosthetic fitter visit the patient before discharge. Letting women know that a wide variety of prostheses is available, such as soft forms and self-adhering forms that come in many colors and textures, is important. Stylish and specially designed lingerie and bathing suits are also available. Nurses who practice in the outpatient setting (e.g., ambulatory care or surgeons' offices) find that having a sample breast prosthesis and mastectomy bra to use during teaching is useful.

Psychosocial Recovery

Detailed discussions of psychological reaction and support programs for patients with breast cancer are found elsewhere in the text. Specific preoperative discussions, in which clinicians can engage with their patients, include attention to the emotional impact of the initial diagnosis, treatment of breast cancer, and acknowledgment that the surgical experience marks the beginning of a long recovery period. Other psychosocial strategies include helping patients to reframe their time sequence; reorder priorities about work, family, and social activities; and use short-term thinking (e.g., taking one day at a time and thinking through the process of the events of the week and time it takes to accomplish tasks). Nurses, in particular, can work with patients to develop a realistic expectation of the time frame for physical recovery, redistribute household tasks, develop a realistic plan for child care, ask for assistance, and anticipate a time to return to work.

PATIENT CARE MANAGEMENT DURING RADIATION THERAPY

Education

Teaching patients about radiation therapy ideally begins during the consultation visit, in which the role of radiation therapy in the overall treatment plan, additional diagnostic studies needed, and treatment planning are discussed. Patients may be apprehensive about starting radiation and may express many psychosocial concerns and fears.[11] Topics to discuss about radiation treatment planning include the rationale for simulation, the need to minimize radiation dose to vital organs such as the lung and heart, and the construction of immobilization devices made of styrofoam to keep the limbs in consistent position during treatment. In preparation for simulation, clinicians can emphasize that patients need to plan at least an hour or longer for simulation, be prepared to feel some discomfort while lying on a hard simulation table, understand that the radiation therapist will place a permanent tattoo or skin markings (the size of a freckle) directly on the skin surface to help reproduce the treatments on a daily basis, and realize that simulation is *not* a radiation treatment.

After simulation is completed, patients receive an appointment to start 5-day-per-week treatment. Patients find it helpful to have the radiation oncology nurse "walk through" a typical day's or week's treatment to get a mental picture of what the experience will be like.[12] A useful patient tip to reduce confusion with procedures is to keep a daily diary of activities and appointments. The first treatment generally takes approximately 30 to 45 minutes; subsequent treatments take approximately 15 minutes. Patients often feel uncomfortable while lying on a hard treatment table. They may be disconcerted by the sounds of the radiation treatment machine. Patients need reassurance that, although they will be alone in a room during treatment, the radiation therapists will be in contact with them via screen monitor and intercom. Although some patients find the treatment room a sterile environment, many radiation oncology departments have updated their treatment room decor with serene colors and pictures and provide soothing music to help allay patients' anxiety. Some patients prefer to bring a tape or compact disk player to listen to their own music during treatment.

Symptom Management during Radiation Therapy

Symptom management includes teaching about the potential side effects of radiation therapy, self-care measures to manage the side effects, and management of the overall radiation therapy experience. The acute physical side effects of radiation therapy are skin reactions,[12–20] fatigue,[20–29] and arm discomfort.

Skin Effects

Radiation-induced skin effects range from slight peeling, dryness, tanning, itchiness, and breast tenderness and fullness to moist desquamation.[12–20] The severity of skin reactions is related to radiation factors (total dose, fractionation, energy beam, and volume of tissue treated) and patient factors. Risk factors for enhanced acute skin effects include larger breast size, previous or concurrent chemotherapy, nutritional state, presence of intercurrent disease, and older age. Particularly susceptible areas of skin breakdown include the inframmary fold and supraclavicular areas.

Teaching patients self-care skin management during radiation ideally begins before or at the start of treatment. The radiation oncology team examines patients for acute side effects on a weekly basis and as needed as therapy progresses. Patients can work with their radiation oncology team by informing them of specific skin care products or preparations, ointments, or creams that they are using or plan to use. In addition, a wide variety of teaching booklets and institution-specific guides are available on skin care management. Although there are variations in practice, some general teaching guidelines for skin care during radiation therapy are listed in Table 2.

Fatigue

Fatigue is the most prevalent symptom of cancer and treatment, with up to 95% of patients affected.[20–31] Fatigue can be a chronic problem that results from several etiologies (i.e., treatment, pathophysiologic, behavioral, and emotional). It occurs during treatment and persists even after treatment ends. Cancer patients report that fatigue has a negative influence on quality of life (QOL) because it can impair the ability to function or maintain daily routines (because of weakness and lack of energy), influence emotional reaction (e.g., sadness, irritability), and interrupt work schedules (because of poor attention or concentration). Although rest can restore a normal level of functioning in the healthy individual, this restorative capacity is diminished in cancer. Table 3 outlines the potential impact of fatigue.

Patients who receive radiation therapy report a usual pattern of fatigue that gradually rises by the third week of treatment and slowly declines after the end of therapy. Some

TABLE 2. *Skin care interventions during radiation therapy*

Side effect	Onset after start of radiation therapy (wk)	Appearance/presentation	Intervention
Erythema	2	Mild redness progressing to bright redness; mild to moderate discomfort	Clean skin with unscented soap Use lukewarm water in shower and bath Lubricate skin with water-based moisturizer that contains no perfumes Do not use deodorant in underarm of treated breast Wear loose-fitting cotton garments and avoid wool and other scratchy fabrics against skin Protect radiated skin from sun, wind, and temperature extremes
Hyperpigmentation	2	Mild to deep tanning; more pronounced in dark-skinned patients; dark brown dots on skin surface	Same as above
Folliculitis	2	Itchy skin; red dots appear in sternal, infraclavicular, and supraclavicular areas	Apply cool, wet packs to skin Oatmeal colloidal-based soap Antihistamine for generalized itching can be taken at bedtime 0.5% corticosteroid cream to affected area; apply thin layer after radiation treatment Unscented moisturizer Aloe vera gel
Dryness or dry desquamation	2–3	Dry, flaking, peeling skin; accompanies folliculitis; most often occurs in supraclavicular areas	Unscented moisturizer Aloe vera gel
Moist desquamation	4–5 wk; may occur after XRT during chemotherapy	Moist peeling of skin; denuded areas exposed; associated with moderate discomfort, particularly in inframammary fold	Clean area with quarter-strength hydrogen peroxide solution Keep area dry with a soft dressing Moisture vapor–permeable dressing can be applied Do not use tape directly on area of skin breakdown NSAID for moderate to severe discomfort
Breast fullness or heaviness			Use firm, athletic support bra

NSAID, nonsteroidal antiinflammatory drug; XRT, radiation therapy.
Adapted from ref. 12.

patients experience less fatigue on weekends, when radiation is not delivered.

Despite the prevalence of cancer-related fatigue, Vogelzang et al.[23] found that fatigue was seldom discussed by oncologists. In a telephone survey using a random sample of 419 cancer patients, 200 primary caregivers, and 197 oncologists (unrelated to the patients), 78% of patients indicated that they experienced fatigue during treatment. Thirty-two percent experienced fatigue daily, and 32% reported that fatigue significantly affected their daily routines. Oncologists reported that pain had a greater adverse effect than fatigue (61% versus 37%); however, patients felt that fatigue adversely affected their lives more than pain (61% versus 19%). Fifty percent of patients did not discuss treatment options with their oncologists, and only 27% reported that their oncologists recommended treatment for fatigue.

Three common approaches to fatigue management are pharmacology (erythropoietin), exercise, and education.[28,29] Erythropoietin is produced in the peritubular interstitial cells of the kidney and in the hepatocytes and is responsible for enhancing the proliferation of erythroid progenitor cells in the bone marrow.[30] It has been used to reduce or eliminate transfusion requirements in patients with anemia secondary to chemotherapy treatment or the disease.

Nonpharmacologic approaches include education about fatigue, its occurrence, and activity and rest patterns; stress management; and nutrition, sleep, and energy conservation. Several researchers have tested different exercise rehabilitation programs in the management of fatigue in breast cancer.[22,32,33] Although the programs differ in the type of exercise (e.g., muscle toning and strengthening, exercise cycling, walking exercise, aerobic dancing, Outward Bound–type and other

TABLE 3. *Impact of fatigue*

Dimension	Potential impact
Emotional	Mood alteration (e.g., depression, irritability, decreased patience); decreased coping ability, decreased motivation
Cognitive	Decreased directed attention; impaired thinking, attention, and concentration; decreased ability to make decisions
Activities	Impaired performance; reduced ability to set goals, plan, initiate, or persist in activities that require effort; decreased activity; decreased movement; low energy levels; other physical distress; sleep/rest disturbance
Family	Parenting, relationships, and/or sexuality role changes
Sociocultural	Decreased social functioning, social withdrawal, changes in nature of interactions, cultural expectations, withdrawal, isolation, dependence on others
Occupational/ role	Absenteeism, lack of concentration
Symptoms	Adherence to treatment regimen
Spiritual	Quality of life, meaning, suffering

From ref. 20, with permission.

wilderness activities) either alone or in combination with support (individual or group), the exercise programs stress self-care and self-motivation in managing fatigue.

Psychosocial and Family Support

Radiation treatments require daily visits over a 4- to 5-week period, which may require some adjustment in work, family, and social patterns. Patients may need assistance in reorganizing work schedules to accommodate daily treatment. Strategies include scheduling radiation treatment at either the beginning or end of the work day, shortening the work day if possible, or even taking a leave of absence during radiation. Because of the daily imposition of the radiation treatment schedule, some patients may need assistance with home management or child care, or both. Some patients may require assistance in traveling to and from daily treatment.

PATIENT CARE MANAGEMENT DURING CHEMOTHERAPY

Education

Patients often experience intense fear, anxiety, and uncertainty on the first day of chemotherapy. These strong emotional feelings can be diffused by having the patient meet with an oncology nurse before treatment and by providing the opportunity to ask questions and tour the treatment facility. Patients also benefit from frequent contact with their oncology nurse either in person or by telephone. At the initial meeting, an oncology nurse can also assess the patient to identify any psychosocial factors that may predispose her to noncompliant behaviors during chemotherapy and to assess her potential risk for chemotherapy-related side effects. A patient's ability to cope with the demands of chemotherapy can vary based on age, concurrent life stressors, and emotional disposition. For example, patients may be more willing to endure debilitating side effects when the treatment goal is curative. On the other hand, patients who are receiving therapy for metastatic disease may be more physically debilitated, emotionally vulnerable, and less willing to cope with the effects of chemotherapy.

Symptom Management during Chemotherapy

Physical distress is a major concern for women who are receiving adjuvant chemotherapy.[34–37] The most common physical symptoms experienced are nausea and vomiting (N and V), hair loss, fatigue, and weight gain. In addition, the management of infusional catheters and decreasing risk of extravasation are important aspects of care. Side effects that occur more often with high-dose chemotherapy include mucositis, immunosuppression, hemorrhagic cystitis, and neurotoxicity.

Nausea and Vomiting

N and V has been one of the most common, severe, and debilitating side effects of chemotherapy.[38–46] Chemotherapy-induced N and V can be divided into three categories: acute (during treatment), delayed (occurs more than 24 hours after therapy), and anticipatory (a classic conditioned response as a result of inadequate antiemetic therapy). The risks for N and V are related to the type and dose of chemotherapy used and individual patient factors. The emetogenic potential of chemotherapeutic agents is classified from high to low. Typical chemotherapeutic agents used to treat breast cancer, such as cisplatin, cyclophosphamide, doxorubicin, and methotrexate, have moderate to high emetogenic potential.

Patient factors that increase risk for N and V include female gender, younger age, previous chemotherapy, and history of motion sickness.[42–44] Patients who are chronic alcohol users are generally considered at lower risk. Although several antiemetic regimens are available, they must be individualized for each patient.[45] Inadequate control of N and V during treatment can lead to anticipatory N and V (ANV), which is inherently more difficult to manage.[45]

The serotonin antagonists, used either alone or in combination with corticosteroids, have led to a substantial improvement in the control of severe N and V.[38–44] These agents are highly selective for 5HT3 receptors and have no action at dopamine receptors. These agents are best used in highly emetogenic chemotherapeutic regimens. Their efficacy is no different than that of standard antiemetics with low to moderate emetogenic chemotherapy. Because these agents are associated with higher costs, their use with low to moderately emetogenic chemotherapy is not advised. The serotonin antagonists do not have the extrapyramidal reactions associated with the dopamine antagonists. Side effects include headache and constipation and, less commonly, dizziness. Although the serotonin antagonists have many advantages, Wickham[44] does not recommend that they be used for multiple daily dosing or for delayed N and V.

Other common antiemetic agents are the dopamine antagonists (i.e., metoclopramide, phenothiazines, and butyrophenones), corticosteroids, benzodiazepines, and cannabinoids. Central acting agents, such as the phenothiazines and metoclopramide, have untoward side effects, including sedation, dizziness, and extrapyramidal reactions.[45] In addition, they are associated with anticholinergic effects, such as dry mouth and constipation. Use of the dopamine antagonists alone or in combination help relieve N and V in patients who are taking chemotherapeutic agents that have low to moderate emetogenicity. They may also be useful in delayed N and V.

Corticosteroids are useful in helping to control N and V with moderately emetogenic chemotherapy. Their mechanism of action is unknown but is thought to have central and peripheral effects.[45] Dexamethasone also enhances the effect of the serotonin antagonists when given in combination. The benzodiazepines have modest antiemetic effects and help to relieve anxiety and agitation associated with N and V. Nonpharmacologic interventions for N and V that have been used as an adjunct to pharmacologic measures include behavioral interventions (e.g., hypnosis, passive relaxation), acupressure, and dietary modifications.[45]

With delayed N and V, the serotonin antagonists have not shown consistent efficacy compared to that seen with metoclopramide and dexamethasone. Benzodiazepines have shown some efficacy in ANV. ANV is less likely to occur in patients who are receiving short term adjuvant chemotherapy.[44] However, it can occur in patients with metastatic disease who are receiving ongoing therapy. ANV symptoms are difficult to manage; thus, emphasis is needed on tailoring antiemetic regimens to individual patient needs early in the disease process.

Alopecia

Alopecia includes body hair loss (facial, including eyelashes and eyebrows, axillary, and pubic). Patients report that hair loss is one of the most distressing side effects of chemotherapy.[46,47] Although a mastectomy scar is devastating, hair loss can be publicly stigmatizing. Hair loss is often viewed as an assault to one's physical appearance, body image, self-esteem, and sexuality. Even though patients may cognitively prepare themselves for loss of their hair, the actual occurrence is most often a difficult emotional experience.

Chemotherapeutic agents can cause either partial or complete atrophy of the hair root bulb with constriction of the hair shaft, which can break easily. Agents have a differential ability to induce hair loss based on their routes of administration, dosing schedules, and peak blood levels. For example, doxorubicin is the chemotherapeutic agent most commonly linked with alopecia. Patterns of doxorubicin-associated hair loss generally occur 2 to 3 weeks after initial treatment, with continued hair loss occurring over time. On the other hand, paclitaxel (Taxol)-associated hair loss often occurs dramatically and suddenly. Methotrexate-fluorouracil is associated with minimal hair loss, and oral cyclophosphamide causes generalized hair thinning, particularly at the crown.

Patient teaching should stress and reassure that hair loss is temporary. Useful interventions for hair loss include the following:

Before hair loss occurs:

- Cut hair in a manageable and easy-to-maintain style before chemotherapy.
- Use a mild, protein-based shampoo and conditioner.
- Use an electric hairdryer on its lowest setting.
- Avoid electric curlers and curling irons, hair spray, and hair dye that may increase the fragility of hair.
- Avoid excessive brushing and hair combing.
- Purchase a wig to fit one's normal hair color and style.
- Consider accessing the American Cancer Society's program called "Look Good...Feel Better," for additional tips on managing hair loss (1-800-ACS-2345 or http://www.cancer.org).

After hair loss occurs:

- Protect exposed scalp from excessive temperature changes.
- Use emollient or lotion to moisturize scalp.
- Reduce scalp itching by using an oatmeal-based colloidal soap.
- Use scarves and turbans as an alternative to wigs.

Fatigue

Several studies evaluated fatigue during adjuvant therapy for breast cancer.[48–51] Berger[49] describes a pattern of fatigue, activity, and rest in 72 women aged 30 to 69 who were receiving chemotherapy for stage I or II breast cancer (see Table 3). She used the Piper Fatigue Scale to measure fatigue 48 hours after each treatment and at treatment cycle midpoints for three cycles and wrist actigraphs to measure activity and rest cycles for 96 hours at each treatment and for 72 hours at each cycle midpoint. Findings showed that total and subscale fatigue scores were significantly different over time, with scores higher at treatment and lower at cycle midpoints. A mirror image pattern of fatigue and activity levels was significantly different over time. Berger's findings suggest a roller-coaster pattern to fatigue and rest in subjects who are undergoing chemotherapy for breast cancer.

Beisecker et al.[34] interviewed 21 women after adjuvant chemotherapy for breast cancer to identify whether they had persistent side effects after treatment. Hair loss, fatigue, nausea, infections, and low blood counts were the most frequently reported problems during the first interviews. Six months later, hair problems, fatigue, weight gain, menopausal problems, emotional problems, and nail problems were most often reported. Most patients did not expect to experience chemotherapy-related problems 6 months after ending treatment.

Hann et al.[50] evaluated the severity of fatigue and its impact on QOL in 43 women who had undergone bone marrow transplantation (BMT) for breast cancer compared to a group of women of similar age with no cancer history. Subjects completed measures of fatigue, anxiety, depression, and sleep habits. Women who had completed BMT for breast cancer reported significantly more frequent and severe fatigue than women with no cancer history. In addition, fatigue had a significant impact on daily functioning and QOL in BMT recipients. Fatigue after BMT for breast cancer was related to treatment factors and psychosocial factors (i.e., anxiety, depressive symptoms, and sleep difficulties).

Interventions for chemotherapy-related fatigue are similar to general fatigue management guidelines identified earlier in this chapter under Symptom Management during Radiation Therapy.

Weight Gain

Weight gain occurs in 50% to 90% of women who receive adjuvant therapy.[52–54] Weight gain of up to 15 to 20 pounds is particularly problematic among premenopausal women. Although the underlying mechanisms of energy imbalance are unknown, they are considered multifactorial, including a combination of decreased physical activity, increased dietary intake, taste changes, mild nausea relieved by eating, hormonal changes, and psychological distress. Helpful interventions to manage weight gain include teaching about nutrition (e.g., examining eating patterns and food choices) and regular exercise.

Management of Vascular Access Devices

Central venous catheters and vascular access devices (VADs) have led to increased comfort and ease during chemotherapy and blood product administration.[55] Several VADs are readily available, and the choice depends on the specific need for chemotherapy and blood products and length of time required for VAD. The various types of VADs available include tunneled central venous catheters (e.g., Hickman, Groshong), peripherally inserted central catheters, implantable ports, and peripheral ports, which are used for long-term continuous or intermittent therapy. Peripheral needles and peripheral catheters are generally selected for short-term access. Management of VADs requires knowledge of their selection, placement, port insertion care, accessing, flushing, site care, troubleshooting, and repair.[55] Efforts are being made to standardize care of VAD; however, individual institutions generally follow specific guidelines in their use. Patient factors must also be considered. For example, external devices must be flushed, cleaned, and cared for, and thus, the patient's ability to understand instructions and properly care for the catheter and purchase supplies is important.

Occlusion and infection are the complications that occur with VADs. Intraluminal catheter occlusion or the inability to withdraw blood or infuse fluid is the general result of a blood clot, precipitant, or unknown cause.[55] When this occurs with a port, the general cause is improper placement of the needle in the septum rather than the portal. Although the risk of infection is less with a VAD, they can nevertheless become locally infected at the catheter exit site. Symptoms include redness, warmth, swelling, and discomfort. Management requires culture and appropriate antibiotics.

Minimizing Extravasation

Extravasation is defined as "the accidental injection or leakage of drugs into the perivascular or subcutaneous spaces during an intravenous administration."[56–58] It is a serious complication that causes pain, swelling, erythema, paresthesias, and ulceration of tissue. The reported incidence of extravasation ranges from 0.01% to 6.00%.[56] Factors that influence the degree of extravasation include the type of vesicant, dose, and concentration. Chemotherapeutic agents are classified as either vesicants (drugs that cause tissue damage if extravasated) or irritants (drugs that cause redness and inflammatory reaction at the injection site without necrosis or ulceration). Chemotherapeutic agents that are classified as vesicants are the anthracyclines, actinomycin D, vinca alkaloids, mitomycin C, and nitrogen mustard.[56–58] Because vesicants cause extensive tissue damage, major efforts are made to prevent its occurrence. In cases in which extravasation occurs, antidotes differ depending on the chemotherapeutic agent. For example, isotonic sodium thiosulfate is the antidote of choice for alkylating agents, and hyaluronidase is the antidote of choice for vinca alkaloid extravasation.[56]

Irritants include fluorouracil, mitoxantrone, and etoposide. Irritants are more readily metabolized, removed from the injection site, and excreted than vesicants. Assessment parameters to differentiate extravasation from irritation or flare reaction include pain, redness, ulceration, swelling, and blood return. Different practices exist in the administration of vesicant chemotherapy. These include timing of vesicant administration, side arm administration, direct push administration, use of antecubital fossa, and use of large- versus small-gauge needles.[57] Regardless of practice, an extravasation kit should be readily available and generally includes 10% or 25% sodium thisulfate, hyaluronidase (stored in refrigerator), 5- and 10-mL syringes, sterile water, sterile saline, and 19- and 25-gauge needles.[57]

Institutional policies regarding VAD and extravasation guidelines, cytotoxic drug handling guidelines, and patient education guidelines are necessary components to minimize complications related to VADs and extravasation.[55–57]

Psychosocial Support

Of the breast cancer treatments, psychosocial response during chemotherapy is generally considered the most difficult to manage. The associated acute physical side effects, combined with the longer duration of chemotherapy, contribute to a deeper psychological burden compared to the effects from radiation therapy or surgery alone. Patients need encouragement to pace their activities, incorporate their treatment into their daily family and work routines, and, most of all, ask for assistance when they need it. Many patients appreciate the support they receive from others who have had or are going through similar experiences. Others take comfort in their family and interpersonal relationships. Some patients search the Web and find sites that have chat rooms dedicated to individuals affected by breast cancer. Most patients prefer to maintain a normal lifestyle during chemotherapy. They may continue to work as long as they desire and may request a treatment schedule that permits recovery from side effects on days off from work. Other patients may request that their chemotherapy treatment be given on weekends or evenings. Clinicians support patients by accommodating reasonable requests as much as possible.

PATIENT CARE MANAGEMENT IN ADVANCED DISEASE

Symptom Management

Symptoms that occur with high-dose chemotherapy are similar to the previously described chemotherapy side effects but are more intense. Depending on the chemotherapy regimen, additional side effects, such as mucositis, hemorrhagic cystitis, and neurotoxicity, may occur.

Mucositis

Mucositis is a general term that refers to an inflammation of the mucosa. The incidence of chemotherapy-induced mucositis rises with high-dose chemotherapy.[58–60] Agents that are considered highly stomatotoxic include the antimetabolites, antitumor antibiotics, plant alkaloids, and taxanes. Patient factors that are considered to raise the risk of developing mucositis include older age, alcohol and tobacco use, poor oral hygiene, poor nutritional status, use of ill-fitting dentures, and compromised renal function.

The risk of developing stomatitis varies by patient and drug regimens.[58–60] Generally, the consistent use of an oral care regimen offers the best protection against mucositis. Pretreatment strategies to prevent and decrease the incidence of oral complication include a baseline oral assessment, treatment of preexisting dental disease, and patient education.[58] Effective oral care protocols include a combination of a cleaning method, use of lubricants, measures to relieve pain and inflammation, and measures to prevent or treat infection.[58] Table 4 outlines oral care protocols for management of mucositis.

TABLE 4. *Interventions for stomatitis*

Potential stomatitis
- Assess oral cavity daily.
- Use routine oral hygiene:
  - Use oral care in the morning and at bedtime.
  - Use soft toothbrush and nonastringent fluoride toothpaste; floss with unwaxed dental floss.
  - Avoid alcohol-containing mouthwashes.
  - Apply lip lubricant.
- Use oxidizing agent as needed for mucolytic areas:
  - Rinse mouth with sodium bicarbonate solution (1 tsp in 8 oz water).
  - Rinse mouth with warm water and saline.
- Use prophylactic chlorhexidine mouth rinse (for high-risk patients).

Mild or moderate stomatitis
- Assess oral cavity twice a day.
- Continue oral care as above:
  - Increase frequency.
  - Alternate oxidizing agent with warm saline if crusts are present.
  - Omit flossing if gums bleed or are painful.
  - Remove and clean dentures; replace only for meals.
- Assess for evidence of infections: Any suspicious lesions should undergo culture assay.
- Apply topical anesthetics before meals and as needed:
  - Lidocaine hydrochloride viscous 2% or 5%:
    - Apply directly to lesion.
    - Dilute in 1 tbsp saline; swish and spit.
  - Benzocaine (Cetacaine or Hurricane) spray; use one or two sprays as needed.
  - Stomatitis cocktail (equal parts lidocaine viscous, diphenhydramine elixir, and Maalox, well shaken): Swish and spit 15 to 30 mL every 4 hours as needed. Swish and swallow if throat is sore.
  - Zilactin (tannic acid 7%, hydroxypropyl cellulose; available without a prescription): Apply directly to lesion.
  - Benzocaine (Oratect) gel: Apply topically directly to lesion.
  - Dyclonine (Dyclone) 0.5–1% solution: Swish and spit 15 mL (also available as extra-strength Sucrets lozenges or spray).
- Use oral analgesics for systemic pain control.
- Adapt diet to ensure adequate nutrition and hydration:
  - Eat soft, bland, nonirritating foods.
  - Take high-protein nutritional supplements.
  - Maintain adequate fluid intake.
- Patients at home with moderate to severe mucositis require frequent communication by phone and office visits as needed.

Severe stomatitis
- Assess oral cavity every 8 hours.
- Assess for evidence of infection: Any suspicious lesions should undergo culture assay.
- Clean the mouth every 2 hours:
  - Alternate warm saline mouthwash with antifungal or antibacterial oral suspension.
  - Rinse with oxidizing agent for mucolytic areas.
- Avoid trauma to the gums; use toothettes if bleeding occurs.
- Maintain integrity of the lips with a lubricant.
- Avoid wearing dental prostheses.
- Continue with local and systemic measures to ensure comfort, nutrition, and hydration.

Hemorrhagic Cystitis

Patients who receive dose intensification therapy are at high risk of developing hemorrhagic cystitis. Symptoms range from microscopic hematuria to frank bleeding and are usually associated with cyclophosphamide.[60] Maintaining adequate hydration of at least 80 ounces of fluid daily and patient education are key factors in preventing this side effect. High-risk patients require hyperhydration, frequent voiding, dipstick testing, and diuresis. Patients should also be instructed to report dysuria, bladder irritation, or suprapubic pain to their care providers.

Neurotoxicity

Patients who receive vincristine, vinblastine, cisplatin, 5-fluorouracil, and paclitaxel are at risk for neurotoxic complications.[61,62] Peripheral, cranial nerve, and autonomic neuropathies are dose-limiting factors associated with vinca alkaloids. Vinca alkaloids can affect specific cranial nerves, causing ptosis, diplopia, facial nerve palsies, and jaw pain. Peripheral neuropathies present with loss of sensation that begins at the fingertips and spreads to the wrist or begins at the toes and spreads to the ankles. An objective early sign is loss of Achilles tendon reflex. With additional therapy, progressive muscle pain, weakness, motor changes, and hypersensitivity to heat and intolerance to cold can occur.[61] Acute cerebellar dysfunction can occur in high-risk individuals, such as the elderly, and with bolus administration of 5-fluorouracil. Effects are dose-limiting and are reversible after medication is withdrawn. Neurotoxicities that patients on paclitaxel experience include numbness and paresthesias in the hands and feet, which can worsen over time with treatment. After treatment is completed, neurotoxicity slowly improves. Autonomic neuropathies associated with vinca alkaloids range from mild constipation to paralytic ileus. For high-risk individuals, such as the elderly and analgesic users, preventive measures include a stool softener, dietary modification, and increasing fluids. Patients need instructions to report changes in bowel habits early so that appropriate measures can be instituted. Alterations in dosing are considered appropriate when the patient is unable to perform fine coordinated movements such as buttoning clothes or writing, or if she experiences muscle pain. Therapy can be reinstituted at a lower dose when symptoms abate. However, symptoms may not completely disappear.

PATIENT CARE MANAGEMENT WITH HORMONAL THERAPY

Education

Several hormonal agents are used in adjuvant or advanced treatment for breast cancer.[63–68] These agents include antiprogestins, progestins, aromatase inhibitors, luteinizing hormone–releasing hormone agonists, androgens, and tamoxifen analogues (toremifene). Some hormonal therapies, such as tamoxifen and toremifine, are used as first-line therapy for pre- and postmenopausal women with estrogen receptor–positive, progesterone receptor–positive tumors. Other hormonal agents, such as megestrol acetate and anastrozole, are used as second-line treatments for postmenopausal women, whereas hormonal agents such as luteinizing hormone–releasing hormone agonists (e.g., goserelin) are used as second-line therapy in premenopausal women.

Symptom Management

Patients may have many questions about the selection of hormonal therapy and the associated side effects. Common side effects of the different hormonal agents are similar and include hot flushes, vaginal dryness or discharge, nausea, weight gain and fluid retention, and headache. Side effect management is directed at symptomatic relief based on the particular hormonal agent used.[63–68]

Psychosocial Support

QOL issues in advanced breast cancer are major concerns.[63,65] Understandably, patients are devastated by the news of recurrence and may have major fears of disfigurement, abandonment, and death. Other patients describe a profound sense of anger and loss on learning of their recurrence. At the same time, the patient can be given information about what treatment options are available and what to expect, and a reasonable discussion about the patient's recovery from treatment and length of survival can take place. Managing treatment of recurrence is balanced against QOL issues.

PATIENT CARE MANAGEMENT DURING THE AFTER-TREATMENT SURVIVAL PERIOD

Education

The end of treatment is associated with a decline in physical side effects, such as N and V, hair loss, and bone marrow depression. It is also associated with a return to some semblance of order and routine. However, breast cancer survivors often experience many physical and psychosocial adjustments after treatment ends.[69–73] Physiologic effects that can persist include fatigue and amenorrhea, with resulting infertility and menopausal symptoms in younger women.[74] Psychosocial adjustments may be marked by feelings of sadness, grief, loss, emotional letdown, and uncertainty over the future. Furthermore, social adjustments and concerns about managing relationships with spouses or significant others, children, family members, and friends[75–77]; sexuality issues; dealing with work and insurance concerns; and the existential focus of finding meaning in the experience of breast cancer are very real and expected tasks of managing illness demands in the aftertreatment period.[72]

Psychosocial Support

Responses of Spouse or Significant Other

Breast cancer exerts its effect on the spouse or significant other particularly during active treatment.[69,75–82] Family research indicates that spouses assume many of the daily home responsibilities during active treatment. However, when treatment ends, the responsibilities shift back to patients. Rarely does a diagnosis of breast cancer lead to major disruption of a marital or intimate relationship. Relationships that were stable before the diagnosis tend to remain stable after treatment. Conversely, relationships that were marked by discord continue to experience strain after treatment ends. Although patients may take advantage of the social support groups available for breast cancer survivors, spouses and significant others do so less often. One promising avenue for spouses to find information and exchange concerns is through Web-based discussions and chat rooms dedicated to breast cancer survivors. A listing of breast cancer–related Web sites is contained in Table 5.

Children's Concerns

Mothers with breast cancer report a variety of concerns about their children, ranging from daily disruptions (becoming sick during chemotherapy) to existential questions about dying and leaving the children behind.[81,82] The day-to-day concerns center on how to talk to their children about breast cancer without frightening them unnecessarily. A child's strengths and vulnerabilities, cognitive capacities, developmental level, age, and gender are the major influence of children's responses to a mother's breast cancer.[78] Hoke[78] suggests several intervention strategies in working with children: (a) Maintain clear and open communication with children about cancer, (b) share information and feelings about the disease, and (c) correct children's beliefs about cancer and allay unnecessary fears.

TABLE 5. *Breast cancer resources and referral Web sites*

Resource	Web site
American Cancer Society National Office 1599 Clifton Road, NE Atlanta, GA 30329, (800)-ACS-2345	http://www.cancer.org The American Cancer Society (ACS) home page includes information about the society and its purpose, mission, research, and grant opportunities. The site also includes information on ACS publications and resources for patients and families. The site contains specific information about breast cancer.
American Society of Clinical Oncology 225 Reinekers Lane, Suite 650 Alexandria, VA 22314 (703)-299-0150; Fax: 703-299-1044 asco@asco.org	http://www.asco.org This home page is aimed primarily at the American Society of Clinical Oncology membership. ASCO Online is an interactive resource for oncology professionals and cancer patients.
American Society of Plastic and Reconstructive Surgeons 444 E. Algonquin Road Arlington Heights, IL 60005 (800)-635-0635	http://www.plasticsurgery.org This site focuses on plastic and reconstructive issues.
American Society of Therapeutic Radiation Oncology	http://astro.org
Association of Oncology Social Work	http://www. medsch.wisc.edu/aosw/aoswhello.html The Association of Oncology Social Work (AOSW) is a nonprofit international organization dedicated to the enhancement of psychosocial services to people with cancer and their families. The AOSW Web page is a resource for its members, clients, and families and others interested in the psychosocial factors of the cancer experience.
Avon's Breast Cancer Awareness Crusade	http://www.avoncrusade.com Avon's Breast Cancer Awareness Crusade addresses concerns of women, with particular attention to low-income, minority, and older women. Information about breast cancer education and early-detection screening services. The Web site contains information of interest to health professionals and the public.

continued

TABLE 5. *Continued*

Resource	Web site
Breast Cancer Action 55 New Montgomery Street, Suite 323 San Francisco, CA 94105 (415)-243-9301; Fax: (415)-243-3996 bcaction@hooked.net	http://www.med.stanford.edu/bca/ This Web site includes more information about breast cancer action and serves as a resource specific to breast cancer.
Breast Cancer Information Clearinghouse	http://www.nysernet.org/bcic This site includes breast cancer–specific patient education materials, statistical information, links to national and federal organizations, and relevant state and federal legislation about breast cancer.
BreastCancer.Net	http://www.breastcancer.net This Web site includes services, news, and articles related to breast cancer and posts links to these stories on the site. It also links to many other breast cancer sites.
CancerCare Inc. 1180 Avenue of the Americas New York, NY 10036 (800)-813-HOPE	http://www.cancercareinc.org CancerCare Inc. provides assistance to people with any type of cancer, at any stage of illness. The Web site includes specific resources for breast cancer.
National Action Plan on Breast Cancer U.S. Public Health Services Office on Women's Health Department of Health and Human Services Room 718F 200 Independence Avenue, SW Washington, DC 20201 (202)-401-9587; Fax: (202)-401-9590 info@napbc.org	http://www.napbc.org The National Action Plan on Breast Cancer (NAPBC) is a private/public partnership dedicated to speeding the progress toward eradicating breast cancer.
National Alliance of Breast Cancer Organizations 9 East 37th Street, 10th Floor New York, NY 10016 (800)-719-9154; Fax: (212)-689-1213 NABCOinfo@aol.com	http://www.nabco.org The National Alliance of Breast Cancer Organizations (NABCO) is a network of breast cancer organizations. This site contains information on resources, clinical trials, support groups, and other topics related to breast cancer.
National Breast Cancer Coalition 1707 L Street, NW, Suite 1060 Washington, DC 20036 (202)-296-7477; Fax: (202)-265-6854	http://www.natlbcc.org The National Breast Cancer Coalition is a grassroots advocacy effort whose mission is to eradicate breast cancer through action and advocacy. Its Web site includes information on political agenda and legislative activities.
National Cancer Institute Cancer Information Service (800)-4-CANCER; Fax: (301)-402-5874 CancerNetComments@icic.nci.nih.gov	http://cancernet.nci.nih.gov CancerNet provides cancer information from the National Cancer Institute's (NCI) International Cancer Information Center and Office of Cancer Communications.
National Coalition for Cancer Survivorship 1010 Wayne Avenue, 5th Floor Silver Spring, MD 20910 (301)-650-8868; Fax: (301)-565-9670	http://www.cancsearch.org The National Coalition for Cancer Survivorship (NCCS) is a nationwide network of organizations and individuals who provide cancer support and information about all types of cancer. The Web site includes information about the organization, survivorship issues, media alerts, conferences and events, and links to cancer sites including breast cancer. Information is also available in Spanish.
National Lymphedema Network 2211 Post Street, Suite 404 San Francisco, CA 94115-3427 Hotline: (800)-541-3259 or (415)-921-1306; Fax: (415)-921-4284	http://www.wenet.net/~lymphnet/ The National Lymphedema Network (NLN) provides education and assistance about the prevention and management of primary and secondary lymphedema.

continued

TABLE 5. *Continued*

Resource	Web site
North American Menopause Society Post Office Box 94527 Cleveland, OH 44101 (216)-844-8748; Fax: (216)-844-8708 info@menopause.org	http://www.menopause.org The North American Menopause Society (NAMS) provides a forum for the discussion of human female menopause. Web site includes useful information about NAMS, publications, education, frequently asked questions (FAQs), and links.
OncoLink	http://cancer.med.upenn.edu The University of Pennsylvania Cancer Resource Web site has links and resources for oncology professionals and patients. Breast cancer information can be accessed. In addition, the site contains information on FAQs, conferences, financial issues, patient education materials, and news groups.
ONS Online Oncology Nursing Society 501 Holiday Drive Pittsburgh, PA 15220-2749 (412)-921-7373; Fax: (412)-921-6565	http://www.ons.org The Oncology Nursing Society (ONS) is a national organization of more than 25,000 registered nurses and other health care professionals dedicated to excellence in patient care, teaching, research, administration, and education in oncology. ONS collaborates with many nursing and health-related organizations throughout the world to educate health care professionals, facilitate information sharing among nurses, and provide state-of-the-knowledge cancer care resources.
SHARE: Self-Help for Women with Breast or Ovarian Cancer 1501 Broadway, Suite 1720 New York, NY 10036 (212)-382-2111; Fax: (212)-869-3431; Hotlines: Breast, (212)-382-2111; ovarian, (212)-719-1204; Spanish, (212)-719-4454	http://www.noah.cuny.edu/providers/share.html SHARE provides women with breast or ovarian cancer, and their families and friends, emotional and social support services.
Sisters Network National Headquarters 8787 Woodway Drive, Suite 4207 Houston, TX 77063 (713)-781-0255; Fax: (713)-780-8998 sistersnet@aol.com	http://users.aol.com/sistersnet/sis.html Sisters Network is a national African-American breast cancer survivors support group dedicated to understanding breast cancer in the African-American community. Web site includes information on its creed, local chapters, and news articles.
Susan G. Komen Breast Cancer Foundation LBJ Freeway, Suite 370 Dallas, TX 75244 (800)-IM-AWARE; Fax: (972)-385-5005	http://www. breastcancerinfo.com BreastCancerInfo.com is an on-line breast cancer information service provided by the Susan G. Komen Breast Cancer Foundation. Visitors to the site can obtain information about the Komen Foundation, Race for the Cure, grant information, and other breast cancer resources.
Y-ME National Breast Cancer Organizations 212 W. Van Buren Street Chicago, IL 60607-3908 (800)-221-2141; Fax: 312-294-8597 24-hour toll-free hotlines: English, (800)-221-2141; Spanish, (800)-986-9505 info@y-me.org	http://www.y-me.org The Y-ME National Breast Cancer Organization provides services through national hotlines, open door groups, early-detection workshops, and its local chapters. This home page provides specific links to breast health, breast cancer, advanced disease, family issues, and Y-ME newsletters.
YWCA Encore Program National Headquarters 726 Broadway, New York, NY 10003 (212)-614-2700	Provides support and rehabilitative exercise for women with breast cancer at various YWCA locations across the United States.

Adapted from Dow KH. *Pocket guide to breast cancer.* Sudbury, MA: Jones & Bartlett, 1999.

Adjustment to Work

Work issues can be major hurdles in adjustment after breast cancer.[80–82] Breast cancer survivors may desire to continue working or may seek new work or professional employment after treatment ends. The worry about health insurance and benefits continues to be a high-priority concern. Several cancer advocacy organizations, particularly the National Coalition for Cancer Survivorship, have excellent pamphlets and books that discuss insurance, employment, legal, and financial matters, all of which are of high concern to cancer survivors.

Meaning in Illness

Patients have used many resources and avenues in helping themselves to manage the breast cancer survival experience. Some become active in breast cancer advocacy; some volunteer at a local cancer organization, giving talks, meeting other breast cancer survivors, and coaching others through the experience; and some choose to spend time with close family and friends. The means are as varied and as individual as the women themselves. The main point to convey to other breast cancer survivors is that there *is* life after cancer. Although life may be different than before the breast cancer experience, it can be an inherently fulfilling and satisfying experience. Women can choose to dwell on the negative aspects, but in many breast cancer survivors' published experiences, rewards are described that were unforeseen or unknown at the time of their diagnosis.[1] Only in reflecting on their experiences were they able to identify them.

SUMMARY

In summary, the human dimension of living through and beyond the breast cancer experience is more than management of acute physical side effects. It is the careful attention to *persons* with breast cancer—their unique personalities, preferences, choices, decisions, experiences, and insights—that gives meaning, shape, and form to the illness and disease. On a day-to-day basis, oncology nurses are a vital component to the oncology team, helping to coordinate patient care, manage symptoms and psychosocial distress, manage the daily patient ebb and flow, evaluate QOL outcomes, and add the critical dimension of caring to oncology care.

REFERENCES

1. Leigh S. Choice and decision making in women with breast cancer. In: Dow KH, ed. *Contemporary issues in breast cancer*. Sudbury, MA: Jones & Bartlett, 1996:143.
2. Pierce PF. Deciding on breast cancer treatment: a description of decision behavior. *Nurs Res* 1993;42:22.
3. Monson M, Harwood K. Helping women select primary breast cancer treatment. *Am J Nurs* 1998;8[Suppl]:3.
4. Johnson J, Roberts C, Cox C, Reintgen D, et al. Breast cancer patients' personality style, age, and treatment decision making. *J Surg Oncol* 1996;63:183.
5. Neill K, Armstrong N, Burnet C. Choosing reconstruction after mastectomy: a qualitative analysis. *Oncol Nurs Forum* 1998;25:743
6. Beaver K, Luker K, Owens G, et al. Treatment decision making in women newly diagnosed with breast cancer. *Cancer Nurs* 1996;19:8.
7. Frogge M, Kalinowski B. Surgical therapy. In: Groenwald S, Frogge M, Yarbro C, Goodman M, eds. *Cancer nursing: principles and practice*, 4th ed. Sudbury, MA: Jones & Bartlett, 1997:229.
8. Kwekkeboom K. Postmastectomy pain syndromes. *Cancer Nurs* 1996;19:37.
9. Smith J, Miller L. Management of patients with cancer-related lymphedema. *Oncology Nursing: Patient Treatment and Support* 1998;5:1.
10. Kalinowski B. Lymphedema. In: Groenwald S, Frogge M, Yarbro C, Goodman M, eds. *Cancer symptom management*, 2nd ed. Sudbury, MA: Jones & Bartlett, 1999:819.
11. Porock D. The effects of preparatory patient education on the anxiety and satisfaction of cancer patients receiving radiotherapy. *Cancer Nurs* 1995;18:206.
12. O'Rourke N, Robinson L. Breast cancer and the role of radiation therapy. In: Dow KH, ed. *Contemporary issues in breast cancer*. Sudbury, MA: Jones & Bartlett, 1996;59.
13. Mazanec S. Breast cancer. In: Dow KH, Bucholtz JD, Iwamoto R, Fieler V, Hilderley L, eds. *Nursing care in radiation oncology*, 2nd ed. Philadelphia: WB Saunders, 1997;101.
14. Porock D, Kristjanson L, Nikoletti S, Cameron F, Pedler P. Predicting the severity of radiation skin reactions in women with breast cancer. *Oncol Nurs Forum* 1998;25:1019.
15. Bentzen S, Overgaard J. Patient-to-patient variability in the expression of radiation-induced normal tissue injury. *Semin Radiat Oncol* 1994;4:69.
16. Sitton E. Early and late radiation-induced skin alterations part I: mechanisms of skin changes. *Oncol Nurs Forum* 1992;19:801.
17. Sitton E. Early and late radiation-induced skin alterations part II: nursing care of irradiated skin. *Oncol Nurs Forum* 1992;19:907.
18. Archambeau J, Pezner R, Wasserman T. Pathophysiology of irradiated skin and breast. *Int Radiat Oncol Biol Phys J* 1995;31:1171.
19. Dunne-Daly CF. Skin and wound care in radiation oncology. *Cancer Nurs* 1995;18:144.
20. Sitton E. Managing side effects of skin changes and fatigue. In: Dow KH, Bucholtz JD, Iwamoto R, Fieler V, Hilderley L, eds. *Nursing care in radiation oncology*, 2nd ed. Philadelphia: WB Saunders, 1997;80.
21. Greenberg D, Sawicka J, Eisenthal S, Ross D. Fatigue syndrome due to localized radiation. *J Pain Symptom Manage* 1992;7:38.
22. Mock V, Hassey Dow K, Meares C, et al. Effects of exercises on fatigue, physical functioning, and emotional distress during radiation therapy for breast cancer. *Oncol Nurs Forum* 1997;24: 991
23. Vogelzang NJ, Breitbart W, Cella D, et al. Patient, caregiver, and oncologist perceptions of cancer-related fatigue: results of a tri-part assessment survey. *Semin Hematol* 1997; 34:3[Suppl 2]:4.
24. Blesch KS, Paice JA, Wickham R, et al. Correlates of fatigue in people with breast or lung cancer. *Oncol Nurs Forum* 1991;18:81.
25. Winningham M, Nail LM, Burke MB, et al. Fatigue and the cancer experience: the state of knowledge. *Oncol Nurs Forum* 1994;21:23.
26. Cimprich B. Symptom management: loss of concentration. *Sem Oncol Nurs* 1995;11:279.
27. Nail L, Winningham ML. Fatigue and weakness in cancer patients: the symptom experience. *Semin Oncol Nurs* 1995;11:272.
28. Graydon J, Bubela N, Irvine D, Vincent L. Fatigue-reducing strategies used by patients receiving treatment for cancer. *Cancer Nurs* 1995;18:23.
29. Miaskowski C. Nursing and medical interventions for cancer-related fatigue. In: Miaskowski C, ed. *Proceedings of access for success: managing fatigue*. San Francisco: Ortho-Biotech, 1997:18.
30. Johnston E, Crawford J. The hematologic support of the cancer patient. In: Berger A, Portenoy R, Weissman D, eds. *Principles and practice of supportive oncology*. Philadelphia: Lippincott–Raven, 1998:549.
31. Young-McCaughan S, Sexton DL. A retrospective investigation of the relationship between aerobic exercise and quality of life in women with breast cancer. *Oncol Nurs Forum* 1991;18:751.
32. Friendenreich CM, Courneya KS. Exercise as rehabilitation for cancer patients. *Clin J Sport Med* 1996;6:237.

33. Schwartz A. Patterns of exercise and fatigue in physically active cancer survivors. *Oncol Nurs Forum* 1998;25:485.
34. Beisecker A, Cook MR, Ashworth J, et al. Side effects of adjuvant chemotherapy: perceptions of node-negative breast cancer patients. *Psychooncology* 1997;6:85.
35. Jacobsen PB, Bovbjerg GH, Redd WH. Anticipatory anxiety in women receiving chemotherapy for breast cancer. *Health Psychol* 1993;12:469.
36. Greene D, Nail L, Fieler V, Dudgen D, Jones LA. Comparison of patient reported side effects during three chemotherapy regimens for breast cancer. *Cancer Pract* 1994;2:57.
37. Coates A, Abraham S, Kaye S, et al. On the receiving end—patient perceptions of the side effects of cancer chemotherapy. *Eur J Cancer Clin Oncol* 1983,19:203.
38. Pisters KM, Kris MG. Management of nausea and vomiting caused by anticancer drugs: state of the art. *Oncology* 1992;6:99.
39. Gregory RE, Ettinger DS. 5-HT3 receptor antagonists for the prevention of chemotherapy-induced nausea and vomiting: a comparison of their pharmacology and clinical efficacy. *Drugs* 1998;55:173.
40. Levitt M, Warr D, Yelle L, Rayner HL, Lofters WS, Perrault DJ, et al. Ondansetron compared with dexamethasone and metoclopramide as antiemetics in the chemotherapy of breast cancer with cyclophosphamide, methotrexate, and fluorouracil. *N Engl J Med* 1993: 328:1081.
41. Harvey RD III, Lindley CL. Serotonin antagonists: an update. *Cancer Pract* 1998;6:133.
42. Cubeddu LX, Hoffman IS, Fuenmayor NT, Finn AL. Antagonism of serotonin S3 receptors with ondansetron prevents nausea and emesis induced by cyclophosphamide-containing chemotherapy regimens. *J Clin Oncol* 1990;8:1721.
43. Nolte MJ, Berkery R, Pizzo B, et al. Assuring the optimal use of serotonin antagonist antiemetics: the process for development and implementation of institutional antiemetic guidelines at Memorial Sloan-Kettering Cancer Center. *J Clin Oncol* 1998;16:771.
44. Morrow GR, Roscoe JA, Kirshner JJ, Hynes HE, Rosenbluth RJ. Anticipatory nausea and vomiting in the era of 5-HT3 antiemetics. *Support Care Cancer* 1998;6:244.
45. Wickham R. Nausea and vomiting. In: Groenwald S, Frogge M, Goodman M, Yarbro C, eds. *Cancer symptom management*, 2nd ed. Sudbury, MA: Jones & Bartlett, 1996:218.
46. Cline BW. Prevention of chemotherapy induced alopecia: a review of the literature. *Cancer Nurs* 1984;6:221
47. Howser D. Alopecia. In: Groenwald S, Frogge M, Goodman M, Yarbro C, eds. *Cancer symptom management*, 2nd ed. Sudbury, MA. Jones & Bartlett, 1996:261.
48. Ferrell BR, Grant M, Dean GE, Funk B, Ly J. "Bone tired": the experience of fatigue and its impact on quality of life. *Oncol Nurs Forum* 1996;23:1539.
49. Berger AM. Patterns of fatigue and activity and rest during adjuvant breast cancer chemotherapy. *Oncol Nurs Forum* 1998;25:51.
50. Hann DM, Jacobsen PB, Martin SC, Kronish LE, Azzarello LM, Fields KK. Fatigue in women treated with bone marrow transplantation for breast cancer: a comparison with women with no history of cancer. *Support Care Cancer* 1997;5:44.
51. Messias D, Yeager K, Dibble S, Dodd M. Patients' perspectives of fatigue while undergoing chemotherapy. *Oncol Nurs Forum* 1997;24:43.
52. Demark-Wahnefried W, Rimer BK, Winer EP. Weight gain in women diagnosed with breast cancer. *J Am Diet Assoc* 1997;97:519.
53. Cheney CL, Mahloch J, Freeny P. Computerized tomography assessment of women with weight changes associated with adjuvant treatment for breast cancer. *Am J Clin Nutr* 1997;1:141.
54. Goodwin P, Esplen MJ, Butler K, et al. Multidisciplinary weight management in locoregional breast cancer: results of a phase II study. *Breast Cancer Res Treat* 1998;48:53.
55. Reymann P. Chemotherapy: principles of administration. In: Groenwald S, Frogge M, Goodman M, Yarbro C, eds. *Cancer nursing: principles and practice*, 3rd ed. Sudbury, MA: Jones & Bartlett, 1993:293.
56. McDonald A. Skin ulceration. In: Groenwald S, Frogge M, Goodman M, Yarbro C, eds. *Cancer symptom management*, 2nd ed. Sudbury, MA: Jones & Bartlett, 1996:364.
57. Powel L. *Cancer chemotherapy guidelines and recommendations for practice*. Pittsburgh: Oncology Nursing Press, 1996.
58. Smith S, Teresi M. Acute leukemias. In: Dipiro J, Talbert R, Yee G, Matzke G, Wells B, Post L, eds. *Pharmacotherapy: a pathophysiologic approach*. Stamford, CT: Appleton & Lange, 1997:2603.
59. Larson PJ, Miaskowski C, MacPhail L, et al. The PRO-SELF Mouth Aware program: an effective approach for reducing chemotherapy-induced mucositis. *Cancer Nurs* 1998;21:263.
60. Carl W. Oral complications of local and systemic cancer treatment. *Curr Opin Oncol* 1995;7:320.
61. Weiss HD, Walker MD, Wiernick PH. Neurotoxicity of commonly used antineoplastic agents. *N Engl J Med* 1974;291:75.
62. Martoni A, Zamagn C, Gheka A, Pannuti F. Antihistamines in the treatment of taxol induced paroxysitic pain. *J Natl Cancer Inst* 1993;85:676.
63. McEvilly JM, Dow KH. Treating metastatic breast cancer: principles and current practice. *Am J Nurs* 1998;[Suppl]:26.
64. Wasaff B. Current status of hormonal treatments for metastatic breast cancer in postmenopausal women. *Oncol Nurs Forum* 1997;24:1515.
65. Dow KH, Cloutier A. Current treatment of advanced breast cancer. In: Dow K, ed. *Contemporary issues in breast cancer*, special ed. Sudbury, MA: Jones & Bartlett, 1996:281.
66. Wood W. Newer developments in the management of advanced breast cancer. *Oncology* 1998;[Suppl]:131.
67. Goss P. Anastrazole: a new selective nonsteroidal aromatase inhibitor. *Oncology* 1997;11:1697.
68. Buzdar A, Hortobagyi G. Tamoxifen and toremifine in breast cancer: comparison of safety and efficacy. *J Clin Oncol* 1998:16:348.
69. Northouse LL, Laten D, Reddy P. Adjustment of women and their husbands to recurrent breast cancer. *Res Nurs Health* 1995;18:515.
70. Ganz PA, Coscarelli A, Fred C, Kahn B, Polinsky ML, Petersen L. Breast cancer survivors: psychosocial concerns and quality of life. *Breast Cancer Res Treat* 1996;38:183.
71. Ferrell BR, Grant MM, Funk BM, Otis-Green SA, Garcia NJ. Quality of life in breast cancer survivors: implications for developing support services. *Oncol Nurs Forum* 1998;25:887.
72. Dow KH, Ferrell BR, Leigh S, Ly J, Gulasekaram J. Quality of life in long-term survivors of breast cancer. *Breast Cancer Res Treatment* 1996;261.
73. Wilmoth MC, Ross JA. Women's perception: breast cancer treatment and sexuality. *Cancer Pract* 1997;5:353.
74. Dow KH, Harris JR, Roy C. Pregnancy after breast conserving surgery and radiation therapy. *J Natl Cancer Inst Monogr* 1994;16:131.
75. Hilton BA. Issues, problems, and challenges for families coping with breast cancer. *Semin Oncol Nurs* 1993;9:88.
76. Northouse LL. The impact of cancer in women on the family. *Cancer Pract* 1995; 3:134.
77. Zahlis EH, Shands ME. The impact of breast cancer on the partner 18 months after diagnosis. *Semin Oncol Nurs* 1993;9:83.
78. Hoke L. When a mother has breast cancer: parenting concerns and psychosocial adjustment in young children and adolescents. In: Dow K, ed. *Contemporary issues in breast cancer*. Sudbury, MA: Jones & Bartlett, 1996:173.
79. Hymovich DP. Child-rearing concerns of parents with cancer. *Oncol Nurs Forum* 1993;20:1355.
80. Berry DL. Return-to-work experience of people with cancer. *Oncol Nurs Forum* 1993;20:905.
81. Satariano WA, DeLorenze GN. The likelihood of returning to work after breast cancer. *Public Health Rep* 1996;111:236.
82. Hoffman B. *A cancer survivor's almanac: charting your journey*. Minneapolis: Chronimed Publishing, 1996.

Diseases of the Breast, 2nd ed.,
edited by Jay R. Harris.
Lippincott Williams & Wilkins, Philadelphia © 2000.

CHAPTER 67

Rehabilitation Management: Restoring Fitness and Return to Functional Activity

Lynn H. Gerber and Elizabeth M. Augustine

Historically, rehabilitation was sought for patients with breast cancer only if they had significant edema or frozen shoulder. Occasionally, patients who had severe pain or bony instability caused by metastatic disease involving bone, or those who were in need of a crutch, walker, or brace when they had an unstable spine or lower extremity, were referred for assistance.

Much has changed since the 1980s, when rehabilitative treatments were directed at crises or specific upper extremity needs, such as shoulder motion and limb compression for edema. Modern clinical practice requires that intervention be provided at multiple stages of breast cancer, as needed, and that it include education and preventive measures as well as restoration of or substitution for a variety of functions.

The needs of breast cancer patients are broad and span multiple stages of the illness. These individuals are likely to benefit from a comprehensive management program designed to provide early education and intervention for edema prevention and management, treatment of shoulder pain and dysfunction, counseling and recommendations for adaptation for change in body image requiring the use of breast prostheses or reconstruction, treatment to assist in the preservation or restoration of physical activity for daily routines and avocational activity, and nonpharmacologic management of pain.

When breast cancer is detected early, its treatment often has minimal impact on function. Nonetheless, not all patients are diagnosed early in their course; hence, educating them about self-monitoring for possible recurrence and taking a proactive role for a healthy lifestyle is very important in the total management. Recurrence, if it occurs, can sometimes be treated successfully, allowing patients to live for long periods of time, albeit with disability. These individuals often require ongoing supportive care, symptom relief, and education about maintaining independence in daily activity. Table 1 summarizes some of these issues.

L. H. Gerber: Rehabilitation Medicine Department, Georgetown University Medical Center, Washington, D.C.

E. M. Augustine: Physical Therapy Section, Warren G. Magnuson Clinical Center, National Institutes of Health, Bethesda, Maryland

APPROACH TO THE REHABILITATIVE MANAGEMENT OF BREAST CANCER

The most frequently seen physical problems in patients with breast cancer include incisional pain, shoulder pain and dysfunction, and limb edema. Upper extremity weakness occurs but is usually self-limited and quite mild. Concerns about body image and the ability to return to the prediagnosis level of function often cause anxiety, sleeplessness, and despair. Treatments that require radiation or chemotherapy, or both, often cause fatigue and nausea, which may increase the level of anxiety and despair. The disruption of normal routines at work, home, or play presents significant problems that often require support and treatment. The rehabilitation team frequently assists in the management of all of these problems.[1]

Data indicate that the greater the number of arm problems, the more psychological distress will occur.[1]

Some of these issues are most pressing during the pretreatment phase and others as the course progresses. We have identified five phases of disease, each with its own issues, that may be amenable to rehabilitation interventions (Table 2).

The diagnostic/predefinitive treatment phase is one in which the patient can benefit from interventions designed to educate her about the disease, what her choices are for treatment, and how to assess changes in function. Symptoms of anxiety that may occur during this phase are usually related to the patient's uncertainty about the future and her ability to remain independent.

The treatment phase requires interventions to help restore and maintain shoulder mobility and activity pertaining to self-care, mobility, and control of pain.

The postdefinitive treatment phase requires education about preserving function and returning to normal activity, dispelling myths about the "to dos" and the "can't dos." During this phase, the patient should be instructed in what to monitor, when to call for help, and how to advocate for her own well-being in the areas of pain, strength, range of motion (ROM), stamina, and edema. The goals are to maxi-

TABLE 1. *Rehabilitation-related issues for cancer patients*

Phase of breast cancer	Patient needs	Symptoms	Impact of symptoms
I. Pretreatment and evaluation	Information about Treatment options Impact of illness	Pain Anxiety	Daily routines Sleep Fatigue
II. Treatment	Information Support Help with daily routines (e.g., vocational, home)	Pain Anxiety Shoulder mobility, wound/skin care	Daily routines Sleep/stamina Self-care Comesis
III. Posttreatment	Support Rehabilitation interventions	Pain, anxiety/depression, shoulder mobility, edema, fatigue/stamina	Sleep/fatigue Activities of daily living Vocational/ avocational Cosmesis
IV. Recurrence	Education Support	Pain Anxiety/depression Fatigue/stamina Edema Bony instability	Sleep disturbance Disability Disruption of routines Cosmesis
V. End of life	Education Support	Pain Fatigue	Dependence

mize activities and to be able to return to a more predictable level of performance at work, home, and play.

The phase in which breast cancer has recurred is, in many ways, similar to the initial phase in terms of reviewing treatment options and their risks. The impact of having a recurrence, how it is treated, and what are the sequelae of treatment are the issues that must be better described and understood. The maintaining of functional activity and rebuilding stamina and strength, controlling pain, and assuring self-advocacy are the important issues during this phase.

During the last phase, end-of-life issues are usually centered around educating the patient and her family about the future course of the disease and its impact on function. Rehabilitation specialists provide assistance in the use of nonpharmacologic management of pain (e.g., heat, cold, transcutaneous electrical nerve stimulator units), providing comfort and symptom relief. Treatment is aimed at maintaining independence and quality in daily activity. Counseling and support are provided for end-of-life issues, when requested.

REHABILITATION AND TREATMENT

Preoperative Evaluation

One preoperative visit (30 to 60 minutes) provides the rehabilitation specialist with valuable baseline information

TABLE 2. *Five phases of disease*

Phase of disease	Issues for rehabilitation professionals to address
I. Diagnosis to treatment planning	1. What to expect with respect to the impact of breast cancer treatment on function 2. Understanding function and how to preserve it 3. Comprehensive rehabilitation preoperative evaluation [e.g., range of motion (ROM), activities of daily living (ADL), strength]
II. Treatment	1. Evaluation of the effects of treatments on function (surgical, chemotherapy, radiation, biological agents) 2. Preserving and restoring function through exercise, edema management, and increased activity 3. Controlling pain using heat, cold, and transcutaneous electrical nerve stimulators
III. Posttreatment	1. Developing and supporting a program to help restore daily routines 2. Educating patient about what to monitor (e.g., strength, ROM, edema, pain) 3. Supervising a maintenance program of exercise and edema management
IV. Recurrence	1. Educating patient about impact of recurrence and its treatment on function 2. Educating patient about what to monitor in the context of her new clinical status 3. Supervising the patient in an appropriate maintenance program 4. Assisting the patient in maintaining activity and quality of life
V. End of life	1. Educating patient and family in mobility training, good body mechanics, and assistive devices 2. Pain management (nonpharmacologic treatment) and symptom control 3. Maintaining independence and quality of life

TABLE 3. *Treatment/education checklist for breast surgery physical therapy*

Educated/discussed with patient
- Sensation changes expected
- Lymphedema precautions
- Prosthesis information
- Posture realignment
- Shoulder movement guidelines
- Lifting precautions (<5 lb for 2 wk) (<10 lb for 6 wk)
- General conditioning recommendations
- Exercise guidelines if receiving radiation treatment
- Breast self-examination and its importance
- Self-monitoring of edema
- Relaxation techniques

Patient taught and performed
- Elevation/positioning of involved upper extremity
- Pumping exercises
- Deep-breathing exercises (emphasizing upper chest and rib cage expansion)
- Cervical range-of-motion exercises
- Shoulder shrugs/retractions
- Elbow flexion/extension/supination/pronation
- Active shoulder range-of-motion exercises (avoid incisional stretch pain)
- Home exercise program
- Other

that can become very important for the patient's overall functional outcome, especially regarding shoulder function and possible postoperative management of lymphedema. Patient education, which can decrease the patient's anxiety regarding postoperative rehabilitation and cosmesis, should take place at this time. Table 3 includes a checklist of patient education topics that are useful for those undergoing breast surgery. It should be noted that, although preoperative bilateral upper extremity circumferential girth measurements are taken, some women experience postoperative lymphedema in the ipsilateral chest wall or remaining breast tissue (lumpectomy) before it is ever manifested in the arm. These patients should be instructed to contact their physician or a rehabilitation specialist, or both, as soon as possible for treatment and instruction in lymphatic drainage massage. Early detection and early intervention minimize the adverse effects of lymphedema.[2,3] For more information on lymphedema management, see Chapter 69.

Treatment

Staging of the breast cancer determines what is needed for medical management. The goals for management of breast cancer are threefold: (a) preserve life, (b) minimize recurrence, and (c) provide best functional and cosmetic results. Table 4 lists recommendations for rehabilitation interventions during oncologic treatment. Medical treatments for breast cancer present a variety of clinical problems that may have functional impact and may respond to different rehabilitation interventions.

Common problems include arm swelling, breast/chest wall swelling, shoulder ROM deficits, cording, weakness in hand grip strength or shoulder girdle strength, scapular winging, shoulder stiffness, postural changes, chest wall tenderness, cervical or upper trapezius pain, and pain in the arm, including numbness along the inner aspect of the arm. Associated symptoms often include depression, anxiety, and fatigue. Perception of loss of self-efficacy is also experienced.

The program developed at the National Institutes of Health is comprehensive and was developed after many years of clinical experience with patients with breast cancer. All patients who undergo mastectomy or axillary dissection are referred to rehabilitation. The patients are provided standard treatment, for which progressive arm mobility is the goal (Table 5). We also attempt to control shoulder girdle and chest wall pain and upper extremity edema to promote full functional recovery.[4] All patients receive encouragement and education regarding the benefits of continuing to live a healthy lifestyle and maintaining aerobic fitness. Table 6 represents a summary of our approach to comprehensive rehabilitation for the patient diagnosed with breast cancer.

Today, many managed care programs offer axillary dissection as an outpatient surgical procedure and aspirate seromas as needed. Also, many managed care programs do not routinely refer breast cancer patients for postoperative rehabilitation. Studies indicate that early postoperative rehabilitation intervention improves functional outcomes.[4,5] If a patient experiences any of the previously mentioned signs or symptoms, she is likely to benefit from treatment, and she should be referred to a rehabilitation specialist for appropriate intervention.

During surgery for axillary lymphadenectomy, trauma to the long thoracic nerve can occur, which can result in weakness of the serratus anterior (SA) muscle. Scapular winging is an early clue to SA muscle weakness. Early detection and intervention can lead to full recovery of the SA muscle with resultant scapular stability by 6 months.[6]

Because the patient with SA palsy is unable to complete full shoulder ROM in an upright position, she is instructed in an exercise program in the supine position to provide stability to the scapula and eliminate the weight of her arm. The patient should continue ROM and strengthening exercises in the supine position until the SA has regained functional strength. Without these instructions, the patient will experience increasing shoulder tightness, pain, and frustration as she attempts unsuccessfully to regain normal shoulder function.[6]

Another condition that can occur after axillary lymphadenectomy is the development of superficial cordlike structures along the medial aspect of the upper arm and over the anterior elbow. These fibrous bands are believed to be sclerosing lymphatics. They may occur in the axilla or olecranon. They can cause pain and limit shoulder flexion and abduction when the elbow is fully extended or may limit elbow extension. These symptoms are self-limited. The cords can break spontaneously or during a treatment session, when the therapist gently applies manual traction to them. Often, a popping sound can be heard when the cords break, and con-

TABLE 4. *Rehabilitation interventions during oncologic treatment*

Oncologic treatment	Recommended rehabilitation during treatment[a]
Cyclophosphamide	Because of frequently observed fatigue, anorexia, and nausea, the following interventions are recommended: an exercise program to improve endurance to perform activities of daily living (ADL), weightbearing activities to prevent osteoporosis, relaxation therapy.
Methotrexate	Because of frequently observed fatigue, nausea, and stomatitis, the following interventions are recommended: an exercise program to improve endurance to perform ADL, relaxation therapy.
5-Fluorouracil	Because of frequently observed fatigue, ataxia, and photosensitivity, the following interventions are recommended: balance and gait training, mobility aids, exercise program to improve endurance to perform ADL, relaxation therapy.
Vincristine	Because of frequently observed fatigue, depression, confusion, and neurotoxicity (temporary paresthesiae, motor weakness, loss of deep tendon reflex), the following interventions are recommended: balance and gait training, mobility aids, hand therapy for fine motor activities, exercise program to strengthen muscles and improve endurance to perform ADL, relaxation therapy, pain management [transcutaneous electrical nerve stimulators (TENS)], sensory stimulation for dysesthesias.
Doxorubicin	Because of the frequently observed fatigue, nausea, vomiting, stomatitis, and cardiotoxicity (cardiac arrhythmias, cardiomyopathy), the following interventions are recommended: carefully supervised exercise program to improve endurance to perform ADL, instruct patient to monitor cardiac status, relaxation therapy.
Tamoxifen	Because of the frequently observed fatigue, hot flashes, nausea, vomiting, weight gain, and pain in existing soft-tissue/bony lesions, the following interventions are recommended: exercise program for weight control and to improve endurance to perform ADL, relaxation therapy, pain management (TENS).
Prednisone	Because of the frequently observed edema (moon face, truncal obesity), muscle weakness and atrophy (high doses), osteoporosis, and glucose intolerance, the following interventions are recommended: edema management, exercise program for strengthening and weight control and increasing bone mineral, possible glucose regulation.
Radiation therapy	Because of the frequently observed fatigue, loss of elasticity and contractility leading to fibrosis of muscle and contractures, and osteopenia, the following interventions are recommended: exercise program to maintain range of motion and prevent contracture and osteoporosis, instruction in activities to avoid/prevent pathologic fractures.
Bone marrow transplant	Because of the frequently observed fatigue, social isolation, loss of lean body mass, and soft-tissue contractures, the following interventions are recommended: carefully supervised exercise program to improve strength and endurance and increase lean mass.

[a]Effects of oncologic interventions that might impact on function and be amenable to treatment.

sequently an increase in shoulder ROM will be noted.[7] These are avascular structures and do not bleed when ruptured.

Because the intercostobrachial and medial brachial cutaneous nerves can be damaged during axillary lymphadenectomy, it is not uncommon for patients to experience medial arm pain and paresthesia. Although the intensity of these symptoms will subside over time, the medial arm numbness may be permanent.

TABLE 5. *Recommended postoperative shoulder mobilization schedule*

Postoperative day	Flexion (degrees)	Abduction (degrees)	Internal and external rotation (degrees)
1–2[a]	40	40	To tolerance
3[a]	45	45	To tolerance
4–6[a]	45–90	45	To tolerance
7	To tolerance	To tolerance	To tolerance
Drains out[b]	To tolerance	To tolerance	To tolerance

[a]Gentle accessory mobilization of glenohumeral joint may also be included.
[b]Active assistive range-of-motion exercises are added or an overhead pulley is used at this time when needed.

Because of the morbidity associated with axillary lymphadenectomy, oncologists are attempting to find less invasive procedures for breast cancer staging, such as the sentinel node biopsy.[8]

The cancer management team should be well acquainted with the needs of the patient undergoing radiation. Close monitoring is needed to prevent potential sequelae of radiation, which include local erythema and possible burn, local edema in the radiation field, and limb edema. In addition, shoulder mobility may be influenced by the radiation field and dosimetry. All patients who undergo radiation therapy for breast cancer should be instructed in a daily home exercise program to maintain their shoulder ROM and strength. (Normal ROM for shoulder abduction is 180 degrees, and patients require at least 110 degrees of shoulder abduction to receive radiation to the axilla.) Without this daily stretching program, radiation-induced fibrosis can occur and cause contractures that result in permanent physical disability.

Ideally, the patient should be seen once or twice by a rehabilitation specialist during the course of radiation ther-

TABLE 6. *Summary of recommendations for rehabilitation treatments*

Problem	Preoperative evaluation	Postoperative evaluation				
		0–2 wk	2–12 wk	3–6 mo	6–12 mo	>1 yr
Edema	Obtain baseline measurements. If edema present, determine cause.	Instruct in preventive arm care. If edema present, 2–4 cm without erythema: Treat and instruct patient in LDM; low-stretch compression bandaging, exercises; fit with ready-made compression sleeve. If edema present, >4 cm without erythema: same as 2–4 cm; use compression pump after LDM with pressures ≤45 mm Hg. Any, with erythema, Rx: antibiotics.	Same as 0–2 wk.	Same as 0–2 wk. Depending on severity, patient may require custom-made compression sleeve. Instruct patient to bandage at night and wear compression sleeve during the day and when flying.	Same as 3–6 mo. With pain, rule out metastasis.	Same as 3–6 mo. With pain, rule out metastasis.
Shoulder motion	Obtain baseline measurements. If <145 degrees of flexion or abduction <60 degrees of ER/IR, Rx: Heat and ROM exercise. Precautions must be taken for proper arm position intra-operatively.	See Table 5.	Begin use of pulley. If <145 degrees of flexion or abduction <60 degrees of ER/IR: Use heat, ice (except when patient is being actively irradiated). Active and passive stretch. If no progress by week 8, add NSAIDs to regimen and check monthly.	Determine ROM. If <160 degrees of flexion, 145 degrees of abduction, 60 degrees of ER/IR, Rx: ROM exercises with assistance from physical therapist.	Determine ROM. If <160 degrees of flexion, 145 degrees of abduction, or 60 degrees of ER/IR, and if ROM exercises not effective, Rx: Scan, NSAIDs, intraarticular steroids.	Same as 6–12 mo.
Muscle strength	Obtain baseline measurement of shoulder complex strength, particularly stabilizers of scapula.	Evaluate strength. If weakness, especially serratus anterior, support scapula with patient in supine position during exercises.	Evaluate strength of shoulder girdle muscle. Strength should be returning by end of this period. Maintain ROM. If weakness, continue to support scapula during exercises.	Evaluate strength of shoulder girdle muscles. If abnormal strength, determine cause. Postoperative weakness should be resolved by 6 mo.	Same as 3–6 mo.	Same as 3–6 mo.
Prosthesis	NA	Fluff or, when wound heals, permanent prosthesis.	Same as 0–2 wk.	Consider reconstruction.	Same as 3–6 mo.	Same as 3–6 mo.
Psychological support	Orientation to surgery, radiation, and common postoperative problems.	Support group and relaxation techniques, if appropriate.	Same as 0–2 wk.	Same as 0–2 wk.	Same as 3–6 mo.	Same as 3–6 mo.

ER, external rotation; IR, internal rotation; LDM, self–lymphatic drainage massage; NA, not applicable; NSAIDs, nonsteroidal antiinflammatory drugs; ROM, range of motion; Rx, therapy.

TABLE 7. *Patient education*

Monitor shoulder range of motion
Monitor girth in limb/remaining breast tissue/chest wall
Daily stretching exercises
Dos and don'ts

apy to monitor compliance and progress with the home exercise program. Regaining full ROM is often difficult if there has been significant loss due to immobilization after axillary dissection and radiation. Patient education before discharge from rehabilitation is extremely important in empowering an individual to be independent in self-management (Table 7).

Fatigue frequently accompanies radiation treatment, during which patients often observe loss of energy and inability to carry out their normal activity. The impact that radiation and chemotherapy have in general tends to place obstacles in the path of continued active lifestyle. Prolonged bed rest or inactivity during this time can cause deconditioning and result in orthostatic hypotension, ataxia, decreased cardiac stroke volume, and muscle atrophy. Hence, the rehabilitation team should address the needs of individuals for activity, determine their aerobic capacity, and provide treatment to help support this during and after treatment. The specifics of the treatment should be tailored to the needs of the patient and her existing medical condition. The appropriate level of fitness has to be established based on the individual's needs and desires.

Exercise can increase a patient's strength, endurance, sense of wellness, and functional abilities.[9–11] A 1998 study of physically active cancer survivors, who spent an average of 9 hours a week exercising, found that by reducing the intensity, frequency, or duration, they could continue to work out during medical treatment for their cancer. For them, moderate exercise was an intervention to reduce cancer-related fatigue.[12] However, contraindications to exercise exist (Table 8).

During prolonged hospitalization for chemotherapy or bone marrow transplant, a comprehensive therapeutic recreation program provides the patient with an active means to reduce anxiety, boredom, depression, disorientation, or isolation. After an informal interview, the recreation therapist can plan for the patient's specific leisure needs during this extended period of time. When patients participate in pleasant leisure activities, they are not focusing on their cancer treatment or side effects. In fact, many patients who participate in craft activities begin to focus on making gifts for friends and family before their discharge from the hospital.[13]

Some patients want to take a more active holistic approach to their cancer treatment and request instruction in relaxation therapy or guided imagery, or both, from the recreation therapists at the National Institutes of Health. Patients feel empowered with this noninvasive, self-enriching adjunct therapy when incorporated with their standard medical treatment. Participation in these nonmedical techniques allows the patient to refocus from illness to wellness and also encourages her to take more responsibility for her health and a healthy lifestyle.[14]

Breast Reconstruction

Many women who undergo a mastectomy opt for breast reconstruction surgery. The transverse rectus abdominis myocutaneous flap has become the most common surgical procedure for breast reconstruction. However, specific postoperative complications after this procedure include decreased abdominal muscle strength, abdominal wall hernias, and low back pain. Atelectasis, pulmonary emboli, and deep vein thrombosis are rare but potential postoperative complications. Patients who undergo a transverse rectus abdominis myocutaneous flap procedure should be referred for postoperative rehabilitation to improve trunk strengthening, improve posture and body mechanics, and reduce low back pain. Patients should be instructed not to perform lifting or sit-ups until 6 weeks after surgery.[15]

MYTHS

Patients are given precautions immediately after surgery; unfortunately, they are often not revisited after the surgical site has healed. Consequently, these precautions become a

TABLE 8. *Contraindications to rehabilitation intervention (or significant modifications to an exercise program)*

Acute infections and fevers
Hematocrit <25% (shortness of breath governs level of activity)
Platelets <5,000 (spontaneous bleeding can occur)
Platelets 5–20,000 (minimal injury can cause bleeding)
Metastatic bony lesions with >50% cortex involved
Large pleural effusions
Recent premature ventricular contractions
Tachycardia
Ascites (severe)
Complications from radiation therapy (local skin changes, seromas)

TABLE 9. *Myths*

I can never lift anything heavier than 10 lb.
I cannot lift objects over my head.
I can never play tennis or be physically active.
There's nothing you can do about lymphedema.
Lymphedema develops in every woman who undergoes an axillary lymph node dissection.
I cannot go out in the sun.
Lymphedema only develops in women who undergo surgery for a mastectomy.
Lumpectomy never develops in women who undergo surgery for a lumpectomy.

TABLE 10. *Dos and don'ts for the limb at risk of developing lymphedema*

Practice good skin hygiene (keep skin clean, supple, and moist).
Avoid trauma to the skin (cuts, sunburns, insect bites).
Wear gloves while gardening or washing dishes.
Don't use saunas or hot tubs.
Wear a compression sleeve during airplane flights.[a]
Avoid binding or squeezing the affected arm (wear loose jewelry, loose sleeves; no injections, blood draws, or blood pressure taken on affected arm).
Redness, warmth, swelling; see your physician as soon as possible.

[a]Casley-Smith J. *Modern treatment for lymphoedema.* Adelaide, Australia: Lymphoedema Association of Australia, 1997:126.

way of life for the patient, even if they are no longer appropriate or accurate (Table 9). The adherence to these may interfere with the patient's attempts to achieve her highest level of function. Lack of education of the patient regarding the potential development of lymphedema after treatment for breast cancer contributes to the formation of additional myths (see Table 9). Referral to a rehabilitation specialist for education and intervention can help to eliminate these myths and allow the patient to return to normal activity.

Although lymphedema does not develop in all women who have been treated for breast cancer, all women should be educated about protecting the limb at risk. We advocate that the patient receive a list of "dos and don'ts" (Table 10) soon after surgery, as well as additional information on the etiology and management of lymphedema. With good self-monitoring, the patient can seek early intervention at the first signs and symptoms of lymphedema and consequently minimize its adverse effects.[16]

Although it is important to bring observations of limb girth changes, as well as weakness, pain, and restricted movement, to the attention of health care professionals, these symptoms often resolve with therapy.[17] Lymphedema is the only sequelum whose incidence increases over time.[18]

REFERENCES

1. Maunsell E, Brisson J, DeSchenes L. Arm problems and psychological distress after surgery for breast cancer. *Can J Surg* 1993;36:315.
2. Rockson S, Miller L, Senie R, et al. Diagnosis and management of lymphedema. *Cancer* 1998;83[Suppl 12]:2882.
3. Clarysse A. Lymphoedema following breast cancer treatment. *Acta Clin Belg* 1993;15[Suppl]:47.
4. Lotze MT, Duncan MA, Gerber LH, et al. Early vs. delayed shoulder motion following axillary dissection. *Ann Surg* 1981;193:288.
5. Healey J. Role of rehabilitation medicine in the care of the patient with breast cancer. *Cancer* 1971;28:1666.
6. Duncan MA, Lotze MT, Gerber LH, Rosenberg SA. Incidence, recovery, and management of serratus anterior muscle palsy after axillary node dissection. *Phys Ther* 1983;63:1243.
7. Wood C, Gerber L. Rehabilitation of the patient with breast cancer. In: Lippman M, Lichter A, Danforth D, eds. *Diagnosis and management of breast cancer*. Philadelphia: WB Saunders, 1988:457.
8. Krag D, Weaver D, Ashikaga T, et al. The sentinel node in breast cancer. *N Engl J Med* 1998;339:941.
9. Winningham ML. Walking program for people with cancer. *Cancer Nurs* 1991;14(5):270.
10. Winningham ML, MacVicar MG, Bondoc M, et al. Effect of aerobic exercise on body weight and composition in patients with breast cancer on adjuvant chemotherapy. *Oncol Nurs Forum* 1989;16:683.
11. Johnson JB, Kelly AW. A multifaceted rehabilitation program for women with cancer. *Oncol Nurs Forum* 1990;17:691.
12. Schwartz AL. Patterns of exercise and fatigue in physically active cancer survivors. *Oncol Nurs Forum* 1998;25:485.
13. O'Connell S. Recreation therapy: reducing the effects of isolation for the patient in a protected environment. *Child Health Care* 1984;12(3):118.
14. Post-White J, Johnson M. Complementary nursing therapies in clinical oncology practice: relaxation and imagery. *Dimens Oncol Nurs* 1991;5(2):15.
15. Monteiro M. Physical therapy implications following the TRAM procedure. *Phys Ther* 1997;77:765.
16. Carter BJ. Women's experiences of lymphedema. *Oncol Nurs Forum* 1997;24(5):875.
17. Gerber L, Lampert M, Wood C, et al. Comparison of pain, motion and edema after modified radical mastectomy vs. local excision with axillary dissection and radiation. *Breast Cancer Res Treat* 1992;21:139.
18. Hladiuk M, Huchcroft S, Temple W, Schnurr BE. Arm function after axillary dissection for breast cancer: a pilot study to provide parameter estimates. *J Surg Oncol* 1992;50:47.

Diseases of the Breast, 2nd ed.,
edited by Jay R. Harris.
Lippincott Williams & Wilkins, Philadelphia © 2000.

CHAPTER 68

Psychosocial Issues and Interventions

Julia H. Rowland and Mary Jane Massie

Breast cancer, the most common form of cancer among American women, will be diagnosed in a projected 175,000 women in in the year 2000; fewer than 43,000 women will die of the disease, based on the currently flat incidence and the declining mortality rates. Although an exact understanding of the causes and control of breast cancer continues to elude researchers, rapid advances in detection and treatment have led to increases in the disease-free survival among women diagnosed with breast cancer.[1–3] The majority of women diagnosed can expect to be cured of or live for long periods with their disease. However, unlike treatment for other chronic diseases, such as diabetes and heart disease, the treatments for cancer are more toxic and intensive. In fact, the general trend since the late 1980s has been to increase the use of adjuvant therapy and the dosages administered in women's care.[4] The result is increasing demands not only on patients' physical reserves, but also on their psychological and social resources to survive and manage illness.

Specific developments in breast cancer care have drawn attention to the key role of psychosocial factors in prevention, detection, treatment, and outcome.[5] Improvements in and broader use of screening mammography have led not only to an increase in numbers of women whose cancers are diagnosed at earlier stages, but also to questions of who gets screened and who does not. The greater availability of options for surgical management (e.g., lumpectomy plus irradiation versus mastectomy with or without breast reconstruction with implants or autologous tissue, or both) has expanded the woman's role in the decision-making process. More extensive use of aggressive multimodal treatment regimens has increased sensitivity to issues of patient-doctor and family communication and patient adherence. Finally, the identification of genetic markers of breast cancer risk and the evaluation of chemopreventive agents have raised awareness of the psychological toll on unaffected women who are at increased risk for this disease, sometimes referred to as the "worried well."[6]

All of these changes have occurred in the context of greater demand by patients for involvement in their own care, consumer activism, attention to ethical and informed consent issues, use of quality of life assessment in treatment outcomes, and, most recently, emphasis on cost efficacy in care. The consequence of these changes is a growing demand for medical professionals to recognize and address the psychosocial impact of breast cancer across the continuum of care.

Although breast cancer is a major stress for any woman, there is great variability in women's psychological responses. This chapter outlines the normal and abnormal responses to breast cancer and factors that may increase a woman's risk for poor adaptation. In addition, because of their growing importance, the role of family in women's adaptation and special concerns related to sexual functioning and survivorship are addressed.

FACTORS THAT AFFECT PSYCHOLOGICAL IMPACT

Three sets of factors contribute to psychological response: the sociocultural context in which treatment options are offered, the psychological and psychosocial factors that the woman and her environment bring to the situation, and the medical factors or physical facts the woman must confront in terms of disease stage, treatment, response, and clinical course (Table 1). To provide comprehensive care to every woman, each of these areas must be assessed and, when encountered, problems must be addressed across the illness trajectory.

Sociocultural Context and Decision Making

To understand and interpret the data on women's responses to breast cancer, an appreciation of the context within which diagnosis and treatment occur, both medically

J. H. Rowland: Office of Cancer Survivorship, Division of Cancer Control and Population Sciences, National Cancer Institute, Bethesda, Maryland

M. J. Massie: Barbara White Fishman Center for Psychological Counseling, Department of Psychiatry and Behavioral Sciences, Memorial Sloan-Kettering Cancer Center, New York, New York

TABLE 1. *Factors that contribute to the psychological responses of women to breast cancer*

Current sociocultural context, treatment options, and decision making
Changes in surgical and medical management from a uniform approach
Breast-conserving management; introduction of sentinel node biopsies and neoadjuvant therapy; more therapeutic options and acknowledged uncertainty
Social attitudes
Public figures openly sharing their breast cancer experience
Autobiographic accounts of and "how to" guides for treatment of breast cancer in popular press
Ethical imperative for patient participation in treatment issues; legal imperative for knowledge of treatment options
Variations in care by ethnicity, location, age
Public awareness of treatment and research controversies; advocacy for more funding and lay oversight
Psychological and psychosocial factors
Type and degree of disruption in life cycle tasks caused by breast cancer (e.g., marital, childbearing)
Psychological stability and ability to cope with stress
Prior psychiatric history
Availability of psychological and social support (partner, family, friends)
Medical factors
Stage of cancer at diagnosis
Treatment(s) received: mastectomy/lumpectomy and radiation, adjuvant chemotherapy, hormonal therapy, bone marrow transplant
Availability of rehabilitation
Psychological (partner, support groups)
Physical (reconstruction; arm mobility and lymphedema prevention)
Psychological support provided by physicians and staff

and socially, is critical. The broader changes in public attitudes toward cancer over the twentieth century are reviewed elsewhere.[7] Several specific changes that have taken place in the scientific understanding of and medical approach to breast cancer in the 1980s and 1990s have had a significant impact on how this disease is viewed by the public. Primary among these changes have been growing attention to the patient's role in decision making across the course of cancer care, increased demand for and greater public involvement in the assessment of research into the prevention and treatment of breast cancer, and more federal support for research on the psychosocial and behavioral aspects of cancer.

The importance of patient involvement in treatment choices is the result of the broader range of options offered at time of diagnosis and greater intensity of treatments recommended for the majority of women, even those with early-stage disease, as well as increased public demand for informed consent. Women with a diagnosis of breast cancer are aware of the plurality of views about primary breast cancer treatment. Most recognize that no "best" treatment exists, that they have options, and that their preference can be considered in the decision. Women are often provided with survival statistics associated with each mode of treatment, although physicians may vary in the emphasis placed on them. The increased dialogue between physician and patient about treatment reduces some of the common stresses faced by women treated prior to the late 1970s when there was little discussion about management of the disease. However, the new psychological burden of responsibility for making the right choice can increase anxiety at a time when it is already great. Women often talk about their experience as one in which they felt they "had to become a breast cancer expert overnight."

Over the course of initial care, women face three major decision points. The first of these is at the time of initial discovery of the lump. Most women consult their gynecologist or a trusted and accessible physician when they find a lump (64% to 70% of which are found by women themselves).[8] How quickly a woman decides to seek evaluation of her lump or to follow up on a recommended course of action depends on a number of variables, including sociodemographic status; knowledge, attitudes, and beliefs about cancer; personality and coping styles; and the nature of the existing doctor-patient relationship.[9] It is well established that the earlier her tumor is detected, the more likely a woman's breast cancer is to be curable. However, presence of advanced disease does not always imply delay.[10] Furthermore, responsibility for delay may rest with the physician, the woman, or both. One study suggests that survival rates are higher in women who themselves delayed diagnosis than in women whose physicians were responsible for the delay.[11] In cases in which delay has occurred, a woman's response, including feelings of guilt over her role in the delay, anger at her physician's role, or both, can interfere with her ability to adapt to treatment. Helping her to focus on the fact that she is receiving care now and deferring exploration of what impact, if any, delaying diagnosis may have had can be important in enabling a woman to engage in the recovery process.

At the time of consultation with a surgeon, the woman is faced with her second set of decisions: whether to accept a one- or two-step procedure; if given a choice, whether to undergo mastectomy or lumpectomy plus irradiation; and whether to seek a second opinion or care elsewhere. In 18 states, the law and clinical practice dictate that the surgeon must inform the woman that she has the option of a two-stage surgical procedure, which separates the diagnostic biopsy from the primary treatment procedure. In these states, the two treatment options of mastectomy or lumpectomy with irradiation must be presented as well, although how this is done varies widely by state.[12] Some insurance carriers mandate a second opinion before the performance of any elective procedure. Research has shown that these laws make a difference; in those states that mandate informed decision making, more women receive lumpectomy.[13,14] At the same time, although these policies provide a valuable impetus for women to obtain thorough medical evaluation and information, they also serve to introduce other sets of opinions. The woman whose second or third opinion differs dramatically has the difficult task of deciding which physician she trusts and which treatment plan to accept.[15] Meanwhile, considerable time can be lost. For surgeons who see a patient who has visited multiple other consultants, it may be important to help set a limit on further information gathering. This can be done very concretely by recommending that she set a date after which to stop her search or by which time she should be scheduled for surgery.

Beginning in the early 1990s, a number of cancer centers across the United States have developed multidisciplinary breast clinics to address the need for women to seek opinions from diverse specialists. In these centers, women are usually seen after their initial biopsy and meet with a surgeon, medical oncologist, and irradiation oncologist and, in some centers, other breast specialists, including a pathologist, radiologist, plastic surgeon, mental health professional, and clinical research nurse. The concept behind this one-stop visit is to provide the woman with information about all of her treatment options in a comprehensive setting and to outline for her treatment that can be tailored to her specific cancer as well as personal needs. Clinical experience and patients' comments suggest that such programs are helpful in reducing the stress experienced by women around decision making and facilitating information gathering. However, studies have yet to be conducted that clearly demonstrate the benefits of this approach compared with the more common practice of multiple consultations. Development by Whelan et al.[16] of a decision board for use in the decision-making process offers another format for communicating information about treatment options. This tool outlines for women the risks and benefits of different surgical treatment options, providing standardized information about each that can be used to supplement the patient-physician dialogue.

During the diagnostic workup, the woman must cope simultaneously with the need to keep her distressing emotions of anxiety and fear within tolerable limits while making the difficult decision about treatment for a potentially fatal disease. To accomplish this, she must assimilate new medical information that, in itself, produces anxiety. One study has shown that, before and after breast biopsy, anxiety and information overload compromise some women's decision-making abilities, making informed decisions difficult, even at best.[17] Valanis and Rumpler[18] note that a woman's previous experiences and her personal and demographic characteristics, as well as those of her social support network (family and friends) and her physician, influence her treatment selection. Research and clinical observation indicate that the time between diagnosis and initiation of treatment is one of the most stressful periods in the breast cancer experience, preceded in degree of stress only by the period of waiting for surgical or other test results.[19]

The legal climate that dictates that full and complete disclosure of information be given by the doctor in a uniform manner to all women fails to take into account the wide variation in women's reactions to the information and the range of ways of dealing with the decisions about treatment. Ideally, the method of giving information should be individualized for each patient. Emphasis on informed decision making places a heavy responsibility on the physician to be cognizant of the individual patient's physical and psychological needs and to tailor the discussion and recommendations with that in mind. At times, it may mean tempering a woman's demands for unrealistic treatment, acquiescing to another woman's desire to defer a final decision to her physician or significant other, or, in some cases, reassuring a woman that she need not reach a decision instantly but has a few days to research her options and come to an appropriate choice. (A broader review of women's response styles and physician-patient communication issues is provided elsewhere.[20–22])

Some women faced with breast cancer find themselves emotionally paralyzed by the decision-making process. They may be overwhelmed by the knowledge that they have breast cancer and by its potential threat to their lives. For these women, even the options are too painful to consider. They often benefit from referral for psychiatric consultation. It is helpful for them to have the pressure temporarily removed by postponing surgery and to be able to review the events and possible treatments in a setting in which they can express concerns and fears and identify the reasons for their response. A useful exercise is for the mental health consultant or specially trained nurse clinician to take them, step by step, through each treatment option, asking at each juncture, "How would you respond to that?" By this method, with reduced anxiety, it usually becomes clear that certain aspects of one or the other treatment are more acceptable to the patient. These women can then return to their surgeon ready to proceed with treatment.

Although many women report the decision-making process as being highly stressful, research indicates that women who are given a choice about treatment do the same as or better psychologically than those who are not.[23–26] Other studies show that the quality of physician communication during this phase is a critical determinant of subsequent psychological well-being in breast cancer patients.[27] Finally, although most women confronted with breast cancer want to have information, clinicians need to be aware that not all women wish to make the final decision about treatment.[28–30] A woman's need for information must be assessed separately from her desire to participate in or delegate treatment choice. Whatever the process, it is important to note that physician recommendation continues to play a critical role in women's choice of treatment and, contrary to popular belief, may be more important to younger patients than older.[31]

Reflecting on the impact that greater public awareness of the triumphs and controversies in breast cancer research has on affected women is instructive. On the negative side, publicized concern over such issues as the safety of silicone implants or validity of clinical trial data caused fear, rage, and confusion for women who felt that their treatment or lives were affected. Other women, striving to put their cancer behind them, note that news of breast cancer seems everywhere in the media, serving as a constant reminder of past illness and future risk. Interpreting reported results for women and providing reassurance to them about their continued well-being have become additional tasks for treating clinicians.

At the same time, disclosure of research information may be encouraging to many women, as with the news of tamoxifen's efficacy as a chemopreventive agent. The availability, as well as the perceived lack of information, has empowered a sector of the population, including consumers and providers, to become increasingly vocal advocates for more and better breast cancer research. The effect of this latter movement has been growing attention to the need for more research on prevention, methods to improve treatment outcomes, funding to achieve these goals, and substantial consumer participation in the entire process. Included in this is emphasis on the role that psychosocial factors play in breast cancer risk, detection, and survival. Importantly, this movement has resulted in greater opportunity for physician-patient dialogue and teamwork in facing the challenges of breast cancer care.

Psychological Variables

In her now classic review, Meyerowitz[32] delineated the psychosocial impact of breast cancer in three broad areas: psychological discomfort (anxiety, depression, and anger), changes in life patterns (consequent to physical discomfort, marital or sexual disruption, and altered activity level), and fears and concerns (mastectomy/loss of breast, recurrence, and death). Although women diagnosed today may have many more treatment options, the psychological concerns remain the same. In addition to these variables, the life stage at which the cancer occurs, previous emotional stability (personality and coping style), and presence of interpersonal support should be included.

Age, or the point in the life cycle at which breast cancer occurs, and what social tasks are threatened or interrupted are of prime importance.[33,34] Concerns about the threat to life and future health, as well as fears of potential disfigurement, disability, and distress associated with treatment, are common to all women faced with a diagnosis of breast cancer. However, these may be more pronounced in younger women. Mor et al.[35] highlight several factors that may put younger women at greater risk for problems in adapting. These include the "off-timedness" of a diagnosis in the younger patient; disruption of primary role as caregiver and, increasingly, as "breadwinner"; and the woman's perception of having more to lose (including career and chance to see offspring grow). An estimated 14% of breast cancers occur in women younger than 45 years of age, with most of these (78%) in individuals between the ages of 35 and 44 years.[36] Although premenopausal women constitute a small proportion of those diagnosed with breast cancer, the special issues related to their cancer risk, survival, and care were the focus of a conference sponsored by the National Cancer Institute.[37] Some researchers have suggested that the older patient may experience less distress because of greater familiarity with medical settings.[38] At the other end of the spectrum, breast cancer diagnosed in a woman older than 80 years may be experienced in the presence of other major losses, particularly of spouse, and concurrent chronic medical conditions. Such realities, coupled with findings indicating that older women are significantly less likely to receive appropriate surgical care or rehabilitation,[39] suggest that patients at both ends of the developmental continuum are at particular risk for problems in adapting to breast cancer. Finally, although the threats to body image, sense of femininity, and self-esteem may be greater in younger women, particularly those who are single or without a partner, it is important to note that these threats also may be concerns of older women. This is increasingly expected to be the case as our population of "young old" grows.

The second variable contributing to adaptation relates to the patient herself—that is, her personality and coping patterns. Each woman has her own style of adaptation to stress, which is a remarkably abiding quality. Studies of breast cancer patients suggest that women who use an active, problem-solving approach to the stresses of illness exhibit less distressed mood and better adaptation.[40–42] In addition, because adaptation to illness is necessarily a dynamic process, those who exhibit flexibility in their efforts cope better. For example, Glanz and Lerman[5] note that, although information-seeking and problem-solving skills may be critical during treatment planning, use of denial and avoidant coping strategies during active chemotherapy or irradiation may be more helpful in reducing or minimizing treatment side effects. The relative efficacy of each style thus may be situation-specific.[43] Finally, women who are able to draw on and use available social resources and support adapt better as well.[44,45] By contrast, women at risk for poor coping are those who exhibit a passive, helpless, hopeless, or pessimistic stance in the face of illness; are rigid in their use of coping strategies; and tend to be socially isolated or to reject help when it is offered. Further studies suggest that women who exhibit a pattern of active "fighting spirit" to their disease not only have better quality of life but also may survive longer than women who appear to "give up."[46,47]

In the context of any discussion of coping responses, it is important to note that the relationship between attitudes and cancer survival, as well as risk, has become a growing area of public interest and psychooncologic research. Because breast cancer is a prevalent neoplasm and one with great psychological impact, the possible role of psychological variables in risk and survival has been explored extensively. The question of a potential role for emotions in vulnerability to breast cancer and its progression has received much attention in the public press. Many women express concern that they "brought it on themselves" or that their attitude is bad and that they or their lifestyle may be making the cancer worse. In a study of what women attributed to having caused their breast cancer, Taylor et al.[40] found that 41% of their well-educated sample felt that they were responsible for the development of the disease and that stress was a major contributor to its development. In research at Georgetown University among women 4 to 12 months after treatment for node-negative breast cancer, 44 of 151 patients interviewed (29%) indicated that they felt that stress or emotions, or both, contributed to their illness; 21% felt that such factors played a major role in disease onset.[19]

The belief that they may be responsible for their own illness and its outcome has become an added psychological burden for many women with breast cancer. Indeed, it is a hazard for those who, based on these beliefs, seek questionable and unproved therapies as primary treatment for their breast cancer, either never starting or discontinuing conventional treatments. Publication in the public media of early and controversial findings about emotions in breast cancer is a growing concern. For these reasons, oncologists should be familiar with the status of psychological research in breast cancer risk and survival to answer their patients' questions on the subject and provide clarification and reassurance. For an extensive review of the research on psychological factors in cancer risk and survival, the reader is referred to reviews by Fox,[48] Bovbjerg and Valdimarsdottir,[49] and Mulder et al.[50]

Prior personal association with breast cancer also can influence adjustment. The memory of a mother, sister, or grandmother's death from breast cancer, or that of a close friend or colleague, makes the diagnosis seem far more ominous and may result in greater levels of psychological distress during and after treatment. Some women with a high investment in their bodies cannot tolerate even the idea of loss or damage to a breast. Such women are at risk for delay in seeking consultation when a symptom occurs; they may also be at risk for problems in adaptation after treatment, particularly if attempts to preserve cosmetic appearance are less successful than expected or must be abandoned because of extent of disease.

Finally, adjustment depends on the response from other significant people, first and foremost from spouse or partner, but also from family and friends. Because of the importance of social support to women's adaptation, this is addressed at greater length in the section Role and Care of the Family.

Prolonged anxiety or depression is not an expected reaction to a cancer diagnosis.[51–53] Of the 49 studies of the prevalence of depression in adults with cancer published between 1967 to 1993, 17 examined women with breast cancer.[54] Reported rates of depression in these 17 studies range from 1.5% to 50.0%. Most of this variance can be attributed to the lack of standardization of methodology and diagnostic criteria. The common stress reactions around the time of diagnosis and during early treatment can be quickly evaluated and managed by the patient's physician, nurse, or specially designated cancer counselor. However, some women have greater problems and can benefit from psychological management by psychiatrists and psychologists, who often are collaborating members of the treatment team (Table 2).

TABLE 2. *Women with breast cancer who should be considered for psychiatric evaluation*

Those who present with current symptoms or a history of
- Depression or anxiety
- Suicidal thinking (attempt)
- Substance or alcohol abuse
- Confusional state (delirium or encephalopathy)
- Akathisia from neuroleptic antiemetics
- Mood swings, insomnia, or irritability from steroids

Those who
- Have a family history of breast cancer
- Are very young, old, pregnant, nursing, single, or alone
- Are adjusting to multiple losses and managing multiple life stresses
- Seem paralyzed with cancer treatment decisions
- Fear death during surgery or are terrified by loss of control under anesthesia
- Request euthanasia
- Seem unable to provide informed consent

Consultation usually is requested for women with the following characteristics: at high genetic risk for breast cancer and who request prophylactic mastectomy, cancer phobic and considering prophylactic mastectomy, unable to make a decision about treatment, or with a psychiatric history of an anxiety or depressive disorder, substance abuse, or other mental illness. The patient who is a management problem for the physician and staff, or who is unable to comply with hospital rules, also needs psychiatric consultation. Rarely are patients so depressed that they are frankly suicidal during evaluation and treatment. However, if suicidal thinking is expressed, a formal psychiatric evaluation should be requested. Patients who have questionable ability to consent to treatment or who refuse treatment (secondary to mental retardation or severe psychiatric symptoms) require careful evaluation.

During workup or during the perioperative period, many patients have anxiety or insomnia that interferes with their usual functioning. Physicians can prescribe low-dose anxiolytic medication (e.g., lorazepam, 0.25 to 1.0 mg orally t.i.d.; alprazolam, 0.5 mg orally t.i.d.; or clonazepam, 1.0 mg orally b.i.d.) to reduce symptoms to a manageable level. Hypnotics (e.g., tirazolam, 0.125 to 0.250 mg orally) are particularly useful during the perioperative period. The antidepressant trazodone is strongly sedating and in low doses (50 to 100 mg orally at bedtime) is helpful in the treatment of the depressed cancer patient with insomnia or in the patient who requests a hypnotic that has no habituating properties. When anxiety and insomnia cannot be controlled with these medications, or when surgical or medical staff observe a significant degree of depression manifesting as frequent crying episodes, irritability, inability to concentrate, or remarks indicating hopelessness or helplessness or suicidal thoughts, psychiatric consultation is indicated. Psychiatric consultants use the crisis intervention model of support that combines support of the patient and evaluation and support of her significant others. Anxiolytic, hypnotic, or antidepressant medication, along with emotional support, usually restores a woman to her prior level of function. The newer selective serotonin reuptake inhibitors (SSRIs; i.e., fluoxetine, paroxetine, and sertraline) are the antidepressants prescribed first in cancer settings, because they have fewer sedative and autonomic effects than the tricyclic antidepressants. All SSRIs can cause sexual dysfunction (anorgasmia in women), a side effect that often leads to cessation of the drug. Clinicians have also noted that the SSRIs may reduce the frequency and intensity of hot flashes in the prematurely menopausal woman with breast cancer; this effect is independent of antidepressant effect.[55]

Medical Variables

The stage of breast cancer at diagnosis, the treatment required, the prognosis, and the rehabilitative opportunities available constitute the medical variables that influence psychological adjustment. Central, however, is a woman's relationship to a supportive surgeon, radiotherapist, or oncologist, who, ideally, is sensitive to her individual concerns, communicates clearly, and monitors emotional as well as physical well-being. The expanded length and intensity of treatments, and the recognition that women treated for breast cancer must be followed for the remainder of their lives, have placed an added burden on health care providers, who are expected to provide support across the course of care, often involving years of follow-up. The office or clinic nurse and treatment staff become the patient's "second family." Receptionists and radiotherapy technicians additionally contribute actively to the social environment that the patient experiences. Some clinicians and staff welcome this added demand, but others are not comfortable with the expected intimacy and care, particularly around psychosocial issues. One model to address this demand involves training nurse clinicians to provide continuity of care and to serve as patient advocates. Other models include screening patients for psychosocial needs and then triaging them to care and assigning specific support or assessment tasks on the basis of staff interest and expertise.[56,57] Depending on the types of medical interventions experienced, the problems faced by women may vary.

Mastectomy

Because it was for so long the standard treatment for breast cancer, and continues to be recommended for large numbers of women, there is considerable research on the impact of loss of one or both breasts on women's physical, social, and emotional functioning. Among the effects documented are feelings of mutilation and altered body image, diminished self-worth, loss of a sense of femininity, decrease in sexual attractiveness and function, anxiety, depression, hopelessness, guilt, shame, and fear of recurrence, abandonment, and death.[32,58] Although mourning for the loss of a cherished body part and the threat to life are universal, the extent to which other sequelae are experienced appears variable. Early research indicated that up to 46% of women studied experienced some degree of social or emotional impairment in the early course of treatment.[59] However, a large prospective study found that women who are well adjusted before they have a mastectomy, and whose disease is in an early stage, can expect at one year to have a quality of life equal to that of unaffected peers, a finding later replicated in other controlled studies.[60,61] In addition to more advanced disease, other predictors of poorer adaptation in the large prospective study were additional concurrent illness or stress, expectation of poor support from others, and a tendency to perceive events in life as less under one's own control. A 1996 study suggests that, although most women report improvement in emotional and physical well-being over time, for a significant minority (20% to 30%) problems may persist beyond 2 years after treatment.[62] However, a woman's persistent issues generally have less to do with the type of surgery received and more to do with her personal and social characteristics and the adjuvant therapy given. Issues related to the latter are discussed in more detail in the treatment-specific chapters and in the Breast Cancer Survivors section in this chapter.

Prophylactic Mastectomy

A discussion of the psychological impact of mastectomy would not be complete without a comment on the role of and women's response to prophylactic mastectomy. Prophylactic mastectomy has long been used as a means of reducing the risk of recurrence of breast cancer in the contralateral breast, particularly among women at increased risk for a second malignancy. It is unknown, however, how often this type of surgery is performed in the context of diagnosed breast cancer. One survey of Maryland surgeons reports that approximately 3% of all mastectomies performed may have been done for prophylactic reasons.[63] Although 85% of plastic surgeons agreed with the statement that bilateral prophylactic mastectomy has a role in the management of women at high risk of breast cancer, only 47% of general surgeons and 38% of gynecologists concurred. Unknown in this survey was the estimated proportion of women undergoing prophylactic surgery who were already diagnosed with breast cancer or who were currently disease free but considered themselves at high risk. Interest in prophylactic mastectomy has intensified in the wake of the identification of genetic markers of breast cancer risk. In a study of genetic testing in family members with hereditary breast-ovarian cancer, Lerman and colleagues[64] report that 2 of 12 women (17%) found to be *BRCA1* gene carriers intended to have mastectomies. Although it is expected that growing numbers of women may request and undergo prophylactic mastectomies, information about the actual rate of breast cancer occurrence (or recurrence) in populations of women who have received this treatment is just beginning to appear.[65] What is clear is that this remains a highly controversial procedure.[66,67] (For a more detailed review of the surgical issues and genetic counseling challenges, see Chapters 17 and 18.)

The relative paucity of information about physical and psychosocial outcomes makes decision making around prophylaxis very difficult. Some data suggest that psychological and sexual problems in women so treated may approximate those seen in mastectomy samples.[68,69] In our centers, surgeons routinely refer for psychological consultation women who are considering prophylactic surgery. These visits are not for the purpose of determining who should or should not have surgery. Rather, they are designed to ensure that a woman contemplating this option has had the opportunity to consider and ask questions about the potential impact of surgery on social (in particular, partner relationships), emotional, and sexual functioning, as well as its likely impact on physical appearance and well-being. Such interviews are helpful to women in evaluating the role that fear of cancer or recurrence or interpretation of personal risk may play in their decision and, if appropriate, in guiding further clarification of actual risk status and alternatives to prophylactic surgery. One study has shown that women at high risk of cancer who are undergoing prophylactic surgery were satisfied with their decision, although comfort with reconstruction was mixed.[70] This same study found that factors influencing selection of surgery included breast cancer–related worry, history of breast biopsies, and subjective breast cancer risk. A second study involving 817 women reported that 5% had later regrets about the surgery.[71] In this research, women cited their physician's recommendation as being the most important factor in the decision-making process, followed by family pressure and their own research. Our clinical experience suggests that most women undergoing prophylactic mastectomy at major cancer centers do so only after careful consideration of their options; these are rarely hasty decisions, particularly among women who are making this choice as a means of primary versus secondary prevention. As with adaptation to other surgeries, however, support of significant others is likely very important in ensuring satisfaction with choice and outcome. Clearly, this is an area in which additional careful research on the decision-making process and outcomes for women being treated is needed.

Based on scientific evidence that systemic versus more extensive local management therapy was more critical to survival, there has been a dramatic shift away from more radical surgical approaches to breast cancer.[72] This also has been advanced by the hope that, by sparing breast tissue, much of the psychosocial morbidity associated with the disease could be reduced.

Breast-Conserving Therapy (Lumpectomy and Irradiation)

Since 1980, more than three dozen studies have examined the differences on social, emotional, and sexual functioning among women undergoing mastectomy versus breast-conserving therapy (BCT) or lumpectomy with irradiation.[73] Despite the variability in methods used, the early pattern of results was very consistent: Women who received BCT were less self-conscious, had a better body image, reported greater satisfaction with sexual activity, and manifested a somewhat better overall adjustment. In particular, women in the conservation group felt they were less sexually inhibited, had sex more frequently, and reported that their husbands were more sexual and affectionate than did women undergoing mastectomy.

Although the overall data suggest that women who receive BCT have, as a group, adapted well,[73–75] three important criticisms have been leveled at this research. First, most of these studies evaluated women within the first year and often the first few months of their treatment. Thus, whether these early differences would persist over time was not known. Indeed, some evidence suggests that women in the conservation group fare no differently from,[76,77] or may do worse than, their mastectomy peers in the long term.[78] Second, in the majority of the studies conducted, women undergoing each option were self-selected, raising concern about potential presurgical differences or selection bias. The few exceptions to this were the studies by Schain et al.,[79,80] de Haes and Welvaart,[81] Fallowfield et al.,[82] and Lasry et al.[83] In each of these studies, the women were randomized to receive either mastectomy or BCT. The data of Schain's[79,80] group and those of de Haes and Welvaart[81] indicate more positive feelings about body image among the BCT group but little difference with respect to the other parameters measured. In contrast, Fallowfield et al.[82] found no significant differences between the groups; if anything, the lumpectomy group appeared to fare somewhat worse. The data of Lasry et al.[83] fell in between: Lumpectomy patients had a better body image than mastectomy patients, but women who received irradiation exhibited higher levels of depression. A further, or third, confound to interpretation of the results of the studies is that younger women, already at increased risk for psychosocial problems in adaptation to breast cancer by virtue of age and developmental stage disruption, tend to select breast conservation.

Given the expected dramatic emotional benefit that saving the breast was expected to provide women, the differences seen are less than might have been predicted.[84,85] In some cases, although statistically significant, the differences observed do not appear to be clinically significant. It is important to be aware that breast conservation is not a psychosocial panacea[78]; rather, it serves to provide a woman with options in her care that may facilitate her particular adaptation.

Two critical factors that continue to influence the surgical decision-making process are attitudes about cancer and irradiation. The thought of leaving tumor cells in the breast is intolerable for some women, who feel more secure with mastectomy. Other women fear irradiation or are unable to devote 6 weeks to daily irradiation therapy treatments because of family or work demands or distance from a treatment center.

Personality characteristics also influence a woman's decision. Women who select BCT over mastectomy have been found to be more concerned about insult to body image and more dependent on their breasts for self-esteem and believe they would have had difficulty adjusting to loss of the breast to mastectomy.[23,86,87] In contrast, patients who choose mastectomy perceive the breast containing cancer as an offending part that should be removed, and they are more fearful of the side effects of irradiation. Whereas it has been suggested that older women may be more likely to select mastectomy,[87] some concern exists that this may reflect as much a bias in the provision of treatment options as personal preference.[88]

Since the mid-1980s, the number of women undergoing BCT has steadily increased. In one large retrospective survey among 1,096 women treated between 1991 and 1996 for early-stage breast cancer, 61.8% had received BCT.[89] Although what percentage of women nationally are offered a choice is unclear, in one prospective study of women who were, almost one-half (49%) chose conservation.[90] These figures are comparable with patterns of care in other large cancer centers, as well as those reported abroad. In their survey of consultant surgeons in Great Britain, Morris et al.[91] found that only 39.1% would perform mastectomy, whereas 64.4% would perform BCT. Most surgeons in this study also said they would offer a choice of treatments.

Although many American women have routinely been given a choice between BCT or mastectomy since the mid- to late-1980s, this is mandated by fewer than one-half the states. Further, little is understood about *how* women make their decisions. It is likely that a significant proportion of decisions are made based on the nature of the care that is available.[13,14,39] For women diagnosed in communities that are removed from major medical centers, mastectomy may simply be a more practical and safe treatment choice. Another deciding factor may be the availability of high-quality irradiation therapy. Restricted access to implants as well as to plastic surgeons who have extensive experience with transverse rectus abdominis myocutaneous (TRAM) flap reconstruction, has already limited the availability of reconstructive options. Cultural and ethnic values may also direct or even dictate choice, although the role of these is poorly understood.[92] Research and clinical experience suggest that physician recommendation continues to exert the most significant influence on treatment choice for the majority of women.

Clinical experience indicates that many women who are treated by BCT alone, with no adjuvant chemotherapy, may not feel the emotional effect of the experience until they begin the daily routine of radiotherapy. Spared the loss of their breast, these women often feel they should be grateful and not complain. Evidence exists that they elicit, or at least perceive themselves as receiving, less emotional support from others than women undergoing mastectomy.[78] It is often only when the irradiation starts, with daily visits to the clinic, exposure to others with cancer, cumulative fatigue, and realization of what they have gone through, that patients react with distress. Physicians and staff should be aware of these delayed reactions, because they, too, may perceive these women as having less severe psychological trauma. It has become clear that women undergoing irradiation are at higher risk of psychological disturbance, in particular depressive symptoms, than has been assumed.[83,93] Although these may be because of the side effects of irradiation, which may vary widely in the degree of discomfort and fatigue produced, mood states need to be monitored.

Women undergoing irradiation therapy experience initial anxiety, which is usually allayed after a few treatments. It often returns, however, as end of treatment approaches, because of fear of regrowth of tumor without treatment, as well as in anticipation of the loss of close observation and frequent visits with the doctor and staff. To ease the transition, patients should be made aware of when treatment will end and of the common paradoxic increase in distress. Reassurance should be provided about staff availability by telephone contact and by systematic scheduling of follow-up appointments. Fears of disease recurrence remain high in many women and reach distressing levels before follow-up visits and scans and while waiting for test results. Anxiety returns to usual levels with news of normal findings.

When discussing women's reactions to irradiation, one additional factor that is important to consider is the risk for upper extremity lymphedema (UEL). The proportion of women affected by this problem has decreased dramatically, largely with the use of less radical node dissection practices and routine encouragement of arm rehabilitation exercises and skin precautions. In addition, broader adoption of sentinel node biopsies for a number of women may reduce further the risk of later UEL. However, although certainly less common than in the days of more radical surgery, risk of UEL remains a problem for some women after treatment for breast cancer.[94] Women undergoing irradiation and surgical resection of axillary lymph nodes are at highest risk for development of UEL.[95–97] These problems can occur immediately after treatment or years later.[98] The actual proportion of women in whom UEL will develop remains unclear, with estimates ranging from as low as 4% to as high as 72%.[99] For these women, the impact on emotional, social, and physical functioning can be profound. The few studies that examined psychosocial functioning in this area report high levels of anxiety, depression, social inhibition, sexual dysfunction, and disability.[99–102] In at least one study, no association was seen between severity of UEL, duration, and psychological distress.[99] However, variables that have been found to increase a woman's risk for problems in functioning include pain, lack of social support, and avoidant coping. In addition, women with UEL in their dominant hand tend to have more difficulties than women whose nondominant arm is affected.[99] For women in whom arm swelling develops, prompt intervention that includes not only physical rehabilitation but also education, consideration of pain medication, emotional support, counseling, and, as appropriate, referral for sexual counseling is warranted.

Reconstruction

The Food and Drug Administration hearings, opened in November 1991, on the safety of silicone gel–filled breast implants brought to the attention of the public and the medical community several important questions: How many women seek implants, what are the benefits of their use, and what are the medical risks associated with these devices? These questions were no more keenly felt than among the estimated one-half million breast cancer survivors with implants. Winer et al.,[103] in a study conducted in the wake of these hearings, found that 55% of women who had undergone breast reconstruction with silicone implants in an earlier period (1985 to 1990) were worried about the safety of these devices. Significantly, however, 76% of these women also reported that reconstruction was important in helping them cope with their cancer.

Although many clinicians believe that the medical questions have been answered,[104] others do not. For example, it is still unknown what percentage of the women who choose or undergo mastectomy do so with the intention of seeking reconstruction. In the 10 years before the implant hearings, national figures suggested that as many as 30% of eligible patients might pursue breast reconstruction.[105] It is clear that the number of breast reconstructions declined after the hearings because of women's fears and the restricted access to needed devices, as well as to the demands placed on physicians and patients involved with implants to participate in extensive follow-up studies. However, postmastectomy breast reconstruction continues to be an important rehabilitative option pursued by a significant subset of women undergoing mastectomy. In the study by Ganz et al.[89] of women treated in Los Angeles and the greater Washington, D.C., areas for early-stage breast cancer, 41.7% of women who received a mastectomy went on to have breast reconstruction.

Although breast reconstruction after cancer has been available far longer than breast conservation, few studies have systematically examined the psychosocial impact of mastectomy alone compared with mastectomy plus reconstruction. This is in contrast to the larger number of studies that have examined mastectomy versus BCT outcomes. Only four studies have been conducted in which women selecting each of the three different surgical options (lumpectomy versus mastectomy alone versus mastectomy with reconstruction) were compared.[23,75,106,107] All of this research involved implant populations, and in only one study were women undergoing reconstruction evaluated separately from those who received mastectomy. In this latter study, which looked only at body image and self-esteem, breast conservation patients reported more positive body image than either mastectomy or immediate reconstruction groups.[107] Interestingly, this difference was not significant for the delayed reconstruction group, suggesting that these women may use a different standard for comparison. No differences were seen between groups on self-esteem, which was uniformly high.

Three empiric studies have appeared comparing women who receive conservation to those who undergo mastectomy with reconstruction. The first of these included a small sample ($n = 9$) and found no differences between groups in quality of life, mood, marital satisfaction, or sexual satisfaction 1 year after surgery.[108] A Japanese study compared 42 women with breast conservation to 48 women undergoing immediate reconstruction with myocutaneous flaps.[109] No differences in sexual satisfaction or fear of recurrence were found between groups an average of 3 years after surgery. Conservation group members were less self-conscious about their appearance and stated that they would be more likely to choose the same treatment again than women in the reconstruction group. In a later retrospective study, 72 women who had partial mastectomy were compared with 146 women who had undergone immediate reconstruction, predominantly with implants, an average of 4 years after surgery.[110] No differences were observed between groups in overall psychosocial adjustment to illness, body image, or satisfaction with relationships or sexual life. However, women who had breast reconstruction reported less frequent breast caressing and more loss of pleasure with this activity. They also tended to be less likely to achieve orgasm with noncoital sexual stimulation. Factors predictive of greater psychosocial distress included a conflicted marriage, feeling unattractive, sexual dissatisfaction, less education, and treatment with chemotherapy.

In the largest prospective study to date, the psychological variables associated with who does and does not seek reconstruction, and women's responses to reconstruction, were examined.[111] A total of 150 women seeking consultation for reconstruction after mastectomy were evaluated along surgical and psychological parameters; 83 of the 117 women undergoing reconstruction were reassessed postoperatively. In addition, a matched comparison sample of 50 women who had not sought reconstruction was studied.[112] The results of this research can be summarized as follows: First, women seeking consultation for reconstruction were psychologically well adjusted, high functioning, and, importantly, appeared functionally no different than their peers who were not seeking this surgery. Second, for women undergoing breast reconstruction, the net effect of the surgery was to increase observed and stated satisfaction with levels of psychological, social, and sexual function. More than 80% stated that they were happy or absolutely delighted with the overall results, and most found that the surgical results met or surpassed their expectations. However, women who pursued reconstruction primarily to please others, or with the expectation of improving sexual and social relations, were at risk of disappointment. Time since cancer surgery also modified response, such that the farther the woman was since mastectomy, the greater her satisfaction with the overall results. Third, comparisons between women who consulted and went on to have reconstruction and those who sought consultation but opted not to pursue additional surgery suggested that women who are at increased risk for subsequent emotional or surgical disappointment after reconstructive procedures may select themselves out at the time of consultation. Similar findings have been reported in other study samples.[113–117] This study was helpful in dispelling some of the myths about who seeks reconstruction and why. The reasons most frequently cited for seeking surgery in our study and that of others were to be rid of the prosthesis, to feel whole again, to reestablish symmetry, and to diminish self-consciousness about appearance. As reflected in age range of women interviewed (28 to 68), it also brought attention to the fact that attractiveness is not primarily a concern of younger women; older women may react as strongly as younger women to breast loss.

Because most of the earlier research among women undergoing reconstruction was conducted at a time when mastectomy was still the primary treatment of choice, how many of these women might have selected breast conservation had it been available to them is not clear. At the same time, many women may select mastectomy precisely because they feel reconstruction will provide an acceptable cosmetic outcome, while avoiding the more limited surgery and irradiation. Clearly, these studies need to be replicated in the context of more recent treatment changes, including the shift to use of saline versus silicone implants.[118] They also need to be expanded to address cultural and ethnic issues, as it is clear that cultural beliefs and practices influence women's choice of options and outcomes.[119–121]

Additional research on the impact on functioning, controlling for extent of surgery performed, is also needed. Only one study has examined the effect of nipple-areolar reconstruction on satisfaction with outcome.[122] In this report, the 33 women in the nipple-added group reported significantly greater satisfaction with the overall breast reconstruction, size, softness, and sexual sensitivity of the reconstruction and greater satisfaction with appearance in the nude than the 26 women without a nipple. They also showed more symptomatology on a psychiatric distress scale. As the authors point out, these data need to be interpreted with some caution. All of these assessments were made after completion of surgery. It is possible that higher satisfaction in the nipple-added group also may reflect the fact that they were more satisfied with the original reconstructive effort independent of addition of a nipple. In addition, because the nipple-added group was significantly younger than the no-nipple group, their young age rather than the effect of surgery may have put them at increased risk for emotional problems. Few studies have specified how much additional surgery was performed to achieve good symmetry.

In addition to local treatment choice (e.g., BCT versus mastectomy with or without reconstruction), the impact on psychosocial function of timing and type of reconstruction performed has been examined.

Timing of Reconstruction: Immediate versus Delayed

Physician support for immediate reconstruction (versus delayed, which is that performed more than a week after mastectomy) is based on the perception of the absence of medical contraindications to immediate reconstruction and anticipation of significant benefits to the woman in sparing her the pain of disfigurement and loss that accompany mastectomy.[123] The American Society of Plastic and Reconstructive Surgeons reports that, of reconstructions performed in 1990 by member surgeons, 38% were immediate and 62% delayed.[105] In a retrospective sample of 149 women undergoing surgery between 1989 to 1993 in two large metropolitan areas (Los Angeles and Washington, D.C.), more than 75% had immediate reconstruction.[124]

Research with women undergoing immediate reconstruction has shown not only high levels of patient satisfaction with surgical results but also significantly less psychosocial morbidity than in those who undergo mastectomy alone.[123,125–128] Patients undergoing immediate reconstruction were less depressed and experienced less impairment of their sense of femininity, self-esteem, and sexual attractiveness than their peers who delayed or did not seek reconstruction. However, as with findings on lumpectomy versus mastectomy, researchers have noted that initial differences in adjustment may be minimal and disappear over time.[127] Furthermore, at least one study has suggested that satisfaction with technical aspects of the reconstructive outcome may be slightly lower among women undergoing earlier versus delayed reconstruction.[111] This may reflect the fact that women with immediate reconstruction compare the result with their original breast, whereas those undergoing delayed surgery use the mastectomy site as their basis for comparison. In addition, although Schain et al.[127] suggest that immediate reconstruction does not interfere with the necessary mourning process associated with threat to life and breast loss, clinicians have reported this as a problem in long-term follow-up of these patients. It is an issue that bears further study.

Type of Reconstruction: Implant versus Transverse Rectus Abdominis Myocutaneous Flap

Research evaluating the psychosocial outcomes for women undergoing reconstruction using abdominal flaps (TRAM surgery) is just becoming available.[129–131] An early study by McCraw et al.[130] reported that TRAM flap patients had fewer complications, higher overall satisfaction, and fewer complaints of pain, asymmetry, or inconvenience than those who received implants. In a small sample study comparing TRAM ($n = 8$) to implant ($n = 14$) groups, Cederna et al.[131] found that women undergoing TRAM flap reconstruction were significantly more satisfied with how their breast felt and tended to be happier with the cosmetic result. However, the TRAM flap group also experienced greater psychological, social, and physical impairments as a result of their surgery. These investigators note that lack of public familiarity with the TRAM surgery and its more complex nature may pose social problems for these patients. Specifically, women may worry about what others think of their pursuit of this option or about how others might respond to the physical results (e.g., when changing in a locker room). When asked, 87% of the TRAM group and 71% of the implant group said they would undergo the same reconstructive surgery if they had to choose again. In our own research, we looked at 146 women undergoing reconstruction; 94 (64%) had an implant, and 51 (35%) underwent autologous tissue reconstruction (TRAM flap).[124] No differences were seen between groups in satisfaction with the appearance or feel of their breasts or the overall impact of breast cancer on their sex lives, although there was a consistent tendency for the women with TRAM reconstructions to report greater comfort and satisfaction. In addition, women who had an implant were significantly more worried about having a problem with their reconstruction in the future; 25% of women with implants indicated they worried a fair amount to very much about the future versus only 8% of the TRAM group.

Use of autologous tissue for reconstruction has the advantage of eliminating many of the medical (e.g., rejection, encapsulation, altered mammographic imaging) and device-related (e.g., rupture, deflation, leakage) problems associated with implants. The cosmetic outcomes also can be as good as or better than those achieved with implants. On the negative side, these procedures require lengthy exposure to anesthesia, major abdominal surgery (with consequent abdominal wall compromise), and, although reportedly low, risk for failure. Because long-term follow-up data on the cosmetic and physical sequelae associated with such reconstruction are still limited, it is difficult to provide women with information on which to make their decisions.

Regardless of the type of reconstructive surgery proposed or selected, women need to be well informed about what to expect. Key concerns of women about reconstruction include the cost of the surgery; the length of time under anesthesia; the number of procedures required; the cosmetic results achievable; and the safety of the techniques used in both potential for complications and, in the case of implants, risk of masking recurrent cancer or promoting recurrent autoimmune disease.[132] Surgeons differ in their approach to informing women about cosmetic results. Some prefer to use written materials only, and others show pictures of reconstructed breasts, whereas many use some combinations of these approaches and, at times, may refer a woman to a previously reconstructed patient for more details. In our own research and that of others, several additional issues appeared of importance in counseling women who were considering or undergoing these procedures.[111,132–134] These include the need for discussion of all facets of the surgical steps (including number and length of hospitalizations and follow-up office visits/procedures) as well as a thorough review of the nature and timing of any planned symmetry and nipple reconstruction procedures.

Adjuvant Chemotherapy

The news that adjuvant chemotherapy is needed demands psychological adjustment to yet another treatment modality. This involves a lengthened treatment period and awareness of the threat to life implicit in the need for systemic therapy. Some women in this group describe their early weeks of treatment as having been characterized by "one piece of bad news after another." Deciding whether to undergo adjuvant treatment, and, if more than one treatment is proposed, which drugs or protocol, constitutes the third decision point in the course of cancer.

Anticipation of chemotherapy can be difficult. Women's fears of the side effects arise from knowledge of the distressing sequelae of chemotherapy. Because many women with node-negative early-stage breast cancer now receive some form of adjuvant therapy, the association of these treatments with "more serious disease" has diminished. Women who are anticipating and undergoing adjuvant therapy are told the specific drugs they will receive and the transient nature of drug side effects. Despite having fears, few women refuse treatment, and most comply with their regimen.[135] Reactive anxiety and depression should be treated to assist in the woman's adjustment.

Meyerowitz et al.[136] studied women with breast cancer during chemotherapy and 2 years after they completed it. Among those who were disease free at 2 years, 23% reported difficulty with personal and family relationships during treatment, and 44% had continuing physical problems 2 years later. Despite this, 89% stated that they would recommend adjuvant chemotherapy to friends in a similar situation. Many reported that they had coped with treatment by "staying busy," "getting information about the treatment," and "keeping a positive, hopeful outlook." In this study 41% of women reported that the treatment had been easier than they expected. Clinical experience suggests that some women cope with the short-term adverse psychological effects by focusing on delayed benefits (e.g., reassurance that they have done everything possible to eradicate their disease).

Nausea and vomiting, once common side effects of adjuvant chemotherapy, feared and dreaded by patients, are now well controlled with pharmacologic and behavioral interventions.[137] However, three additional troublesome side effects of adjuvant therapy that have psychological consequences have received less attention. These include hair loss, weight gain, and problems with concentration. Although anticipated, the impact of alopecia for women undergoing chemotherapy is often devastating. Some women report this as more distressing than the breast surgery itself, in part because it is a visible indicator of disease, but also because it is overtly disfiguring. In our own research, women rated hair loss as being as distressing as learning of their diagnosis.[19] Early discussion of the expected changes, information about wigs, and referral to the American Cancer Society and the cosmetics industry–sponsored *Look Good . . . Feel Better* program can help reduce distress caused by hair loss.[138]

The cause of weight gain remains unclear.[139] A study by Huntington[140] revealed that 50% of patients gained more than ten pounds. No difference was found by treatment regimen [CMF (cyclophosphamide, methotrexate, and 5-fluorouracil) versus CMF plus vincristine and prednisone], estrogen receptor status, age, or menopausal status, although a decrease in activity level was found in those who experienced weight gain. At least one study has shown that weight may be negatively associated with mortality,[141] and another has implicated dietary intake as a factor in increased mortality.[142] The added insult to self-esteem posed by significant weight gain suggests that more attention should be paid to this problem. The introduction of exercise programs during chemotherapy is increasingly being considered, along with nutritional guidance.[143]

Difficulty with concentration and memory is also reported by many women undergoing chemotherapy. Not well researched or clearly documented, these symptoms may be associated with the stress of illness, antiemetic drugs, the chemotherapy itself, and possibly with hormonal changes secondary to chemotherapy-induced menopause.[144] Preliminary research suggests that a dose-effect relationship exists between the adjuvant regimen used and the degree of cognitive impairment. In their study, van Dam et al.[145] reported that 34% of women undergoing high-dose chemotherapy showed signs of cognitive impairment, compared to 17% of women who received standard therapy and only 9% of a control group of women with no adjuvant therapy. Ganz[146] has suggested that cognitive dysfunction may become a dose-limiting toxic effect. She argues for the need to further examine the interrelationship between hormonal status and cognitive functioning as well as the potential effects of antiestrogen treatments. In the same vein, it is possible that some of the more persistent neuralgias and arthralgias being observed by women exposed to paclitaxel (Taxol) may result in the establishment of dose limitations for this therapy.

A final troublesome effect of chemotherapy in younger women is premature menopause.[147] The threatened or actual loss of fertility and acute onset of menopause anticipated with adjuvant treatment often cause distress in the woman who is premenopausal at diagnosis. The hot flashes, night sweats, vaginal dryness, and atrophy caused by chemotherapy-induced menopause produce severe discomfort. The latter symptoms can lead to dyspareunia. Although instruction in the use of vaginal lubricants is helpful, thinning of the vaginal mucosa may still result in irritation on intercourse. A further effect of chemotherapy is loss of libido likely associated with a reduction in circulating androgens.[148] For many women, loss of desire is the most difficult sequela to treat. In these cases, use of androgen supplements can be considered.[148,149] With the advent of sildenafil citrate (Viagra), another option may be available for patients to enhance sexual functioning, although use of this drug in women is not yet well researched.

Although longitudinal data are lacking, it can be expected that early loss of ovarian function also increases the risk in these young patients of later morbidity associated with osteoporosis and cardiovascular disease.[150,151] In a randomly selected survey of 224 breast cancer survivors, differences were found in women's concerns about these health issues by menopausal status.[152] Premenopausal women were more concerned about osteoporosis (82% versus 66% for postmenopausal) and heart disease (92% versus 73%) and that estrogen replacement therapy might precipitate cancer recurrence (98% versus 73%). At the same time, they were more willing to consider estrogen replacement therapy under medical supervision (59% versus 40%). Discussion of these issues early in the course of care and referral for evaluation for risk and intervention is appropriate. Although estrogen replacement in these women remains controversial, proponents for its use from both physician and survivor groups are increasing, and it is being investigated.[153,154] (See also Chapter 70 on management of menopausal symptoms.)

Psychological preparation for chemotherapy is essential and should incorporate patient educational materials, nursing input, and an outline by the physician of the disease and treatment-related expectations. It is equally important to anticipate and plan for emotional reactions to ending treatment when, as with radiotherapy, fears of recurrence peak. Our clinical experience suggests that women experience more severe reactive anxiety and depression during this part of the treatment than at an earlier period, perhaps because of their greater awareness of prognosis. One symptom in particular that may continue to distress patients long after treatment has ended is fatigue. Noted clinically, the prevalence and etiology of posttreatment fatigue has become a new direction of research.[155,156] In one sample of 60 women, 87.5% reported fatigue as a serious and unexpected side effect of chemotherapy.[157] Although careful workup to rule out underlying depression or any medical cause of persistent fatigue is warranted, many women benefit from reassurance that it may take months, not weeks, before they feel that their energy is back to preillness levels.

Adjuvant Hormonal Therapy

Increasing use of tamoxifen in the adjuvant setting has drawn attention to the psychological and sexual impact of hormonal therapies. Although used more commonly for postmenopausal patients, tamoxifen is sometimes given to premenopausal women as part of their adjuvant therapy. Research has shown that tamoxifen, although an antiestrogen, may have weak estrogenic effects on the vaginal mucosa.[158] Some older women find that the associated increase in hot flashes with use of this drug is a side-limiting factor. By contrast, we have had some younger patients report that tamoxifen provides relief from their vaginal dryness and loss of libido that accompany chemotherapy-induced premature menopause. Concern has also been raised about an increased incidence of depression seen in association with the use of tamoxifen.[159,160] Reports of a small but unexpected number of deaths due to tamoxifen-related uterine cancer, as well as concern over ocular toxicities with prolonged use, have made many patients and physicians anxious about continued or long-term use of this drug.[161–163] (See Chapter 37 for discussion of appropriate monitoring for these potential complications.) A variety of hormonal manipulations are given for recurrent disease, including tamoxifen, megestrol acetate, progestins, aminoglutethimide, luteinizing-hormone–releasing-hormone (LHRH) analogues, and estrogens. Aminoglutethimide has been associated with severe vaginal atrophy.[164] Megestrol acetate (Megace) increases appetite and results in significant weight gain for many women. As noted earlier, alterations in appearance due to hormonal therapy may result in embarrassment and loss of self-esteem. Counseling around expected changes is important.

Bone Marrow Transplant

The application of bone marrow transplant (BMT) in the setting of solid tumors, such as ovarian and breast cancer took off in the mid-1980s. Although much has been written about the psychological stages in, and patients' adaptation to, BMT, this research has focused largely on samples of patients treated for hematologic cancers with allogeneic transplants.[165,166] Long-term follow-up of patients undergoing BMT suggests that, although most patients do well, 15% to 20% may continue to experience distress and might benefit from psychological or psychiatric intervention. At least one study reports that, despite the additional strain and longer hospitalization associated with BMT, no difference could be seen in psychological or social functioning between BMT survivors and those treated with conventional chemotherapy alone.[167] To what extent this is true for women with breast cancer who are undergoing these procedures with the benefit of growth factor support, effective antiemetics, and shorter hospitalization is not known. A shift to use of largely outpatient administration of high-dose chemotherapy with autologous peripheral stem cell rescue has decreased considerably the burden for women treated. One study has suggested that women who choose to pursue this aggressive approach may feel that they have something critical to live for; often, this is dependent family.[168] What is clear is that, as with other intensive therapies, the toll on quality of life is often high. Ensuring that psychological support is provided across the course of transplant and follow-up is critical. Regardless of whether psychiatric problems alter survival, they can dramatically impact quality of survival and should be rapidly diagnosed and treated.[169]

Advanced Disease

Supportive care for patients with advanced breast cancer is aimed at comfort and control of symptoms. Different metastatic sites, especially bone, lungs, and brain, present special supportive problems. Bone pain is often difficult to control, and confusional states must be monitored and treated. As discussed under Interventions, the use of support groups may influence quantity as well as quality of survival significantly in this group of women.

Advanced care is often provided at home with support from the family or in a hospice setting (see Chapter 65). Central to the success of a home care program is a sense of continuity of care with physicians and staff and continued support of family and friends. Psychiatric consultation should be considered when distress (anxiety and depression) is not responsive to the usual supportive measures. It is extremely helpful to have a psychiatric consultant who is knowledgeable about the problems faced by women with breast cancer, ideally as a member of a multidisciplinary team.[170]

Among the psychiatric symptoms of most concern, anxiety and depression are the most frequently occurring and the most disabling. Depression may reach significant proportions. Although suicide is unusual, suicidal ideation is common. A management approach that combines psychological support with psychopharmacologic use of antidepressants and mood stabilizers is often helpful. The SSRIs—fluoxetine, sertraline, and paroxetine—are the antidepressants prescribed first in cancer settings. Dosages for fluoxetine and paroxetine start at 5 or 10 mg per day and can be increased to 20 mg per day. Sertraline is started at 25 mg per day and titrated slowly to an effective dose (50 to 150 mg per day). Bupropion is considered if patients have a poor response to a reasonable trial of other antidepressants. Its activating profile makes it useful in lethargic, medically ill patients; it should be avoided in patients with a history of seizure disorder or brain tumor and in those who are malnourished. Bupropion SR (slow release) may be helpful for patients who want to discontinue tobacco smoking. Use of carbamazepine as a mood stabilizer can be problematic in cancer patients because of its bone marrow–suppressing properties. Although valproic acid has not been studied in this population, it is better tolerated than carbamazepine. Anxiety may be high and distressing, especially in the presence of hypoxia or prolonged pain. Anxiolytic drugs, particularly clonazepam and lorazepam, are helpful for control of symptoms. It is best to give these drugs at regular intervals initially to achieve control, thereafter tapering the dose or prescribing the drug on an as-needed basis. In general, if given control of their own dose initially, women take too little to be effective. Agitated behavior associated with metabolic encephalopathy, resulting often from hypercalcemia or associated with narcotic or steroid side effects, may require control by administration of a neuroleptic in small doses.

Because it is such a prevalent concern in more advanced stages of disease, attention to pain is important in the management of care.[171] Cancer patients who experience pain are more likely to exhibit higher levels of mood disturbance and functional disability than are those who have little or no pain.[172] Spiegel and Bloom[173] found that for women with metastatic breast cancer, beliefs about the meaning of the pain in relation to the illness predicted level of pain better than site of metastasis. Glajchen et al.[174] found that 64% of patients surveyed cited communication barriers as an impediment to pain relief. Attitudinal barriers to compliance with medical treatment were cited by more than one-half the respondents, including stoicism and fear of narcotic addiction. Thus, addressing the meaning and response to pain from the perspective of the patient is as important as an explanation of proposed control techniques.

INTERVENTIONS

The use and variety of psychosocial interventions applied in the cancer setting in general, and in breast cancer care in particular, have grown in the 1990s.[175–177] Although varying greatly by type (e.g., individual versus group), orientation (e.g., behavioral versus cognitive versus supportive), duration (time limited versus open ended), and timing (e.g., before, during, or after treatment), as well as target populations served (early versus advanced, younger than 40 versus older, partnered versus single, or mixed), the fundamental purpose of interventions developed has been the same: to provide each woman with the skills or resources necessary to cope with her illness and improve the quality of her life. The various types of psychosocial interventions in use in the cancer setting are well reviewed in the section on interventions (Part X) in the 1998 volume *Psycho-Oncology*, edited by J. Holland, and published by Oxford University Press. The vast majority of these have been developed specifically for or included breast cancer patients. Two meta-analyses examining the efficacy of psychosocial and educational programs in cancer provide more specific information on the relative impact of such interventions on patients' medical and psychosocial outcomes.[178,179] Detailed review of the use of different interventions in the care of breast cancer patients is beyond the scope of this chapter. However, three points must be made regarding the use of such programs in the overall care of breast cancer patients and families.

First, taken as a whole, researchers have found that patients who received an intervention designed to improve knowledge or coping or to reduce distress do better than those who do not. Specifically, patients provided or randomized to some form of individual or group intervention experienced less anxiety and depression,[180,181] had an increased sense of control,[182] improved body image,[183] reported greater satisfaction with care[184] and better sexual function,[185,186] and exhibited improved medication adherence.[187] Importantly, in no studies to date have women who received additional help fared worse than their "standard care" peers.

Second, use of psychosocial interventions is increasing.[188,189] This reflects not only patient demand for supportive care but also growing recognition that addressing psychosocial issues may improve outcomes for patients. In their seminal study, Spiegel et al.[190] found that women with metastatic breast cancer who participated in a year of weekly supportive-expressive group therapy that included instruction in self-hypnosis for pain ($n = 50$) survived an average of 18 months longer from time of randomization compared with a control group ($n = 36$). No studies have examined patients' use of these services in the wake of their expanded availability.

Third, although it might be argued that an individually tailored invention should result in the best outcome for any given patient, this may not be suitable or even desirable in all cases. Most cancer patients resist being singled out for individual therapy and feel burdened by any label that might suggest that they are mentally ill and not simply medically ill. Furthermore, increasing evidence shows that participation in group activity offers a uniquely supportive and normalizing experience for many cancer patients struggling to deal with the realities of their new or continued status as cancer survivors. In studies that have specifically compared use of individual to group interventions, groups were as effective as individual counseling or support in reducing patient distress.[183,184] Krupnick et al.[191] have developed a model that uses groups to educate and support patients across the course of care that can be tailored to the needs of the oncology community being served.

Key to the development of an effective intervention is the recognition that, for many women, cancer represents a transitional event. As defined by Andrykowski et al.,[192] this is "a traumatic event that alters an individual's assumptive world with the potential to produce long-lasting changes of both a positive as well as negative nature." As such, the primary goal in any intervention is to use this teachable moment to help minimize the negative and enhance the positive impact of illness on recovery and well-being.

SPECIAL ISSUES

Three changes in how breast cancer is diagnosed and treated have important ramifications for clinicians in their management of patients. These include increased awareness of the familial nature of breast cancer, greater involvement of family in patient care, and growing attention to the impact of breast cancer treatment on women's sexual functioning. Psychological issues related to being at genetic risk for breast cancer are covered in Chapter 17. In the remaining sections, the special issues related to the care of other family members and the role of sexual quality of life in rehabilitation are reviewed. In addition, a final section touches on the burgeoning interest in and information on the well-being of our growing population of breast cancer survivors.

Role and Care of the Family

Research into the impact of social support and health blossomed in the 1980s and 1990s.[193,194] A positive relationship between social support and health or illness outcome is a consistent finding.[195–197] This has been no more dramatically illustrated than in the context of breast cancer, in which adequate social support has been found to be not only integral to positive adjustment[198] but also to length of survival.[190,199,200] For most patients, primary support comes from the family. At the same time, however, new stresses have taxed this resource. Greater demands on family decision making, the lengthened course of treatment with more aggressive therapies, and shift of care into the outpatient setting have served to place renewed focus on the family in the management of care.

When people are ill, they tend to feel less in control, less powerful, and more inferior, especially when they must rely on others. At the same time, serious illness of any kind increases the ill person's need for closeness to others to counteract feelings of insecurity and vulnerability. The need for love and support often heightens in patients over time, as a reaction to the effects of disease and treatment and the fear that they will no longer be loved or cared for. Fears of abandonment and rejection, experienced by other critically ill patients, are often keenly felt by the cancer patient. Absence of social support or loss of a significant person who withdraws during the patient's illness becomes an additional stressor that may be more emotionally painful than the illness itself.[201]

Active involvement of the family clearly serves a range of patient needs, from the most basic—namely, provision of emotional support (the "psychic fuel" that keeps a patient going)—to the practical (e.g., transportation to therapy sessions and financial resources to support these services), to the more abstract (e.g., providing meaningful roles and hence functional goals toward which the patient can strive). The oncology team may count on the family member to be an advocate, a care provider, and a one-person cheering section on behalf of the patient.

Despite the recognized importance of the role of partners and family in caring for women with breast cancer, this subject has been the focus of few studies. Work by Wellisch et al.[202] indicates that involvement of the husband in the decision-making process, hospital visitation, early viewing of scars, and early resumption of sexual activity are important for optimal functioning of couples. Open dialogue would appear to be critical to this process. Sabo et al.[203] found that the tendency for some men to assume a "protective guardian" stance was sometimes a deterrent to effective and open communication. Maguire[204] found that husbands of mastectomy patients reported more distress than a control group of husbands whose wives had benign breast disease up to a year after surgery. Similarly, Baider and Kaplan-DeNour[205] report that patients and partners experienced moderate degrees of emotional distress related to mastectomy. Further, they found that patients' and husbands' levels of adjustment were significantly related; if one partner was experiencing difficulties in adjustment, the other was also likely to be having problems. Northouse[206] reports that when asked what helped them cope with illness during hospitalization and 1 month later, both patients and husbands identified emotional support, information, attitude, and religion as being important factors. In Northouse's research, patients and partners who reported higher levels of social support reported fewer adjustment difficulties at 3 and 30 days after surgery. However, younger couples may be at particular risk for problems.[207]

The vital nature and complexity of the relationship of spouse or partner and family to patient well-being are no more obvious than when this system goes awry. When such situations occur, it is critical to remember that support is a two-way street; the source of the problem may arise in the provider of support (family member) as well as in the recipient and commonly involves both.[208,209] The impact of cancer can be as devastating to a family member as to the patient herself. Spouses may feel angry, ashamed, and vulnerable to illness themselves. Clinicians who work with families of cancer patients suggest that they may at times need to be viewed as second-order patients. Furthermore, their needs may vary across the course of illness and recovery.[210] Seeing that partners have a support network and chance to air conflicting emotions can be critical to ensuring that they will be available to patients when needed. Toward this end, it is helpful for staff to acknowledge the difficult task faced by family members, to provide opportunities for them to talk about questions and reactions both with the patient and alone, and to ensure that backup supports are available and that provision is made to give family members relief, especially if care is going to be complex or long term. It is also important to permit family members to limit care to those areas in which they are most comfortable and effective.

The traumatic effect on children, both sons and daughters, is great when the mother develops breast cancer. Behavioral disorders, conflicts with parents, and regressive and acting-out behaviors in children have been seen to increase during a parental illness.[211–215] Lichtman et al.[216] noted deterioration of the mother-child relationship in 12% of women with breast cancer whom they studied. Problems were more likely to arise in those situations in which the mother had a poor prognosis, extensive surgery, poor psychological adjustment, or, to a smaller extent, difficulty in adjusting to chemotherapy or radiotherapy. A prior history of parent-child conflicts also placed the relationship at risk during the mother's illness. Mothers' relationships with their daughters were significantly more stressed than those with their sons. Daughters were more likely to show signs of fearfulness, withdrawal, and hostility, emanating, perhaps, from their greater fears of developing the disease and the greater demands placed on the daughters. These findings parallel those reported by Litman[212] and Wellisch,[217] who noted that mothers rely more often on daughters than on sons during illness and that adolescent daughters may be particularly vulnerable to disruption in their lives.

The monitoring of all children, especially when the mother's breast cancer is advanced, is important. The opportunity for parents to discuss how and what to tell their children about the mother's illness early in the course of care is also important and should include advice on tailoring these conversations to meet appropriate developmental needs of their offspring. A number of books,[218–220] as well as a publication of the National Cancer Institute, *When Someone in Your Family Has Cancer*, may be useful in this process.

Finally, concern about what impact breast cancer may have on a mother's survival may be complicated by worry about its meaning for an offspring's future well-being. As 70% of women diagnosed have no known risk factors for development of breast cancer, they are the first in their family to have the disease. Many of these women report feeling guilty at having "brought the disease into the family." At the same time, adult offspring, in particular daughters, may feel angry about or frightened by the potential implications of their mother's illness on their risk of disease. With the growth of high-genetic-risk clinics, attention has focused on the overall psychological adjustment and quality of life of female first-degree relatives of patients. These patterns of response in female family members warrant special attention, as excessive psychological distress potentially can interfere not only with family function but also adherence to subsequent breast cancer screening, an issue addressed in greater detail in Chapter 17.

A number of books are now available that may be helpful to women and their families dealing with the challenges imposed by breast cancer. These include Kathy LaTour's *Breast Cancer Companion* (William Morrow & Co., 1993), Wendy Harpham's *After Cancer* (W. W. Norton & Co., 1994), and Andy Murcia and Bob Stewart's *Man to Man* (St. Martin's Press, 1990). Each is thoughtfully written, highlights the problems that families can expect, and provides resources for dealing with these. Another excellent reference is the *Breast Cancer Resource List*, which is published annually by the National Alliance of Breast Cancer Organizations, located in New York City (1-888-80-NABCO). In addition, the National Coalition for Cancer Survivorship, based in Silver Spring, Maryland (301-650-9127), has produced a volume edited by Barbara Hoffman, entitled *A Cancer Survivor's Almanac: Charting the Journey*, which, as its title implies, discusses the practical problems that arise from diagnosis through survivorship and offers solutions to each.

Quality of Life and Sexual Functioning

Although extensive research has been done on the psychosocial consequences of breast cancer, little of this work addressed the impact of disease and treatment on sexual functioning. Early studies focused on loss of breast and its impact on sexual relationships. These older, longitudinal studies, conducted among women treated with radical or modified radical mastectomy, reported significant sexual problems in 30% to 40% of samples assessed.[32,221,222] However, studies have since shown that the sexual disruption that occurs is independent of type of surgical treatment.[74,78,88,223] In her 1991 review of the effect of breast cancer on sexuality, body image, and intimate relationships, Schover[224] noted the lack of detail and specificity of available data on sexuality after breast cancer treatment, with most studies limiting the assessment to overall satisfaction or information on the frequency of intercourse. She observed that the premature and severe menopausal impact of systemic therapy may be the "most common culprit in causing sexual dysfunction." As observed earlier in this chapter, with increasing numbers of women receiving adjuvant chemotherapy or hormonal therapy, this less-explored area of sexual morbidity is receiving greater attention.

In their review of sexuality and cancer in women, Schultz et al.[225] describe the range of psychological reactions to cancer that threaten sexual function, including threats to (a) sexual identity and self-esteem, such as disturbances of mood, gender, and sexual identity and body image; (b) personal control over body functions, such as disease-related symptoms (e.g., pain, fatigue, nausea) that interfere with or inhibit sexual functioning; (c) intimacy, such as loss of social contacts that have potential for intimate physical expression, the disintegration of established patterns of achieving physical pleasure and intimacy, or myths related to contagion; and (d) reproductive function, such as the direct impairment of fertility or the fear of recurrence with pregnancy. In addition to these psychological reactions, some women experience less joy and vigor, as well as an underlying uncertainty about their health and the vulnerability of their bodies to further assault.[226] All of these factors affect sexual response in the breast cancer survivor.

In research conducted by Ganz et al.,[227,228] 227 patients with early-stage breast cancer were assessed at four points in time during the first year after surgery; some of these women were reassessed at 2 years (n = 69) or 3 years (n = 70) after surgery. Their data suggest that a subset of women may be at risk for psychosexual distress after treatment. Specifically, 1-year problems and frequencies for the at-risk group included not feeling sexually attractive (54%), not being interested in having sex (44%), decreased frequency of sexual intercourse (58%), difficulty in becoming sexually aroused (42%), difficulty with lubrication (50%), and difficulty in achieving orgasm (41% low risk and 56% at risk). Of the 70 women assessed at 3 years, 43% continued to be uncomfortable with body changes, 47% reported lack of interest in sex, and many continued to experience specific sexual dysfunction, including difficulty with arousal (48%), lubrication (64%), and orgasm (52%). Important in their research was the finding that survivors appear to attain maximum recovery from the physical and emotional trauma by 1 year after surgery. Furthermore, despite relatively good physical and emotional recovery, a number of problems persist beyond 1 year, in particular those associated with sexual rehabilitation.

The emotional distress, pain, fatigue, and insult to the patient's body image and self-esteem caused by the diagnosis and treatment of breast cancer can damage sexual functioning, even among individuals who had a strong and satisfying sexual relationship before illness. When illness occurs in the context of preexisting problems or before relationships are fully established, the outcome may be devastating. Despite heightened sensitivity to sexual issues, in practice, provision of effective sexual interventions remains highly variable, in part because of staff avoidance.

Auchincloss[229] found that staff resistance or reluctance to address patients' sexual concerns clusters around four broad themes. First, many professionals whose focus is on treatment and management of illness believe that the sexual consequences of treatment are not their concern. Auchincloss argues strongly that, as with any other side effect of treatment, the responsibility for monitoring sexual sequelae rests with the oncology team. Second, many staff members are reluctant to raise the topic of sex, because they believe that little information is available to remedy problems. This attitude is being slowly replaced as education about effective therapies for problems such as vaginal dryness, painful intercourse, and lack of desire becomes more broadly acknowledged and available. Nursing researchers have frequently been leaders in this area.[230] Third, belief that the patient is principally (or solely) concerned with her cancer prevents other staff from raising sexual issues. Work by Vincent et al.[231] challenges the accuracy of this perception. In their study, 80% of patients interviewed desired more information about sexual issues, although 75% expressed reluctance to broach the subject themselves. Finally, some staff members may simply be too embarrassed to discuss sex. Auchincloss[229] stresses that with time, education, patience, and practice, most health professionals can come to believe that they have something to offer patients who are anxious, distressed over new problems, and unsure of how to go about asking for help. Caregivers should be reassured that patients often feel an enormous sense of relief to have a problem acknowledged and to know that it is not uncommon and that help is available through suitable referral.

Because work such as that done by Ganz et al.[223,227,228] indicates that sexual problems tend to worsen, not improve, over time, sexual rehabilitation needs to start early. Ideally, this should occur before treatment starts for those patients for whom specific impairment of sexual function can be anticipated (e.g., premature menopause in the pre- or perimenopausal woman). Raising the topic of sexual function early, by letting the patient know it is an appropriate focus of concern and that the health care provider is willing to discuss it, opens the door for future dialogue in this area. It also helps to ensure that problems with sexual function will be addressed. The dialogue should include a brief social and sexual history with attention to the woman's particular concerns and needs. Auchincloss[229] cautions, however, against initiating sexual discussions during periods of acute stress (e.g., treatment setbacks, recurrences, family or work crises) and places a high premium on finding a private space for conducting such interviews. Some teams may wish to designate one staff member to initiate conversations or to follow up on those introduced by the primary physician. The primary nurse often is best suited for this position. Establishing this role is important, because it is as undesirable to have everyone asking about sexual function as to have no one inquire about this area. When specific questions arise, the nurse needs to know what the patient has been told and by whom so as to focus questions for patients, direct their inquiries to the appropriate staff member, clarify or reinforce information provided, and serve as an advocate for the patient. Above all, team members should know about efforts in this area and coordinate their input with that of others.

A number of specific sexual problems encountered by women have been raised earlier in the Adjuvant Chemotherapy section. It is beyond the scope of this chapter to detail the additional types of problems that may occur or their treatment. However, a number of resources are available in the growing field of sexual rehabilitation of cancer patients.[232,233] A manual for patients, entitled *Sexuality and the Woman Who Has Cancer and Her Partner*, is available through the American Cancer Society (1-800-ACS-2345). In addition, a small number of programs around the country train sex counselors and therapists. For women with more difficult sexual problems, or long-standing issues further compounded by treatment, referral to a qualified sex therapist should be considered. Names of trained professionals for referral or workshop purposes can be obtained from most major cancer centers, if nearby, or your local Cancer Information Service (1-800-4-CANCER).

Breast Cancer Survivors

Already, breast cancer survivors represent the largest constituency of the cancer survivorship community.[234] Few words may be more terrifying for a woman to hear than, "You have breast cancer." Many women state that they do not remember their physicians telling them anything else once this statement had been made. Nevertheless, research suggests that the majority of women recover and are doing well 1 year after diagnosis. Although women vary widely in their response to diagnosis and treatment, research is beginning to show that once treatment is over, most women return to lives that are as full as and often richer personally than before their illness; in many cases, survivors' functioning was found to be better than that of control or comparison samples of unaffected peers.[62,89,223,235–240] Many breast cancer survivors report taking better care of themselves in the wake of cancer, with particular focus on adopting healthier lifestyles, reducing stress, eating better, and exercising regularly. In general, these new studies have led clinicians to realize that concern about high rates of subsequent impairment in treated women may have been exaggerated. Our own work and that of others have shown that breast cancer does not appear to lead to the development of a posttraumatic stress disorder in significant numbers of women.[19,241] Striking to many clinical researchers involved in the conduct of long-term follow-up studies is the enormous resilience evidenced by women. In the words of one survivor, "It sure has a way of putting your life's priorities in order! Shame it had to happen, but in many ways my life is better. No longer a workaholic, more loving, kinder to others, much more spiritual. Spend much more time with family. More comfortable and 'centered' in my life. Fell in love with my husband all over again."[223] Also impressive has been the willingness of women to share important details about their cancer experience and recovery. Whereas some of the willingness to share is driven by altruistic motives and the hope of many survivors to improve the lives of women who will be diagnosed and treated after them, it also stems from a desire to bring to the attention of the medical community the need to document and, when needed, address the potential late effects of breast cancer on women's lives into the future.

Although concern about disease recurrence may diminish over time, for most breast cancer survivors, this never truly goes away. In our research among women on average 3 years after diagnosis, 42% said they worried a fair amount to very much that the cancer would come back.[223] Part of this residual anxiety may be attributable to the fact that breast cancer survivors understand that their cancer could recur at any time after treatment and that medical follow-up must continue for life. Greater attention in the general medical community to the potential physical late effects of treatment will likely generate new information for women into the future. Persistent problem areas reported by women include fatigue, dealing with menopausal symptoms, coming to terms with body image changes, and negotiating strategies to reduce risk for work and health insurance discrimination. In addition to providing valuable data on the health-related quality of life outcomes for women treated, the growing population of survivors has created a resource both for other survivors and for those who are newly diagnosed with breast cancer. Use of experienced veteran-to-rookie counselors and role models can provide a vital complement to the comprehensive care of patients.

SUMMARY

Breast cancer remains the most common tumor in women; it has a unique and, at times, complex psychological impact, but one to which psychologically healthy women respond well without the development of serious psychological symptoms. Increased use in primary treatment of breast-conserving and reconstructive procedures is reducing the negative effect on self-image and body image. However, ethical and legal constraints relating to treatment options have added substantially to decision-making dilemmas and to fears of recurrence, which may persist for an indefinite period. As newer therapies, such as intensive chemotherapy and peripheral stem cell rescue, are introduced, research on their immediate and delayed psychosocial impact are needed. Broader dissemination of information from the psychological studies of adaptation to the available treatment options can help in efforts to determine the best treatment to meet patients' physical and emotional needs. Sufficient data exist to indicate that addressing the psychosocial and psychosexual needs of breast cancer patients improves quality of survival and may even enhance length of survival. Finally, with the increasing demand for their involvement in care, special attention must be directed to the psychological well-being of the immediate relatives of women with breast cancer, especially their partners and offspring.

In closing, clinicians should be reminded that their relationship with a given patient often remains paramount above all the considerations outlined previously. A physician's style, behavior, attitudes, and beliefs can dramatically affect a woman's experience. Toward this end, it is important for the health care professional to see himself or herself as part of the treatment. By engaging a patient and being respectful and observant of her needs (and those with whom she presents), clinicians can increase the opportunity to minimize psychological trauma, enhance treatment adherence, and obtain the best possible outcome for each woman treated.

MANAGEMENT PRINCIPLES

- Although most women diagnosed and treated for breast cancer do well psychologically and socially, one-fourth of women with breast cancer have psychological symptoms that warrant psychiatric intervention.
- Clues to identifying women with psychological distress include previous treatment for depression or anxiety, symptoms of depression and anxiety that seem out of the "normal" range, and psychological symptoms that are worsening over time.
- The diagnosis and treatment of breast cancer causes a psychological toll for all women; recovery from physical and emotional symptoms usually occurs gradually during the 12 months after the completion of cancer treatment. Tell your patients that their asking for psychological help is a sign of strength, not weakness.
- Consider using brief, easily scored psychiatric symptom rating scales periodically across the course of care to help you identify women who are most in need of psychological treatment.
- Symptoms of anxiety and insomnia during the diagnostic, pretreatment, and treatment phases often can be rapidly and effectively treated with low-dose anxiolytics and hypnotics.
- Symptoms of depression should be evaluated by a psychiatrist or a psychologist; safe and effective antidepressants are available for women.
- Inform women who are receiving dexamethasone that it can cause psychological symptoms (anxiety, depression, mood swings); ask women to report these symptoms if they occur, because they can be rapidly and effectively treated.
- The oncologist can play an important role in encouraging the patient's early resumption of sexual activity after breast surgery or chemotherapy. Encourage the patient's partner to attend diagnostic planning and follow-up visits. Sometimes partners need referral for psychological support so they can better support your patient.

- Psychological symptoms such as anxiety are common at the conclusion of cancer treatment. Women feel vulnerable and less protected when not being seen regularly by their irradiation or medical oncologist. Invite women to schedule a return follow-up visit at the conclusion of treatment if they have questions and feel they could benefit from emotional support.
- Menopausal symptoms are highly distressing for many women. Mood swings, irritability, insomnia, and hot flashes can be effectively treated with a variety of anxiolytic and antidepressant medications. Refer women who have symptoms to a psychiatrist for evaluation.
- Offer psychological support services to *all* women (availability of support services varies depending on your location and type of practice).
- Psychological support comes in many forms (e.g., individual counseling, leader-led group, leaderless group) and is delivered by many professionals (psychiatrists, psychologists, social workers, nurses, and members of the clergy). Encourage your available psychosocial support members to become active participants of your interdisciplinary team. By doing this, they will serve you and your patients better.
- Women value communication with their physicians. The most satisfied patients are those who feel they were compassionately warned about potential side effects of treatment.
- Be aware that some women emotionally "sail" through treatment; symptoms develop in some of these women at the anniversary of their diagnosis or during the following year. Ask women during their 1-year follow-up visits how they are doing emotionally and refer as appropriate.

REFERENCES

1. *1999 Cancer facts and figures*. Atlanta: American Cancer Society, 1999.
2. Hankey BF, Miller B, Curtis R, Kosary C. Trends in breast cancer in younger women in contrast to older women. *J Natl Cancer Inst Monogr* 1994;16:7.
3. Early Breast Cancer Trialists' Collaborative Group. *Treatment of early breast cancer. Vol. 1. Worldwide evidence 1985-1990*. Oxford, UK: Oxford University Press, 1990.
4. Norton L. Evolving concepts in the systematic drug therapy of breast cancer. *Semin Oncol* 1997:24[Suppl 10]:S10.
5. Glanz K, Lerman C. Psychosocial impact of breast cancer. A critical review. *Ann Behav Med* 1992;14:204.
6. Lerman C, Rimer BK, Engstrom PF. Cancer risk notification: psychosocial and ethical implications. *J Clin Oncol* 1991;9:1275.
7. Holland JC. Societal views of cancer and the emergence of psycho oncology. In: Holland JC, ed. *Psycho-oncology*. New York: Oxford University Press, 1998:3.
8. Rosato FE, Rosenberg AL. Examination techniques: role of the physician and patient in evaluating breast diseases. In: Bland KI, Copeland EM III, eds. *The breast. Comprehensive management of benign and malignant diseases*. Philadelphia: WB Saunders, 1991:409.
9. Holland JC. Fears and abnormal reactions to cancer in physically healthy individuals. In: Holland JC, Rowland JH, eds. *Handbook of psychooncology: psychological care of the patient with cancer*. New York: Oxford University Press, 1989:18.
10. Robinson E, Mohilever J, Zidan J, Sapir D. Delay in diagnosis of cancer. Possible effects on the stage of disease and survival. *Cancer* 1984;54:1454.
11. Zidan J, Mohilever J, Sapir D, Robinson E. Statistical analysis of patients referred to the Northern Isreal Oncology Center. *Harefuah* 1982;102:415.
12. Nayfield SG, Bongiovanni CG, Alciati MH, Fischer RA, Bergner L. Statutory requirements for disclosure of breast cancer treatment alternatives. *J Natl Cancer Inst* 1994;86:1202.
13. Nattinger AB, Gottlieb MS, Veum J, Yahnke D, Goodwin JS. Geographic variation in the use of breast-conserving treatment for breast cancer. *N Engl J Med* 1992;326:1102.
14. Farrow DC, Hunt WC, Samet JM. Geographic variation in the treatment of localized breast cancer. *N Engl J Med* 1992;326:1097.
15. Rowland JH, Holland JC. Psychological reactions to breast cancer and its treatment. In: Harris JR, Hellman S, Hendersen IC, Kinne DW, eds. *Breast diseases*, 2nd ed. Philadelphia: JB Lippincott, 1991:849.
16. Whelan T, Levine MN, Gafni A, et al. Mastectomy or lumpectomy? Helping women make informed choices. *J Clin Oncol* 1999 (*in press*).
17. Scott DW. Anxiety, critical thinking and information processing during and after breast biopsy. *Nurs Res* 1983;32:24.
18. Valanis BG, Rumpler CH. Helping women to choose breast cancer treatment alternatives. *Cancer Nurs* 1985;8:167.
19. Green BL, Rowland JH, Krupnick JL, et al. Prevalence of posttraumatic stress disorder in women with breast cancer. *Psychosomatics* 1998;39:102.
20. Hack TF, Degner LF, Dyck DG. Relationship between preferences for decisional control and illness information among women with breast cancer: A quantitative and qualitative analysis. *Soc Sci Med* 1994;39:249.
21. Emanuel EJ, Emanuel LL. Four models of the physician-patient relationship. *JAMA* 1992;267:2221.
22. Siminoff LA. Cancer patient and physician communication: progress and continuing problems. *Ann Behav Med* 1989;11:108.
23. Ashcroft JJ, Leinster SJ, Slade PA. Breast cancer-patient choice of treatment: preliminary communication. *J R Soc Med* 1985;78:43.
24. Morris J, Royle GT. Offering patients a choice of surgery for early breast cancer: a reduction in anxiety and depression in patients and their husbands. *Soc Sci Med* 1988;26:583.
25. Glynn Owens R, Ashcroft JJ, Leinster SJ, Slade PD. Informal decision analysis with breast cancer patients: an aid to psychological preparation for surgery. *J Psychosoc Oncol* 1987;5:23.
26. Fallowfield LJ, Hall A, Maguire GP, Baum M. Psychological outcomes of different treatment policies in women with early breast cancer outside a clinical trial. *BMJ* 1990;301:575.
27. Lerman C, Daly M, Walsh WP, et al. Communication between patients with breast cancer and health care providers. Determinants and implications. *Cancer* 1993;72:2612.
28. Petrisek AC, Laliberte LL, Allen SM, Mor V. The treatment decision-making process: age differences in a sample of women recently diagnosed with nonrecurrent, early stage-breast cancer. *Gerontologist* 1997;37:598.
29. Bilodeau BA, Degner LF. Information needs, sources of information, and decisional roles in women with breast cancer. *Oncol Nurs Forum* 1996;23(4):691.
30. Deber RB, Kraetschmer N, Irvine J. What role do patients wish to play in treatment decision making? *Arch Intern Med* 1996;156:1414.
31. Johnson JD, Roberts CS, Cox CE, et al. Breast cancer patients' personality style, age and treatment decision making. *J Surg Oncol* 1996;63:183
32. Meyerowitz BE. Psychosocial correlates of breast cancer and its treatment. *Psychol Bull* 1980;87:108.
33. Rowland JH. Developmental stage and adaptation: adult model. In: Holland JC, Rowland JH, eds. *Handbook of psycho-oncology: psychological care of the patient with cancer*. New York, Oxford University Press, 1989:25.
34. Harrison J, Maguire P. Influence of age on psychological adjustment to cancer. *Psychooncology* 1995;4:33
35. Mor V, Malin M, Allen S. Age differences in the psychosocial problems encountered by breast cancer patients. *Monogr Natl Cancer Inst* 1994;16:191.
36. Valentgas P, Daling JR. Risk factors for breast cancer in younger women. *Monogr Natl Cancer Inst* 1994;16:15.
37. Breast cancer in younger women. Proceedings of a conference held at the National Institutes of Health, Bethesda, January 28, 1993. *J Natl Cancer Inst Monogr* 1994;16.
38. Ganz PA, Schag CC, Heinrich RL. The psychosocial impact of cancer in the elderly: a comparison with younger patients. *J Am Geriatr Soc* 1985;33:429.

39. Hynes DM. The quality of breast cancer care in local communities: implications for health care reform. *Med Care* 1994;32:328.
40. Taylor SE, Lichtman RR, Wood JV, Bluming AZ, Dosik GM, Leibowitz RL. Illness-related and treatment-related factors in psychological adjustment to breast cancer. *Cancer* 1985;55:2506.
41. Hilton BA. The relationship of uncertainty, control, commitment, and threat of recurrence to coping strategies used by women diagnosed with breast cancer. *J Behav Med* 1989;12:39.
42. Watson M, Greer S. Personality and coping. In: Holland JC, ed. *Psycho-oncology*. New York: Oxford University Press, 1998:91.
43. Suls J, Feltcher B. The relative efficacy of avoidant and non-avoidant coping strategies: a meta-analysis. *Health Psychol* 1985;4:249.
44. Rowland JH. Interpersonal resources: social support. In: Holland JC, Rowland JH, eds. *Handbook of psychooncology: psychological care of the patient with cancer*. New York: Oxford University Press, 1989:58.
45. Helgeson V, Cohen S. Relation of social support to adjustment to cancer: reconciling descriptive, correlational, and intervention research. *Health Psychol* 1996;15:135.
46. Morris T, Pettingale KW, Haybittle JL. Psychological response to cancer diagnosis and disease outcome in patients with breast cancer and lymphoma. *Psychooncology* 1992;1:105.
47. Dean C, Surtees PG. Do psychological factors predict survival in breast cancer? *J Psychosom Res* 1989;33:561.
48. Fox BH. Psychosocial factors in cancer incidence and prognosis. In: Holland JC, ed. *Psycho-oncology*. New York: Oxford University Press, 1998:110.
49. Bovbjerg DH, Valdimarsdottir HB. Psychoneuroimmunology: implications for psycho-oncology. In: Holland JC, ed. *Psycho-oncology*. New York: Oxford University Press, 1998:125.
50. Mulder CL, Van der Pompe G, Spiegel D, et al. Do psychosocial factors influence the course of breast cancer? A review of recent literature, methodologic problems and future directions. *Psychooncology* 1992;1:155.
51. Fertig DL. Depression in patients with breast cancer: prevalence, diagnosis, and treatment. *The Breast Journal* 1997;3:292.
52. McDaniel JS, Musselman DL, Porter MR, et al. Depression in patients with cancer. Diagnosis, biology and treatment. *Arch Gen Psychiatry* 1995;52:89.
53. van't Spijker A, Trijsburg RW, Duivenvoorden HJ. Psychological sequelae of cancer diagnosis: a meta-analytical review of 58 studies after 1980. *Psychosom Med* 1997;59:280.
54. DeFlorio M, Massie MJ. A review of depression in cancer: gender differences. *Depression* 1995;3:66.
55. Loprinzi CL, Pisansky TM, Fonseca R, et al. Pilot evaluation of venlafaxine hydrochloride for the therapy of hot flashes in cancer survivors. *J Clin Oncol* 1998;16:2377.
56. Zabora JR. Screening procedures for psychosocial distress. In: Holland JC, ed. *Psycho-oncology*. New York: Oxford University Press, 1998:653.
57. Payne DK, Hoffman RG, Theodoulou M, et al. Screening for anxiety and depression in women with breast cancer. Psychiatry and medical oncology gear up for managed care. *Psychosomatics* 1999;40:64.
58. Moyer A, Salovey P. Psychosocial sequelae of breast cancer and its treatment. *Ann Behav Med* 1996;18:110.
59. Irvine D, Brown B, Crooks D, Roberts J, Browne G. Psychosocial adjustment in women with breast cancer. *Cancer* 1991;67:1097.
60. Psychological Aspects of Breast Cancer Study Group. Psychological response to mastectomy: a prospective comparison study. *Cancer* 1987;59:189.
61. Hughson AV, Cooper AF, McArdle CS, et al. Psychosocial consequences of mastectomy: levels of morbidity and associated factors. *J Psychosom Med* 1988;32:383.
62. Saleeba AK, Weitzner MA, Meyers CA. Subclinical psychological distress in long-term survivors of breast cancer. *J Psychosoc Oncol* 1996;14(1):83.
63. Houn F, Helzlsouer KJ, Friedman NB, Stefanek ME. The practice of prophylactic mastectomy: a survey of Maryland surgeons. *Am J Public Health* 1995;85:801.
64. Lerman C, Narod S, Schulman K, et al. BRCA1 testing in families with hereditary breast-ovarian cancer. A prospective study of patient decision making and outcomes. *JAMA* 1996;275:1885.
65. Hartmann LC, Schaid DJ, Woods JE, et al. Efficacy of bilateral prophylactic mastectomy in women with a family history of breast cancer. *N Engl J Med* 1999;340:77.
66. Lopez MJ, Porter KA. The current role of prophylactic mastectomy. *Surg Clin North Am* 1996;76:231.
67. King MC, Rowell S, Love SM. Inherited breast and ovarian cancer: what are the risks? What are the choices? *JAMA* 1993;269:1975.
68. Meyer L, Ringberg A. A prospective study of psychiatric and psychosocial sequelae of bilateral subcutaneous mastectomy. *Scand J Plast Reconstr Surg* 1986;20:101.
69. Gyllenskold K, Glaumann B. A pilot study of some psychological aspects of subcutaneous mastectomy. *Scand J Plast Reconstr Surg* 1985;19:283.
70. Stefanek ME, Helslsouer KJ, Wilcox PM, Houn F. Predictors of and satisfaction with bilateral prophylactic mastectomy. *Prev Med* 1995;24:412.
71. Borgen PI, Hill ADK, Tran KN, et al. Patient regrets after prophylactic mastectomy. *Ann Surg Oncol* 1998;5:603.
72. *Breast conservation versus mastectomy: patient survival in day-to-day medical practice and in randomized studies*. Washington: US General Accounting Office, Nov 15, 1994.
73. Moyer A. Psychosocial outcomes of breast-conserving surgery versus mastectomy: a meta-analytic review. *Health Psychol* 1997;16:284.
74. Kiebert GM, de Haes JC, van de Velde CJH. The impact of breast-conserving treatment and mastectomy on the quality-of-life of early-stage breast cancer patients: a review. *J Clin Oncol* 1991;9:1059.
75. Fallowfield LJ. Psychosocial adjustment after treatment for early breast cancer. *Oncology* 1990;4:89.
76. Maunsell E, Brisson J, Deschenes L. Psychological distress after initial treatment for breast cancer: a comparison of partial and total mastectomy. *J Clin Epidemiol* 1989;42:765.
77. Omne-Ponten M, Holmberg L, Sjoden P-O. Psychosocial adjustment among women with breast cancer stages I and II: six-year follow-up of consecutive patients. *J Clin Oncol* 1994;12:1778.
78. Levy SM, Haynes LT, Herberman RB, et al. Mastectomy versus breast conservation surgery: mental health effects at long-term follow-up. *Health Psychol* 1992;11:349.
79. Schain W, Edwards BK, Gorrell EV, et al. Psychosocial and physical outcomes of primary breast cancer therapy: mastectomy vs. excisional biopsy and irradiation. *Breast Cancer Res Treat* 1983;3:377.
80. Schain WS, d'Angelo TM, Dunn ME, et al. Mastectomy versus conservative surgery and radiation therapy: psychosocial consequences. *Cancer* 1994;73:1221.
81. de Haes JC, Welvaart K. Quality of life after breast cancer surgery. *J Surg Oncol* 1985;28:123.
82. Fallowfield LJ, Baum M, Maguire GP. Effects of breast conservation on psychological morbidity associated with diagnosis and treatment of early breast cancer. *BMJ* 1986;293:1331.
83. Lasry J-CM, Margolese RG, Poisson R, et al. Depression and body image following mastectomy and lumpectomy. *J Chron Dis* 1987;40:529.
84. Zevon MA, Rounds JB, Karr J. Psychological outcomes associated with breast conserving surgery: a meta-analysis. Paper presented at the eighth annual meeting of the Society of Behavioral Medicine, Washington, DC; March 1987.
85. Fallowfield LJ, Hall A. Psychosocial and sexual impact of diagnosis and treatment of breast cancer. *Br Med Bull* 1991;47:388.
86. Margolis GJ, Goodman RL, Rubin A, Pajac TF. Psychological factors in the choice of treatment for breast cancer. *Psychosomatics* 1989;30:192.
87. Wolberg WH, Tanner MA, Romsaas EP, et al. Factors influencing options in primary breast cancer treatment. *J Clin Oncol* 1987;5:68.
88. Ganz PA. Treatment options for breast cancer—beyond survival. *N Engl J Med* 1992;326:1147.
89. Ganz PA, Rowland JH, Meyerowitz BE, Desmond KA. Impact of different adjuvant therapy strategies on quality of life in breast cancer survivors. *Recent Results Cancer Res* 1998;152:396.
90. Wolberg WH. Surgical options in 424 patients with primary breast cancer without systemic metastases. *Arch Surg* 1991;126:817.
91. Morris J, Royle GT, Taylor I. Changes in the surgical management of early breast cancer in England. *J R Soc Med* 1989;82:12.
92. Long E. Breast cancer in African-American women. *Cancer Nurs* 1993;16:1.
93. Monroe AJ, Biruls R, Griffin AV, et al. Distress associated with radiotherapy for malignant disease: a quantitative analysis based on patients' perceptions. *Br J Cancer* 1989;60:370.
94. Farncombe M, Daniels G, Gross L. Lymphedema: the seemingly forgotten complication. *J Pain Symptom Manage* 1994;9:269.
95. Markowski J, Wilcox JP, Helm PA. Lymphedema incidence after specific postmastectomy therapy. *Arch Phys Med Rehabil* 1981;62:449.
96. Kissin MW, Della Rovere GQ, Easton D, Westbury G. Risk of lymphedema following the treatment of breast cancer. *Br J Surg* 1986; 73:580.

97. Larson D, Weinstein M, Goldberg I, et al. Edema of the arm as a function of the extent of axillary surgery in patients with stage I-II carcinoma of the breast treated with primary radiotherapy. *Int J Radiat Oncol Biol Phys* 1986;12:1575.
98. Brennan MJ, Weitz J. Lymphedema thirty years after radical mastectomy. *Am J Phys Med Rehabil* 1992;71:12.
99. Passik SD, Newman ML, Brennan M, Tunkel R. Predictors of psychological distress, sexual dysfunction and physical functioning among women with upper extremity lymphedema related to breast cancer. *Psychooncology* 1995;4:255.
100. Passik SD, Newman ML, Brennan M, Holland J. Psychiatric consultation for women undergoing rehabilitation for upper-extremity lymphedema following breast cancer treatment. *J Pain Symptom Manage* 1993;8:1.
101. Maunsell E, Brisson J, Deschenes L. Arm problems and psychological distress after surgery for breast cancer. *Can J Surg* 1993;36:315.
102. Tobin M, Lacey HJ, Meyer L, Mortimer PS. The psychological morbidity of breast cancer-related arm swelling. *Cancer* 1993;72:3248.
103. Winer EP, Fee-Fulkerson K, Fulkerson CC, et al. Silicone controversy: a survey of women with breast cancer and silicone implants. *J Natl Cancer Inst* 1993;85:1407.
104. Angell M. Shattuck lecture: evaluating the health risks of breast implants: the interplay of medical science, the law, and public opinion. *N Engl J Med* 1996;334:1513.
105. American Society of Plastic and Reconstructive Surgeons. 1990 Statistics. Arlington Heights, IL: American Society of Plastic and Reconstructive Surgeons, 1991.
106. Margolis G, Goodman RL, Rubin A. Psychological effects of breast-conserving cancer treatment and mastectomy. *Psychosomatics* 1990;31:33.
107. Mock V. Body image in women treated for breast cancer. *Nurs Res* 1993;42:153.
108. Pozo C, Carver CS, Noriega V, et al. Effects of mastectomy versus lumpectomy on emotional adjustment to breast cancer: a prospective study of the first year postsurgery. *J Clin Oncol* 1992;10:1292.
109. Noguchi M, Kitagawa H, Kinoshita K, et al. Psychologic and cosmetic self-assessments of breast conserving therapy compared with mastectomy and immediate breast reconstruction. *J Surg Oncol* 1993;54:260.
110. Schover LR, Yetman RJ, Tuason LJ, et al. Partial mastectomy and breast reconstruction: a comparison of their effects on psychosocial adjustment, body image, and sexuality. *Cancer* 1995;75:54.
111. Rowland JH, Holland JC, Chaglassian T, Kinne D. Psychological response to breast reconstruction. Expectations for and impact on postmastectomy functioning. *Psychosomatics* 1993;34:241.
112. Rowland JH, Dioso J, Holland JC, Chaglassian T, Kinne D. Breast reconstruction after mastectomy: who seeks it, who refuses? *Plast Reconstr Surg* 1995;95:812.
113. Goin JM, Goin MK. Breast reconstruction after mastectomy. In: Goin JM, Goin MK. *Changing the body: psychological effects of plastic surgery*. Baltimore: Williams & Wilkins, 1981:163.
114. Clifford E. The reconstruction experience: the search for restitution. In: Georgiade NG, ed. *Breast reconstruction following mastectomy*. St. Louis, MO: Mosby, 1979:22.
115. Houpt P, Dijkstra R, Storm van Leeuwen JB. The result of breast reconstruction after mastectomy for breast cancer in 109 patients. *Ann Plast Surg* 1988;21:517.
116. Gilboa D, Borenstein A, Floro S, Shafir R, Falach H, Tsur H. Emotional and psychosocial adjustment of women to breast reconstruction and detection of subgroups at risk for psychological morbidity. *Ann Plast Surg* 1990;25:397.
117. Teimourian B, Adham M. Survey of patients' response to breast reconstruction. *Ann Plast Surg* 1982;9:321.
118. Fee-Fulkerson K, Conaway MR, Winer EP, et al. Factors contributing to patient satisfaction with breast reconstruction using silicone implants. *Plast Reconstr Surg* 1996;97:1420.
119. Filiberti A, Tamburini M, Murru L, et al. Psychologic effects and esthetic results of breast reconstruction after mastectomy. *Tumori* 1986;72:585.
120. Mueller SC, Cioroiu M, LaRaja RD, Rothenberg RE. Postmastectomy breast reconstruction: a survey of general and plastic surgeons. *Plast Reconstr Surg* 1988;82:555.
121. van Dam FS, Bergman RB. Psychosocial and surgical aspects of breast reconstruction. *Eur J Surg Oncol* 1988;14:141.
122. Wellisch DK, Schain WS, Noone RB, Little JW. The psychological contribution of nipple addition in breast reconstruction. *Plast Reconstr Surg* 1987;80:699.
123. Noone RB, Frazier TG, Hayward CZ, Skiles MS. Patient acceptance of immediate reconstruction following mastectomy. *Plast Reconstr Surg* 1982;69:632.
124. Rowland J, Meyerowitz B, Ganz P, et al. Body image and sexual functioning following reconstructive surgery in breast cancer survivors (BCS). *Proc Am Soc Clin Oncol* 1996;15:124(abst 163).
125. Dean C, Chetty U, Forrest APM. Effects of immediate breast reconstruction on psychosocial morbidity after mastectomy. *Lancet* 1983;1:459.
126. Stevens LA, McGrath MH, Druss RG, Kister SJ, Gump FE, Forde KA. The psychological impact of immediate breast reconstruction for women with early breast cancer. *Plast Reconstr Surg* 1984;73:619.
127. Schain WS, Wellisch DK, Pasnau RO, Landsverk J. The sooner the better: a study of psychological factors in women undergoing immediate versus delayed breast reconstruction. *Am J Psychiatry* 1985;142:40.
128. Wellisch DK, Schain WS, Noone BR, Little JW. Psychosocial correlates of immediate versus delayed reconstruction of the breast. *Plast Reconstr Surg* 1985;76:713.
129. Franchelli S, Leone MS, Berrino P, et al. Psychological evaluation of patients undergoing breast reconstruction using two different methods: autologous tissues versus prostheses. *Plast Reconstr Surg* 1995;95:1213.
130. McCraw JB, Horton CE, Grossman JAI, et al. An early appraisal of the methods of tissue expansion and the transverse rectus abdominis musculocutaneous flap in reconstruction of the breast following mastectomy. *Ann Plast Surg* 1987;18:93.
131. Cederna PS, Yates WR, Chang P, et al. Postmastectomy reconstruction: comparative analysis of the psychosocial, and cosmetic effects of transverse rectus abdominus musculocutaneous flap versus breast implant reconstruction. *Ann Plast Surg* 1995;35:458.
132. Schain WS, Jacobs E, Wellisch DK. Psychosocial issues in breast reconstruction: intrapsychic, interpersonal, and practical concerns. *Clin Plast Surg* 1984;11:237.
133. Winder AE, Winder BD. Patient counseling. Clarifying a woman's choice for breast reconstruction. *Patient Educ Couns* 1985;7:65.
134. Matheson G, Drever JM. Psychological preparation of the patient for breast reconstruction. *Ann Plast Surg* 1990;24:238.
135. Taylor SE, Lichtman RR, Wood JV. Compliance with chemotherapy among breast cancer patients. *Health Psychol* 1984;3:553.
136. Meyerowitz BE, Watkins IK, Sparks FC. Psychosocial implications of adjuvant chemotherapy: a two year follow-up. *Cancer* 1983;52:1541.
137. Morrow GR, Roscoe JA, Hickok JT. Nausea and vomiting. In: Holland JC, ed. *Psycho-oncology*. New York: Oxford University Press, 1998;476.
138. Manne SL, Girasek D, Ambrosino J. An evaluation of the impact of a cosmetics class on breast cancer patients. *J Psychosoc Oncol* 1994;12:83.
139. Denmark-Wahnefried W, Winer EP, Rimer BK. Why women gain weight with adjuvant chemotherapy for breast cancer. *J Clin Oncol* 1993;11:1418.
140. Huntington M. Weight gain in patients receiving adjuvant chemotherapy for carcinoma of the breast. *Cancer* 1985;65:572.
141. Senie RT, Rosen PP, Rhodes P, Lesser ML, Kinne DW. Obesity at diagnosis of breast carcinoma influences duration of disease-free survival. *Ann Intern Med* 1992;116:26.
142. Hebert JR, Hurley TG, Ma Y, Hampl JS. The effect of dietary exposures on recurrence and mortality in early stage breast cancer. *Breast Cancer Res Treat* 1998;51:17.
143. Winningham ML, MacVicar MG, Bondon M, et al. Effect of aerobic exercise on body weight and composition in patients with breast cancer on adjuvant chemotherapy. *Oncol Nurs Forum* 1989;16:683.
144. Wieneke MH, Dienst ER. Neuropsychologic assessment of cognitive functioning following chemotherapy for breast cancer. *Psychooncology* 1995;4:61.
145. van Dam FS, Schagen SB, Muller MJ, et al. Impairment of cognitive function in women receiving adjuvant treatment for high-risk breast cancer: high-dose versus standard-dose chemotherapy. *J Natl Cancer Inst* 1998;90:210.
146. Ganz PA. Cognitive dysfunction following adjuvant treatment of breast cancer: a new dose-limiting toxic effect [Editorial]? *J Natl Cancer Inst* 1998;90:182.
147. Schover LR. Sexuality and body image in younger women with breast cancer. *Monogr Natl Cancer Inst* 1994;16:177.
148. Kaplan JS. A neglected issue: the sexual side effects of current treatments for breast cancer. *J Sex Marital Ther* 1992;18:3.

149. Sherwin BB. A comparative analysis of the role of androgen in human male and female sexual behavior: behavioral specificity, critical thresholds, and sensitivity. *Psychobiology* 1988;16:416.
150. Henderson BE, Paganini-Hill A, Ross RK. Decreased mortality in users of estrogen replacement therapy. *Arch Intern Med* 1991;151:75.
151. Dupont WD, Page DL. Menopausal estrogen replacement therapy and breast cancer. *Arch Intern Med* 1991;151:67.
152. Vassilopoulou-Sellin R, Zolinski C. Estrogen replacement therapy in women with breast cancer: a survey of patient attitudes. *Am J Med Sci* 1992;304:145.
153. Vassilopoulou-Sellin R, Theriault RL. Randomized prospective trial of estrogen-replacement therapy in women with a history of breast cancer. *J Natl Cancer Inst Monogr* 1994;16:153.
154. Cobleigh MA, Berris RF, Bush T, et al. Estrogen replacement therapy in breast cancer survivors. A time for change. *JAMA* 1994;272:540.
155. Smets EM, Garssen B, Schuster-Uitterhoeve AL, de Haes JC. Fatigue in cancer patients. *Br J Cancer* 1993;68:220.
156. Andrykowski MA, Curran SL, Lightner R. Off-treatment fatigue in breast cancer survivors: a controlled comparison. *J Behav Med* 1998;21:1
157. Tierney A, Leonard R, Taylor J, et al. Side effects expected and experienced by women receiving chemotherapy for breast cancer. *BMJ* 1991;302:272.
158. Mortimer JE, Boucher L, Baty J, et al. Effect of tamoxifen on sexual functioning. *J Clin Oncol* 1999;17:1488.
159. Cathcart CK, Jones SE, Pumroy CS, et al. Clinical recognition and management of depression in node negative breast cancer patients treated with tamoxifen. *Breast Cancer Res Treat* 1993;27:277.
160. Duffy LS, Greenberg DB, Younger J, Ferraro MG. Iatrogenic acute estrogen deficiency and psychiatric syndromes in breast cancer patients. *Psychosomatics* 1999;40:304.
161. van Leeuwen FE, Benraadt J, Coebergh JW, et al. Risk of endometrial cancer after tamoxifen treatment of breast cancer. *Lancet* 1994;343:448.
162. Uziely B, Lewin A, Brufman G, Dorembus D, Mor-Yosef S. The effect of tamoxifen on the endometrium. *Breast Cancer Res Treat* 1993;26:101.
163. Pavlidis NA, Petris C, Briassoulis E, et al. Clear evidence that long-term, low-dose tamoxifen treatment can induce ocular toxicity. *Cancer* 1992;69:2961.
164. *Physician's desk reference*, 49th ed. Oradell, NJ: Medical Economics Company, 1995:878.
165. Andrykowski MA. Psychosocial factors in bone marrow transplantation: a review and recommendations for research. *Bone Marrow Transplant* 1994;13:357.
166. Ahles TA, Tope DM, Furstenberg C, et al. Psychologic and neuropsychologic impact of autologous bone marrow transplantation. *J Clin Oncol* 1996;14:1457.
167. Lesko LM, Ostroff JS, Mumma GH, Mashberg DE, Holland JC. Long-term psychological adjustment of acute leukemia survivors: impact of bone marrow transplantation versus conventional chemotherapy. *Psychosom Med* 1992;54:30.
168. Yellen SB, Cella DF. Someone to live for: social well-being, parenthood status, and decision-making in oncology. *J Clin Oncol* 1995;13:1255.
169. Jenkins PL, Lester H, Alexander J, Whittaker J. A prospective study of psychosocial morbidity in adult bone marrow transplant recipients. *Psychosomatics* 1994;35:361.
170. Hoffman RS. The psycho-oncologist in a multidisciplinary breast treatment center. In: Cooper CL, ed. *Stress and breast cancer*. New York, John Wiley and Sons, 1988:171.
171. Breitbart W, Payne DK. Pain. In: Holland JC, ed. *Psycho-oncology*. New York: Oxford University Press, 1998:450.
172. Massie MJ, Holland JC. The cancer patient with pain: psychiatric complications and their management. *J Pain Symptom Manage* 1992;7:99.
173. Spiegel D, Bloom JR. Group therapy and hypnosis reduce metastatic breast carcinoma pain. *Psychosom Med* 1983;4:333.
174. Glajchen M, Peyser S, Calder K, Blum D. Multidimensional management of cancer pain. In: Holland JC, Lesko LM, Massie MJ, eds. *Current concepts in psycho-oncology IV. Syllabus of the postgraduate course*. New York: Memorial Sloan-Kettering Cancer Center, 1991:263(abst).
175. Trijsburg RW, van Knippenberg FCE, Rijpma SE. Effects of psychological treatment on cancer patients: a critical review. *Psychosom Med* 1992;54:489
176. Andersen BL. Psychological interventions for cancer patients to enhance the quality of life. *J Consult Clin Psychol* 1992;60:552.
177. Fawzy FI, Fawzy NW, Arndt LA, Pasnau RO. Critical review of psychosocial interventions in cancer care. *Arch Gen Psychiatry* 1995;52:100.
178. Meyer TJ, Mark MM. Effects of psychosocial interventions with adult cancer patients: a meta-analysis of randomized experiments. *Health Psychol* 1995;14:101.
179. Devine EC, Westlake SK. The effects of psychoeducational care provided to adults with cancer. Meta-analysis of 116 studies. *Oncol Nurs Forum* 1995;22:1369.
180. Maguire P, Tait A, Brooke M, Thomas C, Sellwood R. The effects of counseling on the psychiatric morbidity associated with mastectomy. *BMJ* 1980;281:1454.
181. Spiegel D, Bloom JR, Yalom I. Group support for patients with metastatic cancer. *Arch Gen Psychiatry* 1981;38:527.
182. Bloom JR, Ross RD, Burnell G. The effect of social support on patient adjustment after breast surgery. *Patient Couns Health Educ* 1978;1:50.
183. Farash JL. Effects of counseling on resolution of loss and body image disturbance following mastectomy. *Dissertation Abstracts International* 1979;39:4027.
184. Cain EN, Kohorn EI, Quinlan DM, Latimer K, Schwartz PE. Psychosocial benefits of a cancer support group. *Cancer* 1986;57:183.
185. Capone MA, Good RS, Westie KS, Jacobson AF. Psychosocial rehabilitation of gynecologic oncology patients. *Arch Phys Med Rehabil* 1980;61:128.
186. Telch CF, Telch MJ. Group coping skills instruction and supportive group therapy for cancer patients: a comparison of strategies. *J Consult Clin Psychol* 1986;54:802.
187. Richardson JL, Shelton DR, Krailo M, Levine AM. The effect of compliance with treatment on survival among patients with hematologic malignancies. *J Clin Oncol* 1990;8:356.
188. Presberg BA, Levenson JL. A survey of cancer support groups provided by National Cancer Institute clinical and comprehensive centers. *Psychooncology* 1993;2:215.
189. Coluzzi PH, Grant M, Doroshow JH, et al. Survey of the provision of supportive care services at National Cancer Institute-designated cancer centers. *J Clin Oncol* 1995;13:756.
190. Spiegel DS, Bloom JR, Kraemer HC, Gottheil E. Effect of psychosocial treatment on survival of patients with metastatic breast cancer. *Lancet* 1989;2:888.
191. Krupnick JL, Rowland JH, Goldberg RL, Daniel UV. Professionally led support groups for cancer patients: an intervention in search of a model. *Int J Psychiatry Med* 1993;23:275.
192. Andrykowski MA, Curran SL, Studts JL, et al. Psychosocial adjustment and quality of life in women with breast cancer and benign breast problems: a controlled comparison. *J Clin Epidemiol* 1996;49:827.
193. Wortman CB. Social support and the cancer patient. Conceptual and methodologic issues. *Cancer* 1984;53:2339.
194. Helgesen V, Cohen S, Fritz HL. Social ties and cancer. In: Holland JC, ed. *Psycho-oncology*. New York: Oxford University Press, 1998:99.
195. Cohen S, Syme SL, eds. *Social support and health*. New York: Academic Press, 1985.
196. Reifman A. Social relationships, recovering from illness, and survival: a literature review. *Ann Behav Med* 1995;17:124.
197. Cohen S, Wills TA. Stress, social support and the buffering hypothesis. *Psychol Bull* 1985;98:310.
198. Nelles WB, McCaffrey RJ, Blanchard CG, Ruckdeschel JC. Social supports and breast cancer: a review. *J Psychosoc Oncol* 1991;9:21.
199. Funch DP, Marshall J. The role of stress, social support and age in survival from breast cancer. *J Psychosom Res* 1983;27:77.
200. Waxler-Morrison N, Hislop TG, Mears B, Kan L. Effects of social relationships on survival for women with breast cancer: a prospective study. *Soc Sci Med* 1991;33:177.
201. Dunkel-Schetter C, Wortman C. The interpersonal dynamics of cancer: problems in social relationships and their impact on the patients. In: Friedman JS, DiMatteo RM, eds. *Interpersonal issues in health care*. New York: Academic Press, 1982:69.
202. Wellisch DK, Jamison KR, Pasnau RO. Psychosocial aspects of mastectomy. II. The man's perspective. *Am J Psychiatry* 1978;135:543.
203. Sabo D, Brown J, Smith C. The male role and mastectomy: support groups and men's adjustment. *J Psychosoc Oncol* 1986;4:19.
204. Maguire P. The repercussions of mastectomy on the family. *Int J Fam Psychiatry* 1981;1:485.

205. Baider L, Kaplan-DeNour A. Couples' reactions and adjustment to mastectomy: a preliminary report. *Int J Psychiatry Med* 1984;14:265.
206. Northouse LL. The impact of breast cancer on patients and husbands. *Cancer Nurs* 1989;12:276.
207. Northouse LL. Breast cancer in younger women: effects on interpersonal and family relations. *J Natl Cancer Inst Monogr* 1994;16:183.
208. Fisher JD, Nadler A, Whitcher-Alagna S. Recipient reactions to aid. *Psychol Bull* 1982;91:27.
209. Coyne JC, Wortman CB, Lehman DR. The other side of support: emotional overinvolvement and miscarried helping. In: Gottlieb BH, ed. *Marshaling social support*. Newbury Park, CA: Sage, 1988:305.
210. Hoskins CN, Baker S, Budin W, et al. Adjustment among husbands of women with breast cancer. *J Psychosoc Oncol* 1996;14:41.
211. Wellisch DK. Family relationships of the mastectomy patient: interactions with the spouse and children. *Isr J Med Sci* 1981;17:993.
212. Litman TJ. The family as a basic unit in health and medical care: a social behavioral overview. *Soc Sci Med* 1974;8:495.
213. Lewis FM. The impact of cancer on the family: a critical analysis of the research literature. *Patient Educ Couns* 1986;11:269.
214. Howes MJ, Hoke L, Winterbottom M, Delafield D. Psychosocial effects of breast cancer on a patient's children. *J Psychosoc Oncol* 1994;12:1.
215. Lewis FM, Hammond MA, Woods NF. The family's functioning with newly diagnosed breast cancer in the mother: the development of an explanatory model. *J Behav Med* 1993;16:351.
216. Lichtman RR, Taylor SE, Wood JV, Bluming AZ, Dosik GM, Leibowitz RL. Relations with children after breast cancer: the mother-daughter relationship at risk. *J Psychosoc Oncol* 1984;2:1.
217. Wellisch DK. Adolescent acting out when a parent has cancer. *Int J Fam Ther* 1979;1:238.
218. LeShan E. *When a parent is very sick*. Boston: Little, Brown, 1986.
219. McCue K. *How to help children through a parent's serious illness*. New York: St. Martin's Press, 1994.
220. Harpham WS. *When a parent has cancer: a guide to caring for your children*. New York: Harper Collins, 1997.
221. Maguire GP, Lee EG, Bevington DJ, et al. Psychiatric problems in the first year after mastectomy. *BMJ* 1978;279:963.
222. Morris T, Greer HS, White P. Psychological and social adjustment to mastectomy: a two-year follow-up study. *Cancer* 1977;40:2381.
223. Ganz PA, Rowland JH, Desmond K, et al. Life after breast cancer: understanding women's health related quality of life and sexual functioning. *J Clin Oncol* 1998;16:501.
224. Schover LR. The impact of breast cancer on sexuality, body image, and intimate relationships. *CA Cancer J Clin* 1991;41:112.
225. Schultz WCMW, Van de Wiel HBM, Hahn DEE, et al. Sexuality and cancer in women. *Ann Rev Sexual Res* 1992;3:151.
226. Quigley KM. The adult cancer survivor: psychosocial consequences of cure. *Semin Oncol Nurs* 1989;5:63.
227. Ganz PA, Hirji K, Sim M-S, Schag CAC, Fred C, Polinsky ML. Predicting psychosocial risk in patients with breast cancer. *Med Care* 1993;31:419.
228. Ganz PA, Coscarelli A, Fred C, et al. Breast cancer survivors: psychosocial concerns and quality of life. *Breast Cancer Res Treat* 1996;38:183.
229. Auchincloss SS. Sexual dysfunction in cancer patients: issues in evaluation and treatment. In: Holland JC, Rowland JH, eds. *Handbook of psychooncology: psychological care of the patient with cancer*. New York: Oxford University Press, 1989:383.
230. Knobf MT. Menopause in women with breast cancer. *Innovations in Breast Cancer Care* 1997;2(3):42.
231. Vincent CE, Vincent B, Greiss FC, et al. Some marital-sexual concomitants of carcinoma of the cervix. *South Med J* 1975;68:552
232. Schover LR. *Sexuality and fertility after cancer*. New York: John Wiley and Sons, 1997.
233. Andersen BL, Cyranowski JM. Women's sexuality: behaviors, responses, and individual differences. *J Consult Clin Psychol* 1995;63:891.
234. Andersen BL. Surviving cancer. *Cancer* 1994;74[Suppl 4]:1484.
235. Polinsky ML. Functional status of long-term breast cancer survivors: demonstrating chronicity. *Health Soc Work* 1994;19(3):165.
236. Omne-Ponten M, Holmberg L, Sjoden P-O. Psychosocial adjustment among women with breast cancer stages I and II: six-year follow-up of consecutive patients. *J Clin Oncol* 1994;12:1778.
237. Ellman R, Thomas BA. Is psychological well being impaired in long term survivors of breast cancer? *J Med Screen* 1995;2:5.
238. Dow KH, Ferrell BR, Leigh S, et al. An evaluation of the quality of life among long-term survivors of breast cancer. *Breast Cancer Res Treat* 1996;39:261.
239. Wyatt G, Friedman LL. Long-term female cancer survivors: quality of life issues and clinical complications. *Cancer Nurs* 1996;19:1.
240. Ferrell BR, Grant MM, Funk B, et al. Quality of life in breast cancer survivors as identified by focus groups. *Psychooncology* 1997;6:13.
241. Tjemsland L, Soreide JA, Malt UF. Post-traumatic distress symptoms in operable breast cancer III: status one year after surgery. *Breast Cancer Res Treat* 1998;47:141.

Diseases of the Breast, 2nd ed.,
edited by Jay R. Harris.
Lippincott Williams & Wilkins, Philadelphia © 2000.

CHAPTER 69

Lymphedema

Jeanne A. Petrek and Robert Lerner

Lymphedema develops in approximately 15% to 20% of patients after breast cancer treatment. It is estimated that at least one to two million breast cancer survivors who have had lymphadenectomy are alive today, and 400,000 of them cope daily with the disfigurement, discomfort, and disability of arm and hand swelling. Aside from recurrence, lymphedema is the most dreaded sequela of breast cancer treatment.

Lymphedema is a common and troublesome problem. The cosmetic deformity cannot be disguised with normal clothing, physical discomfort and upper extremity disability are associated with the enlargement, and recurrent episodes of cellulitis and lymphangitis occur frequently in this setting. Added to the physical symptoms is the distress caused unintentionally by clinicians who are interested in cancer recurrence and who trivialize the nonlethal nature of lymphedema. The appearance of arm swelling is more distressing than that of a mastectomy because the latter can be easily hidden, but the disfigured arm or hand is a constant reminder of the disease to the woman herself and a subject of curiosity to others.

The study of the incidence, etiology, and treatment is hampered by the decades-long time course of this complication. Furthermore, lymphedema, along with other quality of life and nonlethal conditions, has not received the attention or the research funding that many other complications of cancer treatment have received. The state of knowledge of lymphedema was reviewed and evaluated at an invited workshop sponsored by the American Cancer Society and the Longaberger Company (Newark, OH) in February 1998 in New York City. Sixty international experts, including the authors, then made recommendations for basic research, clinical practice, public and professional education, and advocacy in the work group reports. The entire proceedings were published as a *Cancer* supplement and are available as a 129-page monograph from the American Cancer Society.[1] This volume concludes with a Lymphedema Resource Guide, listing information on professional organizations addressing lymphedema, lymphedema support groups, online information and groups, suppliers of lymphedema garments and pumps, schools for complex decongestive therapy, and recommended readings.

ANATOMY AND PHYSIOPATHOLOGIC FACTORS

Large molecules that reach the interstitial space by filtration, cellular metabolism, or secretion are removed by the lymphatic system. If large molecules accumulate, as in the case of obstructed transport due to axillary treatment, sufficient effective osmotic pressure develops and results in excessive fluid accumulation in the interstitial space—lymphedema.[2,3] It has been estimated that almost one-half of the total circulating plasma protein is returned daily to the venous system through the lymphatic system by way of the thoracic duct.[4] Lymphatic vessels differ from blood vessels in that the basement membrane is virtually absent. This allows for intercellular diffusion of plasma proteins and lipids that are too large for reabsorption through the walls of the venous capillaries. Normally, lymphatic pressure is zero or negative, but it becomes positive with lymphedema.

The smallest superficial channels, sometimes called *primary* or *initial lymphatics*, are valveless and compose a complex dermal network of capillary-like structures.[5] These drain into secondary lymphatics, larger subdermal channels with valves that run roughly parallel to the superficial veins. The secondary lymphatics drain into a third, deeper layer in the subcutaneous fat just above the fascia. The deeper subcutaneous lymphatics have valves and a muscular layer in the wall for active unidirectional transport.[6] A less elaborate system of lymphatics exists intramuscularly, paralleling the deep arteries and draining the muscle compartment. It is believed that the superficial and deep systems effectively function independently except in abnormal states. Lymphedema is a condition that causes enlargement of the skin and subcutaneous spaces but not the muscular compartment.

PRESENTATION AND PROGRESSION OF LYMPHEDEMA

Lymphedema is the result of a functional overload of the lymphatic system in which lymph volume exceeds transport

J. A. Petrek: Evelyn Lauder Breast Center, Memorial Sloan-Kettering Cancer Center, New York, New York
R. Lerner: Lerner Lymphedema Services, New York, New York

capabilities. The buildup of interstitial macromolecules leads to an increase in oncotic pressure in the tissues, producing more edema. Persistent swelling and stagnant protein eventually lead to fibrosis and provide an excellent culture medium for repeated bouts of cellulitis and lymphangitis. With dilatation of the lymphatics, the valves become incompetent, causing further stasis. The muscle compartments below the deep fascia are spared.

Lymphedema can begin insidiously at variable periods after axillary treatment. The swelling may range from being mild, barely noticeable, in the early stages to a seriously disabling enlargement. A brawny skin appearance develops because of the fibrosclerosis of the skin and subcutaneous tissue. With repeated episodes of cellulitis and lymphangitis, the skin becomes indurated, leathery, and hyperkeratotic.

LYMPHEDEMA ASSESSMENT: PHYSICAL MEASURES AND IMAGING TECHNIQUES

Approximately one-half of patients with documented minimal enlargement (1 to 2 cm) suffer symptoms of "arm heaviness."[7] A simple mail questionnaire found that one-half of the patients who answered said that they had arm swelling but never reported this problem to any doctor.[8] The psychosocial aspects of lymphedema, unforgivably ignored in the past, were reviewed in 1998.[9] Women who have poor social support, pain, lymphedema in the dominant hand, a passive and avoidant coping style, or a combination of these factors, report the highest level of disability.[10]

Three physical measurements of lymphedema are available, including circumferential measurements at various points (with bony landmarks as references), volumetric measurements using limb submersion in water, and skin and soft-tissue tonometry, in which soft-tissue compression is quantified. The physical measurements were reviewed in 1998.[11] The traditional method is the tape-measured arm circumference 10 cm below or 10 cm above either the olecranon or the lateral epicondyle. Such measurements can vary according to the degree of constriction of the soft tissues with the tape. Furthermore, it is wise to measure several circumferences of the lower and upper arm (instead of relying on a single value), because the shape of the arm can differ before and after treatment. Measurement of the arm volume by water displacement is more accurate and results in a single value, but the technique is unwieldy and infrequently used. Furthermore, skin and soft-tissue tonometry has no standardization. Other, more sophisticated, little-used methods include dichromatic differential absorptiometry,[12] computed tomographic scanning,[13] magnetic resonance imaging,[14] and optoelectronic scanning.[15]

No standard degree of enlargement constitutes lymphedema. Although a 2-cm difference between arms is the most common definition, such swelling could be severe in a thin arm and unnoticeable in others. Few people have more than a 2-cm greater circumference in the dominant extremity.[16] Thus, it is important to measure both arms and to do so preoperatively if accurate lymphedema assessment is sought. Although physical measures and imaging techniques provide quantitative assessment of the enlargement, a reliable or standard measure to assess the functional impact of lymphedema does not yet exist.

There has been interest since 1990 in noninvasive and, to some extent, even invasive imaging to diagnose and assess treatment.[17] In particular, lymphoscintigraphy has been used in a preliminary way to predict those at increased risk for lymphedema after axillary treatment,[18,19] with the hope of providing better prevention strategies and more frequent follow-up. Lymphoscintigraphy, dichromatic differential absorptiometry,[12] computed tomographic scanning,[13] and optoelectronic scanning[15] may all become used to direct and evaluate the treatments provided.

INCIDENCE

The reported incidence of lymphedema has varied greatly and depends in part on the methods used to define it, the completeness of the patient population follow-up, and the interval between axillary treatment and measurement. For example, in the first three quarters of the twentieth century, when the Halstedian radical mastectomy and modified radical mastectomy were the only treatments, the incidence of lymphedema in a review by American authors Britton and Nelson[20] ranged between 6.7% and 62.5% among nine reports, and a similar review by British authors Hughes and Patel[21] found a range of 41% to 70% among several reports.

To review the worldwide medical literature for incidence of lymphedema related to breast cancer treatment, a comprehensive computerized search was undertaken by one of us (JAP).[22] Since 1970, 35 reports discussed lymphedema incidence. Of these, seven reports published since 1990 from five countries with the most relevance to current patients were selected and are displayed in Table 1. The incidences will increase over time as lymphedema develops in more and more patients. The reports of Ferrandez et al.[23] and Schunemann and Willich[24] were translated from the French and German, respectively. Because only a few reports state the breast carcinoma treatment of their patient population, it was not possible to include this important variable for all the reports. In Table 1, the majority of patients[25] or all patients[26,27] underwent breast conservation. Nevertheless, by focusing on the latest reports, these seven studies should be most relevant to current patients and their treatments.

All reports on the incidence of lymphedema, including the seven chosen, are retrospective, and the denominator, the number of patients at risk for development of lymphedema in a particular population, is imprecise or unknown. The incidence of the seven selected reports varied from 6%[28] to 30%.[29] The report with the lowest incidence of lymphedema also had the shortest follow-up and included patients who returned to the clinic 12 months after axillary dissection. In this series, the patients were all operated on by the same surgeon.

TABLE 1. *Seven reports published since 1990 on the incidence of lymphedema*

Year	First author/ journal	Country	Type of measurement	Definition	Incidence	Follow-up (F/U)	No. of pts./ source/ treatment yr
1991	Werner[26] *Ther Radiol*	United States	Circumference	≥2.5 cm	19.5%	37 mo[a]	282 Clinic F/U 1980–1989
1992	Ball[28] *Ann R Coll Surg Engl*	England	Circumference Patient report	>3 cm N/A	6% 16%	>12 mo	50 1 surgeon 1982–1990
1992	Ivens[27] *Br J Cancer*	England	Volumetric	>200 mL	10%	2 yr[a]	106 Clinic F/U 1986–1990
1993	Lin[25] *J Clin Oncol*	United States	Circumference	(a) <3 cm (b) 3–4 cm (c) >4 cm	16% 6% 2%	2 yr[a]	283 4 surgeons 1988–1990
1996	Paci[29] *Tumori*	Italy	Circumference	(a) ≤4 cm (b) >4 cm–<8 cm (c) ≥8 cm	8.7% 13.7% 7.9%	5 yr[a]	238 Tumor Registry 1985–1986
1996	Ferrandez[23] *Bull Cancer*	France	Circumference	(a) >3 cm–<10 cm (b) ≥10 cm	14.3% 2.6%	14 mo[a]	683 Clinic F/U 1994
1997	Schunemann[24] *Dtsch Med Wochenschr*	Germany	Circumference	≥2 cm	24%	11 yr[b]	5,868 Clinic F/U 1972–1995

F/U, follow-up; N/A, not available; pts., patients.
[a]Median time F/U.
[b]Total.
From ref. 22, with permission.

ETIOLOGIC FACTORS

Almost all studies [16,27,30–34] have found that the incidence and the degree of lymphedema are correlated with the extent of surgical dissection. In fact, the linear relationship of lymphedema and the extent of dissection can be shown best when the extent of dissection is none, sampling (usually retrieving three to eight lymph nodes), or standard dissection.[31] Two large studies[26,35] could not demonstrate a relationship between extent of dissection and lymphedema; perhaps rather small differences in extent were assessed, for example, adding the highest three to six lymph nodes to a standard dissection.[26] A level I to II or even I-II-III dissection for staging and local control is undertaken for typical cancers with positive lymph nodes, and the scope of the dissection can be fitted to the disease. Preservation of 1 cm of fatty axillary tissue inferior to the vein and all the axillary tissue medial, lateral, and superior to the vein may preserve important lymphatic trunks.

Axillary radiotherapy to the dissected area was a strong predictor of lymphedema in every study that evaluated the issue.[16,31,33,35] Axillary radiotherapy can usually be avoided, even in cases of multiple positive lymph nodes, after a full axillary dissection. Nevertheless, even with only breast-field radiotherapy, some dosage may reach the dissected level I or even II area, depending on radiotherapy technique and patient anatomy. Specific breast radiotherapy techniques with the goal to avoid the dissected axilla and the pathophysiology of radiation-related lymphedema were reviewed in 1998.[36] For precise radiation technique, it is helpful to indicate the extent of the axillary dissection by radiopaque clips so that the surgical boundary is marked. The radiation therapist can then more accurately avoid the dissected area, because it will be seen on the simulation films.

Sentinel lymph node biopsy technology should dramatically decrease the incidence of lymphedema. It is biologically intuitive that excision of one or two sentinel lymph nodes could not result in lymphedema, but this has not yet been reported in the literature. However, the addition of full axillary radiotherapy introduces the risk of lymphedema. It is important to remember that in international series reporting axillary radiotherapy but no axillary surgery, lymphedema incidence ranged from 2% to 5%.[26,27,30,35,36] Therefore, the incidence of lymphedema should be at least that if sentinel lymph node biopsy and axillary radiotherapy are performed. Lymphedema after axillary radiotherapy alone was shown to develop later than that developing after combined axillary surgery and radiotherapy.[27]

Beyond these two factors—extent of surgical dissection and radiation to the axilla—a wide range of possible etiologic factors has not been evaluated systematically. There is little agreement on the several variables that have been studied. Older age at diagnosis was reported to be a significant factor in one study,[32] was unrelated to lymphedema incidence in another,[16] and, curiously, was not noted in others.

A tendency to lymphedema was evident when the dominant hand was on the operated side,[27] but another report[16] could not confirm this. Patient weight (height was not recorded) was a significant factor in two studies,[26,34] but obesity, surprisingly, was not evaluated in other studies. One study of the surgical technique found a higher incidence of lymphedema associated with splitting the pectoralis minor muscle,[30] and two studies correlated lymphedema with greater postoperative fluid formation.[37,38] It is surprising that the incidence of lymphedema after bilateral axillary dissection is not any higher than after unilateral axillary dissection.[22,39]

In sum, etiologic factors for lymphedema have not been well studied. Reasons for the scanty evaluation of lymphedema include (a) the prolonged course for development, (b) lack of contact with the original surgeon or the radiotherapist, and, most important, (c) the fact that lymphedema with other issues concerning quality of life have been viewed as less important for research funding.

PREVENTION OF LYMPHEDEMA AFTER AXILLARY TREATMENT

Because controlling lymphedema requires daily attention and because "curing" lymphedema has not been accomplished, emphasis must be placed on prevention. Nevertheless, without evidence-based knowledge of etiologic lifestyle factors, the list of arm precautions is based on intuitive reasoning. As a background, it is important to remember that each woman has a congenitally different anatomy that is probably prone to degenerative conditions, as is the remainder of the vascular system. (This has been studied thus far in a limited fashion by lymphoscintigraphy.[17–19]) The individual patient factors, combined with axillary treatment factors, must be the main determinants, notwithstanding the fact that lymphedema may occur several years after treatment. Events or activities in subsequent years (and decades) have not been studied enough to state which factors should be avoided.

Arm and hand precautions are loosely based on two overarching principles: (a) Do not increase lymph production, which is directly proportional to blood flow, and (b) do not increase blockage to lymph transport. Heat, such as that in a sauna; significant infections; and vigorous arm exercise increase blood flow in the arm and thereby lymph production. Obstruction of lymph flow may result from tight arm garments or from infections, with ensuing fibrosis and scarring of lymphatic vessels.

To avoid arm swelling or infection, or both, the patient is given the following instructions:

1. Avoid vaccinations, injections, blood pressure monitoring, blood drawing, and intravenous administration in that arm.
2. Avoid puncturing or injuring the skin in any way. Use meticulous skin and nail/cuticle care. Pay immediate attention and use standard first aid care on all small or large injuries. Use topical and systemic antibiotics liberally.
3. Avoid constricting sleeves or jewelry and wear a padded bra strap to avoid constriction.
4. Avoid heat (e.g., sunburns, tanning, baths, sauna).
5. Avoid violent exercises and strenuous exertion. Consider vigorous aerobic arm exercise only when the arm is supported by compression garments.

No data exist to govern any of these recommendations. In the only studies that reported on bilateral axillary dissections, these women had no higher risk of lymphedema over those who had unilateral axillary dissection.[22,39] This calls into question the implication that blood drawing, intravenous administration, blood pressure monitoring, and injections can hasten the development of lymphedema. Data for any of the other arm and hand precautions are even more speculative. Studying the lymphatics of the upper limb after axillary treatment with lymphoscintigraphic techniques is under way and may provide answers about arm and hand precautions.[17] Dynamic as well as static images can be obtained at various levels in the arm and under various standardized conditions (e.g., during and after various periods of rest, during and after exercise).

Research such as this is desperately needed, because all patients are currently instructed in the same arm and hand care precautions, which may be too severe for those at low risk but not aggressive enough for those at the highest risk. Because lymphedema development may occur even several decades[40] after the axillary treatment, patients are admonished to follow these demanding precautions for the remainder of their lives.

TREATMENT

Therapeutic nihilism—that is, no treatment at all—is deplorable although quite common. Too often, a woman is told that she "should be thankful to be alive" and that she "must learn to live with it." The sooner the treatment is started, the less treatment is required to prevent further progression, and the better the ultimate result.

The treatment of established lymphedema has varied from none at all to a host of aggressive surgical procedures. Between the extremes are various combined conservative treatments, the most important of which are elevation, compression garments, centripetal massage and exercises, pneumatic compression devices, and the program known as *CDP*, complete (or complex) decongestive physiotherapy.

Complete Decongestive Physiotherapy

CDP has been widely available in Europe for many years. The program takes into account the fact that lymphedema exists in an entire body quadrant, although it is most distressing in the arm or hand. The program includes skin care; gentle specific massage, known as *manual lymph drainage*;

low-stretch multilayer compression bandaging (followed by a fitted compression garment when edema is reduced); and therapeutic exercises with the garment or bandages in place.

The modification and features of the various CDP programs by Vodder,[41] Leduc et al.,[42] Foldi,[43] and Casley-Smith et al.[44] were reviewed in the 1998 American Cancer Society Workshop on Breast Cancer Treatment–Related Lymphedema. Although the principles followed are the same for each school, the massage techniques vary somewhat in the degree of pressure, motion, and timing of strokes. Additionally, the Leduc technique uses low intermittent pneumatic pressure (less than 40 mm Hg) using mechanical pumps, and the Casley-Smith group uses benzopyrone medication.

The following is the author's program, which is from the Vodder method as modified by the Foldi School. CDP must be done by skilled, specially trained therapists. During phase I (treatment phase), the patient is given one or two daily 75- to 90-minute treatments over 1 to 4 weeks. In phase II (maintenance phase), the patient maintains and optimizes the results by applying some of the techniques learned in the treatment phase, wearing an elastic sleeve during the day, bandaging (as described below) the affected limb overnight, and exercising for 15 minutes a day while wearing the bandages. Phase II is continued indefinitely or until the limb no longer swells.

Each CDP treatment (phase I) consists of four steps:

1. Meticulous skin and nail care, because it can optimize the supple normal skin texture and prevent infections.
2. Manual lymph drainage or manual lymph therapy is a delicate massage technique that stimulates lymph vessels to contract more frequently and that directs and channels lymph and edema fluid toward adjacent, functioning lymph basins. Manual lymph drainage begins with stimulation of the lymph vessels and nodes in unaffected and opposite basins (neck, contralateral axilla, ipsilateral groin). Edema fluid and obstructed lymphatics are made to drain toward functioning lymph basins across the midline of the body, down toward the groin, over the top of the shoulder, around the back, and so forth. Finally, in segmented order, the involved trunk, then shoulder, upper arm, forearm, wrist, and hand should be massaged.
3. Multilayer low-stretch bandaging is done immediately after manual lymph drainage. Bandages are wrapped from the fingertips to the axilla with maximal pressure distally and minimal pressure proximally. This is done by using many layers of minimally elastic cotton bandages, beneath which layers of foam rubber padding are inserted to ensure uniform pressure distribution or to increase pressure in areas that are particularly fibrotic.
4. The bandaged patient is next guided through exercises involving active range of motion with the muscles and joints functioning within the closed space of the bandaging. Isometric exercise is generally avoided.

For the maintenance phase, see Table 2. After volume reduction has been accomplished, ongoing control of edema is continued by well-fitted compressive garments (see next section). These should be measured and fitted only after volume reduction. The patient should be remeasured and the garment replaced every 3 to 6 months. The patient and family will have been trained to continue the maintenance program at home. Follow-up visits to the center usually take place at least at 6-month intervals for measurements and reiteration of any components of the program.

TABLE 2. *Complex decongestive therapy*

Phase I: treatment, 1–4 wk
Meticulous skin and nail care
Manual lymphatic drainage
Low-stretch multilayer bandaging
Physical therapy in bandages
Phase II: maintenance
Meticulous skin and nail care
Low-stretch multilayer bandages worn overnight
Prescribed exercises in bandages
Surgical support garments (30–50 mm Hg)

Although this burgeoning technique appears more successful than other modalities, the availability of patient services and treatment centers that can use CDP is limited. The patient availability[45] and the professional education of therapists[46] were reviewed in 1998. Therapists and physicians are continuously being trained to master CDP techniques at several teaching centers. One of the schools (Lerner Lymphedema Services Academy of Lymphatic Studies) is described in a 1998 study.[47] Results obtained in 2,000 CDP-treated patients are also available.[48]

Elevation and Elastic Garments

The elements and some details of the use are set forth in a 1998 review.[49] Although elevation may be helpful in reducing swelling from lymphedema through use of gravity, it is impractical. A patient with lymphedema should be fitted with an elastic sleeve from wrist to axilla if the edema is mild or when reduction in swelling has occurred. A separate gauntlet or handpiece allows the patient to remove the glove to wash the hands without removing the entire sleeve.

The physician who prescribes the support garment should be aware of the different products available and order the proper compression class. These are as follows:

I. 20 to 30 mm Hg
II. 30 to 40 mm Hg
III. 40 to 50 mm Hg
IV. 50 to 60 mm Hg

For upper extremity lymphedema, a class II or III support is generally required. The person who measures the lymphedematous arm and hand should be trained in fitting such garments and in instructing the patient in proper application.

Often, this task is left to a clerk in a surgical supply store who has no specific training. A statistically significant reduction in edema has been reported in women who wore garments for 6 consecutive hours per day.[50] Using these garments during exercise, physical activity, and air travel is strongly recommended.

Pneumatic Pumps

The older, intermittent, single-chamber, nonsegmented compression pumps provide even pressure throughout the treated arm. However, they also allow some back flow of the lymphatic fluid, which can cause an increase of fluid in the distal arm. Newer devices have multiple chambers and can provide sequential compression. The standard sequential system is a multichamber pump that delivers the compression at the same pressure in each garment section from distal to proximal tissues. The gradient sequential system delivers pressures that differ by approximately 10 mm Hg between each chamber, with the higher pressures delivered to the distal chamber. A minimum of 1 hour per pumping session is required, and lower pressures for longer periods are more effective than higher pressures for a shorter time. The arm should be elevated during pumping.

Individualized and tailored pumping programs for patients cannot be intuited. They require an empiric basis for each woman. Recommendations for use of a particular pump should be based on measurable efficacy and tolerability, as evidenced by serial assessment in that patient. The patient is then educated about the limitations and use of that pump before she is placed on a home program.

The various devices have been reported in several controlled studies[51–55] to reduce lymphedema. Although it is theoretically attractive to use machinery for the pumping action on the arm lymphatics, pumping has not been as clinically effective as would be hoped. Although complex decongestive therapy (see Complete Decongestive Physiotherapy) is quite successful for lymphedema, this treatment requires experienced personnel and an ongoing maintenance program by the patient. It had been hoped that the beneficial effects of CDP could be duplicated by pneumatic compression devices or "pumps."[49] However, the pumps can force protein-rich edema fluid toward the shoulder, an area already congested, but not through the axillary blockage. Lymphedema involves the whole quadrant of the ipsilateral trunk, the area that the obstructed axillary channels would normally drain. In particular, pneumatic compression therapy appears less useful in moderate to advanced lymphedema because of the skin thickening and fibrosis. Rationale and controversies about pumps were reviewed in 1998.[49,56]

Surgical Treatment

Operations to cure lymphedema are cited here mainly for historical interest. Although numerous operations have been proposed to treat chronic lymphedema of the extremity, none has been clinically successful. Surgical approaches can be divided into two categories: physiologic and reductive. Physiologic approaches aim to restore lymphatic flow to the limb either by reconstruction of lymphatic channels or by bridging lymphedematous areas to areas with normal lymphatics, usually by direct microsurgical anastomosis of several lymphatics to veins or by microsurgical bypass procedures. Reductive approaches simply remove excess tissue and edema to reduce the limb to a more functional size. These have included removal of skin and subcutaneous tissue followed by skin grafting (Charles procedure) or staged subcutaneous excision beneath skin flaps (Sistrunk procedure). Since 1990, liposuction was used sporadically, although its efficacy is not known. The state of knowledge for surgical procedures was reviewed in 1998.[49]

Medications

Diuretics are not effective in high-protein edemas such as lymphedema. Although the diuretics can temporarily mobilize water, the osmotic pressure from the increased protein in the interstitial space causes rapid reaccumulation of edema.

Benzopyrones belong to a group of drugs that include the bioflavonoids and the coumarins. The former occur widely in nature, especially in fruits and vegetables. Benzopyrones improve chronic lymphedema[57,58] by stimulating macrophage activity for increased proteolysis and thereby removal of stagnant excess protein in the tissue spaces, resulting in less oncotic pressure and edema fluid. Several European and Australian researchers[59–62] have concluded that 5,6-benzo-[alpha]-pyrone produces a slow reduction of lymphedema and that the drugs should be included in physical rehabilitation programs. The benzopyrones can cause liver toxicity but have no effect on blood coagulation.

In 1993, a randomized, double blind, placebo-controlled crossover trial of 5,6-benzo-[alpha]-pyrone demonstrated its efficacy in an Australian study.[63] Although the effect was mild, it was statistically significant. However, a larger number of study subjects at the Mayo Clinic and elsewhere were reported in 1999 in a study of similar design. No difference was found in results obtained by placebo or by benzopyrone, and liver toxicity developed in 6% of those who received benzopyrone.[64]

MANAGEMENT SUMMARY

- Rehabilitation interventions typically are planned by prescribing physicians in concert with physical and occupational therapists. Other individuals, including nurses and licensed massage therapists, may use these techniques as well if supervised by trained physicians. Therapists should also identify and address pain, limitations in range of motion, and impaired activities of daily living.

- Mild lymphedema (resolves completely overnight):
  1. Counsel: arm and hand precautions, normalize body weight, meticulous arm and hand care.
  2. Elevate; centripetal self-administered massage.
  3. Compression garment, particularly during work, exercise, and air travel.
  4. Intermittent pneumatic pump under guidance of physician.
- Moderate and severe lymphedema:
  1. Referral to a rehabilitation center.
  2. Counsel: arm and hand precautions, normalize body weight, meticulous arm and hand care.
  3. Elevate; centripetal self-administered massage.
  4. Compression garment.
  5. Complete decongestive physiotherapy program.

REFERENCES

1. Petrek JA, Pressman PI, Smith RA. The American Cancer Society lymphedema: results from a workshop on breast cancer treatment-related lymphedema and lymphedema resource guide. *Cancer* 1998;83:2775.
2. Kinmonth JB. *Lymphatics, lymphology and diseases of the chyle and lymph systems*, 2nd ed. London: Edward Arnold, 1982.
3. Mortimer PS. The pathophysiology of lymphedema. *Cancer* 1998;83:2798.
4. Witte MH, Honto D, Witte CL. Clinical and experimental techniques to study the lymphatic system. *Vasc Surg* 1977;11:20.
5. Kubik S, Manestar M. Anatomy of the lymph capillaries and pre-collectors of the skin. In: Bollinger A, Partsch H, Wolfe JN, eds. *The initial lymphatics*. Stuttgart, Germany: Verlag, 1985:66.
6. Koshima I, Kawada S, Moriguchi J, Kajiwara Y. Ultrastructural observations of lymphatic vessels in lymphedema in human extremities. *Plast Reconstr Surg* 1996;97:397.
7. Brennan MJ. Lymphedema following the surgical treatment of breast cancer: a review of pathophysiology and treatment. *J Pain Symptom Manage* 1992;7:110.
8. McCaffrey JF. Lymphedema: its treatment. In: Paterson AHG, Lees AW, eds. *Fundamental problems in breast cancer*. Boston: Martinus Nijhoff Publishing, 1987:259.
9. Passik SD, McDonald MV. Psychosocial aspects of upper extremity lymphedema in women treated for breast carcinoma. *Cancer* 1998;83:2817.
10. Passik SD, Newman M, Brennan M, Tunkel R. Predictors of psychological distress, sexual dysfunction and physical functioning among women with upper extremity lymphedema related to breast cancer. *Psycho-Oncol* 1995;4:255.
11. Gerber LH. A review of measures of lymphedema. *Cancer* 1998;83:2803.
12. Bolin FP, Preuss LE, Beninson J. Di-chromatic differential absorptiometry for assessment of lymphedema. *Int J Nucl Med Biol* 1980;7:449.
13. Stewart G, Hurst PAE, Thomas ML, Burnand KG. CAT scanning in the management of the lymphedematous limb. *Immunol Haematol Res* 1988;2:241.
14. Duwell S, Hagspiel KD, Zuber J, et al. Swollen lower extremity: role of MR imaging. *Radiology* 1992;184:227.
15. Stanton AW, Northfield JW, Holroyd B, Mortimer PS, Levick JR. Validation of an optoelectronic limb volumeter (Perometer). *Lymphology* 1997;30:77.
16. Kissen MW, della Rovere QG, Easton D, et al. Risk of lymphedema following the treatment of breast cancer. *Br J Surg* 1986;7:580.
17. Bourgeois P, Leduc O, Leduc A. Imaging techniques in the upper management and prevention of posttherapeutic upper limb edemas. *Cancer* 1998;83:2805.
18. Carena M, Baiardi P, Saponaro M, et al. Scintigraphic evaluation of predisposition to post-mastectomy lymphedema. In: Lokiec FM, Cluzan RV, Pecking AP, eds. *Progress in lymphology*, 13th ed. Berlin: Springer-Verlag, 1992:325.
19. Pecking AP, Floiras JL, Rouesse J. Upper limb lymphedema's frequency in patients by conservative therapy in breast cancer. *Lymphology* 1996;29[Suppl]:293.
20. Britton RC, Nelson PA. Causes and treatment of post-mastectomy lymphedema of the arm: report of 114 cases. *JAMA* 1962;180:95.
21. Hughes JH, Patel AR. Swelling of the arm following radical mastectomy. *Br J Surg* 1966;53:4.
22. Petrek JA, Heelan MC. Incidence of breast carcinoma-related lymphedema. *Cancer* 1998;83:2776.
23. Ferrandez JC, Serin D, Bouges S. Frequence des lymphoedemes du membre superieur apres traitement du cancer du sein: facteurs de risque: a propos de 683 observations. *Bull Cancer (Paris)*1996;83:989.
24. Schunemann H, Willich N. Lymphodeme nach Mammakarzinom: eine Studie über 5868 Falle. *Dtsch Med Wochenschr* 1997;122:536.
25. Lin PP, Allison DC, Wainstock J, et al. Impact of axillary lymph node dissection on the therapy of breast cancer patients. *J Clin Oncol* 1993;11:1536.
26. Werner RS, McCormick B, Petrek JA, et al. Arm edema in conservatively managed breast cancer: obesity is a major predictive factor. *Ther Radiol* 1991;180:177.
27. Ivens D, Hoe AL, Podd CR, et al. Assessment of morbidity from complete axillary dissection. *Br J Cancer* 1992;66:136.
28. Ball ABS, Fish S, Waters R, Meirion Thomas J. Radical axillary dissection in the staging and treatment of breast cancer. *Ann R Coll Surg Engl* 1992;74:126.
29. Paci E, Cariddi A, Barchielli A, et al. Long-term sequelae of breast cancer surgery. *Tumori* 1996;82:321.
30. Pezner RD, Patterson MP, Hill LR, et al. Arm lymphedema in patients treated conservatively for breast cancer: relationship to patient age and axillary node dissection technique. *Int J Radiat Oncol Biol Phys* 1986;12:2079.
31. Yeoh EK, Denham JW, Davies SA, Spittle MF. Primary breast cancer. *Acta Radiol Oncol* 1986;25:105.
32. Delouche G, Bachelot F, Premont M, et al. Conservation treatment of early breast cancer: long term results and complications. *Int J Radiat Oncol Biol Phys* 1987;13:29.
33. Aitken RJ, Gaze MN, Rodger A, et al. Arm morbidity within a trial of mastectomy and either nodal sample with selective radiotherapy or axillary clearance. *Br J Surg* 1989;76:568.
34. Larson D, Weinstein M, Goldberg I, et al. Edema of the arm as a function of the extent of axillary surgery in patients with stage I-II carcinoma of the breast treated with primary radiotherapy. *Int J Radiat Oncol Biol Phys* 1986;12:1575.
35. Dewar JA, Sarrazin D, Benhamou E, et al. Management of the axilla in conservatively treated breast cancer: 592 patients treated at Institut Gustave-Roussy. *Int J Radiat Oncol Biol Phys* 1987;13:475.
36. Meek AG. Breast radiotherapy and lymphedema. *Cancer* 1998;83:2788.
37. Tadych K, Donegan WL. Postmastectomy seromas and wound drainage. *Surg Gynecol Obstet* 1987;165:483.
38. West JP, Ellison JB. A study of the causes and prevention of edema of the arm following radical mastectomy. *Surg Gynecol Obstet* 1959;109:359.
39. Mortimer PS, Bates SO, Brassington HD, Stanton AWB, Strachan DP, Levick JR. The prevalence of arm lymphedema following treatment for breast cancer. *QJM* 1996;89:377.
40. Brennan MJ, Weitz J. Lymphedema 30 years after radical mastectomy. *Am J Phys Med Rehabil* 1992;71:12.
41. Kasseroller RG. The Vodder school: the Vodder method. *Cancer* 1998;83:2840.
42. Leduc O, Leduc A, Bourgeois P, Belgrado JP. The physical treatment of upper limb edema. *Cancer* 1998;83:2835.
43. Foldi E. The treatment of lymphedema. *Cancer* 1998;83:2833.
44. Casley-Smith JR, Boris M, Weindorf S, Lasinski B. Treatment for lymphedema of the arm—the Casley-Smith method: a noninvasive method produces continued reduction. *Cancer* 1998;83:2843.
45. Thiadens SRJ. Current status of education and treatment resources for lymphedema. *Cancer* 1998;83:2864.
46. Augustine E, Corn M, Danoff J. Lymphedema management training for physical therapy students in the United States. *Cancer* 1998;83:2869.
47. Lerner R. Complete decongestive physiotherapy and the Lerner Lymphedema Services Academy of Lymphatic Studies (the Lerner School). *Cancer* 1998;83:2861.

48. Lerner R. What's new in lymphedema therapy in America? *Int J Angiology* 1998;7:191.
49. Brennan MJ, Miller LT. Overview of treatment options and review of the current role and use of compression garments, intermittent pumps, and exercise in the management of lymphedema. *Cancer* 1998;83:2821.
50. Bertelli G, Venturini M, Forno G, Macchiavello F, Dini D. An analysis of prognostic factors in response to conservative treatment of postmastectomy lymphedema. *Surg Gynecol Obstet* 1992;175:455.
51. Klein MJ, Alexander MA, Wright JM, Redmond CK, LaGasse AA. Treatment of adult lower extremity lymphedema with the Wright Linear pump: statistical analysis of a clinical trial. *Arch Phys Med Rehabil* 1988;69:202.
52. Kim-Sing C, Basco VE. Postmastectomy lymphedema treated with the Wright linear pump. *Can J Surg* 1987;5:368.
53. Pappas CJ, O'Donnell TF Jr. Long-term results of compression treatment for lymphedema. *J Vasc Surg* 1992;16:555.
54. Richmand DM, O'Donnell TF Jr, Zelikovski A. Sequential pneumatic compression for lymphedema: a controlled trial. *Arch Surg* 1985; 120:1116.
55. Zanolla R, Monzeglio C, Balzarini A, Martino G. Evaluation of the results of three different methods of postmastectomy lymphedema treatment. *J Surg Oncol* 1984;26:210.
56. Rinehart-Ayres ME. Conservative approaches to lymphedema treatment. *Cancer* 1998;83:2828.
57. Piller NB, Clodius L. The role of the mononuclear phagocytic system in lymphedema and its relationship with histopathological changes in the functioning of the blood-tissue-lymph system. *Z Lymphol* 1980; 4:35.
58. Casley-Smith JR, Gaffney RM. Excess plasma proteins as a cause of chronic inflammation and lymphedema. *J Pathol* 1981;133:243.
59. Cluzan R, Pecking A. Benzopyrone (Lysedem) double blind crossing over study in patients with secondary upper limb edemas. In: Nishi M, Uchino S, Yabuke S, eds. *Progress in lymphology*, 12th ed. Excerpta Medica International Congress Series 887. Amsterdam: Elsevier, 1990:453.
60. Pecking AP, Fevrier B, Wargon C, Pillion G. Efficacy of Daflon 500 mg in the treatment of lymphedema. *Angiology* 1997;48:1.
61. Casley-Smith JR. There are many Benzo-pyrones for lymphedema. *Lymphology* 1997;30:1.
62. Taylor HM, Rose KE, Twycross RG. A double-blind clinical trial of hydroxyethylrutosides in obstructive arm lymphedema. *Phlebologie* 1993;22[Suppl 1]:190.
63. Casley-Smith JR, Morgan RG, Piller NB. Treatment of lymphedema of the arms and legs with 5,6-benzo-[alpha]-pyrone. *N Engl J Med* 1993;16:329.
64. Loprinzi CL, Kugler JW, Sloan JA, et al. Lack of effect of coumarin in women with lymphedema after treatment for breast cancer. *N Engl J Med* 1999;340:346.

Diseases of the Breast, 2nd ed.,
edited by Jay R. Harris.
Lippincott Williams & Wilkins, Philadelphia

CHAPTER 70

Managing Menopausal Problems

Melody A. Cobleigh

Breast cancer survivors often seek advice about menopausal problems from their oncologists. In addition, oncologists interact with colleagues about their patients' menopausal issues. For these reasons, it is important for oncologists to be knowledgeable about the effects of hormone replacement therapy (HRT) on overall health. The need for up-to-the-minute information is intensified by the plethora of new drugs, the greater frequency with which pharmaceutical companies market directly to the public, and the increasing interest of patients in alternative therapies.

GENERAL CONSIDERATIONS

Changes in Metabolism

One of the most important lessons we can teach our menopausal patients (whether menopause is naturally or chemotherapeutically induced) is that, unless they eat less or exercise more, they will gain weight. Women lose fat-free mass after menopause. They also tend to exercise less during leisure time and experience greater increases in fat mass, fasting insulin levels, and waist-hip ratio. Breast cancer survivors often blame the changing shapes of their bodies on tamoxifen, although double-blind, randomized trials show no difference in weight for placebo- versus tamoxifen-treated patients.[1]

Simply put, postmenopausal women burn fewer calories at rest than premenopausal women, suggesting that estrogen helps to control weight.[2] The suggestion is supported by the postmenopausal estrogen-progesterone intervention trial. In this double-blind, randomized study, women who received a placebo gained significantly more weight than those treated with estrogen.[3] Evidence that weight gain is a significant health concern for breast cancer survivors comes from the Nurses' Health Study, which found that weight gain after menopause increases breast cancer incidence and mortality among women who do not take HRT.[4]

M. A. Cobleigh: Section of Medical Oncology, Rush Presbyterian St. Luke's Medical Center, Chicago, Illinois

Vasomotor Instability

The most common reason that Western women seek hormone intervention at menopause is vasomotor symptoms. As many as 85% experience perimenopausal hot flashes and night sweats, and HRT reduces the number of hot flashes by 80% after 1 month of treatment.[5] Women who undergo premature menopause as a consequence of chemotherapy are more symptomatic from vasomotor instability than their naturally menopausal counterparts, and they are likely to seek medical intervention to alleviate their discomfort. Among breast cancer survivors who had heard or read about HRT, 51% had talked to their doctor about it after their diagnosis.[6] Thirty-one percent were willing to take HRT under medical supervision.

In Southeast Asia, vasomotor symptoms are less frequent (20% to 40%).[7] One reason for the difference may be the difficulty in recognizing symptoms of thermoregulatory imbalance in a warm climate; however, another important explanation may be that Asian diets, which are often rich in phytoestrogens, ameliorate hot flashes.

Nonhormonal remedies for hot flashes include clonidine, which decreases the frequency and severity of hot flashes (Table 1).[8–13] Although statistically significant, the clinical benefit is modest and may be achieved at the expense of constipation, dry mouth, and drowsiness. Another alpha$_2$-adrenoceptor agonist, methyldopa, reduces the frequency of hot flashes significantly but can also be associated with unpleasant side effects (tiredness and dry mouth). Bellergal-S is effective. Plain Bellergal works in the short run but is ineffective after 8 weeks. Vitamin E and dong quai (*Angelica polymorpha*, a plant of the carrot family) are ineffective. In an open-label study, venlafaxine reduced symptoms in 58% of women.[14] A double-blind, placebo-controlled randomized trial is under way.

Progestational Agents for Relief of Hot Flashes

Progestational agents are more effective than placebo in relieving hot flashes[15–19] (Table 2). Physicians seem more comfortable prescribing progestogens than estrogens to

TABLE 1. *Nonhormonal alternatives to hormone replacement therapy for relief of hot flashes*

Authors	Number	Medication	Reduction in hot flashes (%)	
			Treatment	Placebo
Nesheim and Saetre[8]	40	Methyldopa, 250 mg, 1 b.i.d.; increase to 2 b.i.d. if no success	65[a] (45–75)	38 (0–59)
Bergmans et al.[9]	66	Bellergal Retard, 1 b.i.d.	75	68
Lebherz and French[10]	72	Bellergal-S, 1 b.i.d.	60[a]	22
Goldberg et al.[11]	110	Clonidine patch, 0.1 mg/day	44[a]	27
Barton et al.[12]	125	Vitamin E, 400 IU b.i.d.	25	22
Hirata et al.[13]	71	Dong quai, 4.5 g/day	33	29

[a]Significantly better than placebo.

relieve vasomotor symptoms in breast cancer survivors. However, the effect of progesterone on normal and malignant breast cells is unknown. In striking contrast to the endometrium, in which progesterone is associated with reduced proliferation, mitotic activity in breast epithelium peaks during days 23 to 25 of the menstrual cycle. This is shortly after the progesterone peak and the second estradiol peak, suggesting that progesterone, or possibly the combination of estrogen and progesterone, is responsible.[20–22] Progestins have been implicated in the development of breast cancer in humans[23] as well as in experimental animals[24–26] and laboratory cell cultures.[27–29]

Interactions between progestational agents and tamoxifen have not been studied in breast cancer survivors. Clinically, the combination of progestins and tamoxifen is less effective than tamoxifen alone in metastatic breast cancer.[30] Further concerns are raised by the finding that progesterone, given for only 1 week a month, reverses the protective effect of tamoxifen in a rat mammary carcinoma model.[31]

Selective Estrogen Receptor Modulators and Hot Flashes

Raloxifene does not alleviate and may exacerbate hot flashes. In a randomized controlled trial, the incidence of hot flashes was 23% in the placebo group and 26% in the group that received 60 mg raloxifene.[32] Women with "serious" postmenopausal symptoms were excluded from the trial. Leg cramps occurred more commonly among women treated with raloxifene (2.6%) than among those who received placebo (0.7%). Tamoxifen significantly increases the incidence of hot flashes.[33]

Hormone Replacement Therapy and Tamoxifen

Breast cancer survivors who experience severe menopausal symptoms are offered HRT and tamoxifen at the Royal Marsden Hospital.[34] Tamoxifen and HRT appeared to interact favorably in a small subset of participants in the British breast cancer prevention trial.[35] The combination caused a reduction in serum cholesterol, an increase in bone mineral density, and no adverse change in coagulation factors. Participants in the Italian breast cancer prevention trial were allowed to continue HRT along with placebo or tamoxifen. Italian researchers found a statistically significant reduction in breast cancer among those who received HRT plus tamoxifen compared with those who received HRT plus placebo.[36] Neither the British nor the Italian group has studied whether HRT relieves hot flashes in women who are taking tamoxifen. This is the primary objective of the Eastern Cooperative Oncology Group HRT/tamoxifen trial.

TABLE 2. *Placebo-controlled randomized trials of progestational agents for relief of vasomotor symptoms*

Authors	Number	Medication	Reduction in hot flashes (%)	
			Treatment	Placebo
Loprinzi et al.[15]	80	MA	73	26
Morrison et al.[16]	34	MPA	68	20
Albrecht et al.[17]	6	MPA	87	25
Schiff et al.[18]	32	MPA	74	26
Bullock et al.[19]	57	MPA	90	25
	12 placebo	MPA		

MA, megestrol acetate; MPA, medroxyprogesterone acetate.

Maintaining Bone Health

Bone mineral density decreases rapidly during the first 5 years after natural menopause. Osteoporotic fractures are an important cause of morbidity in old age and affect 50% of women older than age 50.[37] Breast cancer survivors are at particular risk because of chemotherapy-induced premature menopause. A prospective study of women who experienced chemical castration from adjuvant chemotherapy showed that bone loss was 9.5% at the lumbar spine and 4.6% at the femoral neck after just 2 years.[38] Thus, it is important to maintain the bone health of postmenopausal women, and several strategies are needed.

Diet and Exercise

Postmenopausal women need 1,500 mg calcium daily. A serving of dairy products, such as a glass of milk or a portion of yogurt, contains 200 mg calcium, and therefore supplements are often necessary. Calcium citrate is better absorbed than calcium carbonate. Vitamin D (800 units per day) is also important, particularly for individuals who are deprived of sunlight. This simple dietary intervention has resulted in reductions of 30% to 70% in fracture rates over 2 to 4 years.[39]

Weight-bearing exercise, such as walking, jogging, or aerobics, should be performed for at least 30 minutes three times a week.

Assessment

A woman's height should be measured not only to enable the physician to accurately calculate body surface area for treatment purposes, but also as a baseline for yearly follow-up of skeletal health. It is not sufficient to ask the patient how tall she is, because she may be unaware that she has already lost height from osteoporosis. A baseline bone mineral density, repeated every 2 years, will show osteopenia before irreparable damage has occurred.

Medication for Prevention of Osteoporosis

HRT has been shown to prevent osteoporosis in a randomized, placebo-controlled trial.[40] Participants assigned to placebo lost an average of 1.8% and 1.7%, respectively, of spine and hip bone mineral density after 3 years. Those assigned to active treatment gained bone mineral density, ranging from 3.5% to 5.0% at the spine and averaging 1.7% at the hip.

Tamoxifen significantly reduces bone loss in postmenopausal breast cancer survivors.[41] A randomized, controlled trial showed that raloxifene protected bone density significantly more than placebo over a 2-year period.[42] (Information on fracture prevention is not yet available.) Participants were postmenopausal and did not have osteoporosis. Breast cancer survivors were excluded, as were women with "serious" postmenopausal symptoms or abnormal uterine bleeding. Although the Food and Drug Administration (FDA) has approved raloxifene (60 mg per day) for prevention of osteoporosis, the drug has not been adequately studied in women with a history of breast cancer.

A randomized, placebo-controlled trial showed that alendronate protected bone significantly more than placebo over a 3-year period.[43] Participants were postmenopausal and did not have osteoporosis and women with major upper gastrointestinal diseases were excluded. Another randomized trial showed that alendronate with HRT was more effective than alendronate alone.[44] The FDA has approved alendronate (5 mg per day) for prevention of osteoporosis.

Medication for Treating Osteoporosis

The reduction in the rate of osteoporotic fracture in HRT users ranges between 30% and 60%.[45,46] A randomized, placebo-controlled trial showed that alendronate progressively increased bone mass in the spine, hip, and total body while reducing the incidence of vertebral fractures and height loss in postmenopausal women with osteoporosis.[47] The FDA has approved alendronate (10 mg per day) for treatment of osteoporosis. A 19% reduction in fractures at the hip, spine, and lower radius almost reached statistical significance at a mean of 4 years of treatment in a tamoxifen breast cancer prevention trial.[33]

Cardiovascular Health

Unless women understand that they are vulnerable to coronary artery disease (CAD), they will be unwilling to make the personal changes necessary to prevent cardiovascular illness. The most important health-related behaviors are to avoid smoking, eat a healthy diet, and exercise moderately to help control weight.

Diet and Dietary Supplements

A balanced diet that is low in saturated fat helps control blood lipid levels. Observational studies suggest that consumption of 400 to 800 units of vitamin E daily exerts a protective effect against CAD.[48]

The relationship between homocysteinuria and premature vascular occlusive disease was discovered in patients with a rare inborn error of metabolism. The discovery led to the hypothesis that elevated blood homocysteine levels may be a risk factor for CAD. Dietary supplementation with folate alone or folate plus vitamins B_6 and B_{12} reduces homocysteine levels.

Epidemiologic information suggests that supplemental intake of folate and vitamin B_6 above the current recommended dietary allowance is important for primary prevention of CAD among women. The adjusted odds ratio for CAD among women who consume a daily multiple vitamin is 0.76.[49] Supplementation is especially important among women who regularly consume alcoholic beverages. In this group, the adjusted odds ratio for CAD among those who take a multiple vitamin supplement daily is 0.22.

Premature Menopause

CAD is an insidious and potentially fatal consequence of menopausal estrogen decline. Because the treatment of breast cancer in young women can precipitate premature menopause, its ovarian toxicity is a matter of serious concern. Even though adjuvant chemotherapy causes premature ovarian failure,[50] it is prescribed more often than it used to be, based on favorable outcomes for women with small invasive but node-negative disease.[51–53] However, review of the role of premature menopause in CAD found an increased risk in women with early menopause.[54] Evidence that HRT can reduce this effect of early menopause comes from the Nurses' Health Study, in which women who underwent surgical menopause and received HRT had a significantly lower risk of cardiovascular disease than those with surgical menopause who did not receive HRT.[55]

Most node-negative women are cured of breast cancer, and death from nonneoplastic conditions is common. Moreover, cardiovascular disease is the most common cause of noncancer deaths even in patients who did not receive chemotherapy and thus did not undergo premature menopause.[56] As more node-negative women receive adjuvant chemotherapy, we must acknowledge the possibility that early chemotherapy-mediated gains in survival from breast cancer may be overshadowed by later increases in mortality from cardiovascular and osteoporotic events. That is, women may survive their breast cancers only to succumb to more common, but delayable, afflictions. The latest meta-analysis does not yet suggest, with 15 years of follow-up, that there is an increase in non–breast cancer mortality in women who have received chemotherapy.[57] However, node-positive women represent the overwhelming majority in the study, and breast cancer mortality may obscure such an analysis.

The National Surgical Adjuvant Breast and Bowel Project B-20 trial showed that chemotherapy regimens that do not cause ovarian failure are useful as adjuvant therapy.[58] Premenopausal, node-negative, estrogen receptor–positive patients benefited significantly from tamoxifen plus methotrexate, 5-fluorouracil, and leucovorin, a regimen that does not cause premature ovarian failure.[50] This regimen compared favorably with tamoxifen plus cyclophosphamide, methotrexate, and 5-fluorouracil, a chemotherapy regimen known for significant ovarian toxicity.[50]

Aspirin

Aspirin is an option for prevention in postmenopausal women at high risk for cardiovascular disease. High-risk subjects include those with acute or prior myocardial infarction, a history of stroke or transient ischemic attack, unstable or stable angina, vascular surgery, angioplasty, atrial fibrillation, valvular heart disease, or peripheral vascular disease. Treatment with 75 to 325 mg per day offered significant protection against myocardial infarction, stroke, and death in a meta-analysis of randomized trials.[59]

Statins

Drug therapy for hypercholesterolemia, particularly for women, has remained controversial because of insufficient clinical evidence that treatment enhances survival; however, some reports showed important benefits. In the Scandinavian simvastatin study, women randomly assigned to simvastatin had an absolute 35% reduction in major coronary events compared with placebo-treated women.[60] Another placebo-controlled trial in healthy middle-aged women with average cholesterol (C) and low-density lipoprotein-C and with below-average high-density lipoprotein-C levels showed that lovastatin offered significant benefit in primary prevention of acute coronary events.[61]

Estrogen and Selective Estrogen Receptor Modulators

HRT reduces CAD significantly. Women who undergo natural menopause and take HRT experience a 30% to 70% reduction in heart attack.[45,62,63] A randomized trial showed that 60 mg raloxifene favorably altered biochemical markers of cardiovascular risk. It reduced low-density lipoprotein, fibrinogen, and lipoprotein (a) significantly more than placebo over a 6-month period in healthy postmenopausal women.[64] Information on prevention of myocardial infarction is not yet available. Breast cancer survivors were excluded from the trial, as were women with serious postmenopausal symptoms or abnormal uterine bleeding. Although HRT had no effect on fibrinogen and raised triglycerides significantly, it proved superior to raloxifene in raising high-density lipoprotein and in lowering lipoprotein (a) and PAI-1.

The effects of selective estrogen receptor modulators (SERMs) on lipid profiles are remarkably similar (Table 3). It is therefore notable that no decrease in cardiovascular events has been observed in the Oxford overview analysis of

TABLE 3. *Effects of selective estrogen receptor modulators on blood lipids*

	Good change	HRT[65]	Tamoxifen[65]	Raloxifene[64]	Toremifene[65]	Soy phytoestrogens[66]
LDL-C	↓	↓	↓	↓	↓	↓
HDL-C	↑	↑	↔	↔	↑	↑
Triglycerides	↓	↑	↑	↔	↔	↓
Lp(a)	↓	↓	↓	↓	↓	
Apo A-I	↑	↑	↔	↔	↑	↑
Apo B	↓		↓	↓	↓	
PAI-1	↓	↓		↔		
Fibrinogen	↓	↔	↔[67]	↓		

HDL, high-density lipoprotein; HRT, hormone replacement therapy; LDL, low-density lipoprotein; Lp, lipoprotein; ↑, increase; ↓, decrease; ↔, no change.

adjuvant tamoxifen trials.[67] This is not surprising, because the beneficial effect on atherogenesis attributable to alteration of lipoproteins in primates accounts for only approximately one-third of the overall benefit seen with HRT.[68]

Soybean Phytoestrogens

Soybean phytoestrogens have the same beneficial effects as conjugated equine estrogen (CEE) on plasma lipid and lipoprotein concentrations in postmenopausal primates, except for their effect on triglycerides and apo A-1, which is more favorable.[69] In addition to their lipid-altering effects, soy phytoestrogens, like estrogen, mediate favorable effects on coronary arteries directly. They cause vasodilatation and reduce uptake of lipid in the intima of the coronary artery.[69] No randomized study of soybean phytoestrogens has yet evaluated the rate of myocardial infarction.

Alzheimer's Disease

A 1998 meta-analysis of case-controlled and cohort studies found a 29% reduction in risk of dementia among estrogen users.[70] However, the findings of the studies were heterogeneous, and the authors advised awaiting results of the Women's Health Initiative before prescribing HRT for this indication.

Conspicuously missing in discussions about SERMs is whether they are agonists or antagonists for the brain. Long-term studies of cognitive function in women who are treated chronically with these agents will be important in understanding this potential interaction. Meanwhile, the increase in hot flashes, a central nervous system–mediated effect that is associated with some SERMs, is cause for concern.

Endometrium and Vagina

Neither soybean phytoestrogens nor raloxifene is uterotrophic.[71] Tamoxifen stimulates the endometrium, and women who take it for 5 years have a 1% incidence of endometrial carcinoma. These cancers are stage I and curable by hysterectomy when women are carefully followed by their gynecologists.[33]

Vaginal symptoms are common among breast cancer survivors. Estrogen relieves these symptoms and has been approved by the FDA for treatment of atrophic vaginitis but not for women with a history of breast cancer. Some physicians are more willing to prescribe vaginal estrogen-containing creams than oral estrogens, not realizing that vaginal administration according to the dose recommendation of the package insert raises serum estrogen levels 16- to 20-fold higher than oral administration of the same dose.[72–74]

A 1994 study evaluated low-dose conjugated estrogens (0.3 mg three times a week for 6 months). It revealed satisfactory relief of symptoms in 95% of cases. The vaginal maturation index improved significantly, and no changes in serum estrogen levels occurred. Endometrial biopsies revealed proliferation in only one case.[75]

An estradiol-releasing vaginal ring produced impressive relief of urogenital atrophy in 222 women.[76] The total dose of estradiol during a 12-week period was 0.8 mg. There was no significant change in plasma sex hormone–binding globulin or estradiol. Estrone levels increased by approximately 300 pmol per L to approximately 900 pmol per L but remained below the postmenopausal range (<1,400 pmol/L). Endometrial thickness was not increased after 6 months of treatment in a subset of 30 women who were studied.

A prospective, randomized, open-label trial compared a nonhormonal, local, bioadhesive vaginal moisturizer (Replens) with vaginal estrogen cream (Premarin).[77] Replens improved vaginal health, although to a lesser extent than did Premarin cream. Replens improved vaginal moisture, fluid volume, elasticity, and pH despite a lack of cornification. Because the study did not include quality of life measures, it provides no evidence of how changes in the vagina correlated with symptom relief. If Replens is prescribed, it should be used three times a week for at least a month.

Replens has also been compared with a lubricating (hydroxymethylcellulose, glycerine-delta lactone, hydrogenated palm oil glyceride, and water) product.[78] Both products lessened vaginal dryness and dyspareunia. Dong quai was ineffective in a randomized double-blind trial.[13]

Coagulation

Raloxifene, according to the package insert, is contraindicated in women with active venous thromboembolic events or a history of such events, including deep vein thrombosis, pulmonary embolism, or retinal vein thrombosis. Tamoxifen also causes thrombophlebitis in approximately 1% of women who take it for 5 years. This complication is largely limited to postmenopausal women.[33]

Colon Cancer

Two prospective cohort studies showed that HRT reduced the incidence of colon cancer.[79,80] A third prospective study proved that fewer colon adenomas occurred in HRT users.[81] Of note is that colon cancer is a common second primary malignancy among node-negative breast cancer survivors.[56] Long-term follow-up of adjuvant tamoxifen studies has shown no increase in colon cancer.[67]

Breast Tissue

The best information about the effect of HRT on normal breast tissue comes from a longitudinal evaluation of surgically postmenopausal cynomolgus macaques.[82] These animals share 98% of their DNA with *Homo sapiens*, and

TABLE 4. *Meta-analyses of breast cancer incidence among hormone replacement therapy users versus nonusers*

Authors	Relative risk (RR) any use	95% Confidence interval (CI)	RR longer vs shorter	95% CI
DuPont and Page[88]	1.07	1.00–1.15	Can't conclude	
Steinberg et al.[89]	1.0		1.3 after 15 yr	1.2–1.6
Armstrong[90]	1.01	0.95–1.08	No effect	
Grady and Ernster[91]	No increase		1.25	
Sillero-Arenas et al.[92]	1.06	1.00–1.12		
Colditz et al.[93]	1.02	0.93–1.12		

females are similar to women in their reproductive physiologic and anatomic features.

CEE has a mammotropic effect on the mammary glands of macaques, resulting in greater thickness and epithelial hyperplasia. Combined continuous HRT has a greater effect than CEE alone. Combined HRT also causes down-regulation of estrogen and progesterone receptors. CEE and combined continuous HRT cause increased proliferative activity as measured by Ki67 staining.

Interpretation of Mammograms

Concern has been raised about whether HRT increases breast density, thereby delaying the diagnosis of breast cancer. A prospective blinded trial showed an upward shift in mammographic density for 24% of patients, a downward shift in 12%, and no change in 63%. Baseline density was significantly correlated with risk of mammographic degradation. That is, women who had the least dense breast tissue on mammograms were most likely to experience a change that made their mammograms more difficult to interpret.[83] Women who experienced an upward shift in mammographic density on HRT were also likely to have breast pain.[84]

A nested case-control study of mammograms performed on 1,104 women, with radiologists blinded to the treatment regimen, showed that change was related to type of HRT. Women who consumed no HRT, estrogen alone, cyclic estrogen plus progesterone, and continuous combined estrogen plus progesterone showed a 3.1%, 4.7%, 9.6%, and 27.5% incidence of mammographic degradation, respectively.[85] The majority of these changes were considered "slight." Corresponding mammographic improvements occurred in 9.6%, 12.5%, 12.6%, and 3.9%, respectively.

Hormone Replacement Therapy and Second Breast Cancers

Concern over HRT-induced new breast cancers must be addressed in any trial of replacement therapy for breast cancer survivors, especially because a personal history of breast cancer is a strong risk factor for subsequent development of primary breast cancer.[86] The annual incidence of new primary breast cancers among breast cancer survivors is 14 per 1,000, compared with 2 per 1,000 in the general population.[87] The association between HRT and risk of breast cancer remains controversial, although more than 50 studies and six meta-analyses have been published since 1980[88–93] (Table 4).

Collectively, the studies do not show a consistently increased risk of breast cancer among women who have ever used HRT. Studies that controlled for screening showed no difference in relative risk between cases and control subjects.[94] This suggests that a detection bias may be operating in some studies that report an increased risk of breast cancer among HRT users. Importantly, low-dose CEE (0.625 mg per day) for several years did not appreciably increase the risk of breast cancer.

Although having ever used HRT does not appear to substantially increase the risk of breast cancer, a concern remains that selected subgroups will be adversely affected. For example, some studies have suggested that long-term use (10 to 15 years or more) increases the risk of breast cancer. Although the results are based on small numbers of cases (because relatively few women have used HRT for 15 or more years), the findings are of concern.

A possible confounding factor in these studies is the finding that consumption of alcohol while using HRT increases absorption of estrogen significantly (threefold).[95] Thus, it will be important to control for alcohol consumption in future analyses.

Although the preponderance of evidence shows that short-term use (fewer than 10 years) of HRT does not appear to cause breast cancer in healthy women, it is possible that women with a personal history of breast cancer may be more susceptible to tumor-promoting effects of estrogen. Tamoxifen reduces the risk of contralateral breast cancers in women with a history of breast cancer,[96] and it reduces the incidence of invasive breast cancer during short-term follow-up of high-risk women.[33] Thus, it is possible that tamoxifen administered with HRT may attenuate any potential cancer-promoting effect of estrogen on breast cells. Interestingly, the prognosis of women with breast cancer who received HRT before diagnosis is better than that of women with no recorded exposure[97–104] (Table 5).

These findings of apparently protective effects may arise from confounding factors, including the possibility that HRT may promote development of estrogen-dependent breast cancers that wither on estrogen withdrawal. Another hypothesis is that HRT may stimulate growth of existing cancers, bring-

TABLE 5. *Relative risk of mortality from breast cancer among hormone replacement therapy users compared with those who have never used hormone replacement therapy in cohort studies*

Authors	No. of breast cancers	Relative risk	95% Confidence interval	*p* value
Persson et al.[97]	634	0.5	0.4–0.6	
Gambrell[98]	256	0.53		<.007
Hunt et al.[99]	50	0.55	0.28–0.96	
Henderson et al.[100]	Not stated	0.81		>.05
Criqui et al.[101]	42	0.73[a]	0.44–1.22	
Ewertz et al.[102]	1,684	1.07	0.88–1.30	
Willis et al.[103]	1,469[b]	0.84[c]	0.75–0.94	
Colditz et al.[104]	1,935	1.14[d]	0.85–1.51	
		0.8[e]	0.60–1.07	

[a]Cancer mortality.
[b]Breast cancer deaths.
[c]All cause mortality.
[d]Current users.
[e]Prior users.

ing them to light sooner. Nevertheless, the data are coherent in that they suggest that women who have used HRT and who develop breast cancer are not at increased risk of dying from breast cancer. Indeed, they may have a better prognosis than women who have never used HRT.

Reactivation of Dormant Tumor Cells

The overriding concern among breast cancer survivors considering HRT is that it might hasten their demise. Although limited, there are reports of stimulation of breast cancer in women given hormones.[105–109] A significant increase has been reported in tritiated thymidine incorporation in skin metastasis among women treated with "physiologic doses" of intramuscular estradiol and progesterone.[105]

Fabian et al.[106] used suppositories to obtain elevated serum levels of estradiol in women with stage IIIB breast cancer. Biopsies before and after HRT revealed that estrogen receptor–positive breast cancers had a significant increase in S-phase fraction and proliferative index.

HRT withdrawal resulted in regression of metastatic breast cancer in four women.[107] Two cases of primary tumor regression after discontinuation of HRT have been described.[108,109] Alternate interpretations of these results have been presented.[110]

CONCLUSIONS

Ultimately, the question of how HRT affects mortality from all causes among breast cancer survivors can only be answered by a prospective, randomized trial that requires thousands of women. Many questions exist, and it is premature to mount such a trial without pilot data. Will oncologists accept such trials? Will breast cancer survivors participate in randomized trials of HRT? What are the baseline quality of life measurements in these women? How are they affected by HRT, especially tamoxifen users? What is the proper dose of HRT in tamoxifen users? These questions and many others should be answered before larger trials are planned.

The beneficial effects of HRT on quality of life are indisputable. The impact on overall health is favorable as well. Theoretical concern over activating dormant tumor cells is counterbalanced by existing clinical evidence.[111] Oncologists and their patients need more research like the prospective clinical trial of HRT in breast cancer survivors being conducted by Sellin et al. The primary end point of that trial is osteoporosis prevention. Another trial is being conducted by the Eastern Cooperative Oncology Group and will be open to women who have vasomotor or vaginal symptoms and are taking tamoxifen. They will be randomly assigned to receive HRT or placebo. Primary end points include accrual rate and symptom relief. The Southwest Oncology Group will study the effects of megestrol acetate at two doses and compare them with those of placebo in women with vasomotor symptoms. These clinical trials and others that are planned in Canada and Europe will provide valuable pilot information for the design of larger phase III studies.

ACKNOWLEDGMENT

The author gratefully acknowledges Ms. Joan David for editorial assistance.

REFERENCES

1. Fisher B, Costantino J, Redmond C, et al. A randomized clinical trial evaluating tamoxifen in the treatment of patients with node-negative breast cancer who have estrogen-receptor-positive tumors. *N Engl J Med* 1989;320:479.
2. Poehlman ET, Toth MJ, Gardner AW. Changes in energy balance and body composition at menopause: a controlled longitudinal study. *Ann Intern Med* 1995;123:673.
3. The Writing Group for the PEPI trial. Effects of estrogen or estrogen/progestin regimens on heart disease risk factors in post-

menopausal women: the Postmenopausal Estrogen/Progestin Interventions (PEPI) Trial. *JAMA* 1995;273:199.
4. Huang Z, Hankinson SE, Colditz GA, et al. Dual effects of weight and weight gain on breast cancer risk. *JAMA* 1997;278:1407.
5. Sporrong T, Hellgran M, Samsioe G, Mattsson LA. Comparison of four continuously administered progestogen plus oestradiol combinations for climacteric complaints. *Br J Obstet Gynecol* 1988;95:1042.
6. Couzi RJ, Helzlsouer KJ, Fetting JH. Prevalence of menopausal symptoms among women with a history of breast cancer and attitudes toward estrogen replacement therapy. *J Clin Oncol* 1995;13:2737.
7. Boulet MJ, Oddens BJ, Lehert P, Vemer HM, Visser A. Climacteric and menopause in seven south-east Asian countries. *Maturitas* 1994;19:157.
8. Nesheim BI, Saetre T. Reduction of menopausal hot flushes by methyldopa. *Eur J Clin Pharmacol* 1981;20:413.
9. Bergmans MGM, Merkus JM, Corbey RS, Schellekens LA, Ubachs JM. Effects of bellergal retard on climacteric complaints: a double-blind, placebo-controlled study. *Maturitas* 1987;9:227.
10. Lebherz TB, French L. Nonhormonal treatment of the menopausal syndrome. *Obstet Gynecol* 1969;33:795.
11. Goldberg RM, Loprinzi CL, O'Fallon JR, et al. Transdermal clonidine for ameliorating tamoxifen-induced hot flashes. *J Clin Oncol* 1994;12:155.
12. Barton DL, Loprinzi CL, Quella SK, et al. Prospective evaluation of vitamin E for hot flashes in breast cancer survivors. *J Clin Oncol* 1998;16:495.
13. Hirata JD, Swiersz LM, Zell B, Small R, Ettinger B. Does dong quai have estrogenic effects in postmenopausal women? A double-blind, placebo-controlled trial. *Fertil Steril* 1997;68:981.
14. Loprinzi CL, Pisansky TM, Fonseca R, et al. Pilot evaluation of venlafaxine hydrochloride for the therapy of hot flashes in cancer survivors. *J Clin Oncol* 1998;16:2377.
15. Loprinzi CL, Michalak JC, Quella SK, et al. Megestrol acetate for the prevention of hot flashes. *N Engl J Med* 1994;331:347.
16. Morrison JC, Martin DC, Blair RA, et al. The use of medroxyprogesterone acetate for relief of climacteric symptoms. *Am J Obstet Gynecol* 1980;138:99.
17. Albrecht BG, Schiff I, Tulchinsky D, Ryan KJ. Objective evidence that placebo and oral medroxyprogesterone acetate therapy diminish menopausal vasomotor flushes. *Am J Obstet Gynecol* 1981;139:631.
18. Schiff I, Tuschinsky D, Cramer D. Oral medroxyprogesterone acetate in the treatment of postmenopausal symptoms. *JAMA* 1980;244:1443.
19. Bullock JL, Massey FM, Cambrell RD Jr. Use of medroxyprogesterone acetate to prevent menopausal symptoms. *Obstet Gynecol* 1975;46:165.
20. Longacre TA, Bartow SA. A correlative morphologic study of human breast and endometrium in the menstrual cycle. *Am J Surg Pathol* 1986:10:382.
21. Potten CS, Watson RJ, Williams GT, et al. The effect of age and menstrual cycle upon proliferative activity of the normal human breast. *Br J Cancer* 1988;58:163.
22. Anderson TJ, Battersby S, King RJB, McPherson K, Going JJ. Oral contraceptive use influences resting breast proliferation. *Hum Pathol* 1989;20:1139.
23. Bergkvist L, Adami Ho, Person I, et al. Prognosis after breast cancer diagnosis in women exposed to estrogen and estrogen-progestogen replacement therapy. *Am J Epidemiol* 1992;130:221.
24. Huggins C, Yang NC. Induction and extinction of mammary cancer. *Science* 1962;137:257.
25. Diamond JE, Hollander VP. Progesterone and breast cancer. *Mt Sinai J Med* 1979;46:225.
26. Jordan VC, Lababidi MK, Langan-Fahey S. Suppression of mouse mammary tumorigenesis by long term tamoxifen therapy. *J Natl Cancer Inst* 1991;83:492.
27. Kordon E, Lanari C, Meiss R, Elizalde P, Charreau E, Pasqualini CD. Hormone dependence of a mouse mammary tumor line induced in vivo by medroxyprogesterone acetate. *Breast Cancer Res Treat* 1990;33.
28. Hissom JR, Moore MR. Progestin effects on growth in the human breast cancer cell line T47D. Possible therapeutic implications. *Biochem Biophys Res Commun* 1987;45:706.
29. Braunsberg H, Coldham NG, Wong W. Hormonal therapies for breast cancer: can progestogens stimulate growth? *Cancer Lett* 1986;30:213.
30. Mouridsen HT, Elleman K, Mattsson W. Therapeutic effect of tamoxifen vs tamoxifen combined with medroxyprogesterone acetate in advanced breast cancer in postmenopausal women. *Cancer Treat Rep* 1979;63:171.
31. Gibson DFC, Johnson DA, Langan-Fahey SM, Lababidi MK, Wolberg WH, Jordan VC. The effects of intermittent progesterone upon tamoxifen inhibition of tumor growth in the 7,12-dimethylbenzanthracene rat mammary tumor model. *Breast Cancer Res Treat* 1993;27:283.
32. Delmas PD, Mitlak BH, Christiansen C. Effects of raloxifene in postmenopausal women [Letter]. *N Engl J Med* 1988;338:1313.
33. Fisher B, Costantino JP, Wickerham DL, et al. Tamoxifen for prevention of breast cancer: report of the national surgical adjuvant breast and bowel project P-1 study. *J Natl Cancer Inst* 1998;90:1371.
34. Powles TJ, Hickish T, Casey S, O'Brien M. Hormone replacement after breast cancer. *Lancet* 1993;342:60.
35. Chang J, Powles TJ, Ashley SE, et al. The effect of tamoxifen and hormone replacement therapy on serum cholesterol, bone mineral density and coagulation factors in healthy postmenopausal women participating in a randomized, controlled tamoxifen prevention study. *Ann Oncol* 1996;7:671.
36. Veronesi U, Maisonneuve P, Costa A, et al. Prevention of breast cancer with tamoxifen: preliminary findings from the Italian randomized trial among hysterectomized women. *Lancet* 1998;352:93.
37. Jones G, Nguyen T, Sambrook PN, Kelly PJ, Gilbert C, Eisman JA. Symptomatic fracture incidence in elderly men and women: the Dubbo Osteoporosis Epidemiologic Study (DOES). *Osteoporosis Int* 1994;2:277.
38. Saarto T, Blomqvist C, Valimaki M, Makela P, Sarna S, Elomaa I. Chemical castration induced by adjuvant cyclophosphamide, methotrexate and fluorouracil chemotherapy causes rapid bone loss that is reduced by clodronate: a randomized study in premenopausal breast cancer patients. *J Clin Oncol* 1997;15:1341.
39. Prince RL. Diet and the prevention of osteoporotic fractures. *N Engl J Med* 1997;336:701.
40. The writing group for the PEPI trial. Effects of hormone therapy on bone mineral density. *JAMA* 1996;276:1389.
41. Love RR, Mazess RB, Barden HS, et al. Effects of tamoxifen on bone mineral density in postmenopausal women with breast cancer. *N Engl J Med* 1992;326:852.
42. Delmas PD, Bjarnason NH, Mitlak BH, et al. Effects of raloxifene on bone mineral density, serum cholesterol concentrations, and uterine endometrium in postmenopausal women. *N Engl J Med* 1998;337: 1641.
43. McClung M, Clemmesen B, Daifotis A, et al. Alendronate prevents postmenopausal bone loss in women without osteoporosis. *Ann Intern Med* 1998;128:253.
44. Hosking D, Chilvers CE, Christiansen C, et al. Prevention of bone loss with alendronate in postmenopausal women under 60 years of age. *N Engl J Med* 1998;338;485.
45. Grady D, Rubin SM, Petitti DB, et al. Hormone therapy to prevent disease and prolong life in postmenopausal women. *Ann Intern Med* 1992;15:1016.
46. Kiel DP, Felson DT, Anderson JJ, et al. Hip fracture and the use of estrogens in postmenopausal women. *N Engl J Med* 1987; 317:1169.
47. Liberman UA, Weiss SR, Broll J, et al. Effect of oral alendronate on bone mineral density and the incidence of fractures in postmenopausal osteoporosis. *N Engl J Med* 1995;333:1437.
48. Stampfer MJ, Hennekens CH, Manson JE, Colditz GA, Rosner B, Willett WC. Vitamin E consumption and the risk of coronary disease in women. *N Engl J Med* 1993;328:1444.
49. Rimm EB, Willett WC, Hu FB, et al. Folate and vitamin B_6 from diet and supplements in relation to risk of coronary heart disease among women. *JAMA* 1998;279:359.
50. Bines J, Oleske DM, Cobleigh MA. Ovarian function in premenopausal women treated with adjuvant chemotherapy for breast cancer. *J Clin Oncol* 1996;14:1718.
51. Mansour EG, Gray R, Shatila AH, et al. Efficacy of adjuvant chemotherapy in high-risk node-negative breast cancer. *N Engl J Med* 1989;320:485.
52. The Ludwig Breast Cancer Study Group. Prolonged disease-free survival after one course of perioperative adjuvant chemotherapy for node-negative breast cancer. *N Engl J Med* 1989;320:491.
53. Fisher B, Redmond C, Dimitrov NV, et al. A randomized trial evaluating sequential methotrexate and fluorouracil in the treatment of patients with node-negative breast cancer who have estrogen-receptor-negative tumors. *N Engl J Med* 1989;320:474.
54. Barrett-Connor E, Bush TL. Estrogen and coronary heart disease in women. *JAMA* 1991;265:1861.

55. Stampfer MJ, Colditz GA, Willett WC, et al. Postmenopausal estrogen therapy and cardiovascular disease. Ten-year follow-up from the nurses' health study. *N Engl J Med* 1991;325:756.
56. Rosen PP, Groshen S, Kinne DW, et al. Factors influencing prognosis in node-negative breast carcinoma: analysis of 767 T1N0M0/T2N0M0 patients with long-term follow-up. *J Clin Oncol* 1993;11:2090.
57. Early Breast Cancer Trialists' Collaborative Group. Tamoxifen for early breast cancer: an overview of the randomised trials. *Lancet* 1998;351:1451.
58. Fisher B, Dignam J, Wolmark N, et al. Tamoxifen and chemotherapy for lymph node-negative, estrogen receptor-positive breast cancer. *J Natl Cancer Inst* 1997;89:1673.
59. Antiplatelet trialists' collaboration. Collaborative overview of randomized trials of antiplatelet therapy—I: prevention of death, myocardial infarction and stroke by prolonged antiplatelet therapy in various categories of patients. *BMJ* 1994;308:81.
60. Scandinavian Simvastatin Survival Study Group. Randomized trial of cholesterol lowering in 4444 patients with coronary heart disease: the Scandinavian Simvastatin Survival Study (4S). *Lancet* 1994;344:1383.
61. Downs JR, Clearfield M, Weis S, Whitney E, Shapiro DR, Beere PA, et al. Primary prevention of acute coronary events with Lovastatin in men and women with average cholesterol levels. *JAMA* 1998;279:1615.
62. Barrett-Connor E, Bush TL. Estrogen and coronary heart disease in women. *JAMA* 1991;265:1861.
63. Cardiovascular implications of estrogen replacement therapy. *Obstet Gynecol* 1990;75[Suppl 4]:18S–25S.
64. Walsh BW, Kuller LH, Wild RA, et al. Effects of raloxifene on serum lipids and coagulation factors in healthy postmenopausal women. *JAMA* 1998;279:1445.
65. Saarto T, Blomqzist C, Ehnholm C, Taskinen RM, Elomaa I. Antiatherogenic effects of adjuvant antiestrogens: a randomized trial comparing the effects of tamoxifen and toremifene on plasma lipid levels in postmenopausal women with node-positive breast cancer. *J Clin Oncol* 1996,14:429.
66. Anderson JW, Johnstone B, Cook-Newell ME. Meta-analysis of the effects of soy protein intake on serum lipids. *N Engl J Med* 1995;333:276.
67. Decensi A, Bonanni B, Guerrieri-Gonzaga A, et al. Biologic activity of tamoxifen at low doses in healthy women. *J Natl Cancer Inst* 1998,90.1461.
68. Clarkson TB, Cline JM, Williams JK, Anthony MS. Gonadal hormone substitutes: effects on the cardiovascular system. *Osteoporos Int* 1997;7[Suppl 1]:S43.
69. Anthony MS, Clarkson TB, Hughes CI Jr, Morgan TM, Burke GL. Soybean isoflavones improve cardiovascular risk factors without affecting the reproductive system of peripubertal rhesus monkeys. *J Nutr* 1996;126:43.
70. Yaffe K, Sawaya G, Lieberburg I, Grady D. Estrogen therapy in postmenopausal women: effects on cognitive function and dementia. *JAMA* 1998;279:688.
71. Anthony MS, Clarkson TB, Hughes CI Jr, Morgan TM, Burke GL. Soybean isoflavones improve cardiovascular risk factors without affecting the reproductive system of peripubertal rhesus monkeys. *J Nutr* 1996;126:43.
72. Schiff I, Wentworth B, Koos B, Tulchinsky D, Ryan KJ. Effect of estradiol administration on the hypogonadal woman. *Fertil Steril* 1978;30:278.
73. Mattsson LA, Cullberg G. Vaginal absorption of two estradiol preparations. *Acta Obstet Gynecol Scand* 1983;62:393.
74. Heimer GM. Estradiol in the menopause. *Acta Obstet Gynecol Scand* 1987;139[Suppl]:23P.
75. Handa VL, Bachus KE, Johnston WM, Robboy SJ, Hammond CB. Vaginal administration of low-dose conjugated estrogens: systemic absorption and effects on the endometrium. *Obstet Gynecol* 1994; 84:215.
76. Smith P, Heimer G, Lindskog M, Ulmsten A. Oestradiol-releasing vaginal ring for treatment of postmenopausal urogenital atrophy. *Maturitas* 1993;16:145.
77. Nachtigall LE. Comparative study: Replens versus local estrogen in menopausal women. *Fertil Steril* 1994;61:178.
78. Loprinzi CL, Abu-Ghazaleh S, Sloan JA, et al. Phase III randomized double-blind study to evaluate the efficacy of a polycarbophil-based vaginal moisturizer in women with breast cancer. *J Clin Oncol* 1997;15:969.
79. Cable E, Miracle-McMahill H, Than MJ, Heath C. Estrogen replacement therapy and risk of fatal colon cancer in a prospective cohort of postmenopausal women. *J Natl Cancer Inst* 1995;87:517.
80. Grodstein F, Martinez ME, Platz EA, et al. Postmenopausal hormone use and risk for colorectal cancer and adenoma. *Ann Intern Med* 1998;128:705.
81. Potter JK, Bostick RM, Grandits GA, et al. Hormone replacement therapy is associated with lower risk of adenomatous polyps of the large bowel: the Minnesota Cancer Prevention research unit case-control study. *Cancer Epidemiol Biomarkers Prev* 1996;5:779.
82. Cline JM, Soderqvist G, von Schoultz E, Skoog L, von Schoultz B. Effects of hormone replacement therapy on the mammary gland of surgically postmenopausal cynomolgus macaques. *Am J Obstet Gynecol* 1996;174:93.
83. Laya MB, Gallagher JC, Schreiman JS, et al. Effect of postmenopausal hormonal replacement therapy on mammographic density and parenchymal pattern. *Radiology* 1995;196:433.
84. McNicholas MMJ, Heneghan JP, Milner MH, et al. Pain and increased mammographic density in women receiving hormone replacement therapy: a prospective study. *AJR Am J Roentgenol* 1994;163:311.
85. Persson I, Thurfjell E, Holmberg L. Effect of estrogen and estrogen-progestin replacement regimens on mammographic breast parenchymal density. *J Clin Oncol* 1997;15:3201.
86. Kelsey JL, Berkowitz GS. Breast cancer epidemiology. *Cancer Res* 1988;48:5615.
87. Harvey EB, Brinton LA. Second cancer following cancer of the breast in Connecticut, 1935–1982. In: Boice JD Jr, Storm HH, Curtis RE, eds. *Multiple primary cancers in Connecticut and Denmark*. National Cancer Institute monograph 68. Washington: Government Printing Office, 1985:99. [NIH publication no 85-2714].
88. DuPont WD, Page DL. Menopausal estrogen replacement therapy and breast cancer. *Arch Intern Med* 1991;151:67.
89. Steinberg KK, Thacker SB, Smith SJ, et al. A meta-analysis of the effect of estrogen replacement therapy on the risk of breast cancer. *JAMA* 1991;265:1985.
90. Armstrong BK. Oestrogen therapy after the menopause—boon or bane? *Med J Aust* 1988;148:213.
91. Grady D, Ernster V. Invited commentary: does postmenopausal hormone therapy cause breast cancer? *Am J Epidemiol* 1991:134:1396.
92. Sillero-Arenas M, Delgado-Rodriguez M, Rodrigues-Canteras R, et al. Menopausal hormone replacement therapy and breast cancer: a meta-analysis. *Obstet Gynecol* 1992;79:286.
93. Colditz GA, Egan KM, Stampfer MJ. Hormone replacement therapy and risk of breast cancer; results from epidemiologic studies. *Am J Obstet Gynecol* 1993;168:1473.
94. Henrich JB. The postmenopausal estrogen/breast cancer controversy. *JAMA* 1992;268:1900.
95. Ginsburg ES, Mello NK, Mendelson JK, et al. Effects of alcohol ingestion on estrogens in postmenopausal women. *JAMA* 1996;276:1747.
96. Nayfield SG, Karp JE, Ford LG, et al. Potential role of tamoxifen in prevention of breast cancer. *J Natl Cancer Inst* 1991;83:1450.
97. Persson I, Yuen J, Bergkvist L, Schairer C. Cancer incidence and mortality in women receiving estrogen and estrogen-progestin replacement therapy—long-term follow-up of a Swedish cohort. *Int J Cancer* 1996;67:327.
98. Gambrell DR. Proposal to decrease the risk and improve the prognosis in breast cancer. *Am J Obstet Gynecol* 1984;150:119.
99. Hunt K, Vessey M, McPherson K, Coleman M. Long-term surveillance of mortality and cancer incidence in women receiving hormone replacement therapy. *Br J Obstet Gynecol* 1987;94:620.
100. Henderson BE, Paganini-Hill A, Ross RK. Decreased mortality in users of estrogen replacement therapy. *Arch Intern Med* 1991;151:75.
101. Criqui MH, Suarez L, Barrett-Connor E, et al. Postmenopausal estrogen use and mortality. *Am J Epidemiol* 1988;128:606.
102. Ewertz M, Gillanders S, Meyer L, Zedeler K. Survival of breast cancer patients in relation to factors which affect the risk of developing breast cancer. *Int J Cancer* 1991;49:526.
103. Wilis DB, Calle EE, Miracle-McMahill HL, Heath Jr CW. Estrogen replacement therapy and risk of fatal breast cancer in a prospective cohort of postmenopausal women in the United States. *Cancer Causes Control* 1996;7:449.
104. Colditz GA, Hankinson SE, Hunter DJ, et al. The use of estrogens and progestins and the risk of breast cancer in postmenopausal women. *N Engl J Med* 1995;332:1589.

105. Dao TL, Sinha DI, Nemoto T, Patel J. Effect of estrogen and progesterone on cellular replication of human breast tumors. *Cancer Res* 1982;42:359.
106. Fabian CJ, Kimler BF, McKittrick R, et al. Recruitment with high physiological doses of estradiol preceding chemotherapy: flow cytometric and therapeutic results in women with locally advanced breast cancer—a Southwest Oncology Group Study. *Cancer Res* 1994;54:5357.
107. Dhodapkar MV, Ingle JN, Ahmann DL. Estrogen replacement therapy withdrawal and regression of metastatic breast cancer. *Cancer* 1995; 75:43.
108. Powles TJ, Hickish T. Breast cancer response to hormone replacement therapy withdrawal. *Lancet* 1995;346:1442.
109. Harvey SC, DiPiro PJ, Meyer JE. Marked regression of a nonpalpable breast cancer after cessation of hormone replacement therapy. *AJR Am J Roentgenol* 1996;167:394
110. Cobleigh MA. Hormone replacement therapy in breast cancer survivors. In: Harris JR, Lippman ME, eds. *Diseases of the breast updates.* Cedar Knolls, NJ: Lippincott–Raven Healthcare, 1997; 1:1.
111. Eden JA, Bush T, Nand S, Wren BG. The Royal Hospital for Women Breast Cancer Study—a case-controlled study of combined continuous hormone replacement therapy amongst women with a personal history of breast cancer. *Menopause* 1995;2:67.

Diseases of the Breast, 2nd ed.,
edited by Jay R. Harris.
Lippincott Williams & Wilkins, Philadelphia © 2000.

CHAPTER 71

Reproductive Issues

Harold J. Burstein and Eric P. Winer

Surveillance data indicate that nearly one-fourth (23.5%) of all breast cancer cases are diagnosed in women younger than age 50 years, accounting for an estimated 41,800 cases in the United States in 1997.[1] Although breast cancer is less common in women younger than age 40 years, there are still 9,000 women in their 20s and 30s who are diagnosed with breast cancer each year. Many of these younger premenopausal women and a substantial number of women older than 40 years of age are concerned about the impact of their disease and treatment on subsequent fertility. A reasonable estimate is that each year, 15,000 to 20,000 newly diagnosed breast cancer patients will have fertility concerns as they contemplate treatments.

Several social and medical trends have heightened interest in fertility and reproductive health among breast cancer survivors. First, women are having children at a later age, increasing the number of women diagnosed with breast cancer who still wish to bear one or more children. Second, risk factors for breast cancer, including nulliparity and higher socioeconomic status, are often associated with an interest in childbearing at later ages. Third, the increase in screening mammography in women in their 40s is likely to result in a larger number of breast cancer diagnoses in women who may still be planning subsequent pregnancies. Finally, treatments that have implications for fertility, including chemotherapy and hormone therapy, are being offered with greater frequency to almost all breast cancer patients, enlarging the pool of patients who must contend with these issues. Reproductive issues are clearly important in the long-term physical and psychosocial well-being of breast cancer survivors.

This chapter discusses the impact of breast cancer treatment on fertility and reproductive health, as well as strategies for facilitating pregnancy after treatment. The management of menopause in breast cancer survivors, including the role of hormone replacement therapy, as well as pregnancy and breast cancer, are covered in separate chapters.

H. J. Burstein: Dana-Farber Cancer Institute, Harvard Medical School, Boston, Massachusetts

E. P. Winer: Department of Medicine, Harvard Medical School, Department of Breast Oncology, Dana-Farber Cancer Institute, Boston, Massachusetts

NORMAL REPRODUCTIVE FUNCTION AND MENOPAUSE

The primordial germ cells appear in the fetus 3 weeks into gestation and by 6 weeks' gestation have migrated into the primary sex cords. By 20 weeks, 7 million oogonia are present; that number declines to 700,000 oocytes at the time of birth and 200,000 at puberty.[2] Of these, only 400 mature and ovulate over the course of a woman's life. The rest progressively undergo atresia because of inadequate stimulation from follicle-stimulating hormone (FSH). With the onset of puberty, women begin having monthly menstrual cycles, during which a follicle matures and ovulates under the influence of cyclical hormonal physiology.[3] The follicular phase of the menstrual cycle is of somewhat variable duration, beginning on the first day of menstruation and extending to the time of ovulation. The luteal phase of the cycle is of relatively constant duration and is defined as the time between ovulation and the onset of menstruation. In the follicular phase, follicles are recruited, and estrogen production from the ovary increases. The midcycle surge in FSH and luteinizing hormone (LH) induces ovulation. Thereafter, ovarian estrogen, in concert with progesterone produced by the corpus luteum, causes feedback inhibition of FSH and LH. In the absence of fertilization, progesterone and estrogen levels fall in the late luteal phase, inducing uterine bleeding. Ovarian follicles typically are recruited for maturation 85 days before ovulation. Damage or disruption of the maturing follicles would be expected to cause temporary amenorrhea; damage to the primordial follicles would cause more permanent amenorrhea. Oocyte maturation depends on oocyte function and the function of granulosa cells, which support the maturing oocyte. Toxicity to either cell population prevents follicle maturation and eventually causes depletion of ovarian reserve.

As women reach ages 40 to 45, the menstrual cycle tends to become less regular in length. Although women continue to ovulate, circulating levels of estrogen and progesterone are lower, contributing to variability in menstrual cycles.[4] Compensatory changes gradually produce a rise in FSH to offset the loss of estrogen and progesterone secretion. With time, the finite stock of oocytes is further depleted, and the ovarian follicles fail to respond to stimulation, leading to menopause.[5]

Age at natural menopause follows a normal distribution, with menopause occurring between ages 45 and 55 years in the vast majority of women; the median age is 51. Premature menopause—onset at age younger than 40 years—affects 4% of the female population. The endocrine hallmarks of menopause reflect hypergonadotropic hypogonadism: lack of ovarian synthesis of estrogen (although estrogen is still synthesized by peripheral aromatization of androgens), absence of progesterone, and rises in FSH and LH levels caused by loss of negative feedback inhibition. Pathologic analysis of the ovary after menopause reveals fibrotic tissue and absence of follicles.

Fertility declines with age, beginning considerably earlier than the onset of menopause.[6] Impaired intrinsic oocyte function,[7] an increase in the spontaneous abortion rate,[8] and a greater proportion of anovulatory cycles all contribute to the decline in fertility with advancing age. By contrast, age-related changes in the uterus have only modest effects on fertility, enabling older women to sustain pregnancies achieved with assisted reproductive technology. Approximately three-fourths of all premenopausal breast cancer cases occur in women between the ages of 40 and 50 years. For these women, fertility is already beginning to wane at the time of cancer diagnosis.

TABLE 1. *Effect of chemotherapeutic agents on ovarian function*

Definite impairment
- Cyclophosphamide
- L-Phenylalanine mustard (L-PAM; melphalan)
- Thiotepa
- Busulfan
- Procarbazine
- Chlorambucil
- Cisplatin, carboplatin

Rare or unlikely impairment
- Methotrexate
- Fluorouracil (note: effect of chronic oral administration not known)
- Corticosteroids

Unknown effect, considered less likely to cause impairment
- Vinorelbine, vinblastine, vincristine
- Doxorubicin, epirubicin, other anthracyclines
- Etoposide
- Bleomycin

Unknown effect
- Paclitaxel
- Docetaxel
- Gemcitabine

CHEMOTHERAPY-INDUCED AMENORRHEA

Different types of cancer therapy, including radiation treatment, surgery, chemotherapy, and hormonal treatments, can affect gonadal function.[9] Among breast cancer patients, surgical or radiation damage to the ovary is not an issue unless the very purpose of the procedure is ovarian ablation. However, chemotherapy and tamoxifen can affect ovarian function. For patients with advanced disease, the impact of systemic therapy on fertility may be troubling to the patient but is generally not a paramount concern. On the other hand, loss of fertility is often an important consideration in selecting adjuvant treatment programs for younger women.

The impact of chemotherapy on the ovary is principally a function of the type of chemotherapy, the cumulative dose, and the age of the patient.[10–12] Of the commonly used agents (Table 1), alkylators are most clearly associated with ovarian dysfunction. Platinum analogues have also been found to impair menstrual function in some women.[13–15] Antimetabolites, such as methotrexate and 5-fluorouracil, are not believed to interfere with ovarian function, and the effect of many other agents has not been clearly delineated. Pathology studies from animal models of chemotherapy-induced gonadal damage and from patients demonstrate ovarian fibrosis and depletion and destruction of follicles from chemotherapy[16,17]; granulosa cells and follicular development appear to be affected.[18] Endocrine evaluation of patients treated with chemotherapy reveals hypergonadotropic hypogonadism, with elevated circulating levels of FSH and LH and low levels of estrogen.[19–23] Thus, chemotherapy-induced ovarian failure is a direct consequence of toxicity to the ovary and is not mediated through other mechanisms.

Specific chemotherapy regimens for treating breast cancer cause predictable rates of ovarian failure. The frequency of amenorrhea with a given agent or regimen depends on the age of the patient and the cumulative exposure to the agent(s). In almost all instances, younger women are less likely to have permanent amenorrhea than older women. The median age of the development of amenorrhea from chemotherapy ranges from 38 to 46 years in most reports; by contrast, the median age for women in whom amenorrhea does not develop is 33 to 35 years.[11] The incidence of ovarian failure associated with commonly used regimens is listed in Table 2. With CMF (cyclophosphamide, methotrexate, 5-fluorouracil) administered for 6 months, the risk of ovarian failure is approximately 35% in women younger than age 40 versus 90% in women

TABLE 2. *Incidence of chemotherapy-related amenorrhea after adjuvant treatment for breast cancer*

		Incidence of amenorrhea (%)		
Regimen	Duration (mo)	Age <40 yr	Age >40 yr	Mean age ~40 yr
None[24,25]		4–6	20–25	
CMF-based[26–30]	1	14	34	
	6	31–38	81–96	69–90
	12	51–77	83–98	
L-PAM ± F[31]	24	20–22	60–76	
FAC[34]	24	9	NA	
FEC[35]	6	23	89	
AC[29,30,32]	3	13	57–63	34–60
MF[32]	6			9–13

A, doxorubicin; E, epirubicin; C, cyclophosphamide; F, 5-fluorouracil; L-PAM, L-phenylalanine mustard; M, methotrexate; NA, not available.

TABLE 3. *Incidence of chemotherapy-related amenorrhea after adjuvant treatment for breast cancer among women aged younger than 30 years*

Regimen	Duration (mo)	Incidence (%)	Reference
CMF	6	19	Valagussa et al.[33]
FAC-based	Variable	0	Hortobagyi et al.[36]
FEC	4–5	0	Weber et al.[35]

A, doxorubicin; C, cyclophosphamide; E, epirubicin; F, 5-fluorouracil; M, methotrexate.

older than age 40.[24–30] In contrast, ovarian failure is seen in fewer than 15% of women younger than 40 years of age who receive four cycles of AC (doxorubicin, cyclophosphamide).[29,30,32] For patients younger than age 30 years, the incidence of amenorrhea may be even lower, with some regimens inducing no amenorrhea[33] (Table 3).

Among all age groups, anthracycline-based regimens appear to be associated with less ovarian toxicity than CMF-based regimens (see Tables 2 and 3).[34,35] In general, the cumulative dose of alkylator therapy, particularly cyclophosphamide, is strongly correlated with amenorrhea. Prolonged dosing and higher-dose regimens are associated with higher rates of ovarian failure. The difference in the total dose of cyclophosphamide is likely to be responsible for the lower rate of ovarian failure with anthracycline-based regimens compared with CMF. It is not known what effect the addition or substitution of taxanes in adjuvant chemotherapy regimens will have on ovarian function.

Although older women develop amenorrhea after lower cumulative doses than younger women, prolonged dosing can cause amenorrhea in younger women as well. The mean time to onset of amenorrhea is 4 to 5 months for woman younger than 40 years and 2 to 3 months for older women. Recovery of menstrual function after temporary amenorrhea occurs in some patients; age is again an important factor, as is dose of cyclophosphamide. Although roughly one-half the women younger than age 40 years may regain some menstrual function, the percentage is much lower in older women.

High-dose chemotherapy with bone marrow transplant for hematologic disorders is associated with a very high rate of ovarian failure.[37–39] It should be assumed that the vast majority of women who receive high-dose chemotherapy with stem cell or bone marrow support for breast cancer experience permanent amenorrhea. Occasionally patients, particularly women younger than age 25 years at the time of treatment, resume menstrual cycles after treatment, and pregnancies have been reported in women after bone marrow transplant.[40,41] High-dose chemotherapy regimens that do not require stem cell support have been investigated in breast cancer clinical trials. The impact of these regimens on fertility is not known and should be assessed if these regimens enter widespread use.

It is likely that chemotherapy will result in younger age of menopause for women who continue to menstruate during or after chemotherapy. Experience from pediatric oncology indicates that adolescent women who receive chemotherapy but continue to menstruate afterward are nonetheless at higher risk for early menopause.[42] Anecdotal experience in patients with breast cancer suggests that women who received alkylator-based chemotherapy without permanent amenorrhea often experience menopause at younger ages than other family members.

Premature menopause in these women may have implications for family planning after breast cancer. Historically, women have been advised to wait at least 2 years after their breast cancer diagnosis before becoming pregnant.[43] This recommendation stemmed from the greater likelihood of tumor recurrence in the years immediately after diagnosis and the corresponding fact that longer disease-free survival implies less chance of recurrence in the future. It is not clear if or to what extent delaying pregnancy affects the risk of cancer recurrence.[44] For breast cancer survivors who want to have children, deferring pregnancy too long may reduce their chances of conception, as reproductive reserve has been diminished by chemotherapy treatments and the passage of time. Thus, for some patients, it may be prudent to consider pregnancy sooner rather than later after treatment, especially if the woman is at low risk of cancer recurrence.

GONADAL PROTECTION DURING CHEMOTHERAPY

If chemotherapy affects actively proliferating cells, then suppression of proliferative activity in the ovary during chemotherapy might minimize gonadal toxicity. Clinical support for this idea comes from the observation that chemotherapy-related gonadal damage is most apparent in sexually mature, postpubertal individuals; prepubertal boys and girls treated with chemotherapy appear to suffer less gonadal toxicity.[45] Ovarian suppression can be achieved with either chronic gonadotropin-releasing hormone (GnRH) agonist therapy, such as LH-releasing hormone (LHRH; e.g., leuprolide acetate), or with oral contraceptives. Leuprolide has been used to induce amenorrhea in female patients being treated with high-dose chemotherapy who are at risk of menorrhagia in association with thrombocytopenia.[46,47] In animal models, treatment with LHRH agonist therapy can reduce cyclophosphamide-mediated depletion of ovarian follicles and preserve proliferative activity in some species; it is not clear that this translates into persistent fertility and fecundity.[48,49]

Clinical trials in humans have examined the ability of either GnRH agonist or cyclic oral contraceptives to spare chemotherapy-related ovarian damage. These studies have been done on patients with germ cell tumors, lymphoma, or Hodgkin's disease who were younger than breast cancer patients and who received different chemotherapy regimens than are used to treat breast cancer. The results are equivocal; the limited clinical information is presented in Table 4.

TABLE 4. *Trials of ovarian suppression in women receiving chemotherapy*

Diagnosis	Number of patients	Chemotherapy	Intervention	Outcome
Hodgkin's disease[52]	6	MVPP	Oral contraceptives	83% sustained menses compared to none expected
Hodgkin's disease[53]	56	MVPP/TBV	Oral contraceptives	71% of women taking OC continued menstruating compared to 74% of women not taking OC
Lymphoma[54]	16	MOPP/ABV	GnRH agonist	93% sustained menses compared to 39% of historical controls
Hodgkin's disease[55]	18	MVPP	GnRH agonist	50% of women randomized to treatment with GnRH agonist menstruated after chemotherapy compared to 66% of women not treated

GnRH, gonadotropin-releasing hormone.

Several reports indicate that gonadal protection afforded fertility against the MOPP regimen (mechlorethamine, vincristine, procarbazine, prednisone) that historically rendered patients infertile. However, other studies have failed to document any protective effect.[50,51]

GnRH agonist therapy has been used as treatment of breast cancer in the metastatic and adjuvant setting. However, no trials have been reported of prevention of ovarian damage from chemotherapy among breast cancer patients or even among chemotherapy regimens commonly used for breast cancer. In addition to the lack of data on efficacy of gonadal protection, there are reasons to be cautious about this strategy. First, a transient increase in estrogen levels is observed with initiation of GnRH agonist therapy; it is theoretically possible that this estrogen surge could promote tumor growth in a patient with a new breast cancer diagnosis. Second, there may be therapeutic benefits as a result of amenorrhea. Some retrospective analyses have suggested that functional amenorrhea after adjuvant CMF-based chemotherapy is associated with fewer recurrences and an improved overall outcome,[56,57] but this conclusion remains controversial, and these findings may not extend to anthracycline-based regimens.[58] The intergroup trial in which women were randomized to receive CAF (cyclophosphamide, doxorubicin, 5-fluorouracil) chemotherapy with or without an LHRH agonist should provide further insight into these issues. However, it is not clear that gonadal protection in premenopausal breast cancer patients is either feasible or necessarily desirable. Nonetheless, studies that attempt ovarian protection among breast cancer patients are warranted; patients deserve more definitive answers about these important issues. Ideally, any effort to preserve fertility with GnRH agonists should be considered within the context of a clinical trial.

TAMOXIFEN AND FERTILITY

The first human clinical trials of tamoxifen examined its effectiveness as a means of contraception or ovulation induction. Tamoxifen has diverse endocrine and gynecologic effects in premenopausal women, including hyperestrogenemia with normal or slightly elevated FSH levels, and may affect ovarian size and the incidence of ovarian cysts.[59,60] Women on tamoxifen can have normal sustained menstruation, irregular menses, or development of menopause. In large randomized trials that compare tamoxifen to placebo as adjuvant therapy for breast cancer, premenopausal women on tamoxifen report more vaginal discharge, hot flashes, and irregular menses—symptoms suggestive of menopausal changes.[61] In the Royal Marsden chemoprevention trial, premenopausal women given tamoxifen were more than twice as likely to develop amenorrhea as women on placebo.[62] It is not known whether this effect is permanent or whether menses resume with discontinuation of tamoxifen. In one adjuvant trial, most women who developed menstrual dysfunction with tamoxifen resumed normal menses after cessation of therapy.[63] However, 5 years of adjuvant treatment brings every patient closer to onset of natural menopause.

Pregnancy is possible on tamoxifen, but patients who are receiving the medication should be advised against becoming pregnant. No data are available on the effects of tamoxifen on human fetal development or pregnancy outcome. However, in rodent laboratory models, neonatal tamoxifen exposure is associated with genitourinary abnormalities.[64] For these reasons, pregnancy is considered an absolute contraindication to tamoxifen therapy, and clinicians should recommend appropriate means of contraception for women of childbearing age who are taking tamoxifen. Women taking tamoxifen who wish to become pregnant should stop the drug at least 2 months before conception because of its long half-life. As a practical matter, women advised to take 5 years of tamoxifen will face reduced fertility at the end of adjuvant treatment from their own aging.

CONCEPTION AND PREGNANCY AFTER BREAST CANCER

It is important to distinguish the incidence of menstrual dysfunction after breast cancer treatments, which can be determined fairly easily, from the incidence of successful pregnancy, which is very difficult to assess and obviously subject to considerably more variation. Breast cancer survivors may have received treatment that impairs fertility or

TABLE 5. *Reproductive technology: issues for patients with breast cancer*

Method/ technique	Purpose	Exogenous hormone exposure	Delivery rate (non–breast cancer patients)	Issues for breast cancer patients
Ovulation induction	Generate and collect follicles and ova for fertilization and subsequent transfer or storage	Natural cycle—none IVF—variable, possibly including clomiphene (nonsteroidal estrogen), GnRH agonist, human menopausal gonadotropin (Pergonal), human chorionic gonadotropins	 Age <35 yr, 18–22% Age >40 yr, 4–9%	1. Low oocyte retrieval rate 1. Increased oocycte retrieval yield 2. Can be accomplished rapidly (2–6 wk) 3. Unknown risk of hormone exposure, especially before breast cancer treatment 4. Single-collection cycle pregnancy rate of 18%
Cryopreservation	Storage of collected embryos, oocytes, or sperm		Frozen/thawed embryos: 12% Frozen/thawed oocytes: investigational only; limited case reports of success	1. Embryo storage requires identification of sperm donor 2. Collected embryos can be preserved for use after any ovarian failure
Ovum donation	Donated ova are fertilized and implanted into woman with ovarian failure; includes regimen for uterine preparation.	Estrogen, progesterone, GnRH agonist	25–35%; depends more on age of oocyte donor than on age of recipient	1. Allows pregnancy in women after treatment-related menopause 2. Higher spontaneous abortion rate in women after chemotherapy-induced ovarian failure 3. Unknown risk of hormone exposure

GnRH, gonadotropin-releasing hormone; IVF, *in vitro* fertilization.
Note: See refs. 82–84 for details.

may have deferred pregnancy until an older age. Thus, breast cancer patients face a potentially narrower "window of opportunity" to become pregnant. Women older than 35 years without histories of breast cancer are more likely to experience complications of pregnancy, including greater incidence of spontaneous abortion, abnormal labor, adverse consequences of comorbid disease such as diabetes or hypertension, and cesarean section.[65,66] The older patient with a history of breast cancer is likely to face similar difficulties. Fortunately, chemotherapy in the absence of radiation therapy below the diaphragm does not appear to be associated with an increased risk of congenital anomalies in the offspring of cancer survivors.[10,67–70]

Single-institution experiences suggest that between 3% and 11% of women younger than ages 35 to 40 years become pregnant after a breast cancer diagnosis.[24,25,71–74] Population-based studies of women from Scandinavian countries and New Zealand, which included older women up to ages 45 to 50 years, documented a lower pregnancy rate after breast cancer diagnosis, typically 2% to 4%.[75–77] Given the demographics of breast cancer, it is not surprising that most pregnancies occur within 5 years of diagnosis. Studies of women from a variety of North American and European countries reveal that a significant percentage of women (36% to 60%) who become pregnant after breast cancer elect to have an abortion.[78–80] The available literature does not suggest that pregnancy after breast cancer diagnosis adversely affects a patient's cancer prognosis, although this remains a subject of intense discussion and study.[81] A more detailed discussion of this subject can be found in Chapter 44.

REPRODUCTIVE TECHNOLOGY FOR WOMEN WITH BREAST CANCER

Reproductive medicine may be useful for women with infertility either unrelated to their breast cancer or resulting from breast cancer therapy. There are two general categories of such treatments. The first is *in vitro* fertilization (IVF), which involves induction of ovulation, harvesting of oocytes, fertilization of oocytes to form embryos, and reimplantation of embryos into the uterine cavity. This strategy is appropriate for women with infertility but preserved ovarian function, or as a means of obtaining embryos before treatments that threaten to cause ovarian failure. The second category is oocyte or embryo donation, wherein donated oocytes or embryos are implanted into the uterus. This strategy is used for women without ovarian function, such as those with hypergonadotropic hypogonadism after chemotherapy.

A detailed account of assisted reproductive technology is beyond the scope of this chapter.[82–84] Close cooperation with obstetric-gynecologic services is needed for the care of cancer patients who receive such treatments. An overview of the principal methods is presented in Table 5. Women with a personal history of breast cancer may have infertility and become potential candidates for any assisted reproduction techniques. The major theoretical issue raised in these patients is the risk of hormonal exposure on cancer prognosis. Clomiphene-induced ovulation followed by oocyte retrieval and IVF has been successfully performed in women in whom infertility eventually developed after surgery for breast cancer.[85] It is not known whether different induction strategies using human menopausal gonadotropin (Pergonal) or GnRH agonist therapy, or both, instead of the nonsteroidal estrogen clomiphene afford greater or lesser safety for women with histories of breast cancer.

Two unique circumstances arise in caring for women with breast cancer. The first is consideration of attempted oocyte retrieval before systemic therapy for breast cancer, in an effort to preserve embryos for later pregnancies. This has been successfully accomplished with retrieval of oocytes after a natural menstrual cycle[86]; however, the oocyte yield from natural cycle harvest tends to be low, and most non–breast cancer patients undergo induced ovulation with exogenous hormones to optimize the chance of egg recovery. For the patient with breast cancer, the concerns over potential exacerbation of tumor growth from supraphysiologic levels of circulating hormones are compounded, as the woman has not yet received systemic treatment. Additionally, concern exists regarding delaying breast cancer therapy to accomplish the oocyte harvest. A single harvest cycle requires 4 to 6 weeks; multiple cycles are performed under normal circumstances to optimize the likelihood of pregnancy. These theoretical obstacles must be weighed against the patient's wishes, the likelihood of ovarian failure, and the realistic likelihood of successful birth after subsequent IVF.

Oocyte harvest is typically followed by IVF and then cryopreservation of the fertilized embryos. This requires identification of a sperm donor. For some breast cancer patients, a sperm donor may not be readily available or identifiable. The use of unfertilized, cryopreserved oocytes for subsequent thawing, fertilization, and implantation has been reported. However, such procedures must still be considered experimental and to date are associated with a much lower rate of successful pregnancy and delivery than the use of cryopreserved embryos.

The second unique instance arises in women with treatment-related amenorrhea who wish to become pregnant. If these women cannot be induced to ovulate, they are potential candidates for embryo donation from other oocyte or embryo donors. Preparation of the uterus before implantation requires placing patients on cyclic estrogen and progesterone. This strategy has also been successfully performed in women with a history of breast cancer and chemotherapy-induced ovarian failure.[87] The success of embryo and oocyte donation in women with chemotherapy-induced ovarian failure has been compared to that of women with other causes of ovarian failure.[88] Only a small number of women (8) with chemotherapy-related amenorrhea were treated. These women had pregnancy rates that were comparable to those of other patients, but had lower delivery rates (20% versus 26% to 40%) because of a higher rate of spontaneous abortion.

RISKS OF *IN VITRO* FERTILIZATION AND BREAST CANCER

Concerns have existed that the hormonal exposures of IVF, particularly the phase of ovarian stimulation, might affect the risk of breast cancer. Pregnancy itself is associated with marked elevations in circulating hormones, including estrogen and progesterone.[89] Ovulation induction and uterine preparation for embryo implantation require administration of exogenous hormones. Particularly when performed before breast cancer therapy, this raises the theoretical concern of adversely affecting the cancer. These issues are addressed at length in Chapter 70. In the absence of pregnancy, the hormone treatments associated with assisted reproductive techniques are transient and generally of lower magnitude than those seen in pregnant women. Nonetheless, case reports have identified breast cancers arising in patients after IVF, raising questions about the safety of this procedure for breast cancer survivors.[90–93] Several epidemiologic studies have reported breast cancer incidence among women who received IVF treatments, compared to either the general population[94,95] or to control cohorts of infertile women who did not receive IVF therapy.[96,97] These studies have not identified an increased risk of breast cancer among women who received fertility treatments. Although these findings are reassuring, it is not known what effect fertility treatments might have on breast cancer outcomes among patients with a prior cancer diagnosis.

LACTATION AFTER BREAST CANCER THERAPY

Women who undergo breast-conserving surgical treatment may ask about and consider breast-feeding after pregnancy.[98] The extent and location of surgery affect the normal breast anatomy required for successful lactation; resection of centrally located tumors is more likely to impair lactation. Radiation therapy also can affect lactation and is known to cause lobular sclerosis and atrophy within breast tissues.[99] Patients with breast cancer may experience asymmetric breast enlargement during pregnancy, with the treated breast not experiencing hypertrophy.[100] In a single-institution experience, 4 patients were able to lactate from the irradiated breast among 11 patients who became pregnant after breast-conserving surgery and radiation. However, these patients reported difficult lactation from the breast, with reduced milk output and feeding problems, as the baby preferred the untreated breast.[100] A multicenter retrospective review identified 53 women who became pregnant after breast-conserving surgery and radiation treatments. Of these, one-third had some lactation from the affected breast, but only 25% could successfully breast-feed from the treated breast.[101] Again, many of these patients reported low milk output or other feeding difficulties from the irradiated breast.

PSYCHOSOCIAL IMPLICATIONS

No studies have assessed the relative importance of fertility concerns in patients with breast cancer. It is likely that premature menopause has important emotional and social implications that extend beyond the physical and psychological symptoms that result from reduced levels of estrogen. For some women, the loss of fertility may affect feelings of femininity, self-esteem, and identity.[102] These feelings are compounded in women who have grappled with the physical changes brought about by breast cancer surgery and other treatments.[103] The loss of reproductive potential may be disturbing, even to those women who had not planned on having children. For women who were anticipating more children, the loss of childbearing potential may be of even greater magnitude. Furthermore, the diagnosis of breast cancer may, in and of itself, affect a woman's interest in childbearing. A woman who was not previously inclined to have children might find herself more interested than she previously imagined. For some patients, having children after breast cancer connotes a positive outlook on life and a restoration of normal family relationships.[98] Conversely, other women may respond to breast cancer with less interest in childbearing than before. No easy solutions to these concerns exist, but clinicians who care for young women with breast cancer must be aware of these issues and sensitive to the distress that they may cause for some patients.

DIRECTIONS FOR FURTHER RESEARCH

In this area of breast cancer care, the unknown questions greatly exceed the known answers. Several important avenues of research need to be pursued. These include the following:

1. Identification of risk of amenorrhea associated with newer regimens and agents, particularly taxanes, used in adjuvant chemotherapy
2. Examination of the utility of gonadal protection in the preservation of menstrual function among patients who receive chemotherapy
3. Clarification of the risks of reproductive technology in breast cancer survivors
4. Assessment of the long-term physical and psychological impact of premature ovarian failure in women with breast cancer

CONCLUSION

Considerations of reproductive health are important in planning the long-term treatment of younger patients with breast cancer. Treatment-related menopause remains a significant, irreversible side effect of adjuvant chemotherapy, and concerns over fertility may be a guiding force in choosing adjuvant therapies. Issues of reproductive health and childbearing often take on an intensity and acuity at the time of breast cancer diagnosis and can heighten the strain at a difficult time. In most of these instances, the data are relatively sparse, particularly for any given individual who is trying to assess the risks, and the personal choices are of profound importance. Appropriate medical information and counseling, using colleagues from other specialty disciplines when needed, can help patients understand these complex issues, enabling them to make better decisions.

REFERENCES

1. American Cancer Society. *Breast cancer facts and figures*, 1997.
2. Zeleznik AJ, Hillier SG. The ovary: endocrine function. In: Hillier SG, Kitchener HC, Neilson JP, eds. *Scientific essentials of reproductive medicine*. London: WB Saunders, 1996:133.
3. Carr BR. The normal menstrual cycle. In: Carr BR, Blackwell RE, eds. *Textbook of reproductive medicine*, 2nd ed. Stamford, CT: Appleton & Lange, 1998:233.
4. Sherman BW, West JH, Korenman SG. The menopausal transition: analysis of LH, FSH, estradiol, and progesterone during menstrual cycles of older women. *J Clin Endocrinol Metab* 1976;42:629.
5. Walsh BW, Schiff I. Physiology of the climacteric. In: Carr BR, Blackwell RE, eds. *Textbook of reproductive medicine*, 2nd ed. Stamford, CT: Appleton & Lange, 1998:727.
6. Margoulis GB. Effect of aging on fertility and pregnancy. *Semin Reprod Endocrinol* 1991;9:165.
7. Van Blerkom J. Introduction: intrinsic factors affecting the outcome of laboratory-assisted conception in the human. In: Van Blerkom J, ed. *The biological basis of early human reproductive failure*. New York: Oxford University Press, 1994:3.
8. Spira A. The decline of fecundity with age. *Maturitas* 1988;10[Supp 1]:15.
9. Damewood MD, Grochow LB. Prospects for fertility after chemotherapy or radiation for neoplastic disease. *Fertil Steril* 1986;45:443.
10. Reichman BS, Green KB. Breast cancer in young women: effect of chemotherapy on ovarian function, fertility, and birth defects. *J Natl Cancer Inst Monogr* 1994;16:125.
11. Bines J, Oleske DM, Cobleigh MA. Ovarian function in premenopausal women treated with adjuvant chemotherapy for breast cancer. *J Clin Oncol* 1996;14:1718.
12. Hensley ML, Reichman BS. Fertility and pregnancy after adjuvant chemotherapy for breast cancer. *Crit Rev Oncol Hematol* 1998;28:121.
13. Wallace WHB, Shalet SM, Crowne EC, Morris-Jones PH, Gattamaneni HR, Price DA. Gonadal dysfunction due to cis-platinum. *Med Pediatr Oncol* 1989;17:409.
14. Maneschi F, Benedetti-Panici P, Scambi G, Salerno MG, D'Agostino G, Mancuso S. Menstrual and hormone patterns in women treated with high-dose cisplatin and bleomycin. *Gynecol Oncol* 1994;54:345.
15. Culine S, Lhomme C, Kattan J, Michel G, Duvillard P, Droz JP. Cisplatin-based chemotherapy in the management of germ cell tumors of the ovary: the Institut Gustave Roussy experience. *Gynecol Oncol* 1997;64:160.
16. Warne GI, Fairley KF, Hobbs JB, Martini FIR. Cyclophosphamide-induced ovarian failure. *N Engl J Med* 1973;289:1159.
17. Gradishar WJ, Schilsky RL. Ovarian function following radiation and chemotherapy for cancer. *Semin Oncol* 1989;16:425.
18. Ataky K, Moghiss K. Chemotherapy-induced premature ovarian failure: mechanisms and prevention. *Steroids* 1989;54:607.
19. Rose DP, Davis TE. Ovarian function in patients receiving adjuvant chemotherapy for breast cancer. *Lancet* 1977;1:1174.
20. Schulz KD, Schmidt-Rhode P, Weymar P, Kunzig HJ, Geiger W. The effect of combination chemotherapy on ovarian, hypothalamic and pituitary function in patients with breast cancer. *Arch Gynecol* 1979;227:293.
21. Sherman BM, Wallace RB, Jochimsen PR. Hormonal regulation of the menstrual cycle in women with breast cancer: effect of adjuvant chemotherapy. *Clin Endocrinol* 1979;10:287.

22. Samann NA, DeAsis DN, Buzdar AU, Blmenschein TR. Pituitary-ovarian function in breast cancer patients on adjuvant chemoimmunotherapy. *Cancer* 1978;41:2084.
23. Mehta RR, Beattie CW, Das Gupta TK. Endocrine profile in breast cancer patients receiving chemotherapy. *Breast Cancer Res Treat* 1991;20:125.
24. Brincker H, Mouridsen HT, Andersen KW, et al. Castration induced by cytotoxic chemotherapy. *J Clin Oncol* 1989;7:679.
25. Goldhirsch A, Gelber RD, Castiglinoe M. The magnitude of endocrine effects of adjuvant chemotherapy for premenopausal breast cancer patients. The International Breast Cancer Study Group. *Ann Oncol* 1990;1:183.
26. Bianco AR, Del Mastro L, Gallo C, et al. Prognostic role of amenorrhea induced by adjuvant chemotherapy in premenopausal patients with early breast cancer. *Br J Cancer* 1991;63:799.
27. Ludwig Breast Cancer Study Group. A randomized trial of adjuvant combination chemotherapy with or without prednisone in premenopausal breast cancer patients with metastases in one to three axillary lymph nodes. *Cancer Res* 1985;45:4454.
28. Tancini G, Valagussa P, Bajetta E, et al. Preliminary 3-year results of 12 versus 6 cycles of surgical adjuvant CMF in premenopausal breast cancer. *Cancer Clin Trials* 1979;2:285.
29. Cobleigh MA, Bines J, Harris D, SaFollette S, Lincoln ST, Wolter JM. Amenorrhea following adjuvant chemotherapy for breast cancer. *Proc Am Soc Clin Oncol* 1995;14:115.
30. Bryce CJ, Shenkier T, Gelmon K, Trevisan C, Olivotto I. Menstrual dysruption in premenopausal breast cancer patients receiving CMF (IV) vs. AC adjuvant chemotherapy. *Breast Cancer Res Treat* 1998;50:284.
31. Fisher B, Sherman B, Rockette H, et al. l-Phenylalanine mustard (l-PAM) in the management of premenopausal patients with primary breast cancer: lack of association of disease-free survival with depression of ovarian function. *Cancer* 1979;44:847.
32. Colbeigh MA, Bines J, Lincoln ST, Wolter JM. Amenorrhea following adjuvant chemotherapy for breast cancer. *Proc Am Soc Clin Oncol* 1994;13:63.
33. Valagussa P, De Candis D, Antonelli G, Bonadonna G. Reproductive potential after adjuvant chemotherapy for breast cancer. *Recent Adv Cancer Res* 1996;140:277.
34. Sutton R, Buzdar AU, Hortobagyi GN. Pregnancy and offspring after adjuvant chemotherapy in breast cancer patients. *Cancer* 1990;65:847.
35. Weber B, Luporsi E. Ovarian toxicity of breast cancer chemotherapy. *Eur J Cancer* 1998;34[Suppl 5]:S42.
36. Hortobagyi GN, Buzdar AU, Marcus CE, Smith TL. Immediate and long-term toxicity of adjuvant chemotherapy regimens containing doxorubicin in trials at M. D. Anderson Hospital and Tumor Institute. *J Natl Cancer Inst Monogr* 1986;1:106.
37. Sanders JE, Buckner CD, Amos D, et al. Ovarian function following marrow transplantation for aplastic anemia or leukemia. *J Clin Oncol* 1988;6:813.
38. Keilholz U, Korbling M, Dehrentz D, Bauer H, Hunstein W. Long-term endocrine toxicity of myeloablative treatment followed by autologous bone marrow/blood derived stem cell transplantation in patients with malignant lymphohematopoietic disorders. *Cancer* 1989;64:641.
39. Deeg HJ. Delayed complications and long-term effects after bone marrow transplantation. *Hematol Oncol Clin North Am* 1990;4:641.
40. Hinterberger-Fischer M, Kier P, Kalhs P, Marosi C, Geissler K, Schwarzinger I, et al. Fertility, pregnancies and offspring complications after bone marrow transplantation. *Bone Marrow Transplant* 1991;7:5.
41. Gulati S, Van Poznak C. Pregnancy after bone marrow transplantation. *J Clin Oncol* 1998;16:1978.
42. Byrne J, Fears FR, Gail MG, Pee D, Connelly RR, Austin DF, et al. Early menopause in long-term survivors of cancer during adolescence. *Am J Obstet Gynecol* 1992;166:788.
43. Donegan WL. Breast cancer and pregnancy. *Obstet Gynecol* 1977;50:244.
44. Danforth DN. How subsequent pregnancy affects outcome in women with a prior breast cancer. *Oncology* 1991;11(5):23.
45. Rivkees SA, Crawford JD. The relationship of gonadal activity and chemotherapy-induced gonadal damage. *JAMA* 1988;259:2123.
46. Ghalie R, Porter C, Radwanska E, Fitzsimmons W, Richman C, Kaizer H. Prevention of hypermenorrhea with leuprolide in premenopausal women undergoing bone marrow transplantation. *Am J Hematol* 1993;42:350.
47. Laufer MR, Townsend NL, Parsons KE, et al. Inducing amenorrhea during bone marrow transplantation: a pilot study of leuprolide acetate. *J Reprod Med* 1997;42:537.
48. Montz FJ, Wolff AJ, Cambone JC. Gonadal protection and fecundity rates in cyclophosphamide-treated rats. *Cancer Res* 1991;51:2124.
49. Ataya K, Rao LV, Lawrence E, Kimmel R. Luteinizing hormone–releasing hormone agonist inhibits cyclophosphamide induced ovarian follicular depletion in rhesus monkeys. *Biol Reprod* 1995;52:365.
50. Kreuser ED, Klingmuller D, Thiel E. The role of LHRH-analogues in protecting gonadal functions during chemotherapy and irradiation. *Eur Urol* 1993;23:157.
51. Blumenfeld Z, Haim N. Prevention of gonadal damage during cytotoxic therapy. *Ann Med* 1997:29:199.
52. Chapman RM, Sutcliffe SB. Protection of ovarian function by oral contraceptives in women receiving chemotherapy for Hodgkin's disease. *Blood* 1981;58:849.
53. Redman J, Kirsch J, Zokiner B, Bajorunas D. Ovarian function in women treated with combined modality therapy for clinical stage IA, IIA, and IIIA Hodgkin's disease (HD): ineffectiveness of oral contraceptives in preseving ovarian function. *Proc Am Soc Clin Oncol* 1987;6:195.
54. Blumenfeld Z, Avivii I, Linn S, Epelbaum R, Ben-Shahar M, Haim N. Prevention of irreversible chemotherapy-induced ovarian damage in young women with lymphoma by a gonadotrophin-releasing hormone agonist in parallel to chemotherapy. *Hum Reprod* 1996;11:1620.
55. Waxman JH, Ahmed R, Smith D, Wrigley PFM, Gregory W, Shalet S, et al. Failure to preserve fertility in patients with Hodgkin's disease. *Cancer Chemother Pharmacol* 1987;19:159.
56. Mastro LD, Venturini M, Sertoli RM, Rosso R. Amenorrhea induced by adjuvant chemotherapy in early breast cancer patients: prognostic role and clinical implications. *Breast Cancer Res Treat* 1997;43:183.
57. Powles TJ. Prognostic impact of amenorrhoea after adjuvant chemotherapy. *Eur J Cancer* 1998;34:603.
58. Budman DR, Berry DA, Cirrincione CT, Henderson IC, Wood WC, Weiss RB, et al. Dose and dose intensity as determinants of outcome in the adjuvant treatment of breast cancer. *J Natl Cancer Inst* 1998;90:1205.
59. Obwegeser R, Auerbach L, Kubista E. Gynaecological aspects of tamoxifen treatment in breast cancer patients. *Cancer Treat Rev* 1997; 23:289.
60. Osborne CK. Tamoxifen in the treatment of breast cancer. *N Engl J Med* 1998;339:1609.
61. Sunderland MC, Osborne CK. Tamoxifen in premenopausal patients with metastatic breast cancer: a review. *J Clin Oncol* 1991;9:1283.
62. Chang J, Powles TJ, Ashley SE, Iveson T, Gregory RK, Dowsett M. Variation in endometrial thickening in women with amenorrhea on tamoxifen. *Breast Cancer Res Treat* 1998;48:81.
63. Ribeiro G, Swindell R. The Christie Hospital adjuvant tamoxifen trial—status at 10 years. *Br J Cancer* 1988;57:601.
64. Wolf DM, Jordan VC. Gynecologic complications associated with long-term adjuvant tamoxifen therapy for breast cancer. *Gynecol Oncol* 1992;45:119.
65. Berkowitz GS, Skovron ML, Lapinski RH, Berkowitz RL. Delayed childbearing and the outcome of pregnancy. *N Engl J Med* 1990;322:659.
66. O'Reilly-Green C, Cohen WR. Pregnancy in women aged 40 and older. *Obstet Gynecol Clin North Am* 1993;20:313.
67. Byrne J, Mulvihill JJ, Myers MH, et al. Effects of treatment on fertility in long-term survivors of childhood or adolescent cancer. *N Engl J Med* 1987;317:1315.
68. Blatt J, Mulvihill JJ, Ziegler JL, Young RC, Poplack DG. Pregnancy outcome following cancer chemotherapy. *Am J Med* 1980;69:828.
69. Myers SE, Schilsky RL. Prospects for fertility after cancer chemotherapy. *Semin Oncol* 1992;19:597.
70. Nicholson HS, Byrne J. Fertility and pregnancy after treatment for cancer during childhood or adolescence. *Cancer* 1993;71:3392.
71. Ariel IM, Kempner R. The prognosis of patients who become pregnant after mastectomy for breast cancer. *Int Surg* 1989;74:185.
72. Cooper DR, Butterfield J. Pregnancy subsequent to mastectomy for cancer of the breast. *Ann Surg* 1970;171:429.
73. Malamos NA, Stathopoulos GP, Keramoploulos A, Papadiamantis J, Vassilaros S. Pregnancy and offspring after the appearance of breast cancer. *Oncology* 1996;53:471.
74. Petrek JA. Pregnancy safety after breast cancer. *Cancer* 1994;74:529.
75. Von Schoulz E, Johansson H, Wilking N, Rutqvist LE. Influence of prior and subsequent pregnancy on breast cancer prognosis. *J Clin Oncol* 1995;13:430.

76. Lathaby AE, O'Neill MA, Mason BH, Holdaway IM, Harvey VJ. Overall survival from breast cancer in women pregnant or lactating at or after diagnosis. *Int J Cancer* 1996;67:751.
77. Kroman N, Jensen MB, Melbye M, Wohlfahrt J, Mourisden HT. Should women be advised against pregnancy after breast-cancer treatment? *Lancet* 1997;350:319.
78. Rissanen PM. Pregnancy following treatment of mammary carcinoma. *Acta Radiol Ther Phys Biol* 1969;8:415.
79. Mignot L, Morvan F, Berdah J, et al. Grossesses apres cancer du sein traite. *Presse Med* 1986;15:1961.
80. Collichio FA, Agnello R, Staltzer J. Pregnancy after breast cancer: from psychosocial issues through conception. *Oncology* 1998;12:759.
81. Surbone A, Petrek JA. Childbearing issues in breast carcinoma survivors. *Cancer* 1997;79:1271.
82. Winkel CA, Fossum GT. Current reproductive technology: considerations for the oncologist. *Oncology* 1993;7(3):40.
83. Laufer N, Simon A, Hurwitz A, Glatstein IZ. In vitro fertilization. In: Seibel MM, ed. *Infertility,* 2nd ed. Stamford, CT: Appleton & Lange, 1997:703.
84. Steinkampf MP, Hammond KR, Blackwell RE. Ovulation induction. In: Carr BR, Blackwell RE, eds. *Textbook of reproductive medicine*, 2nd ed. Stamford, CT: Appleton & Lange, 1998:565.
85. El Hussein E, Tan SL. Successful in vitro fertilization and embryo transfer after treatment of invasive carcinoma of the breast. *Fertil Steril* 1992;58:194.
86. Brown JB, Modell E, Obasaju M, Ying YK. Natural cycle in-vitro fertilization with embryo cryopreservation prior to chemotherapy for carcinoma of the breast. *Hum Reprod* 1996;11:197.
87. Sauer MV, Paulson RJ, Lobo RA. Successful pre-embryo donation in ovarian failure after treatment for breast carcinoma. *Lancet* 1990; 335:723.
88. Sauer MV, Paulson RJ, Ary BA, Lobo RA. Three hundred cycles of oocyte donation at the University of Southern California: assessing the effect of age and infertility diagnosis on pregnancy and implantation rates. *J Assist Reprod Genet* 1994;11:92.
89. Casey ML, MacDonald PC, Simpson ER. Endocrinological changes of pregnancy. In: Wilson JD, Foster DW, eds. *Williams textbook of endocrinology,* 8th ed. Philadelphia: WB Saunders, 1992:977.
90. Laing RW, Glaser MG, Barrett GS. A case of breast carcinoma in association with in vitro fertilization. *J Royal Soc Med* 1989;82:503.
91. Brzezinski A, Peretz T, Mor-Yosef S, Schenker JG. Ovarian stimulation and breast cancer: is there a link? *Gynecol Oncol* 1994;52:292.
92. Arbour L, Narod S, Glendon G, et al. In-vitro fertilisation and family history of breast cancer. *Lancet* 1994;344:610.
93. Jourdain O, Avril A, Mauriac L. Breast cancer and in vitro fertilization: about 32 cases. *Eur J Obstet Gynecol* 1996;67:47.
94. Venn A, Watson L, Lumley J, Giles G, King C, Healy D. Breast and ovarian cancer incidence after infertility and in vitro fertilisation. *Lancet* 1995;346:995.
95. Duckitt K, Templeton AA. Cancer in women with infertility. *Curr Opin Obstet Gynecol* 1998;10:199.
96. Rossing MA, Daling JR, Weiss NS, Moore DE, Self SG. Risk of breast cancer in a cohort of infertile women. *Gynecol Oncol* 1996;60:3.
97. Braga C, Negri E, La Vecchia C, Paraaini F, Dal Masa L, Franceschi S. Fertility treatment and risk of breast cancer. *Human Rep* 1996;11:300.
98. Dow KH, Harris JR, Roy C. Pregnancy after breast conserving surgery and radiation therapy for breast cancer. *J Natl Cancer Inst Monogr* 1994;16:131.
99. Schnitt SJ, Connolly MD, Harris JR, Cohen RB. Radiation-induced changes in the breast. *Hum Pathol* 1984;15:545.
100. Higgins S, Haffty BG. Pregnancy and lactation after breast-conserving therapy for early-stage breast cancer. *Cancer* 1994;73:2175.
101. Tralins AH. Lactation after conservative breast surgery combined with radiation therapy. *Am J Clin Oncol* 1995;18:40.
102. Notman MT. Reproduction and pregnancy: a psychodynamic developmental perspective. In: Scotland NL, ed. *Psychiatric aspects of reproductive technology*. Washington: American Psychiatric Press, 1990:13.
103. Schover LR. Sexuality and body image in younger women with breast cancer. *J Natl Cancer Inst Monogr* 1994;16:177.

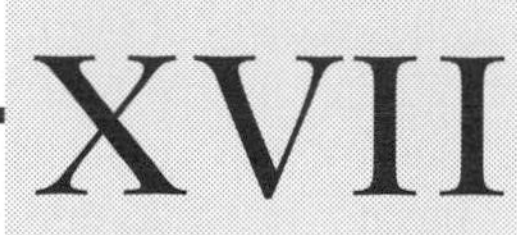

XVII

Diseases of the Breast, 2nd ed.,
edited by Jay R. Harris.
Lippincott Williams & Wilkins, Philadelphia © 2000.

Medicolegal Considerations

CHAPTER 72

Medicolegal Aspects of Breast Cancer Evaluation and Treatment

R. James Brenner

Although the clinical practice of medicine includes many internal forms of quality assurance and accountability, the external or public forum for accountability is found in the legal system and courts. When patients perceive that their medical care has been improper, they may pursue such claims by filing a lawsuit. Lawsuits occur for many reasons, but the most common reason for a claim of malpractice is a form of civil law or "tort" law called *negligence*, in which a physician's conduct is questioned as departing from a standard of care involving the exercise of ordinary skill and care that would be reasonably applied by other physicians in similar circumstances.[1] The breach of this "duty" to the patient, if it bears a substantially causative relation (called *cause in fact* and *proximate cause*) to a patient's injury, may permit the patient to sue for damages, usually in the form of money, for the legal purpose of restitution, not punishment.[2]

Delay in diagnosis of breast cancer, according to a national study in 1995 by a consortium of physician-owned insurance carriers, the Physicians Insurers Association of America (PIAA), is the most common reason that physicians are sued and the second leading cause of overall indemnity payments.[3] Public awareness of the ability to intercept the natural history of this disease in many cases; contingency fees afforded attorneys who represent a large number of women suffering from this disease, often at a relatively early age; and preventable patterns of practice likely contribute to observed claims of malpractice and loss of chance for survival.

Although an adverse event or outcome often triggers the filing of a lawsuit, it is the conduct of the physician that is at issue. The test of such conduct is "reasonableness" as defined by actual laws (statutes) or prior case decisions that have been commented on by higher or appellate courts. The

R. J. Brenner: Department of Radiology, University of California, Los Angeles, UCLA School of Medicine, Los Angeles, California; Department of Breast Imaging, Eisenbery Keefer Breast Center, John Wayne Cancer Institute, St. John's Health Center, Santa Monica, California

Mammography Quality Standards Act of 1992[4] is an example of the former; the common notions of standards of care as established by expert consultants to the court during trial are an example of the latter. This chapter examines several areas of legal exposure in the evaluation of patients for and with breast cancer, attempting to identify circumstances in which knowledge of expected conduct can be translated into risk management strategies.

PATIENT EVALUATION: CLINICAL STANDARDS AND RISK MANAGEMENT

History-taking and physical examination involve subjective and objective impressions and have been labeled both art and science. Such services are provided by primary care physicians and consultants. The definition of *primary care*, having evolved in a managed care era, customarily includes general medical practitioners (internal medicine, family practice) as well as obstetricians and gynecologists. This role has also been assumed by general and even other specialty surgeons, as well as radiologists, when breast care is provided by such physicians under circumstances in which the patient is not under the care of another physician.[5] Regardless of specialty, the duty of the primary care physician is to perform a reasonable physical examination and reasonably evaluate the patient's history (possible signs or symptoms of breast cancer). The parameters of a reasonable examination of the breast are beyond the scope of this discussion and are reviewed in Chapter 3 and elsewhere.[6] The examination needs to be thorough, including not only the entire breast, but also the axillary and clavicular nodal regions; regularly scheduled; and adequately documented. The more deliberate the evaluation, the easier it is to evaluate in a medical or medicolegal context; if proper care is rendered, this ease benefits the caregiver. For example, the diffuse "nodularity" of fibrocystic changes is of less clinical concern than a "nodule," which may connote a dominant mass.

In this regard, emphasis on the medical record and documentation is warranted. The institution of a medical malpractice lawsuit for delay in diagnosis of breast cancer occurs when a patient discovers or has reason to discover that there may have been an unreasonable delay in arriving at this diagnosis resulting from the conduct of those responsible for her care.[7] This event usually triggers a "statute of limitations," a concept that is discussed in the section Fraud. The discovery of breast cancer frequently follows a series of clinical interactions between the physician and patient, after which time the actual filing of the malpractice suit may be further delayed by 1 to 2 years. Consequently, the precise details of the clinical visits, which occurred long before the lawsuit, will likely be unknown to the patient and treating physician, or at least subject to different recollections.

The medical record is the customary manner by which the clinical examination and history-taking are documented. Although it is technically hearsay and subject to exclusion as evidence during trial, the medical record is considered a usual exception to the hearsay rules and thus admissible in court.[8] Although such records can be refuted during trial testimony, admissibility is predicated on the presumption by courts that the record is a valid and reliable indicator of what transpired during the patient visit, so long as it reflects a regular and customary entry proximately following the examination.

A well-documented medical record can thus substantiate and evidence reasonable care. As such, the record should be complete, organized, sequential, accurate, and legible. Vague descriptions of physical findings instead of objective parameters are ill advised. Although physicians often believe that they can escape accountability by vague notes, the converse is more likely. Ambiguity invites misinterpretation and affords an aggrieved plaintiff the opportunity to contend that the examination was not only suboptimally conducted, but also that vaguely defined physical findings were in fact significant and not properly managed. In addition to the example of nodule versus nodularity discussed previously, consider one appellate case in which the patient contended that a lump that was not removed was a cancer, with the medical record sufficiently clear to indicate that the eventual cancer in fact arose in a location inconsistent with the lump detected and documented earlier; the defendant physician prevailed.[9] Conversely, in the absence of such documentation, plaintiffs have prevailed under similar circumstances.[10] More often than not, well-documented deliberate care provides a basis for asserting reasonable conduct.[11]

Busy practices may find physicians struggling to document all instruction parameters thoroughly. Certain mechanisms may facilitate the accomplishment of goals without unnecessary hardship. Preprinted or stamped diagrams of the breast and nodal regions may provide a rapid basis for documenting clinical findings with near-anatomic reproducibility. Mnemonics, so long as they are used in a regular and appropriate manner, can be entered into the chart notes as evidence that certain elements of the history and patient instructions have been accomplished and committed to the record (P. Birney, Esq., *personal communication*, 1995).

Medical records, in addition to personal notes, serve many risk management purposes. The record provides documented communication to others, such as consulting physicians, insurance companies, and utilization review boards. Because photocopies of such records are often required, record entries should be made in black or dark-blue pen and in regular sequential order, with single-line entries receiving both date and personal identifying verification. Transcribed notes, when placed into the medical record, should be proofread. These elements of medical record keeping are applicable to all medical personnel and care. Delayed alteration of such records, for whatever motivation, should not occur, as the perception of altering medical records after litigation is perceived by most juries as being a basis for compromising the credibility of the physician, regardless of the circumstances, and often leads to a plaintiff verdict. If errors are detected at subsequent dates, additional entries with appropriate explanations should be entered into the record, again in sequential order.

The initial evaluation of a patient with "lumpy" breasts may be difficult, and the clinician is often prompted to assign an immediate benign or malignant impression to a given area prematurely. This approach invites overuse of surgical intervention and imaging and delayed interception of breast cancer. In such a context, repeat short-term interval clinical examinations may provide a more rational basis for deciding between continued surveillance or intervention.[12] This approach has been advocated for probably benign, clinically occult, mammographically detected lesions and has been used successfully in practice.[13,14] The medical record may be useful for documenting doubtful areas of concern and corroboration of the absence of worsening changes over time or, alternatively, provide a basis for earlier detection of an emerging abnormality. Such documentation becomes especially useful if a lesion arises in an area distinct from that in which physical findings were nonspecific and unchanging or improving.

When an area of concern is defined clinically, further evaluation is indeed necessary. This does not necessarily translate into biopsy, although biopsy may be a favored alternative. Although the concept of further evaluation is beyond the scope of this discussion, certain principles should be noted. Many courts have indicated that a diagnostic mammography study may be an important component of such further evaluation.[15,16] Appropriate referral, including surgical referral, may also be in order, and a "duty to refer" exists under conditions that require surgery. Unless care for the patient is clearly transferred to a referral source, a process that needs to be documented, the primary care physician maintains responsibility for following the patient's course. This requires reconciling data provided by imaging and pathology service consultations. In like manner, responsibility for appropriate surgical removal of a lesion lies in the purview of the surgeon, who should reconcile radiologic, clinical, and pathologic findings in deciding future patient management. After the diagnosis of cancer, future management should be under the supervision of a designated individual, whether it is the surgical or medical oncologist, primary care physician, or other treating physician.

ELEMENT OF DUTY: A VARIABLE CONCEPT

The discussion of negligence involved the establishment of a duty of reasonable conduct, the breach of which created a basis for legal liability. The element of duty should be seen as a variable or dynamic component rather than a static one. This may seem obvious, given the different presentations of patients to the clinical physician. The concept warrants further discussion, however. Judge Learned Hand, one of the leading jurisprudential commentators regarding tort law, attempted to define *standard of care* mathematically (in discussing requirements for informed consent) as the product of two factors: the likelihood of an untoward event and the severity of such an event.

In evaluating patients for breast cancer, age-related incidence, family history, or prior proliferative breast disease with atypia or lobular carcinoma *in situ* may become part of the equation.[17–20] Periodicity of screening or other surveillance may be predicated on the age of the patient or additional emerging paradigms regarding genetic status (e.g., *BRCA1*, *BRCA2*); small foci of intraductal cancer treated by excision alone may likewise influence risk assessment of the untoward event of breast cancer.[21]

Inherent in the discussion of duty and causation is another legal concept, *foreseeability*. In assessing negligence, the court focuses on the conduct of the defendant, not on the consequences of such conduct. The patient who presents for the first time with metastatic disease and who is referred immediately for interventional therapy has little legal standing for malpractice, even though her disease is diagnosed at a late stage and her prognosis may be poor. Rather, the issue of foreseeability arises when the patient presents to the clinician with nonspecific complaints that may or may not be related to cancer. The operative standard for the clinical assessment can be stated thus: Is it reasonably foreseeable that a specific area of concern represents a breast cancer?

A practical lesson derived from this legal issue is that areas of concern to the patient or physician should be discussed with the patient and that such discussion should be documented. This applies to diagnosis and therapy. For situations in which chemoprevention or chemotherapeutic trials are the basis for management decisions, the potential and limitations of each approach needs to be documented. Surveillance strategies require not only diligence on the part of the physician, but also reasonable compliance by the patient. Most states possess statutes or laws embodied in business and professional codes that are in consonance with appellate court decisions indicating a responsibility of the patient to comply with a physician's recommendations, so long as the latter were properly communicated. Such communication is often the subject of litigation, as the law sees the physician as having superior knowledge that needs to be communicated in lay terms. At times, especially when difficult subjects are being discussed, it may be useful to include family members in such a dialogue; these circumstances often occur when patients are contemplating therapy for newly diagnosed breast cancer, at which time fear and anxiety understandably distract attention. Because estates of decedent patients may also sue a physician for unreasonable communication of prognosis that requires undue hardships in resolving the patient's affairs, such family discussion becomes even more important when the patient has a poor prognosis.[22]

SCREENING AND DIAGNOSTIC MAMMOGRAPHY

The duty to order screening mammography is controversial by virtue of varying interpretations of clinical trials as well as conflict among specialty society recommendations. Although no appellate court has ruled on this matter as a standard of care, the use of screening mammography is raised at trial and has two potential considerations in risk management. The first is that emerging practice standards or critical pathways that invoke evidence-based reporting of statistically significant improved survival from screening of women between 40 and 69 years of age provide a basis to challenge the physician who does not subscribe to such guidelines.[23] A derivative issue is often raised that such studies have only selected this defined population, and women with risk factors who are either older or younger than evidence-based screening trial populations should undergo screening. The latter argument is buttressed by the higher incidence of breast cancer in the elderly population; the former is subject to controversial risk analysis, discussed in Element of Duty: a Variable Concept. The second issue relates to the availability of experts who will testify that cancers discovered clinically would have been detected earlier had a screening mammography study been performed. Although it is likely that this position is true in many cases, it is difficult to ascertain for any given set of circumstances. Clearly, the obtaining of the earlier mammography study either obviates this position or in fact permits earlier intervention.[24]

Screening mammography is performed as a universally prescribed two-view examination, the intent of which is to include all or as much breast tissue as possible to detect potential signs of malignancy in an asymptomatic population. Diagnostic mammography accomplishes this same goal but is often attended by additional ancillary procedures (e.g., special x-ray views, sonography) that also evaluate specific clinical signs or symptoms of breast cancer or abnormalities detected on screening mammography. Thus, a history and physical examination preceding the mammography study are preferred to ensure proper scheduling and to direct the radiologist's attention to areas of clinical concern; it should be recalled that screening mammography is often reasonably performed without an on-site physician, because the protocol for obtaining images is standardized.[25,26] Nonetheless, many patients are evaluated by the clinician only after mammography has been performed, inviting two potential problems.

The first problem is that the clinician may discover an abnormality that is unknown to the patient who has undergone screening mammography, thus rendering the imaging examination suboptimal for the particular circumstances. Subthreshold mammographic features may rise to areas of suspicion based on the clinical findings.[27] In fact, this situation can be remedied by having the clinician request immediate reevaluation. The second potential problem for patients who schedule their own mammography studies ("self-initiated studies") before clinical examination is a false sense of confidence that may emerge with a negative mammography result and a delay in clinical evaluation of a lump that may develop soon after the mammography examination.[5] Screening for breast cancer is not synonymous with mammographic screening, and several studies, including notably the Breast Cancer Detection Demonstration Project, have documented the complementary roles of clinical examination and mammography in detecting breast cancer.[28] This false sense of confidence has been observed in other screening trials, with a resultant delay in diagnosis of clinical breast cancer.[29]

The mammography examination, especially the interpretation, is not tantamount to an automated, reproducible blood test, but results are often received by patients and referring physicians as being entirely objective. In fact, imaging interpretation has a subjective component, just as physical examination does. Clinicians should be familiar with the center to which they refer patients for studies in terms of interpretive ability and should consider second opinions in difficult cases.[30] A minimum outcome analysis by imaging centers is required by federal statute.[4]

LAWSUIT: RECEIVING A SUMMONS AND COMPLAINT

Patient motivations for filing medical malpractice lawsuits against physicians are multifactorial and include the need for money, anger, perceptions of poor patient-physician communication, encouragement by family and acquaintances, the need for information, suspicion of cover-ups, the desire to seek revenge, the desire to protect others from harm, and frustration over the inaccessibility of physicians who would listen to and consider problems.[31,32] The image of the hurried physician incorporates many of these issues and becomes increasingly problematic in a managed care environment. In this regard, the relationship of the physician to the physician assistant is worth review. Although the use of physician assistants may be appropriate in a variety of circumstances, equivocal clinical findings may be sufficient reason for reevaluation by the clinician to corroborate a management plan.[33]

Regardless of the reasons for the lawsuit, the receiving of a summons and complaint triggers a cascade of intellectual and emotional responses by the defendant physician. These responses need to be self-contained, and the physician is advised to "freeze the past action in place and time."[34] The matter should be referred immediately to the physician's insurance carrier and the risk manager of the practice, an effort often required by the terms of the liability contract. The carrier ordinarily assigns administrative personnel and a defense attorney to the case.

The temptation to discuss the particular facts of the case with colleagues and especially patients should be resisted. Once a malpractice claim is filed, all such discussions are "discoverable" under oath. The substance of a seemingly innocuous conversation can be raised at trial, unless the conversation occurs in the presence of the defense attorney under specific circumstances. Physicians are ill advised to believe they can "quash" a complaint by trying to reason with the patient or attorney. The formal complaint is often drafted with the assistance of a prewritten "form" manual used by attorneys and often contains strong language that seems unnecessarily offensive to the defendant. Physicians should read such complaints with the assistance of trained personnel or at least understand that the language used contains required terms of art that appear exaggerated and harsh.

The period after the filing of a legal complaint is known as *discovery*, a time during which interrogatories or questionnaires, requests for medical records and other documents, and depositions or legal testimony are obtained. By these mechanisms, both plaintiff and defendant attorneys learn about the facts of the case and strategize their respective positions. Discovery may extend for more than a year. Offers of settlement may be considered; requirements regarding acceptance of such settlement offers vary with individual liability policies. Any transference of money, by settlement, verdict, forgiving of payment due, or other, must be reported to the National Practitioner Data Bank.

Court trials are concerned with determining questions of fact disputed by the parties, the "trier of fact" being either a judge or jury (notwithstanding alternative dispute resolution methods, such as mediation or arbitration). For situations in which questions of law occur, appellate courts may revisit the facts and comment on standards of conduct. In this manner, court "dicta" have been available to analyze certain acceptable forms of conduct, many of which have been included in this chapter. Every effort must be made to prevail at trial, as appellate court review of medical malpractice cases for delay in diagnosis of breast cancer is very uncommon. Unless a jury or judge's verdict is believed to be extraordinarily irreconcilable, trial verdicts are rarely reviewed and overturned.[35]

Physicians are often used by the courts as expert witnesses to help establish recognized standards of care. Although the legal system refers to this as an *objective standard*, often the concept of objective is more illusory than standard; expressed statutes or laws are less subject to interpretation. Defendants may even be named as experts if they maintain sufficient credentials to warrant such a designation. Regular appointments to (academic) centers of excellence or publications in peer-reviewed journals of materials that are relevant to the case considered may be useful in establishing the basis and reasonableness of a given approach. The increasing role of specialty society standards or practice guidelines will likely influence considerably the evidence for standards of care in court. Because they almost always represent consensus statements that are not subject to cross-examination, they are frequently excluded from direct evidence at trial as "hearsay." However, they can be used as part of the basis or foundation for expert testimony, with consequent impact on jury considerations. In addition, they have been used during negotiated settlements.[36]

An unnecessary result of the legal adversarial approach to dispute resolution has been for experts to insist that only one approach is feasible, buttressed in part when they cite published practice standards, although even published standards may vary. This situation has caused at least one researcher to question whether expert witnesses act as partisans who think it is their job to win the case.[37] The inclusion of previously overlooked legal aspects of medical practice in educational curricula may help to alleviate this problem.[38] It should be noted that, under the "two schools of thought" doctrine, courts accept conduct at variance to espoused positions, even if supported by published standards, in which a reasonable basis for such conduct can be persuasively shown.

OTHER LEGAL ACTIONS

Fraud

Intentional misrepresentation is a problem for which criminal and civil penalties apply. In 1999, even negligence has been the basis for federal investigation of "fraud and abuse" claims, a subject as serious for practicing physicians as its civil counterpart but beyond the scope of this discussion. Rather, civil fraud has current relevance as it impacts the principle of statutes of limitation. The filing of a lawsuit must be completed within a time frame (usually 1 to 2 years) defined by when a patient discovers a wrongful act (negligence) or should reasonably have discovered such act. The rationale for such statutes of limitations is also beyond the scope of this discussion but includes the reliability of accessing information and testimony within a time frame reasonably proximal to the lawsuit. If material or significant information is deliberately withheld or is misrepresented to the patient, such statutes of limitations may be extended or "tolled" and consequently may subject the physician to unending legal exposure for a given episode. Although efforts are often extended with best intentions to mitigate the anxiety of a patient who has discovered that she has breast cancer, the physician must be careful when relating the facts relevant to her care. Medical ethics dictate such standards, but the anxiety and fear imposed by the delayed discovery of breast cancer may prompt actions that, subject to interpretation, may expose the physician to unnecessary and severe legal consequences. Other technical legal doctrines, such as "continuous care," may also extend the period of legal exposure for the defendant but have only indirect relevance to risk management strategies.

Duty to Refer and Negligent Referral

When a clinical situation presents sufficient complexity that proper management is beyond the reasonable expertise of the treating physician, a duty exists to refer the patient to an appropriate physician or facility. If a physician refers a patient to such other party that the referring physician knows or has reason to know is unable to reasonably care for the patient and an untoward event occurs, then legal action may be brought not only against the second treating physician but also against the referring physician for "negligent referral." What constitutes such "reason to know" is a factual determination for the court. Although no prescriptive guidelines can be clearly made, suspension of medical staff privileges for serious offenses or extenuating economic relationships may be factors to consider.

Abandonment

The legal relationship of the patient and physician is not one of parity. A patient may elect to discontinue care from a physician at any time and for any reason, and if the physician is aware of such termination of care, the circumstances should be documented in the medical record, with record of the communication to the patient acknowledging this result. When a physician terminates a relationship with a patient for any reason, sufficient transfer of care must be accomplished and documented, with the requirements increasing depending on the acuity of a clinical condition. The causes for a breakdown in patient-physician relationships are variable, and it may not be in the best interest of either party to maintain a relationship under adversarial circumstances. This is often the case when the patient elects to bring legal action against a physician. It should be remembered that nonpayment for past services is not a sufficient legal basis for not providing appropriate care or for transference of care.

OUTCOMES REVIEW: SETTLEMENTS AND CASES

The cost of malpractice insurance for a physician varies among different states and specialties. One of the more significant elements in determining rates is the presence of statutes limiting recovery for so-called compensatory damages of pain and suffering secondary to the delay in diagnosis of breast cancer. In addition, state courts may vary in assessing damages to be awarded secondary to the future loss of chance of survival. Finally, provisions of the Employment Retirement Insurance Recovery Act have traditionally protected payors from large tort liabilities, shifting the burden of negligence to the physician even when resource limitations have been imposed by the third-party payor. This situation, which has become more noticeable in a managed care environment, has begun to be attacked in court by state legislatures (Texas and Missouri, as of this writing) and is being addressed in Congress. Physicians should be aware that denial of reimbursement will not excuse them from the "tort" liability to the patient under the common-law notions of negligence.

The rationale for assigning malpractice rates based on practice experience is a subject of ongoing evaluation.[39,40] It has been estimated that for every $100 paid to a physician, $11 is allocated for malpractice insurance.[41] Most of this money results not in direct patient compensation but is directed to administrative costs and lawyer fees. Health care reform cannot alleviate these burdens as much as modified practice patterns that avoid common mishaps in clinical work. The above discussion has been directed toward anticipating such areas of exposure and suggesting parameters for reasonable conduct. This discussion looks retrospectively at studies evaluating conduct to reinforce the importance of practice patterns already considered.

TABLE 1. *Claims counts and indemnity by specialty*

Specialty	No. of claims	Total indemnity ($)	Average indemnity ($)
Radiology	165	30,079,579	182,300
Obstetrics and gynecology	154	42,736,849	277,512
Family practice	113	19,744,677	174,732
Surgical specialty	97	24,922,537	256,933
Internal medicine	61	10,760,277	176,397
Pathology	11	3,799,502	345,409
Other physician	31	5,084,276	164,009
Corporation	30	8,155,226	271,841
Hospital	13	1,528,167	117,551
Total	**675**	**146,811,040**	**217,498**

The PIAA Breast Cancer Study of 1995, mentioned earlier, reviewed a total of 487 claims for delayed diagnosis of breast cancer, repeating their study initially done in 1990 and coming to many of the same conclusions.[3] On average, 1.88 physicians were included in lawsuits for negligence of cases reported. Primary care physicians were named most often, followed by radiologists in the 1990 study, although this order was reversed in the 1995 study. Consequently, the PIAA and American College of Radiology conducted a separate study to look at the specific reasons that radiologists were being sued, the most common including poor image quality of the mammographic study, not obtaining additional views when necessary, and poor communication of positive results.[42] Average indemnity payments for all physicians was variable; the frequency and awards are reviewed in Table 1. The study also observed an inverse relationship between age and indemnity payments, perhaps related to (a) increased awards for younger women whose earning capacities are threatened more significantly; (b) firmer breasts among young women that are more difficult to examine, together with a perceived lower index of suspicion by clinicians in this age group; and (c) attorney selection of cases in which remuneration for services is usually based on a contingency fee or percentage of the total award[34,43] (Tables 2 and 3).

TABLE 2. *Percentage of claimants by menopausal status*

Status	Claimants (%)	
	1990	1995
Premenopausal	66.9	54.9
Perimenopausal	7.7	9.0
Postmenopausal	25.4	36.1

TABLE 3. *Comparative average indemnity by claimant age*

Age (yr)	Indemnity ($) 1990	1995
20–29	286,000	375,000
30–39	330,000	358,000
40–49	194,000	334,000
50–59	135,000	262,000
60–69	73,000	197,000
70+	102,000	118,000

TABLE 4. *Reasons for delay in diagnosis*

Reason	Frequency
Physical findings failed to impress	169
Failure to follow up with patient	150
Negative mammographic report	125
Mammogram misread	110
Failure to do proper biopsy	110
Delay in or failure to consult	75
Failure to react to mammogram	60
Distracted by other health problems	55
Repeat examinations did not arouse suspicion	55
Failure to order mammogram	54
Inadequate communication	51
Poor examination by physician	50

Pain was a presenting symptom in slightly more than 27% of cases in the 1990 study and 9.2% of cases in 1995, but, given the high prevalence of this symptom among women without breast cancer, this parameter is difficult to assess. Indices of suspicion for cancer presenting as focal pain or a painful mass may need to be higher than traditional notions suggest or at least prompt evaluation for a reasonable alternative source of pain. As expected, the most common reason for allegation of malpractice is failure to respond to a clinical complaint of a mass, with or without nodal enlargement and with or without pain. Indeed, 21.4% of patients had no clinical findings, and it is not known whether the mammography study was abnormal or allegations of malpractice were made for the general reasons discussed earlier in this section. Physicians should note the observed incidence of reasons for delay in diagnosis (Table 4), recognizing that significant features that "failed to impress" the treating physician and reliance on a negative mammography report for a woman with a dominant mass are circumstances in which remedial management approaches will succeed in avoiding future liability. The average delay in diagnosis was 14 months. A 1998 Colorado Supreme Court decision addressed liability with respect to time of delay and, while permitting trial courts to exercise discretion, upheld a 92-day delay of final diagnosis—after a failed first excisional biopsy—as a basis for negligence.[43]

The findings of the PIAA have been corroborated by a summary of appellate decisions during the past 25 years.[44,45] Liability is likely to increase, if only because the frequency of breast examination and screening mammography is increasing, although this trend may not be immediately realized, as the length of time between which an adverse event occurs and is reviewed at the appellate level may be 10 years.[44,45]

A multitude of other areas affect exposure for medical malpractice, perhaps two of the more prominent ones being the failure to obtain sufficient informed consent and suing for risk of recurrence. With courts more willing to accept what a reasonable patient expects to be told about a procedure rather than what a reasonable physician should disclose, proper communication between patients and providers becomes even more important. Courts are divided on awarding damages for risk of recurrence (or cancerphobia), sometimes requiring that the plaintiff must show that it is more likely than not that cancer will in fact recur.[43,46]

SUMMARY

Experience and expertise in evaluating women for breast cancer are only as effective as their reasonable application in clinical practice. This latter parameter is the basis for legal accountability and the focus of practice patterns suggested in this chapter. Documentation is the essence of risk management in which a reasonable patient history and clinical examination have been performed. Appropriate referral and follow-up demonstrate deliberate management and avoid overuse of resources as well as delayed diagnosis. Ordering of screening mammography may not only conform to standards of practice espoused by many experts, but may also defeat speculation that a lesion could have been detected earlier. When unanticipated circumstances emerge, management needs to be reassessed and discussed with the patient. Perhaps the most powerful advice the author has given in clinical practice is, "When business as usual is not business as usual, don't treat it like business as usual." If subject to legal action, health care personnel need to be sensitive to the careful response required and the need to coordinate it with legal counsel. Physicians may not always be able to prevent adverse outcomes, but practice patterns that are validated by sound medical principles provide the most successful approach for reducing the complications of breast cancer and defeating improper legal redress.

REFERENCES

1. *Skettington v Bradley*, 366 Mich 552, 115 NW 2d 393 (1962).
2. Brenner RJ. Medicolegal aspects of screening mammography. *AJR Am J Roentgenol* 1989;153:53.
3. Physicians Insurers Association of America. *Breast cancer study: June 1995*. Washington, DC: Physicians Insurers Association of America, 1995.
4. Mammography Quality Standards Act, Publ L No. 102-359 (1992).
5. Monsees B, Destouet JM, Evens RG. The self-referred mammography patient: a new responsibility for radiologists. *Radiology* 1988; 166:691.
6. Foster RS Jr. Limitations of physical examination in the early diagnosis of breast cancer. *Surg Oncol Clin North Am* 1994;3:55.

7. *Steingart v White*, 198 Cal App 331, 496 Cal Rptr 678 (1988).
8. Fed R Evid 808(6).
9. *Dentimann v Flanary*, 86 Wis 2d 728 (1979).
10. *Deburkarte v Louvar*, 393 NW 2d 131 (Ia 1986).
11. *Chudson v Ratra*, 76 Md App 753 (1988).
12. Brenner RJ. Breast cancer evaluation: medical-legal and risk management considerations for the clinician. *Cancer* 1994;74[Suppl 1]:486.
13. Brenner RJ, Sickles EA. Acceptability of periodic follow-up as an alternative to biopsy for mammographically detected lesions interpreted as probably benign. *Radiology* 1989;171:645.
14. Sickles EA. Periodic follow-up of probably benign mammographic lesions: results for 3184 consecutive cases. *Radiology* 1991;179:463.
15. *Beckcomb v United States*, 584 F Supp 1471 (ND NY, 1984).
16. *Barrenbrugge v Rich*, 141 Ill App 3d 1046, 490 NE 3d 1368 (1986).
17. Kerliskowske K, Grady D, Barclay J. Positive predictive value of screening mammography by age, family history of breast cancer. *JAMA* 1993;270:2444.
18. Dupont WD, Page DL. Risk factors for breast cancer in women with proliferative breast disease. *N Engl J Med* 1985;312:146.
19. Colditz GA, Willet WC, Hunter DJ, et al. Family history, age, and risk of breast cancer: prospective data from the Nurses' Health Study. *JAMA* 1993;270:338.
20. vanDyck JAAM, Petronella GMP, Hendricks JHCL. Age-dependent growth rate of primary breast cancer. *Cancer* 1993;71:35.
21. Brenner RJ. Medical-legal aspects of ductal carcinoma in situ. In: MJ Silverstein, ed. *Ductal carcinoma in situ of the breast.* Baltimore, MD: Williams & Wilkins, 1997:617.
22. *Arato v Avedon*, Calif Supr Ct No so29049 (1993).
23. Hendrick RE, Smith RA, Rutledge JH, et al. Benefit of screening mammography in women aged 40–49: a new meta-analysis of radomized controlled trials. *J Natl Cancer Inst* 1997;22:87.
24. Brenner RJ. Breast cancer, breast imaging, and malpractice [Editorial]. *Breast Disease: A Yearbook Quarterly* 1995;6:15.
25. Bird RE, McLelland R. How to initiate and operate a low-cost screening mammography center. *Radiology* 1986;161:43.
26. Sickles EA, Wever WN, Galpin HD, et al. Mammographic screening: how to operate successfully at low cost. *Radiology* 1986;160:95.
27. Moskowitz M. The predictive value of certain mammographic signs in screening for breast cancer. *Cancer* 1983;51:1007.
28. Seidman H, Gelb SK, Silverberg E, et al. The Breast Cancer Detection Demonstration Project: end results. *CA Cancer J Clin* 1987;37:1.
29. Kopans DB, Feig SA. The Canadian national breast screening study: a critical review. *AJR Am J Roentgenol* 1993;161:755.
30. Brenner RJ. Evolving medical-legal concepts for clinicians and imagers in the evaluation of breast cancer. *Cancer* 1992;69[Suppl 7]:1850.
31. Waitzkin H. Doctor-patient communication: clinical implications of social science research. *JAMA* 1984;252:2441.
32. Kickson GB, Clayton GW, Githens PB, et al. Factors that prompted families to file medical malpractice claims following personal injuries. *JAMA* 1992; 267:1359.
33. *Montgomery v South Philadelphia Medical Group Inc.*, 656 A2d 1385 (Pa. Super Ct 1996), *reargument denied*, (1995).
34. Brenner RJ. Mammography and malpractice litigation: current status, lessons, and admonitions. *AJR Am J Roentgenol* 1993;161:931.
35. *Livengood v Kerr*, 391 SE 2d 371 (W Va 1990).
36. Hyams AL, Brandenburg JA, Lipsitz SR, et al. Report to physician payment review commission practice guidelines and malpractice litigation. Boston: Harvard School of Public Health, Department of Health Policy and Management, 1994.
37. Brent RL. The irresponsible expert witness: a failure of biomedical graduate education and professional accountability. *Pediatrics* 1982;70:754.
38. Beninger PR, Beninger ES, Fitzgerald FT. Survey on views and knowledge of house officers on medical legal issues. *J Med Edu* 1985;60:481.
39. Rolph JE, Kravitz RI, GoGuigan K. Malpractice claims data as a quality improvement tool: is targeting effective? *JAMA* 1991;266:2093.
40. Sloan FA, Mergenhagen PM, Buatick WB, et al. Medical malpractice experience of physicians: predictable or haphazard? *JAMA* 1989;262: 3291.
41. Domenici PV, Koop CE. Sue the doctor? There's a better way. *New York Times* June 6 1991:A19, A25.
42. Brenner RJ, Lucey LL, Smith JJ, et al. Radiology and medical malpractice claims: a report on the Practice Standards Claims Survey of the Physicians Insurers Association of America and the American College of Radiology. *AJR Am J Roentgenol* 1998;171:19.
43. *Boryla v Pash*, 937 P2d 813 (Col App 1996), *reversed*, 96 SC 735 (1998).
44. Kern KA. Causes of breast cancer malpractice litigation: a 20-year civil court review. *Arch Surg* 1992;127:542.
45. Brenner RJ. Breast cancer and malpractice: a guide to the physician. In: Brenner RJ, ed. *Seminars in breast disease* Philadelphia: WB Saunders, 1998;1:3.
46. *Potter v Firestone Tire & Rubber Co.*, 863 P2d 795 (Cal 1993).

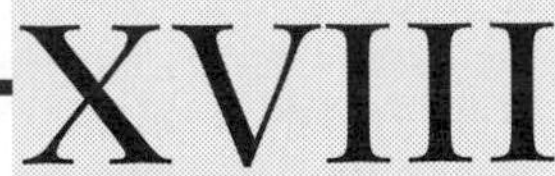

Diseases of the Breast, 2nd ed.,
edited by Jay R. Harris.
Lippincott Williams & Wilkins, Philadelphia © 2000.

Basic Tools for Advancing Knowledge in Breast Cancer

CHAPTER 73

Techniques in Molecular Biology

David Malkin and Hilmi Ozcelik

Since the initial identification and characterization of the double helix structure of deoxyribonucleic acid (DNA) in 1953, an explosion of knowledge has occurred in the field of molecular biology, the study of living organisms in terms of the properties of their constituent molecules. Of course, the concept that such molecules existed was critical to the establishment of Mendel's basic laws of genetics, established more than a century earlier. Mendel identified the *gene* as the most basic unit of genetic information. It was not until 1945, however, that Emil Schrödinger promoted the view that the laws of physics, which were until then thought to be accountable for many natural phenomena, might be inadequate to explain the fundamental properties of genetic material. In particular, the ability to maintain absolute stability from generation to generation appeared to defy established physical principles. "We shall assume the structure of the gene to be that of a huge molecule, capable only of discontinuous change, which consists in a rearrangement of the atoms and leads to an isomeric molecule. The rearrangement [mutation] may affect only a small region of the gene, and a vast number of different rearrangements may be possible."[1] Thus, physical theory attracted many physicists to study biology and molecular biology when these fields were in their infancy.

A gene does not function autonomously but relies heavily on its abilities to interact with other cellular components. Although the "average" gene is in fact a huge molecule, it nevertheless represents only part of a vast length of genetic material known as the *genome*, which contains many genes. Of the 50,000 to 100,000 genes that are thought to compose the human genome, only a small fraction have been isolated, and fewer still have a known function. Each gene is a nucleic acid sequence of the DNA molecule that carries the information defining a particular polypeptide (protein). The search for and characterization of each gene and its encoded protein have constituted a fairly tedious process, carried out in innumerable laboratories, that has relied on various labor-intensive but highly effective molecular biological techniques. A concerted international effort has led to initiation

D. Malkin: Department of Pediatrics, University of Toronto Faculty of Medicine; Division of Hematology-Oncology, Research Institute, The Hospital for Sick Children, Toronto, Ontario, Canada

H. Ozcelik: Department of Laboratory Medicine and Pathobiology, University of Toronto; Department of Pathology and Laboratory Medicine, Mount Sinai Hospital, Toronto, Ontario, Canada

of the Human Genome Project, the ultimate goal of which is to define the human genome and to use this information, as well as the application of molecular techniques, to solve fundamental problems of biology and human disease.

This chapter outlines and updates some of these molecular biological techniques as they might apply to diseases of the breast. None of these techniques is particularly unique to this group of disorders, and virtually all have been used in many biological systems, ranging from the most primitive unicellular organisms to complex vertebrates, including humans. The chapter also describes the use of these techniques to increase our understanding of the flow of genetic information in normal and pathologic cellular pathways, and of the interactive nature of these biological processes. A more detailed description of many of these techniques and their molecular foundation can be found in various textbooks.[1–4]

The reader is initially introduced to some general concepts of the basic elements of molecular analysis: the gene, DNA, ribonucleic acid (RNA), and protein. This discussion is followed by an outline of the most commonly used and well-established fundamental molecular techniques and an evaluation of novel techniques of detection for molecular genetic aberrations at each of these genetic targets. Techniques that are currently being evaluated, that are available only at selected research facilities, and for which clinical applications are still being developed are briefly discussed, although it is possible that as they translate from the research and development realm to common practice, they could supplant current technology. Finally, some of the methods used for genetic manipulation are discussed, and their applications to the understanding of biological functions are evaluated.

The applications of molecular biology theory and techniques will lead medical sciences into the next century. It will be imperative that all clinicians have at least a fundamental understanding of molecular biology so that they can effectively interact with molecular biologists and develop preventive and therapeutic applications to their full potential in the alleviation or elimination of many human diseases.

GENERAL CONCEPTS

Deoxyribonucleic Acid

The genetic code that defines the uniqueness of all organisms is carried in the ordered sequence of nucleotides that makes up the general structure of DNA. In the nucleus, DNA is condensed into chromatin along a chromosome. In humans, if each DNA molecule were unwound and laid end to end, the DNA from one cell would be a meter long. An important feature of the structure of the DNA molecule is that it is independent of the particular sequence of its component nucleotides. Although the particular sequence may in fact affect the gross molecular structure and conformation of the molecule, the sequential code of nucleotides ultimately dictates the sequence of amino acids that forms the corresponding polypeptide, or protein. The relation between the DNA sequence and the corresponding sequence of the protein is called the *genetic code*. The primary sequence of its constitutive amino acids dictates the structure or enzymatic activities of each unique protein. Characteristic segments within the nucleotide sequences are often similar, or even identical, between genes encoding proteins with similar biological functions. In addition, certain sequences are conserved phylogenetically through the animal or plant kingdoms. Such conservation is thought to indicate that these regions are important in the function of the protein. Other regions of the DNA molecule contain nucleotide sequences that are recognized as binding sites for molecules that regulate functions of DNA sequences upstream or downstream of that particular region.

Each nucleic acid consists of a chemically linked sequence of four subunits, each of which is composed of a nitrogenous base, a pentose sugar, and a phosphate group. The *pyrimidines* and *purines* represent the two types of nitrogenous bases. Adenine and guanine are the two purines and are found in RNA and DNA; cytosine and thymine are the two pyrimidines found in DNA, whereas cytosine and uracil are the pyrimidines found in RNA. The bases are usually referred to by their first letters: A,G,C,T, and U. Two types of pentose are found in nucleic acids. In DNA, it is 2-deoxyribose, whereas in RNA, ribose is the sugar. The base-sugar-phosphate–linked group is called a *nucleotide*, and these nucleotides represent the building blocks from which the nucleic acids are constructed. Thus, the nucleotides are linked to form a polynucleotide chain, referred to as the backbone of the molecule.

As originally demonstrated by Watson and Crick in 1953,[5] DNA is a double-stranded helix in which only two types of nucleotide base pairings can occur: adenine with thymine and guanine with cytosine. The model requires the two polynucleotide chains to run in opposite directions, one strand running in the 5' to 3' and the other in the 3' to 5' direction.

The complementarity of base pairing explains three important characteristics of DNA structure and function. First, as outlined previously, it is the basis on which the linear arrangement of nucleotides on the one DNA strand specifies with absolute fidelity the structure and sequence on the opposite strand.

Second, the complementarity of the double helix provides DNA with the ability to encode its own replication. Each of the parental strands can act as a template for synthesis of a complementary daughter strand. In a zipperlike fashion, the two parental strands separate so that each becomes a template. Each daughter duplex is identical to the original parent. In this manner, the original nucleotide sequence can be replicated again and again. It is this principle that was the basis for the development of the polymerase chain reaction (PCR) technique that has revolutionized molecular biology. The complex interaction of enzymes that unwind strands, remove nucleotides, add nucleotides, and "correct" errors of pairing are described in detail in most genetics and biochemistry textbooks and are beyond the scope of this chapter.

Third, the complementary DNA sequence indirectly mediates the synthesis of proteins. In any given region of the genome, only one of the two strands of DNA encodes a protein. For this reason, the genetic code is written as a sequence of bases rather than as base pairs. The code is read in groups of three consecutive nucleotides, each group representing one amino acid. Each trinucleotide sequence is termed a *codon*. The triplet code is outlined in Table 1. The starting point at which the codons are read (in a 5' to 3' direction) represents the way in which nucleotide sequence can be altered by the insertion or deletion of a single base. The resulting *frameshift* leads to the generation of a completely different reading frame that would alter the entire amino acid sequence and function of the protein.

Mutations of the DNA sequence can lead to altered protein structure, which can lead to altered or abrogated protein function. In this manner, many protein functions have been elucidated from the position of the mutations within their encoding DNA sequence. Spontaneous mutations, resulting from normal cellular mechanisms or random interactions with environmental factors (mutagens), occur as characteristic background rates in all organisms. Such mutations are necessarily rare events, and particularly damaging ones are selected against during evolution. Treatment of cells and tissues with mutagens, either *in vitro* or *in vivo*, can induce mutations.

Any base pair of the DNA molecule can be mutated. Two principal mechanisms exist that lead to the occurrence of a point mutation, which changes a single base pair. Either a chemical modification of the DNA directly changes one base to a different base, or an error of DNA replication leads to the incorrect base insertion into the polynucleotide chain during DNA synthesis. Two terms are used to describe the types of base changes. *Transitions* represent the substitution of one pyrimidine for another or of one purine for another. *Transversions*, which are generally less common, represent the substitution of a purine for a pyrimidine or vice versa. Rarely, mutagens are analogues of the usual bases, such as bromouracil, which is an analogue of thymine. Base analogues may be inappropriately incorporated into the DNA strand in place of one of the regular bases. The ambiguous pairing properties of these analogues permit the base to change its structure and thus pair with a selection of potential bases. In each replicating cycle of the duplex, the mistaken incorporation can occur as long as the analogue is present. For the most part, point mutations do not induce a frameshift as do insertions or deletions. If the point mutation leads to the substitution of a particular amino acid with a termination codon, however, the encoded protein may be prematurely truncated and its function altered or completely destroyed.

Chemical modification of one of the four bases can also lead to functional alteration of the DNA molecule. The most commonly modified base is 5-methylcytosine, which is generated by the enzymatic addition of a methyl group to a small proportion of the cytosine residues of DNA. These

TABLE 1. *Genetic code*

RNA codons	Amino acid	Abbreviations	
GCA, GCC, GCG, GCU	Alanine	ala	A
AGA, AGG, CGA, CGC, CGG, CGU	Arginine	arg	R
GAC, GAU	Aspartic acid	asp	D
AAC, AAU	Asparagine	asn	N
UGC, UGU	Cysteine	cys	C
GAA, GAG	Glutamic acid	glu	E
CAA, CAG	Glutamine	gln	Q
GGA, GGC, GGG, GGU	Glycine	gly	G
CAC, CAU	Histidine	his	H
AUA, AUC, AUU	Isoleucine	ile	I
UUA, UUG, CUA, CUC, CUG, CUU	Leucine	leu	L
AAA, AAG	Lysine	lys	K
AUG	Methionine	met	M
UUC, UUU	Phenylalanine	phe	F
CCA, CCC, CCG, CCU	Proline	pro	P
AGC, AGU, UCA, UCC, UCG, UCU	Serine	ser	S
ACA, ACC, ACG, ACU	Threonine	thr	T
UGG	Tryptophan	trp	W
UAC, UAU	Tyrosine	tyr	Y
GUA, GUC, GUG, GUU	Valine	val	V
UAA, UAG, UGA	Stop		

sites then become hot spots for spontaneous point mutations, which are exclusively G-C to A-T transitions. DNA replication itself does not maintain the presence of methylcytosine. Rather, the methyl group needs to be added to each successive generation. As with point mutations, insertions, or deletions, base pair methylation can be reversed. In this manner, modification of the DNA sequence can occur after it has been synthesized. After a mutation has passed through one generation of replication, however, it inevitably becomes a permanent part of the genetic information.

Mutations in DNA are not completely random events. Some sites are more frequently mutated than expected from a random distribution, whereas other codons or nucleotides are rarely altered. The hot spots for mutations vary and depend on the inducing mutagen. Not all hot spots are sites for all types of mutation. Furthermore, not all DNA mutations actually result in a detectable change in phenotype. Such mutations are referred to as *silent mutations*. They may involve base changes that do not alter the amino acid coded for in the corresponding protein. Other silent mutations do change the amino acid, but the switch does not affect the protein's activity. Rarely, although one mutation may in itself significantly alter protein function, the occurrence of a second mutation elsewhere in the DNA sequence might compensate for this effect and restore the protein's integrity.

The complementary nature of the double helix, the ordered sequence of nucleotides, and the naturally occurring means by which DNA is altered provide the biochemical bases for the principal techniques of recombinant DNA technology.

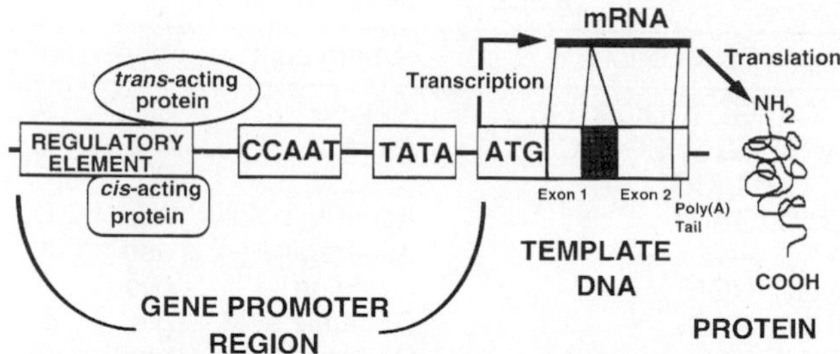

FIG. 1. DNA is transcribed to RNA and translated to protein. Regulatory elements and the CCAAT and TATA boxes are involved in the positive and negative signaling of the initiation of transcription from the start codon ATG. Introns are spliced out from the precursor messenger RNA (mRNA) recognized by specific sequences at the splice-donor and splice-acceptor sites. A stop codon and poly(A) tail at the end of the gene delineate the termination of the template DNA. mRNA is translated into protein in a process mediated by ribosomes moving along the mRNA in a 5' to 3' direction.

Ribonucleic Acid

Several complex steps are required for genetic information contained within the DNA nucleotide sequence to be converted successfully to a functionally intact protein. It is the *transcription* of the genome into RNA that reflects much of the complexity of this system.

RNA is synthesized from the DNA template (Fig. 1). Although they are almost always single stranded, RNA molecules do have complex structures. They frequently have short double-helical regions, which form when two sections of an RNA nucleotide chain lie in a hairpin fold in the correct "antiparallel" orientation for base pairs. The tertiary structures of certain RNA species, particularly transfer RNA (tRNA, described later in this section), are important to their ultimate function. The four bases in the RNA polynucleotide chain are A, G, C, and U. Although, like DNA, base pairings are usually A-T and G-C, weaker G-U pairings occasionally can be identified.

RNA polymerase II is the enzyme principally involved in the transcription of genes from DNA sequence into RNA. The RNA copy of the DNA that is to become protein is termed *messenger RNA* (*mRNA*). This RNA sequence is complementary to the template strand and identical to the coding strand of DNA. The starting point of transcription occurs at the promoter region of the gene (see Fig. 1). The promoter sequence actually surrounds the first base pair that is to be transcribed into RNA. The promoter's function is to be recognized by proteins that control the rate and degree of transcription. In this way, promoters and adjacent transcription control sites differ from other nucleotide sequences, the primary roles of which are exerted through transcription or translation. The information for promoter function is provided directly by DNA sequence, and its structure represents the actual signal. Conservation of bases over only very short consensus sequences is typical of these regulatory sites. Most promoters have a *TATA box*, usually located approximately 25 base pairs upstream of the starting point. This A-T base pair element tends to be surrounded by G-C–rich sequences. The fixed position of the TATA box is critical to the positioning of the RNA polymerase. Another important sequence approximately 70 bases upstream of the starting point is the *CAAT box*. This region plays an important role in determining the efficiency of the promoter but does not appear to play a role in promoter specificity. Other upstream elements have been characterized and are known to modify the rate of transcription from specific promoters in either a positive or negative way. They act, therefore, to regulate gene expression during embryologic development and cellular differentiation. From the promoter region, the RNA polymerase enzyme travels along the template, synthesizing RNA, until it reaches a *terminator* sequence (see Table 1). It might seem that RNA polymerase transcribes genes in an indiscriminate fashion, but other proteins, known as *transcription regulators*, ensure when particular genes are ready for transcription. For a short stretch, as the RNA polymerase moves along the unwinding DNA molecule, the DNA is in a single-stranded conformation. Within a few bases (as soon as the enzyme has passed by), the DNA duplex reforms. In this fashion, the integrity of the DNA molecule is maintained during transcription.

The nucleic acid sequence of the gene includes not only the *coding region* found in the mRNA, which corresponds to the amino acid sequence of the protein, but also additional intervening sequences that lie within the coding region, thus interrupting the sequence that represents the protein. Thus, the *exons* are the regions of the gene represented in the mRNA, whereas *introns* are regions that are absent from the mRNA. The process in which introns are removed from the RNA to yield an mRNA that consists only of exons is known as *RNA splicing*. This processing of the gene and RNA occurs in the nucleus. In addition to splicing out of the introns, a series of some 200 adenine residues is added to the terminal end of the mRNA molecule, which is then said to be *polyadenylated*. Subsequently, the mRNA is transported to the cytoplasm and translated into protein.

Translation of mRNA to protein occurs on the ribosomes within the cell. Each ribosome consists of two subunits, which contain several proteins in association with a long RNA molecule known as *ribosomal RNA*. The generation of the protein's polypeptide change is mediated by yet another small RNA species, termed *transfer RNA* (*tRNA*). A tRNA is able to recognize only the one amino acid to which it is covalently linked. The tRNA contains a trinucleotide sequence, the anticodon, which is complementary to the codon that represents the amino acid. The anticodon allows the tRNA to recognize the codon through complementary base pairing. The ribosome moves along the mRNA, permitting sequential amino acids to be assembled into protein.

As noted earlier (see Table 1) the relation of triplet codons to their respective amino acids is referred to as the genetic code. Because any of the four possible nucleotides can

TABLE 2. *Characteristics of some restriction sites*

Recognition sequence and cleavage points	Restriction endonuclease	Characteristics
... ↓ ... GG CC ...CC↑GG...	*Hae*III	4 bases, flush ends
... ↓ ... GTT ACC ...CAA↑TTG...	*Hpa*I	6 bases, flush ends
... ↓ ... TCG A ...A GC ↑ T...	*Taq*I	4 bases, cohesive ends
...↓ ... GAATTC ... CTTAAG↑...	*Eco*RI	6 bases, cohesive ends
... ↓ ... CTPy PuAC ...GAPu↑PyGT...	*Hind*II	6 bases, ambiguity, cohesive ends
... ↓ ... G ANT C ...C TNA↑G...	*Hinf*I	5 bases, ambiguity, cohesive ends

N, any nucleotide; Pu, purine (A, G); Py, pyrimidine (C, T).

occupy any of the three positions of the codon, there are 4^3, or 64, possible trinucleotide sequence combinations. There are therefore more codons than the 20 amino acids from which proteins are synthesized. This apparent discrepancy is resolved by the observation of *degeneracy*; that is, almost every amino acid is represented by several codons. Only methionine and tryptophan carry unique trinucleotide sequences. Similar amino acids are represented by related codons, presumably in an attempt to minimize the effects of mutations. Three codons (UAA, UAG, and UGA) are used specifically to terminate protein synthesis, and one of these stop (termination) codons marks the end of every gene. Ultimately, the order of the amino acids in a protein confers its three-dimensional conformation and its biological and biochemical activities. Alteration of the amino acid sequence almost invariably alters these characteristics.

Restriction Fragments

On isolation of a segment of DNA, a critical step in obtaining its sequence is to generate a nucleotide map. The identification of *restriction enzymes* that recognize specific short DNA sequences and cleave the DNA strands at those particular sites was a critical development for this technique. These restriction enzymes are produced by bacteria as part of a restriction-modification system that protects the organism from invasion by foreign DNA. Several hundred restriction enzymes that recognize more than 150 specific nucleotide sequences have been identified. Each restriction enzyme recognizes a specific target in double-stranded DNA, usually a sequence of four to six base pairs, and the enzyme cuts the DNA at each point at which its target sequence occurs. Different enzymes recognize different target sequences, although some enzymes recognize the same sites (Table 2). When a panel of enzymes is used to cut DNA, the resulting identification of points of breakage represents a *restriction map*. The distances between breaks varies depending on the sequence of the DNA. In a DNA molecule of random nucleotide sequences, a six-base recognition sequence for a restriction enzyme would be expected to occur once in every 4,096 bases (i.e., 1 in 4^6 bases). Thus, in human DNA, which is approximately 3×10^9 base pairs long, this enzyme would cut the DNA into several million fragments. These fragments can be separated by size using *gel electrophoresis*. In this technique, the cut DNA is placed at the top of a gel made of either agarose or polyacrylamide. As an electrical current is passed through the gel, each fragment moves down the gel at a rate that is inversely proportional to the log of its molecular weight. Because DNA is negatively charged, it tends to migrate to the positive electrode. The DNA fragments can be visualized with ultraviolet light after the gel is stained with ethidium bromide, which intercalates between DNA base pairs and fluoresces when exposed to ultraviolet light. The series of bands that is generated is calibrated against a standard restriction digest of known molecular size. Each band corresponds to a fragment of particular size. The data from this restriction digest can be used to construct a (relatively primitive) map of the original fragment of DNA with which one started. By introducing other enzymes in a sequential fashion, one can generate more complex and accurate maps.

Restriction Fragment–Length Polymorphisms

The coexistence of more than one genetic variation in the population constitutes a *genetic polymorphism*. Any site at which multiple alleles exist as stable components in the population is, by definition, polymorphic. Because the DNA sequence at these sites varies, the restriction maps of the DNA sequences are also distinguishable from each other. Restriction maps of different individuals are therefore useful to detect genomic polymorphisms, which are identified as a change in the pattern of fragments produced by cleavage with a restriction enzyme. When a restriction site is present in one individual and absent in another, the extra cleavage in the first generates two fragments, whose additive size corresponds to the single fragment in the second genome. It is thought that most restriction site polymorphisms in the genome do not actually affect the phenotype. The genetic mutation, usually a point mutation, does not alter the amino acid sequence of the encoded protein. In addition, restriction site polymorphisms frequently occur in intronic sequences that are not known to be associated with any biological function.

The difference in restriction maps between two individuals is known as a *restriction fragment–length polymorphism* (*RFLP*). It can be used as a genotypic genetic marker in the same way as phenotypic markers. Often, recombination frequency can be measured between a restriction marker and a visible phenotypic marker and thus provides the basis for linking genetic loci at the molecular level to a particular phenotype. Thus, if a restriction marker is associated with a phenotypic characteristic, the restriction site must be located near or at the gene responsible for the phenotype. Several such disease-associated genes might be in this region so that, although genetic mapping cannot prove that any particular gene is responsible for the disease, it can exclude target or candidate genes. The high frequency of genetic polymorphisms in the human genome means that each individual has a unique constellation of restriction sites. The *haplotype* of that individual refers to the particular combination of sites found in a specific region.

The mapping of RFLPs has led to the construction of a linkage map for the entire human genome. This map is being used to localize a wide variety of genes associated with human disease. One example has been the localization of a breast cancer susceptibility locus (*BRCA1*) to a region of approximately five centimorgans on chromosome 17q21[6–8] and *BRCA2* on chromosome 13q24, which ultimately led to the cloning of these genes. The use of RFLP mapping assisted in narrowing the region to a manageable length whereby classic cloning techniques could be used to isolate actual genes.

FUNDAMENTAL TECHNIQUES

Polymerase Chain Reaction

Most genes of interest are present as a single copy or, at most, as a few copies, in the human genome. If 10 μg of DNA were used as a template for Southern blot analysis, as little as 10^{-5} μg of the specific gene might be detected. Thus, even when radioactive phosphorous or biotin is used to label probes,

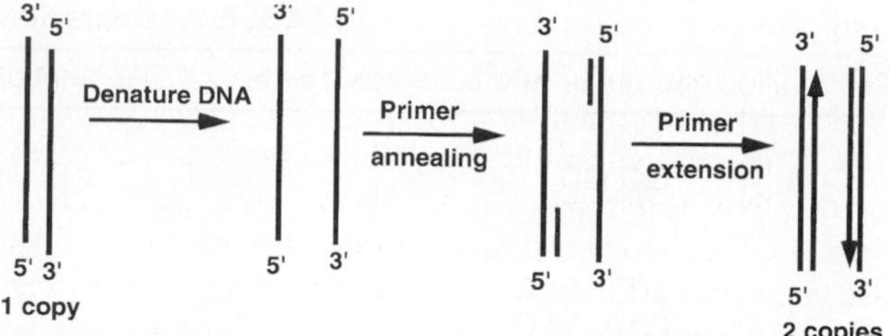

FIG. 2. The principle of the polymerase chain reaction. Three steps in each cycle are denaturation of the double-stranded DNA, annealing of sequence-specific primers to opposite ends of the target region, and extension of the primers with a temperature-stable DNA polymerase. Recognition of the sequence generates copies of the DNA between the primers in an exponential manner: Repeat for n cycles yields approximately 2^n copies.

up to a week's exposure would be required to visualize specific bands. PCR, described in 1987,[9] is a powerful procedure that allows selected regions of the genome to be amplified by a factor of 10^6 or more in an *in vitro* reaction. Although PCR is a conceptually simple procedure that has now been completely automated in its execution, it depends on knowledge of the exact DNA sequence of at least part of the region to be amplified. The procedure is graphically represented in Fig. 2. It is essentially a series of three-step cycles, with the cycles repeated 20 to 40 times to give an exponential increase of the product. At 100% efficiency in each cycle, a double-stranded DNA segment would be predicted to yield 2^{20} (more than 10^6) copies after 20 cycles. In practice, however, efficiencies are less than 100%. Nevertheless, it is relatively easy to produce 10^6 to 10^8 copies of a DNA template in a few hours.

The essential requirement for PCR is a pair of oligonucleotides, or primers, complementary to nucleotide sequences at the ends of the double-stranded DNA fragment that is to be amplified. These primers can be as short as 12 or as long as 60 base pairs. They are synthesized on machines that chemically bond successive nucleotides to produce the desired nucleic acid. One artificially generated primer is made to be complementary to a selected end of the sense strand, and the other is made to be complementary to a selected end of the antisense strand. The amplified region therefore lies between these two selected ends. It is possible to amplify several kilobases of DNA using this technique.

The PCR reaction is catalyzed by a thermostable bacterial polymerase derived from *Thermus aquaticus* (*Taq* polymerase). The series of steps shown in Fig. 2 ultimately yields an amplified fragment corresponding to the target sequence that can be visualized by gel electrophoresis.

It is possible to analyze RNA by PCR; however, it is first necessary to convert the RNA to DNA using the retroviral enzyme reverse transcriptase. The DNA is then amplified in the same manner as described in Fig. 2. The major difficulty with analysis of RNA is the requirement that the sample be fresh. The ubiquitous presence of RNA-degrading enzymes (RNases) often disrupts the molecule sufficiently that a viable template is not available.

PCR has revolutionized molecular diagnosis and recombinant DNA technology. It has been applied to genetic screening for mutation detection, detection of residual disease in patients after cancer therapy, diagnosis based on specific genetic markers, and generation of probes for various other molecular biological techniques, including many of those described here.

Gene Mutation Analysis

Deoxyribonucleic Acid Sequencing

DNA sequencing is one of the fundamental tools in the biological sciences. The ultimate definition of a gene mutation, often initially detected through a deletion or by screening, is in the determination of the exact alteration in the nucleotide sequence. The power of DNA sequence analysis is in the ability of polyacrylamide gels to resolve nucleic acid fragments that differ in length by only a single base.[10] DNA sequencing is achieved by using a single-stranded or double-stranded template, and it is the former method, described by Sanger et al. in 1977[11] (termed *chain-termination DNA sequencing*), that is used most commonly. This technique involves the synthesis of a DNA strand by a DNA polymerase *in vitro* using a single-stranded DNA template. The reaction is performed simultaneously in four tubes, each of which contains a mixture of nucleotides. Synthesis is initiated only at the site at which an oligonucleotide primer anneals to the DNA template. The DNA polymerase catalyses the sequential addition of the appropriate nucleotide to the growing chain. Synthesis is terminated by the incorporation of a nucleotide analogue that cannot support continued elongation of the DNA molecule; hence, the name *chain termination*. The chain-temination nucleotide analogues are the 2',3'-dideoxynucleoside 5'-triphosphates (ddNTPs) that lack the 3'-OH group necessary for DNA elongation. Four separate reactions (A, C, G, and T) are performed, each with a different ddNTP, to give complete sequence information. The DNA fragments that act as sequence templates are typically radiolabeled by either tagging the nucleotides or primers with ^{35}S. The reaction products are then separated by size in adjacent lanes of a high-resolution denaturing polyacrylamide gel and detected using autoradiography. The sequence is interpreted from the pattern of alternating bands in the lanes that correspond to the terminal base of the fragment (Fig. 3). The accuracy of DNA sequencing is high and can be improved by independently sequencing both strands of a DNA molecule. Any sites at which complementarity is lost are identified as possible sequencing errors, and these can be confirmed on resequencing.

Commonly, the DNA template for sequencing is formed when the product of PCR amplification of the fragment of interest is cloned into a plasmid vector. Multiple clones must be sequenced, however, to compensate for the possible errors introduced by the *Taq* polymerase used in the PCR. To overcome this problem, direct sequencing of PCR products is preferred, and many methods have been described.[1] The advent of automated sequencing instruments based on laser-fluorescence technology has replaced radioactive labels and autoradiography. A particularly important strategy takes advantage of the spectral discrimination that is possible with fluorescence to permit all four sequencing reactions to be separated by electrophoresis in a single lane. Four different fluorophores are attached to the oligonucleotide primer, which then becomes attached to the polynucleotide product of the extension reaction. Each reaction (A, G, C, T) is represented by a distinct dye. The products of each reaction are combined and then separated by electrophoresis in a single lane similar to that in conventional DNA sequencing. During the electrophoresis, a laser scans a fixed position near the bottom of the gel detecting fluorescence in the dye primers. A high-sensory detector measures the fluorescence as the tagged DNA bands migrate past this point in the gel. The DNA sequence is determined by the temporal order of the colored bands as they pass through the detector. These data are stored, analyzed, and converted to conventional DNA sequence by a computer (Fig. 4).

After DNA sequences are generated, they are entered into one or more of several internationally available computer databases. These permit other investigators to perform homology comparisons among proteins and nucleic acids

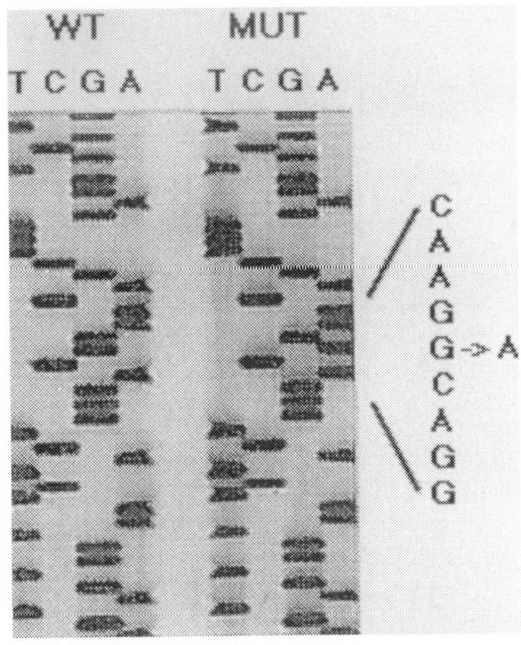

FIG. 3. DNA single-strand sequence. Each band represents the next in the sequence of bases that make up the nucleotide sequence. Each lane is dedicated to one of the four nucleotides. The three-base sequence CGG (left) represents arginine, which becomes glutamine with one base change (right). A, adenine; C, cytosine; G, guanine; MUT, mutant; T, thymine; WT, wild type.

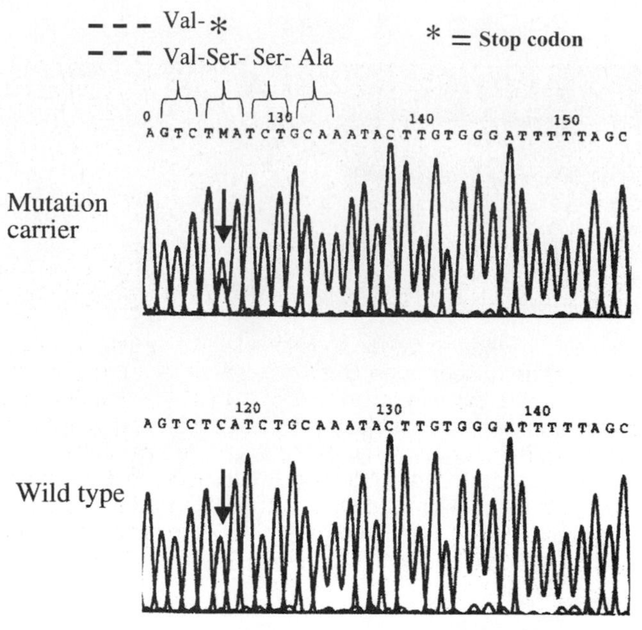

FIG. 4. Automated sequencing of a region in exon 11 of the *BRCA2* gene. Each peak represents nucleotides that make up this stretch of DNA. The lower panel is a sequence of a wild-type DNA sample. The sequence of a mutation carrier in the upper panel contains a double peak (*arrow*) in which the nucleotide "C" at position 6137 is converted to a "G." This C → G change causes the conversion of the amino acid serine to a stop codon, resulting in premature termination of the protein. The presence of a "C" nucleotide in addition to the mutated "G" implies that only one copy of the two *BRCA2* alleles is mutated in this individual.

that have already been entered, provide others with access to the data, and permit interesting regions of the genes to be screened for functionally important domains.

Single-Strand Conformational Polymorphism Analysis

To determine the frequency and characteristics of gene mutations, it is often necessary to analyze large numbers of samples concurrently. Studies of this magnitude have been made practical by the introduction of screening techniques that allow rapid and efficient determination of DNA sequence alterations without the need to sequence the entire gene of interest.

One such method for localizing single base pair differences in a DNA segment is single-strand conformational polymorphism (SSCP) analysis[12,13] (Fig. 5). This technique relies on the property that folding of single-stranded nucleic acid sequences is determined by weak stabilizing forces, such as base stacking and intrastrand pairing, which depend on single nucleotide interactions. Changes in environmental conditions (including temperature and the presence of a denaturant) are likely to result in a conformational change, which is detected in SSCP analysis on a polyacrylamide gel as an alteration in mobility of the polynucleotide strand. It has been shown that the pattern of band separation is generally reproducible for specific mutations; certain mutations are more readily identifiable under more or less stringent electrophoretic conditions. SSCP can identify more than 85% of known mutations with a very low false-negative rate. The sensitivity of the method decreases with increased size of the PCR product, a factor that can occasionally be overcome by restriction digestion of a larger amplification fragment before electrophoresis.[14–16] For SSCP analysis and denaturant gradient gel electrophoresis (described in the following section), the assay determines the existence of a sequence difference within the fragment. The precise nature of the fragment must ultimately be determined by sequencing.

Denaturant Gel Electrophoresis

An alternative screening technique to SSCP is denaturant gradient gel electrophoresis (DGGE).[17] This and similar methods, including constant denaturant gel electrophoresis,[18,19] rely on strand dissociation of DNA fragments in discrete sequence-dependent melting domains. Under the correct denaturing conditions, the DNA strand is left unfolded to a particularly minor or major degree. This dissociation causes a disruption in mobility, which is visible as

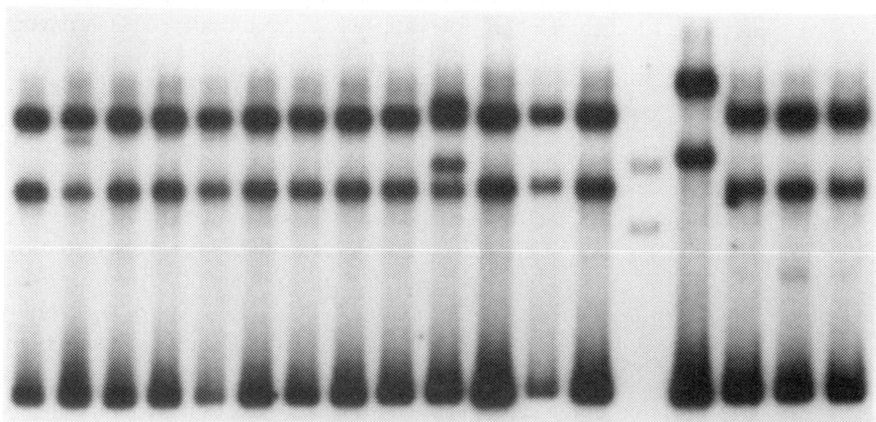

FIG. 5. Single-strand conformational polymorphism analysis of a 235 base pair fragment encompassing exon 7 of the p53 gene in genomic DNA extracted from 18 tumors. Extra bands or band shifts in lanes 2, 10, 14, and 15 indicate probable gene sequence alterations that can then be confirmed by DNA sequencing. The technique is qualitative and does not itself identify the precise nature of the base pair alteration.

with SSCP on an acrylamide gel that contains a gradient of denaturant. A long GC-rich region (GC clamp) attached to one end of the fragment holds that end together and increases resolution. By selecting a specific denaturant concentration based on computer-generated melting curves, maximum separation between wild-type and mutant fragments can be achieved. When normal and mutant fragments are present in the sample, heteroduplex formation between these noncomplementary species is often observed as multiple bands. Even with the advent of direct and automated sequencing, the ease and low expense of these screening techniques make them extremely valuable tools for the molecular biologist in the localization of potential base pair alterations in any gene.

Heteroduplex Analysis

Heteroduplex, a PCR-based technique, is similar to SSCP except that it has the advantage of being sensitive enough to detect single base substitutions in a large tract of DNA.[20,21] Because of its efficiency and simplicity, it is particularly valuable in the detection of nucleotide insertions or deletions, or both, which can be notoriously difficult to detect in a mixture of wild-type and mutant DNA. This method also detects changes on the basis of heteroduplex formation because of the presence of both wild-type and mutant gene sequences in the sample. Primers are used to amplify a region of a gene in which the known mutation occurs. Heteroduplex formation is carried out by subjecting PCR-amplified fragments to heat denaturation, during which DNA molecules are separated into their single-strand forms, and followed by a cooling-down step in which single-stranded molecules reanneal to form double-stranded molecules. In mutation carriers, during the reannealing process some mutated PCR products form incomplete pairing with the wild-type sequences. This is detected on a nondenaturing polyacrylamide gel, in which the mismatched heteroduplex molecules migrate much more slowly than the wild-type homoduplex molecules (Fig. 6).

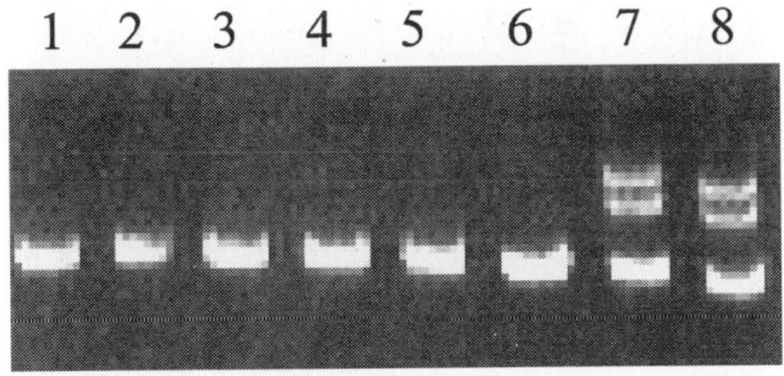

FIG. 6. The heteroduplex analysis of the hereditary breast and ovarian cancer gene *BRCA2*. A small region of *BRCA2* that contains the site for the common 6174T mutation has been amplified and subjected to nondenaturing polyacrylamide gel electrophoresis. The polymerase chain reaction (PCR) products in lanes 1 through 6 represent PCR products from individuals with wild-type sequences for this mutation, whereas lanes 7 and 8 represent PCR products from individuals who are carriers of the *BRCA2* 6174delT mutation.

Gene Products

Southern Blot Analysis

As DNA sequencing and PCR revolutionized the ability to accurately detect the most minute base pair alterations and to manipulate nucleic acid fragments, the Southern blot provided a powerful tool with which to yield a physical position to a DNA fragment of interest. It is a procedure of such wide applicability that it came to bear the name of its inventor, Ed Southern. The Southern blot[22] procedure is outlined in Fig. 7. A sample of genomic DNA, usually 5 to 10 μg, is initially digested by one or more restriction enzymes and resolved in one dimension by agarose gel electrophoresis. Low–molecular-weight DNA, representing small fragments, tends to run farther into the gel than high–molecular-weight fragments. After electrophoresis, the gel is incubated in an alkaline solution, which denatures the DNA strands embedded within. Because DNA fragments cannot be handled directly on an agarose gel, the DNA is transferred (blotted) to a solid matrix, on which hybridization reactions can occur. Nitrocellulose membranes confer a particular ability to trap single-stranded, size-sorted DNA fragments. The DNA is immobilized on the membrane by being baked in an oven. This filter, or blot, can now be placed in a hybridization solution with a radioactively labeled probe that has been rendered single stranded by rapid boiling. Only fragments that are complementary to a particular probe hybridize with it. This hybridization can be visualized through autoradiography. Each complementary sequence gives rise to a band at a position on the gel that is determined by the size of the DNA fragment. The size of the DNA fragments can be estimated by correlating the observed band positions with marker DNA fragments of known molecular weight. The amount of DNA in the sample can be estimated by the intensity of the autoradiographic signal.

Southern blotting permits a particular sequence of DNA to be detected by hybridization in the midst of innumerable DNA fragments. The technique detects large deletions and insertions as represented by the presence of junction fragments or changes in band intensities on the blots. It should be noted that, as long as some of the sequence of the probe is complementary to the target, it will hybridize. The probe also will hybridize satisfactorily to fragments of DNA that it only partly covers, yielding several fragments after Southern blotting. If they alter the restriction sites that were originally used to digest the genomic DNA, point mutations in the DNA fragment can also be inferred.[23] Southern blot analysis has also been used to identify related genes, such as oncogenes, in cells of different species. For example, when DNA

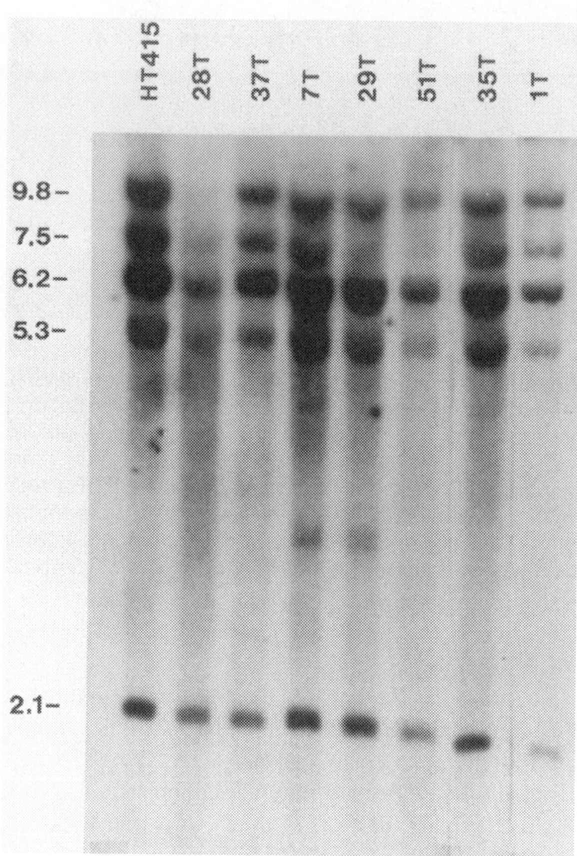

FIG. 7. Southern analysis of a series of breast cancer tumors for the presence of estrogen receptors reveals a normal pattern in lane 1 (HT415) and loss of alleles in three samples (28T, 29T, and possibly 51T) as represented by deletion of specific bands. A probe labeling a ubiquitous DNA species of 2.1 kb demonstrates the consistency of DNA concentration from sample to sample. (Courtesy of Dr. Irene Andrulis, Samuel Lunenfeld Research Institute, Toronto.)

fragments from several species are digested with a restriction enzyme, run on an agarose gel, blotted, and hybridized with a mouse probe, the probe recognizes homologous sequences not only of mouse DNA, but also of the DNA in the other species. Similarities in these gene sequences are shown by the presence of bands on the autoradiograph in lanes from each DNA sample. The implication of such a "zoo blot" is that the fragments of DNA have been conserved through evolution and presumably represent functionally important regions of the genome.

Protein Truncation Test

The protein truncation test (PTT) is a powerful technique for the rapid detection of mutations in large, multiexonic genes, in which a large fraction of mutations result in premature termination of the corresponding protein product.[24] Such mutations can be deletion or insertion of small sequences, nonsense mutations, or splice error mutations. One of the main advantages of the PTT assay is the ability to analyze large stretches of coding sequences ranging from one to three kilobases, a feature not possible with SSCP or denaturant gradient gel electrophoresis. Furthermore, PTT detects larger deletions, including partial or complete deletions of small exonic sequences that may result from genomic deletions or splicing errors. One limitation of PTT is the inability to detect single base substitutions that lead to missense codon changes. PTT is widely used, in conjunction with sequencing, in the detection of mutations in hereditary breast and ovarian cancer genes *BRCA1* and *BRCA2*. PTT is a PCR-based technique in which either DNA or cDNA can be used as a template. The primers are designed to PCR amplify a region of the gene of interest in frame with its protein translation sequence. One of the primers on the 5' end of the fragment is designed to have a linker sequence containing necessary signals for *in vitro* RNA and protein synthesis. PCR products are placed in an *in vitro* transcription/translation system, in the presence of a ^{35}S–labeled amino acid. RNA polymerase recognizes and binds to the transcription promoter sequence within the linker region of the PCR product, hence synthesizing RNA molecules that are complementary to the PCR product. Simultaneously, ribosomes in the extract recognize and bind the ribosome-binding site, thereby initiating protein synthesis from the RNA molecules. During protein synthesis, the labeled amino acids are incorporated into the newly synthesized proteins, allowing their discrimination from the existing proteins of the cell extract. During this reaction, PCR products from the individuals with two copies of wild-type sequences result in a protein of expected size. However, PCR products amplified from individuals with truncating mutations in one copy of the gene will result in a shorter protein in addition to the wild type. This occurs because the truncation mutation introduced into the transcribed RNA causes a premature termination signal for protein synthesis.

After the transcription/translation reaction, the synthesized protein products in each individual sample are subjected to electrophoresis in a manner similar to Western blotting. This system can detect the presence of truncation mutations by separating the synthesized proteins according to their molecular weight. Because the truncated proteins are smaller in size, they migrate faster than wild-type proteins and are detected as shorter bands (Fig. 8).

Pulse-Field Gel Electrophoresis

Methods of gene analysis to deal with fragments larger than 20 kilobases (kb) have been developed that use alterations in the electrical field applied to the DNA that increase the resolution of these large fragments. Basically, pulses of current rather than a constant field are used. This pulse-field gel electrophoresis (PFGE) causes the DNA molecules to align in a linear fashion within the field. The size range in

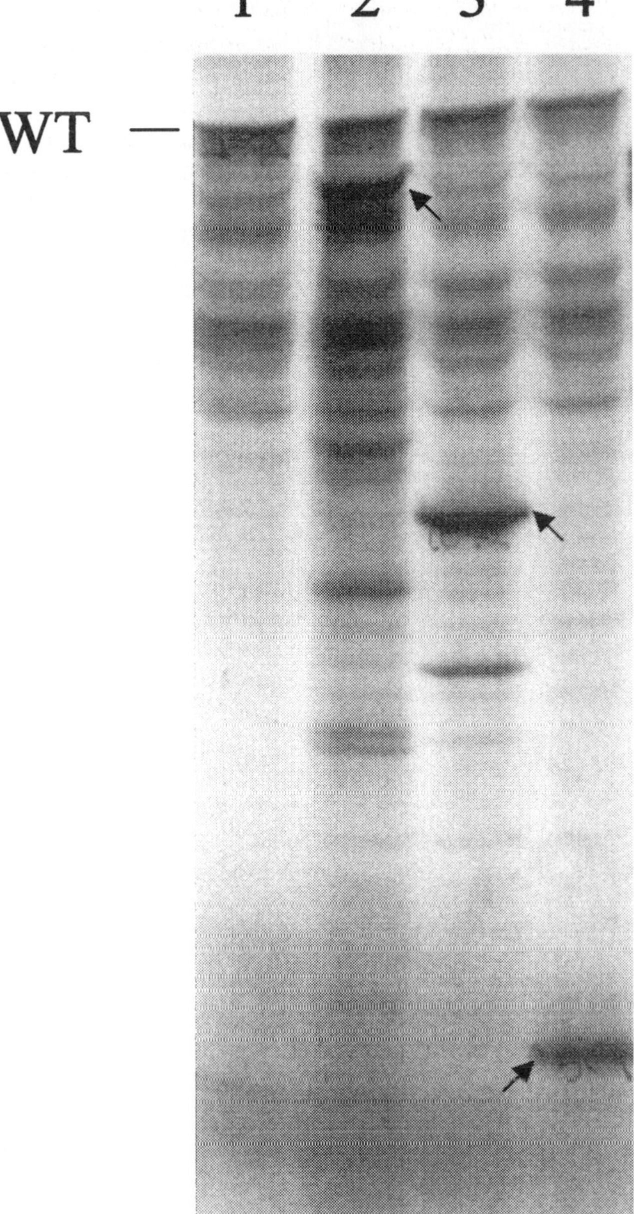

FIG. 8. Protein truncation test of the hereditary breast and ovarian cancer gene *BRCA1*. A region in exon 11 of *BRCA1* has been analyzed in four individuals using genomic DNA obtained from peripheral leukocytes. WT, wild-type protein products (expected size). The truncated protein products are detected in individuals in lanes 2 to 4 (*arrows*). The different sizes of truncated proteins imply that these individuals carry truncation mutations at different regions of the gene.

which fragments resolve depends on the position of electrode placement and the duration of the pulses. By using some of the variations of PFGE, it is possible to separate fragments as large as 7×10^6 base pairs. The use of restriction endonucleases that recognize larger sequences (eight base pair sequences) yields a manageable number of fragments that can be probed with the DNA sequence of interest. The ability of PFGE to resolve large fragments has permitted construction of physical maps of genomes from primitive organisms and of small chromosomes. The genome of *Escherichia coli*, which is approximately 10×10^6 base pairs long, has been mapped in this fashion,[25] as have the maps of other bacterial, yeast, and mammalian chromosomes, including human.[26]

Northern Blot Analysis

Northern blotting or *transfer* is a variation of the Southern technique, differing in that mRNA is the target material for hybridization. The sequence of manipulation is similar to that used for Southern blotting, but there are some important differences. First, fragmentation of RNA is usually not necessary, because mRNA species are already in the size range that is appropriate for electrophoresis and transfer. Second, denaturation of the molecule is required before transfer to disrupt the secondary structure of the unique mRNA species. Without this step, the structure would probably interfere with electrophoretic separation. The electrophoresis itself is also done under denaturing conditions to maintain the looser structure. Third, special precautions must be used in extracting and manipulating the RNA to avoid ubiquitous RNases from destroying the molecule and rendering the Northern analysis uninterpretable. The initial agarose gel electrophoresis usually indicates whether the RNA quality is adequate for analysis.

The size of the RNA sample that is probed can be estimated by correlating the band positions on the gel with marker RNA fragments of known molecular weight in a manner similar to that used for DNA fragments on a Southern blot. An estimate of the amount of RNA in the sample is estimated from the intensity of the autoradiographic signal. Thus, Northern analysis can show quantitative and qualitative information on steady-state mRNA transcripts and can identify the presence of amplified gene expression. This has been applied to MYCN expression in different clinical stages of neuroblastoma or hybrid transcripts in rearranged genomic loci, such as the novel *BCR-ABL* transcript that is expressed in chronic myelogenous leukemia and represents the molecular alteration of the t(9;22) chromosomal translocation.[27,28]

RNase Protection Analysis

Northern analysis provides data on the approximate size of an mRNA transcript but does not indicate the 5' or 3' ends with any precision or provide information on the exon-intron structure of the DNA template from which the mRNA is derived. The nuclease S_1 protection assay, or RNase protection assay, is one method to accomplish this and can also be used to better quantify particularly minute amounts of RNA. The basic method involves the protection of double-stranded hybrids from the degrading action of nucleases. A

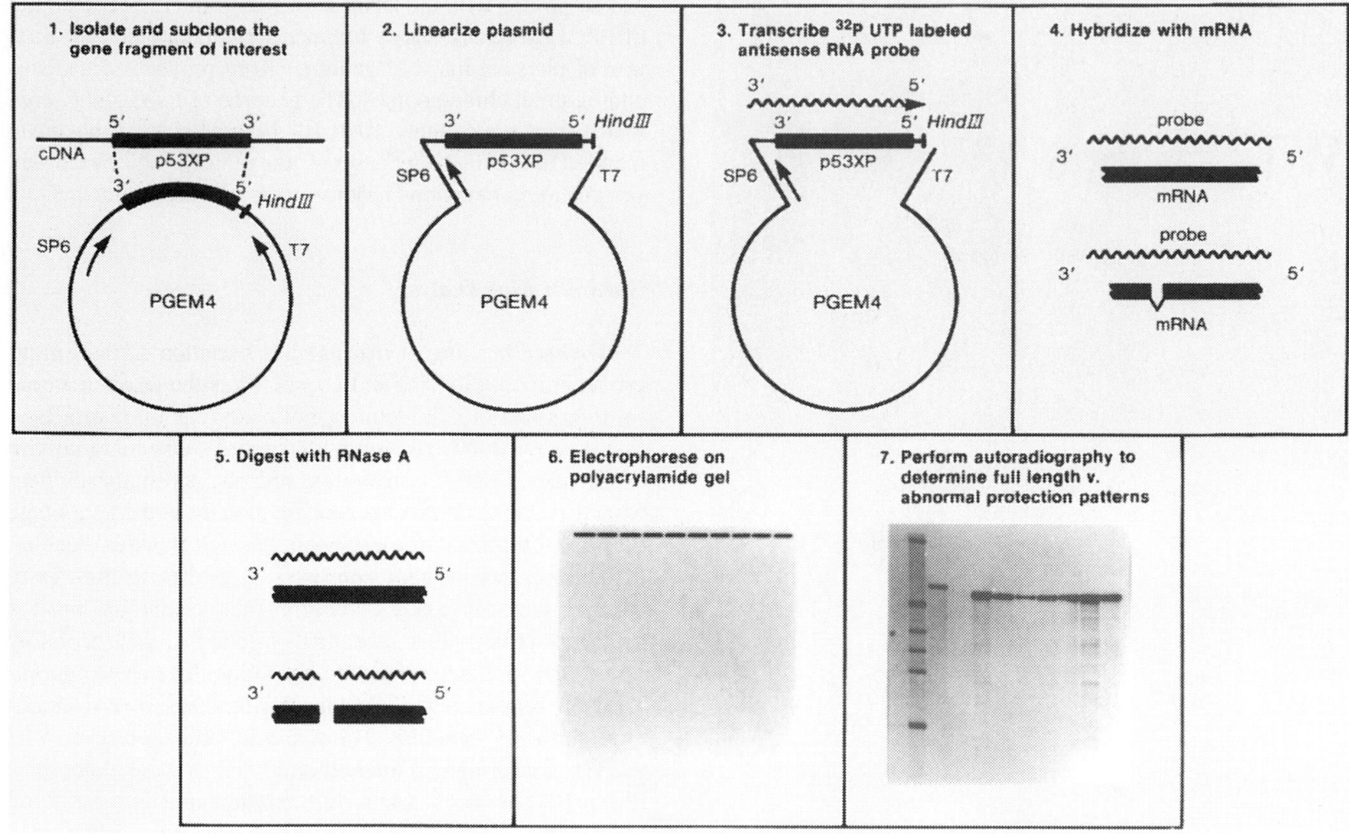

FIG. 9. Schematic representation of RNase protection analysis to determine full-length message versus abnormal patterns. See text for details. (Courtesy of Dr. Carolyn Felix, Children's Hospital of Philadelphia.)

hybrid is formed between mRNA and a complementary DNA probe. The addition of nucleases specifically degrades single-stranded DNA of RNA and leaves double-stranded structures intact. These complexes are then analyzed by polyacrylamide gel electrophoresis (Fig. 9). The extent to which the RNA protects the radiolabeled DNA probe from degradation indicates the structure of the RNA. Because conditions for annealing RNA to DNA are highly selective, S_1 nuclease protection analysis is very sensitive. If sufficient amounts of RNA are available, one mRNA molecule in 100 cells can be detected.

Western Blot Analysis

To follow convention, the electrophoretic blotting technique used to detect and analyze proteins has been designated *Western analysis*. Protein isolated from tissues, blood, or cells is subjected to electrophoresis on polyacrylamide gels that often contain a detergent to separate the molecules by their molecular weight. The separated protein is then transferred to a filter using high-voltage electrophoresis. Enzyme-linked or isotopically labeled antibodies that are species-specific are applied to the filter. After their specific protein is recognized, the antibodies bind, and the protein antibody bands can then be visualized by either autoradiographic or calorimetric methods.[29,30]

In Situ *Hybridization*

The technique of *in situ* hybridization (ISH) is based on the principle that a labeled nucleic acid probe, when rendered single stranded by heat denaturation, binds specifically to complementary sequences in fixed tissue or on a spread of denatured metaphase chromosomes. After binding has occurred and excess labeled probe has been removed, the location of the probe can be visualized by either radiographic or fluorescein-based methods, depending on what tag was used on the probe. Nonisotopic methods of labeling probes have been developed to eliminate numerous methodologic disadvantages of use of the traditional radiographic tritium. Fluorescent ISH is a modification in which the signal can be visualized after hybridization by either fluorescent microscopy or laser-scanning confocal microscopy. This technique is more rapid, less labor intensive, and less prone to scatter than isotope-based ISH. Furthermore, using different fluorochromes for different probes, it is possible to perform two-color or multicolor fluorescence. In this manner, the relative positions of probes can be deduced. This tool becomes

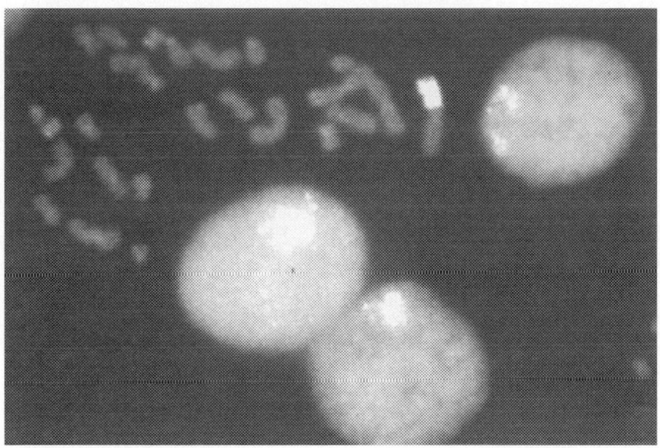

FIG. 10. Fluorescent *in situ* hybridization analysis of tumors. Neuroblastoma with 70 copies of N-*myc* present as a homogeneously staining region on chromosome 4. In the interphase nuclei of the tumor, the yellow-green domain of amplified DNA can easily be seen (*white areas*). The N-*myc* probe is labeled with biotin and detected with avidin conjugated to a yellow fluorochrome. The preparation is counterstained with propidium iodide, giving the red fluorescence of DNA (*grey areas*). (Courtesy of Dr. Jeremy Squire, Ontario Cancer Institute.)

particularly valuable when mapping the relative chromosomal positions of different, closely spaced genes (Fig. 10).

For ISH to succeed, it is critical that the target nucleic acid be retained intact *in situ*, that it not be degraded by nucleases, and that it be accessible for hybridization to the probe. Maximal sensitivity of ISH can be significantly limited by the level of nonspecific background staining. The specificity of the binding of the probe and target binding is influenced by the stringency with which the probe is washed after hybridization occurs, as well as by the extent of similarity between the probe and sequences related to but distinct from the target sequence. Resolution of the signal of probe-target binding can vary from subcellular localization, or even subnuclear localization, to greater than the cell diameter. The specific technique is frequently modified to optimize the degree of the signal for the particular target to be identified.

Microarrays

The study of breast cancer will likely benefit from a new and exciting field termed *functional genomics*. High-throughput technologies, such as cDNA microarrays,[31] are already being used to profile gene expression alterations in human cancers.[32] Essentially, cDNA microarrays contain thousands of particular cDNAs arrayed at high density on glass microscope slides that are then hybridized with labeled cDNA from two different sources, namely, the normal tissue and the tumor tissue. cDNA microarrays can be applied to many investigations and have already been used in a spectrum of applications as a gene discovery tool to a cancer classification tool based on the specific expression pattern of selected genes in particular malignant tissues. Novel software has been developed to extract biologically relevant information from the vast quantities of data produced by microarray experiments.[33] cDNA microarray technology has not only improved the speed with which cancer-associated genes are identified but has also revolutionized the way we think about and investigate the genome-wide expression patterns of genes in cancer.

CLONING GENES

Molecular cloning is the isolation and amplification of specifically defined DNA fragments. It involves the manipulation of DNA with various enzymes followed by isolation of the desired nucleic acid sequence by screening of the DNA with specific probes. In addition to the restriction endonucleases described under Restriction Fragments that are important in cutting DNA into several fragments, a group of enzymes known as *ligases* are of critical importance in cloning experiments. DNA ligase reseals the cohesive ends of two DNA fragments. The third ingredients in cloning procedures are constructs called *vectors*, which are primarily plasmids and bacteriophage DNA. Vectors have been designed that allow expression of mRNA and protein products encoded by the cloned fragment. Figure 11 outlines the procedure of genomic cloning of small fragments of DNA into a vector. Essentially, genomic DNA is cut into

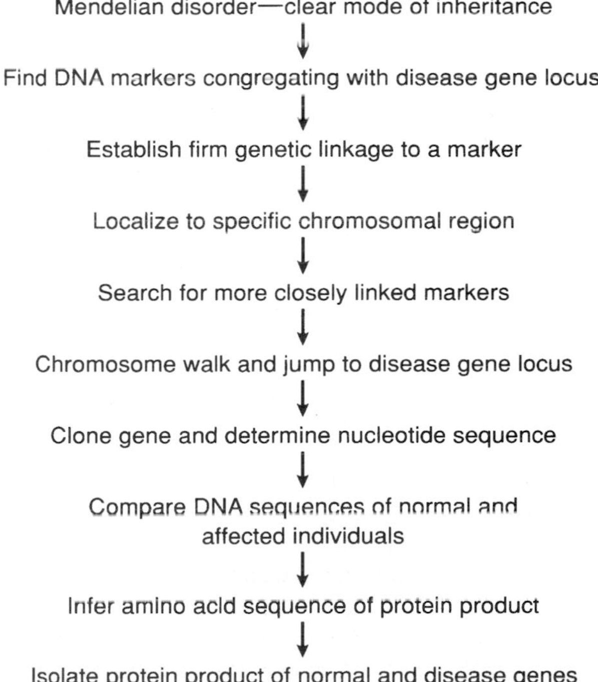

FIG. 11. Reverse genetics, or positional cloning, is represented in a flow diagram in which the clinical observation of a Mendelian disorder, such as hereditary early-onset breast cancer, ultimately yields cloning of a responsible gene and protein. Isolation of the protein is a critical step in understanding the pathogenesis of the disease.

fragments by the addition of restriction enzymes. These fragments can then be specifically ligated into a vector containing a site that has also been cut with restriction enzymes and that is able to accept the foreign DNA. After being transferred into a bacterium such as *E. coli*, small plasmids, which are circular DNA molecules, use the enzymes of the organism to replicate separately (autonomously) from the bacterial chromosome. Plasmids often contain drug-resistance genes, which render the bacterium that harbors the plasmid resistant to antibiotics such as ampicillin or kanamycin. If the foreign DNA that has been ligated into the plasmid positionally disrupts the drug-resistance gene, recombinant DNA (i.e., bacterial plasmids with foreign DNA inserts) can be isolated. This is because only plasmids with disrupted drug-resistance genes are sensitive to the antibiotic. Commercially available plasmids also use the LACZ gene as a marker for the presence of inserts. Typically, the bacteria are grown on X-gal, an artificial substrate for the LACZ-encoded enzyme, and in the presence of an LACZ gene promoter, bacteria with intact plasmids produce blue colonies on agar. In areas in which the plasmids have incorporated foreign DNA, the colonies are white. A combination of drug resistance and color selection can be used to select for bacteria that carry a DNA insert of interest.

Unfortunately, plasmids do not accommodate large vectors; for these, the development of bacteriophage vectors has been significant. These are capable of accepting DNA fragments of up to 20 kb. To handle even larger sizes of DNA, fragments are incorporated into specialized vectors, such as cosmids or yeast artificial chromosomes. The former have the part of the plasmid genome that allows autonomous replication and the phage sequences required for packaging into the phage virion.[34] The average insert size for a yeast artificial chromosome is 350 kb, which represents a huge increase on the maximal insert size of a plasmid vector.

A key step in the cloning of novel genes is the initial preparation of *libraries*, or banks of recombinant vectors, in which all the original inserted DNA sequences that correspond to the complete genome are represented at least once. In practice, such an all-inclusive library is difficult to achieve, and several different libraries may be required to augment the chances of complete representation. Two types of libraries are commonly used. The first is prepared from genomic DNA, which is first digested with a rare cutter-restriction enzyme. After being mixed with a similarly precut vector, the DNA fragments are allowed to be ligated into the vector, and the plasmids are plated with susceptible bacteria on agar. Bacteria infected with the vector are lysed, and clear areas known as *plaques* form on the agar surface. The surface can then be screened with a probe to detect the desired recombinant DNA clone. This screening process is similar to the Southern blotting technique. The colonies, or plaques, are transferred to membranes, which are then treated to denature the DNA and hybridized with the single-stranded probe. Positive spots are detected by autoradiography and, when the filter is overlaid on the agar plate, the corresponding colony containing the DNA insert can be identified. This technique can identify one recombinant molecule among millions of host genomic fragments. The colony with the relevant DNA insert can be grown to microgram or gram quantities for further analysis, which usually includes DNA sequencing to confirm the presence of the potentially novel gene. As one might expect, these DNA libraries can be reused indefinitely, using different probes that recognize different DNA sequences to isolate other DNA segments and genes.

The second, and particularly powerful, method of cloning is to develop a cDNA library. For this method, mRNA that has been isolated from specific cells or tissue is reverse transcribed to single-stranded DNA copies. DNA polymerase is used to generate double-stranded DNA fragments, which are then cloned into vectors. A particular advantage to cDNA libraries is that they are limited to only the transcribed portion of genes. They are therefore much less complex than genomic libraries. They provide amplified copies of specific sequences representative of the particular tissue or cell from which they have been derived.

Cloning genes whose protein products are unknown and whose existence is often inferred solely through a disease phenotype is more difficult than when at least part of the sequence is known. In these cases, reverse genetics or positional cloning is required. This tedious process is initiated by establishment of genetic linkage to DNA markers, followed by mapping of the whole set of markers to a specific region of the chromosome. More closely linked markers are then sought that ideally bracket the disease gene locus. These close markers can then provide the starting points for sophisticated manipulations, including chromosome walking and jumping, in which successive sequences between markers are examined for functional genes. After a candidate gene is identified, it can be cloned and sequenced and its function deduced from structural homologies with other known proteins. This approach was used to clone the *BRCA1* gene that has been implicated in the predisposition to early-onset hereditary breast and breast-ovarian cancer.[6–8,35,36]

The ultimate step in the confirmation that an isolated gene is important in the development of disease is the demonstration that the gene has a specific sequence difference between affected and unaffected individuals. The identification of point mutations in the coding region of the *p53* tumor-suppressor gene in affected members of families with Li-Fraumeni syndrome who are at particularly high risk for the development of various cancers, including breast cancer, exemplifies the candidate gene approach to characterization of a disease gene.[37,38]

The eventual cloning of the entire human genome represents a major undertaking of the Human Genome Project. It is expected that the identification and characterization of these genes will lead to an explosion of research into the functional properties of the proteins that they encode. It is hoped that eventually, with the advent of genetic therapeutic technology, this work will lead directly to intervention strategies and the prevention or successful treatment of various human diseases.

GENETIC MANIPULATION

Transgenic Animals

Organisms that carry genetic material that has been artificially introduced into the germ line are said to be *transgenic*. The inserted transgene may be a segment of genomic DNA from either a homologous or heterologous species or even from lower organisms, including prokaryotes and viruses. Cotransfer of regulatory sequences with the gene permits directed expression of the transgene in specific cells or tissue types; sometimes, when less specific expression is desired, ubiquitous regulatory sequences are used.

Three basic mechanisms have been developed for the introduction of foreign genes into the germ line:

1. DNA can be injected directly into the pronucleus of a mouse embryo using a microscope that permits manipulation of the embryo.
2. Retroviral vectors can carry the foreign gene and transfer it into the embryo in a "controlled" infection.
3. Embryonic stem (ES) cells can be manipulated to act as carriers of the transgene into the recipient blastocyst cells (see the following section).

After any of these forms of microinjection is completed, the embryos that carry the transgene are transplanted into pseudopregnant foster mothers. At birth, DNA is extracted from the offspring and assayed for the presence of the introduced foreign DNA. Assuming that the transgene does not alter the fertility of the offspring, they can then be bred, so that a certain fraction of the positive animals ultimately carries the transgene in the germ line, with the newly acquired trait frequently being transmitted through a classic Mendelian pattern of inheritance.

The transgene is usually subject to normal gene regulation, and the introduction of the foreign DNA can often lead to the development of novel phenotypes. Ectopic or increased expression of certain oncogenes and aberrant expression of tumor-suppressor genes often generate phenotypes that become models for understanding the function of the gene and its encoded protein. Stable lineages of transgenic mice have been developed that express oncogenes and present reproducible preneoplastic or neoplastic phenotypes. When driven by a promoter of mouse mammary tumor viruses, c-*myc* transgenic mice develop mammary adenocarcinomas, whereas under the regulation of an immunoglobulin promoter, the same transgene yields pre-B and B-cell lymphomas. This observation shows the direct association of the expression of these genes with the development of their respective tumors.[39] It is also possible that the abnormal expression of the gene in certain tissues or cell types is not associated with an altered phenotype, indicating the absent role of the gene in the malignant transformation of that tissue.

Embryonic Stem Cell Transfer and "Knockout" Mice

A powerful technique for the introduction of foreign genes into the germ line and generation of transgenic mice takes advantage of cultured ES cells. These are pluripotent cells derived from the mouse blastocyst (the early stage of embryonic development that precedes implantation of the fertilized egg in the uterus). The ES cells can be altered *in vitro* and then reunited with the blastocyst cells to form chimeric animals. Genes are transferred into the ES cells by electroporation, chemical methods, or microinjection. When the donor carries an additional genomic sequence, such as a drug-resistance marker or a particular enzyme, the cells that have incorporated the desired gene can be selected. PCR can also be used to assay the transfected ES cells for successful integration of the donor DNA. After the ES cells have reunited with the recipient blastocyst, some tissues derived from the chimera are of blastocyst origin, whereas others are derived from the injected ES cells. To determine whether the ES cells contributed to the germ-line lineage, the chimeric mouse is crossed with a mouse that lacks the donor trait. Any progeny that carry the trait must be derived from germ cells descended from the injected ES cells. In other words, the entire mouse has been derived from an original ES cell.

Among the most sophisticated applications of this approach is the introduction of a gene that undergoes homologous recombination with a target gene. In this manner, the normal function of a gene can be disrupted, or *knocked out*, and animal models of the consequences of such knockouts can be developed. An example of this process is the generation of mice that are homozygous or heterozygous for deficient p53 function. These mice have an increased and more rapid tendency to develop various tumors, including adenocarcinoma of the breast.[40] Often, however, the mouse phenotype of a gene knockout does not follow the predicted spectrum of tumors, perhaps reflecting cross-species variations, or the presence of modifier genes that modulate the expression of the deficient genes. Thus, *BRCA1* knockout mice do not have a particularly high propensity for the development of breast cancer. As the molecular pathways and other genes involved in carcinogenesis are characterized, it may become possible to more precisely mimic the molecular defects in animal model systems.

Gene Therapy

Mouse models are an important tool in the development of gene therapy protocols and the eventual correction of genetic defects or reversion of malignant transformation. Because the goal of gene therapy is to introduce a gene into a patient's body to replace or repair defective gene function, many of the principles developed in the study of transgenic animals may find their application in humans.[41] The most difficult problem to overcome in the translation of preclinical and animal studies of gene therapy into effective clinical protocols is the development of efficient means of gene transfer. For example, although retroviral vectors carrying transgenes are able to transduce nearly all target cells, their entry into cells depends on the presence of appropriate receptors on the target cell, most of which are not known. Furthermore, it may be necessary to induce cell mitosis to assist viral integration into the DNA of the target cell. Finally, it is often difficult to maintain more than transient integration of viral DNA, because the retroviruses are themselves unstable in the milieu of the host cell.

Since 1994, significant advances in the technical aspects of gene transfer have occurred, and early clinical trials for solid tumor gene therapy are under way. Perhaps the most difficult challenge is that few human disorders, including malignant and nonmalignant diseases of the breast, result from single gene defects. Until effective methods of multigene therapy are developed, it is unlikely that this modality of treatment will find universal use. It is nevertheless important to remember that the double helix was discovered less than one-half century ago. There is still every reason to maintain unmitigated optimism that the technical and theoretical developments in molecular biology will ultimately lead to the better prevention, screening, treatment, and cure of human disease.

ACKNOWLEDGMENTS

This investigation was supported by grant no. 3128, awarded by the National Cancer Institute of Canada, with funds from the Terry Fox Foundation. D. Malkin is a Research Scientist of the NCIC.

REFERENCES

1. Lewin B. *Genes* VI (6th ed). New York: Oxford University Press, 1998.
2. Watson JD, Hopkins NH, Roberts JW, et al. *Molecular biology of the gene*, 4th ed. Menlo Park, CA: Benjamin Cummings, 1997.
3. Alberts B, Bray D, Lewis J, et al. *Molecular biology of the cell*, 3rd ed. New York: Garland, 1994.
4. Sambrook J, Fritsch EF, Maniatis T. *Molecular cloning: a laboratory manual*, 2nd ed. Cold Spring Harbor, NY: Cold Spring Harbor Laboratory, 1989.
5. Watson JD, Crick FH. Molecular structure of nucleic acids: structure for deoxyribonucleic acid. *Nature* 1953;171:964.
6. Hall JM, Lee MK, Newman B, et al. Linkage of early-onset familial breast cancer to chromosome 17q21. *Science* 1990;250:1684.
7. Easton DF, Bishop DT, Ford D, et al. Genetic linkage analysis in familial breast and ovarian cancer: results from 214 families. *Am J Hum Genet* 1993;52:678.
8. Albertsen HM, Plaetke R, Ballard L, et al. Genetic mapping of the BRCA1 region on chromosome 17q21. *Am J Hum Genet* 1994;54:516.
9. Mullis KB, Faloona FA. Specific synthesis of DNA in vitro via a polymerase-catalysed chain reaction. *Methods Enzymol* 1987;155:335.
10. Maxam AM, Gilbert W. A new method for sequencing DNA. *Proc Natl Acad Sci U S A* 1977;74:560.
11. Sanger F, Nicklen S, Coulson AR. DNA sequencing with chain-terminating inhibitors. *Proc Natl Acad Sci U S A* 1977;74:5463.
12. Orita M, Iwahana H, Kanazawa H, et al. Detection of polymorphisms of human DNA by gel electrophoresis as single-strand conformation polymorphisms. *Proc Natl Acad Sci U S A* 1989;86:2766.
13. Iwahana H, Yoshimoto K, Itakara M. Detection of point mutations by SSCP of PCR-amplified DNA after endonuclease digestion. *Biotechniques* 1992;12:64.
14. Yap EP, McGee JO. Nonisotopic SSCP detection in PCR products by ethidium bromide staining. *Trends Genet* 1992;8:49.
15. Makino R. F-SSCP: fluorescence-based SSCP analysis. *PCR Methods Applic* 1992;2:10.
16. Ainsworth PJ, Surh LC, Coulter MMB. Diagnostic single strand conformational polymorphism (SSCP): a simplified non-radioisotopic method as applied to Tay-Sachs B1 variant. *Nucleic Acids Res* 1991;19:405.
17. Myers RM, Maniatis T, Lerman LS. Detection and localization of single base changes by denaturing gradient gel electrophoresis. *Methods Enzymol* 1987;155:501.
18. Sheffield VC, Cox DR, Lerman LS, et al. Attachment of a 40-base pair G+C–rich sequence (GC-clamp) to genomic DNA fragments by the polymerase chain reaction results in improved detection of single-base changes. *Proc Natl Acad Sci U S A* 1989;262:63.
19. Hovig E, Smith-Sorensen B, Brogger A, et al. Constant denaturant gel electrophoresis, a modification of denaturing gradient gel electrophoresis, in mutation detection. *Mutat Res* 1991;262:63.
20. White MB, Carvalho M, Derse D, et al. Detecting single base substitutions as heteroduplex polymorphisms. *Genomics* 1992;12:301.
21. Ozcelik H, Antebi Y, Cole DEC, Andrulis IL. Heteroduplex and protein truncation analysis of the BRCA1 185delAG mutation. *Hum Genet* 1996;98:310.
22. Southern EM. Detection of specific sequences among DNA fragments separated by gel electrophoresis. *J Mol Biol* 1975;98:503.
23. Cooper DN, Youssoufian H. The CpG dinucleotide and human genetic disease. *Hum Genet* 1988;78:151.
24. Roest PAM, Roberts RG, Sugino S, et al. Protein truncation test (PTT) for rapid detection of translation-terminating mutations. *Hum Mol Genet* 1993;2:1719.
25. Smith CL, Econome JG, Schutt A, et al. A physical map of the Escherichia coli K12 genome. *Science* 1987;236:1448.
26. O'Brien SJ. *Genetic maps 1987: a compilation of linkage and restriction maps of genetically studied organisms*, vol 4. Cold Spring Harbor, NY: Cold Spring Harbor Laboratory, 1987.
27. Shtivelman E, Lifshitz B, Gale RP, et al. Fused transcripts of *ABL* and *BCR* genes in chronic myelogenous leukemia. *Nature* 1986;315:556.
28. Grosveld G, Verwoerd T, Van Agthoven T, et al. The chronic myelocytic cell line K562 contains a breakpoint in bcr and produces a chimeric bcr/c-abl transcript. *Mol Cell Biol* 1986;6:607.
29. Towbin H, Staehelin T, Gordon J. Electrophoretic transfer of proteins from polyacrylamide gels to nitrocellulose sheets: procedure and some applications. *Proc Natl Acad Sci U S A* 1979;76:4350.
30. Burnette WN. "Western blotting" electrophoretic transfer of proteins from sodium dodecylsulfate polyacrylamide gels to unmodified nitrocellulose and radiographic detection with antibody and radioiodinated protein A. *Ann Biochem* 1981;112:195.
31. Schena M, Shalon D, Davis RW, et al. Quantitative monitoring of gene expression patterns with a complementary DNA microarray. *Science* 1995;270:467.
32. DeRisi J, Penland L, Brown PO, et al. Use of a cDNA microarray to analyse gene expression patterns in human cancer. *Nat Genet* 1996;14:457.
33. Eisen MB, Spellman PT, Brown P, et al. Cluster analysis and display. *Genetics* 1998;95:14863.
34. Saito I, Stark GR. Charomids: cosmid vectors for efficient cloning and mapping of large or small restriction fragments. *Proc Natl Acad Sci U S A* 1986;83:8664.
35. Miki Y, Swensen J, Shattuck-Eidens D, et al. A strong candidate for the breast and ovarian cancer susceptibility gene BRCA1. *Science* 1994;266:66.
36. Futreal PA, Liu Q, Shattuck-Eidens D, et al. BRCA1 mutations in primary breast and ovarian carcinomas. *Science* 1994;266:120.
37. Malkin D, Li FP, Strong LC, et al. Germ line p53 mutations in a familial syndrome of breast cancer, sarcomas and other neoplasms. *Science* 1990;250:1233.
38. Srivastava S, Zou ZQ, Pirollo K, et al. Germ line transmission of a mutated p53 gene in a cancer-prone family with Li-Fraumeni syndrome. *Nature* 1990;348:747.
39. Wang TC, Cardiff RD, Zukerberg L, et al. Mammary hyperplasia and carcinoma in MMTV-cyclin D1 transgenic mice. *Nature* 1994;369:669.
40. Donehower LA, Harvey M, Slagle BL, et al. Mice deficient for p53 are developmentally normal but susceptible to spontaneous tumours. *Nature* 1992;356:215.
41. Mulligan RC. The basic science of gene therapy. *Science* 1993;260:926.

Diseases of the Breast, 2nd ed.,
edited by Jay R. Harris.
Lippincott Williams & Wilkins, Philadelphia © 2000.

CHAPTER 74

Techniques in Breast Cancer Clinical Trials

Rebecca S. Gelman

TECHNIQUES IN CLINICAL TRIALS

The statistical techniques that are relevant for design and analysis of clinical trials are usually taught in 10 to 20 graduate-level courses. New statistical methods are appearing in the medical literature more rapidly after publication in the statistical literature than they were in the 1970s, making it impossible to squeeze even a very superficial survey of relevant techniques into a single course or book. As stated in a 1994 article[1] in the *Journal of the American Medical Association*, "...already the standard methods taught in an introductory [statistics] course would leave a reader unable to judge a high percentage of articles published in the *New England Journal of Medicine*, and that proportion is likely to increase with time."

This chapter might also leave a reader unable to judge the quality of a high percentage of literature reports on breast cancer trials. A single book on clinical trials[2–9] can be compared to a beginning course in cooking. A successful cooking course can teach a student to prepare one particular (and simple) dinner for friends, a successful clinical trials book may teach a student to design and analyze one particular (and simple) clinical trial. In this analogy, a chapter about clinical trials should be considered an antacid. It doesn't teach anyone how to cook or how to appreciate good cooking. It merely ameliorates some of the symptoms caused by bad cooking or overconsumption. Unfortunately, the indigestion caused by clinical trials is more varied than the indigestion caused by food and can't always be treated by a single brand of antacid. The indication for this chapter is indigestion caused by controversies in statistical power and confidence intervals, survival analysis, trial monitoring, and meta-analysis.

QUANTIFICATION OF TREATMENT DIFFERENCES: POWER AND CONFIDENCE INTERVALS

Power

Here is a common cause of indigestion. A journal article on one randomized trial states that treatment C is associated with significantly longer survival than treatment D, but another article on a similar trial states that treatment C and D do not differ in survival. How do we explain these inconsistent results? A clinician might look first at the authors of the two articles and decide which are more experienced or reliable. Or the clinician might look at specifics of eligibility and at the patient mix on the two trials. A statistician will most likely look first for statements about the power of the two trials. People who read the medical literature should be interested in the statistical power of clinical trials because there are two major explanations for a comparison that fails to be statistically significant:

1. The null hypothesis is true. (In breast cancer, the most common null hypothesis amounts to a statement that two treatments have the same effect on some specified outcome measure.)
2. The alternative hypothesis is true, but the trial did not have enough power to detect this.

Thus, if readers do not know the power of the trial, they cannot choose the most likely explanation for a nonsignificant comparison. People who plan clinical trials are interested in power because no one wants to do all the work involved in conducting a trial if it is highly likely to have an ambiguous result. What is power?

One can think of a statistical test as a type of diagnostic test. In both cases, we are trying to find out about "the true state of the world." For example, does patient P really have disease D, or is treatment C really associated with longer survival than treatment D? (For this example, assume that the null hypothesis of the study is that treatments C and D have the same survival, and the alternative hypothesis is that C has longer survival.) We try to predict the true state of the world from test results (e.g., a blood glucose level 2 hours after eating or the value of a log rank test of survival). Usually, these results are compared to a single cutoff value, such as 130 mg per dL for the blood glucose level or 3.84 for the log rank test. (In these examples, high numbers are predictive for the patient's having diabetes or for the treatments' having different survival.) Either test could have a false-positive result: A nondiabetic patient could have a high glucose level, or two similar treatments could have a large log

R. S. Gelman: Departments of Biostatistics and Radiation Oncology, Harvard School of Public Health, Harvard Medical School, Boston, Massachusetts

rank value. For the statistical test, the probability of a false-positive result is called the *significance level* or *p value*. (For the diagnostic test, one minus the probability of a false-positive result is called the *specificity*.) Either test could have a false-negative result: A diabetic patient could have a low glucose level, or two treatments could have a log rank value near zero even if treatment C truly is associated with longer survival than treatment D. In both cases, one minus the probability of a false-negative result is called the *sensitivity* of the test. For the statistical test, this value is more commonly called the *power* of the clinical trial.

Not all diagnostic tests have the same sensitivity, and not all clinical trials have the same power. It is desirable to have a large power, and most investigators would consider a power less than 80% to be inadequate (because it would correctly decide in favor of the alternative hypothesis fewer than four times out of five when the alternative is true). Larger powers than this (e.g., 90% or 95%) are appropriate for clinical trials whose results would affect large numbers of future patients, because in such a case an error in deciding which treatment is better would affect more people.

The calculation of power is based on three quantities: the size of the relevant treatment effect, the largest tolerable probability of a false-positive result (the significance level), and the effective sample size. The relevant *treatment effect* is either the smallest treatment difference it is clinically important to detect (for a trial with the alternative hypothesis that treatments are different) or the largest difference that is clinically unimportant (for a trial with the alternative hypothesis that treatments are equivalent). How the difference is expressed depends on the endpoint chosen, the difference measure used, and the statistical test to be used; "difference" here need not be subtraction, but could be a ratio or a more complicated expression. It is important that the difference specified be clinically relevant (would this much of an improvement be important to the patient?) and scientifically realistic (based on past studies of these and other treatments, is it reasonable to expect these treatments to differ this much in effect?). For instance, a 40% increase in response rate (e.g., from 50% to 90%) in a trial of two combination chemotherapies for metastatic breast cancer would be highly unusual, and therefore such a large difference would not be realistic. Similarly, a doubling of median survival time in a trial of adjuvant breast cancer therapy would also be unrealistic. In addition, the relevant treatment effect refers to the effect in the "average" patient, *not* the effect in a patient who completes all therapy as specified in the protocol.

The most common *significance level* in the medical literature is .05, but there is nothing magic about this particular number (although a few journal editors have mistakenly made it sacred by demanding that each published article contain at least one *p* value <.05). In trials whose results affect large numbers of future patients, a smaller significance level (e.g., .01 or even .001) might be appropriate. In equivalence trials, a larger significance level (e.g., .10 or .20) is frequently considered tolerable to obtain a larger than usual power (e.g., .95); it is really a question of which error is considered more disastrous and whether a 1 in 20 chance of a disastrous outcome is considered small enough. If the nonequivalence of treatments A and B is only possible if B is better than A, then a one-sided significance level is used (e.g., when A is placebo and B is a treatment without any possible detrimental effect). Otherwise, a two-sided significance level is used. Generally, a two-sided calculation should be done, unless a significant result in one direction (e.g., A better than B) would be ignored and would not be reported as an important difference.

The *effective sample size* is determined by which endpoint is being studied. For example, in a study of response percents, the effective sample size is the number of patients included in the analysis; in a study of time to event (e.g., death) the effective sample size is the number of events (e.g., deaths) that have been observed. (The number of patients who have died is always smaller than the number of patients entered in the trial multiplied by the death rate as read from an actuarial curve, unless all patients still alive have follow-up longer than the last death time.) In planning a clinical trial based on time to event, one must estimate the number of events that will have occurred at the time of analysis. In reporting a trial, one knows the actual number of events that have occurred. The difference between these two numbers (expected and actual number of events) can make a slight difference between planned power and power calculated at time of analysis. (For formulas, graphs, and computer programs to calculate power for differences in response percent, see [10–12], and for time-to-event comparisons, see [13–19].)

Table 1 shows how the power of a particular clinical trial depends on the relevant endpoint and difference measure. [This example is based on results from an International Breast Cancer Study Group (IBCSG) trial.[20]] All the power calculations assume the same number of randomized patients (2,000), the same duration of accrual (2 years), the same median follow-up (5 years), the same two-sided significance level (.05), the same statistical test (log rank), and the same statistical distribution for time to event (negative exponential). The size of the treatment effect is measured in three ways that are common in breast cancer literature: the difference between treatments in the percent of patients who have the event within the first 5 years of follow-up, the ratio of the average hazard rates over the first 5 years, and the odds ratio at 5 years. (*Hazard rate* is the instantaneous risk of the event, which is mathematically equivalent to the derivative of the log of cumulative percent survival. The *odds ratio* is the ratio of failure percents divided by the ratio of nonfailure percents. To many people, the hazard ratio and odds ratio numbers in Table 1 seem to represent a bigger treatment difference than the numbers for difference in failure percents. However, the three numbers in each row are merely different ways to quantitate the identical difference between treatments. In any trial in which a small percentage of patients have had the event of interest, the difference in failure percents looks small when compared to the equiva-

TABLE 1. *Power for various endpoints based on International Breast Cancer Study Group III*

Endpoint	5-yr failure-free % Observation	5-yr failure-free % CMFpT	Difference in 5-yr failure-free %	Hazard ratio	Odds ratio	Power
Disease-free interval	0.31	0.66	0.35	2.8	4.3	0.88
Disease-free survival	0.30	0.57	0.27	2.1	3.1	0.74
Systemic disease-free survival	0.37	0.58	0.21	1.8	2.4	0.46
Survival (breast cancer deaths only)	0.61	0.76	0.15	1.8	2.0	0.16
Survival (all deaths)	0.59	0.70	0.11	1.5	1.6	0.11

CMFpT, cyclophosphamide, methotrexate, 5-fluorouracil, prednisone, tamoxifen.
Note: Assuming 2,000 patients, 2 years of accrual, and 5-year median follow-up.

lent hazard ratio or odds ratio.) From Table 1, we might conclude that the trial has adequate power for reasonable treatment differences in some endpoints (e.g., disease-free interval) but not others (e.g., systemic disease-free survival and overall survival).

Several surveys[21–25] of the medical literature have shown that most trials do not have enough patients to have a good chance of detecting even large differences in treatment outcome, let alone reasonable differences. Zelen et al.[22] surveyed articles on randomized trials that appeared in *Cancer* between 1977 and 1979 and found the median trial size to be 50 per treatment. Mosteller et al.[23] reviewed cancer trials referenced in the 1978 book *Randomized Trials in Cancer: A Critical Review by Sites*[24] and found 108 randomized breast cancer trials with a median size of 45 per treatment. In the small survey the author conducted in 1987,[25] the median accrual for randomized trials in metastatic breast cancer was 57 per treatment; the median accrual for randomized adjuvant trials was 190 per treatment. These surveys probably overestimate the median size of clinical trials, because small "negative" trials do not always get published. To put these surveys in perspective, Table 2 uses the methods given in two references[12,17] to calculate what differences would have an 80% chance of being detected as significant in trials with various numbers of patients per treatment. For example, it would take 100 patients per treatment to have a power of 80% to detect a difference in true response percents of approximately 20% (50% on one arm and 71% on the other), yet many published trials accrue only one-half this many patients. The survival example assumes a negative exponential survival curve (which may not be appropriate for adjuvant breast cancer[26,27]), that the worse treatment is associated with a median survival of 10 years, and that accrual takes 2 years. It also assumes that there are either 3 years or 8 years of additional follow-up after accrual ends (for a 5-year or 10-year study, respectively). Not until the sample size reaches 500 does the detectable difference become at all reasonable (e.g., 15 versus 10 years). Many would argue that even 2,000 patients per treatment are not enough, because a 1-year improvement in median survival time would be of great clinical importance in a disease that kills approximately 50,000 women a year in the United States.

TABLE 2. *Differences that could be detected with significance level .05 and power 0.80*

No. of patients per treatment	Larger response percent if lower one is: 50%	Larger response percent if lower one is: 70%	Longer median survival in years if shorter one is 10 yr, accrual takes 2 yr, and additional F/U is: 3 yr	Longer median survival in years if shorter one is 10 yr, accrual takes 2 yr, and additional F/U is: 8 yr
25	89%	99.8%	180	44
50	79%	93%	44	26
100	71%	87%	26	19
200	65%	83%	19	16
500	59%	78%	15	13
1,000	56%	76%	13	12
2,000	55%	74%	12	11.5

F/U, follow-up.

There is no standard place in which one can find power statements in a medical journal article. The power of a trial can be given in the materials and methods section, the results section, or the discussion. It is often completely absent, especially in trials that have significant results (in which case the probability of a false-negative result is not directly relevant). However, for purposes of comparing different trials in the literature, and for gauging how well a trial was planned, it would be useful to include statements about power in all articles on clinical trials.

Confidence Intervals

An X% confidence interval for a parameter is an interval that has the property that, if the trial is replicated identically many times, X% of such confidence intervals will include the true parameter value. Of course, in actual practice, no trial is replicated exactly, and therefore the more common interpretation is that the X% confidence interval from a particular trial has an X% chance of containing the true parameter. The ends of the confidence interval are called *confidence limits*. The true parameter is never observed but, rather, is estimated from the data. A very common parameter for use with confidence intervals is the mean. For example, one may read that "the average [an estimate of mean] number of bone scans a patient has during the first 5 years of follow-up is 6, with a 95% confidence interval [for the true mean] of 3 to 7." Another common parameter for use with confidence intervals is the true percent. For example, one may read that "there was 70% response [the observed percent, an estimate of true percent] on this therapy, with 95% confidence interval [for the true percent] of 46% and 88%." (The phrases about "observed" and "true" parameters are often omitted, because they are assumed to be understood.) A common misperception is that confidence intervals are always symmetric about the observed parameter (e.g., average ± twice standard deviation). In fact, confidence intervals are symmetric only when the true distribution of the parameter is symmetric, and this is often not the case with biological measurements. Confidence intervals for percents are often approximated by Gaussian (i.e., normal) distributions, but these approximations are very inaccurate if the number of patients they are based on is fewer than 30 or for any number of patients if the percent being estimated is not between 20% and 80%. The confidence interval for a mean is Gaussian if the sample size is large enough, but means are not often used in breast cancer clinical trials (and are inappropriate for time-to-event data because of censoring). The confidence interval for median survival is seldom symmetric, because the survival distribution is almost never symmetric.

Confidence intervals are easiest to calculate if the underlying distribution is Gaussian, in which case the interval is symmetric, and this has resulted in the vast overuse of Gaussian confidence limits (and hence the high prevalence of symmetric confidence intervals) in the medical literature. However, as many investigators have noted, "the experimental fact is that for most physiologic variables the distribution is smooth, unimodal, and skewed, and that mean ± two standard deviations do not cut off the desired 95%."[28]

One can also make confidence intervals for treatment differences (or ratios or more complicated functions) of a parameter; for example, "The observed treatment difference in percent response was 8%, with 95% confidence interval [for the true difference] of 1% to 12%." If one did a test of how far this difference in percent is from zero, then a trial that had a 95% confidence interval that does not include zero would also find the difference to be significantly different from zero with a two-sided p value of less than .05. (However, the usual test of a difference in response percent is the Fisher exact test,[29] which is not a test of how far the difference is from zero and does not correspond to a confidence interval for this difference.) At any rate, because confidence interval percent corresponds to a significance level, it is clear that there is nothing sacred about a 95% confidence interval, just as there is nothing sacred about a 5% significance level. There are times when a 99% or a 90% confidence interval is more relevant; however, the most common confidence interval in use in the medical literature is 95%.

Some authors and journal editors[6,30] have stated that confidence intervals are a better way to summarize results of a clinical trial than hypothesis tests (and significance levels and power). Two main reasons are given for this attitude: A confidence interval reminds the reader that parameter estimates from a study are only estimates and have variability associated with them, and a confidence interval gives the reader an idea of the likely magnitude of a parameter, whereas a hypothesis test tells the reader only that one particular value (often zero) is or is not very likely. In one of the above examples, the difference in response percent was significantly greater than 0, with p less than .05. Even the estimated difference (8%) does not help the reader who would not choose the treatment with higher observed response unless it was very likely to increase true response percent by at least 5% (perhaps because that treatment has more toxicity or is more inconvenient). If provided with the 95% confidence interval of 1% to 12%, this reader would know that he or she should not yet make the treatment with the higher observed response percent the standard. On the other hand, if the 95% confidence interval were 6% to 24%, the reader would be justified in switching treatments.

Three main disadvantages exist for confidence intervals in clinical trials, however. The first is that they are made for *parameters*, and they usually correspond to *parametric tests*—that is, tests based on the known mathematical distribution of a particular parameter. Yet the majority of tests used in clinical trials are *nonparametric*, because no one knows the true mathematical distribution of most of the parameters of interest (e.g., median survival, or the percent of patients who survive longer on treatment A than on treatment B). It is very unlikely that a clinical trial will be large enough to adequately test a particular distribution assumption, precisely because the interesting significance levels correspond to values in the tails (ends) of a distribution (e.g., the most extreme 5%), and distributions that are very similar in the middle may easily be very different in the tails. It is true that most nonparametric tests could be turned into confidence intervals by using computer-intensive methods (e.g., the bootstrap[31]), but these confidence intervals are for parameters that may not have intuitive appeal (e.g., the truncated integral of the product of the cumulative survival on treatment A times the derivative of the cumulative survival on treatment B).

A second disadvantage of a confidence interval is that it applies to a single parameter. Most distributions that seem to fit real data can differ in several parameters. One can do multiple simultaneous confidence intervals for several parameters, or one can calculate confidence regions for two (or three) parameters. One can even calculate confidence curves for censored survival curves, although there is no straightforward generalization for the difference between censored survival curves. Although these extensions of confidence intervals maintain their first advantage (reminding a reader that estimates have variability), it is not clear that they always maintain the second advantage (giving the reader the idea of likely magnitude of a parameter).

The third disadvantage is that confidence intervals for treatment differences are often difficult to compute and do not have simple formulas. The difference between two Gaussian distributions is another Gaussian distribution, which greatly simplifies the calculation of the confidence interval. However, the Gaussian distribution is almost unique in this respect. The difference between two binomial distributions is not binomial; the difference between two negative exponential distributions is not negative exponential, and so on.

These disadvantages do not mean that confidence intervals should be abandoned in clinical trials. If only to emphasize that estimates have statistical variability, it would be best for each estimate reported to have some sort of confidence interval reported with it. This is because humans seem to have a tendency to underestimate statistical (and biological) variation. Most people who are told that a 20-patient trial had a 20% response percent assume that the true response percent is somewhere between 15% and 25%; in fact, this is close to a 28% confidence interval (and would not cover the true response percent 72% of the time). The 95% confidence interval is 6% to 44%. However, because the confidence intervals corresponding to the most common statistical tests used in clinical trials are difficult to calculate and interpret for the reasons given previously, it is not necessary for every test to be accompanied by a confidence interval.

ANALYSIS OF SURVIVAL DATA

Estimation

In a clinical trial, the outcome variable may be the time between two events. Examples are survival (time from randomization or diagnosis to death), disease-free survival (time from primary treatment to first metastases or recurrence or death), and duration of response (time from first documentation of partial response to first documentation of relapse). In all of these measures, the date of the first event is known for all patients; the date of the second event is unknown for some patients, either because no information is available or because the event has not yet occurred for these patients. Such patients are said to be censored for survival; the time from the first date to the date last known to be free of the second event is called the *censored survival time*.

To estimate the survival curve of a group of patients, one typically uses either the life table (also called the *actuarial method*)[2,32–35] or the modification of that method proposed by Kaplan and Meier.[36–39] These methods assume that the censored patients are just like the uncensored patients in their true survival experience and that the mechanism causing patients to have censored survival times is statistically independent of their true survival times. When the mechanism that causes censoring is related in any way to the patients' true survival times, the actuarial method is inappropriate or misleading. Two examples are patients who are lost to follow-up (and therefore censored) for reasons related to therapy or disease status and patients who are censored for death from the cause of primary interest because they die from competing causes. One cannot say *a priori* how patients lost to follow-up affect the analysis. It may sometimes be advisable to count patients who are lost because they are too sick to continue on study as "failures," rather than censored observations. One can also accommodate this type of censoring by making mathematical assumptions about the nature of the relationship between survival and censoring,[40] but these assumptions are usually difficult to check.

The setting in which competing causes result in censoring a patient for the event of interest can arise when deaths not attributable to cancer are counted as censored or when the endpoint is local recurrence and the occurrence of distant recurrence or death leads to censoring. One approach[41] to this problem is to reorient the analysis to first analyze time to first unfavorable event. If no difference is seen in the distribution of this time, then one analyzes type of first unfavorable event (e.g., local failure versus distant failure versus death). When such compound endpoints are unacceptable, specific mathematical assumptions about the relationship between types of failure may allow actuarial-type estimates to be computed.[42]

Comparing the Survival Times of Two Groups of Patients

Deciding whether one of two treatments is associated with better survival time would not be easy, even if the two true survival curves were exactly known. Although it is possible to obtain consensus about which of two integers is larger, it may be difficult or impossible for a group of people to agree on which of two curves is "better." For example, treatment A could be associated with higher early mortality but lower late mortality than treatment B, or treatment C could be associated with a higher proportion of patients surviving at each follow-up time than treatment D even though, if we restrict our attention to those patients who survive 5 years or more, treatment D is associated with a higher proportion surviving at each follow-up time (this situation is sometimes referred to as *crossing hazard rates*). In either setting, it is difficult to designate a "better" treatment. The problem of comparing two curves becomes even more difficult when the curves are estimated from data because of the sampling variability that must be considered. In addition, the estimate of the late part of the curve is always less reliable than the estimate of the earlier part. A data set with many censored values exacerbates this problem.

Sometimes survival curves appear to differ early in the follow-up period and then seem to come together, as in Fig. 1A. Sometimes the opposite happens: The curves are very similar at first and only differ later in the follow-up period, as in Fig. 1B. Not all statistical tests are equally effective in these two situations. This means that a test that is likely to produce a significant result in comparing the curves in Fig. 1A might be very unlikely to produce a significant result in

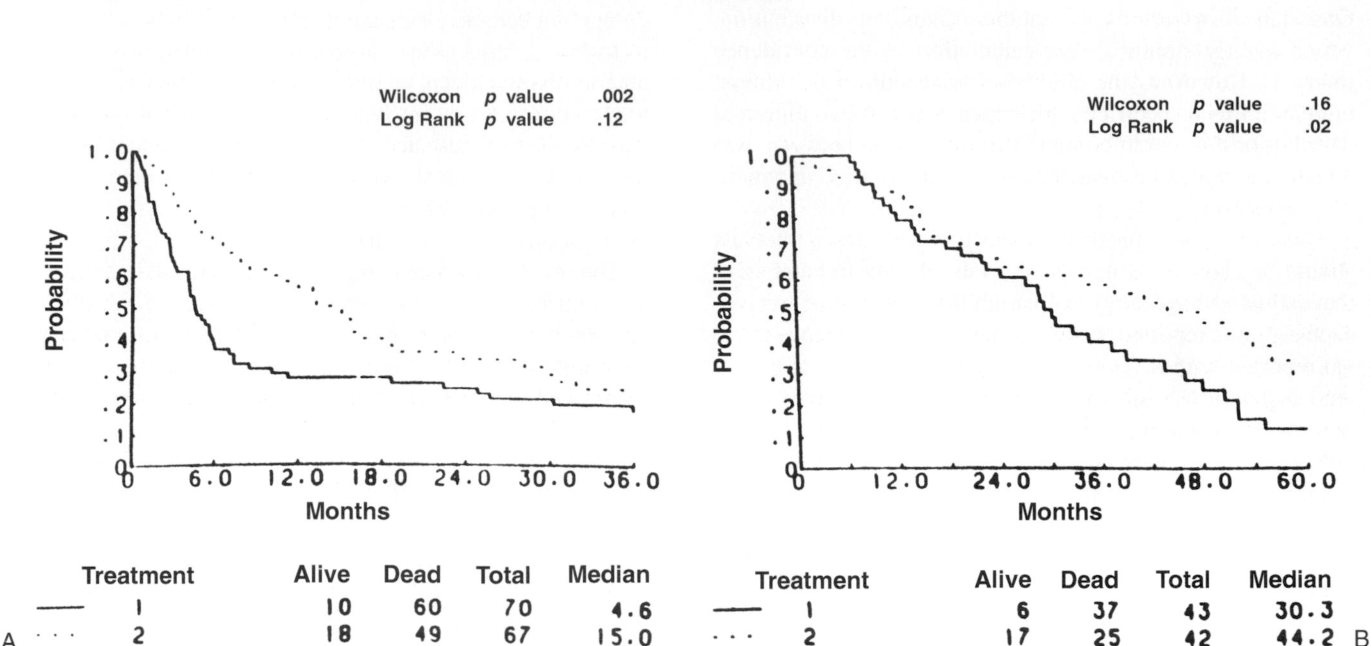

FIG. 1. A: Example of survival curves that separate and then come together. **B:** Example of survival curves that are together and then separate.

comparing the curves in Fig. 1B. Before a trial begins, one must decide which type of survival difference (early or late) would be of most interest and choose the test statistic accordingly. It would be misleading and inappropriate to try several tests and report the most significant or to choose the test after viewing the data.

Two of the most commonly used tests of differences in survival curves are the log rank test (variations are known as the *proportional hazards test*, the *Mantel-Haenszel test*, the *generalized Savage test*, or the *exponential order scores test*[39,43–45]) and the generalized Wilcoxon test (variations are known as the *Gehan modification of the Wilcoxon test*, the *Gilbert modification of the Wilcoxon test*, and the *Breslow test*[46–49]). The distributions of these test statistics follow approximate χ^2 distributions. The generalized Wilcoxon test is relatively more sensitive to differences in survival distributions that occur earlier in time, and the log rank test is relatively more sensitive to differences that occur later in time. As Fleming et al.[50] and Lagakos[51] point out, both statistics can be expressed as the weighted sum of statistics from a series of 2 × 2 contingency tables, with each table corresponding to the number of deaths and number of patients at risk at each observed death time.

If the mechanism that causes censoring is related to the true survival time, the generalized Wilcoxon and the log rank tests give incorrect significance levels. In a randomized trial, a necessary (but not sufficient) condition for independent censoring is identical follow-up and data collection schedules for both regimens. Planning such identical data collection is not always enough. In a multiinstitutional study of a 6-month induction regimen versus a 16-month induction regimen for metastatic breast cancer,[52] the outcome variable of interest was time to failure. Institutions would often wait until the end of the induction period to submit data unless the failure was noted earlier. This is called the *bad news first* phenomenon, because failures are reported in a more timely manner than is follow-up on nonfailed patients. This resulted in dependent censoring, with far more patients on the 16-month regimen censored when the first analysis was performed at the end of the accrual period. The log rank test calculated at that time was nonsignificant; median survival was estimated as 4.0 months on the shorter regimen and 4.7 months on the longer regimen. Analysis of the data available a year after accrual ended showed median survival to be 5.7 months on the shorter regimen and 10.2 months on the longer regimen, a significant difference. Had censoring been independent of survival, the log rank test performed when accrual ended would have detected the significant difference in survival.

MONITORING

Bias and Validity

There is a well-known adage[53] that "power tends to corrupt, and absolute power corrupts absolutely." Having spent several pages arguing that large statistical power is desirable, how can the author apply this statement to clinical trials? A large, and hence powerful, trial that controls most bias is good. A large, and hence powerful, trial that does not control bias is bad, because it will be more readily believed than a small trial, even though the results are mostly owing to bias rather than the true state of the world. The term *bias* refers to any factor other than treatment and chance that might influence outcome. Various categorizations of bias have been made.[54,55] A short list includes selection bias (e.g., poorer-risk patients choosing a less toxic treatment or physicians putting poorly compliant patients on a less toxic treatment), eligibility bias (e.g., patients unable to start adjuvant chemotherapy within a month of mastectomy being excluded from analysis of that regimen but "control" patients having no such reason for exclusion), diagnostic bias (as diagnostic and staging tests get better, survival appears to improve within each stage even if overall survival remains the same), bias due to changes in definitions (especially of endpoints) of follow-up of ancillary therapy or supportive care, and bias due to regression to the mean (e.g., metastatic patients starting a new treatment when they have new or worsening symptoms; some of these patients will appear to respond simply because their bad symptoms were a transient phenomenon).

Bias affects internal and external validity of a trial. *Internal validity* refers to the quality of comparisons done within the trial's population (most important, comparisons of outcome variables in various treatment groups). *External validity* determines how generalizable the trial results are, because it refers to how similar the study patients, treatments, follow-up, and other procedures are to usual care in some well-specified subset of patients with breast cancer. Even a trial with little external validity, but decent internal validity, provides useful information on treatment comparisons, although it may require a verification study or a "translational" study before a new treatment is adopted as standard.

Several design features that can help control bias are clear definitions of eligibility and endpoint variables (including toxicity), institutional logs to document what types of patient are not entering the trial, randomization, blinding of the patient to which treatment she is receiving, blinding of the person collecting endpoint data to which treatment the patient is receiving, and specifying the same follow-up schedule for all patients. Unfortunately, designing a good trial is not enough; some monitoring is necessary to ensure that the design is working as planned.

Monitoring is also important for preserving the power of a trial. For example, a trial may be planned to have 80% power to detect a difference between treatments A and B assuming that 90% of the patients actually receive the treatment to which they are randomized. If only 50% of the patients receive their randomized treatment (and 50% receive the other treatment on the trial), the trial will have zero power (because the treatment mix in the two groups is identical); the power is larger than zero but less than 80% for "noncompliance" between 50% and 90%. If there is a group of ineligible patients for whom it is known *a priori* that neither treatment "works," then these patients will not contribute to power (even if randomized) and the effective sample size does not include them; therefore, power will be lower than expected if many such ineligible patients are enrolled. If endpoints are vaguely defined, then random noise in coding them will also decrease power. To prevent any of these three situations, it is necessary to monitor these features over the course of a trial, with adjustment of sample size or procedures as needed to maintain power.

Types of Monitoring

Attention has focused[56] on the auditing policies of groups that conduct clinical trials; that is, how often and for what percent of patients and data items the data on forms or in a computer database are compared to the patient's medical record. [Paradoxically, the National Surgical Adjuvant Breast Project (NSABP) problem that precipitated the interest in auditing was *not* discovered on an audit but through a simple comparison of dates on different forms.] The National Cancer Institute requires that each institution participating in a clinical oncology group have an on-site audit at least once every 3 years, although the number of patients and trials in the audit varies. However, auditing is not the only form of monitoring.

Monitoring can also include periodic examination of whether a physician, institution, clinic, or laboratory qualifies to participate in a trial (e.g., has a properly constituted Institutional Review Board, passes quality control tests, is licensed or certified by the relevant group); questioning during the randomization phone call to establish whether a patient is eligible; review of clinic logs or the conduct of surveys to determine what types of eligible patients are not being asked to participate in a study; computer or visual checks of data provided for completeness and reasonableness and for consistency over time (sometimes called *logical checks*); periodic production of tables of accrual and toxicity and balance of prognostic factors; workshops to discuss common data abstraction problems and evaluate whether there are major misunderstandings about eligibility requirements, informed consent, randomization procedures, endpoint definitions, toxicity definitions, or reporting procedures; double-keying or other methods of preventing data entry errors; checks that treatment is not begun before patient consent and randomization; pill counts or analysis of blood samples to see how much drug a patient is taking (or whether she is taking drugs from treatment arms to which she was not randomized); medical reviews of the judgment calls of primary physicians (e.g., eligibility, whether toxicity is related to treatment, tumor response); the requirement that two (or more) local physicians examine the patient and agree on eligibility or endpoints; centralized review of pathology or scans or other patient materials; statistical evaluation of whether variation is larger than expected (e.g., institutional differences in patient mix or endpoints) or whether variation is smaller than expected (e.g., a too-perfect linear relation within patient between time and some laboratory value); and statistical review of the assumptions on which sample size was based, as well as formal sequential analysis of results.[57–61]

Some have argued that most clinical trials are burdened by too much monitoring, not only because of costs, but also because monitoring can harm the external validity of a trial, because physicians in practice who use the results of clinical trials and patients treated in accordance with such results are seldom subject to any (let alone so much) checking.[56,62] Others seem to believe that fraud, error, and sloppiness are widespread in clinical trials and that results should not be believed unless all possible steps are taken to weed them out.[8] (Surveys of monitoring results in clinical oncology groups have shown that fraud is the rarest problem, affecting fewer than 0.5% of patients and fewer than 0.1% of endpoint evaluations and that sloppiness is the most common problem,[56,63] but this may not be true in other cancer trials.) The author believes that an attitude between these two extremes is justifiable. Clinical trials should be subject to more monitoring than general practice. On the other hand, the amount of effort expended in monitoring any aspect of a trial should be proportional to how much error in that aspect would affect the internal validity of the trial. Consideration of a few aspects is given below.

Monitoring of Eligibility

Some investigators[64] believe that all patients entered on a randomized study, whether eligible or not, should be included in the analysis ("intent-to-treat" analysis). If this is done, there is little reason to spend much time verifying eligibility. The arguments in favor of general inclusion are that, on average, randomization should distribute these ineligible patients equally to all treatments, some statistical tests (especially permutation tests) would not be exactly correct without including all patients, the number of "mistakes" made in entering an ineligible patient in the trial is likely to underestimate the number of "mistakes" made in treating unsuitable patients when the therapy becomes standard, and the enrollment of ineligible patients can help determine that eligibility criteria were too strict.[65] Other investigators[66] believe that ineligible patients should not be included in the analysis. Their arguments are that there is no clearly defined group to whom the results of the therapies in ineligible patients can be extrapolated, knowing randomization balances "on average" is small comfort when the trial winds up with an imbalance of ineligible patients, the efficacy of breast cancer therapy on a patient who does not have breast cancer simply is not relevant to decisions about the treatment's efficacy in breast cancer (although toxicity may be relevant), and the effects of breast cancer therapy on a breast cancer patient whose concomitant diseases are contraindications for the therapy are not important in deciding on the benefit of the therapy in patients without contraindications. The most helpful literature reports are those that analyze the trial both ways: with and without the ineligible patients. Second in terms of helpfulness are reports that omit only patients with the most extreme types of ineligibility (e.g., those in whom the major endpoint could not be defined or those in whom one of the treatments would be on the border of malpractice because of the high probability of serious toxicity).

In any case, if a patient is omitted from analysis because of ineligibility, it is the responsibility of the authors of the article to convince the reader that the determination of eligibility was unbiased, because biased eligibility determination decreases the internal validity of a trial. To be unbiased, the eligibility determination must *not* depend in *any* way on the treatment assignment (e.g., randomizing at time of mastectomy to chemotherapy or observation and requiring only the chemotherapy patients to be able to start therapy within 3 weeks) or the outcome (e.g., the patient must receive two cycles of phase II therapy to be "evaluable" for response).

In the 1990s, some attempt was made to lessen eligibility requirements in breast cancer clinical trials, precisely to make such trials more generalizable. (Indeed, the part of the NSABP controversy involving nonfraudulent randomization of patients more than a month after primary diagnosis seems moot, because that group and most others have extended the permissible time period in more recent trials.) To the extent that the fewer eligibility requirements remaining in more recent protocols are increasingly likely to represent proven and serious medical contraindications for the trial therapies, it may be more important now to monitor eligibility because of ethical considerations.

Monitoring of Randomization

Randomization is the main way to eliminate conscious and unconscious bias in treatment comparisons. It also balances, on average, the treatments in a trial with respect to known and unknown prognostic factors. (The phrase *on average* means that there will be balance among treatments for all factors if an infinitely large number of trials study the same issue.) Randomization is a process by which treatments are assigned to patients by a chance mechanism such that each patient has a particular prespecified probability of being assigned to each treatment in the trial. (Usually, these prespecified probabilities are equal, because for a fixed total accrual, trials with equal numbers of patients on each treatment have the most power. However, it is possible to have unequal probabilities.) One important feature of randomization is that neither the physician nor the patient knows which treatment the patient will receive before the patient is entered in the trial. Any other arrangement would not eliminate the possibility that the choice of entering the trial was influenced by the treatment assignment.

It has been argued[67] that few patients are willing to be randomized if the process is completely explained to them, and thus randomization itself decreases the external validity of a trial. However, in a disease as heterogeneous as breast cancer, nonrandomized trials are subject to so much bias and imbalance in unknown prognostic factors that they lack internal validity, making external validity a moot point. For example, even the best historically controlled study can be misleading. Pocock[68] examined 19 instances in which a clinical trials group used the same treatment in two consecutive trials: "If historical comparisons of this type are without bias, one would not expect any notable difference in survival for two groups that receive the same treatment. In fact, the 19 changes in death rate ranged from -46% to +24%, and in four instances the difference was statistically significant (each $p < .02$)." Similar examples exist in the breast cancer literature.[69–71] The reliability of historical controls is challenged even more directly when the results of historically controlled trials show significant differences[72] that are not verified by the results of randomized trials.[73]

Monitoring Treatment Compliance

Treatment compliance can be easy to monitor (e.g., documenting that the patient was injected once with the trial vaccine) or complicated to monitor (e.g., deciding if the dose modifications in a yearlong seven-drug chemotherapy were justified by patient toxicity). For some trials, treatment compliance can affect power and generalizability. However, to estimate the effect of compliance on these topics, it is not necessary for all patients to be monitored, but only that a large enough sample be monitored to estimate degree and percent of compliance. To preserve internal validity of a trial, noncompliers should never be omitted from analysis. This is because it is impossible to prove that the decision to depart from protocol guidelines was unaffected by the patient's treatment assignment or outcome. As an example, many studies involving placebos, including the NSABP B-05 adjuvant trial of L-phenylalanine mustard versus placebo,[74] have shown that patients who take full-dose placebo have better outcomes than those who are less compliant on their placebo regimen. Thus, it would obviously be a mistake to omit less compliant patients from chemotherapy arms but not observation arms.

With the exception of bone marrow transplant regimens, most breast cancer chemotherapy is given to outpatients rather than to inpatients, and surgery also involves much less inpatient time than it did in 1980. This, combined with the trend in the 1990s toward more complicated treatments, has made monitoring therapy increasingly difficult. Many protocols now state that treatment modification algorithms are "guidelines" rather than "rules." There is still a role for close monitoring of treatment in phase I and early phase II trials, but it is hard to justify phase III trials unless the primary scientific question involves dose or schedule.

Use of Monitoring Results

Some types of monitoring are educational or corrective in and of themselves—for example, the keeping of clinic logs to see what types of patients are not approached to participate in trials, workshops to discuss common data abstraction problems, and double-keying to prevent data entry errors. Other types of monitoring require plans on how to use the results—for example, amending the protocol to clarify definitions and procedures, scheduling extra workshops, penalizing noncompliant physicians or institutions, reporting suspected fraud to relevant bodies, or modifying the sample size.

It is important to note that most mistakes and sloppiness detected by monitoring that affect internal validity tend to make the treatments in a randomized trial look more similar with respect to endpoints than they really are; that is, they will lower power. Such mistakes usually do *not* make treatments look more different than they really are. This is because, even though some errors may occur more on one treatment than another, there are so many different types of errors that they tend to be distributed on both treatments, just by chance. How a trial was monitored is thus more of an issue in trials that report treatment equivalence than in trials that report treatment difference.

Data Safety and Monitoring Boards and Group Sequential Statistical Designs

All National Cancer Institute–funded cooperative groups[75] and some clinical trials at individual cancer centers, drug companies, and non-U.S. clinical oncology groups have Data Safety and Monitoring Boards (DSMBs, sometimes called *Data Monitoring Committees*) whose job it is to periodically monitor the results of randomized trials. These boards are usually composed of clinicians, statisticians, ethicists, and patient representatives who are not participating in the trials being monitored but who are expected to be familiar with current results in the relevant field and other concurrently running trials. The job of such a board includes monitoring accrual rates, toxicities, and statistical analyses of outcome variables. The board might make suggestions for improving accrual rates, changing protocol design to decrease the number of patients needed, or closing a poorly accruing study. It might make suggestions for closer surveillance of toxicity; for changing treatment dose, schedule, supportive care, or consent forms; for terminating accrual of particular types of patients; or for closing the entire trial based on unusual types or frequencies of toxicity in the trial being monitored or in similar trials. The board might also make suggestions for changing the trial's design based on interim analysis showing that types of patients entered or frequency of endpoints differs from original assumptions. It might decide that one or more arms of a trial should cease accrual because of unexpectedly large treatment differences in the primary endpoint or, conversely, because it is highly unlikely that treatments will be deemed significantly different if the trial were continued. In most cases, DSMBs monitor a trial not only while it is open to accrual, but also after accrual ends but before the endpoint results of the trial are first published; few DSMBs

TABLE 3. *Sequential designs*

	Ignore multiple testing problems		Pocock		O'Brien and Fleming	
K	Nominal *p* value	Cum prob reject null[a]	Nominal *p* value	Cum prob reject null[a]	Nominal *p* value	Cum prob reject value[a]
1	.05	.05	.0158	.0158	.000005	.000005
2	.05	.08	.0158	.0275	.00125	.00126
3	.05	.11	.0158	.0365	.0085	.00891
4	.05	.13	.0158	.0439	.0226	.0256
5	.05	.14	.0158	.0500	.0414	.0500

K = 5, two-sided test, equal increment in events.
[a]Cumulative probability of rejecting the null.

continue to monitor a trial after its first publication. DSMBs were initiated to balance the ethical need to decrease the risks of patients entering the trial and to minimize the number of patients exposed to inferior treatment(s) on the trial, the widespread desire to publish trial results as soon as possible, the observed tendency of clinicians to change the type of patient entered in a trial and the length of time that patients are left on their assigned treatments if early (and nonsignificant) results are made public, and the increased probability that a trial that is analyzed often will have a spuriously significant result.

The last problem is similar to the multiple comparisons problem. If one simply chooses the cutoff (i.e., significance level) for a statistical test so that the probability of a false-positive result on a single test is .05, but one then does the test several times in the course of monitoring the study, the overall probability of a false-positive result increases dramatically, as shown in Table 3 for a trial with four interim analyses and one final analysis.[76] One statistical difficulty in ameliorating this problem is that sequential tests of treatment differences are not usually independent, and the test statistics have to be redefined[77] to have "independent increments." Another difficulty is that few investigators are willing to increase by much the maximum accrual goal of a trial (i.e., the accrual if it does not terminate early) to account for multiple interim analyses. A third difficulty is that, for the overall probability of a false-positive result (i.e., erroneously declaring the treatments to be significantly different at either some interim analysis or at the final analysis) to be only p (e.g., .05), each of the sequential tests (including the final one) must be done at a cutoff corresponding to false-positive probabilities q_i which are much smaller than p (the q_i are sometimes called *nominal p values*).

A number of methods exist for choosing these sequential cutoffs (in the statistical literature, this is called *calculating the stopping boundary* or *deciding on an alpha-spending function*). Pocock[59] suggested that all the q_i should be equal. This has the advantage of simplicity, but to obtain an overall false-positive probability of .05, the q_i for the final statistical test (and the interim tests) is .0158 for five tests and smaller when the number of analyses is larger than five. Hence, many clinical trials (e.g., those with a p value for the final analysis between .0158 and .05) would be declared significant if they had no interim analyses, but must be declared nonsignificant because five interim analyses were done. In addition, either the power of a trial with a Pocock design is far lower than it would be without the interim analyses, or the sample size must be increased considerably to maintain the power.[78]

The only way to have a q_i for the final planned analysis be closer to the overall false-positive probability of p is to make the q_is at earlier interim analyses much smaller. This means that the observed treatment difference early in the monitoring must be very large to result in early termination of the trial, and thus the probability of terminating the trial early even if the alternative hypothesis is true is very small. One popular method of choosing the q_is was proposed by O'Brien and Fleming.[60] Table 3 also shows the Pocock and O'Brien-Fleming q_is as well as the cumulative probability of stopping early for a trial with four interim analyses and one final analysis. There are many other possible stopping rules.[76]

There are also methods[79] for stopping a trial early if there is so little difference between the treatments that further accrual or follow-up, or both, is not expected to result in a significant difference. (Obviously, such methods are not used on equivalence trials, for which the main goal is to show that treatment differences are small.) The argument for such early termination is more economic than ethical: It is assumed that money can be saved (and used for other trials) if the study is stopped early. Tsiatis and Rosner[61] showed that for one cooperative group (the Eastern Cooperative Oncology Group), most of the gains from sequential monitoring were expected to come from the early termination of trials that showed no difference (57 studies, 170 years of follow-up saved) rather than from early termination of trials showing a difference (9 studies, 21 years of follow-up saved). However, it should be remembered that most of the economic savings come from trials that terminate accrual early, *not* from trials that terminate follow-up "early" but terminate after accrual ends. This is because most groups continue to follow patients in trials that end early (for survival, late toxicities, and even late recurrence). Trials in patients with newly diagnosed breast cancer usually accumulate few of the primary endpoints (recurrences or deaths) before accrual ends, and therefore if they are terminated early for lack of a difference, it is usually after accrual has ended. It is often argued that there is some benefit in continuing trials that do not currently show a difference, either to detect possible late differences or to obtain better estimates of risks and benefits for each treatment on the trial. Because the argument for early termination of such trials is not ethical, this type of early termination is more controversial than early termination for large treatment differences.

None of the above discussions should be taken as implying that DSMBs always do what the trial's original design of sequential outcome monitoring suggests they should do. Statistical arguments based on interim analyses are only part of what a DSMB considers in deciding whether to terminate a trial. Other considerations include (but are not limited to) assessments of the reliability of early data and the representativeness of early trial enrollees, biological considerations of how the treatments are assumed to work, and the existence and status of other similar trials. There has been at least one trial (in melanoma) for which the publication[80] indicates that the DSMB decided not to stop and publish the trial when the sequential design indicated a significant difference, but kept the trial in blinded follow-up for another year. In a May 1998 public workshop on DSMBs held at the Harvard School of Public Health, two examples of breast cancer trials that were not terminated according to the original sequential monitoring designs were presented. The Cancer and Leukemia Group B (CALGB) adjuvant breast cancer trial of maintenance paclitaxel (Taxol) versus observation after cyclophosphamide and doxorubicin closed early (and was reported at the American Society of Clinical Oncology[81]) before the original monitoring plan suggested stopping. The NSABP trial P-01 of tamoxifen versus placebo[82] in women without breast cancer (but who were at high risk of developing breast cancer) crossed the originally planned stopping boundary several DSMB meetings before the trial results were made public.

Monitoring and Publishing of Trials after First Publication on Outcome

Some of the statistical techniques for adjusting for multiple interim analyses *before* the planned final analysis (and, usually, publication) have been discussed previously. At this time, there are no widely accepted statistical techniques for adjusting for multiple analyses (and publications) *after* the first publication on outcome. Yet most groups consider it their duty to follow patients for toxicity, recurrence, and death long after the first publication and to publish results from such long-term follow-up (whether they agree with earlier published results or not).

The author believes that such long-term follow-up and publications are of great value in clarifying the relative benefits of treatments for breast cancer. One statistical reason for this is that benefit in an "early" endpoint (e.g., response in a metastatic trial, time to recurrence in an adjuvant trial, or acute toxicity in either) does not necessarily imply benefit in "late" endpoints (e.g., time to relapse in a metastatic trial, survival in an adjuvant trial, or lower risk of leukemia in either), and patients and clinicians need to know about all of the endpoints to weigh risks and benefits.

Another statistical reason is that no single family of mathematical formulas fits the survival curves of breast cancer patients treated with each of the available therapies. (If there were such a single family, the parameters of the mathematical formulas could be estimated from early survival data and used to accurately predict the rest of the survival curve. Because we would be able to accurately predict the whole survival curve for each of the treatments in a randomized trial, we would be able to predict their long-term difference from early data.) Even worse, there are cases in which survival curves are identical for the first 5 (or 10 or 15) years and differ thereafter. Thus, it is not our lack of mathematical sophistication that prevents us from finding such a family of formulas. It is a biological fact that early data on a breast cancer survival curve are not sufficient to predict the rest of the curve. (The same is true of time to recurrence, time to relapse, or any of the other common breast cancer endpoints.)

It should be noted that most trials are planned (both sample size and sequential monitoring) assuming that the time-to-event endpoint has the negative exponential distribution. This distribution is mathematically the simplest of all possible survival distributions, because it has a constant hazard (instantaneous probability of death). Thus, two treatments that have negative exponential survival distributions will always (through the whole of the survival curves) have a constant ratio of hazards (usually called the *hazard ratio*). Most breast cancer trials are analyzed using the log rank test.[43] This is partly because the log rank test puts more weight on differences later in the survival curve than some other tests, such as the Wilcoxon,[46,51] and most investigators are more interested in late differences (and possible cures) than in early differences. The log rank test does not require proportional hazards, but it has the largest power when hazards are proportional. It can be viewed as testing the difference between weighted average hazard functions. Thus, two curves that separate early and then come together (as in Fig. 1A) usually are not (at the end of follow-up) significantly different using the log rank test. Two curves that separate early and then become parallel may also fail to be significant using the log rank test. The proportional hazards model[83] (also called the *Cox model*) is based on the assumption of proportional hazards. (Curves that are not negative exponential can have proportional hazards, but it turns out that power results based on the negative exponential distribution are a good estimate for power results based on these other proportional hazards curves.)

In a design based on the log rank test and negative exponential distributions (whether it is fixed sample design with only one analysis or sequential design with many), early and late events count the same in the sense that the times of final analyses (and interim, if relevant) are based on the number of observed deaths. A trial with a large number of patients accrued quickly might accumulate the necessary number of events for a final analysis in a year or two, whereas a trial with either a small number of patients or a slow accrual might take a decade or more to accumulate the necessary number of events. The first trial might be reported as having a significant log rank test, and the second trial might be reported as having a nonsignificant log rank test even if they use the same treatments on the same patients, have the same reported power and design, and have the same number of events on treatment A and the same number of events on treatment B. The problem is that the two survival distributions do not have proportional hazards. The trial with large and quick accrual is based on a smaller portion of the curves than the trial with small or slow accrual. Similarly, a single trial that is reported to have a significant difference in an early publication may be reported to have a nonsignificant difference in a later publication. This occurred in an International Breast Cancer Study Group node-negative trial of one course of perioperative chemotherapy versus no chemotherapy, first reported[84] to have significant disease-free survival benefit at a median follow-up of 3.5 years (hazard ratio, 0.77; $p = .04$) and later reported[85] to have a nonsignificant disease-free survival difference at a median follow-up of 9 years (approximate hazard ratio, 0.90; $p = .24$). The change could go the other way, from nonsignificant to significant, as in an International Breast Cancer Study Group node-positive trial of one course of perioperative chemotherapy versus perioperative chemotherapy plus 6 months of adjuvant chemotherapy, first found at a median follow-up of 3 years to have no survival difference (approximate hazard ratio, 1.06; $p = .34$ for this comparison; data from group annual report) and then found[86] to have a significant difference at a median follow-up of 8 years (approximate hazard ratio, 1.34; $p = .003$). However, the change from nonsignificance to significance is often caused by an increase in power (due to an increase in the number of failures or deaths) rather than a change in hazard ratios over time.

Is there any guidance as to when in follow-up the significance level of a comparison might be more stable? It is tempting to conclude that the significance level at 2 or 3 years frequently disagrees with later significance levels. There may be some "biological" explanations of the instability at 2 to 3 years. Cooperative oncology groups[87] and tumor registry studies[88,89] have found that annual hazard rates of recurrence and death reach peaks at approximately 2 to 3 years of follow-up; by merely delaying the peak slightly, a treatment could appear to have a very beneficial hazard ratio if analyzed at 2 to 3 years. Also, it could be that some therapies are more likely to have an effect in patients who are not expected to respond in this early peak, and other therapies have more of an effect on patients who are not expected to respond after this peak. In addition, at least one trial from the Eastern Cooperative Oncology Group in postmenopausal node-positive patients has reported[90] that treatment affected the hazards only during the time the chemotherapy was being administered (6 months) and not after chemotherapy was discontinued, but the residual effects on the overall hazard ratio and significance level persisted for 2 years.

It should be noted that the adjuvant breast cancer trials that changed category (from significant to nonsignificant or vice versa) generally have been published with comments about the changing results—but not in the same journal as the original publication. It is difficult to convince journals to accept "follow-up" publications when conclusions change and even more difficult when conclusions do not change. It would be very useful to clinicians and researchers if medical journals would not only accept such follow-up publications but also institute mandatory short updates on clinical trials of chronic diseases (maybe once every 5 years) that would briefly reiterate earlier results.

META-ANALYSIS: STATISTICAL METHODS FOR COMBINING DATA FROM DIFFERENT STUDIES

It is not unusual for a clinical question in breast cancer to be associated with several separate but very similar randomized trials. The results of the separate trials are often not identical and can be contradictory. Hence, medical journals include many breast cancer literature reviews that attempt to draw overall conclusions from the wealth of published reports. In the 1980s and 1990s, the case has been made that in a common disease such as breast cancer, treatments of only small to moderate benefit could prolong many lives.[91] Very large numbers of patients are required to detect small to moderate treatment differences (see Table 2), and one way of obtaining large numbers is to combine the data from many moderate-sized trials.

Combined Group Analysis and Stratified Tests

Some of the literature reviews[92–94] use statistical methodology to combine data. In 1976, Glass[95] coined the term *meta-analysis* to describe the use of such statistical methodology. The terms *overview, pooled analysis*, and *combined analysis* were used earlier and continue to be popular.[91,96] The statistical methods used differ primarily in how much homogeneity of studies is assumed. Conceptually, the simplest way of combining data from several randomized trials using the same two treatments (call them *A* and *B*) and the same outcome variable would be to combine all data on patients treated with A, to combine all data on patients treated with B, and then to compare these two large groups using a statistical test. Let us call this *combined group analysis*. This method assumes complete homogeneity between trials. However, it could very easily happen that some trials show A better than B and some show B better than A, whereas the combined group analysis shows no difference at all between A and B. In this case, the combined group analysis could be very misleading, and an analysis of why the trials differ in results would be much more informative. The power of the analysis could be improved by treating the individual trials as strata and using a stratified test. Stjernsward[92] used a stratified chi-square test on 5-year survival percents to evaluate the benefit of adjuvant radiotherapy for breast cancer. The Oxford overview[94] used a stratified log rank test to evaluate (separately) adjuvant chemotherapy and adjuvant hormonotherapy in breast cancer.

Combining *p* Values

A simpler and cruder way of combining studies involves combining results rather than patient data. L. H. C. Tippet,[97] R. A. Fisher,[98] and K. Pearson[99] independently proposed methods of combining "*p* values" in 1931 to 1933. The simplest of these methods is the sign test. Suppose there are five trials comparing A with B and that in all five, a survival analysis shows A better than B (although not necessarily significantly better). Under the null hypothesis that A and B are associated with the same survival, the probability that five out of five trials would favor A is $(.5)^5 = .03125$. This is evidence that A is associated with longer survival than B. In general, if there are a total of n trials and A appears to be better in k of them, the p value associated with this distribution of trial results is the probability that one observes k successes in n trials of a binomial random variable with a probability of success of .5. This probability can be read directly from a table of binomial probabilities.[100] This method has been used by Stjernsward and Day[93] in combining evidence from trials of adjuvant radiotherapy. Its advantages are that it is simple to calculate and the data needed for its calculation are always available in published reports of clinical trials. Its disadvantages are that all trials are equally weighted (i.e., a trial of 5 patients followed for 2 years counts the same as a trial of 5,000 patients followed for 10 years) and that no estimate of the size of the treatment effect is obtained. In either a stratified test or the combined group analysis, the result of each trial is weighted proportionally to the number of events (e.g., death or response) in the trial. Hence, the stratified tests and the combined group tests are more sensitive to small differences than the sign test. In addition, both stratified tests and combined group tests produce estimates and confidence intervals for the treatment effect.

Random Effects Models

Stratified tests and the sign test assume that some measure of treatment difference is approximately the same for all trials. Although homogeneity of differences is a more reasonable assumption than homogeneity of outcomes within treatment groups, it has often been criticized.[101–104] There is a group of models, called *random effects models*,[105] that allow one to test whether the treatment differences are more heterogeneous than could be expected from the sizes of the trials and, if so, to account for this "extra" variation in a stratified test. Himmel et al.[106] used such a model in analyzing published reports of adjuvant chemotherapy in breast cancer. Random effects models, by using larger variance estimates for some trials, result in less significant p values, on average, than the stratified test described previously (sometimes called *fixed effects models*). Berlin et al.[107] compare the results of 22 meta-analyses analyzed by the stratified log rank test of Peto[94] and the random effects model of DerSimonian and Laird.[105] In the 14 meta-analyses that both methods agreed in classifying as nonheterogeneous, the two methods chose the same 5 to be significant and resulted in very similar p values for all 14. Of the remaining eight heterogeneous meta-analyses, two were found to be nonsignificant by both methods. However, three of the six meta-analyses found significant by the Peto method were found to be nonsignificant by the DerSimonian and Laird method. Hence, one advantage of the random effects models is that they are less likely to declare treatment A to be significantly better than treatment B if the trials in the meta analysis are too heterogeneous to justify this. One disadvantage of random effects models is that they assume that the trials being analyzed represent a random sample of all such trials that could be done. This is clearly not the case; the design and the results of earlier trials affect the design of later trials.

Time Heterogeneity

Heterogeneity of differences over time should be considered in combining data from many studies when the outcome variable used is the time until an event for example, survival time. Even if one is willing to assume homogeneity of differences over trials, one may not be willing to assume homogeneity of differences over time. This is the same problem of nonproportional hazards discussed in the section Monitoring and Publishing of Trials after First Publication on Outcome. In addition, many established prognostic factors[108] do not have a constant effect on the hazard of recurrence or death, so that the "average" benefit of treatments that are truly of benefit to only some patient subgroups would also be expected to change over time. If either of these assertions is true, then combining data from trials with different lengths of follow-up could be misleading. Also, it may be that the trials followed longest are not typical of the studies being combined. If so, the results of the combined analysis might change drastically when more follow-up is obtained on recently started trials.

Publication Bias

The widespread discussion of meta-analysis that followed the first presentation of breast cancer adjuvant chemotherapy and hormonotherapy overviews has had some useful ancillary results in the areas of publication bias, quality of clinical trials, the arithmetic construct, and comparisons of meta-analyses. The dangers of reviewing only published studies have been clearly stated,[109] and in one case[110] (ovarian cancer) the conclusions from reviewing only published studies have been shown to differ from the conclusions drawn when all available studies are reviewed. The problem is that trials with no significant treatment differences, especially trials too small to have adequate power, are less likely to be published than are trials with a significant treatment difference.[111] Increased discussion of such "publication bias" may lead to more complete registries of clinical trials,[110] the organization of "public record" journals to ensure publication of at least minimal data on all randomized trials, and the development of better methods for estimating the effect of unavailable data on the conclusions of literature reviews.[109]

Arithmetic Constructs

The term *arithmetic construct* has been used[112] to refer to the fallacy of assuming that a trial that randomizes the treatment consisting of A plus B against treatment with only A is estimating the same treatment B "effect" as a trial that randomizes B against observation (or placebo). As two counterexamples, it should be considered that although breast cancer patients treated with radiation-induced castration plus prednisone may have better outcomes than patients treated with radiation-induced castration alone,[113] and although patients treated with CMF (cyclophosphamide, methotrexate, 5-fluorouracil) plus prednisone may have better outcomes than patients treated with CMF,[114] prednisone alone still may have no antineoplastic effect in breast cancer. After the original presentation of the breast cancer adjuvant treatment overview, it was pointed out that estimates of the magnitude of tamoxifen benefit came from combining trials of tamoxifen versus no systemic adjuvant therapy with trials of chemotherapy plus tamoxifen versus chemotherapy alone. The subsequent publication[115] summarized the effects of tamoxifen separately for these two types of trials. The arithmetic construct is a potential problem in interpreting the conclusions of many clinical trials, not just in interpreting a meta-analysis. The examples of fallacious conclusions using the arithmetic construct that were published in the wake of the adjuvant therapy overview may help physicians recognize this type of logical fallacy wherever it occurs.

Comparison of Meta-Analyses: Hypothesis Formation

Some investigators believe that the main benefit of overviews is that the evaluation of the arithmetic construct and other trial differences can lead to the formation of important hypotheses that deserve further study. For example, if a meta-analysis of treatment Y in premenopausal patients showed that Y was not of benefit, and a meta-analysis of treatment Y in postmenopausal patients showed Y to be of benefit, reasonable investigators would try to hypothesize why the difference occurred. Some would argue that the large number of subsets of interest in breast cancer make meta-analyses mandatory, because no trial has a large enough accrual to evaluate treatment differences in each of these subsets. The problem is that inconsistent definitions, different percentages of misclassification, and incomplete availability of all prognostic variables can make the results of such subset analyses extremely dubious.[116] It is very important to realize that studies comparing meta-analyses are subject to all the biases that occur when nonrandomized treatments are compared. Selection bias undoubtedly exists.[117] Even if all trials have the same eligibility criteria, the patients who enter a trial of X versus control will differ from the patients who enter a trial of A plus X versus A.[118] The patients who enter the first trial of X versus Y will differ from the patients who enter subsequent trials of X versus Y, particularly if some results of the first trial are known when the subsequent trials start. There are also sources of bias that are likely to be bigger in comparisons of meta-analyses than in comparisons of two nonrandomized treatments: quality bias (one type of trial may by chance be associated with a higher loss to follow-up or more misclassification errors), geographic bias (the types of patients, the treatments available to them, and the factors that influence their agreement to randomization may differ by location, whereas many historical control studies of treatments are restricted to one hospital), and competing risk bias (the effects of breast cancer treatment may differ in populations at very different risks of noncancer death, whether "effects" are evaluated by comparing treatments using deaths from all causes or only breast cancer–related deaths).

Given these biases, comparisons of meta-analyses are useful to the extent that they encourage the formation of testable hypotheses, the keeping of patient logs and other methods of assessing how patients are selected for trials, and the standardization of collection of data items and follow-up. Comparisons of meta-analyses are detrimental to the extent that they are treated as hypothesis tests.

Comparison of Meta-Analyses and Single Clinical Trials

Meta-analyses are by nature retrospective, because at least some results of some of the included clinical trials are known at the time the meta-analysis is done. Most well-known proponents of meta-analysis agree that the gold standard of clinical research is the large-scale clinical trial, not meta-analysis (e.g., Sacks et al.,[96] Chalmers et al.,[111] Wittes,[119] Hennekins et al.,[120] Demets[121]). Many argue that meta-analyses should be used in hypothesis formation rather than hypothesis testing, so that a successful meta-analysis is one that is followed by a large randomized trial.[122,123] A large randomized trial has often been the result of cardiac meta-analyses. For example, in the mid-1980s, an overview[124] of 6,000 patients on 33 trials of fibrinolytic drugs given within 24 hours of the start of myocardial infarction symptoms indicated a statistically significant survival benefit, which led to the design and activation of two very large trials that verified this benefit (GISSI-2 with 37,000 randomized patients and ISIS-2 with 17,000 patients randomized to four treatments). As another example,[125] eight trials of a 24-hour infusion of magnesium in a total of 3,000 patients with myocardial infarctions showed a statistically significant benefit in 1-month mortality, which was not substantiated by a later randomized trial (ISIS-4 with 58,000 patients and a slightly detrimental effect of the drug on 1-month mortality).

Up to now, breast cancer meta-analyses not only have not resulted in new randomized trials, they have also resulted in early termination of ongoing trials.[126] Even Collins et al.,[127] who once stated that meta-analyses are the only practical way to evaluate treatments with "moderately sized benefits" urge that "future trials . . . should plan to obtain sufficient number of events to contribute substantially to such overviews. In many cases, this implies the need for randomized trials that are much larger than is currently standard."

Simon[128] has pointed out that "research reviews have always been regarded as subjective; the determination of what evidence is relevant . . . is not straightforward" and that this same critique applies to meta-analyses. The problem according to Demets[121] is that "procedures for deciding what to combine are not yet adequately developed." Deciding whether the studies included in a meta-analysis are all apples, apples and oranges, or apples and oranges and carrots and airplanes requires a careful evaluation of the treatments involved, the patient populations represented, the quality of the trials, and the medical context during which the trials were performed.[129] There are no general rules for what is "similar enough."

It can be argued that any multicenter (or even multidoctor) clinical trial is also a matter of mixing apples and oranges. However, a single clinical trial probably has a log order[130] less heterogeneity than a meta-analysis, on average, and this should keep the carrots and airplanes out of the fruit salad. For this reason, the author agrees with those who believe that meta-analyses are very useful for hypothesis generation, but that for deciding on the relative effectiveness of two treatments, there is no substitute for large, well-designed clinical trials. The Oxford overview of adjuvant breast cancer therapy has been invaluable in encouraging international cooperation, obtaining data on almost all known relevant trials and thus eliminating publication bias, and forming important hypotheses with regard to length of tamoxifen treatment or the relative benefits of hormonotherapy and chemotherapy in various patient subgroups. To quote Dr. DeMets, it is now time to "spend our creative energies designing simpler, larger multicentre or multi-country studies with common protocols [and] standardized therapy."[121]

ACKNOWLEDGMENT

This investigation was supported by grant CA-06516, awarded by the National Cancer Institute, Department of Health and Human Services.

REFERENCES

1. Altman DG, Goodman SN. Transfer of technology from statistical journals to the biomedical literature: past trends and future predictions. *JAMA* 1994;272:129.
2. Pocock SJ. *Clinical trials: a practical approach.* New York: John Wiley and Sons, 1983.
3. Buyse ME, Staquet MJ, Sylvester RJ, eds. *Cancer clinical trials: methods and practice.* Oxford, UK: Oxford University Press, 1984.
4. Miké V, Stanley KE, eds. *Statistics in medical research.* New York: John Wiley and Sons, 1982.
5. Friedman LM, Furberg CD, DeMets DL. *Fundamentals of clinical trials*, 3rd ed. New York: Springer, 1998.
6. Dawson-Saunders B, Trapp RG. *Basic and clinical biostatistics*, 2nd ed. Norwalk, CT: Appleton & Lange, 1989.
7. Shapiro SH, Louis TA. *Clinical trials.* New York: Marcel Dekker, 1983.
8. Spilker B. *Guide to clinical trials.* New York: Raven Press, 1991.
9. Piantadosi S. *Clinical trials: a methodologic perspective.* New York: John Wiley and Sons, 1997.
10. Fleiss JL. *Statistical methods for rates and proportions.* New York: John Wiley and Sons, 1981:38-48, 260.
11. Feigl P. A graphical aid for determining sample size when comparing two independent proportions. *Biometrics* 1978;34:111.
12. Casagrande JT, Pike MC, Smith PG. The Power function of the exact test for comparing two binomial distributions. *Appl Stat* 1978;27:176.
13. George SL, Desu MM. Planning the size and duration of a clinical trial studying time to some critical event. *J Chron Dis* 1974;27:15.
14. Peto R, Pike MC, Armitage P, et al. Design and analysis of clinical trials requiring prolonged observation of each patient. *Br J Cancer* 1976;34(Part I):585, 1977;35(Part II):1.
15. Lesser ML, Cento SJ. Tables of power for the F-test for comparing two exponential survival distributions. *J Chron Dis* 1981;34:533.
16. Schoenfeld DA, Richter JR. Nomograms for calculating the number of patients needed for a clinical trial with survival as an endpoint. *Biometrics* 1982;38:163.
17. Bernstein D, Lagakos SW. Sample size and power determination for stratified clinical trials. *J Stat Comput Simul* 1978;8:65.
18. Lehmann EL. *Nonparametrics: statistical methods based on ranks.* San Francisco: Holden-Day, 1975:69.
19. Freedman LS. Tables of the number of patients required in clinical trials using the logrank test. *Stat Med* 1982;1:121.
20. Gelber RD, Geldhirsch A. Methodology of clinical trials: investigating endocrine mechanisms in breast cancer. In: Cavalli F, ed. *Endocrine therapy of breast cancer.* New York: Springer-Verlag, 1986:51.
21. Freiman JA, Chalmers TC, Smith H, et al. The importance of beta, the type II error, and sample size in the design and interpretation of the randomized controlled trial. *N Engl J Med* 1978;290:690.
22. Zelen M, Gehan E, Glidewell O. Biostatistics. In: Hoogstraten B, ed. *Cancer research: the impact of the cooperative groups.* New York: Mason Publishing, 1980:291.
23. Mosteller F, Gelbert JP, McPeek B. Reporting standards and research strategies for controlled trials. *Control Clin Trials* 1980;1:37.
24. Staquet MJ, ed. *Randomized trials in cancer: a critical review by sites.* New York: Raven Press, 1978.
25. Gelman R, Zelen M. Interpreting clinical data. In: Harris JR, Hellman S, Henderson IC, Kinne DW, eds. *Breast diseases.* Philadelphia: JB Lippincott, 1987:706.
26. Gore SM. Assessing methods—transforming the data. *BMJ* 1981;283:548.
27. Blackwood JM, Seelig RF, Hutter RV, Rush BF Jr. Survival distribution in breast cancer. *Surgery* 1977;82:443.
28. Elveback LR, Guillier CL, Keating FR Jr. Health, normality, and the ghost of Gauss. *JAMA* 1970;211:69.
29. Fisher RA. *Statistical methods for research workers*, 12th ed. Edinburgh, UK: Oliver & Boyd, 1954.

30. Gardner MJ, Altman DG. CIs rather than P values: estimation rather than hypothesis testing. *BMJ* 1986;292:746.
31. Hall P. *The bootstrap and edgeworth expansion*. New York: Springer-Verlag, 1992:96.
32. Gelman RS, Zelen M. Interpreting clinical data. In: Harris JR, Hellman S, Hendersen IC, Kinne DW, eds. *Breast diseases*, 1st ed. Philadelphia: JB Lippincott, 1987:708.
33. Berkson J, Gage RP. Calculation of survival rates for cancer. *Mayo Clin Proc* 1950;25:270.
34. Cutler SJ, Ederer F. Maximum utilization of the life table method in analyzing survival. *J Chron Dis* 1958;8:699.
35. Kaplan EL, Meier P. Nonparametric estimation from incomplete observations. *J Am Stat Assoc* 1958;53:457.
36. Gelber RD, Zelen M. Planning and reporting of clinical trials. In: Calabresi P, Schein PS, Rosenberg SA, eds. *Medical oncology: basic principles and clinical management of cancer*. New York: Macmillan, 1985:418.
37. Lee ET. *Statistical methods for survival analysis*. Belmont, CA: Wadsworth, 1980.
38. Gross AJ, Clark VA. *Survival distributions, reliability applications in the biomedical sciences*. New York: John Wiley and Sons, 1975:23.
39. Marubini E, Valsecchi MG. *Analysing survival data from clinical trials and observational studies*. New York: John Wiley and Sons, 1995.
40. Lagakos SW, Williams JS. Models for censored survival analysis: a cone class of variable sum models. *Biometrika* 1978:65:181.
41. Gelman R, Gelber R, Henderson IC, et al. Improved methodology for analyzing local and distant recurrence. *J Clin Oncol* 1990;8:548.
42. Prentice RL, Kalbfleisch JD, Peterson AV, et al. The analysis of failure times in the presence of competing risks. *Biometrics* 1978;34:541.
43. Peto R, Peto J. Asymptotically efficient rank test procedures. *J R Stat Soc A* 1972;135:185.
44. Savage IR. Contributions to the theory of rank order statistics. *Ann Math Stat* 1956;27:590.
45. Mantel N. Evaluation of survival data and two new rank order statistics arising in its consideration. *Cancer Chemother Rep* 1966;50:163.
46. Gehan EA. A generalized Wilcoxon test for comparing arbitrarily singly-censored data. *Biometrika* 1965;52:203.
47. Elandt-Johnson RC, Johnson NL. *Survival models and data analysis*. New York: John Wiley and Sons, 1980:225.
48. Breslow N. A generalized Kruskal-Wallis test for comparing K samples subject to unequal patterns of censorship. *Biometrika* 1970; 57:579.
49. Tarone RE. On the distribution of the maximum of the logrank statistic and modified Wilcoxon statistic. *Biometrics* 1981;37:79.
50. Fleming TR, Green SJ, Harrington DP. Performing serial testing of treatment effects. In: Baum M, Kay R, Scheurlen H, eds. *Clinical trials in early breast cancer*, 2nd Heidelberg Symposium. Basel, Switzerland: Berkhauser-Verlag, 1982:469.
51. Lagakos SW. Inference in survival analysis: nonparametric tests to compare survival distribution. In Mike V, Stanley KE, eds. *Statistics in medical research: methods and issues with applications in cancer research*. New York: John Wiley and Sons, 1982:340.
52. Gelman R. Effects of reporting lags on interim inferences from clinical trials. In: Baum M, Kay R, Scheurlen H, eds. *Clinical trials in early breast cancer*, 2nd Heidelberg Symposium. Basel, Switzerland: Berkhauser-Verlag, 1982:175.
53. Dalberg JEE. (Lord Acton), letter to Bishop Modell Creighton, 1887.
54. Sackett DL. Bias in analytic research. *J Chron Dis* 1978;32:51.
55. Feinstein AR. *Clinical epidemiology: the architecture of research*. New York: Saunders, 1985.
56. Cohen J. Clinical trial monitoring: hit or miss. *Science* 1994;264: 1534.
57. Wald A. *Sequential analysis*. New York: Wiley, 1947.
58. Bross I. Sequential medical plans. *Biometrics* 1952;8:188.
59. Pocock SJ. Interim analyses for randomized clinical trials: the group sequential approach. *Biometrics* 1982;38:153.
60. O'Brien PC, Fleming TR. A multiple testing procedure for clinical trials. *Biometrics* 1979;35:549.
61. Rosner GL, Tsiatis AA. The impact that group sequential tests would have made on ECOG clinical trials. *Stat Med* 1989;8:505.
62. Peto R, Collins R, Gray R. Large-scale randomized evidence: large, simple trials and overviews of trials. *Ann N Y Acad Sci* 1994;703:314.
63. Weiss RB, Vogelzang NJ, Peterson BA, et al. A successful system of scientific data audits for clinical trials, a report from CALGB. *JAMA* 1993;270:459.
64. Armitage P. Exclusions, losses to follow-up, and withdrawals in clinical trials. In: Shapiro SA, Louis TA, eds. *Clinical trials: issues and approaches*. New York: Marcel Dekker, 1983.
65. Falkson G, Gelman R, Falkson CI, et al. Factors predicting for response, time to treatment failure, and survival in women with metastatic breast cancer treated with DAVTH: a prospective ECOG study. *J Clin Oncol* 1991;9:2153.
66. Sacket DL. On some prerequisites for a successful clinical trial. In: Shapiro SH, Louis TA, eds. *Clinical trials*. New York: Marcel Dekker, 1983.
67. Hellman S, Hellman DS. Of mice but not men: problems of the randomized clinical trial. *N Engl J Med* 1991;324:1585.
68. Pocock SJ. Letter, Randomized clinical trials. *BMJ* 1977;1:1661.
69. Tormey D, Gelman R, Falkson G. Prospective evaluation of rotating chemotherapy in advanced breast cancer. *Am J Clin Oncol* 1983;6:1.
70. Fisher B, Redmond C. Studies of the NSABP. In: Salmon SE, Jones SE, eds. *Adjuvant therapy of cancer*. New York: Elsevier-Dutton Holland, 1977:67.
71. Fisher B, Redmond C, Fisher ER. A summary of findings from NSABP trials of adjuvant therapy. In: Salmon SE and Jones SE, eds. *Adjuvant therapy of cancer*, 4th ed. New York: Grune & Stratton, 1984:185.
72. Gutterman JU, Cardenas JO, Blumenschein GR, et al. Chemoimmunotherapy of disseminated breast cancer: prolongation of remission and survival. *BMJ* 1976;2:1222.
73. Muss HB, Richards F, Cooper MR, et al. Chemotherapy vs. chemoimmunotherapy with methanol extraction residue of bacillus Calmette-Geurin in advanced breast cancer: a randomized trial by the Piedmont Oncology Association. *Cancer* 1981;47:2295.
74. Redmond C, Fisher B, Wieand HS. The methodologic dilemma in retrospectively correlating the amount of chemotherapy received in adjuvant therapy protocols with disease-free survival. *Cancer Treat Rep* 1983;67:519.
75. Nowak R. Problems in clinical trials go far beyond misconduct. *Science* 1994;264:1538.
76. Fleming TR, Harrington DP, O'Brien PC. Designs for group sequential trials. *Control Clin Trials* 1984;5:348.
77. Tsiatis AA. Repeated significance testing for a general class of statistics used in censored survival analysis. *J Am Stat Assoc* 1982;77:855.
78. Wang SK, Tsiatis AA. Approximately optimal one-parameter boundaries for group sequential trials. *Biometrics* 1987;43:193.
79. Pampallona S, Tsiatis AA. Group sequential designs for one-sided and two-sided hypothesis testing with provision for early stopping in favor of the null hypothesis. *J Stat Planning Inf* 1994;42:19.
80. Kirkwood JM, Strawderman MH, Ernstoff MS, Smith TJ, Borden EC, Blum RH. Interferon alfa-2b adjuvant therapy of high-risk resected cutaneous melanoma: the Eastern Cooperative Oncology Group Trial EST 1684. *J Clin Oncol* 1996;14:7.
81. Henderson IC, Berry D, Demetri G, et al. Improved disease-free and overall survival from the addition of sequential paclitaxel but not from the escalation of doxorubicin dose level in the adjuvant chemotherapy of patients with node-positive primary breast cancer. *Proc ASCO* 1998;17:101(abst).
82. Fisher B, Costantino JP, Wickerhan DL, et al. Tamoxifen for prevention of breast cancer. *J Natl Cancer Inst* 1998;90:1371.
83. Cox DR. Regression models and life tables. *J R Stat Soc B* 1972; 34:187.
84. Ludwig Breast Cancer Study Group. Prolonged disease-free survival after one course of perioperative adjuvant chemotherapy for node-negative breast cancer. *N Engl J Med* 1989;320:491.
85. The International Breast Cancer Study Group. The best available adjuvant treatments are within the framework of clinical trials. *Isr J Med Sci* 1995;31:144.
86. Goldhirsch A, Gelber RD, Castiglione M, et al. Past and future projects of the International Breast Cancer Study Group. *Cancer* 1994;74:1139.
87. Saphner T, Tormey DC, Gray R. Annual hazard rates of recurrence for breast cancer after primary therapy. *J Clin Oncol* 1996;14:2738.
88. Brinkley D, Haybittle JL. The curability of breast cancer. *Lancet* 1975;2:95.
89. Gore S, Langlands A, Pocock S, Kerr G. Natural history of breast cancer. *Recent Results Cancer Res* 1982;80:134.
90. Taylor SG IV, Kalish LA, Olson JE, et al. Adjuvant CMFP versus CMFP plus tamoxifen versus observation alone in postmenopausal, node-positive breast cancer patients: three-year results of an Eastern Cooperative Oncology Group study. *J Clin Oncol* 1985;3:144.

91. Peto R. Statistical aspects of clinical trials. In: Halnan KE, ed. *Treatment of cancer*. London: Chapman and Hall, 1982:867.
92. Stjernsward J. Decreased survival related to irradiation postoperatively in early operable breast cancer. *Lancet* 1974;1:1285.
93. Stjernsward J, Day N. Rebuttal of two articles by Dr. Levitt et al. *Cancer* 1977;40:381.
94. Early Breast Cancer Trialists' Collaborative Group. Effect of adjuvant tamoxifen and of cytotoxic therapy on mortality in early breast cancer: an overview of 61 randomized trials among 28,896 women. *N Engl J Med* 1988;319:1681.
95. Glass GV. Primary secondary and meta-analysis of research. *Educ Res* 1976;5:3.
96. Sacks HS, Barrier J, Reitman D, et al. Metaanalyses of randomized controlled trials. *N Engl J Med* 1987;316:450.
97. Tippet LHC. *The method of statistics*. London: Williams and Norgate, 1931.
98. Fisher RA. *Statistical methods for research workers*, 4th ed. London: Oliver and Boyd, 1932.
99. Pearson K. On a method of determining whether a sample of given size n is supposed to have been drawn from a parent population having a known probability integral has probably been drawn at random. *Biometrika* 1933;25:379.
100. Beyer WH, ed. *CRC handbook of tables for probability and statistics*, 2nd ed. Boca Raton, FL: CRC Press, 1983:194.
101. Levitt SH, McHugh RB. Early breast cancer and post-operative irradiation [Letter]. *Lancet* 1975;1:1258.
102. Levitt SH, McHugh RB, Song CW. Radiotherapy in the post-operative treatment of operable cancer of the breast II. *Cancer* 1976;39:933.
103. Levitt SH, McHugh RB. Reply to rebuttal letter by Drs. Stjernward and Day. *Cancer* 1977;40:382.
104. Goodman SW. Have you ever seen a meta-analysis you didn't like? *Ann Intern Med* 1991;114:244.
105. DerSimonian R, Laird N. Meta-analysis in clinical trials. *Control Clin Trials* 1986;7:177.
106. Himmel HN, Liberati A, Gelber RD, et al. Adjuvant chemotherapy for breast cancer: a pooled estimate based on results from published randomized control trials. *JAMA* 1986;256:1148.
107. Berlin JA, Laird NM, Sacks HE, et al. A comparison of statistical methods for combining event rates from clinical trials. *Stat Med* 1989;8:141.
108. Gray RJ. Flexible methods for analyzing survival data using splines, with applications to breast cancer prognosis. *J Am Stat Assoc* 1992;87:942.
109. Begg CB. A measure to aid in the interpretation of publicised clinical trials. *Stat Med* 1985;4:1.
110. Simes RJ. Publication bias: the case for an international registry of clinical trials. *J Clin Oncol* 1986;4:1529.
111. Chalmers TC, Leven H, Sacks HS, et al. Meta-analysis of clinical trials as a scientific discipline. I: Control of bias and comparison with large co-operative trials. *Stat Med* 1987;6:315.
112. Gelber RD, Goldhirsch A. The concept of an overview of cancer clinical trials with special emphasis on early breast cancer. *J Clin Oncol* 1986;4:1696.
113. Meakin JW, Alt WEC, Beale FA, et al. Ovarian irradiation and prednisone following surgery and radiotherapy for carcinoma of the breast. *Breast Cancer Res Treat* 1983;3[Suppl]:45.
114. Tormey DC, Gelman R, Band PR, et al. Comparison of induction chemotherapies for metastatic breast cancer. *Cancer* 1982;50:1235.
115. Early Breast Cancer Trialists' Collaborative Group (EBCTCG). *Treatment of early breast cancer*. Vol 1. Oxford, UK: Oxford University Press, 1990.
116. Gelber RD, Goldhirsch A. Interpretation of results from subset analyses within overviews of randomized clinical trials. *Stat Med* 1987;6:371.
117. Norton L. Commentary. *Stat Med* 1987;6:333.
118. Gelber RD. Discussion. *Stat Med* 1987;6:379.
119. Wittes RE. Discussion. *Stat Med* 1987;6:277.
120. Hennekens CH, Buring JE, Hebert PR. Implications of overviews of randomized trials. *Stat Med* 1987;6:397.
121. Demets DL. Methods for combining randomized clinical trials: strengths and limitations. *Stat Med* 1987;6:341.
122. Furberg CD, Morgan TM. Lessons from overviews of cardiovascular trials. *Stat Med* 1987;6:295.
123. Collins R. Discussion. *Stat Med* 1987;6:338.
124. Fibrinolytic Therapy Trialists' Collaborative Group. Indications for fibrinolytic therapy in suspected acute myocardial infarction. *Lancet* 1994;343:311.
125. Teo KK, Yusuf S, Collins R, et al. Effects of intravenous magnesium in suspected acute myocardial infarction: overview of randomized trials. *BMJ* 1991;303:1499.
126. Norton L. Discussion. *Stat Med* 1987;6:289.
127. Collins R, Gray R, Godwin J, Peto R. Avoidance of large biases and large random errors in assessment of moderate treatment effects: the need for systemic overviews. *Stat Med* 1987;6:245.
128. Simon R. The role of overviews in cancer therapeutics. *Stat Med* 1987;6:389.
129. Wittes RE. Problems in the medical interpretation of overviews. *Stat Med* 1987;6:269.
130. Wittes RE. Discussion. *Stat Med* 1987;6:278.

CHAPTER 75

Diseases of the Breast, 2nd ed.,
edited by Jay R. Harris.
Lippincott Williams & Wilkins, Philadelphia © 2000.

Techniques in the Assessment of Quality of Life

May Lin Tao and Patricia A. Ganz

TECHNIQUES (OR METHODS) IN THE ASSESSMENT OF QUALITY OF LIFE

Cancer clinical trials have traditionally evaluated the efficacy of a new intervention by measuring prolongation of life or disease control. Owing to advances in the social sciences, the methods for measuring outcomes such as quality of life (QOL) have flourished. As a result, we are witnessing a new generation of clinical studies that incorporate symptomatic relief and QOL measures as important end points.[1] This new effort is driven by the increased value that clinicians, patients, and health policymakers place on QOL outcomes in evaluating treatment options for patient management, individual patient decision making, and resource allocation. Breast cancer is one of the most commonly studied diseases in this regard. This chapter discusses the conceptualization and definition of QOL, describes the properties of a good QOL instrument, reviews types of available instruments for measuring QOL in patients with breast cancer, discusses some factors in selection of the appropriate instrument(s), and presents key contributions of QOL research studies in breast cancer patients and survivors.

CONCEPTUALIZATION AND DEFINITION OF HEALTH-RELATED QUALITY OF LIFE

Health service researchers and clinicians have long struggled to precisely define QOL or, more specifically, health-related QOL. In the context of health care, discussion of QOL generally refers to health-related QOL, acknowledging that there are valued aspects of life, including freedom, finances, job, and housing, that influence but are somewhat distinct from personal health status. Regardless of debates on the exact definition, general agreement exists that QOL should be conceptualized as a multidimensional construct, affected by treatment and disease, that includes critical domains of physical functioning (performance of self-care activities, mobility, physical activities, and role activities, such as work or household responsibilities), somatic symptoms (related to the disease, such as pain or dyspnea, or caused by therapy, such as nausea, hair loss, or premature menopause), psychological well-being (anxiety or depression related to the disease or its treatment), social functioning (disruptions of usual social interactions), and general health perception (global self-assessment of health).[1] Additional considerations may include other relevant health-related domains, such as sexuality, body image, treatment satisfaction, and spiritual well-being. Individual dimensions within QOL may have different levels of importance depending on the patient population; for example, pain is more likely a pressing concern for a woman with metastatic breast cancer than for a woman with ductal carcinoma *in situ*. In addition, specific dimensions that are most affected may vary with time, which may or may not be reflected as a change in overall QOL depending on the fluctuations of and interactions with other domains. For these reasons, consideration of relevant component dimensions should inform choice and design of QOL assessment methods in clinical trials and research studies.

Cella et al.[2] have proposed a definition in which QOL "refers to patients' appraisal of and satisfaction with their current level of functioning compared to what they perceived to be possible or ideal." This definition emphasizes the subjectivity of QOL assessments and the value or preference given to a person's current health state, as influenced by experiences, beliefs, and expectations. Because expectations of health and ability to cope with limitations affect a person's perception of health, two people with the same disability may have drastically different assessments of their QOL. This definition also supports the consensus that QOL should, whenever possible, be rated by the patient rather than a clinician or proxy. Information from an observer, although important for its own essential validity, is likely to be biased by the observer's own values and does not usually agree strongly with the patient's self-ratings.[2]

M. L. Tao: Department of Radiation Oncology, University of California, Los Angeles, UCLA Medical Center, Los Angeles, California

P. A. Ganz: University of California, Los Angeles, UCLA Schools of Medicine and Public Health, Los Angeles, California; Division of Cancer Prevention and Control Research, Jonsson Comprehensive Cancer Center, Los Angeles, California

PROPERTIES OF A GOOD QUALITY OF LIFE INSTRUMENT

Use of a well-tested scale with sound psychometric properties is essential for collection of high-quality outcome data and meaningful conclusions. An understanding of the psychometric aspects of a QOL measurement tool can assist the researcher in the appropriate interpretation of results, minimizing poorly founded conclusions. The test theory underlying QOL instrument development demands careful conceptual and methodologic construction and adherence to rigorous criteria for evaluation.[3] A carefully constructed instrument goes through many, often iterative, stages of item generation; elimination of redundant, irrelevant, and insensitive items; and revisions. The dimensions of the scale must then be determined and tested, a process that is integral to formatting and presentation. Finally, evaluation of psychometric properties must be conducted. The two primary components of the psychometric evaluation process are reliability and validity. Reliability reflects how free the tool is from measurement error—that is, the consistency with which a method assigns scores to subjects. Accordingly, a reliable tool must reproducibly assign the same score, given that a patient's health status remains unchanged. The two most common ways of testing reliability are (a) test-retest, in which the subject is readministered the instrument at a second point in time during a stable health state and scores are compared, and (b) internal consistency, which refers to the similarity of responses to items within the same domain, determined by calculating the average of all the correlations between each item and the total score (Cronbach's alpha coefficient).

Validity of an instrument is the degree to which the tool measures what it purports to measure. Determination of an instrument's validity is the evidence to support inferences that are made based on instrument scores—that is, accuracy of interpretation and the appropriate application of score results. The most rigorous approach to establishing validity is called *construct validity*. This involves an understanding of an instrument's underlying construct, a theoretically derived notion of what the instrument is meant to measure, thereby allowing hypotheses or predictions about how the instrument being tested should behave—for example, how it relates to other measures. For instance, an instrument is "discriminative" if it can detect differences in groups of subjects who are known to be clinically distinct: those receiving a toxic chemotherapy regimen compared to those receiving a minimally toxic regimen. Alternatively, "convergent validity" is supported when a scale measuring emotional function correlates highly with an existing measure of emotional function in the same population.

Other key properties of a QOL instrument are responsiveness and interpretability. The goal of an evaluative instrument is to measure how much QOL has changed over time. Often, scales are tested in cross-sectional studies and lack data on responsiveness—that is, sensitivity to change over time in individuals. Measures that are highly reliable may not detect small but important differences over time. This is a critical property if the study's intention is to measure improvement in QOL with treatment. Finally, meaningful interpretation of an instrument score requires assignment of a clinically relevant marker state or description of health state changes that are familiar to readers for a given incremental score change within subjects or between subjects. Although studies often report statistically significant changes or differences in scores, readers may be left with little information on the clinical relevance, thereby limiting their ability to use such information in counseling patients or evaluating the worth of an intervention. Growing experience with QOL instruments and conscientious reporting of clinical descriptions associated with score changes will improve the interpretability of QOL measures in time.

TYPES OF APPROACHES TO MEASUREMENT OF QUALITY OF LIFE IN BREAST CANCER PATIENTS

In general, QOL survey instruments are self-administered questionnaires that have undergone rigorous reliability and validity testing. This form of QOL measurement has its roots in the fields of social science research and psychometrics. Another approach is utility measurement, which is derived from economic and decision theory and is related to cost-effectiveness or cost-utility analysis.[4] This approach determines an individual's preference for a particular health state by a single summary score along a continuum that usually extends from death to perfect health (0 to 1.0). This application is detailed in Chapter 76.

The expanded pool of psychometrically evaluated survey instruments for use with breast cancer patients includes the following basic types, as categorized by scope: (a) generic health status measures: developed to make comparisons across populations with different clinical conditions, both sick and healthy, but may be less responsive; (b) generic cancer-specific instruments: appropriate for all cancer patients; (c) cancer site– or disease-specific instruments: designed for populations of a specific cancer type; and (d) condition- or symptom-specific instruments: ranging from comprehensive checklists addressing disease symptoms as well as treatment toxicities to more focused scales specifically on pain or nausea and vomiting[5] (Table 1). Specific instruments, although limited in scope, have potential for increased responsiveness as a result of tapping domains that are not only specifically germane to the patients under study but also to areas of routine interest to caring clinicians. Given this broad array of available tools, researchers and clinicians can use a single instrument or a battery of instruments in performing QOL assessment. Although many cancer-specific instruments are comprehensive and cover several dimensions, there is sometimes a bias toward one or two concepts, and one instrument may not adequately cover all dimensions

TABLE 1. *Instruments used to measure quality of life in cancer patients*

- Generic health status instruments
  - Medical Outcomes study instruments (MOS SF-20 and SF-36)[27]
  - McMaster Health Index questionnaire[28]
  - Sickness Impact Profile[29]
- Generic cancer-specific instruments
  - Functional Assessment of Chronic Illness Therapy (FACIT, formerly FACT)[30]
  - European Organization for Research and Treatment of Cancer Quality of Life Questionnaire (EORTC-QLQ)[31]
  - Cancer Rehabilitation Evaluation System (CARES)[32]
  - Functional Living Index–Cancer[33]
  - Southwest Oncology Group (SWOG) questionnaire[34]
- Cancer site-specific instruments
  - Breast Cancer Chemotherapy questionnaire[35]
  - Linear Analogue Self-Assessment (LASA) for Breast Cancer[36]
  - Site-specific modules for the FACIT and EORTC-QLQ (including breast site)[37,38]
  - International Breast Cancer Study Group (IBCSG) questionnaire[14]
- Symptom-oriented scales
  - Rotterdam symptom checklist[39]
  - Memorial Pain Assessment Card[40]
  - Morrow Assessment of Nausea and Emesis (MANE)[41]
  - Breast Cancer Prevention Trial (BCPT) symptom checklist[10]

For a comprehensive guide of available instruments for measuring quality of life, refer to ref. 42.
Adapted from ref. 5.

of interest, or component subscales may have uneven psychometric properties (e.g., low reliability in a domain of particular interest). Scales should be carefully reviewed, keeping in mind the goals of assessment. The use of a battery of instruments—that is, a combination of global scales and subscale components—may enrich assessment by tailored supplementation of areas of interest. Limitations, however, include the variety in response formats of various instruments and multiplicity of scores, aggravating interpretation and analyses.

Selection of a QOL tool for research or clinical use should be based on its content relevance to the questions of interest, as well as on the practical considerations of the evaluation setting. Factors to consider include (a) the need for comprehensive multidimensional assessment of QOL versus directed symptom monitoring only; (b) appropriateness of tool(s) for the target population (e.g., cultural relevancy, readability); (c) determination of an acceptable level of patient burden (considering length of instrument and medical condition of patients); (d) level of resources for data collection, management, and analysis; (e) feasibility of instrument administration, data collection, and quality monitoring if done in a multicenter setting versus single center (i.e., proper infrastructure to support QOL assessment component of study); and (f) known psychometric properties of the instrument for the purposes of study (e.g., prior demonstration of reliability, validity, and responsiveness in the target population or, if a longitudinal study, suitability for repeated use with a methodology for tracking).

A wide variety of reliable and valid instruments are available, and those responsible for the design of clinical trials must become more knowledgeable about them to perform QOL assessment. Repeated use of a single familiar instrument can substantially limit the value of QOL assessment. Proper preparatory work in determining which instrument(s) are most likely to answer expected QOL outcomes maximizes the contribution of QOL assessment in evaluating a treatment.

Beyond the clinical trial setting, it is now becoming increasingly feasible and desirable to implement routine QOL assessment into clinical practice. Computerized scoring methods[6] and new software for computerized administration and generation of reports[7] are now available for many instruments. These approaches can facilitate the collection of outcome data and permit feedback of the information to practitioners in a busy clinic or office. Evaluation in a clinical setting requires additional attention to the validity of alternative modes of administration and documentation of sufficiently high reliability to evaluate individual data (e.g., Cronbach's alpha score greater than 0.9). Potential uses of such data include screening a patient for QOL concerns to provide individual clinical intervention or to design larger-scale intervention programs, measuring outcomes of care, and monitoring quality assurance. Patients may perceive direct benefit by productive and efficient use of their waiting room time and greater likelihood that QOL concerns will be recognized and attended to by their physicians and nurses.

QUALITY OF LIFE ASSESSMENT AS AN OUTCOME IN RESEARCH ON BREAST CANCER PATIENTS AND SURVIVORS

QOL outcome information is emerging from randomized clinical trials as either an important secondary end point in conjunction with standard response and survival data or as a primary end point, particularly when palliation is the treatment goal. Exemplifying this emphasis are the National Cancer Institute of Canada's requirements that QOL end points be used in all its phase III clinical trials[8] and the U.S. Food and Drug Administration's mandate that new cancer therapies must either show a benefit in survival or QOL.[9]

In addition, well-designed descriptive research studies, which often use more extensive assessment with multiple tools, have provided important clinical information on the impact of disease and therapies on QOL during active treatment and long-term follow-up. Descriptive studies can lead to the development and implementation of intervention studies and provide important information that can help patients choose among treatment options based on their preferences. The integration of QOL end points into clinical research has the potential to provide important insight into the impact of breast cancer diagnosis and therapy in a variety of target populations, ranging from healthy women at high risk for breast cancer to those with advanced metastatic disease or long-term survivors. As shown in the spectrum of research studies and clinical trials discussed below, choice of instruments and design of QOL assessment methods require an understanding and careful consideration of the purpose of the study, setting of evaluation, resources available, and target population.

Experience from the Breast Cancer Prevention Trial, using scannable forms with user-friendly format, supports the feasibility of collecting baseline QOL data in a large, multicenter chemoprevention trial.[10] This study not only used the Medical Outcomes study SF-36, a generic health status measure that allowed comparison to the U.S. general population norms, but also included a mood scale, a symptom checklist, and specific questions regarding sexual problems to address potential physical and psychological side effects related to the use of tamoxifen. Follow-up studies on the significance of any adverse effects on QOL related to tamoxifen use in this initially healthy, high-functioning population will better inform the risks to benefits ratio of preventive treatment.

In a descriptive, prospective, longitudinal study, Ganz et al.[11] evaluated 109 women with early-stage breast cancer treated with either mastectomy or breast-conserving therapy and reported no significant differences in QOL, mood disturbance, performance status, or global adjustment between the two groups during the year of follow-up after primary treatment. Although those who underwent mastectomy reported more difficulties with clothing and body image, these findings apparently did not influence mood or overall QOL. Several other research and clinical trial studies have confirmed these results.[12] These findings allow clinicians to reassure women that these two surgical approaches for breast cancer provide similar results with regard to survival as well as changes in life patterns and fears or concerns. The critical clinical message is that physicians need to assess patient preferences in discussing treatment options without making assumptions that a woman characterized by factors including her age, marital status, and ethnicity will make a particular choice. For example, even if medically appropriate, breast conservation may not always be the suitable option. Some women may be so overwhelmed with the anxiety of possible recurrence in the breast that remains intact that mastectomy with or without reconstruction may be the better avenue.

The International Breast Cancer Study Group has developed a QOL assessment approach suitable for conducting large-scale cross-cultural trials to evaluate the impact of adjuvant systemic therapy for breast cancer.[13,14] These investigators balanced the priorities of psychometric rigor and feasibility in designing QOL assessment for their study setting. Their QOL assessment is purposely less comprehensive and is restricted to a few key indicators that have been shown to be relevant for treatment comparisons based on previous breast cancer studies, patient preferences, and expert judgment. They have demonstrated the feasibility and validity (including responsiveness) of a select set of single-item linear analogue self-assessment scales as indicators of components of QOL. In its current form, the assessment tool includes global indicators of well-being, functioning, and health perception (physical well-being, mood, perceived adjustment/coping, social support, and overall health) and specific indicators of symptoms of disease and treatment (appetite, nausea and vomiting, tiredness, hot flushes, and restriction in arm movements). By performing longitudinal assessment, these investigators demonstrated that the adverse effects of chemotherapy on patients' QOL were transient and minor compared to patients' overall ability to adapt and cope after diagnosis and surgery.[13] Preliminary results from the ongoing International Breast Cancer Study Group trial IX show that the specific indicators of symptoms and toxicities were responsive and served as important complements to the global measures. The specific measures distinguished different profiles of changes over time, reflecting the different side effects for chemotherapy, endocrine therapy, and surgery.[14]

In another multicenter clinical trial, Coates et al.[15] evaluated the efficacy of intermittent versus continuous chemotherapy in women with advanced metastatic breast cancer. Primary end points were response rate and survival, with QOL as a secondary end point. Given the limited resources available for data collection and the relatively poor performance status of the patients (40% with Eastern Cooperation Oncology Group performance status 2 or less), QOL assessment was performed using a relatively brief battery of six single-item linear analogue self-assessment scales on physical well-being, mood, pain, nausea and vomiting, appetite, and global QOL. The major findings were that patients who received continuous therapy had a better response rate and longer time to progression and, contrary to their *a priori* hypothesis, also had better QOL. The higher objective response rate was associated with improved QOL rather than increased toxicity. Baseline scores and subsequent changes in QOL were also independent prognostic factors in the proportional-hazards models of subsequent survival, supporting the validity of these simple QOL measures and the potential prognostic importance of QOL data.[16]

Despite being plagued by difficulties with patient attrition and noncompliance with QOL data collection in several clinical centers, the study by Coates et al.[15] is notable as one of the first clinical trials to incorporate QOL assessment along with traditional end points. Their results yield important information that clinicians can use in counseling patients with advanced metastatic breast cancer who are about to start chemotherapy treatment. Given the absence of significant difference in survival, the QOL results in this trial provide the most compelling evidence that continuous chemotherapy is superior to an intermittent course for metastatic breast cancer. Active research continues in the development of more effective cytotoxic agents for advanced breast cancer. In this process, a continued focus on the impact of new systemic regimens on QOL will serve to further optimize the care of women with poor-prognosis disease.

When the primary goal of treatment is symptom palliation and not prolongation of life, the use of a QOL end point is most appropriate. For example, in a randomized clinical trial on the benefit of oral pamidronate in breast cancer patients with bony metastases, von Holten-Verzantvoort et al.[17] demonstrated improvement in selective aspects of QOL, namely bony pain and mobility impairment, as a result of treatment. In this trial, reduction of skeletal complications was associated with improvements in QOL.

For those women who make the transition from patient to survivor, potential residual or long-term effects of breast cancer and its treatment need to be addressed. This need is becoming increasingly urgent as the number of breast cancer survivors being seen by primary care physicians reaches record numbers. Two long-term follow-up studies indicate that breast cancer survivors who remain disease-free after primary treatment report overall QOL outcomes comparable to those of healthy age-matched control subjects.[18,19] One of these studies notes that although breast cancer survivors had more frequent arm problems and less satisfaction with sexual life, global impairment (with regard to physical health, functional status, psychological distress, and social functioning) was not apparent.[18]

The other descriptive follow-up study used a comprehensive battery of instruments that included standardized measures that have been used in healthy populations of middle-aged and elderly women as well as new questions tailored to explore study-specific issues.[19] The result was an extremely comprehensive, purposefully redundant survey battery with particular emphasis on sexual functioning, body image, and partner relationships as important, relatively unexplored dimensions of QOL for long-term survivors. For women who are either newly diagnosed or about to complete therapy, the results from both these studies offer reassurance that overall they are likely to adjust well to their experience. The investigators of the latter study did, however, identify certain groups of survivors at increased risk for poorer sexual functioning—that is, women younger than 50 years of age who were no longer menstruating and women of all ages who had received chemotherapy. These findings stress the importance of physicians' inquiring about menopausal symptoms and provision of symptomatic management or counseling.

Although there remain settings in which QOL is an important end point, they are relatively unexplored. In general, clinical trial situations in which QOL assessment may play a critical role are (a) when a treatment is unlikely to provide a substantial overall survival benefit and benefits are likely related to comfort or functional preservation and (b) situations in which toxicities of treatment may be tremendous or greatly unbalanced compared to the alternative, despite potential survival or tumor control benefit. For example, it is expected that sentinel lymph node biopsy, as an alternative to axillary lymph node dissection, will result in similar prognostic information and improved QOL. Axillary lymph node dissection has long been a standard component of treatment of breast cancer, providing prognostic information and local control benefit. However, the associated morbidity (pain, paresthesias, arm dysfunction) can be disabling. A 1998 study examining patients' preferences regarding the trade-offs between risks and benefits of axillary lymph node dissection found that, for the majority of women, the value of prognostic information outweighed the risks of arm dysfunction.[20] Sentinel lymph node biopsy is a promising new alternative to axillary lymph node dissection, yielding similar prognostic information with likely a reduction in acute and long-term morbidity.[21] It remains to be seen, however, how the expected reduction in arm dysfunction translates into actual improvement in subjective health status.

Women with advanced breast cancer are more frequently receiving high-dose chemotherapy followed by bone marrow or stem cell transplantation. This strategy is also being used more frequently as an adjuvant therapy in women with stage II disease and extensive axillary node involvement. As a result, there is considerable interest in QOL effects of such intensive therapy. Descriptive studies suggest that after autotransplant for breast cancer, many women have significantly compromised functioning in multiple domains that appears to be related to their clinical course, such as longer hospital stay, time to engraftment, and severity of symptoms.[22,23] Structured interviews with these women also reveal that they are wrestling with many other life concerns, such as worries about their job, finances, health and life insurance, and future plans, further taxing their ability to enjoy life.[23]

Another 1998 study assessed the cognitive dysfunction associated with high-dose chemotherapy, using as comparison and control groups women with breast cancer who had received standard-dose chemotherapy or no chemotherapy, respectively.[24] The authors used a battery of neuropsychological tests, interviewed women regarding their cognitive problems, and also included standardized QOL measures. They demonstrated a trend toward greater cognitive impairment with higher-intensity therapy: an 8.2 times higher risk of cognitive impairment (32% prevalence) for those who received high-dose therapy compared to the control group versus a 3.5-fold increased risk of impairment compared to those who received standard-dose chemotherapy. Although this was a small study, it raises important questions about the long-term toxicities of high-dose chemotherapy, indicating that greater attention needs to be given to the potential for serious impact on level of functioning and QOL after high-dose therapy. Ongoing phase III studies comparing autotransplant to conventional therapies have incorporated QOL measures, and we await future reporting of these prospective studies.[25] Still relatively unknown are the long-term sequelae and QOL of women who have undergone high-dose chemotherapy and have a sustained disease-free state. Preliminary results from at least one such study indicate early decrement in QOL (at 3 months' follow-up) after autotransplant compared to conventional dose therapy. However, this improves with longer follow-up, and by one year, there are few differences in survivors.[26]

CONCLUSION

Health care consumers, providers, researchers, and insurers are now demanding to know more about the outcomes of cancer care than survival data alone. This may be particularly true for breast cancer, in which the incidence is rising, media attention has heightened, and the survivor pool has become more vocal. Resource constraints do not permit assessment of QOL in all clinical and research settings. However, many studies will have important value added by the inclusion of a QOL assessment. We can expect results of more ongoing studies that will add to our growing body of knowledge about QOL after breast cancer.

REFERENCES

1. Ganz PA, Moinpour CM, Cella DF, Fetting JH. Quality-of-life assessment in cancer clinical trials: a status report. *J Natl Cancer Inst* 1992;84:994.
2. Cella DF, Cherin EA. Quality of life during and after cancer treatment. *Compr Ther* 1988;14(5):69.
3. Tulsky DS. An introduction to test theory. *Oncology* 1990;4(5):43.
4. Torrance GW. Measurement of health state utilities for economic appraisal. *J Health Econ* 1986;5:1.
5. Ganz PA. Quality of life measures in cancer chemotherapy: methodology and implications. *Pharmacoeconomics* 1994;5(5):376.
6. Schag CAC, Heinrich RL. Development of a comprehensive quality of life measurement tool: CARES. *Oncology* 1990;4(5):135.
7. Taenzer PA, Speca M, Atkinson MJ, et al. Computerized quality of life screening in an oncology clinic. *Cancer Pract* 1997;5(3):168.
8. Osoba D. The Quality of Life Committee of the Clinical Trials Group of the National Cancer Institute of Canada: organization and functions. *Qual Life Res* 1992;1:211.
9. Johnson JR, Temple R. Food and Drug Administration requirements for approval of new anticancer drugs. *Cancer Treat Rep* 1985;69:1155.
10. Ganz PA, Day R, Ware JE Jr, Redmond C, Fisher B. Base-line quality-of-life assessment in the National Surgical Adjuvant Breast and Bowel Project Breast Cancer Prevention Trial. *J Natl Cancer Inst* 1995;87(18):1372.
11. Ganz PA, Schag CAC, Lee JJ, Polinsky ML, Tan SJ. Breast conservation versus mastectomy: is there a difference in psychological adjustment or quality of life in the year after surgery? *Cancer* 1992;69:1729.
12. Kiebert GM, de Haes JC, van de Velde CJA. The impact of breast-conserving treatment and mastectomy on the quality of life of early stage breast cancer patients: a review. *J Clin Oncol* 1991;9:1059.
13. Hurny C, Bernhard J, Coates AS, et al. Impact of adjuvant therapy on quality of life in women with node positive operable breast cancer. *Lancet* 1996;347:1279.
14. Bernhard J, Hurny C, Coates AS, et al. Quality of life assessment in patients receiving adjuvant therapy for breast cancer: the IBCSG approach. The International Breast Cancer Study Group. *Ann Oncol* 1997;8:825.
15. Coates A, Gebski V, Stat M, et al. Improving the quality of life during chemotherapy for advanced breast cancer: a comparison of intermittent and continuous treatment strategies. *N Engl J Med* 1987;317:1490.
16. Coates A, Gebski V, Signorini D, et al. Prognostic value of quality of life scores during chemotherapy for advanced breast cancer. Australian New Zealand Breast Cancer Trials Group. *J Clin Oncol* 1992;10(12):1833.
17. van Holten-Verzantvoort AT, Zwinderman AH, Aaronson NK, et al. The effect of supportive pamidronate treatment on aspects of quality of life of patients with advanced breast cancer. *Eur J Cancer* 1991; 27(5):544.
18. Dorval M, Maunsell E, Deschaenes L, Brisson J, Maasse B. Long term quality of life after breast cancer: comparison of 8-year survivors with population controls. *J Clin Oncol* 1998;16(2):487.
19. Ganz PA, Rowland JH, Desmon K, Meyerowitz BE, Wyatt GE. Life after breast cancer: understanding women's health-related quality of life and sexual functioning. *J Clin Oncol* 1998;16(2):501.
20. Galper SD, Lee S, Troyan S, Kaelin CM, Harris JR, Weeks JC. Patient preferences for axillary lymph node dissection. *Proc Am Soc Clin Oncol* 1998;17:423a(abst).
21. Krag D, Weaver D, Ashikaga T, et al. The sentinel node in breast cancer: a multicenter validation study. *N Engl J Med* 1998;339:941.
22. Hann DM, Jacobsen PB, Martin SC, et al. Quality of life following bone marrow transplantation for breast cancer: a comparative study. *Bone Marrow Transplant* 1997;19(3):257.
23. McQuellon RP, Craven B, Russell GB, et al. Quality of life in breast cancer patients before and after autologous bone marrow transplantation. *Bone Marrow Transplant* 1996;18(3):579.
24. van Dam FS, Schagen SB, Muller MJ, et al. Impairment of cognitive function in women receiving adjuvant treatment for high risk breast cancer: high dose versus standard dose chemotherapy. *J Natl Cancer Inst* 1998;90(3):210.
25. Vahdat L, Antman K. High-dose chemotherapy with autologous stem cell transplantation support for breast cancer. *Curr Opin Hematol* 1997;4(6):381.
26. Winer ED, Herndon J, Peters UP, et al. Quality of life in patients with breast cancer randomized to high dose chemotherapy with bone marrow support versus intermediate dose chemotherapy: CALGB 9066 (Companion protocol to CALGB 9082). *Proc Am Soc Clin Oncol* 1999;18:1593(abst).
27. Ware JE Jr, Sherbourne CD. The MOS 36-item short-form health survey (SF-36). I: Conceptual framework and item selection. *Med Care* 1992;30:473.
28. Chambers LW. The McMaster Health Index Questionnaire: an update. In: Walker SR, Rosser RM, eds. *Quality of Life Assessment: key issues in the 1990s*. Dordrecht, The Netherlands: Kluwer Academic Publishers, 1993:131.
29. Bergner M, Bobbit RA, Carter B, Gilson BS. The Sickness Impact Profile. Development and final revision of a health status measure. *Med Care* 1981;19:787.
30. Cella DF, Tulsky DS, Gray G, et al. The Functional Assessment of Cancer Therapy (FACT) Scale: development and validation of the general measure. *J Clin Oncol* 1993;11:570.
31. Aaronson NK, Ahmedzai S, Bergman B, et al. The European Organization for Research and Treatment of Cancer Quality of life QLQ-C 30: a quality of life instrument for use in international clinical trials in oncology. *J Natl Cancer Inst* 1993;85:365.
32. Ganz PA, Schag CAC, Lee JJ, Sim MS. The CARES: a generic measure of health-related quality of life for patients with cancer. *Qual Life Res* 1992;1:19.
33. Schipper H, Clinch J, McMurray A, Levitt M. Measuring the quality of life in cancer patients: the functional living index-cancer: development and validation. *J Clin Oncol* 1984;2:472.
34. Moinpour CM, Hayden KA, Thompson IM, Feigl P, Metch B. Quality of life assessment in Southwest Oncology Group trials. *Oncology* 1990;4(5):79.
35. Levine MN, Guyatt GH, Gent M, et al. Quality of life in stage II breast cancer: an instrument for clinical trials. *J Clin Oncol* 1988;6(12):1798.
36. Selby PJ, Chapman JAW, Etazadi-Amoli J, Daley D, Boyd NF. The development of a method for assessing the quality of life of cancer patients. *Br J Cancer* 1984;50:13.
37. Brady MJ, Cella DF, Mo F, et al. Reliability and validity of the Functional Assessment of Cancer Therapy-Breast (FACT-B) quality of life instrument. *J Clin Oncol* 1997;15:974.
38. Sprangers MA, Groenwold M, Arraras JI, et al. The European Organization for Research and Treatment of Cancer breast cancer-specific quality of life questionnaire module: first results from a three county field study. *J Clin Oncol* 1996;14(10):2756.
39. de Haes JC, Van Knippenberg FCE, Nejit JP. Measuring psychological and physical distress in cancer patients: structure and application of the Rotterdam Symptom Checklist. *Br J Cancer* 1990; 62:1034.
40. Fishman B, Pasternack S, Wallenstein SL, Houde RW, Holland JC, Foley KM. The Memorial Pain Assessment Card. A valid instrument for the evaluation of cancer pain. *Cancer* 1987;60:1151.
41. Morrow GR. A patient report measure for the quantification of chemotherapy induced nausea and emesis: psychometric properties of the Morrow Assessment of Nausea and Emesis (MANE). *Br J Cancer* 1992;19[Suppl]:S72.
42. McDowell I, Newell C. *Measuring health: a guide to rating scales and questionnaires*, 2nd ed. New York: Oxford University Press, 1996.

Diseases of the Breast, 2nd ed.,
edited by Jay R. Harris.
Lippincott Williams & Wilkins, Philadelphia © 2000.

CHAPTER 76

Techniques Used in the Assessment of Cost-Effectiveness

James A. Hayman and Jane C. Weeks

Despite the influence of managed care, health care costs in the United States continue to rise. Given this environment, purchasers and consumers of health care services are increasingly interested in knowing that they are receiving value for their health care dollars. This is especially true for conditions such as breast cancer, which are relatively common and expensive to treat. According to 1993 estimates from the National Cancer Institute, approximately $5.6 billion was spent in 1990 on the treatment of breast cancer, making it the single most expensive malignancy to treat in the United States.[1]

Cost-effectiveness analysis (CEA) is the most commonly used method for assessing whether the benefits of an intervention justify its costs. A number of CEAs of various interventions used in the diagnosis and treatment of breast cancer have been performed and are appearing with increasing frequency in the literature. It is also likely that the influence of these analyses will continue to grow. Accordingly, it is important that clinicians who care for patients with breast cancer have a basic understanding of the methodology used in performing these analyses.

In this chapter, we provide an overview of the methods used in performing CEAs. We begin by defining what a CEA is, highlighting the theoretical underpinnings of the approach. Second, we describe the methods commonly used to estimate the costs and benefits used in these analyses and, in the process, define the various types of clinical economic analyses. We then compare and contrast the various sources of data used in these analyses and explain the role of decision analytic computer modeling in performing CEAs. Finally, we discuss the issues of sensitivity analysis and discounting. Throughout the chapter, we illustrate various points with examples taken from published CEAs that relate to breast cancer.

J. A. Hayman: Department of Radiation Oncology, University of Michigan Hospital, Ann Arbor, Michigan

J. C. Weeks: Department of Medicine, Harvard Medical School, Department of Adult Oncology, Dana-Farber Cancer Institute, Boston, Massachusetts

WHAT IS A COST-EFFECTIVENESS ANALYSIS?

By definition, a CEA estimates the additional cost per unit benefit associated with the use of a given intervention as compared to the most reasonable alternative. The intervention under investigation could be for prevention, screening, diagnosis, or treatment. The result of a CEA is generally expressed in the form of a ratio that is calculated by dividing the difference in cost between the two competing strategies by the difference in benefit. If an intervention is more effective and less costly than the most reasonable alternative, it is clearly preferred, and there is no need for a CEA. Similarly, an intervention that is less effective and more costly than the alternative should not be used under any circumstances. The results of a CEA are most valuable when an intervention is more effective and more costly than the most reasonable alternative, the most common scenario for new drugs and interventions. The lower the ratio of the incremental cost of this intervention to its benefit, the more value the therapy offers for the cost and the more appealing it is as an addition to the medical armamentarium.

Two key properties of CEAs should be noted. First, CEAs are incremental. The cost-effectiveness of an intervention can only be judged relative to some alternative intervention. The intent of CEAs is not to estimate the cost of an intervention per unit benefit, but rather to estimate how much *more* the intervention will cost per unit benefit as compared to the alternate strategy. An incremental approach is appropriate because, if the proposed strategy is not pursued, some alternative strategy will necessarily be used instead. Even if the alternative is a "no test" or "no treatment" strategy, costs and benefits are still associated with its use. Second, the choice of the alternative strategy is critical. Ideally, it should be the strategy most likely to have been pursued had the intervention under study not been available. For example, if chemotherapy for premenopausal patients with node-positive, estrogen receptor–positive breast cancer were not available, it is likely that hormonal therapy would be used in its place. Accordingly, hormonal therapy, not observation, would be the most appropriate comparator for a CEA of chemotherapy in this setting. In practice, the choice of the alternative can have a significant impact on the value of the cost-effectiveness ratio.

THEORIES AND ASSUMPTIONS UNDERLYING USE OF COST-EFFECTIVENESS ANALYSES

The fundamental question being addressed by CEAs is how best to allocate resources when the budget for health care is not unlimited. One answer to this question is to allocate funds so as to maximize the health of the entire target population, without regard to the impact on any given individual or subgroup. This approach, grounded in the philosophy of utilitarianism, has as its goal "the greatest good for the greatest number." Allocation of resources following strict utilitarian principles would require cost-effectiveness data on all health care interventions.[2] First, CEAs of all the interventions competing for funding would be performed. The interventions could then be ranked in a "league" table, from the most cost-effective (i.e., the intervention with the lowest cost-effectiveness ratio) to the least cost-effective (i.e., the intervention with the highest cost-effectiveness ratio). The available money could then be allocated first to the intervention at the top of the list, then to progressively less cost-effective interventions, until all the money was spent. Using such an approach, those interventions above the cut-off point would be fully funded, whereas those below it would receive no funding at all. In practice, using cost-effectiveness data in this prescriptive fashion is rarely advocated. The importance of considering other factors, the most important being the relative value that society places on certain segments of the population (e.g., children or an identifiable patient in need of a potentially lifesaving procedure) is widely recognized.[3] Therefore, CEAs are best viewed as valuable decision aids to policy makers facing the complex and inherently political process of allocating resources among competing medical interventions.

Although explicit rationing of health care is relatively uncommon in the United States, virtually all health care payers place some limits on the extent and types of services they will cover. Such decisions reflect an implicit societal acceptance of the fact that some services do not produce sufficient benefits to justify the associated costs. The amount of benefit a society demands for its health care dollar varies by the wealth and priorities of the society. This level can be inferred from an examination of interventions, ranked by cost-effectiveness ratios, that are deemed "reasonable" by payers in a specific society. In the United States, this threshold appears to be at least $50,000 per year of life saved and perhaps as high as $100,000. Therefore, if the cost-effectiveness ratio of an intervention is less than $50,000 per year of life saved, it is generally considered cost-effective, and if it is more than $100,000, it is considered cost-ineffective.

IDENTIFYING AND MEASURING COSTS

The first step in performing a CEA is to correctly identify and measure the relevant costs associated with the use of each intervention. These costs should include not only any up-front costs associated with administering a test or treatment but also any downstream costs that might be incurred in further evaluating a positive or negative test, performing routine follow-up, managing treatment-related complications, or caring for progressive disease.

Three major categories of costs should be considered in CEAs.[4] The first category, direct medical costs, is costs incurred in the provision of medical care. Examples include professional physician costs; facility costs associated with procedures such as mammography, surgery, or radiation therapy; and pharmacy costs for chemotherapy. The second category is direct nonmedical costs, which include expenses for items and services that are nonmedical but are required as a result of the disease or treatment. Examples include the cost of transportation to and from the hospital, special diets, or child care during clinic visits. The third category is cost of time that patients expend in seeking and receiving medical care. Two other types of costs could theoretically be included in a CEA, so-called productivity costs and intangible costs. Productivity and intangible costs are estimates of the monetary value of years of life lost and of pain and suffering caused by a particular illness, respectively. Not surprisingly, both of these types of costs can be extremely difficult to estimate. In addition, because survival and quality of life are already captured in the denominator of the cost-effectiveness ratio (see the next section), it is recommended that these two types of costs not be included in the numerator as well, because this would constitute double counting.[4]

What types of costs to include in a given CEA depends on the perspective taken for the analysis. Going from broadest to narrowest, possible perspectives include: (a) society's, (b) the health care sector's, (c) a provider's (e.g., hospital, department, physician), (d) a payer's (e.g., employer, government, insurance company, health maintenance organization), and (e) the patient's perspective. Analyses from a societal perspective include all costs, regardless of who bears them. In all other perspectives, some costs are excluded. In analyses from an insurer's perspective, for example, all costs paid by others, including hospitals' unreimbursed costs and patients' out-of-pocket costs, are excluded. Although rarely performed, CEAs from the patient's perspective are possible and would only include time, transportation, and any out-of-pocket costs, including premiums, deductibles, and copayments, paid by the patient. It is generally recommended that the societal perspective be included as at least one of the perspectives considered in all CEAs to facilitate comparisons between studies and to inform decision making about the allocation of societal resources.[5] However, analyses from other perspectives may be more informative for particular audiences (e.g., a health maintenance organization making decisions about its benefits package).[6] Because of the ease of using reimbursement as a proxy for costs, the payer's perspective is often adopted. No matter which perspective is chosen, it is crucial that it always be identified explicitly.

Once the relevant costs to be included in the analysis have been identified, the next step is to estimate their value. This is generally accomplished by establishing the number of units of each resource consumed (e.g., number of mammograms, surgeries, cycles of chemotherapy, fractions of radiation therapy, etc.) and the unit cost of each resource. Total costs can then be estimated by multiplying the number of units of each resource consumed by the appropriate unit cost and summing all the products.

Ideally, unit cost estimates should reflect the true cost of resources consumed. In the past, the most common strategy for estimating unit costs was to rely on charges as a proxy for costs.[7] However, this approach has fallen out of favor, because it has been shown that charges are influenced by government regulations, market forces, and cost shifting, and therefore they often bear little resemblance to true costs.[8] Alternative, commonly used sources of unit cost estimates are payments, especially Medicare payments. Not only are payments relatively easily obtained, but they also represent the true cost of a given unit of resource to the payer. Another approach that can be used to generate unit cost estimates is to convert charges to costs with Medicare cost-to-charge ratios, conversion factors that must be calculated by all Medicare providers. Finally, sophisticated cost-accounting techniques can be used to allocate the appropriate proportion of labor, depreciation, and overhead costs to a given procedure.

The most precise method for estimating professional costs is to perform detailed time and motion analyses.[9] Alternatively, these costs can be estimated by multiplying the number of professional relative value units for a given procedure by an estimate of the cost per relative value unit. Drug costs can be estimated from average wholesale price or acquisition cost. For estimating patients' unit time costs, it has been recommended that hourly age- and gender-specific wage rates, available from the U.S. Census Bureau, be used.[4] Lastly, it is also important that all unit costs in an analysis be estimated in constant dollars (e.g., 1996) using the medical consumer price index to remove the impact of inflation.

Which methods should be used to estimate the costs for a particular CEA? One could argue that those methods that result in the most precise cost estimates are preferred. However, considerable time and effort may be required to collect exhaustive, accurate cost data. This investment may be unnecessary for certain costs if it can be demonstrated that the results of the analysis do not vary significantly with the precision of the estimates used (see Sensitivity Analysis). In general, the more sensitive the results of a CEA are to a particular cost component, the more effort should be expended to accurately estimate its magnitude.

IDENTIFICATION AND MEASUREMENT OF BENEFITS

Theoretically, *any* clinically meaningful measure of benefit can be used in the denominator of the cost-effectiveness ratio. Examples include the cost per cancer prevented by the use of prevention strategies such as tamoxifen or *BRCA* testing, the cost per cancer detected by a screening intervention such as mammography,[10–12] the cost per delayed diagnosis for a diagnostic procedure such as sestamibi,[13] or the cost per local failure averted by the addition of radiation therapy after lumpectomy.[14] However, if the results of an analysis are to be useful in allocating resources among interventions for diverse conditions (e.g., breast cancer, coronary artery disease, asthma) with various intentions (e.g., prevention, early detection, treatment), the benefits must be measured in units that are not condition- or intervention-specific. One commonly used generic measure of benefit is years of life saved (YOLS).[15,16] However, this measure fails to consider the fact that medical interventions may have important clinical effects that are not associated with prolonged survival. Such quality of life effects would include the anxiety resulting from a falsely positive mammogram, the toxicity of chemotherapy or radiation therapy, or the distress associated with a local or distant recurrence. For that reason, there is a growing consensus that the optimal measure of benefit for CEA is the quality-adjusted life year (QALY), a single measure that captures length and quality of life.[4]

QALYs are essentially the area under the curve of survival plotted against QOL. In other words, each period of survival is weighted by the QOL during that period. Periods can be identified by the calendar (e.g., the first month after diagnosis of breast cancer, the second month, and so forth) or by particular health states (e.g., treatment with toxicity, well without evidence of recurrence, recurrence, death). Each period is then weighted by a period-specific estimate of the quality of life based on the strength of one's preference for life in that period or state. These weights are termed *utilities* and are generally measured on a scale ranging from 0 to 1, in which 0 is defined as being equivalent to death and 1 as being equivalent to optimal health (see Sources of Data for Cost-Effectiveness Analyses).[17] To calculate the number of QALYs associated with a particular life course, the number of years or months spent in each health state is multiplied by the utility for that health state, and the products are summed (Fig. 1).

It is also possible to measure the benefits of medical interventions in financial units, such as dollars. For example, one could ask subjects how much they would be willing to pay for a given improvement in their health or use other techniques to assign a monetary value to a year of life saved. The strategy of valuing all benefits in monetary terms is the norm in industrial and business applications. However, it is both difficult and ethically complex to assign a dollar value to medical benefits, and as a result, it is much more common in clinical economic analyses to measure benefits in units such as YOLS or QALYs.

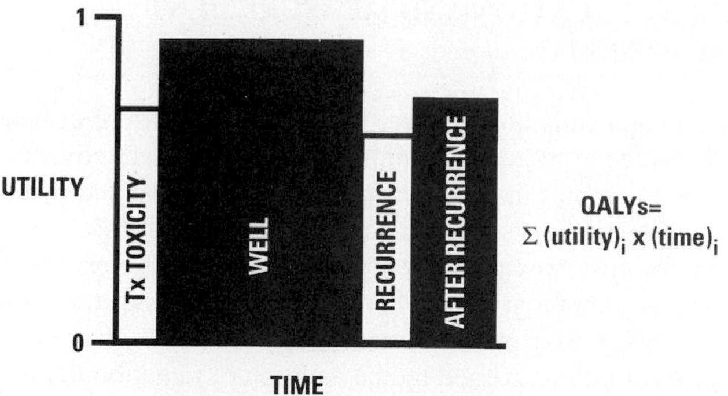

FIG. 1. Imagine that after initiation of a particular treatment, patients can enter four possible health states: They all experience toxicity during treatment (Tx TOXICITY), they can be well without evidence of recurrence (WELL), they can experience a recurrence (RECURRENCE), they can experience a remission (AFTER RECURRENCE), and they all eventually die. To calculate the quality-adjusted life years (QALYs) associated with this strategy, one could first plot each health state on a graph that has utility plotted on the y axis and time in years plotted on the x axis, multiply the number of years spent in each health state by its utility (i.e., calculate the area associated with each health state), and then sum the products. Accordingly, the number of QALYs associated with the strategy is the total area under the curve.

TYPES OF ECONOMIC ANALYSIS

The manner in which benefits are measured in an economic analysis determines what type of analysis it is (Fig. 2). In the simplest type of economic analysis, a *cost-minimization analysis*, the benefits of two or more interventions are assumed to be equivalent. The costs are then compared, the magnitude of the difference reported in dollars, and the strategy with the lowest cost identified as the preferred choice. This approach was adopted by Munoz et al.[18] in a cost-minimization analysis of modified radical mastectomy versus lumpectomy and radiation therapy for the treatment of early-stage breast cancer. They assumed that the two treatment strategies had equivalent outcomes, both in terms of survival and quality of life; found the cost of mastectomy to be lower than that of the breast-conserving approach; and concluded that mastectomy was the preferred strategy. However, although it is true that no difference in survival has been found between the two approaches, there is evidence to suggest that differences in quality of life exist, so that a cost-minimization approach may not fully capture the nature of the trade-offs involved in this decision.

Cost-effectiveness analysis is the term that is used to describe any incremental economic analysis in which the difference in costs appears in the numerator and the difference in benefits, measured in natural units, appears in the denominator. For example, a CEA might report the cost per year of life saved with adjuvant chemotherapy. *Cost-utility analyses* are one specific type of CEA, in which benefits are measured in QALYs. Accordingly, the results of cost-utility analyses are reported in dollars per QALY, and the lower the ratio, the more cost-effective the intervention. A number of the CEAs that pertain to breast cancer have in fact been cost-utility analyses.[7,14,19–23] In the final type of economic analysis, *cost-benefit analysis*, benefits are measured in monetary terms. A cost-benefit ratio consists of a difference in costs (measured in dollars) in the numerator and a difference in benefits (measured in dollars) in the denominator. The result is thus unitless. Any intervention for which the ratio is less than 1 is considered cost-beneficial. Alternatively, incremental costs can be subtracted from incremental benefits; if this difference is positive, the intervention is cost-beneficial.

The recent Panel on Cost-Effectiveness in Health and Medicine identified cost-utility analyses as the preferred type of economic analysis for use in evaluating health care interventions.[4] This preference reflected the Panel's consensus that QALYs are the most comprehensive and clinically meaningful of the possible measures of benefit. To illustrate how a cost-utility ratio is calculated, we use data from a cost-utility analysis of adjuvant chemotherapy in premenopausal women with node-negative breast cancer[7] (Table 1). In their analysis, Hillner et al.[7] estimated that the addition of chemotherapy would result in an increase in life expectancy of 0.9 years (19.5 years with chemotherapy minus 18.6 years without it) at an added cost of \$6,545 (\$26,385 for the strategy involving chemotherapy minus \$19,840 without it). Had they chosen to measure benefit solely in YOLS, the incremental cost-effectiveness ratio would have been \$6,545 divided by 0.9 years, or \$7,272 per

Type of Analysis	Units of Cost	Units of Benefit	Results
Cost-minimization	$	Assumed to be identical	$
Cost-effectiveness	$	Any effect of interest (e.g., YOLS)	$/Unit of effect
Cost-utility	$	QALYs	$/QALY
Cost-benefit	$	$	$ or unitless ratio

FIG. 2. Types of cost-effectiveness analyses. QALY, quality-adjusted life years; YOLS, years of life saved.

TABLE 1. *Calculating the cost-effectiveness and cost-utility ratios for adjuvant chemotherapy in premenopausal women with node-negative breast cancer*

	Cost ($)	Life expectancy (yr)	Cost/ YOLS ($)	QALYs	Cost/ QALY ($)
Treatment with adjuvant chemotherapy	26,385	19.5	—	11.030	—
Treatment without adjuvant chemotherapy	19,840	18.6	—	10.605	—
Incremental increase with addition of chemotherapy	6,545	0.9	7,272	0.425	15,400

QALY, quality-adjusted life year; YOLS, years of life saved.

YOLS. However, by using QALYs as their outcomes measure to perform a cost-utility analysis, the incremental benefit after the addition of chemotherapy fell from 0.9 years to 0.425 QALYs (11.030 QALYs with chemotherapy minus 10.605 QALYs without it). Accordingly, the incremental cost-utility ratio for adjuvant chemotherapy in this setting was $6,545 divided by 0.425 QALYs, or $15,400 per QALY.

SOURCES OF DATA FOR COST-EFFECTIVENESS ANALYSES

To a large degree, CEAs are ultimately judged on the validity of the data used in the analysis. As noted previously, up to three distinctly different types of data are required to perform CEAs: clinical outcome data, utilities, and resource utilization data. Given the variety of data needed, it is not surprising that the data used in CEAs are often obtained from several different sources.

Clinical outcome data form the foundation on which all CEAs are built. Without solid clinical data, a valid analysis cannot be performed. The incremental impact of an intervention on patients' survival is the single most important piece of clinical data. With this information, the difference in life expectancy between competing interventions can be calculated to estimate benefits in terms of YOLS or QALYs. Depending on the type of interventions being investigated and type of analysis being performed, incidence rates, sensitivities and specificities, local and distant recurrence rates, and complication rates may also be needed. These clinical outcome data are useful insofar as they are required to estimate the time spent in the relevant health states when benefits are being measured in QALYs and to help identify when downstream costs are incurred.

Sources of clinical outcome data for performing CEAs include randomized clinical trials, meta-analyses, prospective nonrandomized trials, and retrospective analyses. If investigators choose to use data from a randomized trial, it is important that they choose the trial(s) that is (are) most relevant to the interventions and patient populations under investigation. When performing a cost-utility analysis of radiation therapy after lumpectomy, Hayman et al.[19] chose to use data from the National Surgical Adjuvant Breast and Bowel Project B-06 trial rather than from the other four randomized trials, because it used the type of breast-conserving surgery used most commonly in the United States (i.e., lumpectomy), had the broadest entry criteria in terms of tumor size and nodal status, included patients who had received chemotherapy, and had the longest follow-up. When the randomized trials report conflicting results or when the individual trials lack the statistical power to detect small differences, data from meta-analyses are useful. For example, data from meta-analyses have been used in CEAs of chemotherapy and hormonal therapy in premenopausal women[24] and of mammography for women aged 40 to 49.[15] Unfortunately, such high-quality efficacy data do not exist for many interventions or patient populations; therefore, data from nonrandomized studies or estimates based on "expert judgment" must be used. For example, Hillner et al.[21] had to rely on case series combined with expert opinion in evaluating the cost-effectiveness of autologous bone marrow transplantation for metastatic breast cancer.

To perform a cost-utility analysis, data are also needed on how alternative strategies affect patients' quality of life. Since the 1970s, significant strides have been made in defining health-related quality of life and its constituent domains and in developing valid and reliable instruments to measure it (see Chapter 75). However, as noted previously (see Identification and Measurement of Benefits), quality of life is incorporated into CEAs in the form of utilities and, unfortunately, none of the quality of life questionnaires commonly used in oncology (e.g., MOS SF-36,[25] FACT[26]) generates utilities. There are two basic strategies for collecting utilities: direct elicitation or use of a health index. In direct elicitation, the respondent completes a standard structured interview that elicits his or her preference for a health state by asking what risk of death or decrease in length of life he or she would accept to improve it. Alternatively, respondents can complete a health index (a series of descriptive items on different domains of quality of life), and a conversion formula is then applied to assign a utility score to his or her unique set of responses.[27–30] This formula reflects the values placed on the different domains and levels of quality of life by a reference population.

In both cases, the final utility score reflects the preferences of an individual, or group of individuals, about tradeoffs between length and quality of life. Considerable controversy exists about whose preferences these should be. To date, most cost-utility analyses have relied on physicians or nurses, or both, to provide expert estimates of the utilities for different health states.[7,14,20,23,24] The principal appeal of this approach is that providers are familiar with the nature of the quality of life effects of disease and treatment, and it is a relatively simple matter to ask them to imagine a particular health state and to evaluate it. However, it has been shown that there are systematic differences between providers' utilities and those of patients. Therefore, many believe that patients are the optimal source of utility data for CEAs, arguing that they are the ultimate experts on the true quality of life in a given health state. Although this is undoubtedly true, there are strong theoretical grounds for obtaining utilities for CEAs from a general community sample instead. The Panel on Cost-Effectiveness in Health and Medicine argued that CEA is a tool to be used in allocating society's resources and that society's preferences should guide that decision making.[4] Consensus has not yet been reached on this issue, and the literature on cost-effectiveness in breast cancer includes examples of both approaches. In their cost-utility analysis of breast-conserving surgery and radiation therapy as compared to mastectomy, Norum et al.[22] used the EuroQoL instrument, a health index with preference weights obtained from a general population sample, to estimate the incremental increase in utility with the use of breast-conserving therapy. In contrast, Hayman et al.[19] used direct utility elicitation techniques among 97 women with breast cancer to assess utilities for the relevant health states in a cost-utility analysis of radiation therapy after breast-conserving surgery.

To estimate costs for CEAs, unit cost estimates and data on resource use are required. As noted previously (see Identifying and Measuring Costs), several methods exist for estimating unit costs for facility, professional, pharmaceutical, time, and transportation-related resources. However, accurate data on resource use are much more difficult to obtain. Because resource use has rarely been collected prospectively during clinical trials, most CEAs use much less reliable data. Common strategies include estimating resource usage by examining utilization for a very small number of patients and assuming that these rates are widely applicable[21] or using "expert judgment" to estimate usage for a "typical" patient undergoing a "typical" course of treatment.[7,19]

Ideally, the clinical outcome data, utilities, and resource utilization data used in a CEA should come from randomized clinical trials. If estimates of the difference in outcomes between alternative strategies are obtained from randomized trials, they will be unconfounded by known and unknown prognostic factors and will therefore reflect the true effects of the interventions themselves rather than patient selection. To provide all the data needed for a CEA, a randomized trial would need to collect not only the conventional end points including survival and local and distant recurrence rates but also utilities and resource use. Utilities would need to be measured at baseline, at regular intervals during routine follow-up, and at the time of a change in disease status (e.g., recurrence) using either a rating scale or health index. Data on the consumption of direct medical and nonmedical resources that are known to be costly would also need to be tracked during treatment and follow-up. The resulting data would provide unconfounded estimates of the incremental effects of the strategy examined as well as a measure of the variability of these effects. It would thus be possible to determine whether the differences between outcomes were statistically significant and to construct confidence intervals around estimates of differences in cost and effectiveness as well as the cost-effectiveness ratio.

Such intensive data collection is obviously very expensive. However, there are other drawbacks to relying on randomized clinical trials for data on CEAs. Because of restrictive eligibility criteria and patient self-selection, trial participants tend to be younger, to have less comorbid disease, and to be more compliant than other cancer patients. As a result, a distinction is often made in the health services research literature between "efficacy" and "effectiveness." *Efficacy* and *effectiveness* are defined as the extent to which medical interventions achieve health improvements under ideal and real practice conditions, respectively. Although data on the effectiveness of an intervention are what are truly required for CEA, they are rarely available because it is considered unethical to perform another randomized trial under relaxed conditions when efficacy has already been established in a tightly controlled randomized trial. Therefore, in most CEAs it is just assumed that efficacy and effectiveness are equivalent. Finally, because randomized trials often require more tests and procedures than are typically performed in routine practice, cost estimates derived from trials may be distorted.

Nevertheless, because of their ability to control for confounding, randomized clinical trials provide the highest-quality data for CEAs. However, a review of the published literature quickly reveals a heavy reliance on lower-quality data. The reasons are largely practical. First, there are still many situations in which the efficacy of an intervention used in a particular setting for a particular patient population has not been tested in a randomized trial. Second, although clinical data are often available from randomized trials, cost and utility data have rarely been collected prospectively as part of such trials. Third, CEAs require data on all outcomes until death. Given the relatively long natural history of breast cancer, unless patients participating in the trial have a very poor prognosis, the necessary data are not available. Therefore, because it is extremely uncommon that all the data necessary to perform a CEA are available from a single source, techniques are needed that are capable of combining all of this information and simulating a randomized clinical trial. Decision analysis techniques, especially Markov modeling, can provide a means for combining this information and performing a CEA over any time period.

USE OF DECISION ANALYSIS AND COMPUTER MODELING IN COST-EFFECTIVENESS ANALYSES

The most common approach to cost-effectiveness modeling is to construct a computer simulation of patients moving

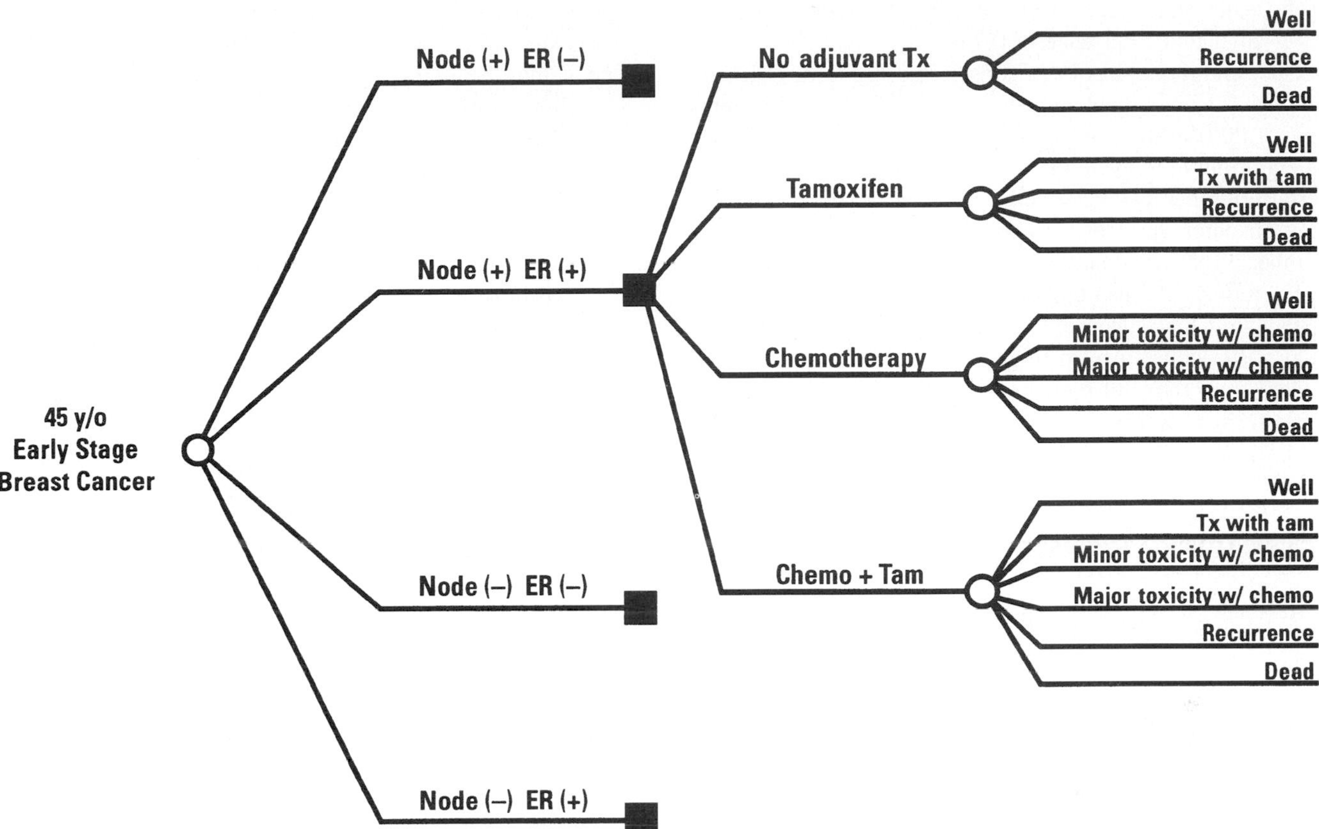

FIG. 3. Decision tree representing the outcomes and decisions faced by a 45-year-old woman recently diagnosed with early-stage breast cancer as described by Smith et al.[24] The *open circles* represent chance events, and the *closed squares* represent decisions. For clarity, the tree has only been extended out for the node-positive, estrogen receptor (ER)–positive subgroup of patients. The branches for the other three subgroups of patients are identical. Chemo, chemotherapy; Tam, tamoxifen; Tx, treatment. (From ref. 24, with permission.)

through successive health states, known as a *Markov model*.[31,32] The first step in constructing a Markov model is to clearly define the initial clinical scenario. For example, in their decision analysis examining the cost-effectiveness of chemotherapy and hormonal therapy for the treatment of premenopausal women with early-stage breast cancer, Smith and Hillner[24] define the clinical scenario as follows: "A 45-year-old woman has early-stage breast cancer that is node-positive (or node-negative) and ER-positive (or ER-negative)." The next step is to identify the relevant alternatives for patients in this scenario. Often, these choices are outlined in a decision tree (Fig. 3).

The next step is to identify all the relevant health states that patients could pass through after a given intervention. Theoretically, patients pass through an infinite number of health states. However, in practice, reality can usually be reasonably approximated by a small number of health states. For example, in their model, Smith and Hillner[24] used the following temporary and chronic recurring health states: "well," "treatment with tamoxifen," "minor toxicity with chemotherapy," "major toxicity with chemotherapy," "first recurrence," "after first recurrence," "second recurrence," "after second recurrence," "third recurrence," and "dead." These outcomes can also be summarized in the decision tree (see Fig. 3).

The next step is to determine how patients will be allowed to transition between the different states in the model. For example, once patients have entered the "after first recurrence" state, they can stay in that health state or transition into the "second recurrence" or "dead" state, but they cannot enter the "well" state again. The probability that a patient in one health state will transition to another during a defined period of time is then set. Accordingly, events (e.g., first recurrence) are modeled as transitions (e.g., from "well" to "first recurrence") using the available data. The defined period of time is known as the *Markov cycle*, and its length should be determined by the clinical situation. Given the relatively prolonged natural history of breast cancer, most published Markov models have used cycle lengths of 1 year.[7,19] The last step in creating each model is to assign the relevant costs to each health state (e.g., "well" assigned cost of routine follow-up, "first recurrence" assigned cost of salvage chemotherapy) and, if a cost-utility analysis is being performed, to assign utilities to each health state (e.g., "well" = 1.00, "first recurrence" = 0.70, "after first recurrence" = 0.75).[24]

Once the model has been constructed, a Markov simulation is performed by placing an imaginary cohort of patients (e.g., 1,000) in the starting health state (e.g., "Tx toxicity") and continuing to cycle them through the model either for a certain number of cycles (e.g., ten 1-year cycles) or until they all enter the "dead" state. The model then tracks the number of patients residing in each health state during each cycle, multiplies this number by the costs and utilities associated with that state, and sums the products. Finally, the total costs incurred by patients after one strategy are subtracted from those of patients followed with the alternative strategy and divided by the difference in benefits (e.g., QALYs) to produce the cost-utility ratio.

SENSITIVITY ANALYSIS

Because the creation of Markov models often requires the use of simplifying assumptions and point estimates of the costs and benefits associated with an intervention, a sensitivity analysis, also known as a "what if . . ." analysis, should be performed to evaluate the robustness of the cost-effectiveness ratio. The relevant issue is not whether such uncertainties exist but whether they could have a meaningful impact on the results of the analysis. Sensitivity analyses are performed by repeating the analysis while the relevant cost, efficacy, utility estimates, or a combination of these are varied over plausible ranges. This can be done by varying the estimates singly (one-way sensitivity analysis) or simultaneously (multiway sensitivity analysis), by determining how high or low the value of a parameter would have to be for an intervention to reach the threshold of cost-effectiveness (threshold analysis), by setting all estimates to values that most bias the analysis either for or against the proposed intervention (best-case and worst-case scenario analysis), or by sampling from a known distribution to generate confidence intervals around results (e.g., Monte Carlo simulation). Examples of all these types of sensitivity analyses can be found in CEAs of interventions that deal with breast cancer. If the cost-effectiveness ratio does not change significantly when a given estimate is varied through a clinically realistic range, the analysis is said to be "insensitive" to this estimate, indicating that the specific value chosen for this estimate is essentially irrelevant. Sensitivity analyses can also help to identify the key variables that are most influential in determining the magnitude of the cost-effectiveness ratio. Future research can then be directed at obtaining more precise estimates of these variables.

DISCOUNTING

Typically, the costs and benefits associated with an intervention do not all occur immediately. Instead, they are often spread over a long period of time. For example, the costs associated with screening mammography accrue up-front, and it may be many years before women experience any benefit in terms of survival.[15] In general, patients and payers are not indifferent to the timing of these events. If given a choice, most patients would prefer to experience all the benefits of treatment as soon as possible, deferring any diminished quality of life due to recurrence or toxicity for as long as possible. Payers would also prefer to postpone paying for any tests or treatments for as long as possible. In economics, this phenomenon is known as *time preference*. In general, the costs and benefits of oncologic interventions tend to occur early and late, respectively, whereas most patients' and payers' time preferences for costs and benefits tend to be late and early, respectively. To adjust for these differences in timing, it is generally recommended that an economic technique known as *discounting* be used. The present value (PV) of costs and benefits experienced "n" years in the future can be calculated using the following equation:

$$PV = \frac{\text{Value at n years}}{(1 + \text{discount rate})^n}$$

where the discount rate is the real rate of return on a risk-free investment (e.g., U.S. Treasury bonds). According to this equation, as costs and benefits occur further and further in the future, their present value decreases exponentially. Some controversy exists concerning whether both costs and benefits should be discounted and what discount rate should be used. In general, it is recommended that both costs and benefits be discounted and that a baseline discount rate of 3% be used in all CEAs. However, because of uncertainty about these recommendations, it is also suggested that the discount rate be varied between 0% and 7% as part of the sensitivity analysis.[4]

CONCLUSION

CEAs will be used increasingly often to evaluate whether the benefits of competing prevention, screening, diagnosis, and treatment strategies are sufficiently large to justify the costs. It is therefore important that the physicians who care for patients with breast cancer become more familiar with the techniques used in performing CEAs so that they can critically evaluate the quality of such analyses. Although many analyses have already been performed, there are still many instances in breast cancer management in which the cost-effectiveness of interventions remains unknown.

REFERENCES

1. Ziegler J. New database allows researchers to evaluate cancer care costs. *J Natl Cancer Inst* 1993;85(5):351–352.
2. Weinstein MC, Stason WB. Foundations of cost-effective analysis for health and medical practices. *N Engl J Med* 1976;296:716–721.
3. Detsky AS, Naglie IG. A clinician's guide to cost-effectiveness analysis. *Ann Intern Med* 1990;113:147–154.

4. Weinstein MC, Siegel JE, Gold MR, Kamlet MS, Russell LB. Recommendations of the panel on cost-effectiveness in health and medicine. *JAMA* 1996;276(15):153–1258.
5. Russell LB, Gold MR, Siegel JE, Daniels N, Weinstein MC. The role of cost-effectiveness analysis in health and medicine. *JAMA* 1996;276(14):1172–1177.
6. Kattlove H, Liberati A, Keeler E, Brook RH. Benefits and costs of screening and treatment for early breast cancer. Development of a basic benefit package. *JAMA* 1995;273(2):142–148.
7. Hillner BE, Smith TJ. Efficacy and cost effectiveness of adjuvant chemotherapy in women with node negative breast cancer. A decision-analysis model. *N Engl J Med* 1991;324(3):160–168.
8. Finkler SA. The distinction between costs and charges. *Ann Intern Med* 1982;96:102–109.
9. Perez CA, Kobeissi B, Smith BD, Fox S, Grigsby PW, Purdy JA, et al. Cost accounting in radiation oncology: a computer-based model for reimbursement. *Int J Radiat Oncol Biol Phys* 1993;25(5):895–906.
10. Brown J, Bryan S, Warren R. Mammography screening: an incremental cost effectiveness analysis of double versus single reading of mammograms [see comments]. *BMJ* 1996;312(7034):809–812.
11. Moskowitz M, Fox SH. Cost analysis of aggressive breast cancer screening. *Radiology* 1979;130(1):253–256.
12. Plans P, Casademont L, Salleras L. Cost-effectiveness of breast cancer screening in Spain. *Int J Technol Assess Health Care* 1996;12(1):146–150.
13. Hillner BE. Decision analysis: MIBI imaging of nonpalpable breast abnormalities. *J Nucl Med* 1997;38(11):1772–1778.
14. Liljegren G, Karlsson G, Bergh J, Holmberg L. The cost-effectiveness of routine postoperative radiotherapy after sector resection and axillary dissection for breast cancer stage 1. Results from a randomized trial. *Ann Oncol* 1997;8(8):757–763.
15. Salzmann P, Kerlikowske K, Phillips K. Cost-effectiveness of extending screening mammography guidelines to include women 40 to 49 years of age. *Ann Intern Med* 1997;127(11):955–965 [Published erratum appears in *Ann Intern Med* 1998 May 15;128(10):878. See comments].
16. Messori A, Becagli P, Trippoli S, Tendi E. Cost-effectiveness of adjuvant chemotherapy with cyclophosphamide+methotrexate+fluorouracil in patients with node-positive breast cancer. *Eur J Clin Pharmacol* 1996;51(2):111–116. [Published erratum appears in *Eur J Clin Pharmacol* 1997;51(5):427].
17. Torrance GW. Measurement of health state utilities for economic appraisal. *J Health Econ* 1986;5:1–29.
18. Munoz E, Shamash F, Friedman M, Tiecher I, Wise L. Lumpectomy vs mastectomy: the cost of breast preservation for cancer. *Arch Surg* 1986;121:1297–1301.
19. Hayman J, Hillner B, Harris J, Weeks J. Cost-effectiveness of routine radiation therapy following conservative surgery for early-stage breast cancer. *J Clin Oncol* 1998;16(3):1022–1029.
20. Desch CE, Hillner BE, Smith TJ, Retchin SM. Should the elderly receive chemotherapy for node-negative breast cancer? A cost-effectiveness analysis examining total and active life-expectancy outcomes. *J Clin Oncol* 1993;11(4):777–782.
21. Hillner BE, Smith TJ, Desch CE. Efficacy and cost-effectiveness of autologous bone marrow transplantation in metastatic breast cancer: estimates using decision analysis while awaiting clinical trial results [see comments]. *JAMA* 1992;267(15):2055–2061.
22. Norum J, Olsen JA, Wist EA. Lumpectomy or mastectomy? Is breast conserving surgery too expensive? *Breast Cancer Res Treat* 1997; 45(1):7–14.
23. Yee GC. Cost-utility analysis of taxane therapy. *Am J Health Syst Pharm* 1997;54[24 Suppl 2]:S11–S15.
24. Smith TJ, Hillner BE. The efficacy and cost-effectiveness of adjuvant therapy of early breast cancer in premenopausal women. *J Clin Oncol* 1993;11(4):771–776.
25. Ware JEJ. In: SF-36 health survey: manual and interpretation guide. Boston, MA: The Health Institute, 1994.
26. Cella DF, Tulsky DS, Gray G. The functional assessment of cancer therapy scale: development and validation of the general measure. *J Cancer Oncol* 1993;11:570–579.
27. Kaplan RM. Quality of life assessment for cost/utility studies in cancer. *Cancer Treat Rev* 1993;19[Suppl A]:85–96.
28. Weeks J, O'Leary D, Fairclough D. The Q-TILITY INDEX: a new tool for assessing quality of life and utilities in clinical trials and clinical practice. *Proc Am Soc Clin Oncol* 1994;13:436.
29. Torrence GW, Boyle MH, Horwood SP. Application of multi-attribute utility theory to measure social preferences for health states. *Oper Res* 1982;30:1043–1069.
30. The EuroQol Group. EuroQol—a new facility for the measurement of health related quality of life. *Health Policy* 1990;16:199–208.
31. Beck JR, Pauker SG. The Markov process in medical prognosis. *Med Decis Making* 1983;3:419–458.
32. Sonnenberg FA, Beck JR. Markov models in medical decision making: a practical guide. *Med Decis Making* 1993;13:322–338.

Index

Page numbers followed by *f* refer to figures; those followed by *t* refer to tables.